CONVERSION OF POUNDS AND OUNCES TO GRAMS FOR PEDIATRIC WEIGHTS

Pounds	Ounces 0	1	2	3	4	5	6	7
0	—	28	57	85	113	142	170	198
1	454	482	510	539	567	595	624	652
2	907	936	964	992	1021	1049	1077	1106
3	1361	1389	1417	1446	1474	1503	1531	1559
4	1814	1843	1871	1899	1928	1956	1984	2013
5	2268	2296	2325	2353	2381	2410	2438	2466
6	2722	2750	2778	2807	2835	2863	2892	2920
7	3175	3203	3232	3260	3289	3317	3345	3374
8	3629	3657	3685	3714	3742	3770	3799	3827
9	4082	4111	4139	4167	4196	4224	4252	4281
10	4536	4564	4593	4621	4649	4678	4706	4734
11	4990	5018	5046	5075	5103	5131	5160	5188
12	5443	5471	5500	5528	5557	5585	5613	5642
13	5897	5925	5953	5982	6010	6038	6067	6095
14	6350	6379	6407	6435	6464	6492	6520	6549
15	6804	6832	6860	6889	6917	6945	6973	7002
16	7257	7286	7313	7342	7371	7399	7427	7456
17	7711	7739	7768	7796	7824	7853	7881	7909
18	8165	8192	8221	8249	8278	8306	8335	8363
19	8618	8646	8675	8703	8731	8760	8788	8816
20	9072	9100	9128	9157	9185	9213	9242	9270
21	9525	9554	9582	9610	9639	9667	9695	9724
22	9979	10007	10036	10064	10092	10120	10149	10177

CONVERSION OF POUNDS AND OUNCES TO GRAMS FOR PEDIATRIC WEIGHTS—*CONT'D*

Pounds	Ounces 8	9	10	11	12	13	14	15
0	227	255	283	312	330	369	397	425
1	680	709	737	765	794	822	850	879
2	1134	1162	1191	1219	1247	1276	1304	1332
3	1588	1616	1644	1673	1701	1729	1758	1786
4	2041	2070	2098	2126	2155	2183	2211	2240
5	2495	2523	2551	2580	2608	2637	2665	2693
6	2948	2977	3005	3033	3062	3090	3118	3147
7	3402	3430	3459	3487	3515	3544	3572	3600
8	3856	3884	3912	3941	3969	3997	4026	4054
9	4309	4337	4366	4394	4423	4451	4479	4508
10	4763	4791	4819	4848	4876	4904	4933	4961
11	5216	5245	5273	5301	5330	5358	5386	5415
12	5670	5698	5727	5755	5783	5812	5840	5868
13	6123	6152	6180	6209	6237	6265	6294	6322
14	6577	6605	6634	6662	6690	6719	6747	6776
15	7030	7059	7087	7115	7144	7172	7201	7228
16	7484	7512	7541	7569	7597	7626	7654	7682
17	7938	7966	7994	8023	8051	8079	8108	8136
18	8391	8420	8448	8476	8504	8533	8561	8590
19	8845	8873	8902	8930	8958	8987	9015	9043
20	9298	9327	9355	9383	9412	9440	9469	9497
21	9752	9780	9809	9837	9865	9894	9922	9950
22	10206	10234	10262	10291	10319	10347	10376	10404

Essentials of Pediatric Nursing

Essentials of Pediatric Nursing

LUCILLE F. WHALEY, R.N., Ed.D.

Specialist, Parent-Child Nursing;
Professor Emeritus,
San Jose State University,
San Jose, California

DONNA L. WONG, R.N., M.N., P.N.P.

Nurse Counselor in Private Practice;
Consultant, Department of Education,
Saint Francis Hospital
Tulsa, Oklahoma

Third Edition

with 563 illustrations

THE C. V. MOSBY COMPANY

ST. LOUIS ◆ BALTIMORE ◆ TORONTO 1989

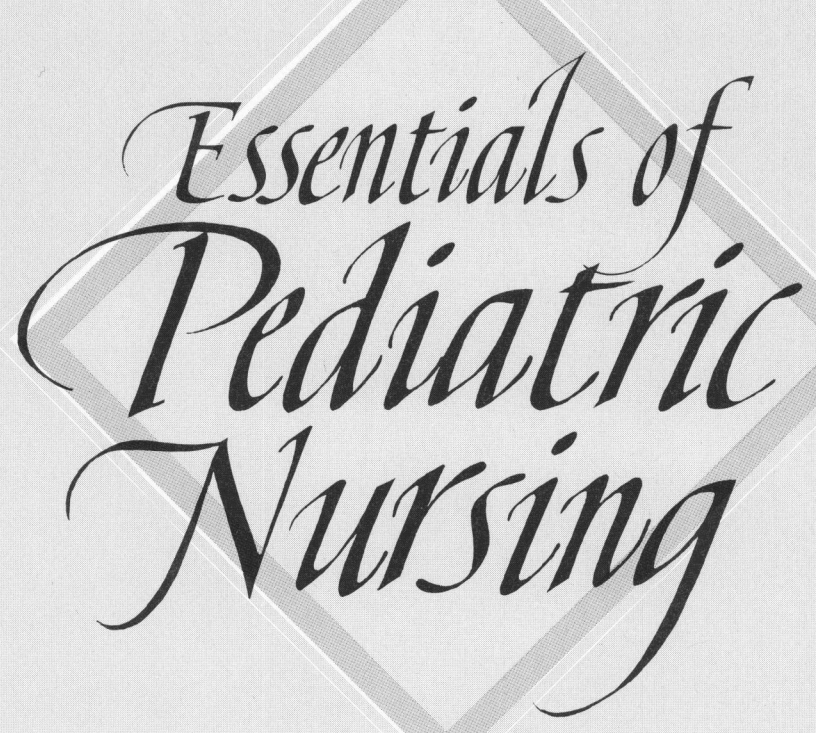

Mosby

Editors: Linda L. Duncan, William G. Brottmiller
Assistant Editor: Joanna May
Project Manager: Carlotta Seely
Production Editors: Jeanne Genz, Cynthia Miller
Manuscript Editors: Linda Bradford, Radhika Rao Gupta
Christine O'Neil, Mary P. Tait
Book Design: Diane Beasley
Cover Design: Liz Fett

Third edition

Printed in the United States of America

The C.V. Mosby Company
11830 Westline Industrial Drive, St. Louis, Missouri 63146

Library of Congress Cataloging in Publication Data

Whaley, Lucille F.
Essentials of pediatric nursing.

Includes bibliographies and index.
1. Pediatric nursing. I. Wong, Donna L.
II. TITLE. [DNLM: 1. Pediatric Nursing.
WY 159 W522e]
RJ245.W46 1989 610.73′62 88-13676
ISBN 0-8016-2879-2

C/VH/VH 9 8 7 6 5 4 3 2 1

◆

To my mother
Isabella Fillmore
and to my brother
Earl B. Fillmore

LUCILLE F. WHALEY

◆

To *Ting* and *Rudy*
for the love and support
that makes it all possible

And to my daughter, *Nina,*
whose commitment to her goals
is an inspiration to me

DONNA L. WONG

Preface

Philosophy and Organization

The third edition of this book maintains the same general philosophy and purpose as the first and second editions—the promotion of optimum health and development for infants and children at any stage of wellness or illness. The emphasis is again on providing the reader with the basic information that is essential to the delivery of safe, comprehensive, and holistic nursing care to children and their families.

In general, the basic organization and presentation of content have been preserved from previous editions. The early chapters of the book emphasize normal growth and maturation and some common health and developmental problems encountered at various age levels. Later chapters focus on serious health problems of infants and children that frequently require hospitalization and/or home care. The role of the nurse in all aspects of health care and maintenance is emphasized throughout.

However, unlike previous editions, a major organizational feature of this edition is the use of the nursing process as a framework for presenting nursing care. An additional chapter outlines the five steps of the nursing process and discusses their application to pediatric nursing care. In this chapter and throughout the text the definition, identification, and application of nursing diagnoses are emphasized. The philosophy that nursing diagnoses are reserved only for patient problems that nurses are capable of treating independently is demonstrated in the revision of the Summaries of Nursing Care. Now titled Nursing Care Plans, nursing interventions are differentiated according to those relating to nursing diagnoses and those relating to medical management. For those conditions in which a Nursing Care Plan is not included, the nursing diagnoses are listed in a separate box. Only nursing diagnoses approved by the North American Nursing Diagnosis Association, including those accepted at the Eighth Conference, are used in the Nursing Care Plans and elsewhere in the text. Diagnostic nomenclature revised by NANDA in September 1988 is used throughout this text. The organizational framework for nursing diagnoses is based on Functional Health Patterns.

A unique feature of the nursing process is the use of both observational guidelines and expected outcomes in the evaluation of nursing care. The observational guidelines are included to help the reader identify methods of evaluating whether the goals or expected outcomes are achieved.

Most of the nursing care related to health problems and to major discussions—such as care of the low-risk or high-risk newborn, the hospitalized child, and the child with chronic, terminal, or disabling conditions—appear in the nursing process format. Because adequate discussion of each step of the nursing process requires considerable space and repetition, less common conditions or disorders involving more medical than nursing care are not organized according to the nursing process but in the same structure as used in previous editions. This decision also allowed us to maintain a manageable book size despite the addition of numerous new features and expanded discussions of material that were necessary for this revision.

The units and their respective chapters reflect the organization of wellness to illness. Unit I introduces the reader to health promotion, including an overview of childhood mortality and morbidity, evolution of child care, and the role of pediatric nurses in health care delivery systems. The presentation of the nursing process prepares the reader for its continued application to nursing care of children throughout the remainder of the book.

Unit II presents an overview of the child's development from a longitudinal perspective as a background for more detailed discussions of growth with a horizontal view. The child is shown in relation to his cultural, religious, and social environment, with emphasis on the influence of the family.

Unit III provides an introduction to the principles and skills of nursing assessment. Guidelines and techniques for communicating with children and families are discussed, as well as history taking, family assessment, and nutritional assessment. Assessment includes observation, physical and behavioral assessment, and developmental screening techniques.

Unit IV is devoted to the stresses of the newborn period, the time of greatest risk to survival. Units V, VI, and VII present detailed discussions of the major developmental stages that were introduced in Unit II and some of the health problems commonly associated with each age level. Unit VIII is concerned with the child who has special health or developmental problems but who has the same developmental needs as other children.

Units IX through XIII describe the various types of serious health problems in children. Unit IX sets the focus of the succeeding chapters with its discussion of the needs and concerns of the hospitalized child and his family and the safe and competent implementation of hospital and home care procedures.

In Units X through XIII the biologic-dysfunctional frameworks allow for a conceptual approach to common symptoms and therapies as well as a discussion of the distinctive manifestations of specific disorders. The nursing process framework used in selected health problems places the emphasis on the nurse's role in health care management. Special physiologic or emotional problems related to specific age-groups are incorporated when appropriate. As always, the reader is expected to apply the basic concepts of growth and development introduced in the early units when formulating individualized nursing care plans.

Special Features

The third edition incorporates several new features to both expand the coverage of nursing of infants, children, and their families and to facilitate the use of the text. In addition to the necessary updating of disease management and therapy, such as acquired immune deficiency syndrome, some content has been expanded and some has been reduced or deleted. Although there has always been a strong emphasis on the family as the unit of care, the sections on cultural, religious, and family influences on health care have been considerably enlarged and are now discussed in two separate chapters. A special section on family assessment has also been included. To emphasize care components that are directed toward family members, the subheading Family Support has been added under Nursing Considerations.

Genetic and prenatal influences on health and development have been reduced or eliminated; basic terms and patterns of inheritance are now in the appendix. The chapters on growth and development for each age-group have been retitled to reflect the increased emphasis on health promotion and reorganized to present a uniform approach. Information on home care has been added to several sections of the book—as part of discharge planning for the hospitalized child in Chapter 20, following the discussion of all procedures in Chapter 21, and with several disorders that require home care, such as infantile apnea, cystic fibrosis, and asthma.

To assist the reader to consolidate content, numerous new tables and boxes have been incorporated into the book. For example, clinical manifestations and many nursing diagnoses are listed in box form for ready visibility, and more disorders appear in tables instead of narrative form. Numerous ***Nursing Guidelines***, such as promoting parent-infant attachment, relieving colic, and cast care, have been highlighted in boxes. Content on emergency treatment of some common or life-threatening conditions has been outlined in a special ***Emergency Treatment*** box, which is clearly designated by a colored tab on the page, and a list of these boxes is included on the inside front cover. As mentioned previously, Summaries of Nursing Care, now called ***Nursing Care Plans***, have been revised to incorporate nursing diagnoses, goals, implementation, and expected patient/family outcomes.

A number of vignettes describing nurse-child-family interaction appear as ***Therapeutic Dialogues***, and helpful ***Nursing Tips*** are included throughout the book. Each chapter begins with ***Learning Objectives***, as in the previous edition, but now also concludes with a ***Summary*** and a list of ***Key Concepts***, which emphasize important information. ***Study Questions and Activities*** are provided to encourage the reader to become actively involved in the content areas and to facilitate learning.

In an effort to provide readers with the most current and valuable information possible, we have taken care to expand and update the reference and bibliography sections. We have continued to divide bibliography entries according to subject, and have also added a color tab to these pages making it easier for readers to locate resources of interest.

Canadian Content

In this edition we have made reference to Canadian statistics regarding infant and child health in Chapter 1. In addition, we have included numerous Canadian service organizations throughout the text. We appreciate the wide usage of our book in Canada and hope that these supplements are of value to the Canadian reader.

Teaching/Learning Package

For the third edition of our text we are pleased to offer an extensive number of ancillary products for instructors and students to use in class and clinical settings.

Instructor's manual. This valuable resource manual follows the textbook chapter by chapter and includes learning objectives, audiovisual and supplementary materials, and recommendations for guest lecturers.

Study guide. This comprehensive and challenging study guide presents overviews and objectives for each chapter along with study activities and outside readings and resources.

Overhead transparencies. One hundred two-color transparency acetates that focus on key material in the text assist instructors in increasing student understanding.

MicroTest II. This computerized testbank, for use with IBM PC and Apple IIe, II+, and IIc, includes over 300 multiple choice questions and a user's manual so that the reader can add, delete, or rearrange items from any part of the text.

CAI software. This unique interactive disk covers care of the child and family with chronic illness. The disk presents self-assessment questions, a review of concepts, clinical simulations, and a post-test.

Acknowledgments

We wish to express our appreciation to those persons who offered comments, suggestions, and assistance with this revision. We are especially grateful to two individuals who joined us in the actual revision of sections of this book. Christina Algiere Kasprisin, R.N., M.S., Quality Attainment Coordinator–Nursing, Saint Francis Hospital, and Assistant Clinical Professor, University of Oklahoma College of Nursing, Tulsa, Oklahoma, wrote the original chapter on the nursing process. The basis for the material in this chapter was the developmental work done at Saint Francis Hospital as a joint effort of the department of nursing and the department of education. We acknowledge the work of the Professional Nursing Project members and the chairperson, Dr. Patricia A. Muller, in sharing this information with our readers and in providing time and support to the continued advancement of professional nursing practice. Donna P. Smith, R.N., M.S., Nurse Consultant, former Assistant Professor of Nursing, University of Tulsa, Tulsa, Oklahoma, revised the chapters on the cultural, religious, and family influences on the child. We value their contribution to this edition and look forward to their continued association with us in future editions.

We also appreciate the efforts of Bernard Rosner, Ph.D., Associate Professor of Preventive Medicine and Clinical Epidemiology (Biostatistics), Harvard Medical School, for compiling the blood pressure percentiles from the Second Task Force on Blood Pressure Control in Children into tabular form for our use on the inside front cover. We are grateful to the National Heart, Lung, and Blood Institute for granting us permission to use these data.

We again extend thanks to those institutions that have welcomed us to the units providing care to infants and children: Saint Francis Hospital, Tulsa, Oklahoma; Arkansas Children's Hospital, Little Rock, Arkansas; Children's Hospital of Wisconsin, Milwaukee, Wisconsin; Miami Children's Hospital, Miami, Florida; Children's Hospital National Medical Center, Washington, DC; Santa Clara Valley Medical Center, San Jose, California; and El Camino Hospital, Mt. View, California. We are most grateful to the library staffs at Santa Clara Valley Medical Center; Stanford University Medical Center, Palo Alto, California; and especially Peggy Cook at Hillcrest Medical Center, Tulsa, Oklahoma, for their efforts in the extensive research needed to update the material.

We are indebted to all the children and families who have allowed us to take photographs and to the persons who have generously provided new photographs for this volume: John Roy, Saint Francis Hospital, Tulsa, Oklahoma; Roy Garibaldi, San Lorenzo, California; Department of Audio-Visual Services, University of Kansas Medical Center, Kansas City, Kansas; Kiyo Sato-Viacrucis; and Ting Kin Wong. Numerous individuals assisted in organizing photography sessions, and we especially thank Diane Bannon, Betty Ann Chaze, Kathy Clarke, Shannon Filosa, Sharon Glass, Lorrie Greylak, Marilyn Knoy, Karen Mueller, Donna Smith, Neala Watkins, and Kathleen Whaley for their efforts.

We again wish to express our gratitude to the editorial and production staffs with whom we were directly involved at The C. V. Mosby Company, specifically Linda Duncan, Alison Miller, William Brottmiller, Joanna May, and Carlotta Seely. Their dedication to incorporating our ideas into a polished product is most appreciated.

No book can be completed without the cooperation, encouragement, and sacrifices of our families. Although it is impossible to describe the full extent of their patience and devotion, we are forever grateful for their presence in our lives. We thank Bert, Kathleen, and Maureen Whaley, Ting and Nina Wong, and Rudolph Mitchko for their love and forbearance. Last of all we again thank each other for the shared excitement of exploration and the stimulation and mutual esteem associated with this collaboration.

LUCILLE F. WHALEY
DONNA L. WONG

Reviewers

A number of colleagues provided reviews of specific content areas. Their constructive criticisms and suggestions have been invaluable in ensuring accurate and up-to-date material that reflects current clinical practice. To the following individuals we express our sincere gratitude.

Rojann R. Alpers, R.N., M.S.
Lecturer, College of Nursing,
University of Iowa,
Iowa City, Iowa

Barbara M. Artinian, Ph.D., R.N.
Professor of Nursing,
Azusa Pacific University,
Azusa, California

Connie Morain Baker, M.S.
Child Life Coordinator,
Children's Hospital of Oklahoma,
Oklahoma City, Oklahoma

R. Stanley Baker, M.D.
Clinical Staff,
Central Ear Research Institute,
Oklahoma City, Oklahoma

Ruth Bindler, R.N., M.S.
Associate Professor,
Intercollegiate Center for Nursing Education of Washington State University,
Spokane, Washington

Marion E. Broome, Ph.D., R.N.
Associate Professor, Parent-Child Nursing;
Director, Center for Nursing Research,
School of Nursing, Medical College of Georgia,
Augusta, Georgia

Pamelia L. Butler, R.N., M.S., J.D.
Associate Dean and Associate Professor,
College of Nursing and Applied Health Sciences,
The University of Tulsa,
Tulsa, Oklahoma

Linda Chase, R.N., B.S.N.
Clinical Nurse Specialist,
University of Iowa Hospitals and Clinics,
Iowa City, Iowa

Lynn Clutter, R.N., M.S.N.
Parent and Child Consultant;
Formerly Clinical Nurse Specialist, Educator, Department of Pediatrics,
City of Faith,
Tulsa, Oklahoma

Martha J. Craft, Ph.D., R.N.
Associate Professor, College of Nursing,
University of Iowa,
Iowa City, Iowa

Shirley A. Corbett, R.N., M.S.N., M.Ed., C.P.N.P.
Nursing Faculty,
Broward Community College,
Pompano Beach, Florida

Judith Ann Davis, R.N., C.S., M.S.N.
Clinical Instructor, Pediatrics,
San Francisco State University,
San Francisco, California

Janet A. Deatrick, R.N., Ph.D.
Assistant Professor, Center for Nursing,
Northwestern University,
Evanston, Illinois

Nancy C. Endress, R.N., M.S.N.
Instructor, Parkland College,
Champaign, Illinois

Sally Fisher, R.N., O.C.N.
Pediatric Cancer Nurse,
Natalie Warren Bryant Cancer Center,
Saint Francis Hospital,
Tulsa, Oklahoma

Terry Fugate, R.N., B.S.N.
Formerly Adjunct and Associate Faculty,
School of Nursing,
Texas Tech University Health Sciences Center,
Lubbock, Texas

Mollie L. Hall, R.N., B.S.N.
Enterostomal Therapy Nurse,
Saint Francis Hospital,
Tulsa, Oklahoma

Deborah Croome Hancock, R.N., M.N.
Formerly Visiting Assistant Professor,
School of Nursing,
University of North Carolina–Greensboro,
Greensboro, North Carolina

Mary L. Henley, R.N.
Research Nurse and Clinic Coordinator,
Tulsa Cystic Fibrosis Center,
Oklahoma University/Tulsa Medical College,
Tulsa, Oklahoma

Caryn Hess, R.N., M.S.
Formerly Assistant Professor, College of Nursing,
University of Oklahoma,
Tulsa, Oklahoma

Marguerite M. Jackson, R.N., M.S., C.I.C.
Director, Medical Center Epidemiology Unit,
University of California,
San Diego, California

Nyla Juhl, R.N., Ph.D.
Chair, Family and Community Nursing,
College of Nursing, University of North Dakota,
Grand Forks, North Dakota

Christina Algiere Kasprisin, R.N., M.S.
Quality Attainment Coordinator,
Saint Francis Hospital;
Assistant Clinical Professor,
University of Oklahoma College of Nursing,
Tulsa, Oklahoma

Duke O. Kasprisin, M.D.
Chief Medical Officer, American Red Cross,
Blood Services Oklahoma Region,
Tulsa, Oklahoma

Charmaine Kleiber, R.N., M.S., C.P.N.P.
Clinical Nurse Specialist,
University of Iowa Hospitals and Clinics,
Iowa City, Iowa

Linda C. Kinrade, R.N., P.N.P., M.N.
Professor, Department of Nursing,
California State University,
Hayward, California

John C. Kramer, M.D.
Director, Tulsa Cystic Fibrosis Center;
Clinical Professor of Pediatrics,
Oral Roberts University and
Oklahoma University/Tulsa Medical College,
Tulsa, Oklahoma

Wendy D.E. Low, R.N., B.S.N., M.Ed.
Instructor, Department of Nursing,
Vancouver, Community College–Langara Campus,
Vancouver, British Columbia, Canada

Gale E. Manke, R.N., M.S.N.
Teaching Associate, College of Nursing,
University of Arizona,
Tucson, Arizona

Charlotte Marcoux, R.N., M.S.
Nutritional Support Clinician,
Saint Francis Hospital,
Tulsa, Oklahoma

Mary Courtney Moore, R.N., R.D., M.S.N.
Graduate Student,
Department of Molecular Physiology and Biophysics,
Vanderbilt University,
Nashville, Tennessee

Kristie Nix, R.N., M.S.
Associate Professor, College of Nursing,
University of Tulsa;
Formerly President of BELT (Buckle Every Little Tot),
Tulsa, Oklahoma

Kim L. Ong, M.S., R.Ph.
Staff Pharmacist, El Camino Hospital,
Mountain View, California

Darlene W. Perkins, R.N., M.S.
Formerly Pediatric Instructor,
College of Nursing, Northeastern University,
Boston, Massachusetts

Cathey Pielsticker, R.N., B.S.N., C.D.E.
Program Manager, Diabetes Center,
Saint Francis Hospital,
Tulsa, Oklahoma

Sharon L. Pontious, Ph.D., R.N.
Assistant Dean,
College of Nursing and Allied Health,
University of Texas at El Paso,
El Paso, Texas

Cecelia Shaw, R.N.C, B.S.N., O.C.N.
Clinical Supervisor/Research Coordinator,
Cancer Care Associates,
Tulsa, Oklahoma

Perle L. Slavik, R.N., M.A.
Lecturer, College of Nursing,
University of Iowa,
Iowa City, Iowa

Deborah Gharst Terry, R.N., M.S.
Instructor, College of Nursing,
The Ohio State University,
Columbus, Ohio

Joanne A. Ulmer, R.N., M.N.
Nursing Instructor,
Florence-Darlington Technical College,
Florence, South Carolina

Ruth E. VanderVeen, R.N., M.N.Sc.
Staff Nurse, Critical Care Nursing Pool,
Arkansas Children's Hospital,
Little Rock, Arkansas

Gayle P. Varnell R.N., M.S.N., C.P.N.P.
Nursing Instructor,
El Centro College–Brookhaven Satellite,
Dallas, Texas

Patty Villarreal, R.N., M.S.
Associate Professor, School of Nursing,
University of Texas Health Science Center,
San Antonio, Texas

Laura J. Wright, R.N., M.S.N.
Executive Director,
Northeast Home Health Care/Wyoming
Home Health Care,
Greeley, Colorado

Contents

Essentials of Pediatric Nursing

UNIT

I

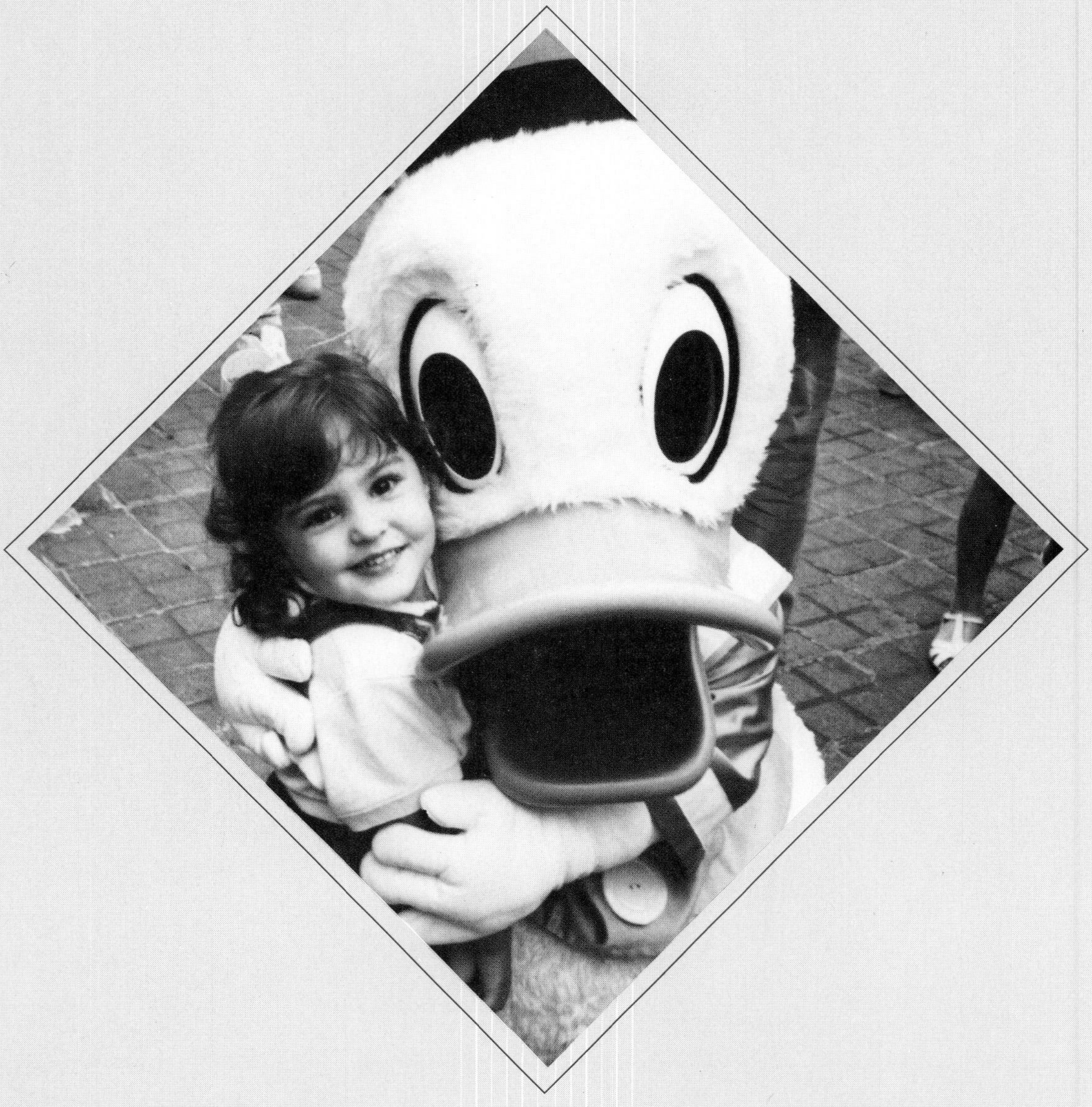

Children, Their Families, and the Nurse

Nursing care of infants and children requires a basic understanding of child health, both from a historical view and from current knowledge of the conditions most likely to adversely affect children's physical and mental well-being. Nurses need to be aware of their unique roles in providing pediatric care, as well as the application of the nursing process in the care of these special clients.

Chapter 1, *Perspectives of Pediatric Nursing,* directs the focus for the remainder of the book, which emphasizes a child- and family-centered approach rather than a disease-centered approach to nursing of infants and children. Childhood health is viewed from the perspective of mortality and morbidity trends at various ages. A historical overview of child health care in the United States is given to serve as a basis for understanding the changes that have occurred in pediatrics. The pediatric nurse is viewed as a person who can work effectively with infants and children and who can help create the kind of conditions in which others, particularly the parents, can function more effectively in child care.

Chapter 2, *Nursing Process in Care of the Child and Family,* presents an overview of the nursing process as it applies to pediatric nursing. The five basic steps of the nursing process are discussed with special emphasis on the identification of nursing diagnoses. This chapter provides the foundation for the integration of the nursing process and nursing care plans throughout the text.

CHAPTER 1

Perspectives of Pediatric Nursing

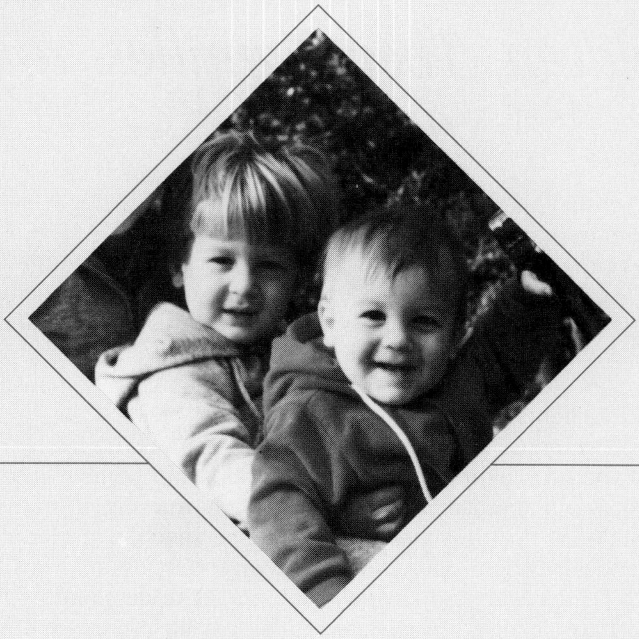

LEARNING OBJECTIVES

On completion of this chapter the reader will be able to:

- Define the terms *mortality* and *morbidity*
- Identify two ways that knowledge of mortality and morbidity can improve child health
- List three major causes of death during infancy, early childhood, later childhood, and adolescence
- List two major causes of illness during childhood
- Outline four events that were significant in the evolution of child health care in the United States
- Describe five broad functions of the pediatric nurse in promoting the health of children

*H*ealth care of children has changed dramatically in the past century. It has paralleled society's change from a view of children as "miniature adults," whose value to the community was measured in productivity, to recognition and appreciation of children as unique individuals with special needs and qualities. The focus in their care has shifted from treatment of disease to prevention of illness and promotion of health. Nurses are no longer solely involved in episodic care of children during an acute illness. They are increasingly responsible for providing comprehensive, distributive care that attempts to meet the needs of children and their families.

This chapter presents an overview of child health through discussion of past and present trends in childhood mortality and morbidity and the significant historical events that shaped present pediatric health care. It discusses the role of the pediatric nurse in both traditional and extended-role situations and emphasizes the benefit of primary nursing.

◆ *Health during Childhood*

Health is a complex phenomenon. As defined by the World Health Organization (WHO), it is "a state of complete physical, mental, and social well-being and not merely the absence of disease." Despite this broad definition, however, health is traditionally assessed by observing *mortality* (death) and *morbidity* (illness) over a period of time. Therefore the *presence* of disease becomes a prime indicator of health.

Information concerning mortality and morbidity is of importance to nurses. Such data yield significant information about (1) the causes of death and illness, (2) high-risk age-groups for certain disorders or hazards, (3) advances in treatment and prevention, and (4) specific areas of health counseling. Statistics enumerating incidence according to race demonstrate that health care is not equally benefiting all segments of society. Nurses who are aware of such information can better guide their planning and delivery of care.

MORTALITY

Figures describing rates of occurrence for events such as death in children are often referred to as *vital statistics. Mortality* statistics describe the incidence or number of individuals who have died over a specific period of time. They are usually presented as rates per 100,000 because of their lower frequency of occurrence. Such rates are calculated from a sample of death certificates.

Infant Mortality

Infant mortality rate is defined as the number of deaths per 1000 live births during the first year of life. It may further be divided into *neonatal* (under 28 days of life) and *postneonatal* (28 days to 11 months) mortality. In the United States there has been a dramatic decrease in infant mortality during the 1900s. At the beginning of the twentieth century the rate was about 200 infant deaths per 1000 live births. In 1985 the number had dropped to an estimated 10.6 deaths per 1000 live births, the lowest rate ever recorded in the United States. This decrease has primarily resulted from infectious disease control and nutritional advances during the early twentieth century, the advent of antibiotic, antibacterial agents in the middle of the century, and recent improvements in perinatal care. However, from a worldwide perspective, the United States lags significantly behind other well-developed countries. In 1985 it ranked nineteenth among the 20 countries with the lowest infant death rates, with Japan having the lowest rate (Table 1-1). This is far behind neighboring countries such as Canada, which ranked sixth.

◆ TABLE 1-1 ◆

Infant Mortality for 20 Countries with Population over 2 Million, 1985 (rate per 1,000 live births)

Country	Rate
Japan	5.5
Finland	6.3
Sweden	6.7*
Switzerland	6.9
Hong Kong	7.5
Canada	7.9
Denmark	7.9
Netherlands	7.9*
France	8.0
Norway	8.5
German Federal Republic	8.9
Ireland	8.9*
Singapore	9.3*
United Kingdom	9.3
Belgium	9.4*
German Democratic Republic	9.6
Australia	10.0
Spain	10.5
United States of America	10.6
New Zealand	10.8*

From Wegman, M.E.: Annual summary of vital statistics—1986, Pediatrics **80**(6):826, 1987.
*Provisional data.

Birth weight is considered the major determinant of neonatal death in the developed countries of the world. The relationship between birth weight and mortality is such that the lower the birth weight, the higher the mortality. The relatively high incidence of very-low-birth-weight infants in the United States is considered a key factor in its higher neonatal mortality rates when compared to other countries.

While there has been a steady and significant decline in infant mortality, the number of deaths occurring at this age is still proportionately high when compared with death rates at other ages (Table 1-2). This is true of other countries, such as Canada (Table 1-3). In the United States and Canada the death rate for infants under 1 year is greater than the rates for individuals ages 1 through 54 years. It is not until age 55 and over that the death rate begins to exceed the rate for infants.

During the first half of the 1900s, neonatal mortalities had not shown the remarkable reduction observed in infant mortality. In the early 1960s attention focused on perinatal health care in an effort to decrease the number of deaths. As a result, neonatal mortality declined from 20.0 per 1000 in 1950 to 7.0 per 1000 in 1984 (Hughes and others, 1987). This has largely resulted from better treatment of premature infants and perinatal illnesses, particularly respiratory and gastrointestinal problems. As Table 1-4 demonstrates, most of the 10 leading causes of death during infancy continue to occur during the perinatal period. The first 4 causes—congenital anomalies, sudden infant death syndrome, respiratory distress syndrome, and disorders related to short gestation and unspecified low birth weight—accounted for over 50% of all deaths of infants under 1 year in 1985.

While a number of perinatal problems have benefitted from improved treatment, congenital anomalies continue

TABLE 1-2

Death Rates by Age, United States, 1986 (estimated rates per 100,000)

Age (years)	Rate
Under 1 year	1036.7
1-4 years	50.8
5-14 years	26.4
15-24 years	102.6
25-34 years	130.2
35-44 years	212.5
45-54 years	504.6
55-59 years	981.8
60-64 years	1,544.0
65-69 years	2,257.2
70-74 years	3,456.6
75-79 years	5,173.0
80-84 years	8,197.3
85 years and over	15,291.1

From National Center for Health Statistics: Annual summary of births, marriages, divorces, and deaths: United States, 1986. Monthly vital statistics report **35**(13):14, DHHS Pub. No. (PHS) 87-1120, Aug. 24, 1987.

TABLE 1-3

Death Rates for Children, Canada, 1985 (rates per 1,000 population)

	Rate		
Age (years)	Total	Male	Female
Under 1	8.0	8.7	7.1
1-4	0.4	0.5	0.4
5-9	0.2	0.3	0.2
10-14	0.3	0.3	0.2
15-19	0.7	1.0	0.4
20-24	0.9	1.4	0.4

From Vital statistics, vol. 1: Births and deaths: 1985, Statistics Canada, Minister of Supply and Services, 1985, pp. 46 and 48.

TABLE 1-4

Leading Causes of Death in Infants under 1 Year of Age, United States, 1985 (rate per 100,000 live births)

Rank	Causes of Death	Rate
1	Congenital anomalies	227.7
2	Sudden infant death syndrome	141.3
3	Respiratory clusters syndrome	98.2
4	Disorders relating to short gestation and unspecified low birthweight	86.6
5	Newborn affected by maternal complications of pregnancy	35.5
6	Intrauterine hypoxia	30.8
7	Infections specific to the perinatal period	25.4
8	Newborn affected by complications of placenta, cord, and membrane	23.7
9	Accidents and adverse effects	23.7
10	Pneumonia and influenza	18.7

From National Center for Health Statistics: Advance report of final mortality statistics, 1985. Monthly vital statistics report **36**(5):39, suppl. DHHS Pub. No. (PHS) 87-1120, Aug. 28, 1987.

to be a leading cause of infant mortality, accounting for over 20% of those deaths. The incidence of the majority of birth defects has remained substantially the same and unlike all other causes of infant death, the rate is similar for blacks and whites. This suggests that genetics, rather than environment, plays the major role in the etiology of congenital anomalies (Wegman, 1986) and suggests the need for discovering and implementing improved prevention strategies (Kalter and Warkany, 1983).

When infant death rates are categorized according to race, a disturbing difference is seen. The infant mortality rates for whites are considerably lower than for all other races in the United States, with blacks having almost twice the rate for whites. Although the birth rate of both groups has declined, the gap has remained fairly constant. One encouraging note is that the gap in mortality rates between all nonwhite races has been narrowing. Since the Indian Health Service assumed responsibility for the health of Native Americans in 1955, infant mortality has declined by 75% (Indian Health Services, 1984). This improvement, however, is primarily due to declines in the neonatal mortality rate. The postneonatal death rates for Native Americans remains twice as high as in the white race. This suggests that Native American infants leave the hospital healthy but go to unsafe environments, which decrease their chances of survival past the first year. This phenomenon is not unique to the United States because postneonatal mortality rates for Northwest Ontario Indians are reported to be four times the Canadian all-race rate (Honigfeld and Kaplan, 1987).

Childhood Mortality

After 1 year of age there is a dramatic change in the causes of death in both the United States and Canada, with injuries (accidents) being the leading cause until people reach their early forties. In addition, the incidence of injuries has not shown the dramatic declines seen in other areas of childhood mortality. Some of the reasons include (Committee on Trauma Research, 1985):

1. Injury has traditionally been regarded as an unavoidable accident or a behavioral problem, rather than a health problem. The term *accident* suggests a chaotic, random event that occurs by "luck" or "chance"; the term *injury* is preferred because it connotes a sense of responsibility and control. (The term *injury,* rather than *accident,* is used throughout the text.)
2. Injury control, including research, has not received high priority or sufficient financial support. No central agency coordinates or is responsible for reducing the incidence of injuries.
3. Research on injuries has not been based on a theoretical framework, as has been done with diseases. There is a need to view injuries in terms of *host,* the affected person, *environment,* the time and place, and *agent,* the object that is the direct cause.

As Tables 1-5 and 1-6 illustrate, injuries account for nearly half of all childhood deaths from ages 1 to 14 years. In young adults ages 15 to 24, injuries, homicide,

TABLE 1-5

Leading Causes of Death in Children at Selected Age Intervals, United States, 1983 (rates per 100,000)

Ages 1-4	Rate	Ages 5-14	Rate	Ages 15-24	Rate
All causes	51.4	All causes	26.3	All causes	95.9
Accidents	20.0	Accidents	12.5	Accidents	48.4
Congenital anomalies	5.9	Cancer	3.5	Suicide	12.9
Cancer	3.8	Congenital anomalies	1.4	Homicide	12.1
Homicide	2.1	Homicide	1.2	Cancer	5.4
Heart disease	2.4	Heart disease	0.9	Heart disease	2.8

From National Center for Health Statistics: Advance report of final mortality statistics, 1983. Monthly vital statistics report **36**(5):20 Suppl. DHHS Pub. No. (PHS) 87-1120, Aug. 28, 1987.

TABLE 1-6

Mortality from Leading Types of Injuries, United States, 1980 (rates per 100,000 population in each age-group)

	Age (years)			
Type of Accident	**Under 1**	**1-4**	**5-14**	**15-24**
Males				
All causes	1217.9	63.2	32.4	140.3
Accidents (all types)	29.2	25.9	16.9	74.8
Motor vehicle	5.3(3)*	8.7(1)	4.4(1)	52.6(1)
Drowning†	2.4(5)	6.3(2)	0.9(4)	7.4(2)
Fires and burns	3.3(4)	5.1(3)	1.2(2)	1.2(5)
Firearms	—	—	1.0(3)	2.4(3)
Ingestion of food/object	6.1(1)	1.0(4)	—	—
Mechanical suffocation	5.6(2)	—	—	—
Falls	—	0.8(5)	0.3(5)	—
Poisoning	—	—	—	1.5(4)
Accidents as percent of all deaths	2.4%	41%	52%	53%
Females				
All causes	982.1	48.2	21.0	50.7
Accidents (all types)	22.6	17.5	8.3	21.7
Motor vehicle	5.0(1)	6.2(1)	4.6(1)	17.2(1)
Drowning	2.4(5)	3.2(3)	0.9(4)	0.7(3)
Fires and burns	3.3(4)	4.1(2)	1.2(2)	0.8(2)
Firearms	—	—	0.2(2)	0.2(5)
Ingestion of food/object	4.1(2)	0.6(5)	—	—
Mechanical suffocation	3.8(3)	—	—	—
Falls	—	0.8(4)	0.1(5)	—
Poisoning	—	—	—	0.7(3)
Accidents as percent of all deaths	2.3%	36%	40%	43%

Modified from National Center for Health Statistics, Public Health Service, U.S. Department of Health and Human Services, as cited in Accident Facts, Chicago, 1986, National Safety Council.
*Indicates rank among the leading types of accidents.
†Exclusive of deaths in water transportation.

and suicide are responsible for about 75% of all deaths. The pattern of deaths caused by injuries, especially from motor vehicles, drowning, and burns, is remarkably consistent in most Western countries, such as the United States and Canada.

Table 1-6 compares the leading causes of accidental deaths for each age-group according to sex. The overwhelming cause of death in American and Canadian children over 1 year is motor vehicle fatalities, including passenger, pedestrian, bicycle, and motorcycle deaths (Fig. 1-1). Even though the *percentage* of infants dying from motor vehicle injuries is small compared to the total number of deaths in that age-group, infants less than 6 months of age are at highest risk for motor vehicle passenger deaths. Factors that may be responsible are the greater frequency of their being held on an adult's lap or being placed on the front seat (Pless and Stulginskas, 1982).

From 1978 to 1982 nearly 3400 child passengers un-

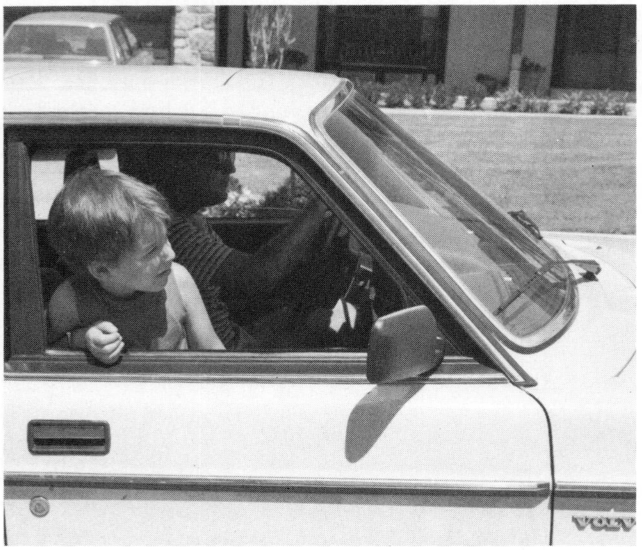

FIG. 1-1 Motor vehicle injuries are the leading cause of death in children over age 1 year.

der 5 years of age were killed in traffic injuries, and an additional 250,000 in this age-group were injured. Tragically, it is estimated that up to 90% of the fatalities and 67% of the disabling injuries could have been prevented by the proper use of child safety restraints (National Transportation Safety Board, 1983). One encouraging note is that the incidence of vehicular injuries, especially among young children, has been declining, probably as a result of child passenger restraint laws. Currently, all states in the United States and most provinces in Canada have enacted legislation requiring young children to be properly restrained in motor vehicles (LaPierre and Aylwin, 1985).

When accidental deaths are compared according to sex and age, the causes of death differ. Drowning and burns are the second and third leading causes of death in boys aged 1 to 14, but the order is reversed in girls (Fig. 1-2). In addition, firearms are a major cause of death in males but not in females (Fig. 1-3). During infancy, more males succumb to death from aspiration than do females (Fig. 1-4). More than half of all poisonings occur in children under 2 years of age (Fig. 1-5). By age 4 to 5 years, nonintentional poisonings are uncommon. Another increase in poisoning occurs in the 15- to 24-year age-group, and it is the fourth leading cause of death from injury. Poisoning is typically intentional and usually represents death from suicide (especially females) or drug abuse.

Analyzing deaths from specific types of injuries by age and sex is useful in identifying high-risk groups. It is also clear from a comparison of accidental deaths to other causes of childhood mortality that the greatest promise for improving childhood survival lies in preventing injuries. Certainly nurses play a major role in providing anticipatory guidance to parents and older children regarding hazards during each age period. In each succeeding chapter discussing health promotion, there is a lengthy discussion of injury prevention.

The total number of deaths is also significant when each age-group is compared (Table 1-7). The school-age

A

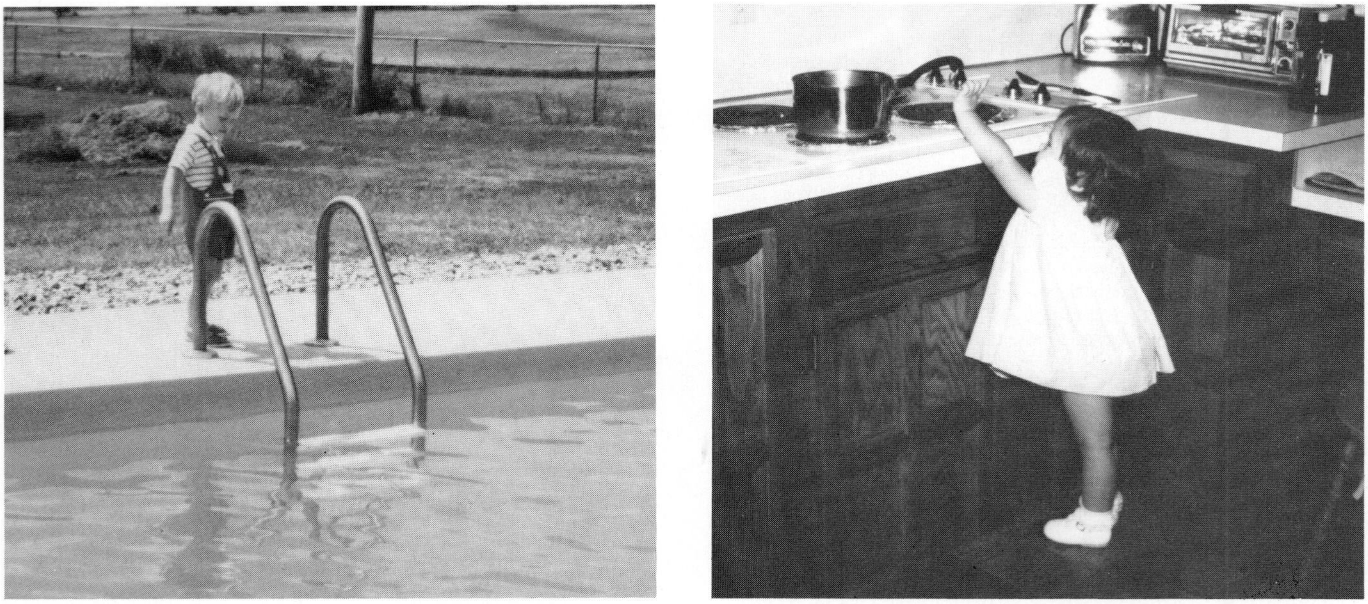

B

FIG. 1-2 A, In children ages 1 to 14 years, drowning is the second leading cause of death in boys and the third in girls. **B,** In children ages 1 to 14 years, burns are the second leading cause of death in girls and the third in boys.

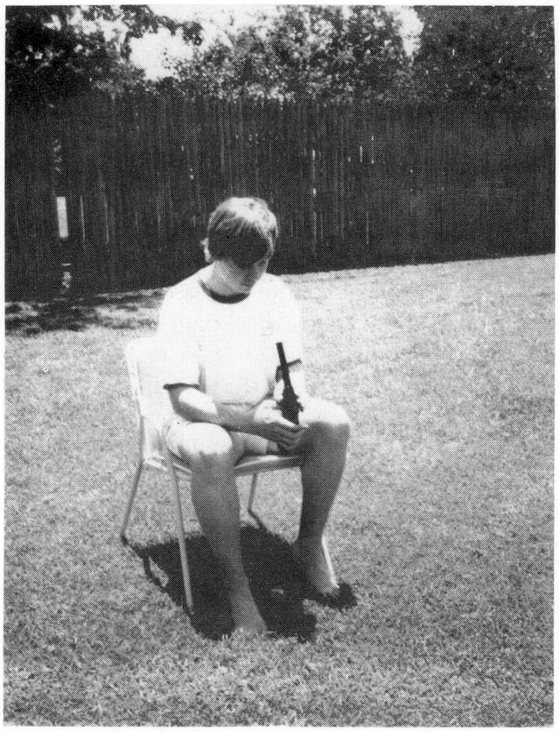

FIG. 1-3 Improper use of firearms is the fourth leading cause of death in boys and girls ages 5 to 14 years and the third cause in boys age 15 to 24.

years have the lowest incidence of fatalities. H there is a sharp rise during later adolescence, when in addition to injuries, the next two leading causes of death, suicide and homicide, are also potentially preventable. Violent deaths have been steadily increasing among all groups of children. In the age-group 15 to 19, there has been a three to four times rate of increase since 1950, and the rate for the age-group 10 to 14 is also increasing. Part of the reason for this in young children is more accurate identification of child abuse. Among adolescents, it may reflect an unhealthy preoccupation with violence and unresolved social tensions. In Canada the suicide rate for the 15 to 19 age-group has more than quadrupled since 1961 (LaPierre and Aylwin, 1985). Prevention lies in a better understanding of the social and psychologic factors that lead to the high rates of suicide and homicide. Nurses need to be aware of young people who are depressed, repeatedly in trouble with the criminal justice system, or associated with groups known to be violent. Prevention requires identification of these youngsters and therapeutic intervention by qualified professionals.

The general trend in racial differences that occurs in infant mortality is seen in childhood deaths. As Table 1-7 demonstrates, for all ages and for both sexes (except males 15 to 20 years) whites have fewer deaths. The accidental death rate for Native American children ages 1 to 4 years is 3 times the average rate. For all ages and

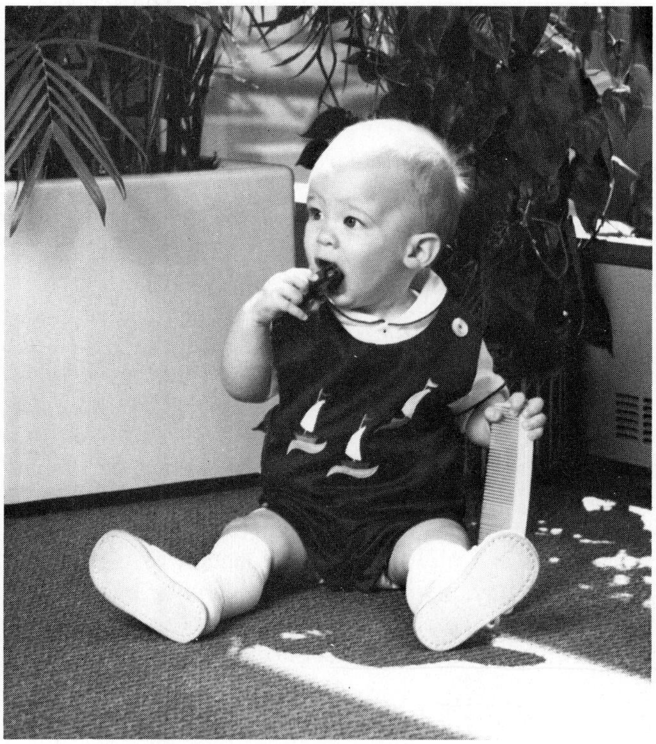

FIG. 1-4 Aspiration is the leading cause of death from injury in infants, especially in males.

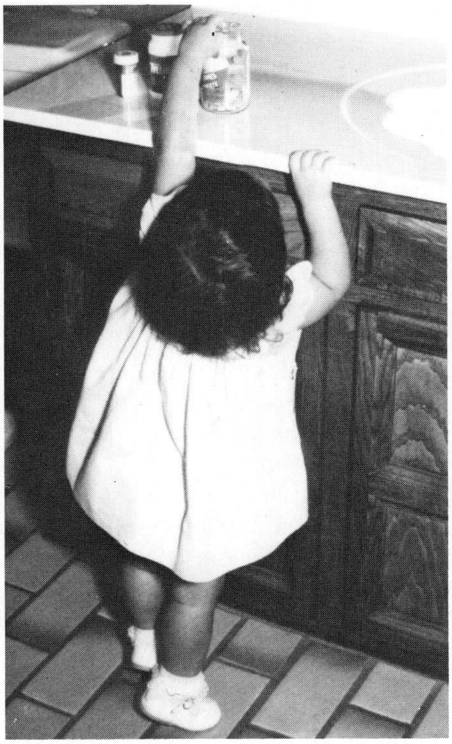

FIG. 1-5 Poisoning causes a considerable number of injuries in children under 4 years of age but is the fourth leading cause of death (usually from suicide) in both sexes ages 15 to 24.

TABLE 1-7

Number of Children Dying at Selected Age Intervals According to Sex and Race, United States, 1985 (of 100,000 born alive)

Age Interval (years)	White		All Other	
	Male	Female	Male	Female
Under 1	1,038.9	786.9	1,888.0	1,550.3
1-4	52.4	39.7	82.8	64.6
5-9	26.0	19.2	38.0	29.4
10-14	33.8	19.7	39.4	24.0
15-19	113.7	47.0	119.2	44.6

From National Center for Health Statistics: Annual report of final mortality statistics, 1985. Monthly vital statistics report **36**(5):12, Suppl. DHHS Pub. No. (PHS) 87-1120. Aug. 28, 1987.

racial groups the number of male deaths outnumber female, especially during the later adolescent years. The lowest death rate occurs during the school-age years.

The absence of infectious diseases as a leading cause of death in the age-groups over 5 years is testimony to the role that antibiotic/antibacterial agents and immunizations have played in the declining death rates and the specific causes of death. More effective treatment of severe infections has resulted in other disorders becoming more prominent in the list of leading killers. Most notable among these are the neoplasms. Cancer is the leading cause of death from disease in children ages 3 to 14 years. About 6600 new cases are diagnosed annually and an estimated 1800 deaths occur each year. About half of these are from leukemia, the most common form of cancer in the age-groups up to 9 years. Due to advances in diagnosis and treatment, the mortality for cancer in children has declined from 8.3 per 100,000 in 1950 to 3.6 in 1985 (Cancer Facts and Figures, 1988).

MORBIDITY

Morbidity statistics describe the prevalence of a specific illness in the population at a particular time. These are generally presented as rates per 1000 population because of their greater frequency of occurrence. Unlike mortality statistics, morbidity is very difficult to define and measure. Morbidity may denote acute illness, chronic disease, or disability. The source of data also greatly influences the resulting statistics. Common sources include reasons for visits to physicians, diagnosis for hospital admission, or household interviews. The following discussion is intended to present an overview of illness in children from a variety of perspectives.

Childhood Morbidity

Acute illness may be defined as symptoms severe enough to limit activity or require medical attention. According to the National Health Survey, children under 5 years of age have about 3.5 acute illnesses per year with 8.8 days of restricted activity. Children ages 5 to 14 years have 2.9 episodes and 9.4 days of disability. As a general rule, acute illness is less frequent in children under 6 months of age, increases thereafter until age 3 or 4 years, and then gradually decreases throughout middle and older childhood. There is a slight peak again during the first year or two of school, probably as a result of increased exposure to new contagions (Green and Haggerty, 1984).

Infections account for nearly 80% of all childhood illnesses, and respiratory infections lead the list, occurring two to three times as often as all other illnesses combined. The chief illness of childhood is the common cold. One third of all children have at least one episode of some other infection, such as gastrointestinal infection, annually as well. Similar patterns are seen in Canadian children.

From the perspective of seeking medical care, more children from white families have acute illnesses than those from black families. However, the illnesses reported by black parents are more likely to be severe. This is probably in part a result of different attitudes toward health care. For most American children in the middle and upper socioeconomic levels, serious physical illness is an uncommon event, but for those from underprivileged environments, serious physical disease occurs with higher frequency.

Another area of morbidity is chronic disorders, which may be roughly defined as conditions that persist for more than 3 months. Statistics regarding the prevalence of chronic disorders are discussed in Chapter 18.

Probably the most important aspect of morbidity is the degree of disability it produces. Disability can be measured in days off from school or days confined to bed. It can be the result of acute or chronic disorders. On an average, a child loses 5.3 days of school per year because of injury or illness. Girls miss somewhat more school than boys; however, boys are more likely to miss school because of injuries. Of all children under 17 years of age, over 95% are not disabled in any way. About 2% have mild disability, another 2% have moderate disability, and 0.2% are severely disabled (Pless, 1987).

While childhood is a time of relative health, it is the rare child who never becomes ill. Most children experience one or more episodes of acute illness annually and may be disabled for a short period of time. The rapidity with which children become ill is often a source of great anxiety for parents, who fear that the illness is serious. Part of nurses' intervention is education of parents regarding the usual types of childhood illness and recognition of those symptoms requiring treatment, such as signs of respiratory distress or dehydration. Certainly, nurses should also be aware of signs of potentially fatal illnesses. However, the future progress in decreasing childhood morbidity, as in childhood mortality, rests more on parent education than on miraculous discoveries such as the antibiotic. Nurses play a vital role in advancing child care through health promotion.

The New Morbidity

In addition to disease and injury, children face other problems that can significantly alter their health. These include behavioral, social (family), and educational problems that are sometimes referred to as the new morbidity. Estimates on the incidence of these problems vary, but they represent at least 5% and as much as 25% to 30% in specific age-groups, social classes, and medical facilities. Although no conclusive characteristics have been identified for children with new-morbidity problems, some findings are significant in terms of defining a high-risk group. These include children (1) from the lowest socioeconomic strata, (2) ages 7 to 14 years, (3) of male gender, (4) from one-parent families, (5) with a presenting complaint of a chronic physical disorder, (6) with reading skills below grade level, and (7) with higher rates of school absenteeism (Goldberg and others, 1984; Nader and others, 1981).

EVOLUTION OF CHILD HEALTH CARE IN THE UNITED STATES

Children in colonial America were born into a world with many hazards to their health and survival. Epidemics were common and no control or treatment was known. Physicians were few and only a small number had any formal training. Midwives also were untrained, usually practicing because of past experiences. Books providing information on child care and feeding were scarce and, when available, were useful only to a minority of literate parents.

Medical care by physicians was limited to wealthy European families who lived in or could travel to more developed cities. Children who lived on farms were cared for mainly by another family member or by a competent neighbor. Traveling medicine men, with their various forms of quackery, were common. Black children who were bought as slaves or born to slaves had only as much care as their owner was able or willing to provide. Native American children were treated for disease according to the tradition of each tribe, which was often a mixture of medicine, magic, and religion. With the colonization of America the Indians were exposed to many new diseases.

Statistics on childhood mortality during the colonial period are largely unavailable. Epidemic diseases were prevalent, however, and included smallpox, measles, mumps, chickenpox, diphtheria, yellow fever, cholera, and whooping cough, but the disease that surpassed all others as a cause of childhood death was dysentery. Sometimes entire families succumbed to this illness. Other major contributors to childhood illness and death were tuberculosis, nutritional diseases, and accidents (Schmidt, 1976). Accidents included skull fractures from playing in the streets; burns from open fireplaces, candles, and gunpowder; scalds resulting from falling into open kettles of boiling milk, water, and chocolate; and drownings from falling into unprotected wells (Cone, 1976).

Although scientific knowledge was accumulating, especially from work done in Europe, there were no organized efforts in the United States to apply that knowledge to the care of the sick. It was not until the Industrial Revolution was well underway in the nineteenth century that the consequences of childhood illness and injury and the effects of poverty and neglect became more widely recognized. The end of the nineteenth century is often regarded as the dark age of pediatrics, and the first half of the twentieth century is regarded as the dawn of improved health care for children.

The study of pediatrics began in the last half of the 1800s, under the influence of a Prussian-born physician, Abraham Jacobi (1830-1919). Because of his many accomplishments, he is referred to as the Father of Pediatrics. With several other physicians he pioneered in the scientific and clinical investigation of childhood diseases. One achievement was the establishment of "milk stations," where mothers could bring sick children for treatment and learn the importance of pure milk and its proper preparation. The crusade for pure milk helped bring the dairy industry under legal control and led to the establishment of infant welfare stations. The remarkable decline in infant mortality since 1900 has been achieved through prevention and health-promoting measures such as improved sanitation and pasteurization of milk. Before these regulations existed, the unsanitary milk supply was a chief source of infantile diarrhea and bovine tuberculosis. Cows were often kept in filthy stables and fed garbage and distillery wastes. Milk from cows that were fed distillery wastes was reported to make infants "tipsy." Some of the cows were so diseased with tuberculosis that they had to be raised on cranes to be milked (Cone, 1976).

Arising about the same time as these developments was the increasing concern for the social welfare of children, especially those who were homeless or employed as factory laborers. The work of one such reformer, Lillian Wald (1867-1940), founder of the Henry Street Settlement in New York, led President Theodore Roosevelt to call the first White House Conference on Children in 1909. It focused on care of dependent children and attempted to address the deplorable working conditions of many youngsters. As a result of this conference, the U.S. Children's Bureau was established under the jurisdiction of the Department of Labor, since at that time laws to regulate child labor were seen as the greatest need. Later, the Bureau was placed under the Department of Health, Education and Welfare (now the Department of Health and Human Services). White House conferences have been held approximately every 10 years to address the welfare, health, education, social, economic, and psychologic needs of children.

Wald's work has had far-reaching effects on child health and nursing. She started visiting nurse services in New York City and was instrumental in establishing the role of the first full-time school nurse. An outgrowth of nursing involvement in school health was the development of pediatric courses and specialized clinical experience in schools of nursing.

As more causes of disease were identified, there was an emphasis on isolation and asepsis. In the early 1900s children with contagious diseases were isolated from adult patients. Parents were prohibited from visiting because they might transmit disease to and from the home. Even toys and personal articles of clothing were kept from the child. It was not until the 1940s and the famous work of Spitz and Robertson on institutionalized children that the effects of isolation and maternal deprivation were recognized. This brought forth a surge of interest in the psychologic health of children and resulted in changes for hospitalized children, such as rooming in, sibling visitations, child life (play) programs, prehospitalization preparation, parent education, and hospital schooling.

On a national level the establishment of the Children's Bureau in 1912 marked the beginning of a period of studies on economic and social factors related to infant mortality, maternal deaths, and maternal and infant care in rural areas, all of which created the basis for stimulating better standards of care for mothers and children. This helped lead to the first Maternity and Infancy Act (Sheppard-Towner Act) in 1921 and to a much broader Maternal and Child Health program under Title V of the Social Security Act in 1935. The program consisted of three proposals: (1) aid to dependent children; (2) maternal and child health services, including Crippled Children's Services (CCS); and (3) child welfare services. The first programs provided by Title V were prenatal and postnatal clinics, child health clinics, and training of professional personnel.

Since 1935 numerous other federal programs have been developed. The Select Committee on Children, Youth and Families report, "Federal Programs Affecting Children" (U.S. House, 1984), lists 71 federal programs. Some of those that have had a major impact on maternal and child health include:

1. **Medicaid.** In 1965 Medicaid was created under Title XIX of the Social Security Act to reduce financial barriers to health care for the poor. It is the largest maternal-child health program. A major project under Medicaid is the Child Health Assessment Program (CHAP), which provides services for a large number of pregnant women and children.
2. **Aid to Families with Dependent Children.** Aid to Families with Dependent Children (AFDC) was established by the Social Security Act of 1935 as a cash grant program to enable states to aid needy children without fathers.
3. **MCH Services Block Grant.** The Maternal and Child Health (MCH) Services Block Grant provides health services to mothers and children, particularly those with low income or limited access to health services. Its primary purposes are to reduce infant mortality, reduce the incidence of preventable disease and handicapping conditions among children, and increase the availability of prenatal, delivery, and postpartum care to eligible mothers.
4. **Alcohol, Drug Abuse, and Mental Health Block Grant.** Established by the Omnibus Budget Reconciliation Act of 1981, the block grant provides funds to states for (1) projects to support prevention, treatment, and rehabilitation related to substance abuse and (2) grants to community mental health centers for the identification, assessment, and treatment of severely mentally disturbed children and adolescents.
5. **Social Services Block Grant.** Established under Title XX of the Social Security Act, this block grant provides states with funds for child daycare, protective and emergency services, counseling, family planning, home-based services, information and referral, and adoption and foster care services.
6. **Women, Infants, and Children.** In 1974 the Special Supplemental Food Program for Women, Infants, and Children (WIC) was started. It provides nutritious food and nutrition education to low-income, pregnant, postpartum, and lactating women and to infants and children up to age 5. Other nutrition programs include Food Stamps, National School Lunch Program, School Breakfast program, and Child Care Food Program, which provides financial assistance for nutritious meals to children in daycare centers, family and group daycare homes, and Head Start centers.
7. **Education for All Handicapped Children Act (P.L. 94-142).** In 1975 P.L. 94-142 was passed to provide a free appropriate public education to all handicapped children from ages 3 to 21 and to provide for those supportive services (speech, counseling, and so on) that ensure the benefit of special education.
8. **Education of the Handicapped Act Amendments of 1986 (P.L. 99-457).** In 1986 P.L. 99-457 was passed to allow for the provision of federal funding to states to develop and implement a statewide, comprehensive, coordinated, and multidisciplinary program of early intervention services for handicapped infants and toddlers and their families.

One of the most drastic changes in health care delivery has been the establishment of a prospective payment system based on diagnosis related groups (DRGs). The DRG categories allow pretreatment (prospective) billing for almost all United States hospitals reimbursed by Medicare. With hospitals now financially responsible when Medicare patients exceed the allotted admission stay, more patients are being discharged early. This has created an immense need for home care and other sources of community-based services. The exact impact DRGs will have on pediatric care is uncertain, but because the containment of health care cost is a national priority, it is inevitable that some form of prospective payment will affect children. Nurses need to be aware of the changing economics and prepared to meet the challenges.

◆ *Pediatric Nursing*

Nursing of infants and children is consistent with the definition of nursing as "the diagnosis and treatment of human responses to actual or potential health problems" (Nursing, 1980). Its purpose is to promote the highest possible state of health in each child. It consists of preventing disease or injury; assisting children, including those with a permanent handicap or health problem, to achieve and maintain an optimum level of health and development; and treating or rehabilitating children who have health deviations.

ROLE OF THE PEDIATRIC NURSE

Pediatric nurses are involved in every aspect of a child's growth and development. Nursing functions vary according to regional job structures, individual education and experience, and personal career goals. Just as clients (children and their families) present a vast and unique background, so it is that each nurse will bring to the clients an individual set of variables that will affect their relationship. No matter where pediatric nurses practice, their primary concern is the welfare of the child and family.

Family Advocacy

Although the nurse is responsible to self, the profession, and the institution of employment, the primary responsibility is to the recipients of nursing services, the child and family. The nurse must work with members of the family, identifying their goals and needs, and plan interventions that best meet the defined problems. As a consumer advocate the nurse must strive to ensure that families are aware of all available health services, informed adequately of treatments and procedures, involved in the child's care when possible, and encouraged to change or support existing health care practices. The pediatric nurse is aware of the United Nations Declaration of the Rights of the Child (see box) and practices within these guidelines to ensure that every child receives optimum care. As child advocate the nurse utilizes this knowledge to adapt care for the child's optimum physical and emotional well-being. Examples of this may be fostering the parent-child relationship during hospitalization, preparing the child before any unfamiliar treatment or procedure, allowing the child privacy, providing play activities for expression of fear, aggression, or loss of control, and respecting cultural differences related to feeding or child-rearing practices.

The nurse is aware of the needs of children and works with all caregivers to ensure that these fundamental requirements are met. This often necessitates that the nurse expand the boundaries of practice to less traditional settings. As a child advocate the nurse may be involved in education, political/legislative change, rehabilitation, screening, administration, and even engineering and architecture. Regardless of how removed from direct patient care individual nurses become, they continue to foster health care practices that promote the optimum well-being of children by incorporating knowledge of child growth and development into particular roles of practice.

At times, the role of family advocate conflicts with other roles of the nurse, such as those imposed by the institution. Inflexible rules, regulations designed for purposes of administration rather than optimum child welfare, and relationships with other professionals who are not knowledgeable of children's needs can create tremendous conflicts and challenges for the nurse who is dedicated to caring for the family in light of individual needs. Although there are rarely easy solutions to such dilem-

United Nations' Declaration of the Rights of the Child

All children need:
- To be free from discrimination
- To develop physically and mentally in freedom and dignity
- To have a name and nationality
- To have adequate nutrition, housing, recreation and medical services
- To receive special treatment if handicapped
- To receive love, understanding, and material security
- To receive an education and develop his/her abilities
- To be the first to receive protection in disaster
- To be protected from neglect, cruelty and exploitation
- To be brought up in a spirit of friendship among people

Code for Nurses

1. The nurse provides services with respect for human dignity and the uniqueness of the client unrestricted by considerations of social or economic status, personal attributes, or the nature of health problems.
2. The nurse safeguards the client's right to privacy by judiciously protecting information of a confidential nature.
3. The nurse acts to safeguard the client and the public when health care and safety are affected by the incompetent, unethical, or illegal practice of any person.
4. The nurse assumes responsibility and accountability for individual nursing judgments and actions.
5. The nurse maintains competence in nursing.
6. The nurse exercises informed judgment and uses individual competence and qualifications as criteria in seeking consultation, accepting responsibilities, and delegating nursing activities to others.
7. The nurse participates in activities that contribute to the ongoing development of the profession's body of knowledge.
8. The nurse participates in the profession's efforts to implement and improve standards of nursing.
9. The nurse participates in the profession's efforts to establish and maintain conditions of employment conducive to high-quality nursing care.
10. The nurse participates in the profession's effort to protect the public from misinformation and misrepresentation and to maintain the integrity of nursing.
11. The nurse collaborates with members of the health professions and other citizens in promoting community and national efforts to meet the health needs of the public.

American Nurses' Association, 1976, 1985. Reproduced with permission of the American Nurses' Association.

mas, the nurse can use the professional code of ethics for guidance. A code of ethics provides one means for professional self-regulation. The Code for Nurses (see box on p. 11) focuses on the nurse's accountability and responsibility to the client and emphasizes the nursing role as an independent professional role that upholds its own legal liability.

Illness Prevention/Health Promotion

The emerging trends toward health care have been prevention of illness and maintenance of health, rather than treatment of disease or disability. Nursing has kept pace with this change, especially in the area of child care. In 1965 specialized programs for pediatric nurse associates/practitioners began to develop that have led to several specialized ambulatory or primary care roles for nurses. The thrust of these programs has been to educate nurses beyond the basic preparational stage in areas of child health maintenance in order for all children to receive high-quality care. An outgrowth of the practitioner programs has been expanded programs for school nurse practitioners.

Obviously, the thrust of these nurse practitioner programs is prevention. However, preventive care is not limited to them. Every nurse involved with child care must practice within the overall dimension of preventive health. Regardless of the identified problem, the role of the nurse is to plan care that fosters every aspect of growth and development. Based on a thorough assessment process, problems related to nutrition, immunizations, safety, dental care, development, socialization, discipline, or schooling frequently become obvious. Once the problem is identified, the nurse acts to intervene directly or to refer the family to other health persons or agencies.

The best approach to prevention is education and anticipatory guidance. In this book each chapter on growth and development includes sections on anticipatory guidance. With an appreciation of the hazards or conflicts of each developmental period, the nurse is able to guide parents regarding childrearing practices aimed at preventing potential problems.

Prevention involves less obvious aspects of child care. Besides preventing physical disease or injury, the nurse's role is also to promote mental health. For example, it is not sufficient to administer immunizations without regard for the psychologic trauma associated with the procedure. Optimum health involves the practice of good medicine with a humane approach to health care; the nurse is often the one professional capable of ensuring "humanity."

Health Teaching

Health teaching is inseparable from family advocacy and prevention. Health teaching may be a direct goal of the nurse, such as during parenting classes, or may be indirect, such as informing parents and children of a diagnosis or medical treatment, encouraging children to ask questions about their bodies, referring families to health-related professional or lay groups, supplying patients with appropriate literature, and providing anticipatory guidance.

Health teaching is often one area in which nurses feel competent because it involves transmitting information rather than receiving messages, translating them, and planning intervention. In other words, it is a concrete, structured, or incidental type of communication as opposed to other, emotionally laden, nondirected types of interaction. However, the nurse focuses on giving appropriate health teaching with generous feedback and evaluation to promote learning.

Support/Counseling

Attention to emotional needs necessitates support and sometimes counseling. Frequently, the role of child advocate or health teacher is supportive by the very nature of the individualized approach. Support can be offered in many ways, the most common of which include listening, touching, and physical presence. The last two are most helpful with children because they facilitate nonverbal communication.

Counseling involves a mutual exchange of ideas and opinions that provides the basis for mutual problem solving. Although it is similar to health teaching, its focus is broader and more intense because it frequently implies some crisis or upsetting event that needs intervention. It involves support as well as teaching, techniques to foster expression of feelings or thoughts, and approaches to help the family cope with stress. Although counseling is often the role of more specialized nurses, counseling techniques are discussed in various sections of the text to help students and nurses cope with immediate crises and refer families for additional professional assistance.

Therapeutic Role

The most basic of all nurses' roles is the restoration of health through caregiving activities. Nurses are intimately involved with meeting the physical and emotional needs of children, including feeding, bathing, toileting, dressing, security, and socialization. They are primarily responsible for instituting physicians' prescriptions; they are also held singularly accountable for their own actions and judgments regardless of written orders.

A significant aspect of the therapeutic role is continual assessment and evaluation of physical status. Only when aware of normal findings can the nurse intelligently identify and document deviations. In addition the pediatric nurse never loses sight of the individual child's emotional and developmental needs, which can significantly influence the course of the disease process.

Restoration frequently implies habilitation and rehabilitation. Through expanding roles nurses are increasingly responsible for health care of children with disabilities. For example, school nurses or pediatric nurse practitioners are involved in programs for severely developmentally disabled children in order to facilitate their attendance in regular classes.

Coordination/Collaboration

Nurses, as members of the health team, collaborate and coordinate their services with other professionals' activities. Working in isolation does not serve the child's best interest. First, the concept of "holistic care" can only be realized through a unified interdisciplinary approach. Second, aware of individual contributions and limitations to the child's care, the nurse must collaborate with other specialists to provide for high-quality health services. Failure to recognize limitations can be nontherapeutic at best and destructive at worst. For example, the nurse who feels competent in counseling when really inadequate in this area may not only prevent the child from dealing with a crisis but may also retard his future success with a qualified professional.

Even nurses who practice in geographically isolated areas widely separated from other health professionals cannot be considered independent. Every nurse works interdependently with the child and family, collaborating on needs and interventions so that the final care plan is one that truly meets the child's needs. Unfortunately, this is one aspect of collaboration and coordination that is lacking in health care planning. Often numerous disciplines work together to formulate a comprehensive approach without consulting with clients regarding their ideas or preferences. The nurse is in a vital position to include consumers in their care, either directly or indirectly, by communicating their thoughts to the group.

Research

Practicing nurses rarely consider themselves researchers, yet they are the individuals most likely to observe human responses to health and illness. Unfortunately few nurses systematically record or analyze such observations. For example, pediatric nurses devise innovative methods to encourage children to comply with treatments. Only if these interventions are shared with other nurses, especially through publications, can a body of knowledge on nursing practice develop.

Research also implies a questioning of *why* something is effective and *if* there is a better approach. Evaluation is essential to the nursing process, and research is one of the best evaluators. Therefore nurses need to be more involved in research and in applying research findings to their practice. Throughout the text research relevant to nursing of children and families is incorporated as appropriate. Research findings are presented to encourage nurses to base their practice on theoretical foundations, not intuition, and additional questions may be proposed in the hope of stimulating research in a particular area.

Health Care Planning

So far, the discussion of the nurse's role has been viewed through the nucleus of a family. However, the nursing role is far more extensive and includes the community or society as a whole. Traditionally nurses have been involved in public health care, either on a distributive or on an episodic basis. Rarely, however, have nurses been involved in health care planning, especially on a political or legislative level. Their role must also involve the decision-making body of government. Nursing, as the largest health profession, needs to have a voice, especially as family/consumer advocate. This does not mean that the nurse must hold public office. Rather it refers to knowledge and awareness of community needs, interest in government formulation of bills and support of politicians to assure passage (or rejection) of significant legislation, and active involvement in groups dedicated to the welfare of children, such as professional nursing societies, parent-teacher organizations, parent support groups, religious affiliations, and voluntary organizations.

Health care planning involves not only providing new services but also promoting the highest quality of existing ones. Nursing needs to ensure the excellence of its own profession through each individual member, who practices according to the Code of Ethics and Standards of Practice. Pediatric nurses are obligated to follow the Standards of Maternal and Child Health Nursing Practice (see the boxed material, p. 14). Each standard is followed by rationale and pertinent assessment factors. Nurses should also help, through education, role modeling, and supervision, to make certain their colleagues implement the standards.

Throughout the text the highest standards of nursing practice are continually reflected in the emphasis on thorough assessment, focus on scientific rationale as the basis for care, summary of nursing care goals and responsibilities, and comprehensive discussion of growth and development. Family-centered principles are continually evident in the consideration of dynamics affecting the child, parents, siblings, and extended family members. The nurse is viewed as a vital component of the health care delivery system. Although nursing functions are clearly outlined, nursing responsibilities must be equally emphasized. It is hoped that the roles briefly described here will be studied, practiced, and implemented to the benefit of all children.

Future Trends

The present shift in focus from treatment of disease to promotion of health is likely to further expand nurses' roles in ambulatory care, with prevention and health

American Nurses' Association Standards of Maternal and Child Health Nursing Practice

Standard I
The nurse helps children and parents attain and maintain optimum health.

Standard II
The nurse assists families to achieve and maintain a balance between the personal growth needs of individual family members and optimum family functioning.

Standard III
The nurse intervenes with vulnerable clients and families at risk to prevent potential developmental and health problems.

Standard IV
The nurse promotes an environment free of hazards to reproduction, growth and development, wellness, and recovery from illness.

Standard V
The nurse detects changes in health status and deviations from optimum development.

Standard VI
The nurse carries out appropriate interventions and treatment to facilitate survival and recovery from illness.

Standard VII
The nurse assists clients and families to understand and cope with developmental and traumatic situations during illness, childbearing, childrearing, and childhood.

Standard VIII
The nurse actively pursues strategies to enhance access to and utilization of adequate health care services.

Standard IX
The nurse improves maternal and child health nursing practice through evaluation of practice, education, and research.

From American Nurses' Association: Standards of Maternal and Child Health Nursing Practice, American Nurses' Association, Kansas City, 1983.

teaching receiving a major emphasis. As prospective payment becomes a certainty in pediatric care, the need for home care and community health services will necessitate that nurses become more independent and highly skilled beyond the traditional care settings. Both of these trends are illustrated throughout the book with increased emphasis on prevention through anticipatory guidance, child health and family assessment, and discharge planning and home care.

Technologic advances will also influence pediatric nurses' roles. Increasing technical skills related to patient care, as well as the demand for computer knowledge in the work setting, are inevitable future trends. As more positions are created in the health care system that do not require a nursing background, such as "patient care educator," nurses will be required to continually update their knowledge and prove their unique contribution. While such demands may appear overwhelming, they also provide challenge and creativity.

PRIMARY NURSING

Inherent in the decision-making process is accountability. Nurses are responsible for their actions, both in the legal and ethical senses. Part of the trend in nursing practice is a deeper commitment to accountability. One of the outgrowths of this has been the movement toward *primary nursing*. Primary nursing involves 24-hour responsibility and accountability by one nurse for the care of a small group of patients. The primary nurse becomes the bedside nurse, with few if any duties delegated to other staff. If responsibilities are shared, it is usually with an associate primary nurse who maintains continuity of care when the primary nurse is not on duty.

One of the traditional problems with primary nursing is providing consistency in scheduling the same nurse and associate. An approach that minimizes this difficulty is to designate one primary nurse and as many associates as are needed to ensure that the same group of nurses care for the child. This *primary core team* necessitates that at least one nurse is assigned to the patient for each shift and that additional nurses are assigned for these individuals' days off. By identifying the core team for a specific period in advance, all the nurses working with the child can plan care jointly, with the primary nurse maintaining overall responsibility.

The philosophy of primary care is supported throughout the discussion of nursing of children. In some instances the one-to-one relationship between child and nurse is emphasized because of its therapeutic benefit, such as in nonorganic failure to thrive. However, primary nursing is universally a supportive intervention in pediatric nursing because it provides a consistent caregiver for the child and focuses on the family unit as an integral component in the planning and implementation of care.

SUMMARY

Mortality and morbidity statistics reflect the health of children by describing the leading causes of death, illness, or disability among the various age-groups. The leading cause of death in infants is congenital anomalies and among children past 1 year of age is injuries. Infections are the chief cause of morbidity.

Advances in child care began in the late 1800s in the United States, and the dramatic decline in infant mortality has been through measures such as improved sanitation, pasteurization of milk, and use of antibiotics and immunizations. Today the greatest promise for lowering infant death lies in preventing low birth weight and for decreasing childhood death is injury prevention. Concern also centers on social problems, such as child abuse and neglect, childhood adjustment disorders, and learning disorders.

As pediatric health concerns have broadened, so have nursing roles. There is movement away from traditional hospital care for acute illness to expanding roles in illness prevention and health promotion. Individual accountability for quality patient care is reflected in primary care models that incorporate the family as the patient.

KEY CONCEPTS

- Health, as defined by WHO, is "a state of complete physical, mental, and social well-being and not merely the absence of disease."
- Although the infant mortality rate in the United States is at an all-time low, the United States lags significantly behind most other well-developed countries.
- Birth weight is the leading determinant of neonatal death in developed countries.
- Injuries are the leading cause of death in children over age 1 year.
- Childhood morbidity, although difficult to define, encompasses acute illness, chronic disease, and disability.
- Eighty percent of childhood illnesses are attributable to infections, with respiratory infections occurring two to three times as often as all other illnesses combined.
- The "new morbidity," or "pediatric social illness," refers to behavioral, social, and educational problems that can significantly alter a child's health.
- The study of pediatrics began in the last half of the 1800s, under the influence of Abraham Jacobi, who is referred to as the Father of Pediatrics.
- The work of Lillian Wald, a social reformer, has had far-reaching effects on child health and nursing. She started visiting nurse services in New York City and was instrumental in establishing the role of the first full-time school nurse.
- The pediatric nurse's roles include family advocacy, illness prevention/health promotion, health teaching, support/counseling, therapeutic role, coordination/collaboration, research, and health care planning.
- With the shift in focus from treatment of disease to promotion of health, nurses' roles may expand in ambulatory care, with emphasis on prevention and health teaching.
- Primary nursing involves care and accountability by one nurse for a small patient population.

STUDY QUESTIONS AND ACTIVITIES

1 In the clinical setting, compile a record of the admissions, noting the children's age, sex, and diagnosis. At the end of the experience, analyze the list for trends: are the sexes and age-groups (infancy, toddler, preschool, school-ager, and adolescent) equally represented, do different age-groups have a predominant type of diagnosis, what proportion of admissions are due to injuries?

2 Interview a school nurse in an elementary and high school and a teacher (a nurse if available) in a daycare center to identify the types of injuries seen in these age-groups.

3 Discuss with the hospital social worker the types of federal programs that serve children. Interview two families who receive benefits from these programs and evaluate the adequacy of the program for the family.

4 Observe nurses functioning in three different pediatric settings (for example, staff nurse, school nurse, public health nurse) and compare their activities to the pediatric nursing roles described in this chapter. What roles are common to all three, which ones differ, what roles are not demonstrated?

5 Observe a pediatric unit that implements primary nursing. Identify the strengths and weaknesses of primary nursing from the observations and from discussions with two nurses and two families on the unit.

REFERENCES

Cancer facts and figures–1988, New York, 1987, American Cancer Society, Inc.

Committee on Trauma Research, Commission on Life Sciences, National Research Council and the Institute of Medicine: Injury in America: a continuing public health problem, Washington, DC, 1985, National Academy Press.

Cone, T.E., Jr.: Highlights of two centuries of American pediatrics, 1776-1976, Am. J. Dis. Child. **130:**762-775, 1976.

Goldberg, I.R., and others: Mental health problems among children seen in pediatric practice: prevalence and management, Pediatrics **73**(3):278-292, 1984.

Green, M., and Haggerty, R.: Episodic problems. In Green, M., and Haggerty, R., editors: Ambulatory pediatrics III, Philadelphia, 1984, W.B. Saunders Co.

Honigfeld, L., and Kaplan, D.: Native American postneonatal mortality, Pediatrics **80**(4):575-578, 1987.

Hughes, D., and others: The health of America's children, Washington, DC, 1987, Children's Defense Fund.

Indian Health Service Chart Book Series, June 1984, U. S. Department of Health and Human Services, Public Health Service, Health Resources and Services Administrations.

Kalter, H., and Warkany, J.: Congenital malformations: etiologic factors and their role in prevention, part I, N. Engl. J. Med. **308:**424-431, Feb. 1983; part II, **308:**491-497, March 1983.

LaPierre, L., and Aylwin, H.: Canadian youth perspective on their health, Canada, 1985, Minister of Supply and Services.

Nader, P., and others: The new morbidity: use of school and community health care resources for behavioral, educational and social-family problems, Pediatrics **67**(1):53-60, 1981.

National Transportation Safety Board: Safety study: child passenger protection against death, disability, and disfigurement in motor vehicle accidents, Washington, DC, 1983, U.S. Government Printing Office.

Nursing: a social policy statement, Kansas City, MO, 1980, American Nurses' Association.

Pless, I.: Morbidity and mortality among the young. In Hoekelman, R.A., editor: Primary pediatric care, St. Louis, 1987, The C.V. Mosby Co.

Pless, I., and Stulginskas, J.: Accidents and violence as a cause of morbidity and mortality in childhood, Adv. Pediatr. **29:**471-495, 1982.

Schmidt, W.M.: Health and welfare of colonial American children, Am. J. Dis. Child. **130:**694-701, 1976.

U.S. House of Representatives, Select Committee on Children, Youth, and Families: Federal programs affecting children, Washington, DC, 1984, U.S. Government Printing Office.

Wegman, M.E.: Annual summary of vital statistics—1986, Pediatrics **80**(6):817-827, 1987.

Restorative Role
1st. Problem-Solving Method = (Nrsg Process)

BIBLIOGRAPHY

Mortality and Morbidity

Canada Year Book 1988, Minister of Supply and Services.

Collins, J.: Persons injured and disability days due to injuries, United States, 1980-1981, Vital and Health Statistics, Series 10, No. 149, DHHS Pub. No. (PHS) 85-1577, National Center for Health Statistics, Public Health Service, Washington, DC, March 1985.

Graham, G.: Poverty, hunger, malnutrition, prematurity, and infant mortality in the United States, Pediatrics **75**(1):117-125, 1985.

Guyer, B., and Gallagher, S.S.: An approach to the epidemiology of childhood injuries, Pediatr. Clin. North Am. **32**(1):5-15, 1985.

Jason, J., Gilliland, J.C., and Tyler, C.W., Jr.: Homicide as a cause of pediatric mortality in the United States, Pediatrics **72**(2):191-197, 1983.

National Center for Health Statistics: Health, United States, 1984, DHHS Pub. No. (PHS) 85-1232, 1984.

Rivara, F.: Epidemiology of childhood injuries, Am. J. Dis. Child. **136:**399-405, 1982.

Rivara, F.: Traumatic deaths of children in the United States: currently available prevention strategies, Pediatrics **75**(3):456-462, 1985.

Shapiro, S., and others: Changes in infant morbidity associated with decreases in neonatal mortality, Pediatrics **72**(3):408-415, 1983.

Starfield, B.: Psychosocial and psychosomatic diagnoses in primary care of children, Pediatrics **66**(2):159-163, 1980.

Withrow, C., and Fleming, J.W.: Pediatric social illness: a challenge to nurses, Issues Compr. Pediatr. Nurs. **6:**261-275, 1983.

Evolution of Child Health Care

Bloch, H.: Jewish children in colonial times, Am. J. Dis. Child. **130:**711-713, 1976.

Brodie, B.: Children: a glance at the past, MCN **7**(4):219-225, 1982.

Coleman, J.R., and Smith, D.S.: DRGs: opportunity or crisis? Pediatr. Nurs. **10**(5):321-323, 1984.

Cone, T.E., Jr.: History of American pediatrics, Boston, 1980, Little, Brown & Co.

Donahue, M.P.: Nursing: the finest art, an illustrated history, St. Louis, 1985, The C.V. Mosby Co.

Fleming, J.: Maternal-child nursing in the decade ahead, MCN **10**(6):369-376, 1985.

Gleeson, S.V.: Public sector perspective: potential nursing services in mental retardation, Pediatr. Nurs. **13**(2):81-83, 1987.

Mitchell, K., and Hargin, R.: Our children: an economic priority, Pediatr. Nurs. **11**(2):82, 1985.

P.L. 99-457: Landmark legislation, ACCH Network **5**(4):1-3, 1987.

Radbill, S.X.: Reared in adversity: institutional care of children in the 18th century, Am. J. Dis. Child. **130:**751-761, 1976.

Rush, D.: National WIC evaluation, Pediatr. Health Currents **26**(4):17-20, 1986.

Sayre, J.W., and Sayre, R.F.: American children and the "children of nature," Am. J. Dis. Child **130:**716-723, 1976.

Scott, R., and Winston, M.: The health and welfare of the black family in the United States, Am. J. Dis. Child **130:**704-707, 1976.

Shaffer, F.A.: DRGs: history and overview, Nurs. Health Care **4**(7):388-396, 1983.

Wallace, H.: Maternal-child health before and after Title V, Public Health Currents **25**(4):15-18, 1985.

Pediatric Nursing

Andreoli, K.G., and Guillory, M.M.: Arenas for practicing health promotion, Fam. Community Health **5**(4):28-40, 1983.

Arbeiter, J.S.: The big shift to home health nursing, RN **47**(11):38-45, 1984.

Boehm, S.: Research as a basis for changing nursing practice, Top. Clin. Nurs. **7**(2):39-44, 1985.

Brown, B., and Chard, M.: Nurse practitioners: a review of the literature, 1965-1979, American Nursing Association Pub. **I-VIII:**1-24, 1980.

Chaisson, G.M.: Patient education: whose responsibility is it and who should be doing it? Nurs. Adm. Q. **4:**1-11, 1980.

Dailey, C.P.: Teaching parents and children preventive health behaviors, Fam. Community Health **7**(4):34-43, 1985.

Gurile, P., and Harter, I.: Getting standards off the shelf and into practice, J. Pediatr. Nurs. **2**(5):295-301, 1987.

Gurile, P., and Harter, I.: Testing child health standards in a clinical setting, J. Pediatr. Nurs. **2**(5):302-307, 1987.

Laffrey, S.: Health promotion: relevance for nursing, Top. Clin. Nurs. **7**(2):29-38, 1985.

Lane, K., and Peppe, K.: Where are the standards? J. Pediatr. Nurs. **2**(5):291-294, 1987.

Meister, S.: Building bridges between practice and health policy, MCN **10**(3):155-157, 1985.

McClowry, S.: Research and treatment: ethical distinctions related to the care of children, J. Pediatr. Nurs. **2**(1):23-29, 1987.

Oberst, M.: Integrating research and clinical practice roles, Top. Clin. Nurs. **7**(2):45-53, 1985.

CHAPTER 2

Nursing Process in Care of the Child and Family

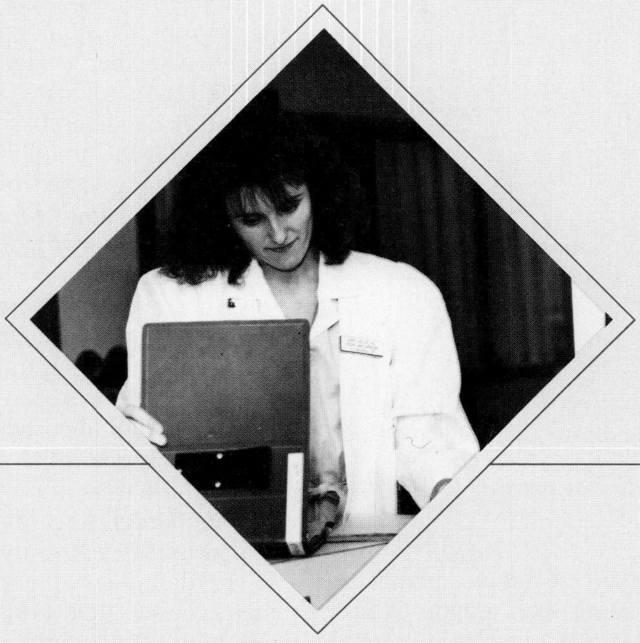

LEARNING OBJECTIVES

On completion of this chapter the reader will be able to:

- List the five steps of the nursing process
- Differentiate among different types of assessment: *comprehensive, screening,* and *focused*
- Define each of the eleven Functional Health Patterns
- Define *nursing diagnosis*
- Describe the five steps in developing a goal/outcome
- Differentiate *standard nursing care plan* from *individualized plan of care*

A systematic thought process is essential to a profession. It assists the professional in meeting the needs of the client. The nursing process is the framework for the practice of professional nursing. It is a method of problem identification and problem solving that describes what the nurse actually does. The five-step model that is accepted as the nursing process is: assessment, diagnosis (problem identification), planning (with outcome development), implementation, and evaluation. The second step of the nursing process, nursing diagnosis, is the naming of the child/family's problem in common nursing language. The North American Nursing Diagnosis Association (NANDA) is responsible for the clinical testing and approval of proposed nursing diagnoses. The nursing process can be envisioned as a continuous cycle. The nurse continually assesses the child and family. The data gathered must be compared with the expected information. The nurse then proceeds with the plan of care or modifies it accordingly. When evaluation is performed, patient status is reassessed and a new cycle begins (Fig. 2-1). In pediatric nursing the nurse must be alert to specific nursing diagnoses for the child as well as for the family. In some instances the only problems

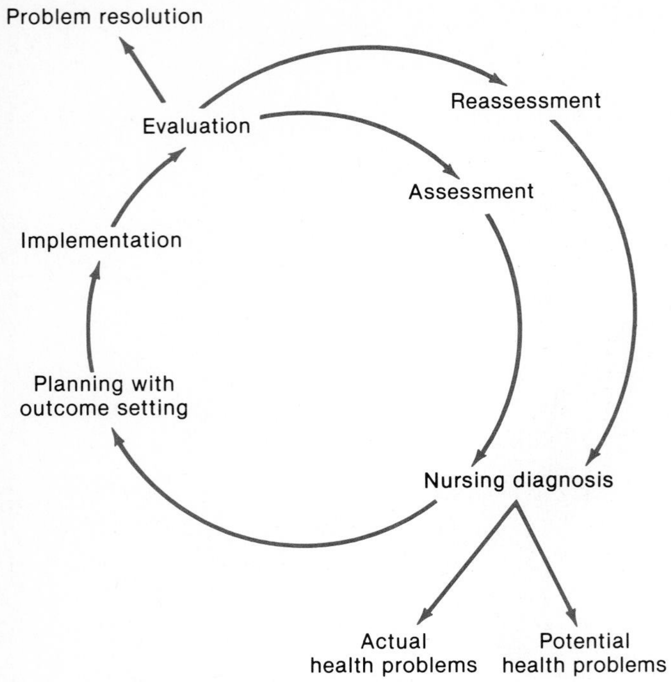

FIG. 2-1 Stages of the nursing process.

identified may be those that apply to family members rather than to the pediatric patient. Such diagnoses include alterations in family process and in parenting. Consequently the family unit must always be viewed as the patient. However, in the nursing of adults family members may be less directly involved in the patient's care.

ASSESSMENT

Nursing assessment is the foundation of the nursing process and the cornerstone of professional nursing practice. It is the deliberate and systematic collection of data from a variety of sources (see box). All clients must be assessed from the physiologic, psychologic, and environmental perspectives. This thorough assessment should be performed periodically on children and their families. The specific setting in which the nurse practices will influence how comprehensive the assessment will be, but all areas should be included (see also History taking, Chapter 6). There are three levels of assessment: comprehensive, screening, and focused (see box).

A *comprehensive* assessment is one in which all the above areas are thoroughly assessed. When a comprehensive assessment is impractical or inappropriate, a *screening* assessment is indicated. This assessment supplies the data necessary to provide basic safe nursing care. For example, a screening assessment may be indicated in the case of a newly admitted critically ill patient because attention must be devoted to preserving and maintaining life. The comprehensive assessment can be deferred until the child's condition has stabilized. Another indication for screening is the ambulatory surgery patient who is comprehensively assessed by the referring health care provider prior to being admitted to the outpatient setting. If a dysfunctional area is observed, an in-depth *focused* assessment for that area should be performed.

Most nurses find it helpful to base nursing process on a framework that facilitates the collection, organization, and use of data. That framework can be formatted in several different ways, and examples have included a systems approach focused on physiologic data, a format based on Maslow's hierarchy of needs, and assessments based on the work of nursing theorists such as Roy, Johnson, and Orem. Regardless of the organizing framework, a nursing perspective must be used.

The definition of nursing proposed by the American Nurses Association (1980) in its social policy statement and incorporated into many state nurse practice acts states in part: *the practice of the profession of nursing as a registered professional nurse is defined as diagnosing and treating human responses to actual or potential health problems.* To identify these human responses, a framework is needed that enables the nurse to focus on how the individual can function within the given environment. Both NANDA (1987) and Gordon (1987) have developed frameworks incorporating the nursing diagnoses. NANDA bases its framework on human response patterns and Gordon on functional health patterns. Gordon's framework consists of 11 categories that encompass all human activities. The descriptions of the functional health patterns are presented in Table 2-1. The nurse assesses the patient within each pattern to determine the adequacy of the functioning of the child and the family. Gordon's framework is used throughout this text.

Sources for Data Collection

Interview/health history:
- Child
- Family
- Significant individuals

Observation of social interactions
Developmental assessment
Physical assessment
Laboratory data
Consultation with other health professionals

Types of Assessment

Comprehensive	Thorough assessment of child and family.
Screening	Answers to selected questions from each area obtained to determine if more information is needed.
Focused	In-depth assessment performed in a particular area when screening assessment indicates problem may exist.

TABLE 2-1

Functional Health Patterns

Functional Health Pattern	Description
Health Perception-Health Management Pattern	Perceptions related to general health management and preventive practices
Nutritional-Metabolic Pattern	Intake of food and fluids related to metabolic requirements
Elimination Pattern	Regularity and control of excretory functions, bowel, bladder, skin, and wastes
Activity-Exercise Pattern	Activity patterns that require energy expenditure and provide for rest
Sleep-Rest Pattern	Effectiveness of the sleep and rest periods
Cognitive-Perceptual Pattern	Adequacy of language, cognitive skills, and perception related to required or desired activities; includes pain perception
Self-Perception–Self-Concept Pattern	Beliefs and evaluation of self-worth
Role-Relationship Pattern	Family and social roles, especially parent-child relationships
Sexuality-Reproductive Pattern	Problems or potential problems with sexuality or reproduction
Coping-Stress Tolerance Pattern	Stress tolerance level and coping patterns, including support systems
Value-Belief Pattern	Values, goals, or beliefs that influence health-related decisions and actions

From Gordon, M.: Nursing diagnosis: process and application, ed. 2, New York, 1987, McGraw-Hill Book Co.

During the assessment period the nurse seeks information to describe and explain the difficulties and strengths of the child and family. The nurse must be able to effectively communicate with both the child and family. Obtaining a complete assessment from a pediatric client presents numerous challenges. The very young child cannot answer questions and may not be able to localize signs and symptoms to aid in the physical exam. The older school-age child may be embarrassed and relucant to give information with parents present. For these reasons the nurse must look for subtle changes in behavior that may indicate physical distress as well as the need for privacy. The preadolescent and adolescent should be interviewed both with and without the parents to determine the perspectives of all concerned. The teenager and the parent may have different opinions on how each is functioning. (For a detailed discussion of communication with parents and children, see Chapter 6.)

As the nurse proceeds through the assessment phase, combining interview skills with physical assessment, cues are identified. A *cue* is information that influences decisions. When a cue is given by the patient, the nurse can decide to collect additional information or to use the cue directly in diagnostic judgment. The initial nursing assessment is complete when (1) the nurse has baseline data about the child and family, (2) the health care needs are evaluated, (3) the areas that interfere with the child and family's functioning are identified, and (4) a statement is made about any problems that exist.

After the initial assessment is completed, all cues must be evaluated. The patient's response should be compared with the expected response considering cultural/ethnic variables. Each piece of data should provide information relative to a judgment about the functioning of the client.

NURSING DIAGNOSIS

The second stage of the nursing process is problem identification and nursing diagnosis. At this point the nurse must interpret and make decisions about the data gathered. The nurse then organizes or clusters the data into similar categories to identify significant areas.

Once the cues have been clustered, the nurse makes one of the following decisions:

1. No dysfunctional health patterns are evident; no interventions are indicated
2. Potential dysfunctional health problems exist; interventions are needed to facilitate health promotion
3. Actual dysfunctional health patterns are evident; interventions are needed to facilitate health promotion

The nursing diagnosis is the naming of the cue clusters that are obtained during the assessment phase. The term *nursing diagnosis* is reserved for patient problems that ". . . nurses by virtue of their education and experience are capable and licensed to treat" (Gordon, 1976).

Nursing diagnoses do *not* describe everything that nursing does. Nursing practice consists of three dimensions: dependent, interdependent, and independent activities. These three dimensions are characterized by the legally defined areas of nursing responsibility. *Dependent activities* are those areas of nursing practice that hold the nurse accountable for implementing the prescribed medical regime. *Interdependent* activities are those areas of nursing practice in which medical and nursing responsi-

*Nursing Diagnoses According to Functional Health Patterns**

Health Perception–Health Management Pattern (HP-HMP)
Altered health maintenance
Health-seeking behaviors (specify)
Noncompliance (specify)
Potential for infection
Potential for injury
Potential for poisoning
Potential for suffocation
Potential for trauma

Nutritional-Metabolic Pattern (N-MP)
Altered nutrition: less than body requirements
Altered nutrition: more than body requirements
Altered nutrition: potential for more than body requirements
Altered oral mucous membrane
Fluid volume deficit (1)
Fluid volume deficit (2)
Fluid volume excess
Hyperthermia
Hypothermia
Impaired skin integrity
Impaired swallowing
Impaired tissue integrity
Ineffective breastfeeding
Ineffective thermoregulation
Potential altered body temperature
Potential fluid volume deficit
Potential for aspiration
Potential impaired skin integrity

Elimination Pattern (EP)
Altered patterns of urinary elimination
Bowel incontinence
Colonic constipation
Constipation
Diarrhea
Functional incontinence
Perceived constipation
Reflex incontinence
Stress incontinence
Total incontinence
Urge incontinence
Urinary retention

Activity-Exercise Pattern (A-EP)
Activity intolerance
Altered growth and development
Altered (specify type) tissue perfusion (renal, cerebral, cardiopulmonary, gastrointestinal, peripheral)
Bathing/hygiene self-care deficit
Decreased cardiac output
Diversional activity deficit
Dressing/grooming self-care deficit
Dysreflexia
Fatigue
Feeding self-care deficit
Impaired gas exchange
Impaired home maintenance management
Impaired physical mobility (level 0 to 4)†
Ineffective airway clearance
Ineffective breathing pattern
Potential activity intolerance
Potential for disuse syndrome
Toileting self-care deficit

Sleep-Rest Pattern (SRP)
Sleep pattern disturbance

Cognitive-Perceptual Pattern (CPP)
Altered thought processes
Chronic pain
Decisional conflict (specify)
Knowledge deficit (specifiy)
Pain
Sensory/perceptual alterations (specify) (visual, auditory, kinesthetic, gustatory, tactile, olfactory)
Unilateral neglect

Self-Perception–Self-Concept Pattern (SP-SCP)
Anxiety
Body image disturbance
Fear
Hopelessness
Personal identity disturbance
Powerlessness
Self-esteem disturbance
  Chronic low self-esteem
  Situational low self-esteem

Role-Relationship Pattern (RRP)
Altered family processes
Altered parenting
Altered role performance
Anticipatory grieving
Dysfunctional grieving
Impaired social interaction
Impaired verbal communication
Parental role conflict
Potential altered parenting
Potential for violence: self-directed or directed at others
Social isolation

Sexuality-Reproductive Pattern (SxRP)
Altered sexuality patterns
Rape-trauma syndrome
Rape-trauma syndrome: compound reaction
Rape-trauma syndrome: silent reaction
Sexual dysfunction

Coping–Stress Tolerance Pattern (CSTP)
Defensive coping
Family coping: potential for growth
Impaired adjustment
Ineffective denial
Ineffective family coping: compromised
Ineffective family coping: disabling
Ineffective individual coping
Post-trauma response

Value-Belief Pattern (VBP)
Spiritual distress (distress of the human spirit)

*Nursing diagnoses include those approved by the North American Diagnosis Association in 1988. Functional Health Patterns from Gordon (1987) and personal communication, 1988. Abbreviations shown here are used to designate Functional Health Patterns in Nursing Care Plans.
†Suggested code for functional level classification: 0 Completely independent; 1 Requires use of equipment or device; 2 Requires help from another person for assistance, supervision, or teaching; 3 Requires help from another person and equipment or device; 4 Is dependent, does not participate in activity.

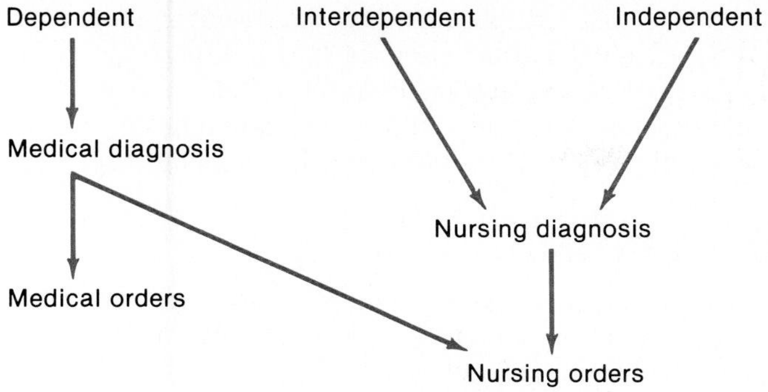

FIG. 2-2 Domains of professional nursing practice. (Modified from the Professional Nursing Project, Saint Francis Hospital, Tulsa, OK, 1985.)

bility and accountability overlap and require collaboration between the two disciplines. *Independent* activities are those areas of nursing practice that are the direct responsibility of the nurse. Nursing diagnoses reflect the interdependent and independent dimensions of nursing (Saint Francis Hospital, 1985), (Fig. 2-2).

Problem

The nursing diagnosis is composed of three components: problem, etiology, and signs and symptoms (often referred to as "PES"). The first—the problem statement—describes the child's response to health pattern deficits in the child, family, or community. This is the patient's response to disturbances of life processes, patterns, functions, or development, including those occuring secondary to disease. In this text the problem statement is written using NANDA diagnostic categories, which are listed within Gordon's 11 functional health patterns (see box).

Not all children will have actual health problems. Some may have a potential health problem, which is a risk state requiring nursing intervention to prevent the development of an actual problem. Potential health problems indicate the presence of *risk factors* that predispose a child and family to a dysfunctional health pattern and are limited to individuals who have a greater number of risk factors than the population as a whole. Risk factors, which are the signs indicating a potential health problem, are potential causes. Intervention is directed toward reducing risk factors. To differentiate actual from potential health problems, the word *potential* is included in the nursing diagnosis statement, for example: *potential altered parenting: knowledge deficit.*

The statement of a nursing diagnosis may not be a "problem." The nurse may write a positive nursing diagnosis, such as a statement from the diagnostic categories noting that the patient has developed adaptive responses to a health problem that the nurse wishes to support or facilitate. An example is "anticipatory grieving." "Dysfunctional grieving," on the other hand, is a maladaptive response that the nurse would attempt to modify.

Etiology

The second component of the PES format, the etiology, describes the physiologic, situational, and maturational factors that cause the problem or influence its development. The etiology may be behaviors of the patient, factors in the environment, or an interaction of both. The etiology is written using NANDA diagnostic categories, for example, *Noncompliance related to powerlessness.* However, this may not always be possible because of the relatively recent development of the diagnostic categories. In using the PES format it is important that the nurse not link the problem statement and etiology with words that imply cause and effect. Etiologies are probable causes; using words that imply cause and effect can result in legal or professional difficulties. Although a direct cause-and-effect relationship may not be involved, the etiology does influence the problem. Therefore the phrase "related to" is used to indicate a relationship between the problem and its etiology.

Differentiating among various etiologies is critically important because *interventions to alter the health problem are directed toward the etiology.* This is a primary concept in understanding nursing process and the PES format. For example, a problem statement of *Noncompliance in dietary restrictions* could have various etiologies. Examples of the etiologic factors include: (1) knowledge deficit, (2) denial of illness, (3) low economic resources, and (4) cultural conflict. Interventions for a knowledge deficit would be very different from interventions for low economic resources.

Not only is differentiation between etiologies critically important, so is being *specific* about the etiology. For example, if the nursing diagnosis is *Noncompliance to dietary restrictions related to knowledge deficit,* the nurse might intervene in varying ways, depending on whether the knowledge deficit is associated with (1) an inability to read, (2) a lack of educational materials, or (3) a lack of practice in menu planning. When the etiology is a broad category such as knowledge deficit, the nurse must investigate further to clarify the origin of the etiology. If the case of the knowledge deficit is an inability to read, then nonwritten patient education material may be needed. If the dietary alterations are complex, practice in menu planning may be necessary. For example, in one family with a child who had congestive heart failure, the origin of the knowledge deficit was an inability to plan meals that were low in sodium. The nursing interventions were directed at teaching the mother as well as the grandmother (who cared for the child during the day) what foods to prepare and having them compile sample menus.

Although nursing interventions are directed at the etiology, the problem statement does *influence* interventions. For example, with the nursing diagnoses of *Social isolation related to impaired physical mobility, level 3* and *Constipation related to impaired physical mobility, level 3,* the interventions are directed at the impaired mobility. However, the focus (or outcome) of mobilizing the patient is different. In the first nursing diagnosis, interventions address the movement of the patient into a social environment. Interventions for the second diagnosis address the need for a high-fiber diet and increased fluids.

At times the etiology of the problem statement is unknown. The use of the term *unknown etiology* in the diagnostic statement alerts the nurse and other members of the nursing staff to perform further assessment for etiological factors. The inclusion of signs and symptoms substantiates the identification of the problem. For example, *Altered parenting related to unknown etiology: history of child abuse, delayed growth and development in child.* Just as the medical profession treats symptomatically for an unknown etiology, the nursing profession directs care at the presenting signs and symptoms until an etiology is identified.

Signs and Symptoms

The third component, signs and symptoms, refers to a cluster of cues and/or defining characteristics that are derived from patient assessment and indicate actual health problems. The defining characteristics are observable when the health problem is present. When a defining characteristic is essential for the diagnosis to be made, it is considered critical. These critical defining characteristics help differentiate between diagnostic categories. For example, in deciding between the diagnostic categories of fear and anxiety, the major defining characteristic of the diagnostic category "fear" is the ability to identify the object of fear. If the child and family cannot identify the source of the feeling of dread, then "anxiety" may be the more appropriate choice for a nursing diagnosis.

Defining characteristics are derived from initial and ongoing patient assessment and may be included in the signs and symptoms to clarify problems and etiologies in the nursing diagnosis. Signs and symptoms are usually documented with assessment data and are not necessarily included in the nursing diagnosis statement. Signs and symptoms are in the nursing diagnosis statement only when needed for clarity, such as in the following example: *Ineffective individual coping, related to pain/refusing to move, apprehensive of anyone jarring bed, rapid pulse, irritable, improved behavior after analgesic administered.* The signs and symptoms clarify the child's behavioral manifestations to the pain and the response to pharmacologic intervention. This information is helpful in directing nursing care; for example, it indicates that better pain management is needed.

Since the nursing diagnoses must be amenable to nursing care, medical diagnoses such as anemia or congestive heart failure are not directly treated by the nurse. The patient may have the nursing diagnosis of ineffective parenting only with etiologies such as knowledge, which are responsive to nursing interventions.

Not all patient problems lend themselves to nursing diagnoses. Consequently the patient will require many nursing interventions, such as the administration of medications, that are dictated by the medical diagnoses. When a child is diagnosed as having congestive heart failure, the nurse automatically performs an assessment and monitors the child with special attention to the cardiac status. This is the interdependent domain of nursing.

PLANNING

Once the diagnoses and patient problems have been identified, a plan of care is developed and outcomes or goals are established. The *outcome* is the projected change in a patient's health status, clinical condition, or behavior that occurs after nursing interventions. The ultimate goal of nursing care is to convert the nursing diagnoses or clinical problem into a desired health state. This must be established before the interventions can be developed.

Many factors are considered when the outcomes are developed. The outcome must be patient centered and individualized according to the capabilities and limitations of the child and family. Unreasonable or unrealistic outcomes will only ensure the failure of the nursing plan of care. The ideal way to determine outcomes is in a conference with the family and child, if appropriate. In this setting all significant persons can agree on what is to be done, learned, or experienced. The final test of the projected outcome is that it must be observable and measurable. This is essential so that the plan of care can be evaluated. The box below illustrates the development of outcomes.

Developing the Outcome

1. Focus on the problem statement of the nursing diagnosis.
2. Using measurable verbs, describe the desired patient's behavior or change in clinical status.
3. Add modifiers that describe what, where, how, and when.
4. Add the achievement time.
5. Examine the statement. Determine if it is measurable, realistic, and achievable.

Examples of Outcome Statements

Measurable Verbs	Modifiers	Achievement Time
Demonstrate	Correct handwashing technique	After watching film twice
Walk	Three times around the nurse's station	24 hours after surgery
Eat	Two high-fiber foods	Each meal
Administer	Correct insulin dose	By discharge
Drink	200 ml fluids	Per day

Modified from Saint Francis Hospital: Professional nursing project manual, Tulsa, OK, 1985, Saint Francis Hospital.

While developing the appropriate outcomes, the nurse must determine the priorities of care. Foremost is the need to stabilize the child physiologically; then other problems may be addressed. The time interval that defines this nurse-patient relationship will influence what outcomes may be expected. Long-term goals are viewed as the desired health status for the child and family and require considerable time to be realized. Short-term goals, those goals that can usually be met within hours or days, can be incremental points toward the long-term goal or an end in themselves in certain health situations. Regardless of whether the goals are long or short term, nursing interventions should be goal directed. This enables the patient to receive the maximum benefit from nursing care.

Nursing Care Plans

The end point of the planning phase is the development of the nursing plan of care. The nursing care plans in this text provide guidelines for the care of children and families with a particular problem. *Standard care plans are plans that are sufficiently broad to account for situations that may develop in patients with particular problems.* For this reason the care plans often have numerous nursing diagnoses. These possible nursing diagnoses can guide patient observation and data collection in monitoring the development of adverse reactions. *Individualized care plans are plans that are concerned with only those diagnoses that apply to the particular patient situation.* Consequently, in actual practice all the problems presented in a standard care plan may not occur. On the average in clinical practice, the child and family will have three nursing diagnoses (NANDA, 1987). When a standard nursing care plan is used as a guide in developing an individualized plan of care, the problems not pertinent to the situation should be eliminated and the outcomes individualized to the specific situations. The characteristics of standard and individualized nursing care plans are compared in Table 2-2. However, before implementation begins, nursing interventions must be developed to meet the expected outcomes and nursing goals.

Nursing goals are broad statements that can apply to any number of individuals sharing a similar problem. Some examples of general nursing goals are "increase fluid intake," "ambulate patient," "support family." *Nursing interventions,* sometimes referred to as *nursing actions* or *nursing orders,* are specific directives for nursing care that are carried out to help the particular patient move from the present state to the state described in the projected outcomes. The objective of the nursing intervention is to direct individualized care to a patient.

In developing nursing interventions, the nurse, child, and family are all important components in the planning process. Selected resource persons may be called in; for example, the clinical nurse specialist, dietitian, physical therapist, social worker, chaplain, or physician.

There are a number of patient and family factors to consider in developing nursing interventions. Some of these are:

- Knowledge, skills, and abilities of the child and family
- Child's and family's perception of health
- Ethnic and cultural factors
- Access to needed resources and/or support people
- Financial resources
- Compensatory mechanisms currently used

In determining the nursing interventions it is important to be aware of the impact that the problem will have on both the child and family. The assessment data should be reviewed and discussed with the family to determine how much time and energy is available for investment in health promotion activities. The child and family with a chronic disorder must value having the disorder under control. The child may see the benefits as increased time with peers or decreased hospitalizations. If control is valued, there is a greater likelihood that the desired behaviors will be incorporated into the child's life-style. The

TABLE 2-2

Characteristics of Standard and Individualized Nursing Care Plans

	Standard Care Plan*	Individualized Care Plan
1. Assessment	Information is specific only to problem	Information specific to both identified problem and the child and family
2. Nursing diagnosis	All probable nursing diagnoses with general etiologic factors are considered	Only nursing diagnoses specific to the child and family are considered; the cause of the disease directs actual plan of care
3. Planning	Goals are broad and represent nursing goals	Goals are specific and reflect patient outcomes
4. Implementation	Nursing interventions are broad and applicable to most patients with problem	Nursing interventions are specific and provide direction for nursing care of individual patient
5. Evaluation	Progress the patient is *expected* to make is identified	Progress the patient has actually made toward the outcome is identified

*Describes format used in nursing care plans in the text that may differ from other types of standardized nursing care plans.

family's economic level must be taken into consideration; this includes any financial problems that may occur and any resources or assistance that can be used. Ethnic and cultural factors can also influence the outcome attainment. For example, in ethnic groups that use soy sauce routinely as a seasoning for food, adherence to a low-sodium diet may be very difficult.

There are nurse factors that will influence the translation of a nursing goal into a nursing intervention. These include creativity in finding ways to help a patient carry out a necessary activity and the ability of the rest of the staff to carry out the nursing interventions. For example, is the nursing intervention practical and able to be carried out within the time frame available? To meet the objective of providing individualized care to the patient and/or family, the intervention should be creative yet realistic. An essential component of implementing the plan of care is the cooperation of all involved staff. The need for consistency in care planning is illustrated in the following example.

Many diverse factors influence nursing care. These include nurses' strongly held personal beliefs and their ethnic or cultural backgrounds. Philosophic differences among members of the nursing staff created many difficulties in planning care for one chronically ill child. He would stay up until early morning watching television and playing games with the nursing staff when the unit was quiet. As a result, often he would sleep late in the morning, miss meals, and be too tired for the necessary physical and respiratory therapy. These difficulties were presented at a patient care conference (Fig. 2-3). At this time the nursing staff agreed to develop a contract with the patient, one that *all* would adhere to. A reasonable bedtime and awakening time were agreed on, and the patient received certain privileges for keeping to the schedule. For this patient the conference and the written plan of care that was established provided the staff with the structure needed to change the child's behavior. (For an in-depth discussion of the chronically ill child, see Chapter 18.)

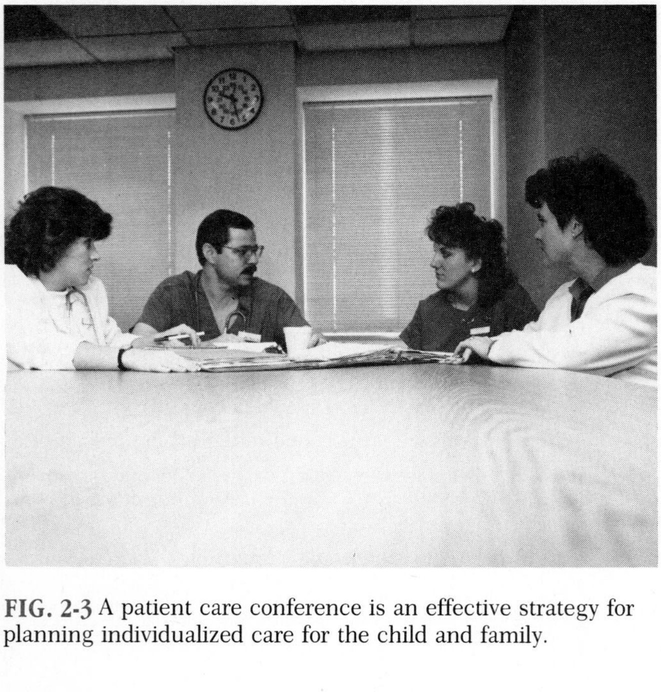

FIG. 2-3 A patient care conference is an effective strategy for planning individualized care for the child and family.

Nursing interventions depend on the causes of the nursing diagnosis or patient problem and the desired outcomes. Nursing interventions should also be designed to direct observation and care to the medical diagnoses. The nurse may determine that more frequent vital-sign measurement may be required. A nursing order will ensure that this is interpreted and carried out with regard to the child's condition. In order to translate the nursing goal into a nursing intervention, the nurse must have data from the patient to answer these questions: What? When? How often? How long? Where? For example, if a nursing goal is to increase fluid intake, the interventions might state "increase fluid to at least 2000 ml in 24 hours. 1000 ml, 7-3; 800 ml, 3-11; 200 ml, 11-7. Child likes orange and apple juice, dislikes carbonated beverage. Offer fluids qh from 0900 to 2100."

The nurse generates and evaluates ideas for nursing interventions and selects those that have the greatest probability of success. Nursing interventions should not be focused on the symptoms of the disorder. Interventions at the symptom level may help temporarily, but seldom solve the underlying problem. Routine interventions should not be used without considering individual patient needs and converting them to specific outcomes. The physician's orders should not be reworded (Saint Francis Hospital, 1985).

Nursing interventions should be written both for patient and nurse behaviors. The most important interventions should be placed first, based on priority of patient needs. The interventions should be reviewed with the patient and family so that they can have a feeling of control. As nurses increase their knowledge about a client, nursing interventions, including collaboratory and coordinating activities, may need to be revised. Suggestions from dietitians, social workers, or physical therapists should be considered when writing nursing interventions. Education needs or referral to an outside agency are also incorporated into discharge planning.

IMPLEMENTATION

Implementation is the actual delivery of nursing care to the patient. This phase of the nursing process puts the nursing and medical plan of care into operation. The nurse's activities are guided by the nursing and medical diagnoses as well as by the patient's current status. For example, the nurse provides the patient with the assistance needed for activities of daily living, hygiene, and safety precautions.

The interventions performed span the three domains of nursing practice: dependent, interdependent, and independent. In the dependent domain the nurse implements the direction/orders of the responsible professional.

However, in all domains nursing judgment is necessary to determine if the order is appropriate for the patient. This involves both an assessment of the patient and an understanding of the intervention.

The interdependent and independent domains of nursing are usually governed by nursing interventions, but some physicians may provide direction in the interdependent area.

During the implementation phase the nurse should use each interaction with the child and family to continue assessing and reassessing nursing diagnoses and plan of care. Interventions such as baths, which require prolonged patient contact, are especially valuable for validating data with the patient.

The implementation of the care plan should be documented in the patient's written record. Interventions can be charted on the flow record and the patient's response should be charted in the progress note. Once the nursing interventions have been implemented, they need to be continually assessed to provide feedback and to evaluate whether they need modification. Assessing the patient's progress toward the projected outcomes enables the nurse to evaluate the effectiveness of the orders. If the nursing interventions have been effective, the signs and symptoms used to diagnose the problem should be changed, outcomes should be achieved, and the patient should be moving toward the time when termination of the nurse-patient relationship will take place and discharge to the home setting or other health care facility will occur.

EVALUATION

The final step of the nursing process is evaluation. Although it sounds easy, evaluation is a very difficult process without measurable outcomes. Effectively evaluating a patient requires several steps (Carnevali, 1983). First, criteria and standards are established that can be used to guide observations to determine patient progress in terms of the diagnoses and goals. For a child with nonorganic failure to thrive (NFTT), criteria might include a daily weight change. Second, the nurse observes the patient to determine what skills and knowledge have been mastered. This involves assessing feeding behaviors and parent-infant interactions. Third, these observed data are compared with the expected outcomes and the amount of progress recorded. For example, for a child with NFTT, actual weight gain is compared with an expected 1 ounce per day. If the patient is not achieving the expected outcomes, the care plan must be assessed to determine what obstacles, if any, exist.

DOCUMENTATION

Documentation is a vital part of the nursing process and is essential for evaluation. Although the nurse can assess and identify problems, plan and implement without documentation, evaluation is best performed with written evidence of progress toward outcomes. However, there should be evidence of the nursing process in the patient's written record. The initial assessment must be recorded, followed by evidence of the diagnostic process. A thorough assessment, followed by the identification-of-problem statement and the supporting data, is required. Then the written plan of care should be made available. All nursing interventions are recorded as they are performed, with the patient response to these interventions. Finally, the evaluation is documented in order to compare current patient status against expected patient outcomes.

The nursing process has become an integral part of professional practice. The Joint Commission on Accreditation of Healthcare Organizations has also incorporated the nursing process into the accreditation process. The fifth standard on which nursing service is evaluated states: "Individualized, goal directed nursing care is provided to patients through the use of the nursing process" (JCAH, 1987). The Joint Commission is actively involved in accrediting many health care providers. Currently hospitals, nursing homes, ambulatory services, and home health agencies can choose to be accredited by this group.

SUMMARY

The nursing process is the framework for professional nursing practice. It is composed of five steps: assessment, problem identification/nursing diagnosis, planning, implementation, and evaluation. To facilitate nursing practice, a framework that is oriented toward the human responses to actual or potential health problems must be used. Gordon's 11 functional patterns describe human functioning. Therefore by assessing each pattern the nurse can determine where problems exist. Once nursing diagnoses have been formulated, a plan of care can be designed and implemented. The evaluation stage measures the child's and/or family's progress toward the established outcomes.

When the patient has been thoroughly assessed and his problems identified, a plan of care established, implemented, and evaluated, then quality nursing care is being delivered. The nursing process combines the art and science of nursing.

KEY CONCEPTS

- The nursing process is the orderly systematic method of determining the client's problems, making plans to solve them, initiating the plan or assigning others to implement it, and evaluating the extent to which the plan was effective in resolving the identified problems.
- Assessment is the deliberate and systematic collection of data.
- Problem identification is the analysis of assessment data to determine what areas of dysfunction or potential dysfunction exist.
- Nursing diagnoses are client problems that nurses, by virtue of their education and experience, are able and licensed to treat.
- Planning is the development of outcomes or nursing goals and interventions to meet them.
- Outcome development involves five steps. These are (1) focusing on the problem statement; (2) describing the child's desired behavior after nursing care—with a measurable verb; (3) adding modifiers that describe what, where, how, and when; (4) setting the achievement time; and (5) reviewing the outcome to ensure that it is measurable, realistic, and achievable.
- Implementation is the actual delivery of nursing care to the child and family.
- Evaluation is the comparison of the child's status with the expected outcomes.

STUDY QUESTIONS AND ACTIVITIES

1 Perform a screening assessment on a patient. Identify areas where a focused assessment may be indicated.
2 Select any two of the following goals or outcomes and write nursing interventions for them: alleviate pain; educate regarding low-sodium diet; increase activity; provide diversional (play) activity, support family.
3 Develop an individualized nursing care plan for a child and family. Compare and contrast this care plan with the comparable nursing care plan found in this text. For example, compare an individualized plan for a child with acute respiratory infection with the standardized one on pp. 696-698.
4 Review any five nursing care plans in the text. Are there certain nursing diagnoses that appear consistently? What could be a rationale for their frequency?

REFERENCES

American Nurses Association: Nursing: a social policy statement, Kansas City, MO, 1980, The Association.

Carnevali, D.L.: Nursing care planning: Diagnosis and management, ed. 3, Philadelphia, 1983, J.B. Lippincott Co.

Gordon, M.: Nursing diagnosis and the diagnostic process, Am. J. Nurs. **76:**1298-1300, 1976.

Gordon, M.: Nursing diagnosis process and application, ed. 2, New York, 1987, McGraw-Hill Book Co.

Joint Commission on Accreditation of Hospitals: AMH 88 accreditation manual for hospitals, Chicago, 1987, The Commission.

Kelly, L.Y.: Dimensions of professional nursing, ed. 5, New York, 1985, Macmillan Publishing Co.

North American Nursing Diagnosis Association: Classification of nursing diagnosis, Proceedings of the seventh conference, ed. A.M. McLane, St. Louis, 1987, The C.V. Mosby Co.

Saint Francis Hospital: Professional nursing project, Tulsa, OK, 1985.

BIBLIOGRAPHY

Baer, C.: Nursing diagnosis, Top. Clin. Nurs., **5**(4):1-103, 1984.
Brooks, E.: The starting point, Nurs. Manage. **14**(6):35-37, 1983.
Bulechek, G.M., and McCloskey, J.C.: Nursing interventions: treatments for nursing diagnoses, Philadelphia, 1985, W.B. Saunders Co.
Carpenito, L.J.: Nursing diagnosis application to clinical practice, Philadelphia, 1982, W.B. Saunders Co.
Case, B.A., and Rooney, D.S.: Planning patient care strategies, Nurs. Manage. **13**(4):23-26, 1982.
Fortin, J.D., and Robinow, J.: Legal implications of nursing diagnoses, Nurs. Clin. North. Am. **14:**553-561, 1979.
Gamberg, D., and others: Outcome charting, Nurs. Manage. **12**(10):36-38, 1981.
Gordon, M.: Manual of nursing diagnosis, New York, 1987, McGraw-Hill Book Co.
Griffith-Kennedy, J.W., and Christensen, P.J.: Nursing process application of theories, frameworks, and models, ed. 2, St. Louis, 1986, The C.V. Mosby Co.
Guzzetta, C.E., and Dossey, B.M.: Nursing diagnosis: framework, process, and outcome, Heart Lung **12:**281-291, 1983.
Hauck, M.R., and Roth, D.: Application of nursing diagnoses in a pediatric clinic, Pediatr. Nurs. **7:**49-52, 1984.
Mallick, M.J.: Nursing diagnosis and the novice student, Nurs. Health Care **4:**457-458, 1983.
Mayers, M.G.: A systematic approach to the nursing care plan, ed. 3, Norwalk, CT, 1983, Appleton-Century-Crofts.
McCloskey, J.C., and Grace, H.K.: Current issues in nursing, Boston, 1985, Blackwell Scientific Publications.
Potter, P.A., and Perry, A.G.: Fundamentals of nursing: concepts, process, and practice, St. Louis, 1985, The C.V. Mosby Co.
Rhodes, A.M.: Contents of nurses' detailed notes, MCN **12**(3):61, 1987.
Shamansky, S., and Yanni, C.R.: In opposition to nursing diagnoses: a minority opinion, Image **15**(2):47-50, 1983.
Stevens, B.J.: Nursing theory, ed. 2, Boston, 1984, Little, Brown & Co.
Walker, L., and Nicholson, R.: Criteria for evaluating nursing process models, Nurse Educator **5:**8-9, 1980.
Warren, J.L.: Accountability and nursing diagnosis: J. Nurs. Admin. **13**(10):34-37, 1983.
Wright, D.: An introduction to the evaluation of nursing care: a review of the literature, J. Adv. Nurs. **9:**457-467, 1984.

UNIT
II

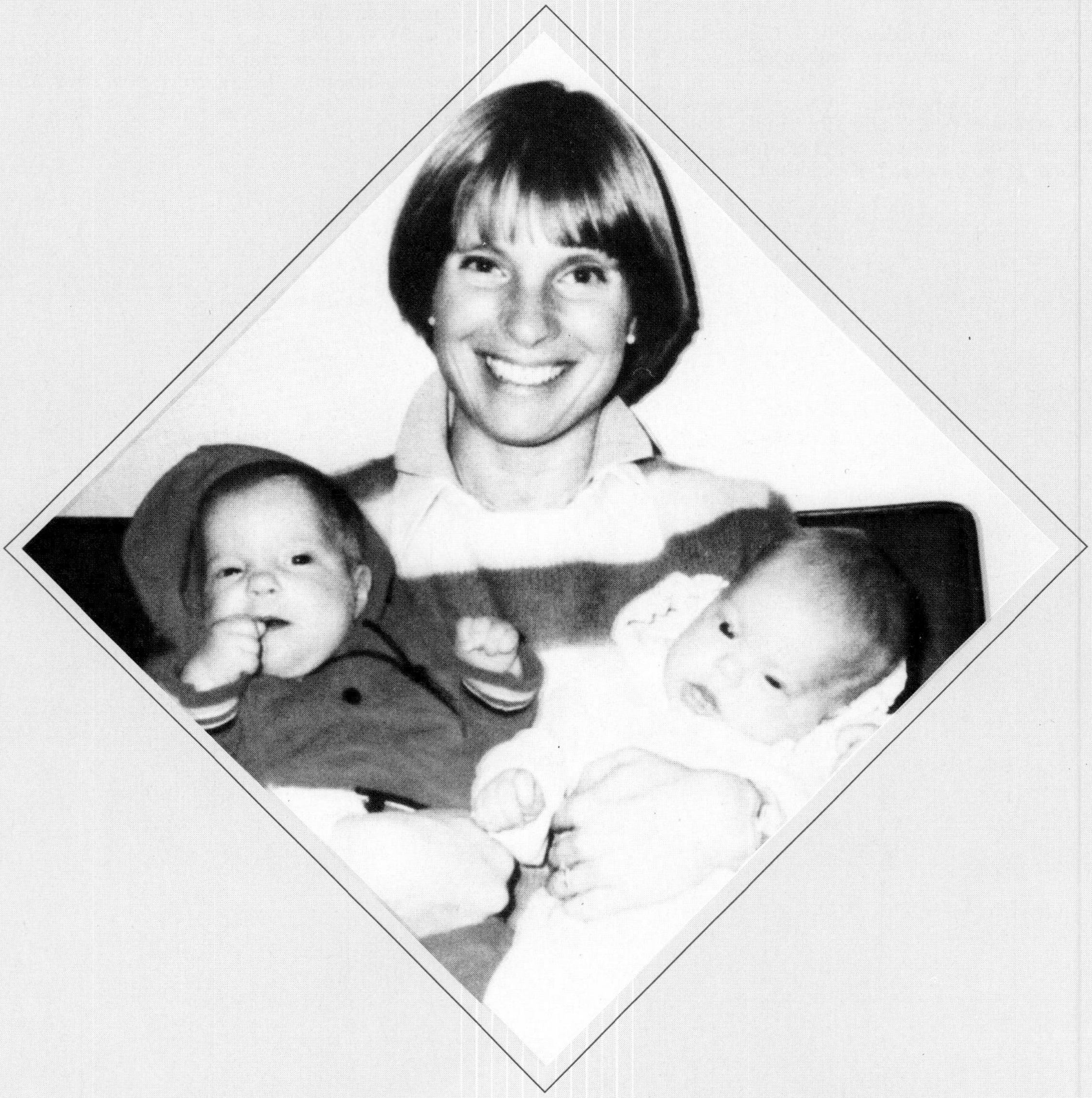

Psychosocial and Developmental Influences on the Child and Family

The ultimate goal of infant and child care is the promotion of optimum health and development for children at any stage of health or illness. To accomplish this purpose nurses need an understanding of children and the way in which they grow and relate with significant persons in their environment, as well as an awareness of the multiple factors that contribute to the uniqueness of each child. To assess and evaluate the health and development of children, it is essential to be aware that the child is in the process of becoming.

Chapter 3, *Social, Cultural, and Religious Influences on the Child and Family,* considers the ways in which the societal and cultural background of the family affects children, their health, and their relationships. The emphasis is on differences in health practices, environmental influences, and perspectives on health and health care providers.

Chapter 4, *Family Influences on Health Promotion of the Child and Family,* is concerned with children in their family setting. It includes selected family theories, family constellations, and the way in which the family influences development. The child's place within the family is examined with emphasis on the role of family members in shaping the child's attitudes and behavior.

Chapter 5, *Developmental Influences on Child Health Promotion,* provides a vertical or longitudinal view of the alterations that take place during growth and development and serves as a preface to the horizontal age-specific discussions in the chapters on health promotion. The discussion presents a brief overview of the major theories of development and factors that affect the growth and health of children, as well as the unique needs of children.

CHAPTER 3

Social, Cultural, and Religious Influences on the Child and Family

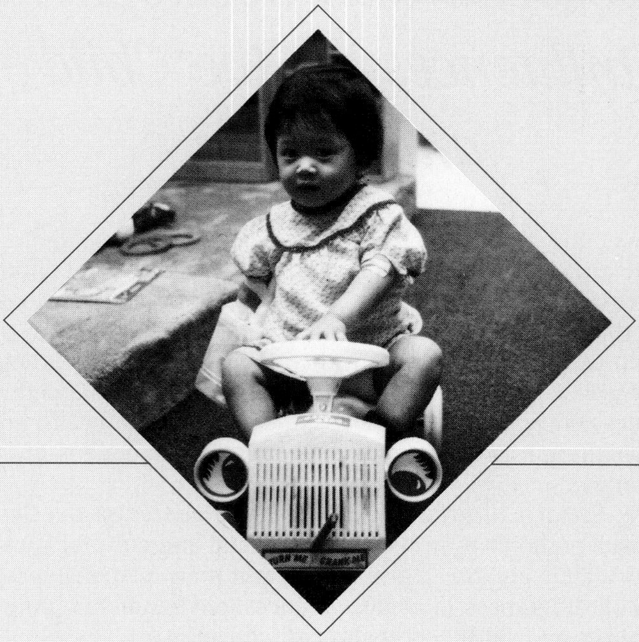

LEARNING OBJECTIVES

On completion of this chapter the reader will be able to:

- Define *culture*, *culture shock*, *ethnicity*, and *race*
- Describe the subcultural influences on child development in the areas of socialization, education, and aspiration
- Compare and contrast the advantages and disadvantages encountered in the educational system by children from lower- and middle-class backgrounds
- Characterize family life in present-day America
- Identify four common diseases or disorders that affect certain ethnic or cultural groups
- Identify areas of potential conflict of values and customs for a nurse interacting with a family from a different cultural/ethnic group
- Describe three religious groups whose beliefs significantly affect their health practices

The future of any society depends on its children. If it is to survive, the society must make provision for their care, nurture, and socialization. Cultural survival depends on whether the customs and values of the culture are transmitted from one generation to the next through the medium of the family. The culture into which children are born outlines the roles of their parents, structures their relationships with other people, and determines much of the behavior they acquire. A holistic view of any child requires nurses to develop some understanding of how culture contributes to the development of social and emotional relationships and influences childrearing practices and attitudes toward health. This includes awareness of the nurse's own cultural frame of reference and a concerted effort to recognize and appreciate the views and beliefs of health care recipients.

◆ Culture

Culture is the acquired knowledge people use to interpret experience and generate behavior and differs from both race and ethnicity. *Race* is defined as a division of mankind possessing traits that are transmissible by descent and sufficient to characterize it as a distinct human type; one classification of race is Caucasoid, Negroid, and Mongoloid. *Ethnicity* is the affiliation of a set of persons who share a unique cultural, social, and linguistic heritage. *Socialization* is the process by which children acquire the beliefs, values, and behaviors considered desirable or appropriate by the culture.

A culture is composed of individuals who share a set of values, beliefs, practices, and information that is learned, integrative, social, and satisfying. Culture is not a surface veneer that covers a basic outlook shared by all human beings but an ingrained orientation to life that serves as a frame of reference for individual perception and judgment. People from one culture differ from those in other cultures in the ways they think, solve problems, perceive, and structure the world. Essentially, culture is the way of life of a group of people that incorporates experiences of the past, influences thought and action in the present, and transmits these traditions to future group members. Adaptation is necessary, however, for the culture to survive in an ever-changing world. Consciously and unconsciously, the members abandon, modify, or assume new patterns to meet the needs of the group.

The culture in which children are reared determines the type of food they will eat, the language they will speak, the ideals of behavior they will follow, and the way they will conduct themselves in social roles. To be acceptable members of the culture, children must learn how the culture expects them to behave toward others in the group. In turn, they learn how they can expect others to behave toward them.

Related to the large culture are many *subcultures*, each with an identity of its own. Subcultural influences will be discussed in more detail later in the chapter.

Cultures and subcultures contribute to the uniqueness of child members in such a subtle way and at such an early age that children grow up to feel that their beliefs, attitudes, values, and practices are the "correct" or "normal" ones; those of other cultures may be viewed as "deviant" or "wrong." A set of values learned in childhood is apt to characterize children's attitudes and behavior for life, guiding their long-range strivings and monitoring their short-range, impulsive inclinations. Thus every ongoing society socializes each succeeding generation to its cultural heritage.

The manner and sequence of the growth and development phenomenon are universal and fundamental features of all children; however, the variations in behavioral responses that children display to similar events are believed to be determined by cultures. Inborn temperament and modes of behavior that prompt children to behave in their own preferred and highly individual manner may be in harmony or in conflict with the culture. Such forces as heredity and maturation impose limits on the influence that parents and other social groups may bring to bear.

The culture fosters and reinforces those behaviors deemed desirable and appropriate; it attempts to depress or extinguish those at conflict with cultural norms. Some cultures encourage aggressive behaviors in their children; others favor amiability and compliance. Some foster individual resourcefulness and competition; others emphasize cooperation and submission to group interest. Cultures may also differ in whether status in the group is based on age or on skill. Even children's play and their types of games are culturally determined. In some cultures children play in groups composed of members of the same sex; in others they play in mixed-sex groups. In some cultures team games predominate; in others most play is limited to individual games.

Standards and norms vary from culture to culture and location to location; a practice that is accepted in one area may meet with disapproval or create tension in another. The extent to which cultures tolerate divergence from the established norm varies among cultures and subcultural groups. Although conformity provides a degree of security, it is a decided deterrent to change.

SOCIAL ROLES

Much of children's self-concept is derived from their ideas about their social roles. Roles are cultural creations; therefore, the culture prescribes patterns of behavior for persons in a variety of social positions. All persons who hold similar social positions have the obligation to behave in a particular manner. A role prohibits some behaviors and allows for others. Because it delineates and clarifies roles, the culture is a significant influence on the development of children's self-concept, that is, the attitudes and beliefs they have about themselves.

A social group consists of a system of roles carried out in both primary and secondary groups. A *primary group* is characterized by intimate, continued face-to-face contact, mutual support of the members, and the ability to order or constrain a considerable proportion of individual members' behavior. Two such groups are the family and the peer group, both of which exert a great deal of influence on the child. Some communities (for example, contemporary rural, religious, or ethnic communities) also exert a strong primary group influence. All members know each other, most belong to the same subgroups, and all are concerned about each member's behavior. There is considerable support among the community members and little conflict of values. Relatives are likely to live close together, allowing young members ample opportunity to observe and absorb the practices and customs of the culture. Any member of the community feels justified in evaluating and censuring the conduct of another member.

Secondary groups are groups that have limited, intermittent contact and in which there is generally less concern for members' behavior. These groups offer little in terms of support or pressure toward conformity except in rigidly limited areas. Examples of secondary groups are professional associations and church organizations (also considered in relation to subgroups). The childrearing orientation in a secondary-group environment, such as urban communities, differs considerably from that of a primary-group community. An urban community is dynamic and rapidly changing; therfore, many of the traditional behaviors and values do not meet its needs. Consequently parents are often uncertain about what to teach their children. They may wish to rear their children with values consistent with their own, but the differences in experience between the generations are too great. As a result, they often grant their children autonomy in some areas of decision making early in the developmental process, and other secondary groups assume a greater influence. The children are exposed to an assortment of social groups with diverse sets of values and expectations. None of the groups is highly dominant in its influence; therefore, the children are exposed to an eclectic set of values, some in agreement and some at conflict with the others. From these they must ultimately select those that they determine to be best for them and adopt them to form a consistent set of roles and behaviors to be incorporated into the self-concept.

Guilt and Shame Orientation

Conditioning children to feel either guilt or shame for misdeeds is a technique used by a culture to control social behavior—to internalize the norms and expectations of others. Some cultural groups value a well-developed conscience (superego) and condition their children to feel guilt following wrongdoing. The offenders get an uncomfortable physical feeling and want to purge themselves. Since guilt is based within the individual, successful conditioning produces self-regulated persons who punish themselves without their being caught in the act of wrongdoing.

In many cultural groups guilt is lacking and social controls are based on the use of shame. The offenders do not want anyone to see them when they have been found guilty of a wrongful deed. Sometimes children in these groups learn that anything is acceptable as long as one is not caught; the shame results when the forbidden act is found out by others.

Although both techniques are used by members of both primary- and secondary-group communities, shame is apt to be more successful in a primary-group community because most behaviors are quite public. In secondary-group communities it is less effective; persons are not as apt to be caught and, if caught, can withdraw and join a group that is unaware of the misdeed.

Guilt probably has a greater influence on behavior in urban communities, although many authorities believe that the trend in urban America is shifting away from a guilt orientation. Rapid changes in the American culture leave parents unsure of their own values; therefore, much of their function is abandoned to the school and peers. Peers are notorious for the use of shame as a disciplinary technique.

SUBCULTURAL INFLUENCES

Except in rare situations, children grow and develop in a blend of cultures and subcultures, those smaller groups within a culture that possess many characteristics of the larger culture while contributing their own particular values. In a large, complex society such as the United States, different groups have their own set of standards, values, and expectations within the collective ways of the large culture. Although many cultural differences are related to geographic boundaries, subcultures are not always restricted by location.

Children's membership in a cultural subgroup is, for the most part, involuntary. They are born into a family with a specific ethnic and/or racial heritage, socioeconomic level, and religious beliefs. Although in the complex American society there are countless subcultures and considerable variation in the way of life, those subcultures that seem to exert the greatest influence on childrearing are ethnicity, social class, and occupational role. Additionally, schools and peer group subcultures are strong influences in the socialization of the child.

Ethnicity

Ethnicity is the classification of or affiliation with any of the basic groups or divisions of mankind or any heterogeneous population differentiated by customs, characteristics, language, or similar distinguishing factors. Ethnic differences extend to many areas and include such manifestations as family structure, language, food preferences, moral codes, and expression of emotion.

To establish their place in the group, children learn how to adhere to a mode of behavior that is in accordance with standards distinctive to the group and learn how they can expect others to behave toward them. They take their cues from observing and imitating those to whom they are exposed. For example, children of a racial minority form a perception of their role as a group member by observing the manner in which role models within the subgroup respond to treatment by people outside the subgroup. When they see group members display an attitude of inferiority, they assume this to be the appropriate behavior. These perceptions are then incorporated into their own self-concept.

In the United States the cross-cultural lines are becoming blurred as subcultures are assimilated and blended into the larger culture (Fig. 3-1). Although ethnic differences in childrearing are probably diminishing, they remain important. It is particularly difficult for persons to attempt to maintain an identity with a subculture while living and conforming to the requirements of the

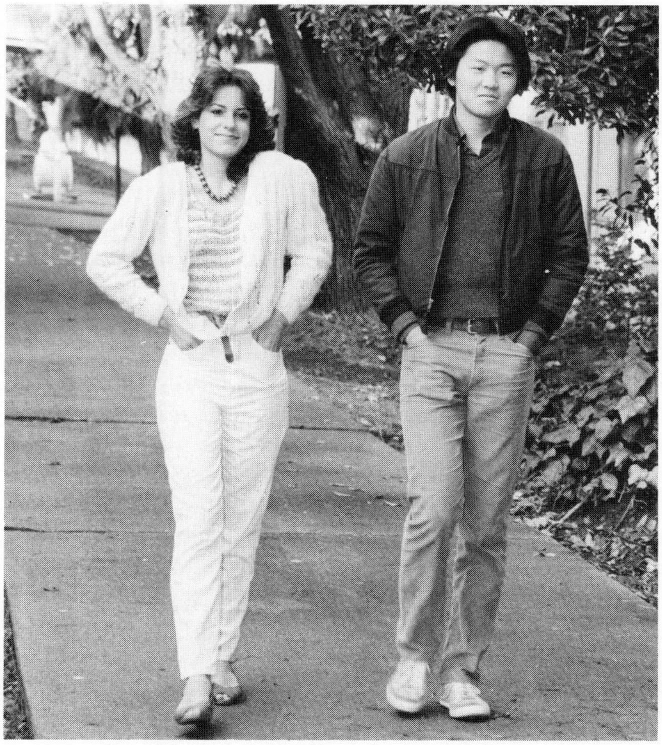

FIG. 3-1 Youngsters from different cultural backgrounds interact within the larger culture.

larger culture. The values of the commercial and educational systems of the dominant culture are often in conflict with those of the minority culture. Consequently children reared in this environment are confused about roles and values, and they usually adopt those of the more influential or higher-status culture. Youth, in particular, are influenced by the locally dominant group.

Ethnocentrism. Ethnocentrism is the emotional attitude that one's own ethnic group is superior to that of others, that one's values, beliefs, and perceptions are the correct ones, and that the group's ways of living and behaving are the best way. This inherent attitude implies that all other groups are inferior and tends to bias one's understanding of the behaviors of others.

Social Class

Those who have made extensive studies conclude that although there are exceptions, probably the greatest influence on childrearing practices and their consequences is the social class of the family into which a child is born. Differences in childrearing goals and practices as well as attitudes toward health have been found to be greater between social classes than between races or ethnic groups. In America social class and socioeconomic level are essentially synonymous, inasmuch as the factors by which a social class are defined are education, occupation, area of residence, and family income. Since children are reared differently by parents who vary in respect to these factors, social class can be expected to produce substantial variation in their upbringing.

Lower and working class. The uncertainty of their life leads members of the lower classes to be present oriented, that is, to take advantage of gratification when possible. This orientation is distinctly different from that of the middle class, who are willing to delay gratification to achieve a long-term goal.

Children in lower-class families encounter major educational disadvantages, reflected in the high incidence of academic failure and attendant dropout rate. Some of the major educational disadvantages encountered by lower-class children include:

- Parents value the concrete and tangible rather than the abstract and are therefore less inclined to encourage these qualities in their children
- Parents are less likely to read to the child or encourage educational play due to their own educational level
- No role models are available to support the value of education
- Inadequate funding and/or poor quality of education exists in neighborhood schools
- Poor health and inadequate nutrition of the children is common
- Limited communication skills, such as simple grammar, inability to express abstractions, and ethnic dialects hamper interactions with teachers from middle-class backgrounds

Lower- and working-class parents are tradition oriented, stressing obedience and conformity to parental values and external regulations. The most frequently used form of discipline for undesirable behavior is physical punishment. Parents are usually less interested in the direction of children's activities than with conduct; they are more concerned that children stay out of trouble.

With better job security through unionization, unemployment compensation, and other welfare features, some segments of the lower classes are finding life more predictable. They are less apt to seize gratifications lest the opportunity vanish and are beginning to develop long-range goals, including an increased interest in education for their children.

Middle and upper class. Children from these classes live in an enriched environment that provides material comforts and broader opportunities. The parents are usually educated, and other authority figures such as teachers with whom the children are routinely in contact are usually from a middle-class background and have activities and expectations for the children that are similar to those of the parents. Parents have occupations that require judgment, creativity, and resourcefulness, and these attributes are fostered in their children.

Middle-class parents are future oriented, have higher educational and occupational aspirations for their children, and use long-range planning to meet these goals (Shaffer, 1985). Middle-class parents encourage their children in activities that foster achievement, such as dancing lessons, athletics, and scouting, in the belief that this will make them well-rounded, self-directed adults.

In the area of discipline, middle-class parents are more

apt to make use of manipulative techniques such as reasoning and drawing on the child's sense of guilt. They tend to scold and use isolation rather than physical punishment. There is more concern regarding the *intent* of the act than the *consequence* of the act.

It is believed that upper-class parents are more permissive and foster desirable behavior through positive reinforcement. However, much of the actual child care in upper-class families is delegated to surrogates, such as housekeepers, governesses, or private schools. The parent serves as an arbitrator between the children and the servants.

Poverty

A subcultural influence closely related to but different from social class is the condition known as poverty. It is a relative concept and is usually associated with the general standards of a population. An *absolute standard* of poverty attempts to delimit a basic set of resources needed for adequate existence; a *relative standard* reflects the median standard of living in a society. That is, what appears to be deprivation in one area may be a standard or norm in another.

The term *poverty* implies both visible and invisible impoverishment. *Visible poverty* refers to lack of money or material resources, which includes insufficient clothing, poor sanitation, and deteriorating housing. *Invisible poverty* refers to social and cultural deprivation such as limited employment opportunities, inferior educational opportunities, lack of or inferior medical services and health care facilities, and an absence of public services.

The very poor in the society who consistently exist on or below the poverty level live in a perpetual state of despair. Their limited skills give them no bargaining power in the job market, and the education needed to improve their status is beyond them. The poor desire better things for their children but are trapped in a circular pattern that perpetuates their life condition. Their powerlessness to control their fate or condition is a source of fatalism and resignation that is characteristic of the group in general. Optimism, when it is manifest, is more likely to be expressed in terms of luck or chance. This fatalistic attitude is a significant impediment to occupational and educational aspirations. It also inhibits them from seeking health care or practicing preventive health care measures. For example, if someone is injured or killed in an automobile accident, it is considered bad luck, not something they could have prevented by wearing a seat belt.

Factors related to poverty. Throughout the United States there are groups of people, geographically segregated, who constitute what is known as "pockets of poverty." These are seen in the dense urban areas, such as the ghettos, and many rural areas, especially those that are geographically isolated from the needed facilities and services. The nonurbanized regions identified as poverty areas in the United States are Appalachia, the deep South, the lower Southwest, and northern New England.

Certain ethnic or racial groups are overrepresented in the impoverished population. The most obvious of these are the blacks, Latinos, and Native Americans. One of the most disadvantaged groups are migrant Latino farm workers and their children. The low position of these families on the economic scale and their rootless, mobile existence subjects them to inadequate sanitation, substandard housing, social isolation, and lack of educational and medical facilities. This life-style is especially deleterious to the children. For example, children are apt to live in a number of localities and attend a variety of schools in the course of a year with no continuity in either education or health care. Because both parents work in the fields, children receive little adult supervision; therefore, accident rates are high and meals are erratic. Except where prohibited by law, children are even recruited to work in the fields along with the adults. Some migrants have a home base to which they return at the end of a growing season; others travel continuously, migrating north in summer and south in winter.

Affluence

On the opposite end of the socioeconomic spectrum are the children of affluent members of society. Although they can live within the warmth of a positive family relationship, many of them appear to be just as deprived as poverty-stricken children. Wealth does not provide protection against many of life's problems and disappointments, especially in the area of parent-child relationships. Like their counterparts in the poverty groups, children of the affluent suffer from discrimination, inadequate parenting, or unsatisfactory role models.

Children of the wealthy suffer most from lack of parental contact. There may be long separations from loving, caring parents because of social or business interests. Some have a cold, sometimes hostile parent, who is rarely available to the children. Even their places of residence contribute to their isolation and loneliness. Purchased parent surrogates, including servants, sports professionals (such as tennis or swimming instructors), and private school personnel, provide them with adult companionship and authority. The children of the wealthy are especially subject to psychologic problems, and emotional abuse is not uncommon.

Many children from wealthy families, like those from poor families, seem to thrive and flourish, making positive contributions to their families and society. However, a large number grow up to display a lack of motivation or self-discipline and boredom. They are suspicious of others, finding it difficult to believe they are liked for themselves and not for their money or position, and they do not trust others enough to enter into true friendships. Affluent children may also fail to acquire skills related to responsibilities and finances.

Occupation

Many authorities believe that the occupational environment of the family head correlates more closely than does social class with the direction of childrearing and the values parents attempt to convey to their children. There appear to be differences in the way of life between "individuated-entrepreneurial" and "welfare-bureaucratic" occupations (Leslie, 1982). Entrepreneurial occupations include the smaller and more traditional enterprises, such as small businesses, sales, and professionals such as medicine, that require self-reliance and independence. Income depends on hard work, individual initiative, and risk taking.

The concept of welfare-bureaucracy is based on large organizational structures. Bureaucracy implies specialization and supervision governed by a set of rules; welfare refers to the job security offered by the organization. In organizational occupations the risk taking is minimum and there is more adjustment to and dependence on others.

Entrepreneurs believe the world to be more harsh than do organizational workers and they rear their children in a more authoritarian manner. They emphasize self-control, self-denial, and responsible independence with a vigorous and control-oriented approach to life. Organizational parents tend toward a more permissive childrearing style that fosters passivity, dependency, and some degree of impulse expression. A concern for group approval (outer-directedness) takes precedence over development of the individual (inner-directedness).

The social values of the family are also related to social class differences in occupation. Parents in middle-class occupations that require initiative, independent judgment, and the ability to deal with others promote self-direction in their children. Working-class occupations are generally those that require conformity and obedience, values that are emphasized by working-class parents.

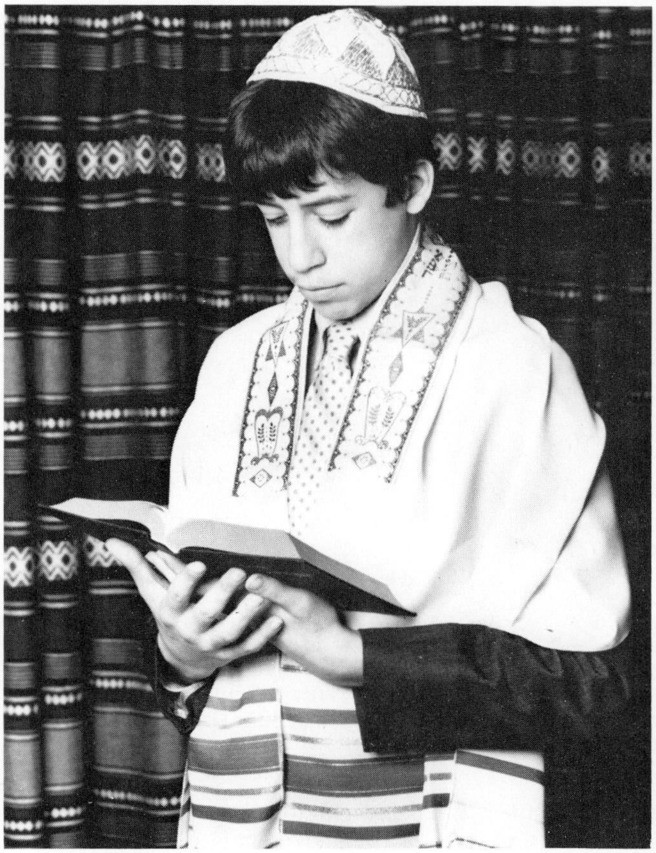

FIG. 3-2 A boy during his bar mitzvah ceremony.

Religion

Probably the most influential factor in shaping the culture of the United States is the Judeo-Christian faith. Many immigrants came to the country for religious freedom and established a religious and moral atmosphere that persists today.

The religious orientation of the family dictates a code of morality and influences the family's attitudes toward education, male and female role identity, and beliefs regarding their ultimate destiny (Fig. 3-2).

It may also determine the school that the children attend, the companions with whom they associate, and often their mate selection.

In some cultures, such as the Oneida and Amish communities, the religious beliefs are the basis of a common way of life that is a totally individualistic life-style.

Schools

Next to the family the schools exert the major force in providing continuity between generations by conveying a vast amount of culture from the older members to the young. In this way children are prepared to carry out the traditional social roles they are expected to assume as adults in society. School rules and regulations regarding attendance, authority relationships, and the system of sanctions and rewards based on achievement transmit to the child the behavioral expectations of the adult world of employment and relationships. School is often the only institution in which children systematically learn about the negative consequences of behaviors that deviate from social expectations. Teachers are expected to stimulate and guide the intellectual development of children and their sense of esthetics and to foster their capacity for creative problem solving. Through education individuals in the lower classes are offered the opportunity for further education and the capacity to move up in the social strata.

Traditionally the socialization process of school has begun when the child enters kindergarten or first grade. Today, with 11 million mothers of preschool children working outside the home, this socialization process begins much earlier for a significant number of children in a variety of daycare settings.

Peer Cultures

Peer groups also have an impact on the socialization of children (Fig. 3-3). Peer relationships become increasingly important and influential as children proceed

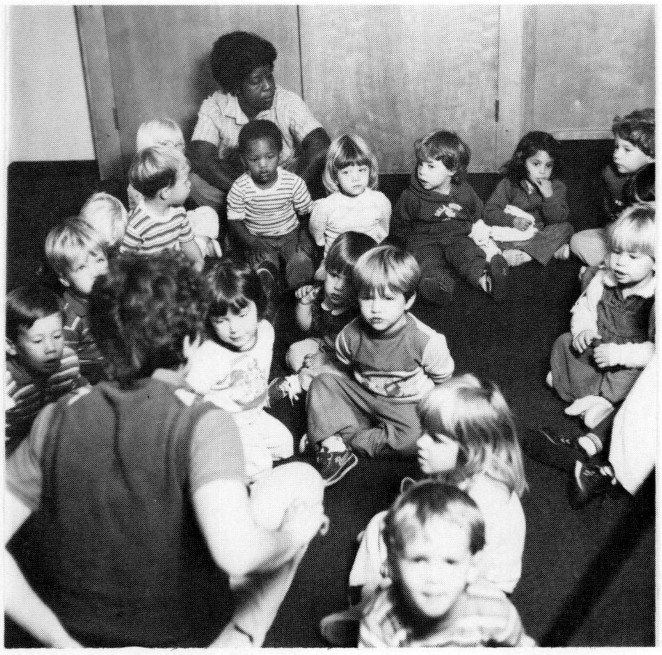

FIG. 3-3 Children from a variety of cultural and ethnic backgrounds begin to socialize in the daycare setting.

through school. In school children have what can be regarded as a culture of their own. It is most apparent in the school and in the unsupervised play group. The play group presents this culture in a much purer form than does the school, which is partly produced by adults.

During their lives children are exposed to value systems such as those of the family, ethnic group, and social class. In peer-group interaction they are confronted with a variety of these sets of values. The values imposed by the peer group are especially compelling because children must accept and conform to them in order to be accepted as members of the group. When the peer values are not too different from those of family and teachers, the mild conflict created by these small differences serves to separate children from the adults in their lives and to strengthen the feeling of belonging to the peer group.

The kind of socialization provided by the peer group depends on the special subculture that develops from the background, interests, and capabilities of its members. Some groups support school achievement, others focus on athletic prowess, and still others are decidedly antithetic to educative goals. Scholastic achievement is strongly related to the value system of the peer groups. Many conflicts between teachers and students and between parents and students can be attributed to fear of rejection by peers.

Although it has neither the traditional authority of the parents nor the legal authority of the schools for teaching information, the peer group manages to convey a substantial amount of information to its members, especially about taboo subjects, such as sex and drugs. Through peer relationships, children learn ways in which to deal with dominance and hostility and to relate with persons in positions of leadership and authority. Another function of the peer subculture is to relieve boredom and to provide recognition that individual members do not receive from teachers and other authority figures.

The peer-group culture has secrets, mores, and codes of ethics with which they promote feelings of group solidarity and detachment from adults. They have traditions and folkways that are transferred from "generation to generation" of school children and that have a great influence over the behavior of all members of the group. There are age-related games and other activities and, as children move from one level to the next, folkways of the younger group are discarded as those of the new are adopted. For example, a school-age child rides a bicycle to school; the high school student prefers to drive a car. As they advance children are forward oriented only—they look forward with anticipation but look backward with contempt.

Biculture

Some children are exposed to the values, role relationships, and life-styles of two cultures—a virtual "straddling" of two cultures.

This background is usually not a significant factor until children enter school. Children of one culture must unlearn some of the established practices of the culture in order to become socialized in the other, especially in role relationships. For example, Latino children are taught to look away when scolded; in U.S. schools the teacher expects direct eye contact—"Look at me when I speak to you." Children learn new roles and social behavior more rapidly than their adult counterparts.

This biculture is particularly marked in language differences. The bilingual child is said to be at a disadvantage in school situations of the dominant culture, especially a culture in which there is controversy over bilingual education. On the one hand those supporting bilingual education adhere to the principle that children will understand more readily and perform more realistically (especially in testing situations) if learning is directed in their own language; others contend that children living in a dominant culture should adopt the ways of that culture, including language.

CULTURAL SHOCK

The term *cultural shock* describes the "feelings of helplessness and discomfort and a state of disorientation experienced by an outsider attempting to comprehend or effectively adapt to a different cultural group because of differences in cultural practices, values, and beliefs" (Leininger, 1978). This state occurs with both clients and health care providers who move from one culture to another culture or setting. It can happen to persons who immigrate to a new country (such as the Asian refugees) or persons from a subcultural group who must adjust to the ways of an unfamiliar subgroup (such as children entering the school subculture or clients who enter the hospital subculture). Habits and customs (such as different role behaviors or etiquette) and differences in attitudes and beliefs are puzzling to the stranger in the new environment. The outsider experiences an intense sense of isolation and feelings of loneliness and nonrelatedness. Cultural shock is characterized by the inability to respond to or function in a new or strange situation.

THE CHILD AND FAMILY IN AMERICA

America is an aggregate of numerous Old and New World cultures that are blended with the unique heritage of pioneering frontiersmen. The frontier background of the American culture has contributed to the overall orientation to life and childrearing. There has always been a basic optimistic view of the world, a belief that things can be better and that the children can and will be better off than the parents. This hopeful outlook and a general future orientation together with the possibility of upward social mobility have created a pervasive overall attitude of optimism. Increasing development of self-confidence and autonomy in children is fostered and encouraged. Children are generally permitted a greater degree of freedom than in more tradition-oriented cultures, where a child born in one social class will remain in that class for his lifetime.

Family life in America is characterized by increasing geographic and economic mobility. Here there is less reliance on tradition, families are fragmented, and there is limited opportunity to transmit and acquire the traditional and accepted customs of a culture. Consequently young adults rely to a greater extent on the professed experts, peers, and the mass media for acquisition of acceptable patterns of behavior, including childrearing practices. Conflicting information can be a source of confusion and frustration as parents attempt to determine the comparatively stable, essential components of the culture and transmit these to their children.

Children in America grow up with a number of adults who differ from one another but who all provide input to them as role models, teachers, and standards for behavior. Most of the children live in some form of nuclear family located in sharply differentiated neighborhoods determined by income and ethnic status within a highly technical, largely urban society. Class differences in childrearing still persist, but they are becoming less divergent as a result of the increased homogeneity of the culture.

Minority-Group Membership

In addition to the problems and risks encountered by all children in the course of development, a small percentage of children are particularly vulnerable to hostility, derogation, and discrimination from children and adults of the majority group. America abounds with racial, ethnic, and religious minority groups. Although the effects of a minority status can apply to any of them, the greatest impact is on blacks, the largest minority.

Studies in the past indicate that early in life children become aware of their racial or ethnic status and of the discriminatory attitudes of the majority culture toward their group. The direct effects of discrimination are anger and low self-esteem, which become manifest in a variety of behaviors. Inner conflicts and suppressed hostility that focus children's attention inward may be factors in the failure of many children to achieve in other areas.

Because of many other factors, for most blacks membership in the black minority also implies membership in the lower levels of social structure. This lower-class, lower-caste status is often characterized by broken homes, dominance of maternal authority, impoverished and deteriorating neighborhoods, environmental encouragement of delinquency, and frequently parent-child friction and antagonism.

Evidence indicates that changes in attitudes are slowly taking place in some groups and in some places. With growing awareness, interest, and understanding by increasing numbers of the majority group, accompanied by the recent emergence of racial and ethnic pride, minority-group children are becoming more secure and confident in their racial or ethnic identity.

◆ *Cultural Influences on Health Care*

Cultural beliefs and practices are an important part of data gathering in the nursing assessment. Nurses continually encounter beliefs and practices that may facilitate or impede nursing interventions, including attitudes toward family planning, food habits, and folkways that are firmly entrenched in the culture. The language of the client may be different from that of the larger culture, or there may be regional or ethnic peculiarities in the use of basic English. Subcultural influences, such as some religious beliefs and practices, may be in conflict with standard health practices and therapeutic interventions.

SUSCEPTIBILITY TO HEALTH PROBLEMS

Some groups of people are more susceptible and others more resistant to certain illnesses than are persons from other groups. An innate susceptibility is acquired through generations of evolutionary changes that take place within constrained or segregated populations. The proximity to disease, environmental factors, and the general physical status are significant factors associated with health problems.

Hereditary Factors

The genetic constitution of individuals as groups influences the degree to which they are susceptible to a specific disorder. It may be the result of an inherent lack of resistance to a disease organism, a trait that is an advantage in one environment but which places the possessor at a disadvantage in another, or it may be the consequence of intermarriage within a relatively narrow range of geographic, ethnic, or religious restrictions.

A geographic constraint is illustrated by the classic example of the common communicable disease rubeola. The rubeola virus, or the populations that were continually exposed to it, became altered in such a way that the disease was considered to be a universal disease of childhood from which the majority of children suffered without ill effects. When other populations (for example, the inhabitants of the Hawaiian Islands) were exposed to the virus by explorers and missionaries, they experienced a violent response that resulted in high mortality.

Another communicable disease, tuberculosis, appears to be more prevalent in certain ethnic groups such as the Native Americans of the Southwest, Vietnamese immigrants, and Mexican-Americans. In many populations it is difficult to determine how much the increased incidence can be attributed to ethnic factors and how much is related to the life-styles in the lower social strata.

A number of diseases show ethnic or racial differences. For example, Tay-Sachs disease, characterized by early neurologic deterioration and mental retardation, affects primarily Ashkenasi Jewish families, particularly those of Northeastern European origin, while Sephardic Jewish families appear to be no more at risk for the disease than other populations. The incidence of cystic fibrosis is highest in whites, it is almost nonexistent in Orientals, and the rare affected blacks are usually in areas where there is apt to be mixed ancestry. A classic disorder of blacks, especially Africans, is sickle cell disease; however, the incidence of cardiovascular disease, pneumonia, and diabetes is also high among blacks. Racial and ethnic differences are further considered in relation to diseases and defects as they are discussed throughout the book.

Common food items and drugs may cause health problems in certain ethnic groups. For example, persons of Mediterranean, African, Near Eastern, and Asian origin frequently have glucose-6-phosphate dehydrogenase (G-6-PD) deficiency. They may develop acute hemolytic anemia after they ingest fava (horse or broad) beans or certain drugs such as aspirin preparations, sulfonamides, or primaquine. Other groups have a sensitivity to foods containing lactose, which when ingested can cause abdominal distention, flatus, and diarrhea (see p. 322). Unknowing but well-meaning health workers may be responsible for these symptoms in their clients when they prescribe foods containing lactose as sources of nutrients.

Physical characteristics. Among racial groups there are observable differences in physical appearance. The most obvious are skin and hair coloring and texture. Skin color is determined by the amount of melanin pigment present in the skin. Persons from countries located near the equator have darkly pigmented skin, which serves to protect the skin from the year-round exposure to the sun's rays; persons from the northern countries have very light skin, which provides for maximum exposure to the sun's rays (necessary for vitamin D metabolism) during the short daylight hours. There can be wide variations in skin color between these two extremes in terms of geographic origin or from intermixing of dark and light skin color. As a consequence of the dark pigmentation, the detection of skin color changes can be difficult and requires modification of assessment techniques (see Table 7-2).

Variations in the newborn are often related to racial or ethnic origin. For example, newborn infants of Asian and black parents are smaller than infants of white parentage, and bluish pigmented areas (mongolian spots) on the sacral region are a common observation on Oriental, black, Native American, and Mexican-American infants.

Evaluation of stature and body build reveals some racial tendencies. Oriental children are usually smaller at all ages and black children are taller and heavier between ages 5 and 14 than white children of the same age. This difference in stature can lead to misinterpretation of health status and capabilities. A black child who appears normal for his age may, in fact, be underdeveloped when compared to other black children (Bloch, 1983).

Socioeconomic Factors

The most overwhelming adverse influence on health is socioeconomic status. A higher percentage of lower-class individuals are suffering from some health problem at any one time than are those in any other group. The sum of all aspects of their situation contributes to and compounds health problems; this includes crowded living conditions and poor sanitation, which facilitate transfer of disease. There is a higher incidence of lead poisoning in children from lower-class families, where there is more ready access to lead in the environment (see p. 404).

In the lower classes, children are less likely to be immunized against preventable diseases than are children in the upper and middle classes. Lack of funds or inaccessibility to health services inhibits treatment for any but severe illness or injury. Sometimes health care is inadequate because of ignorance. In some areas a disorder is so commonplace that it is looked on as unavoidable; it is not recognized as something that requires (or is amenable to) treatment. The parents may not have information regarding causes, treatment, outcome of the illness, or preventive measures.

When medical care is provided to a migrant family, follow-up care is usually impossible because of their transient life-style. Compliance to medical therapies is primarily related to accessibility and availability. For example, medications provided by health workers are more likely to be taken than those that must be obtained at a pharmacy.

Poor nutrition also accounts for many health problems in the lower classes. Lack of funds and ignorance results in a diet that may be seriously lacking in essential food substances, especially protein, vitamins, and iron. This inadequate diet often leads to nutritional deficiency disorders and growth retardation in children.

Upper- and middle-class parents are more likely to seek treatment for many more types of symptoms than are lower-class parents, and they are more concerned with detecting and preventing illness in their children. The disinclination of lower-class families to use preventive health services is probably another symptom of the fatalistic approach to problems and a time orientation that is concentrated on the present rather than the future. Preventive dental care, immunization, and prenatal care are examples of such health services. The incidence of prematurity is highest in the lower classes. Significantly, lower-class parents have a low participation rate in local health programs and are more likely to practice home treatment.

CUSTOMS AND FOLKWAYS

Nurses are becoming increasingly aware of the need to consider cultural differences in clients when providing health care. An understanding of the various beliefs regarding the causation of illness and disease as well as traditional health practices is essential to successful intervention. The more nurses know about the values, beliefs, and customs of other ethnic groups, the better able they are to meet the needs of these families and to gain their cooperation and compliance.

Relationships with Health Care Providers

The manner of relating with health care providers differs considerably among cultural groups. One area of conflict to some nurses is the attitude toward time and waiting that is part of some cultures. For example, blacks are very flexible in their time orientation; a black family may be late for or miss appointments because other issues take precedence over the appointment and they may not communicate this to the health agency (Bloch, 1983). Hispanics, too, have a very relaxed view of time. Whereas the dominant culture in the United States says that "time flies," the Hispanic says, "time walks." The Japanese, on the other hand, consider time to be valuable and to be used wisely. They tend to be punctual for medical appointments and persistent in following prescribed regimens (Hashizume and Takano, 1983). A Vietnamese family will subordinate time to values considered to be more significant, such as propriety. They may be late for an appointment because of an overextended visit by a friend in their home.

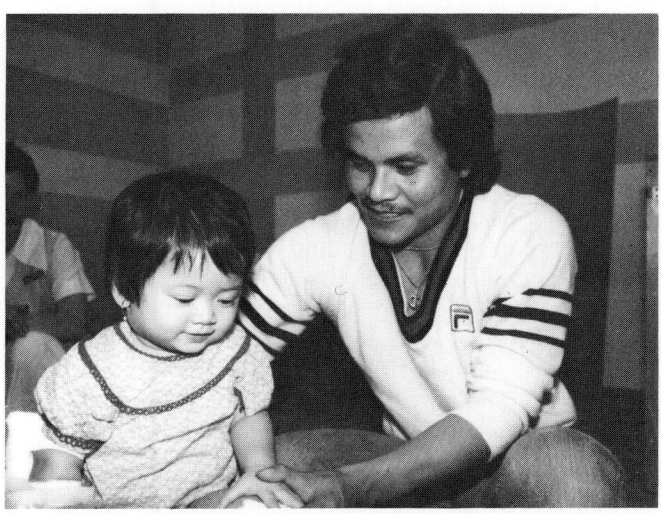

FIG. 3-4 A father with his hospitalized child.

In many cultural groups the mother assumes the responsibility for health care; in others both parents are involved equally in relationships with health workers. A somewhat different approach is apparent in some of the Oriental cultures. For example, the father in Vietnamese families, as unquestioned head of the family, is traditionally the family member who interacts with persons, including health care providers, outside the family unit (Fig. 3-4).

In the Hispanic family the father, as head of the house, makes decisions regarding illness and treatment of family members, but the grandmother in the extended family is consulted regarding child care. Usually the family confers with other members before reaching a decision regarding treatment or hospitalization of a child. The Arab family also relies on others to give advice and guidance in a time of crisis (Meleis, 1981). A Japanese father may appear to be passive and uninvolved but actually is involved according to his own cultural standards (Tseng and others, 1982).

Nurses should make themselves aware of any specific attitudes regarding the manner of approach to a child in a given culture. Navajo Indians do not like a stranger near their infants. It is feared that the stranger may "witch" the child and cause him harm. On the other hand, if a stranger, particularly a woman, lavishes attention on a Latino infant but fails to touch him, he will develop symptoms of the "evil eye" (see p. 41). Vietnamese and Korean families may become upset if a newborn is admired at length for fear the evil spirits will overhear and desire the infant.

Some ethnic groups consider a child's admission to the hospital a family affair, with all members gathering to support and console the child and his parents. In others, such as the Samoan family, the family is willing to relinquish the care of the child to the hospital authority without interference. Their visits with the child are short, although intense, but this behavior may be misinterpreted by the hospital staff as disinterest or abandonment.

Nurses who are members of a majority culture may encounter tension and distrust in a child from a minority culture as a result of the child's learned conception or relationships with other persons in the majority group. Based on these perceptions, minority children often suspect that nurses may have hostile feelings toward them and fear ill treatment. When such children are hospitalized, this feeling compounds the feelings of loneliness, helplessness, and retribution that accompany fearful happenings and separation from families. The reverse situation may be encountered by a nurse from a minority culture attempting to meet the needs of a child who has been conditioned to view the nurse's cultural or ethnic group as inferior.

Communication. Communication may be a source of distress and misunderstanding between persons from different ethnic groups, especially if the languages are different. Ideally, conversations with families who are unable to speak the dominant language are best conducted by a health care worker who speaks the language of the family. If this is not possible, however, it may be necessary to engage the services of an interpreter. However, use of an interpreter can be a source of misunderstanding if the interpreter is unfamiliar with the medical terminology or if there are no corresponding words in the second language to express the ideas and concepts under discussion (see Communicating with families through an interpreter, p. 106).

Some persons with poor or limited language comprehension may simply smile and nod in agreement if they do not understand the questions or directives. It is vital that the family fully understand all implications of a child's care and management before they sign permits for special procedures or assume responsibility for his care. It is not uncommon for a Vietnamese or a Japanese family to indicate "yes" when in fact they mean "no" in order to avoid social disharmony. They tend to use indirectness rather than confrontation and may become evasive when direct questioning makes them feel uncomfortable.

Nonverbal communication is a practiced art in many Native American tribes, and the members are highly sensitive to body language. They emphasize periods of silence to formulate thoughts in preparation for speech and often remain silent after listening to statements by others in order to properly assimilate what has been said. Interruption, interjection, or haste to arrive at abrupt conclusions is perceived as immature behavior.

Eye contact is viewed differently in cultures. It is not uncommon for persons in some ethnic groups to avoid eye contact and become uncomfortable when conversing with health workers. A Vietnamese patient may not look directly into the nurse's eyes, as a sign of respect. Some Native Americans will make eye contact during the initial greeting but continued, unwavering eye contact is considered insulting and disrespectful.

There may be reluctance on the part of families to question or otherwise initiate contact with health professionals. In the Asian cultures, for example, it is considered a sign of disrespect to question those who are viewed as persons of authority. A Japanese family may wait silently rather than ask or question. They believe that the health professionals know best and will meet their needs without being asked (Hashizume and Takano, 1983). It is also important to avoid criticism. Criticism can cause the Japanese American to "lose face," to make him feel ashamed, which is highly undesirable.

It is necessary to speak slowly and carefully, not loudly, when conversing with families who have poor language comprehension. Many persons are able to read and write English better than they can speak or understand it. Also, the dominant language usually takes over in anxiety-provoking situations, even in persons who are able to communicate satisfactorily under ordinary circumstances.

Terms of address and use of first and last names varies among cultures and can create confusion in institutions. For example, in Asian cultures, the family name is given first in respect for the family and the given names follow. Therefore, all siblings in a family have the same first name. Ethiopians use no last names but have a very complex system whereby women retain their last names after marriage and the paternal grandfather's name becomes a child's last name.

The expression of emotion also varies ethnically. In some cultures (for example, persons of Latin or Jewish backgrounds) emotions are expressed openly and members are accustomed to share their sorrows and joys with family and friends. Conversely, Nordic and Asian groups are more restrained in expressing emotion.

Food Customs

Food customs and symbolism of various cultural, ethnic, and religious groups have become an integral part of their lives. Although in a large country such as the United States most persons have adopted the eclectic food habits that have evolved over countless generations, many ethnic and geographic food traditions and preferences are retained. Special holidays, ceremonies, and life experiences such as births, birthdays, weddings, and death are often marked by special food items or feasts. In many cultures specific food practices are followed during pregnancy in the belief that certain foods damage the developing fetus.

The distinctive food customs of ethnic groups are a product of their native environment, determined by availability. Fish is a staple food of persons living near the ocean, such as people from Japan, Polynesia, and Scandinavia. Fruit and vegetable preferences are also directly related to the climate in which these grow naturally or can be cultivated. The types of grain that are ethnically associated are also those that grow best in their native lands. For example, rice is the staple grain of the Orient and Pacific islands, wheat of the temperate climates of Europe, rye in Scandinavia, and corn of the North American Indians. The diet of the Eskimo is predominantly fish and meat, depending on which is the most easily procured in the area. Even in the continental United States there are regional favorites, like rice, hominy grits, and okra in the southern states. In some cultures food is highly spiced, in others foods tend to be bland.

There are a number of restrictions related to food items. Some have a physiologic origin, such as lack of dairy foods in the diets of some persons of African or Asian ancestry in whom a hereditary lactase deficiency prevents digestion of foods containing lactose. Others have religious restrictions, such as kosher foods and food preparation of the Orthodox Jewish faith and the vegetarian diet of Seventh Day Adventists (see Vegetarian diets, p. 311).

Children in a strange environment, such as the hospital, feel much more comfortable when they are served foods to which they are accustomed. The hospital food often tastes strange and bland. The family may be concerned that their child is receiving foods appropriate to their culture and beliefs. Where possible, it is advisable to provide children's ethnic foods or allow families to bring favorite foods that are not available on the hospital menu. Concern for differences in food habits and patterns projects an attitude of respect for the family's ethnic or religious heritage.

HEALTH BELIEFS AND PRACTICES

The nurse encounters people of many different racial and ethnic origins in the process of meeting the health needs of children and families. Some of these families have become so enculturated to the majority culture that their health beliefs and practices are consistent with those of the health care system. There are still numerous families, however, whose traditional practices and beliefs are an integral part of their daily lives. It is important for health care workers to be aware that other people may live by different rules and priorities from those of the health care provider, and these rules and priorities decisively influence health-related behavior.

Health Beliefs

The beliefs related to the cause of illness and the maintenance of health are an integral part of the cultural heritage of families. Often inseparable from religious beliefs, they influence the way that families cope with health problems and the way that they respond to health care providers. Predominant among most cultures are beliefs related to natural forces, supernatural forces, and imbalance between forces.

Natural forces. The most common natural forces held responsible for ill health if the body is not adequately protected include cold air entering the body, impurities in the air, or other natural sources. For example, the Latino or Chinese mother will overdress the infant in an effort to keep cold wind from entering the child's body. The Chinese believe that cold weather, rain, or wind are responsible for "cold" conditions.

In the black culture natural phenomena such as phases of the moon, seasons of the year, and planet positions are believed to affect the body and its processes; therefore, health maintenance is strongly associated with the ability to read "the signs." Most Native Americans consider health to be a state of harmony with nature and the universe.

Supernatural forces. High on the list of causes of illness are forces beyond comprehension and logical explanation. Evil influences such as voodoo, witchcraft, or evil spirits are viewed in some cultures as causes of adverse health, especially those illnesses that cannot be explained by other means.

A health belief that is common among people from Latin American, Mediterranean, Near Eastern, some Asian, and some African societies is the concept of the "evil eye" (*mal ojo* is the Hispanic term). It is part of the concept of health as a state of balance; illness is a state of imbalance (see below). Strength and power are associated with the evil eye; therefore, as long as an individual's strength and weakness remain in balance, he is unlikely to become a victim of the evil eye. Weaknesses are not necessarily physical. For example, an excess of some emotion, such as envy, can create a weakness. Infants and small children, because of immature development of their internal strength-weakness states, are especially vulnerable to the gaze of the evil eye (Pasquale, 1984). Consequently, evil eye serves to rationalize an inexplicable onset of illness in children who display such symptoms as restlessness, crying, diarrhea, vomiting, and fever.

Although seldom expressed to health care providers, the belief that a witch can cast a spell over another person at the request of someone who wishes him ill is found in Hispanic and African cultures. The victim is often tortured in effigy by pins driven into a doll at the location where the intended victim is to be hurt.

Imbalance of forces. The concept of balance or equilibrium is widespread throughout the world. One of the most common imbalances supported by the Hispanic, Filipino, Chinese, and Arab cultures is that which exists between "hot" and "cold." This belief is reputedly derived from Hippocratic theory of humoral pathology, which states that illness is caused by an imbalance of the four humors: phlegm, blood, black bile, and yellow bile. Hot and cold describe certain properties and conditions completely unrelated to temperature. Diseases, areas of the body, foods, and illnesses are classified as either "hot" or "cold." In Chinese health belief the forces are termed *yin* (cold) and *yang* (hot) (Chen-Louie, 1983). In order to maintain health and prevent illness these hot and cold forces must be kept in balance.

Illness is treated by restoring normal balance through the application of appropriate "hot" or "cold" remedies. A "cold" condition such as a respiratory disease is believed to be caused by exposure to cold weather, rain, or cold wind entering the body; it is treated by administration of "hot" foods, herbs, or drugs. Menstruation is considered to be a "hot" condition; therefore, women are cautioned against ingesting "hot" foods that might increase menstrual flow or produce cramping. Ingesting too much of either "hot" or "cold" foods can also be interpreted as a cause of illness.

Health care workers who are aware of this belief are better able to understand why some persons refuse to eat certain foods. It is possible to help families devise a diet that contains the necessary balance of basic food groups prescribed by the medical subculture while conforming to the beliefs of the ethnic subculture.

The hot-cold food classification may have adverse effects. For example, newborn infants are often started on evaporated milk formulas. Evaporated milk is considered to be a hot food while whole milk is viewed as a cold food. Infants tend to develop rashes, which are believed to be caused by "hot" foods; in such cases parents may decide to switch to whole milk. However, parents fear that it is dangerous to change too rapidly, so they often feed the child some type of neutralizing substance, which may create additional health problems. Such a problem might be averted if the family's preference is determined before discharge from the hospital and a formula prescribed that is agreeable to both the family and the physician.

Health Practices

There are numerous similarities among cultures regarding prevention and treatment of illness. All cultures have some types of home remedies that they apply before seeking help from other persons. Within the ethnic community folk healers who are endowed with the ability to "cure" maladies are sought for special situations and when home remedies are unsuccessful. There is the *curandero* (male) or *curandera* (female) of the Mexican-American community whose healing powers are believed to be a gift from God. The Asian consults a herbalist, knowledgeable in medicines, and/or an ethnic physician practiced in Asian therapies, including acupuncture, acupressure, and moxibustion (application of heat). Native Americans consult a variety of healers with specific skills and knowledge. Specialized medicine persons diagnose illness, provide nonsacred treatments (usually by way of massage and herbs), and care for souls. Other specialists perform services or affect cures through spiritual means.

The folk healers are very powerful persons in their community. They "speak the language" of the family who seeks help and often combine their rituals and potions with prayer and entreaties to God. They also are able to create an atmosphere conducive to successful management. Furthermore, they exhibit a sincere interest in the family and their problem.

Often it will be found that the folk remedies are compatible with the medical regimen and can be used as a means to reinforce the treatment plan. For example, most of the foods contraindicated for a person with peptic ulcer are "hot" foods and would be avoided by his belief system. Also, aspirin (a "hot" medication) is an appropriate therapy for "cold" diseases such as the common cold and arthritis. It is not uncommon to discover that a folk prescription has a scientific basis. However, numerous health remedies or preventive practices have no scientific basis, such as the use of *asafetida,* a piece of rotten flesh that looks like a dried sponge and is worn around the neck to prevent contagious diseases. Also, the wearing of copper or silver bracelets to protect the wearer as he grows has no scientific basis. Since they do no harm, these practices should be respected.

To overcome the effect of the evil eye usually requires specialized rituals conducted by the appropriate practitioner. For example, the Chicano curandera ascertains that the condition is truly the result of the evil eye by performing an assessment ritual and, upon a confirmed diagnosis, performs a curative ritual. Sometimes the faith in the folk practitioner delays obtaining needed medical treatment, although the practitioner will usually suggest medical care if his or her ministrations are unsuccessful.

Health practices of different cultures may also present problems of assessment and interpretation. For example, the Vietnamese practice of "coining" may produce welt-like lesions on the child's back when a coin, held on edge, is repeatedly rubbed lengthwise on the oiled skin to rid the body of the disease (Feldman, 1984). Another such custom is the Old World practice of cupping (also practiced by the Vietnamese). A container, such as a tumbler, bottle, or jar, containing steam is placed against the skin surface to "draw out the poison" or other evil. When the heated air within the container cools, a vacuum is created that produces a bruise-like blemish on the skin directly beneath the mouth of the container (Holland and Sweeney, 1985). Both of these remedies can be misdiagnosed as evidence of "child abuse" by uninformed professionals.

Cultural health remedies that are detrimental to health include eating clay or excessive amounts of salt. A mercury compound, *azogue* (the Spanish name for quicksilver), is commonly used in Mexico and sometimes sold illegally to low-income Latino families in the United States as a "remedy" for diarrhea. Alert health care workers know that the drug can cause permanent central nervous system damage. A careful history can reveal these practices, but it may require the collaboration of a folk healer to convince a user to stop the practice.

Faith healing and religious rituals are closely allied with many folk-healing practices. Wearing of amulets, medals, and other religious relics believed by the culture to protect the individual and facilitate healing is a common practice. It is important for health workers to recognize the value of this practice and keep the items where the family has placed them or nearby. It offers comfort and support and rarely impedes medical and nursing care. If an item must be removed during a procedure it should be replaced, if possible, when the procedure is completed. The reason for its temporary removal is explained to the family and they are reassured that their wishes will be respected.

Although most subcultures in the large developed countries have become acculturated to the Western medical system, many still maintain faith in traditional healing practices and practitioners. When the folk practices do not interfere with the welfare of the patient, they need not be discouraged. Often a compromise can be reached that accomplishes the goal of the nurse while it maintains the dignity and self-esteem of the client.

Folklore Related to Prenatal Influences

Since ancient times the striking appearance of abnormal human development has been of concern, as evidenced by descriptions in primitive drawings and on clay tablets, and has served as the origin of numerous legendary and mythologic creatures. Consequently the processes of pregnancy and birth have been surrounded with strongly held beliefs and superstitions that involve taboos and prescriptions for behavior directed toward ensuring the well-being of the unborn child. Even in the face of scientific advances, these superstitions and folkways have survived for generations and may still persist in various forms as part of a cultural heritage.

One of the most universal explanations of defective development has been maternal impressions. It has been a widespread belief that the appearance of the unborn child will be improved if the pregnant woman looks at beautiful people or things. The same concept in reverse has been used to explain birth defects. For example, if a pregnant woman was frightened by a rabbit, it was believed that her child would be born with a cleft (harelip) lip; a microcephalic infant was attributed to the mother's seeing a monkey during pregnancy; and the mother's viewing a person with missing limbs would cause the unborn child to be similarly affected. Activities such as a mother reaching her arms above her head, walking in circles, or tying knots were believed to cause the umbilical cord to be knotted or twisted around the neck of the fetus. Even the shape of birthmarks and other skin defects is sometimes believed to reflect maternal impressions. For example, eating strawberries by the mother is associated with nevi. Articles of apparel or adornment, food cravings, emotions such as fright and anger, undesirable thoughts, and the time and manner of announcing the pregnancy are all believed to influence the well-being of the unborn child.

Expectant mothers who are able to rationalize the illogical nature of the beliefs will, through a normal fear of having an abnormal infant, conform to the superstitions. In most instances these customs are relatively harmless and are not in conflict with sound health practices. However, there are situations when conformity to cultural or subcultural beliefs may compromise the health and well-being of either mother or fetus, for example, the practice of eating clay. Understanding and judicious management on the part of nurses and other health care workers are required to explore with the mother all the ramifications of the practice without creating undue stress and guilt in the mother.

RELIGIOUS BELIEFS

Religion influences the life-style of most cultures. Among many groups illness, injury, or death is believed to be sent by God as a punishment for sin. Some may believe that health workers will be unable to help a person whom God is punishing and may express a fatalistic attitude toward treatment, stating it is "the will of God." Others view it as a test of strength, as the testing of Job in the Bible, and strive to remain faithful and overcome the conflicts.

Nurses need to determine if there are any special considerations, including dietary restrictions, related to spiritual practices that are important to the family. It is comforting to the family of an ill child to have their beliefs recognized and respected. Family members are asked whether they want a clergy member present and whether they prefer hospital staff to call or to do this on their own.

It is also important to determine the wishes of the family regarding baptism, rites or practices related to death, and other religious rituals (such as circumcision, communion, or use of amulets or icons). Religion, which offers families understanding and spiritual support, is a valuable asset to health care. Characteristics of selected religions with beliefs that affect health care are outlined in Table 3-1.

ATTITUDE OF THE NURSE

To begin to understand and to deal effectively with families in a multicultural community or in a unicultural community that is different from one's own, it is most important that nurses be aware of their own attitudes and values regarding a way of life, including health practices. Nurses, too, are a product of their own cultural background and education. Frequently, nurses and other health care workers are not aware of their own cultural values and how those values influence their thoughts and actions. Those who are aware of their own culturally founded behavior are more sensitive to cultural behavior in others. To recognize that a behavior may be characteristic of a culture rather than an "abnormal" behavior places nurses at an advantage in their relationships with families. When nurses respect cultural differences of a family, they are better able to determine whether the behavior is distinctive to the individual or a characteristic of the culture.

Cultural standards and values, the family structure and function, and past experiences with health care influence a family's feelings and attitudes toward health, their children, and health care delivery systems. It is often difficult for nurses to be nonjudgmental and objective in working with families whose behaviors and attitudes differ from or conflict with their own. To be aware of one's own feelings and attitudes as well as to respect those of the family are essential to a helping relationship and achievement of nursing goals. To rely on one's own values and experiences for guidance can result only in frustration and disappointment. It is one thing to know what is needed to deal with a health problem; it is often quite another to implement a fruitful course of action unless nurses work within the cultural and socioeconomic framework of the family.

It is beneficial to make an effort to adapt ethnic practices to the health needs of the family rather than attempt to change long-standing beliefs. To aid their efforts to understand and respect the cultural beliefs of families, nurses should have a readily available resource file containing pertinent information about the cultural and subcultural characteristics of the community in which they practice (for example, traditional practices related to infant feeding practices and the time and manner of weaning and toilet training). Bridging cultural gaps in delivery

Text continued on p. 52.

TABLE 3-1

Religious Beliefs That Affect Nursing Care

Religion	Beliefs about Birth and Death	Beliefs about Diet and Food Practices
Adventist (Seventh Day Adventist; Church of God)	**Birth:** Opposed to infant baptism Baptism in adulthood	Meat prohibited in some groups No alcohol, coffee, or tea
Baptist (27 groups)	**Birth:** Opposed to infant baptism Believers baptize by immersion as adults **Death:** Counsel and prayer with clergy, family, patient	Some groups discourage coffee, tea, and alcohol
Buddhist Churches of America	**Birth:** No infant baptism Infant presentation **Death:** Last rite chanting often practiced at bedside soon after death Priest should be contacted	No requirements or restrictions Some sects are strictly vegetarian Discourage use of alcohol and drugs
Church of Christ Scientist (Christian Science)	**Birth:** No baptism **Death:** No last rites	No requirements or restrictions
Church of Jesus Christ of Latter Day Saints (Mormon)	**Birth:** No baptism at birth Infant is "blessed" by church official at first opportunity after birth (in church) Baptism by immersion at 8 years **Death:** No special rites	Prohibit tea, coffee, alcohol Encourage sparing use of meats Fasting for 24 hours on first Sunday each month (from after evening meal Saturday until evening meal Sunday)
Episcopal (Anglican)	**Birth:** Infant baptism mandatory; urgent if poor prognosis* **Death:** Last rites available but not mandatory	Abstain from meat on fast days May fast on Wednesday, Friday, during Lent, and before Christmas Some fast for 6 hours before receiving Holy Communion
Greek Orthodox	**Birth:** Baptism considered important Performed 40 days after birth If not possible to baptize by sprinkling or immersion, Church allows child baptism "in the air" by moving the child in the form of a cross* as appropriate words are said **Death:** Last rites, administration of Sacrament of Holy Communion Should be performed while dying person is still conscious	Church prescribed fast periods—usually occur on Wednesday, Friday, and during Lent; consist of avoiding meat and (in some cases) dairy products If health compromised, priest may be contacted to convince family to forego fasting
Hindu	**Birth:** No ritual **Death:** Special prescribed rites Priest pours water into the mouth of dead child, ties a thread around neck or wrist to signify blessing (should not be removed) Family washes body and is particular about who touches body	Many dietary restrictions Beef and veal not eaten Some strict vegetarians

Data from Recognizing your patients' spiritual needs, Nursing 77 vol. no. **7**(12):64-68, 1977; Beliefs that can affect therapy, Pediatr. Nurs. **5**(3):40-43, 1979; Carpenito, L.J.: Nursing diagnosis: application to clinical practice, Philadelphia, 1985, J.B. Lippincott Co.; Kozier, B., and Erb, G.: Fundamentals of nursing, ed. 2, Menlo Park, CA, 1983, Addison-Wesley Publishing Co.; Spector, R.E.: Cultural diversity in health and illness, New York, 1979, Appleton-Century-Crofts; personal communications.

Beliefs Regarding Medical Care	Comments
Some believe in divine healing and practice annointing with oil and use of prayer May desire communion or baptism when ill Believe in man's choice and God's sovereignty Some oppose hypnosis as therapy	Sabbath: Saturday for many Accept Bible literally
"Laying on of hands" (some) May encounter some resistance to some therapies such as abortion Believe God functions through physician Some believe in predestination; may respond passively to care	Fundamentalists and conservative groups accept Bible as inspired word of God
Illness believed to be a trial to aid development of soul; illness due to Karmic causes May be reluctant to have surgery or certain treatments on holy days Cleanliness believed to be of great importance Family may request Buddhist priest for counseling	Optimistic outlook; teach ways to overcome fears, anxieties, apprehension
Deny the existence of health crisis; see sickness and sin as errors of mind that can be altered by prayer Oppose human intervention with drugs or other therapies; however, accept legally required immunizations Many adhere to belief that disease is a human mental concept that can be dispelled by "spiritual truth" to extent that they refuse all medical treatment	Many desire services of Practitioner or Reader; will sometimes refuse even emergency treatment until they have consulted a Reader Unlikely to donate organs for transplant
Devout adherents believe in divine healing through annointment with oil and "laying on of hands" by church officials (elders) Medical therapy not prohibited	Married adults wear special undergarments May request Sacrament on Sunday while in hospital Financial support for sick available through well-funded welfare system Discourage cremation Discourage use of tobacco
Some believe in spiritual healing Rite for annointing sick available but not mandatory	Religious icons very important Communion four times yearly: Christmas, Easter, June 30, and August 15; may be mandatory for some
Each health crisis handled by ordained priest; deacon may also serve in some cases Holy Communion administered in hospital Some may desire Sacrament of the Holy Unction performed by priest	Oppose euthanasia Believe every reasonable effort should be made to preserve life until termination by God Discourage autopsies that may cause dismemberment Prefer burial to cremation
Illness or injury believed to represent sins committed in previous life Accept most modern medical practices	Cremation preferred

Continued.

TABLE 3-1

Religious Beliefs That Affect Nursing Care—cont'd

Religion	Beliefs about Birth and Death	Beliefs about Diet and Food Practices
Islam (Muslim/Moslem)	**Birth:** No baptism **Death:** Patient must confess sins and beg forgiveness before death; family should be present Family washes and prepares body, then turns it to face Mecca Only relatives and friends may touch body	Prohibit all pork products Daylight fasting practiced during ninth month of Muhammadan year (Ramadan) Strict Muslims do not use alcohol
Jehovah's Witness	**Birth:** No baptism **Death:** No last rites	Eat nothing to which blood has been added; can eat animal flesh that has been drained
Judaism (Orthodox and Conservative)	**Birth:** No baptism Ritual circumcision of male infants on eighth day; performed by Mohel (ritual circumciser familiar with Jewish law and aseptic technique) Reform Jews favor ritual circumcision, but not as a religious imperative **Death:** Remains are ritually washed by members of the Ritual Burial Society Burial should take place as soon as possible	Numerous dietary kosher laws exist that may be influenced by local practices and family and cultural tradition Allowed only meat from animals that are vegetable eaters, are cloven hoofed, chew their cud, and are ritually slaughtered; fish that have scales and fins Prohibit any combination of meat and milk. Milk products served first can be followed by meat in a few minutes, but milk may not be consumed for several hours after eating meat. Fasting for 24 hours is part of Yom Kipper observance Matzo replaces leavened bread during Passover week
Pentecostal (Assembly of God, Foursquare)	**Birth:** No baptism at birth Baptism by complete immersion after age of accountability **Death:** No last rites	Abstain from alcohol, eating blood, strangled animals, or anything to which blood has been added Some individuals may resist pork
Orthodox Presbyterian	**Birth:** Infant baptism by sprinkling* **Death:** Last rites not a sacramental procedure; scripture reading and prayer	No requirements or restrictions
Roman Catholic	**Birth:** Infant baptism mandatory; especially urgent in poor prognosis, when it may be performed by anyone* **Death:** Rite for Anointing of the sick is mandatory Family or patient may request anointing if prognosis is grave	Fasting or abstaining from meat mandatory on Ash Wednesday and Good Friday; fasting optional during Lent; no meat on Fridays during Lent as general rule Most hospital patients exempt from fasting Some older Catholics may adhere to older rule of eating fish on Friday

*See Baptism, p. 234.

Beliefs Regarding Medical Care	Comments
Faith healing not acceptable unless psychologic condition of patient is deteriorating; performed for morale Ritual washing after prayer; prayer takes place five times daily (upon rising, midday, afternoon, early evening, and before bed); during prayer, face Mecca and kneel on prayer rug	Older Muslims often have a fatalistic view that may interfere with compliance to therapy May oppose autopsy
Adherents are generally absolutely opposed to blood transfusions; individuals can sometimes be persuaded in emergencies May be opposed to modern science, including medicine	Often possible to obtain a court order appointing a hospital official as temporary guardian to consent to a child's transfusion when parents refuse consent Autopsy approved only as required by law
May resist surgical procedures during Sabbath, which extends from sundown Friday until sundown Saturday Seriously ill are exempt from fasting	Oppose all forms of mutilation, including autopsy; body parts not donated or removed, amputated limbs, organs, or surgically removed tissues should be made available to family for burial Donation or transplantation of organs requires rabbinical consent May oppose prolongation of life after irreversible brain damage
No restrictions regarding medical care Deliverance from sickness is provided for in atonement; may pray for divine intervention in health matters and seek God in prayer for themselves and others when ill	Some insist illness is divine punishment; most consider it an intrusion of Satan Practice glossolalia (speaking in tongues)
Communion administered when appropriate and convenient Blood transfusion accepted when advisable Pastor or elder should be called for ill person Believe science should be used for relief of suffering	Full forgiveness granted for any illness connected with a sin
Encourage anointing of sick, although this may be interpreted by older members of church as equivalent to the old terminology "extreme unction" or "last rites"; they may require careful explanation if reluctance associated with fear of imminent death Traditional church teaching does not approve of contraceptives or abortion; however, some clergy advocate more liberal views on these issues	Family may request that major amputated limb be buried in consecrated ground Transplant accepted as long as loss of organ does not deprive donor of life or functional integrity of body Autopsy acceptable Religious articles important

TABLE 3-2

Cultural Characteristics Related to Health Care of Children

Cultural Group	Health Beliefs	Health and Diet Practices
Asian Americans Chinese	A healthy body viewed as gift from parents and ancestors and must be cared for Health is one of the results of balance between the forces of *yin* (cold) and *yang* (hot), energy forces that rule the world Illness caused by imbalance Believe blood is source of life and is not regenerated *Chi* is innate energy Lack of *chi* and blood results in deficiency that produces fatigue, poor constitution, and long illness	Goal of therapy is to restore balance of *yin* and *yang* Acupuncturist applies needles to appropriate meridians identified in terms of *yin* and *yang* Acupressure and *tai chi* replacing acupuncture in some areas Moxibustion is application of heat to skin over specific meridians Wide use of medicinal herbs procured and applied in prescribed ways Folk healers are herbalist, spiritual healer, temple healer, fortune healer Meals may or may not be planned to balance hot and cold Lactose intolerance relatively common Use of condiments, e.g., monosodium glutamate and soy sauce, may create difficulty with some diet regimens, e.g., low salt
Japanese	Three major belief systems: *Shinto* religious influence Humans inherently good Evil caused by outside spirits Illness caused by contact with polluting agents, e.g., blood, corpses, skin diseases Chinese and Korean influence Health achieved through harmony and balance between self and society Disease caused by disharmony with society and not caring for body Portuguese influence Upholds germ theory of disease	Believe evil removed by purification Energy restored by means of acupuncture, acupressure, massage, and moxibustion along affected meridians *Kampō* medicine—use of natural herbs Believe in removal of diseased parts Trend is to use both Western and Oriental healing methods Care for disabled viewed as family's responsibility Take pride in child's good health Seek preventive care, medical care for illness Older persons avoid some food combinations (e.g., milk and cherries, watermelon and crab) and believe pickled plums to have special properties
Vietnamese	Good health considered to be balance between *yin* (cold) and *yang* (hot) Believe person's life has been predisposed toward certain phenomena by cosmic forces Health believed to be result of harmony with existing universal order, harmony attained by pleasing good spirits and avoiding evil ones Belief in *am duc,* the amount of good deeds accumulated by ancestors Many use rituals to prevent illness Practice some restrictions to prevent incurring wrath of evil spirits	Family uses all means possible before using outside agencies for health care Fortune-tellers determine event that caused disturbance May visit temple to procure divine instruction Use astrologer to calculate cyclical changes and forces Regard health as family responsibility; outside aid sought when resources run out Certain illnesses considered only temporary (such as pustules, open wounds) and ignored Seek generalist health healers May use special diets to prevent illness and promote health Lactose intolerance prevalent
Filipino	Believe God's will and supernatural forces govern universe Illness, accidents, and other misfortunes are God's punishment for violations of His will Widely accept "hot" and "cold" balance and imbalance as cause of health and illness	Some use amulets as a shield from witchcraft or as good luck pieces Catholics substitute religious medals and other items

Sources: Bloch, 1983; Chen-Louie, 1983; Chow, 1976; Char, 1981; Ehling, 1981; Greathouse and Miller, 1981; Hashizume and Takano, 1983; Holland and Sweeney, 1985; Hollingsworth, Brown, and Brooten, 1980; Jacques, 1976; Lacay, 1981; Orque, 1983; Sodetaini-Shebata, 1981.

Family Relationships	Communication	Comments
Extended family pattern common Strong concept of loyalty of young to old Respect for elders taught at early age—acceptance without questioning or talking back Children's behavior a reflection on family Family and individual honor and "face" important Self-reliance and self-restraint highly valued; self-expression repressed Males valued more highly than females; women submissive to men in family	Open expression of emotions unacceptable Often smile when do not comprehend	Do not react well to often painful diagnostic workup; are especially upset by drawing of blood Deep respect for their bodies and believe it best to die with bodies intact; therefore may refuse surgery Believe in reincarnation Older members fear hospitals; often believe hospital is a place to go to die Children sometimes breast-fed for up to 4 or 5 years
Close intergenerational relationships Family provides anchor Family tends to keep problems to self Value self-control and self-sufficiency Concept of *haji* (shame) imposes strong control; unacceptable behavior of children reflects on family Many adopt practices of contemporary middle class Concern for child's missing school may result in sending to school before fully recovered from illness	*Issei*—born in Japan; usually speak Japanese only *Nisei, Sansei,* and *Yonsei* have few language difficulties New immigrants able to read and write English better than to speak or understand it Make significant use of nonverbal communication with subtle gestures and facial expression Tend to suppress emotions Will often wait silently	Generational categories: *Issei*—1st generation to live in U.S. *Nisei*—2nd generation *Sansei*—3rd generation *Yonsei*—4th generation *Issei* and *Nisei*—tolerant and permissive childrearing until 5 or 6, then emphasis on emotional reserve and control Cleanliness highly valued Time considered valuable and used wisely Tendency to practice emotional control may make assessment of pain more difficult
Family is revered institution Multigenerational families Family is chief social network Children highly valued Individual needs and interests are subordinate to those of family group Father is main decision maker Women taught submission to men Parents expect respect and obedience from children	Many immigrants are not proficient in speaking and understanding English May hesitate to ask questions Questioning authority is sign of disrespect; asking questions considered impolite Use indirectness rather than forthrightness in expressing disagreement May avoid eye contact with health professionals as a sign of respect	Consider status more important than money Children taught emotional control Time concept more relaxed—consider punctuality less significant than other values, i.e., propriety Place high value on social harmony
Family is highly valued with strong family ties Multigenerational family structure common, often with collateral members as well Personal interests are subordinated to family interests and needs Members avoid any behavior that would bring shame on the family	Immigrants and older persons may not be able to speak or understand English	Tend to have a fatalistic outlook on life Believe time and providence will solve all

Continued.

TABLE 3-2

Cultural Characteristics Related to Health Care of Children—cont'd

Cultural Group	Health Beliefs	Health and Diet Practices
American black	Illness classified as: Natural—affected by forces of nature without adequate protection, e.g., cold air, pollution, food and water Unnatural—evil influences, e.g., witchcraft, voodoo, hoodoo, hex, fix, rootwork; symptoms often associated with eating Believe illness sent by God as punishment, e.g., parents punished by illness or death of child Believe serious illness can be avoided May resist health care because illness is "will of God"	Self-care and folk medicine very prevalent Folk therapies usually religious in origin Attempt home remedies first; poorer people do not seek help until illness serious Usually seek help from: "Old lady"—woman in community with a common knowledge of herbs; consults regarding pediatric care Spiritualist—has received gift from God for healing incurable diseases or solving personal problems; strongly based in Christianity Priest (voodoo priest/priestess)—most powerful healer Root doctor—meet need for herbs, oils, candles, and ointments Prayer is common means for prevention and treatment
Hispanic American Mexican-American (Latino, Chicano, Raza-Latino)	Health beliefs have strong religious association Believe in body imbalance as a cause of illness, especially imbalance between *caliente* (hot) and *frio* (cold) or "wet" and "dry" Some maintain good health is a result of "good luck"—a reward for good behavior Illness prevented by performing properly, eating proper foods, and working proper amount of time; accomplished through prayer, wearing religious medals or amulets, and sleeping with relics at home Illness is a punishment from God for wrongdoing, forces of nature, and the supernatural	Seek help from *curandero* or *curandera*, especially in rural areas Curandero(a) receives his/her position by birth, apprenticeship, or a "calling" via dream or vision Treatments involve use of herbs, rituals, and religious artifacts Practice for severe illness—make promises, visit shrines, offer medals and candles, offer prayers Adhere to "hot" and "cold" food prescriptions and prohibitions for prevention and treatment of illness
Puerto Rican	Subscribe to the "hot-cold" theory of causation of illness Believe some illness caused by evil spirits and forces	Infrequent use of health care systems Seek folk healers—use of herbs, rituals Consult spiritualist medium for mental disorders *Santeria* is system and practitioners are called *santeros* Treatments classified as "hot" or "cold"
Native American (numerous tribes)	Believe health is state of harmony with nature and universe Respect of bodies through proper management All disorders believed to have aspects of supernatural Violation of a restriction or prohibition thought to cause illness Fear of witchcraft May carry objects believed to guard against witchcraft Theology and medicine strongly interwoven	Medicine persons: Altruistic persons who must use powers in purely positive ways Persons capable of both good and evil—perform negative acts against enemies Diviner-diagnosticians—diagnose but do not have powers or skill to implement medical treatment Specialists—use herbs and curative but nonsacred medical procedures Medicine persons—use herbs and ritual Singers—cure by the power of their song obtained from supernatural beings, effect cures by laying on of hands

Family Relationships	Communication	Comments
Strong kinship bonds in extended family; members come to aid of others in crisis Less likely to view illness as a burden Augmented families common (unrelated persons living in same household) Place strong emphasis on work and ambition	Alert to any evidence of discrimination Place importance on nonverbal behavior May use nonstandard English or "black English" Use "testing" behaviors to assess personnel in health care situations before seeking active care May use more paranoid responses than other groups Best to use simple, direct, but caring approach	High level of caution and distrust of majority group Social anxiety related to tradition of humiliation, oppression, and loss of dignity Will elect to retain dignity rather than seek care if values are compromised Strong sense of peoplehood High incidence of poverty Black minister a strong influence in black community Visits by family minister are sought, expected, and valued in helping to cope with illness and suffering
Traditionally men considered breadwinners, women homemakers Males are considered big and strong (*macho*) Strong kinship; extended families include *compadres* (godparents) established by ritual kinship Children valued highly and desired, taken everywhere with family Many homes contain shrines with statues and pictures of saints	May use nonstandard English Most bilingual; many only speak Spanish May have a strong preference for native language and revert to it in times of stress	High degree of modesty—often a deterrent to seeking medical care Youngsters often reluctant to share communal showers in schools Relaxed concept of time—may be late for appointments Magicoreligious practices common May view hospital as place to go to die
Family usually large and home-centered—the core of existence Father has complete authority in family—family provider and decision-maker Wife and children subordinate to father Children valued—seen as a gift from God Children taught to obey and respect parents; corporal punishment to ensure obedience	May use nonstandard English Spanish speaking or bilingual Strong sense of family privacy—may view questions regarding family as impudent	Relaxed sense of time Pay little attention to *exact* time of day Suspicious and fearful of hospitals
Extended family structure—usually includes relatives from both sides of family Elder members assume leadership roles	Most continue to speak their Indian language as well as English Nonverbal communication	Time orientation—present Respect for age Going to hospital associated with illness or disease; therefore may not seek prenatal care since pregnancy viewed as natural process

of health care to children requires the establishment of a close relationship with families and other influential persons in the community (such as the local folk healer) and periodic assessment of one's own attitudes and behaviors and those of other health workers toward people of other racial or ethnic origins.

Some characteristics of selected cultures are outlined in Table 3-2.

SUMMARY

Recognition of the social, cultural, and religious influences on the child and family is an essential component of the nursing process. Cultural differences are not always readily apparent, yet they significantly influence many areas of nursing concern, such as childrearing practices, family structure, educational patterns, occupational aspirations, religious beliefs, communication skills, self-concept development, disease susceptibility, physical characteristics, health beliefs, and diet practices. The nurse who is alert to these influences with every child and family encountered is able to plan and implement an effective plan of care that respects the individuality of cultural heritage.

KEY CONCEPTS

- A culture is composed of individuals with a set of values, beliefs, practices, and information that is learned, integrative, social, and satisfying.
- Nurses have a responsibility to understand the influence of culture, race, and ethnicity on the development of social and emotional relationships, childrearing practices, and attitudes toward health.
- Socialization is the process by which children acquire the beliefs, values, and behaviors considered desirable or appropriate by the culture.
- A child's self-concept evolves from ideas about his social roles.
- Guilt and shame are two behaviors commonly conditioned in children to control social behavior.
- Important subcultural influences on children include ethnicity, social class, poverty, affluence, occupation, religion, schools, peers, and biculture.
- Membership in a minority group presents special challenges for children, although changes in societal attitudes are slowly taking place.
- Cultural shock refers to a person's feeling of helplessness and disorientation while trying to adapt to a different cultural group and its practices, values, and beliefs.
- A child's physical characteristics and susceptibility to health problems are strongly related to ethnic and cultural variations of hereditary and socioeconomic forces.
- Cultural beliefs related to the course of illness and maintenance of health may focus on natural forces, supernatural forces, or imbalance of forces.
- In planning and implementing patient care, nurses need to strive to adapt ethnic practices to the family's health needs rather than attempt to change long-standing beliefs.

STUDY QUESTIONS AND ACTIVITIES

1. Visit a preschool program attended primarily by children from middle-class backgrounds and a program aimed at disadvantaged children, such as Head Start. Compare and contrast observations of cultural differences, such as language skills, interactions with teachers and other children, and play behaviors.
2. Interview parents from a variety of cultural, ethnic, economic, and religious backgrounds to learn about differences in childrearing practices.
3. Select an ethnic group with values and customs that conflict with your own. Use additional resources from the references at the end of this chapter to develop a thorough understanding of that group's beliefs and practices. Develop strategies that might be used to care for a child from that ethnic group in a health care setting.
4. Acquire the recipe for a health remedy from one (or more) families. Determine the essential ingredient. What, if any, scientific basis or known harmful effect can be identified?
5. Interview leaders from two different religious groups as to their beliefs and health practices that may affect nursing care.

REFERENCES

Bloch, B.: Nursing care of black patients. In Orque, M.S., Bloch, B., and Monrroy, L.S.A.: Ethnic nursing care, St. Louis, 1983, The C.V. Mosby Co.

Char, E.L.: The Chinese American. In Clark, A.L., editor: Culture and childrearing, Philadelphia, 1981, F.A. Davis Co.

Chen-Louie, T.: Nursing care of Chinese American patients. In Orque, M.S., Bloch, B., and Monrroy, L.S.A.: Ethnic nursing care, St. Louis, 1983, The C.V. Mosby Co.

Chow, E.: Cultural health traditions: Asian perspectives. In Branch, M.F., and Paxon, P.P., editors: Providing safe nursing care for ethnic people of color, New York, 1976, Appleton-Century-Crofts.

Ehling, M.B.: The Mexican American (El Chicano). In Clark, A.L., editor: Culture and childrearing, Philadelphia, 1981, F.A. Davis Co.

Feldman, K.W.: Pseudoabusive burns in Asian refugees, Am. J. Dis. Child. **138:**768-769, 1984.

Greathouse, B., and Miller, V.G.: The black American. In Clark, A.L., editor: Culture and childrearing, Philadelphia, 1981, F.A. Davis Co.

Hashizume, S., and Takano, J.: Nursing care of Japanese patients. In Orque, M.S., Bloch, B., and Monrroy, L.S.A.: Ethnic nursing care, St. Louis, 1983, The C.V. Mosby Co.

Holland, S., and Sweeney, E.: Vietnamese children and families: the impact of culture, Washington, DC, 1985, Association for Care of Children's Health.

Hollingsworth, A.O., Brown, L.P., and Brooten, D.A.: The refugees and childbearing: what to expect, RN **43**(11):45-48, 1980.

Jacques, G.: Cultural traditions: a black perspective. In Branch, M.F., and Paxton, P.P.: Providing safe nursing care for ethnic people of color, New York, 1976, Appleton-Century-Crofts.

Lacay, G.: The Puerto Rican in mainland America. In Clark, A.L., editor: Culture and childrearing, Philadelphia, 1981, F.A. Davis Co.

Leininger, M.: Transcultural nursing, New York, 1978, John Wiley & Sons.

Leslie, G.R.: The family in social context, ed. 5, New York, 1982, Oxford University Press.

Meleis, A.I.: The Arab American in the health care system, Am. J. Nurs. **81:**1180-1183, 1981.

Orque, M.S., Bloch, B., and Monrroy, L.S.A.: Ethnic nursing care, St. Louis, 1983, The C.V. Mosby Co.

Pasquale, E.A.: The evil eye phenomenon, Home Health Care Nurse **2**(3):32-35, 1984.

Shaffer, D.C.: Developmental psychology: theory, research and application, Monterey, CA, 1985, Brooks/Cole Publishing Co.

Sodetani-Shibata, A.E.: The Japanese American. In Clark, A.L., editor: Culture and childrearing, Philadelphia, 1981, F.A. Davis Co.
Tseng W., and others: Cross-cultural differences in parent-child assessment: U.S.A. and Japan, Int. J. Soc. Psychiatry **28:**305-317, 1982.

BIBLIOGRAPHY

General

Bauwens, E.E., and Anderson, S.: Social and cultural influences on health care. In Stanhope, M., and Lancaster, J.: Community health nursing, St. Louis, 1984, The C.V. Mosby Co.
Beliefs that can affect therapy, Pediatr. Nurs. **5**(3):40-43, 1979.
Bonaparte, B.: Ego defensiveness, open-closed mindedness, and nurses' attitude toward culturally different patients, Nurs. Res. **28:**166-172, 1979.
Brink, P.J.: Value orientations as an assessment tool in cultural diversity, Nurs. Res. **33:**198-203, 1984.
Bullough, V.L., and Bullough, B.: Health care for the other Americans, New York, 1982, Appleton-Century-Crofts.
Carpio, B.: The adolescent immigrant, Can. Nurse **7**(3):27-29, 1981.
Chen-Louie, T.T.: Bicultural experiences, social interactions, and health care implications. In Reinhardt, A.M., and Quinn, M.D., editors: Family-centered community nursing, vol. 2, St. Louis, 1980, The C.V. Mosby Co.
Choi, E.S., and Hamilton, R.K.: The effects of culture on mother-infant interaction, JOGNN **15:**256-261, 1986.
Conatser, C.: Effect of wealth on approach to patient care, J. Assoc. Pediatr. Oncol. Nurses **3**(2):14-19, 1986.
DeGracia, R.T.: Cultural influences on Filipino patients, Am. J. Nurs. **79:**1412-1414, 1979.
Dobson, S.: Bringing culture into care, Nurs. Times **78:**2106-2109, 1982.
Fong, C.M.: Ethnicity and nursing practice, Topics Clin. Nurs. **7**(3):1-10, 1985.
Frenkel, S.I., and others: Does patient contact change racial perceptions? Am. J. Nurs. **80:**1340-1342, 1980.
Germain, C.P.: Cultural concepts in critical care, Crit. Care. Q.**5**(3):61-78, 1982.
Hautman, M.A., and Harrison, J.K.: Health beliefs and practices in a middle-income Anglo-American neighborhood, Adv. Nurs. Sci. **4**(3):49-63, 1982.
Henry, B.M., and DiGiacomo-Geffers, E.: The hospitalized rich and famous, Am. J. Nurs. **80:**1426-1429, 1980.
Johnston, M.: Cultural variations in professional and parenting practices, J. Obstet. Gynecol. Nurs. **9:**9-13, 1980.
Johnston, M.: Folk beliefs and ethnocultural behavior in pediatrics, medicine or magic, Nurs. Clin. North Am. **12:**77-84, 1977.
Kubricht, D.W., and Clark, J.A.: Foreign patients: a system for providing care, Nurs. Outlook **30:**55-57, 1982.
LaFargue, J.P.: Mediating between two views of illness, Topics Clin. Nurs. **7**(3):70-77, 1985.
Lash, M.E.: Community health nursing in a minority setting, Nurs. Clin. North Am. **15**(2):339-348, 1980.
Linley, J.F.: Mothers' attitudes regarding health care for their children, MCN **9:**37-39, 1984.
Lipson, J.G., and Meleis, A.I.: Culturally appropriate care: the case of immigrants, Topics Clin. Nurs. **7**(3):48-56, 1985.
Louie, K.B.: Transcending cultural bias: the literature speaks, Topics Clin. Nurs. **7**(3):78-84, 1985.
Maheady, D.C.: Cultural assessment of children, MCN **11**(2):128, 1986.
Mandelbaum, J.K.: The food square: helping people of different cultures understand balanced diets, Pediatr. Nurs. **9:**20-21, 1985.
Marchant, R.: Caring for hospitalized inner-city children, Pediatr. Nurs. **11:**129-131, 1985.
O'Brien, M.E.: Reaching the migrant worker, Am. J. Nurs. **83:**895-897, 1983.
Orque, M.S., Bloch, B., and Monrroy, L.S.A.: Ethnic nursing care, St. Louis, 1983, The C.V. Mosby Co.
Queen, S.A., Haberstein, R.W., and Quadagno, J.S.: The family in various cultures, New York, 1985, Harper & Row.
Reichenback, M.B.: A framework for the nature and development of health beliefs in children, Matern. Child Nurs. J. **15**(3):119-128, 1986.
Ruiz, M.C.J.: Open-mindedness, intolerance of ambiguity and nursing faculty attitudes toward culturally different patients, Nurs. Res. **30:**177-181, 1981.
Shubin, S.: Nursing patients from different cultures, Nursing 80 **10**(6):78-81, 1980.
Spector, R.E.: Cultural diversity in health and illness, New York, 1979, Appleton-Century-Crofts.
Stern, P.N.: Solving problems of cross-cultural health teaching, Image **13:**47-50, 1981.
Thiederman, S.B.: Ethnocentrism: a barrier to effective health care, Nurs. Pract. **11**(8):52-59, 1986.
Tripp-Reimer, T.: Research in cultural diversity, West. J. Nurs. Res. **6:**353-355, 1984.
Tripp-Reimer, T., Brink, P.J., and Saunders, J.M.: Cultural assessment: content and process, Nurs. Outlook **32:**78-82, 1984.

Religion

Adams, C.E., and others: The effects of religious beliefs on the health care practices of the Amish, Nurs. Pract. **11**(3):58-67, 1986.
Ellis, D.: What happened to the spiritual dimension? Can. Nurs. **76**(9):42-43, 1980.
Gershan, J.A.: Judaic ethical beliefs and customs regarding death and dying, Crit. Care Nurse **5**(1):32-34, 1985.
Kim, M.J., McFarland, G.K., and McLane, A.M., editors: Classification of nursing diagnosis: proceedings of the Fifth National Conference, St. Louis, 1984, The C.V. Mosby Co.
Masulis, K.: When parents refuse treatment for their children . . . Jehovah's Witnesses, J. Christ. Nurs. **4**(2):10-12, 1987.
McDowell, J., and Stewart, D.: Understanding non-Christian religions, San Bernradino, CA, 1982, Here's Life Publishing, Inc.
Roberson, M.H.B.: The influence of religious beliefs on health choices of Afro-Americans, Topics Clin. Nurs. **7**(3):57-63, 1985.
Shelly, J.A.: Spiritual care: planting seeds of hope, Crit. Care Update **9**(2):7-15, 1982.
Sodestrom, K.E., and Martinson, I.M.: Patients' spiritual coping strategies: a study of nurse and patient perspectives, Oncol. Nurs. Forum **14**(2):41-46, 1987.
Stoll, R.T.: Guidelines for spiritual assessment, Am. J. Nurs. **79:**1574-1577, 1979.
Swan, R.: The law should protect all children . . . children in faith-healing sects, J. Christ. Nurs. **4**(2):40, 1987.

Specific Ethnic Groups

Backup, R.W.: Health care of the American Indian patient, Crit. Care Update **7**(2):16-22, 1980.
Brown, B.S.: Growing up healthy: the Chinese experience, Pediatr. Nurs. **9:**255-257, 1983.
Capers, C.F.: Nursing and the Afro-American client, Topics Clin. Nurs. **7**(3):11-17, 1985.
Choi, E.: Unique aspects of Korean-American mothers, JOGNN **15**(5):394-400, 1986.
DeGracia, R.T.: Cultural influences on Filipino patients, Am. J. Nurs. **79:**1412-1414, 1979.
DeGracia, R.T.: Health care of the American Asian patient, Crit. Care Update **6**(12):19-28, 1979.
Desantis, L.: Infant feeding practices of Haitian mothers in South Florida: cultural beliefs and acculturation, Matern. Child Nurs. J. **15:**77-89, 1986.
Drakulic, L., and Tanaka, W.: The East Indian family in Canada. Can. Nurse **7**(3):24-26, 1981.
Egan, M.G.: A family assessment challenge: refugee youth and foster family adaptation, Topics Clin. Nurs. **7**(3):64-69, 1985.
Foreman, J.T.: *Susto* and the health needs of the Cuban refugee population, Topics Clin. Nurs. **7**(3):40-47, 1985.
Gonzales-Swafford, M.J., and Gutierrez, M.G.: Ethno-medical beliefs and practices of Mexican-Americans, Nurs. Pract. **8**(10):29-30, 32, 34, 1983.
Gordon, V.C., Matousek, I.M., and Lang, T.A.: Southeast Asian refugees: life in America, Am. J . Nurs. **80:**2031-2036, 1980.

Grosso, C., and others: The Vietnamese American family . . . and grandma makes three, Am. J. Maternal Child Nurs. **6:**177-180, 1981.

Kwok, A.W.H.: Culture conflict: a study of the problems of Chinese immigrant adolescents in Canada, Can. Nurs. **78**(3):32-34, 1982.

Mardiros, M.: A view toward hospitalization: the Mexican American experience, J. Adv. Nurs. **9:**469-478, 1984.

Marrio, E.B., and Hall, R.R.: Asian family traditions and their influence in transcultural health care delivery, Child. Health Care **15**(3):172-177, 1987.

Meleis, A.I., and Sorrell, L.: Arab American women and their birth experiences, Am. J. Maternal Child Nurs. **6:**171-176, 1981.

Pass, C.M.: Psychological factors, childbearing, and black female adolescents, J. Pediatr. Nurs. **1:**247-259, 1986.

Powers, B.A.: The use of orthodox and black American folk medicine, Adv. Nurs. Sci. **4**(3):35-47, 1982.

Ramirez, A.G.: A media-based acculturation scale for Mexican-Americans: application to public health education programs, Fam. Community Health **9**(3):63-71, 1986.

Richardson, L.: Breakthrough to nursing, Part 2: Folk medicine in a Hispanic population, Imprint **29:**72-77, 1982.

Rosenblum, E.H.: Conversation with a Navajo nurse, Am. J. Nurs. **80:**1459-1461, 1980.

Rosenburg, J.A.: Health care for Cambodian children: integrating treatment plans, Pediatr. Nurs. **12:**118-125, 1986.

Rozendal, N.: Understanding Italian American cultural norms, J. Psychosoc. Nurs. Ment. Health Serv. **25**(2):29-35, 1987.

Satz, K.J.: Integrating Navajo tradition into maternal-child nursing, Image **14:**89-91, 1982.

Tamez, E.G., Familism, machismo, and child rearing practices among Mexican Americans, J. Psychosoc. Nurs. **19**(9):21-25, 1981.

Tripp-Reimer, T.: Barriers to health care: variations in interpretation of Appalachian client behavior by Appalachian and non-Appalachian health professionals, West. J. Nurs. Res. **4:**179-191, 1982.

Zepeda, M.: Selected maternal-infant care practices of Spanish-speaking women, J. Obstet. Gynecol. Nurs. **11:**371-374, 1982.

CHAPTER 4

Family Influences on Health Promotion of the Child and Family

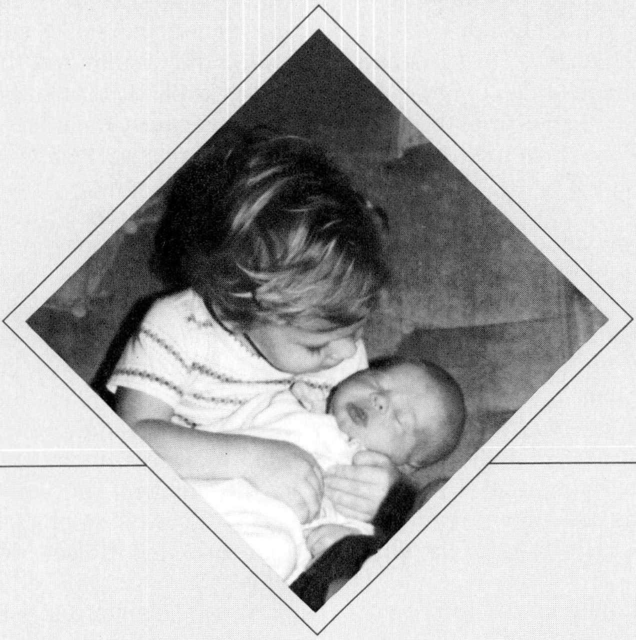

LEARNING OBJECTIVES

On completion of this chapter the reader will be able to:

- Discuss definitions of *family*
- Describe two major family theories
- Identify different family structures found in the United States
- Discuss the effect of family size and configuration on personality development
- Discuss the role transition experienced by new parents
- Explain various parenting behaviors such as parenting styles, disciplinary patterns, and communication skills
- Demonstrate an understanding of special parenting situations such as adoption, divorce, single parenting, stepparenting, and dual-career families

Societies, to maintain and perpetuate themselves, have established institutions designed for the express purpose of rearing and educating their children. The primary institution that accepts this responsibility is the family, and, as the basic interpersonal group, it is a universal characteristic of all human societies. The family provides each newborn member of society with legitimacy, that is, a family connection (usually symbolized by a family name) and an ascribed position in the societal strata.

Although the structure and subordinate goals of the family vary among and within cultures and change at different times and in different places, the overall purpose of the family is to provide for the future of a society and the stability of its culture. During the long time required for human infants to reach a level of independence, individual families assume the responsibility for their rearing, although such families differ considerably in form, complexity, and goals of socialization.

The term *family* has been defined in a number of ways and for a number of purposes according to the individual's own frame of reference, value judgment, or the discipline (Johnson, 1984). Probably one of the most all-encompassing definitions proposed describes family as "the coexistence of more than one human being involving continuous, presumably permanent, sharing of living facilities, a perception of reciprocal obligations, a sense of commonness, and sharing of certain obligations toward each other and toward others" (Mauksch, 1974). Others define family in relation to the persons that comprise the family unit: *consanguinal* (blood relationships), *affinal* (marriage relationships), and *fictive* (invented relationships, such as godparents or groups who call themselves a family).

Traditionally a family has been conceptualized as a group, with the belief that both a mother and father are needed to rear a child. Nearly all societies grant a very high rank to the married status and, although this concept has undergone considerable modification, a great deal of emotion has been generated about some of the newer concepts of family—such as communal families, single-parent families, and homosexual families. To accommodate these and other varieties of family styles, the descriptive term *household* is being used more frequently. Regardless of the definition chosen, a "family" is whatever the client considers it to be.

Although the concept of household is recognized and appreciated, the term *family* will be used consistently throughout this book to indicate the relationships between dependent children and one or more protective adults. It also implies relationships with other dependent selves, that is, siblings. Family members share a sense of belonging to their own family that deeply affects their lives.

Nursing of infants and children is intimately involved with care of the child *and* the family. Consequently, nurses must be aware of the functions of the family, various types of family structures, and theories that provide a foundation for understanding the changes within a family. Since nurses are often the professionals involved in providing anticipatory guidance regarding childrearing, they also need a basic understanding of parenting and special parenting situations. As discussed in Chapter 1 (see Role of the pediatric nurse), nurses working with families have the same responsibilities: as advocate, teacher, counselor, and coordinator. These responsibilities are addressed in this chapter by providing the knowledge to implement such roles, and more specifically throughout the text where appropriate. The critical process of assessment of family function and structure is discussed in the unit on assessment (see pp. 117-122).

◆ *Family Theories*

Numerous theories have been applied to families to describe and predict events and interactions; however, two have been identified that have significant relevance and application to pediatric nursing: *family system theory* and *developmental theory*.

FAMILY SYSTEM THEORY

Family system theory is derived from general system theory, a science of "wholeness" that is characterized by interaction among the components of the system and between the system and the environment. General system theory expanded scientific thought from a simplistic view of direct cause and effect (A causes B) to a more complex and interrelated theory (A influences B, but B also affects A). In family system theory the family is viewed as a system that continually interacts with its members and the environment. The emphasis is on the *interaction* between the members, such that a change in one family member creates a change in other members, which in turn results in a new change in the original member. Consequently, a problem or dysfunction does not lie in any one member but rather in the type of interactions used by the family. Since it is the interactions, rather than individual members, that are viewed as the source of the problem, the family becomes the patient and the focus of care. Examples of the application of family system theory to clinical problems are nonorganic failure to thrive and child abuse. According to system theory, the problem does not rest solely with the parent or child but in the type of interactions between the parent and child, as well as in a host of other factors that affect their relationship.

Understanding system theory and its application to the family requires knowledge of numerous basic definitions and concepts that are beyond the focus of this discussion. However, some general concepts that are unique to this theory and have significance to understanding family dynamics are presented.

The family is viewed as a whole that is different from the sum of the individual members. For example, in a household of parents and one child there are not only three individuals, but also three relationships (or subsystems) that characterize the family system. These include the marital relationship, the mother-child relationship, and the father-child relationship. This concept of nonsummativity—"the whole is greater than the sum of its parts"—implies that, when working with a family, the nurse must be aware of the relationships between family members. To effect positive change in a family it is necessary to work with and through the several subsystems of the family.

Another important concept is that the family is viewed as a highly adaptable unit. When problems exist within the family, change can be effected by altering the interaction or feedback messages that perpetuate disruptive behavior. When the family system is disrupted, change can occur at any point in the system. Consequently, it is not necessary to go back into the family history or an individual's life to find out the "cause" of the problem, as recommended by other theories, such as psychoanalytic theory. In family system theory the emphasis is on what is occurring now in the family and on intervening to change that pattern. This focus allows for sometimes rapid and dramatic changes.

A major factor that influences a family's adaptability is its boundary, an imaginary but very real line that exists between the family and its environment. This boundary or line may be open or closed. If open, the family welcomes input into its system by accepting new ideas, information, resources, and opportunities. This type of family reaches out for help and uses the available support systems. In contrast, a closed family resists input by viewing change as threatening. The family is suspicious of any available support and strives to maintain the family system by avoiding outside influences. Knowledge of boundaries is critical when teaching or counseling families. Although open families are receptive to intervention, closed families typically resist assistance and more effort is required to win their trust and acceptance.

TABLE 4-1

Duvall's Development Stages of the Family

Stages/Tasks
Stage I: Marriage and an independent home: the joining of families
Reestablish couple identity
Realign relationships with extended family
Make decisions regarding parenthood
Stage II: Families with infants
Integrate infants into the family unit
Accommodate to new parenting and grandparenting roles
Maintain the marital bond
Stage III: Families with preschoolers
Socialize children
Parents and children adjust to separation
Stage IV: Families with schoolchildren
Children develop peer relations
Parents adjust to their children's peer and school influence
Stage V: Families with teenagers
Adolescents develop increasing autonomy
Parents refocus on midlife marital and career issues
Parents begin a shift toward concern for the older generation
Stage VI: Families as launching centers
Parents and young adult establish independent identities
Renegotiate marital relationship
Stage VII: Middle-aged families
Reinvest in couple identity with concurrent development of independent interests
Realign relationships to include in-laws and grandchildren
Deal with disabilities and death of older generation
Stage VIII: Aging families
Shift from work role to leisure and semiretirement or full retirement
Maintain couple and individual functioning while adapting to the aging process
Prepare for own death and dealing with the loss of spouse, and/or siblings, and other peers

Modified from Wright, L.M., and Leahey, M.: Nurses and families: a guide to family assessment and intervention, Philadelphia, 1984, F.A. Davis Co.

DEVELOPMENTAL THEORY

Developmental theory is an outgrowth of several theories of development. Foremost among the developers are Duvall (1977), who described eight developmental tasks of the family throughout its life span, derived from Erikson's eight stages of man (see p. 83), and Rogers (1962), who incorporated role theory into the developmental concept. The family is described as a small group, a semiclosed system of personalities that interacts with the larger cultural social system. As an interrelated system, changes do not occur in one part without a series of changes in other parts.

Developmental theory uses a family life-cycle approach to compare the changing structure, function, and roles of the family at various stages of development, focusing on time as the central dimension. The theory delineates developmental tasks for the family much like the individual developmental tasks discussed in relation to personality development. These tasks are defined as those growth responsibilities that arise at a specific stage in the life of the family, which, if successfully achieved, lead to satisfaction and success with later tasks, while failure leads to family unhappiness (Duvall, 1977). These stages are delineated on the basis of transitions and adjustments required by its members at each stage (Table 4-1). Although the family system as a whole is important, it depends on the behavior of its members, and achievement of family developmental tasks at each family life-cycle stage is interrelated with the simultaneous accomplishment of the individual developmental task of each member.

◆ *Family Structure and Function*

Structure is a manner of organization or the arrangement of a number of parts that are interrelated in specified, recurring ways. Function refers to a special duty or performance required in the course of work or activity. The structure of a family may vary according to the composition of its component parts and according to its life-cycle. Both structure and function are altered and modified as the needs of the family change.

FAMILY FUNCTIONS

Authorities agree that families serve society in many ways. They play a vital role in the economy because they produce and consume goods and services. They also are the basic unit for replacing dying members of the society. Furthermore, society, to maintain its continuity, must transmit its knowledge, customs, values, and beliefs to the young. Where children are not an economic necessity, their primary function is to receive and to give love.

Although goals for socialization and childrearing practices differ from one culture to another, in most societies the family appears to have three major objectives in relation to children: caregiving, nurturing, and training.

FAMILY STRUCTURE

The family structure, or family composition, consists of individuals, each with a socially recognized status and position, who interact with one another on a regular, recurring basis in socially sanctioned ways. When members are gained or lost through events (e.g., marriage, divorce, birth, death, abandonment, incarceration), the family composition is altered and roles must be redefined or redistributed.

Traditionally the family structure refers to either *nuclear* or *extended families*. However, family composition has assumed new configurations in recent years, with the single-parent family becoming a prominent form. It is not uncommon for children to belong to several different family groups during their lifetime.

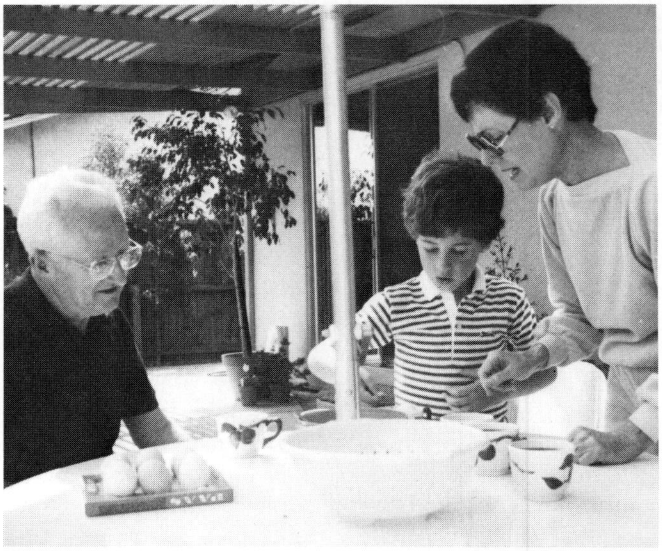

FIG. 4-1 Children benefit from interaction with grandparents even when they do not share the same household.

Nuclear Family

The nuclear, or conjugal, family consists of a husband, a wife, and their children (natural or adopted) who live in a common household. This is the reproductive unit in which the marital tie (legally or otherwise sanctioned) is the chief binding force. A strongly functional nuclear family is the prototype of human relationships and the basic unit from which more complex family forms are composed. In some instances one or more additional persons (e.g., a relative, friend, foster child, or others) may reside in the same household. Some authorities classify childless couples as a nuclear family because it is a conjugal alliance with the theoretic potential for reproduction.

The nuclear family, the predominant structure in America, is more characteristic of an urban, mobile society. It is free to move where there is better financial opportunity. It is not economically bound to a geographic area or dependent on the cooperative efforts of other members. The family members are employed on an individual basis, and economic resources are in the form of money.

Despite this mobility, the majority of nuclear families in America are associated with an extended kinship network of nuclear families living in separate households but in close geographic proximity. This concept, sometimes referred to as a modified extended family, describes a meaningful aspect of daily existence that is reflected in frequent visiting and the exchange of services and financial aid. This family association meets the members' psychologic needs to a greater extent than do experts, friends, or organizations (Fig. 4-1). It is not uncommon for families to reject the opportunity for social or economic advancement rather than leave such kinship associations.

Affiliative relationships. Although the nuclear family is predominantly a legally sanctioned institution, there are a number of families in which the attachment is only affiliative, that is, nonmarital cohabitation. These families consist primarily of two adults, the "couple households" (Macklin, 1980), but may include children. The mother and father live together, often with children from previous matings, and share family responsibilities. However, the family unit is less stable and relationships are subject to change. Instability of the social environment in the home has been associated with juvenile delinquency, which appears to be related to the number of family constellations (changes in the adult members of the household) experienced during childhood. This effect is probably a reflection of repeated adjustment to a variety of authority figures with differing expectations (Mednick and Baker, 1980).

Single-Parent Family

The single-parent family, a result of recent social phenomena, has emerged partially as a consequence of women's rights movements during which more women (and men) have established separate households because of divorce, death, desertion, or illegitimacy. In addition, a more liberal attitude in the courts has made it possible for single persons, both male and female, to adopt children; previously, rigid prerequisites specified that both a father and a mother must be present in the home. Unmarried mothers, choosing to keep and raise their children rather than place them for adoption or marry, are absorbed into the extended family. For instance, in the lower-lower class of the United States, where the incidence of illegitimacy is highest, the maternal grandmother is usually available to care for the children (Whitehead, 1978).

Therefore, with the increased psychologic independence of women as a whole and the increased acceptability of illegitimacy in society, more unmarried women are deliberately choosing mother-child families. The problems of these single-parent families are discussed on p. 70.

Reconstituted Family

Reconstituted families, also referred to as stepfamilies, are those in which one or both of the married adults have children from a previous marriage residing in the household. The term *blended families* or *combined families* more often refers to families composed of parents and the children each of them brings from a previous marriage. It is estimated that one out of every five children is a stepchild (Romanczuk, 1987). The most common stepfamily consists of a mother, her children, and a stepfather (Perkins and Kahan, 1979). The problems of the reconstituted family are further discussed on p. 70.

Extended Family

The extended, or consanguineous, family is one mode of combining nuclear families into larger units through the parent-child relationship. It consists of the nuclear family plus lineal or collateral relatives. More often it is composed of two or more residential units of three or more generations affiliated through extension of the parent-child relationship, that is, grandparents, parents, and grandchildren.

In the extended family childrearing is often a shared responsibility. Relatives are always present and available to help young parents with household chores and child care activities. Daily lives of the children are organized around the needs and requirements of the family with assigned tasks and obligations.

Extended family structure is more functional in areas where land is the basis of wealth and sustenance. Today the best examples of extended family units can be found among successful farmers, Native Americans, and certain recent immigrants. Extended families may form under conditions of either extreme poverty in order to pool resources or extreme wealth in order to consolidate resources.

Alternative Family Structures

Several other family structures exist that are much less common. One of them, *polygamy*, is not legally sanctioned in the United States. In countries where it exists, polygamy is usually accorded a higher status than monogamy. It may be limited to ruling families or to high-status persons and tends to be practiced by a small segment of the population.

Another type of family structure that is relatively uncommon today is the *communal family*. The communal family emerged from a disenchantment with most contemporary life choices. Communal groups share common ownership of property and goods; in cooperatives there is private ownership of property, but certain goods and services are shared and exchanged cooperatively without monetary consideration. There is strong reliance on group members and material interdependence.

Unlike the traditional extended family, nuclear units in a commune may come and go at will. There is no consanguineous tie between the units. The mother-child tie is strong during infancy and early childhood, but many parents are happy to relinquish older children to the care of others. Although the parents maintain primary responsibility for the health and well-being of the children, the children are free to form close relationships with a number of adults in the commune and are encouraged to do so.

A *same-sex*, or *homosexual, family* is one in which there is a marital or common-law tie between two persons of the same sex who have adopted children or in which one or both partners have natural children from a heterosexual mating. Unfortunately little research is available on the spousal unit in same-sex relationships or on the effects of growing up as a child in these households.

Family Structure and Social Class

In family structure, as with other aspects of childrearing, there are greater differences related to social class than any other variable. Although the following discussion may not be representative of families in a particular social class, some commonalities do exist. In the upper-upper class, or the old aristocracy, the nuclear family may be firmly embedded in an extended kinship structure. It is primarily patrifocal in that the older husband-father is the unilateral authority. The family's source of wealth is supervised by male family members, controlled by the eldest, and handed down from one generation to the next.

The tendency in the lower-lower class is toward matrifocal family units. Since the family unit is often torn apart by continual economic stress, the mother-child relationship is the strongest and most intimate tie. There is a higher rate of divorce, illegitimacy, and desertion in this segment of society. Husband and wife are often emotionally separated by unfulfilled expectations. The father, who has few personal or economic assets (and who is more often than not an economic burden), has difficulty establishing a dominant role in the family. In this class the mother is often more easily employed than the father, and she is eligible for welfare benefits when there are minor dependent children; therefore, the mother-child dyad is predominant. Frequently there are three generations—grandmother, mother, and children—living in an extended structure, sharing the economic burden and child care.

Kin ties are stronger among lower- and working-class families than middle-class families. This is particularly true in relation to the kin network among lower-class American blacks where interaction, co-residence, and exchange of mutual aid are stronger than in white families.

◆ *Family Roles and Relationships*

Each individual has a position, or status, in the family structure, and each occupant of a position plays culturally and socially defined roles in interactions within the group. Each family has its own traditions and values and sets its own standards for interaction within and outside the family group. Each determines the experiences the children should have, those they are to be shielded from, and how each of these experiences meets the needs of family members. Where family ties are strong, social control is highly effective, and most members conform to their roles willingly and with commitment.

PARENTAL ROLES

In all family groups the socially recognized status of father and mother exists with socially sanctioned roles that prescribe appropriate sexual behavior and childrearing responsibilities. The guides for behavior in these roles serve to control sexual conflict in society and provide for prolonged care of children. The degree to which parents are committed and the way they play their respective roles are influenced by their own unique socialization experience (see Table 4-1).

Role definitions are changing as a result of the changing economy and the women's liberation movement. Women are achieving equality with men in education, more of them are entering the labor force, and the number of women who choose to have fewer children or none at all is increasing. During childhood, particularly in the upper and middle classes, the trend is toward deemphasizing the basic male-female characteristics of aggression, dependence, and achievement. As the role of the woman changes, there must necessarily be a change in the complementary role of the male. Fathers are taking a more active role in childrearing and household activities, which is most evident in middle-class families. Marital roles, on the other hand, are most segregated in the lower classes. Redefinition of sex roles in the American family is taking place, but a cultural lag of the persisting traditional role definitions creates role conflicts in many of these families.

ROLE LEARNING

Roles are learned through the socialization process. During all stages of development children learn and practice, through interaction with others and in their play, a set of social roles and something of the characteristics of other roles. They behave in patterned and more or less predictable ways because they learn roles that define mutual expectations in typical and recurring social relationships. Role conceptions are transmitted by socializing agents (parents, peers, authority figures) who use positive and negative sanctions to ensure conformity to their norms.

In some cultures the role behavior expected of children conflicts with desirable adult behavior. For example, in the United States children are expected to be submissive in childhood but dominant as adults. This conflict of expectations is known as *role discontinuity*. Other cultures value the same behaviors, such as courage and aggression, both in children and adults; this provides *role continuity*.

Role-structuring initially takes place within the family unit, where the children fulfill a set of roles and respond to the complementary roles of their parents and other family members. The roles of the children are shaped primarily by the parents, who apply direct or indirect pressures in an attempt to induce or force children into the desired patterns of behavior. Each set of parents has their own techniques, and each will determine the course that the process of socialization is to follow (see Shaping behavior, p. 64).

Children respond to life situations according to behaviors learned in reciprocal transactions. As they acquire important role-taking skills, their relationships with others change. They become proficient at understanding others as they acquire the ability to discriminate their own perspectives from those of others. Children who get along well with others and attain status in the peer group have well-developed role-taking skills.

FAMILY SIZE AND CONFIGURATION

The size and composition of the family directly influence child development. No two children grow in exactly the same environment, although identical twins most nearly approximate this. For example, in a nuclear family with two children—even of the same sex—one will live in a family with an older sibling, whereas the other will be reared in a family with a younger sibling. In a family where there is a 10-year age span among the children, one may be born to a 20-year-old mother, the other to a 30-year-old mother. For the child in each situation the environment is different.

Family Size

Parenting practices differ between small and large families. In small families more emphasis is placed on the individual development of the children. Parenting is intensive rather than extensive, and there is constant pressure to measure up to family expectations. Children's development and achievement are measured against that of other children in the neighborhood and social class. In small families there is more democratic participation by the children than in larger families.

Children in a large family are able to adjust to a variety of changes and crises. There is more emphasis on the group and less on the individual (Fig. 4-2). Cooperation is essential, often because of economic necessity. The large number of persons sharing a limited amount of space requires a greater degree of organization, administration, and authoritarian control. The control is wielded by a dominant family member—a parent or an older

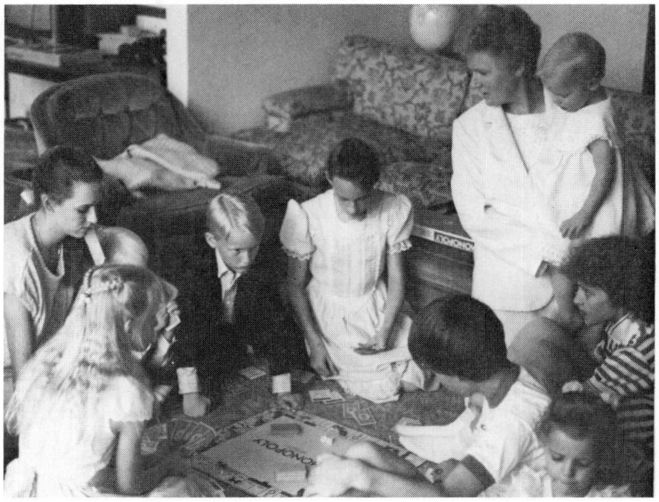

FIG. 4-2 Innumerable relationships and activities are possible in a large family.

Influence of Ordinal Position on Children

Firstborn Children
Are more achievement oriented
Receive more physical punishment
Are allowed to show more aggression to siblings
Have stronger consciences, are more self-disciplined and inner directed
Are prone to feelings of guilt
Identify more with parents than peers
Are subject to greater parental expectations

Middle Children
Have more demands made on them for household help
Are praised less often
Receive less of the parents' time
Learn to compromise and be adaptable
Are less stimulated toward achievement
Are more difficult to characterize due to a variety of positions in family

Youngest Children
Are less dependent than firstborn children
Are less tense, more affectionate, and more good-natured
Tend to identify more with peer group than with parents
Are popular with classmates

Only Children
Resemble firstborn children
Are more mature and cultivated
Experience greater parental pressure for mature behavior and achievement
Demonstrate superiority in language facility
Rarely develop into stereotype of spoiled, selfish child

child. Because the number of children reduces the intimate, one-to-one contact between the parent and any individual child, siblings may turn to each other to have their needs met. Individual children may adopt specialized roles in an attempt to gain recognition in the family.

Discipline is often administered by older siblings in large families. Siblings are usually better attuned to what constitutes misbehavior, and sibling disapproval or ostracism is frequently more meaningful than parental measures. Large families seem to generate a sense of security in the children fostered by sibling support and cooperation. However, adolescents from a large family are more peer oriented than family oriented.

Spacing of Children and Ordinal Position

Age differences between siblings affect the childhood environment but to a lesser extent than does the sex of the siblings. The arrival of a sibling has the greatest impact when a 2- to 4-year difference in age exists. A younger child's self-image is too immature to be threatened, whereas an older child is better able to understand the situation and therefore less likely to see the newcomer as a threat, although he does feel the loss of his only-child status.

In general, the narrower the spacing between siblings, the more the children influence one another, especially in emotional characteristics; the wider the spacing, the greater the influence of the parents. Also, younger children tend to identify with older siblings. Consequently they assume some of the personality characteristics, including sex-role behaviors, of the older child.

It has also been observed for some time that the birth position of children affects their personalities. Parents treat children differently, and sibling interactions are different depending on the children's position within the family. The major influences of ordinal position on children are presented in the boxed material.

Sibling Interaction

Through relationships with siblings, children learn patterns of loyalty, competition, dominance, and other interactional skills. Many factors, such as ordinal position and spacing of siblings as discussed above, may affect the child's view of the world and his relationship with others inside and outside the family.

Sibling rivalry begins at an early age (see p. 349). It has been observed that the character of interactions between children and their parents is much more positive than between siblings (Baskett and Johnson, 1982). Children often talk to, laugh with, and display affection toward their parents, but direct behaviors such as hitting, yelling, and various annoying physical antics toward their siblings. Quarrels are most often initiated by the older sibling and become more frequent and intense as the younger child becomes more mature and is better able to retaliate. Same-sex siblings engage in more positive interaction than cross-sex siblings. Mothers have been observed to direct more attention to the younger sibling who differs in gender from the older one, which may account for the different interaction pattern (Dunn and Kendrick, 1981).

Although competition is commonplace among siblings, especially those who are nearly the same age, there are positive aspects of sibling interactions. Positive social responses outnumber negative ones in total interactions between siblings, and acts of kindness are typically more common than hateful or rivalrous conduct. In many societies older children are the principal caregivers of infants and toddlers, and school-age children often assume some care of younger children in other cultures. Even older preschool children become sources of emotional support to younger ones in situations when parents are not around.

Multiple Births: Twins

The distinctive characteristics of twins have been of special interest to both geneticists and environmentalists in their efforts to obtain information regarding the "nature-nurture" controversy. Regardless of whether they are identical or fraternal, twins share a common environment. Identical (monozygotic) twins are also alike genetically, whereas fraternal (dizygotic) twins share no more genetic similarity than any other pair of siblings.

Twins generally tend to work out a special kind of sibling relationship that is reasonably satisfactory to both. They also demonstrate early independence from parental attention. They develop a remarkable capacity for cooperative play and considerable loyalty and generosity toward each other. It is not uncommon for them to evolve a private language between themselves that may interfere with development of the family language. Fraternal twins, however, especially mixed-sex sets, may behave more like different-age siblings than twins.

Promoting individuality is a complicated process in twins. Early years of togetherness are often the basis of the children's security. To separate them too early may produce unnecessary stresses. The tendency is to foster individual differences as they are evidenced in order to ease the process of separation when it becomes advisable. Unfortunately, twin children are frequently thought of and treated as a unit and efforts they make in the direction of individuality are often impeded by others (Sater, 1979).

Parents of twins have numerous adjustments to make, from difficulty in attachment and bonding (see p. 205) to the stresses of the heavy workload and monetary expenses. The **National Organization of Mothers of Twins Clubs, Inc.*** has local chapters throughout the United States and Canada to offer information and support to parents of twins and is highly recommended as a resource for all new parents of twins. Another Canadian organization offering similar services is the **Parents of Multiple Birth Association.†** The **Twins Foundation‡**—an organization founded by a group of twins and designed to aid twins and other multiples—is recommended for older children.

*5402 Amberwood Lane, Rockville, MD 20853.

†283 7th Ave., Lethbridge, Alta, Canada, T1J 1H6.

‡P.O. Box 9487, Providence, RI 02940-9487.

◆ *Parenting*

Although the impulse for sexual union is spontaneous and not seasonally limited, the union for purposes of procreation can be timed according to needs and desires of the family and based on rational attachment to, and the care and welfare of, another individual. It is a developmental stage in the life cycle, one that may be viewed by the parents as an endurance contest, a dismal failure, or the most rewarding and pleasurable experience of their lives.

MOTIVATION FOR PARENTHOOD

A characteristic in all societies is that adults are expected to become parents and to be gratified by the experience. Pressures of tradition, sentiment regarding the state of motherhood, and religious exhortations to fulfill divine commands of fertility profoundly influence decision making, since conformity to social-role expectations is a strong influence in family planning.

Although many pregnancies are unplanned, there are numerous reasons couples decide to initiate a pregnancy. Many consider children a normal part of marriage, others see them as proof of their adulthood, some desire heirs for the family name and fortune, and a few want to fulfill a parent's wish for grandchildren. Having a child in an attempt to save an unstable marriage is a poor reason, one that usually fails in its goal. However, in most instances the couple has a sincere desire to become parents.

Factors that are likely to influence family size are social class, religion, race, type of conjugal-role relationships, and the social-psychologic aspects of sexual relations. Of course, how effectively the couple practices contraception may determine whether the family size remains as planned. Also, in the case of divorce and remarriage an individual may decide to have more children with the new spouse.

PREPARATION FOR PARENTHOOD

The basic goals of parenting are to promote the physical survival and health of the children, to foster the skills and abilities necessary to be a self-sustaining adult, and to foster behavioral capabilities for maximizing cultural values and beliefs. However, new parents approach parenthood with meager experience and scant knowledge, although no other task can compare, in overall consequences, with that of rearing a human being. Parents learn by trial and error, committing the same mistakes that have been committed by countless other parents, but they somehow manage to accomplish the task, becoming more skilled with each additional child. Tradition rather than rational planning furnishes the chief norms for childrearing. Experience in having been nurtured as a child is an essential component of successful parenting.

Their own parents are probably the only persons that parents observe intimately in the parental role; this results in a *generational continuity*—parents rear their own children in much the same way as they themselves were reared. Other essential skills and knowledge parents need in order to feel more comfortable in the parenting role include a basic understanding of childhood growth and development, bathing, feeding, use of play, and interpersonal communication skills. All of this information is integrated throughout this text.

TRANSITION TO PARENTHOOD

The transition to parenthood is abrupt. Although a couple has anticipated the child's arrival, birth means the sudden imposition of totally dependent care 24 hours a day for the new member of the family. Some have described the birth of an infant as a crisis, and it may very well be a crisis if the event is perceived as disturbing old habits and relationships and eliciting new responses. It requires role changes, destroys or significantly modifies former relationships, and means adjusting to new role realignments. Whereas previously the roles of a couple were husband and wife, they now become, in addition, father and mother. It is difficult to adjust to being parents, but it is a normal human experience and a tool for personal growth.

The birth of an infant is a highly significant event that alters the behavior of both mothers and fathers. No amount of preparation can truly and fully prepare prospective parents for the constant and immediate needs of an infant. Certain factors, however, influence the transition to the parental role. One factor in which the cultural trend has changed in recent years is parental age. The years between 18 and 35 have traditionally been considered the optimum time for childbearing. However, longer life spans, the trend toward dual career marriages, and the desire for financial security before childbearing has increased the age at which parents begin their families, with a substantial rise in the birth rate for women aged 35 to 39 years of age. Research has shown that older mothers are more responsive to their children and appear to derive more pleasure from interactions with their children (Ragozin and others, 1982). Younger mothers, on the other hand, express less favorable attitudes about childrearing and are likely to be less responsive to their infants.

Other factors influencing the transition to the parental role include:

Parents with previous experience, such as another child, appear to be more relaxed and have less conflict in disciplinary relationships, and they are more cognizant of normal growth and development expectations

Fathers who are highly involved with their child often feel more comfortable and successful in the parenting role (Fig. 4-3)

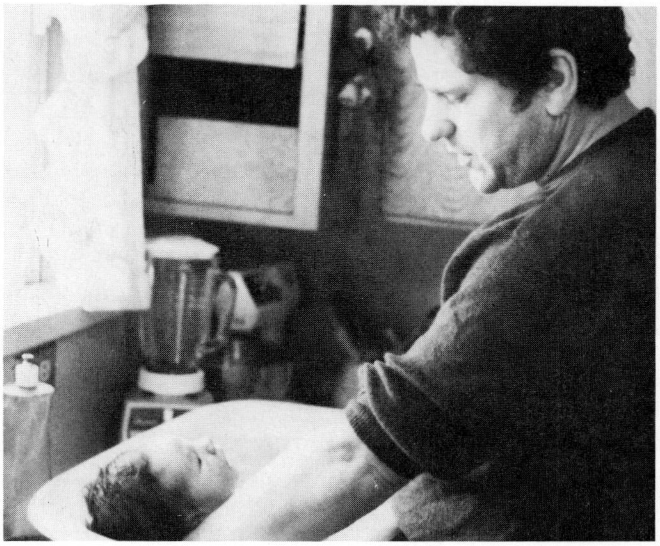

FIG. 4-3 Fathers who assume care of their children may feel more comfortable and successful in their parenting role.

The amount of stress experienced by one or both parents may interfere with their ability to exhibit patience and understanding, or otherwise cope with their children's behavior, than they would at other times

Special characteristics of the infant, such as a temperamentally difficult infant, can cause the parents to lose confidence and doubt their abilities. Also, an infant with special care needs, such as those associated with a disability, can be a significant source of added stress

Marital relationships can have a negative effect on parental transition, as marital tension or strife can alter caregiving routines and interfere with enjoyment of the infant (Belsky, 1981). Conversely, parents who support and encourage one another serve as a positive influence on establishing a satisfying parental role (Crnic and others, 1983)

Support Systems

Successful adaptation to the stress of transition to parenthood involves at least two types of family resources (McCubbin and Paterson, 1982). First are the internal resources of the family, such as *adaptability* and *integration*. Changing from an orderly, predictable life to a relatively disordered, unpredictable one is a universal adaptation families must make. Rigid schedules are impossible to maintain and former activities must be curtailed or abandoned. Adaptation is reflected in learning to be patient, becoming better organized, and becoming more flexible. Integration involves an attempt of the couple to continue some activities in which they were engaged before the advent of parenthood. In this way couples are able to maintain a sense of continuity and appreciate the importance of the husband-wife relationship.

The second kind of resource for coping with stress is

the use of coping strategies that strengthen the organization and functioning of the family. These include the use of community resources, the use of social support, and the adoption of a future orientation. Interpersonal supports that provide information, advice, and caretaking are derived from friends, relatives, and neighbors. Relationships with family, friends, and community are essential. Arranging for time away from the child or children is also beneficial. Fathers can assume care of the family to allow the mother some time to herself at home or away from the home, even for an afternoon or evening. Adoption of a future orientation provides reassurance to parents that things will get better, that they will cope, and that it is realistic to plan for the time when they are able to engage in self-fulfilling activities.

It is also reassuring to know that others experience ambivalent feelings toward parenthood and share the same difficulties and frustrations. Exchanging ideas and experiences with other parents provides an opportunity to voice concerns and to learn new ways of coping with the multiple problems of childrearing. Whether it is family, friends, or community resources, parents need persons to whom they can turn for advice, comfort, and assistance—persons with whom they can share the joys and difficulties of childrearing.

PARENTING BEHAVIORS

Parents' overall acceptance of a child and their disciplinary orientation have a profound impact on the way in which children view themselves and relate with others; adults' attitudes as parents are influenced by their conception of their roles in relation to children. The amount of affection that parents show their children may vary considerably and be influenced by cultural factors and individual differences in the personality and temperament of both the parents and children. How openly or frequently this affection is expressed and the degree to which affection is mixed with feelings of rejection or hostility will differ also. Parents described as warm and nurturant are those who often smile at, praise, and encourage their children while limiting their criticisms, punishments, and signs of disapproval. Children who come from homes in which they are loved and accepted display socially acceptable behavior and are generally good-natured, cheerful, friendly, cooperative, and emotionally stable. Because they are loved and accepted themselves, they are able to form satisfactory relationships with others.

Cool, hostile, or rejecting parents are quick to criticize, belittle, punish, or ignore their children while limiting their expressions of affection or approval. Rejecting parents overtly or covertly express feelings of dislike for the child, indicate that the child is unwanted, or state that caring for the child is burdensome. Children who are rejected develop feelings of insecurity and inferiority; they believe that if they are unworthy of parental love, they must be of no value. Parental styles of control also influence the child's development. The extent to which parents restrict children's behavior or allow them autonomy and freedom significantly affects the psychologic atmosphere in the home. Although there are variations and degrees in parenting styles, they generally fall into one of three main types (see box).

Parental Styles of Control

Authoritarian

Parents control behavior and attitudes through rigid rules and regulations

Often results in rigidly conforming behavior; children tend to be sensitive, shy, self-conscious, retiring, and submissive

Permissive

Parents allow children to regulate their own activity, viewing themselves as resources for the children, not role models

Children are often disobedient, disrespectful, irresponsible, aggressive, and generally defiant of authority

Authoritative

Parents direct their children's behavior and attitudes by emphasizing the reasons for rules but negatively reinforce deviations

Control is firm and consistent but tempered with encouragement, understanding, and security

Children tend to have high self-esteem, are self-reliant, self-assertive, inquisitive, content, and highly interactive with other children

SHAPING BEHAVIOR: DISCIPLINE

Because children live in an organized society, they must be prepared to accept restrictions on their behavior. Discipline is not punishment. Rather it is the teaching of desirable behavior. Children who learn to live within reasonable rules are happier and more secure children. Good discipline provides children with protection from dangers (from within and without) and relieves them of the burden of decisions that they are not prepared to make, yet it permits them to develop independence of thought and action within a secure framework. It allows children to achieve in areas appropriate for mastery at their level, channels undesirable feelings into constructive activity, and teaches children socially acceptable behavior.

Disciplinary Strategies

Parents use various strategies for controlling and shaping behavior. Regardless of the type of discipline used, certain principles are essential in ensuring the efficacy of the approach (see box). Many strategies can be implemented effectively only when principles of consistency and timing are followed. A pattern of intermittent or occasional enforcement of limits actually prolongs the undesirable behavior because children learn that if they are persistent, the behavior is permitted eventually.

To deal with misbehavior, parents need to implement

General Guidelines for Implementing Discipline

Consistency—implement disciplinary action exactly as agreed on and for each infraction
Timing—initiate discipline as soon as the child misbehaves; if delays are necessary, such as to avoid embarrassment, verbally disapprove of the behavior and state that disciplinary action will be implemented
Commitment—follow through with the details of the discipline, such as timing of minutes; avoid distractions that may interfere with the plan, such as telephone calls
Unity—make certain that all caregivers agree on plan and are familiar with the details to prevent confusion and alliances between child and one parent
Flexibility—choose disciplinary strategies that are appropriate to the child's temperament and the severity of the misbehavior
Planning—plan discipline strategies in advance and prepare child if feasible, for example, explaining the use of time-out; for unexpected misbehavior, try to discipline when calm
Behavior-orientation—always disapprove of the behavior, not the child, with such statements as "That was a wrong thing to do. I am unhappy when I see behavior like that."
Privacy—administer discipline in private, especially with older children who may feel ashamed in front of others
Understanding—follow discipline with concern for children's feelings, such as "I am sad that you had to stay at home because you were grounded for breaking the rules"; avoid lecturing or bringing up the infraction once discipline has been implemented
Termination—once the discipline is administered, consider the child as having a "clean slate" and avoid bringing up the incident or lecturing

appropriate disciplinary action. Numerous approaches are available and some have definite advantages over others. The following discussion presents the most common strategies.

Corporal punishment. Corporal punishment most often takes the form of spanking. Based on the principles of aversion therapy, inflicting pain through spanking causes a dramatic decrease in the behavior. However, there are some serious flaws in this approach: (1) it teaches children that violence is acceptable; (2) many times the spanking is the result of parental rage and may physically harm the child; and (3) children become "accustomed" to spanking, requiring more severe corporal punishment each time.

Although there is controversy regarding the use and abuse of corporal punishment, there are some instances when it is effective, especially in children who refuse to listen to verbal commands. For example, slapping the child's hand while saying "No, don't touch" reinforces the meaning of the statement. A good rule when using mild physical punishment is that only one slap is given because the first slap is for the child; additional slaps are for the punisher.

Reasoning and scolding. Reasoning involves explaining why an act is wrong. Although it is always a good practice to explain why limits are being imposed, it is inappropriate to expect young children to understand the explanation.

Reasoning is often combined with scolding, which may sometimes includes shaming the child. For example, the parent may state, "You are a bad boy; I am very disappointed in you." Unfortunately, children take such remarks seriously and personally, believing that *they* are bad. It is important to always disapprove of the *behavior*, not the child, with such statements as, "That was a wrong thing to do. I am disappointed when you act that way." See Therapeutic dialogue.

Reward. Reward is based on *behavior modification theory*—if an act is consistently rewarded, the desired behavior will be strengthened. Using rewards is a positive approach; by encouraging children to behave in specified ways, the tendency to misbehave is lessened. With young children, using stars is a very effective method. For older children, the "token system" is appropriate, especially if a

THERAPEUTIC DIALOGUE

Effective Discipline

Bob, who is 8 years old, has come home late after playing with friends. His father is waiting for him at the front door.

FATHER: Bob, I am concerned about the time. It's a half-hour past the curfew.
BOB: I'm sorry, Dad. I was playing with my friends and I forgot the time.
FATHER: I bet it isn't easy to leave your friends when you are having fun.
BOB: It isn't, Dad. I am so glad you understand.
FATHER: I understand, Son, but I also worry when you are not home. I hope that we can count on your watching the time more closely tomorrow.
BOB: I will, Dad. Thanks for not getting angry.
FATHER: You're welcome, but if we need to talk about this again, we will have to discuss consequences.
BOB: I understand. I will do my best to watch the clock and the sun. As soon as it starts to get dark, I know I should be coming home.

certain number yields a special reward, such as a trip to the movies or a new book. In planning a reward system, the expected behaviors must be clearly explained to the child and the rewards must be reinforcing. A chart should be used to record the stars or tokens and every earned reward promptly given. Verbal approval should always accompany extrinsic rewards.

Ignoring or extinction. Ignoring is based on the behavioral theory that if an act is consistently ignored, the lack of attention will eventually extinguish the behavior. Although this strategy seems very simple, it is extremely difficult to maintain a consistent approach. Parents frequently "give in" and resort to old patterns of discipline, since they lack the perseverance to do nothing. Consequently the behavior is actually reinforced because the child learns that his persistence gained their attention.

Consequences. The strategy of consequences involves allowing children to experience the results of their misbehavior and includes three types:

1. **Natural**—Those that occur without any intervention, such as being late and missing dinner
2. **Logical**—Those that are directly related to the rule, such as not being allowed to play with another toy until the used ones are put away
3. **Unrelated**—Those that are imposed deliberately, such as no playing until homework is completed

Natural or logical consequences are preferred but are effective only when they are meaningful to children. For example, the natural consequence of living in a messy room may do little to encourage cleaning up, but allowing no friends over until the room is neat can be very motivating! Withdrawing privileges and time-out are forms of unrelated consequences. After the child experiences the consequence, the parent should refrain from any comment, because the usual tendency is for the child to try and place blame for imposing the rule.

Time-out. Time-out is actually a refinement of the common practice of "sending the child to his room." It is also based on the premise of removing the reinforcer, that is, the satisfaction or attention the child is receiving from the activity. By being placed in an unstimulating and isolated place, the child becomes bored and consequently agrees to behave appropriately in order to reenter the family group (Fig. 4-4). A rule for the length of time-out is 1 minute per year of age; a kitchen timer, rather than a watch, should be used to record the time. Time-out avoids many of the problems of other disciplinary approaches because no physical punishment is involved, no reasoning or scolding is given, and the parents are usually not present for all of the time-out, which facilitates their ability to consistently apply the punishment.

Contracting. Contracting is a process in which the desired behavior is explicitly outlined in the form of a *written* contract. Based on behavior modification, it is a very effective method of altering behavior, especially with older children who are involved in the process of defining the rules of the agreement. Ideally it should involve tangible rewards, but it may include negative consequences, such as demerits or "checks" for failing to comply. In deciding whether to use positive or negative reinforcers, the nurse should question parents about their opinion regarding powerful motivators for the child. Often the contract includes a commitment from the parent, such as agreeing to stop nagging the child about cleaning his room. Once the contract is implemented, it should be evaluated at the end of the time specified in the agreement and revisions should be made, such as extending the time or terminating the contract. If the contract has not been successful, every effort should be made to ascertain if the goals were realistic, if the time period was sufficient for accomplishing the goal, and if the rewards or consequences were motivating.

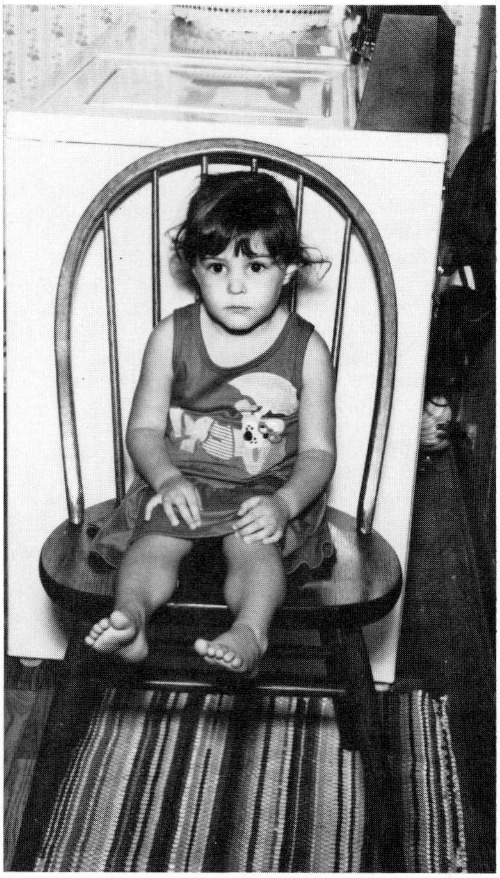

FIG. 4-4 Time-out is an excellent disciplinary strategy for young children. Notice the use of a laundry room as an unstimulating setting for the preschooler.

◆ *Special Parenting Situations*

Parenting is a demanding task under the most ideal circumstances, but when parents and children are faced with situations that deviate from what is considered to be the norm, the potential for family disruption is increased. One of the issues that is encountered frequently is divorce, with accompanying problems of single parenthood and/or reconstituted families. Adoption and dual-career families, too, have special difficulties. The problems associated with children who have an alcoholic parent, a parent with physical disabilities, or an incarcerated parent, especially the mother, are ones that are not addressed in the following discussions but may be topics that the reader may wish to investigate. Special considerations in parenting the child with physical disabilities are discussed in Chapter 18.

PARENTING THE ADOPTED CHILD

Adoptive parents are those who, whatever the motivation, assume the sociologic and ethical responsibility of biologic parents. The ties of affection between them and their children are just as strong as biologic ties.

Most adoptions are by couples who have been unable to have children of their own. Today, however, many people—including single, divorced, and widowed persons—consider adoption for other reasons. There are some who feel a responsibility to provide a home for a child who needs one; others are able to have more children of their own but are seriously concerned about overpopulation and elect to increase their family through adoption; many are families who are finding "room for one more" with whom to share their love. Also, almost half the adoptable children in the United States are adopted by relatives, either extended family members or stepparents. Whatever motivates a couple or a single person to seek adoption as an alternative means to acquire a family, the decision should be based on emotionally healthy needs. The welfare of the child should be the primary consideration in placement.

The Adoptive Family

Most problems faced by adoptive parents are no different from those encountered by natural parents. All parents want to be good parents, but this desire is often intensified in adoptive parents. The mother, in particular, may believe that she must be a better parent than the biologic mother would have been, and if she harbors any feelings about unmarried parents who relinquish children, this may affect her feelings toward the child.

Unlike natural parents who prepare for their child's birth with prenatal classes and support of friends and relatives, adoptive parents have few sources of support and preparation for the new addition to their family. They need information on how to prepare for receiving the infant and instruction on child care. Though the parents may have been waiting years to adopt a child, they may have less than 24 hours notice that they are actually receiving a child (Fig. 4-5). Nurses can refer adoptive parents to state parental support groups such as a state or county welfare office or the **North American Council on Adoptable Children (NACAC)***.

*2001 S St. NW, Washington, DC 20009.

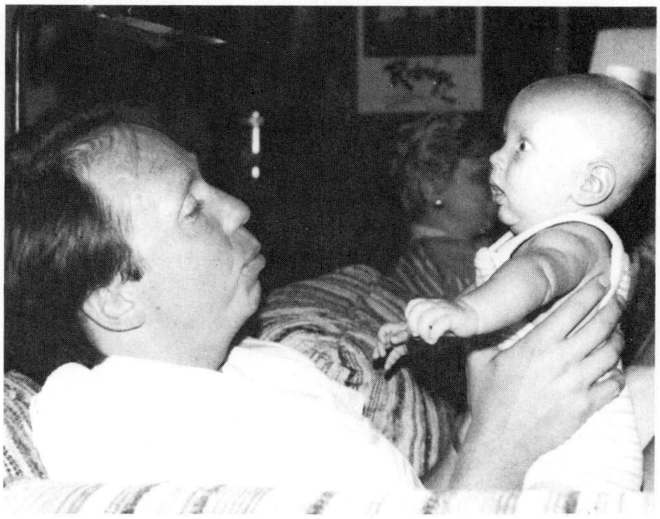

FIG. 4-5 Adoptive parents are often "instant parents." Both they and the child need time to learn about each other.

An initial problem that may be encountered by the adopting family is parent-infant attachment. The difficulties in forming an attachment will depend on the amount of time the infant has spent with earlier caregivers such as the birthmother, nurse, or adoption agency personnel (Clore and Newberry, 1981). Acceptance by extended family members and friends may create additional stresses for the family. This may be a particularly difficult problem when the adopted children are members of different ethnic groups. It should be made clear to everyone that the child is the parents' child, not their "adopted" child.

There are two other areas of special concern to adoptive parents. The first is the task of telling the child that he is adopted. Unfortunately there are no clear-cut guidelines for parents to follow in determining precisely when children are ready for the information, and parents are naturally reluctant to present the child with such unsettling news. However, it is an important aspect of their parental responsibilities, and, although they may be tempted to withhold the fact from the child, it is an essential component of the child's identity.

Parents can anticipate some behavior changes following the disclosure—especially in children who are older. Children may use the fact of their adoption as a weapon to manipulate and threaten parents. There is the inevitable "My real mother would not treat me like this," or "You don't love me as much because I'm adopted." Statements such as these hurt parents and increase their feelings of insecurity so that as parents they may become overly permissive. Adopted children need the same undemanding love as any other child, combined with firm discipline and limit-setting.

The second area of concern special to adoptive parents arises during the adolescent years. The normal confrontations of adolescents and parents may assume more painful aspects in adoptive families. Adolescents may use their adoption as a tool in defying parental authority or as a justification for aberrant behavior. As they attempt to master the task of identity formation, the feeling of abandonment by their natural parents may come to awareness or may be intensified. During this time adopted children may feel the need to discover the identity of their natural parents in order to define themselves and their identity—one of the major tasks of adolescent development. It is important for parents to reassure the youngsters that they understand the feelings of needing to search for one's identity.

Special Adoptive Situations

Unfortunately for persons wishing to adopt a child, the demand for white infants with no physical or mental problems far exceeds the supply. However, it has created an increased opportunity for adoptive parents to provide homes for children with special needs. The additional burdens of care for children with physical or emotional disabilities are no different from those of naturally born children with similar problems, with the possible exception that adoptive parents are aware of the nature of the disabilities before they receive the children. However, adoption of older children and/or those of a different racial or ethnic origin poses some special problems for both parents and children.

Older children. Adopting older children involves a strong commitment on the part of both the adopting family and the adopted child. Children awaiting adoption are usually from foster homes, group homes, or institutions. Several visits of increasing length are usually arranged to allow the child and family to determine whether or not they will be able to make a commitment (Brockhaus and Brockhaus, 1982).

One of the difficulties of rearing adopted older children is helping them to deal with having had another set of parents. In addition to their biologic parents, the children may have lost siblings, grandparents, friends, and personal possessions. Often they have lived in several foster homes in which they formed attachments. They need time and assistance in working through the grief process that is an integral part of any loss. At the same time they must adjust to a new household and relationships. Children who have experienced many losses and disappointments find adjustment more difficult and take a longer period of time to overcome fear of rejection and to develop affectionate ties to the new family. They grieve for those they left behind and may be afraid to love in case they must again move on.

Early in the process of forming lasting relationships the families alter routines and activities to accommodate the children and avoid conflicts. Eventually the parents and the children are unable to maintain the host-house-guest roles and behaviors and begin a stormy period of adjustment. Children continually test families who must repeatedly reassure the children that they are wanted. Children may withdraw or act angry for months. During this time the families may require considerable support and encouragement from sources outside the immediate family unit. Gradually the adopted child begins to develop trust and confidence in the parents and all the members develop into a family unit with autonomy, stability, and identification (Brockhaus and Brockhaus, 1982).

Cross-racial adoption. Adoption of children of racial backgrounds different from that of the family is relatively commonplace. In addition to the problems faced by adopted children of any age, children of a cross-racial adoption must deal with their cultural difference. Parents who adopt such children are urged to preserve the child's racial heritage.

Although the children are full-fledged members of an adopting family and citizens of the adopted country, those with a foreign appearance or other decided racial characteristics may create problems outside the family. Strangers, or even relatives and friends, may make thoughtless comments and talk about the children as though they were not members of the family. It is vital that the family make it clear to others that this is their child and a cherished member of the family.

PARENTING AND DIVORCE

In recent years there has been a marked change in the stability of families that is reflected in increased rates of divorce, single-parenthood, and remarriage. In 1985 the divorce rate for the United States was 5.0 per 1000 total population. Although almost one half of all divorcing couples are childless, over 1 million children experience divorce each year (National Center for Health Statistics, 1987).

During a divorce, parental capacity is often diminished. The parents may be too preoccupied with their own feelings, needs, and life changes to be available and supportive to their children. Newly employed parents, usually mothers, are likely to leave children with new sitters, in strange settings, or alone after school. The parent may also spend more time away from home, searching for or establishing new relationships. Sometimes, however, the adult feels frightened and alone and begins to depend on the child as a substitute for the absent parent. This dependence places an enormous burden on the child.

Common characteristics in the custodial household following separation and divorce include disorder, coercive types of control, inflammable tempers in both parents and children, reduced parental competence, a greater sense of parental helplessness, poorly enforced discipline, and diminished regularity in enforcing household routines. Noncustodial parents also are seldom prepared for the role of visitor and may not have a residence suitable for children's visits. They may be concerned about maintaining the arrangement over the years to follow (Wallerstein, 1983).

Impact of Divorce on Children

The conventional belief has been that unhappily married couples should stay together for the good of the children; yet research indicates that the eventual escape from parental conflict may be the most positive outcome of divorce for many children (Hetherington, 1981). However, in a number of situations the children continue to experience open parental discord for a considerable time following marriage dissolution, which continues to place them at risk for impaired development (Rhyne, 1986).

The impact of divorce on children depends on a variety of factors, including the age and sex of the children, the outcome of the divorce, and the quality of parental care during the years following the divorce. Complications sometimes associated with divorce include efforts on the part of one parent to subvert the child's loyalties to the other, abandonment to other caregivers, and adjustment to a stepparent. In 90% of divorce cases the mother receives custody of the child; this has an effect on the male child's identification with a father figure in addition to all the other ramifications of living in a family without a father or in a single-parent family. Many divorced mothers with small children move in with parents, other relatives, or friends in some kind of dependent or sharing arrangement.

Children may feel a sense of shame and embarrassment concerning the family situation, which may cause them to see themselves as different, inferior, or unworthy of love. Although the social stigma attached to divorce no longer produces the emotions it has in the past, it may still exist in some small towns where attitudes can serve to reinforce children's negative self-image. The lasting effects of divorce depend on the children's and the parents' adjustment to the transition from an intact family to a single-parent family and, often, to a reconstituted family.

Telling the children. Parents are understandably hesitant to tell children about their decision to divorce. Most likely, however, the children are already experiencing vague, uneasy feelings that are more difficult to cope with than being told truthfully about the situation. If possible, the initial disclosure should include both parents and all siblings, followed by later discussions with children individually. Ample time should be set aside for the discussions and they should take place during a period of calm, not after an argument. Parents who physically hold or touch their children provide them with a feeling of warmth that is reassuring. The discussions should include the reason for the divorce—minimizing blame—and reassurance that the divorce is not the fault of the children. Children can have guilt feelings as though they have somehow failed or are being punished for misbehavior. They wonder what role they played in the divorce or failure to keep the family together.

Parents need not fear crying in front of the children; it gives the children permission to cry also. Children need to ventilate their feelings. They normally feel anger and resentment and should be allowed to communicate these feelings without punishment. They also have feelings of terror and abandonment and long for consistency and order in their lives. They need to know where they will live, who will take care of them, if they will be with their siblings, and if there will be enough money to live on. The children may also fear that if the parents stopped loving each other, they could also stop loving them as well (Rhyne, 1986). Their need for assurance of love is tremendous at this time.

Age- and sex-related responses to divorce. A divorce is an unsettling experience and one that few children feel positive about for several years afterward. Previously it was believed that divorce had a greater impact on younger children, but more recent observations indicate that there is little age-related difference in the impact of divorce on children. The feelings and behaviors of children may differ according to age and sex, but all suffer stresses second only to the stress produced by the death of a parent. Even infants suffer from the effects of reduced mothering and possible interference with the attachment process.

Egocentric preschoolers, who see and understand things only in relation to themselves, assume themselves to be the cause of parental distress and interpret the separation as punishment. Moreover, they fear that they may be abandoned by the remaining parent. They may also exhibit regressive behaviors. It is essential to establish some kind of stability for these children and give them frequent, repeated, and concrete explanations of plans.

School-age children are able to deal with parental separation better than younger children even though they feel intense pain, loneliness, and deprivation. Older children are more likely to perceive one parent as responsible or to become angry with both parents. School performance may be affected; therefore teachers and school counselors should be informed of the situation. The children may also exhibit various somatic complaints.

Adolescents may be highly resentful because their lives are already sufficiently difficult and stressful. Although they are able to comprehend the divorce and are less likely to feel responsibility, adolescents find the divorce of their parents extraordinarily painful. The sexual identity of adolescents is affected by disturbed parental relationships, and adolescents are concerned about their own future as a marital partner. They are also anxious about the availability of money for future needs and almost invariably wish for their parents to reunite.

Some observers have noted sex differences in the way children respond to the stress of divorce and living in a single-parent family. Sex differences are more marked when the parental absence occurs early in the child's life and when it is the same-sex parent. Girls from homes where fathers are absent depend more on their mothers and show some anxiety about relationships with males during adolescence. Boys from homes without fathers tend to be less aggressive, more apt to have emotional and social problems, and demonstrate cognitive patterning more similar to that of girls.

Custody and Parenting Partnerships

In 90% of divorce cases the mother still receives custody of the child with visitation agreements for the father. However, more courts are now awarding custody to fathers. Men usually make more money and can offer more material benefits than many women are able to provide. The incidence of delinquent support payments to custodial mothers is a matter of universal concern.

Two other less common custody arrangements are divided custody and joint custody. Divided or split custody means that each parent is awarded custody of one or more of the children, thereby separating siblings. For example, sons might live with the father and the daughters with the mother. In joint custody the parents alternate the physical care and control of the children on a reasonably equitable basis while maintaining shared parenting responsibilities legally. This type of custody arrangement works well for families who live in closer proximity and whose occupations allow an active role in the care and rearing of the children. In a variation of joint custody, the children reside with one parent but both parents are still the children's legal guardians who participate together in childrearing.

Co-parenting offers substantial benefits for the family: children can be close to both parents, and life with each parent can be more normal as opposed to a disciplinarian mother and a fun-and-games father. However, to be successful, the parents must place a high value on the commitment to provide as normal parenting as possible and be able to separate their marital conflicts from the parenting roles. No matter what type of custody arrangement is awarded, the primary consideration is the welfare of the children.

The more financial and emotional support the mother receives from the noncustodial parent, the better she is able to cope with parenting tasks. Custodial mothers who have cordial relationships with their ex-husbands are more sensitive to the needs of the children, and the regular involvement of the father is associated with better adjustment of the children.

In the process of resolution, the single parent must cope with loneliness and fewer family interactions. The feeling of being isolated from all but the children may create parent-child relationships in which the parent and child are either overly attached to each other or in constant conflict. Children feel that the burden of the parent's happiness or unhappiness is on their shoulders.

There is a need on the part of the parent for social contacts and a life separate from the children for the emotional growth of both parent and child. The single parent can find support and encouragement from **Parents Without Partners,*** an organization designed to meet the needs of this increasingly important group. In Canada a similar organization is the **One Parent Families Association.†**

SINGLE-PARENTING

Single-parent status is acquired by means of divorce, separation, death, or through birth or adoption of a child by a single person. Over the past two decades the proportion of children living with two parents has decreased dramatically, while the proportion of children living with only the mother has almost doubled (U.S. Bureau of the Census, 1982). It has been determined that 40% to 50% of children in the United States spend some time in a single-parent home (Hetherington, 1981).

Being the sole provider in all areas of child care places a stress on the parent both economically and emotionally. Many mothers have never worked outside the home or have held only low paying jobs. Following divorce, families headed by mothers must often manage on a fraction of the income to which they were accustomed when the father was present. This frequently necessitates moving to more modest housing in a poorer neighborhood, often away from the friends and neighbors who have been sources of emotional support. When the mother begins to work, she has less time to spend with the children, is frequently fatigued, and can become more erratic and inconsistent in parenting (see Working mothers, p. 71).

Single Fathers

Fathers who have custody of their children have many of the same problems as divorced mothers. They feel overburdened by the responsibility, are depressed, and are concerned about their ability to cope with the emotional needs of the children, especially the needs of the girls (Hetherington, 1981). They find it difficult at first to coordinate household tasks, school visits, and other activities associated with managing a household alone. Fathers often demand more assistance with household tasks and more independence from their children than custodial mothers do, and they are likely to make use of alternative caregiving and support systems.

PARENTING IN RECONSTITUTED FAMILIES

Approximately half of all children from broken homes will experience yet another major change in their lives within 3 years of a divorce—a return to a nuclear family and the sudden acquisition of a stepparent when the custodial parent remarries. The entry of a stepparent into a ready-made family requires adjustments for all the family members. Some obstacles to the role adjustments and the family problem-solving include disruption of previous lifestyles and interaction patterns, complexity in the formation of new ones, and lack of social supports (Nelson and Nelson, 1982). Despite these problems, most children from divorced families want to live in a two-parent home.

*International Headquarters, 7910 Woodmont Ave., Washington, DC 20014. Canadian address: 205 Yonge St., Suite 13, Toronto, Ontario, Canada M5B 1N2.

†2279 Yonge St., Suite 17, Toronto, Ontario, Canada M4P 2C7.

Stepparenting

The role of stepparent is unclear and often confusing. The stereotype of wicked stepmother and cruel stepfather has done little to foster healthy relationships with stepchildren, and stepparents usually go to great lengths in an attempt to avoid this image. They studiously avoid taking sides with stepchildren or minimize involvement with them as much as possible. Sometimes the natural parent at home feels guilty about separating the children from their other parent and restrains the stepparent from an authority position, thus rendering the stepparent powerless in a parental role. Almost always present are the elements of mistrust, fear of failure, and a sense of vulnerability in a reconstituted family.

Many factors that affect childrearing can interfere with the marital relationship between parent and stepparent. The child may serve to constantly remind the parent of the previous relationship; an unresolved relationship between the natural parents may interfere with full development of the new relationship; and the feelings and attitude of the stepchild toward the stepparent may also cause problems.

The stepparent who has replaced a dead parent is in a more difficult position. In this situation guilt and idealization, part of the normal grief process, may become intensified in the children. Overidealization and an attempt to hold onto the dead parent causes some children to make unfair and discriminating comparisons. Probably the best approach on the part of the stepparent is to be frank about the good points of the deceased parent but not to agree with the comparison and avoid defensiveness.

Sources of guidance, education, and support for stepfamilies can be found in numerous publications and from groups such as local chapters of **The Stepfamily Association of America*** and **The Stepfamily Foundation, Inc.**†

PARENTING IN DUAL-CAREER FAMILIES

No change in family life-style has had more impact than the large numbers of women entering the workplace. As women moved away from the traditional homemaker pattern, the numbers of dual-earner families increased dramatically until they now comprise more than half of the married couples in the United States. This trend is unlikely to diminish. As a result, the family is subjected to considerable stress as members attempt to balance occupational demands and family needs. Time demands and scheduling can lead to stress overload in a dual-career family, which can be significantly more intense when there are children. In fact, dual-career couples may increase the strain on themselves in order to avoid creating stress for their children, although there is no evidence to indicate that the dual-career lifestyle, as such, is stressful to children. However, the stress experienced by the parents may affect the children indirectly.

*28 Allegheny Avenue, Suite 1307, Baltimore, MD 21204.
†333 West End Avenue, New York, NY 10023.

Working Mothers

Much has been written and a variety of conclusions drawn regarding the effects of mothers working outside the home. Most mothers work for purely economic reasons, though some work as a response to the boredom of staying at home or to fulfill achievement needs.

Regardless of the mother's motivation, the consensus is that any deleterious effects on the children are related to the *quality* of the mother-child interaction rather than the *quantity* of time spent with the children. Quality time means not only a warm and loving relationship, but time that is stimulating and enriching for both parent and child. Planning time to be alone with the children, engaging in activities that are enjoyable for both, and simply being with the children (even inviting them to assist with tasks) as often as possible constitutes quality time (Fig. 4-6).

The mother's relationship to the rest of the family depends to a large extent on her own feelings and reactions to working and to her job. Although most mothers feel some guilt about leaving their children in the care of others, those who feel secure and happy in their work usually reflect this attitude in the home and in relationships with other members of the family. Sometimes, however, the mother feels guilty about leaving the children so that she can pursue a career or a job, particularly if she enjoys the outside activity. If she compensates for guilt feelings by overindulgence toward the children, they may feel more insecure and take advantage of her vulnerability with demanding behavior. On the whole, children of working mothers are self-reliant, do well in school, and show relatively few ill effects of the separation.

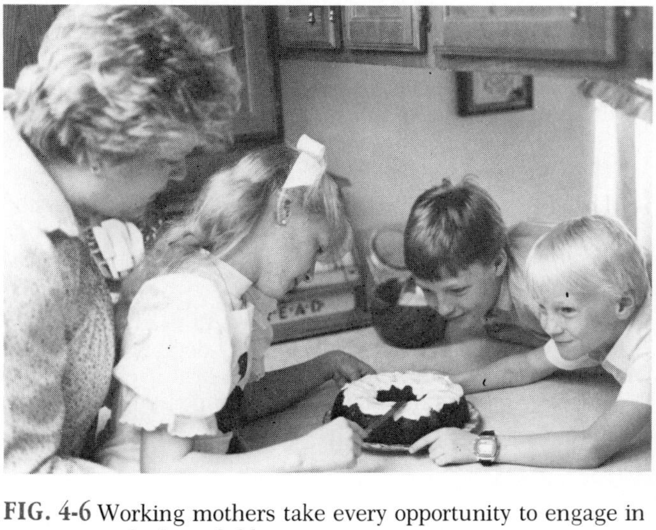

FIG. 4-6 Working mothers take every opportunity to engage in activities with their children.

Many factors are related to the effect that a mother's absence has on the children: the age of the child (very young children feel the impact of the mother's absence more than older children), the attitude of the father toward the wife's employment, the regularity with which she is away from the family, and the availability and quality of substitute child care. Substitute child care, either inside or outside the home, should be selected carefully and evaluated regularly (see p. 373).

SUMMARY

The influence of the family is a major, integral component of a child's development. Numerous everchanging factors such as family structure, size, configuration, parental style, disciplinary methods, and marital relationships interplay to produce a one-of-a-kind, special individual. Nurses must work within the framework of each unique family situation to foster the mental, physical, and emotional health of the child and family in special situations. This includes such situations as adoption; times of upheaval and crisis such as divorce; as well as times of normal developmental change, such as childbearing. A strong knowledge base as to the influences and trends in family life is essential in using the nursing process.

KEY CONCEPTS

- Since there is no agreement about the definition of *family*, a family is what the client considers it to be.
- Two theories that have significant relevance and application to pediatric nursing are family system theory and developmental theory.
- Although the traditional family structure has been nuclear or extended, in recent years other forms, such as the single-parent family, have emerged.
- Family size and positioning within the family structure have a strong impact on a child's development.
- Interpersonal skills and a basic understanding of childhood growth and development are two essential areas of focus for parents.
- Parents tend to predominate in one of three types of parental control: authoritarian, permissive, and authoritative.
- Three areas of special concern to adoptive families include difficulties in initial attachment, the task of telling the children they are adopted, and identity formation during adolescence.
- Marital factors within the home significantly influence a child's development. The impact of divorce on a child depends on age and sex, outcome, and quality of parental care following the divorce.
- Single parenting and stepparenting create adjustment difficulties and add stress to the already-demanding parental role. Significant numbers of children will live in a single-parent or reconstituted family at some point.

STUDY QUESTIONS AND ACTIVITIES

1 Interview a child and a parent from a divorced, single-parent, or reconstituted family. Explore with them the perceived advantages and disadvantages of their family's life-style. What are the similarities and differences in their responses?
2 Attend a preparation for parenthood class. Interview several couples to determine their motivation for becoming parents, and the changes they expect to occur in their life-style.
3 Observe parents and children in a public place such as a park, restaurant, or shopping mall. What types of disciplinary methods are used when the children misbehave? What family member(s) assume(s) the disciplinary role?
4 Interview a mother who is employed full-time outside the home and a mother who is not. Have them outline their daily schedule, especially in relation to child care. How do their schedules differ? Are there specific periods of "quality time" with the children, such as playing or reading together?
5 Interview two children, one from a large family and one who is an only child, regarding the perceived advantages and disadvantages of their ordinal position. Compare their responses to the discussion on ordinal position in this chapter.
6 Locate resources (books, support groups, pamphlets) that would be helpful to children and parents in a divorce or stepparent situation. Review at least two, and list their strengths and weaknesses.
7 List five parental factors that may affect transition to parenthood. Give examples of each that may have a negative or positive influence on parenting.

REFERENCES

Baskett, L.M., and Johnson, S.M.: The young child's interaction with parents versus siblings: a behavioral analysis, Child Dev. **53:**643-650, 1982.

Betsky, J., Early human experience: a family perspective, Dev. Psychol. **17:**3-23, 1981.

Brockhaus, J.P.D., and Brockhaus, R.H.: Adopting an older child—the emotional process, Am. J. Nurs. **82:**288-291, 1982.

Clore, E.R., and Newberry, Y.S.G.: Nurse practitioner guidance for the adoptive family from birth to adolescence, Pediatr. Nurs. **7**(6):16-25, 1981.

Crnic, K.A., and others: Effects of stress and social support on mothers and premature and full-term infants, Child Dev. **54:**209-217, 1983.

Dunn, J., and Kendrick, C.: Social behavior of young siblings in the family context: differences between same-sex and different-sex dyads, Child Dev. **52:**1265-1273, 1981.

Duvall, E.R.: Family development, ed. 5, Philadelphia, 1977, J.B. Lippincott Co.

Espinoza, R., and Newman, Y.: Step-parenting, DHEW Publication No. (ADM)78-579, Washington, DC, 1979, U.S. Government Printing Office.

Hetherington, E.M.: Children and divorce. In Henderson, R.W., editor: Parent-child interaction: theory, research, and prospects, New York, 1981, Academic Press, Inc.

Johnson, R.: Promoting the health of families in the community. In Stanhope, M., and Lancaster, J.: Community health nursing, ed. 2, St. Louis, 1988, The C.V. Mosby Co.

Macklin, E.D.: Nontraditional family forms: a decade of research, J. Marr. Fam. **42:**175-192, 1980.

Mauksch, H.: A social science basis for conceptualizing family health, Soc. Sci. Med. **8:**521-527, 1974.

McCubbin, H.I., and Patterson, J.M.: Family adaptation to crisis. In McCubbin, H.I., Cauble, E., and Patterson, J.M., editors: Family stress, coping, and social support, Springfield, IL, 1982, Charles C Thomas, Publisher.

Mednick, B., and Baker, R.: Consequences of family structure and maternal state for child and mother's development, Final report, NICHD (contract N 01-HD-82807), 1980.

National Center for Health Statistics: Advance report of final divorce statistics, 1985, Monthly Vital Statistics Report **36**(8):1-2, 1987.
Nelson, M., and Nelson, G.K.: Problems of equity in the reconstituted family: a social exchange analysis, Fam. Rel. **31:**223-231, 1982.
Perkins, T.F., and Kahan, J.P.: An empirical comparison of natural-father and stepfather family systems, Fam. Process **18:**175-183, 1979.
Ragozin, A.S., and others: Effects of maternal age on parenting role, Dev. Psychol. **18:**627-634, 1982.
Rhyne, M.C.: Understanding and supporting families in the process of divorce, Nurse Pract., **11**(12):37-51, 1986.
Rogers, R.H.: Improvement in the construction and analysis of family life cycle categories, Kalamazoo, MI, 1962, Western Michigan University.
Sater, J.: Appraising and promoting a sense of self in twins. MCN **4:**218-226, 1979.
Steelman, L.C., and Powell, B.: The social and academic consequences of birth order: real, artifactual, or both? J. Marr. Fam. **47:**117-124, 1985.
U.S. Bureau of the Census: Marital status and living arrangements: March 1981, Curr. Pop. Rep. Series P-20, No. 372, Washington, DC, 1982, U.S. Government Printing Office.
Wallerstein, J.S.: Children of divorce: stress and developmental tasks. In Garmezy, N., and Rutter, M., editors: Stress, coping, and development in children, New York, 1983, McGraw-Hill Book Co.
Whitehead, T.L.: Residence, kinship and mating as survival strategies: a West Indian example, J. Marr. Fam. **40:**817-828, 1978.

BIBLIOGRAPHY

General

Baranowski, E.: Childbirth education classes for expectant deaf parents, MCN **8:**143-146, 1983.
Brandt, M.A.: Consider the patient part of the family, Nurs. Forum **11:**19-23, 1984.
Burr, W.R., and others: Contemporary theories about the family, vol. I, New York, 1979, The Free Press.
Clements, I.W., and Roberts, F.B., editors: Family health: a theoretical approach to nursing care, New York, 1983, John Wiley & Sons, Inc.
Fsife, B.L.: A model for predicting the adaptation of families to a medical crisis: an analysis of role integration, Image **17:**108-112, 1985.
Hymovich, D., and Barnard, M.U.: Family health care, New York, 1979, McGraw-Hill Book Co.
Kaufman, D.H.: An interview guide for helping children make health-care decisions, Pediatr. Nurs. **11:**365-367, 1985.
Klaus, M.H., and Kennell, J.H.: Parent-infant bonding, ed. 2, St. Louis, 1982, The C.V. Mosby Co.
McCubbin, H.I., and Figley, C.R., editors: Stress and the family: coping with normative transitions, New York, 1983, Brunner/Mazel, Inc.
Newman, B.M., and Newman, P.R.: Development through life: a psychosocial approach, ed. 3, Homewood, IL, 1984, The Dorsey Press.
Sciarillo, W.G.: Using Hymovich's framework in the family-oriented approach to nursing care, MCN **5:**242-248, 1980.
Streff, M.B.: Examining family growth and development: a theoretical model, Adv. Nurs. Sci. **3**(4):61-69, 1981.
Wright, L.M., and Leahey, M.: Nurses and families: a guide to family assessment, Philadelphia, 1984, F.A. Davis Co.

Family

Anderson, M.L.: The mental health advantage of twinship, Perspect. Psychiatr. Care **23**(3):114-116, 1985.
Falbo, T.: Only children and interpersonal behavior: an experimental and survey study, J. Appl. Soc. Psychol. **8:**244-253, 1978.
Feetham, S.L.: Family research: issues and directions for nursing. In Werley, H.H., and Fitzpatrick, J.J., editors: Annual review of nursing research, vol. 2, New York, 1984, Springer Publishing Co.
Foley, K.L.: Caring for the parents of newborn twins, MCN **4:**221-226, 1979.
Kidwell, J.S.: Number of siblings, sibling spacing, sex and birth order: their effects on perceived parent-adolescent relationships. J. Marr. Fam. **43:**50-64, 1981.
Stainton, M.C.: The effect of ordinal position or birth order on child development, Nurs. Forum **19**(2):165-179, 1981.

Parenthood and Parenting

Barret, R.L., and Robinson, B.E.: Adolescent fathers: often forgotten parents, Pediatr. Nurs. **12**(4):273-277, 1986.
Benzon, L., and Lastowka, T.: Developing a parent education program in an ambulatory care setting, J. Assoc. Care Child. Hosp. **8:**21-25, 1979.
Brandt, P.A.: Social support and life change during early family development. In Chinn, P.L., and Leonard, K.B.: Current practice in pediatric nursing, vol. 3, St. Louis, 1980, The C.V. Mosby Co.
Brandt, P.A.: Stress-buffering effects of social support on maternal discipline, Nurs. Res. **33:**229-234, 1984.
Briggs, E.: Transition to parenthood, Matern. Child Nurs. J. **8**(2):69-83, 1979.
Cameron, J.: Year-long classes for couples becoming parents, MCN **4:**358-362, 1979.
Damrosch, S.P., Lenz, E.R., and Perry, L.A.: Use of parental advisors in the development of a parental coping scale, Matern. Child Nurs. J. **14**(2):103-109, 1985.
Elkind, D.: David Elkind discusses parental pressures, Pediatr. Nurs. **12**(6):417-418, 1986.
Hanson, S.M.H., and Bozett, F.W.: Fatherhood and changing family roles, Fam. Comm. Health **9**(4):9-21, 1987.
Hollen, P.: Parents' perceptions of parenting support systems, Pediatr. Nurs. **8:**309-313, 1982.
Humenick, S.S., and Bugen, L.A.: Parenting roles: expectation versus reality, MCN **12**(1):36-39, 1987.
Johnston, M.: Cultural variations in professional and parenting patterns, JOGNN **9**(7):9-13, 1980.
Slevin, K.F.: Motherhood, culture, and change, Pediatr. Nurs. **8:**405-408, 1982.
Ventura, J.N.: Parent coping behaviors, parent functioning, and infant temperament characteristics, Nurs. Res. **31:**269-273, 1982.
Webster-Stratton, C., and Kogan, K.: Helping parents parent, Am. J. Nurs. **80:**240-241, 1980.
Wheeler, K.G.: The crisis of the first child. In Chinn, P.L., and Leonard, K.B.: Current practice in pediatric nursing, vol. 3, St. Louis, 1980, The C.V. Mosby Co.

Special Parenting Situations

Brockhaus, J.P.D., and Brockhaus, R.H.: Adopting an older child—the legal process. Am. J. Nurs. **82:**292-294, 1982.
Brown, S.E., and Kelly, P.A.: Responding to a community need: preparation for parenthood for prospective adoptive couples, Fam. Comm. Health **9**(4):77-81, 1987.
Burns, C.E.: The hospitalization experience and single-parent families: a time of special vulnerability, Nurs. Clin. North Am. **19:**285-293, 1984.
Clore, E.R.: The working mother with young children, Child Care Newsletter **4**(1):4-6, 1985.
Coucouvanis, J.A., and Solomons, H.C.: Handling complicated visitation problems of hospitalized children, MCN **8:**131-134, 1983.
Engebretson, J.C.: Stepmothers as first-time parents: their needs and problems, Pediatr. Nurs. **8:**387-390, 1982.
Ganong, L.H., and Coleman, M.: The effects of remarriage on children: a review of the empirical literature, Fam. Rel. **33:**389-406, 1984.
Grief, G.L.: Single fathers rearing children, J. Marr. Fam. **47:**185-191, 1985.
Hanson, S.: Single custodial fathers and the parent-child relationship, Nurs. Res. **30:**202-204, 1981.
Heims, M.: Anticipatory guidance: preventive care for stepfamilies, Oreg. Nurse **51**(2):26, 1986.
Hughes, C.B., and Scoloveno, M.: The single father, Top. Clin. Nurs. **6**(3):1-9, 1984.

Jackson, P.L.: Caring for children from divorced families, MCN **8:**126-130, 1983.

Kutzner, S.K., and Toussie-Weingarten, C.: Working parents: the dilemma of child rearing and career, Top. Clin. Nurs. **6**(3):30-37, 1984.

Leonard, K.B.: The challenge of adoption. In Chinn, P.L., and Leonard, K.B., editors: Current practice in pediatric nursing, vol. 3, St. Louis, 1980, The C.V. Mosby Co.

Meagher, M.A.K.: Separation, divorce, and subsequent coping problems of single-parent families. In Reinhardt, A.M., and Quinn, M.D., editors: Family-centered community nursing: a sociocultural framework, vol. 2, St. Louis, 1980. The C.V. Mosby Co.

Romanczuk, A.N.: Helping the stepparent parent, MCN **12**(2):106-110, 1987.

Reutter, L., and Strang, V.: Yours, mine, and ours: stepparents and their children, MCN **11**(4):264-266, 1986.

Schilling, L.S.: The effects of divorce on children: a perspective for the pediatric health care provider, J. Assoc. Care Child. Health **11:**92-96, 1983.

Sherwen, L.N., Smith, D.W., and Cueman, M.A.: Common concerns of adoptive mothers, Pediatr. Nurs. **10:**127-130, 1984.

Smith, D.W., and Sherwen, L.N.: The bonding process of mothers and adopted children, Top. Clin. Nurs. **6**(3):38-48, 1984.

Stern, P.M.: Conflicting family culture: an impediment to integration in stepfamilies, J. Psychosoc. Nurs. Ment. Health Serv. **20**(10):27-33, 1982.

Sund, K., and Ostwald, S.K.: Dual-earner families' stress levels and personal and life-style–related variables, Nurs. Res. **34**(6):357-361, 1985.

Tankson, E.A.: The single parent. In Johnson, S.H.: Nursing assessment and strategies for the family at risk, ed. 2, Philadelphia, 1986, J.B. Lippincott Co.

Walker, L.O.: Identifying parents in need: an approach to adoptive parenting, MCN **6:**118-123, 1981.

Weinberg, T.S.: Single fatherhood: How is it different? Pediatr. Nurs. **11:**173-175, 1985.

CHAPTER 5

Developmental Influences on Child Health Promotion

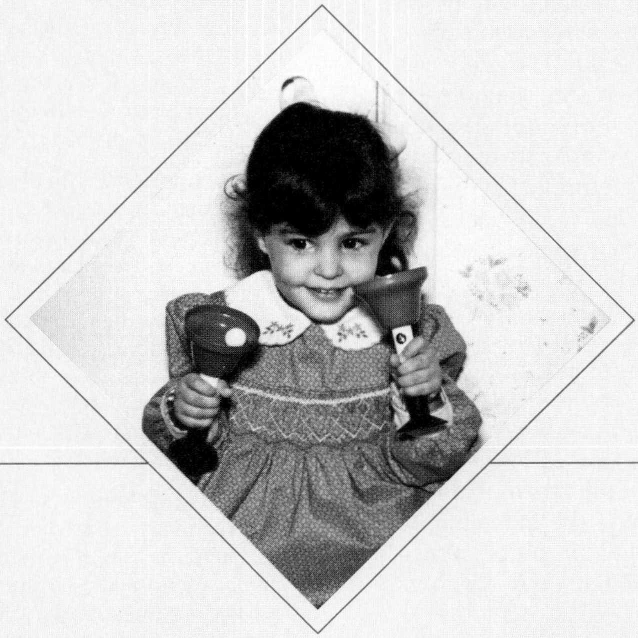

LEARNING OBJECTIVES

On completion of this chapter the reader will be able to:

- Describe major trends in growth and development
- Explain the alterations in the major body systems that take place during the processes of growth and development
- Discuss the development and relationships of cognitive, personality, moral, spiritual, and language development
- Demonstrate an understanding of the role of innate and environmental factors in the physical and emotional development of children
- Describe the role of play in the growth and development of children
- Discuss the basic needs of all children

Growth and development are complex processes involving numerous components that are subject to a wide variety of influences. All facets of the child's body, mind, and personality develop simultaneously, at varying rates and sequences, but not independently. Development of one part may be controlled or influenced by the activity of another part. Physical development proceeds at an orderly rate and sequence, but it is strongly influenced by the environment in which the child grows and develops.

This chapter is devoted to some of the ongoing maturational changes in children from a longitudinal perspective. The reader is introduced to the general progression and flow of developmental changes that take place throughout childhood. Also included are preliminary discussions of some of the major concepts and needs that accompany, are precipitated by, or in some way influence normal development. In subsequent chapters topics introduced here are elaborated in discussions of major developmental stages to provide a holistic view of a child at a specific stage in development.

GROWTH AND DEVELOPMENT

Growth and development, usually referred to as a unit, express the sum of the numerous changes that take place during a lifetime. The entire course is a dynamic process that encompasses several interrelated dimensions.

Growth implies a change in quantity. It results when cells divide and synthesize new proteins. This increase in the number and size of cells is reflected in an increase in the size and weight of the whole or any of its parts.

Maturation, which literally means to ripen, is described as aging or as an increase in competence and adaptability. It is usually used to describe a qualitative change, that is, a change in the complexity of a structure that makes it possible for that structure to begin functioning or to function at a higher level.

Differentiation is primarily a biologic description of the processes by which early cells and structures are systematically modified and altered to achieve specific and characteristic physical and chemical properties. It is sometimes used to describe one of the trends in development, that is, mass to specific.

Development is a gradual growth and expansion. It also involves a change, in this case from a lower to a more advanced stage of complexity. Development is the emerging and expanding of capacities of the individual to provide progressively greater facility in functioning. It is achieved through growth, maturation, and learning.

Stages of Development

Most authorities in the field of child development conveniently categorize child growth and behavior into approximate age stages or in terms that describe the features of an age-group. The age ranges of these stages are admittedly arbitrary and, since they do not take into account individual differences, cannot be applied to all children with any degree of precision. However, this categorization affords a convenient means to describe the characteristics associated with the majority of children at periods when distinctive developmental changes appear and specific developmental tasks* must be accomplished. It is also significant for nurses to know that there are characteristic health problems peculiar to each major phase of development. The sequence of descriptive age periods and subperiods that are used here and elaborated in subsequent chapters includes:

Prenatal period: conception to birth
EMBRYONIC: conception to 8 weeks
FETAL: 8 to 40 weeks (birth)

A rapid growth rate and total dependency make this one of the most crucial periods in the developmental process. The relationship between maternal health and certain manifestations in the newborn emphasizes the importance of adequate prenatal care to the health and well-being of the infant.

Infancy period: birth to 12 or 18 months
NEONATAL: birth to 28 days
INFANCY: 1 to approximately 12 months

The infancy period is one of rapid motor, cognitive, and social development. Through mutuality with the caregiver (mother), the infant establishes a basic trust in the world and the foundation for future interpersonal relationships. The critical first month of life, although part of the infancy period, is often differentiated from the remainder because of the major physical adjustments to extrauterine existence and the psychologic adjustment of the mother.

Early childhood: 1 to 6 years
TODDLER: 1 to 3 years
PRESCHOOL: 3 to 6 years

This period, which extends from the time children attain upright locomotion until they enter school, is characterized by intense activity and discovery. It is a time of marked physical and personality development. Motor development advances steadily. Children at this age acquire language and wider social relationships, learn role standards, gain self-control and mastery, develop increasing awareness of dependence and independence, and begin to develop a self-concept.

Middle childhood: 6 to 11 or 12 years

Frequently referred to as the "school age," this period of development is one in which the child is directed away from the family group and is centered around the wider world of peer relationships. There is steady advancement in physical, mental, and social development with emphasis on developing skill competencies. Social cooperation and early moral development take on more importance with relevance for later life stages. This is a critical period in the development of a self-concept.

Later childhood: 11 to 18 years
PREPUBERTAL: 10 to 13 years
ADOLESCENCE: 13 to approximately 18 years

The tumultuous period of rapid maturation and change known as adolescence has been described in various ways. It is considered a transitional period that begins at the onset of puberty and extends to the point of entry into the adult world—usually high school graduation. Biologic and personality maturation are accompanied by physical and emotional turmoil, and there is redefining of the self-concept. In the late adolescent period the child begins to internalize all the previously learned values and to focus on an individual, rather than a group, identity.

Patterns of Development

There are definite and predictable patterns in growth and development that are continuous, orderly, and progressive. These patterns, which are sometimes referred to as trends or principles, are universal and basic to all human beings. Although they are more apparent with respect to physical growth, most of these patterns apply to psychologic and social growth as well. Growth and development follow predetermined trends in direction, sequence, and pace, but each human being accomplishes these in a manner and time unique to that individual.

Directional trends. Growth and development proceed in regular, related directions or gradients and reflect the

*A developmental task is a set of skills and competencies peculiar to each developmental stage that children must accomplish or master in order to deal effectively with their environment. (From Developmental tasks and education, ed. 3, by Robert J. Havighurst. Copyright © 1972 by Longman, Inc. Reprinted with permission of Longman, New York, and the author.)

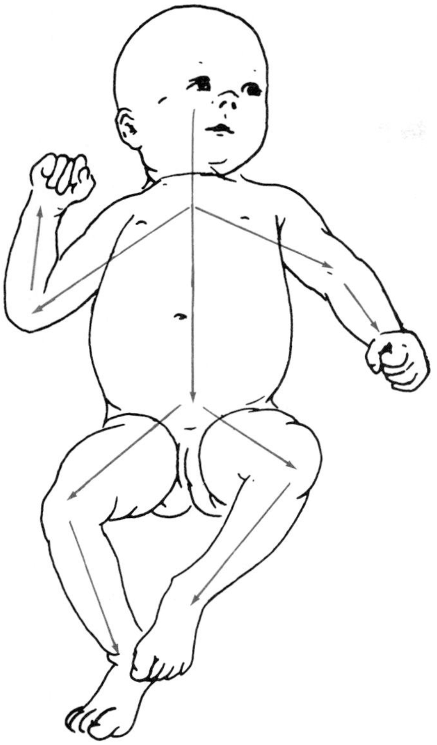

FIG. 5-1 Directional trends in growth.

physical development and maturation of neuromuscular functions (Fig. 5-1). The first pattern is the *cephalocaudal,* or head-to-tail, direction. That is, the head end of the organism develops first and is very large and complex, whereas the lower end is small and simple and takes shape at a later period. The physical evidence of this trend is most apparent during the period before birth, but it also applies to postnatal behavior development. Infants achieve structural control of the head before the trunk and extremities, hold their back erect before they stand, use their eyes before their hands, and gain control of their hands before they have control of their feet.

Second, the *proximodistal,* or near-to-far, trend applies to the midline-to-peripheral concept. A conspicuous illustration is the early embryonic development of limb buds, which is followed by rudimentary fingers and toes. In the infant, shoulder control precedes mastery of the hands, the whole hand is used as a unit before the fingers can be manipulated, and the central nervous system develops more rapidly than the peripheral nervous system.

These trends or patterns are bilateral and appear symmetric—each side develops in the same direction and at the same rate as the other. For some of the neurologic functions, this symmetry is only external because of unilateral differentiation of function at an early stage of postnatal development. For example, by the age of approximately 5 years the child has demonstrated a decided preference for the use of one hand over the other, although previously he had used either one.

The third trend, the *mass to specific* trend (sometimes referred to as differentiation), describes development from simple operations to more complex activities and functions. From very broad, global patterns of behavior, more specific, refined patterns emerge. All areas of development (physical, mental, social, and emotional) proceed in this direction. Generalized development will precede specific or specialized development. Physically there are gross, random muscle movements before fine muscle control takes place. The child will at first run and jump for the sake of motion, but eventually these activities take the more complex form of a race or a game, for example, hopscotch. Infants will respond to people in general before they recognize and prefer their mothers.

Sequential trends. In all dimensions of growth and development there is a definite, predictable sequence. It is orderly and continuous, with each child normally passing through every stage. Children crawl before they creep, creep before they stand, and stand before they walk. Later facets of the personality are built on the early foundation of trust. The child babbles, then forms words and, finally, sentences; writing emerges from scribbling.

Developmental pace. Although there is a fixed, precise order to development, it does not progress at the same rate or pace. There are periods of accelerated growth and periods of decelerated growth. This includes both total body growth and the growth of subsystems. The very rapid growth rate before and after birth gradually levels off through early childhood. The rate is relatively slow during middle childhood, but there is a marked increase at the beginning of adolescence followed by a leveling off in early adulthood. Each child grows at his own pace. Marked individual differences are observed between children as they reach and surmount developmental milestones. Although the sequence remains unchanged, the rate varies with each child.

Sensitive periods. There are limited times during the process of growth when the organism will interact with a particular environment in a specific manner. The terms *critical periods, sensitive periods,* and *optimal periods* have been applied to those times in the lifetime of an organism when it is more susceptible to positive or negative influences.

The quality of interactions during these sensitive periods determines whether the effects on the organism will be beneficial or harmful. For example, physiologic maturation of the central nervous system is influenced by adequacy and timing of contributions from the environment, such as stimulation and nutrition. The first 3 months of prenatal life are sensitive periods for physical growth of the fetus.

Psychologic development also appears to have sensitive periods when an environmental event has maximal influence on the developing personality. For example, primary socialization occurs during the first year when the infant makes the initial social attachments and establishes a basic trust in the world. A warm relationship with a mother figure is fundamental to a healthy personality.

The same concept might be applied to readiness for learning skills such as toilet training or reading. In these instances there appears to be an opportune time when the skill is best learned.

Individual Differences

Each child grows in his or her own unique and personal way. Great individual variation exists in the age at which developmental milestones are reached. The sequence is predictable; the exact timing is not. Rates of growth vary from one individual to another, and measurements are defined in terms of ranges to allow for individual differences among children. Some children are fast growers, others are moderate, and some are slower to reach maturity. For example, periods of fast growth, such as the pubescent growth spurt, may begin earlier or later in some children than in others. Children may grow fast or slow during the spurt and may finish sooner or later than other children. The sex of the child is an influential factor because girls seem to be more advanced in physiologic growth at all ages.

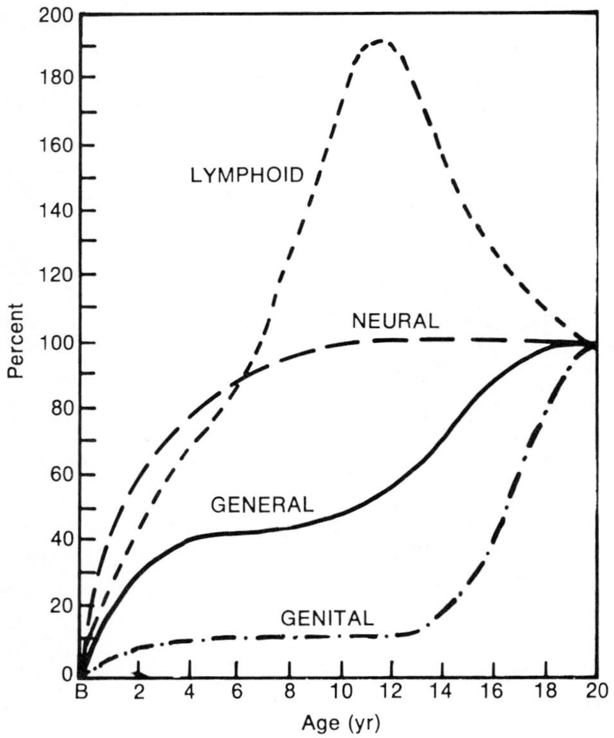

FIG. 5-2 Growth rates for the body as a whole and three types of tissues. *Lymphoid type:* thymus, lymph nodes, and intestinal lymph masses; *neural type:* brain, dura, spinal cord, optic apparatus, and head dimensions; *general type:* body as a whole, external dimension, and respiratory, digestive, renal, circulatory, and musculoskeletal systems. (From Harris, J.A., and others: The measurement of man, Minneapolis, 1930, University of Minnesota Press.)

PHYSICAL DEVELOPMENT

As children grow, their external dimensions change. These changes are accompanied by corresponding alterations in structure and function of internal organs and tissues that reflect the gradual acquisition of physiologic competence. Each part has its own rate of growth, which may be directly related to alterations in the size of the child (e.g., the heart rate). Skeletal muscle growth approximates whole body growth; brain, lymphoid, adrenal, and reproductive tissues follow distinct and individual patterns (Fig. 5-2).

External Proportions

Variations in the growth rate of different tissues and organ systems produce significant changes in body proportions during childhood. The cephalocaudal trend of development is most evident in total body growth as indicated by these changes (Fig. 5-3). During fetal development the head is the fastest growing body part, and at 2 months of gestation the head comprises 50% of total body length. During infancy growth of the trunk predominates; the legs are the most rapidly growing part during childhood; in adolescence, the trunk once again elongates. In the newborn infant, the lower limbs are one third the total body length but only 15% of the total body weight; in the adult the lower limbs comprise one half the total body height and 30% or more of the total body weight. As growth proceeds, the midpoint in head-to-toe measurements gradually descends from a level even with the umbilicus at birth to the level of the symphysis pubis at maturity.

Biologic Determinants of Growth and Development

The most prominent feature of childhood and adolescence is physical growth. Throughout development various tissues in the body undergo changes in growth, composition, and structure. In some tissues the changes are continuous (e.g., bone growth and dentition); in others significant alterations occur at specific stages (e.g., appearance of secondary sex characteristics). When these measurements are compared with standardized norms, a child's developmental progress can be determined with a high degree of confidence (Table 5-1).

Height. Linear growth, or height, occurs almost entirely as a result of skeletal growth and is considered a stable measurement of general growth. Growth in height is not uniform throughout life but ceases when maturation of the skeleton is complete. The maximum growth in length occurs before birth, but the newborn continues to grow at a rapid, though slower, rate.

Weight. At birth, weight is more variable than height and is, to a greater extent, a reflection of the intrauterine environment. The average newborn weighs from 3175 to 3400 g (7 to 7½ pounds). In general, the birth weight doubles by 5 to 6 months of age and triples by the end of

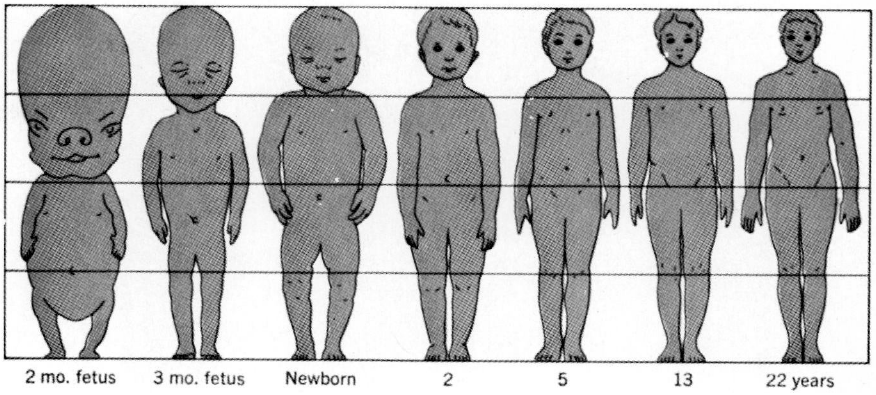

FIG. 5-3 Changes in body proportions from before birth to adulthood. (From Crouch, J.E., and McClintoc, J.R.: Human anatomy and physiology, ed. 2, New York, 1976, John Wiley & Sons, Inc. Reprinted by permission of John Wiley & Sons, Inc.)

the first year. By the end of the second year it usually quadruples. After this point the "normal" rate of weight gain, just as the growth in height, assumes a steady annual increase of approximately 2 to 2.75 kg (4.4 to 6 pounds) per year until the adolescent growth spurt.

Bone age and dentition. Both bone age determinants and state of dentition are used as indicators of development. Since both are discussed elsewhere, neither is elaborated here (see next section for bone age; see p. 80 for dentition).

Skeletal Growth and Maturation

The most accurate measure of general development is skeletal age, the radiologic determination of osseous maturation. Skeletal age appears to correlate more closely with other measures of physiologic maturity (such as onset of menarche) than with chronologic age or height. This "bone age" is determined by comparing the mineralization of ossification centers and advancing bony form to age-related standards.

Bone formation begins during the second month of fetal life when calcium salts are deposited in the intercellular substance (matrix) to form calcified cartilage first and then true bone. There are some differences in this bone formation. In small bones, the bone continues to form in the center and cartilage continues to be laid down on the surfaces. In long bones the ossification begins in the diaphysis (the long central portion of the bone) and continues in the epiphysis (the end portions of the bone).

TABLE 5-1

General Trends in Height and Weight Gain during Childhood

Age	Weight*	Height*
Infants		
Birth-6 months	Weekly gain: 140-200 g (5-7 oz) Birth weight doubles by end of first 6 months†	Monthly gain: 2.5 cm (1 inch)
6-12 months	Weight gain: 85-140 g (3-5 oz) Birth weight triples by end of first year	Monthly gain: 1.25 cm (½ inch) Birth length increases by approximately 50% by end of first year
Toddlers	Birth weight quadruples by age 2½ Yearly gain: 2-3 kg (4½-6½ lb)	Height at age 2 is approximately 50% of eventual adult height Gain during second year: about 12 cm (4¾ inches) Gain during third year: about 6-8 cm (2⅜-3¼ inches)
Preschoolers	Yearly gain: 2-3 kg (4½-6½ lb)	Birth length doubles by age 4 Yearly gain: 5-7.5 cm (2-3 inches)
School-Age Children	Yearly gain: 2-3 kg (4½-6½ lb)	Yearly gain after age 7: 5 cm (2 inches) Birth length triples by about age 13
Pubertal Growth Spurt		
Females—10-14 years	Weight gain: 7-25 kg (15-55 lb) Mean: 17.5 kg (38⅛ lb)	Height gain: 5-25 cm (2-10 inches); approximately 95% of mature height achieved by onset of menarche or skeletal age of 13 Mean: 20.5 cm (8¼ inches)
Males—11-16 years	Weight gain: 7-30 kg (15-65 lb) Mean: 23.7 kg (52⅛ lb)	Height gain: 10-30 cm (4-12 inches); approximately 95% of mature height achieved by skeletal age of 15 years Mean: 27.5 cm (11 inches)

*Yearly height and weight gains for each age-group represent averaged estimates from a variety of sources.
†A study has shown the mean time for doubling of birth weight to be 3¾ months (Neumann and Alpaugh, 1976).

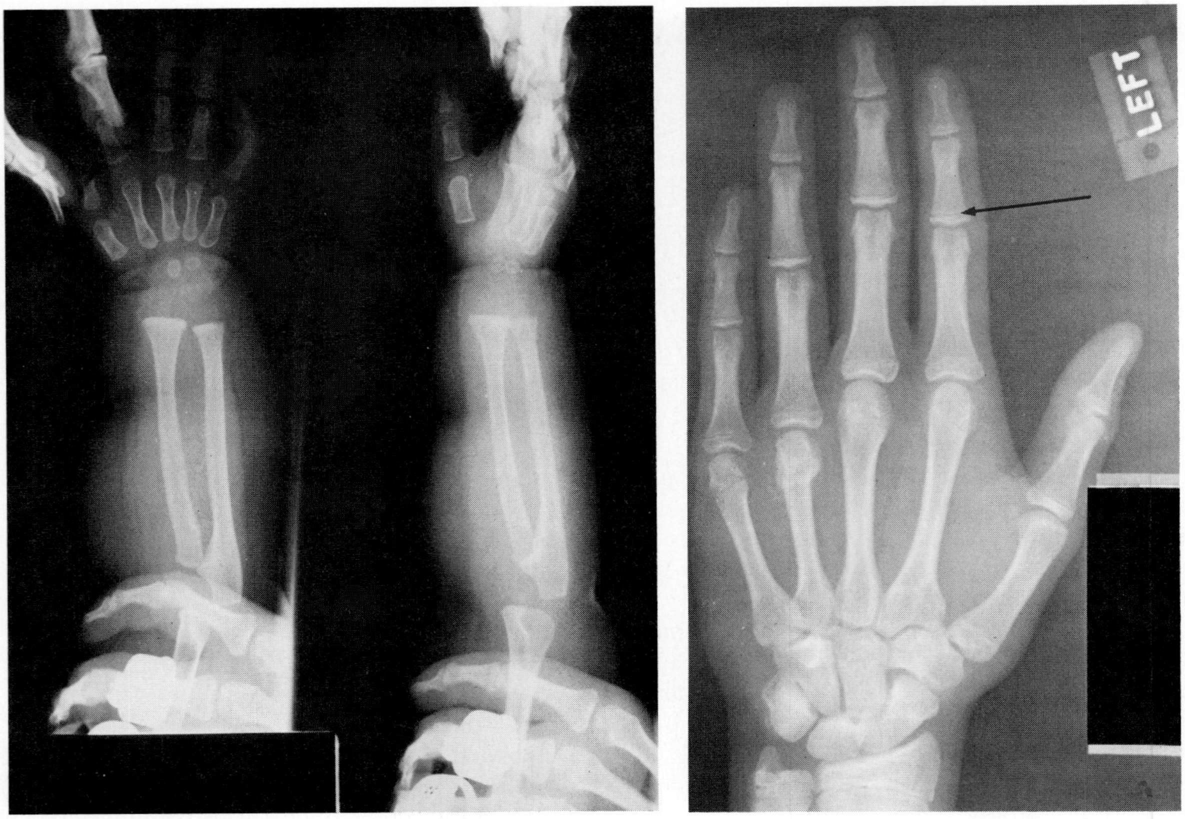

FIG. 5-4 Radiographs illustrating bone age in children. **A,** 8-month-old (note complete ossification in adult fingers holding the child's hand). **B,** 14-year-old; epiphyses visible *(see arrow).*

Between the diaphysis and the epiphysis is an epiphyseal cartilage plate where the active growth in length takes place. Interference with this growth site by trauma or infection can result in deformity.

The first centers of ossification appear in the 2-month-old embryo, and at birth the number is approximately 400, about half the number at maturity. New centers appear at regular intervals during the growth period and provide the basis for assessment of bone age. Postnatally, the earliest centers to appear (at 5 to 6 months of age) are those of the capitate and hamate bones in the wrist. Therefore, radiographs of the hand and wrist provide the most useful areas for screening to determine skeletal age, especially before age 6 years (Fig. 5-4).

Lymphoid Tissues

Lymphoid tissues contained in the lymph nodes, thymus, spleen, tonsils, adenoids and blood lymphocytes follow a growth pattern unlike that of other body tissues. These tissues are small in relation to total body size, but they are well developed at birth. They increase rapidly to reach adult dimensions by 6 years of age and continue to grow. About age 10 to 12 years they reach a maximum development that is approximately twice their adult size. This is followed by a rapid decline to stable adult dimensions by the end of adolescence.

Dentition

Teeth are divided into quadrants of the mandible and maxilla and are named for their location in each quadrant of the dental arch, such as central incisor, lateral incisor, and first and second molars. Teeth are also named after their specific function in the mastication of food. The knife- or scissors-like central and lateral incisors cut the food. The single-pointed cuspids, also called canines, tear the food. The two premolars, called bicuspids because of their two-pointed crown, crush the food. The permanent molars, which have four or five cusps, grind the food.

About the middle of the first year the *primary (deciduous)* teeth begin to erupt, and the total of 20 primary teeth are acquired in characteristic sequence by 30 months of age (see p. 288). The first *secondary (permanent)* teeth erupt at about 6 years of age (see p. 440). The pattern of shedding primary teeth and the eruption of secondary teeth are subject to wide variation among children. However, because of its relative regularity, the eruption of teeth is sometimes used as a criterion for developmental assessment, especially the 6-year molar, which seems to be the most universally consistent in timing. Nonetheless, dental maturation does not correlate well with bone age and is less reliable as an index of biologic age.

Development of Organ Systems

All tissues and organ systems undergo changes during development. Some are striking; others are more subtle. Many have implications for assessment and care. Since the major importance of these changes relates to their dysfunction, the developmental characteristics of various systems and organs are discussed throughout the book as they relate to these areas. Physical characteristics and physiologic changes that vary with age are included in age-group descriptions.

PHYSIOLOGIC CHANGES

Physiologic changes that take place in all organs and systems are discussed as they relate to dysfunction. Others, such as pulse and respiratory rates and blood pressure, are an integral part of physical assessment (see p. 137). In addition, there are changes in basic functions including metabolism, temperature, and patterns of sleep and rest.

Metabolism

The rate of metabolism when the body is at rest (basal metabolic rate [BMR]) demonstrates a distinctive change throughout childhood. It is highest in the newborn infant and is closely related to the proportion of surface area to body mass, which changes as the body increases in size. In both sexes the proportion decreases progressively to maturity and determines the caloric requirements of the child. The basal requirement of infants is about 110 to 120 kcal/kg (50 to 55 kcal/pound) of body weight and decreases to 40 to 50 kcal/kg (18 to 23 kcal/pound) at maturity (Table 5-2). The daily water requirements show a similar modification. Children's energy needs vary considerably at different ages and with changing circumstances. The greatest proportion of calories in infancy is used for basal metabolic needs and growth. The energy requirement to build tissue steadily decreases with age, following the general growth curve; however, exercise needs vary with the individual child and may be considerably more.

TABLE 5-2

Average Daily Requirements for Calories, Protein, and Water through Adolescence

Age (years)	Energy (cal/kg of body weight)	Protein (g/kg of body weight)	Water Requirements per kg per 24 hours (ml)
Infants			
0-½	115	2.2	80-135
½-1	105	2.0	130-135
Children			
1-3	100	1.8	120-100
4-6	85	1.5	100-110
7-10	85	1.2	85-90
Males			
11-14	60	1.0	50-80
15-18	42	0.8	40-50
Females			
11-14	48	1.0	50-80
15-18	38	0.8	40-50

Temperature

Body temperature, reflecting metabolism, displays the same decrement from infancy to maturity (see inside front cover). Following the unstable regulatory ability in the neonatal periods, heat production steadily declines as the infant grows into childhood. Individual differences of ½° to 1° F are normal, and occasionally a child normally displays an unusually high or low temperature. Beginning at approximately 12 years of age, the temperature in girls remains relatively stable, whereas in boys it continues to fall for a few years longer. Females maintain a temperature slightly above that of males throughout life.

Even with improved temperature regulation, infants and young children are highly susceptible to temperature fluctuations. Body temperature responds to changes in environmental temperature and is increased with active exercise, crying, and emotional upset. Infections can cause a higher and more rapid temperature increase in infants and young children than in older children. In relation to body weight, an infant produces more heat per unit than children near maturity. Consequently, during active play or when heavily clothed, an infant or small child is likely to become overheated.

Sleep and Rest

Sleep, a protective function in all organisms, allows for repair and recovery of tissues following activity. As in most aspects of development, there is wide variation between individual children and ages of children in the amount and distribution of sleep. As children mature there is a change in the total time they spend in sleep and in the amount of time spent in deep sleep.

Newborn infants sleep nearly all the time that is not occupied with feeding and other aspects of their care. As infants grow older, total time spent in sleep gradually decreases, they remain awake for longer periods, and they sleep longer at night. During the second year most children sleep through the night and take one or two naps during the day. By the time they are 3 years old, most children have eliminated the second nap; this pattern continues until age 4 or 5. After age 5 the child has usually given up daytime naps except in those cultures in which an afternoon nap or siesta is customary. During ages 5 to 10 sleep time remains relatively constant, then declines sharply during adolescence.

There is a change in the quality of sleep as children mature. The time spent in deep, restful sleep increases from 50% in infancy to 80% in the older child. Spontaneous awakening during sleep is relatively uncommon in childhood and adolescence.

TEMPERAMENT

Temperament is defined as "the manner of thinking, behaving, or reacting characteristic of an individual" (Chess and Thomas, 1985) and refers to the way in which a person deals with life. From the time of birth children exhibit marked individual differences in the way that they respond to their environment and the way others, particularly the parents, respond to them and their needs. Temperament is a categorical term with no implications of good or bad, and most, but not all, children can be placed into one of three common categories based on their overall pattern of temperamental attributes:

1. **The easy child.** Easy-going children are even-tempered, regular and predictable in their habits, and have a positive approach to new stimuli. They are open and adaptable to change, and display a mild to moderately intense mood that is typically positive. Approximately 40% of children fall into this category.
2. **The difficult child.** Difficult children are highly active, irritable, and irregular in their habits. Negative withdrawal responses are typical and they require a more structured environment. These children adapt slowly to new routines, people, or situations. Mood expressions are usually intense and primarily negative. They exhibit frequent periods of crying, and frustration often produces violent tantrums. This group comprises about 10% of children.
3. **The slow-to-warm-up child.** Slow-to-warm-up children typically react negatively and with mild intensity to new stimuli and, unless pressured, adapt slowly with repeated contact. They respond with only mild but passive resistance to novelty or changes in routine. They are quite inactive and moody but show only moderate irregularity in functions. Fifteen percent of children demonstrate this temperament pattern.

Significance of Temperament

There appears to be some relationship between the child's temperament and development of behavior problems. However, any child can develop behavior problems if there is dissonance between the child's temperament and the environment. Demands for change and adaptation that are in conflict with children's capacities can become excessively stressful. However, authorities emphasize that it is not children's temperament patterns that place them at risk but the degree of *fit* between the child and his environment, specifically his parents, that determines the degree of vulnerability. The greater the dissonance between the child's temperament and the ability of the parents to accept and deal with the behavior, the greater the likelihood of subsequent behavior problems. (For example, see Failure to thrive, p. 327.)

Early identification of temperament provides a useful tool for caregivers in anticipating probable areas of difficulty or risk associated with development. For example, "difficult" children may be prone to colic in infancy, active children require more vigilance to prevent injury, and school entry will require different approaches for children with different temperaments.

Several parental questionnaires have been devised to facilitate assessment of temperament. Nurses who employ these assessment tools are better able to help parents interpret their child's behavior and to provide anticipatory guidance regarding numerous aspects of child rearing.

DEVELOPMENT OF MENTAL FUNCTION AND PERSONALITY

Personality and cognitive skills develop in the same manner as biologic growth, and many aspects depend on physical growth and maturation. Personality and cognitive development can be described by predictable age-related stages during which specific changes are assumed to take place. This is not a comprehensive account of the multiple facets of personality and behavior development. These and many other aspects are integrated with the child's emotional and social development in later discussion of various age-groups. Some of the stages of development are outlined in Table 5-3.

Personality Development (Freud)

Freud considered the sexual instincts to be significant in the development of the personality. However, he used the term to describe any *sensual pleasure*. During childhood certain regions of the body assume a prominent psychologic significance as the source of new pleasures and new conflicts gradually shifts from one part of the body to another at particular stages of development. This theory is often termed the *psychosexual* stages of development.

Oral stage (birth to 1 year). During infancy the major source of pleasure-seeking is centered on oral activities such as sucking, biting, chewing, and vocalizing. Children may prefer one of these over the others and the preferred method of oral gratification can provide some indication of the personality they develop.

Anal stage (1 to 3 years). Interest during the second year of life centers in the anal region as sphincter muscles develop and children are able to withhold or expel fecal material at will. At this stage the climate surrounding toilet training can have lasting effects on children's personalities.

Phallic stage (3 to 6 years). During the phallic stage the genitals become an interesting and sensitive area of the body. Children recognize differences between the sexes and become curious about the dissimilarities. This is the period around which the controversial issues of the Oedipus and Electra complexes, penis envy, and castration anxiety are centered.

Latency period (6 to 12 years). During the latency period children elaborate on previously acquired traits and

TABLE 5-3

Summary of Personality, Cognitive, and Moral Development

Stage	Psychosexual Stages (Freud)	Psychosocial Stages (Erikson)	Cognitive Stages (Piaget)	Moral Judgment Stages (Kohlberg)
I Infancy (Birth to 1 yr)	Oral sensory	Trust vs mistrust	Sensorimotor (birth to 18 mo)	
II Toddlerhood (1-3 yr)	Anal-urethral	Autonomy vs shame and doubt	Preoperational thought, preconceptual phase (transductive reasoning) (2-4 yr)	Preconventional level
III Early childhood (3-6 yr)	Phallic-locomotion	Initiative vs guilt	Preoperational thought, intuitive phase (transductive reasoning) (4-7 yr)	
IV Middle childhood (6-12 yr)	Latency	Industry vs inferiority	Concrete operations (inductive reasoning and beginning logic)	Conventional level
V Adolescence (13-18 yr)	Genital	Identity and repudiation vs identity confusion	Formal operations (deductive and abstract reasoning)	Postconventional or principled level

skills. Physical and psychic energy are channeled into acquisition of knowledge and vigorous play.

Genital stage (age 12 and over). The last significant stage begins at puberty with maturation of the reproductive system and production of sex hormones. The genital organs become the major source of sexual tensions and pleasures, but energies are also invested in forming friendships and preparation for marriage.

Personality Development (Erikson)

The personality evolves as children react to their changing bodies and to the environment. The most widely accepted and used theory of personality development is that advanced by Erikson (1963). Although built on Freudian theory, it is known as *psychosocial* development and emphasizes a healthy personality as opposed to a pathologic approach. Erikson also uses the biologic concepts of critical periods and epigenesis, describing key conflicts or core problems that the individual strives to master during critical periods in personality development. Successful completion or mastery of each of these core conflicts is built on the satisfactory completion or mastery of the previous core.

Each psychosocial stage has two components, the favorable and unfavorable aspects of the core conflict, and progress to the next stage depends on resolution of this conflict. No core conflict is ever mastered completely but remains a recurrent problem throughout life. No life situation is ever secure. Each new situation presents the conflict in a new form. For example, when children who have satisfactorily achieved a sense of trust encounter a new experience (for example, hospitalization) they must again develop a sense of trust in those responsible for their care in order to master the situation. Erikson's lifespan approach to personality development consists of eight stages; however, only the first five relating to childhood are included here.

Trust versus mistrust (birth to 1 year). The first and most important attribute to develop for a healthy personality is a basic *trust*. Establishment of basic trust dominates the first year of life and describes all the child's satisfying experiences at this age. Corresponding to Freud's oral stage, it is a time of "getting" and "taking in" through all the senses. It exists only in relation to something or someone; therefore, consistent, loving care by a mothering person is essential to development of trust. *Mistrust* develops when trust-promoting experiences are deficient or lacking or when basic needs are inconsistently or inadequately met. Although there are shreds of mistrust sprinkled throughout the personality, from a basic trust in parents stems a basic trust in the world, other people, and oneself. The result is *faith* and *optimism*.

Autonomy versus shame and doubt (1 to 3 years). Corresponding to Freud's anal stage, the problem of *autonomy* can be symbolized by the holding on and letting go of the sphincter muscles. The development of autonomy during the toddler period is centered around children's increasing ability to control their bodies, themselves, and their environment. They want to do things for themselves, using their newly acquired motor skills of walking, climbing, and manipulating and mental powers of selection and decision making. Much of their learning is acquired through imitating the activities and behavior of others. Negative feelings of *doubt* and *shame* arise when children are made to feel small and self-conscious, when their choices are disastrous, when others shame them, or when they are forced to be dependent in areas in which they are capable of assuming control. The favorable outcomes are *self-control* and *willpower*.

Initiative versus guilt (3 to 6 years). The stage of *initiative* corresponds to Freud's phallic stage and is characterized by vigorous, intrusive behavior, enterprise, and a strong imagination. Children explore the physical world with all their senses and powers. They develop a conscience. No longer guided only by outsiders, there is an inner voice that warns and threatens. Children sometimes undertake goals or activities that are in conflict with those of parents or others, and being made to feel that their activities or imaginings are bad produces a sense of *guilt*. Children must learn to retain a sense of initiative without impinging on the rights and privileges of others. The lasting outcomes are *direction* and *purpose,* the courage to imagine and pursue valued goals.

Industry versus inferiority (6 to 12 years). The stage of *industry* is the latency period of Freud. Having achieved the more crucial stages in personality development, children are now ready to be workers and producers. They want to engage in tasks and activities that they can carry through to completion; they need and want real achievement. Children learn to compete and cooperate with others, and they learn the rules. It is a decisive period in their social relationships with others. Feelings of inadequacy and *inferiority* may develop if too much is expected of them or they believe that they cannot measure up to the standards set for them by others. The ego quality developed from a sense of industry is *competence*—the free exercise of skill and intelligence in the completion of tasks.

Identity versus role confusion (12 to 18 years). Corresponding to Freud's genital period, the development of *identity* is characterized by rapid and marked physical changes. Previous trust in their bodies is shaken, and children become overly preoccupied with the way they appear in the eyes of others as compared with their own self-concept. Adolescents struggle to fit the roles they have played and those they hope to play with the current roles and fashions adopted by their peers, to integrate their concepts and values with those of society, and to come to a decision regarding an occupation. Inability to solve the core conflict results in *role confusion*. The outcome of successful mastery is *devotion* and *fidelity,* the ability to sustain loyalties to others that are freely committed in early adolescence and to values and ideologies that are freely pledged in later adolescence.

Cognitive Development (Piaget)

The term *cognition* refers to the process by which the developing individual becomes acquainted with the world and the objects it contains. Children are born with inherited potentialities for intellectual growth, but they must develop into that potential through interaction with the environment. By assimilating information through the senses, processing it, and acting on it, they come to understand relationships between objects and between themselves and their world. With cognitive development, individuals acquire the ability to reason abstractly, to think in a logical manner, and to organize intellectual functions or performances into higher-order structures.

The best known and most comprehensive theory regarding children's thinking has been developed by the Swiss psychologist Jean Piaget. He believed that there are four major stages in the development of logical thinking. Each stage is derived from and builds on the accomplishments of the previous stage in a continuous, orderly process. The course of intellectual development is both maturational and invariant and is divided into the following stages (these ages are approximate).

Sensorimotor (birth to 2 years). The sensorimotor stage of intellectual development consists of six substages (see p. 276) that are governed by sensations in which simple learning takes place. Children progress from reflex activity through simple repetitive behaviors to imitative behavior. They develop a sense of "cause-and-effect" as they direct behavior toward objects. Problem solving is primarily trial and error. They display a high level of curiosity, experimentation, and enjoyment of novelty and begin to develop a sense of self as they are able to differentiate themselves from their environment. They become aware that objects have permanence—that an object exists even though it is no longer visible (see p. 275). Toward the end of the sensorimotor period children begin to use language and representational thought.

Preoperational (2 to 7 years). The predominant characteristic of the preoperational stage of intellectual development is *egocentricity*. Egocentricity in this sense does not mean selfishness or self-centeredness, but, rather, the inability to put oneself in the place of another. Children interpret objects and events, not in terms of general properties, but in terms of their relationships or their use to them. They are unable to see things from any perspective other than their own; they cannot see another's point of view, nor can they see any reason to do so.

Preoperational thinking is concrete and tangible. Children cannot reason beyond the observable, and they lack the ability to make deductions or generalizations. Thought is dominated by what they see, hear, or otherwise experience. However, they are increasingly able to use language and symbols to represent objects in their environment. Through imaginative play, questioning, and other interacting, they begin to elaborate concepts and to make simple associations between ideas. In the latter stage of this period their reasoning is *intuitive* (for example, the stars have to go to bed just as they do) and they are only beginning to deal with problems of weight, length, size, and time.

Concrete operations (7 to 11 years). At this age, thought becomes increasingly logical and coherent. Children are able to classify, sort, order, and otherwise organize facts about the world to use in problem solving. They develop a new concept of permanence—conservation. That is, they realize that physical factors, such as volume, weight, and number, remain the same even though outward appearances are changed. They are able to deal with a number of different aspects of a situation simultaneously. They do not have the capacity to deal in abstraction; they solve problems in a concrete, systematic fashion based on what they can perceive. Reasoning is inductive. Through progressive changes in thought processes and relationships with others, thought becomes less self-centered.

They can consider points of view other than their own. Thinking has become socialized.

Formal operations (12 to 15 years). Formal operational thought is characterized by adaptability and flexibility. Adolescents can think in abstract terms, use abstract symbols, and draw logical conclusions from a set of observations. They can make hypotheses and test them; they can consider abstract, theoretic, and philosophic matters. Although they may confuse the ideal with the practical, most contradictions in the world can be dealt with and resolved.

Moral Development (Kohlberg)

Children also acquire moral reasoning in a developmental sequence. To understand the stages in the development of moral judgment, it is important to be aware of the relationship to cognitive development and the stages of logical thought as well as to moral behavior.

Moral development is based on cognitive developmental theory and consists of the following three major levels, each of which has two stages (Kohlberg, 1975).

Preconventional level. The preconventional level of moral development parallels the preoperational level of cognitive development and intuitive thought. Culturally oriented to the labels of good/bad and right/wrong, the child integrates these in terms of the physical or pleasurable consequences of his actions.

At first the child determines the goodness or badness of an action in terms of its consequences. He avoids punishment and obeys without question those who have the power to determine and enforce the rules and labels. He has no concept of the basic moral order that supports these consequences.

Later he determines that the right behavior consists of that which satisfies his own needs (and sometimes the needs of others). Although elements of fairness, give and take, and equal sharing are evident, they are interpreted in a very practical, concrete manner without loyalty, gratitude, or justice.

Conventional level. At the conventional stage the child is concerned with conformity and loyalty. He values the maintenance of family, group, or national expectations regardless of consequences. Behavior that meets with approval and pleases or helps others is considered to be good. One earns approval by being "nice." Obeying the rules, doing one's duty, showing respect for authority, and maintaining the social order is the correct behavior. This level is correlated with the stage of concrete operations in cognitive development.

Postconventional, autonomous, or principled level. At the postconventional level the individual has reached the cognitive stage of formal operations. Correct behavior tends to be defined in terms of general individual rights and standards that have been examined and agreed on by the entire society. Although procedural rules for reaching consensus become important with emphasis on the legal point of view, there is also emphasis on the possibility for changing law in terms of societal needs and rational considerations.

The most advanced level of moral development is one in which self-chosen ethical principles guide decisions of conscience. These are abstract and ethical but universal principles of justice and human rights with respect for the dignity of the persons as individuals. It is believed that few persons reach this stage of moral reasoning.

Spiritual Development

Spiritual beliefs are closely related to the moral and ethical portion of the child's self-concept and, as such, must be considered as part of the child's basic needs assessment. Children need to have meaning, purpose, and hope in their lives. Also the need for confession and forgiveness is present, even in very young children. Fowler (1974) has identified stages in the development of faith that are closely associated with and that parallel cognitive and psychosocial development.

Stage 0: Undifferentiated. This stage of development encompasses the period of infancy during which children have no concept of right or wrong, no beliefs, and no convictions to guide their behavior. However, the beginnings of a faith are established with the development of basic trust through their relationships with the primary caregiver.

Stage 1: Intuitive-projective. Toddlerhood is primarily a time of imitating the behavior of others. Children imitate the religious gestures and behaviors of others without comprehending any meaning or significance to the activities. During the preschool years the child assimilates some of the values and beliefs of his parents. Parental attitudes toward moral codes and religious beliefs convey to children what they consider to be good and bad. Children still imitate behavior at this age and follow parental beliefs as part of their daily lives rather than through an understanding of their basic concepts.

Stage 2: Mythical-literal. Through the school-age years, spiritual development parallels cognitive development and is closely related to children's experiences and social interaction. Most have a strong interest in religion during the school-age years. The existence of a deity is accepted and petitions to an omnipotent being are important and expected to be answered; good behavior is rewarded and bad behavior is punished. Their developing conscience bothers them when they disobey. They have a reverence for thoughts and matters and are able to articulate their faith. They may even question its validity.

Stage 3: Synthetic-convention. As children approach adolescence, however, they become increasingly aware of spiritual disappointments. They recognize that prayers are not always answered (at least on their own terms) and may begin to abandon or modify some religious practices. They begin to reason, to question some of the established parental religious standards, and to drop or modify some religious practices.

Stage 4: Individuating-reflexive. Adolescents become more skeptical and begin to compare the religious standards of their parents with others. They attempt to determine which to adopt and incorporate into their own set of values. They also begin to compare religious standards with the scientific viewpoint. It is a time of searching rather than reaching. Adolescents are uncertain about many religious ideas but will not achieve profound insights until late adolescence or early adulthood.

Development of Self-Concept

Self-concept is all the notions, beliefs, and convictions that constitute an individual's knowledge of himself and influence that individual's relationships with others. It is not present at birth but develops gradually as a result of unique experiences within the self, with significant others, and with the realities of the world (Stuart and Sundeen, 1987). Children are continually bombarded by new data to be interpreted and accepted, revised, or rejected. They are strongly influenced by parental attitudes as values are conveyed to them that they interpret as desirable or undesirable.

In infancy the self-concept is primarily an awareness of one's independent existence learned in part as a result of social contacts and experiences with other people. The process becomes more active during toddlerhood as children explore the limits of their capacities and the nature of their impact on others. School-age children are more aware of differences among people, more sensitive to social pressures, and become more preoccupied with issues of self-criticism and self-evaluation. During early adolescence children focus more on physical and emotional changes taking place and peer acceptance. Self-concept is crystallized during later adolescence as the young people organize their self-concept around a set of values, goals, and competencies acquired throughout childhood.

Body image. Body image is a complex phenomenon that evolves and changes during the process of growth and development. Any deviation from the "norm" (no matter how this is interpreted) is cause for concern. The extent to which a characteristic, defect, or disease affects children's body image is influenced by the attitudes and behavior of those around them.

The way children perceive their own bodies is basic to the establishment of an overall identity. Body image begins in infancy, first on a feeling level, then progresses to an interest in individual body parts, which they examine with the same impartial attention they direct toward toys or other objects. By the end of the first year they become aware of themselves as separate from their caregiver and separate from their environment. They can identify body parts and can recognize themselves in a mirror.

Toddlers continually modify the body image they have established as they become more mobile and imitate the behavior of other persons in their world. They learn that they are either a "boy" or a "girl" and gain impressions of themselves from the behavior and comments of other persons in their lives. For example, "Where did you get that curly hair (or dimples)?" They gain increased mastery over their body in performing basic motor skills, in language, and in control of body functions.

During the preschool period children begin to be concerned with what they will become. They continue imitation of parents and other persons in their world. They have no concept of their inner structure. Their awareness of internal organs comes from sensations and discomfort they feel and what they see entering and leaving their bodies. Sex typing and sex-role identification are primary tasks during this time. Children are concerned with their genitals and discover pleasurable sensations by touching and manipulating the genital area. Masturbation is practiced to some extent by all preschool children. They compare their own genitals with those of parents, siblings, and playmates. This is a time when conflicts arise between the gratification received by these activities and the censure they often evoke from parents and society.

The school-age child compares his skills and abilities as well as his physical characteristics with those of his peers. The school-age child is highly concerned about how he looks to others as his social contacts expand. He is acutely aware of physical defects and other deviations from the normal in other persons. The school-age child has countless misconceptions about his inner structure but is interested to learn. Masturbation and sex play are still practiced.

Adolescence is probably the significant period of development for body image formation. The rapid changes of puberty cannot be ignored; they are apparent to the individual and to others. Consequently, an adolescent is forced to alter his body image to accommodate these physical changes. Adolescents focus a great deal of attention on their appearance and make frequent comparisons with their peers and the cultural norms of the society. Identity formation is the prime developmental task of adolescence and any event that alters the body at this time can have a crucial impact on body image construction.

Self-esteem. Self-esteem is a personal, subjective judgment of one's worthiness derived from and influenced by the social groups in the immediate environment and the individuals' perceptions of how they are valued by others. It is a product of both competence and social acceptance that changes with development. Highly egocentric toddlers are unaware of any difference between competence and social approval. Preschool and early school-age children, on the other hand, are increasingly aware of the discrepancy between their competencies and the abilities of more advanced children. The acceptance of adults and peers outside the family group becomes more important to them. Positive feedback enhances their self-esteem; they are vulnerable to feelings of worthlessness and are anxious over failure.

As children's competencies increase and they develop meaningful relationships, their self-esteem rises. Their self-esteem is again at risk during early adolescence when they are defining an identity and sense of self in the context of their peer group. Unless children are continually made to feel incompetent and of little worth, a decrease in self-esteem during vulnerable periods is only temporary.

Language Development

Children are born with the mechanism and capacity to develop speech and language skills. However, they will not speak spontaneously. The environment must provide a means for them to acquire these skills. Speech requires intact physiologic structure and function (including respiratory, auditory, and cerebral) plus intelligence, a need to communicate, and stimulation.

The rate of speech development varies from child to child and is directly related to neurologic competence and intellectual development. Gesture precedes speech, and in this way a small child communicates satisfactorily. As speech develops, gesture recedes but never disappears entirely. At all stages of language development, children's comprehension vocabulary is greater than their expressed vocabulary, and it reflects a continuing process of modification that involves both the acquisition of new words and the expanding and refining of word meanings previously learned. By the time they begin to walk, children are able to attach a name to objects and persons.

The first parts of speech used are nouns, sometimes verbs (for example, go), and combination words (such as bye-bye). Responses are usually structurally incomplete during the toddler period, although the meaning is clear. Next they begin to use adjectives and adverbs to qualify nouns, followed by adverbs to qualify nouns and verbs. Later, pronouns and gender words are added (such as he and she). By the time children enter school they are able to use simple, structurally complete sentences that average five to seven words.

FACTORS THAT INFLUENCE PHYSICAL AND EMOTIONAL DEVELOPMENT

Children are engaged in a continuous and ever-changing series of environmental and interpersonal interactions. It is impossible to include a discussion of all the complex and interrelated factors that influence the development of children as unique individuals. Children are affected by physical factors such as the climate in which they live, physiologic influences such as their innate characteristics and susceptibilities, the value system of their families and culture, and psychologic influences such as the quality of parenting and the number, sex, and personalities of the significant persons in their lives. Some factors that may be facilitated, modified, or otherwise influenced by nursing interventions will be mentioned, although specific activities and elaboration will be discussed elsewhere as appropriate.

Heredity

Inherited characteristics have a profound influence on development. The sex of the child, determined by random selection at the time of conception, directs both his pattern of growth and the behavior of others toward him. In all cultures, attitudes and expectations are different with respect to the sex of the child. Sex plus other hereditary determinants strongly affect the end result of growth and the rate of progress toward it. There is a high correlation between parent and child with regard to traits such as height, weight, and rate of growth. Most physical characteristics, including shape and form of features, body build, and physical peculiarities, are inherited and can influence the way in which children grow and interact with their environment. Many dimensions of personality, such as activity level, responsiveness, and a tendency toward shyness, are also inherited.

Differences in health and vigor of children may be attributed to hereditary traits. An inherited physical or mental defect or disorder will alter or modify a child's physical and/or emotional growth and interactions. The extent to which disabling conditions interfere with the child's growth and well-being will be considered in relation to numerous disabilities throughout the remainder of the book.

Neuroendocrine Factors

Probably all hormones affect growth in some fashion. Growth hormone (somatotropin), secreted by the anterior lobe of the pituitary gland, maintains the normal rate of protein synthesis in the body but produces its main effect on linear growth. An excess of growth hormone can produce a pituitary giant; a deficiency causes pituitary dwarfism. The thyroid hormones (thyroxine and triiodothyronine), secreted by the thyroid gland in response to the stimulation of thyrotrophic hormone, are essential for normal growth. They stimulate general metabolism and are especially important for growth of bones, teeth, and brain. A deficiency of thyroid hormone produces the stunted growth, mental retardation, and other manifestations of hypothyroidism.

The androgens produced and secreted by the adrenal cortex under the stimulation of adrenocorticotropin are responsible for many anabolic effects and for the adolescent growth spurt observed at puberty. These three hormones—somatotrophic hormone, thyroid hormone, and androgens—when given to persons in whom these hormones are deficient, stimulate protein anabolism and thereby produce retention of elements essential for building protoplasm and bony tissue. Other hormones that contribute effects on growth and development include insulin, cortisol, parathyroid hormone, and the sex hormones—testosterone and estrogen.

Nutrition

Nutrition is probably the single most important influence on growth. Dietary factors regulate growth at all stages of development, and their effects are exerted in numerous and complex ways. During the rapid prenatal growth period, faulty nutrition may influence development from the time of implantation of the ovum until birth. During infancy and childhood, the demand for calories is relatively great, as evidenced by the rapid increase in both height and weight. At this time, protein and caloric requirements are higher than at almost any period of postnatal development. As the growth rate slows with its concomitant decrease in metabolism, there is a corresponding reduction in caloric and protein requirement.

Growth is uneven during the periods of childhood between infancy and adolescence when there are plateaus and small growth spurts. The child's appetite will fluctuate in response to these variations until the turbulent growth spurt of adolescence, when adequate nutrition is extremely important but may be subject to numerous emotional influences. Adequate nutrition is closely related to good health throughout life, and an overall improvement in nourishment is evidenced by the gradual increase in size and early maturation of children in this century.

Malnutrition. The term *malnutrition* in its strictest sense is usually used to describe undernutrition, primarily that resulting from insufficient caloric intake. However, malnutrition may result from the following: (1) a dietary intake that is quantitatively or qualitatively inadequate, or both, including overnutrition; (2) disease that interferes with appetite, digestion, or absorption while increasing nutritional requirements; (3) excessive physical activity or inadequate rest; or (4) disturbed interpersonal relationships and other environmental or psychologic factors. Severe malnutrition during the sensitive periods of development, particularly the first 6 months of life, is positively correlated with diminished height, weight, and intelligence scores. Throughout this book, the importance of nutrition as a vital aspect of health promotion during all phases of the illness-wellness continuum is included as it relates to developmental phases and to specific health problems.

Socioeconomic Level

There is evidence to indicate that socioeconomic level has a significant impact on development. At all age levels children from upper- and middle-class families are taller than children from the lower class, and girls from the upper class attain menarche somewhat earlier than those in the lower class.

The cause of these discrepancies is not clear, although nutrition probably plays a prominent role. Poorer families are less likely to consistently provide the food that children need. This is especially critical during the sensitive periods in development. Related factors that might influence nutrition and growth in the lower socioeconomic levels are irregularity of eating, sleeping, and exercising. Also, as a rule, these families have larger numbers of children who must compete with one another for available food supplies.

Disease

Altered growth and development is one of the clinical manifestations in a number of hereditary disorders. Growth impairment is particularly marked in skeletal disorders, such as the various forms of dwarfism and at least one of the chromosomal anomalies (Turner syndrome). Many of the disorders of metabolism, such as vitamin D–resistant rickets, the mucopolysaccharidoses, and the numerous endocrine disorders, interfere with the normal growth pattern. In other disorders the tendency is toward the upper percentile of height, for example, Klinefelter syndrome and Marfan syndrome.

Many chronic illnesses that are associated with varying degrees of growth failure are congenital cardiac anomalies and respiratory disorders such as cystic fibrosis. Any disorder characterized by the inability to digest and absorb body nutrients will have an adverse effect on growth and development. These include the malabsorption syndromes and defects in digestive enzyme systems. Almost any disorder or disease state that persists over an extended period, particularly during a critical period of development, may have a permanent effect on growth.

Interpersonal Relationships

It is well established that relationships with significant others play an important role in development, particularly in emotional, intellectual, and personality development. Not only do the quality and quantity of contacts with other persons exert an influence on the growing child, but the widening range of contacts is essential to learning and the development of a healthy personality.

The mother or mothering person is unquestionably the single most influential person during early infancy. She is the one who meets the infant's basic needs of food, warmth, comfort, and love. She provides stimulation for the child's senses and facilitates his or her expanding capacities. Through her, the child learns to trust the world and feel secure to venture in increasingly wider relationships.

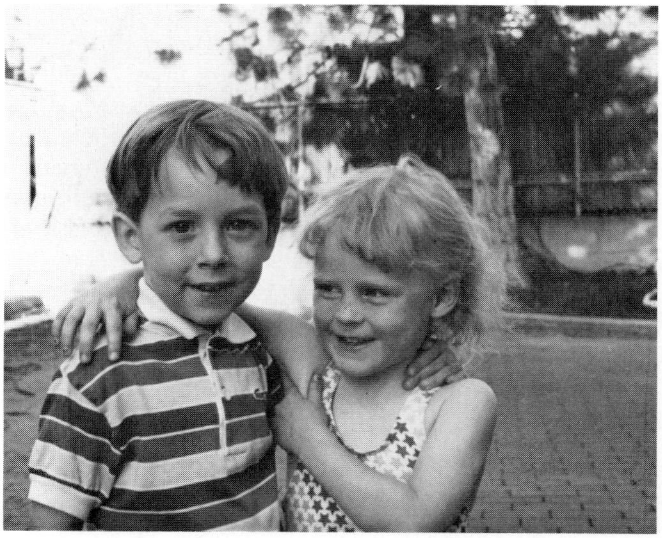

FIG. 5-5 Peers become increasingly important as children develop friendships outside the family group.

The sphere of persons from whom children seek approval widens to include other members of their family, their peers, and, to a lesser extent, other authority figures (for example, teachers). The increasing importance of the peer group in determining the behavior of school-age children and adolescents is well documented (Fig. 5-5).

It is generally the parents who are most influential in assisting the child to assume sex-role identification. Parents define and reinforce acceptable sex-role behavior and provide sex-appropriate role models for the child. In the absence of a sex-role model in the family setting, the child may adopt some characteristics of the opposite sex parent or sibling. Frequently, the child identifies with a teacher or other significant person of the same sex.

Siblings are the child's first peers, and the way in which he learns to relate to them affects later interactions with peers outside the family group. For example, a firstborn child who is accustomed to a position of leadership with siblings will tend to assume the same position with peers; younger children are more often followers. Ease in relationships with peers of the same or opposite sex is frequently associated with similar associations in the home.

Emotional deprivation. The most prominent feature of emotional deprivation, particularly during the first year, is developmental retardation. Much of the information regarding the adverse effects of interpersonal influences on development has been acquired through retrospective studies of gross deprivation and trauma. The most notable instances involved homeless infants who were placed in institutions for care. These infants, who did not receive consistent mothering care, failed to gain weight even with an adequate diet; were pale, listless, and immobile; and were unresponsive to stimuli that usually elicit a response, such as smiling or cooing, in the normal infant. It has been found that if the emotional deprivation continues for a sufficient length of time, the child may not survive infancy.

Although the most remarkable examples of emotional deprivation were first recognized among infants in institutions, the term *masked deprivation* has been used to describe children who are reared in homes where there is a distorted mother-child relationship or otherwise disordered home environment. Infants do not thrive if the mothering person is hostile, fearful of handling them, or indifferent to them and their needs. Such children exhibit poor growth even though apparently free of physical disease. Growth retardation in these children is believed to be caused by a psychologically induced endocrine imbalance that interferes with growth. These same infants and children display "catch-up" growth in a changed environment.

Influence of the Mass Media

There is no doubt that the communications media provide children with a means for extending their knowledge about the world in which they live and have contributed to narrowing the differences between classes.

Reading materials. The oldest of the mass media—books, newspapers, and magazines—contribute to children's competence in almost every direction, as well as providing enjoyment. Recognition of the impact that reading matter in the schools has on the value system and socialization processes has prompted reevaluation of the content of textbooks, for example, the biased presentation of male and female role models, the unrealistic, sugar-coated view of life situations, and the unrealistic, biased history of minority groups.

Fairy tales, for generations the mainstay of young children's literature, for a time suffered condemnation as sexist, overly violent in content, and riddled with unfavorable stereotypes, such as the wicked stepmother, dwarfs, and physical unattractiveness associated with evil. They are now believed to provide an excellent medium for explaining puzzling and important topics such as death, stepparents, and inner feelings and turmoils.

Comic books and other "pulp" reading material have been popular in every generation, usually at the expense of literature provided by schools, libraries, and parents. Many children have nothing else to read. The easy reading, quick action, and adventure in brief episodes seem to fulfill a need for children who are striving to understand both aggression in others and their own impulses. Reading ability, intelligence, and school adjustment apparently have no relationship to the number and type of comic books read. Most comic books appear to be relatively harmless to the majority of children and are in some ways even beneficial. Comic books seem to have only a minor influence on acquisition of beliefs, values, and behaviors. The popularity of this medium has prompted some educators to encourage translations of literature into comic book form in order to stimulate the interest of students in the classics.

Movies. Movies, not closely bound to reality and often portraying an assortment of socially approved behaviors, perhaps make a contribution to children's value systems, but they also provide opportunities for desirable social learning. On the other hand, children, especially adolescents, flock to the "macho" (especially those whose heroes resort to violent resolution of problems and wild car chases), the teenage horror, and teenage sexploitation movies. The carry-over of these influences into daily life and relationships may account, in part, for the increase in violent and promiscuous behavior of young persons.

Television. The medium that is having the most impact on children in America today is television, which has become one of the most significant socializing agents in the life of young children. The content of programs and commercials provides multiple sources for acquiring information, modeling behaviors, and observing value orientations. Besides producing a leveling effect on class differences in general information and vocabulary, TV exposes children to a wider variety of topics and events than they encounter in day-to-day life. Television always has time to talk to children and is a form of access to the adult world.

Much of the adverse influence of TV depends on the

susceptibility of the individual child. Television is a solitary activity and as such increases passivity and decreases physical activity and social interaction. Insecure children with strong feelings of rejection may become addicted to the medium in order to meet a need they are unable to satisfy in other ways. Too often TV can become a substitute for play and other activities.

Most programming stresses the triumph of good over evil, but with an unrealistically rapid resolution of problems, including moral dilemmas, often accompanied by pain or violence. Nor do programs portray the complex internal dynamics that are generally part of children's moral dilemmas. Physical solutions to problems are common with violence as the first alternative for problem solving.

Controversy continues regarding the favorable vs deleterious effects of television viewing. There is ample documentation to implicate television as a source for learning antisocial behavior. For example, it has been shown that viewing violence on television adds aggressive strategies to the children's repertoire of responses. Consequently, in a real-life situation children may imitate the aggressive behavior of television models.

Parents can help children to evaluate the TV violence by pointing out the subtleties that children miss, such as the aggressor's motives, his or her intentions, and the unpleasant consequences that the perpetrators suffer as a result of their aggressive acts. Parents can stress the purpose of the programs—primarily as entertainment—and explain why they like or dislike something on TV, for example, "This show is trying to tell you that crime does not pay and, if one does wrong, one will go to jail." Such discussions can be very effective when begun early and carried out consistently.

On the positive side, television has been shown to be a positive influence on children's abilities to deal with a variety of social issues, such as divorce, the arrival of a new baby, discrimination, honesty, and helpfulness. Children who view educational programming (such as "Mister Rogers' Neighborhood" and "Sesame Street") for a long period of time become more affectionate, considerate, cooperative, and helpful toward their playmates. The ways that racial and ethnic characters are portrayed on television can have an impact on the way the majority culture views minority persons and on the self-image of minority children.

It is clear that parents need to supervise the amount and type of TV programs that their children watch and to teach children how to watch TV. House rules that specify the type and amount of television help children understand limits, and video recorded selections of appropriate programs can be substituted for less desirable offerings. Parents need to carefully monitor cable and other pay TV programming since these popular options present more uncensored programming. Locked boxes are available for cable receivers, which allow families to prevent children from viewing "R" rated or other programs when unsupervised.

Nurses and parents can be powerful forces in influencing the media. They can watch closely for an increase in violence and other undesirable programming and complain if they believe it is not appropriate.

ROLE OF PLAY IN DEVELOPMENT

Through the universal medium of play children learn what no one can teach them. They learn about their world and how to deal with this environment of objects, time, space, structure, and people. They learn about themselves operating within that environment—what they can do, how to relate to things and situations, and how to adapt themselves to the demands society makes on them. It has been said that play is the *work* of the child. In play, children continually practice the complicated, stressful processes of living, communicating, and achieving satisfactory relationships with other people. In addition, while promoting and advancing development and relationships, play is its own reward.

Classification of Play

From a developmental point of view, patterns of children's play can be categorized according to the *content* and the *social character*. In both there is an additive effect. Each builds on past accomplishments, and some element of each is maintained throughout life. At each stage in development the new predominates.

Content of play. Play begins with *social-affective* play, wherein the infant takes pleasure in relationships with people. As adults talk, fondle, nuzzle, and in various ways elicit a response from the infant, he soon learns to provoke parental emotions and responses with such behaviors as smiling, cooing, or initiating games and activities. The type and intensity of the adult behavior with children vary among cultures.

Sense-pleasure play is a nonsocial stimulating experience that originates from outside the individual. Objects in the environment—light and color, tastes and odors, textures and consistencies—attract a child's attention, stimulate his senses, and give pleasure. Pleasurable experiences are derived from handling raw materials (water, sand, food), from body motion (swinging, bouncing, rocking), and from other uses of senses and abilities, such as smelling and humming. Once infants have developed the ability to grasp and manipulate, they persistently demonstrate and exercise their newly acquired abilities through *skill play,* repeating an action over and over again.

One of the vital elements in the child's process of identification is *dramatic* play. It begins in toddlerhood and is the predominant form of play in the preschool child. Once children begin to invest situations and people with meanings and to attribute affective significance to the world, they can pretend and fantasize almost anything. By acting out events of daily life, children learn and practice the roles and identities modeled by the members of their family and society. Their small toys, replicas of the tools of the society in which they live, provide a medium for learning about these adult roles and activities that may be both puzzling and frustrating to them. Interacting with the world is one of the ways in which children get to know it. The simple, imitative, dramatic play of the toddler, such as using the telephone, driving a car, or rocking a doll, evolves into more complex, sustained dramas of the preschooler. These extend beyond common domestic matters to the wider aspects of the world and the society, such as playing policeman, storekeeper, teacher, nurse, and so on. Older children work out elaborate themes, act out stories, and compose plays.

In *unoccupied behavior* children are not playful but focus their attention momentarily on anything that strikes their interest. They daydream, fiddle with clothes or other objects, or walk aimlessly. This differs from onlookers, who actively observe the activities of others.

Very young children participate in simple, *imitative games* such as pat-a-cake and peekaboo. Preschool children learn and enjoy *formal games* that begin with ritualistic, self-sustaining games, such as ring-around-a-rosy and London Bridge, then progress to *competitive games*, such as cards, checkers, or baseball.

Social character of play. The play interactions of infancy are between the child and an adult. Children continue to enjoy the company of an adult but are increasingly able to play alone. As age advances, the interaction with agemates increases in importance and becomes an essential part of the socialization process. Through it, the highly egocentric infant, unable to tolerate delay or interference, ultimately acquires concern for others and the ability to delay gratification or even to reject gratification at the expense of another. A pair of toddlers will engage in a good deal of combat since their personal needs cannot stand delay or compromise. By the time they reach age 5 or 6 years, children are able to arrive at a compromise or make use of arbitration—usually after each child has attempted but failed to gain his own way. Through continued interaction with peers and the growth of conceptual abilities and social skills, children are able to increase participation with others.

Social involvement during play can be categorized by the following:

Onlooker play

In onlooker play the child watches what other children are doing but makes no attempt to enter into the play activity. There is an active interest in observing the interaction of others but no movement toward participating. Watching television is a common example of the onlooker role.

Solitary play

In solitary play children play alone and independently with toys different from those used by other children within the same area. They enjoy the presence of other children but make no effort to get close to or speak to them. Their interest is centered on their own activity, which they pursue with no reference to the activities of the others.

Parallel play

In parallel play children play independently but among other children. They play with toys that are like those that the children around them are using, but as each sees fit, neither influencing nor being influenced by the other children. Each plays beside, but not with, other children. Parallel play is the characteristic play of the toddler, but it may also occur in other groups of any age. Individuals who are engaged in a creative craft with each person separately working on his own project are in parallel play.

Associative play

In associative play children play together and are engaged in a similar or even identical activity, but there is no organization, division of labor, leadership assignment, or mutual goal. There is borrowing and lending of play materials, following one another with wagons and tricycles, and sometimes attempts to control who may or may not play in the group. Each child acts according to his own wishes; there is no group goal. An example of associative play is two children playing with dolls, each borrowing articles of clothing from the other, engaging in similar conversation, but neither directing the other's actions nor establishing rules regarding the limits of the play session. There is a great deal of behavioral contagion—when one child initiates an activity, the entire group follows the example.

Cooperative play

Cooperative play is organized, and the child plays in a group *with* other children. The children discuss and plan activities for the purposes of accomplishing an end—to make something, to attain a competitive goal, to dramatize situations of adult or group life, or to play formal games. The group is loosely formed, but there is a marked sense of belonging or not belonging to the group. The goal and its attainment require organization of activities, division of labor, and playing roles. The leader-follower relationship is definitely established, and the activity is controlled by one or two members who assign roles and direct the activities of the others. The activity is organized to allow one child to supplement another's function in order to complete the goal.

Functions of Play

The specific values of play or the functions that it serves throughout childhood include sensorimotor development, intellectual development, socialization, creativity, self-awareness, and therapeutic and moral value.

Sensorimotor development. Sensorimotor activity is a major component of play at all ages and is the predominant form of play in infancy. Active play is essential for muscle development and serves a useful purpose as a release for surplus energy. Through sensorimotor play children explore the nature of the physical world. Infants gain impressions of themselves and their world through tactile, auditory, visual, and kinesthetic stimulation. Toddlers and preschoolers revel in body movement and exploration of things in space. Children continue to engage in sensorimotor play, although with increasing maturity the play becomes more differentiated and involved. Very young children run for the sheer joy of body movement, and older children incorporate or modify the motions into increasingly complex and coordinated activities such as races, games, roller skating, and bicycle riding.

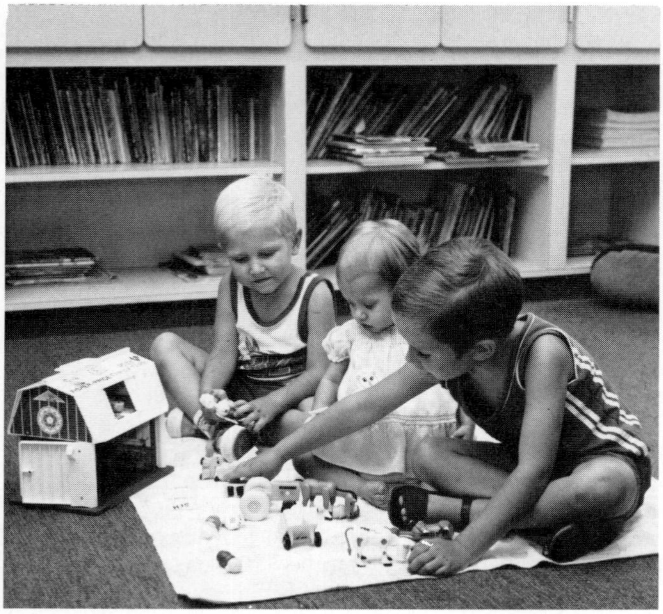

FIG. 5-6 Play helps children comprehend the world in which they live.

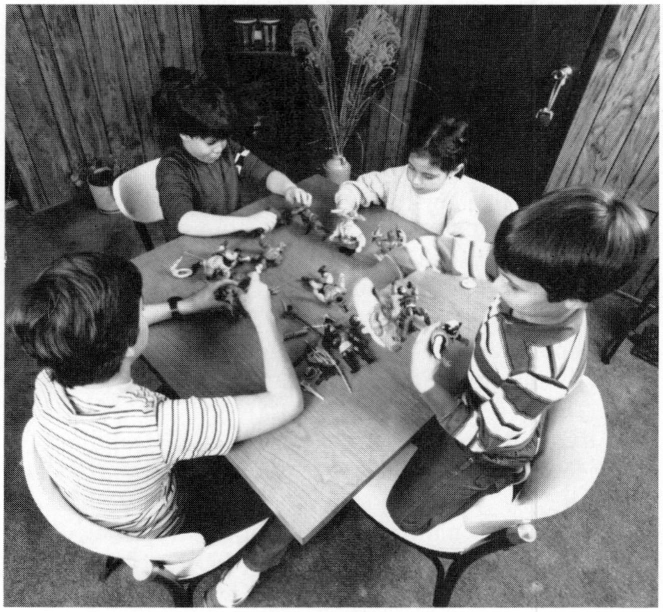

FIG. 5-7 Children show interest and pleasure in the company of others.

Intellectual development. Through exploration and manipulation, children learn colors, shapes, sizes, textures, and the significance of objects. They learn the significance of numbers and how to use them, they learn to associate words with objects, and they develop an understanding of abstract concepts and spatial relationships, such as up, down, under, over, and so on. Activities such as puzzles and games help them to develop problem-solving skills. Books, stories, films, and collections expand knowledge and provide enjoyment as well. Play provides a means to practice and expand language skills. Through play, children continually rehearse past experiences to assimilate them into new perceptions and relationships. Play helps children to comprehend the world in which they live and to distinguish between fantasy and reality (Fig. 5-6).

Socialization. From very early infancy, children show interest and pleasure in the company of others (Fig. 5-7). Their initial social contact is with the mothering person, but through play with other children they learn to establish social relationships and solve the problems associated with these relationships. They learn to give and take, which is more readily learned from critical peers than from the more tolerant adults. They learn the sex role that society expects them to fulfill as well as approved patterns of behavior and deportment. Closely associated with socialization is development of moral values and ethics. Children learn right from wrong, the standards of the society, and to assume responsibility for their actions.

Creativity. In no other situation is there more opportunity to be creative than in play. Children can experiment and try out their ideas in play through every medium at their disposal, including raw materials, fantasy, and exploration. Creativity is stifled by pressure toward conformity; therefore, striving for peer approval may inhibit creative endeavors in the school-age or adolescent child. Creativity is primarily a product of solitary activity, as opposed to group activity. Once children feel the satisfaction of creating something new and different, they transfer this creative interest to situations outside the world of play.

Self-awareness. Beginning with active explorations of their bodies and awareness of themselves as separate from the mother, the process of self-identity is facilitated through play activities. Children learn who they are and what their place is in the world. They become increasingly able to regulate their own behavior, to learn what their abilities are, and to compare their abilities with those of others. Through play, children are able to test their abilities, to assume and try out various roles, and to learn the effect that their behavior has on others.

Therapeutic value. There is no doubt that play is therapeutic at any age. It provides a means for release from the tension and stress encountered in the environment. In play, children can express emotions and release unacceptable impulses in a socially acceptable fashion. Children are able to experiment and test fearful situations and can assume and vicariously master the roles and positions that they are unable to perform in the world of reality. Children reveal much about themselves in play. Through play, children are able to communicate to the alert observer the needs, fears, and desires that they are unable to express with their limited language skills. Throughout their play, children need the acceptance of adults and their presence to help them control aggression and to channel their destructive tendencies.

Guidelines for Toy Safety

When selecting a toy:

Select toys that suit the skills, abilities, and interests of the child.
Select toys that are safe for the specific child; look for a label that indicates the intended age-group. Toys that are safe at one age may not be safe for another.
Make certain all parts are present and directions for use are clear and appropriate to the child.
Check for safety labels such as "flame retardant" or "flame resistant."
Select toys durable enough to survive rough play.
Select toys light enough that they will not cause harm if one falls on a child.
Look for toys with smooth, rounded edges. Avoid toys with sharp edges that can cut or sharp points. Points on the inside of the toy can puncture if the toy is broken.
Avoid toys with any small parts that can be swallowed or aspirated, especially for children under 3 years of age.
Avoid toys with any shooting or throwing objects that can injure eyes. This includes toys into which other missiles, such as sticks or pebbles, might be used as substitutes for the intended projectiles. Arrows and darts used by children should have blunt tips and be manufactured from resilient materials; make certain tips are securely attached.
Make certain that materials in toys are nontoxic.
Avoid toys that make loud noises that might be damaging to a child's hearing. Even some squeaking toys are too loud when held close to the ear.
Remove and discard plastic wrapping from toys that could suffocate a child.
Make certain an older child understands that a toy inappropriate for smaller children should be kept out of the hands of younger brothers and sisters.
Teach the child the proper way to unplug an electric toy—pull on the plug, not the cord.
Teach the child the safe use of utensils that under certain circumstances can cause injury—scissors, knives, needles, heating elements, or loops, long string, or cord (a potential for strangulation in very young children).
Teach children to beware of electrical appliances and even electrically operated playthings. Children are unfamiliar with the hazards of electricity in association with water.
Provide a safe place for the child to store toys.
Select a toy chest or toy box that is ventilated, is free of self-locking devices that could trap a child inside, and has a lid designed not to pinch a child's fingers or fall on a child's head.
Teach the child to store toys safely in order to prevent accidental injury from stepping or falling on a toy.
Check all toys periodically for breakage, loose parts, and other potential hazards.
Check movable parts to make certain they are attached securely to the toy. Sometimes pieces that are safe when attached to the toy become a danger when detached.
Repair or discard broken toys.
Make certain that toys are constructed with nontoxic materials, and use only paint labeled "nontoxic" to repaint toys, toy boxes, or children's furniture.
Sand sharp wooden toys or splintered surfaces smooth.
Examine all outdoor toys regularly for rust and weak or sharp parts that could become a danger to a child.
Maintain toys in good repair, without signs of possible hazards such as sharp edges, splinters, weak seams, rust; keep electrical cords and plugs in good condition.

Moral value. Although children learn at home and at school those behaviors that are considered right and wrong in the culture, the interaction with peers during play contributes significantly to their moral training. Nowhere is the enforcement of moral standards so rigid as in the play situation. If they are to be acceptable members of the group, children must adhere to the accepted codes of behavior of the culture—fairness, honesty, self-control, consideration for others, and so on. Children soon learn that their peers are less tolerant of violations than are adults and that to maintain a place in the play group they must conform to the standards of the group.

Toys

The type of toys chosen by and/or provided for children can facilitate their development in the areas just outlined. Toys that are small replicas of the culture and its tools help them assimilate their culture. Toys that require pushing, pulling, rolling, and manipulating teach them about physical properties of the items and help to develop muscles and coordination. Rules and the basic elements of cooperation and organization are learned through board games.

In providing toys for children it is well to keep in mind that raw materials with which they are able to use their own creativity and imaginations are sometimes superior to ready-made items. For example, building blocks can be used to construct a variety of things, to count, and to learn shapes and sizes. Lewis and Block (1982) outline five ways in which parents can encourage their child's toy play:

1. Realize that play teaches skills and abilities that are the center of intelligence.
2. Play with your child, enroll the child in a play group that meets several times a week, or hire a baby-sitter who can act as a playmate.
3. Do not turn every play activity into an educational lesson.
4. Respect your child's likes and dislikes; remember that learning is best acquired in an enjoyable situation.
5. Observe your child at play so that you come to know favorite types of toys and activities.

Toy safety. Selection of toys and play equipment is a joint effort between parents and children, but evaluation of their safety is the responsibility of the adult. Government agencies do not inspect and police all toys on the market. Therefore adults who purchase, supervise purchases, or allow children to use play equipment need to evaluate such equipment for its safety, including toys that are gifts or those that are purchased by the children themselves (see box). They should also be alert to notices of toys determined to be defective and recalled by the manufacturers. Parents and health workers can obtain information on a variety of recalled products and can report potentially dangerous toys and child products to the **U.S. Consumer Product Safety Commission (CPSC)*** or in Canada, the **Canadian Toy Testing Council.**†

NEEDS OF INFANTS AND CHILDREN

All children are basically alike. They follow the same pattern of development and maturation, whereas, at the same time, their hereditary, cultural, and experiential backgrounds make each a distinct and unique individual. They differ in their rate of growth, their ultimate size and capabilities, and the way in which they respond to their environment. However, regardless of stage of development, state of health, or situation in which encountered, *the child is first of all a child.*

Children need ample physical room in which to grow as well as support from the adults in their environment. Because they do not have the resources for coping with the world, children need to be surrounded by caring people who are willing to share their pleasures and help them through troubling times. Although the emphasis and classification may vary according to the interpreter, the essential needs of children during all stages of development are physical, biologic, and emotional needs, including love, emotional security, discipline, independence, and self-esteem.

Physical and Biologic Needs

First of all, children's basic physical and biologic needs for food, water, air, warmth, elimination, and shelter must be met. Infants, except for limited reflex responses, are totally dependent on adults for satisfaction of even the most basic needs. As development proceeds, children begin to communicate their needs verbally and nonverbally and to assume increasing responsibility for their basic need gratification.

Those who care for children come to understand the physical changes that take place during the process of development and the special needs generated by these changes, for example, the nature and quantity of the food intake, the method and frequency of feeding, and the amount of sleep and activity that change during childhood. Health and safety hazards associated with every phase of development require implementation of measures to provide for the child's physical safety, including prevention of injuries and disease and education of children, families, and communities regarding these potential threats to health and well-being.

Love and Affection

The single most important emotional need of children is to be loved and to feel secure in that love. Children strive above all else to gain the love and acceptance of those who are significant in their lives. When they feel secure in this love they are able to withstand the normal crises associated with growing up and those unexpected crises (such as illness or loss) that are superimposed on the anticipated course of development.

Children cannot receive too much love. However, this love must be communicated to them through words and actions that tell them that they are loved, not for their actions or achievement, but for what they are or simply *because they are.* Although love is closely associated with discipline, independence, and other factors that influence the child's self-concept, it is an undemanding, accepting love that is indispensable to the development of a healthy personality. Unconditional love, freely bestowed, helps establish a sense of security and a positive sense of self within children that will persist throughout their lifetime. It is important that children know they are loved and that whatever happens they can depend on this love. For many children spiritual love is a very significant source of complete undemanding love. Without the security of loving relationships, children may become tense and insecure and develop undesirable behavior patterns as they attempt to obtain that love or try to compensate for its loss.

The primary source of love, particularly during infancy, is the parent, usually the mother, or mothering person. The importance of establishing this early love attachment (or bonding) profoundly influences subsequent interpersonal relationships. With ever-widening relationships, children need the love and acceptance of others. They need to feel they are wanted, accepted, and belong in whatever relationships are important to them at each stage of development.

Parents may truly love their children but be unable to communicate this love to them. Parents who are insecure in their parenting skills frequently seek advice and reassurance from health professionals. Nurses who are aware of indications of parental insecurity will be able to provide assistance and reassurance that can preserve and enhance the parent-child relationship and build a sense of confidence in the parent.

Security

Closely allied to the need for love is the need for a sense of security. As they grow and develop in a complex world, children encounter many threats to their sense of security. Indeed, most behavior problems of childhood are associated with an element of insecurity. Every change in themselves or their environment creates a feeling of uncertainty. Faced with confusing, conflicting adjustments, young children need the security provided by relatively stable situations and dependable human relationships. The degree to which they can cope with these stresses depends on the patience and support they receive from those most closely involved in their care.

There are a multitude of factors that generate a feel-

*CPSC hotline: 1-800-638-CPSC.

†P.O. Box 6014, Stn. J, Ottowa, Ontario, Canada K2A 171.

ing of insecurity in children. Ordinarily the parents, who are sources of comfort, guidance, and encouragement, provide a measure of security in an insecure world. To achieve this security children need the warm acceptance of loving parents, a stable family unit, and judicious handling of stress-provoking situations such as sibling rivalry, relocation to a new neighborhood, and illness in themselves or other members of the family. A disturbed home environment caused by such factors as marital discord, illness of a parent or family member, or death of a family member can shatter their equilibrium.

Infants are disturbed by physical threats, such as hunger, cold, or discomfort. Small children are physiologically disturbed by emotions such as anger, fear, and grief, which they can release only in overt behavior. A measure of relief from these feelings can be obtained by the reassurance that their physical needs will be met, restraints will be placed on their behavior, and expectations that keep pace with their inner controls will be held. Rejection by significant persons, social ineptitude, and physical disabilities often produce insecurity in a child. The number and variety of factors originating within or outside the child are often difficult to determine; therefore, those responsible for the child's care must be alert for cues that reveal threats to this sense of security.

Discipline and Authority

Because children live in an organized society, they must be prepared to accept restrictions on their behavior. Discipline is not punishment. Rather it is the teaching of desirable behavior. Children need to learn the rules governing behavior in the home, the neighborhood, the school, and the community at large. To learn acceptable behavior that permits them to live enjoyably with themselves and others, children need the steady, firm guidance of loving parents and others in authority roles. Good discipline provides children with protection from dangers (from within and without) and relieves them of the burden of decisions that they are not prepared to make, yet allows them to develop independence of thought and action within a secure framework.

Children who learn to live within reasonable rules are happier and more secure. Without the stabilizing influence of controls, children feel uncertain and insecure. Too often, inexperienced and insecure parents fear the loss of a child's love, suffer feelings of guilt over disciplinary action, or may even relinquish their authority to the child. To discipline is to teach reality. Sensible, mature parents establish fair rules and regulations in the home and then see that they are carried out. Parents should never exploit children's love for them as a means to control their children. Children's anxiety lest they lose that love is already great. Discipline based on love of the child and carried out with conviction, confidence, and consistency will produce a self-reliant, buoyant, and self-controlled child.

Dependence and Independence

As children grow and mature, they are increasingly able to direct their own activities and to make more independent decisions. However, there are great fluctuations in their ability to function independently. Even with a compelling inner drive to master and achieve, they are not always able to cope with difficult and frustrating problems or conflicts. All children feel the urge to grow up and move forward toward maturity, but they have at their disposal only those energies that are not being used to maintain their mastery over old conflicts. Independence should be permitted to grow at its own rate.

Periods of regression and dependence are not only normal but are often necessary and helpful. If children feel sufficiently comfortable and content in a situation or relationship and reasonably certain that they can return to this safety and security, they will venture into the untried and untested on their own. If they feel doubtful concerning their abilities to cope, regression to a more comfortable level of competence allows them to replenish their inner resources and prepare to move ahead once again. Independence grows out of dependence; one cannot be considered as distinct from the other.

Children will learn independence of thought and decision making provided the opportunity is not withheld from them. If they are pushed into acting independently before they feel themselves ready, they may withdraw from independence. When they choose not to relinquish the joys of independence and autonomy or move ahead to new worlds of independence, they will dawdle. Parents, teachers, nurses, and others responsible for child care must be able to adjust their expectations and support to meet the child's needs of the moment. It is important to recognize when to help and when not to help children to experiment with their immature and imperfect self-control, when to make demands that require children's utmost ability, and when to allow them to function temporarily on a more immature level. They need these freedoms and controls in the process of becoming mature, self-reliant adults.

Self-Esteem

In order to develop and preserve self-esteem, children need to feel that they are worthwhile individuals who are in some way different from, superior to, and more lovable than any other individual in the world. They need recognition for their achievements and the approval of parents and peers. Parents and other authority figures can foster a positive self-concept by providing appropriate encouragement and recognition for achievement and by discouraging inappropriate behaviors. However, when disapproval is being expressed, it is imperative to convey to a child that it is the *behavior* that is unacceptable, not the child. Constructive communication, such as the use of "I" messages, conveys feeling and needs without destroying the child's self-esteem.

Children who experience warm, affectionate relationships with family, who are accepted by their parents, and who are aware of their parents' positive attitudes toward them are more accepting of themselves. Children who have a strong sense of their own worth are confident, able to initiate activities, explore their environment, and take risks in their behavior when confronted with new or novel situations. They approach tasks and relationships with the expectation that they will be well received and successful. Such is the focus of nursing—to allow children and their families to grow and prosper from their experiences in health and illness.

SUMMARY

Child growth and development are complex processes involving numerous components that are subject to a wide variety of influences. All facets of each child's body, mind, and personality develop simultaneously, although not independently, and emerge at varying rates and sequences. The processes are the same for all children but different for each individual child and are affected by innumerable factors including heredity, environment, and health.

To attain their optimum growth potential children need physical care, security, and an opportunity to play and engage in physical activity. They need a loving family to provide unconditional love, discipline, and appropriate independence. Happy, healthy children grow up with a positive view of themselves and the world around them.

KEY CONCEPTS

- Growth describes a change in quantity and occurs when cells divide and synthesize new proteins.
- Maturation, a qualitative change, describes the aging process or an increase in competence and adaptability.
- Differentiation refers to a biologic description of the processes by which early cells and structures are modified and altered to achieve specific and characteristic physical and chemical properties.
- Development involves change from a lower to a more advanced stage of complexity.
- The five major developmental periods are: prenatal, infancy, early childhood, middle childhood, and later childhood (pubescence and adolescence).
- Growth and development proceeds in predictable patterns of direction, sequence, and pace.
- The directional trends in growth and development are: cephalocaudal, proximodistal, and mass to specific.
- Physical development includes increase in height and weight and changes in body proportion, dentition, and some body tissues.
- The three broad classifications of child temperament are: the easy child, the difficult child, and the slow-to-warm-up child.
- The developmental theories most widely used in explaining child growth and development are Freud's psychosexual stages, Erikson's stages of psychosocial development, Piaget's stages of cognitive development, and Kohlberg's stages of moral development.
- Development of self-concept occurs through a child's interactions and observations of his own experiences with others and with the environment.
- Factors influencing development include heredity, nutrition, disease, socioeconomic status, and interpersonal relationships.
- Play is one of the most important media through which children learn about themselves, others, and their environment.
- In addition to meeting the physical needs of children it is the responsibility of parents and caregivers to provide love and affection, promote physical and emotional security, provide discipline and authority, to allow for independence and dependence, and facilitate the development of a positive self-concept.

STUDY QUESTIONS AND ACTIVITIES

1 Compare two or more children of the same age for similarities and differences in physical, temperamental, and cognitive development.
2 Discuss each of Erikson's psychosocial stages and identify ways in which adults can facilitate a child's mastery of the developmental tasks of these stages.
3 Interview the parent, or parents, of a child in one of the major developmental stages to determine characteristics or behaviors in the child that indicate development of body image. Discuss these findings.
4 Discuss the roles of heredity, nutrition, and socioeconomic level in the development of children.
5 Visit a playground and observe the types of activities in which children of different age-groups are engaged. Determine which function, or functions, each of the observed activities serve in the growth and developmental processes.

REFERENCES

Chess, S., and Thomas, A.: Temperamental differences: a critical concept in child health care, Pediatr. Nurs. **11:**167-171, 1985.

Fowler, J.W.: Toward a developmental perspective on faith, Religious Educ. **69:**207-219, 1974.

Kohlberg, L.: The cognitive-developmental approach to moral education, Phi Delta Kappan **56:**670-677, 1975.

Lewis, M., and Block, J.R.: Toy play. IQ building. Mother's Manual, Sept./Oct., 1982, pp. 31-32.

Neumann, C.G., and Alpaugh, M.: Birth weight doubling time: a fresh look, Pediatrics **57:**469-473, 1976.

Stuart, G.W., and Sundeen, S.J.: Principles and practice of psychiatric nursing, ed. 3, St. Louis, 1987, The C.V. Mosby Co.

BIBLIOGRAPHY

Aquilino, M.L.: Healthy sexual development in childhood, Children's Nurse **4**(5):1-4, 1986.

Betz, C.L.: Faith development in children, Pediatr. Nurs. **7**(2):22-25, 1981.

Brown, C.C., and Gottried, A.W., editors: Play interactions: the role of toys and parental involvement in children's development, Skillman, NJ, 1985, Johnson & Johnson Baby Products Co.

Castiglia, P.T.: Growth and development, J. Pediatr. Health Care **1:**48-49, 1986.

Clark, M.K.: Exercise and physical fitness for good health in children, Children's Nurse **4**(1):1-3, 1986.

Coates, B., Pusser, H.E., and Goodman, I.: The influence of "Sesame Street" and "Mister Rogers' Neighborhood" on children's social behavior in the preschool, Child Dev. **47:**138-144, 1976.
Dashiff, C.J.: Coaching developmental differentiation, Top. Clin. Nurs. **1**(3):11-20, 1979.
Dettmore, D.: Spiritual care: remembering your patients' forgotten needs, Nursing 84 **14**(10):46, 1984.
Endres, J.B., and Rockwell, R.E.: Food, nutrition, and the young child, ed. 2, St. Louis, 1985, The C.V. Mosby Co.
Erikson, E.H.: Childhood and society, ed. 2, New York, 1963, W.W. Norton & Co., Inc.
Gifford, S., and Lieberman, B.I.: Evaluation of growth charts, Issues Compr. Pediatr. Nurs. **4**(2):1-25, 1980.
Grey, M., and Hayman, L.L.: Assessing stress in children: research and clinical implications, J. Pediatr. Nurs. **2:**316-327, 1987.
Lee, J., and Fowler, M.D.: Merely child's play? Developmental work and playthings, J. Pediatr. Nurs. **1:**260-270, 1986.
Lowrey, G.H.: Growth and development of children, ed. 8, Chicago, 1986, Year Book Medical Publishers, Inc.
McCown, D.: TV: its problems for children, Pediatr. Nurs. **5**(2):17-19, 1979.
McCown, D.E.: Moral development in children, Pediatr. Nurs. **10:**42-44, 1984.
Newman, B.M., and Newman, P.R.: Development through life: a psychosocial approach, ed. 3, Homewood, IL, 1984, The Dorsey Press.
Piaget, J.: The theory of stages in cognitive development, New York, 1969, McGraw-Hill Book Co.
Pipes, P.L.: Nutrition in infancy and childhood, ed. 3, St. Louis, 1985, The C.V. Mosby Co.
Pringle, S.M., and Ramsey, B.E.: Promoting the health of children, St. Louis, 1982, The C.V. Mosby Co.
Rothbart, M.K.: Measurement of temperament in infancy, Child Dev. **52:**569-578, 1981.
Rothenberg, M.B.: In my opinion . . . role of television in shaping the attitudes of children, Child. Health Care **13:**148-150, 1985.
Ryan, J.: The neglected crisis, Am. J. Nurs. **84:**1257-1258, 1984.
Selekman, J.: The development of body image in the child: a learned response, Top. Clin. Nurs. **5**(1):13-21, 1983.
Shaffer, D.R.: Developmental psychology: theory, research, and applications, Monterey, CA, 1984, Brooks/Cole Publishing Co.
Shelly, J.A.: Spiritual care: planting seeds of hope, Crit. Care Update **9**(12):7-15, 1982.
Sherwen, L.N.: Separation: the forgotten phenomenon of child development, Top. Clin. Nurs. **5:**1-11, 1983.
Stanwyck, D.J.: Self-esteem through the life span, Top. Clin. Nurs. **6**(2):11-28, 1983.
Stoll, R.I.: Guidelines for spiritual assessment, Am. J. Nurs. **79:**1575-1577, 1979.
Ventura, J.N.: Parent coping behaviors, parent functioning, and infant temperament characteristics, Nurs. Res. **31:**269-273, 1982.

UNIT III

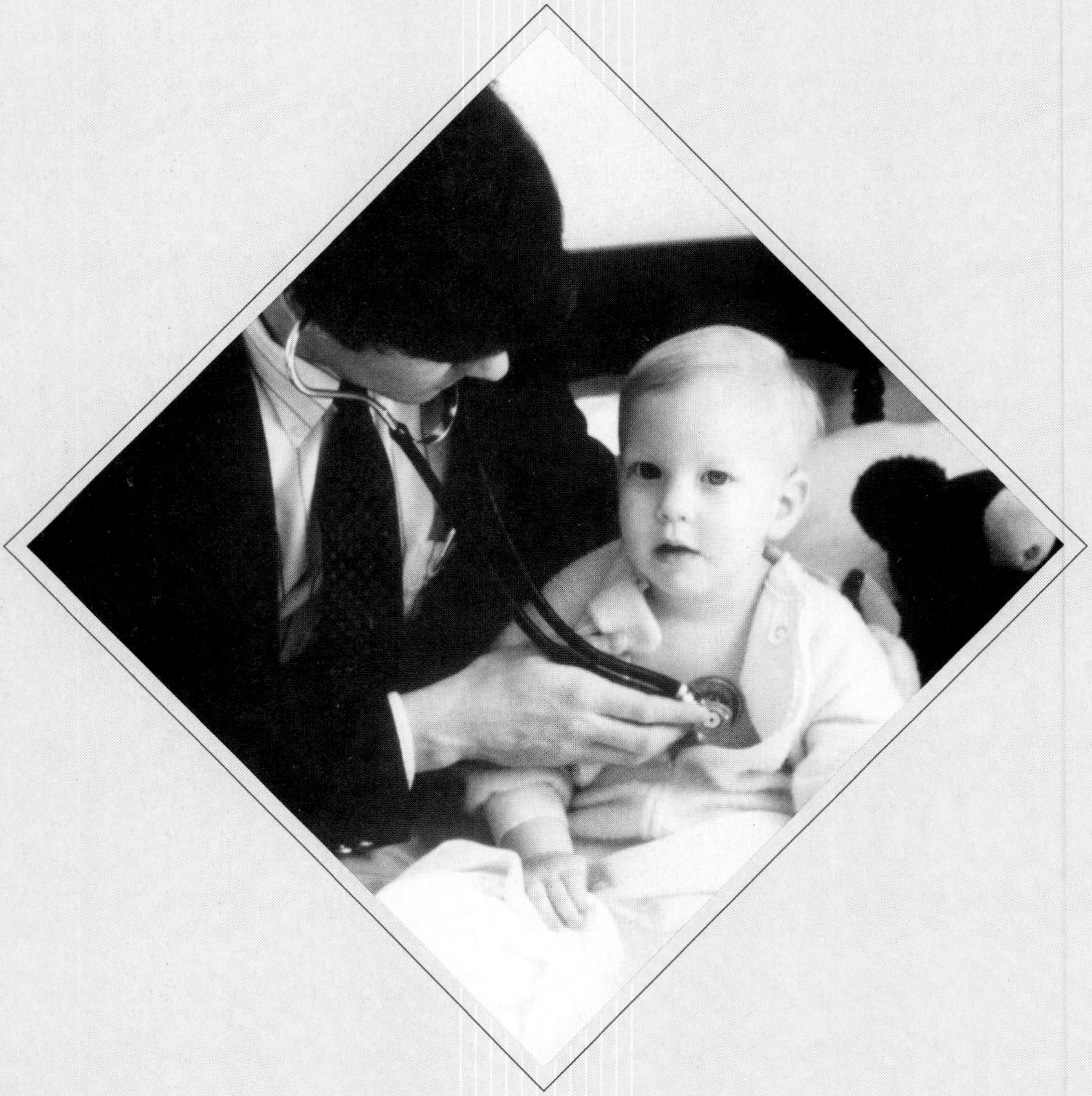

Assessment of the Child and Family

Assessment is fundamental to the nursing process. Establishing a data base on which to formulate a nursing diagnosis, plan interventions, and evaluate outcomes of care is essential whether the nurse is involved with a healthy or ill child. Assessment facilitates identification of present problems and prevention of future ones. Although the assessment process focuses primarily on the child, it permits an exploration into the family dynamics and is often the first clue to cultural, environmental, socioeconomic, or religious traditions that influence the child's total well-being.

Assessment primarily involves some form of communication. Chapter 6, *Communication and Health Assessment of the Child and Family,* is concerned with general aspects of communication as they relate to the nurse, parent, and child. It also discusses the interview process specifically in terms of history taking, with special emphasis on assessment of the family and nutrition.

Chapter 7, *Physical Assessment of the Child,* deals with the procedures and skills required to perform a complete pediatric physical assessment, including sensory and developmental testing. Findings primarily related to normal structure and function are emphasized, with notation of those deviations that require referral and further evaluation.

CHAPTER 6

Communication and Health Assessment of the Child and Family

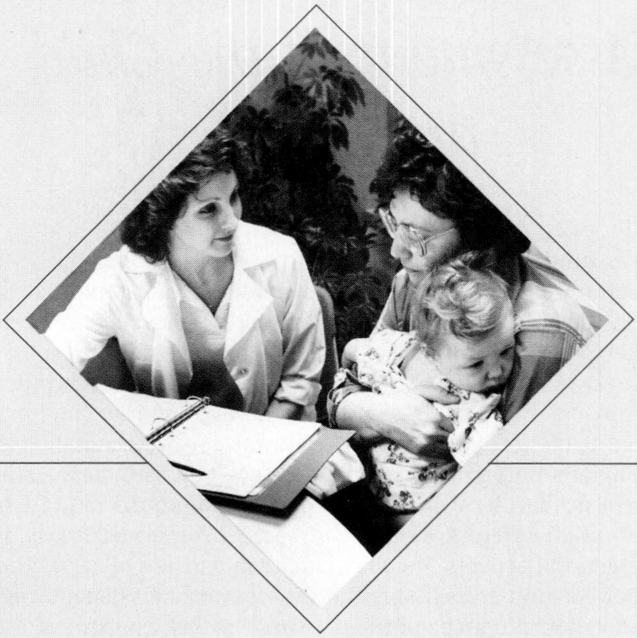

LEARNING OBJECTIVES

On completion of this chapter the reader will be able to:

- Describe guidelines for communication and interviewing
- Identify communication strategies for interviewing parents
- Formulate guidelines for using an interpreter
- Identify communication strategies for communicating with children of different age-groups
- Describe four communication techniques that are useful with children
- State the components of a complete health history
- Describe two strategies for structural and functional assessment of the family
- List three areas that are evaluated as part of nutritional assessment

Communication is essential to the nursing of children and families. It is the most important skill used in assessment of children and their families and the most important feature in forming trusting relationships with them. Communication consists of behaviors by which one person, consciously or unconsciously, affects another. All behavior transmits a message: even the attempt not to communicate creates a particular impression.

This chapter is concerned with the communication process. In the first section guidelines for communication and interviewing are reviewed and specific suggestions for communicating with parents and children are presented. The second section deals with a particular type of interview, the health history. It is presented in detail to give nurses the opportunity to learn to take a history, as well as to facilitate understanding those histories recorded by other health team members. Because of the importance of the family and nutrition in ensuring optimal emotional and physical health, special sections on family and nutritional assessment are included.

◆ *Communication*

The forms of communication may be verbal, nonverbal, or abstract. *Verbal* communication may involve language and its expression, vocalizations in the forms of laughs, moans, or squalls, or the implications of what is not said in light of what has been said. *Nonverbal* communication is often called body language and includes gestures, movements, facial expressions, postures, and reactions. *Abstract* communication takes the form of play, artistic expression, symbols, photographs, and choice of clothing. Because it is possible to exert greater conscious control over verbal communication, it is a less reliable indicator of true feelings, especially with children.

Many factors influence the communication process. To be successful (gratifying), communication must be appropriate to the situation, properly timed, and clearly delivered. This implies that nurses understand and use techniques of effective communication, including listening. Verbal and nonverbal messages must be congruent, that is, two or more messages sent via different levels must not be contradictory.

Nurses need to recognize their own feelings and attempt to recognize those of the persons with whom the communicative interchange takes place. Biases and judgments interfere with all aspects of the process. The tendency to approve or disapprove another's statements inhibits positive reactions. In addition, the transmission and reception of messages may be altered by influences of intimacy or distance, dependence or independence, trust or mistrust, security or insecurity, or caring and not caring on the part of the participants. The value of effective communication is increased understanding between the nurse, the child, and the family. Since nursing of infants and children always involves the inclusion of a caregiver, nurses must be able to communicate not only with children of all ages but with the adults in their lives as well.

VERBAL COMMUNICATION—THE POWER OF WORDS

Words shape reality, and thus they hold tremendous power. A person can change another's perception of reality by the choice of words that are used. For example, if the diagnosis of cancer is always referred to as a tumor, cyst, malignancy, or carcinoma, the person may never really know that he has cancer. Consequently he may assume less responsibility for his care than if he were aware of his condition's seriousness. By learning to recognize how patients and health professionals use language to manipulate reality, one can also learn how to change one's perceptions and communicate more effectively.

Avoidance Language

The most common way that people try to alter reality is by avoiding words that truly describe it. For example, euphemisms such as "passed on" are used instead of the word "death." Avoidance language indicates that a person wants to hide something, particularly his feelings. As a rule, accepting the person's use of euphemisms only serves to perpetuate his fears and never helps him to deal with them. In contrast, use of straightforward, precise, descriptive language lends perspective to the situation and allows the person to discuss his fears. Most often, imagined fears are much worse than reality.

Distancing Language

People may use impersonal words, such as "it" or "others," to shield themselves from the painful reality of a situation. For example, parents may state that they know *someone* with a child who is slow, when they may actually be talking about personal fears regarding *their* child. By realizing that the parents may need to talk about this difficult subject, the nurse can provide sensitive statements that ease them into discussing their situation.

One of the dangers in supporting distancing language is that the person may effectively deny that a problem exists. To return to the previous example, if the issue of retardation is never approached directly but is allowed to be "someone else's problem," the parents may not be able to make decisions for special schools or individualized training.

Sometimes distancing is desirable because the topic may be too painful to discuss directly. The use of the third-person technique (p. 110) may be very therapeutic in allowing an individual the opportunity to indirectly approach a subject and receive feedback but still remain in control.

NONVERBAL COMMUNICATION—PARALANGUAGE

In addition to the spoken word, messages are also relayed through nonverbal means, or paralanguage—the pitch, pause, intonation, rate, volume, and stress apparent in speech. Young children become very adept at understanding paralanguage; long before they know the meaning of words, they sense anxiety or fear by the rise in pitch or the accelerated rate of the parent's voice. By careful observation of the spoken word, nurses can better understand the meaning of another's verbal message and more accurately control their own paralanguage.

Because most people do not exert conscious control over their paralanguage, it is a valuable clue to feelings and concerns. For example, *pausing* may signify a need to formulate thoughts, recall information, or fabricate a story. Frequent pauses often make the speaker sound unsure of himself. Long pauses may mean that the individual needs more information.

Rate is another characteristic that gives unspoken messages. Talking too fast usually makes the speaker sound glib and insensitive. Talking slowly with a firm tone and appropriate pauses conveys authority. Therefore, a person is much more likely to "hear" instructions if the latter approach is used. Children in particular respond attentively to a slow, even, steady voice.

Confirming and Disconfirming Behaviors

People respond to each other through *confirming behaviors,* such as nodding the head, using direct eye contact, repeating or requesting clarification, and making appropriate comments, or *disconfirming behaviors,* such as tapping fingers or a foot, turning away from the speaker, avoiding eye contact, and interrupting (Heineken and Roberts, 1983). Since there is a reciprocal relationship between such behaviors, nurses need to use confirming behaviors to receive confirmation in return. This "mirroring" effect is particularly evident in children because of their sensitivity to nonverbal cues.

◆ *Guidelines for Communication and Interviewing*

Since nurses' effectiveness in practice depends to a large extent on their ability to relate to others, they use the communication process to help children and their parents make use of their professional knowledge and skill. The most widely used method of communicating with parents on a professional basis is the interview process. Interviewing, unlike social conversation, is a specific form of goal-directed communication. As nurses converse with parents, they endeavor to focus on the parents to determine the kind of persons they are, their usual mode of handling problems, whether help is needed, and the way in which parents react to counseling. It requires time and patience to develop interviewing skills. Some of the guiding principles and the obstacles that need to be avoided to facilitate this process are discussed here.

ESTABLISHING THE SETTING

Part of the success in interviewing depends on the type of physical and psychologic setting the interviewer constructs. Appropriate introduction, role clarification, explanation of the reason for the interview, preliminary acquaintance with the family, and assurance of privacy and confidentiality are prerequisites for establishing a setting conducive to communication.

Appropriate Introduction

Nurses should introduce themselves to and ask the name of each family member who is present. During the interview, each person is addressed by name. If there is any question about using the person's first or last name, common courtesy should be the guiding rule. Asking individuals which name they wish to be called conveys respect and communicates a personal interest in them.

At the beginning of the visit, the nurse can include the child in the interaction by asking him his name, age, and other information. Nurses often direct all questions to the adult, even when the child is old enough to speak for himself. This serves to terminate one extremely valuable source of information, the patient himself. When including the child, the general rules for communicating with children are followed (p. 106).

Role Clarification and Explanation of the Interview

During the introduction it is also necessary to clarify the nurse's particular role in the health setting. For example, nurses performing interviews may be pediatric nurse practitioners, inpatient staff nurses, clinic nurses, office nurses, visiting nurses, or school nurses. Since the format resembles a medical history, the nurse needs to clarify the reason for eliciting this information. A parent is much more likely to reveal personal information about the child and family if the relevance and importance of the interview are stressed. If this is not done, parents may refuse to elaborate on certain areas because they feel it has no bearing on the "problem." In addition, since more than one member of the health team may take a history during the course of a hospital admission, it is important to clarify the reason for each interview.

Another reason for role clarification is education of the health consumer. With expanded roles in nursing, it is not unusual for families to think that the examiner is a physician, not a nurse. Role clarification is especially important because some parents may feel deceived if they later are made aware of the nurse's identity. Since the general consumer acceptance of pediatric nurse practitioners has been very favorable, it is also important for them to acknowledge their expertise by emphasizing their role.

Preliminary Acquaintance

To make the family feel at ease and to develop rapport, it is best to begin the interview with some general conversation. The opening statements should be general but still informative. Comments such as "How have things been since your last visit?" "Tell me about Johnny," or (to the child) "What do you think is going to happen today?" allow the parent or child to express his main concern in a casual, relaxed atmosphere.

The preliminary acquaintance conversation also reveals how responsive the informant may be to questions. For example, using open-ended statements, such as "Tell me about the baby," may lead the parent into a lengthy detailed discussion. In this case it may be more beneficial to direct questions toward specific answers in order to avoid irrelevant remarks. At other times a parent may respond to open-ended questions with only minimal information, in which case the continued use of open-ended questions probably reveals more data than "yes" or "no" type questions.

Assurance of Privacy and Confidentiality

The place where the interview is conducted is almost as important as the interview itself. The physical environment should allow for as much privacy as possible and the nurse should keep distractions, such as interruptions, noise, or other visible activity, to a minimum. At times it may be necessary to turn off a television or radio. The environment should also have some play provision for young children to keep them occupied during the parent-nurse interview (Fig. 6-1). Parents who are constantly interrupted by their children are unable to concentrate fully on the questions asked of them and tend to give short answers to terminate the interview as quickly as possible.

Confidentiality is another essential component of the initial phase of the interview. Since the interview is usually shared with other members of the health team or the teacher (as in the case of students), it is the interviewer's responsibility and obligation to inform the parents of the confidential limits of their conversation. If there is any concern regarding confidentiality, such as talking to a parent suspected of child abuse or a teenager contemplating suicide, the nurse must deal with this directly and inform the person that in such instances confidentiality cannot be ensured.

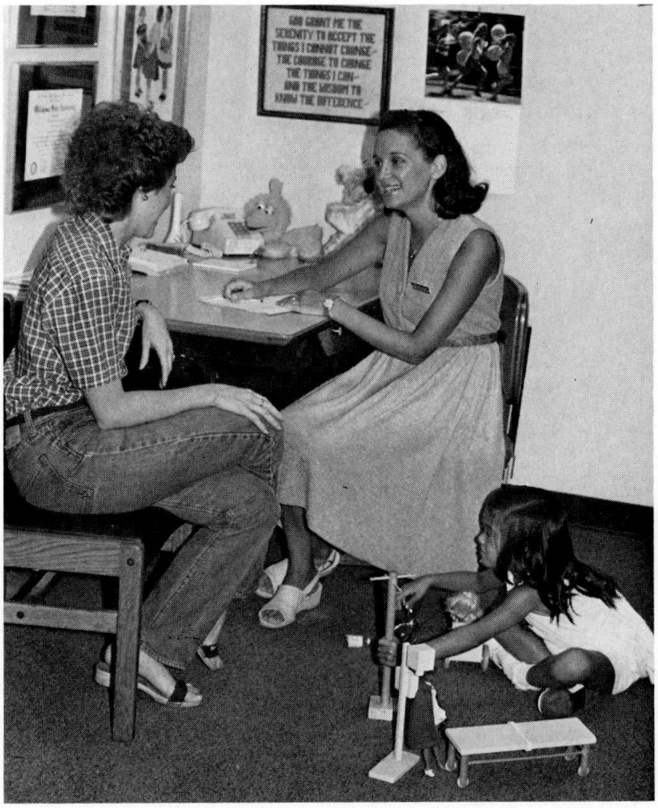

FIG. 6-1 Child plays while nurse interviews parent.

◆ *Communicating with Families*

Communicating with the family is a triangular process involving the nurse, parents, and child. Although the following discussion focuses primarily on this triad, in many circumstances significant others, for example, siblings, relatives, or other caregivers, may be part of the communication process.

COMMUNICATING WITH PARENTS

Although the parent and child are separate and distinct entities, relationships with the child are frequently mediated via the parent, particularly in the case of younger children. For the most part, information about the child is acquired by direct observation or is communicated to the nurse by the parents. Usually it can be assumed that because of the close contact with the child, the information imparted by the parent is reliable. To make an assessment of the child requires input from the child (verbal and nonverbal), information from the parent, and the nurse's own observations, including assessment of the child and interpretation of the relationship between the child and the parent. Counseling and guidance must be directed to the caregiver of infants and small children; when children are old enough to be active participants in their own health maintenance, the parent becomes a collaborator in health care.

Encouraging the Parent to Talk

Interviewing parents not only offers the opportunity to determine the health and developmental status of the child but also offers cues and guides to all those factors that influence the child's life. Whatever the parent sees as a problem should be a concern of the nurse. These problems are not always easy to identify. Nurses will need to be alert for clues and signals by which a parent communicates worries and anxieties. Careful phrasing with broad open-ended questions such as "What is Jimmy eating now?" provides more information than several single-answer questions such as "Is Jimmy eating what the rest of the family eats?"

Sometimes the parent will take the lead without prompting. At other times it may be necessary to direct another question based on an observation such as "Connie seems unhappy today" or "How do you feel when David cries?" If the parent appears to be tired or distraught, the nurse might ask, "What do you do to relax?" or "What help do you have with the children?" A comment such as "You handle the baby very well. What kinds of experience have you had with babies?" to new parents who appear comfortable with their first child gives positive reinforcement and provides an opening for any questions they might have regarding the care of the infant. Often all that is required to keep parents talking is a nod or saying "yes" or "uh-huh" to let them know the nurse is listening and interested.

When attempting to elicit feelings and covert problem areas, it is best to avoid beginning a question with "Does . . .," "Did . . .," or "It's . . .," which usually require only a single response. In addition, asking questions such as "Do you have any problem with your son at school?" subtly implies a lack of parental skills and evokes defensiveness. Instead, it is helpful to say "What . . .," "How . . .," "Tell me about . . .," and to encourage elaboration with "You were saying . . .," "You say that . . .," or reflecting back a key word. Open-ended questions are nonthreatening and encourage description.

Directing the Focus

The ability to direct the focus of the interview while allowing for maximum freedom of expression is one of the most difficult goals in effective communication. One approach is the use of open-ended or broad questions, followed with guiding statements. For example, if the parent proceeds to list the other children by name, the nurse can say, "Tell me their ages, too." If the parent continues on this theme by describing each child in-depth, which is not the purpose of the interview, the focus can be redirected by stating, "Let's talk about the other children later. You were beginning to tell me about Paul's activities at school." This approach conveys interest in the other children but focuses the data collection on the identified patient.

In the event that the parent has suggested that a problem exists with one of the other children, the nurse should reintroduce this subject at the end of the interview to assess the need for further family follow-up. Saying to the parent, "Before, you were mentioning that your older son is having trouble in school. Tell me what you see as the problem," reintroduces this subject but only in terms of the possible problem.

Listening

Listening is the most important component of effective communication. When listening is truly aimed at understanding the client, it is an active process that requires concentration and attention to all aspects of the conversation—verbal, nonverbal, and abstract. A major block to listening is premature judgment.

The attitudes and feelings of the nurse are easily introduced into an interview. Often nurses' perception of a parent's behavior is influenced by their own perceptions, prejudices, and assumptions, which may include racial, religious, and cultural stereotypes. What may be interpreted as passive hostility or disinterest in a parent may be shyness or an expression of anxiety. For example, direct eye contact is frequently regarded as a sign of paying attention. However, in many Native American tribes, looking into another's eyes is considered disrespectful. Therefore, judgments about "listening" need to be made with an appreciation of cultural differences.

Although it is necessary to make some preliminary judgments, the nurse must attempt to "hear" the parent with as much objectivity as possible by clarifying meanings and attempting to see the situation from the parent's point of view. Effective interviewers use conscious control over their reactions and responses and over the techniques they employ.

Use of minimum verbal activity with active listening facilitates parent involvement. Nurses are prone to become quite verbal when health education and advice are indicated. It is tempting to spend time explaining, describing, and interpreting health information when the opportunity presents itself. However, it is possible to provide effective health education by properly timing the information and presenting only as much as is necessary at the moment.

Careful listening facilitates the use of clues, verbal leads, or signals from the interviewee to move the interview along. Frequent references to an area, repetition of certain key words, or a special emphasis on something or someone serve as cues to the interviewer for the direction of inquiry. Concerns and anxieties are usually mentioned in a casual, offhand manner. Even though they are casual, they are of importance and deserve careful scrutiny. This serves to identify problem areas and to pursue the investigation and solution of a problem with systematic questioning. For example, a mother who is concerned about a child's habit of bed-wetting may casually mention that his bed was "wet this morning."

Because the interview is almost always triangular—that is, between the nurse, parent, and child—the parent may wish to convey information in such a way as to prevent the child from hearing it. This requires active listening on the part of the nurse to hear the unspoken message. The following example illustrates this point:

> During a routine health visit the nurse performed a complete history and physical examination on a 4-year-old girl. The child was accompanied by her mother, who appeared to be a reliable, well-informed, and talkative informant. During the child's birth history, the mother gave all the information asked. However, during the family history, the mother stated to the nurse, "I had a hysterectomy 6 years ago." Because the nurse gave no indication of acknowledging the significance of this statement, the mother repeated it, only this time she stressed the "6 years." The nurse, who had not been listening as attentively as she should have, realized that the mother was telling her something very important. The mother raised her eyebrows and gently shook her head "no," warning the nurse not to explore this area too openly. The nurse correctly read the cues and stated, "Let's return to your health history later."
>
> At the completion of the physical examination, the nurse brought the child to the health center's playroom and took the opportunity to investigate this contradictory information of a "4-year-old child born to a woman with a hysterectomy 6 years ago." The mother revealed that this child was adopted. The mother was greatly concerned about the fact that the child was unaware of this and requested the nurse's advice. Fortunately the nurse had "listened" carefully enough to realize the significance of this woman's concern and allowed her the opportunity to discuss it in private.

Listening is also helpful in assessing reliability. For example, the answers elicited at the beginning of the interview may differ from those at the end, when the parent feels more confident in revealing problems. It is important to identify any discrepancies and reintroduce those topics for further investigation.

Using Silence

Silence as a response is often one of the most difficult interviewing techniques to learn. It requires a sense of confidence and comfort on the part of the interviewer to allow the interviewee space in which to think without interruptions. Silence permits the interviewee to sort out thoughts and feelings or to search for responses to questions. It also allows for sharing of feelings in which two or more people absorb the emotion to its depth.

Sometimes it is necessary to break the silence and reopen communication. This should be done in a way that encourages the person to continue talking about what is important to him. Breaking a silence by introducing a new topic or by prolonged talking essentially terminates the interviewee's opportunity to use the silence. Suggestions for breaking the silence include statements such as: "Is there anything else you wish to say?" "I see you find it difficult to continue; how may I help?" or "I don't know what this silence means. Perhaps there is something you would like to put into words but find difficult to say."

Being Empathic

Empathy means feeling and participating in the inner emotions of another while remaining objective. The empathic interviewer attempts to see the world from the interviewee's perspective and to understand him as much as possible. Empathy differs from sympathy, which is subjectively thinking or feeling like the other person. While important and necessary at times, sympathy is not always therapeutic in the helping relationship.

Of the different types of support, such as empathy, encouragement (positive reinforcement in regard to a parent's actions), or reassurance (pacifying a parent's concern or worry), empathy is the most beneficial but least used form. Some individuals are naturally empathic and easily "feel" with another person. However, empathy can be learned by attending to the verbal and nonverbal language of the interviewee. Neurolinguistic programming (NLP) is concerned with the *manner* of accessing and understanding information and is an excellent method of increasing empathic communication. Although people may use all of the following sensory modalities to communicate, usually one modality predominates: visual, auditory, or kinesthetic. The specific sensory mode is identified by observing the type of verbs, adjectives, and adverbs the person uses and then using this mode in responding to the individual. For example, the person using the visual mode may state, "I can't *see* why you have to perform these procedures on my child." A response using the same mode is, "What do you see as the problem?"

Defining the Problem

In order to arrive at a solution to a problem, the nurse and the parent must agree that a problem exists. If neither believes that there is a problem, there is certainly no need to create one. Sometimes the parent may believe that there is a problem that the nurse is unable to see. For example, a mother was overly concerned about every small sniffle, sneeze, or cough in her infant who had been carefully examined and found to be healthy with no evidence of a respiratory problem. On careful questioning, the nurse discovered that a previous child had died of pneumonia in infancy. Consequently the nurse was able to better understand the mother's concern. Once the nurse acknowledges the mother's fear, she can help the mother deal with her special anxieties about her infant and teach her how to recognize when there is need for concern.

Occasionally the nurse identifies a problem that the parent denies exists. In this case the nurse should pursue the situation and either find a way to deal with the situation or enlist the aid of other health team members. For example, the parents of a child with Down syndrome may refuse to believe that their child is different from any other child of the same age. They may say, "He is just a little slow" and "All the child needs to do is to try harder." A child with an obvious behavior problem may be described by the parents as "stubborn." Such statements may be clues that the parents have not progressed past the stage of denial in adjusting to the condition.

Solving the Problem

Once the problem is identified and agreed on by the parent and the nurse, they can begin to arrive at a solution. A parent who is included in the problem-solving process is more apt to follow through with a course of action. Such questions as "What have you tried so far?" or "What have you thought about doing?" provide leads for exploration and give the parents the feeling that their ideas and solutions are worthwhile. These can be followed by "What prevents you from trying that?" "That sounds like a good plan," and "You seem to be stumped. Have you considered trying this?" Such approaches reinforce rather than belittle parents' efforts to solve their problems and encourage active participation.

Sometimes the parents arrive at a solution that the nurse does not consider the best alternative. If it can be ascertained that it will do no harm and if the parents are convinced of its merits, it is usually best to allow them to continue with the plan. A course of action is more likely to be carried out when parents can reach their own conclusions. However, when parental decisions may be hazardous, nurses are obligated to discuss the risks with the family and try to reach a more beneficial solution. Whenever possible, decisions should be theirs with the nurse serving as a *facilitator* in problem solving.

Providing Anticipatory Guidance

The ideal way to handle a problem is to prevent it—to deal with it *before* it becomes a problem. The best preventive measure is anticipatory guidance. One of the most significant areas in pediatrics is injury prevention through appropriate anticipatory guidance. Beginning prenatally, parents need specific instructions on home safety. Because of the child's maturing developmental skills, home safety changes must be implemented early to minimize risks to the child.

Many normal developmental changes can disturb unprepared parents, such as a toddler's diminished appetite, negativism, altered sleeping patterns, and anxiety toward strangers. Such topics are discussed in the chapters on health promotion to provide the nurse with knowledge to counsel parents.

Avoiding Blocks to Communication

There are a number of blocks to communication. Some of the more common blocks include:

- Socializing
- Giving unrestricted and sometimes unasked-for advice
- Offering premature or inappropriate reassurance
- Giving overready encouragement
- Defending a situation or opinion
- Using stereotyped comments or cliches
- Cutting off expression of emotion by asking directed, close-ended questions
- Interrupting and finishing the person's sentence
- Talking more than the interviewee
- Forming prejudged conclusions
- Deliberately changing the focus

Each of these can be corrected by careful analysis of the interview process. One of the best methods for improving interviewing skills is audiotape and/or videotape feedback. With supervision and guidance, the interviewer can recognize the blocks and consciously avoid them.

Communicating with Families through an Interpreter

Sometimes communication is impossible because two people speak different languages. In this case it is necessary to obtain information through a third party, an interpreter. When an interpreter is used, the guidelines in the box should be employed.

The guidelines for using an interpreter apply primarily to the use of an adult interpreter (Kohut, 1975). Often no one other than an older child is available to help translate. In this situation it is important to stress *literal* translation of parent responses. To maximize correct translations, it may be necessary to interrupt the parent and ask the child to translate every few sentences. When children are used as interpreters, the nurse needs to ask questions directed at specific answers and must assess the interpreted translation in terms of nonverbal expressions of communication.

Guidelines for Using an Interpreter

- Explain to interpreter reason for interview and type of questions that will be asked
- Clarify whether a detailed or brief answer is required and whether the translated response can be general or literal
- Introduce interpreter to family and allow some time before actual interview so that they can become acquainted
- Communicate directly with family members when asking questions to reinforce interest in them and to observe nonverbal expressions
- Refrain from interrupting family member and interpreter while they are conversing
- Avoid commenting to interpreter about family members since they may understand some English
- Respect cultural differences; it is often best to pose questions about sex, marriage, or pregnancy indirectly—ask about child's "father" rather than mother's "husband"
- Allow time following interview for interpreter to share something that he or she felt could not be said earlier; ask about interpreter's impression of nonverbal clues to communication and family members' reliability or ease in revealing information
- Arrange for family to speak with same interpreter on subsequent visits whenever possible

COMMUNICATING WITH CHILDREN

Although the greatest amount of verbal communication is usually carried out with the parent, the child should not be excluded during the interview. Periodic attention to infants and younger children through play or by occasionally directing questions or remarks to them makes children participants in the interview. Older children can be actively included as informants.

General guidelines for communicating with children are presented in the box. In addition, some points are elaborated on below. Effective communication requires active effort on the nurse's part to be sensitive to the needs of children at different ages. For example, while young children feel most secure in the presence of their parents, older children may prefer the opportunity to talk alone with the nurse. Specific developmental needs are presented on p. 108.

When relating with children of all ages, it is the nonverbal components of the communication process that convey the most significant messages to them. They are very alert to feelings, attitudes, and surroundings and attach meaning to every gesture and move that is made. This is particularly true with very young children. It is best to avoid rushing in on a child with gestures or with words. The child should be allowed time to make the first move when possible. Sudden or rapid advances are frightening to a child, as are threatening gestures such as facial contortions, including very broad smiles. Although these are usually intended as friendly gestures, they frequently have the opposite effect.

General Guidelines for Communicating with Children

- Allow children time to feel comfortable with the nurse
- Avoid sudden or rapid advances, broad smiles, extended eye contact, or other gestures that may be seen as threatening
- Talk to the parent if child is initially shy
- Communicate through transition objects such as dolls, puppets, or stuffed animals before questioning a young child directly
- Give older children the opportunity to talk without the parents present
- Assume a position that is at eye level with the child
- Speak in a quiet, unhurried, and confident voice
- Speak clearly, be specific, use simple words, and short sentences
- State directions and suggestions *positively*
- Offer choices only when one exists
- Be honest with children
- Allow them to express their concerns and fears
- Use a variety of communication techniques

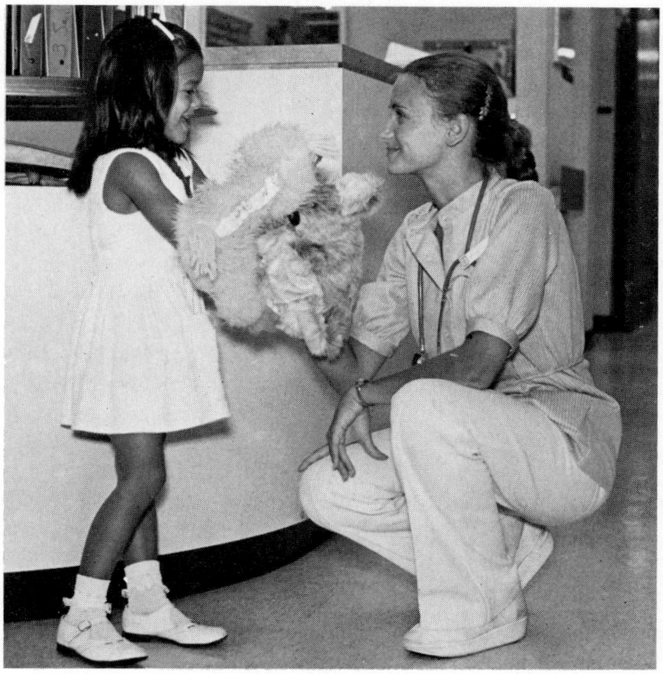

FIG. 6-2 Nurse talks to child using puppets and assumes a position at the child's level.

Children are uncomfortable or even frightened when someone stares at them. It is best to refrain from extended eye contact with a child. Active attempts to make friends with children before they have had an opportunity to evaluate an unfamiliar person tend to increase their anxiety. A helpful tactic is to continue to talk to the child and parent but go about activities that do not involve the child directly, thus allowing him to carry out his observations from a safe position. If the child has a special toy or doll with him, it is helpful to "talk" to the doll first. Also, asking the child simple questions such as, "Does your teddy bear have a special name?" may ease the child into conversation.

Children should be met on their own eye level since communicating down to them emphasizes their smallness. Adults in strange places may assume overwhelming proportions to children who believe themselves to be in helpless positions. Sitting on a low chair, kneeling, squatting, or even sitting on the floor, if appropriate, places the nurse in a more favorable and less threatening position (Fig. 6-2). With very young children every effort is made to preserve physical closeness with the parent. Consequently the entire interview may be done with the child sitting on the parent's lap. Giving the child a toy, bottle, or pacifier helps to quiet him.

With young children much of the nurse's communication centers around gaining the child's cooperation for procedures. When giving directions or suggestions, these are best stated *positively*. An easy way to do this is to avoid using the word "don't." There is more likelihood that a child's cooperation will be gained by saying, "I need you to stay very quiet" rather than "Don't make any noise."

It is confusing to children when they are offered a choice when there actually is none. Again, a positive approach is most successful. For example, when clothes must be removed for an examination, the question "Would you like to take off your dress?" offers the child an alternative she in fact does not have. The statement "We need the dress off so that I can listen to your chest. Shall I help you take it off?" gives the child an explanation, a choice, and some measure of control in the situation.

The nurse should be honest with children and make no promises that are impossible to carry out. To assure them that a procedure, such as an injection, will not hurt is no measure of comfort to children who have either experienced the discomfort previously or who discover that indeed it *does* hurt. Any trust that has been built between the child and the nurse will be damaged by the deception, and the child will be justifiably angry. If children appear upset or concerned, every effort is made to encourage verbalization of feelings.

Children should be told in advance what is going to happen to them. They are fearful of the unknown, and their active imaginations can fantasize images out of proportion to the actual event. Preparation for procedures is discussed in detail in Chapter 21, and developmental considerations are presented below.

Communication Related to Development of Thought Processes

The normal development of language and thought offers a frame of reference in knowing how to communicate with children. Thought processes progress from concrete to functional and finally to abstract, formal operations.

Infancy. Because they are unable to use words, infants primarily use and understand nonverbal communication. Infants communicate their needs and feelings through nonverbal behaviors and vocalizations that can be interpreted by someone who is around them for a sufficient amount of time. Infants smile and coo when content and cry when distressed. Crying is provoked by unpleasant stimuli from inside or outside, such as hunger, pain, body restraint, or loneliness. Adults interpret this to mean that an infant needs something and consequently try to alleviate the discomfort and reduce tension. Crying (or the desire to cry) persists as a part of everyone's communication repertoire.

Infants respond to adults' nonverbal behaviors. They become quiet when they are cuddled, patted, or receive other forms of gentle, physical contact. They derive comfort from the sound of a voice even though they do not understand the words that are spoken. Until infants reach the age where they experience stranger anxiety, they readily respond to any firm, gentle handling and quiet, calm speech. Loud, harsh sounds and sudden movements are frightening.

Older infants' attentions are centered on themselves and their mothers; therefore, any stranger is a potential threat until proved otherwise. Holding out the hands and asking the child to "come" is seldom successful, especially if the infant is with the mother. If infants must be handled, the best approach is simply to pick them up firmly without gestures. It is helpful to observe the position in which the parent holds the infant. Most infants have learned to prefer a particular position and manner of handling. In general, infants are more at ease upright than horizontal. It is also best to hold infants in such a way that they can keep their parents in view. Until they have developed the understanding that an object (in this case the parent) removed from sight can still be present, they have no way of knowing that the object is still there.

Early childhood. Children less than 5 years of age are almost completely egocentric. They see things only in relation to themselves and from their point of view. Therefore, any communication to them should be focused on *them*. They need to be told what they can do or how they will feel. Experiences of others are of no interest to them. It is futile to use another child's experience as an attempt to gain the cooperation of very small children. They should be allowed to touch, examine, and familiarize themselves with articles that will come in contact with them. A stethoscope bell will feel cold; palpating a neck might tickle. Although they have not yet acquired sufficient language skills to express their feelings and wants, toddlers are able to communicate effectively with their hands to transmit ideas without words. They push an unwanted object away, pull another person to show them something, point, and cover the mouth that is saying something they do not wish to hear.

Everything is direct and concrete to small children.

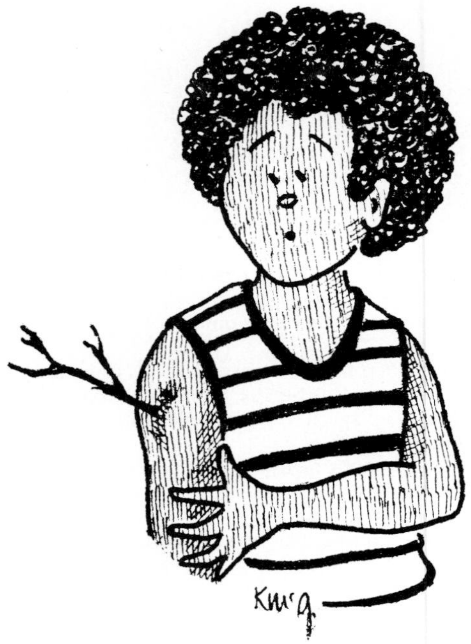

FIG. 6-3 To a young child the expression "a little stick in the arm" is taken literally.

They are unable to work with abstractions and base all deductions on literal formulations. Analogies escape them because they are unable to separate fact from fantasy. For example, they attach literal meaning to such common phrases as "two-faced," "sticky fingers," or "coughing your head off." Children who are told they will get "a little stick in the arm" may not be able to envision an injection (Fig. 6-3). These literal interpretations are an appealing part of this phase of development, but nurses must be aware of inadvertently using a phrase that might be misinterpreted by a small child.

Language is used that is consistent with the child's developmental level. For example, in talking with a young child, it is best to use simple, *short* sentences, repeat words that are *familiar* to the child, and limit descriptions to *concrete* explanations. A general rule for length of a sentence is: one word for each year of age plus one additional word.

Children in this age category assign human attributes to inanimate objects. They endow mechanical devices and instruments with living characteristics. Consequently they fear that these objects may jump, bite, cut, or pinch all by themselves. Children do not know that these devices are unable to perform without human direction. Unfamiliar equipment needs to be simply explained without building the child's fantasies. Understanding comes slowly and is not usually achieved with one explanation, so things should be explained and described over and over again. If the child does understand, he may be seeking affirmation.

School-age years. Children ages 5 to 8 years rely less on what they see and more on what they know when faced with new problems. They want explanations and reasons for everything but require no verification beyond that.

They are interested in the functional aspect of all procedures, objects, and activities. They want to know why an object exists, why it is used, how it works, and the intent and purpose of its user. They need to know what is going to take place and why it is being done to *them* specifically. For example, to explain a procedure such as taking a blood pressure, the nurse might show the child how squeezing the bulb pushes air into the cuff and makes the "silver" in the tube go up. The child should be permitted to operate the bulb. An explanation for the reason might be as simple as, "I want to see how far the silver goes up when the cuff squeezes your arm." Consequently the child becomes an enthusiastic participant. Allowing children to ask questions about what is happening to them and maintaining a permissive atmosphere is conducive to questioning.

Children at this age have a heightened concern about body integrity. Because of the special importance and value they place on their body, they are overly sensitive to anything that constitutes a threat or suggestion of injury to it. This concern extends to their possessions also, so that they may appear to overreact to loss or threatened loss of those objects that they treasure. Helping children to voice their concerns enables the nurse to provide reassurance and to implement activities that reduce their anxiety. For example, if a reticent child fears being the single object of probing inquiry, the nurse can ignore that particular child by talking and relating to other children in the family or group. When the child no longer feels like a single target, he will usually interject his ideas, feelings, and interpretations of events.

Older children have an adequate and satisfactory use of language. They still require relatively simple explanations, but their ability to think concretely can facilitate communication and explanation. Commonly they have sufficient experience with health and health workers to understand what is transpiring and generally what is expected of them.

Adolescence. As children move into adolescence, they fluctuate between child and adult thinking and behavior. They are riding a current that is moving them rapidly toward a maturity that may be beyond their coping ability. Therefore, when tensions rise, they may seek the security of the more familiar and comfortable expectations of childhood. Anticipating these shifts in identity allows the nurse to adjust the course of interaction to meet the needs of the moment. No single approach can be relied on consistently, and one can expect to encounter hostility, anger, bravado, and a variety of other behaviors and attitudes. It is as much a mistake to regard the adolescent as an adult with an adult's wisdom and control as it is to confine to him the concerns and expectations of a child.

Frequently adolescents are more willing to discuss their concerns with an adult outside the family, and they often welcome the opportunity to interact with a nurse. They are extremely susceptible to the advances of anyone who displays a genuine interest in them. However, adolescents are quick to reject persons who attempt to impose their values on them, whose interest is feigned, or who appear to have little respect for who they are and what they think or say.

As with all children, adolescents need to express their feelings. Generally they talk quite freely when given an opportunity. However, what adolescents say cannot always be taken at face value. When emotional factors are involved, the feelings that are interjected into words are as significant as the words that are used. The best way to give support is to be attentive, try not to interrupt, and avoid comments or expressions that convey disapproval or surprise. Prying and asking embarrassing questions should be avoided, and any impulse to give advice should be resisted. Frequently adolescents reveal their feelings or a source of concern or ask a question when they are involved in routine matters such as a physical assessment.

Teenagers characteristically have a language and culture all their own that further sets them apart from others. To avoid misinterpretation, frequent clarification of terms is advisable. Occasionally adolescents are reticent and answer only in monosyllables. Usually this happens when they are opposed to the contact with the nurse or do not yet feel safe enough to reveal themselves. In this instance the best approach is to confine discussions to irrelevant topics to reduce the element of threat until such time as they feel more secure. The nurse must be alert for signals that indicate they are ready to talk. The major sources of concern for adolescents are attitudes and feelings toward sex, relationships with parents, peer-group acceptance, and developing a sense of identity.

Interviewing the adolescent presents some special situations to the interviewer. The first may be whether to talk to the adolescent alone, with the parents, or to each individually. Of course, if the adolescent is alone, there is no question, except that the nurse might want to suggest to the teenager that the nurse talk with the parents at another time. If parents and teenager are together, talking with the adolescent first has the advantage of immediately identifying with the young person, thus fostering the interpersonal relationship. However, talking with the parents initially may provide insight into the family relationship. Whichever decision is made, both parties need an opportunity to be included in the interview. If time constraints are important, such as during history taking, these need to be clarified at the onset to avoid appearing to "take sides" by talking more with one person than the other.

Confidentiality is of great importance when interviewing adolescents. The parents and the teenager need to know the limits of confidentiality, specifically that the young person's disclosures will be kept between him and the nurse. However, exceptions also must be clarified, such as breaking confidence if it is necessary for the welfare of the adolescent, as in the event of suicidal behavior.

Another dilemma in interviewing adolescents is that two views of a problem frequently exist—the teenager's and the parents'. Clarification of the problem is a major task. However, providing both parties with an opportunity to discuss their perceptions in an open and unbiased atmosphere can, by itself, be therapeutic. The nurse, by demonstrating positive communication skills, can help families communicate more effectively.

COMMUNICATION TECHNIQUES

Besides the conventional interviewing methods of reflection, open-ended questions, and prompting statements, a number of other techniques encourage children, and sometimes other individuals, to express their thoughts and feelings in a less direct and confronting manner. The following is a discussion of several verbal and nonverbal approaches that can be helpful in a variety of instances. Throughout the book examples are given that use techniques described here.

Verbal Techniques

A number of verbal techniques can be used to encourage communication. Several of these are techniques that the interviewer can employ to pose questions or concerns in a less threatening manner. Others can be presented as "word games" that are often well received by children.

Third-person technique. The third-person technique involves expressing a feeling in terms of a third person. This technique is less threatening than directly asking a child how he feels, because it gives him the opportunities to agree or disagree without being defensive. For example, the nurse may comment, "Sometimes when a person is sick a lot he feels angry and sad because he cannot do what others can," and either wait silently for a response or encourage a reply with a statement such as, "Did you ever feel that way?" This approach allows the child three choices: (1) to agree and, hopefully, express how he feels, (2) to disagree, or (3) to remain silent, in which case he probably has such feelings but is unable to express them at that time. Demonstrating to parents how useful such techniques are also helps them learn new ways of communicating with the child.

Another variation of the third-person technique is to ask about friends, for example, "Do any of your friends smoke or drink alcohol?" Since peer group activity is a good indicator of the child's activity, this may introduce the topic in such a way that the young person is able to talk about his habits or concerns.

Facilitative responding. Facilitative responding is the careful listening and reflecting back to patients the feelings and content of their statements. Such responses are empathetic, nonjudgmental, and legitimize the person's feelings. The formula for facilitative responses is, "You feel ____________ because ______________" (Henrich and Bernheim, 1981).

For example, if a child states, "I hate coming to the hospital and getting shots," a facilitative response is, "You feel unhappy because of all the things that are done to you." (See also the Therapeutic dialogue on p. 119.)

Storytelling. Storytelling uses the language of the child to probe into areas of his thinking while bypassing conscious inhibitions or fears. Children respond to a variety of storytelling techniques. The simplest is asking a child to relate a story about an event, such as "being in the hospital." Another approach involves showing him a picture of a particular event, such as a child in a hospital with other people in the room, and asking him to describe the scene. Comic strips cut from a newspaper with the words removed are excellent vehicles when the child ascribes his own statements to each comic scene (Epstein, 1975). If the child draws a family or hospital scene, he can fill in short verbal communication above each person, similar to a comic strip theme (Fig. 6-4).

Mutual storytelling involves a more therapeutic approach. It not only serves to uncover the child's thinking but also attempts to change the child's perceptions or fears by retelling a somewhat different story. It is a powerful tool and must be used wisely. It begins by asking the child to tell a story about something, followed by another story told by the nurse that is similar to the child's tale but that has differences that help the child in problem areas. A typical example is the child's story of going to the hospital and never seeing his parents again. The nurse's story is also of a child (using different names but similar circumstances) in a hospital whose parents visit every day, but in the evening after coming home from work. In this way the child's fears of abandonment and separation are handled.

Sometimes children need help in beginning a story with encouragements, such as "Once upon a time . . .,"

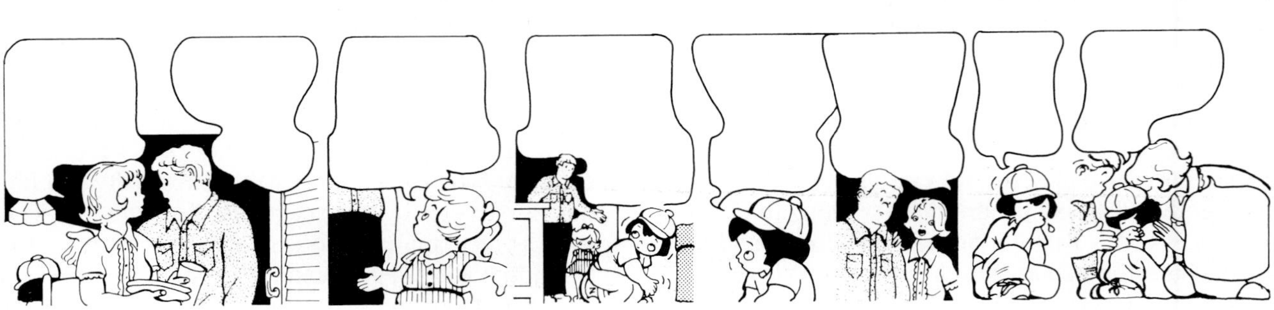

FIG. 6-4 Filling in the blanks on a comic strip is an effective communication technique with older children.

or the use of a tape recorder. For a less verbal child, having him draw pictures or write about an event may help him relate stories.

Bibliotherapy. Bibliotherapy involves the use of books in a therapeutic and supportive process. Its goal is to help the child express feelings and concerns through the familiar activity of being read to or reading to himself. Although it incorporates an educational component, it involves more than using a book for its preparatory value, such as familiarizing a child with hospitalization or a specific procedure. It provides the child with an opportunity to explore an event that is similar to his own but also sufficiently different to allow him to distance himself from it and remain in control. Since children tend to trust the characters in a book, they are able to feel familiar with the content even if they are suspicious of who reads the story. A book is essentially nonthreatening because the child can close it or stop reading it at any time.

"What if" questions. "What if" questions encourage children to explore potential situations and to consider different problem-solving options. For example, the nurse can ask a child, "What if you got sick and had to go to the hospital?" The child's response reveals what he knows already and what he is curious about. His thoughts concerning a new experience are elicited in a nonthreatening manner. This type of communication is excellent for helping children learn coping skills, especially in potentially dangerous situations. For example, parents might ask, "What if a stranger comes to school to pick you up and tells you your mommy is sick?" to prepare a child for appropriate responses.

Three wishes. Another simple device to engage children in conversation is the "three wishes" technique. The nurse asks, "If you could have any three things in the world, what would they be?" One child's answer to this was most revealing. He responded, "I don't want to be sick anymore." When asked about the other two wishes, he replied, "If that one came true, so would every other wish, so I don't have any more." Following this the nurse and boy were able to talk about what being sick meant to him. Although the nurse could not make him better, she was able to make some of the other "wishes" come true. One of them was to arrange for school friends to visit the child during his hospitalization and convalescence at home. Before this conversation the youngster's desire for peer companionship had never been revealed.

Rating scale. There are many applications of the rating scale. Some of them are particularly helpful in encouraging older children to talk. Instead of asking a youngster how he feels, the nurse asks him how his day has been "on a scale from 1 to 10, with 10 being the best." With a reply of "Today is a 2," one can begin exploring why this day rates so poorly. An extension of this is to have the youngster keep a log of each day's rating and expand it into a diary. The use of a rating scale can be helpful in assessing the degree of pain (see p. 591) or emotions such as sadness or happiness.

Word association game. Another approach is the word association game. The nurse can begin by having a list of key words and asking the child to say the first word that he thinks of when he hears the word. It is best to start with neutral words and then introduce more anxiety-producing words, such as illness, needles, hospitals, operation, and so on. The key words should be ones that relate to some significant event in the child's life.

Fill in the blanks. Without directly asking about feelings, one can probe into areas of concern by presenting a statement and having the child complete it. This is particularly useful with older school-age children and adolescents. Some sample statements are:

The thing I like best (least) about school is __________.
The best (worst) age to be is __________.
The most (least) fun thing I ever did was __________.
The thing I like most (least) about my parents is __________.
If I could change one thing about my family, it would be ___.
If I could be anything I wanted, I would be __________.
The thing I like most (least) about myself is __________.

Notice that the beginning statements are more neutral than the last ones, which center on feelings about oneself.

Pros and cons. A somewhat different approach to encouraging exploration of feelings is to select a topic, such as "being in the hospital," and have the child list "five good things and five bad things" about it. This is an exceptionally valuable technique when applied to relationships. For example, family members can be asked to write down five things they like and dislike about each other. In reviewing the lists, each member has the opportunity to discuss his or her feelings in a nonjudgmental atmosphere. However, when this technique is used, the nurse must be able to handle feelings that can surface unexpectedly.

Nonverbal Techniques

Many children and adults find talking about their feelings difficult. For them verbal communication may be more stressful than supportive. Several nonverbal techniques can be used to encourage communication, especially the use of drawing and play in young children.

Writing. An alternative approach to verbal interchange is writing. Some specific suggestions include (1) keeping a journal or diary, (2) writing down feelings or thoughts that are difficult to talk about, (3) writing "letters" that are never mailed (a variation is making up a "pen pal" and writing to him or her), or (4) keeping an account of the child's progress both from a physical and emotional viewpoint.

To initiate a conversation, the nurse can inquire about the writing, possibly even asking to read some of it. Frequently, as a person writes down his ideas, thoughts, or feelings, there is also an urge to discuss them. Once they are written, they are more real and tangible but often less frightening than when kept locked inside the mind.

Drawing. Drawing is one of the most valuable forms of

communication—both nonverbal, from looking at the drawing, and verbal, from the child's story of the picture. Children's drawings tell a great deal about them because they are projections of their personality. A child's drawing is usually of himself, his experience, or those who are significant to him. Besides offering communication about himself, art provides the child with a natural activity that helps him deal with conscious and unconscious feelings.

Drawing can be spontaneous or directed. *Spontaneous drawings* involve giving the child a variety of art supplies (older children like felt-tipped pens) and providing the opportunity to draw. The only encouragement may be the statement, "Draw something for me." *Directed drawing* involves a more specific direction, such as "Draw a person." In isolated figure drawings the child's response tends to be predominantly intellectual in that he will produce a more complete picture with more parts than those he draws in a group picture.

If the child needs encouragement to draw, the "three themes" approach is helpful. It involves writing three statements about the child at the bottom of the paper, for example, "I like playing the piano. I am in the hospital now. My dog's name is Poochie." The child chooses one theme to draw a picture (Fig. 6-5).

Group drawings are highly influenced by the child's feelings and the response is predominantly emotional. Consequently group drawings are highly valuable in disclosing what the child thinks about himself and others. The most valuable group drawing is of the family. A special type is the *kinetic family drawing* (Burns and Kaufman, 1970), in which the child is asked to, "Draw your family doing something." In giving directions, the nurse must be careful to offer only a general statement of encouragement and refrain from suggesting themes. Drawing the family is appropriate for children over 4 years of age. (See also the sociogram, p. 119.)

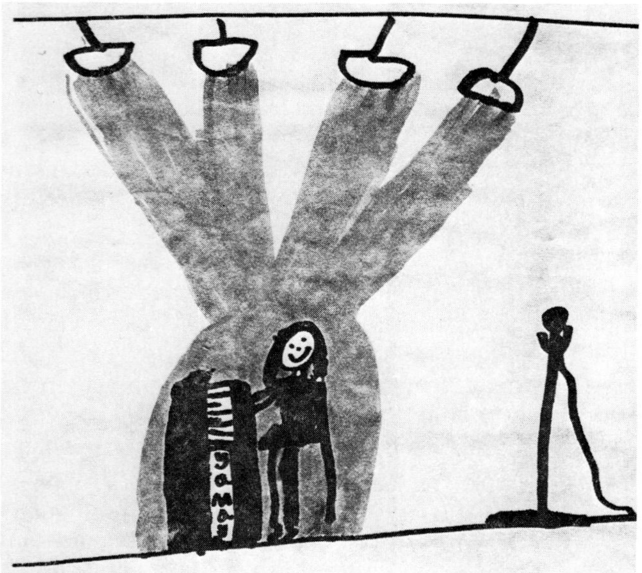

FIG. 6-5 Using the three themes approach, this child chooses to draw herself playing the piano; the spotlights focus on her as the center of attention, which is consistent with her position as an only child in the family.

The basic assumption in interpreting drawings is that the child is revealing something about himself. However, interpretation must be undertaken with an understanding of normal development in art expression. For example, it is normal for a 4-year-old to draw arms attached to a head but highly questionable in a 6-year-old. Understanding how to "read" and use drawings takes considerable time, experience, study, and patience. It is just as dangerous to "read" too much into a drawing and mislabel a person as it is to disregard a drawing as meaningless. When studying a drawing, the nurse must evaluate every detail, as well as relationships of one part to another. It is helpful to label the characters (mother, father, and so on) and to denote the order in which each was drawn.

When evaluating a drawing, the nurse should assess the following features:

1. The size of individual figures (expresses importance, power, authority)
2. The order in which figures are drawn (expresses priority in terms of importance)
3. The child's position in relation to other family members (expresses feelings of status or alliance)
4. The exclusion of a member (may denote feeling of not belonging or desire to eliminate)
5. Accentuated parts (usually expresses concern for areas of special importance, for example, large hands may be sign of aggression)
6. Erasures, shadings, or cross-hatching (expresses ambivalence, concern, or anxiety with particular area)

These suggestions are by no means a complete inventory for analyzing drawing. However, they do provide initial guidelines that can offer much information about the child. One caution is that interpretation must be viewed in light of the child's particular circumstances. For example, while cross-hatching is generally a sign of anxiety, it can also be an attempt to reproduce a design in a particular artistic effect, in which case it has much less significance.

Play. Play is the universal language of children. It is one of the most important forms of communication and can be an effective technique in relating with them. Clues about physical, intellectual, and social developmental progress can often be derived from the form and complexity of a child's play behaviors. Therapeutic play requires little or no equipment and is often used to reduce the trauma of illness and hospitalization, as is discussed in Chapters 20 and 21.

Because their ability to perceive precedes their ability to transmit, small infants respond to activities that register on their senses. Patting, stroking, and other skin play convey messages. Repetitive actions such as stretching an infant's arms out to the side while he is lying on his back and then folding them across his chest or raising and revolving his legs in a bicycling motion will elicit pleasurable sounds. Colorful items to catch the eye or interesting sounds such as a ticking clock, chimes, bells, or singing can be used to attract the child's attention.

Older infants respond to simple games. The old game of peekaboo is an excellent means of initiating communication with infants while maintaining a "safe" nonthreatening distance. After this intermittent eye-to-eye contact, the nurse is no longer viewed as a stranger but as a friend. This can be followed by touch games. Clapping an infant's hands together for pat-a-cake or wiggling his toes for "this little piggy" delights an infant or small child. Much of the nursing assessment can be carried out with the use of games and simple play equipment while the infant remains in the safety of the parent's arms or lap. Talking to a foot or other part of the child's body is another effective tactic.

The nurse can capitalize on the natural curiosity of small children by playing games such as, "Which hand do you take?" and "Guess what I have in my hand" or by manipulating items such as a flashlight or stethoscope. Finger games are very useful. More elaborate materials, such as puppets and replicas of familiar or unfamiliar items, serve as excellent means to communicate with small children. The variety and extent are limited only by the nurse's imagination.

Through play children reveal their perceptions of interpersonal relationships with their family and friends or the hospital personnel. Children may also reveal the wide scope of knowledge they have acquired from listening to others around them. For example, through needle play children may disclose how carefully they have watched each procedure by precisely duplicating the technical skills.

Play sessions serve not only as assessment tools for determining children's awareness and perception of their illness but also as methods of intervention and evaluation. A change in the type of drawing or the theme of the play may indicate progression toward or away from an ability to deal with anxiety.

◆ *History Taking*

This section deals with interviewing as it relates to the health history. The precise depth and extent of a nursing history vary with its intended purpose. The nurse uses judgment in deciding what data are necessary and relevant for the identification of problems or concerns.

The format used resembles a medical history, but the objective of each assessment area is the identification of nursing diagnoses. The value in following the well-established medical approach is that it is systematic and familiar to members of the health team. The categories listed in the box encompass the children's current and past health status and information about their psychosocial environment.

Outline of a Pediatric Health History

Identifying Information
1. Name
2. Address
3. Telephone
4. Birthdate and place
5. Race
6. Sex
7. Religion
8. Nationality
9. Date of interview
10. Informant

Chief Complaint (CC): to establish the major *specific* reason for the child's and parents' seeking professional health attention

Present Illness (PI): to obtain *all* details related to the chief complaint

Past History (PH): to elicit a profile of the child's previous illnesses, injuries, or operations
1. Birth history (pregnancy, labor, and delivery, perinatal history)
2. Previous illnesses, injuries, or operations
3. Allergies
4. Current medications
5. Immunizations
6. Growth and development
7. Habits

Review of Systems (ROS): to elicit information concerning any potential health problem
1. General
2. Integument
3. Head
4. Eyes
5. Ears
6. Nose
7. Mouth
8. Throat
9. Neck
10. Chest
11. Respiratory
12. Cardiovascular
13. Gastrointestinal
14. Genitourinary
15. Gynecologic
16. Musculoskeletal
17. Neurologic
18. Endocrine

Family Medical History (FMH): to identify the presence of genetic traits or diseases that have familial tendencies and to assess exposure to a communicable disease in a family member

Sexual History (SxH): to elicit information concerning the child's sexual concerns and/or activities and any pertinent data regarding adults' sexual activity that influence the child

Family History (FH): to develop an understanding of the child as an individual and as a member of a family and a community
1. Family composition
2. Home and community environment
3. Occupation and education of family members
4. Cultural and religious traditions
5. Family function and relationships

Nutritional Assessment (NA): to elicit information on the adequacy of the child's nutritional intake and need
1. Dietary intake
2. Clinical examination
3. Biochemical analysis

PERFORMING A HEALTH HISTORY

The format used for history taking may be (1) *direct*—the nurse asks the information via direct interview with the informant, or (2) *indirect*—the informant supplies the information by completing some type of questionnaire. The direct method is superior to the indirect approach or a combination of both. However, in view of time constraints, the direct approach is not always practical. If the indirect method is used, it is important to review informants' written responses and question them regarding any unusual answers.

The direct method can lose its value if the nurse asks questions directly from a form. In essence, the parent is completing the form by listening to it rather than by reading it. Using a systematic approach does not imply rote memory of a specific outline. Rather, it denotes the use of categories to define what areas of information are required. If nurses use as a model the basic categories outlined in the box (p. 113) and understand the objective of each, they can then obtain the required information as it arises during the course of the interview. However, the history should be recorded using the specified format.

Identifying Information

Much of the identifying information may already be available from other recorded sources. However, if the parent seems anxious, the nurse may ask about such information to help the parent feel more comfortable.

Informant. One of the important areas under identifying information concerns the informant, the person(s) who furnished the information. The following data about the informant are recorded: (1) who it is (child, parent, or other), (2) an impression of reliability and willingness to communicate, and (3) any special circumstances, such as the use of an interpreter or conflicting answers by more than one person.

Chief Complaint

The chief complaint represents the specific reason for the child's visit to the clinic, office, or hospital. The chief complaint may be viewed as the theme with the present illness as the description of the problem. The chief complaint is elicited by asking open-ended neutral statements or questions, such as, "Tell me what seems to be the matter," "How may I help you?" or "What brings you here?" Labeling-type questions, such as, "How are you sick?" are avoided, since it is possible that the reason for the visit is not because of illness.

Occasionally it is difficult to isolate one symptom or problem as the chief complaint because the parent may identify many. In this situation it is important to be as specific as possible when asking questions. For example, asking informants to state which *one* problem or symptom prompted them to seek help now may help them focus on the most immediate concern.

Present Illness

The history of the present illness* is a narrative of the chief complaint from its earliest onset through its progression to the present. Its four major components are: (1) the details of *onset,* (2) a complete *interval* history, (3) the *present* status, and (4) the reason for seeking help *now*. The focus of the present illness is on all factors relevant to the main problem, even if they have disappeared or changed during the onset, interval, and present.

Analyzing a symptom. Since pain is often the most characteristic symptom denoting onset of a physical problem, it is used as a prototype for analysis of a symptom. Assessment includes (1) type, (2) location, (3) severity, (4) duration, and (5) influencing factors.

The *type* or character of pain should be as specific as possible. However, with young children, it is almost always impossible for them to describe the pain. Asking the parents how they know the child is in pain may help describe its type, location, and severity. For example, a parent may state, "My child must have a severe earache because she pulls at her ears, rolls her head on the floor, and screams. Nothing seems to help."

The nurse can help older children describe the pain by asking them if it is sharp, throbbing, dull, aching, stabbing, and so on. Whatever words they use are recorded in quotes.

The *location* of the pain must also be specific. "Stomach pains" is too general a description. Children can better localize the pain if they are asked to "point with one finger to where it hurts" or to "point to where Mommy would put a Band-Aid." The nurse can also determine if the pain radiates by asking, "Does the pain stay there or move? Show me with your finger where the pain goes."

The *severity* of pain is best determined by finding out how it affects the child's usual behavior. Pain that prevents a child from playing, interacting with others, sleeping, and eating is most often severe. It is preferable to record pain in terms of interference with activity, rather than to quote the parent's or child's adjectives.

Duration of pain should include the duration, onset, and frequency of attacks. It may be necessary to describe this in terms of activity and behavior, such as "pain lasted all night because child refused to sleep and cried intermittently."

Influencing factors are anything that causes a change in the type, location, severity, or duration of the pain. These include (1) precipitating events (those that cause or increase the pain), (2) relieving events (those that lessen the pain, such as medications), (3) temporal events (times when the pain is relieved or increased), (4) positional events (standing, sitting, and lying down), and (5) associated events (meals, stress, and coughing).

*The term *illness* is used in its broadest sense to denote any problem of a physical, emotional, or psychosocial nature. It is actually a history of the chief complaint.

Past History

The past history contains information relating to all previous aspects of the child's health status and concentrates on several areas that are ordinarily deleted in the history of an adult, such as birth history, detailed feeding history, immunizations, and growth and development. Since a great deal of data is included in this section, it is more efficient to use a combination of open-ended and fact-finding questions. For example, the nurse may begin interviewing for each section with an open-ended statement, such as, "Tell me about your child's birth," in order to provide the informant with the opportunity to relate what he or she thinks is most important. Fact-finding questions related to specific details are asked whenever necessary to focus the interview on certain topics.

Birth history. Birth history includes all data concerning (1) the mother's health during pregnancy, (2) the labor and delivery, and (3) the infant's condition immediately after birth. Since prenatal influences have significant effects on a child's physical and emotional development, a thorough investigation of birth history is essential. Since parents may question what relevance pregnancy and birth have on the child's present condition, particularly if the child is past infancy, it is best to explain why such questions are included. An appropriate statement may be: "I will be asking you some questions about your pregnancy and . . . (refer to child by name) birth. Your answers will give me a more complete picture of his overall health."

Because emotional factors also affect the outcome of pregnancy and the subsequent parent-child relationship, it is important to investigate (1) concurrent crises during pregnancy and (2) prenatal attitudes toward the fetus. It is best to approach the topic of parental acceptance of pregnancy through indirect questioning. Asking parents if the pregnancy was planned is a leading statement because they may respond affirmatively for fear of criticism if the pregnancy was unexpected. The nurse can encourage parents to disclose their true reactions by referring to specific facts relating to the pregnancy, such as the spacing between offspring, an extended or short interval between marriage and conception, or the concurrent experience of pregnancy and adolescence. The parent can choose to explore such statements with further explanations or, for the moment, may not be able to reveal such feelings. Silence should alert the nurse to the importance of refocusing on this topic later in the interview.

Dietary history. The dietary history is discussed in detail at the end of this chapter under "Nutritional assessment," page 122.

Previous illnesses, injuries, and operations. When inquiring about past medical illnesses, the nurse can begin with a general statement, such as, "What other illnesses has your child had?" Since parents are most likely to recall serious health problems, it is important to specifically ask about colds, earaches, and common childhood diseases, such as measles, rubella (German measles), chickenpox, mumps, pertussis (whooping cough), diphtheria, scarlet fever, strep throat, tonsillitis, or allergic manifestations.

In addition to illnesses, the parent is asked about injuries that required medical intervention, operations, and any other reason for hospitalization, including the dates of each incident. It is important to focus on injuries such as accidental falls, poisonings, chokings, or burns, since this may be a potential area for parental guidance.

Allergies. Inquiry is needed regarding commonly known allergic disorders, such as hay fever and asthma, as well as unusual reactions to foods, drugs, or contact agents, such as animals, household products, fabrics, or poisonous plants. The parent should describe the allergic reactions to drugs since a known side effect can be confused with an allergic reaction. If the child has a known allergy to antibiotics, it is important to inquire about reactions to specific immunizations, such as measles or rubella, which may contain neomycin.

Current medications. In addition to any drug allergies, the nurse asks about current drug regimens, including vitamins, aspirin, antibiotics, antihistamines, decongestants, or antitussives. All medications are listed, including name, dose, schedule, duration, and reason for administration.

Immunizations. A record of all immunizations or "baby shots" is essential. Since many parents are unaware of the exact name and date of each immunization, the most reliable source of information is a hospital, clinic, or private physician's record. All immunizations and "boosters" are listed, stating (1) the name of the specific disease, (2) the number of injections, (3) the dosage (sometimes lesser amounts are given if a reaction is anticipated), (4) the ages when administered, and (5) the occurrence of any reaction following the immunization. The nurse should also inquire about the previous administration of any horse or other foreign serum, recent administration of gamma globulin or blood transfusion, anaphylactoid reactions to neomycin or chicken eggs, and tuberculin testing. If tuberculin testing was done, the child's positive or negative intradermal reaction is recorded.

Growth and development. The most important previous growth patterns to record are: (1) approximate weight at 6 months, 1 year, 2 years, and 5 years of age, (2) approximate length at ages 1 and 4 years, and (3) dentition, including age of onset, number of teeth, and symptoms during teething. Developmental milestones include: (1) age of holding up head steadily, (2) age of sitting alone without support, (3) age of walking without assistance, (4) age of saying first words with meaning, (5) present grade in school, (6) scholastic grades, and (7) interaction with other children, peers, and adults.

Specific and detailed questions are used when inquiring about each developmental milestone. For example "sitting up" can mean many different activities, such as sitting propped up, sitting in someone's lap, sitting with support, sitting up alone but in a hyperflexed position for assisted balance, or sitting up unsupported with the back slightly rounded. A clue to misunderstanding of the requested activity may be an unusually early age of achievement.

Habits. Habits are an important area to explore because numerous parental concerns may be discovered. They include:

1. Behavior patterns, such as nail-biting, thumb-sucking, pica, rituals ("security" blanket or toy), and unusual movements (head-banging, rocking, overt masturbation, and walking on toes)
2. Activities of daily living, such as hour of sleep and arising, duration of nighttime sleep and naps, type and duration of exercise, regularity of stools and urination, age of toilet training, and occurrences of daytime or nighttime bedwetting
3. Usual disposition as well as response to frustration
4. Use or abuse of alcohol, drugs, coffee, and cigarettes

The last category is primarily applicable to adolescents, although nurses must be aware of the increasing juvenile experimentation and use of potentially harmful substances. If a youngster admits to smoking, drinking, or drug use, a specific average amount, such as one cigarette a week or two cans of beer on weekends, is recorded. A statement such as, "I pop pills once in a while" has tremendously wide variations in meaning. Following this response with, "How many pills and when is once in a while?" may yield a measurable intake of drugs. If older children deny use of such substances, it is advisable to inquire about past experimentation. Asking "You mean you never tried to smoke or drink?" implies that the nurse expects some such activity and consequently is likely to be nonjudgmental of an affirmative answer. The interviewer should also be aware of the confidential nature of such questioning and the adverse effect that the parents' presence may have on the adolescent's willingness to answer.

Review of Systems

Review of systems is exactly what the title implies—a specific review of each body system, similar to the order of the physical examination. Often the history of the present illness provides a complete review of the system involved in the chief complaint. Since asking questions about other body systems may appear unrelated and irrelevant to the parents or child, it is important to precede the questioning with an explanation of why the data is needed (similar to the explanation concerning relevance of birth history) and reassurance that the child's main problem has not been forgotten.

The review of a specific system should begin with a broad statement, such as, "How has your child's general health been?" or "Has your child had any problems with his eyes?" If the parent states that there have been past problems with some body function, this is pursued with an encouraging statement, such as, "Tell me more about that." If the parent denies any problems, it is best to query for specific symptoms, such as, "No headaches, bumping into objects, or squinting?" If the parent reconfirms the absence of such symptoms, positive statements to this effect are recorded in the history, such as, "Mother denies headaches, bumping into objects, or squinting." In this way, anyone who reviews the health history is aware of exactly what symptoms were investigated.

The following is a list of suggested areas for review of each body system or body part. Although medical terminology may be used to record a symptom during the interview, only terms that are clearly understood by the parent or child are used.

general health overall state of health, fatigue, recent and/or unexplained weight gain or loss, period of time for either, contributing factors (change of diet, illness, altered appetite), exercise tolerance, fevers (time of day), chills, night sweats (unrelated to climatic conditions), frequent infections, general ability to carry out activities of daily living

integumentary system pruritus, pigment or other color changes, acne, eruptions, rashes (location), tendency to bruising, petechiae, excessive dryness, general texture, disorders or deformities of nails, hair growth or loss, hair color change (for adolescent, use of hair dyes or other potentially toxic substances, such as hair straighteners)

head headaches, dizziness, injury (specific details)

eyes visual problems (ask about behaviors indicative of blurred vision, such as bumping into objects, clumsiness, sitting very close to the television, holding a book close to the face, writing with head near desk, squinting, rubbing the eyes, bending the head in an awkward position), "cross-eye" (strabismus), eye infections, edema of lids, excessive tearing, use of glasses or contact lenses, date of last optic examination

nose nosebleeds (epistaxis), constant or frequent running or stuffy nose, nasal obstruction (difficulty in breathing), sense of smell

ears earaches, discharge, evidence of hearing loss (ask about behaviors, such as need to repeat requests, loud speech, inattentive behavior), results of any previous auditory testing

mouth mouth breathing, gum bleeding, toothaches, toothbrushing, use of fluoride, difficulty with teething (symptoms), last visit to dentist (especially if temporary dentition is complete), response to dentist

throat sore throats, difficulty in swallowing, choking (especially when chewing food—may be from poor chewing habits), hoarseness or other voice irregularities

neck pain, limitation of movement, stiffness, difficulty in holding head straight (torticollis), thyroid enlargement, enlarged nodes or other masses

chest breast enlargement, discharge, masses, enlarged axillary nodes (for adolescent female, ask about breast self-examination)

respiratory system chronic cough, frequent colds (number per year), wheezing, shortness of breath at rest or on exertion, difficulty in breathing, sputum production, infections (pneumonia, tuberculosis), date of last chest x-ray examination

cardiovascular system cyanosis or fatigue on exertion, history of heart murmur or rheumatic fever, anemia, date of last blood count, blood type, recent transfusion

gastrointestinal system (much of this in regard to appetite, food tolerance, and elimination habits has been asked elsewhere), nausea, vomiting (not associated with eating may be indicative of brain tumor or increased intracranial pressure), jaundice or yellowing skin or sclera, belching, flatulence, recent change in bowel habits (blood in stools, change of color, diarrhea, or constipation)

genitourinary system pain on urination, frequency, hesitancy, urgency, hematuria, nocturia, polyuria, unpleasant odor to urine, force of stream, discharge, change in size of scrotum, date of last urinalysis (for adolescent, sexually transmitted disease, type of treatment; for male adolescent, ask about testicular self-examination)

gynecologic system menarche, date of last menstrual period, regularity or problems with menstruation, vaginal discharge, pruritus, date and result of last Pap smear (include obstetric history as discussed under birth history when applicable); if sexually active, type of contraception

musculoskeletal system weakness, clumsiness, lack of coordination, unusual movements, back or joint stiffness, muscle pains or cramps, abnormal gait, deformity, fractures, serious sprains, activity level

neurologic system seizures, tremors, dizziness, loss of memory, general affect, fears, nightmares, speech problems, any unusual habits

endocrine system intolerance to weather changes, excessive thirst, excessive urination, excessive sweating, salty taste to skin, signs of early puberty

Family Medical History

The family medical history is used primarily for the purpose of discovering the potential existence of hereditary or familial diseases in the parents and child. In general it is confined to first-degree relatives (parents, siblings, and grandparents and their children). Information for each family member includes age, marital status, state of health if living, cause of death if deceased, and any evidence of the following conditions: heart disease, hypertension, cancer, diabetes mellitus, obesity, congenital anomalies, allergy, asthma, tuberculosis, sickle cell disease, mental retardation, convulsions, insanity or other emotional problems, syphilis, or rheumatic fever. The accuracy of the reported disorders is confirmed by inquiring about the symptoms, course, treatment, and sequelae of each diagnosis.

Geographic location. One of the important areas to explore when assessing the family health history is geographic location, including birthplace and travel to different areas in or outside of the country for identification of possible exposure to endemic diseases. Although the primary interest focuses on the child's temporary residence in various localities, the nurse should also inquire about close family members' travel, especially during tours of military service or business trips. Children are especially susceptible to parasitic infestation in areas of poor sanitary conditions and to vector-borne diseases, such as those from mosquitoes or ticks in warm and humid or heavily wooded regions.

Sexual History

Sexual history is an essential component of adolescents' health assessment. It is warranted regardless of their degree of sexual activity since concerns about sexual matters can influence physical and psychologic well-being.

One approach toward initiating a conversation about sexual concerns is to begin with a history of peer interactions. Open-ended statements such as "Tell me about your social life," or "Who are your closest friends?" generally lead into a discussion of dating and sexual issues. To probe further, questions about the adolescent's attitudes on such topics as sex education, "going steady," "living together," and premarital sex can be included. Questions should be phrased to reflect concern and not judgment or criticism of sexual practices.

In any conversation regarding sexual history, the nurse must be aware of the language that is used in either eliciting or conveying sexual information. For example, it is best to avoid asking if the adolescent is "sexually active," since this term is broadly defined. "Are you having sex with anyone?" is probably the most direct and best understood question (Strasburger, 1986). Since homosexual experimentation may occur, all sexual contacts should be referred to in nongender terms, such as "anyone" or "partners," rather than "girlfriends" or "boyfriends."

A detailed account of sexual partners is needed if the patient has a history of, displays any of the symptoms of, or asks for treatment of a sexually transmitted disease. A difficult but necessary part of the interview is to determine the sites of possible infection. Since sexual diseases can be contracted at any of the body orifices, the adolescent should be informed that a sexually transmitted disease can be acquired without visible signs of disease at nongenital sites.

◆ *Family Assessment*

Assessment of the family, both its structure and function, is an essential component of the history-taking process. Because the quality of the functional relationship between the child and family members is a major factor in emotional and physical health, family assessment is discussed separately and in greater detail apart from the more traditional health history.

Family assessment is the collection of data about the composition of the family and the relationships among its members. In its broadest sense the family refers to all those individuals who are significant to the nuclear unit, including relatives, friends, and other social groups, such as the school and church. While family assessment should not be confused with family therapy, it can and frequently is therapeutic. Involving family members in discussing family characteristics and activities often stimulates productive discussion and insight into family dynamics and relationships.

Because of the time involved in performing an in-depth family assessment as presented here, the nurse should be selective in deciding when knowledge of family function may facilitate nursing care. During brief contacts with families a full assessment may not be appropriate and screening with one or two questions from each category may reflect the health of the family system or the potential need for additional assessment.

ASSESSMENT OF FAMILY STRUCTURE

Family structure refers to the composition of the family—who lives in the home and those social, cultural, religious, and economic characteristics that influence the child's and family's overall psychobiologic health (see also Chapter 3 and 4). Since the information elicited in this part of the history is often the most personal and confidential, it is discussed toward the end of the interview, when the nurse-parent-child rapport is well established.

Structural Assessment Interview

The more traditional method of eliciting information on family structure is by interviewing family members. The principal areas of concern are (1) family composition, (2) home and community environment, (3) occupation and education of family members, and (4) cultural and religious traditions.

Family composition. Family composition is primarily concerned with the immediate members of the household but should also include a review of the family's extended support system. For example, in a single-parent family, the household members may consist of the mother and two children, but the mother's parents may be very significant sources of child care and financial support. Although the interview method can be used to collect information about household members—their relationship, ages, and roles within the family, as well as significant individuals outside the family unit—other efficient methods include those discussed under "Structural assessment tools" (p. 119).

In discussing family composition it is sometimes difficult to ascertain the status of the adult relationships. For example, the parent may fail to mention the other parent. In this case the nurse can then ask, "Where is the child's father (or mother)?" It is best to avoid the term *husband* or *wife* because that precludes the existence of nonmarital relationships. If the parent states that the child's father (or mother) is not part of the household, the nurse can explore this by inquiring about the absent person's continued relationship with the child and the presence of any other significant male (or female) within the home. The nurse should also inquire about previous marriages, separations, death of spouses, or divorces. It is important to ask about the children's reaction to any of these events, which usually have a tremendous effect on their general physical and emotional health.

Home and community environment. Information about the home environment includes (1) type of dwelling (private home, apartment, multiple dwelling, or trailer); (2) number of rooms, including sleeping arrangements, floors, and occupants; (3) accessibility of stairs or elevators; (4) adequacy of utilities; (5) safety features (fire escape, guardrails on high-rise windows, smoke detectors, and use of car restraints); and (6) housing problems (insects, poor sanitation, or flaking paint).

Recent stresses or changes in the home should be explored, such as relocation, change in employment status, marital discord or divorce, and addition of a new sibling. If any are identified, the nurse should inquire about the child's adjustment to the change.

Information regarding the community environment may vary according to geographic location, such as an urban or rural setting. It is the nurse's responsibility to have at least a general knowledge of the locality in order to focus questions on specific areas of significance. However, some general topics for investigation include (1) type of neighborhood (residential or industrial, relative age of neighboring families, willingness of neighbors to help one another, interracial or ethnic problems); (2) location of and distance to school; (3) usual transportation to school; (4) availability of age-mates for the child; and (5) available play areas. It is also important to focus on potential dangers in the community environment such as (1) proximity to industrial centers (for example, an asbestos or chemical factory); (2) incidence of crime; and (3) potential sources of injury such as a swimming pool, drainage ditch, or other adjacent body of water, steep hill or cliff, or heavy street traffic.

Occupation and education of family members. The occupational history of the parents consists of more than a listing of their career and place of employment. It should focus on (1) type of activity (manual or sedentary, individual-paced or highly pressured), (2) number of hours away from the home, (3) exposure to environmental hazards (chemicals, coal, radiation, lead, carbon monoxide, or fire), and (4) satisfaction associated with the employment.

The occupational history should also lead into a discussion of the family's financial status. Since some parents may resist disclosing their yearly income, the nurse can assess the adequacy of financial resources by inquiring about source of income when unemployed, usual housing expenses, and expenditures for food, shelter, clothing, and recreation. A general statement, such as, "The cost of living is certainly high today. How do you make ends meet?" may encourage parents to discuss any financial hardships without fear of criticism. The nurse also investigates the type of medical coverage or insurance the family has.

Ascertaining the parents' educational preparation usually follows a discussion of occupation. By the end of the interview the nurse has probably made some personal judgment regarding the parent's level of formal and/or informal education. However, since many people feel embarrassed to admit failure to complete the usual academic learning, it is best to approach the area of years in school indirectly whenever possible. For example, the nurse can ask about the type of training, education, or acquisition of special skills that may be required for the parents' vocation. This information is highly valuable in planning implementation of care (e.g., counseling, guidance, or teaching) and is another reason to refrain from actual intervention until the history (and physical examination whenever warranted) is completed.

Cultural and religious traditions. Knowledge of the family's cultural traditions and religious practices is essential in planning care. The influence of culture and religion on the family is discussed in Chapter 3. Cultural traditions and religious practices that should be assessed in the family history include childrearing beliefs, attitudes toward health care, and personal faith in a deity. Cultural practice in relation to nutrition is discussed on p. 123. The following questions encourage families to verbalize about their heritage:

How do your beliefs regarding ____________ differ from those of your parents?
What special ____________ (name of culture or nationality) traditions do you practice in your home?
What language do you speak in the home?
How are American children different from children in your country?
What is your family's religion?
How is your religion a part of your life?

Structural Assessment Tool

Several structural assessment tools can be used to collect and record data about family composition and environment. Like the interview method, such tools also provide information about relationships, although several additional methods should be used to assess family function.

Sociogram. The sociogram uses a drawing of circles to indicate the significant persons in the individual's life and is appropriate for adults and children as young as 5 years of age. The person is given blank paper and a pencil with the instructions: "Draw a circle to represent you. Around the circle draw circles to represent the most significant persons in your life and label each. Draw the circles in proximity to your circle to represent closeness. For example, the person who is most significant is the circle closest to you." Family members can label the relationships as supportive with a plus sign or negative with a minus sign.

Not only is the sociogram a portrait of the person's significant relationships, it may also uncover unresolved relationships as described in the Therapeutic dialogue (see box and Fig. 6-6). After completing the sociogram, the

THERAPEUTIC DIALOGUE

Using the Sociogram

During a comprehensive well-child visit the nurse requested each family member (mother, father, and 6 year-old son) to draw a sociogram. After each person completed the drawing, the nurse asked them to describe the picture. The drawings included similar people, except for the mother, who drew an unlabeled circle inside her circle (Fig. 6-6). When asked about this circle, the following conversation occurred.

MOTHER: I did not know where to put my daughter, who died at 3 months of age. She was still more like *in* my circle when she died and I guess there is just a hole in my circle now.

NURSE: Tell me about your daughter.

MOTHER: She was born nine months ago with a congenital heart defect and shortly after birth developed congestive heart failure. Her little heart was too small and fragile to keep her alive and she died.

NURSE: Tell me about her being in your circle.

MOTHER: Well, I had carried her inside of me for nine months and after she was born I cared for her every minute of the day. We were never apart. I feel she is still part of my body, but more like a big hole in my heart. (Mother begins to cry.)

NURSE: You feel sadness because she is not here anymore. (Nurse uses facilitative responding (p. 110) to focus on the feelings.)

MOTHER: Yes and nobody understands. (She states this with some anger in her voice and quickly looks at her husband.)

NURSE: Who doesn't understand?

MOTHER: He doesn't (looking at husband). He never talks about our baby and once he said we were better off that she died.

FATHER: That's not fair. I miss her too but I don't want to talk about her because it always makes you cry.

SUMMARY

Following this conversation the mother and father talked together about their feelings, something they had not done previously. The nurse included the child in the discussion and it became clear that he was unsure of why the baby died. Both parents took the opportunity to explain the cause of death to him.

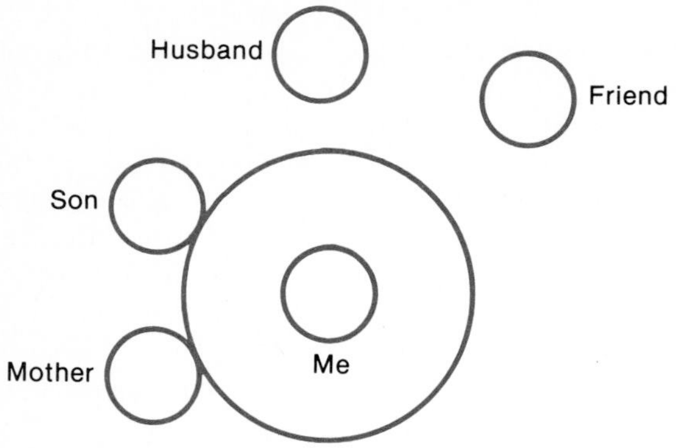

FIG. 6-6 Sociogram of a mother with an unlabeled circle to represent "hole in my circle" after her infant's death.

family can be encouraged to explore their feelings further with questions such as the following:

How would you change the circles to improve relationships?
How do you think you could accomplish these changes?
If one person in the circle were to change, what effect do you think that would have on others in the circle?

ASSESSMENT OF FAMILY FUNCTION

Family function is concerned with how the family behaves toward one another and the quality of the relationships (see also p. 57). It is considered the most important component in determining "family health." Assessment of function requires more skill on the part of the interviewer than does assessment of structure and is best approached after structure is assessed.

Family Function Interview

As in assessment of family structure, the more traditional method of eliciting information on family function is by interviewing family members. The principal areas of concern are characteristics discussed below.

Family interaction and roles. Family interaction refers to the ways family members relate to each other. The chief concern is the amount of intimacy and closeness among the members, especially the spouses. Roles refer to the behaviors of people as they assume different statuses or positions. The more flexibility and sharing of roles, the better family members are able to meet each other's needs. In assessing interactions and roles, general observations are made about the family's response to each other (e.g., cordial, hostile, cool, loving, patient, or short-tempered), obvious roles of leadership versus submission, and support and attention shown to various members.

Asking questions concerning with whom the child shares a room, the child's household chores, and activities the family performs together gives some idea of how the family interacts. It is best to avoid direct questions such as, "How does your family get along with each other?" because the usual response is "OK." An effective way of approaching this topic, especially with adolescents, is use of the third-person technique (see p. 110). The nurse may say, for example, "Teenagers and parents have a way of seeing things differently, especially when it comes to money, dating, clothes, using the car, and curfew. Have you and your parents ever disagreed about such things?" The young person is then allowed an opportunity to present his views because he is aware that the nurse expects such events and is therefore less likely to judge or criticize his response. (For a more detailed discussion of family communication strategies, see pp. 110-113.)

Other assessment questions include:

Who do you talk to when something is bothering you?
Who usually oversees what is happening with the children, such as at school or concerning their health?
How easy or difficult is it for your family to change or accept new responsibilities for household tasks?

Power, decision-making, and problem-solving. Power and control in the family is a critical issue. Clear boundaries of power, that is, shared power by the parents in rearing the children, is essential for family health (Lewis and others, 1979). Knowledge of who has power and how decisions are made usually offers clues to how problems are solved. One of the best methods of collecting data is to offer a hypothetical conflict or problem, such as a child with failing school grades, and ask the family how they would handle this situation. By observing the group dynamics, conclusions can be drawn about how the family typically deals with conflicts or problems.

Assessment questions include:

Who usually makes the decisions in your family?
(Directed to the child) If one parent makes a decision, can you appeal to the other parent to change it?
(Directed to the parents) What input do the children have in making decisions or discussing rules?
Who makes and enforces the rules?
What happens when a rule is broken?

Communication. In interviewing the family the nurse is concerned with the clarity and directness of communication patterns. Clear communication relays messages that are understood by all members. Direct communication is sent to the intended receiver. Assessments are made by observing who speaks to whom, if one person speaks for another or interrupts, if members appear disinterested when certain individuals speak, and if there is agreement between verbal and nonverbal messages. To further assess communication, the nurse can periodically ask family members if they understood what was just said and to repeat the message.

Expression of feelings and individuality. Healthy families allow expression of feelings and promote the development of individuality while encouraging family closeness. There is the space and freedom to grow with the limits and structure needed for guidance. Observing patterns of communication offers clues to how freely feelings are expressed.

Family APGAR

Definition	Functions Measured by the Family APGAR	Relevant Open-Ended Questions
Adaptation is the use of intrafamilial and extrafamilial resources for problem-solving when family equilibrium is stressed during a crisis.	How resources are shared, or the degree to which a member is satisfied with the assistance received when family resources are needed.	How have family members aided each other in time of need? In what way have family members received help or assistance from friends and community agencies?
Partnership is the sharing of decision-making and nurturing responsibilities by family members.	How decisions are shared, or the member's satisfaction with mutuality in family communication and problem-solving.	How do family members communicate with each other about such matters as vacations, finances, medical care, large purchases, and personal problems?
Growth is the physical and emotional maturation and self-fulfillment that is achieved by family members through mutual support and guidance.	How nurturing is shared, or the member's satisfaction with the freedom available within the family to change roles and attain physical and emotional growth or maturation.	How have family members changed during the past years? How has this change been accepted by family members? In what ways have family members aided each other in growing or developing independent life-styles? How have family members reacted to your desires for change?
Affection is the caring or loving relationship that exists among family members.	How emotional experiences are shared, or the member's satisfaction with the intimacy and emotional interaction that exists in the family.	How have members of your family responded to emotional expressions such as affection, love, sorrow, or anger?
Resolve is the commitment to devote time to other members of the family for physical and emotional nurturing. It also usually involves a decision to share wealth and space.	How time (and space and money) is shared, or the member's satisfaction with the time commitment that has been made to the family by its members.	How do members of your family share time, space, and money?

Modified from Smilkstein, G.: The Family APGAR: a proposal for a family function test and its use by physicians, J. Fam. Pract. **6**(6):1231-1239, 1978.

Assessment questions include:

Is it OK to get angry or sad in your house?
Who gets angry most of the time? What do they do?
If you are upset, how do other family members try to comfort you?
Who comforts you?
When you want to do something new, such as try out for a new sport or get a job, what is the family's response (offer assistance, discourage you, or leave it to you to work out)?

Family Function Assessment Tools

In addition to observing and interviewing the family to assess family function, several other methods are available and should be used as needed to obtain a comprehensive assessment. The following section discusses selected instruments that are reliable and valid but require little formal training and minimal time to administer.

Family APGAR. The Family APGAR is a brief screening questionnaire designed to reflect a family member's satisfaction with the functional state of the family (Smilkstein, 1978) (see Appendix A). The acronym APGAR is for Adaptability, Partnership, Growth, Affection, and Resolve (commitment) (see box). It is not related to the Apgar scoring system for newborns, although the acronym was chosen because it is familiar to health professionals. It requires about 5 minutes to complete and can be used by nuclear families, as well as families with alternative life-styles. The questions in the box can be used in the interview without the APGAR ratings to elicit similar types of information.

Home Observation and Measurement of the Environment and Home Screening Questionnaire. Ideally a thorough assessment includes observing the child and family in a variety of settings. Undoubtedly the richest environment for observing a child's development and interactions with family members is the home. Two tools that can be used to assess the child's home environment are the Home Observation for Management of the Environment (HOME)* (Caldwell and Bradley, 1984) and the Home Screening Questionnaire (HSQ)† (Frankenburg and Coons, 1986).† Both are divided into two age-groups—birth to 3 years of age and 3 to 6 years of age. HOME has an additional inventory for elementary age children. HOME (for children from 0 to 3 years) has 45 items in 6 major categories, the form for children from 3 to 6 years consists of 55 items in 8 categories, and HOME (for children from 6 to

*The forms and a comprehensive manual are available for a fee of $12.00; the forms and an administration manual cost $6.00. Both are available from the Bureau of Educational Research, University of Arkansas, 33rd Street and University Avenue, Little Rock, AK 72204.
†The forms and manual are available for a fee from Denver Developmental Materials, Inc., P.O. Box 20037, Denver, CO 80220.

10 years) includes 59 items in 8 categories. Some of the items require direct observation, whereas others necessitate questioning of the parents. Each item receives a "yes" or "no" response. The number of "yes" scores correlates with the amount of appropriate environmental stimulation. Any "no" scores indicate possible areas for intervention and counseling. Use of HOME requires about a 1-hour home visit with both the child and major caregiver.

The HSQ was developed using HOME as a guide. The form for children from 0 to 3 years consists of 30 items plus a checklist of toys available to the child in the home. The form for children from 3 to 6 years has 34 items and a similar toy checklist. The questions are written at approximately a third to sixth grade reading level and, unlike the HOME, can be completed by the parents in any setting in about 15 to 20 minutes. Scoring directions are detailed in the manual and are based on credits for different answers. For each age-group there is a minimum score for determining suspect or nonsuspect results.

◆ *Nutritional Assessment*

A nutritional assessment is an essential part of a complete health appraisal. Its purpose is to evaluate the child's nutritional status, the state of balance between nutrient intake and nutrient expenditure or need. A thorough nutritional status assessment includes: (1) dietary intake, (2) clinical examination, and (3) biochemical analysis.

DIETARY INTAKE

Knowledge of the child's dietary intake is a useful and practical component of a nutritional assessment. However, it is also one of the most difficult factors to assess. Individuals' recall of food consumption, especially amounts eaten, is frequently unreliable. In addition people may be hesitant to reveal their eating patterns if they sense criticism from the nurse. People from different cultures may have difficulty adequately describing the types of food they eat. Despite these obstacles, however, a food intake record is essential. Several methods are available.

Dietary History

Regardless of the format used in recording food intake, every nutritional assessment should begin with a dietary history. The exact questions used to elicit a dietary history vary with the child's age. In general, the younger the child, the more specific and detailed the history should be. The box below provides a sample dietary history for children and gives additional questions on infant feeding.

The broad overview elicited from the dietary history can be helpful in evaluating food frequency records (see box, p. 123). It also is concerned with financial and cul-

Dietary History

What are the family's usual mealtimes?
Do family members eat together or at separate times?
Who does the family grocery shopping and meal preparation?
How much money is spent to buy food each week?
How are most foods prepared—baked, broiled, fried, other?
How often does the family or your child eat out?
  What kinds of restaurants do you go to?
  What kinds of food does your child typically eat at restaurants?
Does your child eat breakfast regularly?
Where does he eat lunch?
What are your child's favorite foods, beverages, and snacks?
  Average amounts consumed or usual size portions?
  Special cultural practices, such as family only eats ethnic food?
What foods and beverages does your child dislike?
How would you describe his usual appetite (hearty eater, picky eater)?
What are his feeding habits (breast, bottle, cup, spoon, eats by self, needs assistance, any special devices)?
Does he take vitamins or other supplements; do they contain iron or fluoride?
Are there any known or suspected food allergies; is your child on a special diet?
Has your child lost or gained weight recently?
Are there any feeding problems (excessive fussiness, spitting up, colic, difficulty sucking or swallowing); any dental problems or appliances, such as braces that affect eating?
What types of exercise does your child do regularly?
Is there a family history of cancer, diabetes, heart disease, high blood pressure, or obesity?

Additional Questions for Infants

What was the infant's birth weight; when did it double, triple?
Was the infant premature?
Are you breast-feeding or have you breast-fed your infant?
  For how long?
If you use a formula, what is the brand?
  How long has the infant been taking it?
  How many ounces does he drink a day?
Are you giving the infant cow's milk (whole, low-fat, skimmed)?
  When did you start?
  How many ounces does he drink a day?
Do you give your infant extra fluids (water, juice)?
If he takes a bottle to bed at nap or nighttime, what is in the bottle?
At what age did you start cereal, vegetables, meat or other protein sources, fruit/juice, finger food, table food?
Do you make your own baby food or use commercial foods, such as infant cereal?
Does the infant take a vitamin/mineral supplement? If so, what type?
Has the infant shown an allergic reaction to any food(s)? If so, list the foods and describe the reaction.
Does the infant spit up frequently, have unusually loose stools, or have hard, dry stools? If so, how often?
How often do you feed your infant?
How would you describe your infant's appetite?

tural factors that influence food selection and preparation. Because cultural practices are very prevalent in food preparation, it is important to consider carefully the kind of questions that are asked and the judgment made in regard to counseling. For example, some cultures, such as Hispanic, black, and Native American, include many vegetables, legumes, and starches in their diet that together provide sufficient essential amino acids, even though the actual amount of meat or dairy protein is low. (See p. 48 for cultural food practices.)

Twenty-four-hour recall. The most common and probably easiest method of assessing daily intake is the 24-hour recall. The child or parent recalls every item eaten in the past 24 hours and the approximate amounts. The 24-hour recall is most beneficial when it is representative of a typical day's intake. Some of the difficulties with a daily recall are the family's inability to remember exactly what was eaten and inaccurate estimation of portion size. To increase accuracy of reporting portion sizes, the use of food models and additional questioning are recommended. In general this method is most useful in providing *qualitative* information about the child's diet.

Food diary. To improve the reliability of the daily recall, the family can complete a food diary by recording every food and liquid consumed for a certain number of days. A 3-day record consisting of 2 weekdays and 1 weekend day is representative for most people. Providing specific charts to record intake can improve compliance. The family should record items immediately after eating.

Food frequency record. A food frequency questionnaire or record provides information about the number of times in a day, week, or month a child consumes items from the four food groups (box below). In general, it provides more of a qualitative overview but has the advantage of avoiding recall based on a "typical" day. It can be especially useful when verifying a food history or diary.

CLINICAL EXAMINATION

A significant amount of information regarding nutritional deficiencies is elicited from a clinical examination, especially from assessing the skin, hair, teeth, gums, lips, tongue, and eyes. Hair, skin, and mouth are vulnerable because of the rapid turnover of epithelial and mucosal

*Food Frequency Record**

Food Group	Number of Servings (day, week)	Serving Size (in cup, tablespoon, or ounce portions)	Food Group	Number of Servings (day, week)	Serving Size (in cup, tablespoon, or ounce portions)
Milk/Cheese Milk Cheese Yogurt Pudding Ice cream Other			**Fruits/Juice** Citrus (orange, grapefruit, tangerine) Noncitrus Other		
Protein Foods Meat Fish Poultry Egg Peanut butter Legumes (dried beans, peas) Nuts Other			**Fats** Butter, oil, margarine, mayonnaise, salad dressing		
Breads/Cereals Bread, tortilla Cooked pasta, rice, hot cereal Dry cereal (not presweetened) Crackers Muffins Other			**Sweets** Soda, punch Cake/cookie, etc. Candy Presweetened cereal		
Vegetables Yellow or orange Green/leafy Other					

*For comparison of actual intake with recommended intake, see Appendix F.

TABLE 6-1

Clinical Assessment of Nutritional Status

Evidence of Adequate Nutrition	Evidence of Deficient or Excess Nutrition	Deficiency/Excess*
General Growth		
Within 5th and 95th percentiles for height, weight, and head circumference	Below 5th or above 95th percentiles for growth	Protein, calories, fats, and other essential nutrients, especially A, pyridoxine, niacin, calcium, iodine, manganese, zinc
Steady gain with expected growth spurts during infancy and adolescence	Absence of or delayed growth spurts; poor weight gain	
Sexual development appropriate for age	Delayed sexual development	
		Excess vitamin A, D
Skin		
Smooth, slightly dry to touch	Hardening and scaling	Vitamin A
Elastic and firm	Seborrheic dermatitis	Excess niacin
Absence of lesions	Dry, rough, petechiae	Riboflavin
Color appropriate to genetic background	Delayed wound healing	Vitamin C
	Scaly dermatitis on exposed surfaces	Riboflavin, vitamin C, zinc
	Wrinkled, flabby	Niacin
	Crusted lesions around orifices, especially nares	Protein and calories Zinc
	Pruritus	Excess vitamin A, riboflavin, niacin
	Poor turgor	Water, sodium
	Edema	Protein, thiamin Excess sodium
	Yellow tinge (jaundice)	Vitamin B_{12} Excess vitamin A, niacin
	Depigmentation	Protein, calories
	Pallor (anemia)	Pyridoxine, folic acid, vitamin B_{12}, C, E (in premature infants), iron Excess vitamin C, zinc
	Paresthesia	Excess riboflavin
Hair		
Lustrous, silky, strong, elastic	Stringy, friable, dull, dry, thin	Protein, calories
	Alopecia	Protein, calories, zinc
	Depigmentation	Protein, calories, copper
	Raised areas around hair follicles	Vitamin C
Head		
Even molding, occipital prominence, symmetric facial features	Softening of cranial bones, prominence of frontal bones, skull flat and depressed toward middle	Vitamin D
Fused sutures after 18 months	Delayed fusion of sutures	Vitamin D
	Hard tender lumps in occiput	Excess vitamin A
	Headache	Excess thiamin
Neck		
Thyroid not visible, palpable in midline	Thyroid enlarged; may be grossly visible	Iodine
Eyes		
Clear, bright	Hardening and scaling of cornea and conjunctiva	Vitamin A
Conjunctiva—pink, glossy	Night blindness	
Good night vision	Burning, itching, photophobia, cataracts, corneal vascularization	Riboflavin
Ears		
Tympanic membrane—pliable	Calcified (hearing loss)	Excess vitamin D
Nose		
Smooth, intact nasal angle	Irritation and cracks at nasal angle	Riboflavin Excess vitamin A
Mouth		
Lips—smooth, moist, darker color than skin	Fissures and inflammation at corners	Riboflavin Excess vitamin A
Gums—firm, coral pink color, stippled	Spongy, friable, swollen, bluish-red or black color, bleed easily	Vitamin C
Mucous membranes—bright pink, smooth, moist	Stomatitis	Niacin

*Nutrients listed are deficient unless specified as excess.

TABLE 6-1

Clinical Assessment of Nutritional Status—cont'd

Evidence of Adequate Nutrition	Evidence of Deficient or Excess Nutrition	Deficiency/Excess*
Tongue—rough texture, no lesions, taste sensation	Glossitis	Niacin, riboflavin, folic acid
	Diminished taste sensation	Zinc
Teeth—uniform white color, smooth, intact	Brown mottling, pits, fissures	Excess fluoride
	Defective enamel	Vitamin A, C, D, calcium, phosphorus
	Caries	Excess carbohydrates
Chest		
In infants, shape is almost circular	Depressed lower portion of rib cage	Vitamin D
In children, lateral diameter increases in proportion to anteroposterior diameter	Sharp protrusion of sternum	
Smooth costochondral junctions	Enlarged costochondral junctions	Vitamin C, D
Breast development—normal for age	Delayed development	See General growth, above, especially zinc
Cardiovascular System		
Pulse and blood pressure (BP) within normal limits	Palpitations	Thiamin
	Rapid pulse	Potassium Excess thiamin
	Arrhythmias	Magnesium, potassium Excess niacin, potassium
	Increased BP	Excess sodium
	Decreased BP	Thiamin Excess niacin
Abdomen		
In young children, cylindric and prominent	Distended, flabby, poor musculature	Protein, calories
	Prominent, large	Excess calories
Older children, flat	Potbelly, constipation	Vitamin D
Normal bowel habits	Diarrhea	Niacin Excess vitamin C
	Constipation	Excess calcium, potassium
Musculoskeletal System		
Muscles—firm, well-developed, equal strength bilaterally	Flabby, weak, generalized wasting	Protein, calories
	Weakness, pain, cramps	Thiamin, sodium, chloride, potassium, phosphorus, magnesium Excess thiamin
	Muscle twitching, tremors	Magnesium
	Muscular paralysis	Excess potassium
Spine—cervical and lumbar curves (double S curve)	Kyphosis, lordosis, scoliosis	Vitamin D
Extremities—symmetric; legs straight with minimum bowing	Bowing of extremities, knock-knees	Vitamin D, calcium, phosphorus
	Epiphyseal enlargement	Vitamin A, D
	Bleeding into joints and muscles, joint swelling, pain	Vitamin C
Joints—flexible, full range of motion, no pain or stiffness	Thickening of cortex of long bones with pain and fragility, hard tender lumps in extremities	Excess vitamin A
	Osteoporosis of long bones	Calcium Excess vitamin D
Neurologic System		
Behavior—alert, responsive, emotionally stable	Listless, irritable, lethargic, apathetic (sometimes apprehensive, anxious, drowsy, mentally slow, confused)	Thiamin, niacin, pyridoxine, vitamin C, potassium, magnesium, iron, protein, calories Excess vitamin A, D, thiamin, folic acid, calcium
	Masklike facial expression, blurred speech, involuntary laughing	Excess manganese
Absence of tetany, convulsions	Convulsions	Thiamin, pyridoxine, vitamin D, calcium, magnesium Excess phosphorus (in relation to calcium)
Intact peripheral nervous system	Peripheral nervous system toxicity (unsteady gait, numb feet and hands, fine motor clumsiness)	Excess pyridoxine
Intact reflexes	Diminished or absent tendon reflexes	Thiamin

tissue. Table 6-1 summarizes clinical signs of possible nutritional deficiency or excess. Few are diagnostic for a specific nutrient and if suspicious signs are found, they must be confirmed with dietary and biochemical data. Generally the clinical examination does not reveal children at risk for a deficiency or excess.

Anthropometry

An essential parameter of nutritional status is anthropometry, the measurement of height, weight, head circumference in young children, proportions, skinfold thickness, and arm circumference. Height and head circumference reflect past nutrition, while weight, skinfold thickness, and arm circumference reflect present nutritional status, especially of protein and fat reserves. Skinfold thickness is a measurement of the body's fat content since approximately one half of the body's total fat stores are directly beneath the skin. The upper arm muscle circumference is correlated with measurements of total muscle mass. Since muscle serves as the body's major protein reserve, this measurement is considered an index of the body's protein stores. Ideally growth measurements are recorded over a period of time, and comparisons are made regarding the *velocity* of growth based on previous and present values. Techniques for anthropomorphic measurement are discussed in Chapter 7.

BIOCHEMICAL ANALYSIS

Numerous biochemical tests are available for assessing nutritional status and include analysis of plasma, blood cells, urine, or tissues from liver, bone, hair, and fingernails. Many of these tests are complicated and are not performed routinely. Common laboratory procedures for nutritional status include measurement of hemoglobin, hematocrit, albumin, creatinine, and nitrogen. Laboratory values for these tests and more specific nutrient measurements are given in Appendix E.

EVALUATION OF NUTRITIONAL ASSESSMENT

After collecting the data needed for a thorough nutritional assessment, the nurse should evaluate the findings to plan appropriate counseling. From the data, the child can be assessed as (1) malnourished, (2) at risk for becoming malnourished, or (3) well nourished with adequate reserves.

The daily food diary is analyzed for inclusion of selections in each of the four basic food groups (see p. 123). For example, if the list includes no vegetables, the nurse should inquire about this rather than assume that the child dislikes vegetables because it could be that none were served on that day. Also the information obtained needs to be evaluated in terms of the family's ethnic practices and financial resources. To encourage increased protein intake with additional meat may be unfeasible for families on a limited budget or in conflict with food practices that use meat sparingly, such as in Asian meal preparation. Consequently, appropriate counseling needs to be based on the specific details of the nutrition history.

Findings from clinical examination and anthropometry are evaluated with the data obtained from the dietary intake. For example, findings suggestive of anemia and a dietary record of iron-poor foods necessitate laboratory analysis of hemoglobin. Any suspicious findings should be appropriately referred for further evaluation.

SUMMARY

Communication is the most important skill nurses use in relating to children and their families. Effective communication must be concerned with establishing an appropriate setting, using effective interviewing skills with parents and children, and recognizing the developmental differences of children at various ages. Several verbal and nonverbal communication techniques can enhance and facilitate the collection of quality information.

The health history is a particular type of interview that is concerned with information about the child's past and present physical, social, and emotional health. The health of the family system is of primary concern and involves an assessment of the structure and function of the family. In addition to the interview, specific tools or instruments can be employed to gain additional information about the family. Lastly, a thorough nutritional assessment includes data obtained from dietary intake history, clinical examination, and selected laboratory tests.

KEY CONCEPTS

- Communication, the most important skill nurses must possess in the care of children, has verbal, nonverbal, and abstract components.
- To effectively establish a setting for communication, the nurse must make an appropriate introduction, clarify her role and the purpose of the interview, and ensure privacy and confidentiality.
- When communicating with parents, the nurse needs to encourage parental involvement, listen carefully, use silence, and be empathic.
- Communication with children must reflect their development stage.
- Verbal communication techniques that have proved to be effective include the third-person technique, facilitative responding, storytelling, bibliotherapy, the use of "what if" questions, and other word games.
- Nonverbal communication with children may take the form of writing, drawing, and play.
- The objectives of performing a health history are to identify pertinent information, determine the chief complaint, analyze the present illness, secure the past history, review biologic systems, and record a family and sexual history.
- Family assessment is the collection of data about family composition and relationships among its members and also focuses on home and community environment, occupation and education, and cultural and religious traditions.

- The family function interview examines interaction and roles, power, decision-making, problem-solving, communication, and expression of feelings and individuality.
- Nutritional assessment is performed by determination of dietary intake, clinical examination, and biochemical analysis.

STUDY QUESTIONS AND ACTIVITIES

1 Interview two families, preferably families with differences in ages of children, socioeconomic status, and ethnic background, and compare the type of responses from each. Consider the following: Do they respond better to open- or closed-ended sentences? What are their concerns regarding their children? How do their cultural traditions affect family function?
2 Interview children in the age-groups of toddler, preschooler, school-ager, and adolescent about a similar topic, such as their favorite activities. Compare the different phrasing of questions that are needed to elicit responses and the types of answers. What developmental characteristics were evident during the interviews?
3 During an interview with a child or family use four of the communication techniques described on pp. 110-113.
4 Conduct and record a complete health history on a child, including assessment of the family and the child's nutritional status. Note the length of time required and those areas of the interview that demanded more skill in the interviewing process.
5 Keep a dietary history of your eating habits using the 24-hour recall, 3-day food diary, and food frequency record. Compare the information obtained from these three methods. What method yielded information that was most representative of your actual eating habits?

REFERENCES

Burns, R.C., and Kaufman, S.H.: Kinetic family drawings, New York, 1970, Brunner/Mazel, Inc.

Caldwell, B., and Bradley, R.: Home observation for measurement of the environment, rev. ed., Little Rock, AR, University of Arkansas, 1984.

Epstein, C.: Nursing the dying patient, Reston, VA, 1975, Reston Publishing Co., Inc.

Frankenburg, W., and Coons, C.: Home Screening Questionnaire: its validity in assessing home environment, J. Pediatr. **108**(4):624-626, 1986.

Heineken, J., and Roberts, F.B.: Confirming, not disconfirming: communicating in a more positive manner, MCN **8**(1):78-80, 1983.

Henrich, A.P., and Bernheim, K.F.: Responding to patients' concerns, Nurs. Outlook **29**(7):428-433, 1981.

Kohut, S.A.: Guidelines for using interpreters, Hosp. Prog. **56**(4):39-40, 1975.

Lewis, J., and others: No single thread: psychological health in family systems, New York, 1976, Brunner/Mazel, Inc.

Smilkstein, G.: The family APGAR: a proposal for a family function test and its use by physicians, J. Fam. Pract. **6**(6):1231-1239, 1978.

Strasburger, V.: The challenge of adolescent medicine in the 1980s, Child Care Newsletter **5**(1):1-3, 1986.

BIBLIOGRAPHY

Communication Strategies

Berg, P.J., Devlin, M.K., and Gedaly-Duff, V.: Bibliotherapy with children experiencing loss, Issues Compr. Pediatr. Nurs. **4**:37-50, 1980.

Brockopp, D.Y.: What is NLP? Am. J. Nurs. **83**(7):1012-1014, 1983.

Cameron, C.O., Juszczak, L., and Wallace, N.: Using creative arts to help children cope with altered body image, Child. Health Care **12**(3):108-112, 1984.

Cassell, E.J.: Learning language skills: changing the words changes the world, Patient Care **14**:126-142, 1980.

Cassell, E.J.: Learning language skills: hear what the patient means, say what you mean, Patient Care **14**:80-90, 1980.

Cassell, E.J.: Learning language skills: untwisting the fibers of "paralanguage," Patient Care **14**:186-204, 1980.

Clutter, L., and others: Communicating effectively with young children, Child. Nurse **5**(4):1-4, 1987.

Clutter, L., and others: Communicating effectively with older children and adolescents, Child. Nurse **6**(1):4-8, 1988.

Crews, N.E.: Developing empathy for effective communication, AORN J. **30**:536, 1979.

DiLeo, J.H.: Interpreting children's drawings, New York, 1983, Brunner/Mazel, Inc.

Faber, A., and Mazlish, E.: How to talk so kids will listen & listen so kids will talk, New York, 1980, Avon Books.

Farr, K.: Communication pitfalls in routine counseling, Pediatr. Nurs. **5**(1):55-57, 1979.

Fosson, A., and Husband, E.: Bibliotherapy for hospitalized children, South. Med. J. **77**(3):342-346, 1984.

Fosson, A., and deQuan, M.M.: Reassuring and talking with hospitalized children, Child. Health Care **13**(1):37-44, 1984.

Gelhard, H.L.: Drawing and development, Pediatr. Nurs. **4**(6):23-25, 1978.

Hahn, K.: Therapeutic storytelling: helping children learn and cope, Pediatr. Nurs. **13**(3):175-178, 1987.

How should patients be addressed? AORN J. **31**:1142-1146, 1980.

Johnson, S.H.: Avoiding communication blocks with high-risk parents, Issues Compr. Pediatr. Nurs. **4**:61-72, 1980.

Jolly, J.D.: Through a child's eyes: the problems of communicating with sick children, Nursing (Oxford) **1**:1012-1014, 1981.

Knowles, R.D.: Building rapport through neuro-linguistic programming, Am. J. Nurs. **83**(7):1010-1014, 1983.

Maheady, D.: Cultural assessment of children, MCN **11**(2):128, 1986.

McLeavey, K.A.: Children's art as an assessment tool, Pediatr. Nurs. **5**(2):9-14, 1979.

Mengel, A.: Getting the most from patient interviews, Nursing 82 **12**(11):46-49, 1982.

Monsen, R.: Phases in the caring relationship: from adversary to ally to coordinator, MCN **11**(5):316-318, 1986.

Pontious, S.L.: Practical Piaget: helping children understand, Am. J. Nurs. **82**(1):114-117, 1982.

Smith, E.C.: Communicating with young children: are you really communicating? Am. J. Nurs. **77**:1966-1967, 1977.

Use C-A-R-E to show your concern, Nursing 87 **87**(9):117, 1987.

Wallace, N.E.: Special books for special children, Child. Health Care **12**(1):34-36, 1983.

Health Interview

Baer, E.D., McGowan, M.N., and McGivern, D.O.: Taking a health history, Am. J. Nurs. **77**(7):1190-1193, 1977.

Brown, M.S., and Murphy, M.A.: Ambulatory pediatrics for nurses, New York, 1979, McGraw-Hill Book Co.

McBride, M.M.: Can you tell me where it hurts? Pediatr. Nurs. **3**(4):7-8, 1977.

Moss, M., and Schleutermann, J.: Assessment of the pediatric client. In Malasanos, L., and others, editors: Health assessment, ed. 3, St. Louis, 1986, The C.V. Mosby Co.

Muscari, M.E.: Obtaining the adolescent sexual history, Pediatr. Nurs. **13**(5):307-310, 1987.

Family Assessment

Bradley, R., and Caldwell, B.: Using the HOME inventory to assess the family environment, Pediatr. Nurs. **14**(2):97-102, 1988.

Calloway, S.: Home Observation for Measurement of the Environment. In Humenick, S., editor: Analysis of current assessment strategies in the health care of young children and childbearing families, Norwalk, CT, 1982, Appleton-Century-Crofts.

Holt, S.J., and Robinson, T.M.: The school nurse's "family assessment tool," Am. J. Nurs. **79**(5):950-953, 1979.

Lewis, J.M.: How's your family? New York, 1979, Brunner/Mazel, Inc.

Meister, S.B.: Charting a family's developmental status—for intervention and for the record, MCN **2**(1):43-48, 1977.

Miller, J., and Janosik, E., editors: Family-focused care, New York, 1980, McGraw-Hill Book Co.

Sedgwick, R., and Hildebrand, S.: Family health assessment, Nurse Pract. **6**(2):37-45, 1981.

Speer, J., and Sachs, B.: Selecting the appropriate family assessment tool, Pediatr. Nurs. **11**(5):349-355, 1985.

Wright, L., and Leahey, M.: Nurses and families: a guide to family assessment and intervention, Philadelphia, 1984, F.A. Davis Co.

Nutritional Assessment

American Academy of Pediatrics Committee on Nutrition: Assessment of nutritional status. In Pediatric nutrition handbook, ed. 2, Elk Grove Village, IL, 1985, The Academy.

Dansky, K.H.: Assessing children's nutrition, Am. J. Nurs. **77**(10):1610-1611, 1977.

Hinson, L.: Nutritional assessment and management of the hospitalized patient, Crit. Care Nurs. **5**:53-60, 1985.

Krause, M.V., and Mahan, L.K.: Food, nutrition, and diet therapy, Philadelphia, 1984, W.B. Saunders Co.

Mahan, L.K., and Rees, J.M.: Nutrition in adolescence, St. Louis, 1984, Times Mirror/Mosby College Publishing.

Pipes, P.L.: Nutrition in infancy and childhood, St. Louis, 1985, The C.V. Mosby Co.

Stuff, J.E., and others: A comparison of dietary methods in nutritional studies, Am. J. Clin. Nutr. **37**:300-306, 1983.

Todd, K.S., Hudes, M., and Calloway, D.H.: Food intake measurement: problems and approaches, Am. J. Clin. Nutr. **37**:139-146, 1983.

Williams, S.R.: Nutrition and diet therapy, ed. 4, St. Louis, 1985, Times Mirror/Mosby College Publishing.

CHAPTER 7

Physical and Developmental Assessment of the Child

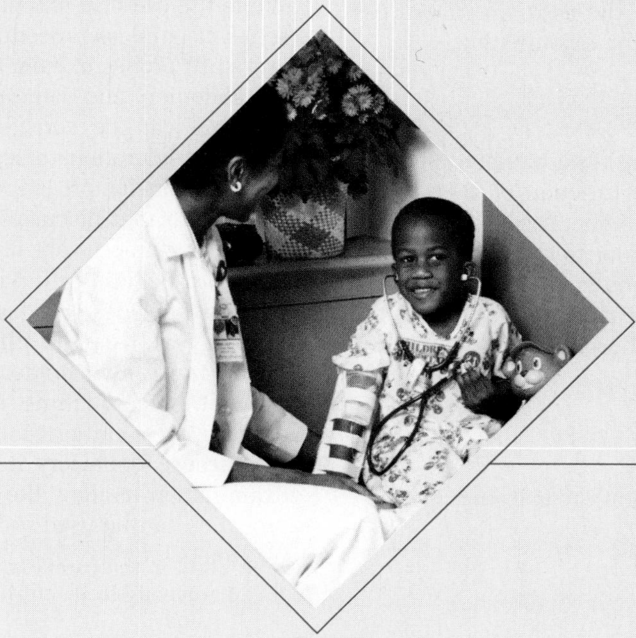

LEARNING OBJECTIVES

On completion of this chapter the reader will be able to:

- Prepare a child for a physical examination based on his developmental needs
- Perform a physical examination in a sequence appropriate to the child's age
- Recognize expected normal findings for children at various ages
- Record the physical examination according to the head-to-toe format
- Perform a developmental assessment using a standard screening test, such as the Denver Developmental Screening Test

Physical assessment is a continuous process that begins during the interview, primarily by use of the tool of inspection or observation, and that continues to some degree throughout the professional relationship. While the format for organization of a systematic approach resembles that of a medical physical examination, the objective of each assessment area is to formulate nursing diagnoses and evaluate the effectiveness of interventions. Although the nurse may diagnose or assist in the establishment of a medical diagnosis, this is secondary to the primary goal of identifying patient problems.

This chapter discusses the influence of age in the preparation of children for physical examination. It also details the performance of the examination and the expected normal findings for children at various ages. It concludes with a discussion of developmental assessment and administration of selected tests, such as the Denver Developmental Screening Test.

◆ *General Approaches Toward Examining the Child*

The physical examination is more than a series of technical maneuvers. It demands the same sensitivity to the child's physical and psychologic needs as any other strange and unfamiliar experience. This discussion is concerned with the sequence of the assessment process and preparation of the child for the examination.

SEQUENCE OF THE EXAMINATION

Ordinarily the sequence for examining patients follows a head-to-toe direction. The main function of such a systematic approach is to provide a general guideline for assessment of each body area in order to minimize omitting segments of the examination. The standard recording of data also facilitates exchange of information among different professionals. The typical organization of a physical examination is listed here:

1. Growth measurements
   a. Height (length)
   b. Weight
   c. Skinfold thickness and arm circumference
   d. Head circumference
2. Physiologic measurements
   a. Temperature
   b. Pulse
   c. Respiration
   d. Blood pressure
3. General appearance
4. Skin
5. Lymph nodes
6. Head
7. Neck
8. Eyes
9. Ears
10. Nose
11. Mouth and throat
12. Chest
13. Lungs
14. Heart
15. Abdomen
16. Genitalia
17. Anus
18. Back and extremities
19. Neurologic assessment
    a. Cerebellar functioning
    b. Reflexes
    c. Cranial nerves
20. Developmental screening

In examining children, this orderly sequence is frequently altered to accommodate the child's developmental needs, although the examination is recorded following the head-to-toe model. Using developmental and chronologic age as the main criteria for assessing each body system accomplishes several goals:

1. It minimizes stress and anxiety associated with assessment of various body parts
2. It fosters a trusting nurse-child-parent relationship
3. It allows for maximum preparation of the child
4. It preserves the essential security of the parent-child relationship, especially with young children
5. It maximizes the accuracy and reliability of assessment findings

PREPARATION OF THE CHILD

While the physical examination is usually thought of as a series of painless procedures, to a child the use of a tight arm cuff, probes in ears, mouth, and rectum, pressing on the abdomen, and listening to the chest with a cold piece of metal can be considerably stressful. Therefore, the same considerations discussed in Chapter 21 for preparing children for procedures should be followed here. In addition to that discussion certain aspects related to the examining process are presented below.

Before beginning the examination the nurse needs to be aware of cues that signal the child's readiness to cooperate, such as the child's willingness to talk to the nurse, make eye contact, accept the offered equipment, allow physical touching, smile, or choose to sit on the examining table rather than the parent's lap. Failure to observe these behaviors indicates a need to postpone the examination to allow the child to "warm up." Several approaches can be used to facilitate this:

1. Talk to the parent while essentially "ignoring" the child; gradually focus on the child or a favorite object, such as a doll
2. Make complimentary remarks about the child's dress and appearance
3. Tell a funny story or play a simple trick
4. Have a nonthreatening friend available, such as a hand puppet to "talk" for the nurse
5. Allow choices whenever possible, such as, "Would you like to sit up on the table or in your mom's lap?"
6. Begin the examination with those activities that can be presented as games, such as tests for the cranial nerves (p. 170) or parts of the Denver Developmental Screening Test (DDST) (p. 171) and end with the more traumatic procedures, such as examining the ears and mouth

Another approach that is effective in preparing the child for the examination is the "paper-doll technique." The child lies supine on the examining table, and his length is measured by marking the end points of the head and heels on the paper. When he sits up, the nurse asks him to look at the two marks and suggests that the rest of him be filled in to see "how big" he is. Children are usually amazed to see their body outline and quickly become absorbed in drawing more parts. Consequently, before areas of the body are assessed, they can be drawn on the "paper doll" and "examined." For example, before auscultating the heart, the nurse can draw in the heart, "listen" to it on the paper, and then say to the child, "Let's listen to your heart and see what sound it makes" (Fig. 7-1). With older children the nurse can use a more detailed drawing to help them learn about their bodies. At the conclusion of the visit the child can bring the paper doll home as a memento of his experience.

Whatever approach is used, statements are made in a

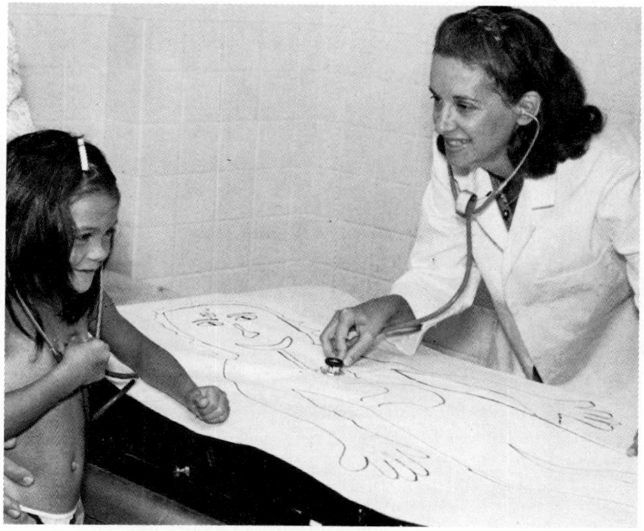

FIG. 7-1 Using paper-doll technique to prepare child.

positive manner and in a tone of voice that says, "I expect you to cooperate." Suggestive statements, such as, "I am going to feel your belly, but it won't hurt," are avoided, since the child immediately assumes it will hurt. Instead the nurse states what is going to be done and offers distractions, such as the Nursing tip on p. 162.

Although the variations in the general approaches are numerous, some of them are elaborated here because they are more common. For example, the suggested sequence may change considerably when the child is in pain or when obvious physical defects are present. In either situation it is preferable to examine the affected area last to minimize distress early in the examination and to focus on normal, healthy, or functioning body parts rather than questionable ones.

Positioning may also be altered because of physical distress. For example, the child who is having difficulty breathing may not be able to lie down, necessitating that as much of the physical examination as possible be performed in a sitting or slightly reclining position or that the examination be completed at another time. On the other hand, the child with abdominal pain may rest most comfortably in a side-lying position with the knees drawn up to the chest and may refuse to sit up or be supine. In this case the examiner may need to gradually ease the child into a supine position with knees and hips flexed to examine the abdomen.

Although parental presence is almost always conducive to a child's cooperation and sense of security, there are occasions when older children prefer to be examined alone. In these instances it is best to request parents to leave the room before the examination begins. When the nurse and child are alone, the nurse can begin to establish rapport on a one-to-one basis by talking to the child and using appropriate preparatory measures rather than immediately initiating the examination. If the nurse

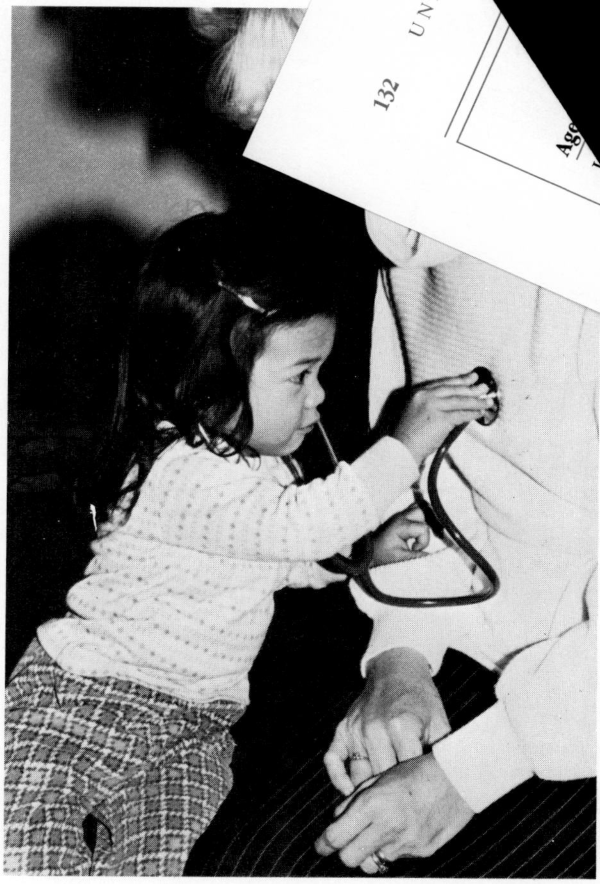

FIG. 7-2 Preparing child for physical examination.

judges that assistance may be needed, another person's help is enlisted.

Table 7-1 summarizes guidelines for positioning, preparing, and examining children at various ages. Since few children fit precisely into one category, it may be necessary to vary the approach after a preliminary assessment of the child's development. Even when the best approach is used, many toddlers are uncooperative and unable to be consoled for much of the physical examination, especially during restrictive procedures. However, some children seem intrigued by the new surroundings and unfamiliar equipment and cooperate with a minimum of resistance. Some preschoolers may require more of the security measures employed with younger children, such as performing the examination on the parent's lap, and less of the preparatory measures, such as playing with the equipment (Fig. 7-2).

◆ *Physical Examination*

Although the approach to and sequence of the physical examination differ according to the child's age, the following discussion outlines the head-to-toe model for physical assessment. It emphasizes normal findings, in-

TABLE 7-1

Age-Specific Approaches to Physical Examination during Childhood

Age	Position	Sequence	Preparation
Infant	Before sits alone: supine or prone, preferably in parent's lap; before 4 to 6 months: can place on examining table After sits alone: use sitting in parent's lap whenever possible If on table, place with parent in full view	If quiet, auscultate heart, lungs, abdomen Record heart and respiratory rates Palpate and percuss same areas Proceed in usual head-toe direction Perform traumatic procedures last (eyes, ears, mouth [while crying], rectal temperature [if taken]) Elicit reflexes as body part examined Elicit Moro reflex last	Completely undress if room temperature permits Leave diaper on male Gain cooperation with distraction, bright objects, rattles, talking Smile at infant; use soft, gentle voice Pacify with bottle of sugar water or feeding Enlist parent's aid for restraining to examine ears, mouth Avoid abrupt, jerky movements
Toddler	Sitting or standing on/by parent Prone or supine in parent's lap	Inspect body area through play: "count fingers," "tickle toes" Use minimal physical contact initially Introduce equipment slowly Auscultate, percuss, palpate whenever quiet Perform traumatic procedures last (same as for infant)	Have parent remove outer clothing Remove underwear as body part examined Allow to inspect equipment; demonstrating use of equipment usually ineffective If uncooperative, perform procedures quickly Use restraint when appropriate; request parent's assistance Talk about examination if cooperative; use short phrases Praise for cooperative behavior
Preschool child	Prefer standing or sitting Usually cooperative prone/supine Prefer parent's closeness	If cooperative, proceed in head-toe direction If uncooperative, proceed as with toddler	Request self-undressing Allow to wear underpants if shy Offer equipment for inspection Briefly demonstrate use Make up "story" about procedure: "I'm seeing how strong your muscles are" (blood pressure) Use paper-doll technique Give choices when possible Expect cooperation; use positive statements: "Open your mouth"
School-age child	Prefer sitting Cooperative in most positions Younger age prefer parent's presence Older age may prefer privacy	Proceed in head-toe direction May examine genitalia last in older child Respect need for privacy	Request self-undressing Allow to wear underpants Give gown to wear Explain purpose of equipment and significance of procedure, such as otoscope to see eardrum, which is necessary for hearing Teach about body functioning and care
Adolescent	Same as for school-age child Offer option of parent's presence	Same as older school-age child	Allow to undress in private Give gown Expose only area to be examined Respect need for privacy Explain findings during examination: "Your muscles are firm and strong" Matter-of-factly comment about sexual development: "Your breasts are developing as they should be" Emphasize normalcy of development Examine genitalia as any other body part; may leave to end

dications for counseling, and general abnormalities that necessitate appropriate referral. While the focus includes all age-groups, the reader is referred to Chapter 8 for a discussion of newborn assessment.

GROWTH MEASUREMENTS

Measurement of physical growth in children is a key element in evaluation of their health status. Physical growth parameters include height (length), weight, skinfold thickness, and head circumference. Values are plotted on growth charts for height, weight, and head circumference, and the child's measurements in percentiles are compared to those of the general population. Although some studies conclude that differences in height and weight among well-nourished children of different ethnic backgrounds are relatively small and that the present growth charts can be used for all racial or ethnic groups with a similar socioeconomic level, others demonstrate that ethnic differences do exist. A comparison of the average growth of American and Chinese children demonstrates that the average height and weight for Chinese children based on growth standards from China (see Appendix D) falls below the 50th percentile on the standard National Center for Health Statistics growth charts.

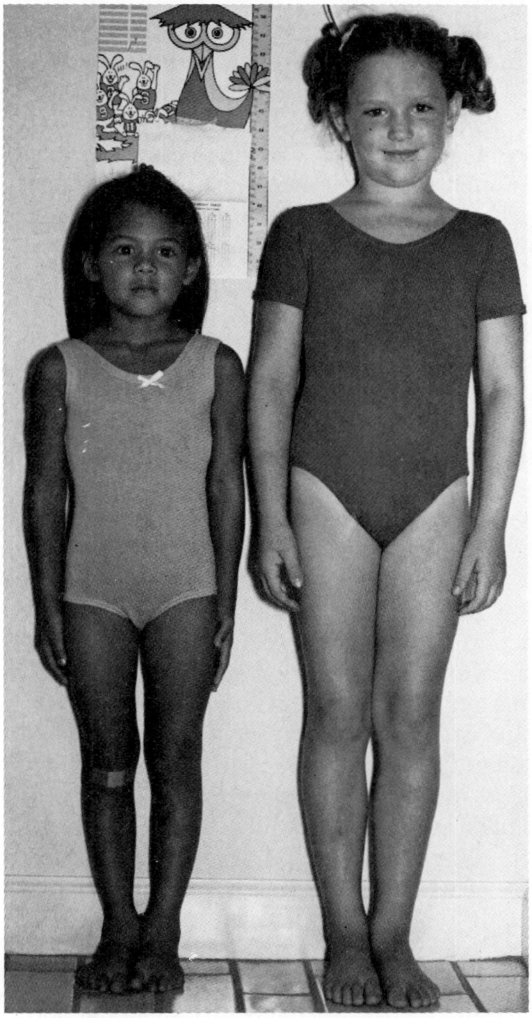

FIG. 7-3 These children of identical age (5-3/4 years) are markedly different in size. The child on the left, of partly Oriental descent, is at 5th percentile for height and weight. The white child on the right is above 95th percentile for height and weight. However, both children demonstrate normal growth patterns.

The most commonly used growth charts in the United States are from the National Center for Health Statistics. They are available for boys and girls ages birth to 18 years and use the 5th and 95th percentiles as criteria for determining which children are outside the normal limits for growth. In general, children whose height or weight falls below the 5th percentile are considered underweight or small in stature; those whose measurements are above the 95th percentile are considered overweight or large in stature.

Overall evaluation of growth requires judgment in interpretation of growth percentiles. Children who fall above or below the standard deviation in both height and weight may not be abnormal but may reflect a genetically large or small frame (Fig. 7-3). Comparing their growth trends with those of their parents and siblings is essential in evaluating adequate growth. Children whose growth may be questionable include:

1. Children whose height and weight percentiles are widely disparate, for example, height in the 10th percentile and weight in the 90th percentile, especially with above average skinfold thickness
2. Children who fail to show the expected gain in height and weight, especially during the rapid growth periods of infancy and adolescence
3. Children who show a sudden increase, except during puberty, or decrease in a previously steady growth pattern

Since growth is a continuous but uneven process, the most reliable evaluation lies in comparison of growth measurements over a prolonged period of time.

Length

Until children are 24 months old, recumbent height or length is measured in the supine position. Because of children's normally flexed position during infancy, measuring length requires full extension of the legs by (1) holding the head in midline, (2) grasping the knees together gently, and (3) pushing down on the knees until the legs are fully extended and flat against the table. If a measuring board is used, the head is placed firmly at the top of the board, and the heels of the feet are placed firmly against the footboard.

If such a measuring device is not available, the child's length is measured by placing him on a paper-covered surface, marking the end points of the top of the head and heels of the feet, and measuring between these two points (Fig. 7-4). For accurate measurement the writing utensil is held at a right angle to the table when the cephalic point is marked and the feet are positioned with

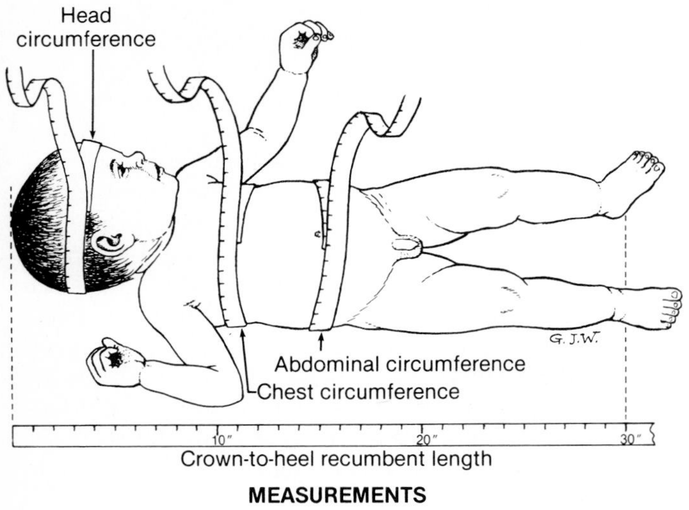

FIG. 7-4 Measurement of head, chest, and abdominal circumference and crown-to-heel (recumbent) length.

the toes pointing directly to the ceiling when the heel point is marked. Regardless of the method used, assistance in holding the child's head in midline is enlisted while the nurse extends the legs and takes the measurements.

Height

Recumbent or standing height may be taken in children who are over 24 months of age, although the latter is the usual procedure for those 3 years of age or older. Standing height is measured by having the child remove his shoes and stand as tall and straight as possible, with the head in midline and the line of vision parallel to the ceiling or floor. The child's back is to the wall or other vertical flat surface, with the heels, buttocks, and back of the shoulders touching the wall. Any flexion of the knees, slumping of the shoulders, or raising of the heels of the feet is checked and corrected.

Height is measured by placing a firm, flat surface against the vertex or crown of the head. The movable measuring rod of platform scales is accurate only if it maintains a parallel position to the floor and rests securely on the topmost part of the head. Another method for measuring height is to attach a paper or metal tape or a yardstick to the wall, position the child adjacent to the device, and place a thick object, such as book, on the head, making sure that the object rests firmly against the wall to form a right angle. The point of juncture of the underside of the book and the tape or yardstick is marked. For the most accurate height a wall mounted unit (Stadiometer) may be used (see Fig. 28-1). Height or stature should be measured to the nearest 1 mm or ⅛ inch.

Weight

Weight is measured using an appropriate-sized beam balance scale that measures weight to the nearest 10 g or ½ ounce for infants and 100 g or ¼ pound for children. Before children are weighed, the scale is balanced by setting it at zero and noting if the balance registers exactly in the middle of the mark. If the end of the balance beam rises to the top or bottom of the mark, more or less weight, respectively, must be added. Some scales are designed to allow for self-correction, and others need to be recalibrated by the manufacturer. Since the accuracy of scales varies, the same scale should be used for successive measurements.

Measurements should be made in a comfortably warm room. Infants are weighed nude; older children are usually weighed while wearing their underpants or a light gown in order to respect their need for privacy. If the child must be weighed wearing some article of clothing or some type of special device, such as a prosthesis, this is noted when the weight is recorded. Children who are measured for recumbent height are usually weighed on a large platform-type infant scale and placed in a lying-down or sitting position (Fig. 7-5, *A*). When weighing infants, the nurse places the hand slightly above the infant to prevent him from accidentally falling off the scale (Fig. 7-5, *B*). Once the standing height is taken, the weight can be measured on a standing-type upright platform scale. For maximum asepsis, scales are covered with a clean sheet of paper that is changed between each child's measurement.

Skinfold Thickness and Arm Circumference

Measures of relative weight and stature cannot distinguish between adiposity (amount of fatty tissue) or muscularity. One convenient measure of body fat is skinfold thickness, which can be measured with special calipers. The most common sites for measuring skinfold thickness are the triceps (most practical for routine clinical use), subscapula, suprailiac, abdomen, and upper thigh. For greatest reliability the exact procedure for measurement must be followed and the average of at least two measurements of one site recorded. Fig. 7-6 describes the procedure for measurement of triceps skinfold thickness.

Arm circumference is an indirect measure of muscle mass and is also recommended in the evaluation of nutritional status. Measurement of arm circumference follows the same procedure for skinfold thickness except the midpoint is measured with a paper or steel tape. Percentiles for triceps skinfold and arm circumference in children are listed in Appendix D.

Head Circumference

Head circumference is usually taken in all children up to 36 months of age and in any child whose head size is questionable, such as a child with hydrocephalus. The head is measured at its greatest circumference, that is, slightly above the eyebrows and pinna of the ears and around the occipital prominence at the back of the skull (see Fig. 7-4). A paper or metal tape is used since a cloth

A

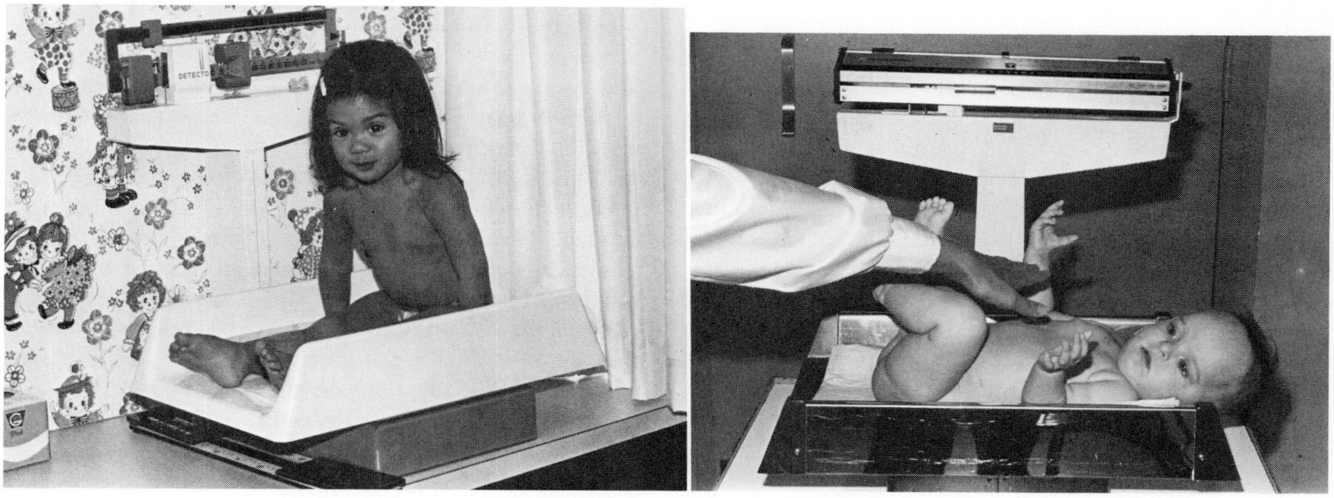

B

FIG. 7-5 A, Toddler on scale. **B,** Infant on scale.

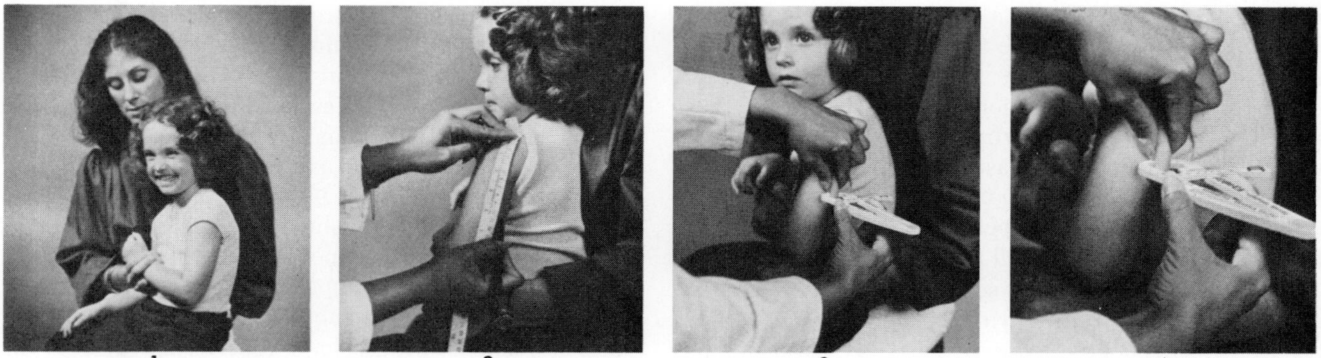

1
For a child, have an attendant hold the child's left hand or forearm with the elbow flexed to approximately 90 degrees and pressed gently against his or her abdomen. The child can be either standing or sitting.

For an infant, have an attendant (preferably the mother) hold the infant in a semi-upright position, with infant's right side next to but not touching mother's body, and with infant's head facing forward. Gently restrain the infant's left hand or forearm with the elbow flexed to approximately 90 degrees and pressed gently against his or her abdomen.

2
Marks are placed at the left acromion (shoulder) and olecranon (elbow). The distance between these marks is measured and the midpoint marked.

3
At a site 1 cm above midpoint, grasp a layer of skin and subcutaneous tissue with the first finger and thumb of one hand, gently pulling it away from the underlying muscle, and continue to hold until measurement is completed.

Place caliper jaws over the skinfold at the midpoint mark and apply pressure with the thumb to align the lines on the caliper. Do not apply excessive pressure.

4
Estimate reading to nearest 1.0 mm, 2 to 3 seconds after aligning lines.

Three readings should be taken, averaged, and recorded. Compare present measurement with previous triceps skinfold measurement(s) to determine possible change.

FIG. 7-6 Measurement of triceps skinfold. (Reprinted with permission of Ross Laboratories, Columbus, OH 43216, from Adipometer Skinfold Caliper and Instruction Chart, 1978, Ross Laboratories.)

tape may stretch and give a falsely small measurement. The head size is plotted on the growth chart under head circumference (see Appendix D). Generally head and chest circumference are equal at about 1 to 2 years of age. During childhood, chest circumference exceeds head size by about 5 to 7 cm (2 to 3 inches). (For the newborn see p. 190.)

PHYSIOLOGIC MEASUREMENTS

Physiologic measurements include temperature, pulse, respiration, and blood pressure. Although not usually recorded on a graph similar to growth charts for determination of percentiles, each physiologic recording is compared with normal values for that age-group (see the inside front cover). In addition, values taken on preceding health visits should be compared with present recordings.

As in most procedures carried out with children, older children and adolescents are treated much the same as are adults. However, special consideration must be given to preschool children, whose fear of mutilation is intensified with any intrusive procedure (p. 370).

For best results in taking vital signs of infants, the usual order of approach is reversed. Respirations are counted first, before the infant is disturbed, the pulse next, and temperature last. If vital signs cannot be taken without disturbing the child, the child's behavior (e.g., crying) is recorded with the measurement.

Temperature

Temperature can be measured at several sites in the body. Temperature measurement using a mercury thermometer is taken by the oral, rectal, or axillary route. The only difference in selection of thermometers is that the rectal type has a more rounded blunt bulb as compared to the oral type, which has a more slender, elongated tip.

Recent substitutes for the mercury thermometer are the electronic thermometer, the tympanic membrane sensor, the plastic strip thermometer, and the digital thermometer. The electronic thermometer is ideally suited to pediatric use because the plastic sheath is unbreakable, the child's mouth can remain open when an oral temperature is taken, and the temperature registers within 60 seconds and is accurate for all three routes.

The tympanic membrane sensor gathers the infrared energy emitted from the tympanic membrane, which serves as an excellent site because both the eardrum and the hypothalamus (temperature-regulating center) are perfused by the same circulation. The covered probe tip is placed gently at the external opening of the auditory canal and a temperature reading is given in only 1 second. Although the sensor is unaffected by cerumen, in the presence of otitis media it measures the local heat from the inflammation rather than core body temperature. Reports on the validity of the device demonstrate that it correlates well with oral, rectal, and axillary measurement of core body temperature (Hancock, 1987).

The plastic strip thermometer changes color in response to sensed temperature changes. The strip is placed on the forehead until a color change occurs. Research on the Clinitest II forehead strip demonstrates that it correlates well with measurements taken with mercury thermometers, although its readings are frequently higher than mercury readings (Martyn and others, 1988).

The digital thermometer consists of a probe that connects to a microprocessor chip. The chip translates the signals into degrees and sends the figure to a digital display. The digital thermometer is more accurate and easier to read, but more expensive, than the mercury or plastic strip thermometer.

Measurement. Although various devices are used to measure body temperature, the following discussion focuses on using mercury thermometers. *Oral temperatures* are taken in children who can be trusted to keep the thermometer under their tongue with their mouth closed without biting on the glass. Some agencies have a specific age for permitting oral temperatures (e.g., after 5 or 6 years, but some younger children can cooperate.

When an oral temperature is taken, the thermometer is placed under the tongue in the right or left posterior sublingual pocket, not in the area in front of the tongue. Contrary to traditional belief, the sublingual site indicates rapid changes in core body temperature better than the rectum. The sublingual area has a rich blood supply derived from the carotid arteries, which are close to the temperature-regulating center in the brain and the central circulation at the heart. However, several factors can temporarily affect the temperature of the mouth, such as hot or cold beverages, smoking, rapid breathing, and possibly oxygen by mask.

Axillary temperatures are often recommended for children who object strongly to a rectal temperature but for whom an oral temperature is not feasible. Axillary temperatures have the advantage of avoiding an intrusive procedure and eliminating the risk of rectal perforation and possible peritonitis, especially in newborn and premature infants. To take an axillary temperature, the thermometer is placed in the axilla with the arm kept close to the child's side (Fig. 7-7, *A*).

Rectal temperatures should be taken only when the oral or axillary route cannot be used, such as in children whose mental age or temperament precludes cooperation and understanding instructions and those who have had oral and axillary injuries or surgery. They are contraindicated in newborns and anyone who has had rectal surgery. One factor affecting the accuracy of rectal measurements is the presence of stool in the rectum.

To take a rectal temperature, the child is placed in a side-lying, supine, or prone position. A convenient position for infants is supine with the knees flexed toward the abdomen (Fig. 7-7, *B*). The position is maintained with one hand while the other hand is used to insert the lubricated bulb of the thermometer a maximum of 2.5 cm (1 inch). Further insertion increases the risk of perforation, because the colon curves at a depth of about 3 cm (1 1/4 inches). It is advisable to cover the penis because this procedure often stimulates urination.

An alternative position that works very well is for the parent to hold the child so that his arms are hugging the parent's neck and his legs are wrapped around the parent's waist. With the child in this straddle position, gently insert the thermometer into the rectum. This approach is effective, especially with toddlers, because it increases the child's security by preserving parental closeness and maintaining an upright position.

No universal agreement exists regarding the length of time mercury thermometers should be kept in place. Recommendations based on research are 7 minutes for an oral reading; 4 minutes for a rectal reading; and 5 minutes for an axillary reading. However, these times may

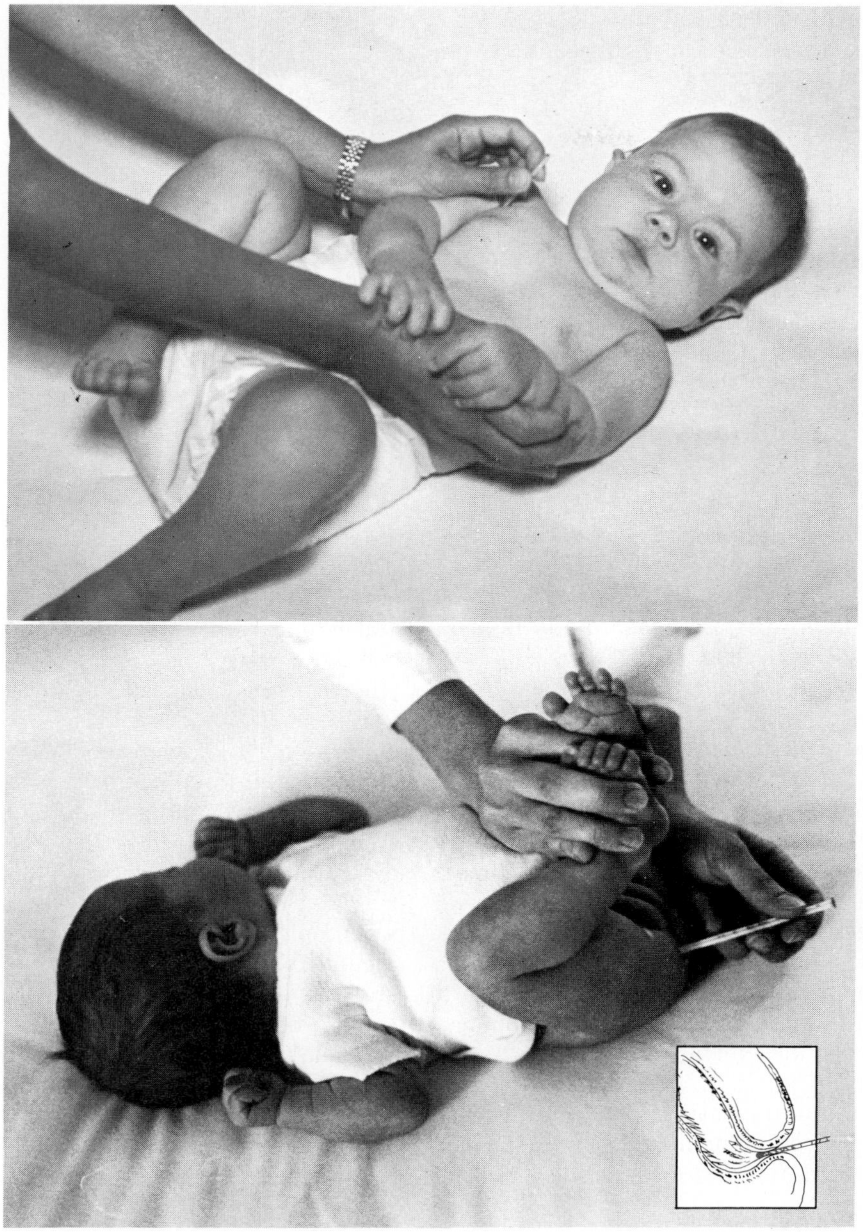

FIG. 7-7 **A,** Position for taking axillary temperature. **B,** Position for taking rectal temperature in infant. Inset of cross-section of rectum illustrates curve at approximately 3 cm from anus.

vary widely within practice settings and may not represent clinically significant differences in temperature readings taken for shorter intervals.

Normal body temperature registers 37.0° C (98.6° F) via the oral route. Traditionally it has been assumed that rectal temperatures are 1° F higher and axillary temperatures 1° F lower than oral temperatures. However, it has been demonstrated that this difference may be considerably less. Because of these variations, the route is charted along with the recorded temperature reading.

A characteristic of some small children is the tendency toward a rapid temperature elevation with the associated risk of precipitating seizures. Whenever a child feels extra warm to the touch, his temperature should be taken, even if it was found to be normal only a short time before. Children under 3 years of age are especially vulnerable to febrile seizures.

Pulse

A satisfactory pulse can be taken radially in children over 2 years of age. However, in infants and young children the apical pulse (heard through a stethoscope held to the chest at the apex of the heart) is more reliable. (See Fig. 7-31 for location of the apex and Fig. 7-32 for location of pulses.) The pulse is counted for 1 full minute in infants and young children because of possible irregularities in rhythm. (See the inside front cover for normal rates for pediatric age-groups.)

Respiration

The respiratory rate is counted in the same manner as it is in the adult patient except that, in infants, the movements are primarily diaphragmatic and, therefore, observed by abdominal movement. Since the movements may be irregular, they should be counted for 1 full minute for accuracy (see also pp. 156 and 157). (See the inside front cover for normal respiratory rates in children.)

Blood Pressure

Blood pressure measurement is part of a routine vital sign determination. Blood pressure should be measured annually in children 3 years of age through adolescence and in children with symptoms of hypertension, children in emergency rooms and intensive care units, and in high-risk infants (Report of the Second Task Force, 1987). Several authorities also recommend routine measurements in low-risk neonates.

A number of devices are available for measuring blood pressure. The most commonly used instruments are the mercury-gravity (use of mercury reservoir) or the aneroid (use of metal bellows) sphygmomanometers. Blood measure can also be measured using electronic devices that employ oscillometric or Doppler techniques. In oscillometry, pressure changes are transmitted through the arterial wall to the pressure cuff, and the oscillations are detected by a sensitive pressure indicator (see Fig. 8-4). The Doppler instrument translates changes in ultrasound frequency caused by blood movement within the artery to audible sound by means of a transducer in the cuff. Such instruments are very useful in measuring blood pressure in infants and have replaced the flush method, which reflects only the *mean* blood pressure (average of systolic and diastolic pressures).

Selection of cuff. Accurate measurement requires the use of an appropriately sized cuff (cuff size refers only to the inner inflatable bladder not the cloth covering). The cuff should be long enough to completely encircle the circumference of the arm with or without overlapping and sufficiently wide to cover approximately 75% of the upper arm between the top of the shoulder and the olecranon. There should be enough room at the antecubital fossa to place the bell of the stethoscope and at the upper edge of the cuff to prevent obstruction of the axilla (Report of the Second Task Force, 1987). Available cuff sizes are listed in the box, although the selection of a cuff must be individualized for each child.

Ill-fitting cuffs are a common cause of incorrect blood pressure readings. A small cuff causes a falsely elevated reading, while a large cuff or compression of the brachial artery by clothing pushed up the arm may result in a lower reading. However, wide cuffs apparently do not cause the low readings observed in adults (Steinfeld and others, 1978). Therefore in choosing cuff sizes, it is preferable to use an oversized cuff rather than an undersized one when the correct size is not available or to use another site that more adequately accommodates the cuff size. For example, radial pressure can be taken when a cuff is too small, such as on an obese adolescent. The largest size arm cuff is placed above the wrist, and the radial artery is used for auscultation or palpation. The systolic pressure in the radial artery is 10 mm Hg lower than in the brachial artery.

Thigh blood pressure can be taken on small children when only large cuffs are available. The cuff is wrapped around the thigh just above the knee and the popliteal artery is auscultated or palpated (Fig. 7-8). Blood pressure in the thigh normally averages 10 mm Hg higher than the arm pressure. A lower pressure in the lower extremities may indicate some interference with circulation such as coarctation of the aorta. A comparison of blood pressure in the arm and leg should be done at least once during early childhood to detect such abnormalities.

Measurement. The technique of blood pressure measurement in children is generally the same as that used for adults. However, some aspects of the procedure require special attention. Because children are easily upset by unfamiliar procedures, every effort is made to prepare them for blood pressure measurement. For children of preschool age and above each step of the procedure is explained and they are told how the cuff will feel, such as a tight feeling or an arm hug. Explanations such as "I want to see how strong your muscle is" or "Let's watch the silver rise in the tube" are especially appealing to young children.

Since the child should be quiet and relaxed during the procedure, blood pressure is measured before any anxiety-producing procedures are performed. Infants and small children may be more quiet if the reading is taken while they are sitting in the parent's lap.

For greatest accuracy the following procedure is recommended (Report of the Second Task Force, 1987):

Commonly Available Blood Pressure Cuffs

Cuff Name*	Bladder Width (cm)	Bladder Length (cm)
Newborn	2.5-4.0	5.0-9.0
Infant	4.0-6.0	11.5-18.0
Child	7.5-9.0	17.0-19.0
Adult	11.5-13.0	22.0-26.0
Large arm	14.0-15.0	30.5-33.0
Thigh	18.0-19.0	36.0-38.0

From Report of the Second Task Force on Blood Pressure Control in Children–1987, Pediatrics **79**(1):1-25, 1987.
*Cuff name does not guarantee that the cuff will be appropriate size for a child within that age range.

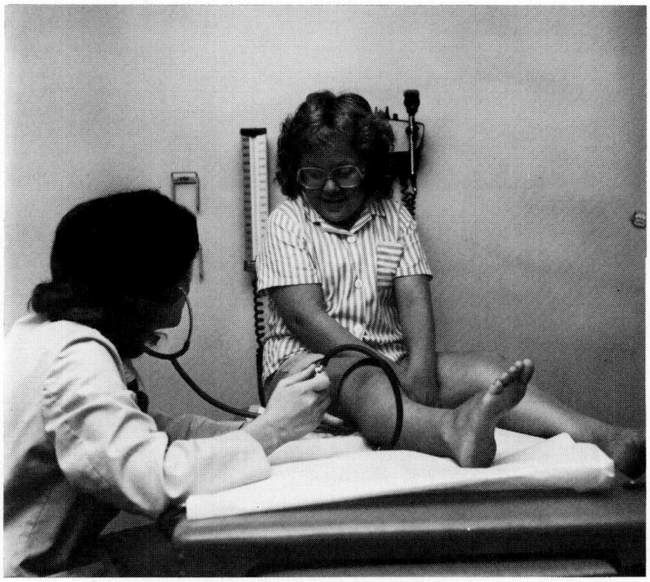

FIG. 7-8 Using the popliteal artery for blood pressure.

1. Use the same position, preferably sitting, and the right arm
2. Position the arm at the level of the heart
3. Rapidly inflate the cuff to about 20 mm Hg above the point at which the radial pulse disappears
4. Release the cuff pressure at a rate of about 2 to 3 mm Hg per second during auscultation of the artery
5. Read the mercury-gravity manometer at eye level
6. Record the systolic value as the onset of a clear tapping sound (first Korotkoff sound)
7. Record the diastolic pressure as both the fourth Korotkoff sound (K4) (low-pitched, muffled sound) and the fifth Korotkoff sound (K5) (disappearance of all sound) along with systolic pressure, limb, position, and cuff size. (For example, BP = 100/60/54 mm Hg, right arm, sitting, with child cuff)

The average blood pressure readings at various ages throughout childhood are listed on the inside front cover. Blood pressure standards use K4 diastolic pressure for infants and children 3 to 12 years and K5 diastolic pressure for adolescents 13 to 18 years. Normal blood pressure is defined as systolic and diastolic pressure less than the 90th percentile for age and sex. However, body size needs to be considered when blood values reach the upper limit, since larger children have higher blood pressures than smaller children of the same age. For example, a tall child whose BP is at the 90th percentile for age is considered normal. Measurements that are above the 90th percentile should be repeated during subsequent visits with every effort made to reduce the child's anxiety (Report of the Second Task Force, 1987).

GENERAL APPEARANCE

The general appearance of the child is a cumulative, subjective impression of the child's physical appearance, state of nutrition, behavior, personality, interactions with parents and nurse (also siblings if present), posture, development, and speech. Although general appearance is recorded in the beginning of the physical examination, it encompasses all the observations of the child during the interview and physical assessment.

Physical Appearance

The description of physical appearance notes the *facies*, the facial expression and appearance of the child. For example, the facies may give clues to children who are in pain, have difficulty in breathing, feel frightened, discontent, or happy, are mentally deficient, or are acutely ill.

Posture, position, and types of *body movement* also are important in the overall assessment of physical appearance. The child with hearing or vision loss may characteristically tilt his head in an awkward position to facilitate perception of sound or sight. The child in pain may favor a body part. The child with low self-esteem or a feeling of rejection may assume a slumped, careless, and apathetic pose or posture. Likewise, a child with confidence, a feeling of self-worth, and a sense of security usually demonstrates a tall, straight, well-balanced posture. Although the nurse observes such "body language," it must not be interpreted too freely but rather recorded objectively.

Hygiene is noted in terms of the child's state of cleanliness, unusual body odor, the condition of the hair, neck, nails, teeth, and feet, and the condition of the clothing. Such observations give excellent clues to possible instances of neglect, inadequate financial resources, housing difficulties (e.g., no running water), or lack of knowledge of children's needs.

Nutrition

General appearance includes an overall impression of the child's state of nutrition. This impression is more than a statement describing body weight or stature, such as "slender and tall." It is an estimation of the quality, as well as the quantity, of nutritional intake. For example, two children can be of the same height and weight, yet one can appear overweight because of flabby, loose skin, while the other child appears strong, robust, and well built because of firm, well-defined musculature.

The nurse's impression of nutritional state should be compared with the parents' history of feeding practices. Discrepancies between the two "impressions" may be a valuable area for nutritional counseling. For example, parents who believe that their child is too thin and eats too little, despite evidence of adequate growth and physical signs of proper nutrition, may find it helpful to keep a daily diary in order to calculate the child's cumulative food intake. When this is done, many parents are surprised at the quantity of food ingested, even though the amounts at each meal or snack are small.

Behavior

Behavior includes the child's personality, level of activity, reaction to stress, requests, frustration, interactions with others (primarily the parent and nurse), degree of alertness, and response to stimuli. Some mental questions that serve as reminders for observing behavior include: What is the child's overall personality? Does he have a long attention span or is he easily distracted? Can he follow two or three commands in succession without the need for repetition? What is his response to delayed gratification or frustration? Does he use eye-to-eye contact during conversation? What is his reaction to the nurse and family members? Is he quick or slow to grasp explanations?

Development

An overall estimate of the child's speech development, motor skills, degree of coordination, and recent area of achievement is recorded under general appearance. The impressions should be documented with screening tests, such as the Denver Developmental Screening Test (DDST) (see p. 171).

SKIN

Skin is assessed for color, texture, temperature, moisture, and turgor. Examination of the skin and its accessory organs primarily involves inspection and palpation. The normal color in light-skinned children varies from a milky-white and rose color to a deep-hued pink color. Dark-skinned children, such as those from Native American, Hispanic, or black descent, have inherited various brown, red, yellow, olive-green, and bluish tones in their skin. Oriental persons have skin that is normally of a yellow tone.

Several variations in skin color can occur and some of these variations warrant further investigation. The types of color change and their appearance in children with light or dark skin are summarized in Table 7-2.

Normally the skin of young children is smooth, slightly dry to the touch, not oily or clammy, and of even exterior temperature. Skin temperature is evaluated by symmetrically feeling each part of the body and comparing upper areas with lower ones. Any difference in temperature is noted.

Tissue turgor refers to the amount of elasticity in the skin. It is best determined by grasping the skin on the

TABLE 7-2

Differences in Color Changes of Racial Groups

Color Change	Description	Appearance in Light Skin	Appearance in Dark Skin
Cyanosis	A bluish tone through skin reflects reduced (deoxygenated) hemoglobin	Bluish tinge, especially in palpebral conjunctiva (lower eyelid), nail beds, earlobes, lips, oral membranes, soles, and palms	Ashen gray lips and tongue
Pallor	Paleness may be a sign of anemia, chronic disease, edema, or shock	Loss of rosy glow in skin, especially face	Ashen-gray appearance in black skin More yellowish-brown color in brown skin
Erythema	Redness may be result of increased blood flow from climatic conditions, local inflammation, infection, skin irritation, allergy, or other dermatoses or may be caused by increased numbers of red blood cells as a compensatory response to chronic hypoxia	Redness easily seen anywhere on body	Much more difficult to assess; rely on palpation for warmth or edema
Ecchymosis	Large, diffuse areas, usually black and blue in color, are caused by hemorrhage of blood into skin; are typically result of injuries	Purplish to yellow-green areas; may be seen anywhere on skin	Very difficult to see unless in mouth or conjunctiva
Petechiae	Same as ecchymosis except for size: small, distinct pinpoint hemorrhages 2 mm or less in size; can denote some type of blood disorder, such as leukemia	Purplish pinpoints most easily seen on buttocks, abdomen, and inner surfaces of the arms or legs	Usually invisible except in oral mucosa, conjunctiva of eyelids, and conjunctiva covering eyeball
Jaundice	Yellow staining of the skin usually caused by bile pigments	Yellow staining seen in sclera of eyes, skin, fingernails, soles, palms, and oral mucosa	Most reliably assessed in sclera, hard palate, palms, and soles

abdomen between the thumb and index finger, pulling it taut, and quickly releasing it. Elastic tissue immediately assumes its normal position without residual marks or creases. In children with poor skin turgor the skin remains suspended or tented for a few seconds before slowly falling back on the abdomen. Skin turgor is one of the best estimates of adequate hydration and nutrition.

Accessory Structures

Inspection of the accessory structures of the skin may be performed while the skin is being examined or when the scalp and extremities are being assessed.

Hair. The hair is inspected for color, texture, quality, distribution, and elasticity. Children's scalp hair is usually lustrous, silky, strong, and elastic. Genetic factors affect the appearance of hair. For example, the hair of black children is usually curlier and coarser than that of white children. Hair that is stringy, dull, brittle, dry, friable, and depigmented may suggest poor nutrition. Any bald or thinning spots are recorded. Loss of hair in infants may indicate lying in the same position and may be a clue for counseling parents concerning the child's stimulation needs.

The hair and scalp are inspected for general cleanliness. Various ethnic groups condition their hair with oils or lubricants, which, if not thoroughly washed from the scalp, clog the sebaceous glands, causing scalp infections. The hair and scalp are also examined for lesions, scaliness, evidence of infestation, such as lice or ticks, and signs of trauma, such as ecchymosis, masses, or scars.

In older children who are approaching puberty, growth of secondary hair is noted as a sign of normally progressing pubertal changes. Precocious or delayed appearance of hair growth is noted because, although not always suggestive of hormonal dysfunction, it may be of great concern to the early- or late-maturing adolescent.

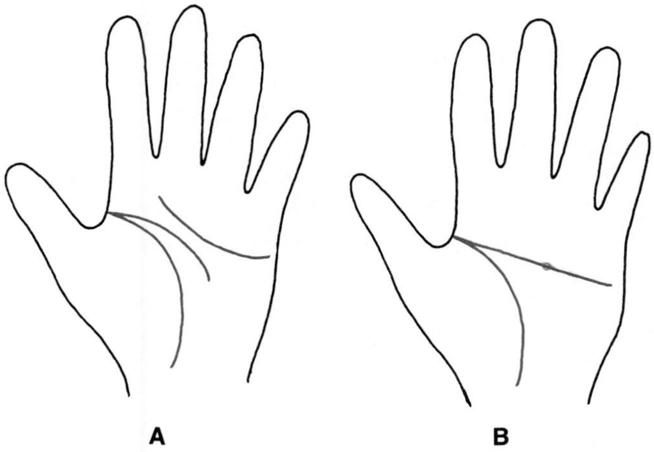

FIG. 7-9 Examples of flexion creases on palm. **A,** Normal; **B,** simian crease.

Nails. The nails are inspected for color, shape, texture, and quality. Normally the nails are pink, convex in shape, smooth, and hard but flexible (not brittle). The edges, which are usually white, should extend over the fingers. Dark-skinned individuals may have more deeply pigmented nail beds. Short, ragged nails are typical of habitual biting. Uncut, dirty nails are a sign of poor hygiene.

Dermatoglyphics. Each individual has a distinct set of handprints and footprints created by epidermal ridges and creases formed in the third month of prenatal life and cracks that develop subsequently throughout a lifetime. The patterns, or *dermatoglyphics,* are unique to the individual and vary a great deal in detail and complexity. The palm normally shows three flexion creases (Fig. 7-9, *A*). In some situations the two distal horizontal creases are fused to form a single horizontal crease called a *single palmar crease* or *simian crease* (Fig. 7-9, *B*), which is noted in almost all conditions that are caused by chromosomal abnormalities. If grossly abnormal lines or folds are observed, the nurse should sketch a picture to describe them and refer the finding to a specialist for further investigation.

LYMPH NODES

Lymph nodes are usually assessed when the part of the body in which they are located is examined. Although the body's lymphatic drainage system is extensive, the usual sites for palpating accessible lymph nodes are shown in Fig. 7-10.

Nodes are palpated by using the distal portion of the fingers and gently but firmly pressing in a circular motion along the regions where nodes are normally present. During assessment of the nodes in the head and neck, the child's head is tilted upward slightly but without tensing the sternocleidomastoid or trapezius muscles. This position facilitates palpation of the *submental, submaxillary, tonsillar,* and *cervical* nodes. The *axillary* nodes are palpated with the arms relaxed at the side but slightly abducted. The *inguinal* nodes are best assessed with the child in the supine position. Size, mobility, temperature, and tenderness are noted, as well as reports by the parents regarding any visible change of enlarged nodes. In children small, nontender, movable nodes are usually normal. Tender, enlarged, warm lymph nodes generally indicate infection or inflammation proximal to their location. Such findings are reported for further investigation.

HEAD

The head is inspected for general *shape* and *symmetry.* It should be symmetric with frontal, parietal, and occipital prominences. The *face* is inspected for symmetry, movement, and general appearance. Asking the child to "make a face" is a way to assess symmetric movement and disclose any degree of paralysis. Any unusual facial proportion is noted, such as unusually high or low forehead, wide or close-set eyes, or small, receding chin.

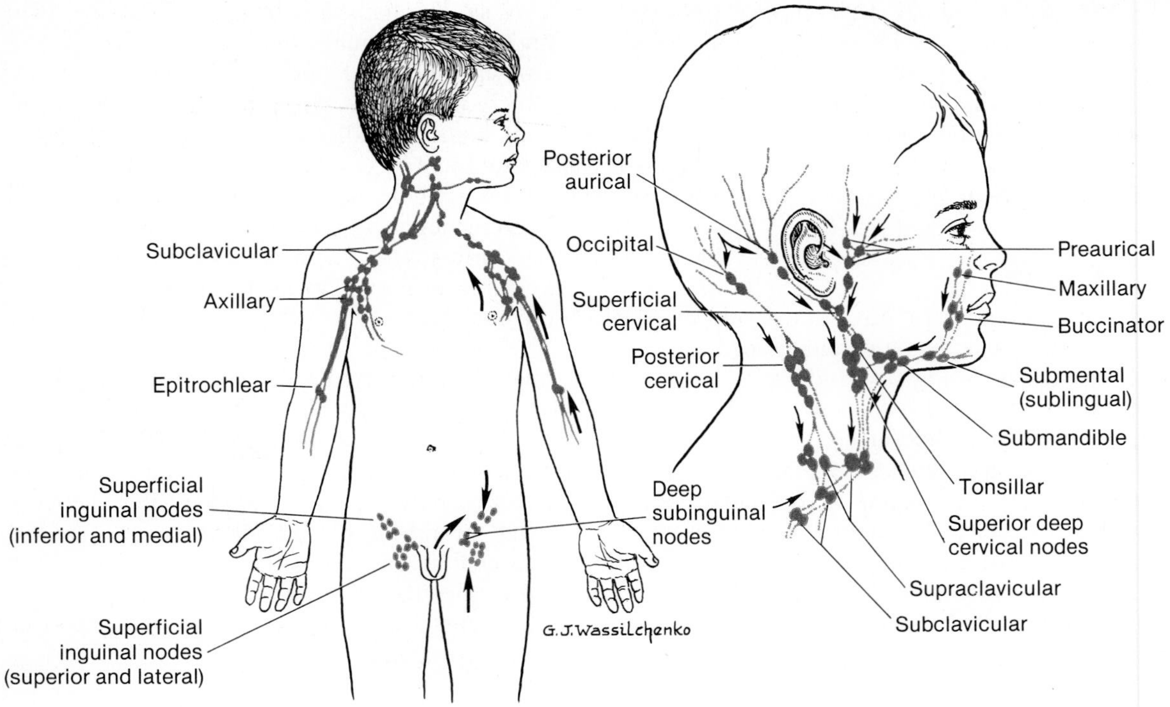

FIG. 7-10 Location of superficial lymph nodes. Arrows indicate directional flow of lymph.

Head control is noted in infants, and head posture is noted in older children. Most infants by 4 months of age should be able to hold the head erect and in midline when in a vertical position. Significant head lag after 4 months of age strongly suggests cerebral injury. Range of motion is evaluated by asking the older child to look in each direction (to either side, up, and down) or manually putting the younger child through each position. Limited range of motion may indicate wryneck, or *torticollis,* a result of injury to the sternocleidomastoid muscle, in which the child holds the head to one side with the chin pointing toward the opposite side.

The skull is palpated for patent sutures, fontanels, fractures, and swellings. The posterior fontanel normally closes by 2 months of age, and the anterior fontanel closes between 12 and 18 months of age (see Chapter 8).

NECK

Beside assessing mobility of the head and neck, the neck is inspected for size and palpated for associated structures. The neck is normally short with skin folds between the head and shoulders during infancy; however, it lengthens during the next 3 to 4 years.

The *trachea* is palpated by placing the thumb and index finger on each side and sliding them back and forth to note any masses. Normally the trachea is in midline. Any shift from midline or questionable masses in the neck are recorded and reported for further investigation.

EYES

Examination of the eyes involves inspection of all exterior structures for size, symmetry, color, and motility, and inspection of the interior surfaces for examination of retinal structures. The latter requires the use of an ophthalmoscope and is a highly skilled procedure. Discussion of the retinal examination includes the basic normal findings that the nurse should be able to discern with some practice in using the ophthalmoscope. The third part of the examination involves vision testing.

Inspection of External Structures (Fig. 7-11)

The *lids* are inspected for proper placement on the eye. When the eye is open, the upper lid should fall between the upper iris and the top portion of the pupil. When the eyes are closed, the lids should completely cover the cornea and sclera.

The general slant of the *palpebral fissures* or lids is inspected. The degree of slant is judged by drawing an imaginary line through the two points of the medial canthus and across the outer orbit of the eyes and aligning each eye on the line. Usually the palpebral fissures lie horizontally. However, in Oriental persons the slant is normally upward.

The lining of the lids, the *palpebral conjunctiva* is also inspected. Examining the lower conjunctival sac is easily accomplished by pulling the lid down while the patient looks up. To evert the upper lid, the child looks down

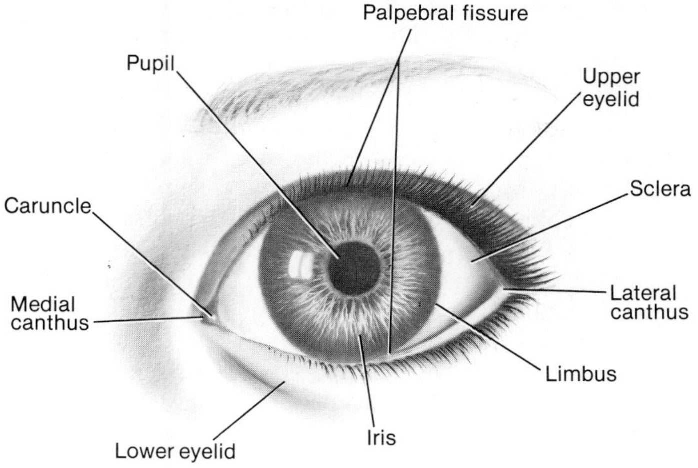

FIG. 7-11 External structures of eye.

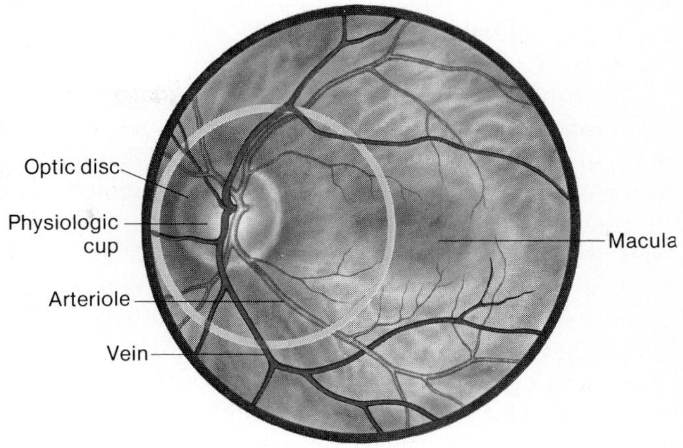

FIG. 7-12 Structures of the fundus. The interior circle represents the appropriate size of the area seen with the ophthalmoscope.

while the nurse holds the upper lashes and gently pulls *down* and *forward*. Normally the conjunctiva appears pink and glossy. Vertical yellow striations along the edge are the meibomian or sebaceous glands near the hair follicle. Located in the inner or medial canthus and situated on the inner edge of the upper and lower lids is a tiny opening, called the lacrimal punctum. Any excessive tearing or inflammation of the lacrimal apparatus should be noted.

The *bulbar conjunctiva,* which covers the eye up to the limbus or junction of the cornea and sclera, should be transparent. The *sclera* or white covering of the eyeball should be clear. Tiny black marks in the sclera of heavily pigmented individuals are normal.

The *cornea,* or covering of the iris and pupil, should be clear and transparent. Any opacities are recorded since they can be signs of scarring or ulceration, which can interfere with vision. The best way to test for opacities is to illuminate the eyeball by shining a light at an angle (obliquely) toward the cornea.

The *pupils* are compared for size, shape, and movement. They should be round, clear, and equal. The nurse tests their *reaction to light* by quickly shining a source of light toward the eye and removing it. As the light approaches, the pupils should constrict; as the light fades, the pupils should dilate. *Accommodation,* or the focusing ability of the eyes to produce clear vision at different distances, is tested by having the child look at a bright, shiny object at a distance and quickly moving the object toward the face. The pupils should constrict as the object is brought near the eye. The normal findings when examining the pupils may be recorded as *PERRLA,* which means "pupils equal, round, react to light and accommodation."

The *iris* is inspected for color, size, and clarity. Permanent eye color is usually established by 6 to 12 months of age. As the iris and pupil are inspected, the *lens* is also examined. Normally the lens is not visible through the pupil.

Inspection of Internal Structures

The ophthalmoscope permits visualization of the interior of the eyeball with a system of lenses and a high-intensity light. The lenses permit clear visualization of eye structures at different distances from the nurse's eye and correct visual acuity differences in the examiner and child. Use of the ophthalmoscope requires practice to know which lens setting produces the clearest image.

The ophthalmic and otic head are usually interchangeable on one "body" or handle, which encloses the power source, either disposable or rechargeable batteries. The nurse should practice changing the heads, which snap on and are secured with a quarter turn, and replacing the batteries and light bulbs. Nurses who are not directly involved in physical assessment are often responsible for assuring that the equipment functions properly.

Preparing the child. The child is prepared for the ophthalmic examination by showing him the instrument, demonstrating the light source and how it shines in the eye, and explaining the reason for darkening the room. For infants and young children who do not respond to such explanations, it is best to try and use distraction to encourage them to keep their eyes open. Forcibly parting the lids results in an uncooperative, watery-eyed child and a frustrated nurse. Usually, with some practice, the nurse can elicit a red reflex almost instantly while approaching the child and may also gain a momentary inspection of the blood vessels, macula, or optic disc.

Fundoscopic examination. Fig. 7-12 illustrates the structures of the back of the eyeball or the *fundus.* In examining the interior of the eye, the nurse inspects the red reflex, the optic disc, the macula, and the blood vessels. It is important to remember that the ophthalmoscope permits only a small area of visualization. In order to perform an adequate examination, the nurse must move the ophthalmoscope systematically around the fundus to locate each structure.

The fundus derives its orange-red color from the inner two layers of the eye, the choroid and the retina, which are immediately apparent as the *red reflex*. The intensity of the orange-red color increases in darkly pigmented individuals. A brilliant, uniform red reflex is an important sign, because it virtually rules out almost all serious defects of the cornea, aqueous chamber, lens, and vitreous chamber. Any dark shadows or opacities are recorded because they usually indicate some abnormality in any of these structures.

As the nurse approaches the child with the ophthalmoscope, the most conspicuous feature of the fundus is the *optic disc,* the area where the blood vessels and optic nerve fibers enter and exit from the eye. The color of the disc is creamy pink; it is lighter in color than the surrounding fundus. It derives its color from the rich capillary network. It is normally round or vertically oval. Its size is important because other structures of the fundus are measured in relationship to the disc's diameter (DD). Most discs have a small, pale depression in their center, called the *physiologic cup* or *depression,* which represents the blind spot of the retina. It is not always visible but, when large enough to be seen, should not extend to the disc margin.

After the optic disc is located, the area is inspected for *blood vessels*. The central retinal artery and vein appear in the depths of the disc and emanate outward with visible branching. The *veins* are darker in color and about one fourth larger in size than the *arteries*. Normally the branches of the arteries and veins cross each other.

About 2 DD temporal to the disc is the *macula,* the area of the fundus with the greatest concentration of visual receptors. It is about 1 DD in size and darker in color than the fundus (red reflex) or optic disc. The intensity of the color directly correlates with the individual's skin pigmentation, that is, the darker the skin, the darker the color of the macula. In the center of the macula is a minute glistening spot of reflected light called the *fovea centralis*. It is the area of most perfect vision. If locating the macula is difficult, the child is asked to look directly at the light. However, since this is the most light-sensitive area of the retina, the nurse must be careful to focus on the macula only momentarily.

Vision Testing

Several tests are available for assessing vision. This discussion focuses on four areas of vision testing: (1) binocularity, (2) visual acuity, (3) peripheral vision, and (4) color vision. The reader is referred to Chapter 19 for behavioral and physical signs that indicate visual impairment.

Binocularity. Normally, by the age of 3 to 4 months, children achieve the ability to fixate on one visual field

A

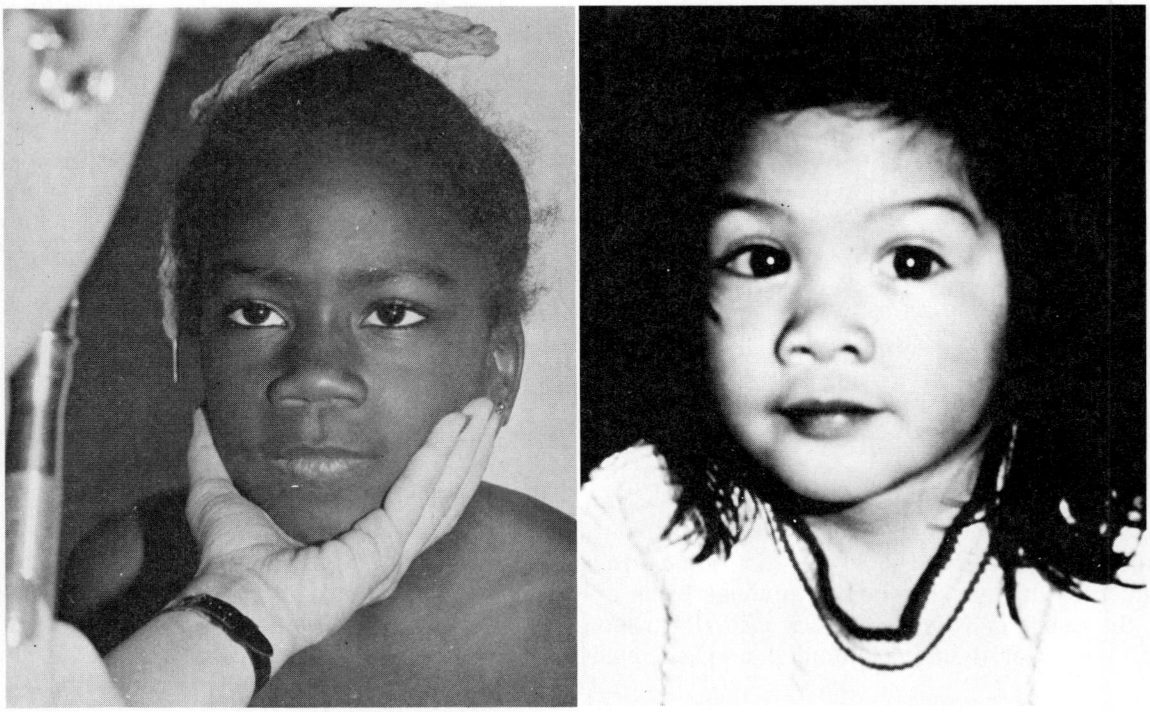

B

FIG. 7-13 A, Corneal light reflex test demonstrating orthophoric eyes. **B,** Pseudostrabimus. Inner epicanthal folds cause eyes to appear malaligned; however, corneal light reflexes fall perfectly symmetrically.

with both eyes simultaneously (binocularity). One of the most important tests for binocularity is alignment of the eyes to detect nonbinocular vision or *strabismus*. In strabismus, or "cross-eye," one eye deviates from the point of fixation. If the malalignment is constant, the weak eye becomes "lazy," and the brain eventually suppresses the image produced by that eye. If strabismus is not detected and corrected by age 4 to 6 years, a type of blindness, called *amblyopia*, may result.

Two tests commonly used to detect malalignment are the corneal light reflex test (also called red reflex gemini test or Hirschberg test) and the cover test. In the *corneal light reflex test* the nurse shines a flashlight or the light of the ophthalmoscope directly into the patient's eyes from a distance of about 40.5 cm (16 inches). If the eyes are *orthophoric* or normal, the light falls symmetrically within each pupil (Fig. 7-13, *A*). If the light falls off center in one eye, the eyes are malaligned. *Epicanthal folds*, excess folds of skin that extend from the roof of the nose to the inner termination of the eyebrow and that partially or completely overlap the inner canthus of the eye, may give a false impression of malalignment (pseudostrabismus) (Fig. 7-13, *B*). Epicanthal folds are frequently found in Oriental children.

In the *cover test* one eye is covered and the movement of the *uncovered* eye is observed when the child looks at a near (33 cm or 13 inches) or distant (50 cm or 20 inches) object. If the uncovered eye does not move, it is aligned. If the uncovered eye moves, a malalignment is present because when the stronger eye is temporarily covered, the weaker eye attempts to fixate on the object.

In the *uncover test* occlusion is shifted back and forth from one eye to the other eye and movement of the *covered* eye is observed as soon as the occluder is removed while the child focuses on a point in front of him. If normal alignment is present, shifting the cover from one eye to the other eye will not cause movement of the covered eye. If malalignment is present, the covered eye will move from its position when covered to a straight position when uncovered. This test takes more practice than the

A

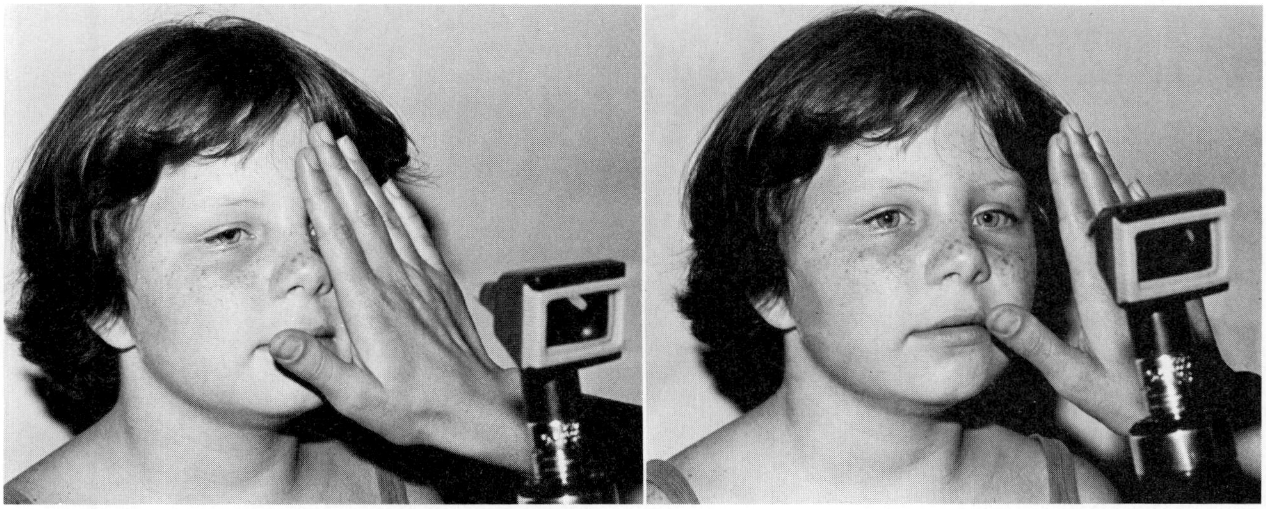

B

C

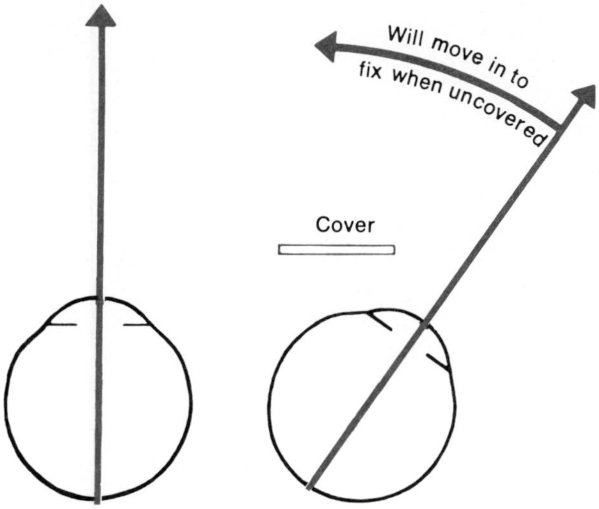

FIG. 7-14 Uncover test for strabismus. **A,** Eye is occluded, child is fixating on light source. **B,** If eye does not move when uncovered, eyes are aligned. **C,** Exophoria. As eye is uncovered, it shifts to fixate on object. (**C** from Prior, J.A., Silberstein, J.S., and Stang, J.M.: Physical diagnosis: the history and examination of the patient, ed. 6, St. Louis, 1981, The C.V. Mosby Co.)

other cover test because the occluder must be moved back and forth quickly and accurately in order to see the eye move. Usually it is easier to perform this test by using one's hand rather than a card or other object such as the occluder (Fig. 7-14). Since deviations can occur at different ranges, it is important to perform the cover tests at both close and far distances.

Visual acuity. Visual acuity refers to the ability to see near and far objects clearly. Several screening tests may be used to test visual acuity. Those that are more commonly employed are discussed below.

Snellen charts. The most common test for measuring visual acuity is the *Snellen letter chart,* which consists of lines of letters of decreasing size (see Appendix C). The person to be tested stands 20 feet from the chart and reads each line. If he can read the 20-foot line, he has 20/20 vision, the accepted standard for normal acuity. If the person can only read the second line, he has 20/100 vision. That means that what he is able to see at a distance of 20 feet, the person with 20/20 or normal eyesight can see at 100 feet. This test is suitable for most children above the second grade who are familiar with the alphabet.

The 20-foot distance for measuring visual acuity is not a strict requirement and young children are often more attentive at closer range. If screening is done at a distance other than 20 feet with the appropriate chart, an equivalent measurement is used. For example, in screening with the 10-foot chart the equivalent measurement for 20/40 is 10/20.

A version of the Snellen letter chart is the *Snellen E Chart,* which uses the capital letter E pointing in four different directions. The child "reads" the chart by showing the direction of the letter E or the "legs of the table" either by pointing with his hand or by verbally identifying the direction, such as "toward the ceiling, floor, window, or wall." Although it is frequently used to test preschoolers, young children may have difficulty with this test because of confusion in identifying the direction rather than inability to see clearly. This can be corrected by giving them a large duplicate letter E and having them turn it to match the letter on the chart. The Snellen E Chart is available for home vision screening from the **National Society to Prevent Blindness,*** which recommends its use for children between preschool and 6 years of age.

The National Society to Prevent Blindness (1982) recommends the following criteria for referring children for a professional eye examination when using the Snellen charts:

1. Three-year-old children with vision in either eye of 20/50 or less (inability to correctly identify one more than half the symbols on the 40-foot line) *or* a two-line difference in visual acuity between the eyes in the passing range; for example, 20/20 in one eye and 20/40 in the other
2. All other ages and grades with vision in either eye of 20/40 or less (inability to correctly identify one more than half the symbols on the 30-foot line)
3. All children who consistently show any of the signs of possible visual disturbances, regardless of visual acuity

*79 Madison Avenue, New York, NY 10016. Also available is an excellent book on vision screening for preschoolers and school age children entitled *Children's Eye Health Guide.*

Blackbird Vision Screening System. To avoid the confusion problems with the Snellen E Chart, the Blackbird Vision Screening Kit was developed by a nurse (Sato-Viacrucis, 1985). The screening system uses a modified E that resembles a bird and a story about the Blackbird to help engage children's attention and teach the bird's flight positions. Testing is done with flash cards and the children are instructed to indicate the direction of the bird's flight. The test is suitable with children as young as 3 years and includes guidelines for screening nonverbal, nonreader, and/or non-English–speaking children. The Blackbird Storybook Home Eye Test can be used by parents and teachers for children ages 2 1/2 years and older (Fig. 7-15).*

Denver Eye Screening Test. Another test that is suitable for children age 2½ years and older is the *Denver Eye Screening Test* (DEST) (see Appendix C). It tests for visual acuity in children 3 years or older by using a single card for the letter E, and it tests from a distance of 15

*Available from Blackbird Vision Screening System, P.O. Box 7424, Sacramento, CA 95826.

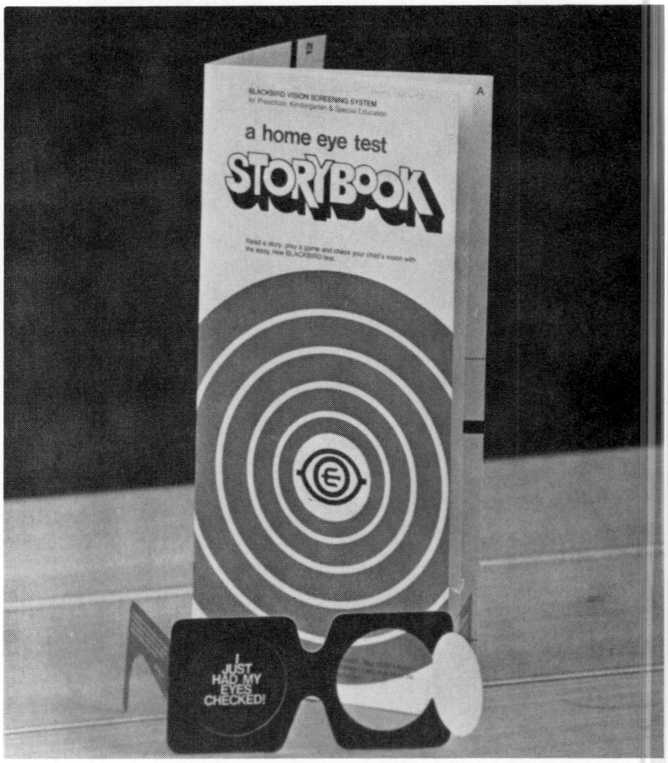

FIG. 7-15 The Blackbird Storybook Home Eye Test. Note the Blackbird symbol in the center circle and the special "eyeglass" occluder.

feet, rather than 20 feet. The large E (20/100) is used primarily for explanation and demonstration of the procedure to the child. The small E (20/30) is used for testing. Failure to correctly identify the direction of the small E over three trials is considered abnormal. As with every other vision screening test, each eye is tested separately.

For children from 2½ to 2 11/12 years of age or those who are untestable with the DEST letter E test, picture cards (or Allen cards) which accompany the DEST are used. Although the DEST is recommended for children beginning at age 30 months, the Allen cards can be used reliably with cooperative children from the age of 24 months. The pictures (a tree, birthday cake, horse and rider, telephone, car, house, and teddy bear) are shown to the child at close range to make certain that he can readily identify them and then are shown at a distance of 15 feet. If the child cannot correctly name three of the seven cards in three to five trials, his performance is considered abnormal.

The DEST also screens children from 6 to 30 months of age who may be at risk for visual problems by testing for (1) fixation (ability to follow a moving light source or spinning toy), (2) squinting (observation of the child's eyes or report by parent), and (3) strabismus (report by parent and performance on cover and pupillary [corneal] light reflex tests). Abnormal findings include failure to fixate, presence of a squint, and/or failing two of the three procedures for strabismus.

Newborn screening. In newborns, vision is tested mainly by checking for *light perception* by shining a light into the eyes and noting responses such as blinking, following the light to midline, increased alertness, or refusing to open the eyes after exposure to the light. Vision can also be tested in an alert newborn by eliciting optokinetic nystagmus, which involves rotating a striped drum in front of his face and noting nystagmus (involuntary rapid eye movement), which indicates that vision is present. A more sophisticated and accurate test is the *visually evoked response (VER),* which is determined by stimulating the eyes with a bright light and recording electrical activity through scalp electrodes placed on the head over the visual cortex.

Peripheral vision. In a child who is old enough to cooperate, peripheral vision, or the visual field of each eye, is estimated. The test is performed by having the child fixate on a specific point directly in front of him as an object, such as a finger or a pencil, is moved from beyond the field of vision into the range of peripheral vision. Each eye is checked separately and for each quadrant of vision. As soon as the child sees the object, he tells the nurse to stop moving it. At that point the angle from the anteroposterior axis of the eye (straight line of vision) to the peripheral axis (point at which the object is first seen) is measured. Normally the child sees about 50 degrees upward, 70 degrees downward, 60 degrees nasalward, and 90 degrees temporally. Limitations in peripheral vision may be indicative of blindness from damage to structures within the eye or to any of the visual pathways.

Color vision. Another important test is for color vision. It is estimated that from 8% to 10% of white males and less than half that percentage of black males have inherited the X-linked disorder known as *color vision deficit* (less acceptable term, *color blindness*). From 0.5% to 1% of white females are affected. Although the severity of impaired perception of color varies considerably, the two most common types are (1) confusion of gray with pink or pale blue with green, and (2) confusion of gray with pale purple or green. In most of these individuals, the color vision deficit causes no major problems. However, some of the difficulties encountered by individuals with more severe deficits may be inability to distinguish amber or red traffic lights, failure to see a red brake light on the rear of a car, difficulty in distinguishing green traffic lights from certain types of incandescent street lamps, and a poor sense of color coordination of clothing. For school-age children with color vision deficits the greatest difficulty lies in performance of academic skills that use color as a visual aid. Adolescents with color vision deficits may be ineligible for certain vocational opportunities, such as electronics, photography, printing, interior decorating, pharmaceuticals, textiles, police work, and for several types of military service (Kovalesky, 1985).

The tests available for color vision include the *Ishihara test* and the *Hardy-Rand-Rittler* (HRR) *test*. Each consists of a series of cards (pseudoisochromatic) on which is printed a color field composed of spots of a certain "confusion" color. Against the field is a number or symbol similarly printed in dots but of a color likely to be confused with the field color by the person with a color vision deficit. As a result the figure or letter is invisible to an affected individual but is clearly seen by a person with normal vision. By using the HRR test, which uses symbols rather than numbers, reliable testing can be done on children as young as 3 years of age (Kovalesky, 1985). Nurses administering the test must be familiar with the testing materials and should be able to inform the parents of the disorder's effects on practical areas of living, its genetic transmission, and its irreversibility.

EARS

Like the eyes, examination of the ears involves inspection of the external auditory structures, visualization of the internal landmarks using a special instrument called the otoscope, and screening for hearing ability.

Inspection of External Structures

The entire external earlobe is called the *pinna* or *auricle* and is located on each side of the head. The *height* alignment of the pinna is measured by drawing an imaginary line from the outer orbit of the eye to the occiput or most prominent protuberance of the skull. The top of the pinna should meet or cross this line. The *angle* of the pinna is measured by drawing a perpendicular line from the imaginary horizontal line and aligning the pinna next to this

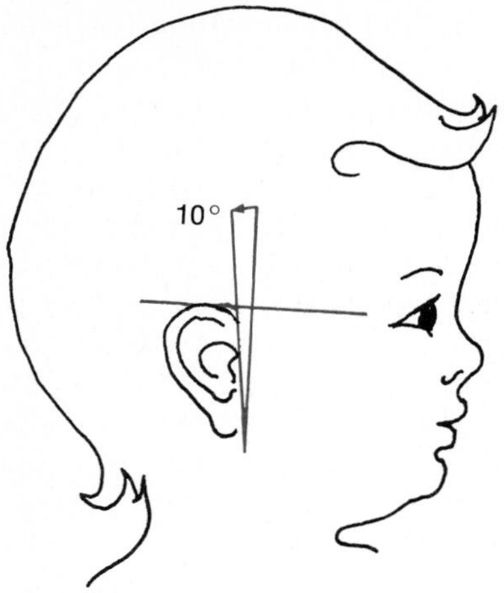

FIG. 7-16 Ear alignment.

mark. Normally the pinna lies within a 10-degree angle of the vertical line (Fig. 7-16). If it falls outside this area, the deviation is recorded.

Normally the pinna extends slightly outward from the skull. Except in newborn infants, ears that are flat against the head or protruding away from the scalp may indicate problems. Flattened ears in infants may suggest a frequent side-lying position and, just as with isolated areas of hair loss, may be a clue to investigating parents' understanding of the child's stimulation needs.

The *skin* surface around the ear is inspected for small openings, extra tags of skin, or sinuses. If a sinus is found, a special notation is made, since it may represent a fistula that drains into some area of the neck or ear. Cutaneous tags represent no pathologic process but may cause parents concern in terms of the child's appearance.

The ear is also assessed for general *hygiene*. An otoscope is not necessary for looking into the external canal to note the presence of cerumen, a waxy substance produced by the ceruminous glands in the outer portion of the canal. Cerumen is usually yellow-brown and soft. If an otoscope is used and any discharge is seen, its color and odor are noted. Care is taken to prevent transmitting potentially infectious material to the other ear or to another child through handwashing and changing otic specula.

Inspection of Internal Structures

The otic head permits visualization of the tympanic membrane by use of a bright light, a magnifying glass, and a speculum. Some otoscopes have an attachment for a pneumonic device to insert air into the canal when a determination of membrane compliance (movement) is needed. The speculum, which is inserted into the external canal, comes in a variety of sizes to accommodate different canal widths. The largest speculum that fits comfortably into the ear is used in order to achieve the greatest area of visualization. The lens or magnifying glass is movable, allowing the examiner to insert an object, such as a curette, into the ear canal through the speculum while still viewing the structures through the lens. The handle is the same as for the ophthalmic head and operates similarly. The nurse should become familiar with the instrument and practice attaching the speculum securely to the otic head.

Positioning the child. Before beginning the otoscopic examination, the nurse positions the child. Older children are usually cooperative and need no type of restraint. They should, however, be prepared for the procedure by allowing them to play with the instrument, demonstrating how it works, and impressing upon them the need to remain still. It may be helpful to let them observe the nurse examine the parent's ear. The nurse can let older children view the inside of the ear. As the speculum is inserted into the meatus, it should be moved around the outer rim to accustom the child to the feel of something entering the ear.

For their protection and safety infants and toddlers cannot be trusted to remain still, regardless of their former degree of cooperation. There are two general positions of restraint. In one the child is seated sideways in the parent's lap with one arm "hugging" the parent and the other arm at his side. The ear to be examined is toward the nurse. With one arm the parent holds the child's head firmly against his or her chest, and with the other arm "hugs" the child, thereby securing the child's free arm. The nurse then examines the ear using the same procedure in holding the otoscope as described in the section that follows (Fig. 7-17, *A*).

The other position involves placing the child on his side or abdomen with his arms at his side and his head turned so that the ear to be examined points toward the ceiling. The nurse leans over the child and uses the upper part of the body to restrain his arms and upper trunk movements and the examining hand to stabilize his head. This position is practical for young infants or older children who need minimal restraining; it may not be feasible for other children who protest vigorously. For safety the nurse should enlist the parent's help in immobilizing the head by firmly placing one hand above the ear and the other on the child's back or side (Fig. 7-17, *B*).

With cooperative children the ear can be examined with the child in a side-lying, sitting, or standing position. One disadvantage to standing is that the child may "walk away" as the otoscope enters the canal. If the child is standing or sitting, proper positioning of the head is essential to achieve a full view of the membrane. The head is tilted slightly away from the nurse or toward the child's opposite shoulder to bring the drum to a 90-degree angle (Fig. 7-18).

Manipulating the otoscope. With the thumb and forefinger of the free hand, the nurse grasps the auricle. For either of the two positions of restraint, the otoscope is held upside down at the junction of its head and handle with the thumb and index finger. The other fingers are placed against the skull to allow the otoscope to move

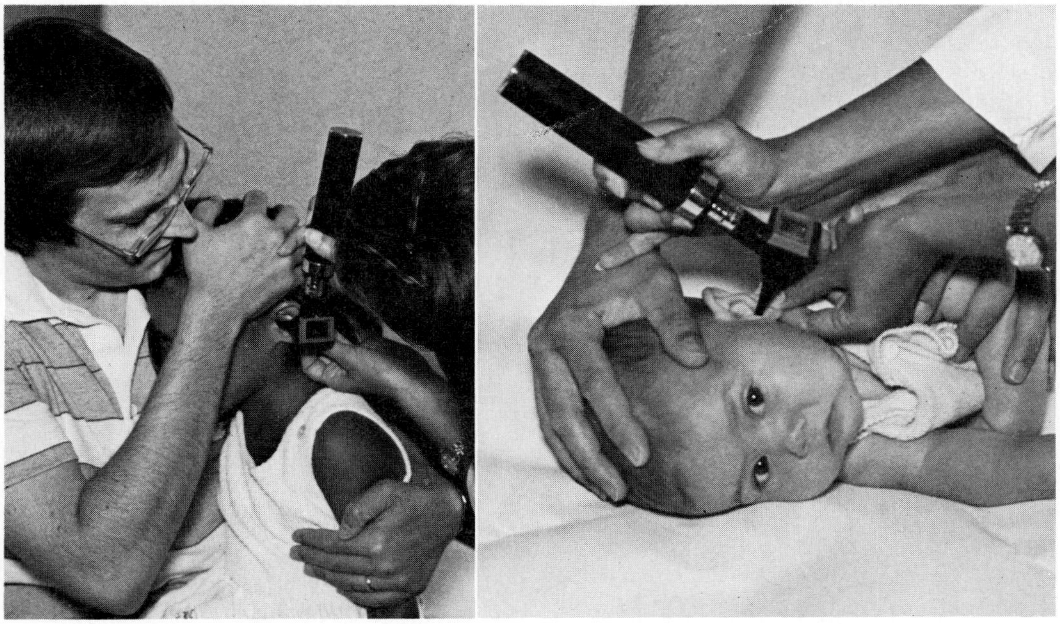

FIG. 7-17 Position for restraining **A,** child, and **B,** infant, during otoscopic examination.

with the child in case he moves suddenly. In examining a cooperative child, the handle is held between thumb and index finger with the otic head upright or upside down. The other fingers are still placed against the child's head to detect unexpected movement (see Fig. 7-18).

Entering the canal. Before introducing the speculum into the canal, the examiner should imagine that the external ear and the tympanic membrane are superimposed on a clock (see Fig. 7-20). The numbers become important geographic landmarks. The speculum is introduced into the meatus between the 3 and 9 o'clock positions in a downward and forward position. Because the canal is curved, the speculum does not permit a panoramic view of the tympanic membrane unless the canal is straightened. In infants the canal curves upward and the tympanic membrane lies almost horizontally along the upper wall of the canal. The pinna must be pulled *downward* and *backward* to the 6 to 9 o'clock range to straighten the canal (Fig. 7-19, *A*).

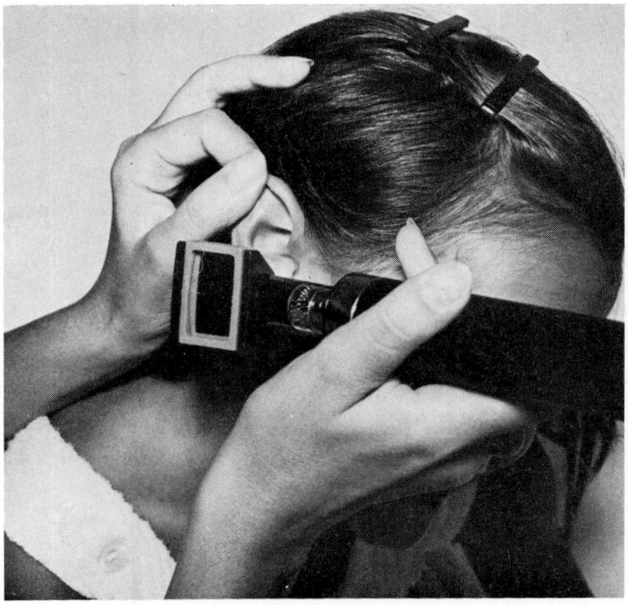

FIG. 7-18 Positioning head by tilting it toward opposite shoulder for full view of tympanic membrane.

With older children, usually those over 3 years of age, the canal curves downward and forward, and the drum, although more vertical, slopes inward and forward. Therefore the pinna is pulled *upward* and *backward* toward a 10 o'clock position (Fig. 7-19, *B*). If there is difficulty in visualizing the membrane, reposition the head, introduce the speculum at a different angle, and pull the pinna in a slightly different direction to bring the drum into view.

In neonates and young infants the walls of the canals are pliable and floppy because of the underdeveloped cartilaginous and bony structures. Therefore the very small (2 mm) speculum usually needs to be inserted deeper into the canal than in older children. Great care must be exercised not to damage the walls or drum. For this reason, only an experienced examiner should insert an otoscope into the ears of very young infants.

Otoscopic examination. As the speculum is introduced into the external canal, the walls of the canal, the color of the tympanic membrane, the light reflex, and the usual landmarks of the bony prominences of the middle ear are noted. Fig. 7-20 illustrates the usual view of the tympanic membrane.

The *walls* of the external auditory canal are usually pink, although they are normally more pigmented in dark-skinned children. Minute hairs are evident in the outermost portion, where cerumen is produced.

The color of the *tympanic membrane* is normally a translucent, light pearly pink or gray. The characteristic tenseness and slope of the tympanic membrane causes the light of the otoscope to reflect at about the 5 or 7 o'clock position. The *light reflex* is a fairly well-defined, cone-shaped reflection, which normally points away from the face.

The *bony landmarks* of the drum are formed by the *umbo,* or long arm of the malleus bone, which appears as a small, round, opaque, concave spot near the center

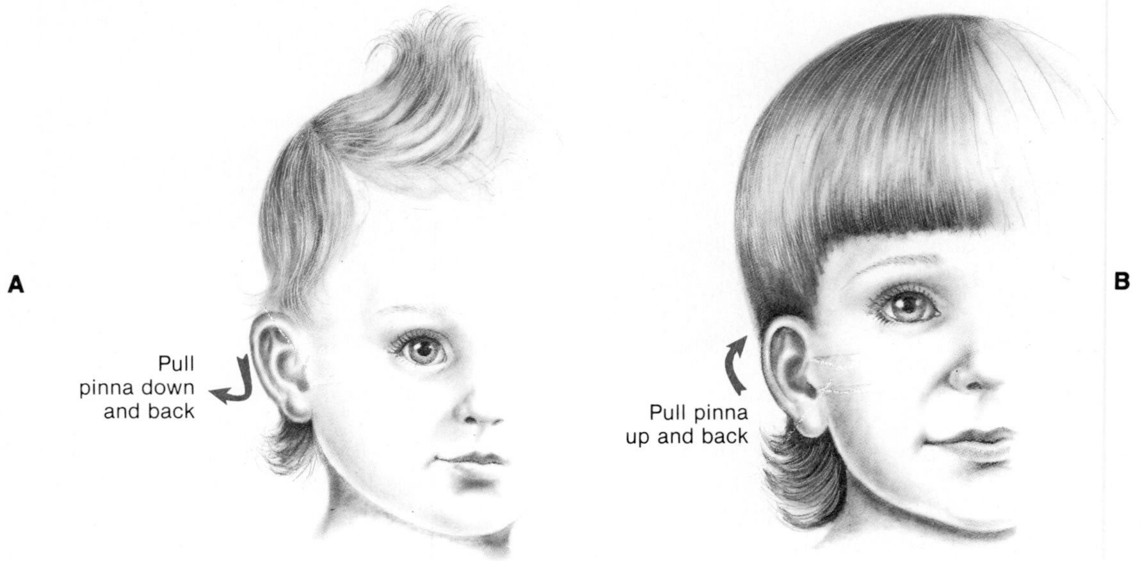

FIG. 7-19 Positioning of eardrum in **A,** infant, and **B,** child over 3 years of age.

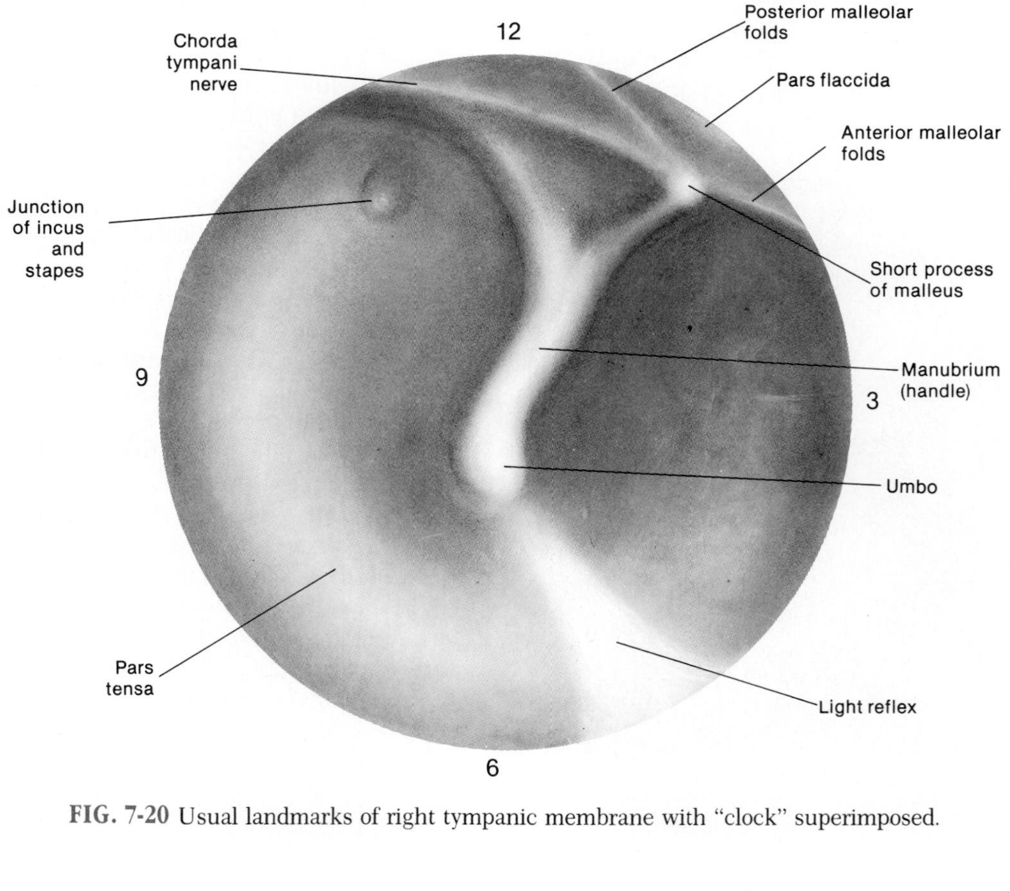

FIG. 7-20 Usual landmarks of right tympanic membrane with "clock" superimposed.

of the drum. The *manubrium,* the long process or handle of the malleus, appears as a whitish line extending from the umbo upward to the margin of the membrane. At the upper end of the long process near the 1 o'clock position is a sharp knoblike protuberance, representing the *short process* of the malleus. Absence of the light reflex or loss of any of these landmarks is always reported for further evaluation.

Auditory Testing

Several types of hearing tests are available. Some of them, such as audiometric testing, use specialized equipment that measures the degree of hearing loss. Others, such as tests for the startle reflex in neonates, are rough estimations of perception of sound. The nurse must operate under a high index of suspicion for those children who may have conditions associated with hearing loss and who may have developed behaviors indicative of auditory impairment. Types, causes, clinical manifestations, and appropriate treatment of hearing loss are discussed in Chapter 19.

Audiometry. In audiometry an electrical audiometer measures the threshold of hearing for pure-tone frequencies and loudness. An audiogram is a record of the audiometric testing. A sound is transmitted to the child's ear and reduced until he indicates the sound is no longer heard. This procedure is repeated for several sounds covering the range found in conversation. In an air conduction audiogram the sounds are transmitted through earphones, which the nurse can describe to young children as part of a "space helmet." With bone conduction the sounds are passed through a plaque placed over the mastoid bone. Since the child is listening to very soft sounds, audiometry may be performed in a soundproof room.

Pure-tone audiometry provides valuable information regarding the severity of the hearing loss, the sound cycles involved, and the possible location of the defect. However, it requires specialized training of personnel, expensive equipment, and cooperation from the child in terms of confirming the perception of sound. For children 24 months to about 5 years *play audiometry* can be implemented to increase cooperation. Based on behavior modification, it involves reinforcement for correct response. Also available is an Audioscope,* which incorporates hearing screening and otoscopy in a single instrument for use with children 3 years and older.

Tympanometry. Another specialized test is *acoustic impedance* measurements or *tympanometry.* This technique measures tympanic membrane compliance (or mobility) and estimates middle ear air pressure. It is suitable for infants, young children, and those who are difficult to test by other methods because little cooperation is necessary, and the procedure is not painful. Like audiometry, this technique requires special equipment, although minimal training is necessary for the procedure. This test detects middle ear disease and abnormalities but does not indicate the degree of hearing loss or the interpretation of sound.

Clinical hearing tests. In newborns, hearing is best determined clinically by eliciting the *startle reflex* (p. 196) and by observing other neonatal responses to loud noises, such as facial grimaces, blinking, gross motor movements, quieting if crying or crying if quiet, opening the eyes, or ceasing sucking activity. An objective sign may be an increase in heart or respiratory rate following a loud noise. Absence of such alerting behaviors suggests a hearing loss.

During infancy the nurse can test hearing by making a noise and noting the child's specific reaction to *localization of sound.* The nurse stands about 18 inches away from the child, to the side, and out of his peripheral field of vision. With the room silent and the child sitting contentedly in his parent's lap, distracted by a toy or other object, the nurse makes a voice sound, such as PS or PHTH, which is high-pitched, or OO, which is low-pitched, rings a bell or a rattle, or rustles tissue paper. The child's response in terms of localizing the sound is compared to the expected age response (see the box). This test is usually inadequate for toddlers and preschoolers because of less cooperation and the learned response to willingly ignore sounds.

Brainstem-evoked response. In an attempt to objectively assess hearing in newborns and other hard-to-test children, a complex and expensive method called brainstem-evoked response audiometry (BSER) has been developed. Through electrode wires attached to the infant's scalp,

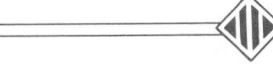

Major Developmental Characteristics of Hearing

Age (weeks)	Development
Birth	Responds to loud noise by startle reflex Responds to sound of human voice more readily than to any other sound Low-pitched sounds, such as lullaby, metronome, or heartbeat, have quieting effect
8-12	Turns head to side when sound is made at level of ear
12-16	Locates sound by turning head to side and looking in same direction
16-24	Can localize sounds made below ear, which is followed by localization of sound made above ear; will turn head to the side and then look up or down
24-32	Locates sounds by turning head in a curving arc Responds to own name
32-40	Localizes sounds by turning head diagonally and directly toward sound
40-52	Learns to control and adjust own response to sound, such as listening for the sound to occur again

Modified from Illingworth, R.S.: The development of the infant and young child, ed. 7, New York, 1980, Churchill Livingstone.

*Manufactured by Welch Allyn, Skaneateles Falls, NY 13153.

electrical or brain wave potentials generated within the auditory system are transmitted to a computer for analysis. Following repetitive acoustic stimulation, the waveforms from a normal sleeping or quiet infant consist of several peaks and valleys that reflect activations of neural structures of the brain. The BSER audiogram is analyzed by a specially trained technician to determine the threshold of hearing response.

Crib-o-gram. The Crib-o-gram,* a neonatal screening tool, analyzes hearing responses by comparing the infant's motor activity before, during, and after a sound is introduced. Both administration of the test and its scoring are totally automated. A motion-sensitive transducer is placed beneath the crib or Isolette mattress, and a microprocessor "reads" the infant's movement. A change in activity that coincides with the test sound is scored as a "pass." The sequence is repeated several times to assure reliability.

Conduction tests. Two tests are also used to distinguish between air and bone conduction—Rinne test and Weber test. In air conduction sound is transmitted to the brain through the external, middle, and inner ear structures. In bone conduction the sound bypasses the external and middle ear and is transmitted to the brain through the mastoid bone to the inner ear structures and auditory nerve. Normally air conduction is considerably better than bone conduction.

In the *Rinne test* the stem of the tuning fork is placed against the mastoid bone until the sound ceases to be audible. It is then moved so that the prongs are held near, but not touching, the auditory meatus. The child should again hear the sound (Rinne positive). If the sound is not again audible (Rinne negative), some abnormality is interfering with the conduction of air through the external and middle ear chambers. This test requires the cooperation and ability of the child to signal when the sound is no longer audible and when it is again heard. It is not useful for most children before preschool age.

*Manufactured by Telesensory Systems, Inc., Palo Alto, CA 94304.

In the *Weber test* the stem of the tuning fork is held in the midline of the head. The child should hear the sound equally in both ears (Weber positive). With air conductive loss he will hear the sound better in the *affected* ear (Weber negative). This test is frequently not suitable for young children because of their difficulty in discriminating between "better, more, or less." Any child who is suspected of a hearing loss because of poor performance using any of these tests is referred for special audiometric testing.

NOSE

The nose, which marks the beginning of the passageway through the respiratory tract, is a sensory organ for olfaction (smell) and an important organ for filtration, temperature control, and humidification of inspired air. Each of these functions depends on the patency of the passageways and on the mucosal lining of the nasal cavity. Inspection is primarily used to assess the external and internal structures.

Inspection of External Structures

The nose is located in the middle of the face just below the eyes and above the lips. Its placement and alignment can be compared by drawing an imaginary vertical line from the center point between the eyes down to the notch of the upper lip. The nose should lie exactly vertical to this line and each side should be symmetric. Its location, any deviation to one side, and asymmetry in overall size and in diameter of the nares (nostrils) are noted. The

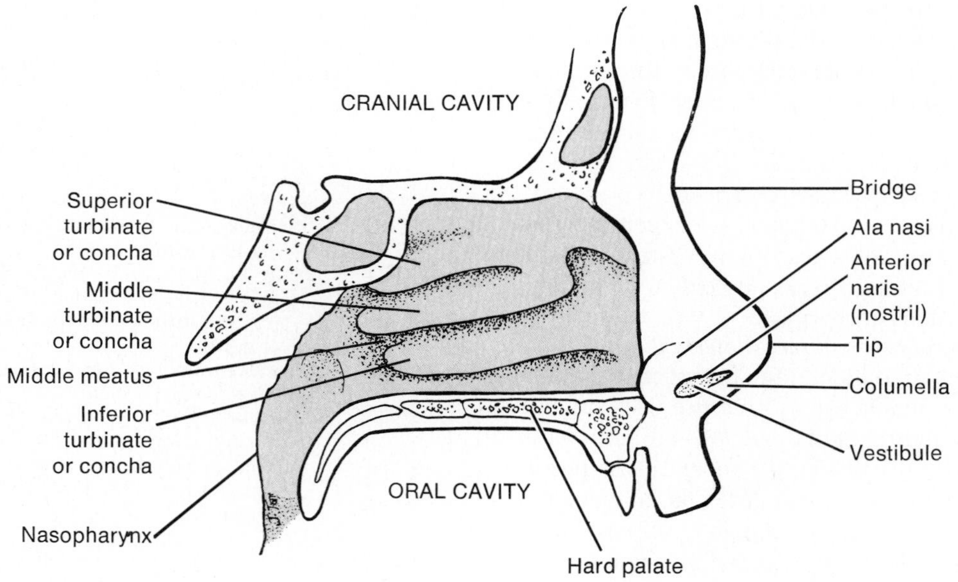

FIG. 7-21 External landmarks and internal structures of nose.

bridge of the nose is sometimes flat in black or Asian children. The alae nasi are observed for any sign of flaring, which may indicate respiratory difficulty. Fig. 7-21 illustrates the usual landmarks used in describing the external structures of the nose.

Inspection of Internal Structures

The anterior vestibule of the nose is inspected by pushing the tip upward, tilting the head backward, and illuminating the cavity with a flashlight or otoscope without the attached ear speculum.

The color of the *mucosal lining,* which is normally redder than the oral membranes, is observed. Any swelling, discharge, dryness, or bleeding are also noted. There should be no discharge from the nose.

On looking deeper into the nose, the nurse inspects the *turbinates* or *concha,* plates of bone that jut into the nasal cavity and are enveloped by mucous membrane. The turbinates greatly increase the surface area of the nasal cavity as air is inhaled. The spaces or channels between the turbinates are called *meatus* and correspond to each of the three turbinates. Normally the front end of the inferior and middle turbinate and the middle meatus are seen. They should be the same color as the lining of the vestibule.

The *septum,* which should divide the vestibules equally, is also inspected. Any deviation is noted, especially if it causes an occlusion of one side of the nose. A perforation may be evident within the septum. If this is suspected, the nurse can shine the light of the otoscope into one naris and look for admittance of light through the perforation to the other nostril.

Since olfaction is an important function of the nose, testing for smell may be done at this point or as part of cranial nerve assessment (see p. 170).

Nursing Tips: Examination of Mouth

To encourage the child to open the mouth for examination:

- Perform the examination in front of a mirror
- Let the child first examine someone else's mouth, such as the parent, the nurse, or a puppet (Fig. 7-22, *A*) and then examine the child's mouth

If the child resists opening the mouth, pinch the nostrils closed; this forces the child to open the mouth to breathe.

MOUTH AND THROAT

With a cooperative child, almost the entire examination of the mouth and throat can be accomplished without the use of a tongue blade. The nurse asks the child to open his mouth wide, requests that he move his tongue in different directions for full visualization, and has him say "Ahh" in order to depress the tongue for full view of the back of the mouth (tonsils, uvula, and oropharynx). For a closer look at the buccal mucosa or lining of the cheeks, the nurse can ask the child to use his fingers to move the outer lip and cheek to one side. Other strategies for encouraging cooperation are listed in the Nursing tips box.

Infants and toddlers, however, usually resist attempts to keep the mouth open. Because it is an upsetting part of the examination, it is performed at the end of the physical examination (along with examination of the ears) or during episodes of crying. However, the use of a tongue blade to depress the tongue is necessary. The tongue blade is placed along the *side* of the tongue; it is not placed in the center back area where the gag reflex is elicited. Fig. 7-22, *B*, illustrates proper positioning of the child for the oral examination.

A

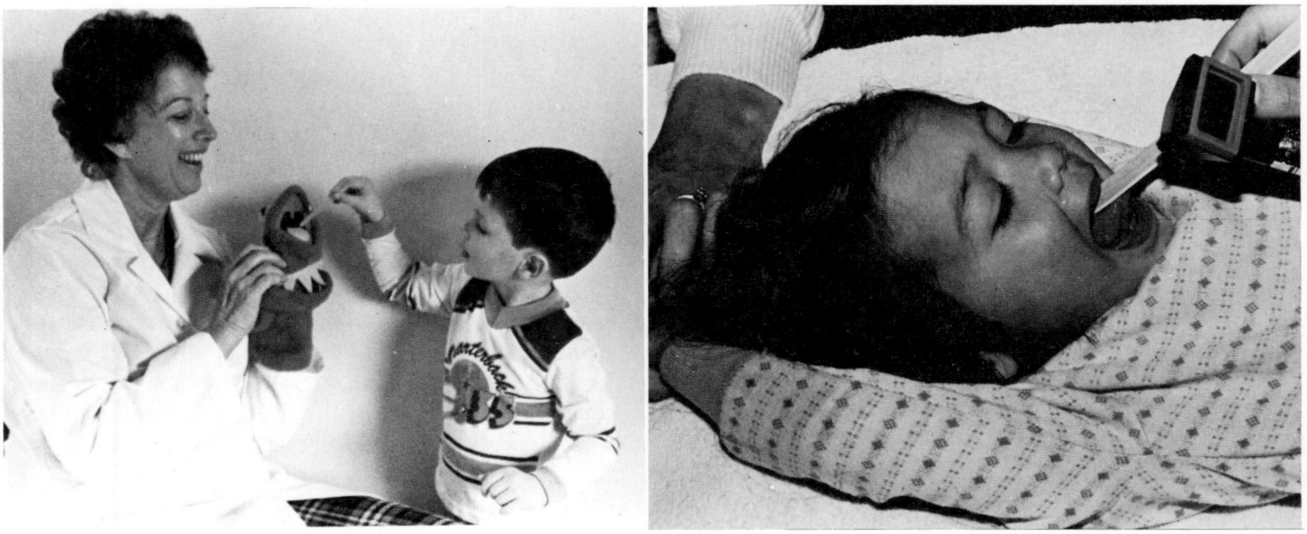

B

FIG. 7-22 A, Encouraging child to cooperate. **B,** Positioning child for examination of mouth.

The major structure of the exterior of the mouth is the *lips*. The lips should be moist, soft, smooth, and pink, the color of a deeper hue than the surrounding skin. The lips should be symmetric when relaxed or tensed. Symmetry is easily assessed when the child talks or cries.

Inspection of Internal Structures

The major structures that are visible within the oral cavity and oropharynx are the mucosal lining of the lips and cheeks, gums or gingiva, teeth, tongue, palate, uvula, tonsils, and posterior oropharynx (Fig. 7-23). All areas lined with *mucous membranes* (inside the lips and cheeks, gingiva, underside of tongue, palate, and back of pharynx) are inspected for color, any areas of white patches or ulceration, bleeding, sensitivity, and moisture. The membranes should be bright pink, smooth, glistening, uniform, and moist.

The *teeth* are inspected for number in each dental arch, for hygiene, and for occlusion or bite. The general rule for estimating the number of temporary teeth in children who are 2 years of age or younger is: *the child's age in months minus 6 months equals the number of teeth.* Discoloration of tooth enamel with obvious plaque (whitish coating on the surface of the teeth) is a sign of poor dental hygiene and indicates a need for dental counseling. Brown spots in the crevices of the crown of the tooth or between the teeth may be caries (cavities). Chalky white to yellow or brown areas on the enamel may indicate fluorosis (excessive fluoride ingestion). Teeth that appear greenish black may be stained temporarily from oral ingestion of supplemental iron. Malocclusion or poor biting relationship of the teeth is also noted.

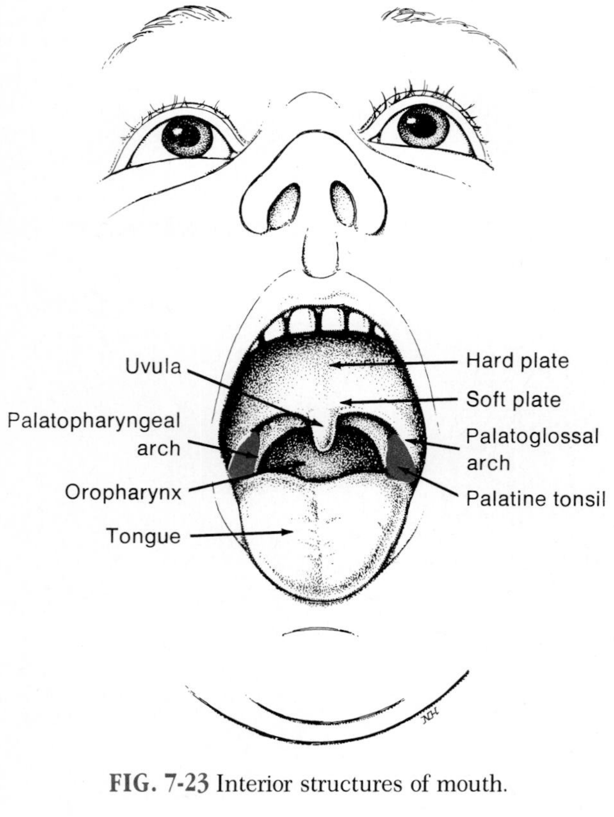

FIG. 7-23 Interior structures of mouth.

The *gums* (gingiva) surrounding the teeth are examined. The color is normally coral pink, and the surface texture is stippled, similar to the appearance of orange peel. In dark-skinned children, the gums are more deeply colored, and a brownish area is often observed along the gum line.

The *tongue* is inspected for the presence of papillae, small projections that contain several taste buds and give the tongue its characteristic rough appearance. The nurse also notes the size and mobility of the tongue. Normally the tip of the tongue should extend to the lips or beyond.

The roof of the mouth consists of the *hard palate,* which is located near the front of the oral cavity, and the *soft palate,* which is located toward the back of the pharynx and which has a small midline protrusion called the *uvula*. Both palates are carefully inspected to be sure that they are intact. The arch of the palate should be dome shaped. A narrow, flat roof or a high, arched palate affects the placement of the tongue and can cause feeding and speech problems. Movement of the uvula should be tested by eliciting a gag reflex. It should move upward to close off the nasopharynx from the oropharynx.

As the recesses of the oropharynx are examined, the size and color of the *palatine tonsils* are also noted. They are normally the same color as the surrounding mucosa, glandular, rather than smooth in appearance, and barely visible over the edge of the palatoglossal arches. The size of the tonsils varies considerably during childhood.

CHEST

Although the thoracic cavity houses two vital organs, the heart and lungs, the anatomic structures of the chest wall are important sources of information concerning cardiac and pulmonary function, skeletal formation, and secondary sexual development. The chest is inspected for size, shape, symmetry, movement, breast development, and the presence of the bony landmarks formed by the ribs and sternum.

The *rib cage* consists of twelve ribs and the sternum, or breast bone, which is located in the midline of the trunk (Fig. 7-24). The *sternum* is composed of three main parts. The *manubrium,* the uppermost portion, can be felt at the base of the neck at the *suprasternal notch.* The largest segment of the sternum is the *body,* which forms the *sternal angle* as it articulates with the manubrium. At the end of the body is a small, movable process called the *xiphoid.* The angle of the costal margin as it attaches to the sternum is called the *costal angle* and is normally about 45 to 50 degrees. These bony structures are important landmarks in the location of ribs and intercostal spaces.

Intercostal spaces are the spaces between the ribs. They are numbered according to the rib directly *above*

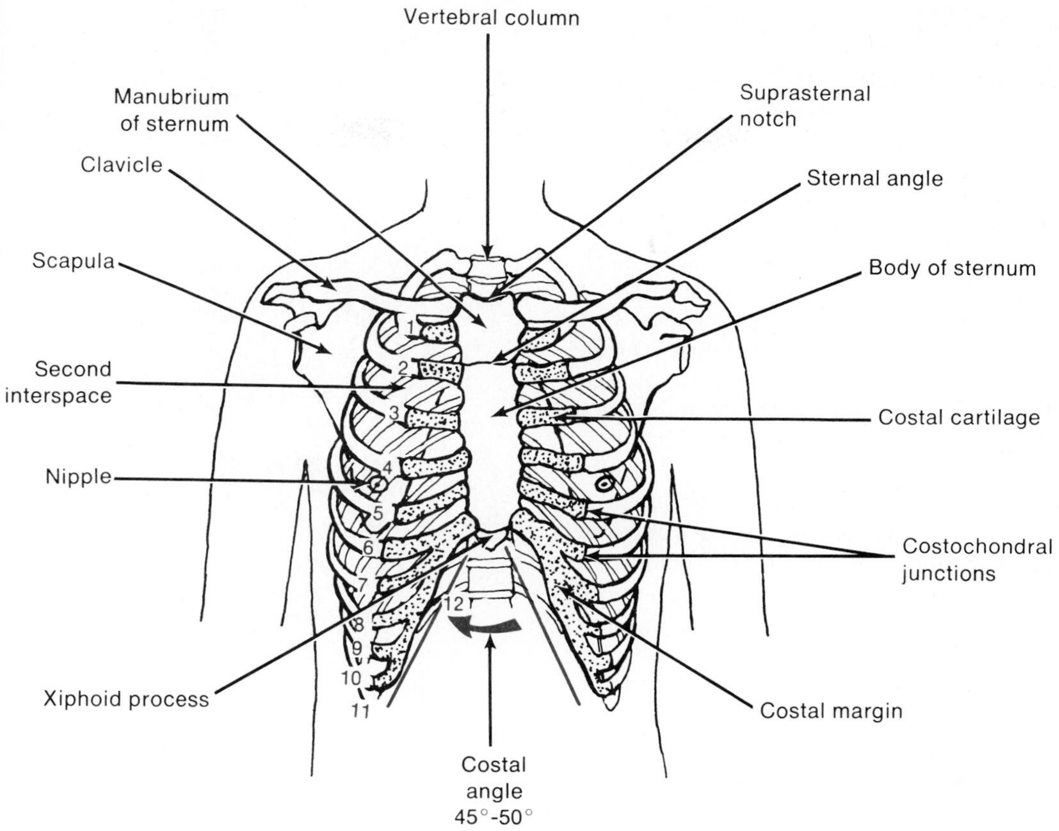

FIG. 7-24 Rib cage.

the space. For example, the space immediately below the second rib is the second intercostal space.

The *thoracic cavity* is also divided into segments by drawing imaginary lines on the chest and back. Fig. 7-25 illustrates the anterior, lateral, and posterior divisions. The nurse should become familiar with each imaginary landmark, as well as with the rib number and corresponding interspace, because they are geographic landmarks for palpating, percussing, and auscultating underlying organs.

The *size* of the chest is measured by placing the measuring tape around the rib cage at the nipple line (see Fig. 7-4). For greatest accuracy two measurements are taken, one during inspiration and the other during expiration, and the average is recorded. Chest size is important mainly in comparison to its relationship with head circumference, which has been discussed on p. 134. Marked disproportions are always recorded because most are caused by abnormal head growth, although some may be the result of altered chest shape, such as barrel chest or pigeon chest.

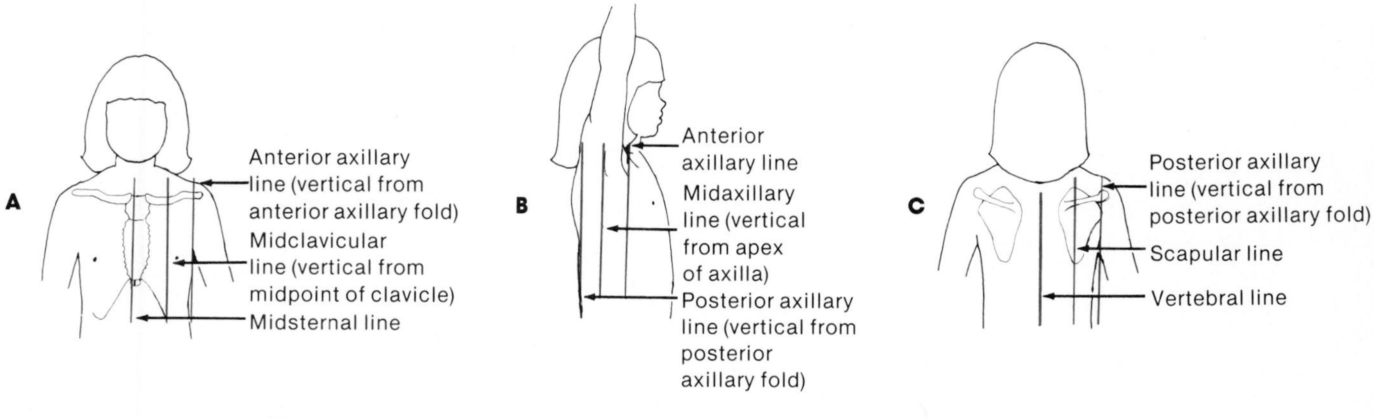

FIG. 7-25 Imaginary landmarks of chest. **A,** Anterior; **B,** right lateral; **C,** posterior.

During infancy the *shape* of the chest is almost circular, with the anteroposterior (front-to-back) diameter equaling the transverse or lateral (side-to-side) diameter. As the child grows, the chest normally increases in the transverse direction, causing the anteroposterior diameter to be less than the lateral diameter. The *angle* made by the lower costal margin and the sternum is noted as well as the junction of the ribs to the costal cartilage (costochondral junction) and sternum, which should be fairly smooth.

Movement of the chest wall is noted. It should be symmetric bilaterally and coordinated with breathing. During inspiration, the chest rises and expands, the diaphragm descends, and the costal angle increases. During expiration, the chest falls and decreases in size, the diaphragm rises, and the costal angle narrows (Fig. 7-26). In children under 6 or 7 years of age, respiratory movement is principally abdominal or diaphragmatic. In older children, particularly females, respirations are chiefly thoracic. In either type, the chest and abdomen should rise and fall together. Any asymmetry of movement warrants referral for further investigation.

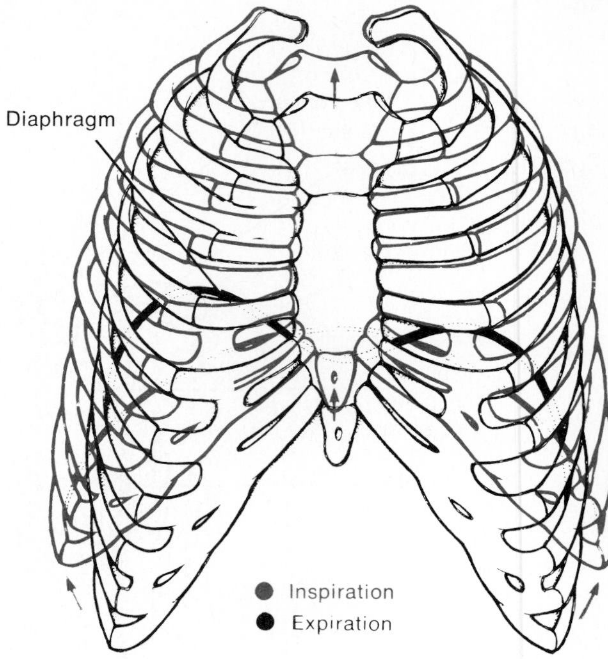

FIG. 7-26 Movement of chest during respiration.

As the surface of the chest is inspected, the position of the *nipples* is observed as well as any evidence of *breast* development. The nipples are normally located slightly lateral to the midclavicular line between the fourth and fifth ribs. The symmetry of nipple placement and the normal configuration of a darker pigmented areola surrounding a flat nipple in the prepubertal child are noted.

Any evidence of pubertal breast development, which usually begins in girls between 10 and 14 years of age, is noted. Precocious or delayed breast development is recorded, as well as evidence of any other secondary sexual characteristics. In males gynecomastia may be caused by hormonal or systemic disorders, but more commonly it is the result of adipose tissue from obesity or a transitory body change during early puberty. In either situation the nurse should investigate the child's feelings regarding breast enlargement.

In adolescent females who have achieved sexual maturity, the breasts are palpated for evidence of any masses or hard nodules. This opportunity should also be taken to discuss the importance of routine breast self-examination. Although carcinoma of the breast is rare in women under 20 years of age, it is advisable to stress the value of routine breast self-examination so that it becomes a practiced habit during later years.

LUNGS

Examination of the lungs involves the skills of inspection, palpation, percussion, and auscultation. The most important of these is auscultation. Assessment of the lungs requires knowledge of their location and of their relationship to the rib cage (Fig. 7-27).

The lungs are situated inside the thoracic cavity, with one lung on each side of the sternum. Each lung is divided into an *apex*, which is slightly pointed and rises above the first rib; a *base*, which is wide and concave and rides on the dome-shaped diaphragm; and a body, which is divided into *lobes*. The right lung has three lobes: the upper, middle, and lower. The left lung has only two lobes, the upper and lower, because of the space occupied by the heart.

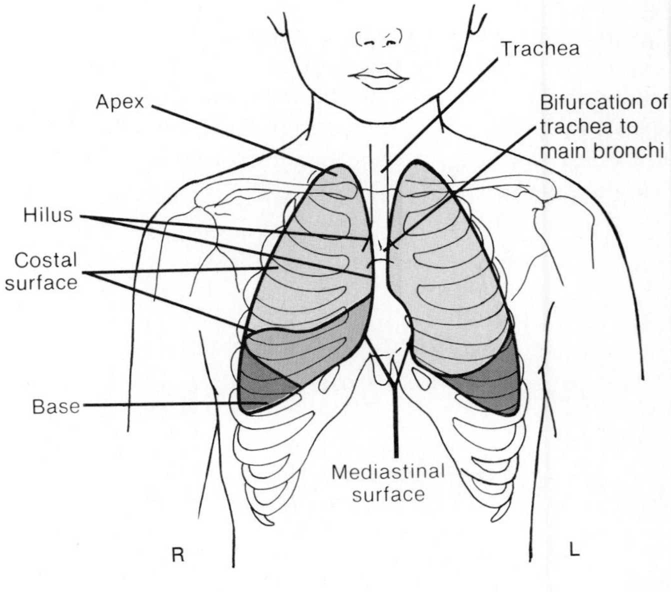

FIG. 7-27 Location of lobes of lungs within thoracic cavity.

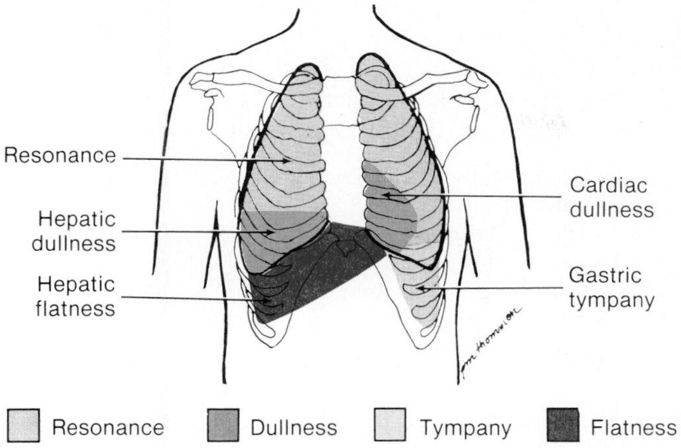

FIG. 7-28 Percussion sounds found in normal thorax.

Inspection of the lungs primarily involves observation of respiratory movements, which are discussed on p. 138. Respirations are evaluated for rate (number per minute), rhythm (regular, irregular, or periodic), depth (deep or shallow), and quality (effortless, automatic, difficult, or labored). The character of breath sounds is noted, such as noisy, grunting, snoring, or heavy.

Respiratory movements are felt by placing each hand flat against the back or chest with the thumbs in midline along the lower costal margin of the lungs. The child should be sitting during this procedure and, if cooperative, should take several deep breaths. During respiration the nurse's hands will move with the chest wall. The amount and speed of respiratory excursion is evaluated and any asymmetry of movement is noted.

In percussing the chest, the anterior lung is percussed from apex to base, usually with the child in the supine or sitting position. Each side of the chest is percussed in sequence in order to compare the sounds. When percussing the posterior lung, the procedure and sequence are the same, although the child should be sitting.

Fig. 7-28 illustrates the usual percussion sounds within the anterior thorax. *Resonance* is heard over all the lobes of the lungs that are not adjacent to other organs. *Dullness* is heard beginning at the fifth interspace in the right midclavicular line. Percussing downward to the end of the liver, the sound becomes *flat,* because the liver no longer overlies the air-filled lung. *Cardiac dullness* is felt over the left sternal border from the second to the fifth interspace medially to the midclavicular line. Below the fifth interspace on the left side, *tympany* results from the air-filled stomach. Deviations from expected sounds are always recorded and reported.

Auscultation

Auscultation involves using the stethoscope to evaluate breath sounds. Breath sounds are best heard if the child inspires deeply. The child can be encouraged to "take a big breath" by following a demonstration of "breathing in through the nose and out through the mouth." Younger children respond well to activities such as making a pinwheel spin, "smelling" an artificial flower, or "blowing out" the light of the otoscope (Fig. 7-29).

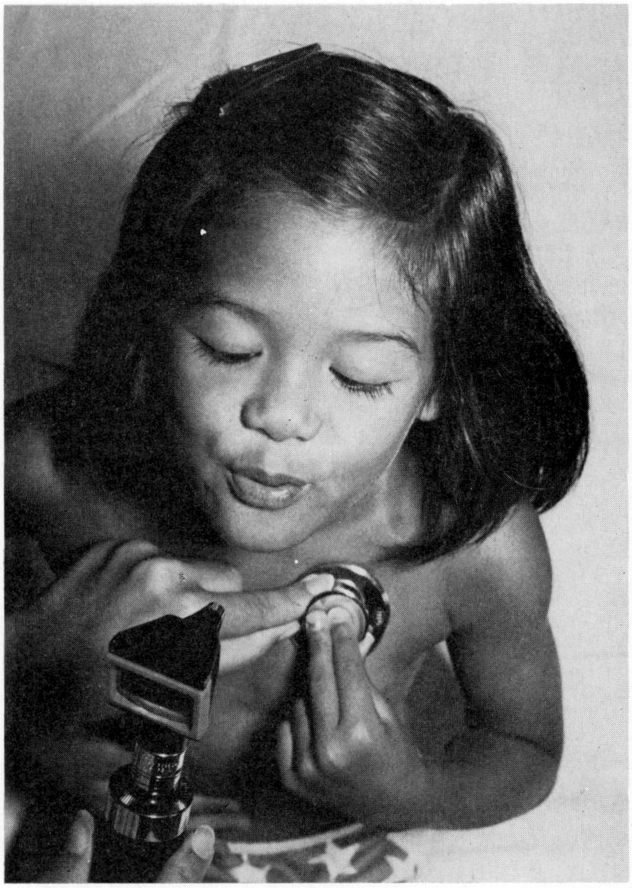

FIG. 7-29 Auscultating lungs while child "blows out" otoscope light.

In the lungs, breath sounds are classified as vesicular, bronchovesicular, or bronchial. They are described below:

Vesicular breath sounds, heard over entire surface of lungs, with exception of upper intrascapular area and area beneath manubrium; inspiration is louder, longer, and higher-pitched than expiration; sound is soft, swishing noise

Bronchovesicular breath sounds, normally heard over manubrium and in upper intrascapular regions where trachea and bronchi bifurcate; inspiration is louder and higher in pitch than in vesicular breathing

Bronchial breath sounds, heard only over trachea near suprasternal notch; almost reverse of vesicular sounds; inspiratory phase is short and expiratory phase is longer, louder, and of higher pitch

Absent or diminished breath sounds are always an abnormal finding warranting investigation. Fluid, air, or solid masses in the pleural space all interfere with the conduction of breath sounds. Diminished breath sounds in certain segments of the lung can alert the nurse to pulmonary areas that may benefit from postural drainage and percussion. Increased breath sounds following pulmonary therapy indicate improved passage of air through the respiratory tract.

Various pulmonary abnormalities produce *adventitious sounds* that are not normally heard over the chest. These are not alterations of normal breath sounds but sounds that occur in addition to normal or abnormal breath sounds. They are classified into two main groups: *rales* or *crackles*, which result from the passage of air through fluid or moisture, and *rhonchi*, which are sounds produced as air passes through narrowed passageways, regardless of the cause, such as exudate, inflammation, spasm, or tumor. Considerable practice with an experienced tutor is necessary to differentiate the various types of rales and rhonchi. Often it is best to describe the type of sound heard in the lungs rather than to try and label it correctly. Any abnormal sounds are always reported for further medical evaluation.

HEART

Examination of the heart involves the skills of inspection, palpation, percussion, and auscultation, although the last is the most significant. Knowledge of the location of the heart in relation to the rib cage is essential for evaluating and describing findings. Fig. 7-30 illustrates the usual position of the heart in the thorax.

The heart is situated like a trapezoid:

vertically along the right sternal border (RSB) from the second to the fifth rib

horizontally (long side) from the lower right sternum to the fifth rib at the left midclavicular line (LMCL)

diagonally from the left sternal border (LSB) at the second rib to the LMCL at the fifth rib

horizontally (short side) from the RSB and LSB at the second intercostal space

The *base* of the heart is actually the top of the trapezoid or the pulmonic and aortic areas. The *apex* is located at the left midclavicular line and fifth intercostal space or mitral area. The heart of the infant is more horizontally positioned; therefore, the apex is higher than (third to fourth intercostal space) and to the left of the midclavicular line (Fig. 7-31). The apical impulse, or *point of maximum impulse* (PMI) (the area where the heartbeat is the loudest), is normally located at the apex.

Inspection is best done with the child sitting in a semi-Fowler position. The nurse should look at the anterior chest wall from an angle and compare both sides of the rib cage to each other. Normally they should be symmetric. In children with thin chest walls, the PMI is sometimes apparent as a pulsation. Noting the location of the impulse gives some indication of the size and positioning of the heart.

Palpation is useful in determining the size of the heart by feeling for the point of maximum impulse. It is felt by placing the fingertips or the palmar aspect of the fingers and hand at the fifth intercostal space and left midclavicular line. At this point in the examination other pulses may also be palpated, noting symmetry of pulsations (Fig. 7-32). Percussion is used mainly to determine the size of the heart by outlining its borders. Dullness is normally heard over the left area of the heart and partially over the right.

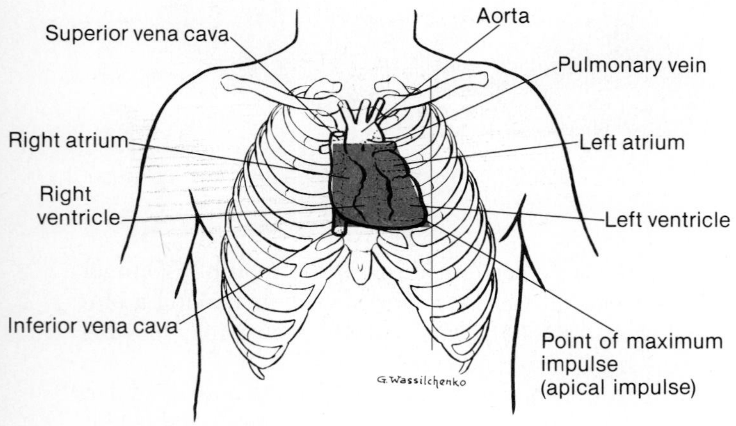

FIG. 7-30 Position of heart within thorax.

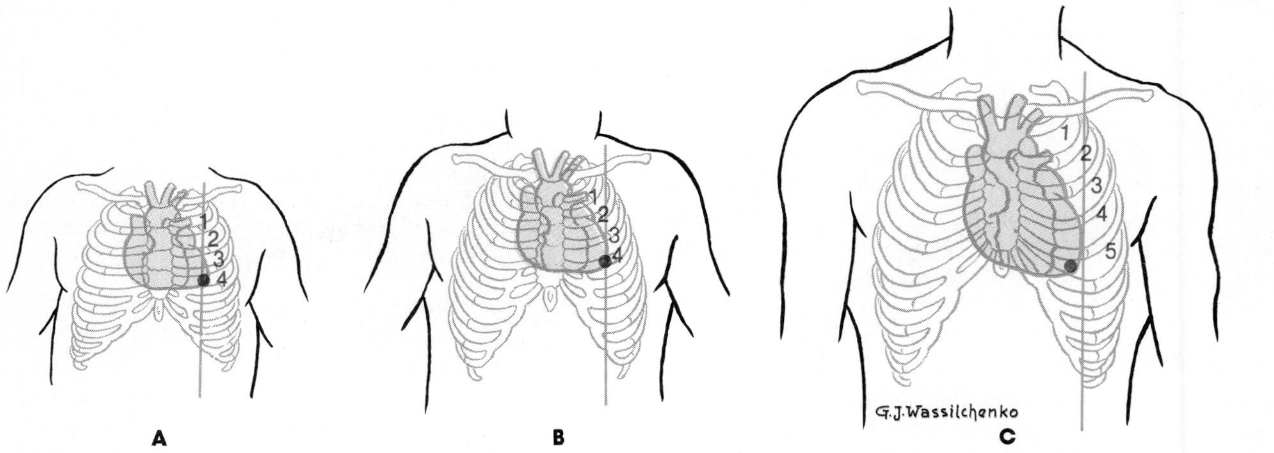

FIG. 7-31 Location of apex of heart. **A,** Infant; **B,** child; **C,** adult.

Auscultation

Auscultation involves listening for heart sounds with the stethoscope; it is similar to the procedure used in assessing breath sounds.

Origin of heart sounds. The heart sounds are produced by the opening and closing of the valves and the vibration of blood against the walls of the heart and vessels. Normally two sounds—S_1 and S_2—are heard, which correspond respectively to the familiar "lub dub" often used to describe the sounds. S_1 is caused by the closure of the *tricuspid* and *mitral valves* (sometimes called the atrioventricular valves). S_2 is the result of the closure of the *pulmonic* and *aortic* valves (sometimes called semilunar valves). Normally there is an audible pause or split between the two sounds that widens during inspiration. *Physiologic splitting* is a significant normal finding that should be elicited. *Fixed splitting,* in which the split in S_2 does not change during inspiration, is an important diagnostic sign of atrial septal defect and is always reported for further evaluation.

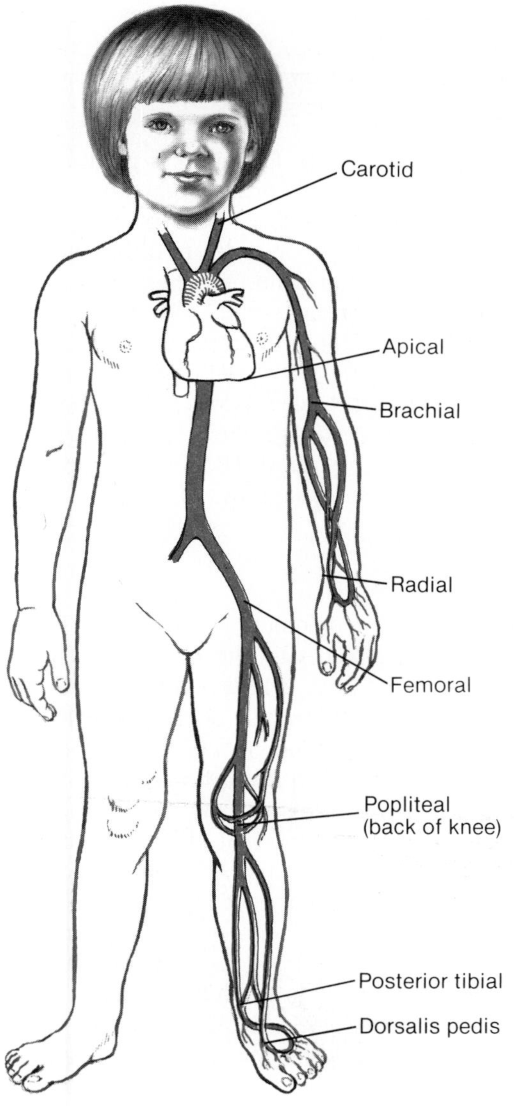

FIG. 7-32 Location of pulses.

Nursing Tip: Heart Sounds

To distinguish between S_1 or S_2 heart sounds, simultaneously palpate the carotid pulse with the index and middle finger and listen to the heart sounds; S_1 is synchronous with the carotid pulse.

Two other heart sounds—S_3 and S_4—may be produced. S_3 is normally heard in some children and young adults but is considered abnormal in older individuals. S_4 is rarely heard as a normal heart sound; usually it indicates the need for further cardiac evaluation.

Another important category of heart sounds is *murmurs*. Murmurs are produced by vibrations within the heart chambers or in the major arteries from the back and forth flow of blood. The description and classification of murmurs are skills that require considerable practice and training. The nurse should consult with a physician whenever a murmur is identified or suspected.

Differentiating normal heart sounds. Fig. 7-33 illustrates the approximate anatomic position of the valves within the heart chambers. It is important to note that the anatomic location of valves does not correspond to the area where the sounds are heard best. The auscultatory sites are located in the direction of the blood flow through the valves.

Normally S_1 is louder at the apex of the heart in the mitral and tricuspid area, and S_2 is louder near the base of the heart in the pulmonic and aortic area. The nurse listens to each sound by inching down the chest in the sequence outlined in Table 7-3. (If there is difficulty in deciding which sound is S_1 or S_2, see Nursing tip box.)

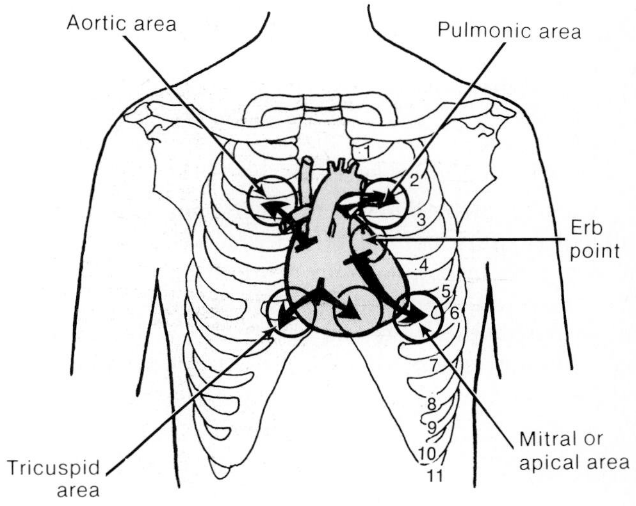

FIG. 7-33 Direction of heart sounds for anatomic valve sites and areas (circled) for auscultation.

TABLE 7-3

*Sequence of Auscultating Heart Sounds**

Auscultatory Site	Chest Location	Characteristics of Heart Sounds
Aortic area	Second right intercostal space close to sternum	S_2 heard louder than S_1; aortic closure heard loudest
Pulmonic area	Second left intercostal space close to sternum	Splitting of S_2 heard best, normally widens on inspiration; pulmonic closure heard best
Erb point	Second and third left intercostal space close to sternum	Frequent site of innocent murmurs and those of aortic or pulmonic origin
Tricuspid area	Fifth right and left intercostal space close to sternum	S_1 heard as louder sound preceding S_2 (S_1 synchronous with carotid pulse)
Mitral or apical area	Fifth intercostal space, left midclavicular line (third to fourth intercostal space and lateral to left midclavicular line in infants)	S_1 heard loudest; splitting of S_1 may be audible because mitral closure is louder than tricuspid closure S_3 heard best at beginning of expiration with child in recumbent or left side-lying position, occurs immediately after S_2, sounds like word "Ken-tuc-ky" S_1 S_2 S_3 S_4 heard best during expiration with child in recumbent position (left side-lying position decreases sound), occurs immediately before S_1, sounds like word "Ten-nes-see" S_4 S_1 S_2

*Use both diaphragm and bell chestpieces when auscultating heart sounds. Bell chestpiece is necessary for low-pitched sounds of murmurs, S_3, and S_4.

In addition to the sites listed in Table 7-3, the following areas should also be ausculated for sounds, such as murmurs, which may radiate to these sites: sternoclavicular area above the clavicles and manubrium, area along the sternal border, area along the left midaxillary line, and area below the scapulae.

The heart is auscultated with the child in at least two positions, sitting and reclining. Both the diaphragm and bell chestpieces are used when listening to each auscultatory area. The diaphragm chestpiece is better for the detection of high-pitched sounds, such as S_1 and S_2. The bell chestpiece is used for low-pitched sounds, such as S_3, S_4, or murmurs.

Heart sounds are evaluated for:

1. **Quality,** which should be clear and distinct, not muffled, diffuse, or distant
2. **Intensity,** especially in relation to location or auscultatory site
3. **Rate,** which should be the same as the radial pulse
4. **Rhythm,** which should be regular and even

A particular arrhythmia that occurs normally in many children is *sinus arrhythmia,* in which the heart rate increases with inspiration and decreases with expiration. This can be differentiated from a truly abnormal arrhythmia by having the child hold his breath. In sinus arrhythmia cessation of breathing causes the heart rate to remain steady.

ABDOMEN

Examination of the abdomen involves the usual four skills, except that the order of their use is significantly changed. Inspection is followed by auscultation, percussion, and then palpation. Palpation is performed last because it may distort the normal abdominal sounds. The nurse must have knowledge of the anatomic placement of the abdominal organs in order to differentiate normal, expected findings from abnormal ones (Fig. 7-34).

For descriptive purposes the abdominal cavity is divided into four quadrants by drawing a vertical line midway from the sternum to the pubic symphysis and a horizontal line across the abdomen through the umbilicus. Each section is named as follows: right upper quadrant (RUQ), right lower quadrant (RLQ), left upper quadrant (LUQ), and left lower quadrant (LLQ).

Inspection

The *contour* of the abdomen is inspected with the child erect and supine. Normally the abdomen of infants and young children is quite cylindric and, in the erect position, fairly prominent because of the physiologic lordosis of the spine. In the supine position the abdomen appears flat. A midline protrusion from the xiphoid to the umbilicus or pubic symphysis is usually *diastasis recti,* or failure of the rectus abdominis muscles to join in utero. In a healthy child a midline protrusion is usually a variation of normal muscular development. During adolescence the usual male and female contours of the pelvic cavity change the shape of the abdomen to form characteristic adult curves, especially in the female.

The condition of the *skin* covering the abdomen is noted. It should be uniformly taut, without wrinkles or creases. Sometimes silvery, whitish striae are seen, especially if the skin has been stretched as in obesity. Superficial veins are usually visible in light-skinned, thin in-

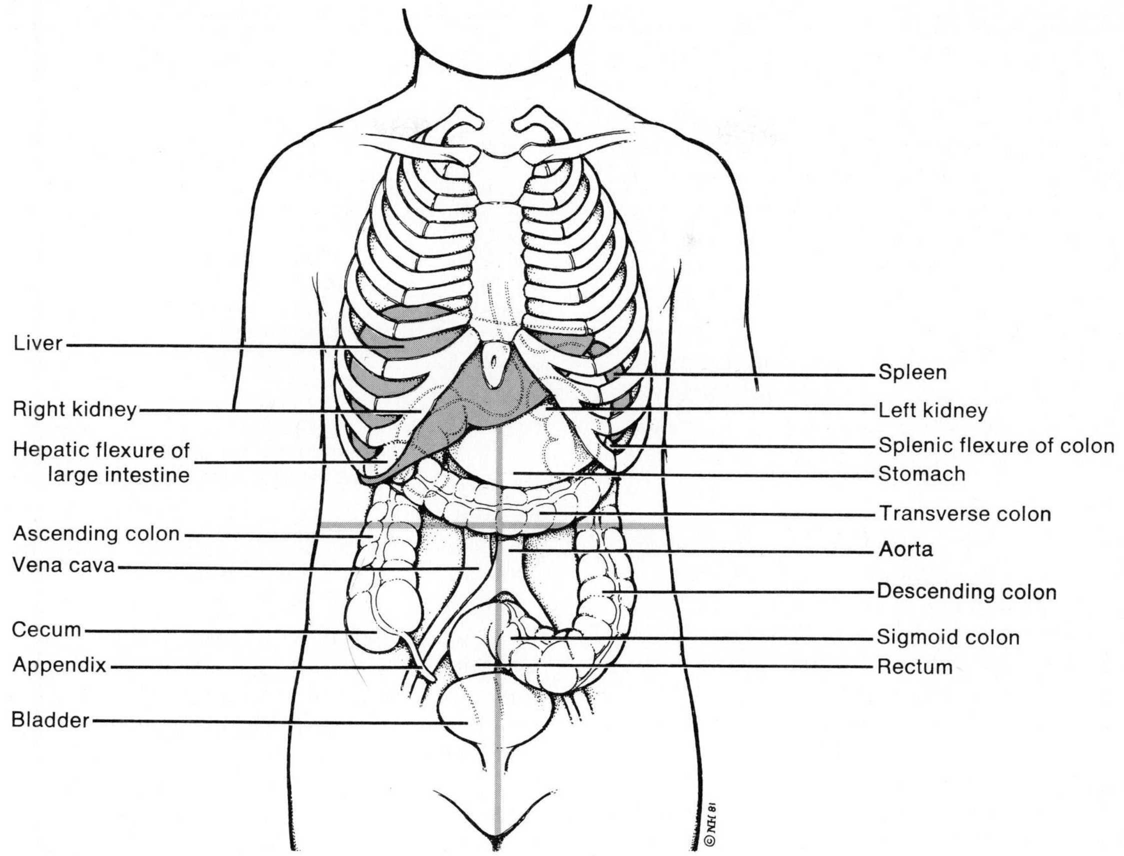

FIG. 7-34 Anatomy of major organs within the abdominal cavity. (For illustrative purposes pancreas, small intestine, and gallbladder are not shown.) Red lines divide the abdominal cavity into quadrants.

fants, but distended veins are an abnormal finding.

Movement of the abdomen is observed. Normally chest and abdominal movements are synchronous. In infants and thin children, *peristaltic waves* may be visible through the abdominal wall; these always warrant careful evaluation. They are best observed by standing at eye level to and across from the abdomen.

The *umbilicus* is examined for size, hygiene, and evidence of any abnormalities, such as hernias. The umbilicus should be flat or only slightly protruding. If a herniation is present, the sac is palpated for abdominal contents and the approximate size of the opening is estimated. Umbilical hernias are common in infants, especially in black children.

Hernias can exist elsewhere on the abdominal wall, such as in the inguinal or femoral region (Fig. 7-35). An *inguinal hernia* is a protrusion of peritoneum through the abdominal wall in the inguinal canal. It occurs most often in males, is frequently bilateral, and may be visible as a mass in the scrotum. It is palpated by sliding the little finger into the external inguinal ring at the base of the scrotum and asking the child to cough. If a hernia is present, it will hit the tip of the finger. If the child is too young to cough, he can be given a balloon to blow up.

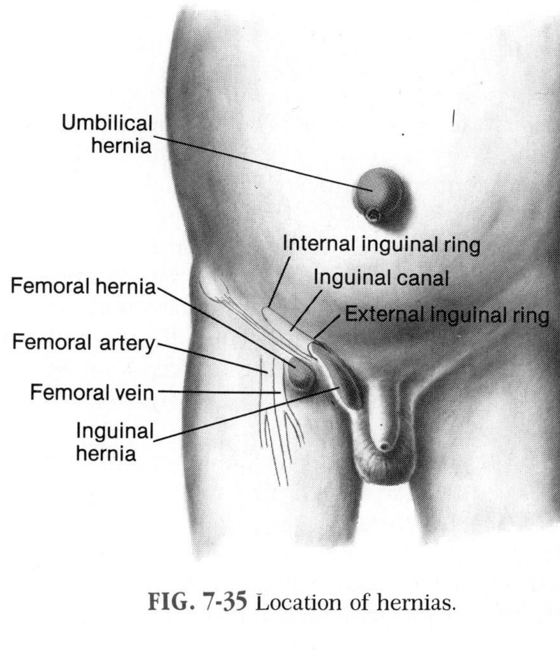

FIG. 7-35 Location of hernias.

Just trying to inflate the balloon raises the intra-abdominal pressure sufficiently to demonstrate the presence of an inguinal hernia.

A *femoral hernia,* which occurs more frequently in girls, is felt or seen as a small mass on the anterior surface of the thigh just below the inguinal ligament in the femoral canal (a potential space medial to the femoral artery). Its location can be estimated by placing the index finger of the right hand on the child's right femoral pulse (left hand for left pulse) and the middle ring finger flat against the skin toward the midline. The ring finger lies over the femoral canal, where the herniation occurs. Palpation of hernias in the pelvic region, particularly inguinal ones, is often part of the examination of genitalia.

Nursing Tips: Avoiding Tickling Sensation

To minimize the sensation of tickling during palpation:
- Have children "help" with the palpation by placing their hand over the palpating hand
- Have them place their hand on the abdomen with the fingers spread wide apart and palpate between their fingers
- Distract them with statements such as "I am trying to feel what you ate today"
- Maintain conversation about their eating habits to distract them from the palpation

Auscultation

The most important finding to listen for is *peristalsis* or *bowel sounds,* which sound like short metallic clicks and gurgles. Their frequency per minute should be recorded (for example, 5 bowel sounds/minute). Bowel sounds may be stimulated by stroking the abdominal surface with a fingernail. Absent bowel sounds or hyperperistalsis is recorded and reported, since either usually denotes an abdominal pathologic condition.

Percussion

Percussion of the abdomen is performed in the same manner as percussion of the lungs and heart (see Fig. 7-28). Normally dullness or flatness is heard on the right side at the lower costal margin because of the location of the liver. Tympany is typically heard over the stomach on the left side and usually in the rest of the abdomen. An unusually tympanitic sound, like the beating of a tight drum, usually denotes air in the stomach, a common cause of which is mouth breathing.

Palpation

Two types of palpation are performed, superficial and deep. In *superficial palpation* the nurse lightly places the hand against the skin and feels each quadrant, noting any areas of tenderness, muscle tone, and superficial lesions, such as cysts.

Since superficial palpation is often perceived as tickling, several techniques can be used to minimize this sensation (see Nursing tips box). Admonishing the child to stop laughing only draws attention to the sensation and decreases cooperation. Positioning the child supine with the legs flexed at the hips and knees helps relax the abdominal muscles.

Deep palpation is used for palpating organs and large blood vessels and for detecting masses and tenderness that were not discovered during superficial palpation. If the child complains of abdominal pain, that area of the abdomen is palpated last. Palpation usually begins in the lower quadrants and proceeds upward to avoid missing the edge of an enlarged liver or spleen. Except for palpating the liver, successful identification of other organs, such as the spleen, kidney, and part of the colon, requires considerable practice with tutored supervision.

The lower edge of the *liver* is sometimes felt in infants and young children as a superficial mass 1 to 2 cm (0.4 to 0.8 inch) below the right costal margin (the distance is sometimes measured in fingerbreadths). If the liver is 3 cm (1.2 inches) or 2 fingerbreadths below the costal margin, it is considered enlarged, and this finding is referred to a physician. Normally the liver descends during inspiration as the diaphragm moves downward. This downward displacement should not be mistaken as a sign of liver enlargement.

The *spleen* is palpated by feeling it between the hand placed against the back and the other hand placed on the left upper quadrant. It is much smaller than the liver and positioned behind the fundus of the stomach. The tip of the spleen is normally felt during inspiration as it descends within the abdominal cavity. It is sometimes palpable 1 to 2 cm below the left costal margin in infants and young children. A spleen that is more than 2 cm below the right costal margin is enlarged and is always reported for further investigation.

The *bladder* may be palpated slightly above the pubic symphysis in infants and young children. It descends deeper into the pelvic cavity during adolescence, when it is not felt except if distended.

Other anatomic structures that are sometimes palpable in children include the kidney, cecum, and sigmoid colon. Although these structures are not routinely felt, the nurse should be aware of their relative location and characteristics in order not to mistake them for abnormal masses. Any questionable mass must be referred to a physician before it can be ruled out as benign.

During palpation of the abdomen the *femoral pulses* are felt by placing the tips of two or three fingers (index, middle, and/or ring) along the inguinal ligament about midway between the iliac crest and pubic symphysis. Both pulses are felt simultaneously to make certain that they are equal and strong (Fig. 7-36). Absence of femoral pulses is a significant sign of coarctation of the aorta.

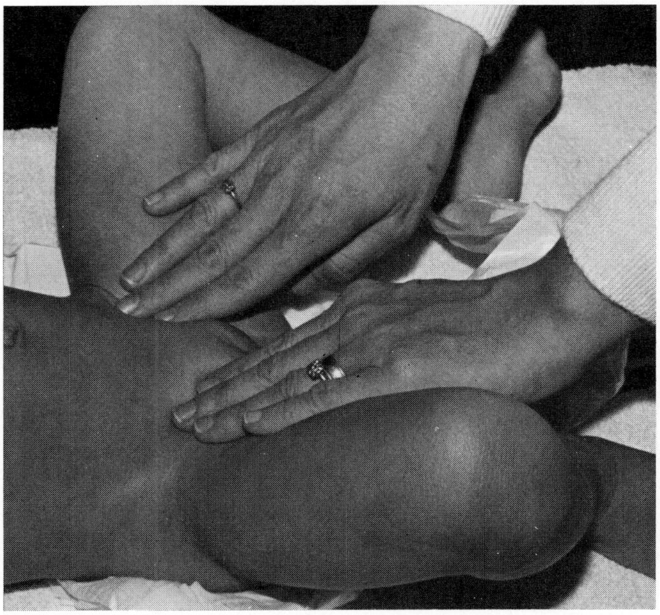

FIG. 7-36 Palpating for femoral pulses.

GENITALIA

Examination of genitalia conveniently follows assessment of the abdomen while the child is still supine. In adolescents inspection of the genitalia may be left to the end of the examination. The best approach is to examine the genitals matter-of-factly, placing no more emphasis on this part of the assessment than on any other segment. It helps to relieve children's and parents' anxiety by telling them the results of the findings as the nurse proceeds, for example, by stating, "Everything looks fine here." If the nurse finds it necessary to ask questions, such as about discharge or difficulty in urinating, consideration for the youngster's privacy should be observed by covering the lower abdomen with the gown or underpants. Examination of the genitalia provides an excellent opportunity for the nurse to elicit sexual concerns (see Therapeutic dialogue).

In examining the genitalia of adolescents the nurse should wear gloves to guard against infection from sexually transmitted disease. It might be helpful for the adolescent to know that this also prevents skin-to-skin contact. Each step of the examination is explained before it is performed, such as checking the scrotum for an inguinal hernia. If the male has an erection during the examination, the nurse assures him that this is a normal involuntary physiologic response to touch and proceeds with the remainder of the examination.

The examination of female genitalia is limited to inspection and palpation of external structures. If a vaginal examination is required, an appropriate referral is made unless the nurse is qualified to perform the procedure.

Male Genitalia

The external appearance of the genitalia is noted (Fig. 7-37). The size of the *penis* is generally small in infants and young boys, until puberty, when it begins to increase in

THERAPEUTIC DIALOGUE

Sexual Concerns during Adolescence

Following examination of the genitalia, the nurse comments to a 13-year-old girl, "Everything looks fine here. You are becoming a young woman. Are there any questions you would like to ask about how you are developing?"

ADOLESCENT: No. (Eyes are downcast; face has a sad expression.)

NURSE: During this time many young people have a lot of questions, but they are embarrassed to ask them. Have you ever felt that way? (Nurse uses third-person technique; see p. 110.)

ADOLESCENT: Yes. (Eyes look teary.)

NURSE: I think that this is very difficult for you to talk about. The tears are hard to hold back, aren't they?

(Adolescent begins to cry, nurse moves closer to her, and hands her a tissue.)

NURSE: Sometimes talking helps. I am here to listen.

ADOLESCENT: Most of my friends have their period and have boyfriends. I don't have either.

SUMMARY

With the adolescent's admission of her concerns, the nurse and teenager were able to discuss different rates of growth, both physically and emotionally. The nurse also suggested that the youngster talk with her mother about her worries. The mother, who had been in the room but had not joined in the discussion, expressed that she too had menstruated late and had felt left out among her peers. She encouraged her daughter to talk with her more because she did understand some of the pains of growing up.

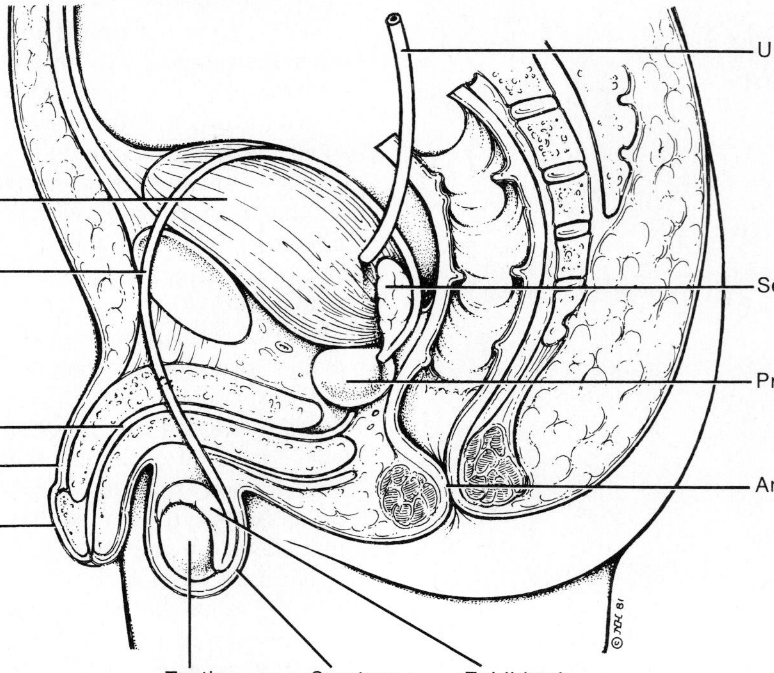

FIG. 7-37 Major structures of genitalia in circumcised prepubertal male.

both length and width. The nurse should be familiar with normal pubertal growth of the external male genitalia in order to compare the findings with the expected sequence of maturation.

The *glans* (the head of the penis) and the *shaft* (the portion between the perineum and prepuce) are examined. If the child is uncircumcised, the *prepuce* or foreskin covers the glans. In infants the prepuce is tight and should not be retracted for examination. In children the foreskin should be gently retracted for examination of the glans and the meatus.

The *urethral meatus* is carefully inspected for location and evidence of discharge. Normally it is centered at the tip of the glans.

Hair distribution is also noted. Normally before puberty no pubic hair is present. Soft downy hair at the base of the penis is an early sign of pubertal maturation. In older adolescents hair distribution forms a diamond-shaped pattern from the umbilicus to the anus.

The location and size of the *scrotum* are noted. The scrota hang freely from the perineum behind the penis and the left scrotum normally hangs lower than the right. In infants the scrota appear large in relation to the rest of the genitalia. The skin of the scrotum is loose and highly rugated (wrinkled). During early adolescence the skin normally becomes redder and coarser. In dark-skinned children the scrota are usually more deeply pigmented.

Palpation of the scrotum includes identification of the testes, epididymis, and, if present, inguinal hernias. The two *testes* are felt as small ovoid bodies, about 1.5 to 2 cm (0.6 to 0.8 inch) long—one in each scrotal sac. They do not enlarge until puberty, when they approximately double in size.

Palpating for the presence of the testes requires an understanding of the normal anatomy and physiology of the coverings of the testes and scrotal sac. The scrotum and testes are surrounded by the cremasteric fascia, which extends to the cremaster muscle. The muscle attaches to a point in the abdomen and extends downward along the inner surface of the thigh. The muscle or *cremasteric reflex* is stimulated by cold, touch, emotional excitement, or exercise. When contracted, the muscle pulls the testes higher into the pelvic cavity. Therefore the nurse must be careful not to elicit this reflex.

Several measures are useful in preventing the cremasteric reflex during palpation of the scrotum. First, the hands should be warm, not cold. Second, if old enough, the child is examined while sitting in a tailor or "Indian" position, which stretches the muscle, preventing its contraction (Fig. 7-38, *A*). Third, the normal pathway of ascent of the testes can be blocked by placing the thumb and index finger over the upper part of the scrotal sac along the inguinal canal (Fig. 7-38, *B*). If there is any question concerning the existence of two testes, the index and middle fingers are placed in a scissors fashion to separate the right and left scrotum. If after using these techniques the testes have not been palpated, the nurse should palpate the inguinal canal and perineum to locate masses that may be undescended testes. Although undescended testes may descend at any time during childhood and are checked at each visit, failure to palpate testes is reported.

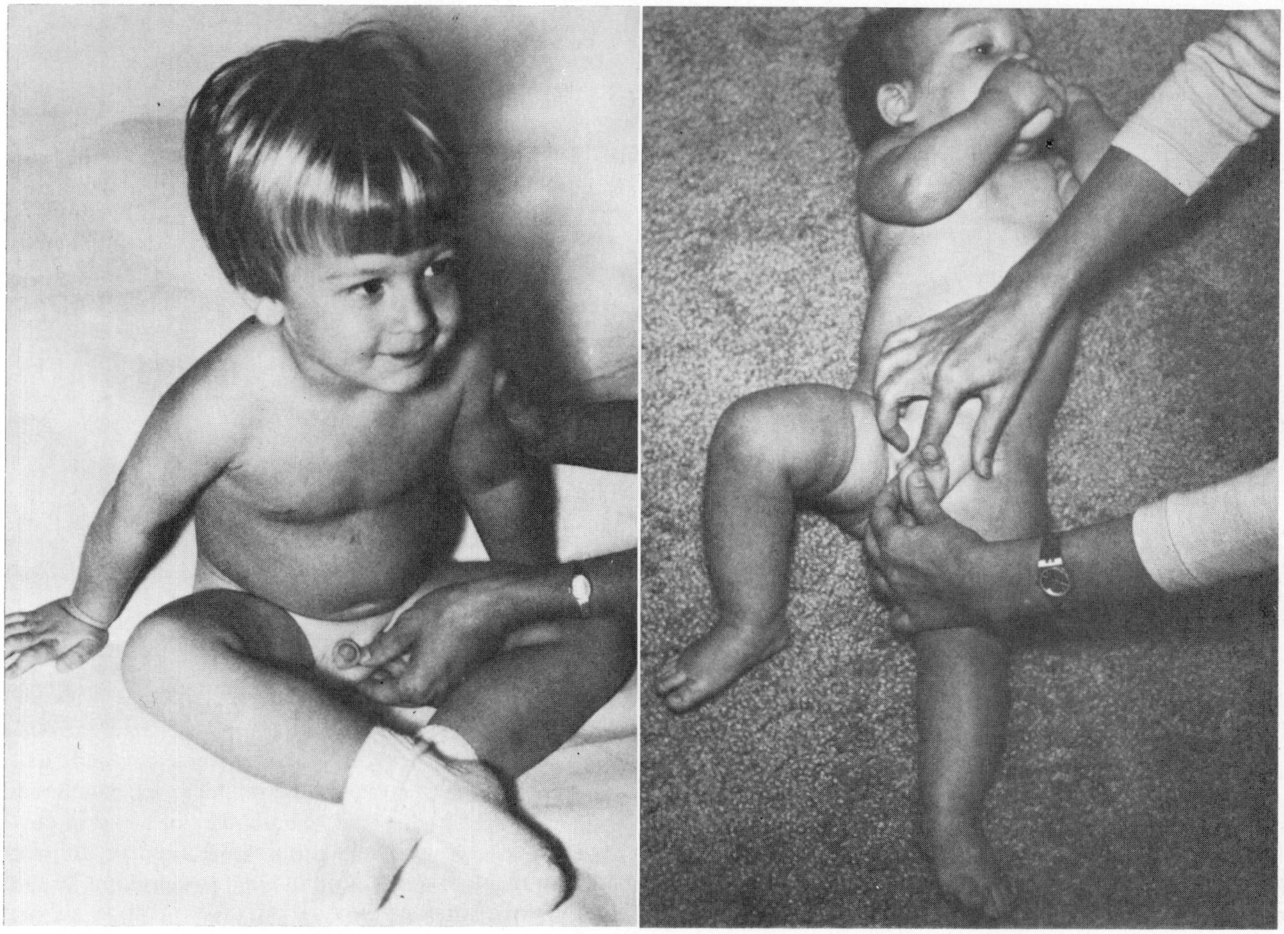

FIG. 7-38 A, Preventing the cremasteric reflex by having the child sit in "tailor" position. **B,** blocking inguinal canal during palpation of scrotum for descended testes.

Female Genitalia

A convenient position for examination of the genitalia involves placing the young child in a semireclining position on the parent's lap with the feet supported on the nurse's knees as the nurse sits facing the child. The child's attention is diverted from the examination by instructing her to try to keep the soles of her feet pressed together. The labia majora are held between the thumb and index finger and retracted outward in order to expose the labia minora, urethral meatus, and vaginal orifice.

The female genitalia are examined for size and location of the structures of the *vulva* or *pudendum* (Fig. 7-39). The *mons pubis* is a pad of adipose tissue over the symphysis pubis. At puberty the mons is covered with hair, which extends along the labia. The usual pattern of female *hair distribution* is an inverted triangle. The appearance of soft downy hair along the labia majora is an early sign of sexual maturation.

The size and location of the *clitoris* are noted. It is a small erectile organ located at the anterior end of the labia minora. It is covered by a small flap of skin, the *prepuce*.

The *labia majora* are two thick folds of skin running posteriorly from the mons to the posterior commissure of the vagina. Internal to the labia majora are two folds of skin called the *labia minora*. Although the labia minora are usually prominent in the newborn, they gradually atrophy, which makes them almost invisible until their enlargement during puberty.

The inner surface of the labia should be pink and moist. The size of the labia and any evidence of fusion, which may suggest male scrota, are noted. Normally no masses are palpable within the labia.

The *urethral meatus* is located posterior to the clitoris and is surrounded by Skene glands and ducts. Although not a prominent structure, the meatus appears as a small V-shaped slit. The nurse notes its location, especially if it opens from the clitoris or inside the vagina. The glands, which are common sites of cysts and sexually transmitted lesions, are gently palpated.

The *vaginal orifice* is located posterior to the urethral meatus. Its appearance is variable depending on individual anatomy and sexual activity. Ordinarily examination of the vagina is limited to inspection. In virgins a thin

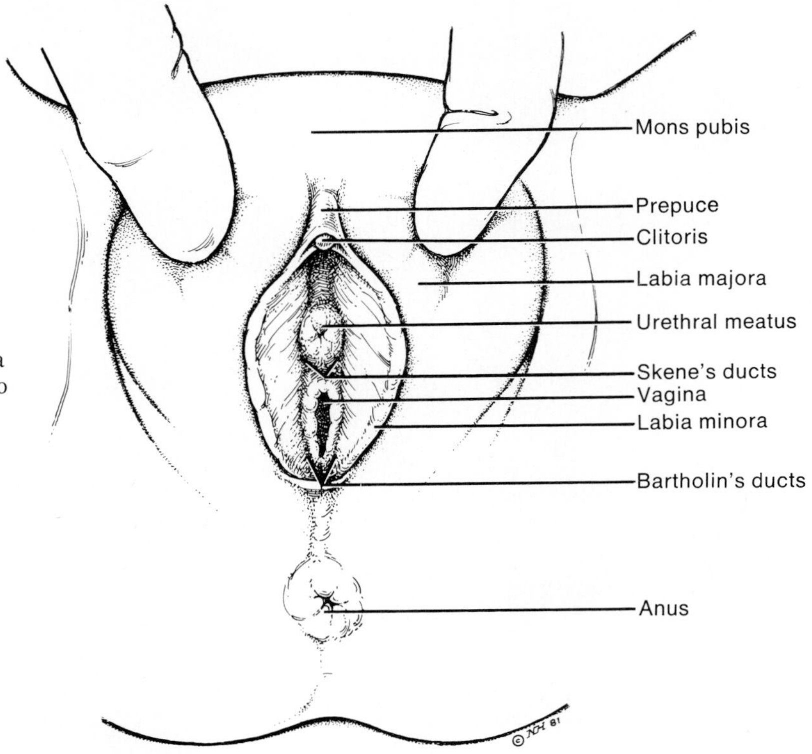

FIG. 7-39 External structures of genitalia in prepubertal female. Labia are spread to reveal deep structures.

crescent-shaped or circular membrane, called the *hymen,* may cover part of the vaginal opening. At times it completely occludes the orifice. After rupture, small rounded pieces of tissue called *carunculae* remain.

Surrounding the vaginal opening are *Bartholin glands,* which secrete a clear, mucoid fluid into the vagina for lubrication during intercourse. The ducts are palpated for cysts. The discharge from the vagina, which is usually clear or white, is also noted.

ANUS

Following examination of the genitalia, the anal area is easily examined, although the child should be placed on the abdomen. The general firmness of the *buttocks* and symmetry of the gluteal folds are noted. The tone of the anal sphincter is assessed by eliciting the *anal reflex.* Scratching or gently pricking the anal area results in an obvious quick contraction of the external anal sphincter.

BACK AND EXTREMITIES

Examination of the back and extremities is concerned with inspection of the spine, legs, arms, hands, feet, joints, and muscles. Certain specific tests are used to screen for scoliosis, pedal reflexes, and muscle strength.

Spine

The general *curvature* of the spine is noted. Normally the back of a newborn is rounded or C-shaped from the thoracic and pelvic curves. The development of the cervical and lumbar curves approximates development of various motor skills, such as cervical curvature with head control, and gives the older child the typical double-S curve.

Marked curvatures in posture are abnormal (see Fig. 30-17). *Scoliosis,* lateral curvature of the spine, is an important childhood problem, especially in females. Although scoliosis may be identified by observing and palpating the spine and noting a sideways displacement, more objective tests include:

1. With the child standing erect, clothed only in underpants (and bra if older girl), observe from behind, noting asymmetry of the shoulders and hips
2. With the child bending forward so that the back is parallel to the floor, observe from the side, noting asymmetry or prominence of the rib cage

A slight limp, a crooked hemline, or complaints of a sore back are other signs and symptoms of scoliosis.

The *back,* especially along the spine, is inspected for any tufts of hair, dimples, or discoloration. *Mobility* of the vertebral column is easily assessed in most children because of their propensity for constant motion during the examination. However, mobility can be tested by asking the child to sit up from a prone position or to do a modified sit-up exercise.

Extremities

Each extremity is inspected for symmetry of length and size; any deviation is referred for orthopedic evaluation. The fingers and toes are counted to be certain of the nor-

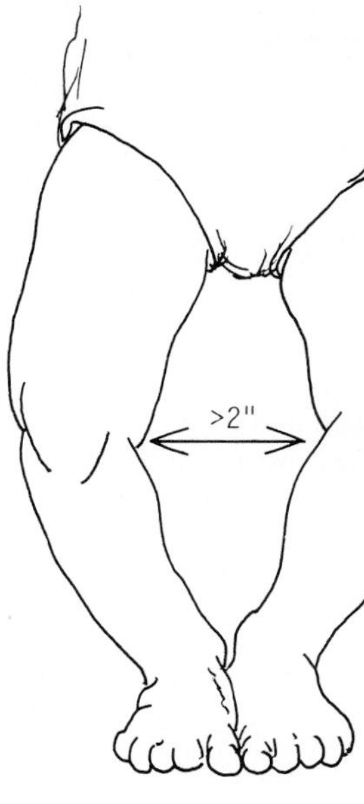

FIG. 7-40 Bowleg.

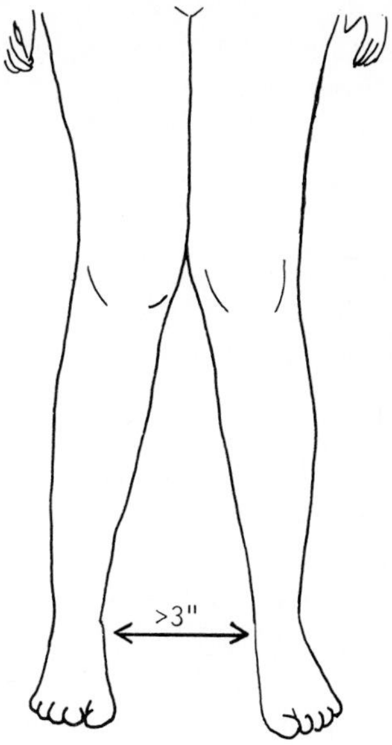

FIG. 7-41 Knock-knee.

mal number. This is so often taken for granted that an extra digit (polydactyly) or fusion of digits (syndactyly) may go unnoticed.

The arms and legs are inspected for *temperature* and *color,* which should be equal in each extremity, although the feet may normally be colder than the hands.

The *shape* of bones is assessed. Several variations of bone shape may be observed in children. Although many of them cause parents concern, most are benign and require no treatment. *Bowleg,* or *genu varum,* is lateral bowing of the tibia. It is clinically present when the child stands with the medial malleoli (rounded prominence on either side of the ankle) in apposition and the space between the knees is greater than approximately 5 cm (2 inches) (Fig. 7-40). Toddlers are usually bowlegged after beginning to walk until all their lower back and leg muscles are well developed. Unilateral or asymmetric bowlegs that are present beyond the age of 2 to 3 years, particularly in black children, may represent pathologic conditions requiring further investigation.

Knock-knee, or *genu valgum,* appears as the opposite of bowleg, in that the knees are close together but the feet are spread apart. It is determined clinically by using the same method as for genu varum but by measuring the distance between the malleoli, which normally should be less than 7.5 cm (3 inches) (Fig. 7-41). Knock-knee is normally present in children from about 2 to 7 years of age. Knock-knee that is excessive, asymmetric, accompanied by shortened stature, or evident in a child nearing puberty requires further evaluation.

Next the *feet* are inspected. Infants' and toddlers' feet appear flat because the foot is normally wide and the arch is covered by a fat pad. Development of the arch occurs naturally from the action of walking. Normally at birth the feet are held in a valgus (outward) or varus (inward) position. To determine whether a foot deformity at birth is the result of intrauterine position or development, the outer, then inner, side of the sole is scratched. If the foot position is self-correctable, it will assume a right angle to the leg. As the child begins to walk, the feet turn outward less than 30 degrees and inward less than 10 degrees.

Toddlers have a "toddling" or broad-based gait, which facilitates walking by lowering the center of gravity. As the child reaches preschool age, the legs are brought closer together. By school age the walking posture is much more graceful and balanced.

The most common gait problem in young children is pigeon toe or toeing in, which usually results from torsional deformities, such as internal tibial torsion (abnormal rotation or bowing of the tibia). Tests for tibial torsion include measuring the thigh-foot angle, which requires considerable practice for accuracy.

The *plantar* or *grasp reflex* is elicited by exerting firm but gentle pressure with the tip of the thumb against the lateral sole of the foot from the heel upward to the little toe and then across to the big toe. The normal response in children who are walking is flexion of the toes. *Babinski sign,* dorsiflexion of the big toe and fanning of the other toes, is normal during infancy but abnormal after about 1 year of age or when locomotion begins (see Fig. 8-9).

Joints

The joints are evaluated for *range of motion.* Normally this requires no specific testing if the nurse has been observant of the child's movements during the examination. However, the hips should be routinely investigated in infants for congenital dislocation. Signs of congenital hip dislocation are discussed on p. 1031. Any evidence of joint immobility or hyperflexibility is reported.

The joints are routinely palpated for *heat, tenderness,* and *swelling*. These signs, as well as redness over the joint, warrant further investigation.

Muscles

Symmetry and quality of muscle development, tone, and strength are noted. *Development* is observed by looking at the shape and contour of the body both in a relaxed and tensed state. *Tone* is estimated by grasping the muscle and feeling its firmness when it is relaxed and contracted. A common site for testing tone is the biceps muscle of the arm. Children are usually willing to "make a muscle" by clenching their fist.

Strength is estimated by having the child use an extremity to push or pull against resistance, as in the following examples:

Arm strength: Child holds his arms outstretched in front of him and tries to raise the arms while downward pressure is applied.
Hand strength: Child shakes hands with nurse and squeezes one or two fingers of the nurse's hand.
Leg strength: Child sits on a table or chair with the legs dangling and tries to raise the legs while downward pressure is applied.

Symmetry of strength is estimated in the extremities, hands, and fingers. Evidence of paresis or weakness is reported.

NEUROLOGIC ASSESSMENT

The assessment of the nervous system is the broadest and most diverse part of the examining process since every human function, both physical and emotional, is controlled by neurologic impulses. Much of the neurologic examination has already been discussed, such as assessment of behavior, sensory testing, and motor functioning. The following focuses on a general appraisal of cerebellar functioning, deep tendon reflexes, and the cranial nerves.

Assessment of neurologic function requires the use of a few additional tools. A reflex hammer, which has a small rounded rubber head, is used to test deep tendon reflexes. A pin and cotton are useful when testing sensory function. For the assessment of the cranial nerves, some flavors to taste and some odors to smell are necessary.

Cerebellar Functioning

The cerebellum controls balance and coordination. Much of the assessment of cerebellar functioning is included in observing the child's posture, body movements, gait, and development of fine and gross motor skills. Tests such as balancing on one foot and heel-to-toe walk on the Denver Developmental Screening Test assess balance. *Coordination* is tested by asking the child to reach for a toy, button his clothes, tie his shoes, or draw a straight line on a piece of paper, provided he is old enough to be expected to do each of these activities. Coordination can also be tested by any sequence of rapid successive movements, such as quickly touching each finger with the thumb of the same hand.

Tests for cerebellar function that can be performed as games include:

1. **Finger-to-nose test:** with the child's arm extended, ask the child to touch his nose with the index finger both with his eyes open and then closed
2. **Heel-to-shin test:** with the child standing, have him run the heel of one foot down the shin or anterior aspect of the tibia of the other leg, both with his eyes opened and then closed
3. **Romberg test:** with the eyes closed, have the child stand with his heels together; falling or leaning to one side is abnormal and is called *Romberg sign*

School-age children should be able to perform these tests, although preschoolers normally can only bring the finger within 5 to 7.5 cm (2 to 3) inches of their nose. Difficulty in performing these exercises indicates poor sense of position (especially with the eyes closed) and incoordination (especially with the eyes opened).

Reflexes

Testing reflexes is an important part of the neurologic examination. Persistence of primitive reflexes, loss of reflexes, or hyperactivity of deep tendon reflexes is usually the result of a cerebral insult. This discussion is primarily concerned with reflexes found in children past infancy. The primitive reflexes of the newborn are discussed in detail in Chapter 8 under physical assessment of the neonate.

Reflexes can be elicited by using the rubber head of the reflex hammer, flat of the finger, or side of the hand. If the child is easily frightened by equipment, it is best to use one's hand or finger. Although testing reflexes is a simple procedure to perform, the child may inhibit the reflex by unconsciously tensing the muscle. The nurse should try to distract younger children with toys or by talking to them. Older children can concentrate on the exercise of grasping their two hands in front of them and trying to pull them apart. This diverts their attention away from the testing and causes involuntary relaxation of the muscles.

Deep tendon reflexes are stretch reflexes of a muscle. The most common deep tendon reflex is the *knee jerk,* or *patellar reflex* (this is sometimes called the *quadriceps reflex*). The reflexes normally elicited are described in Figs. 7-42 to 7-45. Any diminished or hyperreflexic response is reported for further evaluation.

Cranial Nerves

Assessment of the cranial nerves is an important area of neurologic assessment (Table 7-4). With older children most of the tests can be made into games and, because

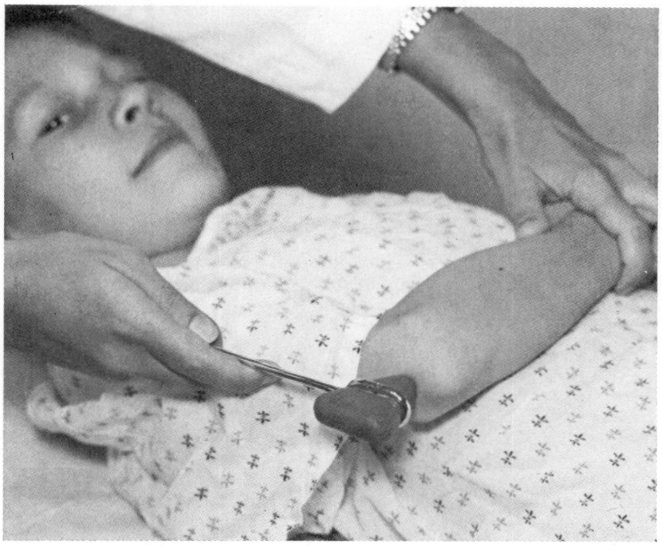

FIG. 7-42 Testing for triceps reflex. Child is placed supine, with the forearm resting over the chest, and triceps tendon is struck. Alternate procedure: Child's arm is abducted, with upper arm supported and forearm allowed to hang freely. Triceps tendon is struck. Normal response is partial extension of forearm.

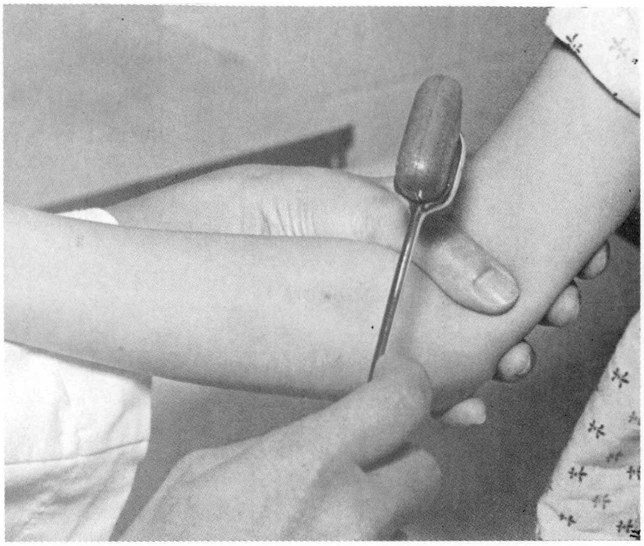

FIG. 7-43 Testing for biceps reflex. Child's arm is held by placing partially flexed elbow in examiner's hand with thumb over antecubital space. Examiner's thumbnail is struck with hammer. Normal response is partial flexion of forearm.

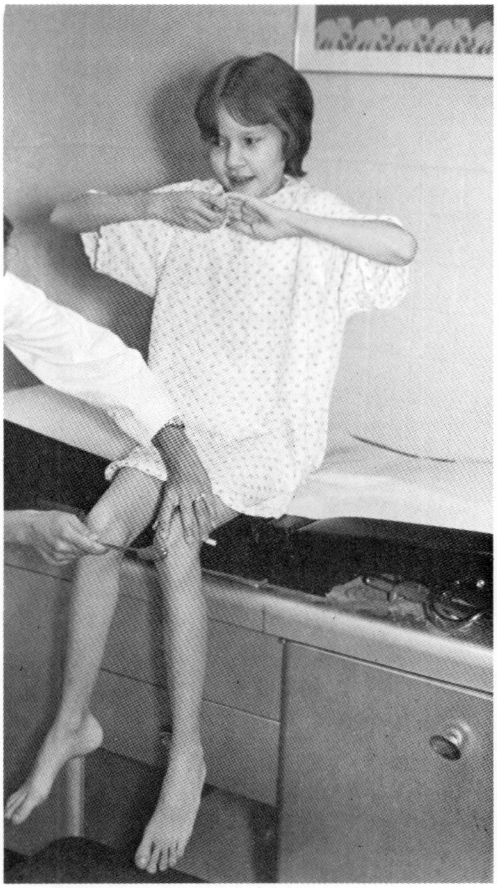

FIG. 7-44 Testing for patellar, or knee jerk, reflex, using distraction. Child sits on edge of examining table (or on parent's lap) with lower legs flexed at knee and dangling freely. Patellar tendon is tapped just below kneecap. Normal response is partial extension of lower leg.

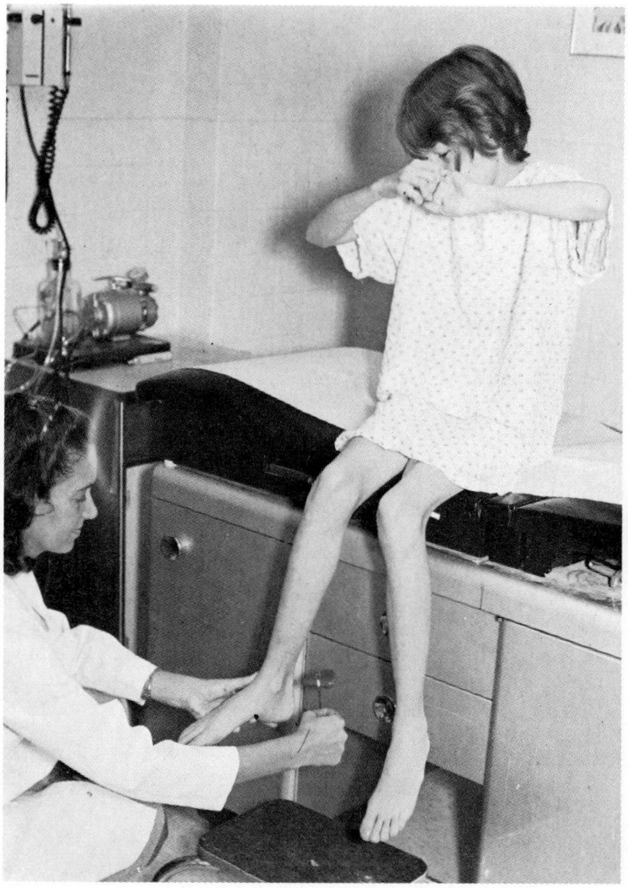

FIG. 7-45 Testing for Achilles reflex. Same position employed in eliciting knee jerk reflex is used. Foot is supported lightly in examiner's hand, and Achilles tendon is struck. Normal response is plantar flexion of foot (foot pointing downward).

TABLE 7-4

Assessment of Cranial Nerves

Cranial Nerve	Distribution	Test
I—Olfactory (S)*	Olfactory mucosa of nasal cavity	With his eyes closed, have child identify odors such as coffee, alcohol from a swab, or other smells; test each nostril separately
II—Optic (S)	Rods and cones of retina, optic nerve	Check for perception of light, visual acuity, peripheral vision, color vision, and normal optic disc
III—Oculomotor (M)*	Extraocular muscles of eye Superior rectus (SR)—moves eyeball up and in Inferior rectus (IR)—moves eyeball down and in Medial rectus (MR)—moves eyeball nasally Inferior oblique (IO)—moves eyeball up and out	Have child follow an object (toy) or light in the six cardinal positions of gaze (see Fig. 7-46)
	Pupil constriction and accommodation	Perform PERRLA (see p. 143)
	Eyelid opening	Check for proper placement of lid (see p. 142)
IV—Trochlear (M)	Superior oblique muscle (SO)—moves eye down and out	Have child look down and in (see Fig. 7-46)
V—Trigeminal (M, S)	Muscles of mastication	Have child bite down hard and open his jaw; test symmetry and strength
	Sensory: face, scalp, nasal and buccal mucosa	With his eyes closed, see if child can detect light touch in the mandibular and maxillary regions Test corneal and blink reflex by touching cornea lightly (approach child from the side so that he does not blink before cornea is touched)
VI—Abducens (M)	Lateral rectus (LR) muscle—moves eye temporally	Have child look toward temporal side (Fig. 7-46)
VII—Facial (M, S)	Muscles for facial expression	Have child smile, make funny face, or show his teeth to see symmetry of expression
	Anterior two thirds of tongue (sensory)	Have child identify a sweet, sour, or bitter solution; place each taste on anterior section and sides of protruding tongue; if child retracts tongue, solution will dissolve toward posterior part of tongue
	Nasal cavity and lacrimal gland, sublingual and submandibular salivary glands	Not tested
VIII—Auditory, acoustic, or vestibulocochlear (S)	Internal ear	Test hearing; note any loss of equilibrium or presence of vertigo
IX—Glossopharyngeal (M, S)	Pharynx, tongue	Stimulate the posterior pharynx with a tongue blade; the child should gag
	Posterior one third of tongue (sensory)	Test sense of taste on posterior segment of tongue
X—Vagus (M, S)	Muscles of larynx, pharynx, sensory fibers of root of tongue, heart, lung, and some organs of gastrointestinal system	Note hoarseness of the voice, gag reflex, and ability to swallow Check that uvula is in midline; when stimulated with a tongue blade, should deviate upward and to the stimulated side
XI—Accessory (M)	Sternocleidomastoid and trapezius muscles of shoulder	Have child shrug his shoulders while applying mild pressure; with the hands placed on his shoulders, have child turn his head against opposing pressure on either side; note symmetry and strength
XII—Hypoglossal (M)	Muscles of tongue	Have child move tongue in all directions; have him protrude the tongue as far as possible; note any midline deviation Test strength by placing tongue blade on one side of tongue and having child move it away

*S—sensory; M—motor.

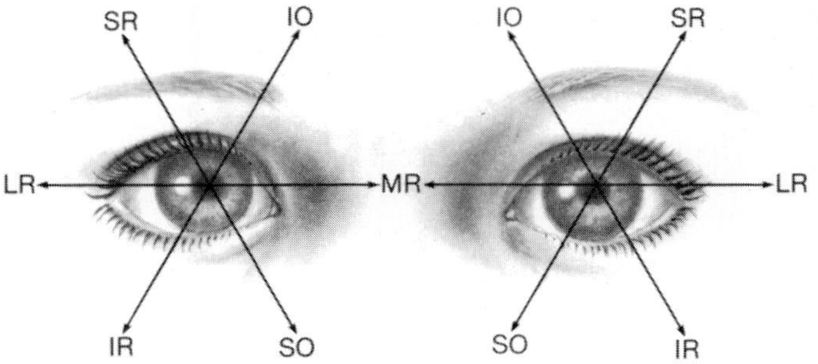

FIG. 7-46 Testing cardinal positions of gaze.

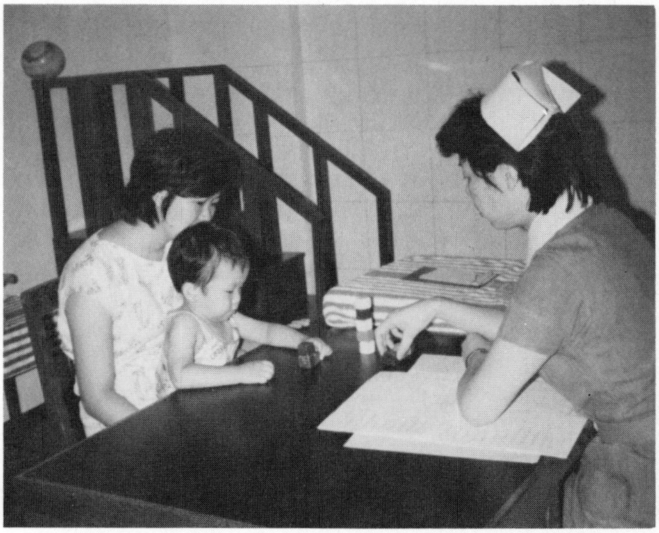

FIG. 7-47 When administering the DDST, the nurse must consider cultural variations that may erroneously label the child delayed.

no traumatic equipment is used, may encourage trust and security at the beginning of the examination. However, if the nurse is familiar with the functions of each nerve, much of the testing can be included when each "system" is examined, such as tongue movement and strength, gag reflex, swallowing, and position of the uvula during examination of the mouth.

◆ *Developmental Assessment*

One of the most essential components of a complete health appraisal is assessment of developmental functioning. *Screening procedures* are designed to identify quickly and reliably those children whose developmental level is below normal for their age and who, therefore, require further investigation. They also provide a means of recording objective measurements of present developmental functioning for future reference. In this discussion the nurse's role is viewed primarily in terms of screening.

Although screening tests are an effective method of applying the knowledge of children's expected rate of development to a large segment of the population, they are only as successful as the individuals' expertise in administering them. Since many of the screening tests are devised to be used by paraprofessionals, there are inherent risks in screening if such individuals are not properly trained or supervised. For example, false-positives can label the child as developmentally delayed and cause problems that otherwise might not have existed. It is the responsibility of the nurse to ensure that screening tests are properly administered and that the results are correctly interpreted. The complexity of mental and physical health can never be measured by any one index. Evaluation of the child's total well-being is the result of evaluating data from a comprehensive history, physical examination, and developmental screening.

DENVER DEVELOPMENTAL SCREENING TEST

The most widely used screening test for assessing a young child's development is the *Denver Developmental Screening Test (DDST)* and the *Revised Denver Developmental Screening Test (DDST-R)* (see Appendix C). The tests are composed of four major categories: personal-social, fine motor–adaptive, language, and gross motor and are applicable for children from birth through 6 years of age. The age divisions are monthly until age 24 months and then every 6 months until 6 years of age. Allowances are made for infants who were born prematurely by subtracting the number of months of missed gestation from their present age and testing them at the adjusted age. For example, a 9-month-old infant who was born 4 weeks prematurely is tested at an 8-month level.

The results of the DDST and DDST-R compare favorably to other psychometric tests. However, one weakness of the test is its limitations in terms of predictive validity with lower socioeconomic groups and children of different cultural backgrounds. For example, Southeast Asian children have demonstrated delays in the areas of personal-social development because of lack of familiarity with games like pat-a-cake and in language because of differences in word usage, such as absence of plurals (Miller, Onotera, and Deinard, 1984). The more protective parental attitude of Southeast Asians toward the young child may also prevent early learning of self-help skills (Fung and Lau, 1985). Several of these variations were noted also in native African children (Olade, 1984). Such cultural differences must be considered when administering the test to prevent erroneous labeling of the child as "developmentally delayed" (Fig. 7-47).

The major differences between the original DDST and the DDST-R are the arrangement of items on the form and the scoring. On the original form, items are scored as "P" for pass, "F" for fail, or "R" for refusal. On the DDST-R only the items passed are scored. The revised DDST-R has been found to have several advantages over the original form: (1) it is easier to use, especially for those not trained with DDST, (2) it facilitates using the short DDST (see p. 173), (3) it provides a more dynamic representation of the child's development because the form resembles a growth curve, and (4) subsequent testing of the child requires administering only those items not previously scored with a "P" that are to the left of the child's age line (Frankenburg and others, 1981). However, the instruction manual* uses the original form for training; therefore this form may be more familiar to practitioners.

The DDST is designed for administration by both professionals and paraprofessionals and takes about 15 to 20 minutes to complete. The kits for testing include a red wool ball, raisins, a small, clear bottle with a 5/8-inch opening, a rattle with a narrow handle, eight 1-inch square blocks in red, blue, yellow, and green colors, a small bell, a tennis ball, and a pencil.

Each item is designated by a bar that represents the ages at which 25%, 50%, 70%, and 90% of the tested population could perform the particular item. Scoring is based on the number of *delays,* which are defined as "failure to perform an item which is passed by 90% of the children who are of the same age or any item which falls completely to the *left* of the age line." *Abnormal* is determined by either:

1. Two or more sectors with two or more delays
2. One sector with two or more delays plus one or more sectors with one delay and, in that same sector, no passes through the age line

Questionable is determined by either:

1. One sector with two or more delays
2. One or more sectors with one delay and in that same sector no passes through the age line

Children are considered *untestable* when the number of refusals is large enough to cause the test result to be questionable or abnormal *if* the refusals are scored as failures. *Normal* is determined by any score that does not meet these other criteria.

Guidelines for Administration

Although it is not the purpose of this discussion to detail the instruction manual, there are some points concerning preparation, administration, and interpretation of the DDST that necessitate emphasis. Before the test is begun, both the child and parent need an explanation. For parents this means clarifying that the DDST is *not* an intelligence test but a method of helping the nurse observe what the child can do at this age. It is best to deemphasize the word *test* while emphasizing that the child is *not* expected to perform each item on the sheet.

The parent is told before the screening begins that the results of the child's performance will be explained after all the items have been concluded. It is the nurse's responsibility to properly inform parents of any testing or screening procedure before its administration so that they are fully aware of its purpose and intent.

The nurse prepares toddlers and preschoolers for the test by presenting it as a game. Frequently the DDST is an excellent way to begin a health appraisal because it is nonthreatening, requires no painful or unfamiliar procedures, and capitalizes on the child's natural activity of play. Since children are easily distracted, it is best to perform the test quickly and to present only one toy from the kit at a time. After that toy's purpose is concluded, such as building a tower of blocks or identifying its color, the toy is placed back in the bag and another one is brought out for testing purposes. Other temporary factors that may interfere with the child's performance include fatigue, illness, fear, hospitalization, separation from the parent, or general unwillingness to perform activities asked. In addition, undiagnosed mental retardation, hearing loss, vision loss, neurologic impairment, or a familial pattern of slow development greatly influences the child's performance.

Following completion of the DDST, the parent is asked if the child's performance on the test was typical of his behavior at other times. If the parent replies affirmatively and if the child's cooperation was satisfactory, the nurse explains the results, emphasizing all successful items first, then those items failed but which the child was not expected to pass, and finally those items that were delays.

In explaining a normal score, the nurse should focus on how well the child performed and should reinforce the parents' efforts in satisfactorily stimulating their child. Although one does not wish to encourage parents to teach their child skills in order to pass the test, the DDST can be used to guide parents toward those activities that are appropriate, although not necessarily expected, for the child's age. For example, although not all 3-year-old children can button their clothes or dress with supervision only, the nurse can inquire if the parent has presented such opportunities to the child. If the parent has not, the nurse can state that this is an activity that some 3-year-old children can perform, especially if encouraged and helped to do so.

In explaining delays, the nurse carefully notes the parent's response, especially casual acceptance, such as, "He'll catch up." Since all children with questionable or abnormal results should be rescreened before referral for diagnostic testing, some of the parents' more serious questions, such as, "Does this mean my child is retarded?" can be deferred until the next screening session. The nurse must be aware of personal anxieties during these situations and refrain from giving glib reassurances, such as, "I'm sure he will do better the next time." Rather, parents' questions should be answered honestly yet with appropriate flexibility and concern (see Therapeutic dialogue on p. 545).

If the parents reply that the child's performance was not typical of his usual behavior, it is best to defer any scoring or discussion of the test results with the parents, especially if the refusals yield a questionable or abnormal

*Forms and instruction manual are available from Denver Developmental Materials, Inc., P.O. Box 20037, Denver, CO 80220.

rating. In this case the DDST is rescheduled for a time when the child is more likely to cooperate.

SHORT DDST

Several other screening tests are available. One is the short DDST. Using the short DDST form, only the three items immediately to the left of the age line, but not intersecting the line, in each of the four sectors are administered. If all 12 items are passed, the child receives no further testing until the next scheduled visit. However, if one or more items are failed or refused, then the full DDST is administered while the child is in the test setting. The major advantages of the short DDST are that it takes less time (5 to 7 minutes) and that the second stage testing can be done immediately if needed.

REVISED DENVER PRESCREENING DEVELOPMENTAL QUESTIONNAIRE

Another prescreening test is the *Revised-Denver Prescreening Developmental Questionnaire (R-PDQ)*. It is designed to identify those children ages 3 months to 6 years who require a more thorough screening with the DDST. It has the advantage of being very rapid and easy to administer. Parents answer questions about their child's development; the questions describe tasks that are performed by 90% of children at a younger age than the child being screened. Children with a score of 1 or no delays are nonsuspect, but those with a score of 2 or more delays are suspect and are tested with the full DDST (Frankenburg, 1986).

SUMMARY

Physical examination involves a number of important skills, such as inspection, palpation, percussion, and auscultation, and the use of special equipment to thoroughly assess all body functions. With children certain modifications in the sequence of and approach to the examination are necessary to reduce the anxiety associated with certain procedures. Developmental assessment is a unique feature of the appraisal process with young children and requires judgment in administering various screening tests and interpreting their results.

KEY CONCEPTS

- The traditional head-to-toe sequence of physical examination is frequently altered in children to reduce their anxiety and obtain more accurate findings.
- Growth measurements during the physical examination focus on length, height, weight, skinfold thickness, and arm and head circumference. Assessment of growth is measured against standard growth charts to determine a child's status in comparison with other children of his age.
- Measurements of temperature, pulse, respiration, and blood pressure constitute the physiologic approach to assessment.
- The general appearance of a child is a cumulative, subjective impression of physical appearance, state of nutrition, behavior, personality, interactions with parents and nurse, posture, development, and speech.
- Assessment of the skin, which primarily involves inspection and palpation, focuses on color, texture, temperature, moisture, and turgor. The nurse needs to be aware of both physiologic and ethnic factors that may affect these areas.
- In assessment of the lymph nodes, the nurse examines, by palpation, the part of the body in which the glands are located.
- The head is inspected for shape and symmetry.
- Assessment of the neck includes palpation of the trachea and thyroid gland.
- Examination of the eyes includes placement and alignment, inspection of external and internal structures, and vision testing.
- Ears are examined for placement and alignment, inspection of external and internal structures, and auditory testing.
- The lungs are examined by methods of inspection, palpation, percussion, and auscultation.
- Auscultation is the most important procedure for examining the heart.
- Abdominal assessment follows an orderly sequence of inspection, auscultation, percussion, and palpation, since the latter may distort normal abdominal sounds.
- Examination of the genitalia may be anxiety-provoking in the child, and the nurse must avoid any transference of anxiety.
- Neurologic assessment addresses behavior; motor, sensory, and cerebellar functioning; reflexes; and cranial nerves.
- The Denver Developmental Screening Test, the most widely used assessment tool, is composed of four categories: personal-social, fine motor–adaptive, language, and gross motor.

STUDY QUESTIONS AND ACTIVITIES

1 Perform a complete physical examination on a toddler and a school-age child. Compare the children's responses to the examining procedures and the alterations in sequence to accommodate each child's needs.
2 Record the physical examination using the head-to-toe format.
3 Perform a short form and the complete DDST on a child under 6 years of age. Compare the amount of testing time required for each. Score the short form to determine if the longer version would have been required.
4 Observe specialized sensory testing, such as audiometry, brainstem or visually evoked potentials, and otokinetic nystagmus, and describe the indications for their use and the training required to perform them.

REFERENCES

Frankenburg, W.K.: Revising the Denver Prescreening Developmental Questionnaire, Early Childhood Update **2**(1):1-3, 1986.

Frankenburg, W.K., and others: The newly abbreviated and revised Denver Developmental Screening Test, J. Pediatr. **99**(6):995-999, 1981.

Fung, K., and Lau, S.: Denver Developmental Screening Test: cultural variables, J. Pediatr. **106**(2):343, 1985.

Hancock, L.A.: FirstTemp, J. Pediatr. Health Care **1**(3):163-163, 1987.

Kovalesky, A.: Nurses' guide to children's eyes, New York, 1985, Grune & Stratton, Inc.

Martyn, K., and others: Comparison of axillary, rectal and skin-based temperature assessment in preschoolers, Nurs. Pract. **13**(4):31-36, 1988.

Miller, V., Onotera, R., and Deinard, A.: Denver Developmental Screening Test: cultural variations in Southeast Asian children, J. Pediatr. **104**(3):481-482, 1984.

National Society for the Prevention of Blindness, Inc.: Children's eye health guide, New York, 1982, The Society.

Olade, R.A.: Evaluation of the Denver Developmental Screening Test as applied to African children, Nurs. Res. **33**(4):204-207, 1984.

Report of the Second Task Force on Blood Pressure Control in Children-1987, Pediatrics **79**(1):1-25, 1987.

Sato-Viacrucis, K.: The evolution of the Snellen E to the Blackbird, School Nurse, pp. 18-19, Spring 1985.

Steinfeld, L., and others: Sphygmomanometry in the pediatric patient, J. Pediatr. **92**(6):934-938, 1978.

BIBLIOGRAPHY

Physical Examination

Alexander, M.M., and Brown, M.S.: Physical examination. Part 12. Examining the chest and lungs, Nursing 75 **5**(1):44-48, 1975.

Alexander, M.M., and Brown, M.S.: Physical examination. Part 13. Examining the abdomen, Nursing 76 **6**(1):65-70, 1976.

Alexander, M.M., and Brown, M.S.: Physical examination. Part 14. Male genitalia, Nursing 76 **6**(2):39-43, 1976.

Alexander, M.M., and Brown, M.S.: Physical examination. Part 16. The musculoskeletal system, Nursing 76 **6**(4):51-56, 1976.

Alexander, M.M., and Brown, M.S.: Physical examination. Part 17. Performing the neurological examination, Nursing 76 **6**(6):38-43, 1976.

Alexander, M.M., and Brown, M.S.: Physical examination. Part 18. Neurological examination, Nursing 76 **6**(7):50-55, 1976.

Barrus, D.H.: A comparison of rectal and axillary temperatures by electronic thermometer measurement in preschool children, Pediatr. Nurs. **9**(6):424-425, l983.

Behee-Miller, B.: Basic principles of measurement, Child. Nurs. **4**(4):1-3, 1986.

Bowers, A., and Thompson, J.: Clinical manual of health assessment, ed. 2, St. Louis, 1984, The C.V. Mosby Co.

Brown, M.S., and Alexander, M.M.: Physical examination. Part 15. Female genitalia, Nursing 76 **6**(3):39-41, 1976.

Brown, M.S., and Murphy, M.A.: Ambulatory pediatrics for nurses, ed. 2, New York, 1980, McGraw-Hill Book Co.

Caufield, C.: A developmental approach to hearing screening in children, Pediatr. Nurs. **4**(2):39-42, 1978.

Chard, M.: An approach to examining the adolescent male, MCN **1**(1):41-43, 1976.

Church, J.L., and Baer, K.J.: Examination of the adolescent—a practical guide, J. Pediatr. Health Care **1**(2):65-72, 1987.

Cohen, S.: Patient assessment: examination of the female pelvis. Part I, Am. J. Nurs. **78:**1717-1746, 1978.

Cohen, S.: Patient assessment: examination of the male genitalia, Am. J. Nurs. **79:**689-712, 1979.

Cohen, S.: Patient assessment: examining joints of the upper and lower extremities, Am. J. Nurs. **81:**763-786, 1981.

Delancy, V.L., and North, C.: Skin assessment, Top. Clin. Nurs. **5**(2):5-10, 1983.

Dessertine, P.S.: Those neglected heart sounds, Pediatr. Nurs. **3**(1):18-20, 1977.

DiChiara, E.: A sound method for testing child's hearing, Am. J. Nurs. **84**(9):1104-1106, 1984.

Dossey, B.: Perfecting your skills for systematic patient assessments, Nursing 79 **9**(2):42-45, 1979.

Dunn, B.H.: Components of musculoskeletal examination, Orthop. Nurs. **1**(6):33-36, 1982.
Egan, D., and Brown, R.: Vision testing of young children in the age range 18 months to 4-1/2 years, Child Care Health Dev. **10:**381-390, 1984.
Eoff, M.J., and Joyce, B.: Temperature measurements in children, Am. J. Nurs. **81:**1010-1011, May 1981.
Eoff, M.J., Meier, R.S., and Miller, C.: Temperature measurement in infants, Nurs. Res. **23:**457-460, Nov./Dec. 1974.
Erickson, R.: Oral temperature differences in relation to thermometer and technique, Nurs. Res. **29**(3):157-164, 1980.
Erickson, B.: Detecting abnormal sounds, Nursing 86 **16**(1):58-63, 1986.
Gemberling, C.L.: The adolescent gynecologic examination: an overview, J. Pediatr. Nurs. **1**(3):141-151, 1987.
Harris, J.A.: Pediatric abdominal assessment, Pediatr. Nurs. **12**(5):355-362, 1986.
Holland, S.H.: 20/20 vision screening, Pediatr. Nurs. **8**(2):81-87, 1982.
Hutchfield, K., and Crump, A.: Holding children for examination, Nursing (Oxford) **1:**1003-1005, March 1981.
Johnson, J.L., and others: The school nurse's role in vision screening for the difficult-to-test student, J. Sch. Health **53**(6):345-349, 1983.
King, R.C.: Examining the thorax and respiratory system, RN **45:**55-63, 1982.
Linley, J.: Screening children for common orthopedic problems, Am. J. Nurs. **87**(10):1312-1316, 1987.
Mitchell, J.R.: Male adolescents' concern about a physical examination conducted by a female, Nurs. Res. **29**(3):165-169, 1980.
Moss, J.R.: Helping young children cope with the physical examination, Pediatr. Nurs. **7**(2):17-20, 1981.
Moss, J.R.: Predicting young children's cooperation with the physical examination, Pediatr. Nurs. **9**(3):188-190, 1983.
Pickwell, S.: Primary health care of Indochinese refugee children, Pediatr. Nurs. **8**(2):104-107, 1982.
Rieser, P.: Role of the school nurse in the assessment of linear growth, Commun. Nurs. Forum **4**(1):1-12, 1987.
Saul, L.: For CE credit: heart sounds and common murmurs, Am. J. Nurs. **83**(12):1679-1689, 1983.
Schweiger, J., Lang, J., and Schweiger, J.: Oral assessment: how to do it, Am. J. Nurs. **80**(4):654-663, 1980.
Seidel, H., and others: Mosby's guide to physical examination, St. Louis, 1987, The C.V. Mosby Co.
Smith, C.E.: Abdominal assessment—a blending of science and art, Nursing 81 **11**(2):42-49, 1981.
Smith, C.E.: With good assessment skills you can construct a solid framework for patient care, Nursing 84 **14**(12):26-31, 1984.
Smith, C.E.: Assessing the liver, Nursing 85 **15**(7):36-37, 1985.
Thomson, L.R.: Understanding tympanometry, Pediatr. Nurs. **8**(3):193-197, 1982.
Walleck, C.: A neurological assessment procedure that won't make you nervous, Nursing 82 **12**(12):50-56, 1982.
Wong, D.L.: The paper-doll technique, Pediatr. Nurs. **7**(6):39-40, 1981.
Yoos, L.: A developmental approach to physical assessment, MCN **6**(3):168-170, 1981.
Younger, J.: Detecting visual problems in children, Pediatr. Nurs. **5**(6):50-51, 1979.

Developmental Assessment

Bradshaw, M.M.: Denver Developmental Screening Test. In Humenick, S.S., editor: Analysis of current assessment strategies in the health care of young children and childbearing families, Norwalk, CT, 1982, Appleton-Century-Crofts.
Castiglia, P.T., and Petrini, M.A.: Selecting a developmental screening tool, Pediatr. Nurs. **11**(1):8-17, 1985.
Harris, C.: Assessment of children's behavior. In Hall, S., editor: Nursing assessment and strategies for the family at risk, ed. 2, Philadelphia, 1986, J.B. Lippincott Co.
Lynn, M.R.: Update: the Denver Developmental Screening Test, J. Pediatr. Nurs. **2**(5):348-531, 1987.
Medenwald, N.A., and others: Is the DDST as good as you think it is? Pediatr. Nurs. **4**(5):53-55, 1978.
Meisels, S.J.: Uses and abuses of developmental screening and school readiness testing, Young Child. **42**(2):4-8, 1987.
O'Pray, M.: Developmental screening tools: using them effectively, MCN **5**(2):126-130, 1980.

UNIT IV

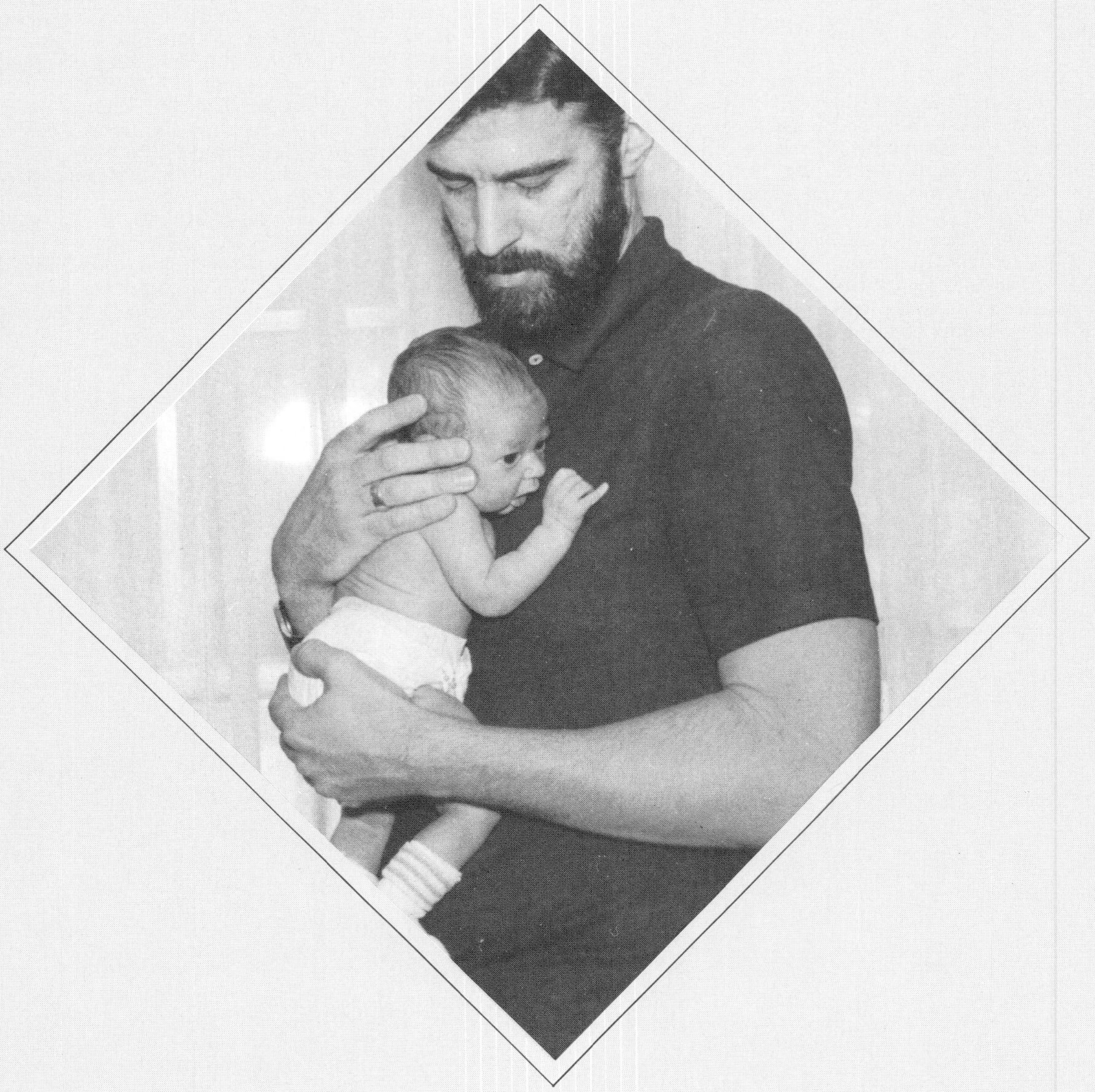

The Newborn

Probably no event is more dramatic or miraculous than the birth of a child. It is the culmination of a 9-month gestation period during which the fetus prepares for extrauterine existence and the parents prepare for the addition of a totally dependent member to their lives. At the time of delivery profound physiologic and psychologic reactions occur that further ready the child and parents for this experience.

In most instances the birth and the perinatal period are uneventful and infants return home with their parents to begin developing as vital, healthy, and loved children. Chapter 8, *Health Promotion of the Newborn and Family,* is concerned with infants' normal adjustment to extrauterine life, their physiologic status at birth, and the nursing knowledge required to care for them at and immediately following delivery, to perform a newborn assessment, and to promote parent-infant attachment. Chapter 9, *Health Problems of the Newborn,* deals with problems encountered during the neonatal period, including birth trauma, congenital defects, physiologic derangements, perinatal infection, and dysmaturity. The concept of high risk is introduced and focuses on identification and assessment of high-risk neonates, problems common to them because of their high-risk status, and supportive care of the child and family throughout this ordeal.

CHAPTER 8

Health Promotion of the Newborn and Family

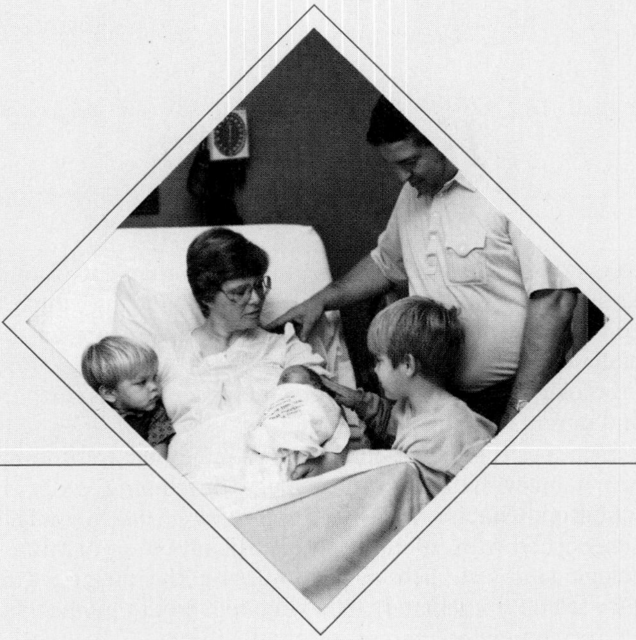

LEARNING OBJECTIVES

On completion of this chapter the reader will be able to:

- Identify the principal cardiorespiratory changes that occur during transition to extrauterine life
- Identify the immature physiologic functioning of each body system and its significance to nursing care of the newborn
- Perform an initial and transitional assessment of the newborn based on the Apgar score and periods of reactivity
- Perform a newborn physical assessment based on recognition of expected normal findings
- Outline a nursing care plan for the newborn in the nursery
- Assess and promote parent-infant attachment behaviors

Childbirth is an intense and exhausting physiologic and emotional experience for mothers and newborns (neonates). Even when this process progresses normally, neonates are required to withstand extreme changes as they leave a completely life-sustaining environment and enter a variable atmosphere that demands profound physiologic alteration for survival. The neonatal or perinatal period, the interval from viability until 28 days after birth, presents the greatest risk to newborns. In the United States, for example, about three quarters of all deaths during the first year of life occur during these 4 weeks.

The nurse's role is one of supporting the family and infant through the birth process, preventing physiologic complications in the neonate's adjustment to extrauterine life, and promoting the attachment process between child and parents. Expert technologic and psychologic nursing care during the immediate postpartum period lays a strong foundation for healthy parent-child development.

◆ *Adjustment to Extrauterine Life*

The most profound physiologic change required of the neonate is transition from fetal or placental circulation to independent respiration. The loss of the placental connection means the loss of complete metabolic support, the most important and essential function being the supply of oxygen and the removal of carbon dioxide. The normal stresses of labor and delivery produce alterations of placental gas exchange patterns, acid-base balance in the blood, and cardiovascular activity in the infant. Factors that interfere with this normal transition or that increase fetal asphyxia (a condition of hypoxemia, hypercapnia, and acidosis) will affect the fetus's adjustment to extrauterine life.

IMMEDIATE ADJUSTMENTS

The newborn's adjustment to extrauterine life is a complex physiologic process. The first 24 hours are the most critical because during this time respiratory distress and circulatory failure can occur rapidly and with little warning. There is a higher incidence of death during these initial 24 hours than during the entire succeeding perinatal period.

Respiratory System

The most critical and immediate physiologic change required of the newborn is the onset of breathing. The stimuli that help initiate the first respiration are primarily chemical and thermal. *Chemical* factors in the blood like low oxygen, high carbon dioxide, and low pH initiate impulses that excite the respiratory center in the medulla. The primary *thermal* stimulus is the sudden chilling of the infant who leaves a warm environment and enters a relatively cooler atmosphere. This abrupt change in temperature excites sensory impulses in the skin that are transmitted to the respiratory center.

The significance of *tactile* stimulation is questionable. Probably descent through the birth canal and normal handling during delivery have some effect on initiation of respiration. Slapping the infant's feet or buttocks has no beneficial effect. However, it can waste precious time in the event of respiratory difficulty and can cause additional damage if cerebral trauma has occurred.

The initial entry of air into the lungs is opposed by the surface tension of the fluid that filled the fetal lungs and the alveoli. However, fetal lung fluid is removed by the lymphatic vessels and pulmonary capillaries. Some fluid is also removed during the normal forces of labor and delivery. As the chest emerges from the birth canal, fluid is squeezed from the lungs through the nose and mouth. Following complete delivery of the chest, a brisk recoil of the thorax occurs. Air enters the upper airway to replace the lost fluid. In cesarean birth the chest is not compressed and the newborn may need additional respiratory support.

In the alveoli the surface tension of the fluid is reduced by *surfactant*, a substance produced by the alveolar epithelium that coats the alveolar surface. The effect of surfactant in facilitating breathing is discussed in relation to respiratory distress syndrome (see p. 243).

Circulatory System

Equally important as the initiation of respiration are the circulatory changes that allow blood to flow through the lungs. These changes, which occur more gradually, are the result of shifts in pressure in the heart and major vessels from increased pulmonary and systemic blood volume secondary to decreased pulmonary vascular resistance and increased systemic vascular resistance. The transition from fetal circulation to postnatal circulation involves the functional closure of the fetal shunts, the foramen ovale, the ductus arteriosus, and eventually the ductus venosus. (For a review of fetal circulation see Chapter 24.)

Once the lungs are expanded, the inspired oxygen dilates the pulmonary vessels, which decreases pulmonary vascular resistance and consequently increases pulmonary blood flow. As the lungs receive blood, the pressure in the right atrium, right ventricle, and pulmonary arteries decreases. At the same time there is a progressive rise in systemic vascular resistance from the increased volume of blood through the placenta at cord clamping. This increases the pressure in the left side of the heart. Since blood flows from an area of high pressure to one of low pressure, the circulation of blood through the fetal shunts is reversed.

The most important factor controlling ductal closure is the increased oxygen concentration of the blood. Secondary factors are the fall in endogenous prostaglandins and acidosis. The foramen ovale closes functionally at or soon after birth. The ductus arteriosus is closed functionally by the fourth day. Anatomic closure takes considerably longer. Failure of the ducts to close results in congenital heart defects (see Chapter 24).

Because of the reversible flow of blood through the ducts during the early neonatal period, functional murmurs are occasionally heard. In conditions such as crying or straining the increased pressure shunts unoxygenated blood from the right side of the heart across the ductal opening, causing transient cyanosis.

PHYSIOLOGIC STATUS OF OTHER SYSTEMS

The major life-dependent physiologic changes in the cardiovascular and respiratory systems of the newborn have already been discussed. However, all of the body systems undergo some change, and most are immature at birth. Each should be observed closely for proper functioning and adjustment to extrauterine life.

Thermoregulation

Next to establishing respiration, heat regulation is most critical to the newborn's survival. Although the newborn's capacity for heat production is adequate, several factors predispose to excessive heat loss:

1. The newborn's large surface area facilitates heat loss to the environment, although this is partially compensated by the newborn's usual position of flexion, which decreases the amount of surface area exposed to the environment
2. The newborn's thin layer of subcutaneous fat provides poor insulation for conservation of heat
3. The newborn's mechanism for producing heat is different from the adult, who can increase heat production through shivering. The chilled neonate cannot shiver but produces heat through nonshivering thermogenesis, which involves increased metabolism and oxygen consumption

The principal thermogenic sources are the heart, liver, and brain. However, there is an additional source unique to the newborn known as *brown adipose tissue (BAT)*, or *brown fat*. Brown fat, which owes its name to its larger content of mitochondrial cytochromes, has a greater capacity for heat production through intensified metabolic activity than does ordinary adipose tissue. Heat generated in the brown fat is distributed to other parts of the body by the blood, which is warmed as it flows through the layers of this tissue. Superficial deposits of brown fat are located between the scapulae, around the neck, and behind the sternum. Deeper layers surround the kidneys, trachea, esophagus, some major arteries, and adrenals. The location of the brown fat may explain why the nape of the neck often feels warmer than the rest of the infant's body.

Although newborns' ability to conserve heat is usually a matter of concern, they also can have difficulty dissipating heat in an overheated environment, which increases the risk of hyperthermia.

Hemopoietic System

The blood volume of the newborn depends on the amount of placental transfer of blood. The blood volume of the full-term infant is about 80 to 85 ml per kg of body weight. Immediately after birth the total blood volume averages 300 ml, but depending on how long the infant is attached to the placenta, as much as 100 ml can be added to the blood volume. Blood values for the newborn are listed in Appendix E.

Fluid and Electrolyte Balance

Changes occur in the total body water volume, extracellular fluid volume, and intracellular fluid volume during the transition from fetal to postnatal life. At birth the total weight of the infant is 73% fluid, as compared to 58% in the adult. The infant has a proportionately higher ratio of extracellular fluid than the adult and consequently has a higher level of total body sodium and chloride and a lower level of potassium, magnesium, and phosphate.

Gastrointestinal System

The ability of the newborn to digest, absorb, and metabolize foodstuff is adequate but limited in certain functions. Enzymes are adequate to handle the proteins and simple carbohydrates (monosaccharides and disaccharides), but deficient production of pancreatic amylase impairs utilization of complex carbohydrates (polysaccharides). Deficiency of pancreatic lipase limits absorption of fats, especially with ingestion of foods with high saturated fatty acid content, such as cow's milk.

The liver is the most immature of the gastrointestinal organs. The activity of the enzyme *glucuronyl transferase* is reduced, which affects the conjugation of bilirubin with glucuronic acid and contributes to the physiologic jaundice of the newborn. The liver is also deficient in forming plasma proteins. The decreased plasma protein concentration probably plays a role in the edema usually seen at birth. Prothrombin and other coagulation factors are also low. The liver stores less glycogen at birth than later in life. Consequently the newborn is prone to hypoglycemia, which may be prevented by early feeding.

Some salivary glands are functioning at birth, but the majority do not begin to secrete saliva until about the age of 2 to 3 months, when drooling is frequent. Stomach capacity is limited to about 90 ml; thus the infant requires frequent small feedings. Emptying time is short, about 2½ to 3 hours, and peristalsis is rapid. These two factors accelerate the transit time of food passing through the stomach and colon. During the early weeks of life the newborn may have a bowel movement after each feeding.

The infant's intestine is longer in relation to body size than that in the adult. Therefore there are a larger number of secretory glands and a larger surface area for absorption as compared to the adult's intestine. There are rapid peristaltic waves and simultaneous nonperistaltic waves along the entire esophagus. These waves, combined with an immature relaxed cardiac sphincter, make regurgitation a common occurrence.

Progressive changes in the stooling pattern indicate a properly functioning gastrointestinal tract. The infant's first stool is the sticky and greenish black *meconium*, which is composed of amniotic fluid and its constituents, intestinal secretions, shed mucosal cells, and possibly blood (ingested maternal blood or minor bleeding of alimentary tract vessels). Passage of meconium should occur within the first 36 hours.

Usually by the third day after the initiation of feedings, *transitional stools* appear. They are greenish brown to yellowish brown in color, less sticky than meconium, and may contain some milk curds. By the fourth day a typical *milk stool* is passed. In breast-fed infants the stools are yellow to golden in color and pasty in consistency. They have a peculiar odor, similar to that of sour milk. In infants fed cow's milk formula, the stools are pale yellow to light brown, are firmer in consistency, and have a more offensive odor.

Breast-fed infants usually have more stools than do bottle-fed infants. The stool pattern can vary widely; six stools a day may be normal for one infant, whereas a stool every other day may be normal for another.

Renal System

All structural components are present in the renal system, but there is a functional deficiency in the kidney's ability to concentrate urine and to cope with conditions of fluid and electrolyte stress, such as dehydration or a concentrated solute load.

Total volume of urine per 24 hours is about 200 to 300 ml by the end of the first week. However, the bladder voluntarily empties when stretched by a volume of 15 ml, resulting in as many as 20 voidings per day. The first voiding should occur within 24 hours. The neonate's urine is colorless and odorless and has a specific gravity of about 1.020.

Integumentary System

At birth all the structures within the skin are present, but many of the functions of the integument are immature. The two layers of the skin, the epidermis and dermis, are loosely bound to each other and are very thin. Slight friction across the epidermis, such as from rapid removal of adhesive tape, can cause separation of these layers and blister formation. The transitional zone between the cornified and living layers of the epidermis is effective in preventing fluid from reaching the skin surface.

The *sebaceous glands* are very active late in fetal life and in early infancy because of the high levels of maternal androgens. They are most densely located on the scalp, face, and genitalia and produce the greasy vernix caseosa that covers the infant at birth. Plugging of the sebaceous glands causes milia (tiny white papules).

The *eccrine glands,* which produce sweat in response to heat or emotional stimuli, are functional at birth, and palmar sweating on crying reaches levels equivalent to that of anxious adults by 43 weeks of gestation. Observing palmar sweating is helpful in the assessment of pain. The eccrine glands produce sweat in response to higher temperatures than those required in adults, and the retention of sweat may result in miliaria (minute vesicles and papules, sometimes called "prickly heat"). The *apocrine glands* remain small and nonfunctional until puberty.

The growth phases of hair follicles usually occur simultaneously at birth. During the first few months the synchrony between hair loss and regrowth is disrupted, and there may be overgrowth of hair or temporary alopecia. Boys' hair grows faster than girls' hair, and in both sexes scalp hair growth is slower at the crown.

Because melanin is low at birth, newborns are lighter skinned than they will be as children. Consequently, they are more susceptible to the harmful effects of the sun and require adequate protection.

Musculoskeletal System

At birth the skeletal system contains larger amounts of cartilage than ossified bone, although the process of ossification is fairly rapid during the first year. The nose, for example, is predominantly cartilage at birth and is frequently flattened by the force of delivery. The six skull bones are relatively soft and are separated only by membranous seams. The sinuses are incompletely formed in the newborn.

Unlike the skeletal system, the muscular system is almost completely formed at birth. Growth in the size of muscular tissue is caused by hypertrophy, rather than hyperplasia, of cells.

Defenses Against Infection

The infant is born with several defenses against infection. The first line of defense is the *skin* and *mucous membranes,* which protect the body from invading organisms. The second line of defense is the *reticuloendothelial system,* which produces several types of cells capable of attacking a pathogen. The neutrophils and monocytes are phagocytes, which means they can engulf, ingest, and destroy foreign agents. Eosinophils also probably have a phagocytic property, since they increase in number in the presence of foreign protein. The lymphocytes (T- and B-cells) are capable of being converted to other cell types, such as monocytes and antibodies. Although the phagocytic properties of the blood are present in the infant, the inflammatory response of the tissues to localize an infection is immature.

The third line of defense is the formation of specific *antibodies* to an antigen. This process requires exposure to various foreign agents for antibody production to occur. Infants are generally not capable of producing their own gamma globulins until the beginning of the second month of life, but they receive considerable passive immunity in the form of IgG from the maternal circulation and from human milk (see p. 201). They are protected against most major childhood diseases, including diphtheria, measles, poliomyelitis, infectious hepatitis, and rubella for about 3 months, provided the mother has developed antibodies to these illnesses.

Endocrine System

Ordinarily the endocrine system of the newborn is adequately developed, but its functions are immature. For example, the posterior lobe of the pituitary gland produces limited quantities of antidiuretic hormone (ADH) or vasopressin, which inhibits diuresis. This renders the young infant highly susceptible to dehydration.

The effect of maternal sex hormones is particularly evident in the newborn because it causes a miniature puberty. The labia are hypertrophied and the breasts may be engorged and secrete milk during the first few days of life. Female newborns sometimes have pseudomenstruation, which usually disappears by 2 to 4 weeks of age, from the sudden drop in the level of progesterone and estrogen.

Neurologic System

At birth the nervous system is incompletely integrated but sufficiently developed to sustain extrauterine life. Most neurologic functions are primitive reflexes. The autonomic nervous system is crucial during transition because it stimulates initial respirations, helps maintain acid-base balance, and partially regulates temperature control.

Myelination of the nervous system follows the cephalocaudal-proximodistal laws of development and is closely related to observed mastery of fine and gross motor skills. Myelin is necessary for rapid and efficient transmission of some, but not all, nerve impulses along the neural pathway. The tracts that develop myelin earliest are the sensory, cerebellar, and extrapyramidal tracts. This accounts for the acute senses of taste, smell, and hearing and the perception of pain in the newborn. All cranial nerves are present and myelinated except for the optic and olfactory nerves.

Sensory Functions

The newborn's sensory functions are remarkably well developed and have a significant effect on growth and development, including the attachment process.

Vision. At birth the eye is structurally incomplete. The ciliary muscles are immature, limiting the ability of the eyes to accommodate and focus on an object for any length of time. The infant can track and follow objects. The pupils react to light, the blink reflex is responsive to a minimal stimulus, and the corneal reflex is activated by a light touch. Tear glands usually do not begin to function until 2 to 4 weeks of age.

The newborn has the ability to focus momentarily on a bright or moving object that is within 20 cm (8 inches) and in the midline of the visual field. In fact the infant's ability to fixate on coordinated movement is greater during the first hour of life than during the succeeding several days. Visual acuity is reported to be between 20/100 and 20/400, depending on the vision measurement techniques.

The infant also demonstrates visual preferences: medium colors (yellow, green, pink) over bright (red, orange, blue) or dim colors; black and white contrasting patterns, especially geometric shapes and checkerboards; large objects with medium complexity rather than small, complex objects; and reflecting objects over dull ones.

Hearing. Once the amniotic fluid has drained from the ears, the infant probably has auditory acuity similar to that of an adult. The neonate is able to detect a loud sound of about 90 decibels and reacts with a startle reflex. The newborn's response to sounds of low frequency versus those of high frequency differs; the former, such as the sound of a heartbeat, metronome, or lullaby, tends to decrease an infant's motor activity and crying, whereas the latter elicits an alerting reaction. There is also an early sensitivity to the sound of human voices, though not specifically speech sounds. For example, infants younger than 3 days of age can discriminate the mother's voice from that of other females. As early as age 2 weeks the infant may stop crying to listen to the sound of a voice.

The internal and middle ear are large at birth, but the external canal is small. The mastoid process and the bony part of the external canal have not yet developed. Consequently, the tympanic membrane and facial nerve are very close to the surface and can be easily damaged.

Smell. Research conducted on newborns' ability to smell demonstrates that they respond differently to various odors. Newborns react to strong odors such as alcohol or vinegar by turning their heads away. Breast-fed infants are able to smell breast milk and will cry for their mothers when the breasts are engorged and leaking. Infants are also able to differentiate the breast milk from their mother or from other females by smell, and maternal odors are believed to influence the attachment process.

Taste. The newborn has the ability to distinguish between tastes. Various types of solutions elicit differing gustofacial reflexes. A tasteless solution elicits no facial expression, a sweet solution elicits an eager suck and a look of satisfaction, a sour solution causes the usual puckering of the lips, and a bitter liquid produces an angry, upset expression. During early childhood the taste buds are distributed mostly on the tip of the tongue.

Touch. At birth the infant is able to perceive tactile sensation in any part of the body, although the face (especially the mouth), hands, and soles of the feet seem to be most sensitive. There is increasing documentation that touch and motion are essential to normal growth and development. Gentle patting of the back or rubbing of the abdomen usually elicits a calming response from the infant. However, painful stimuli, such as a pinprick, will elicit an angry, upsetting response.

◆ *The Newborn and Family*

The newborn depends completely on others for every aspect of care. Although parents are ultimately responsible for this care, nurses usually assume a major caregiving role while the infant is in the nursery. During this brief period, they can involve the family in learning about the physical and emotional needs of the newborn. By helping the family discover the infant's unique adaptive and coping abilities, nurses can also positively influence the attachment process between child and parents.

NURSING CARE OF THE NEWBORN AND FAMILY

Nursing care of the newborn and family involves a wide range of skills to ensure safe and optimal care to both the infant and the family. Although most of the care is routine, nurses need to maintain a high index of suspicion for possible physical problems in the newborn and potential areas of concern regarding emotional bonding. With increasingly shorter postpartum admissions, the accomplishment of thorough newborn assessment and parent teaching has become a challenge.

ASSESSMENT

The newborn requires thorough, skilled observation to ensure a satisfactory adjustment to extrauterine life. Physical assessment following delivery can be divided into three phases: (1) the initial assessment using the Apgar scoring system, (2) transitional assessment during the periods of reactivity, and (3) periodic assessment through systematic physical examination. In addition, the nurse must be aware of those behaviors that signal successful attachment between the infant and parents. Awareness of the expected normal findings during each assessment process helps the nurse recognize any deviation that may prevent the infant from progressing uneventfully through the early postnatal period.

Initial Assessment: Apgar Scoring

The most frequently used method to assess the newborn's immediate adjustment to extrauterine life is the Apgar scoring system. The score is based on observation of heart rate, respiratory effort, muscle tone, reflex irritability, and color (Table 8-1). Each item is given a score of 0, 1, or 2. Evaluations of all five categories are made at 1 and 5 minutes after birth and are repeated until the infant's condition stabilizes. Total scores of 0 to 3 represent severe distress, scores of 4 to 6 signify moderate difficulty, and scores of 7 to 10 indicate absence of difficulty in adjusting to life.

Transitional Assessment: Periods of Reactivity

The newborn exhibits behavioral and physiologic characteristics that can at first appear to be signs of stress. However, during the initial 24 hours, changes in heart rate, respiration, motor activity, color, mucus production, and bowel activity occur in an orderly, predictable sequence that is normal and indicates lack of stress.

For 6 to 8 hours after birth, the newborn is in the *first period of reactivity*. During the first 30 minutes the infant is very alert, cries vigorously, may suck his fist greedily, and appears very interested in his environment. At this time his eyes are usually open, suggesting that this is an excellent opportunity for mother, father, and child to see each other. Because he has a vigorous suck, this is also an opportune time to begin breast-feeding. He will usually grasp the nipple quickly, satisfying both mother and infant. This is particularly important for nurses to remember, because after this initially highly active state the infant may be quite sleepy and uninterested in sucking. Physiologically the respiratory rate during this period is as high as 80 breaths/minute, rales may be heard, heart rate reaches 180 beats/minute, bowel sounds are active, mucous secretions are increased, and temperature may decrease.

After this initial stage of alertness and activity, the infant's responsiveness diminishes. Heart and respiratory rates decrease, temperature continues to fall, mucus production decreases, and urine or stool is usually not passed. The infant is in a state of sleep and relative calm. Any attempt to stimulate him usually elicits a minimal response. This second stage of the first reactive period lasts 2 to 4 hours. Because of the continued decrease in body temperature, undressing or bathing should be avoided during this time.

The *second period of reactivity* begins when the infant awakes from this deep sleep, lasts about 2 to 5 hours, and provides another excellent opportunity for child and parents to interact. The infant is again alert and responsive, heart and respiratory rates increase, the gag reflex is active, gastric and respiratory secretions are increased, and passage of meconium frequently occurs. This period is usually over when the amount of respiratory mucus has decreased. Following this stage is a period of stabilization of physiologic systems and vacillating pattern of sleep and activity.

TABLE 8-1

Infant Evaluation at Birth—Apgar Scoring System

	0	1	2	Comments
Heart rate	Absent	Slow (less than 100 beats/min)	Greater than 100 beats/min	Apical pulse counted for 1 minute
Respiratory effort	Absent	Slow or irregular	Good; crying lustily	Respiratory rate counted for 1 minute
Muscle tone	Limp	Some flexion of extremities	Active motion; well flexed	Attempts to extend extremities met with resistance
Reflex irritability	No response	Grimace	Cough or sneeze; vigorous cry	Response to slapping sole of foot with palm of hand
Color	Blue or pale	Body pink, extremities blue	Completely pink	Few newborns completely pink at birth

TABLE 8-2

States of Sleep and Activity

State/Behavior	Duration	Implications for Parenting
Regular Sleep		
Closed eyes Regular breathing No movement except for sudden bodily jerks	4-5 hr/day, 10-20 min/sleep cycle	External stimuli do not arouse infant Continue usual house noises Leave infant alone, if sudden loud noise awakens infant and he cries
Irregular Sleep		
Closed eyes Irregular breathing Slight muscular twitching of body	12-15 hr/day, 20-45 min/sleep cycle	External stimuli that did not arouse infant during regular sleep may minimally arouse him Periodic groaning or crying is usual; do not interpret as an indication of pain or discomfort
Drowsiness		
Eyes may be open Irregular breathing Active body movement	Variable	Most stimuli arouse infant Pick infant up during this time rather than leave in crib
Alert Inactivity		
Responds to environment by active body movement and staring at close-range objects	2-3 hr/day	Satisfy infant's needs such as hunger Place infant in area of home where activity is continuous Place toys in crib or playpen Place objects within 17.5-20 cm (7-8 inches) of infant's view
Waking and Crying		
May begin with whimpering and slight body movement Progresses to strong, angry crying and uncoordinated thrashing of extremities	1-4 hr/day	Remove intense internal or external stimuli Stimuli that were effective during alert inactivity are usually ineffective Rock and swaddle to decrease crying

Behavioral Assessment

Another important area of assessment is observation of behavior. It is becoming increasingly apparent that infants' behavior helps shape their environment. Their ability to react to various stimuli affects how others relate to them. The principal areas of behavior for newborns are sleep, wakefulness, and activity, such as crying.

One method of systematically assessing the infant's behavior is the use of the *Brazelton Neonatal Behavioral Assessment Scale (BNBAS)* (Brazelton, 1984). The BNBAS is an interactive examination that measures several aspects of infant behavior. It is generally used as a research or diagnostic tool and requires special training. However, it may also be used to help parents focus on their infant's individuality and to develop a deeper attachment to their child.

Sleep, wakefulness, and crying. Newborns begin life with a systematic schedule of sleep and wakefulness that is initially evident during the periods of reactivity. Following this initial period, it is not unusual for the infant to sleep almost constantly for the next 2 to 3 days in order to recover from the exhausting birth process.

Five distinct states comprise the infant's sleep; these are summarized in Table 8-2. The cycle of these sleep states is highly variable and is based on the number of hours an infant sleeps per day, which may range anywhere from 10½ to 23 hours, with an average of 16½ hours. Generally about 75% of the infant's sleep is in the irregular state.

The newborn should begin extrauterine life with a strong, lusty cry. The sounds produced by crying can be described as hunger, anger, pain, and "bid for attention" cries. Discomfort (pain) sounds initially consist of gasps and cries in which the consonant "H" is clearly distinguishable. The duration of crying is as highly variable in each infant as is the duration of sleep patterns. Some newborns may cry as little as 5 minutes or as much as 2 hours or more per day.

Behavioral states can be influenced by environmental stimuli. Feeding usually terminates the crying when hunger is the cause. However, an awake infant exhibits more motor activity before feeding than after. Swaddling or wrapping an infant snugly in a blanket promotes sleep as well as maintains body temperature. Rocking the infant reduces crying and induces quiet alertness or sleep.

Assessment of Attachment Behaviors

One of the most important areas of assessment is careful observation of those behaviors that are thought to indicate the formation of emotional bonds between the newborn and family, especially the mother. Such behaviors include the *en face* position, undressing and touching the infant, smiling, kissing, and talking to the infant, and holding, rocking and cradling the child close to the body (Avant, 1982) (see box). However, because assessment is closely related to interventions that promote attachment, for example, encouraging these behaviors in parents, the

Guidelines for Assessing Attachment Behavior

When the infant is brought to the parents, do they reach out for the child and call the child by name?

Do the parents speak about the child in terms of identification—whom the infant looks like; what appears special about their child over other infants?

When parents are holding the infant, what kind of body contact is there—do parents feel at ease in changing the infant's position; are fingertips or whole hands used; are there parts of the body they avoid touching or parts of the body they investigate and scrutinize?

When the infant is awake, what kinds of stimulation do the parents provide—do they talk to the infant, to each other, or to no one; how do they look at the infant—direct visual contact, avoidance of eye contact, or looking at other people or objects?

How comfortable do the parents appear in terms of caring for the infant? Do they express any concern regarding their ability or disgust for certain activities, such as changing diapers?

What type of affection do they demonstrate to the newborn, such as smiling, stroking, kissing, or rocking?

If the infant is fussy, what kinds of comforting techniques do the parents use, such as rocking, swaddling, talking, or stroking?

major portion of assessing attachment behaviors is discussed on p. 204.

Physical Assessment

An essential aspect of the care of the newborn is a thorough physical assessment that includes estimation of gestational age and physical examination to identify normal characteristics and existing abnormalities. These initial and ongoing assessments are critical to establishing baseline data for planning, implementing, and evaluating care and should be one of the nurse's priorities in caring for the newborn. The discussion of physical examination focuses on normal findings and variations from the norm that require little or no intervention. The reader is encouraged to review the material in Chapter 7 for further discussions of examination techniques. Table 8-3 summarizes physical examination of the newborn.

Examination of newborns generally presents few problems in terms of gaining their acceptance or cooperation. In general it is best to proceed in an orderly head-to-toe progression, with a few exceptions. Since exposing infants to the air when undressing them usually elicits crying, it is best to listen to the heart, lungs, and abdomen first. Head, chest, and length measurements are taken at the same time to record them accurately and to mentally note their relationship to each other. Weight should be taken with the infant fully undressed. If clothing is not removed, the scale is prebalanced to adjust for the excess weight by weighing similar articles of clothing first. If irritability and crying occur during the examination, the newborn can be allowed to suck on a pacifier or on one's gloved finger, which usually quiets the child sufficiently to complete palpation and auscultation. Whether or not all these suggestions are followed is less important than establishing a routine that minimizes delay, haphazard organization, and omission of details.

Assessment of clinical gestational age. Assessment of gestational age is an important criterion because perinatal morbidity and mortality are related to gestational age and birth weight. One of the most frequently used methods of determining gestational age is based on physical and neurologic findings. Although several scales are in current use, the one most commonly used is the Simplified Assessment of Gestational Age (Fig. 8-1, *A*). It assesses six external physical and six neuromuscular signs. Each sign has a number score and the cumulative score correlates with a maturity rating from 26 to 44 weeks (see Maturity rating box on scale). The maturity rating is accurate within ± 2 weeks of the infant's true age.

Assessments can be performed anytime from birth to 42 hours of age, but the greatest reliability is at 30 and 42 hours. By this time the infant has sufficiently stabilized and adjusted following birth, but changes resulting from rapid extrauterine maturation do not interfere with the findings. No matter what scale is used the infant should be examined when alert and with strict adherence to the directions described by the original authors.

In order to facilitate the use of the assessment chart, the following tests and relevant observations are further described:

resting posture With the infant lying in a supine position, the degree of extension and flexion of arms and legs, knees and elbows, and adduction and abduction of hips are evaluated

square window The examiner flexes the forearm with enough pressure to obtain as full a flexion as possible in order to measure the angle between the hypothenar eminence and the ventral aspect of the forearm

recoil The arm is fully flexed for 5 seconds, then extended by traction on foot or hand, and the maximum response is noted. Full flexion is a maximum response. A brisk return to full flexion is characteristic of a full-term infant; the preterm infant displays sluggish return, only random movements, or no movement at all

popliteal angle With the thigh in knee-chest position, the leg is extended by gentle pressure to measure the popliteal angle

scarf sign The examiner attempts to place the infant's hand as far posteriorly across the chest and neck as possible in the direction of the opposite shoulder

heel-to-ear maneuver The infant's foot is drawn as near to the head as possible without force. The degree of extension and the distance between the foot and the head are noted

Weight related to gestational age. The weight of the infant at birth also correlates with the incidence of perinatal morbidity and mortality. Since many infants who weigh less than 2500 g (5½ pounds) are not premature by gestational age, there is often confusion in distinguishing be-

TABLE 8-3

Summary of Physical Assessment of the Newborn

Area	Usual Findings	Comments
General measurements	Head circumference 33-35.5 cm (13-14 inches) Chest circumference 30.5-33 cm (12-13 inches) Head circumference should be about 2-3 cm (1 inch) larger than chest circumference Crown-to-rump length 31-35 cm (12½-14 inches) Crown-to-rump length approximately equal to head circumference Head-to-heel length 48-53 cm (19-21 inches) Birth weight 2700-4000 g (6-9 pounds)	Molding after birth may decrease head circumference Head and chest circumferences may be equal for first 1-2 days after birth
General appearance	Posture—flexion of head and extremities, which rest on chest and abdomen	In frank breech—extended legs, abducted and fully rotated thighs, flattened head, extended neck
Skin	At birth—bright red, puffy, smooth Second to third day—pink, flaky, dry Vernix caseosa Lanugo Edema around eyes, face, legs, dorsa of hands, feet, and scrotum or labia	Other common findings: Neonatal jaundice after first 24 hours Ecchymoses or petechiae caused by birth trauma Milia neonatorum Sudamina
	Normal Color Changes: *Acrocyanosis*—Cyanosis of hands and feet *Cutis marmorata*—Transient mottling when infant is exposed to decreased temperature *Erythema toxicum*—Pink papular rash with vesicles superimposed on thorax, back, buttocks, and abdomen; may appear in 24 to 48 hours and resolves after several days *Harlequin color change*—Clearly outlined color change as infant lies on side; lower half of body becomes pink and upper half is pale *Mongolian spots*—Irregular areas of deep blue pigmentation, usually in the sacral and gluteal regions; seen predominantly in newborns of African, Asian, or Hispanic descent *Telangiectatic nevi ("stork bites")*—Flat, deep pink localized areas usually seen in back of neck	
Head	Anterior fontanel—diamond-shaped 2.5-4.0 cm (1-1¾ inches) at widest part Posterior fontanel—triangular-shaped, 0.5-1 cm (¼-⅜ inch) Fontanels should be flat, soft, and firm	Molding usually follows vaginal delivery Fontanels may bulge because of crying or coughing
Eyes	Lids usually edematous Eyes usually closed Color—slate gray, dark blue, brown Absence of tears Presence of red reflex Corneal reflex in response to touch Pupillary reflex in response to light Blink reflex in response to light or touch Rudimentary fixation on objects and ability to follow to midline	Searching nystagmus or strabismus is common
Ears	Position—top of pinna on horizontal line with outer canthus of eye Startle reflex elicited by a loud, sudden noise Pinna flexible, cartilage present	Inability to visualize tympanic membrane because of filled aural canals Pinna is flat against head
Nose	Nasal patency Nasal discharge—thin white mucus Sneezing	May be flattened and bruised
Mouth and throat	Intact, high-arched palate Uvula in midline Frenulum of tongue Frenum of upper lip Sucking reflex–strong and coordinated with swallowing Rooting reflex Gag reflex Extrusion reflex Absent or minimal salivation Vigorous cry	May see Epstein pearls

TABLE 8-3

Summary of Physical Assessment of the Newborn—cont'd

Area	Usual Findings	Comments
Neck	Short, thick, usually surrounded by skin folds Tonic neck reflex	
Chest	Anteroposterior and lateral diameters equal Slight sternal retractions evident during inspiration Xiphoid process evident Breast enlargement	Secretion of milky substance from breasts is common in some female infants
Lungs	Rate—30-60 breaths/min Respirations chiefly abdominal Cough reflex absent at birth, present by 1-2 days Bilateral bronchial breath sounds	Rate and depth of respirations may be irregular, momentary apneic spells are common
Heart	Rate—120-140 beats/min and regular Apex—third to fourth intercostal space, lateral to midclavicular line S_2 slightly sharper and higher in pitch than S_1	Sinus arrhythmia is common Transient cyanosis is present on crying or straining
Abdomen	Cylindric in shape Liver—palpable 3 cm (about 1 inch) below right costal margin Spleen—tip palpable 1 cm below left costal margin Kidneys—palpable 1-2 cm (⅜ to ¾ inch) above umbilicus Equal bilateral femoral pulses	Umbilical hernia may be present
Female genitalia	Labia and clitoris usually edematous Labia minora larger than labia majora Urethral meatus behind clitoris Hymenal tag Vernix caseosa between labia Urinates within 24 hours	Blood-tinged or milky discharge (pseudomenstruation) may be present
Male genitalia	Urethral opening at tip of glans penis Testes palpable in each scrotum Scrotum large, edematous, and pendulous; usually deeply pigmented in dark-skinned ethnic groups Smegma Urinates within 24 hours	Other common findings: Urethral opening covered by prepuce Inability to retract foreskin Epithelial pearls Erection or priapism Testes palpable in inguinal canal Scrotum small
Back and rectum	Spine intact, no openings, masses, or prominent curves Trunk incurvation reflex Patent anal opening Passes meconium within 36 hours	Mongolian spots
Extremities	10 fingers and toes Full range of motion Nail beds pink, with transient cyanosis immediately after birth Creases on anterior two thirds of sole Sole usually flat Symmetry of extremities Equal muscle tone bilaterally, especially resistance to opposing flexion Equal bilateral brachial and femoral pulses	Other common findings: Partial syndactyly between second and third toes Clinodactyly of second toe with overlapping into third toe Wide gap between first and second toe Deep crease on plantar surface of foot between first and second toes Asymmetric length of toes Dorsiflexion and shortness of first toe
Neuromuscular system	Extremities usually maintain some degree of flexion Extension of an extremity followed by previous position of flexion Head lag while sitting, but momentary ability to hold head erect Able to turn head from side to side when prone Able to hold head in horizontal line with back when held prone	Quivering or momentary tremors are common

tween preterm and small-for-gestational-age infants; fetal growth, gestational age, and fetal maturity are closely related but are not synonymous. Maturity implies functional capacity—the degree to which the neonate's organ systems are able to adapt to the requirements of extrauterine life. Therefore gestational age is more closely related to fetal maturity than is birth weight. Since heredity influences a newborn's size, noting the size of other family members is part of the assessment process.

Classification of infants at birth by both weight and gestational age provides a more satisfactory method for predicting mortality risks and providing guidelines for management of the neonate than estimating gestational age or birth weight alone. The infant's birth weight, length, and head circumference are plotted on standardized graphs that identify normal values for gestational age (Fig. 8-1, *B*). The infant whose weight is appropriate for gestational age (between 10th and 90th percentile) can

ESTIMATION OF GESTATIONAL AGE BY MATURITY RATING

Symbols: X - 1st Exam O - 2nd Exam

NEUROMUSCULAR MATURITY

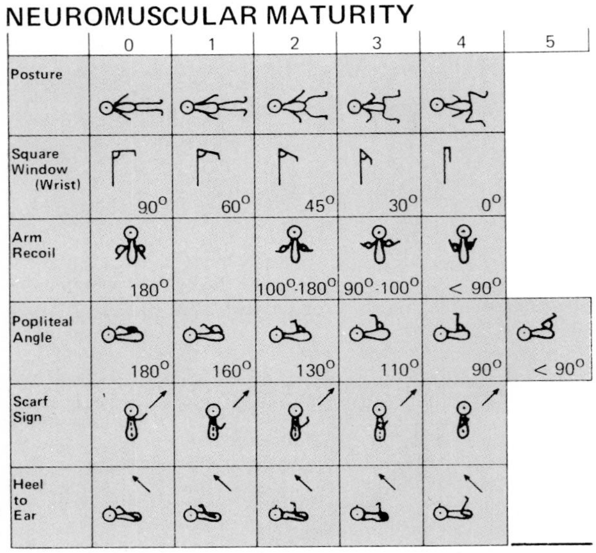

A

PHYSICAL MATURITY

	0	1	2	3	4	5
SKIN	gelatinous red, trans-parent	smooth pink, visible veins	superficial peeling &/or rash, few veins	cracking pale area, rare veins	parchment, deep cracking, no vessels	leathery, cracked, wrinkled
LANUGO	none	abundant	thinning	bald areas	mostly bald	
PLANTAR CREASES	no crease	faint red marks	anterior transverse crease only	creases ant. 2/3	creases cover entire sole	
BREAST	barely percept.	flat areola, no bud	stippled areola, 1–2 mm bud	raised areola, 3–4 mm bud	full areola, 5–10 mm bud	
EAR	pinna flat, stays folded	sl. curved pinna, soft with slow recoil	well-curv. pinna, soft but ready recoil	formed & firm with instant recoil	thick cartilage, ear stiff	
GENITALS Male	scrotum empty, no rugae		testes descend-ing, few rugae	testes down, good rugae	testes pendulous, deep rugae	
GENITALS Female	prominent clitoris & labia minora		majora & minora equally prominent	majora large, minora small	clitoris & minora completely covered	

Gestation by Dates ________ wks

Birth Date ________ Hour ________ am pm

APGAR ________ 1 min ________ 5 min

MATURITY RATING

Score	Wks
5	26
10	28
15	30
20	32
25	34
30	36
35	38
40	40
45	42
50	44

SCORING SECTION

	1st Exam=X	2nd Exam=O
Estimating Gest Age by Maturity Rating	________ Weeks	________ Weeks
Time of Exam	Date ________ Hour ________ am pm	Date ________ Hour ________ am pm
Age at Exam	________ Hours	________ Hours
Signature of Examiner	________ M.D.	________ M.D.

FIG. 8-1 A, Newborn maturity rating. Courtesy Mead Johnson & Co., Evansville, IN. **A,** Scoring section adapted from Ballard, J.L., and others: Pediatr. Res. **11:**374, 1977. Figures adapted from Sweet, A.Y.: Classification of the low-birth-weight infant. In Klaus, M.H., and Fanaroff, A.A.: Care of the high-risk infant, Philadelphia, 1977, W.B. Saunders Co.

be presumed to have grown at a normal rate regardless of the time of birth—preterm, term, or postterm. The infant who is large for gestational age (above 90th percentile) can be presumed to have grown at an accelerated rate during fetal life; the small-for-gestational-age infant (below 10th percentile) can be assumed to have grown at a retarded rate during intrauterine life. Fig. 8-2 illustrates the disparity between birth weights of three preterm infants of the same gestational age of 32 weeks. The infant with a birth weight of 600 g has over a 50% mortality rate, the infant weighing 1400 gm has a 25% to 50% mortality rate, whereas the infant weighing 2750 g has less than a 4% mortality rate. Therefore birth weight influences mortality—the lower the birth weight, the higher the mortality rate.

General measurements. There are several important measurements of the newborn that have significance when compared to each other as well as when recorded

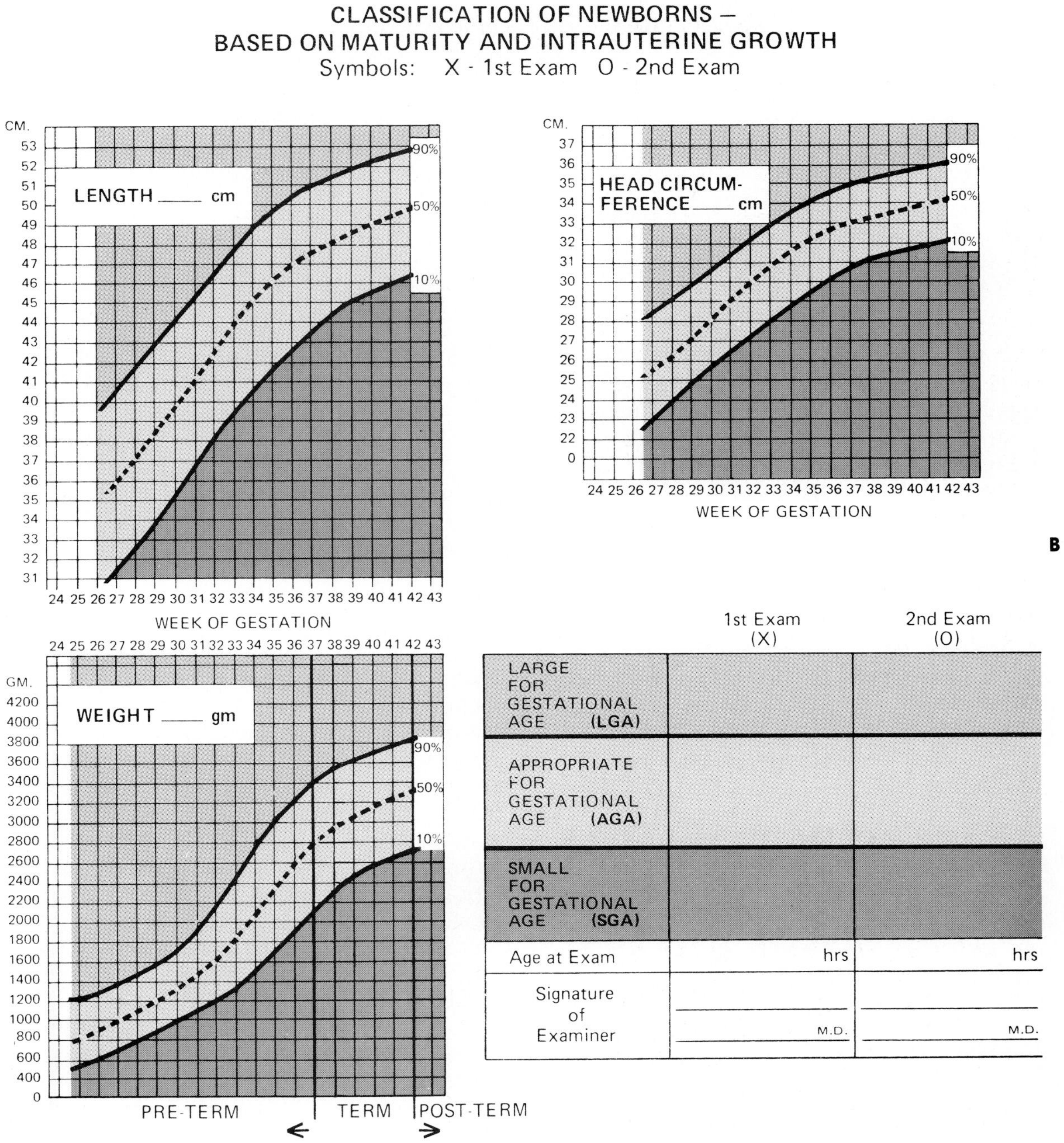

FIG. 8-1, cont'd B, Newborn classification based on maturity and intrauterine growth. **B,** Adapted from Lubchenko, L.C., Hansman, C., and Boyd, E.: J. Pediatr. **37:**403, 1966; Battagia F.C., and Lubchenko, L.D.: J. Pediatr. **71:**159, 1967.

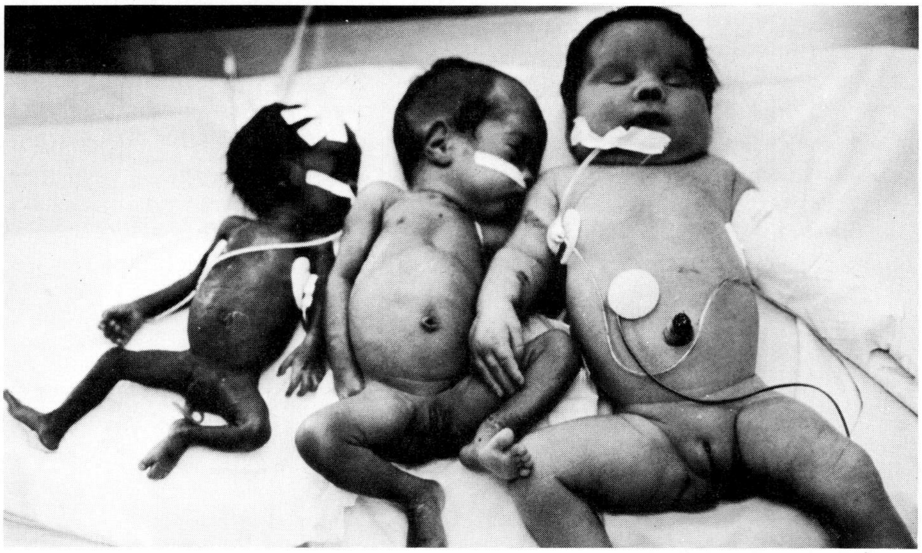

FIG. 8-2 Three babies, same gestational age, weight 600 g, 1400 g, and 2750 g, respectively, from left to right. From Korones, S.B.: High-risk newborn infants: the basis for intensive nursing care, ed. 4, St. Louis, 1986, The C.V. Mosby Co., p. 118.

over time on a graph. For the full-term infant, average *head circumference* is between 33 and 35.5 cm (13 to 14 inches). Head circumference may be somewhat less immediately after birth because of the molding process that occurs during a normal vaginal delivery. Usually by the second or third day the normal size and contour of the skull have returned.

Chest circumference is 30.5 to 33 cm (12 to 13 inches). The usual relationship between head and chest circumference is a difference of about 2 to 3 cm, or 1 inch. Because of the molding of the head during delivery, initially these measurements may appear equal.

Head circumference may also be compared with *crown-to-rump* length, or sitting height (Fig. 8-3). Crown-to-rump measurements are usually 31 to 35 cm (12.5 to 14 inches) and are approximately equal to head circumference. The relationship of the head and crown-to-rump measurements is more reliable than that of the head and chest.

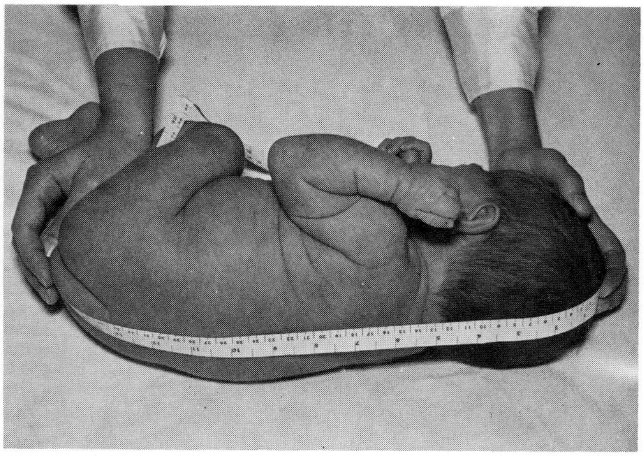

FIG. 8-3 Measurement of crown-to-rump length in newborn.

Head-to-heel length is also measured in the newborn. Because of the usual flexed position of the infant, it is important to extend the leg completely when measuring total body length. The average length of the newborn is 48 to 53 cm (19 to 21 inches).

Body weight is taken soon after birth because weight loss occurs fairly rapidly after birth. Normally the neonate loses about 10% of the birth weight by 3 to 4 days of age because of loss of excessive extracellular fluid, meconium, and limited food intake. The birth weight is usually regained by the tenth day of life. Most newborns weigh 2700 to 4000 g (6 to 9 pounds), the average weight being about 3400 g (7.5 pounds). Accurate birth weights and lengths are important because they provide a baseline for assessment of future growth.

Another category of measurements is vital signs. *Axillary temperatures* are taken because insertion of a thermometer into the rectum can cause perforation of the mucosa (see also p. 136). Core (internal) body temperature varies according to the periods of reactivity but is usually 36.5° to 37.5° C (97.7° to 99.5° F).

Pulse and *respirations* also vary according to the periods of reactivity and to the infant's behaviors but are usually in the range of 120 to 140 beats/minute and 30 to 60 breaths/minute, respectively. Both are counted for a full 60 seconds to detect irregularities in rate or rhythm. Heart rate is taken apically with a stethoscope.

Blood pressure should be taken and is most accurately assessed using oscillometry (Fig. 8-4) (see also p. 138). Comparisons should be made between the blood pressure

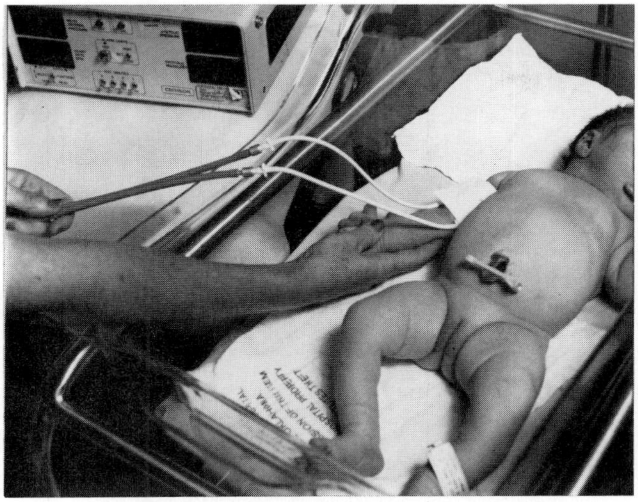

FIG. 8-4 Measurement of blood pressure by oscillometry.

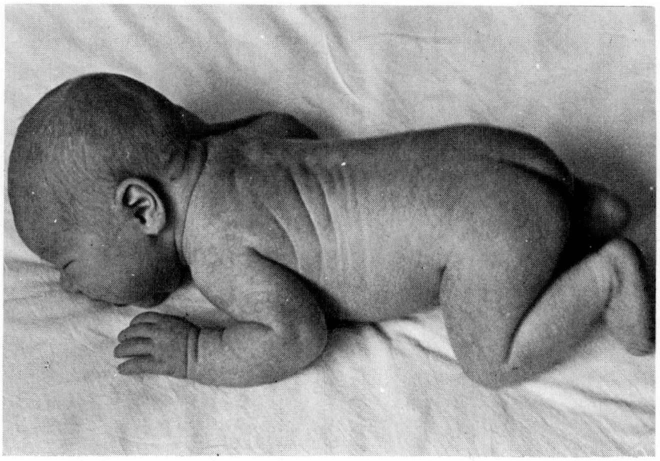

FIG. 8-5 Flexion position of newborn.

in the upper and lower extremities and differences of more than 10 mm Hg reported. At the 50th percentile the systolic blood pressure is 72 mm Hg and diastolic pressure is 50 mm Hg for boys; in girls the systolic pressure is slightly lower (68 mm Hg) (Report of the Second Task Force, 1987).

A suggested schedule for monitoring vital signs is upon the newborn's admission to the nursery and at 4-hour intervals until the signs are stable and then once every 8 hours until discharge (American Academy of Pediatrics, 1988). However, this schedule may vary according to institutional policy. Any change in the infant, such as in color, muscle tone, or behavior, necessitates more frequent monitoring.

General appearance. Before each body system is assessed, it is important to describe the general posture and behavior of the newborn. The overall appearance yields valuable clues to the physical status of the infant.

Posture. In the full-term neonate the posture is one of complete flexion as a result of in utero position (Fig. 8-5). Most infants are born in a vertex presentation with the head flexed and chin resting on the upper chest, arms flexed with hands clenched, legs flexed at knees and the hips, and the feet dorsiflexed. The vertebral column is also flexed. It is important to recognize any deviation from this very characteristic fetal position.

Behavior. The infant's behavior is carefully noted, especially the degree of alertness, drowsiness, and irritability, which are common signs of neurologic problems. Some questions to mentally ask when assessing behavior include:

Is the infant awakened easily by a loud noise?
Is the infant comforted by rocking, sucking, or cuddling?
Do there seem to be periods of deep and light sleep?
When awake, does the infant seem satisfied after a feeding?
What stimuli elicit responses from him?
When disturbed, how much does the infant protest?

Skin. The skin of the newborn is velvety smooth and puffy, especially about the eyes, the legs, the dorsal aspect of the hands and the feet, and the scrotum or labia. Skin color depends on racial and familial background and varies greatly among newborns. In general, the white infant is usually pink to red; the black newborn may appear a pinkish or yellowish brown. Infants of Hispanic descent may have an olive tint or a slight yellow cast to the skin. Infants of Oriental descent may be a rosy or yellowish tan. The color of Native American newborns depends upon the tribe and can vary from a light pink to a dark, reddish brown. By the second or third day the skin turns to its more natural tone and is drier and flakier. Several other color changes that may be noted on the skin are described in Table 8-3.

At birth the skin is covered with a grayish-white, cheese-like substance called *vernix caseosa,* a mixture of sebum and desquamating cells. If it is not removed during the bath, it will dry and disappear by about 24 to 48 hours. A fine, downy hair called *lanugo* is present on the skin, especially on the forehead, cheeks, shoulders, and back. *Milia,* distended sebaceous glands, appear as tiny white papules on the cheeks, chin, and nose. They usually disappear spontaneously in a few weeks. *Sudamina* or *miliaria* are distended sweat (eccrine) glands that cause minute vesicles on the skin surface, especially on the face.

Head. General observation of the contour of the head is important, since molding occurs in almost all vaginal deliveries. In a vertex delivery the head is usually flattened at the forehead, with the apex rising and forming a point at the end of the parietal bones and the posterior skull or occiput dropping abruptly. The usual, more oval contour of the head is apparent by 1 to 2 days after birth. The change in shape occurs because the bones of the cranium are not fused, allowing for overlapping of the edges of these bones to accommodate to the size of the birth

A

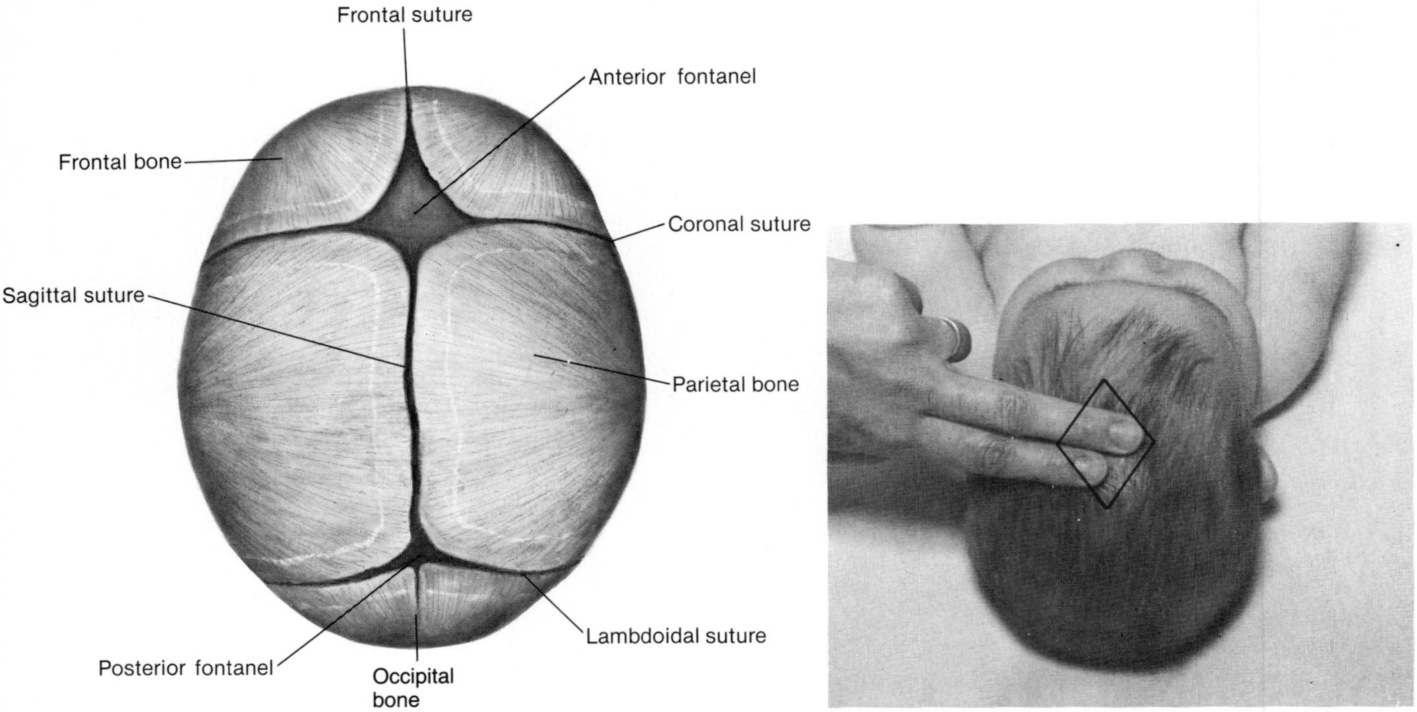

B

FIG. 8-6 **A,** Location of sutures. **B,** Palpating anterior fontanel.

canal during delivery. Such molding does not occur in infants born by cesarean section.

Six bones—the frontal, occipital, two parietals, and two temporals—comprise the cranium. Between the junction of these bones are bands of connective tissue called *sutures*. At the junction of the sutures are wider spaces of unossified membranous tissue called *fontanels*. The two most prominent fontanels in infants are the *anterior fontanel,* formed by the junction of the sagittal, coronal, and frontal sutures, and the *posterior fontanel,* formed by the junction of the sagittal and lambdoid sutures. The location of the sutures is easily remembered because the coronal suture "crowns" the head and the sagittal suture "separates" the head (Fig. 8-6, *A*).

The skull is palpated for all patent sutures and fontanels, noting size, shape, molding, or abnormal closure. The sutures feel like cracks between the skull bones, and the fontanels like wider "soft spots" at the junction of the sutures. These are palpated by using the tip of the index finger and running it along the ends of the bones (Fig. 8-6, *B*).

The anterior fontanel is diamond shaped and measures 4 to 5 cm (about 2 inches) at its widest point (from bone to bone, rather than from suture to suture). The posterior fontanel is easily located by following the sagittal suture toward the occiput. The *posterior fontanel* is triangular-shaped, usually measuring between 0.5 and 1 cm (less than ½ inch) at its widest part. The fontanels should feel flat, firm, and well demarcated against the bony edges of the skull. Frequently pulsations are visible at the anterior fontanel. Coughing, crying, or lying down may temporarily cause the fontanels to bulge and become more taut. However, a widened, tense, bulging fontanel or a markedly sunken, depressed fontanel is always recorded and reported.

The degree of *head control* is also assessed. Although *head lag* is normal in the newborn, the degree of the ability to control the head in certain positions should be recognized. If the supine infant is pulled from the arms into a semi-Fowler position, marked head lag and hyperextension are noted (Fig. 8-7, *A*). However, as the infant is brought forward into a sitting position, the infant will attempt to control the head in an upright position. As the head falls forward onto the chest, many infants will attempt to right it into the erect position. Also, if the infant is held in ventral suspension, that is, held prone above and parallel to the examining surface, the infant will hold the head in a straight line with the spinal column (Fig. 8-7, *B*). When lying on the abdomen, the newborn has the ability to lift the head slightly, turning it from side to side.

Eyes. Since newborns tend to have their eyes tightly closed, it is best to begin the examination of the eyes by observing the lids for edema, which is normally present for the first 2 days after delivery. The eyes are observed for symmetry.

In order to visualize the surface structures of the eye, the nurse holds the infant supine and gently lowers the head. The eyes will usually open, similar to the mechanism of dolls' eyes. The sclera should be white and clear.

A 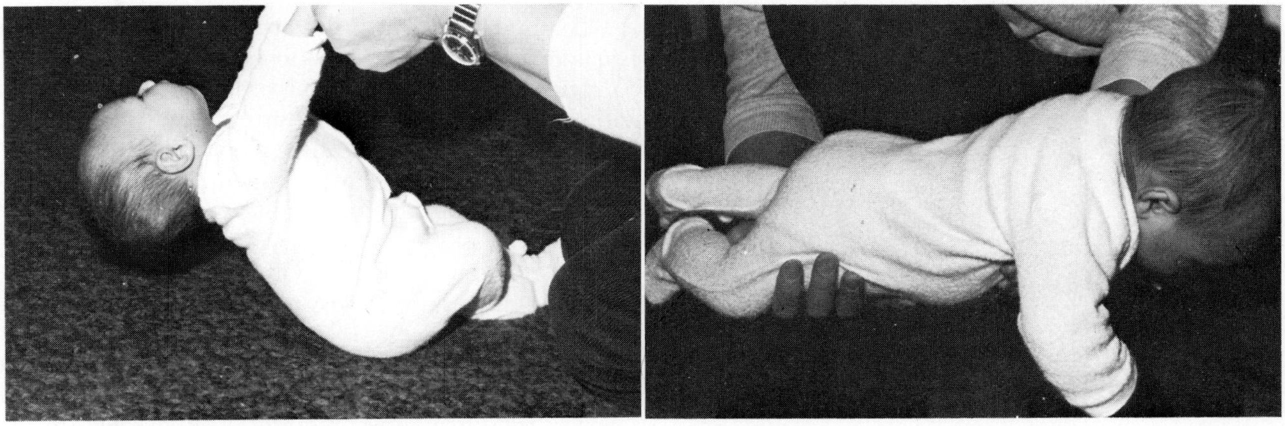 B

FIG. 8-7 Head control. **A,** Inability to hold erect when pulled to sitting position. **B,** Ability to hold erect when placed in ventral suspension.

The cornea is examined for the presence of any opacities or haziness. The *corneal reflex* is normally present at birth but is generally not elicited unless brain or eye damage is suspected. The pupil will usually respond to light by constricting. The pupils are normally malaligned. A searching *nystagmus* or *strabismus* is common. The color of the iris is noted. Most light-skinned newborns have slate gray or dark blue eyes, whereas dark-skinned infants have brown eyes.

A funduscopic examination is quite difficult to perform because of the infant's tendency to keep the eyes tightly closed. However, a red reflex should be elicited.

Ears. The ears are examined for position, structure, and auditory function. The top of the pinna should lie in a horizontal plane to the outer canthus of the eye (see Fig. 7-16). The pinna is often flattened against the side of the head from pressure in utero. An otoscopic examination is ordinarily not performed because the *canals* are filled with vernix caseosa and amniotic fluid, making visualization of the drum difficult.

Auditory ability is assessed by making a sharp, loud noise close to the infant's head and noting the presence of the *startle reflex* (see p. 196) or twitching of the eyelids. Absence of any behavioral response to a sudden noise may indicate congenital deafness and is always reported. In some nurseries auditory screening of newborns considered at risk for hearing loss may be performed. Such infants are those with family history of childhood hearing loss, congenital perinatal infections or bacterial meningitis, malformations of the head or neck, low birth weight, severe asphyxia, or severe hyperbilirubinemia (American Academy of Pediatrics, 1983).

Nose. The nose is usually flattened after birth, and bruises are common. Patency of the nasal canals can be assessed by holding the hand over the infant's mouth and one canal and noting the passage of air through the unobstructed opening. If nasal patency is questionable, it is reported because most newborns are obligatory nose breathers. Thin white mucus is very common in the newborn as is frequent sneezing.

Mouth and throat. External defects of the mouth, such as cleft lips, are readily apparent; however, the internal structures require careful inspection. The palate is normally high arched and somewhat narrow. Rarely teeth may be present. A common finding is *Epstein pearls,* small, white, epithelial cysts along both sides of the midline of the hard palate. They are insignificant and disappear in several weeks.

The frenum of the upper lip is a band of thick, pink tissue that lies under the inner surface of the upper lip and extends to the maxillary alveolar ridge. It is particularly evident when the infant yawns or smiles. It disappears as the maxilla grows.

The *sucking reflex* is elicited by placing a nipple or gloved finger in the infant's mouth. The infant should exhibit a strong, vigorous suck. The *rooting reflex* is obtained by stroking the cheek and noting the infant's response of turning toward the stimulated side and sucking (Fig. 8-8).

The *uvula* can be inspected while the infant is crying and the chin is depressed. However, it may be retracted upward and backward during crying. Tonsillar tissue is generally not seen in the newborn. Natal teeth are seen infrequently and erupt chiefly at the position of the lower incisors. They are reported because most of them are loosely attached, increasing the risk of aspiration.

Neck. Since the newborn's neck is short and covered with folds of tissue, adequate assessment of the neck requires allowing the head to fall gently backward in hyperextension while the back is supported in a slightly raised position. The nurse observes for range of motion, shape, and any abnormal masses.

Chest. The newborn's chest is almost circular because the anteroposterior and lateral diameters are equal. The ribs are very flexible, and slight intercostal retractions are normally seen on inspiration. The xiphoid process is com-

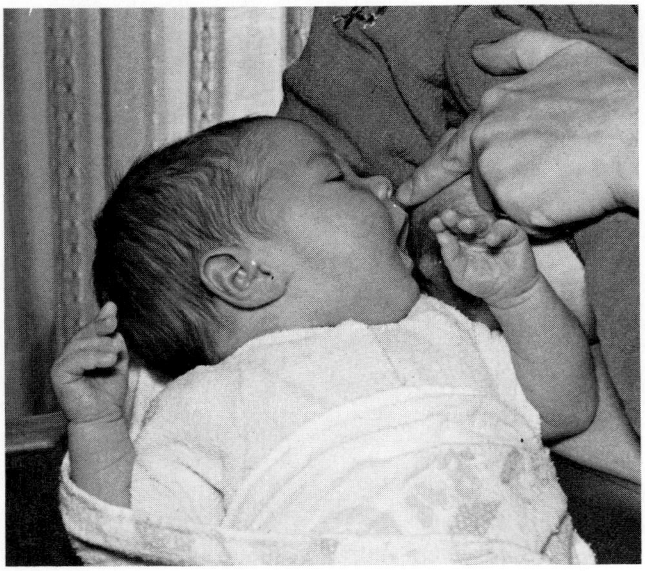

FIG. 8-8 Eliciting rooting reflex.

monly visible as a small protrusion at the end of the sternum. The sternum is generally raised and slightly curved.

The breasts are inspected for size, shape, and nipple formation, location, and number. Breast enlargement appears in many newborns of either sex by the second or third day and is caused by maternal hormones. Occasionally a milky substance sometimes called "witches' milk" is secreted by the infant's breasts by the end of the first week.

Lungs. The normal respirations of the newborn are irregular and abdominal, and the rate is between 30 and 60 breaths/minute. Periods of apnea less than 15 seconds in duration are considered normal. After the initial forceful breaths required to initiate respiration, subsequent breaths should be easy and fairly regular in rhythm. Occasional irregularities occur in relation to crying, sleeping, and feeding.

It is important that the nurse learn to carefully assess the respiratory status of the newborn through observation, since auscultation is difficult because of the small size of the chest and the effective transmission of cardiac and bowel sounds to all parts of the pleural cavity.

Heart. Heart rate should always be auscultated and may range from 100 to 180 beats per minute shortly after birth and, when the infant has stabilized, from 120 to 140 beats per minute. The location of the heart is determined by palpation and auscultation. The *apical impulse* is at the fifth intercostal space, at or near the midclavicular line.

Abdomen. The normal contour of the abdomen is cylindric and usually prominent with visible veins. Bowel sounds are heard a few hours after birth. Visible peristaltic waves may be observed in thin newborns but should not be seen in well-nourished infants.

The umbilical cord is inspected to determine the presence of two arteries, which look like papular structures, and one vein, which has a larger lumen than the arteries and a thinner vessel wall. At birth the cord should appear bluish white and moist. After clamping it begins to dry and appears a dull, yellowish brown. It progressively shrivels in size and turns greenish black.

Palpation is done after inspection of the abdomen. The liver is normally palpable 3 cm (about 1 inch) below the right costal margin. The tip of the spleen can sometimes be felt, but a palpable spleen more than 1 cm below the left costal margin suggests enlargement and warrants further investigation. While both kidneys should be palpated, this maneuver requires considerable practice. When felt, the lower half of the right kidney and the tip of the left kidney are 1 to 2 cm above the umbilicus.

During examination of the lower abdomen, it is particularly important to palpate for femoral pulses, which should be strong and equal bilaterally.

Female genitalia. Normally the labia minora and clitoris are edematous, especially following a breech delivery. However, the labia and clitoris must be carefully inspected to identify any evidence of ambiguous genitalia or other abnormalities. Normally in a female the urethral opening is located behind the clitoris.

A hymenal tag is occasionally visible from the posterior opening of the vagina. It is composed of tissue from the hymen and the labia minora. It usually disappears in several weeks. Generally the vaginal vault is not inspected.

Vaginal discharge (more often seen as a milky secretion than actual blood) may be noted during the first week of life. Fecal discharge from the vaginal opening indicates a rectovaginal fistula and is always reported. Vernix caseosa may be present in large amounts between the labia.

Male genitalia. The penis is inspected for the location of the urethral opening, which is located at the tip. However, the opening may be totally covered by the prepuce, or foreskin, which covers the glans penis. A tight prepuce is a very common finding in the newborn. It should not be forcefully retracted, except to locate the urinary opening. *Smegma,* a white cheesy substance, is commonly found around the glans penis, under the foreskin. Small, white, firm lesions called *epithelial pearls* may be seen at the tip of the prepuce. An erection is common in the newborn.

The scrotum may be large, edematous and pendulous in the full-term neonate, especially in the infant born in breech position. Palpation of the scrotum is routinely performed to detect the presence of testes, which should be descended in the full-term infant (see Fig. 7-38).

Back and rectum. With the infant prone, the spine is inspected. The shape of the spine should be gently rounded, with none of the characteristic S-shaped curves seen later in life. Stroking the back along one side of the vertebral column will cause the infant to move the hips toward the stimulated side *(trunk incurvation reflex)*.

With the infant still prone, symmetry of the gluteal

A 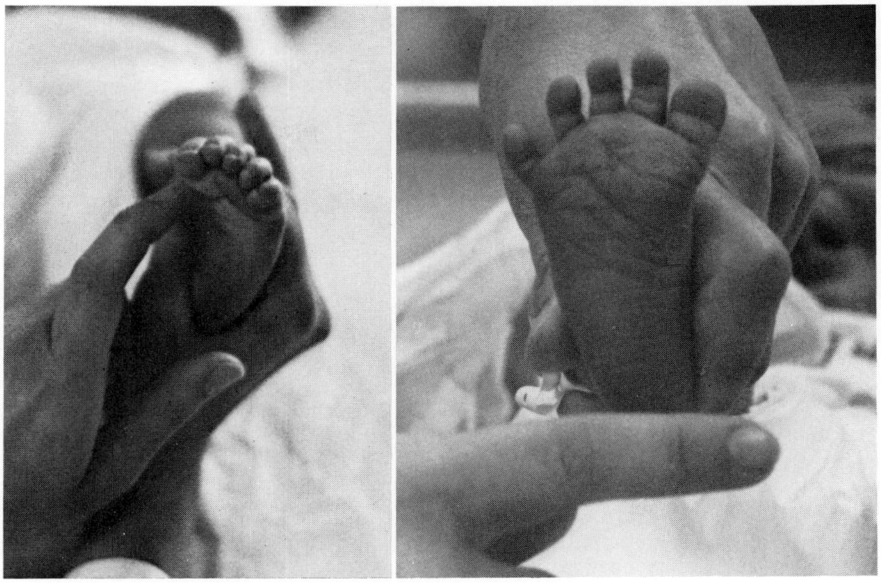 B

FIG. 8-9 A, Plantar or grasp reflex. **B,** Babinski reflex.

folds is carefully noted. Any evidence of asymmetry is reported since it may be a sign of congenital hip dislocation.

Passage of meconium indicates anal patency. If an imperforate anus is suspected and is not readily visible, the little finger (gloved and lubricated) or a rubber catheter should be inserted into the anal opening. Rectal thermometers are not used because of the risk of mucosal perforation (see Fig. 7-7). In addition, the small diameter of the thermometer may pass through even a severely stenotic anus.

Extremities. The extremities are examined for symmetry, range of motion, and reflexes. The fingers and toes are counted, and supernumerary digits *(polydactyly)* or fusion of digits *(syndactyly)* is noted. A partial syndactyly between the second and third toes is a common variation seen in otherwise normal infants. The nail beds should be pink, although slight blueness is evident in acrocyanosis.

The palms of the hands should have the usual creases (see Fig. 7-9). The full-term newborn usually has creases on the anterior two thirds of the sole of the foot. The soles of the feet are flat with prominent fat pads.

Range of motion of the extremities should be observed throughout the entire examination. The hips are rotated to identify a congenital dislocation. With the infant supine, the legs should be flexed *gently* at the hips and knees and abducted to almost 175 degrees. Limitation in abduction often indicates dislocation. Symmetry is noted when the infant moves, particularly when a Moro reflex is elicited.

Muscle tone should also be assessed. By attempting to extend a flexed extremity, the nurse determines if tone is equal bilaterally.

Two reflexes are elicited. The first is the *grasp reflex*. Touching the palms of the hands or soles of the feet near the base of the digits causes flexion or grasping (Fig. 8-9, *A*). The other is the *Babinski reflex*. Stroking the outer sole of the foot upward from the heel across the ball of the foot causes the big toe to dorsiflex and the other toes to hyperextend (Fig. 8-9, *B*).

Neurologic system. Assessing neurologic status is a critical part of the physical assessment of the newborn. Much of the neurologic examination takes place during examination of body systems, such as eliciting localized reflexes and observing posture, muscle tone, head control, and movement. However, several important mass (total body) reflexes also need to be elicited. They are usually left to the end of the examination because they may disturb the infant and interfere with auscultation. These reflexes are described in Table 8-4.

NURSING DIAGNOSIS

A number of nursing diagnoses are prominent in the nursing care of the newborn and family and others specific to individual cases become evident. The most common nursing diagnoses are outlined in the Nursing Care Plan on p. 208.

PLANNING

The main nursing goal for newborns is provision of physical care. For the family the principal goal is promotion of psychologic care. Specifically this involves the following:

1. Maintain a patent airway
2. Maintain a stable body temperature
3. Protect the infant from infection and injury
4. Provide optimum nutrition
5. Promote parent-infant attachment
6. Prepare for discharge and home care

TABLE 8-4

Assessment of Reflexes in the Normal Newborn

Reflex	Expected Behavioral Response	Comments
Moro	Sudden jarring or change in equilibrium causes extension and abduction of extremities and fanning of fingers, with index finger and thumb forming a "C" shape, followed by flexion and adduction of extremities; legs may weakly flex; infant may cry (Fig. 8-10)	Elicit by holding the infant above the examining table in a supine position with one hand beneath the sacrum and the other supporting the upper back and head; the infant's head is then suddenly allowed to fall about 30 degrees Disappears after age 3-4 months, usually strongest during first 2 months
Startle	A sudden loud noise causes abduction of the arms with flexion of the elbows; the hands remain clenched	Disappears by age 4 months
Tonic neck	When infant's head is quickly turned to one side, arm and leg will extend on that side, and opposite arm and leg will flex; posture resembles a fencing position (Fig. 8-11)	Disappears by age 3-4 months, to be replaced by symmetric positioning of both sides of body
Dance or step	If infant is held so that sole of foot touches a hard surface, there will be a reciprocal flexion and extension of the leg, simulating walking (Fig. 8-12)	Disappears after age 3-4 weeks, to be replaced by deliberate movement
Crawling	When infant is placed on abdomen, he will make crawling movements with the arms and legs (Fig. 8-13)	Disappears at about age 6 weeks

IMPLEMENTATION

The following discussion on implementing newborn care focuses on nursing care after the infant has been delivered. Readers who are interested in a more detailed discussion of the birth and immediate care of the neonate are referred to the many excellent maternity texts.

Maintain a Patent Airway

Establishing a patent airway is a primary objective in the delivery room and is the responsibility of the attending physicians and obstetric nurses. However, maintaining a patent airway continues to be a priority goal in the nursery with attention to proper positioning of the infant to facilitate drainage of secretions, especially after feeding (see Fig. 8-17). A bulb syringe is kept near the infant and is used if suctioning is required. To avoid aspiration of amniotic fluid or mucus, the pharynx is cleared first, then the nasal passages. The bulb is compressed *before* insertion to prevent forcing secretions into the bronchi. Used bulb syringes should probably be replaced every 24 hours in the hospital and boiled for 10 minutes before reuse in the home to eliminate bacterial contamination (Patel and others, 1988).

If more forceful removal of secretions is required, mechanical suction is used. The use of the proper size catheter and correct suctioning technique is essential in order to prevent mucosal damage and edema. Gentle suctioning is necessary to prevent reflex bradycardia, laryngospasm, and cardiac arrhythmias from vagal stimulation. Suctioning is performed for 5 seconds with sufficient time between suctioning to allow the infant to reoxygenate (Fuller, 1988). This prevents depletion of the infant's oxygen supply.

In some nurseries the stomach is routinely lavaged to remove amniotic fluid, which may cause abdominal distention and interfere with the establishment of respiration. Passing a catheter to the stomach also rules out esophageal atresia. Vital signs are closely monitored and any indication of respiratory distress is immediately reported.

Maintain Stable Body Temperature

Conserving the newborn's body heat is an important nursing goal. It requires an understanding of the causes of heat loss: evaporation, radiation, conduction, and convection. Nursing care is based on preventing these from occurring.

At birth a major cause of heat loss is *evaporation,* the loss of heat through moisture. The amniotic fluid that bathes the infant's skin favors evaporation, especially when combined with the cool atmosphere of the delivery room. Heat loss through evaporation is minimized by rapidly drying the skin and hair with a warmed towel and placing the infant in a heated environment.

Another major cause of heat loss is *radiation,* the loss of heat to cooler solid objects in the environment that are not in direct contact with the infant. Loss of heat through radiation increases as these solid objects become colder and closer to the infant. The temperature of ambient or surrounding air in the Isolette or incubator essentially has no effect on loss of heat through radiation. This is a critical point to remember when attempting to maintain a constant temperature for the infant because even though the temperature of the ambient air is optimal, the infant can be hypothermic.

An example of radiant heat loss is the placement of the

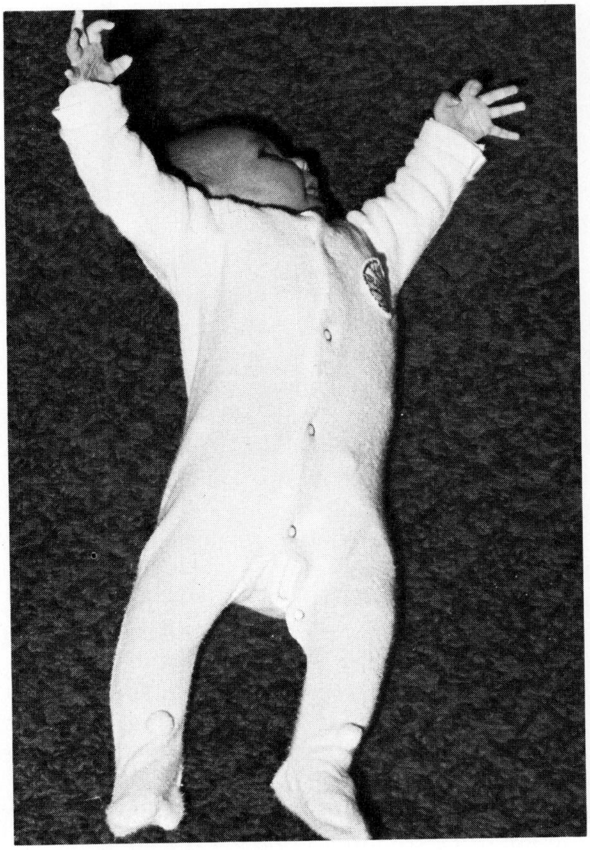

FIG. 8-10 Moro reflex.

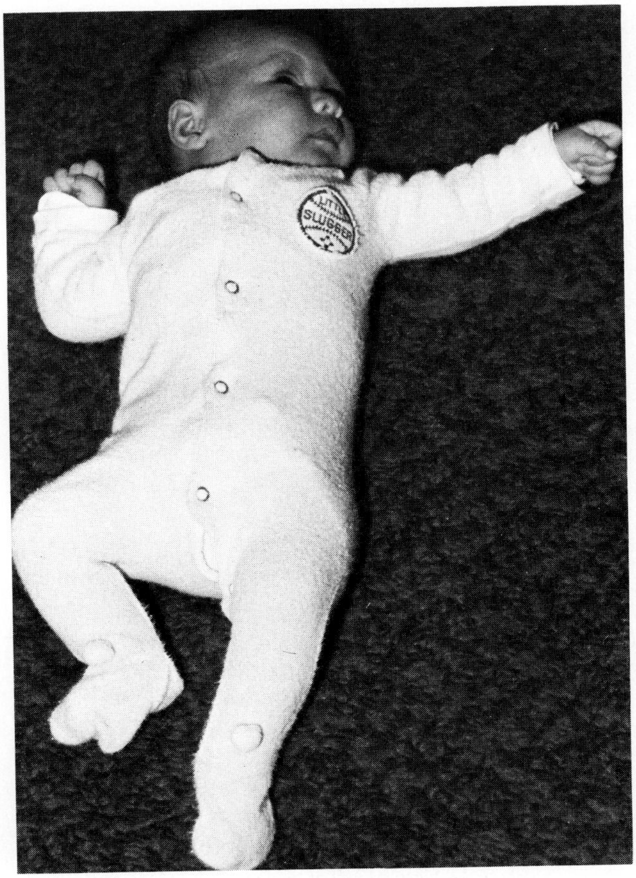

FIG. 8-11 Tonic neck reflex.

FIG. 8-12 Dance reflex.

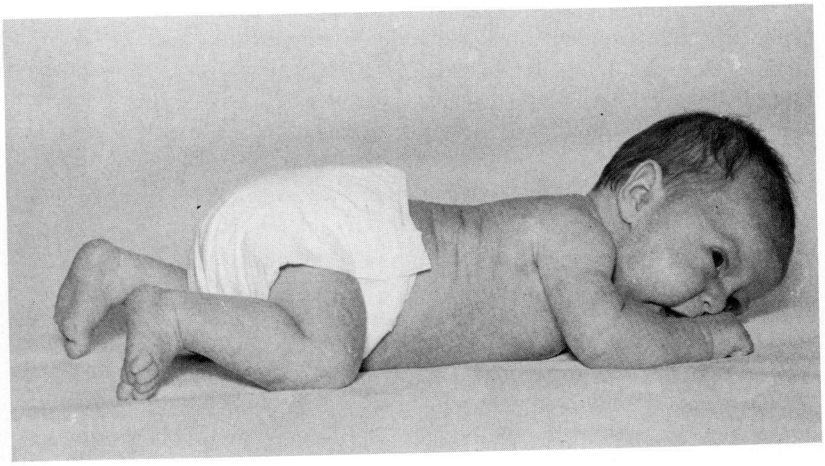

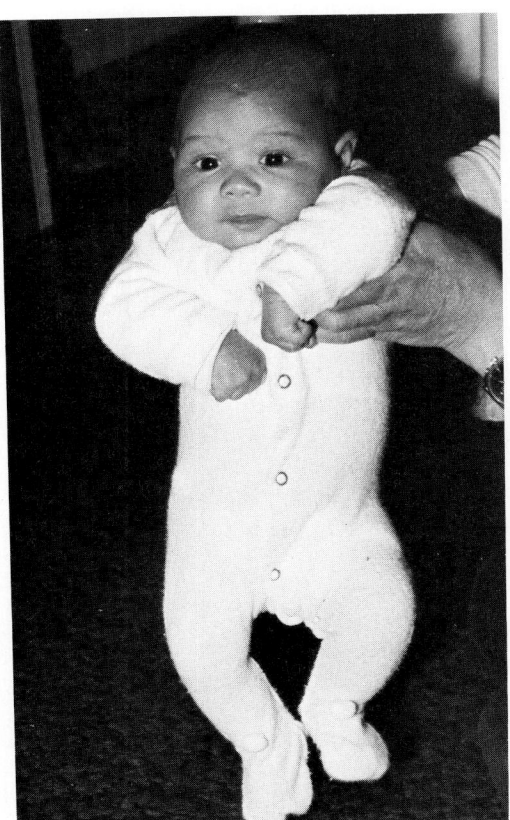

FIG. 8-13 Crawl reflex.

incubator close to a cold window or air conditioning unit. The cold from either source will cool the walls of the incubator and, subsequently, the body of the neonate. To prevent this, the infant is placed as far away as possible from walls, windows, and ventilating units. If heat loss continues to be a problem, a radiant warmer may be placed over the infant or infant and mother.

Heat loss can also occur through conduction and convection. *Conduction* involves loss of heat from the body because of direct contact of skin with a cooler solid object. This can be minimized by placing the infant on a padded, covered surface and by providing insulation through clothes and blankets rather than by placing the infant directly on a hard table. Placing the newborn very close to his mother, such as in her arms or on her abdomen, is physically beneficial in terms of conserving heat as well as fostering maternal attachment.

Convection is similar to conduction, except that heat loss is aided by surrounding air currents. For example, placing the infant in the direct flow of air from a fan or air conditioner vent will cause rapid heat loss through convection. Transporting the neonate in a crib with solid sides reduces airflow around the infant.

Protect From Infection and Injury

The most important practice for preventing cross-infection is thorough handwashing of all individuals involved in the infant's care. Several other procedures to prevent infection include eye care, umbilical care, bathing, and care of the circumcision. Vitamin K is administered to protect against hemorrhage. In addition several safety measures are practiced, particularly in terms of proper identification, and screening tests are used to detect genetic disorders, such as phenylketonuria and hypothyroidism.

Identification. Proper identification of the newborn is the responsibility of the delivery room nurse. However, upon the infant's admission to the newborn care unit the nurse *must* check that two identifying bands are securely fastened, usually on the wrist and ankle, and verify the information (name, sex, mother's admission number, date, and time of birth) against the birth records and the child's actual sex. When the infant is brought to the mother, she should also be asked to verify the information on the identification bands and the child's sex.

Eye care. Prophylactic eye treatment to prevent *ophthalmia neonatorum,* infectious conjunctivitis of the newborn, includes the use of erythromycin (0.5%) or tetracycline (1%) ophthalmic ointment or drops. Although effective against *Neisseria gonorrhoeae,* silver nitrate is not recommended because it does not protect against *Chlamydia trachomatis,* another major cause of ophthalmia neonatorum.

Correct application of the medication is essential for optimum protection and includes the following steps (National Society, 1981):

1. Clean the eyelids with sterile cotton and sterile water if needed
2. Separate lids and apply 2 drops or at least 1 to 2 cm (1/2 inch) of ointment to the conjunctival sac
3. Manipulate lids to ensure spread of the medication
4. Use 2 ampules, one for each eye, or 1 tube per infant, being careful not to touch eyelid or eyeball with the tip of the tube
5. Wipe excess medication from eye 1 minute after application
6. Do not rinse eyes with sterile normal saline solution

Since during the first hour of life a newborn has a greater ability to focus on coordinated movement than at any other time during the next several days and since eye-to-eye contact is considered important in the development of maternal-infant bonding, the routine administration of antibiotics can be postponed up to 1 hour. However, there must be some kind of checklist to ensure that the drug is given as soon as possible.

Bathing. Bath time can be an opportunity for the nurse to accomplish much more than general hygiene. It is an excellent time for observation of the infant's behavior, such as irritability, state of arousal, alertness, and muscular activity.

In hospitals where there is rooming-in of infant and mother, bath time provides an opportunity for the nurse to involve the parents in the care of their child and to learn about his individual characteristics (Fig. 8-14). Parents are encouraged to examine every finger and toe of their infant. Frequently normal variations such as Epstein pearls, mongolian spots, or "stork bites" cause parents undue concern because they are unaware of the insignificance of such findings. Minor birth injuries may

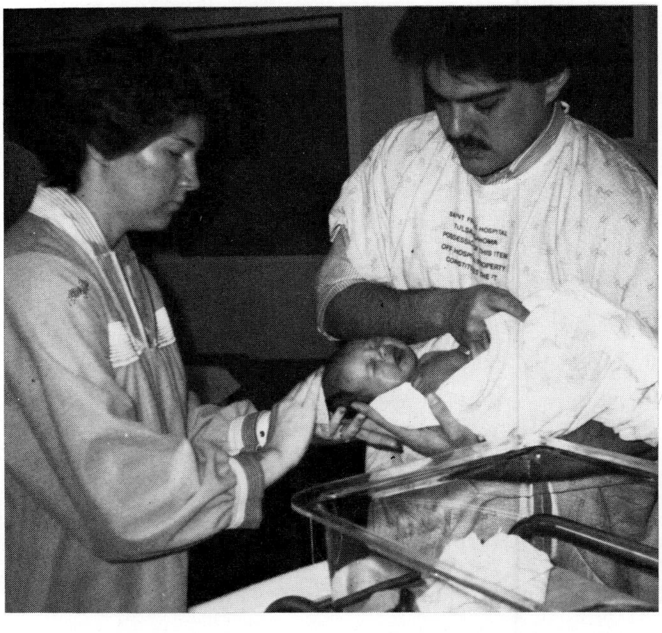

FIG. 8-14 Bath time is an excellent opportunity for parents to learn about their newborn.

appear as major defects to them. Explaining how these occurred and when they will disappear is reassuring to parents. Common variations are discussed further in Chapter 9.

One of the most important considerations in skin cleansing is preservation of the skin's pH, which is about 5 soon after birth. The slightly acidic skin surface has bacteriostatic effects. Consequently, only plain warm water should be used for the bath. Alkaline soaps, such as Ivory, oils, powder, and lotions are not used because they alter the pH, thus providing a better environment for bacterial growth. Talcum has the added risk of aspiration if applied too close to the infant's face.

Bathing should be done in the nursery after the vital signs have stabilized. There is no need to immediately wash a newborn, except to remove the blood from the face and head. Cleansing proceeds in the cephalocaudal direction. A washcloth is used and turned so that a clean part touches the skin with each stroke. The eyes are carefully wiped from the inner to the outer aspect of the lid. The face is cleansed next. The nares are carefully inspected for any crusted secretions. The scalp is usually wiped, although it is sometimes necessary to shampoo the hair. Shampooing is best accomplished by positioning the infant's head over a small basin, lathering the scalp with a mild soap, and rinsing by pouring water from a small vessel over the head into the basin. The rest of the body should be covered during this procedure and the head should be dried quickly to prevent evaporation heat loss. The ears are cleaned with the twisted end of a washcloth, not with a cotton-tipped swab which, if inserted into the canal, can damage the ear.

The rest of the body is washed in a similar manner. Although the infant's skin requires little rubbing for adequate cleansing, certain areas such as the folds of the neck, the axillae, and creases at joints need special attention. The area around the neck is especially prone to a rash from regurgitation of feeding and should be thoroughly washed and dried.

The genitalia of both sexes require careful cleansing. Cleansing of the vulva is done in a front-to-back direction. The bath is a perfect opportunity to stress this part of hygiene to the mother, both for the infant's and for her own protection against urinary tract infection.

Cleansing the male genitalia involves washing the penis and scrotum. Sometimes smegma needs to be removed by wiping around the glans. The foreskin is not retracted because it is normally tight in newborns. If the infant is not to be circumcised, the parents are taught how to cleanse under and around the foreskin by retracting it gently *only* as far as it will go and returning it to its normal position. Leaving the prepuce retracted constricts the blood vessels supplying the glans penis, causing edema.

The buttocks and anal area are thoroughly cleansed of any fecal material. As with the rest of the body, the area is dried to prevent a warm, moist environment that fosters growth of bacteria.

Diapers are applied after the bath. They should fit snugly around the thighs and abdomen to prevent urine from leaking. In males cloth diapers should be folded with extra thickness in the front to provide greater absorbency. In females the placement of the extra fold depends on whether the infant is prone or supine. Diapers are fastened with the back side overlapping the front side to allow full flexion of the hips.

The nurse should discuss the choice of cloth or disposable diapers with parents. Using disposable diapers exclusively is the most expensive method, costing several times more than cloth diapers laundered at home. Diaper service costs vary but may be more than twice as much as the self-laundry method. Over 1 or 2 years the cost or savings can be considerable, particularly if more than one child is wearing diapers. However, some brands of disposable diapers (those containing special material to absorb fluid) may offer advantages of increased wetness control and decreased diaper dermatitis.

Care of the umbilicus. Because the umbilical stump is an excellent medium for bacterial growth, various methods of cord care are practiced, such as the topical application of triple dye (a solution of brilliant green, proflavine hemisulfate, and crystal violet) or of bacitracin ointment. The dye or ointment is applied at the base of the cord with a cotton-tipped applicator and may be reapplied as prescribed by the physician. The diaper is placed below the cord to avoid irritation against the fabric.

Parents are instructed regarding stump deterioration and proper umbilical care. The stump deteriorates through the process of dry gangrene, and when triple dye is used, it falls off in 14 to 17 days. The cord base takes a few more weeks to heal completely. During this time care consists of keeping the cord clean and dry and may include wiping the base with alcohol. Any signs of infection, such as presence of erythema and malodorous, purulent discharge, are reported.

Circumcision. Circumcision is the surgical removal of the foreskin on the glans penis. In the Jewish culture circumcision is performed during a highly significant ceremony called a *berith,* or *brit,* which takes place on the eighth day of life. A rabbi skilled in the procedure usually performs the circumcision. However, in most instances it is routinely done in the hospital by the physician.

There is much controversy regarding the benefits and risks of this widely practiced procedure (see box). The American Academy of Pediatrics (1975) reaffirmed its position that there are no valid medical indications for circumcision of the newborn and that a program of good personal hygiene offers all the advantages of circumcision without the attendant surgical risks. In light of these arguments, parents should be allowed an "informed" choice when considering circumcision.

Circumcision is usually performed in the nursery sometime after birth. It should not be performed immediately after delivery because of the neonate's unstabilized physiologic status and increased susceptibility to stress. Preoperative nursing care includes allowing the

Risks and Benefits of Neonatal Circumcision

Risks	Benefits
Complications: Hemorrhage Infection Dehiscence (separation of approximated edges of skin) Meatitis (from loss of protective foreskin) Adhesions Concealed penis Urethral fistula Meatal stenosis Pain in unanesthetized infants (long-term consequences unknown, but short-term physiologic stresses include increased heart rate, respiratory rate, and blood pressure and decreased oxygen saturation	Prevention of penile cancer and posthitis (inflammation of prepuce) Decreased incidence of balanitis (inflammation of glans) and, possibly, urinary tract infection in infant males Prevention of complications associated with later circumcision Preservation of male's body image that is consistent with peers (in countries where procedure is common)

infant nothing by mouth before the procedure (about 2 hours) to prevent aspiration of vomitus, checking for a signed consent form, and adequately restraining the infant, usually on a special board (Fig. 8-15). All the equipment used for the procedure, such as gloves, instruments, alcohol wipes, dressings, and draping towels, must be sterile.

Circumcision is usually performed without anesthetics, although this practice is being questioned. The American Academy of Pediatrics (1987) recommends the administration of an anesthesic or an analgesic to neonates undergoing surgical procedures using the same guidelines as those used for older patients. The dorsal penile nerve block (injection of lidocaine into the base of the penis) has been shown to be an effective and safe local anesthetic (Maxwell and others, 1987). (See also Nursing tip box.)

The procedure involves freeing the foreskin from the glans penis by using a scalpel, Gomco clamp, or Hollister Plastibell. In the Gomco technique the foreskin is clamped and removed; the clamp crushes the nerve endings and blood vessels, promoting hemostasis. In the Plastibell procedure the foreskin is removed using a plastic ring and a string tied around the foreskin like a tourniquet. The excess foreskin is trimmed. In about 5 to 8 days the plastic ring separates and falls off.

Nursing Tip: Circumcision

Give a pacifier to the unanesthetized infant during circumcision as this may decrease physical distress.

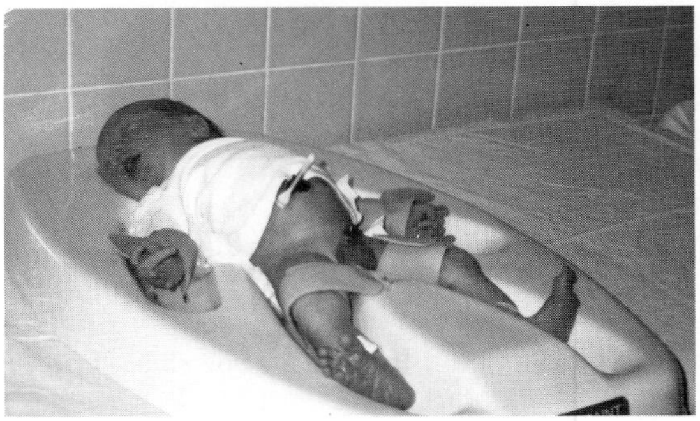

FIG. 8-15 Proper positioning of infant in Circumstraint.

As soon as the procedure is completed, the infant is released from the restraints and comforted. Since parents are often concerned about the infant's well-being during this time, the nurse reassures them that the infant is recovering uneventfully. As soon as the infant is calmed and stabilized, he can be brought to the parents.

Care of the circumcised area depends on the type of procedure. If a clamp was used, a petrolatum gauze dressing may be applied loosely to prevent adherence to the diaper. If the Plastibell was applied, no special dressing is required. Since the area is tender, the diaper is applied loosely to prevent friction against the penis. Normally on the second day a yellowish white exudate forms as part of the granulating process. This is not a sign of infection and should not be forcibly removed. As healing progresses, the exudate disappears. Parents are cautioned to report any evidence of bleeding or unusual swelling to their health professional.

Vitamin K. Shortly after birth, vitamin K is administered intramuscularly to prevent hemorrhagic disease of the newborn. Normally, vitamin K is synthesized by the intestinal flora. However, since the infant's intestine is sterile at birth, and since breast milk contains low levels of vitamin K, the supply is inadequate for at least the first 3 to 4 days. The major function of vitamin K is to catalyze the synthesis of prothrombin in the liver, which is needed for blood clotting and coagulation. The vastus lateralis muscle is the preferred intramuscular injection site because of the absence of other well-developed muscle masses.

Screening for genetic disease. A number of genetic disorders can be detected in the newborn period. Since there is national policy in the United States, the extent of neonatal screening is determined by state laws and voluntary guidelines. Most states require screening for phenylketonuria (PKU) and hypothyroidism (see Chapter 9). Other genetic diseases that may be tested for include galactosemia, maple syrup urine disease, homocystinuria, sickle cell anemia, and thalassemia.

The nurse's responsibility is to educate parents regarding the importance of screening and to collect appropriate specimens at the recommended time. Follow-up of newborns discharged early or born at home is critical to prevent unidentified cases.

Transportation after discharge. An important area of counseling is the safe transportation of the newborn home from the hospital. Ideally this counseling should occur *before* delivery to allow parents an opportunity to purchase a suitable infant car restraint. Parents are more likely to use a restraint if the proper use of one is demonstrated and its necessity is stressed, such as including this recommendation in discharge orders and emphasizing that all states legally require proper restraint of young children. (For a discussion of appropriate car restraints for infants, see p. 298.)

Provide Optimum Nutrition

Selection of a feeding method is one of the major decisions faced by parents. In general there are three acceptable choices: human milk, commercially prepared cow's milk formula, and modified cow's milk. There are significant nutritional, economic, and psychologic advantages and differences among each. Nurses need to be aware of the types of feeding to help parents choose the method that best meets their needs.

Significant nutritional differences exist between human milk and whole cow's milk (see box). While both contain the same amount of fat and provide the same calories, cow's milk contains three times as much protein as human milk, making whole cow's milk unsuitable for infant nutrition. To meet the protein requirement, cow's milk must be diluted, but, when dilute, it does not meet the caloric or fat requirement. Consequently, bottle-feeding using commercially prepared formula or modified evaporated milk is chosen as a substitute if breast-feeding is not selected.

Advantages of Human Milk vs Cow's Milk

- Contains adequate (not excessive) protein
- Contains more lactalbumin (produces easily digested curds) than casein (produces large, hard curds)
- Contains more lactose, which in the gut stimulates growth of microorganisms, which synthesize some B vitamins and produce organic acids that may retard growth of harmful bacteria
- Contains more monounsaturated fatty acids, which enhance absorption of fat and calcium
- Contains adequate (not excessive) minerals with exception of fluoride (low in both)
- Amounts of iron and zinc are low but more readily absorbed
- Contains high calcium and low phosphorus; the reverse ratio in cow's milk promotes calcium excretion, causing tetany
- Contains adequate amounts of vitamins A, B complex, and E; vitamin C content depends on maternal intake; vitamin D is low but more readily absorbed (vitamin C, D, and E are low in cow's milk, but K is higher)
- Contains growth modulators that modify growth or differentiation
- Offers several immunologic benefits: contains various immunoglobins (Ig), especially Ig A; macrophages, granulocytes, T- and B-cell lymphocytes; and other factors that inhibit bacterial growth
- Has laxative effect
- Is economical, readily available, and sanitary
- Has psychologic benefits of close bond between infant and mother during feeding

Breast-feeding. Human milk is the preferred form of nutrition for the infant. In the United States about 60% of newborns in hospitals are breast-fed and there is a continuing trend for more mothers from all socioeconomic levels to breast-feed and to continue breast-feeding longer.

Besides the physiologic advantages of human milk, the most outstanding psychologic benefit of breast-feeding is the close maternal-child relationship. The infant is nestled very close to the mother's skin, can hear the rhythm of her heartbeat, feel the warmth of her body, and sense a peaceful security. The mother has a very close feeling of union with her child and feels a sense of accomplishment and satisfaction as the infant draws milk from her. Some mothers also experience a type of sensation similar to sexual excitement.

Breast-feeding is the most economical form of feeding, although it is not "free" milk because the lactating mother needs a high-protein, high-calorie diet. Breast milk is always available, ready to serve at room temperature, and free of bacterial contamination. There is also less chance of overfeeding and consequent obesity because the infant nurses until satisfied while bottle-fed infants are usually encouraged to finish all their formula. In general, bottle-fed infants gain weight faster than do breast-fed infants.

The few contraindications to breast-feeding include any serious, debilitating maternal illness (such as severe heart disease or advanced cancer), maternal infections (such as sputum-positive tuberculosis, hepatitis B, or acquired immune deficiency syndrome [AIDS]), and galactosemia in the infant. Mastitis (inflammation of the mammary gland) is usually not a contraindication if the discomfort is tolerable. Rarely "breast milk jaundice" may require temporary cessation of breast-feeding (see p. 238).

Probably the greatest disadvantage of breast-feeding to many mothers is the perceived inconvenience of loss of freedom and independence. Being committed to feeding the infant every 2 to 3 hours can be overwhelming, especially to women with multiple responsibilities. Many women resume their careers shortly after their pregnancy and prefer to use bottle-feeding. However, breast-feeding and employment are possible and suggestions for the mother include expressing breast milk for bottle-feeding or using formula feedings during her absence after breast-feeding is well established. Breast-feeding is the preferred form of infant feeding, but a mother's decision regarding her preferences must be supported and respected.

Successful breast-feeding probably depends more on the mother's desire to breast-feed, satisfaction with breast-feeding, and available support systems than on any other factors. Contrary to popular belief, breast-feeding is not instinctive. Mothers need support, encouragement, and assistance during their postpartum hospital stay to enhance their opportunities for success and satisfaction. Certainly, nurses play a very significant role in the breast-feeding decision and must make themselves available to families for guidance and support. Several excellent books (Lawrence, 1985; Riordan, 1983) and organizations* are available as resources for professionals and breast-feeding mothers.

Bottle-feeding. Bottle-feeding generally refers to the use of bottles for feeding commercial or evaporated milk formula rather than using the breast. However, in some instances human milk may be expressed and fed with a bottle. With commercial formulas that closely approximate human milk and greatly improved conditions of sanitation, bottle-feeding is a perfectly acceptable method of feeding.

Commercially prepared formulas (Similac, Enfamil, SMA) are milk-based formulas that have been modified to closely resemble human milk. Although they are not an exact substitute, they do provide an optimum source of nutrition. The formulas are available in three preparations: (1) a ready-to-use form in cans or bottles, (2) a concentrated liquid form that is diluted with an equal amount of water, and (3) a powdered form that must be prepared according to the manufacturer's directions. One consideration in the use of commercially prepared formulas is their cost. Parents should do comparison shopping since one preparation can be considerably more expensive than another.

In the United States only a very small percentage of infants are fed evaporated milk formula. However, it has many advantages over whole milk. It is readily available in cans, needs no refrigeration if unopened, provides a softer, more digestible curd, and contains more lactalbumin and a higher calcium/phosphorus ratio. It is also less expensive than commercial formula. A common rule for preparing evaporated milk formula is diluting the 13-ounce can of milk with 17 ounces of water and adding 1 to 2 tablespoons of sugar or corn syrup.

Evaporated milk must not be confused with condensed milk, which is a form of evaporated milk with 45% more sugar. Because of its high carbohydrate concentration and disproportionately low fat and protein content, condensed milk is not used for infant feeding. Likewise, skim milk should not be used because it is deficient in caloric concentration, significantly increases the renal solute load and water demands, and deprives the body of essential fatty acids.

Feeding techniques. Nurses should not assume that new mothers automatically know how to breast- or bottle-feed their infant. Breast-feeding mothers, in particular, need support and assistance during the early postpartum period to feel comfortable and successful with lactation. Parents who choose bottle-feeding need guidelines in preparing the formula and using feeding techniques to meet both the infant's nutritional and psychologic needs. The following is an overview of the basic techniques of breast- or bottle-feeding. More detailed information, especially on breast-feeding, can be found in the resources footnoted here.

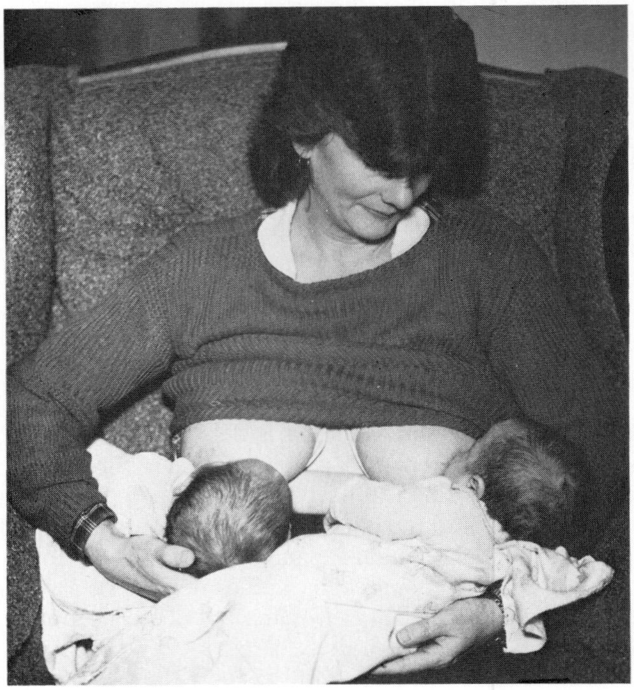

FIG. 8-16 Simultaneous breast-feeding of twins.

During breast-feeding both the infant and mother need to be in a comfortable position that allows for the infant's face to be directly in front of the breast (see Fig. 8-16). The infant cannot swallow if the head is turned to the side. The mother should use two fingers to compress and support the areola for the infant to grasp the entire areola. The breasts should be alternated during the feeding, especially for the newborn. When the infant is finished feeding, suction is released by placing a finger between areola and lips, not by pulling the infant from the breast.

The birth of twins need not create a breast-feeding problem. If both twins are full-term, they can begin feedings immediately after birth (Fig. 8-16).* Simultaneous feeding promotes the rapid production of milk needed for both infants and makes the milk that would normally be lost in the let-down reflex available to one of the twins. When only one infant is hungry, the mother should feed singly. She should also feed each infant on both breasts and avoid favoring one breast for one infant to offer the visual stimulation and exercise that alternating breasts provides.

During bottle-feeding the infant is held close to the body and rocked or cuddled to assure the emotional com-

*La Leche League International, Inc., 9616 Minneapolis Ave., Franklin Park, IL 60131; Box 39, Williamsburg, Ontario, Canada KOC 2HO.

*A helpful booklet for mothers is "Breastfeeding your twins" from Health Education Associates, 211 S. Eastern Rd., Glenside, PA 19038.

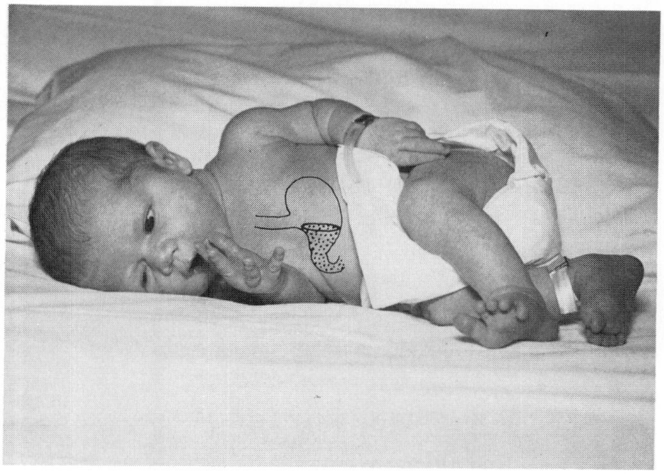

FIG. 8-17 Right side-lying position after feeding.

ponent of feeding. Propping the bottle is discouraged for the following reasons:

1. It denies the infant the important component of close human contact
2. The infant may aspirate formula while sleeping
3. It may facilitate the development of middle ear infections. As the infant lies flat and sucks, milk that has pooled in the pharynx becomes a suitable medium for bacterial growth. Bacteria then enter the eustachian tube, which leads to the middle ear, causing acute otitis media
4. It encourages continuous pooling of formula in the mouth, which can lead to bottle caries when the teeth erupt (see p. 356).

The feeding should not be hurried. Even though the infant may suck vigorously for the first 5 minutes and seem to be satisfied, he should be allowed to continue sucking. Infants need at least 2 hours of sucking a day. If there are six feedings per day, then about 20 minutes of sucking should be allowed at each feeding for oral gratification.

Because infants do not have the motor control to voluntarily push the bottle away when finished, they should be fed only as much as they voluntarily consume to prevent overfeeding. During feedings the bottle is removed and with the infant in an upright position, the back is gently patted to burp or bubble the infant. During breast-feeding bubbling may be done after alternating breasts or at the end of the feeding.

After feedings the infant is positioned on the right side to permit the feeding to flow toward the lower end of the stomach and to allow any swallowed air to rise above the fluid and through the esophagus (Fig. 8-17). This prevents regurgitation and distention. To maintain the side-lying position, a pillow can be propped behind the infant's back.

Preparation of formula. The two traditional ways of preparing formula are the terminal heat method and the aseptic method. In the terminal heat method all the utensils and formula are boiled together for 25 minutes. In the aseptic method the equipment is boiled separately, after which the formula is poured into the bottles.

Because of improved sanitary conditions, neither of these methods is essential. The clean technique is satisfactory. Persons preparing the formula should wash their hands well and then wash all the equipment used to prepare the formula, including the cans of formula or evaporated milk. The formula is prepared and bottled immediately before each feeding. Warming the formula is optional, although many parents prefer to warm it before feeding. Any milk remaining in the bottle after the feeding is discarded, since it is an excellent medium for bacterial growth. Opened cans of formula are covered and refrigerated until the next feeding.

Recommendations for labeling infant formulas require that the directions for preparation and use of the formula include pictures and symbols for nonreading individuals. In addition manufacturers are translating the directions into foreign languages, such as Spanish and Vietnamese, to prevent misunderstanding and errors in formula preparation. It is important to impress upon families that the proportions *must not be altered*—neither diluted to extend the amount of formula nor concentrated to provide more calories.

Feeding schedules. Ideally feeding schedules should be determined by the infant's hunger. Feeding infants when they signal readiness is called *demand feeding*. However, many mothers use *scheduled feedings* arranged at predetermined intervals to meet family routines. Some hospitals routinely feed infants every 4 hours. Although this is satisfactory for bottle-fed infants, it does hinder the breast-feeding process. Since breast-fed infants tend to be hungry every 2 to 3 hours, they should be fed on demand.

Supplemental feedings should *not* be offered to breast-fed infants before lactation is well established because they satiate the infant and cause nipple confusion. Satiated infants suck less vigorously at the breast, and without complete emptying of the ducts milk production is reduced. In addition, the process of sucking from a bottle is different from breast-nipple compression. When infants use the tongue movements needed for bottle-feeding during breast-feeding, they may push the human nipple out of the mouth and incorrectly grasp the areola.

Usually by 3 weeks of age, lactation is well established and a feeding schedule has been formed. Bottle-fed newborns retain about 2 to 3 ounces of formula at each feeding and are fed about six times a day. Breast-fed infants may feed as frequently as 10 to 12 times daily. Larger infants are able to retain increased amounts because of greater stomach capacity; as a result they generally sleep through the night sooner than smaller infants or breast-fed infants.

Promote Parent-Infant Bonding (Attachment)

The process of parenting is based on a mutual relationship between parent and infant. Much of past research on parent-child attachment has focused on the development of "mothering" or maternal attachment to the infant. Current attention focuses on the infant's role in this process. Although the words "bonding" and "attachment" are sometimes referred to as separate phenomena with *bonding* as the development of emotional ties from parent to infant and *attachment* representing the emotional ties from infant to parent, in this discussion the words are used interchangeably to denote both processes.

As more is learned of the complexity of neonates and of their potential for influencing and shaping their environments, particularly their interaction with significant others, it becomes obvious that promoting positive parent-child relationships necessitates an understanding of factors involved in identifying behavioral steps in attachment, variables that enhance or hinder this process, and methods of teaching parents ways to develop a stronger relationship with their children, especially by recognizing potential problems.

Infant behavior. Nurses must appreciate the individuality and uniqueness of each infant. According to the infant's temperament, he will change and shape the environment, which will undoubtedly influence future development. Obviously an infant who sleeps 20 hours a day will be exposed to much fewer stimuli than the infant who sleeps 16 hours a day. In turn, each infant will likely effect a different response from his parents. The infant who is quiet, undemanding, and passive may receive much less attention than the infant who is responsive, alert, and active. Such behavioral characteristics have implications for parenting because forming a relationship is based on responding to reciprocal cues from each individual. The infant who responds to cuddling, smiling, and cooing evokes an attentive, pleasurable response from the parent, which will reinforce such behavior. An infant who stiffens when held, looks away when someone approaches too closely, or cries after feedings typically evokes feelings of rejection, dissatisfaction, and insecurity in the parent that may seriously hinder the attachment process.

Nurses can intervene and positively influence the attachment of parent and child. The first step is recognizing individual differences and explaining to parents that such characteristics are normal. For example, most people believe that infants sleep throughout the day, except for a half-hour feeding. For some newborns this may be true, but for many it is not. Understanding that the infant's wakefulness is part of his body rhythm and not a reflection of inadequate mothering can be crucial in promoting healthy parent-child relationships. Another aspect of helping parents involves supplying guidelines on how to enhance the infant's development during awake periods. Placing the child in a crib to stare at the same mobile every day is not particularly exciting, but carrying him into each room as one does daily chores can be fascinating. Simple suggestions can make life very stimulating for the infant and much more pleasurable and gratifying for the parents (see box).

*How to Make the Infant's World More Exciting**

Infant prefers animated and auditory objects.
Infant enjoys novelty, quickly tires of seeing same objects; mobile should be changed frequently.
Infant prefers to look at medium-intensity colors and contrasting colors, such as black and white.
Infant likes geometric shapes and checkerboards; prefers patterns over straight lines.
Contrasting lights and reflective surfaces such as mirrors are especially interesting.
But most of all, nothing is as fascinating as the human face and voice!

*Objects should be placed about 20 cm (8 inches) away from infant.

Maternal attachment. During pregnancy, and in many cases even before conception occurs, parents develop an image of the "ideal or fantasy infant." The unborn child has an imagined appearance, pattern of behavior, expected accomplishments, and predetermined effect on the life-style of the parents. At birth the fantasy infant becomes the real infant. How closely the dream child resembles the real child will influence the acceptance process. If the parents expected an alert, active infant who sleeps little and enjoys human contact and the real infant fulfills these expectations, the attachment process will be facilitated. If parents imagine that the newborn will sleep most of the time, will need little attention except feeding and diapering, and will not disturb their life-style significantly, the birth of a very active infant may cause considerable conflicts in the emotional bonding.

Assessing such expectations during pregnancy and at the time of the infant's birth will allow nurses to identify discrepancies in the parents' view of the fantasy vs the real child.

The labor process also significantly affects the immediate attachment of mothers to their newborn children. In general the mother's perception of maintaining control during the labor and birth process enhances the initial attachment, which, ideally, should take place during the first hour of life. A feeling of loss of control because of factors such as a long, difficult labor, excessive medication and sedation, or unwanted medical intervention will hinder the initial bonding process. Encouraging mothers to talk about their feelings of loss of control, particularly about the specific event that they perceive caused the lack of self-control, allows them to dissipate the emotional energy investigated in these feelings. It is not until such emotional tensions and anxieties are released that parents can attend to the emotional component of the attachment process.

It is believed that there is a *maternal sensitive period* immediately and for a short time after birth when parents

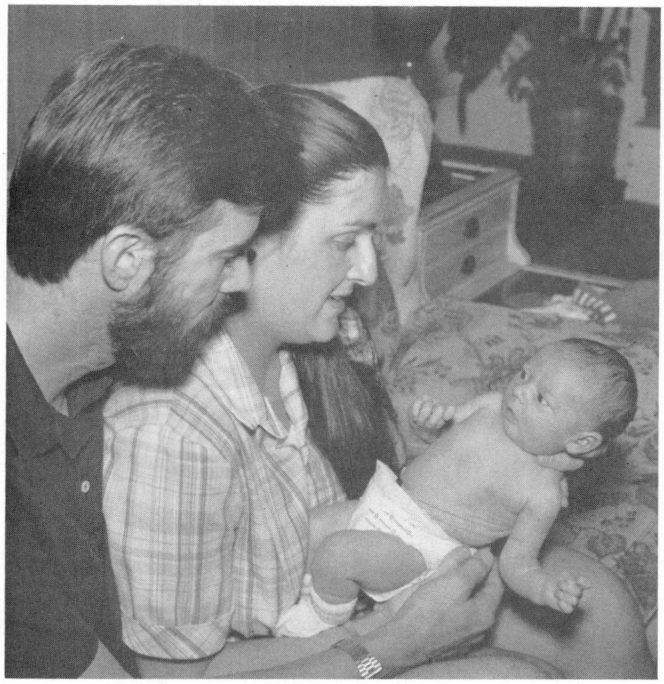

FIG. 8-18 En face position between parents and infant can be significant in attachment process.

have a unique ability to attach to their infants (Klaus and Kennell, 1982). Mothers demonstrate a predictable and orderly pattern of behavior during the development of the attachment process. When mothers are presented with their nude infants, they begin examining the infant with their fingertips, concentrating on touching the extremities, and then proceed to massage and encompass the trunk with their entire hands. Assuming the *en face* position, in which the mother's and the infant's eyes meet in visual contact in the same vertical plane, is significant in the formation of affectional ties (Fig. 8-18).

Although similar patterns of touching have been observed, additional studies demonstrate different patterns for mothers. Consequently nurses must exercise caution in interpreting behaviors such as touching. Observation is important, however, in identifying potential signs of inadequate or delayed mothering. For example, the mother who consistently feeds her infant while holding him at a distance from her body, who supports him with fingertips rather than embracing him in her arms, who does not undress the infant for inspection, and who looks away from the infant most of the time is exhibiting behavior that needs to be assessed more carefully.

Several studies have attempted to substantiate the long-term benefits of providing parents with opportunities to optimally bond with their infant during the initial postpartum period. There has been some evidence that increased parent-child contact at birth encourages prolonged breast-feeding and may minimize the risks of parenting disorders. However, not all studies support the findings relating to parenting disorders, such as child abuse and neglect. In addition, some authorities claim that the emphasis on bonding has been unjustified and may lead to guilt and fear in those parents who did not receive early contact with their infant. Certainly, it should be stressed to parents that although early bonding may be valuable, it does not represent an "all or none" phenomenon. Throughout the child's life there will be multiple opportunities for the development of parent-child attachment. Bonding is a complex process that develops gradually and is influenced by numerous factors.

Another component of successful maternal attachment is the concept of *reciprocity*. As the mother responds to the infant, the infant must respond to the mother by some signal such as sucking, cooing, eye contact, grasping, or molding (conforming to the other's body during close physical contact). Five steps are described in positive mother-infant reciprocity (Brazelton, 1974). The first step is *initiation*, in which interaction between infant and parent begins. Next is *orientation*, which establishes the partners' expectation of each other during the interaction. Following orientation is *acceleration* of the attention cycle to a peak of excitement. The infant reaches out and coos, both arms jerk forward, the head moves backward, the eyes dilate, and the face brightens. After a short time *deceleration* of the excitement and *turning away* occur, in which the infant shifts his eyes away from his mother's and grasps his shirt. During this cycle of nonattention, repeated verbal or visual attempts to reinitiate his attention are ineffective. This deceleration and turning away probably prevent the infant from being overwhelmed by excessive stimuli. In a good interaction both partners have synchronized their attention-nonattention cycles. Parents or other caregivers who do not allow the infant to turn away and who continually attempt to maintain visual contact encourage the infant to turn off his attention cycles and thus prolong the nonattention phase.

Although this description of reciprocal interacting behavior is usually observable in the infant by 2 to 3 weeks of age, nurses can use this information to teach parents how to interact with their infant. Recognizing the attention cycle vs the nonattention cycle and understanding that the latter is not a rejection of the parent is one aspect in helping parents develop competence in parenting.

Monotropy is another component of attachment that has special meaning for health professionals. Monotropy refers to the principle that a person can become optimally attached to only one individual at a time (Klaus and Kennell, 1982). This is very significant in the attachment process that occurs in multiple births. If a parent can form only one attachment at a time, how then can all the siblings of a multiple birth receive optimum emotional care?

Minimal research is available on maternal-twin bonding and the conclusions of different authors vary. Some report that mothers bond equally to each twin at the time of birth, even if one twin is ill (Abbink, 1982). Others suggest that mothers of twins may take months or even years to form individual attachments to each child and even longer if the twins are identical. The mother's separation from a sick twin during the perinatal period can have devastating results, since attachment to the well child occurs quickly but may impede attachment to the other twin (Gromada, 1981).

Nurses can be instrumental in promoting bonding of twins. The most important principle is to assist the parents in recognizing the individuality of the children. The mother should visit with each newborn as much as possible after birth, including a sick infant. Rooming-in and breast-feeding are both feasible and should be encouraged. Any characteristics that are unique to each child are emphasized and each infant is called by name, rather than "the twins." Bonding behaviors are assessed and differences are noted, such as a parent's distinct preference for one twin over the other. In this situation the nurse can gently draw attention to these behaviors and encourage the parent to discuss feelings regarding a multiple birth. The **National Organization of Mothers of Twins Club, Inc.*** and the **Parents of Multiple Birth Association of Canada, Inc.†** can be sources of support to new parents.

Paternal engrossment. Fathers also show specific behaviors during the attachment process, or what has been termed "engrossment," forming a sense of absorption, preoccupation, and interest in the infant. The major characteristics of engrossment include (1) visual awareness of the newborn, especially focusing on the beauty of the child, (2) tactile awareness, often expressed in a desire to hold the infant, (3) awareness of distinct characteristics with emphasis on those features of the infant that resemble the father, (4) perception of the infant as perfect, (5) development of a strong feeling of attraction to the child that leads to intense focusing of attention on him, (6) experiencing a feeling of extreme elation, and (7) feeling a sense of deep self-esteem and satisfaction. These responses are greatest during the early contacts with the infant and are intensified by the neonate's normal reflex activity, especially the grasp reflex, and visual alertness (Greenberg and Morris, 1974).

The development of engrossment has significant implications for nurses. Initially it is imperative that nurses recognize the importance of early father-infant contact in releasing these behaviors. Fathers need to be encouraged to express their positive feelings, especially if such emotions are contrary to the cultural belief that fathers should remain stoic. If this is not clarified, fathers may feel confused and attempt to suppress the natural sensations of absorption, preoccupation, and interest in order to conform with societal expectations.

*5402 Amberwood Lane, Rockville, MD 20853.
†283 7th Ave. South, Lethbridge, Alta, Canada 71J 1H6.

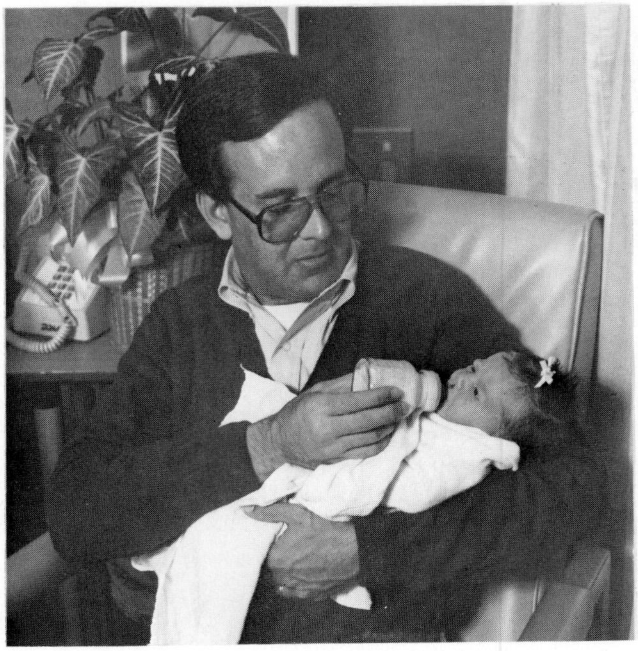

FIG. 8-19 A desire to hold the infant and participate in caregiving activities is an indication of paternal engrossment.

Mothers also need to be aware of the responses of the father toward the newborn, especially since one of the consequences of paternal preoccupation with the infant is less overt attention toward the mother. If both parents are able to share their feelings, each can appreciate the process of attachment toward their child and will avoid the unfortunate conflict of being insensitive and unaware of the other's needs. In addition a father who is encouraged to form a relationship with his newborn is less likely to feel excluded and abandoned once the family returns home and the mother directs her attention toward caring for the infant.

Ideally the process of engrossment should be discussed with parents before the delivery, such as in prenatal classes, to reinforce the father's awareness of his natural feelings toward the expected child. Focusing on the future experience of seeing, touching, and holding one's newborn may also help expectant fathers become more comfortable in accepting their paternal feelings toward the unborn child. This in turn can assist them in being more supportive toward their wives, especially as the labor and delivery event draws near.

At the infant's birth the nurse can play a vital role in assisting the father to release or express engrossment by assessing the neonate in front of the couple; pointing out normal characteristics, especially the grasp reflex; encouraging identification through consistent referral to the child by name; demonstrating whenever necessary the soothing powers of caressing, stroking, and rocking the child; and encouraging the father to cuddle, hold, talk to, or feed the infant (Fig. 8-19) (see Therapeutic dialogue).

THERAPEUTIC DIALOGUE

Encouraging Paternal Engrossment

The nurse brings the newborn to the parents shortly after birth and hands the infant to the father. The father carefully but somewhat unsteadily holds his son.

NURSE: Jonathan is so perfect and beautiful.

FATHER: Yes, but he is so small and fragile.

NURSE: He is small, but you think he is fragile?

FATHER: Yes. I never feel good around babies. They are cute and all, but I am always afraid I will drop them or hurt them.

NURSE: How do you think you could hurt them?

FATHER: I could squeeze them too hard or hurt that soft spot on the head.

NURSE: You are afraid of hurting them because you think they are fragile (nurse uses facilitative responding, p. 110).

FATHER: Yes, I already told my wife that she will have to do everything. She will be a good mother.

NURSE: Mrs. H., what do you think about all of this?

MOTHER: Well, I am a little afraid too but I would like to have some help with the baby. Do you think babies are so fragile?

NURSE: No. They look fragile because they are so small and, of course, they should be handled gently. But they don't break easily and they like firm hugging. Let's look at Jonathan's soft spot.

◆ ◆ ◆

The nurse proceeds to show them the fontanels, explains their purpose, and has the parents feel the head. She explains that the skin over this area is not likely to tear or puncture. She demonstrates the grasp reflex and how the infant's grasp is strong enough for the nurse to pull him slightly forward. She encourages the parents, especially the father, to hold the infant in different positions.

◆ ◆ ◆

FATHER: I never knew those things about the head. And I never knew you could pick up babies so many different ways. Jonathan seems to like being held against my shoulder. I guess that with practice this will feel more natural for me. He really is cute and he has strong hands. I bet he will be a good baseball player.

Fathers are encouraged to be with the mother during labor and delivery and to spend time alone with the mother and newborn after delivery. Whenever possible, the father should "room in" with the mother.

The nurse looks for the same indication of affectional ties from the father as those expected in the mother, such as visual contact in the *en face* position and embracing the infant close to the body. When present, such behaviors are reinforced. If such responses are not obvious, the nurse needs to assess the father's feelings regarding this birth, cultural beliefs that may prevent his emotional expression, and other factors, in order to help him facilitate a positive attachment during this critical period. Literature can also be given to the parents to help them understand the process of attachment and its importance in parent-infant bonding.*

Siblings. Although the attachment process has been discussed almost exclusively in terms of the parents and infant, it is essential that nurses be aware of other family members, such as siblings and members of the extended family, who need preparation for the acceptance of this

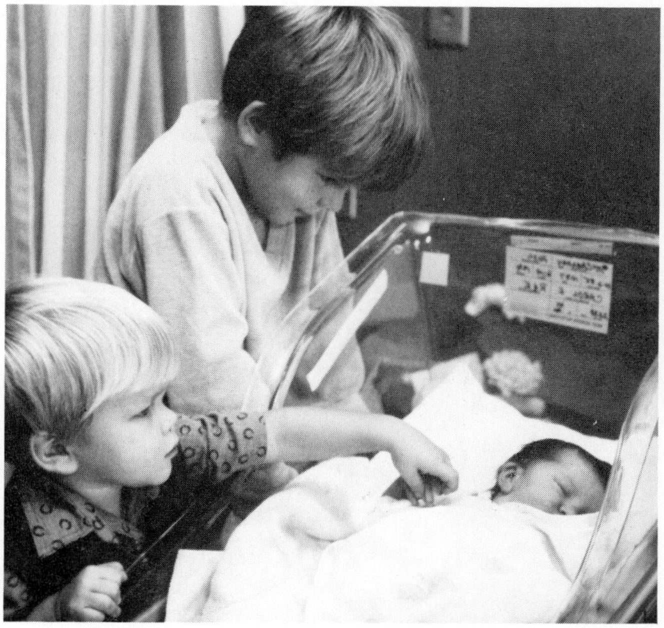

FIG. 8-20 Sibling visitation shortly after birth can be significant in the attachment process.

*A suggested book is *On becoming a family: the growth of attachment,* by T.B. Brazelton, NY, 1981, Dell Publishing Co., Inc.

NURSING CARE PLAN

The Newborn and Family

Nursing Goals	Nursing Interventions	Expected Patient/Family Outcomes
NDx HP-HMP*	**Potential for infection** **Risk factors: deficient immunologic defenses, environmental factors**	
	Transitional Care	
Protect from infection and trauma	Wash hands before and after caring for each infant Never leave infant unsupervised on a raised surface without sides Always close diaper pins and place them away from infant's body Keep pointed or sharp objects out of infant's reach Keep own fingernails short and trimmed; avoid jewelry that can scratch infant	Infant exhibits no evidence of infection or trauma
	Care in Nursery or Mother's Room	
	Check eyes daily for any discharge Ideally, involve mother and father in bathing of infant Clean vulva in posterior direction to prevent fecal contamination of vagina or urethra; stress this to parents While cleaning penis, do not retract foreskin; gently wipe away smegma Maintain asepsis during circumcision If infant has been circumcised, cover area with a petrolatum jelly gauze (if ordered)	Eyes remain clear with no evidence of irritation Genital area is free of irritation
	Keep umbilical stump clean and dry Place diapers below umbilical stump Assess cord daily for odor, color, and drainage	Cord appears dry, surrounding area free of infection
NDx N-MP	**Ineffective thermoregulation** **Risk factor: immature temperature control**	
	Transitional Care	
Maintain stable body temperature	Wrap infant snugly in a warmed blanket Place infant in a preheated environment (under radiant warmer or next to mother) Place infant on a padded, covered surface Keep infant away from drafts, air conditioning vents, or fans Place infant in a recessed cubicle with walls high enough to shield from cross ventilation Warm all objects used to examine or cover infant, for example, place them under radiant warmer Uncover only one area of body for examination or procedures Monitor skin temperature and relate it to ambient air temperature; decreased skin temperature may indicate radiant heat loss Take axillary temperature according to institutional policy or until stable Be aware of signs of hypothermia or hyperthermia Postpone bath for first 4 to 6 hours until temperature stabilizes at 37°C Postpone circumcision until after postnatal recovery period	Infant's temperature remains at optimum level (36.5° to 37.5°C [97.7° to 99.5°F])

*For an explanation of abbreviations, see p. 20.

NURSING CARE PLAN

The Newborn and Family—cont'd

Nursing Goals	Nursing Interventions	Expected Patient/Family Outcomes
	Care in Nursery or Mother's Room	
	Take infant's temperature on arrival at nursery or mother's room and, if stable, proceed according to hospital policy Maintain room temperature between 24° and 25.5°C (75° to 78°F) and humidity about 40% to 50% Dress infant in a shirt and diaper and swaddle in a blanket Prevent chilling of infant during daily bath If there is any question regarding stabilization of body temperature, postpone bath Keep infant's head covered if heat loss is a problem	
ND N-MP Potential altered nutrition **Risk factors: immaturity, parental knowledge deficit**		
	Transitional Care	
Provide optimum nutrition	During first hour after delivery, put infant to mother's breast when possible Postpone bottle-feeding of 5% glucose water until sucking and swallowing are well coordinated Do not offer routine water or supplemental feedings to breast-feeding infants	Infant demonstrates strong suck
	Care in Nursery or Mother's Room	
	Assess strength of suck and coordination with swallowing Bring breast-fed infants to mothers on demand during day and night Offer bottle-fed infants 2 to 3 ounces of formula after they have retained their glucose feeding Support and assist breast-feeding mothers during initial feedings Encourage father to remain with mother to help her and infant with positioning, relaxation, and reinforcement Encourage father to participate in bottle-feeding	Infant receives an adequate amount of nutrients (specify amount and frequency of feedings) Infant loses 10% of birth weight or less
	Place infant on right side after feeding to prevent regurgitation Observe stool pattern	Infant retains feedings
ND A-EP Ineffective airway clearance **Etiology: excess mucus, improper positioning**		
	Transitional Care	
Establish and maintain patent airway	Suction mouth and nasopharynx with bulb syringe as needed Lavage stomach of amniotic fluid and check for tracheoesophageal anomalies (not routinely done in all hospitals) Position infant on side or abdomen with head slightly lower than chest (about 15 degrees) to facilitate drainage of secretions Perform as few procedures as possible on infant during first hour and have oxygen ready for use if respiratory distress should develop Take vital signs according to institutional policy and more frequently if necessary	Breathing is regular and unlabored Respiratory rate is within normal limits (see inside front cover for normal variations) Gastric aspirate is less than 20 ml (if performed)

*Nursing outcome.

Continued.

NURSING CARE PLAN

The Newborn and Family—cont'd

Nursing Goals	Nursing Interventions	Expected Patient/Family Outcomes
	Care in Nursery or Mother's Room	
	Position infant on right side or abdomen after feeding to prevent aspiration Keep diapers, clothing, and blankets loose enough to allow maximum lung (abdominal) expansion Clean nares of any crusted secretions during bath or when necessary Check for patent nares	Airway remains patent
RRP Altered family processes **Etiology: maturational crisis, birth of term infant, change in family unit**		
Facilitate siblings' adjustment to newborn	Allow to visit and touch newborn when feasible Explain physical differences in newborn, such as bald head, umbilical stump and clamp, circumcision Explain to siblings realistic expectations regarding newborn abilities and needs Requires complete care Is not a playmate Encourage siblings to participate in care at home Encourage parents to spend individual time with other children at home	Siblings express interest in newborn and realistic expectations for their age
RRP Potential altered parenting **Risk factors: knowledge deficit, lack of available role models**		
	Transitional Care	
Facilitate parent-infant attachment process	As soon after delivery as possible, allow parents to see and hold infant; place newborn close to face of parents so that visual contact can be established; ensure infant's identity Ideally, perform eye care after initial meeting of infant and parents, usually about 1 hour after birth Identify for parents specific behaviors manifested by infant, for example, alertness, ability to see, vigorous suck, rooting behavior, and attention to human voice	Parents establish contact with infant immediately or soon after birth *ID bracelet is in place Parents demonstrate attachment behaviors, such as touch, eye contact, naming and calling infant by name, talking to infant, participating in caregiving activities Family members avail themselves of needed services
	Care in Nursery or Mother's Room	
	Discuss with parents their expectations of fantasy child vs real child Encourage parents to "talk out" their labor and delivery experience; identify any events that signify loss of control to either parent, especially mother	Family discusses expectations for child and delivery experience
	Identify behavioral steps in attachment process and evaluate those aspects that could be considered positive and those that may represent inadequate or delayed parenting	Parents demonstrate positive attachment behaviors
	Encourage family to call for infant frequently Observe and assess the reciprocity of cues between infant and parent	Parents spend considerable time with infant (specified amount)
	Assist parents in recognizing attention-nonattention cycles and in understanding their significance Assess variables affecting development of attachment through observing infant and parent and interviewing each parent or other significant caregiver	Parents recognize attention-nonattention cycles
	If parent-infant attachment is at risk, refer to appropriate agencies (social services, family and child services, at-risk programs)	Parents avail themselves of resources

*Nursing outcome.

NURSING CARE PLAN

The Newborn and Family—cont'd

Nursing Goals	Nursing Interventions	Expected Patient/Family Outcomes
Prepare for discharge	Instruct in newborn care Feeding (formula or breast) Bathing Umbilical and circumcision care Encourage participation in parenting classes, if offered Discuss importance and proper use of federally approved car restraints Refer to organizations that may rent car restraints	Family demonstrates ability to provide care for infant Family keeps appointments for follow-up care Infant rides home in federally approved car restraint

Nursing interventions related to medical management

Protect from infection and injury
Instill prophylactic eye medication into conjunctival sac of each eye from inner canthus outward; do not irrigate eyes with sterile saline
Administer vitamin K intramuscularly, using vastus lateralis muscle as site of injection
Apply antibacterial agent or alcohol or both to cord as ordered

Assist in identifying congenital disorders
Collect blood specimens for required screening tests

*Nursing outcome.

new child. Young children in particular need sensitive preparation for the birth to minimize sibling rivalry (Fig. 8-20) (see also p. 340).

There is an increasing trend to allow siblings to visit the mother on the postpartum unit and in some instances to hold the newborn. Siblings have even been allowed to witness the birth. However, they need preparation for and support during these events.

Prepare for Discharge and Care at Home

With increasingly shorter postpartum hospitalizations, and the trend towards home deliveries, discharge planning, referral, and home visiting are important components of comprehensive care. First-time as well as "experienced" parents benefit from guidance and assistance with the infant's care, such as breast- or formula-feeding and with the family's integration of a new member, particularly sibling adjustment (see p. 349). To assess and meet these needs, discharge planning *must* begin immediately on admission to the hospital or birthing center. A nursing admission history assists in systematic collection of data to formulate nursing diagnoses and to plan care. This assessment continues throughout the admission and includes the family's support system. Nurses in the birthing, nursery, and postpartum units need to coordinate their assessments for the most effective interventions.

Ideally, the family should receive a home visit shortly after an early discharge to assess their immediate adjustments and deal with their concerns, which commonly relate to breast-feeding, maternal fatigue and depression, bonding, neonatal jaundice, and excessive infant crying (Jansson, 1985).

Professional support for the new family should be continued from the hospital to the home through community services as needed. The concept of family-centered care is practiced when the family receives consistent comprehensive care beginning with preventive prenatal care and continuing through child health maintenance.

EVALUATION

The effectiveness of nursing interventions is determined by continual reassessment and evaluation of care based on the following observational guidelines and expected outcomes:

1. Observe infant's color and respiratory patterns
2. Monitor axillary temperature regularly; observe for signs of chilling, such as skin mottling
3. Observe for any evidence of infection, especially at umbilicus or site of circumcision; check presence of identification bands; check medical record for documentation of prophylactic eye treatment, vitamin K injection, and genetic screening test
4. Monitor daily weight
5. Observe interactions between infant and family members; interview family regarding their feelings toward the newborn
6. Observe parents' ability to provide care for infant; interview parents regarding any concerns about infant's care at home

Expected outcomes:
See Nursing Care Plan, pp. 208 to 211.

SUMMARY

The birth of an infant is a major transitional period for the family. Not only must the newborn's physical needs be met, but the family's attachment to the child must be facilitated. Expert and sensitive nursing care from the time of delivery to discharge from the nursery is essential in meeting these goals. Nurses need to have a knowledge of the physiologic adjustments to extrauterine life that are required of the neonate and those interventions needed to support these adjustments. They must be aware of the usual findings on physical assessment that indicate the infant's normalcy. In addition, they must be able to provide the physical care consistent with the total dependency of the newborn and the psychologic care that promotes positive bonding between the infant and family.

KEY CONCEPTS

- Transition from fetal or placental circulation to independent respiration is the most important physiologic change required of the newborn.
- Chemical and thermal factors help initiate the neonate's first respiration.
- Circulatory changes in the neonate result from shifts in pressure in the heart and major vessels and from functional closures of the fetal shunts.
- The newborn's large surface area, thin layer of subcutaneous fat, and unique mechanism for producing heat predispose the newborn to excessive heat loss.
- The skin and mucous membranes, the reticuloendothelial system, and antibodies are the first, second, and third lines of defense against infection.
- Apgar scoring, the initial assessment of the newborn, focuses on heart rate, respiratory effort, muscle tone, reflex irritability, and color.
- Physical assessment of the newborn includes assessment of clinical gestational age, general measurements, general appearance, and head-to-toe assessment.
- Neurologic assessment focuses on localized reflexes and posture, muscle tone, head control, and movement and is best accomplished during the general physical examination.
- Behavioral assessment is concerned with the newborn's interaction with the environment. The principal areas of behavior for newborns are sleep, wakefulness, and activity, including crying.
- Physical care for the newborn includes maintaining a patent airway, maintaining stable body temperature, protecting from infection and injury, and providing optimum nutrition.
- Breast-feeding is the preferred method of infant nutrition as it offers significant physiologic and psychologic benefits. Bottle-feeding includes the use of commercial or evaporated milk formula and is an acceptable substitute for breast-feeding.
- Although the attachment, or bonding, process primarily affects infants and parents, siblings also play an important role.

STUDY QUESTIONS AND ACTIVITIES

1 Care for a newborn and the parents soon after birth. Describe the physical care needed by the infant to facilitate adjustment to extrauterine life and early signs of maternal/paternal attachment.

2 Perform a transitional and physical assessment and estimate gestational age on a newborn. Record the findings and compare them to the discussion in the text, noting any differences from the normal findings described.

3 Interview two mothers who have selected different feeding methods and describe the reasons why each chose breast-feeding or bottle-feeding. Did the mother who chose bottle-feeding identify a perceived disadvantage to breast-feeding that might have been changed with additional education?

4 Outline a teaching plan for parents on one of the following infant care areas: bathing, breast-feeding, or bottle-feeding.

5 Observe the interactions of various family members (ideally, mother, father, and siblings) to the newborn and record their behaviors, such as touching, talking, inspecting, and comforting. Compare how the behaviors differ among the members.

REFERENCES

Abbink, C.: Bonding as perceived by mothers of twins, Pediatr. Nurs. **8**(6):411-413, 1982.

American Academy of Pediatrics and American College of Obstetricians and Gynecologists: Guidelines for perinatal care, ed. 2, Elk Grove Village, IL, 1988, The Academy.

American Academy of Pediatrics, Committee on Fetus and Newborn: Report of the Ad Hoc Task Force on Circumcision, Pediatrics **56:**610-611, Oct. 1975.

American Academy of Pediatrics, Committee on Fetus and Newborn, and others: Neonatal anesthesia, Pediatrics **80**(3):446, 1987.

Avant, P.K.: A maternal attachment assessment strategy. In Humenick, S.S., editor: Analysis of current assessment strategies in the health care of young children and childbearing families, Norwalk, CT, 1982, Appleton-Century-Crofts.

Brazelton, T.B.: Neonatal behavioral assessment scale, ed. 2, Philadelphia, 1984, J.B. Lippincott Co.

Brazelton, T.B.: Mother-infant reciprocity. In Klaus, M., and others, editors: Maternal attachment and mothering disorders, New Brunswick, NJ, 1974, Johnson & Johnson Baby Products Co.

Fuller, R.: Upper respiratory obstruction in the neonate: a case of neonatal rhinitis, Pediatr. Nurs. **14**(1):30-31, 1988.

Greenberg, M., and Morris, N.: Engrossment: the newborn's impact upon the father, Am. J. Orthopsychiatry **44**(4):520-531, 1974.

Gromada, K.: Maternal-infant attachment: the first step toward individualizing twins, MCN **6**(2):129-134, 1981.

Jansson, P.: Early postpartum discharge, Am. J. Nurs. **85**(5):547-550, 1985.

Klaus, M.H., and Kennell, J.H., editors: Parent-infant bonding, ed. 2, St. Louis, 1982, The C.V. Mosby Co.

Lawrence, R.: Breast-feeding: a guide for the medical profession, ed. 2, St. Louis, 1985, The C.V. Mosby Co.

Maxwell, L., and others: Penile nerve block for newborn circumcision, Obstet. Gynecol. **71**(3):415-419, 1987.

National Society to Prevent Blindness, Committee on Ophthalmia Neonatorum: Prevention and treatment of ophthalmia neonatorum, New York, 1981, The National Society.

Patel, D., and others: Bacterial colonization of plastic bulb syringes, J. Pediatr. **112**(3):466-468, 1988.

Report of the Second Task Force on Blood Pressure Control in Children–1987, Pediatrics **79**(1):1-25, 1987.

Riordan, J.: A practical guide to breastfeeding, St. Louis, 1983, The C.V. Mosby Co.

BIBLIOGRAPHY

Physiologic Status/Assessment of the Newborn

Baron, M., and Tafuro, P.: The extremes of age: the newborn and the elderly, Nurs. Clin. North Am. **20**(1):181-190, 1985.

Cloherty, J.P., and Stark, A.R., editors: Manual of neonatal care, ed. 2, Boston, 1985, Little, Brown & Co.

Davis, V.: The structure and function of brown adipose tissue in the neonate, JOGNN **9**(6):368-372, 1980.

Fanaroff, A., and Martin, R., editors: Neonatal-perinatal medicine: diseases of the fetus and infant, ed. 4, St. Louis, 1987, The C.V. Mosby Co.

The first six hours of life: assessment of risk in the newborn: evaluation during the transitional period, New York, 1980, March of Dimes—Birth Defects Foundation.

Frodi, A.M., and others: Fathers' and mothers' responses to the face and cries of normal and premature infants, Dev. Psychobiol. **14:**490-498, 1978.

Johnson, T.R., and others: Children are different: developmental physiology, ed. 2, Columbus, OH, 1978, Ross Laboratories.

Judd, J.M.: Assessing the newborn from head to toe, Nursing 85 **15**(12):34-41, 1985.

Korones, S.B.: High-risk newborn infants: the basis for intensive nursing care, ed. 4, St. Louis, 1986, The C.V. Mosby Co.

Labson, L.H.: Newborn exam: evaluation in the nursery, Patient Care **17**(10):95-98, 1983.

Lester, B.M.: There's more to crying than meets the ear, Child Care Newsletter **2**(2):1-5, 1983.

Ludington-Hoe, S.M.: What can newborns really see? Am. J. Nurs. **83**(9):1286-1289, 1983.

Marchbanks, P.: Newborn assessment: physical examination. In Humenick, S.S., editor: Analysis of current assessment strategies in the health care of young children and childbearing families, Norwalk, CT, 1982, Appleton-Century-Crofts.

Ruchala, P.: The effect of wearing headcoverings on the axillary temperatures of infants, MCN **10**(4):240, 1985.

Scanlon, J.W., and others: A system of newborn physical examination, Baltimore, 1979, University Park Press.

Scharping, E.M.: Physiological measurements of the neonate, MCN **8**(1):70-73, 1983.

Schiffman, R.F.: Temperature monitoring in the neonate: a comparison of axillary and rectal temperatures, Nurs. Res. **31**(5):274-277, 1982.

Taylor, K.M.: The Apgar scoring system. In Humenick, S.S., editor: Analysis of current assessment strategies in the health care of young children and childbearing families, Norwalk, CT, 1982, Appleton-Century-Crofts.

Taylor, K.M.: Gestational age assessment. In Humenick, S.S., editor: Analysis of current assessment strategies in the health care of young children and childbearing families, Norwalk, CT, 1982, Appleton-Century-Crofts.

Nursing Care of the Newborn

Albers, R.M.: Emotional support for the breast-feeding mother, Issues Compr. Pediatr. Nurs. **5:**109-124, 1981.

American Academy of Pediatrics Policy Statement Based on Task Force Report: The promotion of breast-feeding, Pediatrics **69**(5):654-661, 1982.

Boyer, K.B.: Routine circumcision of the newborn: reasonable precaution or unnecessary risk? J. Nurse Midwife **25:**27-31, 1980.

Boyes, S.M.: AIDS virus in breast milk: a new threat to neonates and donor breast milk banks, Neonatal Network **5**(5):37-39, 1987.

Caravella, S., Clark, D., and Dweck, H.: Health codes for newborn care, Pediatrics **80**(1):1-5, 1987.

Cusson, R.M.: Attitudes toward breast-feeding among female high-school students, Pediatr. Nurs. **11**(3):189-191, 1985.

Field, T., and Goldson, E.: Pacifying effects of nonnutritive sucking on term and preterm neonates during heelstick procedures, Pediatrics **74:**1012-1015, 1984.

Gibbons, M.B.: Circumcision: the controversy continues, Pediatr. Nurs. **10**(2):103-109, 1984.

Grimes, D.A.: Routine circumcision reconsidered, Am. J. Nurs. **1**(80):108-109, 1980.

Gulick, E.: Infant health and breast-feeding, Pediatr. Nurs. **9**(5):359-362+, 1983.

Harris, C.C., and Stern, P.N.: Care of the prepuce in the uncircumcised child: reinforcing nature's laws of health, Issues Compr. Pediatr. Nurs. **5:**233-242, 1981.

Hobbie, C.: Breastfeeding and returning to work, J. Pediatr. Health Care **1**(2):108-109, 1987.

Humenick, S.S., and Van Steenkiste, S.: Early indicators of breast-feeding progress, Issues Compr. Pediatr. Nurs. **6:**205-215, 1983.

Jeffries, R.D.: A short course in breastfeeding, Issues Compr. Pediatr. Nurs. **5:**243-251, 1981.

Lindeke, L., Iverson, S., and Fisch, R.: Neonatal circumcision: a social and medical dilemma, Matern. Child Nurs. J. **12** (1):31-37, 1986.

Lum, B., and Lortz, R.: Reappraising newborn eye care, Am. J. Nurs. **80**(9):1602-1603, 1980.

McDermott, R.J., Wilson, D.D., and Marty, P.J.: Neonatal circumcision, Patient Couns. Health Educ. **3**(4):132-136, 1982.

Pipes, P.L.: Nutrition in infancy and childhood, ed. 3, St. Louis, 1985, The C.V. Mosby Co.

Sasso, S.C.: Erythromycin for eye prophylaxis, MCN **9:**417, 1984.

Schlegel, A.M.: Observations on breast-feeding technique: facts and fallacies, MCN **8**(3):204-208, 1983.

Taylor, L.S.: Newborn feeding behaviors and attaching, MCN **6**(3):201-202, 1981.

Wayland, J.R., and Higgins, P.G.: Newborn circumcision: father's involvement, Pediatr. Nurs. **9**(1):41-42, 1983.

Wink, D.: Getting through the maze of infant formulas, Am. J. Nurs. **85**(4):388-392, 1985.

Wood, C.S., and others: Exclusively breast-fed infants: growth and caloric intake, Pediatr. Nurs. **14**(2):117-124, 1988.

Worthington-Roberts, B.S., Vermeersch, J., and Williams, S.R.: Nutrition in pregnancy and lactation, St. Louis, 1985, Times Mirror/Mosby College Publishing.

Parent-Infant Bonding (Attachment)

American Academy of Pediatrics, Committee on Fetus and Newborn: Postpartum (neonatal) sibling visitation, Pediatrics **76**(4):650, 1985.

Anderson, C.J.: Enhancing reciprocity between mother and neonate, Nurs. Res. **30**(2):89-93, 1981.

Anderson, C.J.: Integration of the Brazelton Neonatal Behavioral Assessment Scale into routine neonatal nursing care, Issues Compr. Pediatr. Nurs. **9**:341-351, 1986.

Beal, J.A.: The Brazelton Neonatal Behavioral Assessment Scale: a tool to enhance parental attachment, J. Pediatr. Nurs. **1**(3):170-177, 1986.

Buckner, E.B.: Use of Brazelton Neonatal Behavioral Assessment in planning care for parents and newborns, JOGNN **12**:26-30, 1983.

Cannon, R.B.: The development of maternal touch during early mother-infant interaction, JOGNN **6**(2):28-33, 1977.

Carter-Jessop, L.: Promoting maternal attachment through prenatal intervention, MCN **6**(2):107-112, 1981.

Cronenwett, L.R., and Kunst-Wilson, W.: Stress, social support, and the transition to fatherhood, Nurs. Res. **30**(4):196-201, 1981.

Cropley, C.: Assessment of mothering behaviors. In Johnson, S.H., editor: Nursing assessment and strategies for the family at risk, ed. 2, Philadelphia, 1986, J.B. Lippincott Co.

Daniels, M.: The birth experience for the sibling: description and evaluation of a program, J. Nurse Midwife **28**(5):15-22, 1983.

Dean, P.G., Morgan, P., and Towle, J.M.: Making baby's acquaintance: a unique attachment strategy, MCN **7**(1):37-41, 1982.

Foley, K.L.: Caring for the parents of newborn twins, MCN **4**(4):221-226, 1979.

Goldberg, S.: Parent-infant bonding: another look, Child Dev. **54**:1355-1382, 1983.

Grace, J.T.: Does a mother's knowledge of fetal gender affect attachment? MCN **9**:42-45, 1984.

Jenkins, R.L., and Westhus, N.K.: The nurse role in parent-infant bonding: overview, assessment, intervention, JOGNN **10**(2):114-118, 1981.

Karraker, K.H.: Adult attention to infants in a newborn nursery, Nurs. Res. **35**(6):358-363, 1986.

Klaus, M., and Kennell, J.: Parent to infant bonding: setting the record straight, J. Pediatr. **102**(4):575-576, 1983.

Lumley, J.: Preschool siblings at birth: short-term effects, Birth **10**(1):11-16, 1983.

Marecki, M., and others: Early sibling attachment, JOGNN **14**(5):418-423, 1985.

Mercer, R.T.: The nurse and maternal tasks of early postpartum, MCN **6**(5):341-345, 1981.

Mitchell, K., and Mills, N.M.: Is the sensitive period in parent-infant bonding overrated? Pediatr. Nurs. **9**(2):91-94, 1983.

Murphy, C.M.: Assessment of fathering behaviors. In Johnson, S.H., editor: Nursing assessment and strategies for the family at risk, ed. 2, 1986, Philadelphia, J.B. Lippincott Co., pp. 36-49.

Nugent, J.K.: The Brazelton Neonatal Behavioral Assessment Scale: implications for intervention, Pediatr. Nurs. **7**(3):18-21, 1981.

Perez, P.: Nurturing children who attend the birth of a sibling, MCN **4**(4):215-217, 1979.

Roberts, F.B.: Infant behavior and the transition to parenthood, Nurs. Res. **32**(4):213-217, 1983.

Tomlinson, P.S.: Fathers' involvement with first-born infants: interpersonal and situational factors, Pediatr. Nurs. **13** (2):101-105, 1987.

Toney, L.: The effects of holding the newborn at delivery on paternal bonding, Nurs. Res. **32**(1):16-19, 1983.

Walker, L.O.: Brazelton Neonatal Behavioral Assessment Scale. In Humenick, S.S., editor: Analysis of current assessment strategies in the health care of young children and childbearing families, Norwalk, CT, 1982, Appleton-Century-Crofts.

Walker, L.O., Crain, H., and Thompson, E.: Mothering behavior and maternal role attainment during the postpartum period, Nurs. Res. **35**(6):352-355, 1986.

Walz, B.L.: Maternal tasks of taking on a second child in the postpartum period, Matern. Child Nurs. J. **12**(3):185-216, 1983.

Weaver, R.H., and Cranley, M.S.: An exploration of paternal-fetal attachment behavior, Nurs. Res. **32**(2):68-72, 1983.

Wieser, M.A., and Castiglia, P.T.: Assessing early father-infant attachment, MCN **9**(2):104-106, 1984.

CHAPTER 9

Health Problems of the Newborn

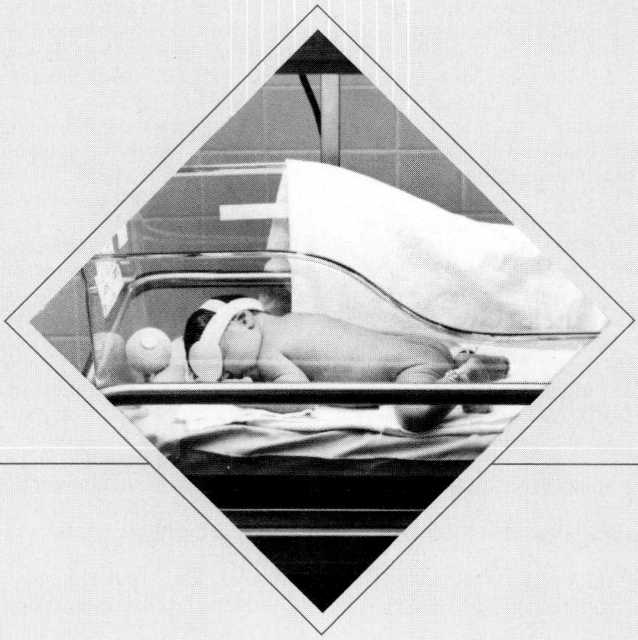

LEARNING OBJECTIVES

On completion of this chapter the reader will be able to:

- Recognize common deviations from the normal expectations in the newborn
- Perform a systematic assessment of an ill newborn
- Outline a general plan of care for a high-risk infant
- Discuss the role of the nurse in facilitating positive parent-child relationships
- Contrast the characteristics of a premature infant and a full-term infant
- Discuss the rationale for screening newborns and for providing genetic counseling for families of a newborn with a hereditary condition
- Modify a general care plan to meet the needs of an infant with a specific high-risk health deviation

Factors that determine the degree to which the newborn adjusts to the extrauterine environment are numerous and varied. Certain factors determine the innate constitutional structure and function of the neonate. These include hereditary characteristics and environmental factors that influence development from the time of conception. The immature physiologic systems of the newborn impose threats to his survival. Although infants are able to survive before the optimum level of maturity has been reached, there is a point at which extrauterine existence is impossible even with excellent, intensive prenatal, intrapartum, and postnatal care. In addition, there are all those factors that produce pathologic conditions in an otherwise normal, full-term infant. These pathologic conditions may be directly related to the birth process or may be postnatal hazards to the newborn. Some of the conditions require no intervention other than careful assessment and continued observation to distinguish them from potential pathologic situations. Others require immediate identification and intervention to prevent future problems. The nurse's ability to recognize such conditions and institute appropriate care significantly affects the neonate's immediate survival and later development.

◆ *Birth Injuries*

Birth injuries that occur during the birth process are most likely to occur when the baby is large, the presentation is breech, forceful extraction is used, or inexperienced practitioners manage the delivery.

Many injuries are minor and resolve spontaneously in a few days; others, although minor, require some degree of intervention. Still others can be very serious, even fatal. Part of the nurse's responsibility is to identify such injuries in order that appropriate intervention can be initiated as soon as possible.

SOFT TISSUE INJURY

Various types of soft tissue injury may be sustained during the process of birth, primarily in the form of bruises and/or abrasions secondary to dystocia. Soft tissue injury usually occurs when there is some degree of disproportion between the presenting part and the maternal pelvis (cephalopelvic disproportion). Application of forceps to facilitate a difficult vertex delivery may produce discoloration or abrasion of the same configuration as the forceps on the sides of the neonate's face. Petechiae or ecchymoses may be observed on the presenting part after a breech or brow delivery. The sudden release of pressure on the head can produce scleral hemorrhages and/or generalized petechiae over the face and head after a difficult or too-rapid delivery. Rarely, lacerations occur during cesarean section.

These traumatic lesions generally fade spontaneously within a few days, without treatment. However, petechiae may be a manifestation of some underlying bleeding disorders and should be evaluated. Nursing care is primarily directed toward assessing the injury and providing an explanation and reassurance to the parents.

HEAD TRAUMA

Trauma to the head that occurs during the birth process is usually benign but occasionally results in more serious injury. The injuries that produce serious trauma, such as intraventricular hemorrhage and subdural hematoma, are discussed in relation to neurologic disturbances (see Chapter 27). Skull fractures are discussed in association with other fractures sustained during the process of birth.

Caput Succedaneum

The most commonly observed scalp lesion is caput succedaneum, a vaguely outlined area of edematous tissue situated over the portion of the scalp that presents in a vertex delivery (Fig. 9-1). The swelling consists of serum or blood, or both, accumulated in the tissues above the

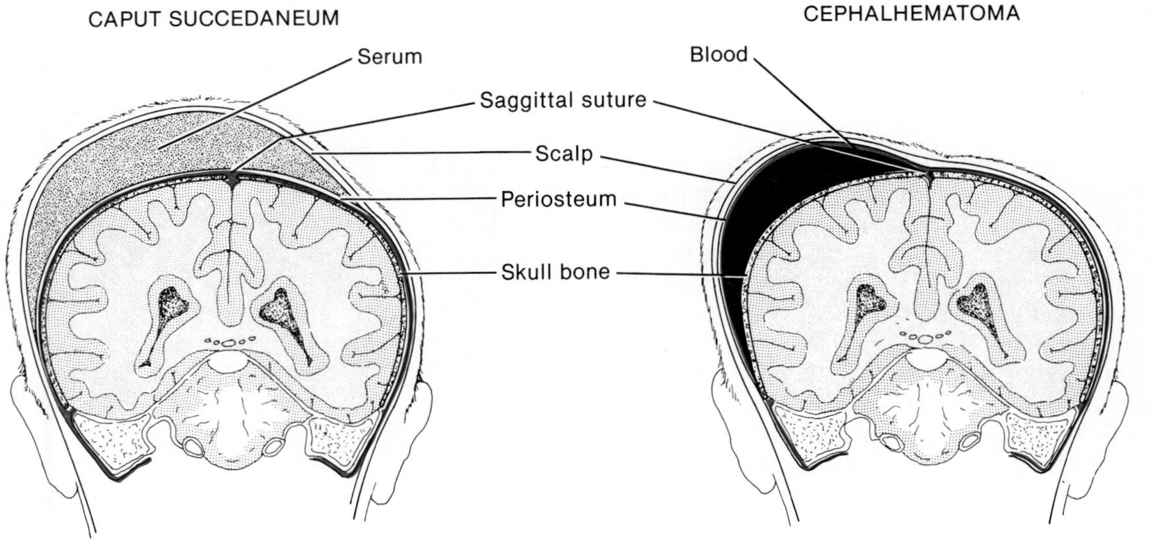

Description: Edema of soft scalp tissue
Manifestations: Ill-defined, soft, nonfluctuant mass; pitting edema
Onset: Within 24 hours after birth

Description: Hematoma between periosteum and skull bone
Manifestations: Well-defined, soft, fluctuant mass
Onset: 24 to 48 hours after birth

FIG. 9-1 Comparison of caput succedaneum and cephalhematoma. (Modified from Bobak, I.M., and Jensen, M.D.: Maternity and gynecologic care: the nurse and the family, ed. 4, St. Louis, 1989, The C.V. Mosby Co.)

bone, and it often extends beyond the bone margins. The swelling may be associated with overlying petechiae or ecchymoses. No specific treatment is needed, and the swelling subsides within a few days.

Cephalhematoma

Infrequently, a cephalhematoma is formed when blood vessels rupture during a difficult labor or delivery, producing bleeding into the area between the bone and its periosteum. The boundaries of the cephalhematoma are sharply demarcated and do not extend beyond the limits of the bone (Fig. 9-1). The cephalhematoma may involve one or both parietal bones. Less frequently, the occipital and, rarely, the frontal bones are affected. The swelling is usually minimal at birth but increases in size on the second or third day.

No treatment is indicated for uncomplicated cephalhematoma, and most lesions are absorbed within 2 weeks to 3 months. Lesions that result in severe blood loss to the area or that involve an underlying fracture require further evaluation and appropriate therapy.

Nursing Considerations

Nursing care is directed toward assessment and observation of the two head injuries and vigilance in observing for possible associated complications such as infection, subdural hematoma, or intraventricular hemorrhage. Because both of these visible injuries resolve spontaneously, parents need reassurance of their usual benign nature.

FRACTURES

Fracture of the clavicle, or collarbone, is the most frequent birth injury. It is often associated with difficult vertex or breech delivery of infants of greater than average weight. The newborn with a fractured clavicle may have no symptoms, but a fracture should be suspected if an infant has limited use of the affected arm, malposition of the arm, asymmetric Moro reflex, focal swelling or tenderness, or cries in pain when the arm is moved. Crepitus (the crackling sound produced by the rubbing together of fractured bone fragments) is often heard on further examination, and radiographs usually reveal a complete fracture with overriding of the fragments.

Fractures of long bones, such as the femur or the humerus, are difficult to detect by radiographic examination. Although osteogenesis imperfecta is a rare finding, a newborn infant with a fracture should be assessed for other evidence of this congenital disorder.

Fractures of the neonatal skull are uncommon. The bones, which are less mineralized and more compressible than bones in older infants and children, are separated by membranous seams that allow sufficient alteration in the head contour so that it adjusts to the birth canal during delivery. Skull fractures usually follow prolonged, difficult delivery or forceps extraction. Most fractures are linear, but some may be visible as depressed indentations resembling a Ping-Pong ball.

Nursing Considerations

Frequently, no intervention may be prescribed other than proper body alignment, careful dressing and undressing of the infant, and handling and carrying that support the affected bone. Occasionally, for immobilization and relief of pain, the arm on the side of the fractured clavicle may be fixed on the body by pinning the sleeve to the shirt or by application of a triangular sling or a figure-8 bandage.

Linear skull fractures usually require no treatment. A Ping-Pong type fracture usually can be decompressed by nonsurgical methods. The infant is carefully observed for signs of cerebral complications. The parents of infants with a fracture of any bone should be involved in caring for the infant during hospitalization as part of discharge planning for care at home.

PARALYSES

Pressure exerted on nerves during a difficult labor can cause injury and paralysis of muscles that they supply. The most frequently observed nerve injuries are those involving the brachial plexus and the facial nerve.

Facial Paralysis

Pressure on the facial nerve during delivery may result in injury to cranial nerve VII. Clinical manifestations are primarily loss of movement on the affected side, such as inability to completely close the eye, drooping of the corner of the mouth, and absence of wrinkling of the forehead (Fig. 9-2). The paralysis is most noticeable when

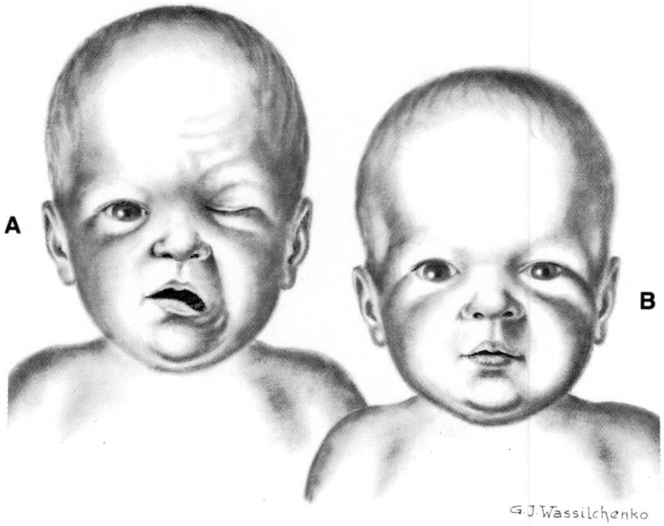

FIG. 9-2 A, Paralysis of right side of face 15 minutes after forceps delivery. Absence of movement on affected side is especially noticeable when infant cries. **B,** Same infant 24 hours later.

the infant cries. No medical intervention is necessary; the paralysis usually disappears spontaneously in a few days, but this may take as long as several months.

Brachial Palsy

Plexus injury results from forces that alter the normal position and relationship of the arm, shoulder, and neck. *Erb palsy* (Erb-Duchenne paralysis), caused by damage to the upper plexus, is usually a result of stretching or pulling away of the shoulder from the head. The less-common lower plexus palsy, or *Klumpke palsy,* results from severe stretching of the upper extremity while the trunk is relatively immobile. The clinical manifestations of Erb palsy are related to the paralysis of the affected extremity and muscles. The arm hangs limp alongside the body and is internally rotated with the wrist pronated (Fig. 9-3). The muscles of the hand are paralyzed in lower plexus palsy, with absence of voluntary movements of the wrist. In severe forms of brachial palsy, the entire arm is paralyzed and hangs limp and motionless at the side.

Treatment of an affected arm is aimed at preventing contractures of the paralyzed muscles and maintaining correct placement of the humeral head within the glenoid fossa of the scapula. Complete recovery from stretched nerves usually takes about 3 months. Avulsion of the nerves may result in permanent damage, requiring surgical and orthopedic intervention.

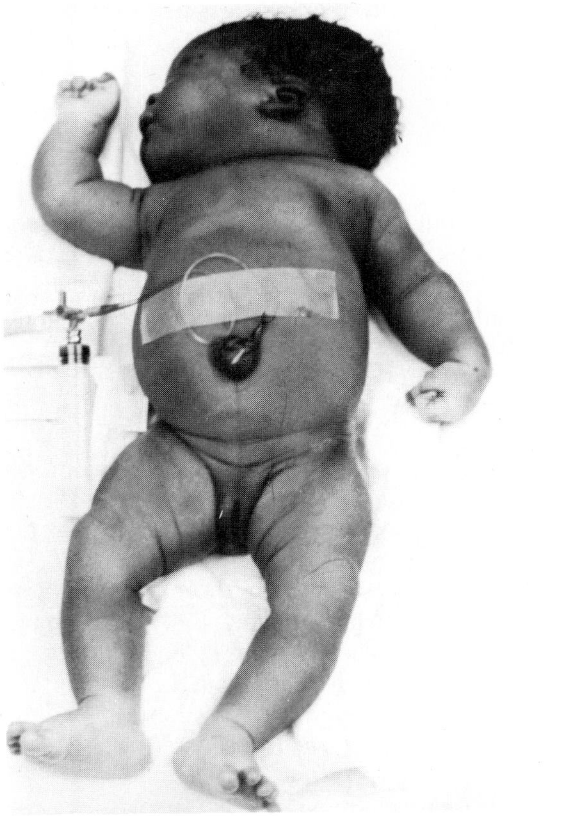

FIG. 9-3 Brachial plexus (Erb) palsy, left sided. Note the extended, internally rotated arm and pronated wrist on the affected side. (From Korones, S.B.: High-risk newborn infant: the basis for intensive nursing care, ed. 4, St. Louis, 1986, The C.V. Mosby Co.)

Phrenic Nerve Paralysis

Phrenic nerve paralysis resulting in diaphragmatic paralysis sometimes occurs in conjunction with brachial palsy. Respiratory distress is the most common and important sign of injury. Because injury to this nerve is usually unilateral, the lung on the affected side does not expand and respiratory efforts are ineffectual. Breathing is primarily thoracic and cyanosis is a prominent sign. Pneumonia is a frequent complication.

Nursing Considerations

Nursing care of the infant with facial nerve paralysis involves aiding the infant to suck and assisting the mother with feeding techniques. If the lid of the eye on the affected side does not close completely, artificial tears can be instilled daily to prevent drying of the conjunctiva and injury to the sclera and cornea. The lid is often taped shut to prevent accidental injury.

Nursing care of the newborn with brachial palsy is concerned primarily with proper positioning of the affected arm. In upper arm paralysis the arm should be abducted 90 degrees with external rotation at the shoulder, 90-degree flexion at the elbow, full supination of the forearm, and slight extension of the wrist so that the palm of the hand is turned toward the face. The position may be maintained with intermittent splinting. The arm should also be put through complete, passive range-of-motion exercises daily to maintain muscle tone and function. When dressing the infant, the nurse should always give special preference to the affected arm. Undressing should begin with the unaffected arm and redressing should begin with the affected arm to prevent unnecessary manipulation and stress on the paralyzed muscles.

The infant with phrenic nerve paralysis requires the same nursing care as any infant with respiratory distress. As with other birth injuries, family members of the infant with paralysis need support and education (see discussion of soft tissue injury). Also, because of the extended treatment for some paralyses, follow-up care is essential.

◆ *Common Problems in the Newborn*

Numerous problems may be encountered in the newborn period. Many are innocuous conditions that are of concern only to the parents; others require intervention to prevent complications. Some are discussed elsewhere, as appropriate, throughout the book; for example, skin manifestations and color changes in the newborn (p. 186).

One of the most common observations in the newborn period is jaundice, but since it can be a high-risk condition also, it is discussed at length under that category later in this chapter.

ERYTHEMA TOXICUM

Erythema toxicum, also known as "flea-bite dermatitis" or *newborn rash,* is a benign, self-limiting eruption of unknown cause that usually appears within the first 2 days of life. The lesions are firm, 1 to 3 mm in diameter, pale-yellow or white papules and/or pustules on an erythematous base, and resemble flea bites. The rash appears most commonly on the face, proximal aspects of the extremities, trunk, and buttocks but may be located anywhere on the body except the palms and soles. The rash is more obvious during crying episodes. There are no systemic manifestations and successive crops of lesions heal without pigmentation. The rash usually lasts about 5 to 7 days. Although no treatment is necessary, parents are usually concerned about the rash and need to be reassured of its benign and transient nature.

CANDIDIASIS

Candida infections, also known as *moniliasis*, are not uncommon in the newborn. *Candida albicans*, the usual organism responsible, may cause disease in any organ system. It is a yeastlike fungus (it produces yeast cells and spores) that can be acquired from a maternal vaginal infection during delivery, by person-to-person transmission (especially poor handwashing technique), or from contaminated hands, bottles, nipples, or other articles. Mucocutaneous, cutaneous, and disseminated candidiasis infections are all observed in this age-group. It is usually a benign disorder in the neonate, often confined to the oral and diaper regions.

Candidal Diaper Dermatitis

The warm, moist atmosphere created in the diaper area provides an optimal environment for candidal growth. The dermatitis appears in the perianal area, inguinal folds, and lower abdomen. The affected area is intensely erythematous, with a sharply demarcated, scalloped edge and frequently with numerous satellite lesions that extend beyond the larger lesion. The usual source of infection is through the gastrointestinal tract when organisms are swallowed from the birth canal during delivery. It may also appear 2 to 3 days following an oral infection.

Therapy consists of applications of an anticandidal ointment, such as nystatin, with each diaper change. The caregiver is taught to keep the diaper area as clean and dry as possible, and good hygienic care is essential to prevent spread. Sometimes the infant is also given an oral antifungal preparation to eliminate any gastrointestinal source of infection (see the section on oral candidiasis).

Oral Candidiasis

Oral candidiasis (thrush) is characterized by white, adherent patches on the tongue, palate, and inner aspects of the cheeks. It is readily distinguished from coagulated milk when attempts to remove the patches are unsuccessful, usually resulting in bleeding from the scraped surfaces. The infant may refuse to suck because of pain in the mouth, but this is infrequent.

The condition tends to be acute in the newborn and chronic in infants and young children, and it appears when the oral flora is altered as a result of antibiotic therapy. Although the disorder is usually self-limiting, spontaneous resolution may take as long as 2 months, during which time lesions may spread to the larynx, trachea, bronchi, and lungs and along the gastrointestinal tract. The disease should always be treated with good hygiene, application of a fungicide, and correction of any underlying disturbance. The source of infection should be identified to prevent reinfection.

Topical application of 1 ml nystatin (Mycostatin) over the surfaces of the oral cavity four times a day or every 6 hours is usually sufficient to prevent spread of the disease or prolong its course. Another effective therapy is application of 1% aqueous gentian violet three times a day. More resistant forms may be treated with fungicides such as amphotericin B (Fungizone), clotrimazole (Lotrimin), or miconazole (Monistat, Micatin) given intravenously or as topical applications.

Nursing Considerations

Nursing care is directed toward preventing spread of the infection and correctly applying the prescribed topical medication. Mycostatin is applied after feedings. The medication is distributed on the surface of the oral mucosa and tongue with an applicator. The remainder of the dose is deposited in the mouth and swallowed by the infant to treat any gastrointestinal lesions. Therapy is continued for about 1 week, even when lesions disappear within a few days.

Clotrimazole or nystatin can also be administered by suppository, which is inserted into the tip of a nipple for the infant to suck. In older children the suppositories can be used as oral "lozenges."

Other measures to control thrush, in addition to good hygienic care, include rinsing the infant's mouth with plain water after each feeding before applying the medication, boiling reusable nipples and bottles for at least 20 minutes after thorough washing (spores are heat resistant), and treating the source.

"BIRTHMARKS"

Discolorations of the skin are very common findings in the newborn infant. (See Skin assessment of the newborn, p. 186). Most, such as mongolian spots or telangiectatic nevi, involve no therapy other than reassurance to parents of their benign nature. Some can be a manifestation of a disease that suggests further examination of the child and other family members (for example, the multiple light-brown *café-au-lait spots* that often characterize the autosomal-dominant hereditary disorder neurofibromatosis and are common findings in Albright syndrome).

Darker and/or more extensive lesions demand further scrutiny, and excision of the lesion is recommended when feasible or excisional biopsy is performed. These include the reddish-brown solitary nodule that appears on the face or upper arm that usually represents a spindle and epithelioid cell nevus (juvenile melanoma); a giant pigmented nevus (bathing trunk nevus); a dark-brown to black, irregular plaque that is at risk of transformation to malignant melanoma; and the dark brown or black macules that become more numerous with age (junctional or compound nevi).

Vascular birthmarks, those orange or light red (salmon patch) or dark red or bluish red (port wine stain) lesions, are permanent lesions that require no treatment and may even become darker in color. Parents may need advice regarding the use of cosmetic coverings (such as Covermark) at a later time when they feel that the child may be adversely affected by the defect. Good results have been achieved with the argon laser treatment but should not be attempted before the age of 13 years because of the risk of scarring in younger children.

Strawberry hemangiomas, those red, rubbery nodules with a rough surface, may not be present at birth but appear at 2 to 4 weeks of age. The parents can be reassured that the lesions (even very large ones) resolve spontaneously during childhood and usually require no treatment. If there is evidence of ulceration on the surface of the lesion, the child should receive systemic antibiotics to prevent infection and subsequent scar formation.

HYPOTONIA (FLOPPY INFANT SYNDROME)

Decreased muscle tone in an infant is not an unusual observation in the newborn nursery and is one of the most common presenting symptoms in neuromuscular disorders. It may also indicate a variety of systemic conditions. The most frequent causes are cerebral trauma or hypoxia at birth and chromosome disorders, particularly Down syndrome.

Hypotonia, sometimes called the *floppy infant syndrome,* is marked by diminished muscle tone and weakness in response to both spontaneous and passive motion and to reflex testing. The infant, placed in a supine position, assumes a characteristic "frog posture" or lies in some other unusual position at rest. Normally, the young infant who is held in ventral suspension, that is, with the examiner's hand supporting the infant under the chest, will respond by slightly raising his head, with his back relatively straight, arms flexed and slightly abducted, and knees partly flexed (see Fig. 8-7, *B*). The hypotonic infant droops over the supporting hand with head and extremities hanging loosely, resembling an inverted U (Fig. 9-4). The muscles feel flabby when palpated and there is marked head lag when the infant is pulled to a sitting position. Poor sucking may be noted.

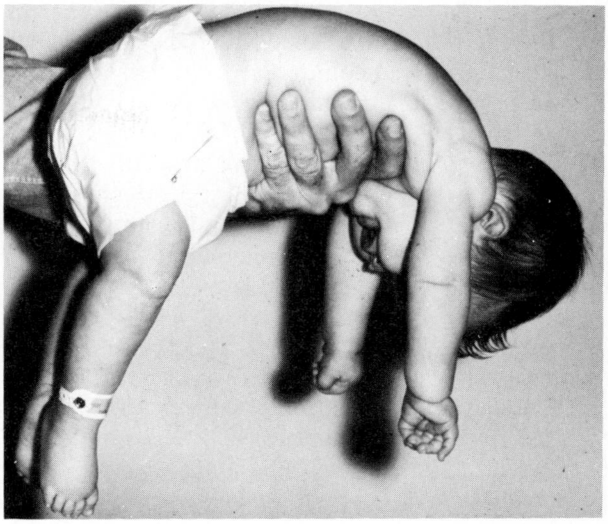

FIG. 9-4 Hypotonicity demonstrated by horizontal suspension in an infant with Werdnig-Hoffman disease. (From Swaiman, K.F., and Wright, F.S.: The practice of pediatric neurology, ed. 2, St. Louis, 1982, The C.V. Mosby Co.)

The management of these infants is determined by the cause of the hypotonia. It is a nurse's responsibility to record and report findings that suggest hypotonia in an infant so that further evaluation can be carried out and therapeutic measures implemented if indicated.

◆ *The High-Risk Newborn and Family*

A high-risk neonate can be defined as the newborn, regardless of gestational age or birth weight, who has a greater than average chance of morbidity or mortality because of conditions or circumstances that are superimposed on the normal course of events associated with birth and the adjustment to extrauterine existence. The high-risk period encompasses human growth and development from the time of viability until 28 days following birth and includes threats to life and health that occur during the prenatal, perinatal, and postnatal periods.

NURSING CARE OF THE HIGH-RISK NEWBORN

In recent years, there has been an increase in the survival rate of newborn infants that has coincided with the establishment of programs directed toward improving the health of mothers, the planned timing of their pregnancies, and the introduction of important new techniques in neonatal care. Many problems can be anticipated before delivery. Prenatal testing and labor monitoring have reduced the incidence of perinatal mortality, and specialized care of the distressed newborn is increasing the survival rate of such infants. If an infant is likely to require special therapy at or soon after birth, plans should be made for delivery to take place at or near a hospital that has the facilities to provide such care. In this way, there is no delay in initiating needed care, and some of the hazards associated with transporting the sick newborn are averted.

ASSESSMENT

At birth the newborn is given a cursory assessment to determine any apparent problems and those that demand immediate attention. This examination is primarily concerned with evaluation of cardiopulmonary and neurologic function. The assessment includes assignment of an Apgar score (see p. 183) and evaluation for pallor, cyanosis, prematurity, any obvious congenital anomalies, or evidence of neonatal disease. If the infant displays any need for intensive care, he is taken immediately to the neonatal intensive care unit (NICU) for initiation of therapy and more extensive assessment, including assessment of gestational age (see p. 185).

The majority of infants requiring specialized care are those who are considered to be outside the normal range for size or gestational age. Intrauterine growth rates are not the same for all infants and other factors (e.g., heredity, placental insufficiency, and maternal disease) influence intrauterine growth and birth weight of the infant. The lowest perinatal mortality is found in full-term infants who weigh between 3500 and 4000 g. Classification of infants outside this optimum status are outlined in the box.

Classification of High-Risk Infants

Classification According to Size

low-birth-weight (LBW) infant An infant whose birth weight is less than 2500 g regardless of gestational age
very-low-birth-weight (VLBW) infant An infant whose weight is less than 1500 g
appropriate-for-gestational-age (AGA) infant An infant whose weight falls between the 10th and 90th percentiles on intrauterine growth curves
small-for-date (SFD) or small-for-gestational-age (SGA) infant An infant whose rate of intrauterine growth was slowed and who was delivered at or later than term; the infant's birth weight falls below the 10th percentile on intrauterine growth curves
intrauterine growth retardation (IUGR) Found in infants whose intrauterine growth is retarded (sometimes used as a more descriptive term for the SGA infant)
large-for-gestational-age (LGA) infant An infant whose birth weight falls above the 90th percentile on intrauterine growth curves

Classification According to Gestational Age

premature (preterm) infant An infant born before completion of 37 weeks of gestation, regardless of birth weight
term infant An infant born between the beginning of the 38 weeks and the completion of the 42 weeks of gestation, regardless of birth weight
postmature (postterm) infant An infant born after 42 weeks of gestational age, regardless of birth weight

Classification According to Mortality

live birth Birth in which the neonate manifests any heartbeat, breathes, or displays voluntary movement, regardless of gestational age
fetal death Death of the fetus after 20 weeks of gestation and before delivery, with absence of any signs of life after birth
neonatal death Death that occurs in the first 28 days of life; early neonatal or postnatal deaths occur in the first week of life
perinatal mortality Describes the total number of fetal and early neonatal deaths per 1000 live births

Neonatal intensive care nursing is a highly specialized area of knowledge and practice that requires lengthy supervised experience to reach a level of competence that permits independent functioning. Neonatal intensive care nursing involves an understanding of neonatal physiology and characteristics, a knowledge of the function and management of a number of mechanical devices and apparatus, the ability to recognize very subtle deviations from the expected, and the ability to implement a judicious course of action.

Some major nursing observations and assessments apply to all high-risk infants, regardless of diagnosis. Therefore, the general aspects of assessment of the high-risk infant will be described briefly here. Many aspects in relation to the care of the newborn were discussed in Chapter 8. Others will be considered throughout the remainder of this chapter and summarized in relation to specific patient problems.

Maintaining detailed, ongoing records of all activities and observations is an important function of nurses in the intensive care setting. Knowledge and operation of complex pieces of equipment and mechanical devices are inherent in the care of the ill neonate. However, sophisticated monitoring and life-support systems cannot replace the vigilance and constant scrutiny of infants by experienced personnel. Subtle changes that are not apparent on mechanical devices can be detected by alert nurses.

Systematic Assessment of the High-Risk Newborn

Nurses are usually responsible for the same infant each day, which allows for more accurate determination of day-to-day progress. During the course of daily care the nurse makes frequent systematic assessments of physical status, since vital signs of small infants change several times in a very few hours.

In the course of an assessment the nurse ascertains that any mechanical apparatus being used is functioning properly and at the correct settings according to the prescribed therapy and the needs of the infant. The assessment of the infant should proceed in a systematic manner. Each nurse develops an approach that is comfortable for him or her and follows the same pattern routinely. An observational assessment is usually performed hourly, or more frequently on very ill infants, and a synopsis is included in the charting. However, any assessment procedures that require that the infant be disturbed should be timed to allow for sufficient rest between assessments.

General Assessment

- Weigh two or three times daily, as ordered.
- Describe general body shape and size, presence and location of edema, amount of body fat.
- Describe any apparent deformities.

Respiratory Assessment

- Describe shape of chest (barrel, concave), symmetry, presence of incisions, chest tubes, or other deviations.
- Describe use of accessory muscles; substernal, intercostal, or subclavicular retractions; nasal flaring.
- Determine respiratory rate and regularity.
- Describe breath sounds: rales, rhonchi, wheezing, wet diminished sounds, areas of absence of sound, grunting.
- Describe secretions.
- Determine whether suctioning is needed.
- Describe cry.
- Describe ambient oxygen and method of delivery; if intubated, describe size of tube, type of ventilator, and settings.

Cardiovascular Assessment

- Determine heart rate and rhythm.
- Describe heart sounds, including any suspected murmurs.
- Determine the point of maximum intensity, the point where the heartbeat sounds loudest (a change in the point of maximum intensity may indicate a mediastinal shift).
- Describe infant's color (may be of cardiac, respiratory, or hematopoietic origin): cyanosis, pallor, plethora, jaundice.
- Determine blood pressure; indicate extremity used.
- Describe peripheral pulses.
- Determine central venous pressure (if central venous pressure line is part of infant's apparatus).
- Describe monitors and their parameters.

Gastrointestinal Assessment

- Determine presence of any indication of abdominal distention: increase in circumference, shiny skin.
- Observe feeding behavior (strength of suck, coordination of sucking and swallowing).
- Determine any signs of regurgitation, especially following feeding; character and amount of residual if gavage fed; if nasogastric tube in place, describe type of suction, drainage (color, consistency, pH, guaiac).
- Describe amount, color, consistency, and odor of any emesis.
- Describe amount, color, and consistency of stools; check for occult blood if indicated by physician's order or appearance of stool.
- Describe bowel sounds: presence or absence.

Genitourinary Assessment

- Describe any abnormalities of genitalia.
- Describe amount (as determined by weight), color, pH, labstick findings, and specific gravity of urine (to screen for adequacy of hydration).
- Check weight (the most accurate measure for assessment of hydration).

Neurologic-Musculoskeletal Assessment

- Describe infant's movements: random, purposeful, jittery, twitching, spontaneous, elicited.
- Describe infant's position or attitude: flexed, extended.
- Describe reflexes observed: Moro, sucking, Babinski, and other expected reflexes.
- Determine level of response.
- Determine changes in head circumference (if indicated).
- Determine pupillary responses.

Temperature Assessment

- Determine axillary temperature.
- Determine relationship to environmental temperature.

Skin Assessment

- Describe any discoloration, reddened area, or signs of irritation, especially where monitoring equipment, infusion lines, or other apparatus comes in contact with skin; also check and note any skin preparation used (e.g., povodine-iodine).
- Determine texture and turgor of skin: dry, smooth, flaky, peeling, etc.
- Describe any rash or skin lesion.
- Determine whether intravenous infusion catheter or needle is in place and observe for signs of infiltration.
- Describe parenteral infusion lines: location, type (arterial, venous, hyperalimentation, central venous pressure); type of infusion and relevant information; type of infusion pump and rate of flow; type of needle (butterfly, Quik-Cath); appearance of insertion site.

The infant's position is changed every 1 to 2 hours, and any significant reaction to the changing process or to a specific position is noted. To conserve the infant's energy, the position changing and periodic treatments should be timed to coincide with an assessment. Much of the assessment can be accomplished without moving the child, but necessary handling is minimum and as atraumatic as possible.

Monitoring Physiologic Data

Most neonates under intensive observation are placed in a controlled thermal environment and monitored for heart rate, respiratory activity, and temperature. The monitoring devices are equipped with an alarm system that indicates when the vital signs are above or below preset limits. However, it is essential to check the heartbeat and compare it with the monitor reading. Proper placement and maintenance of electrodes and their connections are nursing responsibilities. Electrodes are either attached topically to the outer aspects of the chest wall, one on each side, by special electrode paste or jelly and adhesive disks or by needle electrodes inserted intradermally and anchored with Transpore tape.

In the NICU, frequent laboratory examinations are an integral part of the ongoing assessment of infants' progress. Accurate intake and output records are kept on all infants. An accurate output can be obtained by collection of urine in a plastic urine collection bag (see p. 653) or by weighing the diapers, the simplest and least traumatic means of measuring urine output. The preweighed wet diaper is weighed on a gram scale, and the gram weight of the urine is converted directly to milliliters, for example, 25 g = 25 ml. Cotton balls inside the diaper next to the perineum aid in absorbing moisture. Plastic collecting devices can be used when it is necessary to collect urine for laboratory examination. Since the volume normally voided is insufficient to float the standard urometer, a refractometer requiring only a single drop of urine is standard equipment in the NICU. A drop of urine can be easily aspirated with a syringe from the wet diaper or cotton balls.

Blood examinations are a necessary part of the ongoing assessment and monitoring of the sick newborn's progress. The tests most often performed are blood glucose, bilirubin, calcium, hematocrit, and blood gasses. Samples may be obtained from the heel, by venipuncture, or by an indwelling catheter in an umbilical vein, umbilical artery, or peripheral artery. To secure frequent samples for monitoring arterial blood gas levels without repeated arterial punctures, it is preferable to use transcutaneous oxygen measurements—the Po_2 monitor, which measures the partial pressure of oxygen in the blood, or the oxygen saturation monitor or pulse oximeter, which measures the saturation of oxygen in the hemoglobin.

NURSING DIAGNOSES

Many nursing diagnoses may be evident after a careful assessment of the infant at risk. Some apply to all infants; others will vary according to the needs and characteristics of individual infants and their families. The nursing diagnoses that represent general guides for nursing intervention are found in the Nursing Care Plan on pp. 231-233. Since a number of health problems accompany infant immaturity, the nurse is also alert to the possibility of conditions and complications discussed elsewhere in this book.

PLANNING

The nursing plan for the high-risk infant depends to a large extent on the diagnosis of the health problem that places the infant at risk. However, the following are basic to the care of all high-risk infants:

1. Promote respiratory efforts
2. Provide warmth
3. Protect infant from infection
4. Provide hydration and nutrition
5. Conserve energy
6. Prevent other complications—skin care; administration of medications
7. Provide sensory stimulation
8. Promote parent-infant relationships and prepare for home care
9. Support family in the event of neonatal death

IMPLEMENTATION

Nurses in an NICU are vital to the successful operation of the unit. They are subject to stresses not found in many pediatric units. The critical nature of their patients' conditions generates a stressful atmosphere and their care demands constant observation and rapid evaluation and intervention.

Respiratory Support

In care of the high-risk infant, the primary objective is to establish and maintain respiration. Many infants require supplemental oxygen and assisted ventilation. Infants with or without these supportive treatments are positioned to maximum airflow (see Respiratory distress syndrome, p. 243). Other nursing interventions are common to all high-risk infants.

Thermoregulation

After, or concurrent with, the establishment of respiration, the most crucial need of high-risk infants is the application of external warmth. To delay or prevent the effects of cold stress, the infants are placed in a heated environment immediately after birth; they remain there until they are able to maintain thermal stability (balance heat production and conservation with heat dissipation). This is especially important for the preterm infant whose very high skin surface relative to body mass promotes heat loss.

The naked infant is placed in the controlled microenvironment of an Isolette or incubator. A Plexiglas top affords a clear view of the infant from all aspects. There is easy access through portholes that minimize temperature and oxygen loss and a large door that provides a more extensive approach (Fig. 9-5). Maximum accessibility is provided by an open unit with an overhead radiant warming system (Fig. 9-6).

Since overheating produces an increase in oxygen and calorie consumption, the infant is also jeopardized in a hyperthermic environment. A *neutral thermal environment* is one that permits the infant to maintain a normal core temperature, with minimum oxygen consumption and calorie expenditure. The very small infant, especially one with a meager subcutaneous fat layer, can control body heat loss or gain only within a very limited range of environmental temperature.

Consumption of oxygen is minimal at an abdominal skin temperature of 36.5° C (97.7° F). When abdominal skin temperature increases or decreases, the oxygen con-

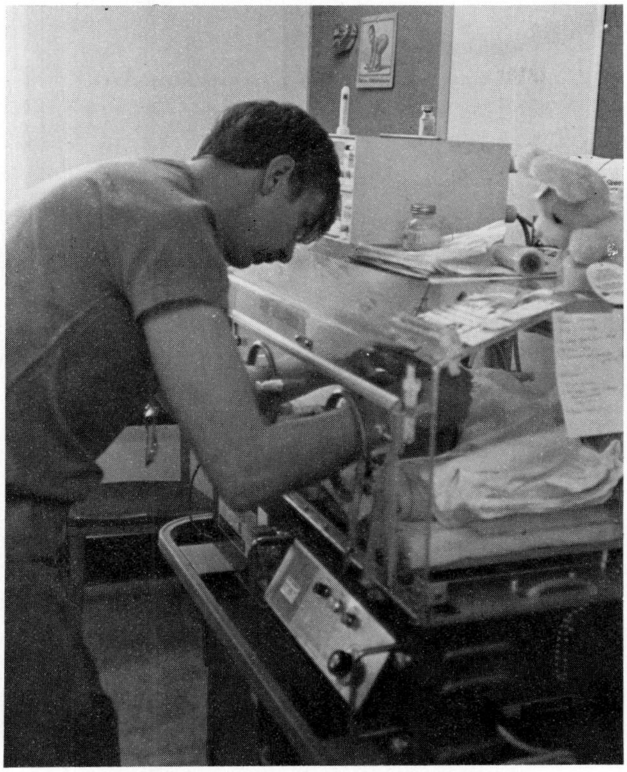

FIG. 9-5 Nurse caring for infant in Isolette.

sumption increases. The range of abdominal temperature that produces a neutral thermal environment is 36.1° to 36.8° C (97° to 98.2° F).

The dressed infant under blankets can maintain a body temperature within a wider range of environmental temperatures; however, the close observations required for most high-risk infants are best accomplished if the infants remain unclothed. When an infant is removed

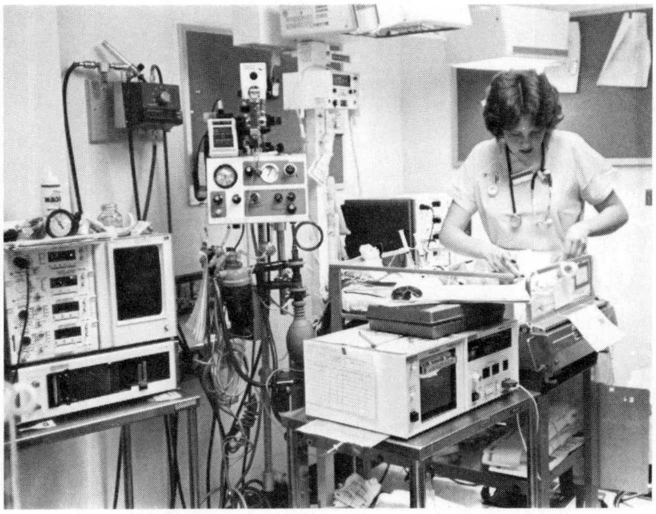

FIG. 9-6 Infant under overhead warming unit.

Nursing Tip: Prevent Heat Loss

Placing a knitted cap or a cap fashioned from a piece of stockinette helps reduce heat loss from the head.

from the warm environment of the Isolette for feeding or cuddling, he is clothed and wrapped warmly in blankets (see Nursing tip: Prevent heat loss).

The most effective means for maintaining the desired range of temperature in the naked infant is by way of a manually adjusted or automatically controlled heat panel or incubator, which adjusts automatically in response to signals from a thermal sensor attached to the abdominal skin. The mechanical temperature reading is periodically verified during routine assessments.

Whereas loss of heat by convection is a constant problem in the open units, radiant heat loss is one of the greatest threats to temperature regulation in the Isolette, since the temperature of circulating air within has no influence on heat loss to cooler surfaces without, such as windows or walls, or on heat loss resulting from a lower nursery temperature. A high-humidity atmosphere provided from an external source such as humidified oxygen or air contributes to body temperature maintenance by reducing evaporative heat loss.

Lining the lower inside of the Isolette with aluminum foil or placing a sheet of clear plastic wrap over the open warmer crib may help prevent heat loss caused by radiation. A plastic bubble wrap, similar to that used as packing material, is sometimes used as a blanket to help preserve heat and prevent fluid loss, especially for infants under a radiant warmer.

Protection from Infection

Protection from infection is an integral part of all newborn care, but preterm and sick neonates are particularly susceptible. The protective environment of a regularly cleaned Isolette provides effective isolation from airborne infective agents. However, thorough, meticulous, and frequent handwashing is the foundation of prevention. This includes *all* persons who come in contact with the infant and his equipment. After handling another infant or equipment, no one ever touches an infant without first washing hands. Personnel with infectious disorders either are barred from the unit until they can no longer transmit the disease to the infants and other personnel or are required to wear suitable shields, such as masks or gloves, to reduce the likelihood of contamination. In some areas annual influenza vaccination is recommended for NICU. Many units have adopted universal precautions as a method of infection control (see p. 645).

In most areas special clothing furnished by the institution is worn by everyone working in the unit. Fresh scrub dresses or suits are put on before entering the unit and are changed any time they become contaminated.

When personnel leave the unit, the scrub clothing is protected by a cover gown that is removed, then discarded in the laundry hamper before the wearer reenters the unit. Anyone entering the unit for a short time, whether or not that person provides any care, must scrub thoroughly and either change to appropriate clothing or wear a cover gown. Parents are taught these precautionary measures and become willing and cooperative allies in protecting their infants from infection.

This practice is not universal, however. As accumulated evidence indicates that special clothing and gowning are ineffective in preventing the spread of infection, many institutions have abandoned the practice (Cloney and Donowitz, 1986).

Hydration

It is not uncommon for high-risk infants to receive supplemental parenteral fluids to supply additional calories, electrolytes, and/or water. Adequate hydration is particularly important in preterm infants because their extracellular water content is higher (70% in full-term infants and up to 90% in preterm infants), their body surface is larger, and the capacity for osmotic diuresis is limited in preterm infants' underdeveloped kidneys. Therefore, these infants are highly vulnerable to water depletion.

A great deal of heat and moisture are lost in rapid breathing, and infants under a radiant warmer or phototherapy lights must be closely observed for signs of dehydration (p. 740). It is important to obtain weights frequently and measure intake and output accurately. In addition, the very small, fragile blood vessels are subject to rupture and subsequent infiltration. Nurses are constantly on the alert for signs of infiltration and evidence of overhydration.

Nutrition

The amount and method of feeding are determined by the size and condition of the infant. The various mechanisms for ingestion and digestion of foods are not fully developed in the preterm infant, and the younger the infant, the greater the problem. The infant's need for rapid growth and daily maintenance must be met in the presence of several anatomic and physiologic handicaps. Although sucking and swallowing are established before birth, coordination of these mechanisms does not occur until approximately 32 to 34 weeks of gestation and they are not fully developed until after birth. Consequently, the preterm infant is highly prone to aspiration, with its attendant dangers.

Very small or ill infants are fed by the parenteral route until their condition is stabilized and their neurologic and physical state permits enteral feedings. Often, enteral feedings must be supplemented by parenteral infusions to ensure an adequate intake of carbohydrates and water.

Although the timing of the first feeding has been a matter of controversy, most authorities now believe that early feeding, usually within 3 to 6 hours after birth, reduces the incidence of complicating factors, such as hypoglycemia and dehydration, and the degree of hyperbilirubinemia. The feeding regimen employed varies from institution to institution. However, the initial enteral feeding is not attempted until infants have adapted to extrauterine existence as evidenced by temperature neutrality, normal breathing, and good color, tone, and cry. The amount, interval, and method of feeding are individualized for each infant.

Nipple feeding. Vigorous infants can be fed from a soft nipple with little difficulty (Fig. 9-7), whereas weaker infants will require alternative methods. Sterile water is offered first, the same as for any newborn, because it causes no pulmonary reaction if aspirated as has been found with both milk and glucose water. The amount to be fed is determined by the infant's size, age, and condition. It is important not to tire the infant or to overtax his capacity to retain the feedings. Usually 15 to 20 minutes is considered to be a maximum feeding time. Vital signs (especially pulse) are taken after feeding to assess the degree of stress to which the infant may have been subjected.

The high-risk infant is often a slow feeder and requires periods of rest and frequent bubbling (burping). When he is unable to tolerate bottle feedings, intermittent feedings by gavage are instituted until he gains enough strength and coordination to handle the nipple. Special formulas are designed for the preterm infant and high-risk infants are often fed breast milk obtained from the infant's mother or a milk bank.

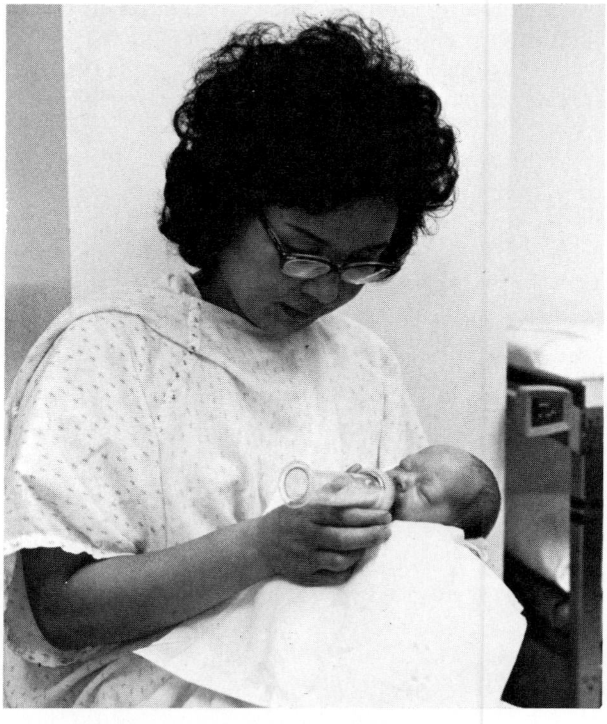

FIG. 9-7 Position for nipple feeding the premature infant.

Sometimes supplementary calories are needed in the form of dietary additives such as Lipomul-Oral or other LBW formulas,* which provide vegetable fat and carbohydrates, and MCT oil,† which provides fat in the form of medium-chain triglycerides. Often, oral feedings are supplemented by parenteral infusions to ensure an adequate intake of carbohydrate and water.

Breast-feeding. Studies indicate that even small preterm infants are able to breast-feed if the infant has adequate sucking and swallowing reflexes and there are no other contraindications, such as facial defects, respiratory complications, or concurrent illness (Meier and Pugh, 1985; Meier and Anderson, 1987). The infants in these studies were developmentally advanced (gestational age 32.5 to 36 weeks) but small (less than 1500 g). During breast-feeding they sucked for a longer period of time and exhibited less evidence of stress (as determined by transcutaneous oxygen measurements, skin temperature, and heart rate) than they did during bottle feeding. It requires more time, patience, and dedication on the part of the mother and the staff to help infants who breast-feed. Because teaching infants to breast-feed after they are accustomed to nipple feeding is difficult, these infants are sometimes given supplementary gavage feedings until they are breast-feeding and gaining weight satisfactorily (Boggs and Rau, 1983).

Gavage feeding. Intermittent gavage feeding is one of the safest means for meeting the nutritional requirements of infants who were born at less than 32 weeks of gestation or infants who weigh less than 1650 g. These infants are usually too weak to suck effectively and are unable to coordinate swallowing. For larger infants who become excessively tired, are listless, or become cyanotic, gavage feeding can be employed as an energy-saving technique.

A 15-inch (37.5 cm), size 5 or 8 French, polyethylene feeding tube is used to instill the formula, and the usual methods for determining correct placement are employed (see p. 680 for technique). Although the more relaxed cardiac sphincter permits easy passage of the tube, there may be changes in heart rate and blood pressure in response to vagal stimulation. The procedure can be accomplished when an infant is supine, prone, or on the right side with the head slightly elevated. It is preferable to insert the tube through the mouth rather than the nares. Nasal insertion obstructs nose breathing and may irritate the delicate nasal mucosa. Passage through the mouth also provides an opportunity to observe the sucking response. The formula is allowed to flow by gravity, and the feeding time should approximate the time required for a nipple feeding.

The intermittent method of gavage feeding stimulates the infant to begin making attempts at sucking and swallowing. The nurse needs to observe premature infants closely for behaviors that indicate readiness to handle bottle-feedings. These include: (1) a strong, vigorous suck, (2) coordination of sucking and swallowing, (3) sucking in response to the gavage tube or other objects placed near the mouth, and (4) wakefulness before and sleeping after feedings. When these behaviors are noted, infants can be challenged with nipple feedings introduced slowly. It is often of value to encourage nonnutritive sucking on a pacifier by infants during gavage feedings. It helps nurses assess the sucking ability of the infants and helps the infants to associate the sucking with the feeling of food in the stomach.

To determine how well the infant tolerates the feedings, the stomach contents are aspirated before each feeding and the residual fluid is recorded and replaced as part of the feeding. Whether or not the amount of the aspirant is deducted from the total feeding varies among units. Some advocate deducting to avoid overdistending the stomach. For example, if the feeding is 25 ml and the aspirant 5 ml, the aspirant is returned plus 20 ml of feeding for a total of 25 ml. Others determine the amount on an individual basis.

Conserve Energy

One of the major goals of care for the high-risk infant is conservation of energy. Much of the care described in this section is directed toward this end, for example, disturbing the infant as little as possible, maintaining a neutral thermal environment, gavage feeding, easing respirations, and judicious application of stimulation techniques. When energy is not expended to cope with efforts to breathe, eat, and alter body temperature, it can be used for growth and development. Diminishing environmental noise levels and shading the infant from bright lights also promotes rest.

Skin Care

The skin of premature infants is characteristically immature relative to that of full-term infants. Because of its increased sensitivity and fragility, it is recommended that no alkaline-base soap or detergent be used that might destroy the "acid mantle" of the skin. The skin is cleansed with plain, clear water or mild, nonalkaline cleanser only two to three times per week. Any topical preparation (including creams, lotions, or medicated ointments) should be carefully assessed for possible toxic effects before it is applied. The increased permeability of the skin facilitates absorption of ingredients. Hexachlorophene has been discontinued as a cleansing agent because of its proven toxic effect. Other germicides (e.g., alcohol or povidone-iodine) are used with caution, and the skin is rinsed after they are used, since these substances may cause severe irritation in low-birth-weight infants.

The skin is easily excoriated and denuded; therefore care must be taken to avoid damage to the delicate structure. The total skin is less thick than that of full-term

*The Upjohn Co., Kalamazoo, MI.
†Mead Johnson & Co., Evansville, IN.

infants and has fewer elastic fibers, and there is less cohesion between the thinner skin layers. Adhesives used after heel sticks or to secure monitoring equipment or intravenous infusions may excoriate the skin or adhere to the skin surface so well that the skin can be separated from understructures and pulled away with the tape. Transpore tape is a tape that can safely be applied directly to the skin of small infants. It is best to first apply a coating of a protective substance to which the adhesive tape is attached, or to use a protective layer of polyurethane elastic film, such as Hollihesive or Op-Site.

It is unsafe to use scissors to remove dressings or adhesive tape from the extremities of very small and immature infants, because it is easy to snip off tiny extremities or nick loosely attached skin. Special care must be exercised in removing tape (see Nursing tip). Solvents used to remove tape tend to dry and burn the delicate skin.

Nursing Tip: Adhesive Tape

Adhesive tape is best removed by applying water-soaked cotton balls to the tape, then lifting the tape *carefully* while applying pressure on the skin directly beneath the tape.

Administration of Medications

Administration of therapeutic agents, such as drugs, ointments, intravenous infusions, and oxygen, requires judicious handling and meticulous attention to details. The computation, preparation, and administration of drugs in minute amounts often require collaboration between nurses to reduce the chance of error. (See section on Administration of medications in Chapter 21, p. 656.)

Oral administration of hyperosmolar solutions presents a potential danger to preterm infants because their immature kidneys are unable to adjust urine concentration to accommodate concentrated or highly diluted substances. More concentrated doses have been administered to ensure that all the medication is ingested, but the practice is questioned. It is now recommended that medications be administered parenterally or sufficiently diluted to prevent complications related to hyperosmolality.

Warnings have also been issued regarding the hazards of bacteriostatic parenteral solutions given to infants. Benzyl alcohol, a common preservative in bacteriostatic water and saline, has been shown to be toxic to newborns and should not be used to dilute or reconstitute medications.

Supportive Care of the High-Risk Infant and Family

The significance of early parent-child interaction and infant stimulation has been documented by reliable research, and nurses, aware of these infant and family needs, must incorporate activities that facilitate family interaction into the nursing care plan.

Neurologic impairment and serious sequelae appear to correlate with the size and gestational age of the infant at birth and with the degree of intensive care instituted. The greater the degree of immaturity, the greater the degree of disability. Small-for-gestational-age infants appear to be less at a disadvantage than appropriate-for-gestational-age infants born early, although both are at a greater disadvantage than normal-weight term infants. There is an increase in the incidence of neurologic sequelae, such as cerebral palsy, attention deficit disorder, visual-motor deficits, and intellectual development, in preterm infants.

Infant stimulation. Recently, attention has been focused on the effects of early stimulation, or lack of it, on both normal and preterm infants. Findings indicate that infants are able to respond to a greater variety of stimuli than had been previously thought. Nurses who are aware of this need can incorporate a stimulation program into the nursing care plan, providing *appropriate* stimuli whenever possible.

Twenty-four-hour surveillance of sick infants implies maximum visibility. However, many units have instigated a program to help establish a night-day sleep pattern by either darkening the room, if the infant's condition allows, covering cribs with blankets, or placing eye patches over the infant's eyes at night. Others believe that rest for these infants is so vital to their growth that the cribs are covered with blankets and infants left undisturbed for 1 hour of every 3 to provide for total rest.

When the condition of an infant is sufficiently advanced to begin a stimulation program, some activities are individualized according to each infant's cues, temperament, state of health, behavioral organization, and particular needs (see p. 183 for stages of alertness). Stimulation periods are shorter than they are for full-term infants; for example, 1 to 2 minutes for visual stimulation, 2 to 3 minutes of voices, and 5 minutes for quiet music. Some suggested activities are outlined in the box. When a stimulation program is implemented, the parents should be involved as early as possible. See the discussion that follows for further suggestions.

Parental involvement. The birth of a premature infant is usually an unexpected and stressful event for which the family is emotionally unprepared. To compound the situation, the precarious nature of the infant's condition engenders an atmosphere of apprehension and uncertainty. The parents see the infant only briefly before he is removed to the intensive care unit or even to another hospital, leaving them with just the recollection of the infant's very small size and unusual appearance. The staff and physician are often guarded in discussing the infant's condition; the parents are continually expecting to hear that the infant has died.

If the infant is to be transported from the hospital in which he was born, the parents need information about the facility to which he is going, including the location,

Interventions for Infant Stimulation

General Guidelines

Offer stimulation only during periods of alertness.
Limit stimulation to one or two types of stimulus per session.
Provide stimulation for short periods.
Space stimulation periods according to infant's tolerance.

Visual Stimulation

Place magazine photographs (black-and-white schematic faces) in visual range (19 to 22 cm) in "en face" position.
Cover mattress with black-and-white patterned material for length of stimulation period.
Provide black-and-white mobiles with varied hanging shapes.
Initiate eye-to-eye contact repeatedly.
Alternate holding black-and-white pattern still and moving it across the infant's visual field.

Tactile Stimulation

Stroke skin slowly and gently in head-to-toe direction.
Provide alternate textures, e.g., sheepskin, satin, velvet.

Auditory Stimulation

Play tape of parents voices.
Play classical music recording or music box (jazz or rock are less effective).
Speak with a variety of voice inflections; alternate adult and baby talk.
Call infant by name at each interaction.

Vestibular Stimulation

Place on waterbed with oscillations and waves per minute determined on an individual basis; alternate oscillation with rest periods.
Rock in chair.
Place in sling and rock.
Provide passive range-of-motion exercise to knee and hip joints.
Close infant's fist around cloth toy.
Lift head to upright position, tip to right and then to left, stopping at midline.

Olfactory Stimulation

Pass open breast milk or formula container under nose.
Pass various sweet-smelling items under nose, e.g., cherry syrup, cinnamon, nutmeg, strawberry extract.

Gustatory Stimulation

Place infant's hand or pacifier in mouth when sucking movements are observed or during gavage feeding.
Place 2 drops of milk in infant's mouth with each tube feeding.

Derived extensively from Chaze, B.A., and Ludington-Hoe, S.M.: Sensory stimulation in the NICU, Am. J. Nurs. **84:**68-71, Jan. 1984.

the care he is expected to receive, the name of his physician, and the telephone number of the nursery. Explanations should be simple, and parents should be given the opportunity to ask questions. Perhaps most important of all, the parents, especially the mother, should be allowed some contact with the infant before transport takes place.

When they visit the infant, parents are usually overwhelmed by the frightening array of equipment and activity, and they need reassurance that the infant is receiving proper care. Once they understand that the infant needs this intensive care, they are content to be kept informed of his condition. It is not necessary to share too much information with the parents, such as very technical information that does not contribute to their understanding. Considering the parents' fears, the nurse can be truthful without being unduly candid regarding the more negative aspects of the child's condition.

There is increasing evidence to indicate that the emotional separation that accompanies the physical separation of mother and infant interferes with the normal maternal-infant attachment process (p. 204). When the infant is sick, the necessary physical separation appears to be accompanied by an emotional estrangement on the part of the mother that may seriously limit her capacity for mothering the infant.

Facilitating parent-infant relationships. The current concept in the comprehensive management of the high-risk newborn is to encourage parental involvement rather than to isolate parents from their infant and his care. Nursing interventions relative to the needs of parents are directed toward assisting them with tasks that must be accomplished during their infant's care. Parents need to:

Realistically perceive their infant's medical condition and needs
Adapt to the infant's hospital environment
Become involved in the infant's care
Assume total responsibility for care upon discharge of the patient
For some families, cope with death of an infant

Preparing the parents to see their infant for the first time is a nursing responsibility. Before the first visit the parents should be prepared for the infant's appearance, the equipment that is attached, and some indication of the general atmosphere of the unit. At the bedside the nurse explains the function of each piece of equipment and the role it plays in facilitating recovery. When possible, some items related to therapy can be removed; for example, phototherapy can be temporarily discontinued and eye patches removed to permit eye-to-eye contact.

Parents will usually appreciate the support of a nurse during the initial visit with the infant, but they should be left alone with the infant for a short time. It is important during the early visits to emphasize positive aspects of the infant's behavior, to help the parents focus on the infant as an individual rather than on the equipment that surrounds him. Most institutions allow parents to visit their infants as often as they wish and encourage them to do so.

Most parents feel very shaky and insecure about initiating interaction with the infant. Nurses can sense the parent's level of readiness and offer encouragement in these first efforts. Parents of premature infants follow the same acquaintance process as do parents of normal infants (Fig. 9-8). They may quickly proceed through the process, or they may require several days or even weeks to complete it. Throughout the parent-infant acquaintance process, the nurse listens carefully to what the parents say, in order to assess their concerns and

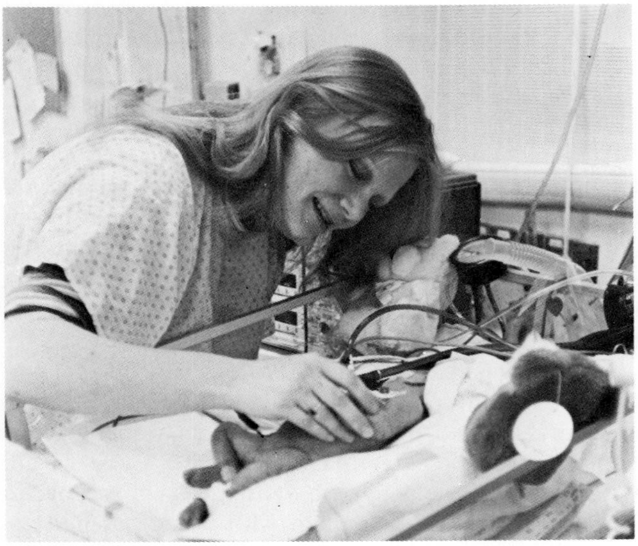

FIG. 9-8 Encouraging interaction of mother and her premature infant facilitates mother-infant attachment process.

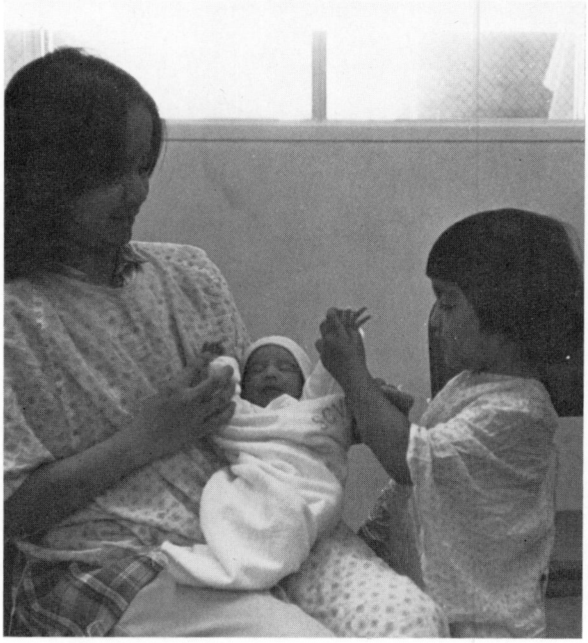

FIG. 9-9 Big sister gets acquainted with the new baby.

their progress toward incorporating the infant into their lives.

Parents are encouraged to bring in clothes and toys for the infant, and the nurse helps the mother set goals for both herself and the infant. Feeding schedules are discussed, and the parents are encouraged to visit at times when they can become involved in the infant's care. Although the advisability of sibling visitation is still a matter of controversy in many neonatal units, the trend is toward allowing siblings into the NICU or as soon as the infant can be transferred to a transitional care unit (Fig. 9-9). Other visitors, such as grandparents, are permitted in most institutions.

Parent support groups have been of immeasurable value to families of infants in neonatal intensive care facilities. Some groups consist of parents who have infants in the hospital and who share the same anxieties and concerns. Other groups include parents who have had the same experiences and who have dealt with the crisis effectively. A national organization, **Parent Care,*** which evolved from a local parents' group, provides information, referrals, and support to parents and professionals concerned with the care of high-risk infants. It also publishes a newsletter and a resource directory.

Preparing for discharge. Parents become very apprehensive as well as excited as time for discharge approaches. They have many concerns and insecurities regarding the care of the infant. Often, all that parents need is reassurance that the behavior about which they are concerned is a normal reaction and that it will disappear as the infant matures (for example, the exaggerated Moro reflex or the inability to coordinate swallowing) or that they will have the support of the nurse during caregiving activities. Knowing that members of the staff are available for telephone or personal contact when the infant goes home provides a measure of security to insecure parents. However, it is the responsibility of the nursing staff to make certain that parents are prepared to care for their infant—emotionally and physically (see also Discharge planning and home care, p. 609).

Neonatal Loss

The precarious condition of many high-risk infants makes death a very real and ever-present possibility. Nurses in the intensive care unit are in an excellent position to prepare the parents for an inevitable death and to facilitate the family's grieving process after an expected or unexpected death. It is important that the staff allow the parents to hold and touch the infant before death and to be provided with an opportunity to see, touch, and hold the infant privately after death if they desire.

A photograph of the infant taken before or after his death is highly desirable. The parents may not wish to see the photograph at the time of death, but to be able to refer to it later will help make the infant seem more real, a part of the normal grief process. Other tangible remembrances of the child can be provided, such as name tags, arm bands, and locks of hair shaved for intravenous insertion or other procedures. If the parents have not done so, they should be encouraged to name the infant.

At least one nurse who is familiar to the family should

*University of Utah Medical Center, 50 North Medical Drive, Room 2A210, Salt Lake City, UT 84132.

NURSING CARE PLAN

The Low-Birth-Weight Infant

Nursing Goals	Nursing Interventions	Expected Patient/Family Outcomes
NDx HP-HMP* Potential for infection **Etiology: deficient immunologic defenses**		
Prevent infection	Carry out meticulous handwashing before handling infant Ensure that all equipment in contact with infant is scrupulously clean or sterile Prevent personnel with infections from coming into direct contact with infant Isolate other infants who have infections	Infant exhibits no evidence of infection
NDx N-MP Ineffective thermoregulation **Etiology: immature temperature control**		
Provide neutral thermal environment	Place infant in humidified Isolette, radiant warmer, or warmly clothed in open crib Monitor temperature hourly in unstable infants (take axillary temperature; check function of Servo-controlled mechanism when used) Check temperature of infant in relation to temperature of heating unit Avoid situations that might predispose infant to chilling, such as exposure to cool air	Infant's temperature remains at optimum level
NDx N-MP Potential fluid volume deficit **Risk factors: physiologic characteristics of preterm infant**		
Maintain hydration	Monitor therapies that increase insensible water loss, e.g., phototherapy Ensure adequate intake Assess state of hydration, e.g., skin turgor, temperature, weight, urine specific gravity	Infant exhibits no evidence of dehydration
NDx N-MP Altered nutrition: less than body requirements **Etiology: inability to ingest nutrients because of weakness**		
Provide nutrition	Bottle-feed infant if strong sucking and swallowing reflexes are present Gavage feed if infant tires easily or has weak sucking, gag, or swallowing reflexes Assist mothers with breast-feeding if feasible and desirable	Infant receives an adequate amount of nutrients Infant demonstrates a steady weight gain
NDx N-MP Potential impaired skin integrity **Risk factors: immature skin structure, immobility**		
Prevent skin breakdown	Cleanse skin with clear water or approved cleanser Avoid use of alkaline-based or hexachlorophene cleansing products or lotions Use Transpore tape only to secure items to the skin Apply protective covering to skin on which tape or adhesive-backed items, e.g., electrodes, may be attached Exert extreme care when performing activities involving skin, e.g., removing dressings, electrodes, tape Place infant on water pillow or fleece Turn at least every 2 hours	Skin remains clean and intact with no evidence of irritation or injury

*For an explanation of abbreviations, see p. 20.

Continued.

NURSING CARE PLAN

The Low-Birth-Weight Infant—cont'd

Nursing Goals	Nursing Interventions	Expected Patient/Family Outcomes
A-EP Ineffective breathing pattern **Etiology: neuromuscular impairment (immature respiratory center), decreased energy, and fatigue**		
Support respiratory efforts	Position for optimum air exchange (head supported when on side) Observe for deviations from desired functioning; recognize signs of distress Suction as necessary to remove accumulated mucus from nasopharynx, trachea, and (where necessary) endotracheal tube Carry out percussion, vibration, and postural drainage to loosen secretions in respiratory tree Prevent aspiration Observe for signs of respiratory distress—nasal flaring, retractions, tachypnea	Breathing is regular and unlabored Respiratory rate is within normal limits (specify)
A-EP Activity intolerance **Etiology: imbalance between oxygen supply and demand**		
Conserve energy	Maintain neutral thermal environment Concentrate activities to allow for longer periods of rest Administer gavage feeding when infant tires easily Ensure minimum handling of infant	Infant rests 1 hour (uninterrupted) at regularly scheduled intervals (specify)
A-EP Altered growth and development **Etiology: preterm birth**		
Facilitate physical adjustments	Assess physiologic status Provide appropriate physiologic support as outlined in appropriate nursing diagnoses	*Physiologic status is determined
Determine physiologic status	Measure infant Assess gestational age based on external characteristics and neurologic signs Weigh daily	*Gestational age of infant is recorded at birth *Any deviation from baseline information is detected early and appropriate action implemented
CPP Sensory-perceptual alterations (visual, auditory, kinesthetic, gustatory, tactile, olfactory) **Etiology: therapeutically restricted environment**		
Provide sensory stimulation	See box on p. 229	Infant responds to appropriate stimuli
RRP Altered family processes **Etiology: situational/maturational crisis, knowledge deficit (birth of a preterm infant)**		
Keep parents informed of infant's progress	Answer questions, allow expression of concern regarding care and prognosis Encourage mother and father to visit and/or call unit Emphasize positive aspects of infant status Be honest but not overly candid or overly optimistic	Parents express feelings and concerns regarding the infant and his prognosis
Facilitate sibling-infant attachment	Allow siblings to visit infant when feasible Explain environment, events, and strange appearance of infant, e.g., why infant cannot come home, "special" bed Provide photos of infant or other items if siblings unable to visit	Siblings visit infant in nursery Siblings exhibit an understanding of explanations (specify) Siblings receive infant-related items (specify)
Prepare for infant's discharge	Assess readiness of family (especially mother) to care for infant Teach necessary techniques and observations Arrange for public health referral if indicated	Family demonstrates the ability to provide care for the infant Family members take advantage of available services

*Nursing outcome.

NURSING CARE PLAN

The Low-Birth-Weight Infant

Nursing Goals	Nursing Interventions	Expected Patient/Family Outcomes
	Reinforce follow-up care Refer to appropriate agencies or services for needed assistance Encourage and facilitate involvement with parent group Teach family infant cardiopulmonary resuscitation technique and response to choking incident	Family members keep appointments for follow-up care
NDA RRP Altered parenting **Etiology: interruption of bonding process**		
Facilitate parent-infant attachment process	Initiate parents' visit as soon as possible Encourage parents to Visit infant frequently Touch, fondle, and caress infant Become actively involved in infant's care Bring clothing to dress up infant as soon as condition permits Reinforce parents' endeavors Be alert to signs of tension in parents Allow parents to spend time alone with infant Help parents interpret infant responses; comment regarding any positive infant response Help parents by demonstrating techniques and offer support	Parents visit infant soon after birth and at frequent intervals Parents relate positively with infant Parents provide care for the infant and demonstrate an attitude of comfort in relationships with the infant

Nursing interventions related to medical management

Support respiratory efforts
- Maintain ambient oxygen at level to ensure satisfactory skin color with minimum respiratory effort and energy expenditure
- Carry out regimen prescribed for supplemental oxygen therapy (maintain ambient oxygen concentration at minimum FiO_2 level to maintain good color and energy expenditure)
- Apply and manage monitoring equipment correctly
- Understand functioning of respiratory support apparatus
  - Assisted ventilation apparatus
  - Controlled ventilation apparatus
  - Insufflation bags with masks and/or endotracheal adaptor
  - Oxygen hoods
  - Humidifier warmers

Provide nutrition
- Maintain parenteral fluid or hyperalimentation therapy as ordered

Maintain hydration
- Regulate parenteral fluids
- Avoid administering hypertonic fluids, e.g., undiluted medications

Monitor physiologic data
- Understand proper function and use of monitoring equipment and maintain at desired settings
  - Apnea monitor
  - Heart rate monitor, including oscilloscope and electrocardiograph printout units
  - Temperature monitor, usually with skin probe
  - Oxygen analyzers
  - Transcutaneous monitors
- Collect specimens
  - Blood for glucose, bilirubin, electrolytes, and pH determinations
  - Blood for hemoglobin, hematocrit, microscopic examination, and culture
  - Urine for laboratory examination
- Take vital signs as ordered (axillary temperature, apical pulse)

Prevent or control infection
- Administer prophylactic antibiotics as ordered

Assist in specific therapies
- Phototherapy—implement and maintain protective measures
- Administer medications as ordered
  - Antibiotics prophylactically or therapeutically
  - Vitamin K to prevent hemorrhage
  - Sedatives, etc., for withdrawal symptoms, seizures, irritability
  - Electrolyte replacement
  - Alkali therapy in acidosis
- Avoid use of substances known to be toxic to premature infants, e.g., benzyl alcohol or other preservatives
- Provide assisted ventilation and therapeutic measures as indicated

be present during discussion of the dead or dying infant. Funeral arrangements should be discussed with parents openly and honestly, since few of them have had experience with this aspect of death. They need to be informed of options available, but it is preferable to encourage a funeral because the ritual provides an opportunity for parents to feel the support of friends and relatives. A clergyman of the appropriate faith should be offered if available.

Before the parents leave the hospital they should be given the telephone number of the unit (if they do not have it) and invited to call any time they have further questions. Many intensive care units make it a point to contact the parents after a neonatal death to assess parents' coping mechanisms and provide support as needed. Several organizations are available to offer support and understanding to families who have lost a newborn, including **Compassionate Friends,*** **S.H.A.R.E. (Source of Help in Airing & Resolving Experiences),**† and **A.M.E.N.D. (Aiding Mothers & Fathers Experiencing Neo-Natal Death).**‡

Baptism. Since most Christian parents wish to have their children baptized if death is anticipated or a decided possibility, this becomes a nursing responsibility. Whenever possible, it is desirable that a representative of the parents' faith—that is, a Roman Catholic priest or a Protestant minister—perform the ritual. When death is imminent, however, a nurse or a physician can perform the baptism by simply pouring water on the infant's forehead (a medicine dropper is a convenient means) while saying, "I baptize you in the name of the Father and of the Son and of the Holy Spirit." Such baptisms may need to be performed for newborns of any gestational age. Baptism is particularly important when the parents are of the Roman Catholic faith. When the faith of the parent is uncertain, a conditional baptism can be carried out by saying, "If you are capable of receiving baptism, I baptize you in the name of the Father and of the Son and of the Holy Spirit." The fact of the baptism is recorded in the infant's chart, and a notice is placed on the crib or Isolette. Parents are informed at the first opportunity.

EVALUATION

The effectiveness of nursing interventions is determined by continual reassessment and evaluation of care based on the following observational guidelines and expected outcomes:

1. Take vital signs at frequent intervals (specify time intervals based on infant's needs); observe respiratory efforts; check functioning of respiratory equipment; review laboratory test results
2. Measure abdominal skin temperature at specified intervals
3. Observe infant's behavior and appearance for evidence of sepsis
4. Assess for hydration; observe the infant during feeding, measure amount of formula consumed; weigh daily or as prescribed
5. Observe the infant's behavior for evidence of fatigue
6. Observe the infant for evidence of any complications (follow assessment guide on p. 223)
7. Observe infant behaviors in response to stimuli
8. Observe parental interaction with the infant; interview family regarding their feelings and concerns and readiness for home care
9. Interview family and observe their behaviors during and after the death of their infant

(See also evaluative criteria for any specific health problem.)

Expected outcomes:
See Nursing Care Plan on pp. 231-233.

◆ *High-Risk Related to Dysmaturity*

The majority of infants classified as being of low birth weight are born before the estimated date of delivery. Although prematurity is encountered more frequently and is a greater threat to life, postmaturity is not without problems.

THE PRETERM INFANT

The terms *preterm* and *premature* are used to describe the infant who is born before the completion of the 37 weeks of gestation, regardless of birth weight. Prematurity accounts for the largest number of admissions to neonatal intensive care units. The incidence of neonatal complications is highest in the preterm (premature) infant, and infants with other high-risk factors—for example, severe congenital defects often found in association with prematurity. Prematurity is generally accepted as the single greatest contributor to infant mortality.

The actual cause of prematurity is not known in most instances. The incidence is lowest in the middle and high socioeconomic classes, in which pregnant women are generally in good health, are well nourished, and receive prompt and comprehensive prenatal care. The incidence is highest in the low socioeconomic class, in which a combination of deleterious circumstances is present. Other factors, such as multiple pregnancies, preeclampsia, and placental accidents that interrupt the normal course of gestation before completion of fetal development, are responsible for a large number of premature births.

The outlook for a premature infant is largely, but not entirely, related to the state of physiologic and anatomic immaturity of the various organs and systems at the time of birth. The infant at term has advanced to a state of maturity sufficient to allow a successful transition to the extrauterine environment. The infant born prematurely must make the same adjustments but with functional im-

*P.O. Box 3696, Oak Brook, IL 60522-3696 or call (312)323-5010; 685 William Ave., Winnipeg, Canada, R3E 022.

†St. Johns Hospital, 800 Carpenter, Springfield, IL 62769 or call (217)544-6464, Ext. 5275.

‡Contact Maureen Connelly, 4324 Berrywick Terrace, St. Louis, MO 63128 or call (314)487-7582.

Clinical Manifestations of Prematurity

Very small, scrawny appearance
Skin—red to pink with visible veins
Fine, feathery hair; lanugo on back and face
Little or no evidence of subcutaneous fat
Head larger in relation to body
Sucking pads prominent
Lies in "relaxed attitude"
Limbs extended
Ear cartilages poorly developed
Few fine wrinkles on palms and soles
Clitoris prominent in female
Scrotum underdeveloped, nonpendulous, with minimal rugae and undescended testes
Lax, easily manipulated joints
Absent, weak, or ineffectual grasping, sucking, and swallowing reflexes
Other neurologic signs are absent or diminished
Unable to maintain body temperature
Dilute urine
Pliable thorax
Periodic breathing, hypoventilation
Frequent episodes of apnea

maturity that is directly related to the stage of development reached at the time of birth. The degree to which the infant is prepared for extrauterine life can be predicted to some extent by weight and estimated gestational age.

Diagnostic Evaluation

On inspection, the premature infant is very small and appears scrawny because of lack of or minimal subcutaneous fat deposits, with a proportionately large head in relation to the body, which reflects the cephalocaudal direction of growth. In contrast to the full-term infant's overall attitude of flexion and continuous activity, the premature infant is inactive and motionless. The common characteristics of preterm infants are outlined in the box; these can be compared with the features of normal and premature infants in Fig. 9-10. (See also Assessment of gestational age, p. 185).

Therapeutic Management

As a consequence of anatomic, physiologic, and biochemical inadequacies, the premature infant is prone to a variety of problems that must be anticipated and managed in the neonatal period. When a preterm infant is anticipated, the intensive care nursery is alerted and a pediatrician, ideally a neonatologist, is present for the delivery. The infant who does not require resuscitation is transferred immediately in a heated Isolette to the intensive care nursery to be weighed and where any necessary therapies are initiated based on the needs of the infant. Resuscitation is conducted in the delivery area until the infant can be safely transported to the intensive care unit.

Subsequent care is determined by the status of the infant. The general care of the preterm infant differs from that of the full-term infant primarily in the areas of respiratory support, temperature regulation, nutrition, susceptibility to infection, activity intolerance, and other consequences of physical immaturity. All are placed in a controlled thermal environment and appropriate measures implemented to protect the infant from infection. An intravenous access is established to provide a means for providing fluids, medication, and (sometimes) nutrition. Most infants require special feeding methods and supplemental calories. Complications, such as hypoglycemia and hypocalcemia, that are frequent in preterm infants are managed according to the specific condition. Respiratory distress syndrome is one of the most common concurrent problems of prematurity and requires respiratory support (p. 243).

Nursing Considerations

The nursing care, like the therapeutic management, is individualized for each infant. Nurses must be aware of the special needs of the preterm infant and must incorporate appropriate interventions to meet these needs. (See nursing care of the high-risk infant, p. 221).

THE POSTMATURE INFANT

Infants born after 42 weeks of gestation, as calculated from the mother's last menstrual period, are considered to be *postmature* or *postterm*, regardless of birth weight. This comprises approximately 12% of all births. The cause of delayed birth is unknown. Some infants are appropriate size for gestational age, but many show the characteristics of intrauterine impoverishment from progressive placental dysfunction. The appropriate-for-gestational-age infants are often indistinguishable in appearance from term infants. Others—most often called *postmature infants*—display the characteristics of infants who are 1 to 3 weeks of age (see box).

There is a significant increase in fetal and neonatal mortality in postterm infants compared to those born at term. They are especially prone to intrauterine hypoxia associated with the decreasing efficiency of the placenta and to the meconium aspiration syndrome. The greatest risk occurs during the stresses of labor and delivery, par-

Clinical Manifestations of Postmaturity

Absence of lanugo
Little if any vernix caseosa, deep yellow or green in color
Abundant scalp hair
Long fingernails
Whiter skin than term newborns
Skin frequently cracked, parchmentlike, and desquamating
Wasted physical appearance
Long, thin appearance

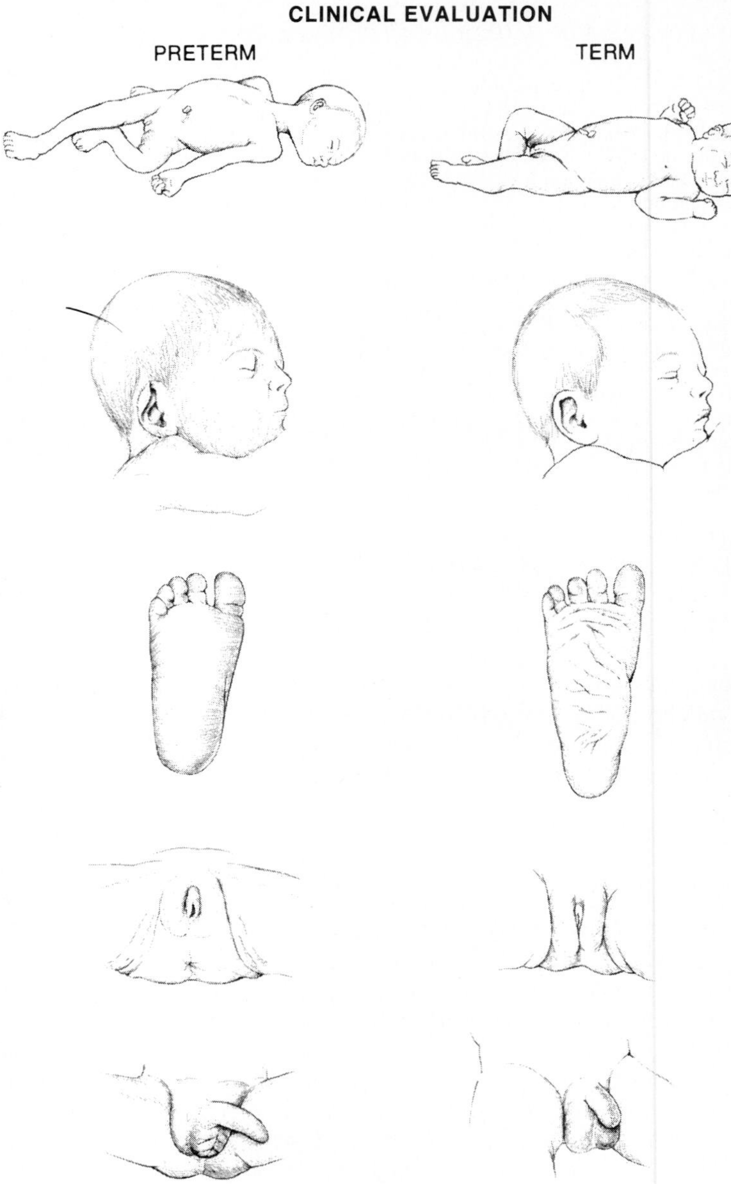

The preterm infant lies in a "relaxed attitude," limbs more extended; his body size is small, and his head may appear somewhat larger in proportion to the body size. The term infant has more subcutaneous fat tissue and rests in a more flexed attitude.

The preterm infant's ear cartilages are poorly developed, and the ear may fold easily; the hair is fine and feathery, and lanugo may cover the back and face. The mature infant's ear cartilages are well formed, and the hair is more likely to form firm separate strands.

The sole of the foot of the preterm infant appears more turgid and may have only fine wrinkles. The mature infant's sole (foot) is well and deeply creased.

The preterm female infant's clitoris is prominent, and labia majora are poorly developed and gaping. The mature female infant's labia majora are fully developed, and the clitoris is not as prominent.

The preterm male infant's scrotum is undeveloped and not pendulous; minimal rugae are present, and the testes may be in the inguinal canals or in the abdominal cavity. The term male infant's scrotum is well developed, pendulous, and rugated, and the testes are well down in the scrotal sac.

ticularly in infants of primigravidas (women delivering their first child). Cesarean section or induction of labor is usually recommended when the infant is significantly overdue.

◆ *High Risk Related to Physiologic Complications*

A number of pathologic processes interfere with the normal course of adjustment to extrauterine life. Some can be attributed directly to mechanical injuries during the birth process (intracranial hemorrhage, meconium aspiration), some are the result of postdelivery disturbances hypoglycemia and hypocalcemia), and others are pathologic variations of certain physiologic peculiarities in some newborn infants (blood incompatibilities).

HYPERBILIRUBINEMIA

The term *hyperbilirubinemia* refers to an excessive accumulation of bilirubin in the blood and is characterized by *jaundice*, or *icterus*, a yellowish discoloration of the skin and other organs. Hyperbilirubinemia is a common

FIG. 9-10 Clinical and neurologic examinations comparing preterm and full-term infants. (From Pierog, S.H., and Ferrara, A.: Medical care of the sick newborn, ed. 2, St. Louis, 1976, The C.V. Mosby Co.)

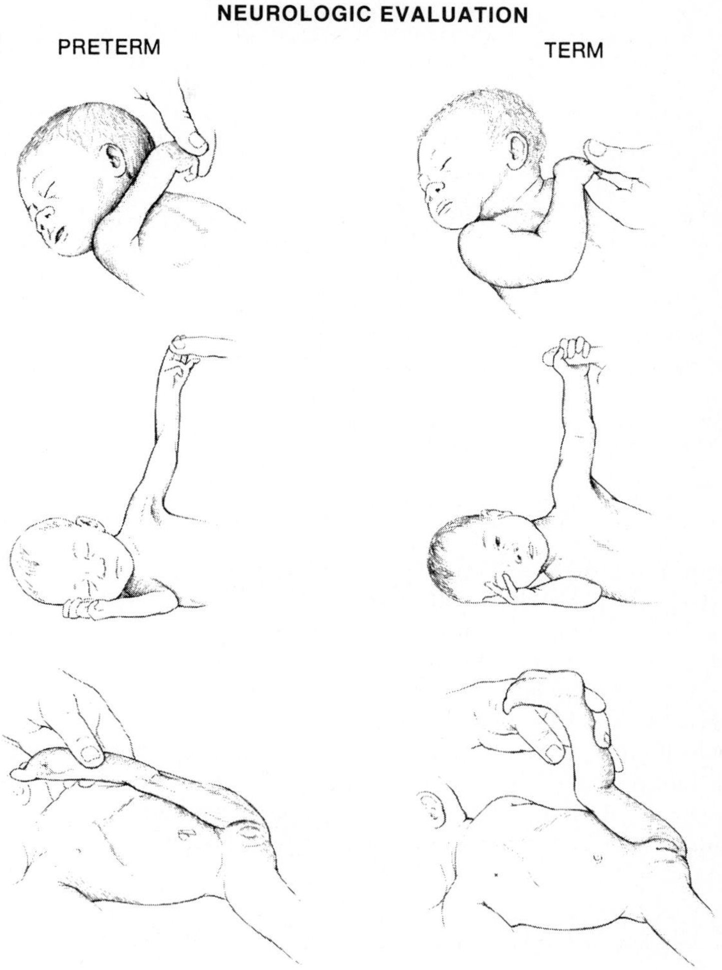

Scarf sign—The preterm infant's elbow may be easily brought across the chest with little or no resistance. The mature infant's elbow may be brought to the midline of the chest, resisting attempts to bring the elbow past the midline.

Grasp reflex—The preterm infant's grasp is weak; the term infant's grasp is strong, allowing the infant to be lifted up from the mattress.

Heel-to-ear maneuver—The preterm infant's heel is easily brought to the ear, meeting with no resistance. This maneuver is not possible in the term infant, since there is considerable resistance at the knee.

finding in the newborn and, in most instances, is relatively benign. However, it can also indicate a pathologic state. Following is a brief description of the pathophysiology of bilirubin production and excretion and a discussion of several disorders that cause hyperbilirubinemia in the newborn.

Pathophysiology

Bilirubin is one of the breakdown products of hemoglobin that results from red blood cell destruction. When red blood cells are destroyed, the breakdown products are released into the circulation where the hemoglobin splits into two fractions, heme and globin. The globin (protein) portion is used by the body, and the heme portion is converted to unconjugated bilirubin, an insoluble substance bound to albumin. In the liver the bilirubin is detached from the plasma protein and, in the presence of the enzyme *glucuronyl transferase,* is conjugated with glucuronic acid to produce a highly soluble substance, bilirubin glucuronide, which is then excreted into the bile.

The normal newborn produces an average of twice as much bilirubin as does an adult because of higher concentrations of circulating erythrocytes and a shorter life

TABLE 9-1

Comparison of Three Types of Unconjugated Hyperbilirubinemia

	Physiologic Jaundice	Breast-Feeding Jaundice	Hemolytic Disease
Cause	Immature hepatic function plus increased bilirubin load from red blood cell hemolysis	Unknown etiology Early: related to fewer calories consumed by infant before mother's milk established Late: factor in breast milk that inhibits bilirubin conjugation	Blood antigen incompatibility causes hemolysis of large numbers of erythrocytes Liver unable to conjugate and excrete excess bilirubin from hemolysis
Onset	After 24 hours (premature infants, before 48 hours)	Early: 3 to 4 days of age Late: 4 to 5 days	During first 24 hours
Peak	Second to third days	Third week	
Duration	Decline fifth to seventh days	Up to 3 to 12 weeks	
Therapy	Phototherapy	Frequent breast-feeding When bilirubin levels reach 15 to 16 mg/100 ml, temporary discontinuation of breast-feeding for 48 hours	Postnatal: exchange transfusion Prenatal: transfusion (fetus) Prevent sensitization (Rh incompatibility) of Rh-negative mother with RhoGam

span of red blood cells (only 60 to 80 days, in contrast to 120 days in the older child and the adult). In addition, the liver's ability to conjugate bilirubin is reduced because of diminished glucuronyl transferase production.

Although the body is normally able to maintain a balance between the destruction of red blood cells and the utilization or excretion of by-products, when developmental limitations or a pathologic process interferes with this balance, bilirubin accumulates in the tissues to produce jaundice. In the newborn, infant hyperbilirubinemia may be the result of:

1. Excess production of bilirubin
2. Disturbed capacity of the liver to conjugate bilirubin
3. Bile duct obstruction (biliary atresia) (see p. 763)

The most common cause of hyperbilirubinemia is the relatively mild and self-limited *physiologic jaundice*, or *icterus neonatorum*. However, it may be the result of a disease process such as hemolytic disease of the newborn or infection. See Table 9-1 for a comparison of the more common causes of hyperbilirubinemia.

Diagnostic Evaluation

Almost all newborns experience elevated bilirubin levels (above the normal value of 0.2 to 1.4 mg/100 ml); however, about half demonstrate observable signs of jaundice (see box). In the newborn, bilirubin levels must exceed 5 mg/100 ml before jaundice or icterus is observable, principally in the sclera, nails, or skin. As a rule, jaundice that appears within the first 24 hours is caused by hemolytic disease of the newborn, sepsis, or one of the maternally derived diseases (p. 256); jaundice that appears on the second or third day, peaks on the second to fourth days, and decreases between the fifth and seventh days is usually the result of physiologic jaundice; jaundice appearing after the third day but within the first week suggests sepsis. Because unconjugated bilirubin is highly toxic to neurons, an infant with severe jaundice is at risk of developing *kernicterus,* severe brain damage resulting from the deposition of unconjugated bilirubin in brain cells when the serum concentration of bilirubin reaches toxic levels, regardless of the cause.

Infants of Oriental descent (including Native Americans) have mean bilirubin levels almost twice those seen in whites or blacks. An increased incidence of hyperbilirubinemia is seen in newborns from certain geographic areas, particularly areas around Greece. Also, approximately 1 in 200 breast-fed infants with no evidence of disease develop hyperbilirubinemia.

Therapeutic Management

The aims of therapy for hyperbilirubinemia are to prevent kernicterus and, in any blood group incompatibility, to reverse the hemolytic process (see p. 242). The main forms of therapy are phototherapy and pharmacologic manage-

Clinical Manifestations of Hyperbilirubinemia

Jaundice—yellowish discoloration of skin
- Bright yellow or orange—unconjugated (indirect)
- Greenish, muddy yellow—conjugated (direct)

Intensity of jaundice
- Unrelated to degree of bilirubinemia
- Determined by serum bilirubin measurements

ment. Exchange transfusion is usually restricted to management of hemolytic disease.

Phototherapy. Phototherapy consists of the application of intense fluorescent light to the infant's exposed skin. Light in the blue and green ranges enhances bilirubin excretion by the process of photoisomerization, which alters the structure of bilirubin to a soluble form for easier excretion. Because blue light alters the coloration of the infant, the normal light of full-spectrum fluorescent bulbs is preferred so that the skin of the infant can be better observed for color, pallor, cyanosis, or other conditions. Although the value of phototherapy in effectively reducing or preventing rising bilirubin levels is well documented, its long-term effects are unclear.

The effectiveness of phototherapy is determined by a decrease in bilirubin levels, usually a fall of 3 to 4 mg/100 ml after 8 to 12 hours of therapy. The infant's total physical status is assessed because suppression of jaundice may mask signs of sepsis, hemolytic disease, or hepatitis.

Because hyperbilirubinemia is a common occurrence among newborns, phototherapy in the home is becoming a widely used alternative means for providing care for some infants. This permits earlier discharge of the infant. However, the practice is not universally endorsed.

Pharmacologic management. Some moderate success has been achieved by the administration of barbiturates, such as phenobarbital, to infants with hyperbilirubinemia to stimulate liver maturation. However, best results are observed when the drug is administered to the mother 1 to 2 weeks before delivery. The effect of treatment is not rapid enough when administered to the infant with hyperbilirubinemia.

Nursing Considerations

The primary nursing consideration is recognizing jaundice and helping to distinguish the benign disorder from a threatening one.

ASSESSMENT

Part of the routine physical assessment includes observing for evidence of jaundice at regular intervals. Jaundice is most reliably assessed by observing the color of the sclera, nails, and skin, including palms, soles, and mucous membranes. Applying direct pressure to the skin, especially over bony prominences such as the tip of the nose or the sternum, causes blanching and allows the yellow stain to be more pronounced. For dark-skinned infants, the color of the sclera, conjunctiva, and oral mucosa is the most reliable indicator. The nurse observes the infant in natural daylight for a true assessment of color. Any neonate who becomes icteric during the first 24 hours of life and has rapidly rising bilirubin levels is referred to the physician for immediate evaluation.

The transcutaneous bilirubin meter is a useful screening device and is used to detect neonatal jaundice in full-term infants. However, phototherapy reduces the accuracy of the instrument; therefore its value is limited to the initial assessment. Institutions in which the device is employed set up their own criteria based on their experience with the particular instrument in use.

Blood samples are also taken for measurement of bilirubin in the laboratory. While blood is drawn the lights should be turned off to avoid a false reading from bilirubin destruction in the test tube.

Nursing Diagnoses: Infant with Hyperbilirubinemia

Potential altered body temperature, increase related to use of phototherapy
Potential fluid volume deficit related to phototherapy
Altered family processes related to situational crisis, prolonged hospitalization of infant

NURSING DIAGNOSES

Based on the nursing assessment a number of nursing diagnoses may be evident (see box). Some are the same as for any high-risk infant; others may be related to concomitant health problems, such as prematurity or sepsis.

PLANNING

The broad objectives for management of hyperbilirubinemia are to:

1. Assist with measures to reduce serum bilirubin levels
2. Prevent complications from therapy
3. Support family

IMPLEMENTATION

The infant who receives phototherapy is placed nude under the fluorescent light and turned frequently to expose all body surface areas to the light. To be effective, light must come in contact with the skin surface. Areas that are protected from the light retain their jaundiced appearance. There is evidence to indicate that a cap, fashioned from stockinette, worn by the infant during phototherapy prevents phototherapy-induced hypocalcemia (Blake, 1983).

Several precautions are instituted to protect the infant during phototherapy. The infant's eyes are shielded by an opaque mask to prevent exposure to the light (Fig. 9-11). The eye shield should be properly sized and correctly positioned to prevent any occlusion of the nares. The infant's eyelids are closed before the mask is applied, since the corneas may become excoriated if they come in contact with the dressing. On each shift, the eyes are checked for evidence of discharge, excessive pressure on the lids, or corneal irritation.

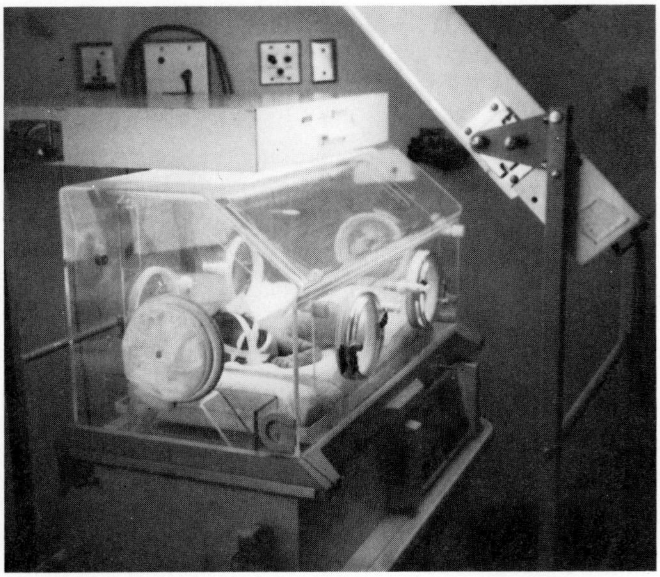

FIG. 9-11 Phototherapy unit with infant in Isolette. Note that the bilirubin lights have been positioned laterally to increase exposure to phototherapy.

At the present time the long-term risks from phototherapy are not known. However, minor side effects do occur and should be observed for and recorded. These include loose greenish stools, hyperthermia, increased metabolic rate, increased evaporative loss of water, and priapism. The temperature is closely monitored to detect early signs of hyperthermia and the skin observed for evidence of dehydration and drying, which can lead to excoriation and breakdown. Oily lubricants or lotions are not used on the skin in order to avoid increased tanning, or a so-called "frying" effect. Infants receiving phototherapy require up to 25% additional fluid volume to compensate for insensible and intestinal fluid loss.

Where home phototherapy is used nurses are actively involved in preparing families for the infant's care and supervising therapy in the home (see also Discharge planning and home care, p. 609).

Family support. Parents need constant reassurance concerning their infant's progress. All the procedures are explained to them so that they are aware of the benefits and risks. For example, they need to be reassured that the naked infant who is under the bilirubin light is warm and comfortable. Parents may be concerned about the blindfolds, since "blindness" is a frightening experience. Blindfolds are removed when the parents are visiting to facilitate the attachment process, and the parents can be reassured that the neonate is accustomed to darkness after months of intrauterine existence and benefits a great deal from auditory and tactile stimulation.

EVALUATION

The effectiveness of nursing interventions is determined by continual reassessment and evaluation of care based on the following observational guidelines and expected outcomes:

1. Observe skin color; review bilirubinometric and/or laboratory findings
2. Observe for signs of neurologic impairment (see Assessment guidelines on p. 223)
3. Check placement of eye shields; observe skin for signs of dehydration; take temperature
4. Interview family members and observe parent-infant interactions

Expected outcomes:

1. Signs of hyperbilirubinemia diminish and/or disappear
2. The infant displays no evidence of neurologic complications
3. The infant exhibits no signs of adverse effects of phototherapy: eyes remain free of irritation, infant remains well hydrated, temperature remains below 38° C (100.4° F)
4. Family members demonstrate an understanding of the disease and its therapy; they interact with the infant appropriately

HEMOLYTIC DISEASE OF THE NEWBORN

Hyperbilirubinemia in the first 24 hours of life is most often the result of hemolytic disease (*erythroblastosis fetalis*, an abnormally rapid rate of red cell destruction). Anemia caused by this destruction stimulates the production of red blood cells, which, in turn, provides increasing numbers of cells for hemolysis. Major causes of increased erythrocyte destruction are isoimmunization (primarily Rh) and ABO incompatibility.

Blood Incompatibility

The membranes of human blood cells contain a variety of antigens, also known as *agglutinogens*, substances capable of producing an immune response if recognized by the body as a foreign substance. It is the reciprocal relationship between the antigens on the red blood cells and the antibodies in the serum that causes agglutination to take place.

In other words, antibodies in the serum of one group (except AB blood group, which contains no antibodies) will produce an agglutination or clumping reaction when mixed with antigens of a different blood group. In the ABO blood group system the antibodies occur naturally. In the Rh system the person must first be exposed to the Rh antigen before significant antibody formation takes place to cause a sensitivity response.

Rh incompatibility (isoimmunization). The Rh blood group consists of several antigens, but for simplicity, only the terms *Rh-positive* (presence of the antigen) and *Rh-negative* (absence of the antigen) are used in this discussion (see recessive inheritance pattern, Appendix B). The presence or absence of the naturally occurring Rh factor determines the blood type. Ordinarily no problems are anticipated when the Rh blood types are the same in both mother and fetus or if the mother is Rh-positive and the infant Rh-negative. Difficulty may arise when the blood

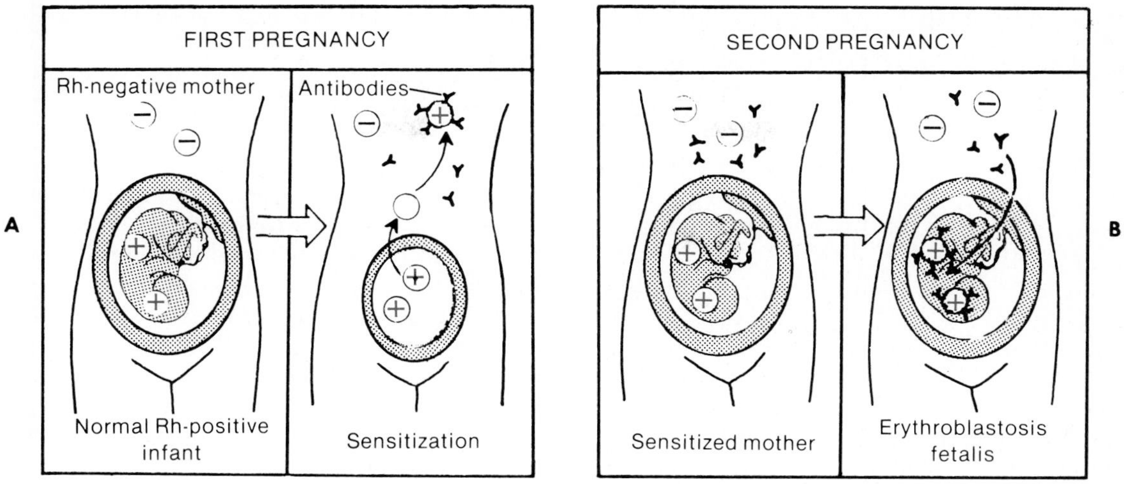

FIG. 9-12 Development of maternal sensitization to Rh antigens. **A,** Fetal Rh-positive erythrocytes enter the maternal system. Maternal anti-Rh antibodies are formed. **B,** Anti-Rh antibodies cross the placenta and attack the fetal erythrocytes.

of the mother is Rh-negative and that of the infant is Rh-positive.

Although the maternal and fetal circulations are separate and distinct, sometimes fetal red blood cells (with antigens foreign to the mother) gain access to the maternal circulation through minute breaks in the placental vessels. The mother's natural defense mechanism responds to these alien cells by producing anti-Rh antibodies (isoimmunization).

Under normal circumstances, this process of isoimmunization has no effect on the fetus during the first pregnancy with an Rh-positive fetus because the initial sensitization to Rh antigens rarely occurs before the onset of labor. However, as larger amounts of fetal blood are transferred to the maternal circulation during placental separation, the maternal immune system is stimulated to form anti-Rh antibodies. During a subsequent pregnancy with an Rh-positive fetus, these previously formed maternal antibodies to Rh-positive blood cells enter the fetal circulation, where they attack and destroy fetal erythrocytes (Fig. 9-12). Since the disease begins in utero, the fetus attempts to compensate for the progressive hemolysis by accelerating the rate of erythropoiesis. As a result, immature red blood cells (erythroblasts) appear in the fetal circulation; hence the term *erythroblastosis fetalis*.

There is wide variability in the development of maternal sensitization to Rh-positive antigens. Sensitization may occur during the first pregnancy if the woman had previously received an Rh-positive blood transfusion. No sensitization may occur in situations where a strong placental barrier prevents transfer of fetal blood into the maternal circulation. In about 10% to 15% of sensitized mothers, there is no hemolytic reaction in the newborn.

In the most severe form of erythroblastosis fetalis, *hydrops fetalis,* the progressive hemolysis causes fetal hypoxia, cardiac failure, generalized edema (anasarca), and effusions of the pericardial, pleural, and peritoneal spaces. The fetus may be delivered stillborn or in severe respiratory distress. Even with immediate exchange transfusions, few of these infants survive.

ABO incompatibility. Hemolytic disease can also occur when the major blood group antigens of the fetus are different from those of the mother. The most common blood group incompatibility occurs between an infant with A or B blood group and a mother with O blood group. (Other possible ABO incompatibilities are listed in Table 9-2.) The naturally occurring anti-A or anti-B antibodies already present in the maternal circulation cross the placenta and attack the fetal red blood cells, causing hemolysis. Usually, however, the hemolytic reaction is less severe than in Rh incompatibility. Since the anti-A or anti-B antibodies are naturally present in the serum, the number of pregnancies is insignificant in the development of ABO incompatibility and preventive measures such as those used in Rh incompatibility are not available.

Diagnostic Evaluation

Diagnosis of isoimmunization before delivery can be made through amniocentesis and analysis of bilirubin levels in amniotic fluid. Increasing bilirubin levels indicate

TABLE 9-2

Potential Maternal-Fetal ABO Incompatibilities

Maternal Blood Group	Fetal Blood Group
O	A or B
B	A or AB
A	B or AB

Clinical Manifestations of Hemolytic Disease

Jaundice appearing shortly after birth during first 24 hours
Hepatosplenomegaly may be evident
Signs of anemia (notably, marked pallor) in severely affected infants

progressive fetal hemolysis and may indicate the need for an intrauterine transfusion or immediate termination of the pregnancy. Erythroblastosis fetalis caused by Rh incompatibility can also be assessed by evaluating rising anti-Rh antibody titers in the maternal circulation (indirect Coombs test).

The disease in the newborn is suspected on the basis of the timing and appearance of jaundice (see box) and can be confirmed postnatally by detecting antibodies attached to the circulating erythrocytes of affected infants (direct Coombs test). The Coombs test is routinely performed on cord blood samples from infants born to Rh-negative mothers.

Therapeutic Management

The primary aim of therapeutic management of isoimmunization is prevention. Postnatal therapy is usually exchange transfusion. Although phototherapy may control bilirubin levels in mild cases, the hemolytic disease may continue, causing severe anemia.

Prevention of Rh isoimmunization. The administration of Rho-immune globulin (RhoGAM*) to all unsensitized Rh-negative mothers after delivery or abortion of an Rh-positive infant or fetus prevents the development of maternal sensitization to the Rh factor. When RhoGAM is given to unsensitized mothers within 72 hours (but possibly as long as 3 to 4 weeks) after delivery or abortion, injected anti-Rh antibodies destroy the fetal erythrocytes passing into the maternal circulation before they are able to exert their immunogenic effect. To be effective, RhoGAM must be administered after the first delivery and repeated after subsequent ones. The administration of RhoGAM at 26 to 28 weeks gestation is also recommended to further reduce the risk of Rh immunization. RhoGAM is not effective against existing Rh-positive antibodies in the maternal circulation.

Exchange transfusion. Exchange transfusion, in which the infant's blood is removed in small amounts (usually 10 to 20 ml at a time) and replaced with compatible blood (such as Rh-negative blood), is a standard mode of therapy for treatment of hyperbilirubinemia and the treatment of choice for hyperbilirubinemia caused by Rh incompatibility. Exchange transfusion removes the sensitized erythrocytes, lowers the serum bilirubin level to prevent kernicterus, corrects the anemia, and prevents cardiac failure. Indications for exchange transfusion include a positive direct Coombs test, hemoglobin concentration of cord blood below 12 g/100 ml, and a bilirubin level of 20 mg/100 ml in the full-term infant or 15 mg/100 ml in the premature infant. An infant born with hydrops fetalis or signs of cardiac failure is a candidate for immediate exchange transfusion with fresh whole blood.

An exchange transfusion is a sterile surgical procedure. A catheter is inserted into the umbilical vein and threaded into the inferior vena cava. Depending on the infant's weight 5 to 20 ml of blood is withdrawn within 15 to 20 seconds and the same volume of donor blood is infused over 60 to 90 seconds. If the blood has been citrated (addition of citrate phosphate dextrose adenine to prevent coagulation), calcium gluconate may be given after infusion of each 100 ml of donor's blood to prevent hypocalcemia.

*Orthodiagnostics, Raritan, NJ.

Nursing Considerations

The initial nursing responsibility is recognizing hyperbilirubinemia. The possibility of hemolytic disease can be anticipated from the prenatal and perinatal history. Prenatal evidence of incompatibility and the laboratory results of the Coombs test are cause for increased vigilance for early signs of jaundice in an infant. Subsequent care is the same as for any high-risk infant. If an exchange transfusion is needed, the nurse prepares the infant and the family and assists the physician with the procedure.

In addition to assisting the physician during the initial stages of the procedure, the nurse keeps accurate records of blood volumes exchanged, including amount of blood withdrawn and infused, time of each procedure, and cumulative record of the total volume exchanged. Vital signs that are monitored electronically are evaluated frequently and correlated with removal and infusion of blood. If signs of restlessness or cardiac arrhythmias occur, the rate of infusion is slowed. Throughout the procedure the infant requires attention to thermoregulation. He should be kept under a radiant warmer, and warmed blankets kept at hand in the event the infant becomes chilled.

After the procedure is completed, the nurse inspects the umbilical site for evidence of bleeding. Usually, the catheter remains in place for use during repeated exchanges. A sterile dressing is applied and checked periodically for evidence of bleeding or infection.

Parents frequently feel guilty because they think they have caused the blood incompatibility. Parents should never be made to feel responsible or negligent. They should be encouraged to verbalize and express their thoughts. Actions that were taken to prevent any problems, such as frequent antepartum examinations and blood tests, should be referred to and praised.

METABOLIC COMPLICATIONS

The stressed newborn infant is subject to a variety of complications related to physiologic function. Prominent among these are fluid and electrolyte derangements (see p. 739), hypoglycemia, and hypocalcemia. Often these complications are associated with other disorders and are difficult to differentiate from other conditions. The major characteristics of hypoglycemia and hypocalcemia are outlined in Table 9-3.

RESPIRATORY DISTRESS SYNDROME

Respiratory distress is common in several neonatal disorders—for example, hypovolemia, hypoglycemia, congenital heart disease, and cerebral hemorrhage. However, the terms *respiratory distress syndrome (RDS), idiopathic respiratory distress syndrome,* and *hyaline membrane disease* (HMD) are most often applied to the severe lung disorder that not only is responsible for more deaths in the pediatric population than any other disease but also carries the highest risk in terms of long-term neurologic complications. It is seen almost exclusively in the preterm infant, the infant of the diabetic mother, and the infant born by cesarean section.

Pneumonia in the newborn period is respiratory distress caused by pathologic organisms. The disease may occur alone or as a complication of HMD. However, because so many of the terms are used interchangeably, for this discussion the more general term *respiratory distress syndrome* will be used except where HMD is particularly applicable.

Pathophysiology

The preterm infant is born before the lungs are fully prepared to serve as efficient organs for gas exchange. Most

TABLE 9-3

Metabolic Abnormalities

	Hypoglycemia	Hypocalcemia
Definition	Blood glucose concentration significantly lower than that in the majority of infants of the same age and weight	Abnormally low levels of calcium in circulating blood
Types	Early transitional neonatal: large or normal-size infants who appear to suffer from hyperinsulinism Classic transient neonatal: infants who suffered intrauterine malnutrition that depleted glycogen and fat stores Secondary: a response to perinatal stresses that increase infant's metabolic needs relative to glycogen stores Recurrent, severe: caused by an enzymatic or metabolic-endocrine defect	Early onset: appears in first 48 hours, appears in preterm infants who experienced perinatal hypoxia Late onset, cow's milk–induced hypocalcemia (neonatal tetany): apparent after first 3 to 4 days (high phosphorus-to-calcium ratio of cow's milk depresses parathyroid activity, reducing serum calcium levels)
Clinical manifestations	Vague, often indistinguishable from other conditions Cerebral signs: jitteriness, tremors, twitching, weak or high-pitched cry, lethargy, limpness, apathy, convulsions, and coma Other: cyanosis, apnea, rapid irregular respirations, sweating, eye rolling, refusal to eat Signs often transient but recurrent	Early onset: jitteriness, apnea, cyanotic episodes, edema, high-pitched cry, abdominal distention Late onset: twitching, tremors, seizures
Laboratory diagnosis	Plasma glucose concentrations less than 35 mg/100 ml in first 72 hours; 45 mg/100 ml thereafter (LBW infants: less than 25 mg/dl)	Serum calcium less than 7 mg/100 ml Ionized calcium less than 3 to 3.5 mg/100 ml
Treatment	Intravenous glucose administration Preventive: early feeding in normoglycemic infants	Early onset: increased milk feedings, administration of calcium supplements (sometimes) Late onset: administration of calcium gluconate orally or intravenously (slowly); vitamin D
Nursing	See Nursing care of the high-risk infant, p. 221 Identify infants with hypoglycemia Reduce environmental factors that predispose to hypoglycemia, e.g., cold stress, respiratory Employ proper feeding techniques Administer glucose as prescribed	See Nursing care of the high-risk infant, p. 221 Identify infants with hypocalcemia Administer calcium as prescribed Observe for signs of acute hypercalcemia, e.g., vomiting, bradycardia Manipulate environment to reduce stimuli that might precipitate a seizure or tremors, e.g., picking up infant suddenly, sudden jarring of crib

full-term infants successfully accomplish the respiratory adjustments required at birth; the premature infant with respiratory distress is unable to do so. The infant with respiratory distress syndrome can develop respiratory insufficiency either acutely (in 30 minutes) or over a period of hours. Usually, the observable signs produced by the pulmonary changes begin to appear in an infant who apparently achieves normal breathing and color soon after birth.

Although a number of factors are involved, most authorities believe that the central factor responsible for this adaptation is normal development of the surfactant system. Surfactant is a surface-active phospholipid secreted by the alveolar epithelium. Acting much like a detergent, this substance reduces the surface tension of fluids that line the alveoli and respiratory passages, resulting in uniform expansion of lungs and maintenance of lung expansion. Without surfactant, the infant is unable to keep the lungs inflated and, therefore, exerts a great deal of effort to reexpand the alveoli with each breath. This inability to maintain lung expansion produces widespread atelectasis, hypoxemia, and hypercapnia.

To compound this situation, increased amounts of lactic acid are formed to produce a metabolic acidosis, and the inability of the atelectatic lungs to blow off excess carbon dioxide produces a respiratory acidosis. The acidosis causes vasoconstriction, which diminishes pulmonary circulation, and materials needed for surfactant production are not circulated to the alveoli. The hyaline membrane, characteristic of the disorder, decreases the elasticity of the lungs, which become stiff and require far more pressure than do normal lungs to achieve an equal amount of expansion. In addition, the characteristically weak chest wall muscles and the highly cartilaginous nature of the rib structure produce an abnormally elastic rib cage.

Clinical Manifestations of RDS

Dyspnea
Tachypnea (up to 80 to 120 breaths/min)
Pronounced substernal retractions (Fig. 9-13)
Fine inspiratory rales heard over both lungs
Audible expiratory grunt
Flaring of the external nares
Cyanosis
As the disease progresses:
- Flaccidity
- Inertness
- Unresponsiveness
- Frequent apneic episodes
- Diminished breath sounds

Severe disease associated with:
- Shocklike state
- Diminished cardiac return
- Low arterial blood pressure

Diagnostic Evaluation

The diagnosis of RDS is made on the basis of clinical manifestations (see box) and radiographic studies. The extent of respiratory and metabolic acidosis is determined by blood gas analysis.

Therapeutic Management

The treatment of the infant with RDS is largely supportive; it includes all the general measures required of any premature infant. General supportive measures include minimal handling and providing adequate caloric intake and hydration. Oral feedings are contraindicated in any situation that creates a marked increase in respiratory rate because of the greater hazards of aspiration. Nutrition is provided by gavage and/or parenteral means.

The specific supportive measures that are most crucial to a favorable outcome are to (1) correct acidosis by intravenous administration of sodium bicarbonate, (2) maintain a neutral temperature environment to conserve utilization of oxygen, and (3) provide oxygen by increasing the ambient oxygen concentration in the Isolette or that delivered via an oxygen hood or by instituting assisted ventilation.

The goals of oxygen therapy are to provide adequate oxygen to the tissues, prevent lactic acid accumulation resulting from hypoxia, and, at the same time, avoid the toxic effects of oxygen—that is, retinopathy of prematurity and pulmonary oxygen toxicity. The most widely used method is assisted ventilation that supports the infant's own respiratory efforts. This method is known as *continuous positive airway pressure (CPAP)* or *continuous positive pressure breathing (CPPB)*. The objective of continuous positive airway pressure is to apply just enough pressure to open and keep open (and yet avoid overdistending) the already expanded alveoli. If the oxygen saturation (Po_2) of the blood cannot be maintained at a satisfactory level and the carbon dioxide level (Pco_2) rises, the infant will require controlled ventilation, usually *positive end-expiratory pressure* or *high-frequency ventilation*, a method that provides a very high respiratory rate with less tracheal pressure.

A new approach to management of RDS is administration of artificial surfactant or surfactant obtained from exogenous sources, such as human amniotic fluid. An even newer method is the use of *extracorporeal membrane oxygenation (ECMO)* with a modified heart-lung machine. The blood is shunted from the right atrium, through an oxygenator outside the body, and returned to the systemic circulation via the aorta, thus allowing the lungs to rest.

Prevention. The most successful approach to prevention of RDS is prevention of premature delivery, especially in elective early delivery and cesarean section. Improved methods for assessing the maturity of the fetal lung by amniocentesis, although not a routine procedure, allow a reasonable prediction of whether the fetus of a high-risk pregnancy is likely to develop RDS. The princi-

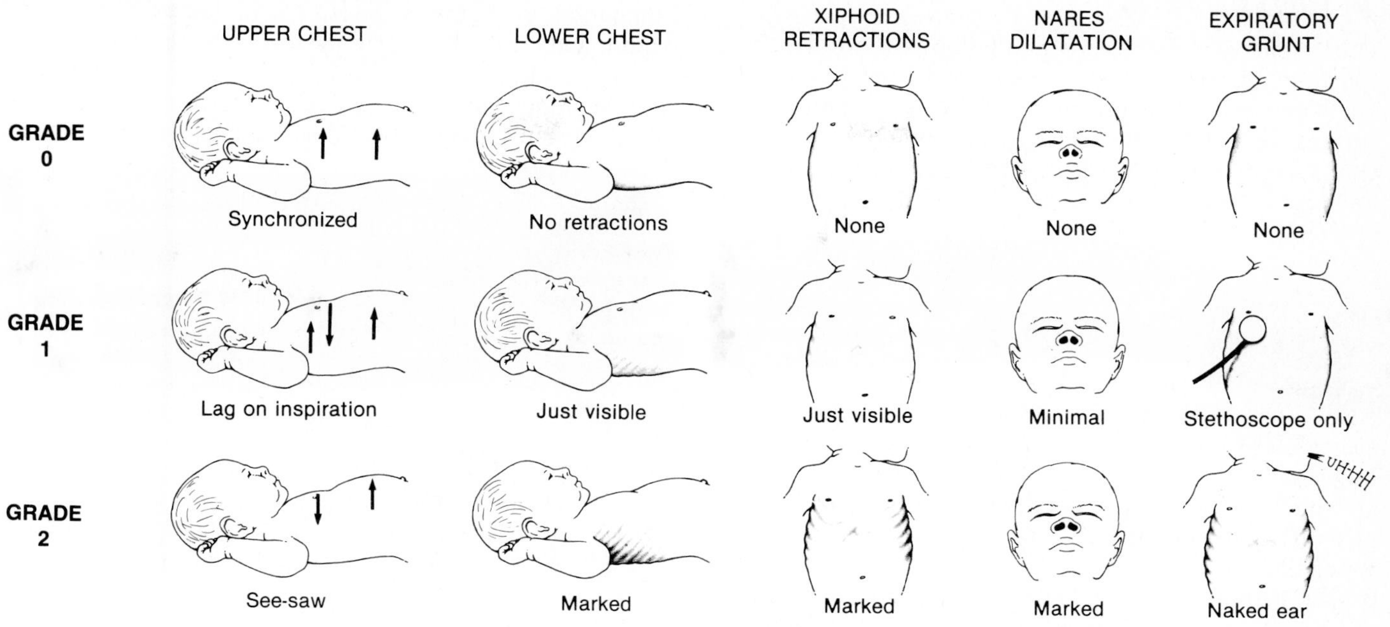

FIG. 9-13 Criteria for evaluating respiratory distress. (From Silverman, W.A., and Andersen, D.H.: Pediatrics **17**:1, 1956; copyright American Academy of Pediatrics, 1956.)

pal tests performed on amniotic fluid are determination of the lecithin/sphingomyelin ratio and prostaglandin levels.

In limited experiments, the administration of corticosteroids to mothers for 24 hours to 7 days prior to delivery has appeared to stimulate surfactant production in the fetus and to reduce the incidence of respiratory distress syndrome. No beneficial effects in the prevention of the disorder have resulted from administration of corticosteroids to infants after birth.

Nursing Considerations

Care of the infant with respiratory distress syndrome includes all the nursing skills required for any high-risk infant. In addition, special skills and observations are required in relation to oxygen administration.

ASSESSMENT

After initial observations that help diagnose the presence of RDS, the most essential nursing function is to observe and assess the infant's response to therapy. Since oxygen concentration and continuous positive airway pressure are prescribed according to the infant's color and blood gas measurements and since the infant's status can change rapidly, frequent monitoring and close observation are mandatory. The amount of oxygen administered is based on these observations.

Arterial samples ($Pa\text{ø}_2$) are drawn from an umbilical artery catheter or from the radial or posterior tibial arteries by needle puncture. For capillary samples, blood is most often collected from the heel. In many instances the noninvasive technique of percutaneous blood gas analysis is employed. These nursing activities are frequently carried out at least every 4 hours on sick infants and as often as every 15 minutes on acutely ill infants.

NURSING DIAGNOSES

Many of the diagnoses associated with any high-risk infant are appropriate for the infant with RDS. Diagnoses that are more specifically related to respiratory distress are listed in the box.

PLANNING

The major objectives of management of the infant with respiratory distress are the same as for any high-risk infant (such as infant and family support) with special emphasis on respiratory needs:

1. Facilitate respiratory efforts
2. Prevent complications

Nursing Diagnoses: Infant with RDS

Ineffective airway clearance related to flexible rib cage, fatigue, weak or absent cough reflex
Ineffective breathing pattern related to increased surface tension of alveoli, flexible rib cage
Impaired gas exchange related to inability to maintain lung expansion, presence of hyaline membrane
Potential for tissue trauma (brain) related to hypoxemia and hypercapnia
Potential for infection, pneumonia related to accumulation of pulmonary secretions

IMPLEMENTATION

Thick, tenacious mucus frequently forms in the respiratory tract, interfering with gas flow and predisposing the infant to obstruction of the air passages, including the endotracheal (ET) tube. Routine suctioning may be required every 2 hours or as needed based on assessment. Care must be exercised, since the procedure may cause bronchospasm or vagal nerve stimulation that can produce bradycardia. When the nasopharyngeal passages, trachea, or endotracheal tube is being suctioned, the catheter should be inserted gently but quickly; then intermittent suction should be applied as the catheter is withdrawn. It is imperative that the time the airway is obstructed by the catheter be limited to no more than 5 seconds. Also, continuous suction removes air from the lungs along with the mucus. The catheter should be inserted to a predetermined depth of 0.5 cm beyond the end of the ET tube to remove accumulated mucous (Kleiber, Krutfield, and Rose, 1988). Sterile normal saline (0.25 to 0.5 ml) instilled in the endotracheal tube before insertion of the suction catheter aids in loosening mucus and removing secretions (see also p. 677).

Removal of secretions can be further facilitated by application of percussion and vibration to the thoracic wall. The technique and positioning for postural drainage, percussion, and vibration are outlined in Chapter 19. The principles are the same, but the cupped hand is much too large to be used on the very small infant (see Nursing tip on percussion). Vibration is even more difficult to accomplish on the infant whose respiratory rate is 60 to 80 breaths/min (see Nursing tip on vibration). When applied to the chest, this provides effective vibrations. Percussion and vibration are performed every 2 hours, with rotation of segments of the lungs that are percussed. The preterm infant is usually unable to tolerate a full regimen each time. The length of time allotted to any given segment is also subject to the infant's tolerance and to the degree of lobar involvement, which is best determined by radiologic evaluation.

The most advantageous positions of the infant for facilitation of an open airway are on the side, with the head supported in alignment by a small folded blanket or towel, and on the back, with a small shoulder roll to keep the neck slightly extended. With the head in the "sniffing" position, the trachea is opened to its maximum; hyperextension reduces the tracheal diameter in the neonate.

Mouth care is especially important when the infant is receiving nothing by mouth, and the problem is often aggravated by the drying effect of oxygen therapy. Drying and cracking can be prevented by good oral hygiene with saline or petroleum jelly. The irritation to the nares or mouth that results from appliances used to administer oxygen may be reduced by the use of antibiotic ointment.

Nursing Tip: Percussion

An effective means for providing percussion is by the use of small plastic cups with padded rims, a small nipple, a stethoscope bell, or a small face mask with the airway opening occluded (Fig. 9-14).

Nursing Tip: Vibration

A helpful aid for performing vibration is an electric toothbrush with foam padding placed over the handle.

EVALUATION

The effectiveness of nursing interventions is determined by continual reassessment and evaluation of care based on the following observational guidelines and expected outcomes:

1. Perform frequent respiratory assessment (see Assessment guidelines, p. 223)
2. Observe infant's behavior; weigh daily or as prescribed, take vital signs and observe for signs of sepsis and respiratory complications (atelectasis, pneumothorax, pneumonia)

Expected outcomes:

1. The infant is able to breathe and maintain optimum blood gas measurements without ventilatory assistance.
2. The infant remains free of complications.

RESPIRATORY COMPLICATIONS

The newborn infant is vulnerable to a variety of pulmonary complications, some requiring oxygen therapy (Table 9-4). For example, the premature infant is subject to periods of apnea, and prenatal distress often causes the

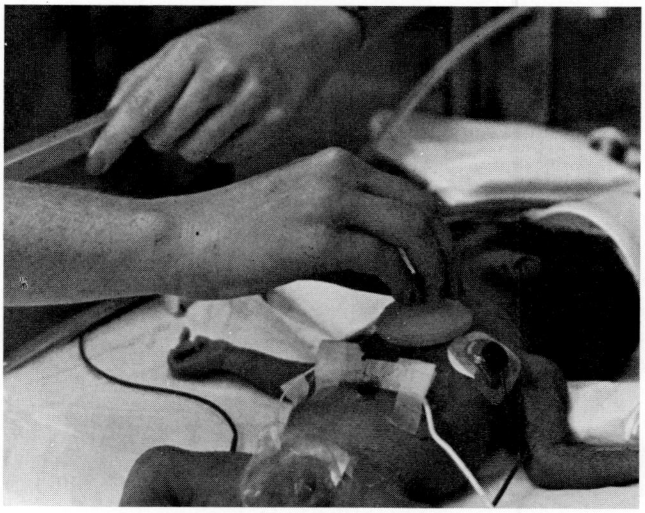

FIG. 9-14 Use of face mask for percussion of infant.

TABLE 9-4

Respiratory Complications

Description	Specific Manifestations	Treatment	Nursing Considerations
Meconium aspiration syndrome (MAS) Aspiration of amniotic fluid containing meconium into fetal or newborn trachea in utero or at first breath	Meconium stained at birth Tachypnea Hypoxia Depressed Hyperventilation (early) Hypoventilation (later)	Vigorous suction of hypopharynx at birth Treat for respiratory distress	See nursing care of infant with respiratory distress syndrome, p. 243
Apnea of prematurity Lapse of spontaneous breathing for 20 or more seconds, followed by bradycardia and color change	Persistent apneic spells	Observe for apnea Administer theophylline	Monitor respiratory and heart rates Observe for presence of respirations Observe color Apply gentle tactile stimulation Suction nose and oropharynx if still apneic Apply artificial ventilation with mask and AMBU with sufficient pressure to lift rib cage Assess for and manage any precipitating factors, e.g., temperature, humidity, distention, ambient oxygen
Pneumothorax Presence of extraneous air in the pleural space as a result of alveolar rupture	Tachypnea Grunting, flaring nares Retractions Absent or diminished breath sounds Shift in point of maximum intensity of heart sounds	Evacuate trapped air from pleural space through chest tubes and water-seal drainage	Maintain close vigilance of infants with respiratory distress or those on assisted ventilation Provide appropriate care of chest drainage apparatus
Bronchopulmonary dysplasia (BPD) A pathologic process related to alveolar damage from lung disease, prolonged exposure to high oxygen concentrations, use of positive-pressure ventilation, and endotracheal intubation	Nonspecific Susceptibility to upper respiratory infections Frequent hospitalization for respiratory dysfunction	Nonspecific Support respiratory efforts Prevent and/or control respiratory infections	Provide opportunities for additional rest, fluids, and calories Provide small, frequent feedings to avoid overextending stomach, which interferes with respiration Observe for signs of over- or under-hydration

fetus to pass meconium, which can be aspirated before or during birth. Oxygen therapy, although lifesaving, is not without its hazards. Positive pressure introduced by mechanical apparatus has created an increase in the incidence of ruptured alveoli and subsequent *pneumothorax* and *bronchopulmonary dysplasia* (*chronic* or *respirator lung disease*). *Retinopathy of prematurity* (*retrolental fibroplasia*) is observed exclusively in premature infants and appears to be in some manner related to oxygen therapy (see Table 9-5).

CARDIOVASCULAR COMPLICATIONS

The most serious cardiovascular disorders of the newborn are the congenital heart defects (p. 787). Other conditions that occur in the newborn period are usually related to prematurity (e.g., anemia, patent ductus arteriosus) or other diseases (e.g., respiratory distress). Hemorrhagic disease of the newborn is related to physiologic characteristics of the newborn and is preventable. Some of these disorders are outlined in Table 9-5.

NEONATAL SEIZURES

Seizures in the neonatal period are usually the clinical manifestation of a serious underlying disease. Therefore, seizures, although not life-threatening as an isolated entity, constitute a medical emergency, because they signal a disease process that may produce irreversible brain damage. Consequently it is imperative to recognize a seizure and its significance so that the cause as well as the seizure can be treated.

TABLE 9-5

Cardiovascular Complications

Description	Clinical Manifestations	Therapeutic Management	Nursing Considerations
Patent ductus arteriosus (PDA) (see p. 790)	Increased Pco_2 Recurrent apnea Bounding peripheral pulses Typical systolic or continuous murmur	Regulate fluids Provide respiratory support Administer indomethacin	See nursing care of the high-risk infant, p. 221 Collect specimens as needed Assess renal function Observe for bleeding tendencies
Persistent pulmonary hypertension (PPH) Severe pulmonary hypertension and large right-to-left shunt through foramen ovale and ductus arteriosus	Hypoxia when agitated Marked cyanosis Tachypnea with grunting and retractions Decreased peripheral pulses	Regulate fluids Give supplemental oxygen Give assisted ventilation Administer vasodilators (sometimes)	See nursing care of high-risk infant, p. 221, infant with respiratory distress syndrome, p. 243 Reduce stress to infant, especially noxious stimuli that cause crying and struggling Decrease physical manipulation and disturbance
Anemia Loss of blood from hemorrhage in organs (during delivery), blood diseases Contributing: decreased fetal hemoglobin and shortened red blood cell survival time in preterm infant	Pallor Dyspnea Tachycardia Tachypnea Diminished activity	Administer iron-fortified formula and/or supplemental iron Transfuse with packed red blood cells for severe anemia	Monitor blood drawn for tests Administer iron as prescribed
Polycythemia/hyperviscosity syndrome Venous hematocrit 65% or greater owing to twin-to-twin or mother-to-fetus transfusion or increased red blood cell production	High incidence of: Cardiovascular symptoms (PPH, cyanosis, apnea) Seizures Hyperbilirubinemia Gastrointestinal abnormalities	Correct metabolic imbalances Implement partial exchange transfusion Provide appropriate therapy for associated problems	See nursing care of high-risk infant and infant with hyperbilirubinemia, p. 236
Hemorrhagic disease of the newborn Bleeding disorder resulting from transient deficiency of vitamin K–dependent blood factors	Oozing blood from umbilicus or circumcision Bloody or black stools Hematuria Ecchymosis Epistaxis	Administer prophylactic vitamin K	Administer vitamin K into vastus lateralis muscle
Retinopathy of prematurity (ROP) Replacement of retina by fibrous tissue and blood vessels	Progressive vascular growth of retina Eventual blindness	Arrest proliferation process—cryotherapy Administer prophylactic vitamin E (sometimes) Use supplemental oxygen judiciously, and monitor carefully	See nursing care of high-risk newborn Monitor oxygen concentration

The causes of neonatal seizures are many and varied including:

metabolic disorders such as hypoglycemia and hypocalcemia

toxic and electrolyte disturbances such as hypernatremia, hyponatremia, narcotic withdrawal, and bilirubin encephalopathy

infections such as bacterial meningitis, sepsis, herpes simplex, and cytomegalic inclusion disease

trauma at birth such as hypoxic encephalopathy and intracranial hemorrhage

congenital malformations such as hydrocephaly and central nervous system agenesis

miscellaneous disorders such as degenerative diseases

Clinical Manifestations of Newborn Seizures or Tremors

1. Types of seizures
   - Subtle seizures—signs may appear alone or in combination
     - Clonic horizontal eye deviation
     - Repetitive blinking or fluttering of eyelids
     - Drooling
     - Sucking or other oral-buccal-lingual movements
     - Arm movements resembling rowing or swimming
     - Leg movements described as pedaling or bicycling
     - Apnea
   - Generalized tonic seizures
     - Usually manifest as extensions of all four limbs, similar to decerebrate rigidity
     - Occasionally upper limbs are maintained in stiffly flexed position resembling decorticate rigidity
     - Appear more frequently in premature infants
   - Multifocal clonic seizures
     - Rhythmic jerking movements, about 1 to 3 per second
     - May migrate randomly from one part of the body to another
     - Simultaneous involvement of separate areas often occurs
     - Convulsive movements may start at different times and at different rates
2. Jitteriness or tremulousness
   - Repetitive shaking of an extremity or extremities
   - Observed with crying, may occur with changes in sleeping state, or may be elicited with stimulation
   - Relatively common in newborn
   - Mild jitteriness may be considered normal during first 4 days of life
   - Can be distinguished from seizures by several characteristics:
     - Not accompanied by ocular movement as are seizures
     - Dominant movement in jitteriness is tremor
     - Seizure movement is clonic jerking that cannot be stopped by flexion of affected limb
     - Jitteriness is highly sensitive to stimulation; seizures are not

The features of neonatal seizures are different from those observed in the older infant or child. The well-organized, generalized tonic-clonic seizures seen in older children are rare in the infant, especially the preterm infant. The seizures may be subtle and barely discernible or grossly apparent (see box).

Diagnostic Evaluation

Early evaluation and diagnosis of seizures are urgent. In addition to a careful physical examination, the pregnancy and family histories are investigated for familial and prenatal causes of seizure activity. Blood is drawn for glucose and electrolyte examination, and cerebrospinal fluid is obtained for examination for gross blood cell count, protein, glucose, and culture. Electroencephalography may help identify subtle seizures but is less helpful in establishing a diagnosis. Other diagnostic procedures such as computed tomography may be indicated.

Therapeutic Management

Treatment is directed toward prevention of cerebral damage and involves correction of metabolic derangements, respiratory and cardiovascular support, and suppression of the seizure activity. The underlying cause is the focus of therapy—for example, glucose infusion for hypoglycemia, calcium for hypocalcemia, and antibiotics for infection. If needed, respiratory support is provided for hypoxia, and anticonvulsants may be administered, especially when the other measures fail to control the seizures. Phenobarbital, given orally or intramuscularly, is the treatment of choice, but the intravenous route is used if seizures are severe and persistent. Other drugs that may be employed are diazepam (Valium), paraldehyde, and phenytoin (Dilantin).

Nursing Considerations

The major nursing responsibilities in the care of the infant with seizures are to recognize when the infant is having a seizure so that therapy can be instituted, to carry out the therapeutic regimen, and to observe the response to the therapy and any further evidence of seizures or other symptoms. Assessment and all other aspects of care are the same as for any high-risk infant. Parents need to be informed of the infant's status, with the nurse reinforcing and clarifying the explanations of the attending physician. The infant's behaviors need to be interpreted to the parents, and the significance of the infant's responses to the treatment must be anticipated and explained. Parents should be encouraged to visit the child and perform the parenting activities consistent with the plan of care. Seizures are a frightening phenomenon and generate a great deal of anxiety and fear, which is easily compounded by the justifiable concern of the staff. Providing support and guidance is an important nursing function.

CEREBRAL COMPLICATIONS

Cerebral injury in newborn infants is not an uncommon observation. Newborn infants are particularly vulnerable to ischemic injury caused by decreased cerebral blood flow subsequent to asphyxia, and preterm infants, with a fragile cerebrovascular network, are highly prone to periventricular or intraventricular hemorrhage. Intracranial hemorrhage as a result of either trauma or hypoxia is a common complication of premature birth. Fragility and increased permeability of capillaries and prolonged prothrombin time predispose the premature infant to trauma when delicate structures are subjected to the forces of labor. The more common cerebral complications are outlined in Table 9-6.

TABLE 9-6

Cerebral Complications

Description	Clinical Manifestations	Therapeutic Management	Nursing Considerations
Hypoxic-ischemic brain injury			
Nonprogressive neurologic (brain) impairment caused by intrauterine or postnatal asphyxia resulting in hypoxemia and/or cerebral ischemia	Appears in first 24 hours after hypoxic episode Seizures Abnormal muscle tone (usually hypotonia) Disturbance of sucking and swallowing Apneic episodes Stupor or coma	Provide vigorous supportive care Provide adequate ventilation Maintain cerebral perfusion Prevent cerebral edema Treat seizures	See nursing care of high-risk infant, p. 221 Observe for signs that indicate cerebral hypoxia Monitor ventilatory and intravenous therapy and nutrition Observe for and manage seizures Support family Provide guidelines for family management of permanent neurologic damage
Periventricular/intraventricular hemorrhage (PVH/IVH)			
Hemorrhage into and around ventricles caused by ruptured vessels as result of an event that increases cerebral blood flow to area	Tense, bulging anterior fontanel Separated sutures Neurologic signs: Twitching Stupor Apnea Seizures Evident on ultrasonography and/or tomography	Supportive care: Provide ventilatory support Maintain oxygenation Regulate fluid and electrolytes, acid-base balance Suppress or prevent seizures	See nursing care of high-risk infant, p. 221 Prevent increased cerebral blood pressure Elevate head Avoid pressure-producing procedures Support family
Intracranial hemorrhage			
Subdural Subarachnoid Intracerebellar	See p. 905	See p. 906	Same as for PVH/IVH

◆ *High Risk Related to Bacterial Infection*

The newborn infant is subject to environmental factors that cause injury or illness. The immature immune system with its inability to localize infection renders the infant especially vulnerable to infectious organisms. Prevention of infection in the newborn, especially the infant who is already compromised by physiologic or structural disorders, is a primary nursing concern.

SEPSIS

Sepsis, or septicemia, refers to a generalized bacterial infection in the bloodstream. Neonates are susceptible to infection because they have diminished nonspecific and specific immunity. Because of the infant's poor response to infectious agents, there is usually no local inflammatory reaction at the portal of entry to signal an infection and the resulting symptoms tend to be vague and nonspecific. Consequently, diagnosis and treatment may be delayed. Skin eruptions in the newborn infant are less common than they are in children. However, because of their immature immune systems, infants are more vulnerable to bacterial invasion, which tends to be more serious and less likely to remain localized.

Sepsis in the neonatal period can be acquired prenatally or during labor, from infected amniotic fluid; across the placenta from the maternal bloodstream; or by direct contact with maternal tissues during the neonate's passage through the birth canal. Postnatal infection is acquired by cross-contamination from other infants, personnel, or objects in the environment, primarily lifesaving apparatus such as mechanical ventilators and indwelling venous and arterial catheters used for infusions, blood sampling, and monitoring vital signs. Neonatal sepsis is most common in the infant at risk, particularly the preterm infant and the infant born after a difficult or traumatic labor and delivery.

Diagnostic Evaluation

A few neonatal infections (for example, pyoderma, conjunctivitis, omphalitis, and mastitis) are easily recognized. However, systemic infections are characterized by very subtle, vague, nonspecific, and almost imperceptible

Clinical Manifestations of Newborn Sepsis

Subtle, vague, and nonspecific signs:
- "Failure to do well"
- "Does not look right"
- Nonspecific respiratory distress

Respiratory distress:
- Apnea
- Irregular, grunting respirations
- Retractions

Gastric distress:
- Vomiting (vomitus may be bile stained)
- Diarrhea
- Abdominal distention
- Absent stools as a result of paralytic ileus
- Poor sucking and feeding

Skin manifestations may include:
- Cyanosis
- Pallor
- Mottling
- Jaundice
- Lesions associated with specific organisms

Central nervous system involvement:
- Irritability
- Apathy
- Tremors
- Convulsions
- Coma
- Signs of increased intracranial pressure related to meningitis, a frequent sequela of sepsis

Fever frequently absent; body temperature commonly normal or suboptimum

Indication of local inflammatory response rare

physical signs. See the accompanying box for some of the usual manifestations observed in newborn sepsis. Repeated blood cultures and analysis of potential primary sources of infection, such as the umbilicus, nasal-oral-pharyngeal cavity, ear canals, skin lesions, cerebrospinal fluid, stool, and urine, identify specific organisms. Direct (conjugated) hyperbilirubinemia is frequently seen in infants with sepsis, particularly of gram-negative origin. Blood studies may show signs of anemia, leukocytosis, or leukopenia. Leukopenia is usually an ominous sign because it is frequently associated with high mortality.

Therapeutic Management

Early recognition and diagnosis and institution of vigorous therapeutic measures are essential to increasing the chance for survival and reducing the likelihood of permanent neurologic damage. Treatment consists of aggressive administration of appropriate antibiotics and supportive therapy, careful regulation of fluids and electrolytes, and temporary discontinuation of oral feedings. Transfusions with polymorphonuclear leukocytes obtained from adult donors have proved to be highly effective in lowering mortality from this disease.

Supportive therapy usually involves administration of oxygen if respiratory distress or cyanosis is evident, adequate hydration with intravenous fluid and electrolytes, and isolation of the infant in an Isolette or incubator. Blood transfusions may be needed to correct anemia or shock, and electronic monitoring of vital signs and regulation of the thermal environment are mandatory.

Nursing Considerations

Nursing care of the infant with sepsis is similar to the care of any high-risk infant. In addition, recognition of the existing problem is of paramount importance; it is usually the nurse who frequently observes and assesses the infant and who recognizes that "something is wrong" with the child. Awareness of the potential modes of transmission allows the nurse to identify those infants more at risk for developing sepsis.

Much of the care of the infant involves the medical treatment directed at illness. Knowledge of the side effects of the specific antibiotic and proper regulation and administration of the drug via the intravenous route are mandatory.

Part of the total care of the infant with sepsis is to decrease any additional physiologic or environmental stress. This includes providing an optimum, thermoregulated environment and anticipating potential problems such as dehydration or anoxia. Another aspect of caring for the infant with sepsis involves observation for signs of meningitis, a frequent sequela of septicemia. The most common indication of meningitis is a full or bulging anterior fontanel (see also p. 916).

A severe complication of sepsis is shock, which is caused by the release of toxins within the bloodstream. Signs of shock are often difficult to distinguish from those of sepsis, such as rapid, irregular respirations and pulse. However, blood pressure usually falls in shock; therefore this measurement should be a part of the infant's routine vital signs.

The newborn with sepsis is usually quite ill. The prognosis varies from patient to patient, but with immediate and vigorous antibiotic therapy, mortality is quite low.

NECROTIZING ENTEROCOLITIS

Necrotizing enterocolitis (NEC) is a serious condition in a premature infant that may go undetected for some time because of the ambiguity of symptoms in the preterm infant and preoccupation with other life-threatening problems by members of the staff. Three factors appear to play an important role in its development: intestinal ischemia, bacterial colonization, and early enteric feeding.

Pathophysiology

The precise cause of the disorder is still speculative, although it appears to occur in an infant whose gastrointestinal tract has suffered a vascular compromise somehow related to an episode of hypoxia or sepsis, or after an exchange transfusion. The reduced blood supply to the in-

Clinical Manifestations of NEC

Nonspecific clinical signs:
- Lethargy
- Poor feeding
- Hypotension
- Vomiting
- Apnea
- Decreased urine output
- Unstable temperature

Specific signs:
- Distended (often shiny) abdomen
- Blood in the stools or gastric contents
- Gastric retention

testines causes damage and death to mucosal cells lining the bowel wall. The intestines are unable to secrete protective mucus; therefore, the unprotected bowel wall is invaded by gas-forming bacteria, producing pneumatosis intestinalis (presence of air in the submucosal or subserosal surfaces of the colon), a consistent and diagnostic finding.

There is a consistent relationship between the development of NEC and feedings of hypertonic formula, but it is unclear whether this is a result of the formula imposing a stress on an ischemic bowel or serving as a medium for bacterial growth.

Diagnostic Evaluation

The diagnosis of NEC is made from observations of physical signs and laboratory and radiographic findings (see box).

Therapeutic Management

Treatment of confirmed necrotizing enterocolitis consists of discontinuation of all oral feedings and starting intravenous fluids, correction of fluid and electrolyte imbalances, institution of abdominal decompression via nasogastric suction, and administration of systemic antibiotics. If there is progressive deterioration under medical management or evidence of perforation, surgical resection and anastomosis are carried out. Extensive involvement may necessitate establishment of an ileostomy or a colostomy.

Nursing Considerations

Nursing responsibilities begin with early recognition of the disease. Because the signs are similar to those observed in many other disorders of the newborn, nurses must be constantly aware of the possibility of this disease and alert to indications of its early development. Checking the abdomen frequently for distention, measuring for residual gastric contents before feedings, and listening for presence of bowel sounds are especially important in detecting the early signs of NEC.

When the disease is suspected, the nurse assists with diagnostic procedures and implements the therapeutic regimen. Vital signs, including blood pressure, are monitored for changes that indicate impending sepsis or cardiovascular shock. It is especially important to avoid taking rectal temperatures because of the increased danger of perforation. To avoid pressure on the distended abdomen, the infant is not diapered or positioned on the abdomen.

Conscientious attention to nutritional and hydration needs is essential, and antibiotics are administered as prescribed. The time at which oral feedings are reinstituted varies considerably but is usually at least 7 days after diagnosis. Plain water or electrolyte solution is given for two feedings, followed by dilute human milk formula. The concentration is gradually increased over 2 to 3 weeks until the infant is again taking full-strength feedings.

The infant who requires surgery is given the same careful care and observation as any infant with abdominal surgery, including colostomy care. Throughout the management of the infant with NEC the nurse is continually alert to signs of complications such as sepsis, disseminated intravascular coagulation, hypoglycemia, and other metabolic derangements.

BULLOUS IMPETIGO

Bullous impetigo (impetigo neonatorum) is a superficial skin infection most often caused by group 2 phage type *Staphylococcus aureus*. It is characterized by the eruption of bullous vesicular lesions on previously untraumatized skin. The lesions may appear on any body surface and sometimes become widespread, but the usual distribution involves the buttocks, perineum, trunk, and face. They vary in size from a few millimeters to several centimeters in diameter, contain turbid fluid, and are easily ruptured. The bullae rupture in 1 to 2 days, leaving a superficial red, moist, denuded area with very little crusting.

Warm saline compresses applied to the lesions are followed by gentle cleansing and application of a topical antibiotic several times a day. Systemic antibiotics and corticosteroids are sometimes administered to small infants and those with widespread lesions. Recovery is usually rapid and uneventful.

Nursing Considerations

Once the diagnosis is suspected, appropriate precautionary measures are instituted to prevent spread of the infection to other infants. Persons who have come in contact with the infant are investigated to determine a possible source of the infecting organism. Other infants in the nursery should be scrutinized for early detection of any signs of infection. Parents and other visitors are in-structured regarding precautions for prevention of infection.

◆ *High Risk Related to Maternal Factors*

Some newborn infants are at risk for disease or abnormal development because of adverse influences present before birth. These factors may be diseases of the mother that are transmitted to the infant (rubella), diseases or deficiencies of the mother that cause chemical or physiologic imbalances in the infant (diabetes mellitus), or chemicals that produce an undesirable effect in the infant (narcotics).

INFANT OF THE DIABETIC MOTHER

Before the introduction of insulin therapy, few women with diabetes were able to conceive, and for those who did, the mortality rates for both mother and infant were high. As a result of effective control of diabetes and an increased understanding of fetal disorders, the morbidity and mortality of infants of diabetic mothers (IDMs) have been significantly reduced.

The severity of the maternal disease affects infant and fetal survival, and there is a relationship between length of gestation and neonatal mortality. There is a higher incidence of stillborn infants in the more severely insulin-dependent women, and their live-born infants appear to be more at risk than those of mothers with less severe diabetic involvement. This risk increases dramatically after 37 weeks of gestation. To ensure the best possible outcome for the infant, tests of fetal well-being are performed routinely during pregnancy, and some mothers are hospitalized at 36 to 37 weeks of gestation for management.

Pathophysiology

Hypoglycemia appears within a short period after birth and is associated with increased insulin activity in the blood. It has been demonstrated that IDMs have hypertrophy and hyperplasia of the pancreatic islet cells and are in a state of hyperinsulinism. It is generally agreed that during fetal life high maternal blood sugar levels provide a continual stimulus to the fetal islet cells for insulin production. This sustained state of hyperglycemia promotes fetal insulin secretion, which ultimately leads to excessive growth and deposition of fat, which probably accounts for the infants who are large for gestational age. When this glucose supply is removed abruptly at the time of birth, the continued production of insulin soon depletes the blood of circulating glucose, creating a state of hypoglycemia within 2 to 4 hours. Sudden drops in blood glucose levels can cause serious neurologic abnormality or death.

All infants of these mothers with poor disease control have a characteristic appearance (see box). Although they are large, these infants are often prematurely born—either because of an elective early delivery or for other reasons. Their appearance has been described as that of a premature infant seen through a magnifying glass (Fig. 9-15).

Clinical Manifestations of IDM

- Large for their gestational age
- Very plump and full-faced
- Liberal coat of vernix caseosa
- Plethora
- Listlessness and lethargy

There is an increase in congenital anomalies, such as heart defects, in this group as well as a high susceptibility to hypoglycemia, hypocalcemia, hyperbilirubinemia, and hyaline membrane disease. No satisfactory explanation has been accepted for all the abnormalities in these infants, although a number of complications may be related to the prematurity factor.

Therapeutic Management

If hypoglycemia is left untreated, it can cause rapid, irreversible central nervous system damage. The most effective management appears to be careful observation of all

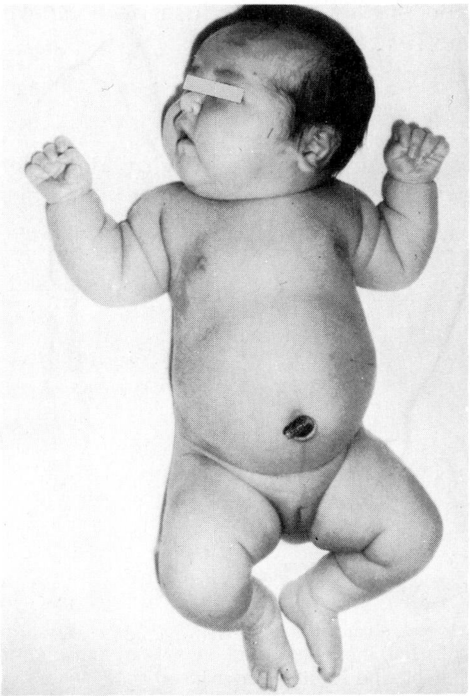

FIG. 9-15 Infant of diabetic mother born at 40 weeks of gestation. Birth weight, 4.7 kg; postnatal age, 1 week. (From Fanaroff, A.A., and Martin, R.J., editors: Behrman's neonatal-perinatal medicine, ed. 3, St. Louis, 1983, The C.V. Mosby Co.)

IDMs in the special-care nursery, with early feeding of 5% to 10% glucose followed by formula, if tolerated. Critically ill infants require intravenous infusions. Frequent determinations of blood glucose levels are needed for the first 2 days of life, to assess the degree of hypoglycemia present at any given time.

Nursing Considerations

Nursing care of IDMs requires observation for signs of complications to which they are more susceptible than other neonates. Hypoglycemia is the most immediate and consistent threat to these infants; therefore, feedings are initiated early and the infant is observed for central nervous system signs such as hyperirritability, tremors, and jitteriness during the early hours of life. Other complications that occur with increased frequency in the IDMs are polycythemia, hyperbilirubinemia, sepsis, and respiratory distress syndrome. Vigilance is needed to detect signs that indicate development of any of these neonatal problems. (See a textbook on maternity nursing for prenatal care and special needs of the mother.)

DRUG-ADDICTED INFANTS

Narcotics, which have a low molecular weight, readily cross the placental membrane and enter the fetal system. When the mother is a habitual user of narcotics, in particular heroin or methadone, the unborn child becomes passively addicted to the drug, which places such infants at risk during the early neonatal period. Some drugs (e.g., cocaine) do not appear to induce neonatal withdrawal (Smith and Deitch, 1987).

Diagnostic Evaluation

Most passively addicted infants of drug-dependent mothers appear normal at birth but begin to exhibit signs of drug withdrawal within 12 to 24 hours if the mother has been taking only heroin. If she has been taking methadone, the signs appear somewhat later, anytime from 1 or 2 days to a week or more after birth. The manifestations become most pronounced between 48 and 72 hours of age and may last anywhere from 6 days to 8 weeks, depending on the severity of the withdrawal.

The clinical manifestations of withdrawal in the neonate, which are predominantly those of autonomic nervous system hyperirritability, may persist for 3 or 4 months. The most common acute signs are outlined in the box. Although infants undergoing withdrawal suck avidly on fists and display an exaggerated rooting reflex, they are poor feeders.

Not all infants of heroin-addicted mothers show signs of withdrawal. Because of irregular and varying degrees of drug use, varying quality of drug, and mixed drug usage by the mother, some infants display mild or variable manifestations. A higher rate of SIDS (p. 330) is reported in these infants than in the general infant population.

It is significant to note that, although passively addicted infants have some tachypnea, cyanosis, and/or apnea, they rarely develop respiratory distress syndrome. Apparently, the heroin or related factors in the intrauterine environment cause accelerated lung maturation in these infants, even in the face of a high incidence of prematurity.

Clinical Manifestations of Newborn Narcotic Withdrawal

- Tremors
- Restlessness and irritability
- Hypertonicity of muscles
- Hyperactive reflexes
- Frequent sneezing
- Frequent yawning
- Low-grade fever
- Tachypnea
- High-pitched, shrill cry
- Uncoordinated, ineffectual sucking and swallowing reflexes
- Regurgitation and vomiting after feedings
- Diarrhea—a later manifestation
- Minimum sleeping
- Sweating
- Seizures

Therapeutic Management

The initial treatment of the infant consists of intramuscular administration of diazepam or phenobarbital followed by oral administration individualized in amount and frequency. If there are gastrointestinal symptoms such as diarrhea, paregoric may be the drug of choice.

Nursing Considerations

The management of the infant of the drug-addicted mother begins with recognizing manifestations that indicate withdrawal. Once the presence of withdrawal is identified in an infant, nursing care is directed toward reducing the stimuli that might trigger hyperactivity and irritability, providing adequate nutrition and hydration, and promoting maternal-infant relationships. Irritable and hyperactive infants have been found to respond to comforting, movement, and close contact. Wrapping the infant snugly to limit his ability to self-stimulate and holding him tightly and arranging nursing activities to reduce the amount of disturbance help to decrease external stimulation.

Loose stools together with poor intake and regurgitation following feeding predispose the infants to malnutrition, dehydration, and electrolyte imbalance that can progress to shock and coma. Frequent measurements of weight, careful monitoring of intake and output, and administration of supplemental parenteral fluids may be

TABLE 9-7

Congenital Disorders Acquired from Maternal Infections

Fetal or Newborn Effect	Comments and Nursing Considerations*
Acquired Immune Deficiency Syndrome (AIDS) (human immunodeficiency virus [HIV])	
Growth failure Prominent boxlike forehead Short nose with flattened columella Well-formed, triangular philtrum Microcephaly Flat nasal bridge Mild upward or downward obliquity of eyes Long palpebral fissures with blue sclerae Patulous lips Ocular hypertelorism	Transmitted: transplacentally; during delivery; in breast milk (highly suggestive) (see also p. 85) No treatment currently available other than supportive care
Coxsackie Virus (group B)	
Poor feeding, vomiting, diarrhea, fever; cardiac enlargement, arrhythmias, congestive heart failure; lethargy, seizures, meningeal involvement	Transmitted: first trimester or late in pregnancy
Chlamydia* Infection *(Chlamydia trachomatis)	
Conjunctivitis, pneumonia	Transmitted: last trimester or intrapartum Apply prophylactic medication to eyes at time of birth Treatment: antibiotics
Cytomegalic Inclusion Disease—CID (cytomegalovirus [CMV])	
Microcephaly, cerebral calcifications, chorioretinitis Jaundice, hepatosplenomegaly Petechial or purpuric rash Neurologic sequelae: seizure disorders, sensorimotor deafness, mental retardation	Transmitted: throughout pregnancy Affected individuals excrete virus Virus detected in urine by electron microscopy Avoid kissing affected child Pregnant women should avoid close contact with known cases Treatment: antimetabolites, antiviral agent
Gonococcal Disease *(Neisseria gonorrhoeae)*	
Ophthalmitis Neonatal gonococcal arthritis, septicemia, meningitis	Transmitted: last trimester or intrapartum Apply prophylactic medication to eyes at time of birth Obtain smears for culture Treatment: penicillin
Hepatitis B (virus)	
May be asymptomatic Acute hepatitis, changes in liver function	Transmitted: transplacentally, contaminated maternal secretions during delivery; possibly through breast-feeding, especially if mother has cracked nipples Treatment: hepatitis B immune globulin to all infants of HBsAg-positive mothers
Herpes, Neonatal (herpes simplex virus)	
Cutaneous lesions: vesicles at 6 to 10 days of age, may be no lesions Disseminated disease: resembles sepsis Visceral involvement: granulomas Early nonspecific signs: fever, lethargy, poor feeding, irritability, vomiting May include hyperbilirubinemia, seizures, flaccid or spastic paralysis, apneic episodes, respiratory distress, lethargy, or coma	History of genital infection in mother/partner in 50% of cases Transmitted: intrapartum either ascending and/or direct contact; incubation period 6 to 10 days Rarely acquired as intrauterine infection during first trimester and intrapartum Cesarean section a preventive measure for mothers with active lesions
Listeriosis *(Listeria)*	
Acquired in late pregnancy: stillborn or acutely ill; may die within an hour after birth Late onset: septicemia; meningitis	Transmitted: transplacentally or by aspiration of secretions at birth Segregate infants until cultures are negative
Rubella, Congenital (rubella virus)	
Eye defects: cataracts (unilateral or bilateral), microphthalmia, retinitis, glaucoma Central nervous system signs: microcephaly, seizures, severe mental retardation Congenital heart defects: patent ductus arteriosus Auditory: high incidence of delayed hearing loss Intrauterine growth retardation Hyperbilirubinemia, spinal fluid abnormalities, thrombocytopenia, hepatomegaly	Transmitted: first trimester; early second trimester Pregnant women should avoid contact with all affected persons, including infants with rubella syndrome Emphasize vaccination of all unimmunized prepubertal children, susceptible adolescents, and adult females of childbearing age Caution women against pregnancy for at least 3 months after vaccination Strict isolation of affected infant

*Isolation precautions depend on institution policy (see p. 645).

Continued.

TABLE 9-7

Congenital Disorders Acquired from Maternal Infections—cont'd

Fetal or Newborn Effect	Comments and Nursing Considerations
Syphilis, Congenital *(Treponema pallidum)*	
Copper-colored maculopapular cutaneous lesions (after 7th day), mucous membrane patches, hair loss, nail exfoliation, sniffles (syphilitic rhinitis), profound anemia, poor feeding, pseudoparalysis of one or more limbs	Transmitted: transplacentally, usually after 18th week of pregnancy Most severe form of syphilis Strict isolation of infant Treatment: penicillin
Toxoplasmosis *(Toxoplasma gondii)*	
Hydrocephaly, cerebral calcifications, chorioretinitis (classic triad) Microcephaly Encephalitis, myocarditis, hepatosplenomegaly, anemia, jaundice, diarrhea, vomiting, seizures, pupura	Transmitted: throughout pregnancy Predominant host for organism is cats May be transmitted through cat feces, poorly cooked or raw infected meat Caution pregnant women to avoid contact with cat feces, e.g., emptying cat litter boxes Treatment: sulfonamides, pyrimethamine
Varicella (Chickenpox) (varicella virus)	
Skin lesions, microcephaly, limb deformities, encephalomyocarditis, visceral involvement	Transmitted: first trimester or intrapartum Isolate infant

necessary in addition to the care ordinarily afforded high-risk newborn infants. Monitoring and recording activity levels and their relationship to other activities, such as feeding and preventing complications, are important nursing functions.

A valuable aid to anticipating problems in the newborn is recognizing drug addiction in the mother. Unless the mother is enrolled in a methadone rehabilitation program, she seldom risks calling attention to her habit by seeking prenatal care. Consequently, the infant and mother are exposed to the additional hazards of obstetric and medical complications. In addition, the nature of heroin addiction predisposes the user to disorders such as AIDS, hepatitis, and foreign body reaction and to the hazards of inadequate nutrition and premature birth. Methadone treatment does not prevent withdrawal reaction in the neonate, but the clinical course may be modified. Planning for follow-up care of the mother and infant is essential.

DISORDERS CAUSED BY MATERNAL INFECTIONS

A variety of disorders have been attributed to maternal infections during a sensitive period of fetal development. The clinical picture of disorders caused by transplacental transfer of infectious agents is not always well defined. One group of microbial agents can cause remarkably similar manifestations, and it is not uncommon to test for all when a prenatal infection is suspected. This is the so-called TORCH complex, an acronym that represents the following infections:

T—toxoplasmosis
O—other
R—rubella
C—cytomegalovirus infection
H—herpes simplex

To determine the causative agent in an infant with symptoms, tests are performed to rule out each of these infections. The "O" category may involve testing for several viral infections and listeriosis. Sometimes "S" is added (TORCHS) to include congenital syphilis. Bacterial infections are not included in the TORCH work-up because they are usually identified by clinical manifestations and readily available laboratory tests. Gonococcal conjunctivitis (ophthalmia neonatorum) has been virtually eliminated by prophylactic measures and is not discussed in this section. AIDS, a growing prenatal and postnatal concern, is discussed on p. 851. The major maternal infections, their possible teratogenic effects, and specific nursing considerations are outlined in Table 9-7.

Nursing Considerations

One of the major goals in the care of infants suspected of having a maternally derived infectious disease is identification of the causative agent. Until diagnosis is established, the infant is isolated from contact with other infants. In suspected cytomegalovirus and rubella infections, pregnant personnel are cautioned to avoid contact with the infant. Herpes simplex is easily transmitted from one infant to another; therefore, risk of cross-contamination should be eliminated.

Special feeding techniques may need to be implemented for infants with feeding difficulties, and infants subject to seizures should be protected from adverse environmental stimuli. Specimens need to be obtained for laboratory examinations, and the infant and parents need to be prepared for diagnostic procedures. When possible, long-term disabilities are prevented by early evaluation and implementation of therapy. If sequelae are inevitable, the family will need assistance in determining how they can best cope with the problems, such as assistance with home care, referral to appropriate agencies, or placement in an institution for care.

◆ *Congenital Abnormalities*

Congenital abnormalities, or birth defects, constitute a large group of defects and disorders that are so variable in type and causation that there is no satisfactory method for classifying them. A few are clearly caused by a single gene. Some of the more common inborn errors of metabolism that are identified in the newborn period as a result of screening are discussed in the following section; others are discussed as appropriate throughout the book; for example, congenital heart disease, skeletal defects, and spina bifida. Some congenital defects are associated with chromosomal abnormalities (see below).

Some congenital malformations are produced by known intrauterine environmental factors, such as maternal exposure to chemical agents. However, many of the more common and severe defects (for example, central nervous system malformations, cataracts, and congenital heart disease) fit in no clearly defined category. There is a high correlation between the incidence of congenital abnormalities and the infant who is small for gestational age. The more severe the growth retardation, the greater the chance of malformation.

CHROMOSOMAL ABERRATIONS

An aberration is defined as a deviation from that which is normal or typical. Chromosome aberrations are deviations in either structure or number of chromosomes, and the consequences in either situation can be readily observed in the affected individual. A structural aberration involves loss, addition, rearrangement, or exchange of some of the genes of a chromosome. Deviations in chromosomal number involve the gain or loss of a chromosome and are designated with the suffix -*somy*. A cell that contains one less than the total number of chromosomes is called a *monosomy* because of the loss of one member of a chromosome pair; a cell containing one more than the total number of chromosomes that results from the addition of an extra member to a normal pair is called a *trisomy*. Most chromosome abnormalities result from abnormal cell division during germ cell formation or early cell division in the zygote. Others are caused by a *translocation* in which two chromosomes become permanently attached. A translocation can be transmitted to the offspring; therefore, referral for genetic counseling is a special consideration for parents of an affected child. Trisomies are the chromosomal aberrations encountered most frequently by health workers.

Both numeric and structural abnormalities of autosomes account for a variety of disorders of infancy and childhood. A few are associated with a group of characteristics that clearly indicate the precise chromosomal anomaly (Table 9-8). The most common is Down syndrome, in which there is a trisomy of the G group chromosome, usually number 21 (see Chapter 19 for a further discussion of Down syndrome). The other known viable autosomal trisomies involve chromosomes 18 and 13. Abnormalities of sex chromosomes are discussed in Chapter 17 (see p. 473).

DEFECTS CAUSED BY CHEMICAL AGENTS

The relationship of the fetal and maternal circulations allows for the interchange of chemical substances across the placental membrane. Many drugs have been sus-

TABLE 9-8

Common Autosomal Aberrations

Syndrome	Chromosomal Abnormality and Nomenclature	Average Incidence (live births)	Major Clinical Manifestations
Cri du chat	Deletion of short arm of B (No. 5) chromosome—46,XY,5p−		Distinctive weak, high-pitched, mewlike cry resembling the cry of a cat; small head; hypertelorism; failure to thrive; severe mental retardation—profound with age
Trisomy 13 (Patau)	Trisomy of group D (No. 13) chromosome—47,XY,13+	1:4000-10,000	Multiple anomalies, including cleft lip and palate (frequently bilateral); ear malformations; microphthalmia; polydactyly; eye defects; mental retardation; early death
Trisomy 18 (Edwards)	Trisomy of group E (No. 18) chromosome—47,XY,18+	1:3500-7500	Deformed and low-set ears; micrognathia; rocker-bottom feet; overlapping (index over third) fingers; prominent occiput; hypertelorism; failure to thrive and early death; mental retardation
Trisomy 21 (Down)	Trisomy of group G (No. 21) chromosome—47,XY,21+ (trisomy); 46,XY,D−,G−(DqGq)+ (translocation); 46,XY/47,XY,21+ (mosaic)	1:650-1100	Brachycephaly with flat occiput; inner epicanthal folds; small ears, nose, and mouth with protruding tongue; muscular hypotonia; broad, short hands with stubby fingers and transverse palmar crease; broad, stubby feet with wide space between big and second toes; mental retardation; variable life expectancy

TABLE 9-9

Congenital Effects of Maternal Ingestion of Alcohol and Smoking

Fetal or Newborn Effects	Comments and Nursing Considerations
Alcohol (Fetal Alcohol Syndrome [FAS])	
Facial features: hypoplastic maxilla, micrognathia, hypoplastic philtrum, short palpebral fissures	Exact quantity of alcohol needed to produce teratogenic effects in fetus is not known
Neurologic: mental retardation, motor retardation, microcephaly, hypotonia	Women with histories of heavy drinking should be counseled regarding risks to fetus
Growth: prenatal growth retardation, persistent postnatal growth lag	Provide mother with resources for treatment to decrease or eliminate alcoholic intake
Maternal Tobacco Smoking	
Fetal growth retardation	Women should be counseled regarding the risk to fetus
Increased perinatal deaths	Provide with resources to help eliminate smoking
Increased spontaneous abortions	
Postnatal: growth and intellectual and emotional developmental deficits	

pected of producing congenital malformations and some have been definitely implicated. It has been estimated that women take an average of four or five drugs—either prescription or over-the-counter preparations—during their pregnancies.

The extent to which chemical agents affect the unborn child depends on the interplay of several factors—the nature of the agent and its accessibility to the fetus, the time of its applications, the level and duration of the dosage, and the genetic makeup of the fetus. To help ensure that fewer women will inadvertently take some chemical that might be harmful to the fetus, labels on medications are now required to include information regarding the possible effects of the drug. The effects of maternal alcohol consumption and tobacco smoking are listed in Table 9-9. All women of childbearing age should be educated regarding these effects with special emphasis placed on pregnant women.

◆ *Inborn Errors of Metabolism*

Inborn errors of metabolism is a term applied to a large number of inherited diseases caused by the absence or deficiency of a substance essential to cellular metabolism, usually an enzyme. When the normal metabolic process is interrupted as a result of a missing enzyme, an accumulation of substances precedes the interruption, the end product of the process is absent, or the process takes an alternate metabolic pathway. The consequence is disease.

CONGENITAL HYPOTHYROIDISM

Congenital hypothyroidism (sometimes called by the undesirable term *cretinism*) may have a number of etiologies and can be either permanent or transient. However, no matter what the cause, the manifestations (see box) and management are similar. In some conditions the thyroid deficiency is severe and manifestations develop early; in others the symptoms may be delayed for months or years.

Diagnostic Evaluation

Several tests are available to assess thyroid activity: measurements of thyroxine (T_4), triiodothyronine (T_3), and thyroid-stimulating hormone (TSH). In congenital hypothyroidism T_4 and T_3 levels are low or borderline. Neonatal screening is now possible with a highly sensitive and specific radioimmunoassay for T_4 or TSH and is mandatory in most states. Diagnosis rests on the detection of a high serum level of TSH and a low level of T_4 during the early days of life.

Therapeutic Management

Treatment involves lifelong replacement therapy with a thyroid hormone preparation to abolish all signs of hypothyroidism and reestablish normal physical and mental development. If treatment is started shortly after birth, normal growth is possible and the chance for normal intelligence is increased. The most signficant factor adversely affecting eventual intelligence appears to be inadequate treatment, which may be related to noncompliance.

Nursing Considerations

The most important nursing objective is early identification of the disorder. Nurses caring for neonates must be certain that screening is performed, especially in infants who are discharged early or born at home. Although the screening test is very specific, some children may not be identified, and nurses in ambulatory settings for well-infant care need to be aware of the earliest signs of the disorder. Parental remarks about an unusually "quiet and good" baby coupled with any of the early physical manifestations should lead the nurse to suspect hypothyroidism and refer the child for specific tests. Unfortunately, many parents harbor guilt about their impressions of the infant before the diagnosis because the child's inactivity may not have alerted them to a problem, with the result that treatment was delayed.

Possible Manifestations of Congenital Hypothyroidism

At Birth	Before 3 Months of Age	Older Child
Gestation >42 weeks	Umbilical hernia	Short stature
Birth weight >4 kg (8.8 lb)	Mottled and dry skin	Infantile proportions persist; length of trunk long relative to legs
Widened posterior fontanelle	Constipation	Decreased metabolic rate; weight gain, often leading to obesity
Hypothermia, 95° F or less	Large tongue	Infantile facial features of myxedema
Peripheral cyanosis	Hoarse	Short forehead
Respiratory distress	Cold to touch	Wide, puffy eyes; wrinkled eyelids
Edema	Excessive sleepiness	Broad, short, upturned nose
Prolonged physiologic jaundice	Difficulty feeding related to lethargy	Large, protruding tongue
Abdominal distention	Minimum crying	Hair often dry, brittle, or lusterless extending far down onto the forehead
Vomiting		Dentition delayed and usually defective
Delayed passage of meconium		Intellectual deficit of varying degrees
Feeding difficulties		
Hypoactivity		

Once the diagnosis is confirmed, parents need an explanation of the disorder, the need for lifelong treatment, and the importance of compliance with the drug regimen. Parents also need to be aware of signs indicating overdose, namely, rapid pulse, dyspnea, irritability, insomnia, fever, sweating, and weight loss. Ideally they should know how to count the pulse and be instructed to withhold a dose and consult the physician if the pulse rate is above a certain value. Signs of inadequate treatment are fatigue, sleepiness, decreased appetite, and constipation.

If the diagnosis was delayed past early infancy, the chance of permanent mental retardation is great. Such parents need the same guidance in caring for their child as do others who have an offspring with cognitive impairment (Chapter 19). They need an opportunity to discuss their feelings regarding late recognition of the disorder. Although treatment will not reverse the intellectual deficit, it may prevent further damage. Genetic counseling is important, especially if the disorder is caused by an inborn error of thyroid hormone synthesis, an autosomal-recessive trait.

PHENYLKETONURIA

Phenylketonuria (PKU) is a genetic disease, inherited as an autosomal-recessive trait (see Appendix B) and caused by the absence of an enzyme that is necessary for the metabolism of the essential amino acid phenylalanine. It is not a common inborn error of metabolism—it affects 1 in every 10,000 to 20,000 live births but is a potentially significant cause of mental retardation. PKU primarily affects whites, with the incidence being highest in people living in the United States or Northern Europe. It is very rare in the African, Jewish, or Japanese populations.

There are a number of variations of disturbed phenylalanine metabolism, or *hyperphenylalaninemia*. But because the variant forms are diagnosed and the patients treated differently, the following discussion is limited to the severe, classic PKU.

Pathophysiology

In PKU the hepatic enzyme *phenylalanine hydroxylase*, which normally controls the conversion of phenylalanine to tyrosine, is absent, resulting in the accumulation of phenylalanine in the bloodstream and urinary excretion of its abnormal metabolites, the phenyl acids (Fig. 9-16). One of these metabolites, phenylpyruvic acid, gives urine the characteristic musty odor associated with this disease and is responsible for the term *phenylketonuria*. In addition to the accumulating phenylalanine, there is an absence of the amino acid tyrosine, which is needed for the formation of the pigment melanin and the hormones epinephrine and thyroxin.

Diagnostic Evaluation

The objective in diagnosing PKU or treating the affected patient is to prevent mental retardation. All the tests for PKU are based on the detection of increasing phenylalanine levels in the blood or characteristic metabolites in the urine. The most reliable test for screening newborns for PKU is the *Guthrie test*, which measures blood phenylalanine levels. When this test is performed reliably, serum phenylalanine levels greater than 4 mg/100 ml (normal = 2 mg/100 ml) can be detected.

The screening test is most reliable if the blood sample is taken after the infant has ingested a source of protein. However, because of early discharge from the hospital, the American Academy of Pediatrics (1982) recommends that (1) the test be performed on all newborns before they leave the nursery, regardless of age, and (2) a repeat blood specimen be obtained by the third week of life from all infants in whom the initial specimen was taken within the first 24 hours of life.

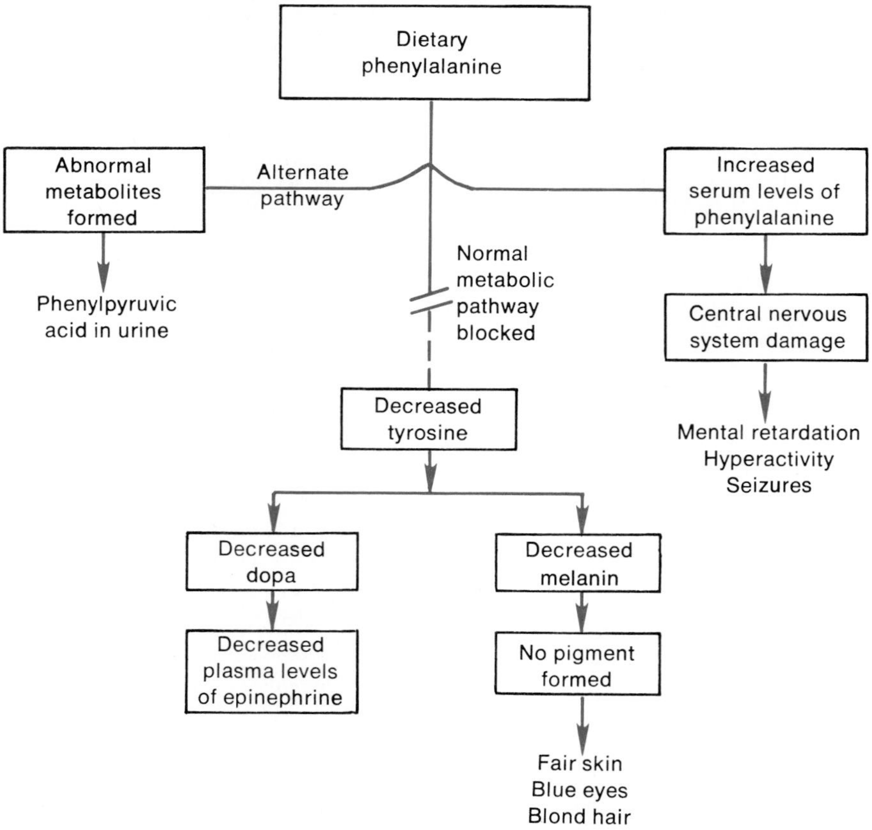

FIG. 9-16 Metabolic error and consequences in phenylketonuria.

Signs of PKU observed in later infancy and childhood are outlined in the box.

Therapeutic Management

Treatment for the infant with PKU is dietary. Since the genetic enzyme is intracellular, systemic administration of phenylalanine hydroxylase is of no value. Phenylalanine cannot be eliminated because it is an essential amino acid for tissue growth. Therefore dietary management must meet two criteria:

1. It must meet the child's nutritional need for optimum growth.
2. It must maintain phenylalanine levels within a safe range.

The diet is calculated to allow 20 to 30 mg of phenylalanine per kilogram of body weight per day, which should maintain blood levels between 3 and 10 mg/100 ml. Significant brain damage usually occurs when levels are greater than 10 to 15 mg/100 ml. At levels less than 2 mg/100 ml the body begins to catabolize its protein stores, resulting in growth retardation.

Since all natural food proteins contain about 15% phenylalanine, specially prepared milk substitutes such as *Lofenalac*,* made from specially treated enzymatic casein hydrolysate, contain 0.4% phenylalanine as well as minerals and vitamins to provide a balanced nutritional formula. Because of the low phenylalanine content of breast milk, total or partial breast-feeding may be allowed, with close monitoring of phenylalanine levels. Because

Clinical Manifestations of PKU (Child)

Blonde hair, blue eyes, and fair skin (commonly)
High susceptibility to eczema and other dermatologic problems
Mental retardation
Failure to thrive
Frequent vomiting
Irritability
Hyperactivity
Unpredictable, erratic behavior
Bizarre or schizoidlike behavior patterns are common
- Fright reactions
- Screaming episodes
- Disorientation
- Failure to respond to strong stimuli
- Catatonic-like positions

Convulsions (severe cases)

*Mead Johnson & Co., Evansville, IN.

levels of tyrosine are also inadequate, this amino acid and several others are supplied to the infant.

Other milk substitutes that contain no phenylalanine are available and allow for a greater variety of exchanges with natural low-phenylalanine foods in the diet and a more normal diet. However, these are not universally recommended for children under 2 years of age. The best time to begin a low-phenylalanine diet is as soon as possible after birth. It is not yet known how long the diet therapy must be continued. At present many centers discontinue the diet when the child is 6 to 8 years old, although many believe that increased phenylalanine levels beyond this age can have neuropsychologic sequelae, such as lowered intelligence quotient and attentional and academic difficulties.

To evaluate the effectiveness of dietary treatment, frequent monitoring of blood phenylalanine levels is necessary. With improved dietary control of PKU, the increased life span of individuals with this disorder presents additional concerns. High phenylalanine blood levels in mothers with PKU affect the normal embryologic development of the fetus. Consequently, the low-phenylalanine diet should be resumed *prior to* pregnancy in affected women.

Nursing Considerations

The principal nursing considerations involve teaching the family regarding the dietary restrictions. Although the treatment may sound simple, the task of maintaining such a strict dietary regimen is very demanding. Foods with low phenylalanine levels, such as vegetables, fruits, juices, and some cereals, breads, and starches, must be measured to provide the prescribed amount of phenylalanine. Most high-protein foods, such as meat and dairy products, are either eliminated or restricted to small amounts. The sweetener aspartame (NutraSweet) must be avoided because it is converted to phenylalanine in the body. Also, the substitutes are quite expensive, adding financial burdens.

Parents need a basic understanding of the disorder and practical suggestions regarding food selection and preparation. The lumpy consistency and distinctive odor and taste of the formula present some difficulties in its preparation. A blender or mixer dissolves the powder more easily, but carrying such equipment is inconvenient when traveling. Although the taste is virtually impossible to camouflage, modifying the flavor with orange Tang, fruit-flavored powdered punch, or strawberry or chocolate powdered flavoring alters the flavor somewhat and provides variety without greatly altering the phenylalanine content. The chocolate-flavored formula can be heated and served as hot cocoa or frozen into popsicles.

As with any hereditary disorder the family should be provided with genetic counseling and follow-up. PKU is a chronic condition; therefore, the principles of care and management are the same as that for any child and family with a chronic illness (see Chapter 18).

GALACTOSEMIA

Galactosemia is an inborn error of carbohydrate metabolism, inherited as an autosomal-recessive trait, in which the hepatic enzyme *galactose-1-phosphate uridyl transferase* is absent, preventing the conversion of galactose to glucose. As galactose accumulates in the blood, several organs are affected. Hepatic dysfunction leads to cirrhosis, resulting in jaundice in the infant by the second week of life. The spleen subsequently becomes enlarged as a result of portal hypertension. Cataracts are usually recognizable by 1 or 2 months of age; cerebral damage, manifested by the symptoms of lethargy and hypotonia, is evident soon afterward. Infants with galactosemia appear normal at birth, but within a few days after ingesting milk, which has a high lactose content, they begin to vomit and lose weight. Drowsiness, nausea, and diarrhea also occur. Death during the first month of life is not infrequent in untreated infants.

Diagnosis of this rare disorder is made on the basis of galactosuria, increased levels of galactose in the blood, or decreased enzyme levels in erythrocytes. Screening tests are available and mandatory in several states.

Treatment of galactosemia is dietary; it consists of eliminating all milk and galactose-containing foods, including breast milk, from the diet. Strict adherence to the diet is necessary for the first 7 to 8 years, followed by a modified regimen throughout life.

Nursing considerations are similar to those for PKU, but dietary restrictions are easier to maintain. However, reading food labels very carefully for the presence of any form of dairy product, such as cream, yogurt, cheese, or butter, is essential. During infancy, soybean-based formulas are used. Many drugs, such as penicillin, contain lactose as fillers and must also be avoided.

GENETIC COUNSELING

Genetic counseling is a communication process concerned with the human problems associated with the occurrence, or risk of occurrence, of a genetic disorder in a family. Nurses in the field of infant and child care continually encounter genetic diseases and families in which there is a risk that a disorder may be transmitted to an offspring. It is a responsibility of nurses to be alert to situations in which persons could benefit from genetic counseling, to become familiar with facilities in their areas where genetic counseling is available, and to learn the basic principles of heredity. In this way they will be able to direct individuals and families to take advantage of needed services and to be active participants in the counseling process.

The success of counseling is measured by the way in which the family utilizes the information presented to them. Maintaining contact with the family or referring the family to an agency that can provide a sustained relationship, usually the public health agency in their locality, is one of the most important aspects of the counseling process. In a disorder such as PKU that requires conscientious diet management, it is important to make certain that the family understands and follows the advice. Children born later must be carefully observed to ensure early detection of symptoms in the event that they have also inherited the disorder.

Psychologic Aspects of Genetic Disease

It requires time and understanding to deal with the emotional tension and anxiety generated in families who are faced with the prospect of a genetic disorder. Knowledge of and the ability to deal with the range of psychologic responses and all their ramifications (such as the grief reaction, guilt, anger, and coping mechanisms) are essential components of the nursing role in genetic counseling.

It is important to stress that there is nothing shameful about an inherited or congenital defect and to emphasize any appropriate remedy. Families have a tendency to be more ashamed of a hereditary disorder than of one caused by self-indulgence, such as obesity or alcoholism. The threat of a hereditary "taint" often creates intrafamily strife, hostility, and marital disharmony, sometimes to the point of family disintegration. Relatives frequently cease reproduction after the diagnosis of a hereditary defect in a member, or the decision to marry may be postponed indefinitely on the basis of a disorder in a relative, even a remote one, of a prospective partner. Although people may understand the situation on an intellectual level, this will not help them on an emotional level. A large and vital part of the nurse's role in genetic counseling is that of a sympathetic and supportive listener.

SUMMARY

In recent years there has been an increase in the survival rate of newborns that has coincided with the development of programs to improve the health of expectant mothers and the timing of their pregnancies and with the introduction of important new techniques in neonatal care. Assessment and prompt intervention in life-threatening emergencies often make the difference between a favorable outcome and a lifetime of disability. Nurses are familiar with the characteristics of newborn infants and recognize the significance of benign and serious deviations from expected observations. They can identify those subtle signs that indicate impending difficulties—color changes, lethargy, poor feeding, altered vital signs, and other unusual behavior. When the need for specialized care is anticipated and planned for, the probability of a successful outcome is increased.

KEY CONCEPTS

- Health problems of the newborn infant may result from hereditary conditions or from prenatal, natal, or postnatal environmental factors.
- Birth injuries are usually those affecting soft tissues, bones, or nervous tissues.
- High-risk neonates are those newborn infants, regardless of gestational age or birth weight, who have a greater than average chance of morbidity or mortality because of conditions or circumstances that are superimposed on the normal course of events associated with birth and adjustment of extrauterine life.
- Appropriate stimulation of infants in the intensive care unit facilitates their growth and maturation.
- Parents are encouraged to interact with their high-risk infants and gradually assume care of the infant when the infant's condition allows and the parents feel comfortable in doing so.
- Hyperbilirubinemia is a common problem in the newborn that results from red blood cell breakdown that exceeds the ability of the immature liver to metabolize and excrete.
- Because of their immature physical status preterm infants need special attention to promote respiratory efforts, maintain body temperature, conserve energy, prevent infection, and provide nutrition.
- Preterm infants are subject to a number of complications including apnea, infection, anemia, respiratory distress syndrome, and intraventricular hemorrhage.
- Sepsis is a serious condition with vague, nonspecific manifestations that render it difficult to distinguish from other conditions in the newborn infant.
- Maternal prenatal conditions are responsible for high-risk health problems in some newborn infants, especially maternal diabetes, physical dependency on drugs, some infections, and ingestion of certain chemical substances.
- The inborn errors of metabolism for which newborns are routinely screened are congenital hypothyroidism, phenylketonuria, and galactosemia.

STUDY QUESTIONS AND ACTIVITIES

1. Observe both a full-term infant and a preterm infant. Compare the similarities and differences between these two infants relative to physical appearance and behavior.
2. Describe the characteristics of low-birth-weight preterm infants that render them vulnerable to physiologic complications and the complications to which they are susceptible.
3. Interview a nurse in an intensive care nursery to determine: (a) what special services, such as parent groups, are available to families of high-risk infants and (b) the policy of the unit regarding family visitation and involvement, including siblings of the infant.
4. Devise a teaching plan for families with an infant being discharged on home phototherapy.
5. Interview the infection control nurse regarding hospital policy for preventing the spread of infectious disease in the nursery.

REFERENCES

American Academy of Pediatrics, Committee on Genetics: New issues in newborn screening for phenylketonuria and congenital hypothyroidism, Pediatrics **69:**104-106, 1982.

Blake, S.: The bright side of phototherapy, MCN **8:**23, 1983.

Cloney, D.L., and Donowitz, L.G.: Overgrown use for infection control in nurseries and neonatal intensive care units, Am. J. Dis. Child. **140:**680-683, 1986.

Kleiber, C., Krutzfield, N., and Rose, E.: Acute histologic changes in the tracheobronchial tree associated with different suction catheter insertion techniques, Heart Lung **17:**10-14, 1988.
Meier, P., and Anderson, G.C.: Responses of small preterm infants to bottle- and breast-feeding, MCN **12:**97-105, 1987.
Meier, P., and Pugh, E.J.: Breast-feeding behavior of small preterm infants, MCN **10:**396-401, 1985.
Smith, J.E., and Deitch, K.V.: Cocaine: a maternal, fetal, and neonatal risk, J. Pediatr. Health Care **1:**120-124, 1987.

BIBLIOGRAPHY

Nursing Care of the High-Risk Infant

Anderberg, G.J.: Initial aquaintance and attachment behavior of siblings with the newborn, JOGNN **17**(1):49-54, 1988.
Anderson, G.C., and others: Effects of time-controlled non-nutritive sucking opportunities, Nurs. Res. **31:**63, 1982.
Bailey, C.F.: Withholding or withdrawing treatment on handicapped newborns, Pediatr. Nurs. **12:**413-416, 1986.
Bethea, S.W.: Primary nursing in the infant special care unit, JOGNN **14:**202-208, 1985.
Blackburn, S., and Lowen, L.: Grandparents in NICUs, MCN **11:**190-192, 1986.
Blackburn, S., and Lowen, L.: Impact of an infant's premature birth on the grandparents and parents, JOGNN **15:**173-178, 1986.
Boggs, K.R., and Rau, P.K.: Breastfeeding the premature infant, Am. J. Nurs. **83:**1437-1439, 1983.
Bull, M.J., and Stroup, K.B.: Premature infants in car seats, Pediatrics **75:**336-339, 1985.
Censullo, M.: Home care of the high-risk newborn, JOGNN **15:**146-153, 1986.
Chaze, B.A., and Ludington-Hoe, S.M.: Sensory stimulation in the ICU, Am. J. Nurs. **84:**68-71, 1984.
Cole, J.G.: Infant stimulation reexamined: an environmental- and behavioral-based approach, Neonatal Network **3**(5):24-31, 1985.
Cole, J.G., and Frappier, P.A.: Infant stimulation reassessed. A new approach to providing care for the preterm infant, JOGNN **14:**471-477, 1985.
Consolvo, C.A.: Relieving parental anxiety in the care-by-parent unit, JOGNN **15:**154-159, 1986.
Consolvo, C.A.: Siblings in the NICU, Neonatal Network **5**(5):7-12, 1987.
Fanaroff, A., and Martin, R., editors: Neonatal-perinatal medicine, ed. 4, St. Louis, 1987, The C.V. Mosby Co.
Gennaro, S.: Anxiety and problem-solving ability in mothers of premature infants, JOGNN **15:**160-164, 1986.
Glass, S.M., and Giacoia, G.P.: Intravenous drug therapy in premature infants: practical aspects, JOGNN **16:**310-318, 1987.
Gunderson, L.P., and Kenner, C.: Neonatal stress: physiologic adaptation and nursing implications, Neonatal Network **6**(1):37-42, 1987.
Haddock, N.: Blood pressure monitoring in neonates, MCN **5:**131-135, 1980.
Harrison, L.L., and Twardosz, S.: Teaching mothers about their preterm infants, JOGNN **15:**165-172, 1986.
Hayes, J.S.: Premature infant development; the relationship of neonatal stimulation, birth condition, and home environment, Pediatr. Nurs. **6**(6):33-36, 1980.
Jenkins, R.L., and Tock, M.K.S.: Helping parents bond to their premature infant, MCN **11:**32-34, 1986.
Johnson, S.H.: The premature infant. In Johnson, S.H., editor: Nursing assessment and strategies for the family at risk, ed. 2, Philadelphia, 1986, J.B. Lippincott Co.
Jacobson, G., and others: Handwashing: ring-wearing and number of microorganisms, Nurs. Res. **34:**186-188, 1985.
Johnson, S.H.: Nursing assessment and strategies for the family at risk, ed. 2, Philadelphia, 1986, J.B. Lippincott Co.
Kennedy, J.: Evacuation of a neonatal unit, Can. Nurse **79:**26-29, 1983.
Knutson, M.G., Biro, P.J., and Padgett, D.: Tracking infants at risk: Washington state's high priority infant tracking system, J. Pediatr. Health Care **1:**180-189, 1987.
Konings, K.: Application of an ostomy pouch to a preterm infant, Neonatal Network **5**(5):49-51, 1987.
Korones, S.B.: High-risk newborn infants: the basis for intensive nursing care, ed. 4, St. Louis, 1986, The C.V. Mosby Co.
Kowba, M.D., and Schwirian, P.M.: Direct sibling contact and bacterial colonization in newborns, JOGNN **14:**412-417, 1985.
Kuller, J.M., Lund, C., and Tobin, C.: Improved skin care for premature infants, MCN **8:**200-203, 1983.
Larrow, L., and Noe, J.M.: Port wine stain hemangiomas, Am. J. Nurs. **82:**786-790, 1982.
Lund, C., and others: Evaluation of a pectin-based barrier under tape to protect neonatal skin, JOGNN **15:**39-44, 1986.
Magyary, D.: Early social interactions: preterm infant-parent dyads, Issues Compr. Pediatr. Nurs. **7:**233-254, 1984.
McClowry, S.G.: Research and treatment: ethical distinctions related to the care of children, J. Pediatr. Nurs. **2:**23-29, 1987.
Merenstein, G.B., and Gardner, S.L.: Handbook of neonatal intensive care, St. Louis, 1985, The C.V. Mosby Co.
Moen, J.E., and others: Axillary versus rectal temperatures in preterm infants under radiant warmers, JOGNN **16:**348-352, 1987.
Moore, M.C.: Total parenteral nutrition for infants, Neonatal Network **6**(2):33-40, 1987.
Nelson, D., Heitman, R., and Jennings, C.: Effects of tactile stimulation on pemature infant weight gain, JOGNN **15:**262-267, 1986.
Oelerich, W.J., and Dombrowski, J.M.: Mini IV patients . . . maximum precautions, RN **44**(9):43-47, 1982.
Penticuff, J.H.: Neonatal nursing ethics: toward a consensus, Neonatal Network **5**(6):7-16, 1987.
Perez, R.H.: Protocols for perinatal nursing practice, St. Louis, 1981, The C.V. Mosby Co.
Rice, B.R., and Feeg, V.D.: First-year developmental outcomes for multiple-risk premature infants, Pediatr. Nurs. **11**(1):30-35, 1985.
Rothenberg, L.S.: To feed or not to feed: that is the question and the ethical dilemma, J. Pediatr. Nurs. **1:**226-229, 1986.
Ruchala, P.: The effect of wearing headcoverings on the axillary temperatures of infants, MCN **10:**240, 1985.
Rushton, C.H.: Promoting normal growth and development in the hospital environment, Neonatal Network **4**(6):21-30, 1986.
Sammons, W.A.H., and Lewis, J.M.: Premature babies: a different beginning, St. Louis, 1985, The C.V. Mosby Co.
Sims-Jones, N.: Back to the theories: another way to view mothers of prematures, MCN **11:**394-397, 1986.
Smith, S.M.: Primary nursing in the NICU: a parent's perspective, Neonatal Network **5**(4):25-27, 1987.
Tucker, S.C.: Dopamine use in neonates, Neonatal Network **6**(2):21-24, 1987.
Umphenour, J.H.: Bacterial colonization in neonates with sibling visitation, JOGNN **9:**73-75, 1980.
VandenBerg, K.A.: Revising the traditional model: an individualized approach to developmental interventions in the intensive care nursery, Neonatal Network **3**(5):32-38, 1985.
Varner, B., Ossenkop, D., and Lyon, J.: Prematures, too, need rooming-in and care-by-parent programs, MCN **5:**431-432, 1980.
White-Traut, R.C., and Tubeszewski, K.A.: Multimodal stimulation of the premature infant, J. Pediatr. Nurs. **1:**90-95, 1986.
Wranesh, B.L.: The effect of sibling visitation on bacterial colonization rate in neonates, JOGNN **11:**211-213, 1982.

Neonatal Loss

Beckey, R.D., and others: Development of a perinatal grief checklist, JOGNN **14:**194-199, 1985.
Bright, P.D.: Adolescent pregnancy and loss, Matern. Child Nurs. J. **16**(1):1-12, 1987.
Brown, S.E.: A case study in death with dignity, Neonatal Network **5**(2):51-54, 1986.
Bryan, E.M.: When a twin dies, Nurs. Times **80**(10):24-26, 1984.
Cordell, A.S., and Apolito, R.: Family support in infant death, JOGNN **10**(4):281-285, 1981.

Gardner, S.L., and Merenstein, G.B.: Helping families deal with perinatal loss, Neonatal Network **5**(2):17-33, 1986.
Gardner, S.L., and Merenstein, G.B.: Perinatal grief and loss: an overview, Neonatal Network **5**(2):7-15, 1986.
Landon-Malone, K.A., Kirkpatrick, J.M., and Stull, S.P.: Incorporating hospice care in a community hospital NICU, Neonatal Network **6**(1):13-19, 1987.
Mahan, C.K., and others: Neonatal death: parental evaluation of the NICU experience, Issues Compr. Pediatr. Nurs. **5**:279-292, 1981.
Thomas, N., and Cordell, A.: The dying infant: aiding parents in the detachment process, Pediatr. Nurs. **9**:355-357, 1983.
Trouy, M.B., and Ward-Larson, C.: Sibling grief, Neonatal Network **5**(4):35-40, 1987.
Wooten, B.: Death of an infant, MCN **6**:257-260, 1981.
Work, R.B.: When we cannot cure, care (Letters to the editor), MCN **8**:111-112, 1983.

Parental Involvement

Arenson, J.: Discharge teaching in the NICU: the changing needs of NICU graduates and their families, Neonatal Network **6**(4):29-30, 47-52, 1988.
Chitwood, L.: A lesson in living, Nursing 84 **14**(1):55-56, 1984.
Eager, M., and Exoo, R.: Parents visiting parents for unequaled support, MCN **5**:35-36, 1980.
Eikner, S.: Dealing with long-term problems: a parent's perspective, Neonatal Network **5**(2):45-49, 1986.
Gennaro, S.: Maternal anxiety, problem-solving ability, and adaptation to the premature infant, Pediatr. Nurs. **11**:343-348, 1985.
Hawkins-Walsh, E.: Diminishing anxiety in parents of sick newborns, MCN **5**:30-34, 1980.
Kelting, S.: Supporting parents in the NICU, Neonatal Network **4**(6):14-18, 1986.
Kemp, V.H., and Page, C.K.: The psychosocial impact of a high-risk pregnancy on the family, JOGNN **16**:232-236, 1986.
Kemp, V.H., and Page, C.K.: Maternal prenatal attachment in normal and high-risk pregnancies, JOGNN **16**:179-184, 1987.
Miles, M.S., and Carter, M.C.: Assessing parental stress in intensive care units, MCN **8**:354-359, 1983.
Montgomery, L.A.V., and Williams-Judge, S.: An anticipatory support program for high-risk parents, Neonatal Network **5**(1):33-35, 1986.
Schraeder, B.D.: Attachment and parenting despite lengthy intensive care, MCN **5**:37-41, 1980.
Solheim, K., and Spellacy, C.: Sibling visitation: effects on newborn infection rates, JOGNN **17**(1):43-48, 1988.
Steele, K.H.: Caring for parents of critically ill neonates during hospitalization: strategies for health care professionals, Matern. Child Nurs. J. **16**(1):13-27, 1987.
Thornton, J., Berry, J., and Dal Santo, J.: Neonatal intensive care: the nurse's role in supporting the family, Nurs. Clin. North Am. **19**:125-137, 1984.
Turley, M.A.: A meta-analysis of informing mothers concerning the sensory and perceptual capabilities of their infants: the effects on maternal-infant interaction, Matern. Child Nurs. J. **14**(3):183-198, 1985.
Whetsell, M.V., and Larrabbee, M.J.: Using guilt constructively in the NICU to affirm parental coping, Neonatal Network **6**(4):21-27, 1988.

Hyperbilirubinemia, Hypoglycemia, and Hypocalcemia

Brucker, M.C., and MacMullen, N.J.: Neonatal jaundice in the home: assessment with a noninvasive device, JOGNN **16**:355-358, 1987.
Carmen, S.: Neonatal hypoglycemia in response to maternal glucose infusion before delivery, JOGNN **15**:319-323, 1986.
Dortch, E., and Spottiswoode, P.: New light on phototherapy: home use, Neonatal Network **4**(4):30-34, 1986.
Hammer, R.M., Bower, E.J., and Messina, L.J.: The prenatal use of Rho(D) immune globulin, MCN **9**:29-31, 1984.
Hartsell, M.B.: Home phototherapy, J. Pediatr. Nurs. **1**:282-283, 1986.
Locklin, M.: Assessing jaundice in full-term newborns, Pediatr. Nurs. **13**:15-19, 1987.
Perry, S.E., Parer, J.T., and Interrisi, M.: Intrauterine transfusion for severe isoimmunization, MCN **11**:182-189, 1986.
Taur, K.M.: Physiologic mechanisms in childhood hypoglycemia, Pediatr. Nurs. **9**:341-344, 1983.

Respiratory Distress Syndrome

Bancalari, E.: Transcutaneous oxygen monitoring: a new wave in newborn care, Contemp. Pediatr. **4**(1):107-110, 1987.
Cohen, M.A.: Transcutaneous oxygen monitoring for sick neonates, MCN **9**:324-330, 1984.
Dingle, R.E., and others: Continuous transcutaneous O_2 monitoring in the neonate, Am. J. Nurs. **80**:890-893, 1980.
Few, B.J.: Neonatal update: surfactant replacement, MCN **12**:129, 1987.
Gerraughty, A.B., and Younie, L.J.: ECMO: the artificial lung for gravely ill newborns, Am. J. Nurs. **87**:655-658, 1987.
Gruden, M.: High-frequency ventilation: an overview, Crit. Care Nurs. **5**:36-40, 1985.
Hartsell, M.: Noninvasive oxygen monitoring, J. Pediatr. Nurs. **2**:64-65, 1987.
Inwood, S., Finley, G.A., and Fitzhardinge, P.M.: High-frequency oscillation: a new mode of ventilation for the neonate, Neonatal Network **4**(5):53-58, 1986.
Kaplow, R., and Fromme, L.R.: Nursing care plan for the patient receiving high-frequency jet ventilation, Crit. Care Nurs. **5**:25-27, 1985.
Karp, T.B., and others: High frequency jet ventilation: a neonatal nursing perspective, Neonatal Network **4**(5):42-50, 1986.
Kling, P.: Respiratory distress syndrome in the tiny baby, Neonatal Network **4**(5):7-13, 1986.
Loper, D.L.: Surfactant replacement therapy, Neonatal Network **4**(5):14-17, 1986.
Mason, T.N.: A hand ventilation technique for neonates, MCN **7**:366-369, 1982.
McBurney, B.H.: The role of the community hospital nurse in supporting parents of transported infants, Neonatal Network **6**(4):60-64, 1988.
McFadden, R.: Decreasing respiratory compromise during infant suctioning, Am. J. Nurs. **81**:2158-2161, 1981.
Nugent, J.: Extracorporeal membrane oxygenation in the neonate, Neonatal Network **4**(4):27-38, 1986.
Oellrich, R.G.: Pneumothorax, chest tubes, and the neonate, MCN **10**:29-35, 1985.
O'Pray, M.: Working with families with infants with respiratory equipment in the home, Issues Compr. Pediatr. Nurs. **10**:113-121, 1987.

Respiratory and Cardiovascular Complications

Foster, S.D.: Indomethacin: pharmacologic closure of the ductus arteriosus, MCN **7**:171, 1982.
Gregory, S.E.B.: Air leak syndromes, Neonatal Network **5**(4):40-46, 1987.
Hazinski, M.F.: New guidelines for pediatric and neonatal cardiopulmonary resuscitation and advanced life support. Part III: Neonatal advanced life support, Pediatr. Nurs. **13**:57-59, 1987.
Jackson, D.F.: Nursing care plan: home management of children with BPD, Pediatr. Nurs. **12**:342-348, 1986.
Kenney, M.M.: Hospital to home: care of the child with a tracheostomy, Neonatal Network **6**(1):21-24, 1987.
Lawson, M.: Persistent pulmonary hypertension of the newborn: current trends in classification and diagnosis, Neonatal Network **6**(1):27-35, 1987.
Shapiro, C.: Retrolental fibroplasia: what we know and what we don't know, Neonatal Network **4**(6):33-44, 1986.
Southwell, S.: Update on the treatment of persistent pulmonary hypertension of the newborn, Neonatal Network **4**(5):19-25, 1986.
Wood, A.F.: Sequelae of perinatal asphyxia, Neonatal Network **5**(5):21-23, 1987.

Cerebral Complications

Brann, A.W., Jr.: Hypoxic ischemic encephalopathy (asphyxia), Pediatr. Clin. North Am. **33:**451-464, 1986.
MacDonald, N.P.: Motor development in premature infants with intracranial hemorrhage, Pediatr. Nurs. **12:**263-267, 1986.
Sommer, C.: Callous nurses, a bewildered mother, a brain-damaged baby, RN **50**(6):48-51, 1987.
Torrence, C.: Neonatal seizures: Part I. A developmental and clinical understanding, Neonatal Network **4**(8):9-15, 1985.

Infections

Gaffney, S.E., and Salinger, L.: Group B streptococcus: the pregnant woman and her neonate, JOGNN **16:**91-96, 1986.
Gennaro, S.: Necrotizing enterocolitis: detecting it and treating it, Nursing 80 **80**(1):52-56, 1980.
Henneberry, C.: Candida sepsis in the very low birthweight infant, Neonatal Network **5**(6):39-45, 1987.
Larson, E.: Rituals in infection control: what works in the newborn nursery? JOGNN **16**(6):411-416, 1987.
Plapp, P.R.: Nursing implications in the early recognition of necrotizing enterocolitis, Issues Compr. Pediatr. Nurs. **4**(2):77-81, 1980.
Strodtbeck, F.: Critical care concepts related to neonatal septicemia and septic shock, Crit. Care Q. **4**(1):71-77, 1981.
Whiteman, L., Wuethrick, M., and Egan, E.: Infants who survive necrotizing enterocolitis, Matern. Child. Nurs. J. **14**(3):123-134, 1985.

Disorders Caused by Maternal Factors

Alexander, L.L.: The pregnant smoker: nursing implications, JOGNN **16:**167-173, 1987.
Boland, M.G., and Klug, R.M.: AIDS: the implications for home care, Am. J. Nurs. **86:**404-411, 1986.
Boyes, S.M.: AIDS virus in breast milk: a new threat to neonates and donor breast milk banks, Neonatal Network **5**(5):37-39, 1987.
Burns, E.M.: Diabetes mellitus and pregnancy, Nurs. Clin. North Am. **18:**673-685, 1983.
Edmondson, K.S.: Acquired immune deficiency syndrome in the neonate, Neonatal Network **6**(4):7-12, 1988.
Enloe, C.F.: How alcohol affects the developing fetus, Nutr. Today, Sept./Oct. 1980, pp. 12-15.
Fuhrmann, K., and others: Prevention of congenital malformations in infants of insulin-dependent diabetic mothers, Diabetes Care **6:**219-223, 1983.
Iazzetti, L.: Nursing management of the pediatric AIDS patient, Issues Compr. Pediatr. Nurs. **9:**119-129, 1986.
Inglis, A.D., and Lozano, M.: AIDS and the neonatal ICU, Neonatal Network **5**(3):39-43, 1986.
Larson, E.: Trends in neonatal infections, JOGNN **16**(6):404-409, 1987.
Lemons, P.M.: Beyond the birth of a defective child, Neonatal Network **5**(3):13-20, 1986.
Lott, J.W.: PKU: a nursing update, J. Pediatr. Nurs. **3:**29-34, 1988.
Lynch, J.M.: Helping patients through the recurring nightmare of herpes, Nursing 82 **12**(10):52-57, 1982.
Merker, L., Higgins, P., and Kinnard, E.: Assessing narcotic addiction in neonates, Pediatr. Nurs. **11:**177-181, 1985.
Stagno, S.: Toxoplasmosis, Am. J. Nurs. **80:**720-722, 1980.
Stephens, C.J.: The fetal alcohol syndrome: cause for concern, MCN **6:**251-256, 1981.
Withers, J., and Bradshaw, E.: Preventing neonatal hepatitis-B infection, MCN **11:**270-272, 1986.
Zigrossi, S.T., and Riga-Ziegler, M.: The stress of medical management on pregnant diabetics, MCN **11:**320-323, 1986.

Inborn Errors of Metabolism

Barnico, L.M., and Cullinane, M.M.: Maternal phenylketonuria: an unexpected challenge, MCN **10:**108-110, 1985.
Coody, D.: Congenital hypothyroidism, Pediatr. Nurs. **10**(5):342-345, 1984.
Hayes, J.S., and others: Managing PKU: an update, MCN **12:**119-123, 1987.
Hurst, J.D., and Stullenbarger, B.: Implementation of a self-care approach in a pediatric interdisciplinary phenylketonuria (PKU) clinic, Pediatr. Nurs. **1:**159-163, 1986.
Kotzer, A.M., and McCabe, E.R.B.: Newborn screening for inherited metabolic disease: principles and practice, Neonatal Network **6**(4):15-19, 1988.
Levy, H.L., and Waisbren, S.E.: Effects of untreated maternal phenylketonuria and hyperphenylalaninemia, N. Engl. J. Med. **309:**1269-1274, 1983.
Messer, S.S.: PKU: a mother's perspective, Pediatr. Nurs. **11:**121-123, 1985.
Sbravati, C., and Fischer, R.G.: What sugar substitutes are available and are there any differences between them? Pediatr. Nurs. **9:**138, 1983.
Schor, D.P.: Phenylketonuria and temperament in middle childhood, Child. Health Care **14**(3):163-167, 1986.
Smith, E.J.: Galactosemia: an inborn error of metabolism, Nurse Pract. **5:**8-9, March/April 1980.

UNIT

V

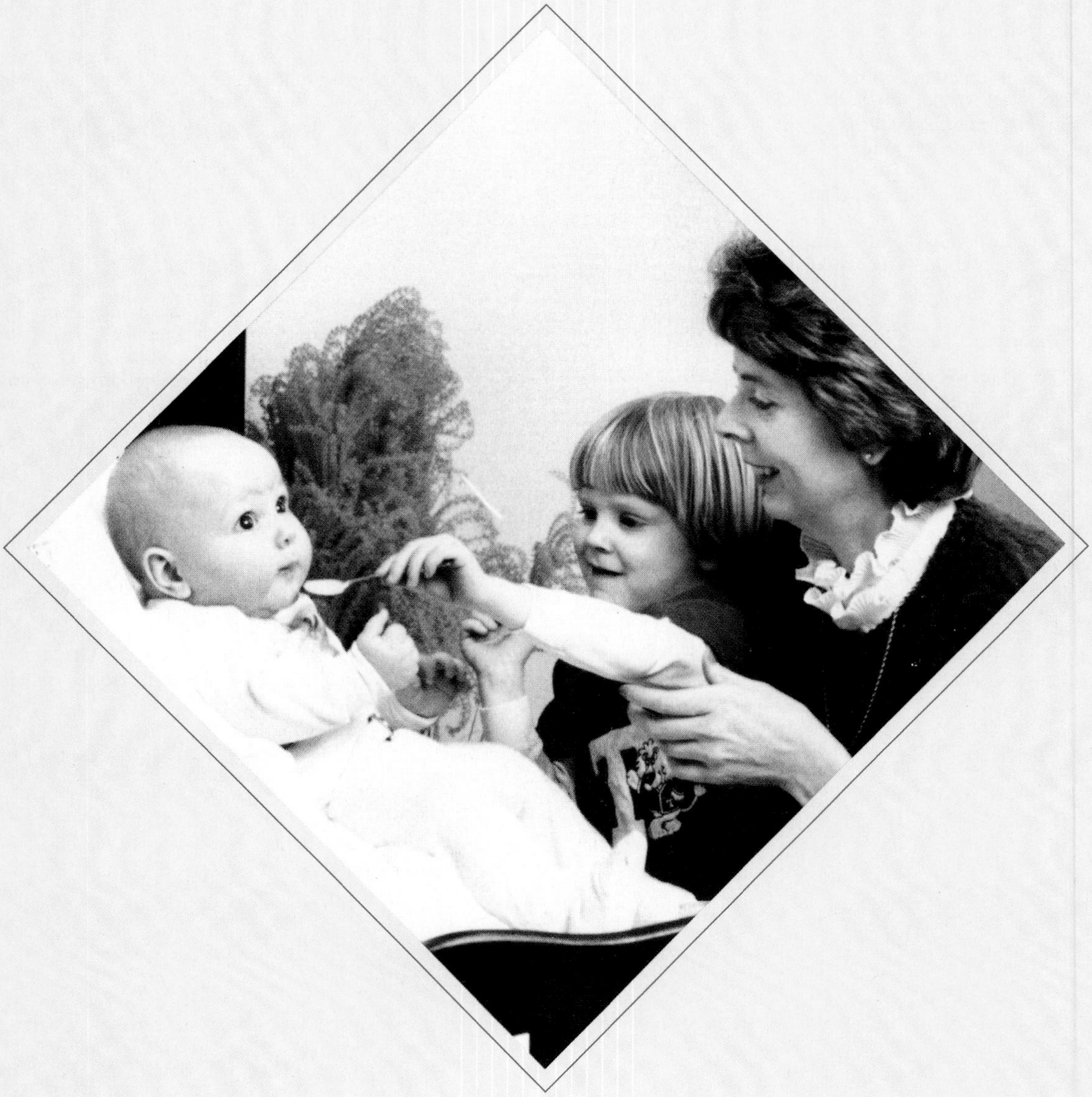

Infancy

The first 12 months of childhood is the period of most rapid gain in physical size and most dramatic achievement in developmental milestones of an individual's entire life. It is marked by an orderly progression of physical, intellectual, and social maturation. It is also a highly vulnerable period for both positive and negative influences governing optimum growth and development.

Chapter 10, *Health Promotion of the Infant and Family,* investigates the infant's biologic, psychosocial, cognitive, and adaptive development. It is concerned with fostering optimum health through anticipatory guidance regarding nutrition, prevention of disease and injury, and promotion of parent-child attachment. Chapter 11, *Health Problems during the First Year,* deals with health problems that commonly occur during the first year, usually as a result of environmental, rather than pathologic, processes, and that therefore are amenable to prevention. It is also concerned with conditions of unknown cause, such as sudden infant death syndrome, which has profound emotional consequences on the developing family.

CHAPTER 10

Health Promotion of the Infant and Family

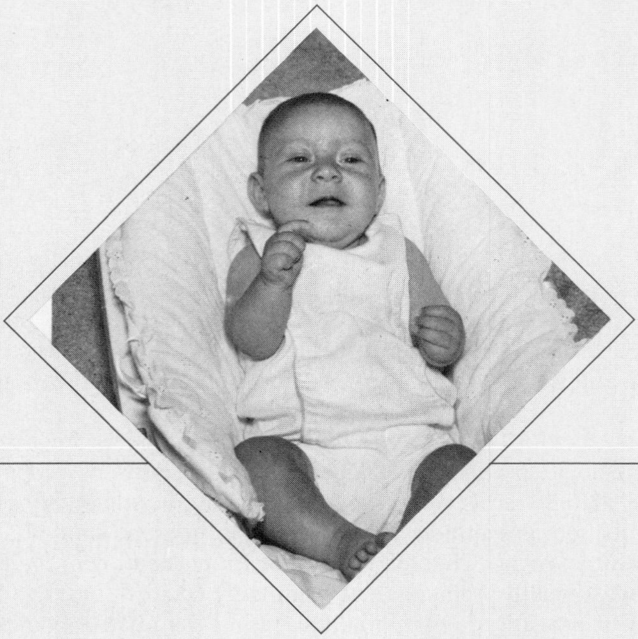

LEARNING OBJECTIVES

On completion of this chapter the reader will be able to:

- Identify the major biologic, psychosocial, cognitive, and social developments during the first year
- Relate parent-child attachment, separation anxiety, and stranger fear to developmental achievements during infancy
- Provide anticipatory guidance to parents regarding common parental concerns during infancy
- Provide parents with feeding recommendations for infants
- Outline immunization requirements during infancy
- List general contraindications, precautions, and administration routes for immunizations
- Provide anticipatory guidance to parents regarding injury prevention based on the infant's developmental achievements

The miracle of birth is surpassed only by the wonder of growth and development unfolding in the succeeding months and years. The biologic growth and developmental maturation of the infant are a study of perfection in nature. The nurse's understanding of these processes is essential to the optimum care of the child and family. To present relevant data for appreciation of growth and development, it is necessary to systematize and categorize the facts into various levels of maturation and age-groups. However, no child is represented in any one table or chart, for each child is as much an individual as the number of variables that influence his existence.

◆ *Promoting Optimum Growth and Development*

General concepts of growth and development, such as stages and patterns of development and individual differences, are discussed extensively in Chapter 5. This chapter is primarily concerned with biologic, psychosocial, cognitive, and social development of the child from 1 to 12 months of age. It also includes a discussion of common parental concerns that are typical of the developmental characteristics of this age-group.

BIOLOGIC DEVELOPMENT

At no other time in life are physical changes and developmental achievements so dramatic as during infancy. All major body systems undergo progressive maturation, and there is concurrent development of skills that increasingly allows infants to respond to and cope with the environment. Acquisition of these fine and gross motor skills occurs in an orderly sequence, following usual cephalocaudal-proximodistal laws.

Proportional Changes

During the first year growth is very rapid, especially during the initial 6 months. Infants gain 680 g (1.5 pounds) a month until age 6 months, when the birth weight has at least doubled. An average weight for a 6-month-old child is 7.26 kg (16 pounds). Weight gain decreases by half that amount during the second 6 months. By 1 year of age the infant's birth weight has tripled for an average weight of 9.75 kg (21.5 pounds).

Height increases by 2.5 cm (1 inch) a month during the first 6 months and by half that amount during each of the second 6 months. Average height is 65 cm (25½ inches) at 6 months and 74 cm (29 inches) at 12 months. By 1 year the birth length has increased by almost 50%. The increase in length occurs mainly in the trunk, rather than in the legs, and contributes to the characteristic physique of the infant (see Fig. 10-6, *E*).

Head growth is also rapid. During the first 6 months head circumference increases approximately 1.5 cm (0.6 inch) a month but decreases to only 0.5 cm (0.2 inch) monthly during the second 6 months. The average size is 43 cm (17 inches) at 6 months and 46 cm (18 inches) at 12 months. By 1 year head size has increased by almost 33%. Closure of the cranial sutures occurs, with the posterior fontanel fusing by 6 to 8 weeks of age, and the anterior fontanel closing by 12 to 18 months of age.

Expanding head size reflects the growth and differentiation of the nervous system. By the end of the first year the brain has increased in weight about two and one half times. The maturation of the brain is exhibited in the dramatic developmental achievements of infancy (see Table 10-3). The primitive reflexes are replaced by voluntary, purposeful movement. New reflexes appear that influence motor development (see Table 10-1).

The chest assumes a more adult contour, with the lateral diameter becoming larger than the anteroposterior diameter. The chest circumference approximately equals head circumference by the end of the first year. The heart grows less rapidly than does the rest of the body. Its weight is usually doubled by 1 year of age, in comparison with body weight, which triples during the same period. The size of the heart is still large in relation to the chest cavity; its width is about 55% of the width of the chest.

Maturation of Systems

Most organ systems change and grow during infancy. The respiratory rate slows somewhat (see inside front cover) and is relatively stable. Respiratory movements continue to be abdominal. Several factors predispose the infant to more severe and acute respiratory problems. The close proximity of the trachea to the bronchi and its branching structures rapidly transmits an infectious agent from one anatomic location to another. The short, straight eustachian tube closely communicates with the ear, allowing infection to ascend from the pharynx to the middle ear. In addition, the immunologic ability of the mucosal lining provides less protection against infection in infancy than during later childhood.

The heart rate slows (see inside front cover), and frequently displays *sinus arrhythmia* (rate increases with inspiration and decreases with expiration). The regularity of the rhythm correlates with the respiratory rate: the faster the respiratory rate, the more regular the heartbeat, and the slower the respiratory rate, the more irregular the heartbeat. Consequently, sinus arrhythmia is most obvious during sleep.

Blood pressure also changes during infancy (see inside front cover). The systolic pressure rises during the first 2 months as a result of the increasing ability of the left ventricle to pump blood into the systemic circulation. Fluctuations in blood pressure occur during varying states of activity and emotion.

Significant hemopoietic changes occur during the first year (Appendix E). Fetal hemoglobin is present for the first 5 months, with adult hemoglobin forming at about 13 weeks of age. Maternal iron stores are present for the first 5 to 6 months and then gradually diminish, which partially accounts for lowered hemoglobin levels toward the end of the first 6 months. *Physiologic anemia* is seen at 2 to 3 months of age because of the decreasing number of red blood cells. This phenomenon is thought to be caused by the suppression of the hemopoietic system from the high level of fetal hemoglobin, which suppresses the production of erythropoietin, a hormone released by the kidney. The occurrence of physiologic anemia is not affected by an adequate supply of iron. However, when erythropoiesis is stimulated, iron supplies are necessary for formation of hemoglobin.

The digestive processes are immature at birth. Saliva is secreted in small amounts, but the majority of all diges-

TABLE 10-1

Neurologic Reflexes That Appear during Infancy

Reflex	Expected Behavioral Response	Age of Appearance (months)
Labyrinth-righting	When infant is in prone or supine position, he is able to raise head	2, strongest at 10
Neck-righting	While infant is supine, head is turned to one side; shoulder, trunk, and finally pelvis will turn toward that side	3, until 24-36
Body-righting	A modification of the neck-righting reflex in which turning hips and shoulders to one side causes all other body parts to follow	6, until 24-36
Otolith-righting	When body of an erect infant is tilted, head is returned to upright, erect position	7-12, persists indefinitely
Landau	When infant is suspended in a horizontal prone position, the head is raised, legs and spine are extended	6-8, until 12-24
Parachute	When infant is suspended in a horizontal prone position and suddenly thrust downward, hands and fingers extend forward as if to protect himself from falling (Fig. 10-1)	7-9, persists indefinitely

tive processes do not begin functioning until age 3 months, when drooling is common because of the poorly coordinated swallowing reflex. The enzyme *ptyalin* (also called amylase) is present in small amounts but usually has little effect on the foodstuff because of the small amount of time the food stays in the mouth. Gastric digestion consists primarily of the action of hydrochloric acid and rennin, an enzyme that acts specifically on the casein in milk to form curds, which are coagulated semisolid particles of milk. The curds cause the milk to be retained in the stomach long enough for digestion to occur.

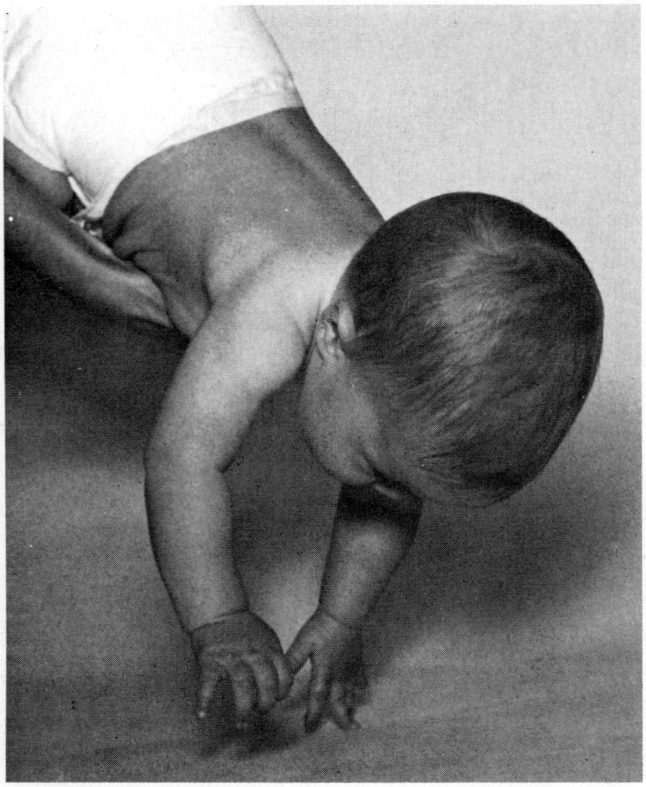

FIG. 10-1 Parachute reflex.

Digestion also takes place in the duodenum, where pancreatic enzymes and bile begin to break down protein and fat. Secretion of the pancreatic enzyme *amylase*, which is needed for digestion of complex carbohydrates, is deficient until about the fourth to sixth month of life. *Lipase* is also limited, and infants do not achieve adult levels of fat absorption until 4 to 5 months of age. *Trypsin* is secreted in sufficient quantities to catabolize protein into polypeptides and some amino acids.

The immaturity of the digestive processes is evident in the appearance of stools. During infancy solid foods, such as peas, carrots, corn, and raisins, are passed incompletely broken down in the feces. Not until the second year are fibrous foods more completely digested. An excess quantity of fiber disposes the child to loose, bulky stools.

The rapid peristaltic activity of the gastrointestinal tract slows down throughout infancy, and the stomach enlarges to accommodate a greater volume of food. By the end of the first year the infant is able to tolerate three meals a day and a before-bedtime bottle, and he may have one or two bowel movements daily. However, any type of gastric irritation causes the transit time to increase above its already rapid rate, making the infant vulnerable to diarrhea, vomiting, and dehydration (see Chapter 23).

Paralleling the ability of the gastrointestinal system to digest and absorb more complex foodstuff is the process of tooth eruption. Tooth eruption occurs in a fairly orderly sequence beginning at about 6 to 7 months of age (see discussion of teething on p. 288).

The immunologic system undergoes numerous changes during the first year. The newborn receives significant amounts of maternal IgG, which confers immunity for about 3 months against antigens to which the mother was exposed. During this time the infant begins to synthesize IgG, and about 40% of adult levels are reached by 1 year of age. Significant amounts of IgM are produced at birth, and adult levels are reached by 9 months of age. The production of IgA, IgD, and IgE is much more gradual, and maximum levels are not attained until early childhood.

During infancy the ability of the skin to contract and shiver in response to cold increases. The peripheral capillaries respond to change in ambient temperature to regulate heat loss. In response to cold, the capillaries constrict, conserving core body temperature and decreasing potential evaporative heat loss from the skin surface. In response to heat the capillaries dilate, decreasing internal body temperature through evaporation, conduction, and convection. Shivering causes the muscles and muscle fibers to contract, generating metabolic heat, which is distributed throughout the body. Accumulation of adipose tissue during the first 6 months serves to insulate the body against heat loss.

At birth there is a shift in the total body fluid of the neonate, resulting in a higher level of intracellular fluid than of extracellular fluid, probably because of the progressive growth of cells at the expense of extracellular fluid. However, the proportion of extracellular fluid, which is composed of blood plasma, interstitial fluid, and lymph, still remains high in comparison to adult levels and predisposes the infant to a more rapid loss of total body fluid and consequently dehydration.

The immaturity of the renal structures also predisposes the infant to dehydration. Complete maturity of the kidney occurs during the latter half of the second year. Prior to this time the filtration capacity of the glomeruli is reduced.

Visual acuity gradually improves and binocular fixation is established. *Binocularity,* or the fixation of two ocular images into one cerebral picture (fusion), begins to develop by 6 weeks of age and should be well established by age 12 months. *Depth perception* (stereopsis) begins to develop by age 7 to 9 months but may exist earlier as an innate safety mechanism against accidental falling.

Fine Motor Behavior

Fine motor behavior includes the use of the hands and fingers in the prehension (grasp) of an object. Grasping occurs during the first 2 to 3 months as a reflex and gradually becomes voluntary. At 1 month the hands are predominantly closed and by 3 months are mostly open. By this time the infant demonstrates a desire to grasp an object, but he "grasps" it more with the eyes than with the hands. If a rattle is placed in his hand, he will actively hold onto it. By 4 months he regards both a small pellet and his hands, then will look from the object to his hands and back again. Hand regard is common at this age because of the limitation of symmetric positioning that prevents the infant from exploring the periphery. Hand regard occurs in children who are blind because it is a developmental process that occurs without visual stimulation. By 5 months the infant is able to voluntarily grasp an object.

Gradually the palmar grasp (using the whole hand) is replaced with a pincer grasp (using the thumb and index finger). By 8 to 9 months the infant uses a crude pincer grasp but by 11 months has progressed to a neat pincer grasp (Fig. 10-2).

By 6 months the infant has increased manipulative skill. He holds his bottle, grasps his feet and pulls them to his mouth, and feeds himself a cracker. By 7 months he transfers objects from one hand to the other, uses one

A

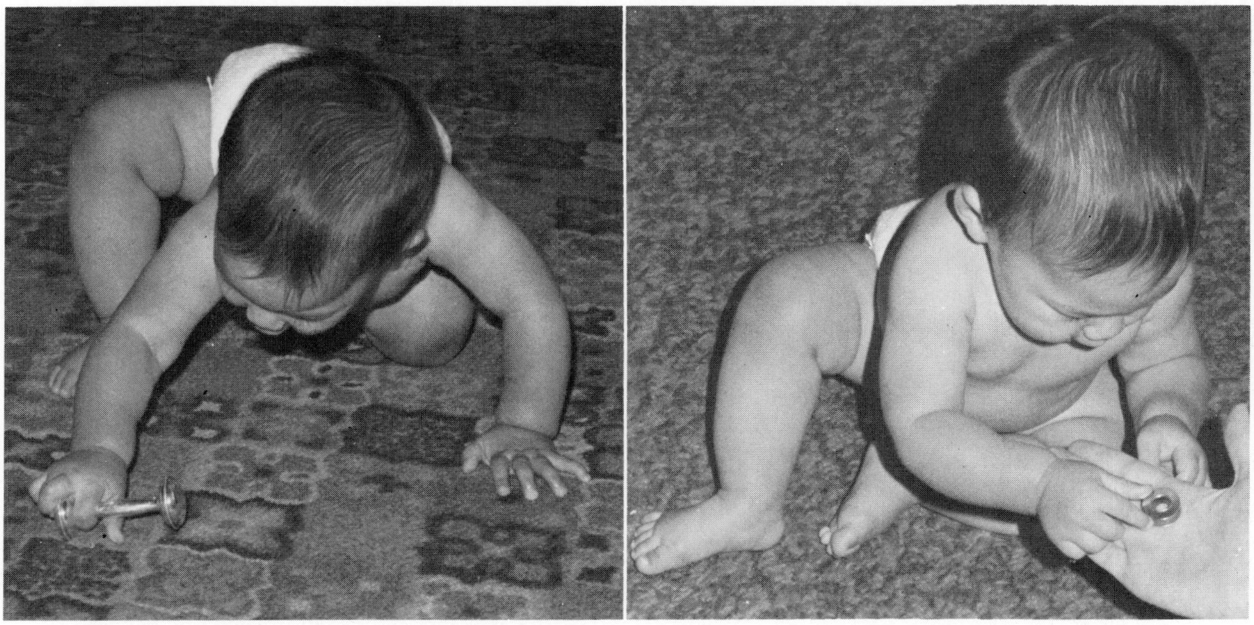

B

FIG. 10-2 A, Crude pincer grasp at 8 to 10 months. **B,** Neat pincer grasp at 10 to 11 months.

hand for grasping, and holds a cube in each hand simultaneously. He enjoys banging objects and will explore the movable parts of a toy.

By 10 months pincer grasp is sufficiently established to enable the infant to pick up a raisin and other finger foods. He can deliberately let go of an object and will offer it to someone. By 11 months he puts objects into a container and likes to remove them. By 1 year the infant tries to build a tower of two blocks but fails.

Gross Motor Development

Gross motor behavior includes developmental maturation in posture, head balance, sitting, creeping, standing, and walking.

Head control. The full-term newborn can momentarily hold the head in midline and parallel when the body is suspended ventrally and can lift and turn the head from side to side when prone (see Fig. 8-7). However, marked head lag is evident when the infant is pulled from a lying

A

B

C

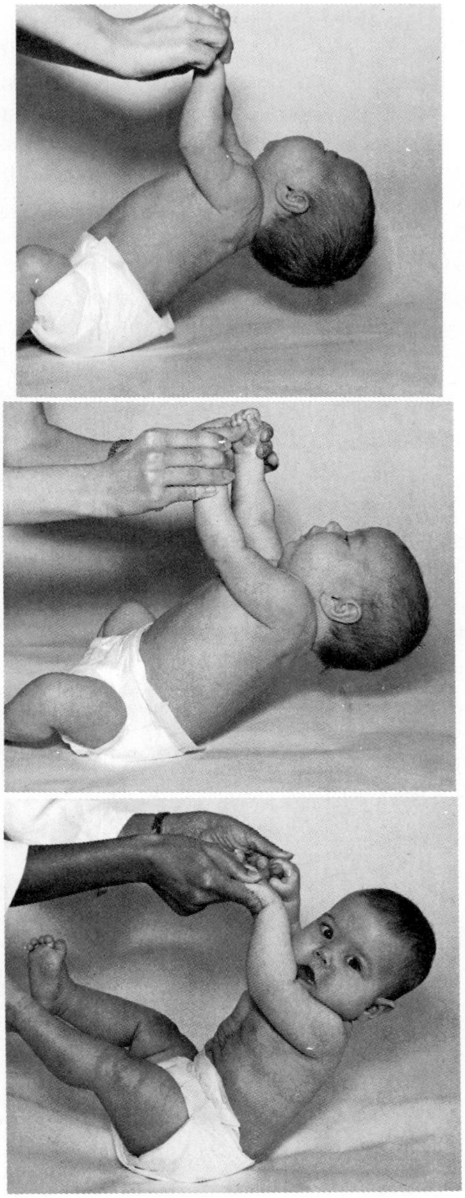

FIG. 10-3 Head control while pulled to sitting. **A,** Complete head lag at 1 month. **B,** Partial head lag at 2 months. **C,** Almost no head lag at 4 months.

A

B

C

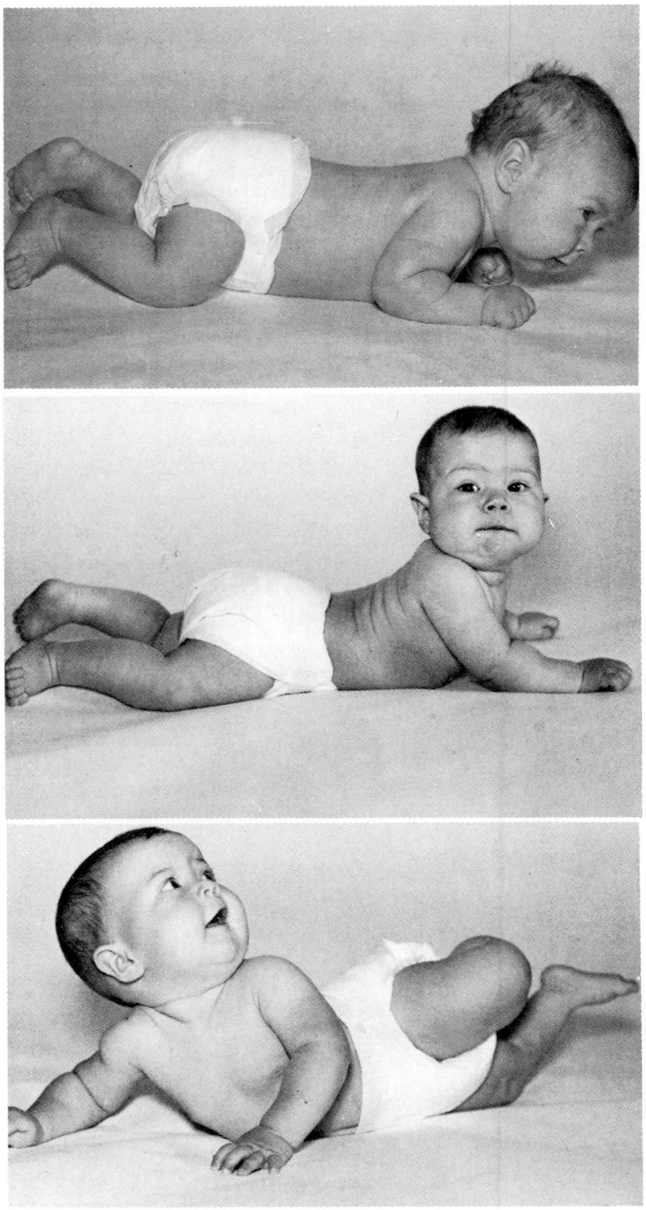

FIG. 10-4 Head control while prone. **A,** Momentarily lifts head at 1 month. **B,** Lifts head and chest 90 degrees and bears weight on forearms at 4 months. **C,** Lifts head, chest, and upper abdomen and can bear weight on hands at 6 months. Note how this position facilitates turning from abdomen to back.

to a sitting position. By 3 months of age the infant can hold his head well beyond the plane of his body, and by 4 months of age he can lift the head and front portion of the chest about 90 degrees above the table, bearing his weight on the forearms. Only slight head lag is evident when the infant is pulled from a lying to a sitting position, and by 4 to 6 months head control is well established (Figs. 10-3 and 10-4).

Rolling over. The newborn may roll over accidentally because of his rounded back. The ability to willfully turn from the abdomen to the back occurs at 5 months and from the back to the abdomen at 6 months. It is noteworthy that the parachute reflex, which elicits a protective response to falling, appears at 7 months.

Sitting. The ability to sit follows progressive head control and straightening of the back as shown in Fig. 10-5. For the first 2 to 3 months the back is uniformly rounded. The convex cervical curve forms at about 3 to 4 months

A B C D E

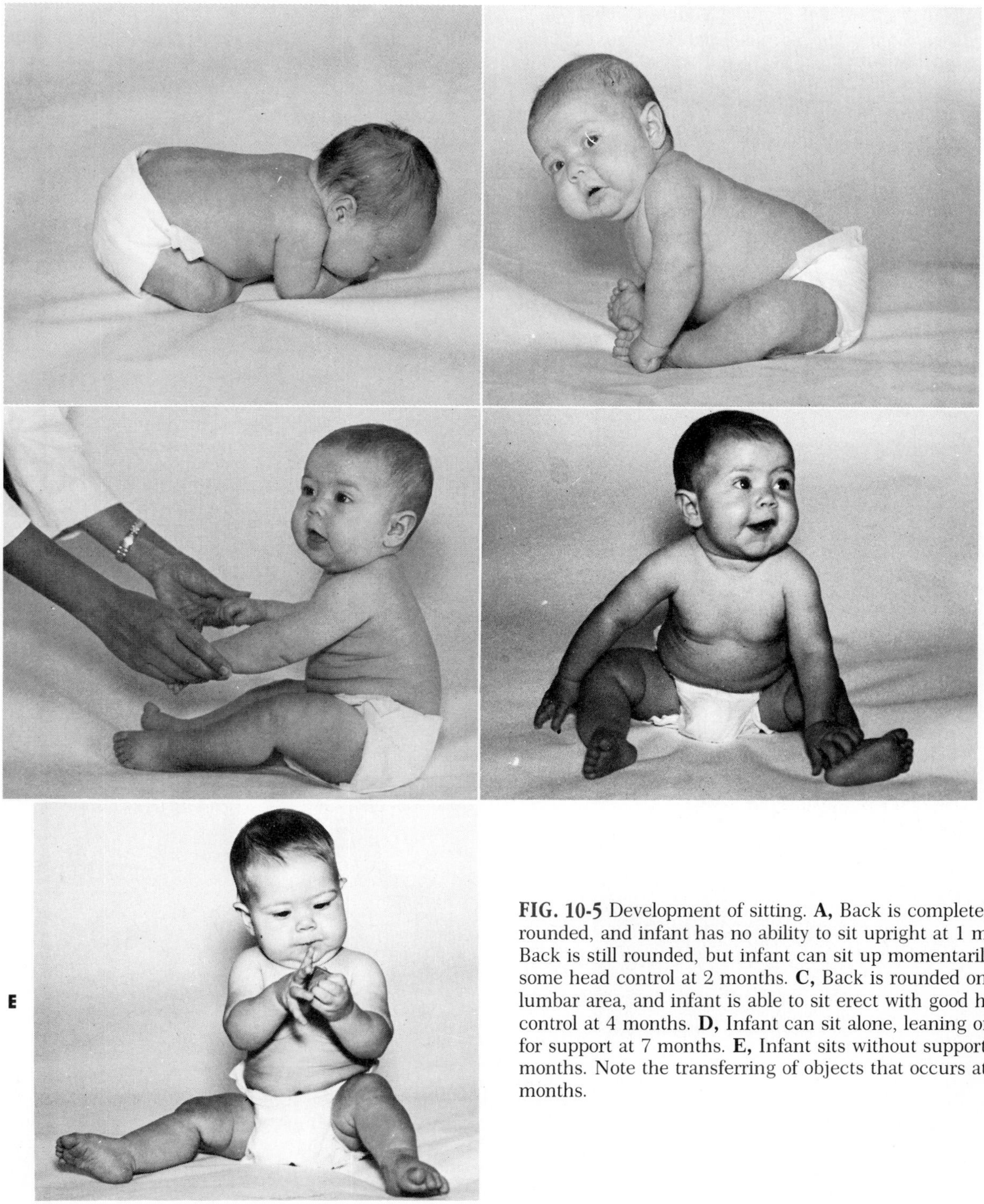

FIG. 10-5 Development of sitting. **A,** Back is completely rounded, and infant has no ability to sit upright at 1 month. **B,** Back is still rounded, but infant can sit up momentarily with some head control at 2 months. **C,** Back is rounded only in lumbar area, and infant is able to sit erect with good head control at 4 months. **D,** Infant can sit alone, leaning on hands for support at 7 months. **E,** Infant sits without support at 8 months. Note the transferring of objects that occurs at 7 months.

when head control is established. The convex lumbar curve appears when the child begins to sit, about age 4 months. As the spinal column straightens, the infant can be propped in a sitting position. By ages 6 to 7 months he can sit alone, leaning forward on his hands for support. By ages 7 to 8 months he can sit well unsupported and begins to explore his surroundings in this position rather than in a lying position.

Locomotion. Locomotion involves acquiring the ability to bear weight, propel forward on all four extremities, stand upright with support, and finally walk alone (Fig. 10-6). By 6 to 7 months the infant is able to bear all his weight. By 9 months he stands holding onto furniture and can pull himself to the standing position but is unable to maneuver himself back down, except by falling. He also can crawl on all fours with his belly on the floor. At first crawling is often in reverse direction because the flexor muscles are stronger than the extensors. At 10 months he steps with one foot and crawls well. By 11 months he creeps (belly off the floor) and walks while holding onto furniture or with both hands held. By 1 year he may be able to walk with one hand held.

PSYCHOSOCIAL DEVELOPMENT

Infants are born with the basic abilities needed for extrauterine survival, such as respiration, thermoregulation, and digestion. However, they cannot survive without a caregiver to provide for their essential needs, such as food, warmth, and security. In addition to their basic needs, which must be supplied for them, infants have certain tasks that they must achieve for themselves during the first year of life. How their needs are met by others greatly determines to what degree they accomplish their tasks.

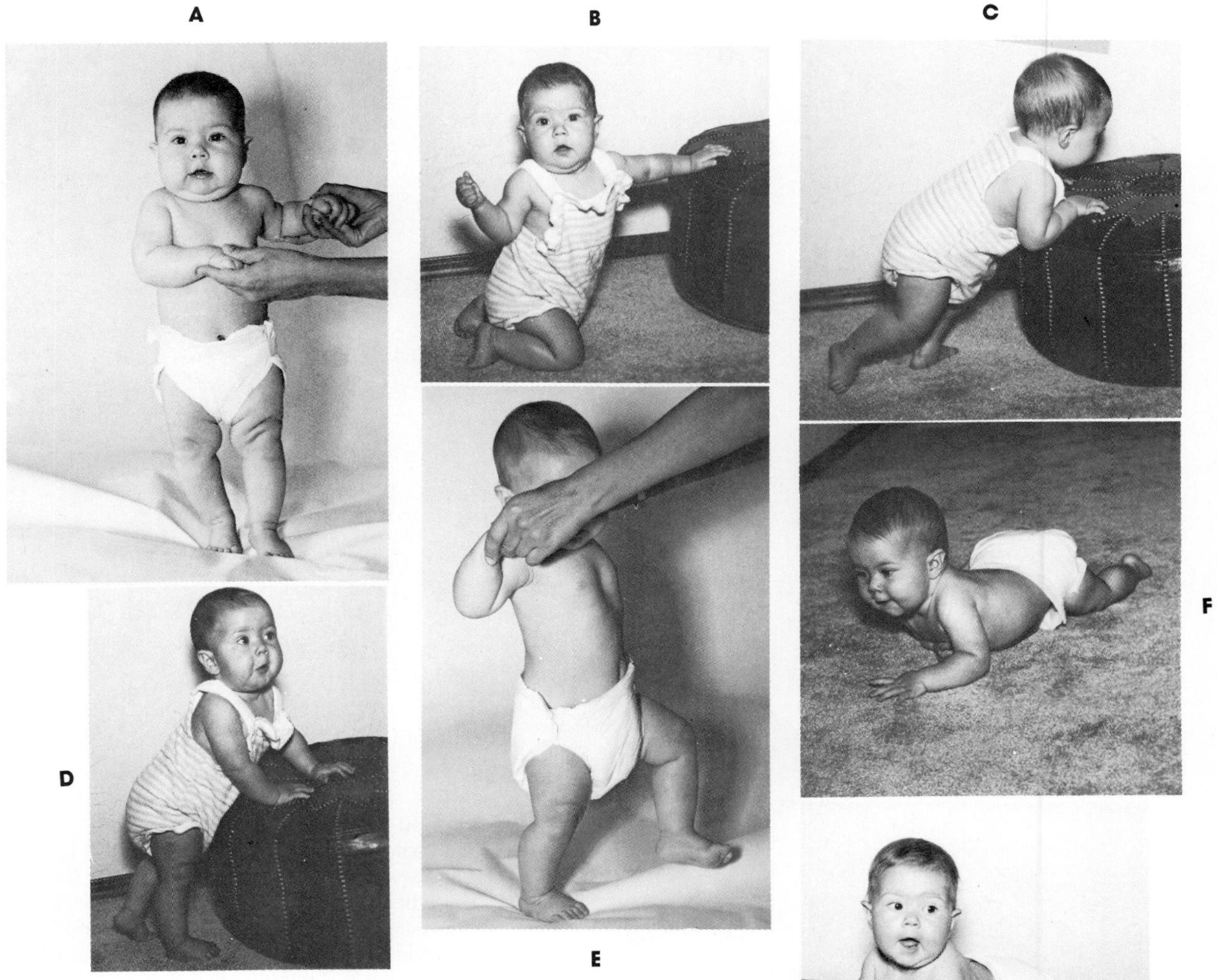
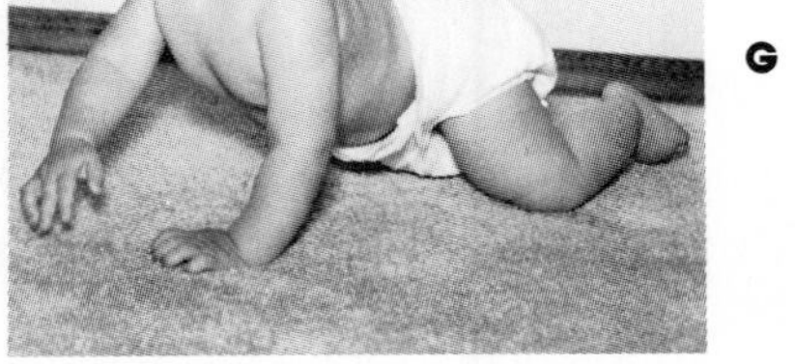

FIG. 10-6 Development of locomotion. **A,** Infant bears full weight on feet by 7 months. **B,** Infant can maneuver from sitting to kneeling position. **C,** Infant can pull self to standing position, and **D,** infant can stand holding onto furniture at 9 months. **E,** While standing, infant takes deliberate step at 10 months. **F,** Infant crawls with abdomen on floor and pulls self forward with hands at 10 months. **G,** Infant creeps on hands and knees at 11 months.

Developing a Sense of Trust (Erikson)

Erikson's phase I (birth to 1 year) is concerned with acquiring a sense of basic *trust* while overcoming a sense of mistrust. The trust acquired in infancy provides a foundation for all the succeeding phases. It allows the infant a feeling of physical comfort and security, which assists him in experiencing unfamiliar, unknown situations with a minimum of fear. The crucial element for the achievement of this task is the *quality* of the mother (caregiver)-child relationship. The provision of food, warmth, and shelter are alone inadequate for the development of a strong ego. The infant and mother must jointly learn to satisfactorily meet their needs in order for mutual regulation of frustration to occur. When this synchrony fails to develop, mistrust is the eventual outcome.

The acquisition of trust involves the libidinal or psychologic energy of the erotic centers of the body, especially the mouth. Erikson has described particular stages in the oral phase. The first social modality is primarily *oral*. During the first 3 to 4 months, food intake is the most important social activity in which the infant engages. The newborn can tolerate little frustration or delay of gratification. Primary *narcissism* (total concern for oneself) is at its height.

However, as bodily processes such as vision, motor movements, and vocalization are better controlled, the infant uses more advanced behaviors to interact with others. For example, rather than crying the infant may put his arms up to signify a desire to be held.

Failure to learn "delayed gratification" leads to mistrust. It can result from too much or too little frustration. If the mother always meets the child's needs before he signals his readiness, the infant will never learn to test his ability to control the environment. If the delay is prolonged, the infant will experience constant frustration and eventually mistrust others in their efforts to satisfy him.

The next social modality involves an incorporative mode of reaching out to others through *grasping*. Initially grasping is reflexive, but even as a reflex it has a powerful social meaning to the parents. The reciprocal response to the infant's grasping is the parents' holding on and touching. There is pleasurable tactile stimulation for both the child and parents.

Tactile stimulation is extremely important in the total process of acquiring trust. In fact, the degree of mothering skill, the quantity of food, or the length of sucking does not determine the quality of the experience. Rather, it is the total nature of the quality of the interpersonal relationship that influences the infant's formulation of trust.

During the second incorporative stage, the more active and aggressive modality of *biting* occurs. The infant learns that he can hold onto what is his own and can more fully control his environment. During this stage the infant may be confronted with one of his first conflicts. If he is breast-feeding, he quickly learns that biting causes withdrawal of the nipple and anxiety in the mother. Yet biting also brings internal relief from teething discomfort and a sense of power or control.

This conflict may be solved in a variety of ways. The mother may wean the infant from the breast and begin bottle-feeding. The infant may learn to bite substitute "nipples," such as a pacifier, and retain pleasurable breast-feeding. The successful resolution of this conflict strengthens the mother-child relationship because it occurs at a time when the infant is recognizing her as the most significant person in his life.

COGNITIVE DEVELOPMENT

Intellectual development is concurrent with biologic, motor, language, and personal-social achievements, many of which must occur before learning can take place. For example, visual ability must be sufficient for the infant to see objects clearly before associations about the object can be made. Learning occurs when behavior changes as a result of experience or growth. As motor function progresses, learning occurs through the infant's more active participation in the environment. The theory most frequently quoted to explain cognition, or the ability to know, is that of Piaget.

The Sensorimotor Phase (Piaget)

The period of birth to 24 months is termed the sensorimotor phase and is composed of six stages; however, inasmuch as this discussion is concerned with ages birth to 12 months, only the first four stages are discussed. The last two stages occur during the toddler period of 12 to 24 months, and are discussed in Chapter 12.

During the sensorimotor phase the infant progresses from reflex behavior to simple repetitive acts to imitative activity. Three crucial events take place during this phase.

First, the infant learns to separate himself from other objects in the environment. He realizes that others besides himself control the environment and that certain readjustments must take place for mutual satisfaction to occur. This coincides with Erikson's concept of the formation of trust and mutual regulation of frustration.

The second major accomplishment is achieving the concept of *permanency*, or the realization that objects that leave one's visual field still exist. A typical example of the development of object permanency is the infant's ability to separate from his parents at bedtime because of his realization that they will be present when he awakens. Eventually he broadens this concept to tolerate brief periods of separation with a different caregiver.

The last major intellectual development of this period is the ability to use symbols or "mental representation." The use of symbols allows the infant to think of an object or situation without actually experiencing it. The recognition of symbols is the beginning of understanding of time and space.

Use of reflexes. The first stage, from birth to 1 month, is identified by the use of reflexes. At birth the infant's individuality and temperament are expressed through the physiologic reflexes of sucking, rooting, grasping, and crying. The repetitious nature of the reflexes is the beginning of associations between an act and a sequential response. When the infant cries because he is hungry, a nipple is put in his mouth, and he sucks, feels satisfaction, and sleeps.

Primary circular reactions. This stage marks the beginning of the replacement of reflexive behavior with voluntary acts. During this period from 1 to 4 months, activities such as sucking or grasping become deliberate acts that elicit certain responses. The infant incorporates and adapts his reactions to the environment and recognizes the stimulus that produced a response. Previously the infant would cry until the nipple was brought to his mouth. Now he will associate the nipple with the sound of the mother's voice. He accommodates this new piece of information and adapts by ceasing to cry when he hears her voice, before he receives the nipple.

Secondary circular reactions. The third stage is a continuation of the previous one and lasts until 8 months of age. In this stage the circular primary reactions are repeated and prolonged for the response that results. Grasping and holding now become shaking, banging, and pulling. Shaking is performed to hear a noise, not solely for the pleasure of shaking. Quality and quantity of an act become evident. "More" or "less" shaking produces different responses. Causality, time, deliberate intention, and one's separateness from the environment begin to develop.

Three new processes of human behavior—imitation, play, and affect—occur. *Imitation* requires the differentiation of selected acts from several events. By the second half of the first year, the infant can imitate sounds and simple gestures. *Play* becomes evident as the infant takes pleasure in performing an act after he has mastered it. Many of the infant's waking hours are absorbed in sensorimotor play. *Affect* is seen as the infant begins to develop a sense of permanency. During the first 6 months the infant believes that an object exists only for as long as he can visually perceive it. In other words, out of sight—out of mind. When the object continues to be present or remembered even though it is beyond the range of perception, affect to external objects is evident. Object permanence is a critical component of parent-child attachment and is seen in the development of stranger anxiety at 6 to 8 months of age (p. 277).

Coordination of secondary schemata and its application to new situations. During the fourth sensorimotor stage, the infant uses previous behavioral achievements primarily as the foundation for adding new intellectual skills to his expanding repertoire. This stage from 9 to 12 months is largely transitional. Increasing motor skills allow for greater exploration of the environment. The child begins to discover that hiding an object does not mean that it is gone and that removing an obstacle will reveal the object

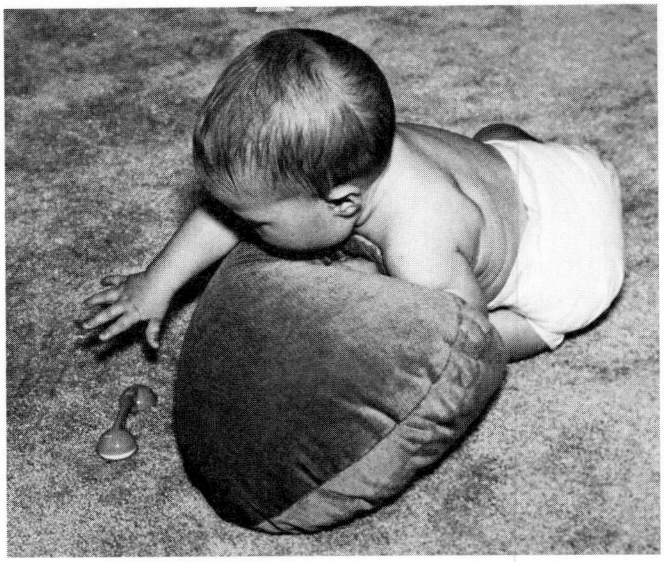

FIG. 10-7 Nine-month-old infant actively searches for object hidden behind pillow.

(Fig. 10-7). This marks the beginning of intellectual reasoning. Furthermore, he can experience an event by *observing* it, and he begins to associate symbols with events, such as "bye-bye" with "Daddy goes to work," but the classification is purely his own. Unlike the second stage, where the infant learned from the type of interaction between objects or individuals, in this stage the child learns from the object itself. Intentionality is further developed in that now the infant will actively attempt to remove a barrier to his desired (or undesired) action. If something is in his way, he will attempt to climb over it or push it away. Previously an obstacle would cause him to give up any further attempt to achieve his desired goal.

DEVELOPMENT OF BODY IMAGE

The development of body image parallels sensorimotor development. Infants' kinesthetic and tactile experiences are the first perceptions of their body and the mouth is the principal area of pleasurable sensations. Other parts of the body are primarily objects of pleasure—the hands and fingers to suck and the feet to play with. As physical needs are met, they feel comfort and satisfaction with their body. Messages conveyed by the caregivers reinforce these feelings. For example, when infants smile, they receive emotional satisfaction from others who smile back.

The development of object permanence is basic to the development of self-image. By the end of the first year infants recognize that they are distinct from their parents. At the same time there is increasing interest in their image, especially in the mirror (Fig. 10-8). As motor skills develop, they learn that parts of the body are useful; for example, the hands bring objects to the mouth and the

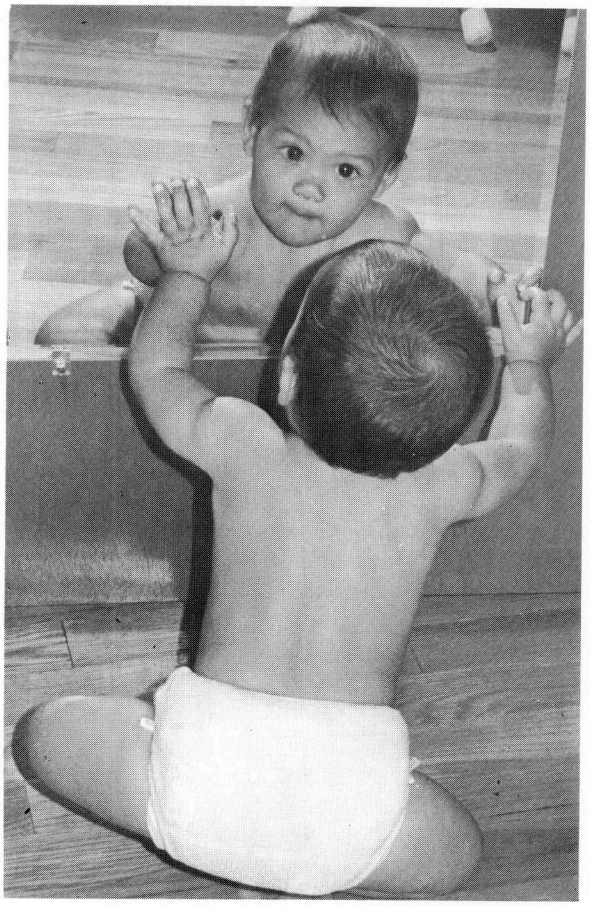

FIG. 10-8 Eight-month-old infant enjoying her image in mirror.

legs help them move to different locations. All of these achievements transmit messages to them.

SOCIAL DEVELOPMENT

Infants' social development is initially influenced by their reflexive behavior, such as the grasp, and eventually depends primarily on the interaction between them and the principal caregivers. Attachment to the parent is increasingly evident during the second half of the first year. In addition, tremendous strides are made in communication and personal-social behavior. Play is a major socializing agent and provides stimulation needed to learn from and interact with the environment.

Attachment

Several components are crucial in the process of attachment. Some of them, such as the maternal sensitive period and paternal engrossment, have been discussed in Chapter 8 and emphasize the importance of the first hour and days of life. The following is a discussion of attachment after the neonatal period. Although the word "mother" is frequently used, it does not refer exclusively to the biologic mother but to the consistent caregiver with whom the child relates more than anyone else. In light of the changing social climate, this may very well be the father. Studies on father-child attachment demonstrate that similar stages occur as with mother attachment (Lincoln, 1984).

During infancy attachment progresses with the child assuming an increasingly significant role. Two components of cognitive development are required for attachment: (1) the ability to discriminate the mother from other individuals and (2) the achievement of object permanence. Both of these processes prepare the infant for an equally important aspect of attachment—separation from the parent.

During the formation of attachment to the parent the infant progresses through four distinct but overlapping stages. For the first few weeks the infant responds indiscriminately to anyone. Beginning at about 8 to 12 weeks of age, the infant cries, smiles, and vocalizes more to the mother than to anyone else but continues to respond to others, whether familiar or not. At about age 6 months the infant shows a distinct preference for the mother. He follows her more, cries when she leaves, enjoys playing with her more, and feels most secure in her arms. About 1 month after showing attachment to the mother, many infants begin attaching to other members of the family, most often the father.

Infants acquire other developmental behaviors that influence the attachment process. These include (1) differential crying, smiling, and vocalization (more to mother than to anyone else), (2) visual-motor orientation (looking more at mother even if she is not close), (3) crying when mother leaves the room, (4) approach through locomotion (crawling, creeping, or walking), (5) clinging (especially in presence of a stranger), and (6) exploring away from mother while using her as a secure base.

Separation anxiety. Between 4 and 8 months the infant begins to have some awareness of self and mother as separate individuals. At this same time object permanence is developing and the infant is aware that the parent can be absent. Consequently, separation anxiety develops and is manifest through a predictable sequence of behaviors.

During the early second half of the first year the infant protests when placed in his crib, and a short time later objects when his mother leaves the room. Subsequently the infant may not notice the mother's absence if he is absorbed in an activity. However, when he realizes her absence, he protests. From this point onward he becomes very alert to her activities and whereabouts. By 11 to 12 months he is able to anticipate her imminent departure by watching her behaviors and begins to protest *before* she leaves. At this point many parents learn to postpone alerting the child to their departure until just before leaving.

Stranger fear. As the infant demonstrates attachment to one person, he correspondingly exhibits less friendliness to others. Between ages 6 and 8 months fear of strangers

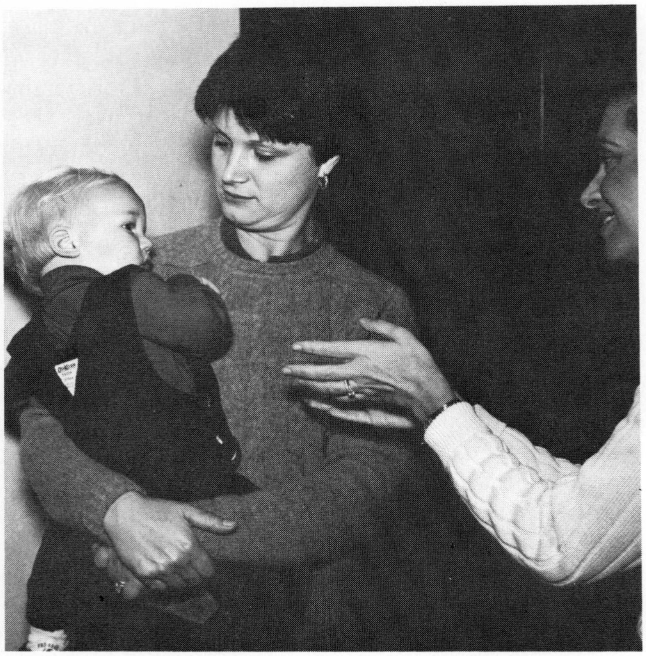

FIG. 10-9 Behaviors related to fear of strangers include clinging to the parent and turning away from the stranger.

and stranger anxiety become prominent and are related to the infant's ability to discriminate between familiar and nonfamiliar people. Such behaviors as clinging to the parent, crying, and turning away from the stranger are common (Fig. 10-9).

Language Development

The infant's first means of verbal communication is crying, and he learns to signal displeasure before pleasure. Vocalizations heard during crying eventually become some syllables and words, for example, the "mama" heard during vigorous crying. The infant vocalizes as early as 5 to 6 weeks of age by making small throaty sounds. By 2 months he makes single vowel sounds, such as *ah, eh,* and *uh.* By 3 to 4 months the consonants *n, k, g, p,* and *b* are added, and the infant coos, gurgles, and laughs aloud. By 8 months he adds the consonants *t, d,* and *w* and combines syllables, such as "dada," but he does not ascribe meaning to the word until ages 10 to 11 months. By 9 to 10 months he comprehends the meaning of the word "no" and obeys simple commands. By age 1 year he can say two to three words with meaning.

During the acquisition of new language skills the child temporarily may give up other recently learned sounds or words. This is often distressing for parents after waiting in anticipation for the words "dada" or "mama." However, these sounds are frequently given up for other vocalizations and may not be repeated for several weeks. It is reassuring for parents to know that the child will again say these words, probably with meaning.

Personal-Social Behavior

Personal-social behavior includes the child's personal responses to the environment. It is the area most influenced by external stimuli but, as in the other fields of behavior, follows certain developmental laws. Personal-social behavior implies communication with self and with others. It is the basis for the successful mastery of skills such as feeding, control of bodily functions, independence, and cooperativeness in play.

Infants have the ability to shape their environment and to elicit certain responses. The newborn shows visual preference for the human face and, as early as 1 week of age, begins to watch his mother intently as she speaks to him. By ages 6 to 8 weeks a social smile in response to pleasurable stimuli is present. This has a profound effect on family members and is a tremendous stimulus for evoking continued responses from others. By 3 months he shows considerable interest in the environment: excitement when a toy is presented, refusal to be left alone, recognition of mother, and demonstration of pleasure by squealing. By 4 months he laughs aloud and enjoys strange, novel stimuli.

By age 6 months the infant is very personable. He plays games such as peekaboo when his head is hidden in a towel, he signals his desire to be picked up by extending his arms, and he shows displeasure when a toy is removed or his face is washed. There is increasing demonstration of his ability to control his environment. The acquisition of fine and gross motor skills allows him much more independence in movement.

By the second half of the first year the infant understands simple discipline, such as the meaning of the word "no" or a scolding remark. He comprehends different facial expressions and is sensitive to emotional changes in others. Imitation and independence are developing during this time. He is learning to feed himself and use a spoon and cup. He can help with dressing by putting his foot out for a shoe or pushing his arm through the sleeve. He not only comprehends the meaning of "no" but also shakes his head to signal his understanding. He can follow simple directions and will gladly perform for others to attract and prolong their attention.

Play

Play mirrors all of the developmental tasks and allows children to experiment safely with their newly learned skills. Play during infancy represents the various social and cognitive modalities proposed by Erikson and Piaget. The infant's activity is primarily narcissistic, revolving around his own body. At 2 months of age the infant will look at his extended hand as if it were an unfamiliar object. At about age 6 months the infant plays with his feet and finds fingers excellent nipple substitutes (Fig. 10-10). During this time the ability to grasp is well under voluntary control, and everything is reached for and brought to the mouth for inquisitive exploration. When the pincer

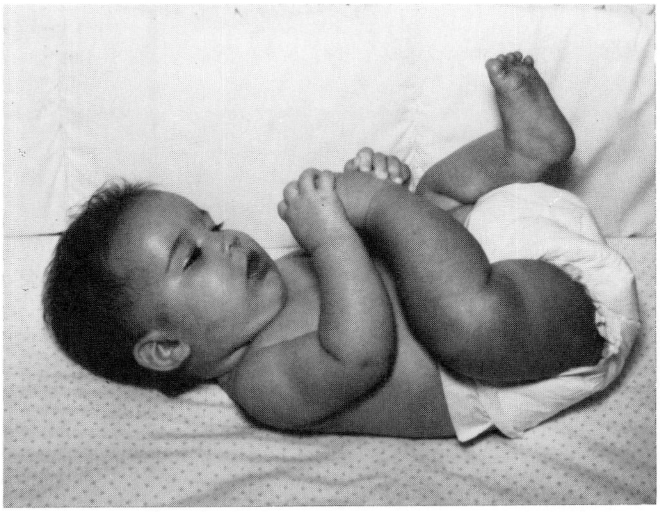

FIG. 10-10 During early infancy body parts are primarily objects of pleasure for the child.

grasp is mastered, the infant is absorbed with growing independence, refusing to allow others to feed him.

Play reflects the infant's social development and his increasing awareness of the environment. From birth to age 3 months the infant's response to the environment is global and largely undifferentiated. Play is dependent; pleasure is demonstrated by a quieting attitude (age 1 month), later by a smile (age 2 months), and then by a squeal (age 3 months). From ages 3 to 6 months the infant shows more discriminate interest in the stimuli presented to him and begins to play alone with a rattle or soft stuffed toy or to play with someone else. There is much more interaction during play. By 4 months of age he laughs aloud, shows preference for certain toys, and is excited when food or a favorite object is brought to him.

By 6 months to 1 year of age, play is much more sophisticated and involves sensorimotor skills. Actual games are played, such as peekaboo, pat-a-cake, verbal repetition, and imitation of simple gestures in response to demonstration. Play is much more selective, not only in terms of specific toys but also in terms of "playmates." Although play is solitary or one-sided, the infant chooses with whom he will interact. At 6 to 8 months of age he usually refuses to play with strangers until he begins to know them. Parents are definite favorites, and he knows how to attract their attention. At 6 months he extends his arms to be picked up, at 7 months he coughs to make his presence known, at age 10 months he pulls the parents' clothing, and at 1 year he calls them by name. This represents a tremendous advance from the newborn who signaled biologic needs by crying to express displeasure.

Stimulation is as important for developmental growth as food is for biologic growth. Knowledge of developmental milestones allows nurses to guide parents regarding proper play for infants. It is not sufficient to place a mobile over a crib and toys in a playpen for a child's optimum social, emotional, and intellectual development. Play must provide interpersonal contact, as well as recreational and educational stimulation. Infants need to be *played with,* not merely allowed *to play*. Although the type of play infants engage in is called *solitary,* this is only a figurative, not literal, term to denote one-sided play. The kind of toys given to the child is much less important than the quality of personal interaction that occurs.

Table 10-2 lists play activities that are appropriate for the developmental level of the infant in view of motor, language, and personal-social achievements. Although the activities are grouped according to the major mode of stimulation provided, there is overlap in many instances. In addition play activities suggested for one age-group may be appropriate for an older age-group but are generally inappropriate for a younger age-group.

TEMPERAMENT

The infant's temperament or behavioral style influences the kind of interaction that occurs between the child and parents and other family members (see general discussion of temperament on p. 82.) In assessing a child's temperament, it is the parents' perception of the child and the degree of *fit* between their expectations and the child's actual temperament that is important. The more dissonance or lack of harmony between the child's temperament and the parent's ability to accept and deal with the behavior, the more risk for subsequent parent-child conflicts.

The Infant Temperament Questionnaire (ITQ) (Carey and McDevitt, 1978) can be used as a screening tool with parents. The questionnaire focuses on nine temperament variables, but the questions relate specifically to activities such as sleep, feeding, play, diapering, and dressing. The scores from the ITQ help identify the child's temperamental style.

With knowledge of the infant's temperament, nurses are better able to guide parents regarding appropriate childrearing techniques. For example, "difficult" children may respond better to scheduled feedings and structured caregiving routines than demand feedings and frequent changes in daily routines. These children sleep less and may need more structured approaches to bedtime to prevent bedtime problems. "Highly distractible" children may require additional soothing measures such as swinging, rocking, or being carried in a pack that the parent wears across the chest or back. Children with "high activity" levels require vigilant watching, and parents need to take extra precautions in safeguarding the home. These children benefit from increased opportunities for gross motor activity to constructively channel their energy.

In addition, appropriate counseling based on awareness of the child's temperament can greatly enhance the quality of interaction between parents and infant. Even just letting parents know that "difficult" traits are innate can greatly relieve feelings of guilt and incompetence.

TABLE 10-2

Play during Infancy

Age (months)	Visual Stimulation	Auditory Stimulation	Tactile Stimulation	Kinetic Stimulation
Suggested Activities				
Birth-1	Look at infant at close range Hang bright, shiny object within 20-25 cm (8-10 in) of infant's face and in midline	Talk to infant, sing in soft voice Play music box, radio, television Have ticking clock or metronome nearby	Hold, caress, cuddle Keep infant warm May like to be swaddled	Rock infant, place in cradle Use carriage for walks
2-3	Provide bright objects Make room bright with pictures or mirrors on walls Take infant to various rooms while doing chores Place him in infant seat for vertical view of environment	Talk to infant Include in family gatherings Expose to various environmental noises other than those of home Use rattles, wind chimes	Caress infant while bathing, at diaper change Comb hair with a soft brush	Use swing Take in car for rides Exercise body by moving extremities in swimming motion
4-6	Place infant so that he can look in mirror Place in front of television with family Give brightly colored toys to hold (small enough to grasp)	Talk to infant, repeat sounds he makes Laugh when he laughs Call him by name Crinkle different papers by his ear Place rattle or bell in hand, show him how to shake them	Give infant soft squeeze toys of various textures Allow to splash in bath Place nude on soft furry rug and move extremities	Use swing or stroller Bounce infant in lap while holding him in standing position Help him roll over Support him in sitting position, let him lean forward to balance himself Put him in an open box and tilt gently
Suggested Toys	Nursery mobiles Unbreakable mirrors See-through crib bumpers Contrasting colored sheets *Tracking tube *Visual panels	Music boxes Musical mobiles Crib dangle bells Small-handled clear rattle *Spin-a-round	Stuffed animals Soft clothes Soft or furry quilt Soft mobiles	Rocking crib/cradle Weighted or suction toy
Suggested Activities				
6-9	Give infant large toys with bright colors, movable parts, and noisemakers Place unbreakable mirror where infant can see self Play peekaboo, especially hiding his face in a towel Make funny faces to encourage imitation Give infant paper to tear, crumple Give ball of yarn or string to pull apart	Call infant by name Repeat simple words such as "dada," "mama," "bye-bye" Speak clearly Name parts of body, people, and foods Tell infant what you are doing Use "no" only when necessary Give simple commands Show how to clap hands, bang a drum	Let infant play with fabrics of various textures Have bowl with foods of different size and textures to feel Let infant "catch" running water Encourage "swimming" in large bathtub or shallow pool Give wad of sticky tape to manipulate	Place infant on floor to crawl, roll over, sit Hold upright to bear weight and bounce Pick up, say "up" Put down, say "down" Place toys out of reach; encourage infant to get them Play pat-a-cake

*These toys, from a specially designed series called Playpath Playthings produced as part of the Johnson & Johnson Baby Products Child Development Program, are available for purchase; information can be obtained by writing to Johnson & Johnson, Grandview Rd., Skillman, NJ 08558.

TABLE 10-2

Play during Infancy—cont'd

Age (months)	Visual Stimulation	Auditory Stimulation	Tactile Stimulation	Kinetic Stimulation
9-12	Show infant large pictures in books Take infant to places where there are animals, many people, different objects (shopping center) Play ball by rolling it to child, demonstrate "throwing" it back Demonstrate building a two-block tower	Read infant simple nursery rhymes Point to body parts and name each one Imitate sounds of animals	Give infant finger foods of different textures Let infant mess and squash food Let him feel cold (ice cube) or warm objects; say what temperature each is Let him feel a breeze (fan blowing)	Give large push-pull toys to encourage walking Place furniture in a circle to encourage cruising Encourage "rough-house" play Turn in different positions
Suggested Toys	Various colored blocks Nested boxes or cups Books with rhymes and bright pictures Strings of big beads Simple take-apart toys Large ball Cup and spoon *Fitting forms Large puzzles	Rattles of different sizes, shapes, tones, and bright colors Squeaky animals and dolls Records with light, rhythmic music *Balls in a bowl	Soft, different textured animals and dolls Sponge toys, floating toys Squeeze toys Teething toys Books with textures and objects, such as fur and zipper	Push-pull toys Baby swing

*These toys, from a specially designed series called Playpath Playthings produced as part of the Johnson & Johnson Baby Products Child Development Program, are available for purchase; information can be obtained by writing to Johnson & Johnson, Grandview Rd., Skillman, NJ 08558.

SUMMARY OF GROWTH AND DEVELOPMENT DURING INFANCY

Knowledge of the developmental sequence allows the nurse to assess normal growth and minor or abnormal deviations, helps parents gain realistic expectations of their child's ability, and provides guidelines for suitable play and stimulation. Because of the complexity of the developmental process during the first 12 months, Table 10-3 is presented to help organize and clarify the data already discussed. Although all milestones are important, some represent essential integrative aspects of development that lay the foundation for the achievement of more advanced skills. These essential milestones are designated by a bullet (•) in the chart. The table represents the *average* monthly age at which various skills are attained. It must be remembered that although the sequence is the same, the rate will vary among children.

COPING WITH CONCERNS RELATED TO NORMAL GROWTH AND DEVELOPMENT

New parents, and some who are experienced, have many concerns about childrearing during the first year. Fears, daycare, discipline, thumb- or pacifier-sucking, and teething, are just a sampling of topics that parents have questions about. Nurses must be aware of these concerns and provide answers that give guidance and help decrease anxiety.

Separation and Stranger Fear

During infancy a number of fears can appear. However, the fear that causes parents most concern is fear related to strangers and separation. Although erroneously interpreted by some as a sign of undesirable, antisocial behavior, stranger fear and separation anxiety are important components of a strong, healthy parent-child attachment. However, this period can present difficulties for parent and child. Parents may be more confined to the home because the infant protests violently against the babysitter. To accustom the infant to new people, parents are encouraged to have close friends or relatives visit often. This provides for other persons with whom the child is comfortable and who can give parents time for themselves.

Infants also need opportunities to safely experience strangers. Usually toward the end of the first year infants begin to venture away from the parent and demonstrate curiosity about strangers. If allowed to explore at their own rate, many infants will eventually "warm up." If parents hold the child away from their face, the infant can observe while maintaining close physical contact. The best approach for the stranger (who may be the nurse) is

Text continued on p. 286.

TABLE 10-3

Summary of Growth and Development during Infancy

Age (months)	Physical	Gross Motor	Fine Motor
1	Weight gain of 150 to 210 g (5 to 7 oz) weekly for first 6 months Height gain of 2.5 cm (1 in) monthly for first 6 months Head circumference increases by 1.5 cm (½ in) monthly for first 6 months Primitive reflexes present and strong Doll's eye reflex and dance reflex fading Obligatory nose breathing (most infants)	•Assumes flexed position with pelvis high but knees not under abdomen when prone (at birth, knees flexed under abdomen) •Can turn head from side to side when prone, lifts head momentarily from bed (Fig. 10-4, *A*) Marked head lag, especially when pulled from lying to sitting position (Fig. 10-3, *A*) Holds head momentarily parallel and in midline when suspended in prone position Assumes asymmetric tonic neck reflex position when supine Makes crawling movements when prone When held in standing position, body limp at knees and hips In sitting position back is uniformly rounded, absence of head control (Fig. 10-5, *A*)	Hands predominantly closed Grasp reflex strong Hand clenches on contact with rattle
2	Posterior fontanel closed Crawling reflex disappears	•Assumes less flexed position when prone—hips flat, legs extended, arms flexed, head to side Less head lag when pulled to sitting position (Fig. 10-3, *B*) Can maintain head in same plane as rest of body when held in ventral suspension When prone, can lift head almost 45 degrees off table When held in sitting position, head is held up but bobs forward (Fig. 10-5, *B*) Assumes asymmetric tonic neck reflex position intermittently	Hands frequently open Grasp reflex fading
3	Primitive reflexes fading	Able to hold head more erect when sitting, but still bobs forward Only slight head lag when pulled to sitting Assumes symmetric body positioning Able to raise head and shoulders from prone position to a 45- to 90-degree angle from table; bears weight on forearms When held in standing position, able to bear slight fraction of weight on legs Regards own hand	•Actively holds rattle but will not reach for it Grasp reflex absent Hands kept loosely open Clutches own hand; pulls at blankets and clothes
4	Drooling begins Moro, tonic neck, rooting, and Perez reflexes have disappeared	•Almost no head lag when pulled to sitting position (Fig. 10-3, *C*) •Balances head well in sitting position (Fig. 10-5, *C*) Back less rounded, curved only in lumbar area Able to sit erect if propped up Able to raise head and chest off couch to angle of 90 degrees (Fig. 10-4, *B*) Assumes predominant symmetric position Rolls from back to side	•Inspects and plays with hands; pulls clothing or blanket over face in play Tries to reach objects with hand but overshoots Grasps object with both hands Plays with rattle placed in hand, shakes it, but cannot pick it up if dropped Can carry objects to mouth
5	Growth rate may begin to decline Beginning signs of tooth eruption	No head lag when pulled to sitting position When sitting, able to hold head erect and steady Able to sit for longer periods when back is well supported Back straight When prone, assumes symmetric positioning with arms extended Can turn over from abdomen to back When supine, puts feet to mouth	•Able to grasp objects voluntarily Uses palmar grasp, bidextrous approach Plays with toes Takes objects directly to mouth Holds one cube while regarding a second

•Milestone that represents essential integrative aspects of development that lay the foundation for the achievement of more advanced skills.

Sensory	Vocalization	Socialization
•Able to fixate on moving object Follows light to midline Quiets when hears a voice	Cries to express displeasure Makes small throaty sounds Makes comfort sounds during feeding	Watches parent's face intently as she or he talks to infant
Binocular fixation and convergence to near objects beginning When supine, follows dangling toy from side to point beyond midline Visually searches to locate sounds Turns head to side when sound is made at level of ear	•Vocalizes, distinct from crying Crying becomes differentiated Coos Vocalizes to familiar voice	•Social smile in response to various stimuli
•Follows object to periphery (180 degrees) •Locates sound by turning head to side and looking in same direction Begins to have ability to coordinate stimuli from various sense organs	•Squeals aloud to show pleasure Coos, babbles, chuckles Vocalizes when smiling "Talks" a great deal when spoken to Less crying during periods of wakefulness	Much interest in surroundings Ceases crying when parent enters room Can recognize familiar faces and objects, such as feeding bottle Shows awareness of strange situations
Able to accommodate to near objects Binocular vision fairly well established Can focus on a 1.25 cm (½-in) block Beginning eye-hand coordination	Makes consonant sounds n, k, g, p, b Laughs aloud Vocalization changes according to mood	Demands attention by fussing; becomes bored if left alone Enjoys social interaction with people Anticipates feeding when sees bottle Shows excitement with whole body, squeals, breathes heavily Shows interest in strange stimuli
Visually pursues a dropped object Able to sustain visual inspection of an object Can localize sounds made below the ear	•Squeals Vowel cooing sounds interspersed with consonant sounds (for example, ah-goo)	Smiles at mirror image Pats bottle with both hands More enthusiastically playful, but may have rapid mood swings Able to discriminate strangers from family Vocalizes displeasure when object taken away

Continued.

TABLE 10-3

Summary of Growth and Development during Infancy—cont'd

Age (months)	Physical	Gross Motor	Fine Motor
6	Birth weight doubled Weight gain of 90 to 150 g (3 to 5 oz) weekly for next 6 months Height gain of 1.25 cm (½ in) monthly for next 6 months Teething may begin with eruption of two lower central incisors ●Chewing and biting occur	When prone, can lift chest and upper abdomen off table, bearing weight on hands (Fig. 10-4, *C*) When about to be pulled to a sitting position, lifts head Sits in high chair with back straight Rolls from back to abdomen When held in standing position, bears almost all of weight Hand regard absent	Resecures a dropped object Drops one cube when another is given Grasps and manipulates small objects Holds bottle Grasps feet and pulls to mouth
7	Eruption of upper central incisors	●When supine, spontaneously lifts head off table ●Sits, leaning forward on both hands (Fig. 10-5, *D*) When prone, bears weight on one hand Sits erect momentarily Bears full weight on feet (Fig. 10-6, *A*) When held in standing position, bounces actively	●Transfers objects from one hand to the other (Fig. 10-5, *E*) Unidextrous approach and grasp Holds two cubes more than momentarily Bangs cube on table Rakes at a small object
8	Begins to show regular patterns in bladder and bowel elimination Parachute reflex appears (Fig. 10-1)	●Sits steadily unsupported (Fig. 10-5, *E*) Readily bears weight on legs when supported; may stand holding on to furniture Adjusts posture to reach an object	Beginning pincer grasp using the index, fourth, and fifth fingers against the lower part of the thumb Releases objects at will Rings bell purposely Retains two cubes while regarding the third cube Secures an object by pulling on a string Reaches persistently for toys out of reach
9	Eruption of upper lateral incisor may begin	Crawls; may progress backward at first Sits steadily on floor for prolonged time (10 minutes) Recovers balance when leans forward but cannot do so when leaning sideways Pulls self to standing position and stands holding onto furniture (Fig. 10-6, *B, C, D*)	●Ability to use thumb and index finger in crude pincer grasp (Fig. 10-2) Preference for use of dominant hand now evident Grasps third cube Compares two cubes by bringing them together
10	Labyrinth-righting reflex is strongest	Crawls by pulling self forward with hands (Fig. 10-6, *F*) Can change from prone to sitting position Pulls self to sitting position Stands while holding onto furniture, sits by falling down Recovers balance easily while sitting While standing, lifts one foot to take a step (Fig. 10-6, *E*)	Crude release of an object beginning Grasps bell by handle

●Milestone that represents essential integrative aspects of development that lay the foundation for the achievement of more advanced skills.

Sensory	Vocalization	Socialization/Cognition
Adjusts posture to see an object Prefers more complex visual stimuli Can localize sounds made above the ear Will turn head to the side, then look up or down	•Begins to imitate sounds •Babbling resembles one-syllable utterances—ma, mu, da, di, hi Vocalizes to toys, mirror image Laughs aloud Takes pleasure in hearing own sounds (self-reinforcement)	Recognizes parents; begins to fear strangers Holds arms out to be picked up Has definite likes and dislikes Begins to imitate (cough, protrusion of tongue) Excites on hearing footsteps Laughs when head is hidden in a towel Briefly searches for a dropped object (object permanence beginning) Frequent mood swings—from crying to laughing with little or no provocation
•Can fixate on very small objects Responds to own name Localizes sound by turning head in a curving arch Beginning awareness of depth and space Has taste preferences	•Produces vowel sounds and chained syllables—baba, dada, kaka Vocalizes four distinct vowel sounds "Talks" when others are talking	•Increasing fear of strangers; shows signs of fretfulness when mother disappears Imitates simple acts and noises Tries to attract attention by coughing or snorting Plays peekaboo Demonstrates dislike of food by keeping lips closed Exhibits oral aggressiveness in biting and mouthing Demonstrates expectation in response to repetition of stimuli
	Makes consonant sounds t, d, and w Listens selectively to familiar words Utterances signal emphasis and emotion Combines syllables, such as dada, but does not ascribe meaning to them	Increasing anxiety over loss of parent, particularly mother, and fear of strangers Responds to word "no" Dislikes dressing, diaper change
Localizes sounds by turning head diagonally and directly toward sound Depth perception increasing	Responds to simple verbal commands Comprehends "no-no"	Parent (mother) is increasingly important for own sake Shows increasing interest in pleasing parent Begins to show fears of going to bed and being left alone Puts arms in front of face to avoid having it washed Is in phase of coordination of secondary schemata and its application to new situations (9 to 12 months)
	•Says dada, mama with meaning Comprehends "bye-bye" May say one word (for example, hi, bye, what, no)	Inhibits behavior to verbal command of "no-no" or own name Imitates facial expressions, waves bye-bye Extends toy to another person but will not release it Looks around a corner or under a pillow for an object Repeats actions that attract attention and cause laughter Pulls clothes of another to attract attention Plays interactive games such as pat-a-cake Reacts to adult anger, cries when scolded Demonstrates independence in dressing, feeding, locomotive skills, and testing of parents Looks at and follows pictures in a book

Continued.

TABLE 10-3

Summary of Growth and Development during Infancy—cont'd

Age (months)	Physical	Gross Motor	Fine Motor
11	Eruption of lower lateral incisors may begin	•Creeps with abdomen off floor (Fig. 10-6, *G*) When sitting, pivots to reach toward back to pick up an object Cruises or walks holding onto furniture or with both hands held	Can hold crayon to make a mark on paper Explores objects more thoroughly (for example, clapper inside bell) Has neat pincer grasp (Fig. 10-2, *B*) Drops object deliberately for it to be picked up Puts one object after another into a container (sequential play) Able to manipulate an object to remove it from tight-fitting enclosure
12	Birth weight tripled Birth length increased by 50% Head and chest circumference equal (head circumference 46.5 cm [18½ in]) Has total of six to eight deciduous teeth Anterior fontanel almost closed Landau reflex fading Babinski reflex disappears Lumbar curve develops, lordosis evident during walking	Walks with one hand held Cruises well May attempt to stand alone momentarily Can sit down from standing position without help	Releases cube in cup Attempts to build two-block tower but fails Tries to insert a pellet into a narrow-neck bottle but fails Can turn pages in a book, many at a time

•Milestone that represents essential integrative aspects of development that lay the foundation for the achievement of more advanced skills.

to talk to the parent, maintain a safe distance from the infant, and avoid gestures, such as holding the arms out and smiling broadly.

Parents also may wonder whether they should encourage the child's clinging, dependent behavior, especially if there is pressure from others who view this as "spoiling." Parents need to be reassured that such behavior is healthy, desirable, and necessary for the child's optimum emotional development. If parents can reassure the infant of their presence, the infant will learn to realize that they are still there even if not physically present. Talking to infants when leaving the room, allowing them to hear one's voice on the telephone, and using transitional objects, such as a favorite blanket or toy, reassures them of the parent's continued presence.

Daycare

For many parents, especially working mothers, the need for locating safe and competent daycare facilities for the infant is an increasingly difficult problem—one that is compounded by the number of mothers working outside the home. Over the past 25 years there has been a marked shift in child care arrangements, with fewer children cared for at home and more children cared for in group centers or other settings.

The basic types of care are in-home care, in either the parent's or the caregiver's home, and center-based care, usually in a daycare center. In-home care may consist of a full-time baby-sitter who lives in the home, a full-time baby-sitter who comes to the home, cooperative arrangements such as exchange baby-sitting, and family daycare. A family daycare home typically provides care and protection for up to five children for part of a 24-hour day. Center-based care usually refers to a daycare facility that provides care for six or more children, for 6 or more hours in a 24-hour day. Work-based group care is another option that is becoming increasingly popular as employers recognize the benefit of quality and convenient child care to their employees.

Nurses play an important role in providing guidance to parents in selecting suitable, well-qualified facilities or individuals to care for their child. The decision to leave an infant in another's care often engenders doubt and guilt

Sensory	Vocalization	Socialization/Cognition
	Imitates definite speech sounds Uses jargon	Experiences joy and satisfaction when a task is mastered Reacts to restrictions with frustration Rolls ball to another on request Anticipates body gestures when a familiar nursery rhyme or story is being told (for example, holds toes and feet in response to "This little piggy went to market") Plays game up-down, "so big," or peekaboo Shakes head for "no"
Discriminates simple geometric forms (for example, circle) Amblyopia may develop with lack of binocularity Can follow rapidly moving object Controls and adjusts response to sound; listens for sound to recur	•Says two or more words besides dada, mama Comprehends meaning of several words (comprehension always precedes verbalization) Recognizes objects by name Imitates animal sounds Understands simple verbal commands (for example, "Give it to me," "Show me your eyes")	Shows emotions such as jealousy, affection (may give hug or kiss on request), anger, fear Enjoys familiar surroundings and explores away from parent Fearful in strange situation, clings to parent May develop habit of "security blanket" or favorite toy Increasing determination to practice locomotor skills

in the parent, despite reassurance that the provision of competent, loving care by someone other than the parent is not detrimental to the child's future development. Therefore any assistance is often appreciated.

Guidelines for selecting daycare facilities are discussed in Chapter 13. The same conscientious attention should be applied to locating competent baby-sitters. References from other employers are essential, and there is no substitute for observing the interaction between the individual and the child. Although very young infants need little if any preparation for the introduction of a new caregiver, older infants may benefit from a gradual placement to reduce stranger fear. At all times the parent should have the right to visit the child, and regular conferences should be established to review the child's progress.

Limit-Setting and Discipline

As infants' motor skills advance and mobility increases, parents are faced with the need to set safe limits (see discussion of nurse's role in injury prevention on p. 298). Although there are numerous disciplinary techniques, some are more appropriate for this age than others. Parents can begin discipline using a negative voice and stern eye-to-eye contact. Although corporal punishment is not recommended, at times *one* slap on the hand or buttocks may be effective in conveying the message that a behavior is unacceptable, especially when the child insists on performing a dangerous activity. Although parents may be concerned with instituting discipline during infancy, it is important to stress that the earlier effective disciplinary methods are employed, the easier it is to continue these approaches.

Thumb-Sucking and Use of Pacifier

Sucking is the infant's chief pleasure, and it may not be satisfied by breast- or bottle-feeding. It is such a strong need that infants who are deprived of sucking, such as those with a cleft lip repair, will suck on their tongue. Some newborns are born with sucking pads on their fingers from in utero sucking activity. Several benefits of nonnutritive sucking have been documented, such as in-

THERAPEUTIC DIALOGUE

Thumb-Sucking

During a well-child visit the nurse observes that the mother persistently takes the thumb out of her 10-month-old daughter's mouth.

NURSE: I can see that Annie likes to suck her thumb.
MOTHER: Too much. I am always trying to discourage her from this habit.
NURSE: You have concerns about her thumb-sucking?
MOTHER: Of course. Her teeth are coming in so nice and straight and I don't want the thumb to make them crooked.
NURSE: Tell me about the thumb making the teeth crooked.
MOTHER: My mother feels that it does. My brother sucked his thumb until he was 2 years old and as a teenager he needed braces. Now I never sucked my thumb and my teeth are straight.
NURSE: I understand how your mother could make that connection. Do you think that teeth can become crooked for other reasons?
MOTHER: I guess so. Why?
NURSE: I asked because your mother is partially right. Thumb-sucking after age 4 can cause dental problems, but teeth can need braces for many other reasons. Babies enjoy sucking. Sometimes, making an issue of the sucking can cause it to last longer. Sucking on a thumb or pacifier is very common in young children, especially in infants. It satisfies their need to suck and helps them to comfort themselves. Let's talk about thumb-sucking at your next visit.
MOTHER: OK. I appreciate our talking about this because my taking the thumb out of her mouth doesn't stop the habit. She often gets angry and cries and I feel upset. For now I'll just let her suck her thumb.

creased weight gain in premature infants and decreased crying (Anderson, 1986).

Problems arise when parents are concerned about sucking of fingers, thumb, or pacifier and attempt to restrain this natural tendency. Before offering advice, nurses should investigate the parents' feelings and base guidance on this information (see Therapeutic dialogue).

In general, there is no need to restrain nonnutritive sucking during infancy. Malocclusion may occur if thumb-sucking persists past 4 years of age or when the permanent teeth erupt. However, there is less dental displacement with the use of a pacifier than with the use of a hard, rigid finger. Pacifiers may also be relinquished earlier than thumbs because they are less readily available. If the child uses a pacifier, safety considerations in purchasing one must be stressed (see p. 300).

To decrease dependence on nonnutritive sucking, sucking pleasure can be increased by prolonging feeding time. A small-holed, firm nipple causes stronger sucking and slower feeding. Also the parent's excessive use of the pacifier to calm the child should be explored. It is not unusual for parents to place a pacifier in the infant's mouth as soon as crying begins, thus reinforcing a pattern of distress-relief.

Thumb-sucking reaches its peak at ages 18 to 20 months and is most prevalent when the child is hungry or tired. Persistent thumb-sucking in a listless, apathetic child always warrants investigation. It may be a sign of an emotional problem between parent and child or of boredom, isolation, and lack of stimulation.

Teething

One of the more difficult periods in the infant's (and parents') life is the eruption of the deciduous (primary) teeth, often referred to as teething. The age of tooth eruption shows considerable variation among children, but the order of their appearance is fairly regular and predictable (Fig. 10-11). The first primary teeth to erupt are the lower central incisors, which appear at approximately 6 to 8 months of age. These are followed closely by the upper central incisors. A quick guide to assessment of deciduous teeth during the first 2 years is: *age of the child in months* $-$ *6* $=$ *number of teeth*.

Teething is a physiologic process, and as the crown of the tooth breaks through the periodontal membrane, some discomfort may be experienced. Some children show minimum evidence of teething, such as drooling, increased finger-sucking, or biting on hard objects. Others are very irritable, have difficulty sleeping, and refuse to eat. Generally signs of illness such as fever, vomiting, or diarrhea are not symptoms of teething but of illness. Continued irritability may be a clue to disturbances other than teething and warrants further investigation.

Inasmuch as teething pain is a result of inflammation, cold is soothing. Giving the child a frozen teething ring or an ice cube wrapped in a washcloth helps relieve the inflammation. Several nonprescription topical anesthetic ointments are available, such as Baby Ora-Jel. If these are used, parents are advised to apply them correctly.

In the event of persistent irritability that affects sleeping and feeding, systemic analgesics, preferably nonaspi-

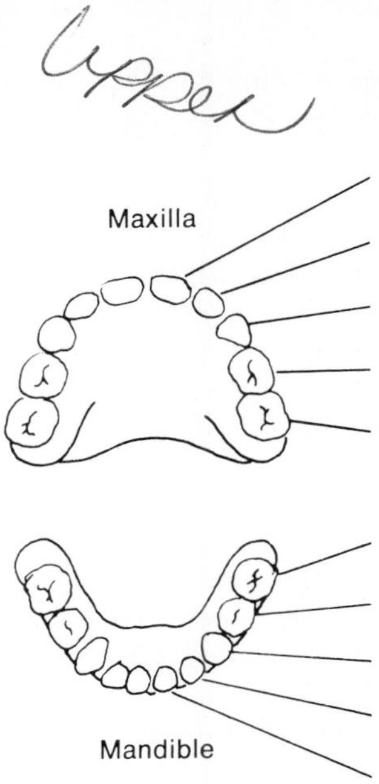

Average age of eruption (mo)	Average age of shedding (yr)
9.6	7.5
12.4	8
18.3	11.5
15.7	10.5
26.2	10.5
26.0	11
15.1	10
18.2	9.5
11.5	7
7.8	6

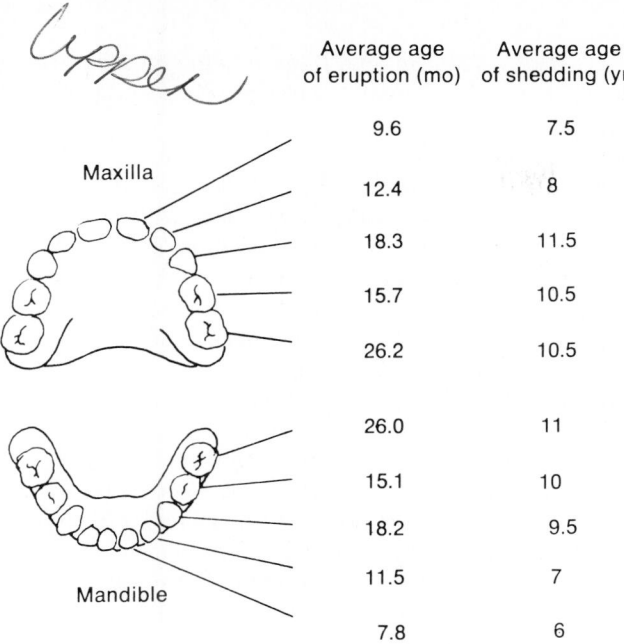

FIG. 10-11 Sequence of eruption and shedding primary teeth.

rin compounds such as acetaminophen, can be given judiciously. Parents should know that this is a temporary measure. The use of teething powders or procedures such as cutting or rubbing the gums with aspirin is discouraged, because ingestion or aspiration of the substance, infection, irritation, or ulceration of the tissue can occur.

Infant Shoes

Many parents are unaware of the type of shoes that is appropriate for the older infant and buy expensive infant shoes because of misleading advertising claims. Inflexible shoes that have hard soles can be detrimental by delaying walking, aggravating intoeing and outtoeing, and impeding the development of supportive foot muscles. Therefore counseling parents regarding footwear should begin when the infant is 6 months old, well before he is standing or walking (Glendon, 1987).

When children begin walking, the main reason for wearing shoes is *protection*. To provide protection, the shoe should retain its fit, be made of durable material with a smooth interior and few construction seams to irritate the skin, and be soft and flexible, especially in the toe area. A high-top shoe is not necessary for support but may be helpful in keeping the foot in the shoe.

A good shoe conforms to the anatomic shape of the foot, with a rounded toe area and sufficient toe room. During weight bearing, there should be at least the space of half the width of the thumbnail, or 1.25 cm (½ inch), between the end of the longest toe and the shoe. Roomy and square-toed socks also allow for proper growth and alignment. Inexpensive but well-constructed flexible sneakers or soft-leather moccasin-type shoes are adequate footgear for walking infants.

Even if the shoes are fitted properly, frequent changes are needed to accommodate the infant's rapidly growing feet. Shoe size changes at approximately 3-month intervals from 12 to 30 months of age; during this time the child's foot should be measured every 2 to 3 months. Curled toes when shoes are removed and redness and irritation of the skin on the bottom of the toes indicate the need for a larger size.

◆ *Promoting Optimum Health during Infancy*

The infant's first year is a time of monumental change and achievement, and the rapidity of the changes can easily overwhelm parents. Each month and phase of development have implications for care of the child. Health promotion during this time involves nutritional guidance, appropriate sleep and activity, proper dental care, prevention of disease through immunization, and provision of a safe environment.

NUTRITION

Ideally, discussion of optimum nutrition should begin prenatally with the decision to breast- or bottle-feed the infant. The choice for either is highly individual and is discussed in Chapter 8. This section is primarily concerned with infant nutrition during the next 12 months, when growth needs and developmental milestones ready the child for introduction of solid foods. Frequently the nurse is asked when to begin feeding solid foods, how to introduce new foods, and what foods are best. A thorough understanding of each of these areas prepares the nurse to answer these questions so that the nutritional needs of each child are met.

The First 6 Months

Human milk is the most desirable and complete diet for the infant for the first 6 months. The normal infant receiving breast milk from a well-nourished mother needs no specific vitamin and mineral supplements, with the exception of fluoride in a dose of 0.25 mg daily (regardless of the fluoride content of the local water supply) and iron by 6 months of age (when fetal iron stores are depleted). Supplements of 400 IU of vitamin D daily may be indicated if the mother's vitamin D intake is inadequate or if the infant does not benefit from adequate ultraviolet light because of dark skin color or little exposure to light (American Academy of Pediatrics, 1980).

An acceptable alternative to breast-feeding is commercial iron-fortified formula. Like human milk, it supplies all the nutrients needed by the infant for the first 6 months. The only supplementation required is 0.25 mg of fluoride if the local water supply is not fluoridated or if the infant is given ready-to-feed formula, which eliminates the use of fluoridated tap water.

If evaporated milk formula is given, supplemental iron, vitamin C, and fluoride (depending on local water supply) are required. Commercially prepared vitamin/iron preparations with or without fluoride are available to meet the specific needs of the infant. Unmodified whole cow's milk, low-fat cow's milk, or imitation milks are not acceptable as a major source of nutrition for infants.

The addition of solid foods before 5 to 6 months is not recommended. During the early months solid foods are not compatible with the gastrointestinal ability and nutritional needs of the infant. For example, feeding solids to the infant exposes him to food antigens that may produce food-protein allergy. Developmentally, the infant is not ready. The extrusion (protrusion) reflex is strong and pushes food out of the mouth. The infant instinctively sucks when given food. Because of his limited range of motor abilities, the infant is unable to deliberately push food away or avoid feeding. Therefore, early introduction of solids is a type of forced feeding.

The Second 6 Months

During the second half of the first year human milk or formula continues to be the primary source of nutrition. If breast-feeding is discontinued, commercial iron-fortified formula should be substituted. Whole cow's milk can be given if the infant is consuming one third of the calories as supplemental foods consisting of a balanced mixture of cereal, vegetables, fruits, and other foods to ensure adequate sources of iron and vitamin C (American Academy of Pediatrics, 1983).

The major change in feeding habits is the addition of solid foods to the infant's diet. Physiologically and developmentally 5 to 6 months is a transition period. By this time the gastrointestinal tract has matured sufficiently to handle more complex nutrients and is less sensitive to potentially allergenic foods. Tooth eruption is beginning and facilitates biting and chewing. The extrusion reflex has disappeared, and swallowing is more coordinated to allow the infant to easily accept solids. Head control is well developed, permitting the infant to sit with support and purposely turn his head away to communicate disinterest in food. Voluntary grasping and improved eye-hand coordination gradually allow the infant to pick up "finger" foods and feed himself. His increasing sense of independence is evident in his desire to hold his own bottle and try to "help" during feeding.

Selection and Preparation of Solid Foods

The choice of foods to introduce first is variable but should be based on the reasons for feeding, such as supplying nutrients not found in formula or breast milk. Cereal is generally introduced first because of its high iron content (7 mg/3 tablespoons of dry cereal). There are several types of commercially prepared infant cereals, such as rice, barley, oatmeal, and high-protein cereals, but rice is usually suggested as an initial food because of its easy digestibility and low allergenic potential.

Cereal is mixed with formula until whole milk is given. If the infant is breast-fed, the cereal is mixed with expressed breast milk or water rather than with cow's milk because the child may be sensitive to cow's milk. If fruit juices have been started, they can be mixed with the dry cereal. The vitamin C content of the juice enhances the absorption of iron in the cereal. Because of their benefit as a source of iron, infant cereals should be continued until the child is 18 months of age.

At the same time solid foods are introduced, fruit juice can be offered for its rich source of vitamin C and as a substitute for milk. Because vitamin C is naturally destroyed by heat, juice is not warmed. Containers of juice are always kept covered and refrigerated to prevent further vitamin loss. Fruit juice is offered from a cup, rather than a bottle, to prevent the development of "nursing bottle" caries (see p. 293).

The addition of other foods is arbitrary. A common sequence is strained fruits followed by vegetables and finally meats. At 6 months foods such as a cracker or zwieback can be offered as a type of finger and teething food. By 8 to 9 months junior foods and nutritious finger foods such as a firmly cooked vegetable, raw pieces of fruit (except grapes), or cheese can be given. By 1 year well-cooked table foods are served.

Commercially prepared baby foods are the most commonly used types of food served to infants in the United States. They are convenient, contain no added salt or sugar, but are relatively expensive. An alternative is preparing baby foods at home, which is a simple and inexpensive process. Fruits and vegetables can be steamed in a small amount of water and pureed in a blender or food processor. Many of them, such as ripe banana, can be mashed fine with a fork. Fruits such as apples or pears require little or no water in the cooking process. Vegetables such as carrots, potatoes, or string beans require additional water in the cooking and blending process. Preferably, home-prepared infant foods should be fresh or frozen, because canned foods, other than those specially prepared for infants, may have excessive sodium or sugar or be a source of lead from the container.

Introduction of Solid Foods

When the spoon is first introduced to the infant, the likelihood is that he will push it away and appear dissatisfied. Some patience and skill are required to overcome this initial response. A small-bowled, straight, and long-handled spoon, similar to a demitasse spoon, allows a small portion of food to be placed toward the back of the tongue. If food is placed on the front of the tongue, it will be pushed out. It is simply scooped up and refed. As the child becomes accustomed to the spoon, he will more eagerly accept the food and will eventually open his mouth in anticipation (or keep it closed in dislike). Since the first intro-

Guidelines for Method of Introducing Solid Foods to Infants

1. Introduce solids when infant is hungry.
2. Begin spoon feeding by pushing food to back of tongue because of infant's natural tendency to thrust tongue forward.
3. Use a small spoon with straight handle; begin with 1 or 2 teaspoons of food; gradually increase to a couple of tablespoons per feeding.
4. Introduce one food at a time, usually at intervals of 4 to 7 days to allow for identification of food allergies.
5. Decrease the quantity of milk as the amount of solid food increases to prevent overfeeding.
6. Do not introduce foods by mixing them with formula in the bottle.

duction of food is a new experience, the spoon feeding should be attempted before or after ingestion of a small amount of breast milk or formula to associate this new experience with a pleasurable and satisfying experience. Trying to introduce a new food *after* the entire milk feeding is usually useless, since the infant is satiated and has no inclination to try something new.

After several spoon feedings, new food can be introduced at the beginning of a meal. It is best to introduce many new foods during the first year when the infant is more likely to eat them because of a hearty appetite resulting from a rapid growth rate.

Each new food is introduced at intervals of 4 to 7 days to allow for identification of food allergies. New foods are offered in small amounts, from 1 teaspoon to 1 to 2 tablespoons. As the amount of solid food increases, the quantity of milk is decreased to less than a liter a day to prevent overfeeding.

Food should not be mixed in the bottle and fed through a nipple with a large hole. This deprives the child of the pleasure of learning new tastes and developing a discriminating palate. It can also cause problems with poor chewing of food later in life since this experience would be lacking. A summary of the principles that govern the introduction of new foods is given in the box.

Weaning

Weaning, the process of giving up one method of feeding for another, usually refers to relinquishing the breast or bottle for a cup. In Western societies this is generally regarded as a major task for infants and is frequently seen as a potentially traumatic experience. It is psychologically significant because the infant is required to give up a major source of oral pleasure and gratification.

There is no one time for weaning that is best for every child, but generally most infants show signs of readiness during the second half of the first year. They have learned that good things come from a spoon. Their increasing desire for freedom of movement may lessen their desire to be held close for feedings. They are acquiring more control over their actions and can easily manipulate a cup to their lips (even if it is held upside down!). Since imitation becomes a powerful motivator by age 8 or 9 months, they enjoy using a cup or glass as others do.

Weaning should be gradual, one bottle- or breast-feeding being replaced at a time. The last feeding to be discontinued is usually the nighttime one. If breast-feeding must be terminated before 5 or 6 months of age, weaning should be to a bottle to provide for the infant's continued sucking needs. If breast-feeding is discontinued later, weaning can be directly to a cup.

Nutritional Counseling

The relatively simple feeding plan for infants, especially during the first 6 months, allows the nurse ample opportunity to educate parents regarding the nutritional needs of their child and to prepare them for the addition of solid foods. A prime consideration of counseling is provision of optimum nutrition. This includes education concerning what infants need and do not need. It may necessitate an introduction to the basic four food groups in order for the parents to wisely select foods for the infant's diet.

Preventing obesity. Besides selection of foods, the nurse must also consider amount of food. The most prevalent nutritional disorder in the United States is overeating, and prevention begins early. From the infant's first feeding parents should allow the child to regulate the amount of formula he desires. No attempt should be made to encourage the infant to finish the last drop or, later, to clean his plate.

Often eating habits are controlled by the sociocultural background of the family, rather than by their knowledge of well-balanced nutrition. Common myths such as "a fat baby is a healthy baby" are difficult to dispel. In some cultures overweight infants are regarded as a sign of good mothering, and any suggestion regarding altering the child's weight is threatening to the parent. Understanding cultural values is important in effecting change through counseling.

A thorough nutritional history is also a prerequisite for counseling. Asking questions such as, "Does your child drink too much milk?" may yield little reliable information. Phrasing the question by saying, "Your child certainly looks well fed; how many bottles of milk a day does he drink?" lessens parents' defensiveness and offers an objective number of ounces. (See also Chapter 6 for a discussion of nutritional assessment.)

If too much formula or milk is the problem, several strategies can be used to reduce their intake (see Nursing tip, p. 292). A commercial formula, Advance,* is also available that provides 20% fewer calories than regular for-

*Manufactured by Ross Laboratories, Columbus, OH.

Nursing Tip: Formula/Milk Intake

To reduce consumption of formula or milk:
- Dilute the feeding
- Substitute water for a bottle of formula
- Use a smaller-hole nipple to prolong sucking with less intake

mula or whole cow's milk. Dietary fat should not be restricted. For example, substituting skim or low-fat milk is unacceptable because the essential fatty acids are inadequate and the solute concentration of protein and electrolytes, such as sodium, is too high. Overall, the objective is not for the infant to lose weight but for his weight gain to slow until it is appropriate for his age and height.

The selection of solid foods is also an important aspect of controlling obesity. Approximately 20% of commercial baby foods contain less than 50 kcal/100 g, whereas another 20% contain more than 100 kcal/100 g. Choosing low-calorie foods can significantly lower the daily calorie intake without actually decreasing the total quantity of food. The selection of sweet foods should be kept to a minimum. This includes not adding additional sugar to the formula or cereal and avoiding finger foods such as cookies. Other foods rich in calories that should be restricted in serving size rather than eliminated include butter, cream, ice cream, pudding, and chocolate.

Parents are also encouraged to interpret the infant's signals of discomfort and intervene in ways other than through feeding. Crying, fussiness, or sucking do not necessarily indicate hunger. Rocking, stroking, holding, and offering a toy or a pacifier may be more appropriate than automatically responding with food.

SLEEP AND ACTIVITY

Sleep patterns vary among infants, and active infants typically sleep less than placid children. Generally by 3 to 4 months of age most infants have developed a nocturnal pattern of sleep lasting from 8 to 10 hours. The total daily sleep is 13 to 15 hours. The number of naps per day varies, but by the end of the year infants may take one or two naps. Breast-fed infants usually sleep for less prolonged periods, especially during the night, than do bottle-fed infants. Because of the trend toward breast-feeding, sleep norms such as those described above, which were based primarily on bottle-fed infants, may no longer be relevant (Elias and others, 1986).

Most infants are naturally active and need no encouragement to be mobile. However, problems can arise when devices such as playpens, strollers, commercial swings, and walkers are used excessively. These restrict movement and prevent infants from exploring and developing gross motor skills. Contrary to popular belief, walkers do not enhance coordination and are dangerous if tipped over or placed near stairs (Reider, Schwartz, and Newman, 1986).

Sleep Disturbances

Concerns regarding sleep are common during infancy. Sometimes they are as basic as parents' questioning the infant's need for additional sleep. In this case it is best to investigate the reason for their concern, stressing the individual needs of each child.

When a sleeping problem is presented, a careful assessment is warranted. Questions regarding the frequency and duration of waking, the usual bedtime routine, the number of nighttime feedings, the perceived problem (e.g., how much disruption does the behavior generate), and the attempted interventions are important in planning effective approaches. A common suggestion to parents is to "let the child cry until falling asleep," but this is very difficult to implement. Once the parents relent and console the child, they have only reinforced the crying. An equally effective but more practical approach is suggested in the Nursing tip (see box).

Nursing Tip: Night Crying

To eliminate night crying:
Let the child cry for progressively longer times between *brief* interventions that consist only of reassurance, not rocking, holding, or using the bottle or pacifier. For example, check on the child every 5 minutes during the first night, and progressively extend this interval by 5 minutes on successive nights.

The best way to prevent sleep problems is to encourage parents to establish bedtime rituals that do not foster problematic patterns. One of the most constructive is placing infants *awake* in their own crib. When infants are accustomed to falling asleep somewhere else, such as their parent's arms, and then being transferred to their crib, they awaken in unfamiliar surroundings and are unable to fall asleep until the routine is repeated. Also, the bed should be used for sleeping only—not as a playpen—so that the child associates the bed with sleep, not with activity (Ferber, 1984).

DENTAL HEALTH

Good dental hygiene begins as soon as the primary teeth erupt. During infancy the teeth are cleaned by wiping them with a damp cloth; toothbrushing is too harsh for the tender gingiva. Fluoride supplements, an essential mineral for building caries-resistant teeth, are prescribed as appropriate for:

- All infants 2 weeks of age or older who live in areas with suboptimum levels of fluoride in the local water supply

- Exclusively breast-fed infants regardless of the fluoride content of the local water supply
- Infants who consume relatively little fluoridated tap water, such as those receiving ready-to-serve formula

Dietary considerations are also important because habits begun during infancy tend to continue into later years. Foods with concentrated sugar should be used sparingly (if at all) in the infant's diet. The practice of coating pacifiers with honey or using commercially available hard-candy pacifiers is discouraged. Besides being cariogenic, honey also may cause infant botulism. Parents need to be counseled regarding the detrimental effects of frequent and prolonged bottle- or breast-feeding during sleep, when the sweet milk or other fluid, such as juice, bathes the teeth, producing *nursing-bottle caries*. (See also Chapter 12 for a more extensive discussion of dental care, including nursing-bottle caries.)

IMMUNIZATIONS

One of the most dramatic advances in pediatrics has been the decline of infectious diseases over the past 40 years because of the widespread use of immunization for preventable diseases. Although many of the presently available immunizations can be given to individuals of any age, the recommended primary schedule begins during infancy and, with the exception of boosters, is completed during early childhood. Therefore the discussion of childhood immunizations for diphtheria, pertussis, tetanus, polio, measles, mumps, rubella, and *Haemophilus influenzae* type b is included under health promotion during the first year. Selected vaccines that are generally reserved for children considered at high risk for the disease are also discussed.

Schedule for Immunizations

The recommended age for beginning primary immunizations of normal infants is 2 months (Table 10-4). Recommended schedules for children not immunized during infancy are included in Table 10-5. Children who began primary immunization at the recommended age but for some reason did not receive all the doses do not have to begin the series again. They receive only those doses that were missed. In situations when there is doubt that the child will return for immunization according to the optimum schedule, DTP, OPV, MMR, and *Haemophilus influenzae* (Hib) vaccine can be administered simultaneously as appropriate to the age and previous vaccination status of the child. DTP, MMR, and Hib are given in separate syringes at different injection sites (American Academy of Pediatrics, 1986).

One major change in the immunization schedule is the discontinuation of routine smallpox vaccination in the United States. This occurred because over a period of years, the risks from receiving the vaccination were greater than the chance of contracting the actual disease. In 1980 the World Health Organization announced the worldwide eradication of smallpox.

Recommendations for Routine Immunizations

Several vaccines are administered to all children in the United States according to the schedules listed in Tables 10-4 and 10-5. The following is a brief description of the immunizations.

Diphtheria. Diphtheria vaccine is commonly administered (1) in combination with tetanus and pertussis vaccines (DTP) for normal children younger than 7 years of age, (2) in a combined vaccine with tetanus (DT) for chil-

TABLE 10-4

Recommended Schedule for Active Immunization of Normal Infants and Children

Recommended Age	Immunization(s)	Comments
2 mo	DTP, OPV	Can be initiated as early as 2 weeks of age in areas of high endemicity or during epidemics
4 mo	DTP, OPV	2-month interval desired for OPV to avoid interference from previous dose
6 mo	DTP (OPV)	OPV is optional (may be given in areas with increased risk of polio exposure)
15 mo	MMR	MMR preferred to individual vaccines; tuberculin testing may be done
18 mo	DTP,*† OPV†	
24 mo	HBPV	
4-6 yr‡	DTP, OPV	At or before school entry
14-16 yr	Td	Repeat every 10 years throughout life

DTP, diphtheria and tetanus toxoids with pertussis vaccine; *HBPV, Haemophilus influenzae* type b polysaccharide vaccine; *MMR*, live measles, mumps, and rubella viruses in a combined vaccine; *OPV*, oral poliovirus vaccine containing attenuated poliovirus types 1, 2, and 3; *Td*, adult tetanus toxoid (full dose) and diphtheria toxoid (reduced dose) in combination.
*Should be given 6 to 12 months after the third dose.
†May be given simultaneously with MMR at 15 months of age.
‡Up to the seventh birthday.
From American Academy of Pediatrics: Report of the Committee on Infectious Diseases, ed. 20, Elk Grove Village, IL, 1986. Copyright American Academy of Pediatrics, 1986.
Author's note: For recommendations for the *Haemophilus influenzae* type b conjugate vaccine, see p. 295.

TABLE 10-5

Recommended Immunization Schedules for Children not Immunized in First Year of Life

Recommended Time	Immunization(s)	Comments
Younger than 7 years old		
First visit	DTP, OPV, MMR	MMR if child ≥15 months old; tuberculin testing may be done
Interval after first visit		
1 mo	HBPV*	For children 24-60 months
2 mo	DTP, OPV	
4 mo	DTP (OPV)	OPV is optional (may be given in areas with increased risk of poliovirus exposure)
10-16 mo	DTP, OPV	OPV is not given if third dose was given earlier
4-6 yr (at or before school entry)	DTP, OPV	DTP is not necessary if the fourth dose was given after the fourth birthday; OPV is not necessary if recommended OPV dose at 10-16 months following first visit was given after the fourth birthday
Age 14-16 yr	Td	Repeat every 10 years throughout life
7 years old and older		
First visit	Td, OPV, MMR	
Interval after first visit		
2 mo	Td, OPV	
8-14 mo	Td, OPV	
Age 14-16 yr	Td	Repeat every 10 years throughout life

DTP, diphtheria and tetanus toxoids with pertussis vaccine; *HBPV, Haemophilus influenzae* type b polysaccharide vaccine; *MMR,* live measles, mumps, and rubella viruses in combined vaccine; *OPV,* oral poliovirus vaccine; *Td,* tetanus toxoid and diphtheria toxoid.
**Haemophilus influenzae* type b polysaccharide vaccine can be given, if necessary, simultaneously with DTP (at separate sites). The initial three doses of DTP can be given at 1- to 2-month intervals; so, for the child in whom immunization is initiated at 24 months old or older, one visit could be eliminated by giving DTP, OPV, MMR at the first visit; DTP and HBPV at the second visit (1 month later); and DTP and OPV at the third visit (2 months after the first visit). Subsequent DTP and OPV 10 to 16 months after the first visit are still indicated.
From American Academy of Pediatrics: Report of the Committee on Infectious Diseases, ed. 20, Elk Grove Village, IL, 1986. Copyright American Academy of Pediatrics, 1986.
Author's note: For recommendations for the *Haemophilus influenzae* type b conjugate vaccine, see p. 295.

dren younger than 7 years of age who have some contraindication for receiving pertussis vaccine, (3) in smaller doses (15% to 20% of that in DTP or DT) with tetanus vaccine (Td) for use in children age 7 years and older, or (4) as a single antigen when combined antigen preparations are not indicated. Although the diphtheria vaccine does not produce absolute immunity, when given according to the recommended schedule, protective antitoxin persists for 10 years or more.

Tetanus. Three forms of tetanus vaccine—tetanus toxoid, tetanus immune globulin (TIG) (human), and tetanus antitoxin (usually horse serum)—are available. Tetanus toxoid is used for routine primary immunization, usually in one of the combinations listed above, and provides protective antitoxin levels for 10 years or more. For wound management, see p. 1073.

Pertussis. Pertussis vaccine is recommended for all children 6 weeks through 6 years of age (up to the seventh birthday) who have no neurologic contraindications to its use. It is not given to children 7 years or older because the risk of receiving the vaccine increases as the incidence, severity, and fatality of the disease decrease.

Polio. The trivalent oral form of poliovirus (TOPV) (developed by Sabin) is recommended for all children younger than 18 years of age who have no specific contraindications to its use, regardless of the number of administrations of inactivated poliovirus vaccine (IPV) (developed by Salk) they have received. For infants and children with immune deficiency diseases and for their siblings, IPV is the vaccine of choice because it has no reported history of causing vaccine-associated paralysis. However, it has the disadvantages of being given by subcutaneous injection and requiring periodic boosters to maintain immunity.

Measles. Because of the presence of maternal antibodies, measles virus vaccine should be delayed until 15 months of age for infants who live in communities where the disease is not prevalent. However, during the course of measles outbreaks, the vaccine can be given anytime after 6 months of age, followed by a second inoculation after age 15 months.

Mumps. Mumps virus vaccine may be given at any time to children between 15 months and 12 years of age who have not had the disease.

Rubella. Rubella is a relatively mild infection in children, but in a pregnant woman it presents serious risks to the developing fetus. Therefore the aim of rubella immunization is actually protection of the unborn child rather than the recipient of the immunization.

Rubella immunization is recommended for all children at 12 months of age or older. If administered in a combined form with measles vaccine, it should be given to

TABLE 10-6

Recommendations for Selected Immunizations

Immunization	Description	Administration/Precautions
Influenza virus vaccine	Affords protection against some strains of influenza Recommended for children 6 months and older with chronic disorders of cardiovascular or pulmonary systems whose severity warranted regular medical care or hospitalization during preceding year. Other eligible children include those with diabetes mellitus, renal dysfunction, anemia, immunosuppression, or those on long-term aspirin therapy	Administered in fall, repeated yearly Intramuscular (preferred) injection (2 doses at least 4 weeks apart for children 12 years or younger; 1 dose for children over 12 years) May be associated with mild flulike symptoms for 1 to 2 days Contraindicated in persons with severe allergy to eggs
Pneumococcal polysaccharide vaccine (Pneumovax; Pne-Immune)	Affords protection against 23 types of *Streptococcus pneumoniae* Recommended for children 2 years and older with sickle cell disease, functional or anatomic asplenia, nephrotic syndrome, and Hodgkin disease prior to beginning cytoreduction therapy	Subcutaneous or intramuscular injection Revaccination is not recommended Contraindicated during pregnancy
Meningococcal polysaccharide vaccine (Menomune)	Affords protection against *Neisseria meningitidis,* serogroups A, C, Y, and W-135 Recommended for children 2 years and older with terminal complement deficiencies and anatomic or functional asplenia	Subcutaneous injection Duration of protection unknown Safety during pregnancy not established
Hepatitis B vaccine (Heptavax-B)	Affords protection against hepatitis B virus (HBV) Recommended for several high-risk groups, especially adults at risk for infection from contaminated blood products; among children, infants born to mothers who are hepatitis B surface antigen (HBsAg) positive	Infants: combined hepatitis B immune globulin (HBIG) and HB vaccine Administered at birth, 1, and 6 months of age Intramuscular injections at separate sites

children at about 15 months of age. Increased emphasis should also be placed on vaccinating all unimmunized prepubertal children and susceptible adolescents and adult women in the childbearing age-group.

***Haemophilus influenzae* type b.** *Haemophilus influenzae* type b (Hib) vaccines provide protection against a number of serious infections caused by Hib, especially bacterial meningitis, epiglottitis, bacterial pneumonia, septic arthritis, and sepsis. Two Hib vaccines are available: the original polysaccharide vaccine and the recently developed conjugate vaccine. Current recommendations for the conjugate vaccine differ from those listed in Tables 10-4 and 10-5 for the polysaccharide vaccine primarily in initial age of administration (18 months rather than 24 months) and includes the following (Recommendation of ACIP, 1988):

- All children at 18 months of age
- Children older than 24 months who have not received the Hib vaccine and who are at increased risk of Hib infection, such as those attending daycare facilities, those with anatomic or functional asplenia such as sickle cell disease, and those with malignancies associated with immunosuppression
- Children between 18 and 24 months of age who received the polysaccharide vaccine
- Children less than 24 months of age who had the disease

Recommendations for Selected Immunizations

Several vaccines have been developed that are reserved for children considered at high risk for the disease. Most of the vaccines are suggested for children with immune deficiencies or asplenia who are more susceptible to infection from the organism than the general population. Selected immunizations are presented in Table 10-6. Others, such as the rabies vaccine, are discussed as appropriate throughout the text.

Reactions

Vaccines are among the safest and most reliable drugs available. However, minor side effects do occur following many of the immunizations, and, rarely, a serious reaction may result.

In general with inactivated antigens, such as DTP and Hib, side effects are most likely to occur within a few hours or days of administration. The common reactions are fever, soreness, redness, and swelling at the site of injection. Pertussis immunization may be associated with more severe reactions such as loss of consciousness, convulsions, and thrombocytopenia.

The live attenuated virus vaccines, such as those for measles, mumps, rubella, and oral poliovirus, may cause possible unfavorable reactions, and "vaccine-associated" disorders can occur for a period of 30 to 60 days. Poliovirus and mumps immunization have essentially no side effects, although a vaccine-associated paralysis rarely occurs from TOPV. Measles is occasionally associated with anorexia, malaise, rash, and fever 7 to 10 days after immunization. Rarely, a subsequent encephalitis may occur. In some children rubella vaccine causes mild rash, arthralgia, and/or paresthesia. However, in adults the reactions can be much more severe and prolonged. This is an additional reason for ensuring that individuals receive this immunization during childhood.

No specific treatment is required for the expected reactions. Acetaminophen given as soon as side effects occur is adequate, and there is evidence that acetaminophen given at the time of DTP vaccination and every 4 to 6 hours for 48 to 72 hours reduces side effects (Recommendation of ACIP, 1987). However, the nurse should advise parents to notify the physician immediately if any unusual symptoms or neurologic sequelae peculiar to pertussis occur.

Contraindications

The general contraindication for all immunizations is a severe febrile illness. This precaution is to avoid adding the risk of adverse side effects from the vaccine on an already ill child or mistakenly identifying a symptom of the disease as having been caused by the vaccine. The presence of minor illnesses, such as the common cold, is *not* a contraindication.

Live-virus vaccines are not given to anyone with an altered immune system because multiplication of the virus may be enhanced, causing a severe vaccine-induced illness. Such children include (1) those with immunologic-deficiency disease, such as leukemia, lymphoma, generalized malignancy, or acquired immune deficiency syndrome (AIDS), and (2) those receiving immunosuppressive therapy, such as steroids, chemotherapy, or radiation. In addition, household contacts of such children should not receive oral poliovirus vaccine because the excreted virus can be communicable to the immunosuppressed child. Another contraindication to live-virus vaccines is the presence of recently acquired passive immunity, including blood transfusions, immunoglobulin, or maternal antibodies. Administration of such vaccines should be postponed until 3 months after passive immunization with immune serum globulin.

Pregnancy is a known contraindication to immunization against mumps, measles, and rubella. In addition these vaccines should not be given to women who are likely to become pregnant within 3 months after vaccination. However, if rubella vaccination is given during pregnancy, it should not be a routine reason for therapeutic abortion since current evidence from women who received the vaccine while pregnant and delivered unaffected offspring indicates that the risk to the fetus is negligible (Hinman, 1985). Oral poliovirus vaccine should also be withheld unless there is risk of exposure during an outbreak of polio.

A final contraindication is a known allergic response to a previously administered vaccine or a substance in the vaccine. If any of the following adverse events occur after combined DTP or single-antigen pertussis vaccination, further immunization with pertussis vaccine is contraindicated: (1) allergic hypersensitivity, (2) fever (temperature 40.5° C [105° F] or greater) within 48 hours, (3) collapse or shocklike state within 48 hours, (4) persistent, inconsolable crying lasting 3 hours or longer or an unusual, high-pitched cry occurring within 48 hours, (5) convulsions within 3 days, or (6) encephalopathy (alterations in consciousnesss with generalized or focal neurologic signs) within 7 days (Recommendation of ACIP, 1985).

Measles, mumps, and rubella virus vaccines contain minute amounts of neomycin, and measles and mumps vaccines, which are grown on chick embryo tissue cultures, may contain substances allergenic to egg-sensitive individuals. However, only a history of anaphylactoid reaction to the antibiotic or to egg is considered a contraindication to their use. To identify the rare child who may not be able to receive the vaccines, a careful allergy history is taken. If the child has a history of anaphylaxis, it is reported to the physician before the vaccine is administered.

Administration/precautions. The principal precautions in administering immunizations include proper storage of the vaccine to protect its potency and following recommended procedure for injection. The meningococcal vaccine and the virus vaccines (except oral polio and influenza) are administered subcutaneously; DTP, influenza, and hepatitis B vaccines are given intramuscularly. The Hib and pneumococcal vaccines may be injected intramuscularly or subcutaneously. Since the total series for routine immunization requires a number of injections, every attempt is made to administer them as painlessly as possible (see Chapter 21).

The DTP vaccines contain an adjuvant aluminum compound that is used to retain the antigen at the injection site and prolong the antigen's stimulatory effect. Because subcutaneous or intracutaneous injection of the adjuvant can cause local irritation, inflammation, or abscess formation, several precautions are suggested to prevent tracking the fluid through the skin (see Nursing tip box).

Nursing Tip: DTP Injection

To minimize local reactions from DTP vaccines:
- Select a needle of adequate length to deposit the antigen deep in the muscle mass
- Inject into the vastus lateralis or ventrogluteal muscle
- Use an air bubble to clear the needle after injecting the vaccine

Note: Changing the needle on the syringe after drawing up the vaccine and before injecting it has not been shown to be effective (Salomon and others, 1987).

TABLE 10-7

Injury Prevention during Infancy

Age: Birth-4 Months

Major Developmental Accomplishments

Involuntary reflexes, such as the crawling reflex, may propel infant forward
May roll over
Increasing eye-hand coordination and voluntary grasp reflex

Injury Prevention

Aspiration
Not as great a danger to this age-group, but should begin practicing safeguarding early (see under 4-7 months)
Never shake baby powder directly on infant; place powder in hand and then on infant's skin; store container closed and out of infant's reach

Suffocation
Keep all plastic bags stored out of infant's reach; discard large plastic garment bags after tying in a knot
Do not cover mattress or pillows with plastic
Use a firm mattress, no pillows, and loose blankets
Make sure crib design follows federal regulations and mattress fits snugly
Position crib away from other furniture
Avoid sleeping in bed with infant
Do not tie pacifier on a string around infant's neck
Remove bibs at bedtime
Drowning—never leave infant alone in bath

Falls
Always raise crib rails; tie them to crib if malfunctioning
Never leave infant on a raised, unguarded surface
When in doubt where to place child, use the floor
Restrain child in the infant seat and never leave him unattended while the seat is resting on a raised surface
Avoid using a high chair until child is old enough to sit well

Poisoning
Not as great a danger to this age-group, but should begin practicing safeguards early (see under 4-7 months)

Burns
Install smoke detectors in home
Use caution when warming formula in microwave oven; always check temperature of liquid before feeding
Check bath water
Do not pour hot liquids when infant is close by, such as sitting on lap
Beware of cigarette ashes that may fall on infant
Do not leave infant in the sun for more than a few minutes
Wash flame-retardant clothes according to label directions
Use cool-mist vaporizers
Do not leave child in parked car
Check surface heat of car restraint before placing child in seat

Motor vehicles
Transport infant in federally approved rear-facing car seat*
Do not place infant on the seat or in lap
Do not place child in a carriage or stroller behind a parked car

Bodily damage
Avoid sharp, jagged objects
Keep diaper pins closed and away from infant

Age: 4-7 Months

Major Developmental Accomplishments

Rolls over
Sits momentarily
Grasps and manipulates small objects
Resecures a dropped object
Has well-developed eye-hand coordination
Can focus on and locate very small objects
Mouthing very prominent

Injury Prevention

Aspiration
Keep buttons, beads, and other small objects out of infant's reach
Use pacifier with one-piece construction and loop handle
Keep floor free of any small objects
Do not feed infant hard candy, nuts, food with pits or seeds, or whole or circular pieces of hot dogs
Do not feed infant while he is lying down
Inspect toys for removable parts
Avoid balloons as playthings
Discard used button-size batteries; store new batteries in safe area
Keep baby powder, if used, out of reach

Suffocation
May begin to teach swimming as part of water safety
Do not tie toys across crib rails

Falls
Restrain in a high chair
Keep crib rails raised to full height

Poisoning
Make sure that paint for furniture or toys does not contain lead
Place toxic substances on a high shelf or in locked cabinet
Hang plants or place on high surface rather than on floor
Avoid storing large quantities of cleaning fluid, paints, pesticides, and other toxic substances
Discard used containers of poisonous substances
Do not store toxic substances in food containers
Know telephone number of local poison control center (usually listed in front of telephone directory)

Burns
Keep faucets out of reach
Place hot objects (cigarettes, candles, incense) on high surface

Motor vehicles
(See under Birth-4 months)

Bodily damage
Give toys that are smooth and rounded, preferably made of wood or plastic
Avoid long, pointed objects as toys
Avoid toys that are excessively loud
Keep sharp objects out of infant's reach

*Car safety instructions for families are available in Wong, D., and Whaley, L.: Clinical handbook of pediatric nursing, ed. 2, Copyright © 1986, The C.V. Mosby Co., St. Louis.

Continued.

TABLE 10-7

Injury Prevention during Infancy—cont'd

Age: 8-12 Months

Major Developmental Accomplishments

Crawls	Throws objects
Stands, holding onto furniture	Able to pick up small objects
Stands alone	Explores by putting objects in mouth
Cruises around furniture	Dislikes being restrained
Walks	Explores away from parent
Climbs	Increasing understanding of simple commands and phrases
Pulls on objects	Helpless in water

Injury Prevention

Aspiration
(See under 4-7 months)

Suffocation
Keep doors of ovens, dishwashers, refrigerators, and front-loading clothes washers and dryers closed at all times
If storing an unused appliance, such as a refrigerator, remove the door
Fence swimming pools; always supervise when near any source of water, such as cleaning buckets
Keep bathroom doors closed

Falls
Fence stairways at top and bottom if child has access to either end
Dress infant in safe shoes and clothing
Avoid walkers, especially near stairs

Poisoning
Administer medications as a drug, not as a candy
Do not administer medications unless so prescribed by a physician
Replace medications and poisons immediately after use; replace caps properly if a child-protector cap is used
Have syrup of ipecac in home; use only if advised

Burns
Place guards in front of or around any heating appliance, fireplace, or furnace
Keep electrical wires hidden or out of reach
Place plastic guards over electrical outlets; place furniture in front of outlets
Keep hanging tablecloths out of reach
Do not allow infant to play with electrical appliance
Apply a sunscreen when infant is exposed to sunlight

Motor vehicles
Do not use adult seat or shoulder belt without federally approved infant car seat
Do not allow to crawl behind a parked car
If infant plays in a yard, have the yard fenced or use a playpen

Bodily damage
Do not allow infant to use a fork for self-feeding
Use plastic cups or dishes
Check safety of toys and toy box
Protect from young children and animals, especially dogs

The manufacturer's package insert specifies proper storage and reconstitution techniques. Nurses are often responsible for the handling of immunizations. For example, if the vaccine is to be refrigerated, it should be stored on a center shelf, not on the door, where frequent temperature increases from opening the refrigerator can alter the vaccine's potency.

Another important nursing responsibility is accurate documentation. Each child should have an immunization record for parents to keep, especially for families who move frequently. This form and the medical record should include the following information: day, month, and year of administration; manufacturer and lot number of vaccine; and the name, address, and title of the person administering the vaccine (National Childhood Vaccine Injury Act, 1988). The medical record should also include evidence that the parent or legal guardian gave informed consent before the immunization was administered.

INJURY PREVENTION

Injuries are a major cause of death during infancy, especially for children 6 to 12 months old. Constant vigilance, awareness, and supervision are essential as the child gains increased locomotor and manipulative skills that are coupled with an insatiable curiosity about the environment. Table 10-7 lists the major developmental achievements of each period during infancy and the appropriate injury prevention plan.

Motor Vehicle Injuries

Automobile injuries are the leading cause of accidental death in children. Infants die mainly from improper restraint within the vehicle. Consequently, all infants, newborns included, must be secured in a federally approved car restraint rather than held or placed on the seat of the car.

A variety of car seats are available for young children. For infants up to 9 kg (20 pounds) the recommended type is a rear-facing molded plastic shell seat or convertible infant-toddler seat that includes a shoulder restraint and uses the car seat belt (Fig. 10-12). In this position the most dangerous forces in a crash are absorbed by the infant's back.

Generally the middle of the back seat is considered the

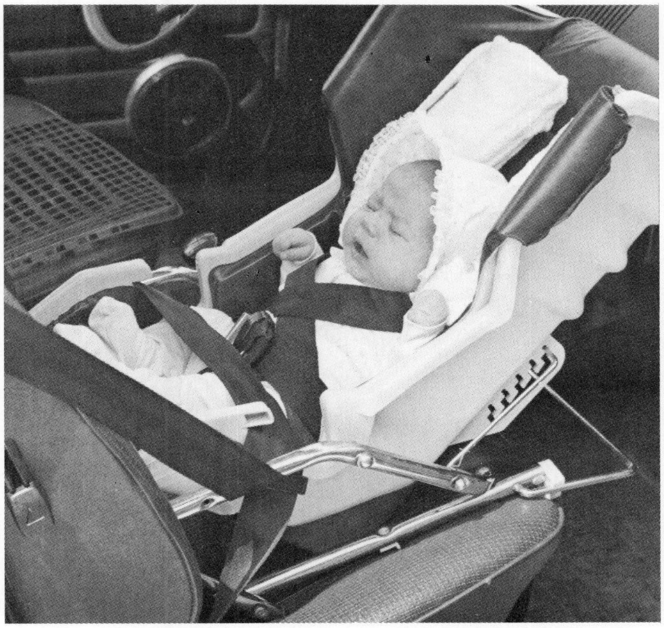

FIG. 10-12 Federally approved infant car restraint. Child's clothing allows proper placement of harness, and rolled blankets on either side of head facilitate proper positioning of child.

safest area of the car. However, with an infant restraint it is preferable to position the child in the front seat, where the driver can observe the infant without having to turn around.

For restraints to be effective they must be used properly. Dressing the infant in an outfit with sleeves and legs allows the harness to be placed correctly. A small blanket or towel rolled tightly can be placed on either side of the head to minimize movement and increase comfort. Although many infant restraints can be recliners, they should only be used in the car in the position specified by the manufacturer. Many of the infant car restraints also serve as baby carriers, a point that should be stressed to parents to encourage their purchasing a suitable restraint. (For further discussion of restraints see Chapter 12.)

Another potential vehicular injury is caused by placing a carriage or stroller behind a car, particularly a car parked in a garage or driveway. It is possible that the driver may not see the small stroller and, while driving in reverse, run over the child. Once the child crawls, he should not be allowed to play in areas where vehicles can be a hazard.

Aspiration of Foreign Objects

Asphyxiation by foreign material in the respiratory tract is the leading cause of fatal injury in males and the second leading cause of fatal injury in females younger than 1 year of age. The size, shape, and consistency of foods or objects are important determinants of fatal obstruction.

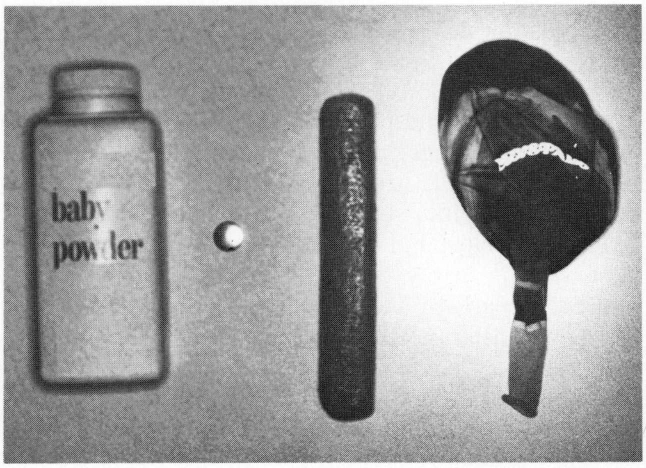

FIG. 10-13 Four common household objects that can be deadly to infants (from left to right): talcum powder, button-size battery, whole hot dog, and balloon.

For example, small (less than 3.2 cm, or 1¼ inches), spheric or cylindric, and pliable objects are most likely to completely obstruct the airway. Unfortunately, common household items can be deadly to infants (Fig. 10-13).

Nonfood items cause the majority of deaths in young children. Balloons, whether partially inflated, uninflated, or popped, cause more deaths in children than any other kind of small object and should be kept away from infants and young children. Another hazard is plastic lining from diapers; the accessibility of the plastic diaper lining both on the infant and/or on dolls is especially dangerous to young children.

As soon as the infant has the ability to find his mouth, he is vulnerable to aspiration of small objects, such as those left within reach or removable parts of objects that may on initial inspection appear safe. Rattles, for example, contain small beads to produce noise. A broken or cracked rattle can be dangerous because the beads can easily be swallowed while the infant has the toy in his mouth. Stuffed animals are another potentially dangerous toy if any of the parts, such as the eyes or nose, are removable buttons or plastic pieces.

All toys must be carefully inspected for potential danger. An active infant can grab a low-hanging mobile and quickly chew off a small piece. As soon as the infant crawls or plays on the floor, the floor must be kept free of any small articles that can be picked up and swallowed, such as coins.

When infant clothes are purchased, the type of closure used should be considered. A front button can easily be pulled off and swallowed. Safety pins for diapers should be kept closed and away from the dressing table. Even though a young infant may not search for them, practicing this good habit from the beginning prevents future injuries.

Food items are the second most common cause of aspiration, and the most frequent offenders are hot dogs, candy, nuts, and grapes (Harris and others, 1984). When new foods are given to the child, nuts, hard candies, or fruits with pits or seeds should be avoided. When traveling, especially in airplanes, or entertaining, snack foods such as peanuts and popcorn should be kept away from young children. If given to young children, hot dogs must be cut into small, irregular pieces rather than served whole or sliced into sections, because their size (diameter), round shape, and consistency allow for complete occlusion of the airway.

Pacifiers can also be dangerous because the entire object may be aspirated if it is small or the nipple and shield may become detached from the handle and become lodged in the pharynx. Improvised pacifiers, such as those commonly made in hospitals from a padded nipple, also present dangers. The nipple may separate from the plastic collar and be aspirated (Millunchick and McArtor, 1986). In addition, parents may continue to offer this pacifier to the infant at home. Safe pacifiers should be of one-piece construction, have a shield or flange that is large enough to prevent entry into the mouth, and have a handle that can be grasped (Fig. 10-14). To prevent the hazards of improvised pacifiers, hospitals should use only safe commercial types.

Another commonly aspirated substance is baby powder, which is usually a mixture of talc (hydrous magnesium silicate) and other silicates. Although the use of talc has been discouraged, it is a common baby care product and can cause severe and often fatal aspiration pneumonia. One of the factors involved in talc aspiration is the similar appearance of baby powder containers and nursing bottles. Talc containers often become favorite playthings and are placed in the mouth. Improper use of powder by sprinkling it directly on the skin creates a cloud of talc dust that is easily inhaled. Parents are advised of the danger of baby powder and discouraged from using it. If they prefer to use a powder, a cornstarch preparation can be substituted. Whenever a powder is used, it should be placed in the hand and then applied to the skin, never shaken directly from the container to the skin. The container is kept closed and immediately stored in a safe place, especially away from curious toddlers who often imitate caregiving activities and may accidentally shake it on the infant.

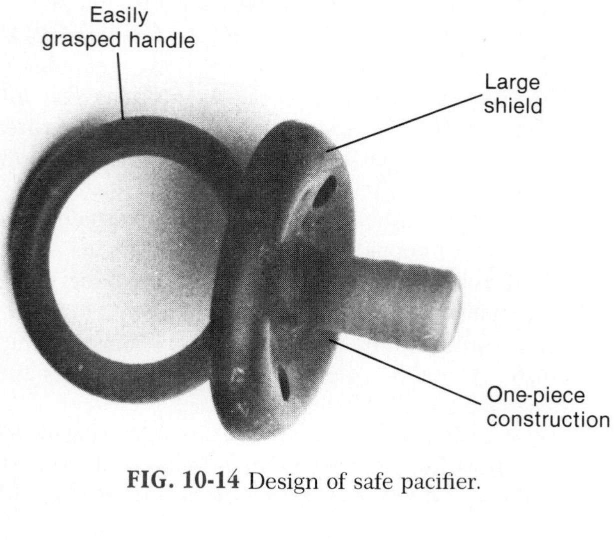

FIG. 10-14 Design of safe pacifier.

Suffocation

Mechanical suffocation is the third leading cause of accidental death in infants and includes suffocation by covering the mouth and nose, by pressure on the throat and chest, and by exclusion of air, such as by refrigerator entrapment.

An infant who is placed in a bed under blankets and sheets that are tucked in can be caught under them and be unable to wriggle free. There are potential dangers in adults sleeping with a small infant because of the possibility of their rolling over and smothering the child. Even though this possibility is slight, the consequent parental guilt if it happens can be devastating.

Another cause of suffocation is plastic bags. Large plastic bags used over garments are very lightweight and can easily and quickly be wrapped around the head of an active infant or pressed against his face. Pillows and mattresses should not be covered with plastic for this reason. Older infants may play with a plastic bag and accidentally pull it over their heads. Because plastic is nonporous, suffocation takes place in a matter of minutes.

Anything tied around the infant's neck can potentially cause strangulation. Bibs should be removed at bedtime, and objects such as pacifiers should never be hung on a string around the infant's neck. This is a common practice in some cultures and can be remedied by attaching a short string tied to a pacifier and pinning the string on the child's shirt.

Toys that have strings attached, such as a telephone, or toys that are tied to cribs or playpens can be hazards because the string can become wrapped around the child's neck or the child can become entrapped in the toy. As a precaution all cords should be less than 30 cm (12 inches) long. Crib toys should be hung high enough that the infant cannot become entangled in them or avoided once the child is able to reach them.

Restraining straps, if applied too loosely or left unfastened, can be a hazard. For example, a child may slide off a high chair beneath the tray and strangle himself on the loose strap. Therefore all straps should be fastened securely.

Infant strangulation may occur if the infant's head becomes caught between the crib slats and mattress or objects close to the crib. According to federal regulation the distance between crib slats should not be more than 2⅜ inches (about 6 cm), roughly the width of three adult fingers. Mattresses and bumper pads should fit snugly against the slats. A general rule is that if two adult fingers can be placed between the mattress and crib side, the mattress is too small. A temporary solution is to place large, rolled towels in the space to create a snug fit. Ideally, information regarding correct crib design should be given prenatally before parents have purchased or borrowed a crib.*

Mesh-sided playpens and cribs can result in death if the sides are left in the lowered position. Infants have suffocated when they fell off the edge of the mattress and the head or chest was compressed between the floorboard and mesh side. Parents should be advised of this danger and encouraged to *always* keep the sides locked securely in the up position whenever the child is in the playpen or crib.

The crib should be positioned away from large furniture, because children who crawl out of the crib may become caught between the two objects. Cribs should also be located away from windows, where drape cords can become wrapped around the infant's neck.

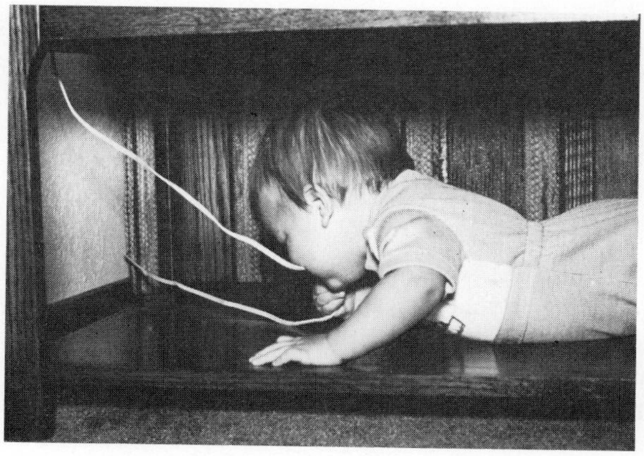

FIG. 10-15 Crawling infants can find hazardous electric wires even in "hidden" areas.

Burns

Burns are often not thought of as a particular danger to infants but are the fourth cause of accidental death. Several important hazards exist, such as scalding from water that is too hot, excessive sunburn, and burns from electrical wires, sockets, and heating elements such as radiators, registers, and floor furnaces. The infant's skin is particularly sensitive to irritation, and the mechanisms for temperature perception are not completely developed. As a general precaution all homes should have smoke alarms installed near the bedroom areas.

Scald burns from hot tap water can be prevented by lowering the hot water heater to a safe temperature of no higher than 49° C (120° F). In addition, the bathwater should be checked before the infant is immersed. If formula or food is warmed in a microwave oven, it must be checked before feeding because the container may remain cool while the contents are hot. Another danger from using a microwave oven to warm a bottle is an explosion from the build-up of steam. Consequently, great caution must be used when warming liquids this way. The handles of cooking utensils should be turned toward the back of the stove. When the infant is underfoot, pouring hot liquids and cooking with hot oil are avoided. Hanging tablecloths are also placed out of the infant's reach.

Sunburn can be a source of a first- or second-degree burn. Exposure to direct sunlight or filtered light through a window should be gradual, about 5 minutes initially. The infant's head should be covered because it represents a large proportion of body surface. Sunscreen agents are helpful and should be applied 20 to 30 minutes before swimming or sweating. Although black-skinned infants burn less readily, their thin skin can become sunburned.

Electrical outlets should be covered with protective plastic caps that prevent the child from sucking on the outlet or putting objects such as hairpins into it (see Fig. 10-17). Live wires are placed out of reach so that curious infants cannot chew on them and break the rubber coating (Fig. 10-15). Infants should not be allowed to play near television sets, stereo units, or other appliances, whether these units are on or off; infants cannot determine when the appliance is safe.

Any heat-producing element should have a guard placed in front of it. Fireplaces should be well screened because they are very appealing and within easy access. Small portable heaters should be placed on a high surface. Floor furnaces should have barrier gates to prevent children from crawling or walking over them. Burning cigarettes, candles, and incense are kept out of reach, and infants should not be held by a smoking adult, because falling ashes are a hazard, especially to the eyes. Heated-mist vaporizers are a source of burns and should not be used. If humidity is needed, only cool-mist vaporizers are safe.

By law all infant sleepwear must be flame retardant. Unfortunately this does not apply to all infant clothing. Flame-retardant fabric must never be viewed as the ultimate protection against burns. Repeated washing reduces the flame-retardant properties, and the use of soap or bleach destroys the protection. Inasmuch as detergent should be used for washing flame-retardant clothing, infants who are sensitive to such wash agents are unprotected when their clothing is washed even with a mild soap. If sleepwear is home sewn, mothers should be advised to look for specially treated flame-retardant fabric.

Another type of thermal injury occurs when children are exposed to excessive heat during confinement in poorly ventilated cars. The practice of leaving the windows open a couple of inches does not appear to be protective. The nurse should caution parents never to leave children in parked cars, especially when the automobile is in direct sunlight.

Children can also be burned by overheated metal hardware and vinyl seats in cars parked in the sun. As a precaution the surface heat of car restraints should be determined before placing children in them. Covering the re-

*The booklet *It Hurts When They Cry* gives basic information on hazards, safety features, and proper use of nursery furniture and equipment. It is available at no charge from U.S. Consumer Product Safety Commission, Washington, DC 20207.

straints and hardware (such as metal latches on seat belts) may be necessary to prevent skin burns. An additional safeguard is buying a light-colored restraint, which absorbs less heat.

Drowning

Drowning is the fifth cause of accidental death in this age-group and can occur in only inches of water. Consequently, infants should never be left unsupervised in a bathtub, hot tub, or near a source of water such as a swimming pool, lake, toilet, or bucket. One way to stress water safety is to teach infants to swim. Infants younger than 6 months of age have two reflexes that enhance swimming. The crawl reflex causes a swimming motion strong enough to propel the infant through water for a short distance. The dive reflex inhibits breathing when the infant is submerged. Most infants, if introduced to the water properly, will not be afraid and can be taught to float and to swim underwater for a few feet. Not until they are 3 or 4 years old can they swim above water for longer distances, because of the proportionately heavy weight of the head. Regardless of swimming instructions, no infant can be expected to learn the elements of water safety or to react appropriately in an emergency. Therefore all young children need to be considered at risk when near water (Fig. 10-16).

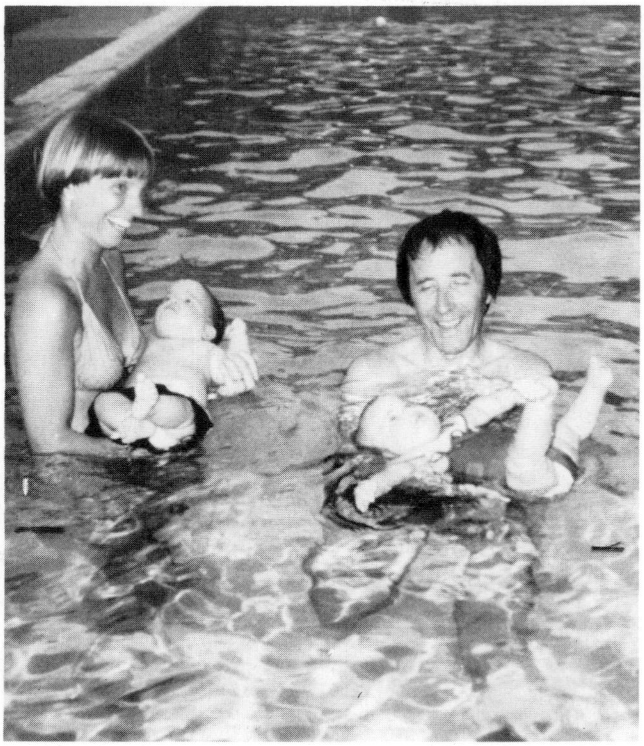

FIG. 10-16 Teaching swimming to infants and young children is one approach to water safety, but infants must always be considered at risk when near any body of water.

Falls

Falls are most common after 4 months of age when the infant has learned to roll over, but they can occur at any age. Newborns are normally active, assume a flexed position, and have crawling and Moro reflexes that can propel them forward. The best advice is never to place a child unattended on a raised surface that has no type of guardrails. When in doubt, the safest place is the floor. Even though young infants cannot climb over a partially raised crib rail, it is best to form a habit of raising the side rail all the way, because someday that infant will be able to climb out. Crib sides should have a latching device that cannot be easily released. Ideally cribs should be placed on carpeted, not hard, floors.

Another danger area for falling is a changing table, which is usually high and narrow. Although these tables have a restraining belt, it is unwise to leave the child unattended even when so restrained. The best way to avoid having to leave is to arrange the area with all necessary articles within easy reach so the child is always in full sight of the caregiver. It only takes a fraction of a second for an infant to fall off. During the latter half of the first year, infants usually resist dressing and diapering and may be difficult to manage. If there is danger that the child is strong enough to resist restraining, he should be changed on the floor.

Infant seats, high chairs, walkers, and swings present additional opportunities for falls. If the infant seat is placed on a table where the infant has an excellent panorama of his environment, he should never be left unrestrained or unattended. The same rule is essential for other baby equipment, particularly when the child has learned to crawl and to stand up. Small infants can slip through a high chair if a protective harness is not used. High chairs are designed for older infants who can sit well and who are tall enough to have the tray at the level of their chest or abdomen. Walkers are responsible for a number of different types of injuries that occur because the walker tipped over or fell down stairs. Parents need to be warned of these dangers and encouraged to keep a constant vigil on their child's activities.

Although the infant begins to develop depth perception by age 9 months, that is no guarantee of his ability to perceive danger. His curiosity may still propel him forward and over, or his immature locomotor skills may be inadequate to keep him from falling even though he is aware of the danger. Infants should not be allowed to crawl unsupervised on any raised surface, near stairs, or near any water reservoir. Gates should be used at the bottom and top of stairs, because both present dangers to the crawling and climbing infant. However, certain types of gates can present hazards. Free-standing enclosures constructed of criss-crossed wood slats that expand and contract can trap the head or neck when children attempt to climb over them. If these types of gates are used, they must be securely fastened to prevent mobility of the slats.

Sometimes even when the environment is made safe

infants may literally trip over their own feet. Slippery socks, hard, slick soles on shoes or rubber soles that can catch, especially on a carpet, and long pants or pajama bottoms can easily upset a child's balance. Such dangers need to be pointed out to parents, especially when the infant is taking his first steps.

Poisoning

The majority of poisonings occur in children younger than 5 years of age. The highest incidence occurs in those in the 2-year-old group, with the second highest incidence in 1-year-old children. The infant who has not learned to crawl is relatively free from danger of poisonous agents by virtue of his confinement. However, once locomotion begins, danger from poisoning is present almost everywhere. There are more than 500 toxic substances in the average home, and about 34% of all poisonings occur in the kitchen.

The major reason for ingestion of poisons is improper storage. Toxic agents placed on a low shelf, table, floor, or unlocked cabinet are accessible to infants. Drugs that are kept in a purse pose additional dangers; if the purse is given to the infant to play with, he may open it and ingest the drug. Another unrecognized hazard is during diaper changes when infants are near many toxic substances such as ointments, creams, oils, and talc. Parents may even hand the infant a potentially poisonous object to quiet him. Such dangers need to be stressed to parents and toys kept at diapering areas to minimize risks.

Poisoning is almost always the result of inadequate supervision, but it may not represent neglect. Children are very fast, and it takes only seconds to eat a bar of soap or a handful of cleanser or detergent. Although infants usually do not possess the manipulative skill to open closed jars, they are amazingly persistent and inventive. For example, an ant trap placed in an out-of-the-way corner is easy for a crawling infant to find.

Plants are another source of poisoning for infants. Plants are frequently placed on the floor, and the leaves or flowers are attractive and easy to pull off. More than 700 species of plants are known to have caused illness or death.

A previously unrecognized danger is ingestion of button-size batteries that are used in devices such as hearing aids, calculators, watches, and cameras. Because they are bright and shiny they are attractive to children. However, they can cause severe morbidity, even death, if lodged in the esophagus. The strong alkali in a battery can leak and cause a severe caustic burn. As a precaution small batteries must be safely stored and discarded where young children cannot easily retrieve them.

The only sure way to prevent poisoning is to remove toxic agents, which means placing them high out of the infant's reach. However, because crawling infants soon become climbing toddlers, it is best to keep all toxic agents, especially drugs, in a locked cabinet. Special plastic hooks can be attached to the inside of cabinet doors to keep them securely closed (see Fig. 10-17). Firm thumb pressure is required to unlatch the hook, and small children are usually unable to manipulate them. Locks are best, but for cleaning agents frequently used, such as under a kitchen sink, hooks are a practical alternative. Impractical suggestions are usually ignored, and some protection is better than none.

With several hundred toxic substances in each house, locking up all potentially toxic substances could present a problem; however, careful planning can help. A large surplus of cleaning agents, furniture polishes, laundry additives, paints, insecticides, and solvents should be avoided. Used poison containers should be promptly discarded and not used to store another poison without adequately marking the package. Inasmuch as young children cannot read, any potentially hazardous substance should not be stored in any type of food container. A popular container used to store toxic liquids is a soda bottle. A child who is unaware of the dangerous contents is a vulnerable victim for poisoning. Parents should know the location of local poison control centers and call them in the event of a suspected poisoning. Emergency measures for poisoning are discussed in Chapter 14.

Bodily Damage

Injuries can occur in numerous ways. Sharp, jagged-edged objects can cause wounds in the skin. Long, pointed articles, such as the common toothpick or fork, can be poked into the eye or ear, causing serious damage. Such articles should be safely stored away from the infant's reach; forks are best avoided for self-feeding until the child has mastered the spoon, usually by age 24 months.

In addition to hazards such as aspiration from toys, small articles can be placed in the ear or nose, and excessive noise from toys can result in sensorineural hearing

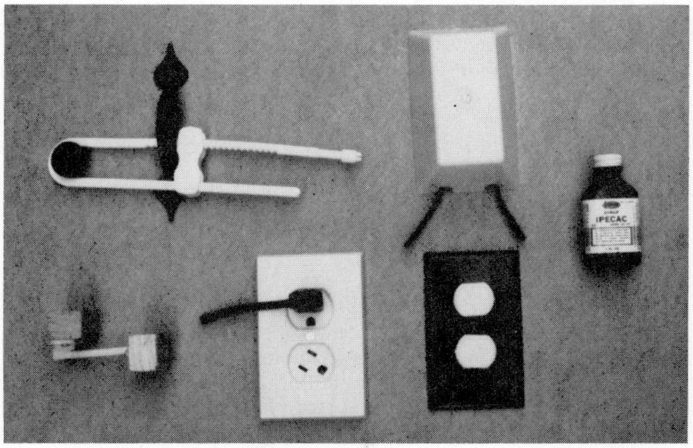

FIG. 10-17 Safety demonstration board (clockwise from lower left): cabinet latch, cabinet lock, shock guard for electrical outlet, syrup of ipecac, and two types of outlet covers (white cover is passive device that automatically covers outlet when plug is removed).

loss. Although toys with the highest noise levels are model airplanes, air guns, toy cap guns, and firecrackers, common squeaking toys used by young children may be harmful if placed close to the ear (Axelsson and Herson, 1985).

Even clothes can present dangers to infants who cannot call attention to the problem. For example, excessively tight bands on socks can cause constriction injuries. Another frequently unrecognized danger to infants is animal attacks and sometimes jealous, older siblings. Helpless infants, as newcomers to the home, can provoke jealousy in the animal or another child. Parents must be constantly vigilant of protecting the child from these potential dangers.

Nurse's Role in Injury Prevention

When the potential environmental dangers to which infants are vulnerable are considered, the task of preventing these injuries only begins to be appreciated. Nurses

Child Safety Home Inventory

Safety: Fire, Electrical, Burns

*Guards in front of or around any heating appliance, fireplace, or furnace
*Electrical wires hidden or out of reach
No frayed or broken wires
*Plastic guards or caps over electrical outlets, furniture in front of outlets
*Hanging tablecloths out of reach and away from open fires
Smoke detectors tested and operating properly
*Kitchen matches stored out of child's reach
Large, deep ashtrays throughout house (if used)
Small stoves, heaters, and other hot objects (cigarettes, candles, coffee pots) placed where they cannot be tipped over or reached by children
Hot water heater set to 125° F or lower
Pot handles turned toward back of stove
No loose clothing worn near stove
No cooking or eating with child nearby or in lap
All small appliances, such as iron, turned off and disconnected when not in use
Cool, not hot, mist vaporizer used
Fire extinguisher available and checked periodically
Electrical fuse box and gas outlet accessible
Family escape plan in case of a fire, and practiced periodically
Telephone number of fire or rescue squad posted near phone

Safety: Poisoning

Toxic substances placed on a high shelf or in locked cabinet
*Toxic plants hung or placed on high surface rather than on floor
Excess quantities of cleaning fluid, paints, pesticides, drugs, and other toxic substances not stored in home
Used containers of poisonous substances discarded where child cannot obtain access
Telephone number of local poison control center posted near phone
Syrup of ipecac in home, with two doses per child
Medicines clearly labeled in childproof containers and stored out of reach; old medicines discarded
Household cleaners, disinfectants, and insecticides kept in their original containers, separate from food and out of reach
Alcoholic beverages stored out of reach
Ashtrays empty or kept out of reach

Safety: Suffocation and Aspiration

*Small objects stored out of reach
*Toys inspected for small removable parts or long strings
*Plastic bags stored away from young child's reach; large plastic garment bags discarded after tying in a knot
*Mattress or pillow not covered with plastic
*Crib design according to federal regulations with snug-fitting mattress
*Crib positioned away from other furniture or windows
*Button-size batteries stored safely and discarded properly, where child will not have access
*Bathroom doors kept closed and toilet seats down
*Faucets turned off firmly
Pool fenced, with locked gate
Proper safety equipment at poolside
Electric garage door openers stored safely and adjusted to raise when door strikes object
*Doors of ovens, trunks, dishwashers, refrigerators, and front-loading clothes washers and dryers closed at all times
*Unused appliance, such as a refrigerator, securely closed with lock or doors removed
*Food served in small noncylindric pieces to young children
*Toy chests with lids that securely lock in open position
*Pails and buckets kept empty
Clothesline above head level

Safety: Bodily Injury

Knives, power tools, and unloaded firearms stored safely or placed in locked cabinet
Garden tools returned to storage racks after use
Pets properly restrained and immunized for rabies
Swings, slides, and other outdoor play equipment kept in safe condition
Yard clear of broken glass, nail-studded boards, and other litter

Safety: Falls

Nonskid mats, abrasive strips, or textured surfaces in tubs and showers
Exits, halls, and passageways in rooms kept clear of toys, furniture, boxes, or other items that could be obstructive
Stairs and halls well lighted, with switches at both top and bottom
Sturdy handrails for all steps and stairways
Nothing stored on stairways
Treads, risers, and carpeting in good repair
Glass doors and walls marked with decals
Safety glass used in doors, windows, and walls
*Gates on top and bottom of staircases
*Guardrails on upstairs windows with locks that limit window opening
*Crib siderails raised to full height; mattress lowered as child grows
*Restraints used in high chairs, walkers, or other baby furniture
Scatter rugs secured in place or used with nonskid backing
Walks, patios, and driveways in good repair

*Safety measures are specific for homes with young children. Appropriate safety measures should be implemented in homes where children reside and visit frequently, such as those of grandparents or babysitters.

must be aware of the possible causes of injury in each age-group to teach *anticipatory* prevention. For example, the guidelines for injury prevention during infancy presented in Table 10-7 should be discussed before the child reaches the susceptible age-group. Preventive teaching ideally occurs during pregnancy. Inasmuch as two thirds of all injuries to children occur in the home, the importance of safety cannot be overemphasized. The box summarizes a home safety inventory plan that can be presented to parents to increase their awareness of danger areas in the home and assist them in implementing safety devices and practices *before* their absence can inflict injury on infants. In addition, displays such as a safety demonstration board (Fig. 10-17) can be helpful in familiarizing parents with inexpensive, commercial devices that can be used in the home to prevent injuries.

Injury prevention requires *protection* of the child and *education* of the parents or caregiver. Nurses in ambulatory care settings, health maintenance centers, or visiting nurse agencies are in a most favorable position for injury education. This does not exclude nurses in inpatient facilities, who could use visiting times as an excellent opportunity for discussing this topic.

One approach to teaching injury prevention is to relate why children in various age-groups are prone to specific types of injuries. Stressing prevention is just as important as emphasizing the *why* of the injury. However, injury prevention must also be practical. For example, suggesting that *all* potentially toxic substances be locked in a cabinet or placed on a high shelf may be so impractical that no change will occur. Asking parents for their ideas leads to realistic suggestions that can be followed. For instance, bathroom cleaning agents, cosmetics, and personal care items can be placed on a top shelf in the linen closet, and towels or sheets can be stored on the lower shelves and floor.

If an injury has occurred, the nurse should not be too quick to admonish the parent. Injuries do not always indicate neglect. It is a difficult task to watch children carefully without overprotecting or unnecessarily confining them. Small falls help children learn the dangers of heights. Touching a hot object once can emphasize to the child the pain of a burn. Allowing children to explore while maintaining *consistent, age-appropriate limits* is sound advice.

Parents need to remember that infants and young children cannot anticipate danger or understand when it is or is not present. A dead electrical wire may present no actual harm, but if the child is allowed to play with it, poor behavior is enforced and will be practiced when the child encounters a live wire. Although it is always wise to explain why something is dangerous, it must be remembered that small children need to be physically removed from the situation.

It is not easy to teach safety, supervise closely, and refrain from saying "no" numerous times a day. Parents become acutely aware of this dilemma as soon as the infant learns to crawl. Preventing injuries to children is usually the first reason for limit setting and discipline, but also to prevent damage to valuable household objects. When small children are in the home, dangerous objects must be removed or guarded and valuable articles placed out of reach. Children, even the youngest crawling infant, will almost always test their parents. It is better to learn a lesson from breaking an inexpensive ashtray than a valuable crystal decanter or by falling off a step stool rather than down a flight of stairs. In either case the lesson is similar, but the price is different.

One additional factor must be stressed concerning injury prevention and education. Children are imitators; they copy what they see and hear. *Practicing safety teaches safety,* which applies to parents and their children and to nurses and their clients. Saying one thing but doing another confuses children and can lead to difficulties as the child grows older.

ANTICIPATORY GUIDANCE—CARE OF FAMILIES

Childrearing is no easy task; it presents challenges to new parents as well as to "seasoned" parents. With society's changing roles and mores, combined with a highly

Parental Guidance during Infant's First Year

First 6 Months

Understand each parent's adjustment to newborn, especially mother's postpartal emotional needs
Teach care of infant and assist parents to understand his individual needs and temperament and that he expresses his wants through crying
Reassure that infant cannot be spoiled by too much attention during the first 4 to 6 months
Encourage parents to establish a schedule that meets needs of child and themselves
Help parents understand infant's need for stimulation in environment
Support parents' pleasure in seeing child's growing friendliness and social response, especially smiling
Plan anticipatory guidance for safety
Stress need for artificial immunization
Prepare for introduction of solid foods

Second 6 Months

Prepare parents for child's "stranger anxiety"
Encourage parents to allow child to cling to mother or father and avoid long separation from either
Guide parents concerning discipline because of infant's increasing mobility
Encourage use of negative voice and eye contact rather than physical punishment as a means of discipline; if unsuccessful, use one slap on the hand
Encourage showing most attention when infant is behaving well, rather than when crying
Teach injury prevention because of child's advancing motor skills and curiosity
Encourage parents to leave child with suitable mother substitute to allow some free time
Discuss readiness for weaning
Explore parents' feelings regarding infant's sleep patterns

mobile population, there is little stability for traditional role models and time-honored methods of raising children. As a result parents look more to professionals for guidance. Nurses are in an advantageous position to render assistance and suggestions. Every phase of a child's life has its particular traumas—toilet training for toddlers, unexplained fears for preschoolers, or identity crises for adolescents. For parents of an infant some challenges center around dependency, discipline, increased mobility, and safety. Major areas for parental guidance during the first year are listed in the box.

SUMMARY

Infancy is the period of the most dramatic developmental progress in physical, psychologic, and cognitive skills during the life span. Each month infants attain new abilities that increase their interaction with the environment. From helpless, completely dependent beings, one-year-old children are mobile, curious, and assertive. They have distinct preferences for significant caregivers, especially the mother, and develop fears of strangers. Such developmental changes bring numerous challenges and concerns to parents, including stranger anxiety, selection of daycare, dealing with habits such as thumb-sucking and pacifiers, and teething.

Health promotion encompasses several critical areas. Nutritional needs change during infancy, as infants cease complete bottle- or breast-feeding for gradual introduction of solid foods during the second half of the year. Parents require guidance in food selection, preparation, and introduction. Infancy is an optimum time to counsel parents regarding healthy dietary habits to avoid underfeeding or overfeeding children.

Prevention of certain diseases begins with routine immunization at 2 months of age. Nurses must be familiar with the recommended schedule and the biologic agents for diphtheria, pertussis, tetanus, measles, mumps, rubella, polio, and *Haemophilus influenzae*. For children at risk for diseases such as influenza virus and hepatitis B, immunization may be given during infancy.

Although injuries do not head the list of infant killers, they are responsible for a significant number of deaths, especially from motor vehicles, aspiration, suffocation, burns, and drowning. Safety education must begin early to eliminate or lessen these hazards from the child's environment.

KEY CONCEPTS

- Biologic development of the child encompasses proportional changes; sensory changes, including binocularity and depth perception; maturation of biologic systems, fine motor development, and gross motor development.
- Erikson's theory of psychosocial development (birth to 1 year) is concerned with acquiring a sense of trust while overcoming a sense of mistrust.
- Piaget's theory of cognitive development, as it applies to the infant, focuses on the sensorimotor phase, which includes the use of reflexes, primary circular reactions, secondary circular reactions, and coordination of secondary schemata and their application to new situations.
- Development of body image begins in infancy; by 1 year of age infants recognize that they are distinct from their parents.
- Social development of the infant is guided by attachment, language development, personal-social behavior, and participation in play.
- Temperament is an important indicator of the kind of interaction that occurs between the child and parents and siblings.
- Parents are faced with many concerns, including infant fears, daycare, limit-setting and discipline, thumb-sucking and pacifier use, teething, and choice of infant shoes.
- Breast milk or formula is the most desirable food for the infant during the first 6 months, followed by gradual introduction of solid food during the second 6 months.
- Infants may be prone to sleep disturbances, and the nurse should instruct the parents, after careful assessment, in adjusting the infant's schedule.
- Fluoride supplements and appropriate dietary intake promote good dental hygiene.
- Recommended routine immunizations include those for diphtheria, tetanus, pertussis, polio, measles, mumps, rubella, and *Haemophilus influenzae* type B.
- Recommended immunizations for selected groups of children are influenza virus, pneumococcal, meningococcal, and hepatitis B vaccines.
- Because injuries are a major cause of death during infancy, parents should be alerted to motor vehicle, aspiration, suffocation, burn, drowning, fall, poisoning, and bodily injuries.

STUDY QUESTIONS AND ACTIVITIES

1 Select three infants of different ages and observe their physical/cognitive abilities. List the observed behaviors in the areas of fine and gross motor skills and language. Compare these with the norms presented in Table 10-3.
2 Interview at least two families with infants who are about 1 year old. Discuss with them any concerns they experienced regarding stranger fear, thumb-sucking or use of pacifier, teething, and weaning.
3 Prepare a teaching plan regarding introduction of solid foods, including food selection, preparation, and method of introduction.
4 Outline an immunization schedule for infants up to 18 months of age. List routes of administration, precautions in administering various vaccines, and possible reactions. Include special immunizations that are recommended for high-risk children.
5 Prepare a teaching plan for injury prevention and identify the ages at which safety precautions for injuries caused by motor vehicles, aspiration, suffocation, burns, drowning, falls, and poisoning should be initiated.

REFERENCES

American Academy of Pediatrics: Report of the Committee on Infectious Diseases, ed. 20, Elk Grove Village, IL, 1986, The Academy.

American Academy of Pediatrics, Committee on Nutrition: The use of whole cow's milk in infancy, Pediatrics **72**(2):253-255, 1983.

Anderson, G.: Pacifiers: the positive side, MCN **11**(2):122-124, 1986.

Axelsson, A., and Jerson, T.: Noisy toys: a possible source of sensorineural hearing loss, Pediatrics **76**(4):574-578, 1985.

Baker, S.P., and Fisher, R.S.: Childhood asphyxiation by choking or suffocation, JAMA **244**(12):1343-1346, 1980.

Carey, W.B., and McDevitt, S.C.: Revision of the infant temperament questionnaire, Pediatrics **61**(5):735-739, 1978.

Elias, M., and others: Sleep/wake patterns of breast-fed infants in the first 2 years of life, Pediatrics **77**(3):322-329, 1986.

Ferber, R.: Diagnosis and treatment of sleep disorders in childhood, Pediatr. Basics **39:**7-14, 1984.

Glendon, M.P.: If the shoe fits . . . wear it, Pediatr. Nurs. **13**(4):230-271, 1987.

Harris, C.S., and others: Childhood asphyxiation by food, JAMA **251:**2231-2235, 1984.

Hinman, A.R.: Prevention of congenital rubella infection: symposium summary, Pediatrics **75**(6):1162-1165, 1985.

Lincoln, L.M.: Fathering and the separation-individuation process, Matern. Child Nurs. J. **13**(2):103-111, 1984.

Millunchick, E., and McArtor, R.: Fatal aspiration of a makeshift pacifier, Pediatrics **77**(3):369-370, 1986.

National Childhood Vaccine Injury Act: requirements for permanent vaccination records and for reporting of selected events after vaccination, MMWR **37**(13):197–200, 1988.

Recommendation of the Immunization Practices Advisory Committee (ACIP): Diphtheria, tetanus, and pertussis: guidelines for vaccine prophylaxis and other preventive measures, MMWR **34**(27):405-426, 1985.

Recommendation of the Immunization Practices Advisory Committee (ACIP): Pertussis immunization: family history of convulsions and use of antipyretics—supplementary ACIP statement, MMWR **36**(18):281-282, 1987.

Recommendation of the Immunization Practices Advisory Committee (ACIP): Update: prevention of *Haemophilus influenzae* type b disease, MMWR **37**(2):13-16, 1988.

Rieder, M.J., Schwartz, C., and Newman, J.: Patterns of walker use and walker injury, Pediatrics **78:**488-493, 1986.

Salomon, M., and others: Evaluation of the two-needle strategy for reducing reactions to DPT vaccination, Am. J. Dis. Child. **141**(7):796-798, 1987.

BIBLIOGRAPHY

Growth and Development

Belfer, M., and Lukens, P.: Body image: impacts and distortions. In Levine, M., and others, editors: Developmental-behavioral pediatrics, Philadelphia, 1983, W.B. Saunders Co.

Castiglia, P.T.: Speech-language development, J. Pediatr. Health Care **1**(3):165-167, 1987.

Chase, R.A., and Rubin, R.R.: The first wondrous year, New York, 1979, Macmillan Publishing Co., Inc.

Erikson, E.: Childhood and society, ed. 2, New York, 1963, W.W. Norton & Co., Inc.

Fraiberg, S.: The magic years, New York, 1968, Charles Scribner's Sons.

Illingworth, R.S.: Development of the infant and young child, ed. 7, New York, 1980, Churchill Livingstone, Inc.

Kaluger, G., and Kaluger, M.F.: Human development: the span of life, ed. 3, St. Louis, 1984, The C.V. Mosby Co.

Knobloch, H., and Pasamanick, B.: Gesell and Amatruda's developmental diagnosis, New York, 1974, Harper & Row, Publishers, Inc.

Lester, B.M.: There's more to crying than meets the ear, Child Care Newsletter **2**(2):1-4, 1983.

Lombardino, L., and others: Evaluating communicative behaviors in infancy, J. Pediatr. Health Care **1**(5):240-246, 1987.

Lowrey, G.H.: Growth and development of children, ed. 8, Chicago, 1986, Year Book Medical Publishers, Inc.

Maier, H.: Three theories of child development, ed. 3, New York, 1978, Harper & Row, Publishers, Inc.

Nelms, B.C.: Attachment versus spoiling, Pediatr. Nurs. **9**(1):49-51, 1983.

Nelms, B.C.: Stress during childhood: long-lasting effects? Pediatr. Nurs. **11**(2):95-98, 1985.

Newman, B., and Newman, P.: Development through life: a psychosocial approach, Homewood, IL, 1984, The Dorsey Press.

Piaget, J.: The construction of reality in the child, New York, 1975, Ballantine Books, Inc.

Reilly, A.P., editor: The communication game, Skillman, NJ, 1980, Johnson & Johnson Baby Products Co.

Sherwen, L.N.: Separation: the forgotten phenomenon of child development, Top. Clin. Nurs. **5**(1):1-11, 1983.

Whitehouse, H.: How infants achieve self-organization and self-confidence: implications for health care professionals and parents, part I, Feelings and Their Medical Significance **29**(5):27-32, 1987.

Zigler, E., and Lang, M.E.: The emergence of "superbaby": a good thing? Pediatr. Nurs. **11**(5):337-342, 1985.

Attachment/Temperament

Als, H.: Assessing infant individuality. In Brown, C.C., editor: Infants at risk, Skillman, NJ, 1981, Johnson & Johnson Baby Products Co.

Blosser, C.: Avoiding potential behavior problems in children, Pediatr. Nurs. **5**(3):11-15, 1979.

Brewer, J.M.H.: The revised infant temperament scale. In Humenick, S.S., editor: Analysis of current assessment strategies in the health care of young children and childbearing families, Norwalk, CT, 1982, Appleton-Century-Crofts.

Carey, W.: Intervention strategies using temperament data. In Brown, C.C., editor: Infants at risk: assessment and intervention, Skillman, NJ, 1981, Johnson & Johnson Baby Products Co.

Chess, S., and Thomas, A.: Temperamental differences: a critical concept in child health care, Pediatr. Nurs. **11**(3):167-171, 1985.

Harris, C.H.: Assessment of children's behavior. In Johnson, S.M., editor: Nursing assessment and strategies for the family at risk, New York, 1986, J.B. Lippincott Co.

Harris, F.G.: Strategies for parenting during the early stages of a child's life, Issues Ment. Health Nurs. **2**(3):71-84, 1980.

Klaus, M.H., and Kennell, J.H., editors: Parent-infant bonding, ed. 2, St. Louis, 1982, The C.V. Mosby Co.

Lamb, J.M.: The rapprochement subphase of the separation-individuation process, Matern. Child Nurs. J. **15**(3):129-138, 1986.

Powell, M.L.: Assessment of infant temperament. In Powell, M.L., editor: Assessment and management of developmental changes and problems in children, ed. 2, St. Louis, 1981, The C.V. Mosby Co.

Roberts, F.B.: Infant behavior and the transition to parenthood, Nurs. Res. **32**(4):213-217, 1983.

Skerrett, K., Hardin, S.B., and Puskar, K.R.: Infant anxiety, Matern. Child Nurs. J. **12**(1):51-59, 1983.

Snyder, C., Eyres, S.J., and Barnard, K.: New findings about mothers' antenatal expectations and their relationship to infant development, MCN **4**(6):354-357, 1979.

Thomas, A., and Chess, S.: Temperament and development, New York, 1977, Brunner/Mazel, Inc.

Ventura, J.N.: Parent coping behaviors, parent functioning, and infant temperament characteristics, Nurs. Res. **31**(5):269-273, 1982.

Concerns Related to Growth and Development

For bibliography on daycare, see Chapter 13.

Alley, J.M., and Rogers, C.S.: Sleep patterns of breast-fed and non-breast-fed infants, Pediatr. Nurs. **12**(5):349-351, 1986.

Bradshaw, T.W.: Teething, Pediatr. Nurs. **7**(3):41-42, 1981.

Chong, A.: Selecting shoes for children, Baby Talk **52**(3):40-42, 1987.

Friman, P.C.: Thumb-sucking in childhood, Feelings and Their Medical Significance **29**(3):11-14, 1987.

Merrifield, E.B., and Ryberg, J.W.: What parents should know about pacifiers, Child. Nurse **3**(4):1-3, 1985.

Musselman, R.J.: Oral facial development and oral habits, Pediatr. Basics **30:**12-14, 1981.

Nutrition

American Academy of Pediatrics, Committee on Nutrition: On the feeding of supplemental foods to infants, Pediatrics **65**(6):1178-1181, 1980.

American Academy of Pediatrics, Committee on Nutrition: Imitation and substitute milks, Pediatrics **73**(6):876, 1984.

American Academy of Pediatrics, Committee on Nutrition: Pediatric nutrition handbook, ed. 2, Elk Grove Village, IL, 1985, The Academy.

American Academy of Pediatrics, Committee on Nutrition: Fluoride supplementation, Pediatrics **77**(5):758-761, 1986.

Anholm, P.C.H.: Breastfeeding: a preventive approach to health care in infancy, Issues Compr. Pediatr. Nurs. **9**(1):1-10, 1986.

Bishop, W.S.: Weaning the breast-fed toddler or preschooler, Pediatr. Nurs. **11**(3):211-214, 1985.

Castiglia, P.T.: Obesity in infants and toddlers, J. Pediatr. Health Care **1**(4):218-220, 1987.

Crummette, B., and Munton, M.: Mothers' decisions about infant nutrition, Pediatr. Nurs. **6**(6):16-19, 1980.

Humphrey, N.: Common questions about breast-feeding, Child. Nurse **3**(2):1-3, 1985.

Lawrence, R.A.: Breast-feeding, ed. 2, St. Louis, 1985, The C.V. Mosby Co.

MacLaughlin, S., and Strelnick, E.G.: Breast-feeding and working outside the home, Issues Compr. Pediatr. Nurs. **7**(1):67-81, 1984.

Pipes, P.L.: Nutrition in infancy and childhood, ed. 4, St. Louis, 1989, The C.V. Mosby Co.

Rogers, C., Morris, S., and Taper, L.: Weaning from the breast: influences on maternal decisions, Pediatr. Nurs. **13**(5):341-345, 1987.

Ross, L.: Weaning practices, J. Nurse Midwife. **26**(1):9-14, 1981.

Satter, E.: Developmental guidelines for feeding infants and young children, Food Nutr. News **56**(4):21-26, 1984.

Wishon, P., and Kinnuk, V.: Helping infants overcome the problem of obesity, MCN **11**(e):118-121, 1986.

Sleep and Activity

Clark, M.K.: Exercise and physical fitness for good health in children, Child. Nurse **4**(1):1-3, 1986.

Edgil, A.E., Wood, K.R., and Smith, D.P.: Sleep problems of older infants and preschool children, Pediatr. Nurs. **11**(2):87-89, 1985.

Osterholm, P., Lindeke, L.L., and Amidon, D.: Sleep disturbance in infants aged 6 to 12 months, Pediatr. Nurs. **9**(4):269-271, 1983.

Romanko, M.V., and Brost, B.A.: Swaddling: an effective invention for pacifying infants, Pediatr. Nurs. **8**(4):259-261, 1982.

Younger, J.B.: The management of night waking in older infants, Pediatr. Nurs. **8**(3):155-158, 1982.

Dental Health

For bibliography, see Chapter 12.

Immunizations

American Academy of Pediatrics, Committee on Infectious Diseases: Prevention of hepatitis B virus infections, Pediatrics **75**(2):362-364, 1985.

American Academy of Pediatrics, Committee on Infectious Diseases: Recommendations for using pneumococcal vaccine in children, Pediatrics **75**(6):1153-1158, 1985.

Bindler, R.M.: Truths and trends in immunization, Child. Nurse **2**(1):1-4, 1984.

Claypool, J.M.: Rubella protection for maternal child health care providers, MCN **6**(1):53-56, 1981.

Hall, C.B.: Influenza: impact and implications for immunization, Immunizations Monitor **1**(1):11-14, 1987.

Hepatitis B vaccine: where to inject it, Am. J. Nurs. **85**(11):1268, 1985.

Longyear, L.A., and Clore, E.R.: Keeping children safe: the *Haemophilus influenzae* type b immunization, J. Pediatr. Health Care **1**(2):73-76, 1987.

Pajares, K.F., Parks, B.R., Jr., and Fischer, R.G.: Rubella vaccination, Pediatr. Nurs. **10**(1):72, 1984.

Recommendation of the Immunization Practices Advisory Committee (ACIP): Inactivated hepatitis B virus vaccine, MMWR **31**(24):317-328, 1982.

Recommendation of the Immunization Practices Advisory Committee (ACIP): Postexposure prophylaxis of hepatitis B, MMWR **33:**285-287, 1984.

Recommendation of the Immunization Practices Advisory Committee (ACIP): Prevention and control of influenza, MMWR **36:**373-387, 1985.

Sklaren, B.C.: The pertussis vaccine: an update, Child. Nurse **4**(3):1-4, 1986.

Whiteman, K.: Why bother about flu shots? Am. J. Nurs. **87**(11):1408-1413, 1987.

Injury Prevention

For additional citations, see bibliography in Chapter 12.

American Academy of Pediatrics, Committee on Accident and Poison Prevention: Injury control for children and youth, Elk Grove Village, IL, 1987, The Academy.

Bass, J.L., and others: Educating parents about injury prevention, Pediatr. Clin. North Am. **32**(1):233-243, 1985.

Bausell, R.B.: A national survey assessing pediatric preventive behaviors, Pediatr. Nurs. **11:**438-442, 1985.

Berger, L.R., and others: Promoting the use of car safety devices for infants: an intensive health education approach, Pediatrics **74**(1):16-19, 1984.

Bergman, A.: Use of education in preventing injuries, Pediatr. Clin. North Am. **29**(2):331-338, 1982.

Dershewitz, R.A., and Christophersen, E.R.: Childhood household safety, Am. J. Dis. Child. **138:**85-88, 1984.

DeSwarte, J.: Nursing's responsibility in promoting the use of car safety seats for children, Home Health Care **2**(1):23-25, 1984.

Gallagher, S.S., Hunter, P., and Guyer, B.: A home injury prevention program for children, Pediatr. Clin. North Am. **32**(1):95-112, 1985.

Greensher, J., and Mofenson, H.C.: Aspiration accidents: choking and drowning, Pediatr. Ann. **12**(10):747-750, 1983.

Hartsell, M.B.: New technology for safety and research, J. Pediatr. Nurs. **2**(3):212-213, 1987.

Holland, S.H.: Car safety for infants, Child. Nurse **2**(5):1-3, 1984.

Surveyer, J.A., and Halpern, J.: Age-related burn injuries and their prevention, Pediatr. Nurs. **7**(5):29-34, 1981.

Wagner, T.J., and Hindi-Alexander, M.: Hazards of baby powder? Pediatr. Nurs. **10**(2):124-125, 1984.

CHAPTER 11

Health Problems during the First Year

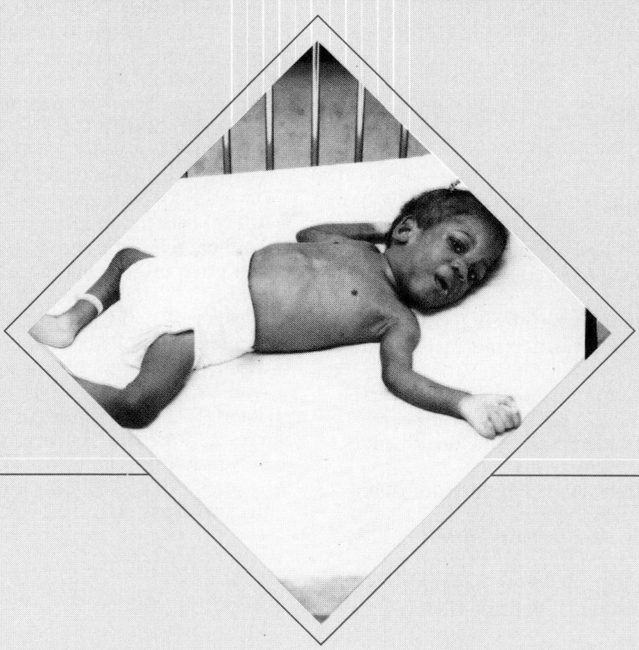

LEARNING OBJECTIVES

On completion of this chapter the reader will be able to:

- Identify children at increased risk of developing nutritional disturbances
- Outline a nutritional counseling plan for vitamin or mineral deficiency and excess
- Outline a dietary plan for parents when the infant is sensitive to milk
- Outline a feeding plan for the child with rumination
- List measures that can be used to alleviate colic
- Identify characteristics of failure-to-thrive children and their families
- Plan nursing care that meets the physical and emotional needs of the failure-to-thrive child and parent
- Provide nursing care that meets the immediate and long-term needs of the family who have lost a child from sudden infant death syndrome
- Identify the stresses and needs of the family whose child is home monitored for apnea
- Identify characteristics of children with autism

The infant's immature physiologic system predisposes him to several potential health problems during the first year. This chapter deals primarily with health problems that are influenced by environmental factors affecting the physical or psychologic development of the child. Some of the problems, such as the nutritional disturbances, have special implications for nurses because they are preventable. Others, such as sudden infant death syndrome, are uncontrollable and unpredictable; however, the intervention needed after the death of the child is crucial for the reintegration of the family. Although several topics discussed here can occur in other age-groups, the greatest significance of these disorders is evident during the early months of life. Prompt awareness and identification of health problems will avert complications in later life. Prevention, whenever possible, rather than treatment should be every health professional's goal in the care of children.

◆ *Nutritional Disturbances*

Malnutrition is a general term that refers to poor or inadequate nutrition. Although it is generally thought of in terms of undernutrition, it also includes overnutrition, which may be manifested as obesity (see p. 480) or hypervitaminosis. Inadequate nutrition is most commonly seen as mineral deficiency, such as iron deficiency anemia (Chapter 25), vitamin deficiencies, or failure to thrive. The most severe states of malnutrition involve the protein and caloric deficiencies, kwashiorkor and marasmus.

VITAMIN DISTURBANCES

True vitamin disturbances are rare in the United States. Subclinical deficiencies are commonly seen, however, especially in lower socioeconomic groups, where dietary intake may be unbalanced. Vitamin deficiencies of the fat-soluble vitamins A and D may occur in malabsorptive disorders. Recently, there has been an increase in vitamin D–deficient rickets. Populations at risk include (1) children born of mothers who are vitamin D deficient, (2) individuals who are exposed to minimal sunlight because of distinctive clothing, housing in areas of high pollution, or dark skin pigmentation, (3) adherents to vegetarian diets that are low in sources of vitamin D, and (4) those who use milk products, such as yogurt or raw cow's milk, as the primary source of milk (Bachrach, Fisher, and Parks, 1979; Saal and others, 1985). Children may also be at risk secondary to disorders or their treatment. For example, children on high-dose salicylate levels, such as for rheumatoid arthritis, may have impaired vitamin C storage (Olness, 1985).

Of equal if not greater concern is the overuse of vitamins. With the addition of vitamins to commercially packaged foods, the potential for hypervitaminosis has escalated, especially when vitamin supplements are used injudiciously. Hypervitaminoses of A and D present the greatest problems because the fat-soluble vitamins are stored in the body. However, it is now well documented that the water-soluble vitamins, B complex and C, can also cause toxicity.

Deficiencies and excesses of vitamins A, B complex, C, D, E, and K are summarized in Table 11-1, and the recommended daily dietary allowances (RDA) are listed in Appendix F. General nursing considerations are discussed on p. 316, and specific interventions are presented in the table.

MINERAL DISTURBANCES

A number of minerals are essential nutrients. The *macrominerals* refer to those with daily requirements greater than 100 mg and include calcium, phosphorus, magnesium, sodium, potassium, chloride, and sulfur. *Microminerals* or *trace elements* have daily requirements less than 100 mg and include several essential minerals and those whose exact role in nutrition is still unclear. The greatest concern with minerals is deficiency, especially iron deficiency anemia (see Chapter 25). However, other minerals that may be inadequate in children's diets include calcium, magnesium, and zinc.

The regulation of mineral balance in the body is a complex process. Dietary extremes of mineral intake can cause a number of mineral-mineral interactions that can result in unexpected deficiencies or excesses. For example, excessive amounts of one mineral, such as zinc, can result in a deficiency of another mineral, such as copper, even if sufficient amounts of copper are ingested. Deficiencies can occur from limited intake of the mineral and also from the interaction of various substances in the diet with minerals. For example, both zinc and calcium are capable of forming insoluble complexes with phytates (found in plant proteins), which can cause a zinc or calcium deficiency. This type of interaction is thought to be important in vegetarian diets.

Deficiencies and excesses of the essential macrominerals and microminerals are summarized in Table 11-2, and the recommended daily dietary allowances (RDA) are listed in Appendix F. General nursing considerations are discussed on p. 316, and specific interventions are presented in the table.

VEGETARIAN DIETS

The importance of vegetarian diets and their relationship to potential nutritional deficiencies in children cannot be overemphasized. The stricter the vegetarian diet, the more difficult it becomes to ensure adequate nutrition for infants and children. The major types of vegetarianism are:

Lacto-ovovegetarians, who exclude meat from their diet but eat milk and eggs and sometimes fish
Lactovegetarians, who exclude meat and eggs but drink milk
Pure vegetarians (vegans), who eliminate any food of animal origin, including milk and eggs
Zen macrobiotics, who are even more restrictive than pure vegetarians in that cereals, especially brown rice, are the mainstay of the diet

Many individuals who are concerned about healthful diets subscribe to vegetarian diets that are not typified by the above categories. Therefore, during nutritional assessment it is necessary to clearly list exactly what the diet includes and excludes.

Text continued on p. 316.

TABLE 11-1

Vitamins and Their Nutritional Significance

Physiologic Functions/Sources	Results of Deficiency or Excess	Nursing Considerations
Vitamin A (retinol)*		
Functions Necessary component in formation of pigment rhodopsin (visual purple) Formation and maintenance of epithelial tissue Normal bone growth and tooth development Needed for growth and spermatogenesis Involved in thyroxine formation ***Sources*** Natural form—liver, kidney, fish oils, milk and nonskimmed milk products, egg yolk Provitamin A (carotene)—carrots, sweet potatoes, squash, apricots, spinach, collards, broccoli, cabbage, artichokes	***Deficiency*** Night blindness Keratinization (hardening and scaling) of epithelium Xerophthalmia (hardening and scaling of cornea and conjunctiva) Phrynoderma (toadskin) Drying of respiratory, gastrointestinal, and genitourinary tracts Defective tooth enamel Retarded growth Impaired bone formation Decreased thyroxine formation	Encourage foods rich in vitamin A, such as whole cow's milk As milk consumption decreases, encourage foods rich in vitamin A
	Excess Early signs—irritability, anorexia, pruritus, fissures at corners of nose and lips Later signs—hepatomegaly, jaundice, retarded growth, poor weight gain, thickening of the cortex of long bones with pain and fragility, hard tender lumps in extremities and occiput of the skull May cause birth defects from excessive maternal intake	Emphasize correct use of vitamin supplements and potential hazards of excess Investigate child's dietary habits to calculate approximate intake; if excessive, remove supplemental source
	NOTE: Overdose only results from ingestion of large quantities of the vitamin, not the provitamin; large amounts of carotene (carotenemia) cause yellow or orange discoloration of the skin (not the sclera, urine, or feces as in jaundice), but none of the above symptoms	Advise parents of the benign nature of carotenemia; treatment is avoidance of excess pigmented fruits or vegetables, especially carrots; skin color returns to normal in 2 to 6 weeks
Vitamin B_1 (thiamine)†		
Functions Coenzyme (with phosphorus) in carbohydrate metabolism Needed for healthy nervous system ***Sources*** Pork, beef, liver, legumes, nuts, whole or enriched grains	***Deficiency*** BERIBERI Gastrointestinal—anorexia, constipation, indigestion Neurologic—apathy, fatigue, emotional instability, polyneuritis, tenderness of calf muscles, partial anesthesia, muscle weakness, paresthesia, hyperesthesia, decreased or absent tendon reflexes, convulsions, and coma (in infants) Cardiovascular—palpitations, cardiac failure, peripheral vasodilation, edema	VITAMIN B COMPLEX Encourage foods rich in B vitamins Stress proper cooking and storage techniques to preserve potency, such as minimal cooking of vegetables in small amount of liquid; storage of milk in opaque container Advise against fad diets that severely restrict groups of food, such as vegetarianism Explore need for vitamin supplements when dieting or when using goat milk exclusively for infant feeding (deficient in folic acid) or when the breast-feeding mother is a strict vegetarian (vitamin B_{12})
	Excess Headache Irritability Insomnia Rapid pulse Weakness	Emphasize correct use of vitamin supplements and potential hazards of excesses
Vitamin B_2 (riboflavin)†		
Functions Coenzyme (with phosphorus) in carbohydrate, protein, and fat metabolism Maintains healthy skin especially around mouth, nose, and eyes ***Sources*** Milk and its products, eggs, organ meats (liver, kidney, and heart), enriched cereals, some green leafy vegetables, legumes	***Deficiency*** ARIBOFLAVINOSIS Lips—cheilosis (fissures at corners of lips), prelèche (inflammation at corners of lips) Tongue—glossitis Nose—irritation and cracks at nasal angle Eyes—burning, itching, tearing, photophobia, corneal vascularization, cataracts Skin—seborrheic dermatitis, delayed wound healing and tissue repair	Same as vitamin B complex
	Excess Paresthesia, pruritus	

*Fat soluble.
†Water soluble.

TABLE 11-1

Vitamins and Their Nutritional Significance—cont'd

Physiologic Functions/Sources	Results of Deficiency or Excess	Nursing Considerations
Niacin (nicotinic acid, nicotinamide)†		
Functions Coenzyme (with riboflavin) in protein and fat metabolism Needed for healthy nervous system, skin, and normal digestion ***Sources*** Meat, poultry, fish, peanuts, beans, peas, whole or enriched grains except corn and rice Milk and its products are sources of tryptophan (60 mg of tryptophan = 1 mg of niacin)	***Deficiency*** PELLAGRA Oral—stomatitis, glossitis Cutaneous—scaly dermatitis on exposed areas Gastrointestinal—anorexia, weight loss, diarrhea, fatigue Neurologic—apathy, anxiety, confusion, depression, dementia Death ***Excess*** Release of vasodilator, histamine (flushing, decreased blood pressure, increased cerebral bloodflow; aggravates asthma) Dermatologic problems (pruritus, rash, hyperkeratosis, acanthosis nigricans) Increased gastric acidity (aggravates peptic ulcer disease) Hepatotoxicity Increased serum uric acid levels Elevated plasma glucose levels Certain cardiac arrhythmias	Same as vitamin B complex
Vitamin B_6 (pyridoxine)†		
Functions Coenzyme in protein and fat metabolism Needed for formation of antibodies, hemoglobin Needed for utilization of copper and iron Aids in conversion of tryptophan to niacin ***Sources*** Meats, especially liver and kidney, cereal grains (wheat and corn), yeast, soybeans, peanuts	***Deficiency*** Scaly dermatitis, weight loss, anemia, retarded growth, irritability, convulsions, peripheral neuritis ***Excess*** Peripheral nervous system toxicity (unsteady gait, numb feet and hands, clumsiness of hands, sometimes perioral numbness) May cause peptic ulcer disease or seizures	Same as vitamin B complex
Folic Acid (folacin; reduced form is called folinic acid or citrovorum factor)†		
Functions Coenzyme for single-carbon transfer (purines, thymine, hemoglobin) Necessary for formation of red blood cells ***Sources*** Green leafy vegetables (spinach), asparagus, liver, kidney, nuts, eggs, whole grain cereals	***Deficiency*** Macrocytic anemia, bone marrow depression, glossitis, intestinal malabsorption ***Excess*** Rare because megadoses not available over the counter May cause insomnia and irritability	Same as vitamin B complex
Vitamin B_{12} (cobalamin)†		
Functions Coenzyme in protein synthesis; indirect effect on formation of red blood cells (particularly on formation of nucleic acids and folic acid metabolism) Needed for normal functioning of nervous tissue ***Sources*** Meat liver, kidney, fish, milk, eggs, cheese, nutritional yeast, sea vegetables	***Deficiency*** PERNICIOUS ANEMIA (one form of deficiency from absence of intrinsic factor in gastric secretions) General signs of severe anemia Lemon yellow tinge to skin Spinal cord degeneration ***Excess*** Excess is rare	Same as vitamin B complex

*Fat soluble.
†Water Soluble.

Continued.

TABLE 11-1

Vitamins and Their Nutritional Significance—cont'd

Physiologic Functions/Sources	Results of Deficiency or Excess	Nursing Considerations
Biotin		
Functions Coenzyme in carbohydrate, protein, and fat metabolism Interrelated with functions of other B vitamins ***Sources*** Liver, kidney, egg yolk, tomatoes, legumes, nuts	***Deficiency*** Deficiency is uncommon because synthesized by bacterial flora ***Excess*** Unknown	Same as vitamin B complex
Pantothenic Acid†		
Functions Coenzyme in carbohydrate, protein, and fat metabolism Synthesis of amino acids, fatty acids, and steroids ***Sources*** Liver, kidney, heart, salmon, eggs, vegetables, legumes, whole grains	***Deficiency*** Deficiency is uncommon because of its multiple food sources and synthesis by bacterial flora ***Excess*** Minimum toxicity (occasional diarrhea and water retention)	Same as vitamin B complex
Vitamin C (ascorbic acid)†		
Functions Essential for collagen formation Increases absorption of iron for hemoglobin formation Enhances conversion of folic to folinic acid Affects cholesterol synthesis and conversion of proline to hydroxyproline Probably a coenzyme in metabolism of tyrosine and phenylalanine May play role in hydroxylation of adrenal steroids May have stimulating effect on phagocytic activity of leukocytes and formation of antibodies Antioxidant agent (spares other vitamins from oxidation)	***Deficiency*** SCURVY Skin—dry, rough, petechiae, perifollicular hyperkeratotic papules (raised areas around hair follicles) Musculoskeletal—bleeding into muscles and joints, pseudoparalysis from pain, swelling of joints, costochondral beading (scorbutic rosary) Gums—spongy, friable, swollen, bleed easily, bluish red or black color, teeth loosen and fall out General disposition—irritable, anorexic, apprehensive, in pain, refuses to move, assumes semi-froglike position when supine (scorbutic pose) Signs of anemia Decreased wound healing	Encourage foods rich in vitamin C Investigate infant's diet for sources of vitamin, especially when cow's milk is principal source of nutrition Stress proper cooking and storing techniques to preserve potency Wash vegetables quickly; do not soak in water Cook vegetables in covered pot with minimal water and for short time; avoid copper or cast iron cookware Do not add baking soda to cooking water Use fresh fruits and vegetables as soon as possible; store in refrigerator Store juice in airtight opaque container
Sources Citrus fruits, strawberries, tomatoes, potatoes, melon, cabbage, broccoli, papaya, mango	Increased susceptibility to infection	In caring for child with scurvy: Position for comfort and rest Handle very gently and minimally Administer analgesics as needed Prevent infection Provide good oral care Provide soft, bland diet Emphasize rapid recovery when vitamin is replaced
	Excess Diarrhea Increased excretion of uric acid and acidification of urine (may cause urate precipitation and formation of oxalate stones) Hemolysis Impaired leukocytosis activity Damage to beta cells of pancreas and decreased insulin production Reproductive failure "Rebound scurvy" from withdrawal of large amounts	Emphasize correct use of vitamin supplement and potential hazards of excess Identify groups at risk for vitamin C supplements; those with thalassemia; those on anticoagulant or aminoglycoside antibiotic therapy

*Fat soluble.
†Water soluble.

TABLE 11-1

Vitamins and Their Nutritional Significance—cont'd

Physiologic Functions/Sources	Results of Deficiency or Excess	Nursing Considerations
Vitamin D_2 (ergocalciferol) and D_3 (cholecalciferol)*		
Functions Absorption of calcium and phosphorus and decreased renal excretion of phosphorus ***Sources*** Direct sunlight Cod liver oil, herring, mackerel, salmon, tuna, sardines Enriched food sources—milk, milk products, cereals, margarine, breads, many breakfast drinks	***Deficiency*** RICKETS Head—craniotabes (softening of cranial bones, prominence of frontal bones), deformed shape (skull flat and depressed toward middle), delayed closure of fontanels Chest—rachitic rosary (enlargement of costochondral junction of ribs), Harrison groove (horizontal depression in lower portion of rib cage), pigeon chest (sharp protrusion of sternum) Spine—kyphosis, scoliosis, lordosis Abdomen—potbelly, constipation Extremities—bowing of arms and legs, knock-knee, saber shins, instability of hip joints, pelvic deformity, enlargement of epiphysis at ends of long bones Teeth—delayed calcification, especially of permanent teeth Rachitic tetany—seizures	Encourage foods rich in vitamin D, especially fortified cow's milk In breast-fed infants encourage use of vitamin D supplements if maternal diet inadequate or infant exposed to minimal sunlight Emphasize importance of exposure to sun as source of vitamin In caring for child with rickets: Maintain good body alignment Reposition frequently to prevent decubiti and respiratory infection Handle very gently and minimally Prevent infection Institute seizure precautions Have 10% calcium gluconate available in case of tetany Observe for possibility of overdose from supplements If prescribed, supervise proper use of orthopedic splints or braces
	Excess Acute—vomiting, dehydration, fever, abdominal cramps, bone pain, convulsions, and coma Chronic—lassitude, mental slowness, anorexia, failure to thrive, thirst, urinary urgency, polyuria, vomiting, diarrhea, abdominal cramps, bone pain, pathologic fractures Calcification of soft tissue—kidneys, lungs, adrenal glands, vessels (hypertension), heart, gastric lining, tympanic membrane (deafness) Osteoporosis of long bones Elevated serum levels of calcium and phosphorus	Same as vitamin A; may include low-calcium diet during initial therapy
Vitamin E (tocopherol)*		
Functions Production of red blood cells and protection from hemolysis Muscle and liver integrity Coenzyme factor in tissue respiration Minimizes oxidation of polyunsaturated fatty acids and vitamins A and C in intestinal tract and tissues ***Sources*** Vegetable oils, wheat germ oil, milk, egg yolk, muscle meats, fish, whole grains, nuts, legumes, spinach, broccoli	***Deficiency*** Hemolytic anemia from hemolysis caused by shortened life of red blood cells, especially in premature infants, and focal necrosis of tissues Causes infertility in rats, but not in humans (does *not* increase human male virility or potency) ***Excess*** Little is known: less toxic than other fat-soluble vitamins but excess of water-soluble preparations has been fatal in premature infants	Initiate early feeding in premature infants; may need supplementation

*Fat soluble.
†Water soluble.

Continued.

TABLE 11-1

Vitamins and Their Nutritional Significance—cont'd

Physiologic Functions/Sources	Results of Deficiency or Excess	Nursing Considerations
Vitamin K*		
Functions	***Deficiency***	
Catalyst for production of prothrombin and blood clotting factors II, VII, IX, and X by the liver	Hemorrhage	Administer prophylactically to newborns Other indications include intestinal disease, lack of bile, prolonged antibiotic therapy; may be used in management of blood-clotting time when anticoagulants such as dicumarol (bishydroxycoumarin), which are vitamin K antagonists, are used
Sources		
Pork, liver, green leafy vegetables (spinach, kale, cabbage), tomatoes, egg yolk, cheese		
	Excess	
	Hyperbilirubinemia in infants Hemolytic anemia in individuals who are deficient in glucose-6-phosphate dehydrogenase	

*Fat soluble.
†Water soluble.

The lacto-ovovegetarian diet is associated with the least deficiencies, although protein intake needs to be monitored. The lactovegetarian diet may also be low in protein, as well as iron. The major deficiencies in the stricter vegetarian diets are inadequate protein for growth, inadequate calories for energy and growth, poor digestibility of many of the natural, unprocessed foods, especially for infants, and deficiencies of vitamin B_{12}, niacin, thiamine, riboflavin, vitamin D, iron, calcium, and zinc. In the United States strict vegetarian diets are common among members of Black Muslim or Seventh Day Adventist faiths.

Nursing Considerations

Identification of nutrient imbalance is the initial nursing goal and requires assessment based on a dietary history and physical examination for signs of deficiency or excess (pp. 122-125). Once assessment data are collected, this information is evaluated against standard intakes to identify areas of concern. The most widely used standard is the Recommended Dietary Allowances (RDA), developed by the National Academy of Sciences, Food and Nutrition Board (see Appendix F). The RDA are not average requirements but recommendations intended to meet the physiologic needs of almost every healthy person. To meet the needs of those with the highest requirements, the RDA will exceed most people's requirements. Therefore, children consuming less than the RDA are not necessarily consuming an inadequate diet, but they are more likely at risk for deficiency than those who are consuming nutrients in amounts equal to the RDA.

Achieving a nutritionally adequate vegetarian diet (with the exception of strictest diets) is not difficult, but it requires careful planning and knowledge of nutrient sources.* For children, the lacto-ovovegetarian diet is nutritionally adequate; however, the vegan diet requires supplementation with vitamins D and B_{12} for children ages 2 to 12 years. Infants should be breast-fed for the first 6 months and preferably for 1 year, be fed solid foods after about 4 months, and receive iron-fortified cereal for at least 18 months. The use of vitamin C juices with foods high in iron will further improve iron absorption. However, breast milk from vegetarian mothers can be deficient in vitamin B_{12}; supplementation of both mother and child is advisable. If cow's or human milk is not given, fortified soy milk is recommended (Fanelli and Kuczmarski, 1983). When solid foods are introduced, the safety and digestibility of the selections must be considered. Raw fruits with seeds, vegetables, and nuts are hazardous for young children because of the danger of aspiration. Beans, grain cereals, and vegetables should be served well cooked and mashed during infancy. A variety of foods should be introduced during the early years to ensure a more well-balanced intake.

To ensure sufficient protein in the diet, foods with incomplete proteins (those that do not have all the essential amino acids) should be eaten at the same meal with other foods that supply the missing amino acids. The three basic combinations of foods consumed by vegetarians that generally provide the appropriate amounts of essential amino acids are:

grains (cereal, rice, pasta) and **legumes** (beans, peas, lentils, peanuts)
grains and **milk products** (milk, cheese, yogurt)
seeds (sesame, sunflower) and **legumes**

*A helpful book for families is *Teddy Bears & Bean Sprouts: The Infant and Vegetarian Nutrition,* which is available from Gerber Products Co., 445 State St., Fremont, MI 49412.

Text continued on p. 321.

TABLE 11-2

Minerals and Their Nutritional Significance

Physiologic Functions/Sources	Results of Deficiency or Excess	Nursing Considerations
Calcium		
Functions Bone and tooth development and maintenance (in combination with phosphorus) Muscle contractions, especially the heart Blood clotting Absorption of vitamin B_{12} Enzyme activation Nerve conduction Integrity of intracellular cement substances and various membranes ***Sources*** Dairy products, egg yolk, sardines, canned salmon with bones, dark-green leafy vegetables, soybeans, dried beans, and peas	***Deficiency*** RICKETS Tetany Impaired growth, especially of bones and teeth ***Excess*** Drowsiness, extreme lethargy Impaired absorption of other minerals (iron, zinc, manganese) Calcium deposits in tissues (renal failure)	Encourage foods rich in calcium, especially dairy products Caution that oxalates in leafy vegetables, oxalates in chocolates, and a high phosphorus intake (especially from carbonated beverages) can decrease calcium absorption Discourage use of whole cow's milk in newborns because the high phosphorus-to-calcium ratio favors excretion of calcium Advise against fad diets, especially those that restrict dairy products Emphasize correct use of calcium supplement, especially the possible interaction between megadoses of calcium and resulting deficiency states of other minerals
Chloride		
Functions Acid-base and fluid balance Enzyme activation in saliva Component of hydrochloric acid in stomach ***Sources*** Salt, meat, eggs, dairy products, many prepared and preserved foods	***Deficiency*** Acid-base disturbances (hypochloremic alkalosis, dehydration); occurs mostly in combination with sodium loss ***Excess*** Acid-base disturbance	Deficiency and excess are unusual; most diets supply adequate chloride (usually in combination with sodium) Disease states such as excessive vomiting can necessitate chloride replacement
Chromium		
Functions Involved in glucose metabolism and energy production ***Sources*** Meat, cheese, whole grain breads and cereals, legumes, peanuts, brewer's yeast, vegetable oils	***Deficiency*** Possible abnormal glucose metabolism ***Excess*** Unknown	No specific recommendations are needed
Copper		
Functions Production of hemoglobin Essential component of several enzyme systems ***Sources*** Organ meats, oysters, nuts, seeds, legumes, corn oil margarine	***Deficiency*** Anemia, leukopenia, neutropenia ***Excess*** Severe vomiting and diarrhea Hemolytic anemia	Deficiency from inadequate food sources is less likely than from excess intake of other minerals, especially zinc and possibly iron; therefore emphasize the correct use of any vitamin supplement Caution against cooking acid foods in unlined copper pots, which can lead to chronic and toxic accumulation of copper

Continued.

TABLE 11-2

Minerals and Their Nutritional Significance—cont'd

Physiologic Functions/Sources	Results of Deficiency or Excess	Nursing Considerations
Fluorine		
Functions Formation of caries-resistant teeth Strong bone development ***Sources*** Fluoridated water and foods or beverages prepared with fluoridated water; fish, tea, commercially prepared chicken for infants	***Deficiency*** Increased susceptibility to tooth decay	In areas with optimally fluoridated water, encourage sufficient intake to supply recommended amount of fluoride (see p. 356) In areas of unfluoridated water or when ready-to-use formula or breast milk are used, stress the importance of fluoride supplements
	Excess FLUOROSIS (mottling and/or pitting of enamel) Severe bone deformities	In areas with excess fluoride in the water, consider the use of bottled water in drinking and possibly cooking to reduce the fluoride intake to safe levels Fluorine has the narrowest range of safe and adequate intake; therefore, stress the importance of storing supplements in a safe area
Iodine		
Functions Production of thyroid hormone Normal reproduction	***Deficiency*** GOITER (enlarged thyroid from decreased thyroxine formation)	Encourage use of iodized salt for individuals living far from the sea
Sources Seafood, kelp, iodized salt, sea salt, enriched bread, milk (from dairy processing)	***Excess*** Unknown from food sources; may occur from ingestion of iodine preparations, such as saturated solutions of potassium iodide (SSKI)	If iodine preparations are in the home, stress the importance of safe storage
Iron		
Functions Formation of hemoglobin and myoglobin Essential part of several enzymes and proteins ***Sources*** Liver, especially pork, followed by calf, beef, and chicken; kidney, red meat, poultry, shellfish, whole grains, enriched cereals and bread, legumes, nuts, seeds, green leafy vegetables, dried fruits, potatoes, molasses, iron-enriched infant formula and cereal	***Deficiency*** ANEMIA (see p. 820)	Encourage foods rich in iron Discourage excessive milk consumption, especially more than 1 liter per day (milk is a very poor source of iron) If iron supplements are prescribed, teach parents factors that affect absorption (see box below)
	Excess Hemosiderosis (excess iron storage in various tissues of the body, especially the spleen, liver, lymph glands, heart, and pancreas) Hemochromatosis (excess iron storage with cellular damage)	Stress the importance of storing iron supplements in a safe area

Factors That Affect Iron Absorption

Increase	Decrease
Acidity (low pH)—administer iron between meals (gastric hydrochloric acid)	Alkalinity (high pH)—avoid any antacid preparation
Ascorbic acid (vitamin C)—administer iron with juice, fruit, or multivitamin preparation	Phosphates—milk is unfavorable vehicle for iron administration
Calcium	Phytates—found in cereals
Tissue need	Oxalates—found in many fruits and vegetables (plums, currants, green beans, spinach, sweet potatoes, tomatoes)
Meat, fish, poultry	Tannins—found in tea, coffee
Cooking in cast iron pots	Tissue saturation
	Malabsorptive disorders
	Disturbances that cause diarrhea or steatorrhea
	Infection

TABLE 11-2

Minerals and Their Nutritional Significance—cont'd

Physiologic Functions/Sources	Results of Deficiency or Excess	Nursing Considerations
Magnesium		
Functions Bone and tooth formation Production of proteins Nerve conduction to muscles Activation of enzymes needed for carbohydrate and protein metabolism ***Sources*** Whole grains, nuts, soybeans, meat, green leafy vegetables (uncooked), tea, cocoa, raisins	***Deficiency*** Tremors, spasm Irregular heartbeat Muscular weakness Lower extremity cramps Convulsions, delirium ***Excess*** Nervous system disturbances due to imbalance in calcium-to-magnesium ratio	Deficiency and excess are unusual, except in disease states such as prolonged vomiting or diarrhea or kidney dysfunction, where replacement may be needed
Manganese		
Functions Activation of enzymes involved in reproduction, growth, and fat metabolism Normal bone structure Nervous system functioning ***Sources*** Nuts, whole grains, legumes, green vegetables, fruit	***Deficiency*** Unknown ***Excess*** Unknown	No specific recommendations are needed
Molybdenum		
Functions Essential component of several oxidative enzymes ***Sources*** Legumes, whole grains, organ meats, some dark green vegetables	***Deficiency*** Very rare; diagnosed in patients on complete total parenteral alimentation ***Excess*** Produces secondary copper deficiency (growth failure, anemia, and disturbed bone development)	No specific recommendations are needed
Phosphorus		
Functions Bone and tooth development (in combination with calcium) Involved in numerous chemical reactions, including protein, carbohydrate, and fat metabolism Acid-base balance ***Sources*** Dairy products, eggs, meat, poultry, legumes, carbonated beverages	***Deficiency*** Weakness, anorexia, malaise, bone pain ***Excess*** Produces secondary calcium deficiency from disturbed calcium-to-phosphorus ratio	Dietary deficiency is uncommon, although prolonged use of antacids can produce deficiency, in which case supplementation is recommended To preserve calcium-to-phosphorus ratio in newborns, discourage use of whole cow's milk
Potassium		
Functions Acid-base and fluid balance (major extracellular fluid areas) Nerve conduction Muscular contraction, especially the heart Release of energy ***Sources*** Bananas, citrus fruit, dried fruits, meat, fish, bran, legumes, peanut butter, potatoes, coffee, tea, cocoa	***Deficiency*** Cardiac arrhythmias Muscular weakness Lethargy Kidney and respiratory failure Heart failure ***Excess*** Cardiac arrhythmias Respiratory failure Mental confusion Numbness of extremities	Dietary deficiency and excess are unlikely, although disease states such as prolonged nausea and vomiting, or the use of diuretics can result in hypokalemia; in such instances, encourage replacement with supplements of rich food sources, such as bananas

TABLE 11-2

Minerals and Their Nutritional Significance—cont'd

Physiologic Functions/Sources	Results of Deficiency or Excess	Nursing Considerations
Selenium		
Functions Antioxident, especially protective of vitamin E Protects against toxicity of heavy metals Associated with fat metabolism	***Deficiency*** Keshan disease—cardiomyopathy in children (found in China)	Deficiency and excess are uncommon in North America, although selenium deficiency can occur in patients on prolonged total parenteral alimentation; in these instances supplementation is required
Sources Seafood, organ meats, egg yolk, whole grain, chicken, meat, tomatoes, cabbage, garlic, mushrooms, milk	***Excess*** Eye, nose, and throat irritation Increased dental caries Liver and kidney degeneration	
Sodium		
Functions Acid-base and fluid balance (major extracellular fluid cation) Cell permeability; absorption of glucose Muscle contraction	***Deficiency*** Dehydration Hypotension Convulsions Muscle cramps	Deficient intake is very rare, although losses secondary to nausea, vomiting, excessive sweating, and use of diuretics can occur and require replacement
Sources Table salt, seafood, meat, poultry, numerous prepared foods	***Excess*** Edema Hypertension Intracranial hemorrhage	Encourage parents to limit excessive use of salt in preparing foods and commercial foods with high sodium content, such as smoked meats
Sulfur		
Functions Essential component of cell protein, especially of hair and skin Enzyme activation Associated with energy metabolism Detoxification of certain chemical reactions	***Deficiency*** Unknown ***Excess*** Unknown	No specific recommendations are needed
Sources Dairy products, eggs, meat, fish, nuts, legumes		
Zinc		
Functions Component of about 100 enzymes Synthesis of nucleic acids and protein in immune system and coagulation Release of vitamin A from liver Improved wound healing with vitamin C ***Sources*** Seafood (especially oysters), meat, poultry, eggs, wheat, legumes	***Deficiency*** Loss of appetite Diminished taste sensation Delayed healing Skin lesions—erythematous, crusted lesions around body orifices Alopecia Diarrhea Growth failure Retarded sexual maturity	Encourage food sources rich in zinc, especially protein Caution that fiber, phytates, oxalates, tannins (in tea or coffee), and iron and calcium adversely affect zinc absorption Recognize groups at risk for zinc deficiency, such as vegetarians and Mexican-Americans, whose diets may have restricted or low meat content and high fiber, phytate content; and patients with malabsorption syndromes
	Excess Vomiting and diarrhea Malaise, dizziness Anemia, gastric bleeding Impaired absorption of calcium and copper	Emphasize correct use of zinc supplements and the possible interaction with other minerals

PROTEIN AND CALORIE MALNUTRITION

Hunger is one of the world's gravest and most prevalent health problems, especially in underdeveloped or third world countries, where in the 1- to 4-year-old age-group the death rate may be 20 to 50 times higher than in the United States. However, even in the United States, the protein and calorie malnutrition (PCM) diseases of kwashiorkor and marasmus occur, primarily (1) as a complication of an underlying disease process, (2) as a result of fad diets, such as some types of vegetarianism, (3) from lack of parental education regarding infant nutrition, (4) from incorrect preparation of formula, such as adding extra water because of ignorance, economic need, or exaggerated concerns about excessive food intake, or (5) from inappropriate management of food allergy, for example, the use of high-fat, low-protein, nondairy creamer as a substitute for milk.

KWASHIORKOR

Kwashiorkor is a deficiency of protein with an adequate supply of calories. The word comes from the Ghan language and means "the sickness the older child gets when the next baby is born." It is an appropriate name because the syndrome develops in the first child, usually between 1 and 4 years of age, when he is weaned from the breast and fed a diet consisting mainly of starch grains or tubers once the second child is born. Such a diet provides adequate calories in the form of carbohydrates but an inadequate amount of high-quality proteins.

The child with kwashiorkor has thin, wasted extremities and a prominent abdomen from edema (ascites). The edema often masks the severe muscular atrophy, making the child appear less debilitated than he actually is. The skin is scaly and dry and has areas of depigmentation. Several dermatoses may be evident, partly resulting from the vitamin deficiencies. Permanent blindness often results from the severe lack of vitamin A. Mineral deficiencies are common, especially iron, calcium, and zinc. The hair is thin, dry, coarse, and dull. Depigmentation is common, and patchy alopecia may occur.

Diarrhea frequently results from a lowered resistance to infection. Gastrointestinal disturbances include reversible fatty infiltration of the liver and atrophy of the acinar cells of the pancreas. Behavioral changes are evident as the child grows progressively irritable, lethargic, withdrawn, and apathetic. Fatal deterioration may be caused by diarrhea and infection or as the result of circulatory failure.

MARASMUS

Marasmus is the result of general malnutrition of both calories and protein. It is a common occurrence in underdeveloped countries during times of drought. In some cultures, adults, especially men, eat first, and the remaining food is often insufficient in quality and quantity for the children.

However, marasmus is usually a syndrome of physical and emotional deprivation that is not confined to geographic areas where food supplies are inadequate. It may be seen in children with failure to thrive, where the cause is not solely nutritional but primarily emotional, and in individuals with an excessive desire for thinness (see Anorexia nervosa, p. 486).

Marasmus is characterized by gradual wasting and atrophy of body tissues, especially of subcutaneous fat. The child appears to be very old; his skin is flabby and wrinkled, unlike the child with kwashiorkor who appears more rounded from the edema. Fat metabolism is less impaired than in kwashiorkor, so that deficiency of fat-soluble vitamins is usually minimal or absent.

The child is fretful, apathetic, withdrawn, and so lethargic that prostration frequently occurs. Intercurrent infection with debilitating diseases, such as tuberculosis, parasitosis, and dysentery, is common.

Therapeutic Management

Treatment of PCM includes providing a diet high in quality proteins and/or carbohydrates, vitamins, and minerals. Electrolyte imbalance requires immediate attention, and parenteral fluid replacement may be necessary initially to correct the dehydration and restore renal function. When oral fluids and food are not tolerated, hyperalimentation is lifesaving. Coexisting problems, such as infection, diarrhea, parasitic infestation, and anemia, require prompt attention for optimum recovery.

Nursing Considerations

Provision of essential physiologic needs, such as rest, individually tailored activity, and protection from infection, is paramount. Since the child is usually weak and withdrawn, he depends on others to feed him. Hygiene may be distressing because of the poor integrity of the skin, and decubiti are a constant threat. Appropriate developmental stimulation should be provided also.

The larger problem is the prevention of these conditions through education concerning the importance of high-quality proteins and adequate carbohydrates. Since children with marasmus may suffer from emotional starvation as well, care should be consistent with care of the child with failure to thrive (p. 327).

FOOD INTOLERANCE

Food intolerance is a broad term that includes any adverse response to food. Although the terms *food allergy* and *food sensitivity* are used interchangeably, food allergy is applied to immediate onset reactions. Food allergies are most common during infancy, and the chief offenders are cow's milk, eggs, and wheat. Food sensitivity usually includes those reactions that are delayed and comprise a complex of symptoms, such as gluten-sensitive enteropathy (celiac disease).

Food intolerance can occur in anyone at any age, and frequently the allergic response is exhibited after the food has been ingested one or more times. Food allergies are common during infancy because the infant is exposed to many new food antigens. Physiologically the intestinal tract is immature and is permeable to many more inadequately catabolized proteins, which, unlike the amino acids that compose them, are capable of producing an allergic response. As the intestinal tract matures, many food allergies disappear.

There is some evidence that nutritional allergies can be delayed and possibly prevented. In families with a history of allergy, mothers may be advised to exclusively breast-feed for 6 months or longer to reduce the child's chances of developing antibodies to cow's milk protein. The mother also needs to avoid ingesting all milk products while breast-feeding and during the last trimester of pregnancy (such mothers usually need calcium supplements). If a child has a strong family history of allergy, certain foods should be avoided during the first year.

Table 11-3 lists common foods that are potentially allergenic. Soy-based formula is recommended as a substitute for cow's milk formulas in infants at risk for developing allergies unless the infant has already manifested an allergy to cow's milk (see treatment of cow's milk sensitivity, below). In addition, if careful schedules are followed in introducing new foods, the offending agent can quickly be identified. If any local inflammation occurs, such as swelling of the lip or urticaria around the mouth, the food must be avoided and is usually not reintroduced for a period of 6 or more months.

TABLE 11-3

Hyperallergenic Foods

Food	Sources
Milk	Ice cream, butter, margarine (if it contains dairy products), yogurt, cheese, pudding, baked goods, wieners, bologna, canned creamed soups, instant breakfast drinks, powdered milk drinks, milk chocolate
Eggs	Mayonnaise, creamy salad dressing, baked goods, egg noodles, some cake icing, meringue, custard, pancakes, French toast, root beer
Wheat	Almost all baked goods, wieners, bologna, pressed or chopped cold cuts, gravy, pasta, some canned soups
Legumes	Peanuts, peanut butter or oil, beans, peas, lentils
Nuts	Some chocolates, candy, baked goods, cherry soda (may be flavored with a nut extract), walnut oil
Fish or shellfish	Cod liver oil, pizza with anchovies, Caesar salad dressing, any food fried in same oil as fish
Chocolate	Cola beverages, cocoa, chocolate-flavored drinks
Buckwheat	Some cereals, pancakes
Pork, chicken	Bacon, wieners, sausage, pork fat, chicken broth
Strawberries, melon, pineapple	Gelatin, syrups
Corn	Popcorn, cereal, muffins, cornstarch, corn meal
Citrus fruits	Orange, lemon, lime, grapefruit; any of these in drinks, gelatin, juice, or medicines
Tomatoes	Juice, some vegetable soups, spaghetti, pizza sauce, and catsup
Spices	Chili, pepper, vinegar, cinnamon

COW'S MILK SENSITIVITY

Cow's milk sensitivity (milk allergy, milk intolerance) is a multifaceted disorder representing adverse systemic and local gastrointestinal reactions to cow's milk protein. It is the most common nutritional allergy during infancy, affecting 0.3% to 7% of all infants. It usually appears within the first 2 months of life following cow's milk feeding. Some newborns and exclusively breast-fed infants may be symptomatic following their first exposure to cow's milk, suggesting placental sensitization in utero or sensitization by cow's milk protein in breast milk from maternal ingestion of milk. Many children who are sensitive to cow's milk can tolerate it by 2 years of age.

Diagnostic Evaluation

Clinical manifestations of milk allergy are generally gastrointestinal disturbances but may include a wide variety of other symptoms (see box). Consequently, there must be a high index of suspicion for milk allergy to correctly identify affected children.

The diagnosis of milk intolerance is initially made from the findings of the history. Preliminary tests include stool analysis for blood, white blood cells, and sugar. To detect sugar (lactose), the stool is tested with Clinitest. A num-

Clinical Manifestations of Cow's Milk Sensitivity

Gastrointestinal	Respiratory	Other signs and symptoms
Diarrhea	Rhinitis	Eczema
Vomiting	Bronchitis	Excessive crying
Colic	Asthma	Pallor (from anemia secondary to chronic blood loss in gastrointestinal tract)
Abdominal pain	Wheezing	
	Sneezing	
	Coughing	

ber of other tests may be performed, such as skin-prick testing and the radioallergosorbent test (RAST) for a specific antigen or the lactose tolerance test or hydrogen breath test for lactase activity. However, the simplest and most frequently used approach is an elimination diet followed by challenge testing, in which the suspect food is ingested in measured amounts to detect resurgence of symptoms. Careful observation of the child is required during a challenge test because of the possibility of anaphylactic shock.

Milk allergy can be mistakenly diagnosed as galactosemia (see p. 261) or as lactose intolerance, a deficiency of the enzyme lactase, which is needed for the digestion of lactose. Lactose intolerance may be present shortly after birth or be manifest later in life. It is more common in those of Mediterranean, African, and Asian extraction and is less prevalent in young children than in adults. The principal manifestations of lactose intolerance include diarrhea, abdominal pain and distension, and flatus shortly after ingesting milk.

Therapeutic Management

Management of milk sensitivity involves elimination of cow's milk. The initial alternative is soy milk, although approximately 1:5 children who are allergic to cow's milk are also sensitive to soy milk. Commercially available soy formulas include Prosobee and Isomil. Commercial formulas that are suitable cow's and soy milk substitutes include Nutramigen and Pregestimil which contain hydrolyzed protein. Goat's milk is not an acceptable substitute because it cross-reacts with cow's milk protein and is deficient in folic acid.

Infants are maintained on the diet until after 1 year of age, when very small quantities of milk are gradually reintroduced. Children with eczema or other allergic disorders may not be given milk for a considerably longer time.

Nursing Considerations

The principal nursing objectives are identification of potential milk sensitivity and appropriate counseling of parents regarding substitute formulas. If milk sensitivity is suspected, finding acceptable substitutions is frequently time-consuming, frustrating, and expensive. Parents are advised to purchase small quantities of the formula and to ask if unused portions can be returned. Frequently when parents are told to try a new formula, they purchase a case rather than a few cans. At the end of the trial period they have a large reserve of unused, costly formulas.

The protein hydrolysate formulas are less palatable than milk-based formulas. Consequently reluctance to accept the new formula may be a problem. This can be overcome by introducing the formula gradually over a few days using 1 ounce of new formula to 7 ounces of old formula, then 2 to 6 ounces, 3 to 4, as needed. Parents also need to be reassured that the infant will receive complete nutrition from the new formula and will suffer no ill effects from the absence of cow's milk.

The nurse also stresses that all associated milk products must be avoided (see Table 11-3). This requires careful reading of all food labels to avoid potential addition of milk products to the prepared food. If the infant is sensitive to soy, parents are advised that it is commonly found in baby junior foods and cereals. Since allergy to one protein may mean allergy to others, particularly egg albumin and wheat, such foods should be restricted from the infant's diet for the first 9 to 12 months of life.

◆ *Feeding Difficulties*

A number of feeding difficulties can occur during the infant's first year. A common cause of feeding problems is improper feeding techniques. A satisfactory feeding requires a number of mechanical skills, such as placing the infant to the breast properly (see p. 202); holding the bottle at an angle that allows fluid, not air, to flow into the nipple; "reading" the infant's cues for burping or satiation; and holding the infant during feeding, rather than propping the bottle. A number of other problems can also occur singly or in combination, such as feeding too much or too little food; feeding too often, especially with breastfeeding, or too infrequently; selecting inappropriate foods for the infant's physiologic and motor development; and incorrectly preparing formula. While such feeding problems are more common in inexperienced parents, they can also occur with seasoned parents who are unprepared for an infant with different needs or less clear cues of hunger or satiation.

All of these feeding problems are easily corrected with guidance and demonstration. Early assessment is essential to prevent complex problems from developing between the parent and child at mealtime. Written guidelines for feeding infants can help new parents experience success with their child. Helpful tips, such as evaluating the effectiveness of burping (see box), should also be shared with parents.

Occasionally, parents perceive that problems exist when in fact they are a normal occurrence, such as spitting up. Other problems such as colic can disrupt a family tremendously, although the problem resolves spontaneously. Still other disorders, such as rumination and failure to thrive, can be fatal even though there may be no organic cause.

> ***Nursing Tip: Burping the Infant***
>
> To check if an infant has burped, place one hand on the infant's abdomen and the other hand on the back and gently jiggle the child. If a splashing sound is not heard, the infant has burped (Temple and Farley, 1983).

REGURGITATION OR "SPITTING UP"

The return of small amounts of food after a feeding is a common occurrence during infancy. It should not be confused with actual vomiting, which can be associated with a number of disturbances, both insignificant and serious (see Chapter 23). For clarification the following terms are defined:

spitting up dribbling of unswallowed formula from the infant's mouth immediately after a feeding

regurgitation the return of undigested food from the stomach, usually accompanied by burping

The insignificance of regurgitation or spitting up should be explained to parents, especially to those who are unduly concerned. It can be reduced by some simple measures, such as frequent burping during and after feeding, minimal handling at feeding and after, and positioning the child on the right side with the head slightly elevated after feeding. See Nursing tip on p. 323 for checking if the infant has burped. To reassure parents that the infant is ingesting sufficient amounts of formula or breast milk, the nurse can suggest that they estimate the volume expelled. For example, a ring of fluid about 6 inches in diameter is only about ½ ounce. The inconvenience of spitting up is managed with use of absorbent bibs on the infant and protective cloths on the parent.

Sometimes, frequent dribbling of formula causes excoriation of the corners of the mouth, chin, and neck. Keeping the area dry promotes healing but can be difficult to maintain. Helpful suggestions include applying a thin film of petrolatum jelly or A and D ointment to the affected areas after cleansing and using absorbent non-plastic-lined terrycloth bibs that are changed frequently.

PAROXYSMAL ABDOMINAL PAIN (COLIC)

Colic is generally described as paroxysmal abdominal pain or cramping that is manifested by loud crying and drawing the legs up to the abdomen. It is more common in infants under the age of 3 months than in older infants and also in infants with "difficult" temperaments. Despite the obvious behavioral indications of pain, the child tolerates the formula well, gains weight, and thrives.

Many theories have been investigated as potential causative factors, such as too-rapid feeding, overeating, swallowing excessive air, improper feeding technique, especially in positioning and burping, and emotional stress or tension between parent and child. While all of these may occur, there is no evidence that one factor is consistently present. Colic may be a sign of cow's milk sensitivity, and there is evidence that eliminating cow's milk products from the diet of lactating mothers can reduce the symptoms. Parental smoking has also been associated with colic. Management of colic should begin with an investigation of such causes.

While colic is considered a minor ailment, a colicky, crying, irritable infant can have an intense emotional impact on parent-child attachment and family relationships.

Nursing Diagnoses: Colic

- Pain related to abdominal spasms
- Sleep-pattern disturbance related to excessive crying
- Potential knowledge deficit related to feeding other child, care skills
- Anxiety related to perceived change in child's health status
- Altered family processes related to temporary family disorganization

Mothers often relate histories of the daily routine that are laden with feelings of frustration, anger, despair, guilt, fatigue, and helplessness. A vicious cycle ensues in which the parent's own anxiety may be transferred to the infant, which further increases his tension, irritability, and crying.

Nursing Considerations

Nurses can play an important role in helping the family cope with the frustrations created by having an infant with colic. Counseling regarding measures to reduce colic and offering support to the family are key elements of nursing care.

ASSESSMENT

The initial step in managing colic is to take a thorough, detailed history of the usual daily events or to ask parents to keep a log for 48 to 72 hours. Areas that should be stressed include (1) diet of the breast-feeding mother, (2) time of day when attacks occur, (3) relationship of the attacks to feeding time, (4) presence of specific family members during attacks, (5) activity of the usual caregiver before, during, and after the crying, (6) smoking habits of family members, and (7) measures used to relieve the crying. Of special emphasis is a careful assessment of the feeding process via *demonstration* by the parent.

NURSING DIAGNOSES

After a thorough assessment of those factors that may influence the development of colic, a number of nursing diagnoses may be evident. However, not all may apply to every family. Examples of nursing diagnoses are listed in the box.

PLANNING

Once the diagnosis of colic is established, a number of goals may be appropriate. For example:

1. Eliminate factors that may aggravate the colic
2. Provide comfort measures for the child
3. Support the parents during the colic period

Nursing Guidelines for Relieving Colic

Place infant prone over a covered hot-water bottle, heated towel, or covered heating pad.
Massage abdomen.
Change the infant's position frequently; walk with him face down with his body across the parent's arm and hand under the abdomen applying gentle pressure (Fig. 11-1).
Use a front carrier for transporting the infant.
Swaddle tightly with a soft, stretchy blanket.
Place in a wind-up swing.
Take for car rides or outside for a change in environment.
Use a commercial device* in the crib that simulates the vibration and sound of a car ride.
Provide smaller, frequent feedings; burp during and after feedings using the shoulder position, and place in an upright seat after feedings.
Introduce a pacifier for added sucking.
Try giving warm, dilute herbal teas using one teaspoon fennel, chamomile, or anise.
In breast-fed infants, have mother avoid all milk products for a trial period.
If household members smoke, avoid smoking near infant; preferably confine smoking activity to outside of home.
If nothing reduces the crying, place infant in crib and allow to cry; periodically hold and comfort child and put down again.

*Sleeplight, Inc., 3613 Mueller Road, St. Charles, MO 63301.

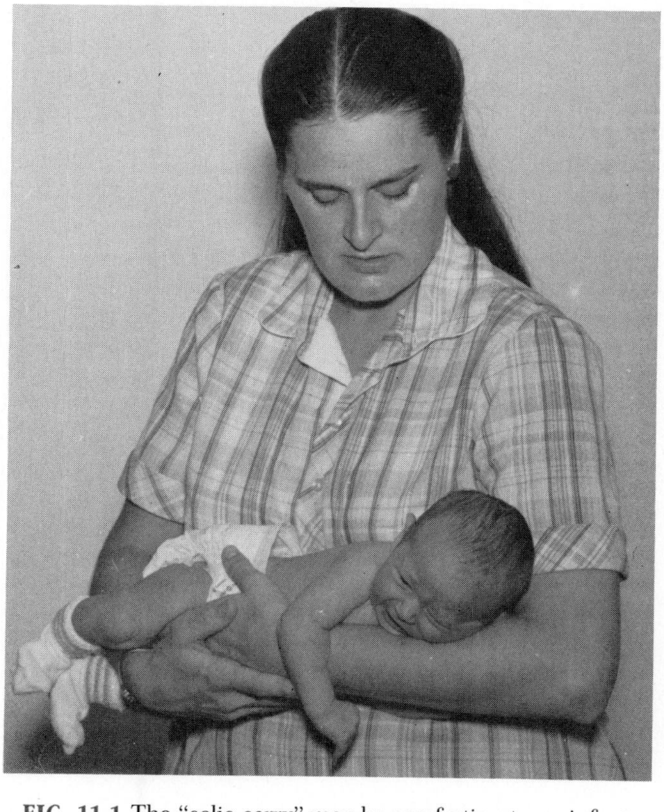

FIG. 11-1 The "colic carry" may be comforting to an infant with colic.

IMPLEMENTATION

In breast-feeding mothers a milk-free di 3) should be followed for a minimum of tempt to reduce symptoms in the infant. cessful, the milk-free diet is continued, alt may need to take calcium supplements. M need to be cautioned about some nondairy creamers that may contain calcium caseinate, a cow's milk protein.

Often no change is required in feeding practices. When no cause can be identified, it is preferable to determine the time of the onset of crying and attempt to manipulate the circumstances associated with it. For example, some infants have episodes of colic around the family's dinnertime, when all household members are home and are often tired, members may be smoking, and the parent is preoccupied with cooking. The overstimulating, more tense atmosphere may upset the infant. Encouraging the parent to prepare food items, such as salad, dessert, or vegetables, for dinner earlier in the day, and feeding the infant in a quieter area of the house may help reverse the environmental conditions that may have provoked the attack of colic. Other approaches for relieving colic are listed in the boxed material.* Parents are encouraged to try as many of them as possible because not all are effective for every infant. Mild sedation may be prescribed but should be delayed until other options are exhausted.

One of the most important areas of nursing concern is the support of parents during the colic period. It is stressed that despite the crying and obvious pain, the infant is doing well. Colic disappears spontaneously, usually by 3 months of age, although guarantees should never be given because it may continue for much longer. The parent should be encouraged to arrange for some free time. Most importantly, it should be emphasized that the colic is not an indicator of poor or inadequate parenting. The parents' negative feelings toward the infant and their insecurities regarding parenting abilities are normal. Parents should be encouraged to talk about them, since active listening may do more to relieve the colic syndrome than offering stereotyped advice, remedies, and glib statements such as, "Don't worry about it; your child will eventually outgrow the colicky spells." (See Therapeutic dialogue, p. 326.)

EVALUATION

The effectiveness of nursing interventions is determined by continual reassessment and evaluation of care based on the following observational guidelines and expected outcomes:

1. Keep a dietary record to chart elimination of offending foods or habits, such as smoking; evaluate feeding technique after teaching parents the correct procedure

*A helpful booklet for families is *Coping with Infant: A Guide for Parents*, which is available from Ross Laboratories, Columbus, OH 43216.

THERAPEUTIC DIALOGUE

Colic

During a routine clinical visit, the nurse is taking a history from the parents of a 2-month-old male infant. While both parents look tired, they have mentioned no concerns until the nurse inquires about the infant's habits.

NURSE: Tell me about the baby's daily habits, such as his routine for feeding, sleeping, awake time, and crying.

MOTHER: He eats about every 4 hours and usually falls asleep after each meal except at dinner. Then he decides it is time to cry and cry and cry.

NURSE: He cries a lot at this time of the day?

FATHER: That's an understatement. Quite frankly, we are at the point where we don't know what to do. Some friends have told us this is colic and not to worry, but just try to live with a screaming baby!

NURSE: It sounds like it has been a difficult time.

MOTHER: Yes. My husband says he hates to come home after work, and yet I cannot wait for him to walk in the door to take the baby for a little while. Is this colic, or are we doing something wrong?

NURSE: From what you have told me about the baby's vigorous eating and his good weight gain, I think it is colic. Tell me about your thoughts regarding doing something wrong.

FATHER: This is our first child, and we know we have a lot to learn. But when nothing you do comforts your child, you cannot help feeling inadequate as a parent.

NURSE: Your feelings are so understandable and typical of parents with a colicky infant. Let's talk more about what you have tried and some things that may help you survive this temporary misery.

MOTHER: Just hearing you say that the colic is temporary and other parents feel the way we do is helpful.

2. List each comfort measure that parents try and the child's response
3. Ask parents to verbalize their feelings about having an infant with colic; also ask if they have arranged for time away from the infant to meet their own needs

Expected outcomes:

1. Factors that aggravate colic are identified and eliminated.
2. Effective comfort measures are implemented.
3. Parents' verbal responses indicate positive feelings toward infant.

RUMINATION

Rumination is the active, voluntary return of swallowed food into the mouth. The food is then rechewed, partially or completely reswallowed, or expelled. In some instances rumination may lead to progressive malnutrition and even death, since considerable food and fluid loss can occur.

Rumination differs from regurgitation, which is involuntary. The ruminating infant makes purposeful movements of the mouth, tongue, and stomach in an attempt to force food back into the oropharynx. On successful regurgitation the infant is obviously satisfied with the activity.

Organic causes for rumination are rarely found, although the possibility of gastroesophageal reflux should be investigated in the differential diagnosis. It may also be seen in children who are profoundly retarded. However, it most often is a result of a disturbance in the parent-child relationship. The factors culminating in the disorder are similar to those described in nonorganic failure to thrive.

Nursing Considerations

The primary objective is to terminate the ruminating behavior and restore normal feeding patterns. This is accomplished through a structured feeding plan. Generally the same guidelines apply to feeding the ruminating child as to feeding the child with nonorganic failure to thrive. In addition, emphasis should be placed on the following areas:

1. Assign the same nurse to feed the child as often as possible. This intervention is even more critical than in failure to thrive.
2. Continue *positive* attention immediately after the feeding, since ruminating infants often vomit after a feeding once they are left unattended.
3. Introduce new foods slowly, with emphasis on texture, consistency, and flavor. These children are often "picky eaters," and new foods introduced too quickly can increase rumination.
4. If acceptance of solids is a problem, give the child a small quantity of milk (or juice), immediately followed by 1 teaspoon of solid food. Begin with pureed food, and once accepted, advance to junior and adult foods. Gradually give fewer sips of milk and more spoonfuls of food until a regular diet for the child's age is achieved.

These children often require prolonged inpatient intervention to reduce their rumination. Positive stimulation programs must accompany the feeding plan. Parents need to be included in learning how to feed the child, and follow-up after discharge is essential to prevent a recurrence of the behavior.

FAILURE TO THRIVE

The term *failure to thrive (FTT)* refers to a state of inadequate growth from inability to obtain and/or use calories required for growth. Failure to thrive has no universal definition, although one of the more common parameters is a weight and sometimes height that fall below the 5th percentile for the child's age. Some authorities prefer the 3rd percentile as a criterion, but the widely used National Center for Health Statistics growth charts include only the 5th, not the 3rd, percentile in their measurements. Growth measurements alone are not used to diagnose children with FTT. Rather, the finding of a persistent deviation from an established growth curve is cause for concern.

Three general categories of failure to thrive have been defined:

organic failure to thrive (OFTT), which is the result of a physical cause, such as congenital heart defects, neurologic lesions, microcephaly, chronic urinary tract infection, gastroesophageal reflux, renal insufficiency, malabsorption syndrome, endocrine dysfunction, or cystic fibrosis.

nonorganic failure to thrive (NFTT or NOFTT), which has a definable cause that is unrelated to disease. NFTT is most often the result of psychosocial factors, such as inadequte nutritional information by the parent, deficiency in maternal care or a disturbance in maternal-child attachment, or a disturbance in separation by the child, leading to food refusal (Egan, Chatoor, and Rosen, 1980). NFTT has been described under a variety of less acceptable names, including maternal deprivation, environmental deprivation, and deprivation dwarfism.

idiopathic failure to thrive, which is unexplained by the usual organic and environmental etiologies but may also be classified as NFTT.

Regardless of the classification a minority of cases (20% to 30%) are found to have organic causes, and the diagnosis of NFTT is usually made on the basis of exclusion of pathophysiologic findings. Unfortunately many of these children are unnecessarily subjected to exhausting, traumatic, and expensive diagnostic procedures. To prevent this, NFTT should be considered *early* in the differential diagnosis, when a careful history and physical examination rule out a gross medical cause. The following discussion is devoted primarily to NFTT.

Prognosis

The prognosis for NFTT is related to the cause. If the parents have simply been ignorant of the infant's needs, teaching may remedy the child's limited caloric intake and permanently reverse the growth failure. However, when the family dysfunction is extensive, the prognosis is uncertain. Many of these children are below normal in intellectual development, have poorer language development and less well-developed reading skills, attain lower social maturity, and have a higher incidence of behavioral disturbances (Oates, Peacock, and Forrest, 1985). Such findings indicate that a long-term plan is needed for the optimum development of these children.

Nursing Considerations

Caring for the child with NFTT presents many nursing challenges, both when treatment takes place in the hospital or home. Providing a positive feeding environment, teaching the parent successful feeding strategies, and supporting the child and family are essential components of care.

ASSESSMENT

Nurses play a critical role in the diagnosis of FTT through their assessment of the child, parents, and family interaction. Knowledge of the characteristics of children with FTT and their families is essential in helping identify these children and hastening the confirmation of a correct diagnosis (see box below). Accurate assessment of initial weight and height and daily weight is mandatory, as well as recording of all food intake. The feeding behavior of the child is documented, as well as the parent-child interaction during feeding, other caregiving activities, and play. Assessing the approximate developmental age should be done on admission by administering the Denver Developmental Screening Test (DDST) or other developmental test. The DDST gives an approximate age for the child's present achievement in gross/fine motor, social-adaptive, and language skills (see p. 171). Only after objective measurements are available can a plan of care for stimulation be planned.

The nursing admission history and ongoing assessment should also focus on the following characteristics that have been identified in many of these children and their parents.

The child. Besides the obvious signs of malnutrition and delayed development, children with NFTT may inter-

Clinical Manifestations of Nonorganic Failure to Thrive

Growth failure—below 5th percentile in height and weight
Developmental retardation—social, motor, adaptive, language
Apathy
Poor hygiene
Withdrawn behavior
Feeding or eating disorders, such as vomiting, anorexia, pica, rumination
No fear of strangers (at age when stranger anxiety is normal)
Avoidance of eye-to-eye contact
Wide-eyed gaze and continual scan of the environment ("radar gaze")
Stiff and unyielding or flaccid and unresponsive
Minimum smiling

act differently from children with OFTT (see box, p. 327). They display intense interest in inanimate objects, such as a toy, but much less interest in social interactions. They are vigilant of people at a distance but become increasingly distressed as they come closer. They dislike being touched or held and avoid face-to-face contact. However, when held, they protest briefly on being put down and are apathetic when left alone.

Frequently there is a history of difficult feeding, vomiting, sleep disturbance, and excessive irritability. Difficulties in infant feeding may include poor appetite, poor suck, crying during feedings, vomiting, hoarding food in the mouth, ruminating after feeding, refusal to switch from liquids to solids, and aversion behavior such as turning from food or spitting food. Ultimately these habit patterns become attention-seeking mechanisms to prolong the attention received at mealtime. In addition, chronic reduction in calories can lead to appetite depression, which compounds the problem.

An outstanding feature of children with NFTT is their irregularity (low rhythmicity) in activities of daily living. Some of these children typify the "difficult" temperament pattern. However, another type is the passive, sleepy, lethargic infants who do not wake up for feedings. Parents who have been advised of "demand feeding schedules" may be unsure of whether to wake the child or let him sleep. Because of their inexperience and lack of guidance, parents may develop a pattern of infrequent feeding that is inadequate to meet the infant's nutritional needs. Such a pattern is particularly detrimental with the breast-feeding infant, where frequent nursing is essential to an adequate milk supply.

It cannot be assumed that such characteristics in a child result in NFTT. Rather, there is probably a complex set of variables that are significant. One may be the degree of *fit* between the child's temperament and that of the parents. Since the personalities of infants can have definite effects on the parent-child attachment process, identifying such situations of disharmony may be one approach toward prevention and anticipatory guidance.

The parents. Some parents are at increased risk for attachment problems because of (1) isolation and social crisis, (2) inadequate support systems, and (3) poor parenting as a child. Other factors that should be considered are lack of education; physical and mental health problems, such as retardation, depression, or drug dependence; immaturity, especially in adolescent parents; and lack of commitment to parenting, such as giving higher priority to career goals.

Frequently these parents and their families are under stress and in multiple chronic emotional, social, and financial crises. Of particular significance is the prevalence of marital discord, including frequent arguments, separations, and reconciliations (Altemeier and others, 1985).

Many of these parents display negative maladaptive feelings toward the infant (see box above). Inadequate feeding and caregiving may be part of an abuse cycle. Ambivalence toward pregnancy can be an early clue when combined with other characteristics of high-risk parents. Being alert to such clues may avert a potential NFTT situation by identifying these parents prenatally and planning interventions aimed at increasing satisfying parenting skills.

Children with NFTT are not limited to lower socioeconomic groups. Although financial crisis generally means "poor," families with adequate monetary resources can be in chronic financial stress if their standard of living exceeds their income. Emotional deprivation, a kind of rejection, can also occur in financially stable homes where all childrearing responsibilities are left to others. Although this is less visible and borders more on emotionally neglected children, such families can include children who are physically and emotionally starved. Refusal to eat may be the child's response to an uncaring environment. It is essential for nurses to set aside stereotypes and prejudices in order to be aware of the potential for existence of such children in *any* family situation.

Parental Maladaptive Behaviors Toward Infant

- Persistent ambivalence or negative feelings about the fetus and the pregnancy during the prenatal period
- Makes no plans for obtaining basic infant supplies
- Appears indifferent to infant at time of delivery; may appear sad or angry; is expressionless
- Makes no effort to establish eye-to-eye contact with infant
- Handles infant only when necessary
- Does not talk to infant
- Makes few or no spontaneous movements with infant
- Asks few questions about care
- Sees infant as ugly, fat, or unattractive
- Displays disgust with infant's drooling and sucking sounds; is revolted by infant's body fluids
- Annoyed with diaper changing
- Perceives infant's odor as revolting
- Holds infant with little support to head and body
- Holds infant away from body during feeding or props bottle for feeding; seldom cuddles infant
- Does not coo or talk to infant
- Refers to infant in an impersonal manner
- Develops inappropriate responses to infant's needs, such as leaving infant in one place for long periods, leaving him alone in room, overfeeding or underfeeding, overstimulating or understimulating infant, forcing or refusing eye contact, bouncing or tickling infant when he is fatigued
- Cannot discriminate between infant's signals for hunger, comfort, rest, body contact
- Is convinced the infant has a defect or disease even when reassured to the contrary
- Makes negative statements regarding parenting role
- Believes the infant is judging him/her and efforts as an adult
- Believes the infant does not love him/her
- Develops paradoxical attitudes and behaviors toward the infant

NURSING DIAGNOSES

A number of nursing diagnoses are prominent in the nursing care of the child with NFTT. The most common nursing diagnoses are outlined in the Nursing Care Plan on p. 331. If an organic cause is found, additional nursing diagnoses may be related to care specific for that disorder, such as heart disease.

PLANNING

Planning needs to begin as soon as possible on admission. The priority nursing goal is providing the infant with sufficient nutrients for growth. More specific nursing care depends on the identified cause of FTT. If an organic etiology is confirmed, care is related primarily to management of the disorder. If the problem is one of inadequate knowledge regarding child feeding, parental education is required. When serious psychosocial factors are involved, hospitalization is needed and additional interventions are required to meet the needs of both the child and family. The following are goals for the hospitalized child with NFTT:

1. Structure a feeding environment that encourages the child to consume adequate calories; provide age-appropriate foods
2. Provide appropriate developmental stimulation for the child
3. Teach parents feeding techniques and other caregiving activities, such as suitable play, that are successful in the hospital
4. Provide a nurturing environment for the parent; make appropriate referrals for supportive services

IMPLEMENTATION

Since part of the difficulty between parent and child was dissatisfaction and frustration, the child should have a consistent primary nurse for all three shifts (Fig. 11-2). Only the same nurse caring for the child over a period of time can learn to perceive the child's cues and reverse the cycle of dissatisfaction, especially in the area of feeding. Since these children are not ill with any physical disorder but debilitated from general malnutrition, they should be placed in a room with noninfectious children of a similar age.

Since many of these children are responding to stimuli that have led to the negative feeding patterns, the first goal is to structure the feeding environment to encourage eating. Initially staff members may need to feed these children to assess thoroughly the difficulties encountered during the feeding process and to devise strategies that eliminate or minimize such problems. During this initial period it may be beneficial for parents not to be present at mealtime. General guidelines for the feeding process include:

1. **Provide a quiet, unstimulating atmosphere.** A number of these children are very distractible, and their attention is diverted with minimal stimuli. Older children do well at a feeding table; younger children should always be held. A single adult in the feeding situation is recommended.
2. **Maintain a calm, even temperament throughout the meal.** Negative outbursts may be commonplace in this child's habit formation. Limits on eating behavior definitely need to be provided, but they should be stated in a firm, calm tone. If the nurse is hurried or anxious, the feeding process will not be optimized.
3. **Talk to the child by giving directions about eating.** "Take a bite, Lisa" is appropriate and directive. The more distractible the child, the more directive the nurse should be to refocus attention on feeding. Positive comments about feeding are actively given.
4. **Follow the child's rhythm of feeding.** The child will set a rhythm when the previous conditions are met.
5. **Develop a structured routine.** FTT children are in particular need of routine feeding patterns. Disruption in their other activities of daily living has great impact on feeding responses, so these should be structured also. The same nurse should feed the child in the same way and place as often as possible. The length of the feeding should also be established (usually 30 minutes).
6. **Be persistent.** This is perhaps one of the most important guidelines. Parents often give up when the child begins negative feeding behavior. Calm perseverance through 10 to 15 minutes of food refusal will eventually diminish negative behavior. Although forced feeding is avoided, "strictly encouraged" feeding is essential.
7. **Maintain a face-to-face posture with the child when possible.** Encourage eye contact and remain with the child throughout the meal.

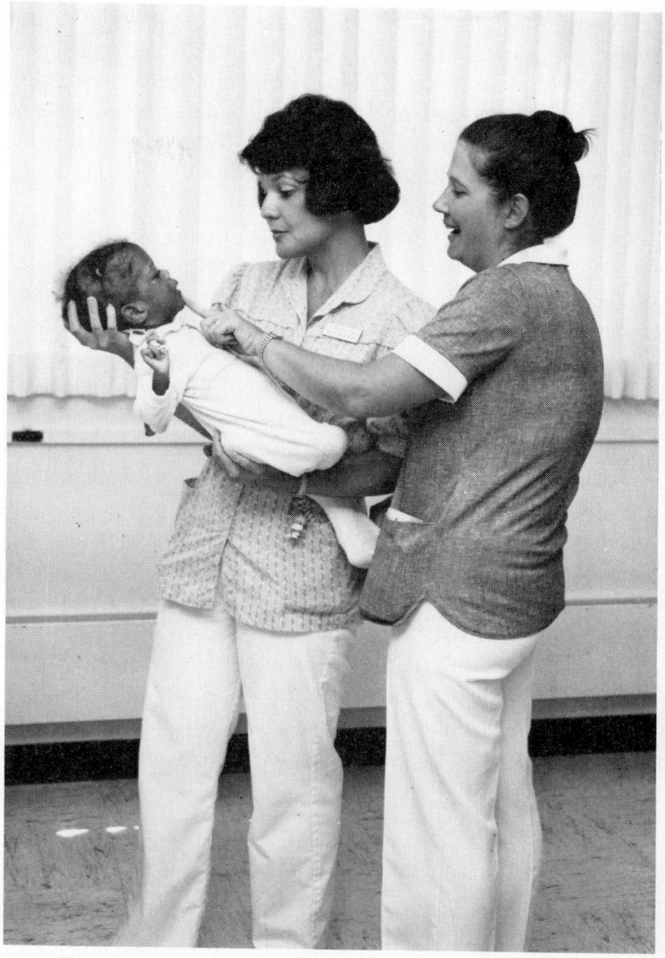

FIG. 11-2 A consistent core of nurses is important in developing trust with infants with nonorganic failure to thrive.

Foods appropriate to the child's age are selected. To increase caloric intake, supplements, such as Polycose, can be added to foods. Often, these children have been exclusively bottle-fed and refuse all solids. In these situations, introduction of solids begins with pureed foods, then junior foods, finger foods, and finally regular table food.

Besides attending to the physical needs of the child, the nurse must plan care for appropriate developmental stimulation. The word "appropriate" is emphasized because it refers to the child's developmental, not chronologic, age. Once an approximate developmental age is established, then a planned program of play is instituted. Ideally a child life specialist should be involved to implement and supervise the stimulation program. Every effort is made to teach the parent how to play and interact with the child.

Nursing care of these children involves a systems approach (see p. 56). In other words, for the entire family to become healthy, each member must be helped to change. To nurture the child back to physical, developmental, and emotional health during his hospitalization while neglecting the emotional needs of the parents does not solve the problem. Therefore, nursing care must also be directed to the parents and siblings. Other significant persons, who can be helped to be more emotionally, physically, and financially supportive to the family unit, can become the emotional reservoir needed by parents to give nurturance to their child. Some hospitals have special programs, such as volunteer foster grandparents. They spend scheduled, consistent periods of time with the infant as a kind of surrogate parent. Mental health services, such as individual or group therapy, may also be beneficial.

Care of the parents is aimed at helping them increase their feelings of self-esteem through positive, successful parenting skills. Initially this necessitates providing an environment in which they feel welcomed and accepted. Because these parents are often distrustful of authority figures, it may take some time before they develop any trust toward the nurse. One approach is to empathize with the parent about the difficulties of child-rearing. For example, the nurse may state that many parents find adjusting to parenthood a trying time or that the demands of caring for an infant can become overwhelming.

Once the parents feel comfortable enough to visit with their infant, teaching infant care techniques is begun through *example* and *demonstration,* not by lecturing. As the nurse perceives the infant's cues, these are emphasized to the parents. For example, during a feeding the nurse might comment that the infant is still hungry because he sucks vigorously and looks at her. When he is satisfied, the nurse points out that the infant is signaling this by releasing the strong suck, closing his eyes, and breathing deeply and more slowly. By example, the child is gently placed in the crib for a nap.

At the same time the parents are offered an opportunity to care for the infant without making demands on them. For example, the nurse suggests that at the next feeding one of the parents offer the child the bottle. Whenever the parents participate, they are praised for their efforts and encouraged to continue caring for the child.

Before discharge, plans are made to continue these interventions at home. A public health referral is made, and if a foster grandparent was included, this person should also visit the family. Social agencies that can provide financial or housing assistance to lessen the stress of everyday life are also contacted.

EVALUATION

The effectiveness of nursing interventions is determined by continual reassessment and evaluation of care based on the following observational guidelines and expected outcomes:

1. Record weight and calorie intake daily; document child's reaction to feeding environment; review notes to see if changes were made as necessary to improve eating and if consistent group of nurses fed child
2. Perform periodic developmental screening tests
3. Document parents' relationship with staff or other supportive individuals. Note length of time parents visit with these people, appointments kept with referral services, and any requests for help
4. Keep a record of all teaching and compare taught skills with parent's actual skills

Expected outcomes:
See Nursing Care Plan, pp. 331-332.

◆ *Disorders of Unknown Etiology*

A number of disorders may occur during early childhood in which the etiology is unknown or speculative. However, two of the disorders, sudden infant death syndrome and autism, occur almost exclusively during infancy and generate tremendous stress for the family. In one, the family must cope with the loss of an infant; in the other the family must deal with the stresses of caring for a severely disturbed child. Competent and sensitive nursing care can relieve some of the emotional burden.

SUDDEN INFANT DEATH SYNDROME

Sudden infant death syndrome (SIDS, cot or crib death) is defined as the sudden death of any infant or young child, which is unexpected by history, and in which a thorough postmortem examination fails to demonstrate an adequate cause for death. It is the leading cause of death in children between the ages of 1 week and 1 year. Table 11-4 summarizes the major characteristics of SIDS.

Possible Etiology

Numerous theories have been proposed regarding the etiology of SIDS; however, the cause is unknown. Of the

NURSING CARE PLAN

The Child with Nonorganic Failure to Thrive

Nursing Goals	Nursing Interventions	Expected Patient/Family Outcomes
HP-HMP Potential for trauma, neglect Risk factors: parenting failure		
Identify parents at risk	Be alert to parental maladaptive behaviors toward the infant (see box, p. 328) Determine extent and quality of parent's mothering Determine if pregnancy was planned or unplanned Determine if there were any disturbing events associated with pregnancy or delivery of the child	†High-risk parents are identified early and appropriate intervention is initiated
Recognize characteristics of parents of failure-to-thrive children	Be alert to the following History of maternal deprivation as a child Low self-esteem; feelings of inadequacy Desire for dependency Loneliness, isolation Limited support system Multiple life crises and stress	†Same as above
Identify children who fail to thrive	Suspect nonorganic failure to thrive in infants and young children who display typical characteristics (see box, p. 327)	†Children are identified and appropriate care is implemented
N-MP Altered nutrition: less than body requirements Etiology: deprivation of necessities, emotional deprivation		
Make feeding a priority goal	Provide unlimited feedings of a regular diet for the age of the child (preferably foods to which the child is accustomed) Avoid interruption of feedings with other activities, such as laboratory examinations or radiography Keep accurate record of intake to ensure ingestion of calculated daily calories Weigh daily and record to ascertain weight gain	Child gains 1 to 2 ounces per day (minimum)
Introduce a positive feeding environment	Assign one nurse for feeding Maintain calm, even temperament; be persistent Provide a quiet, unstimulating environment Hold young child for feeding Maintain eye-to-eye contact with child Talk to child by giving appropriate directions and praise for eating Follow the child's rhythm of feeding Establish a structured routine and follow it consistently	Child responds positively to feeding practices (specify)
CPP Altered growth and development Etiology: socially restricted environment (infant deprivation)		
Provide a nurturing environment for the hospitalized child	Assess child's developmental age Apply primary care concepts to ensure continuity of care with a minimum number of caregivers Provide gentle, sure, and loving handling Perform physical care with as much holding, rocking, and cuddling as the child will respond to Encourage eye-to-eye contact Employ consistent schedule in meeting child's needs for food, hygiene, care, and rest Assign a foster grandparent or child life specialist to child Provide sensory stimulation and play appropriate to the child's developmental level	Child displays a positive response to interventions, e.g., social smile, advanced developmental age

*For an explanation of abbreviations, see p. 20.
†Nursing outcome.

Continued.

NURSING CARE PLAN

The Child with Nonorganic Failure to Thrive—cont'd

Nursing Goals	Nursing Interventions	Expected Patient/Family Outcomes
RRP Altered parenting **Etiology: specify (knowledge deficit, poverty, neglect, etc.)**		
Reduce parental anxiety and provide education	Welcome parents and encourage, but do not push, them to become involved in the child's care Teach parents about the child's physical care, developmental skills, and emotional needs through example, not lecture Afford parents the opportunity to discuss their lives and feelings toward the child Supply emotional nurturance without encouraging dependency Promote parents' self-esteem and confidence by praising their achievements with the child Prepare parents for adjustments with anticipatory guidance	Parents demonstrate the ability to provide appropriate care to the child
Prepare for discharge	Assess home environment and relationships Continue interventions begun in the hospital Establish a consistent contact system through public health nurse Establish an infant stimulation program Provide for stress-relieving services to the family Refer to appropriate agencies for assistance with financial, social, mental health, or other family needs	Child exhibits continued weight gain appropriate for his age Family follows through on programs and activities

leading hypotheses, two are strongly supported by evidence found in many, but not all, SIDS victims. The *hypoxemia hypothesis* suggests that SIDS occurs because of damage to the respiratory control centers in the brain stem as a result of chronic hypoxemia. The *apnea theory* proposes that SIDS victims experience periods of prolonged apnea during sleep and eventually die during one of these episodes because of a failure in the autonomic regulation of breathing. However, infantile apnea (IA) does not cause SIDS. The vast majority of infants with apnea do not die, and only a minority of SIDS victims have documented life-threatening episodes of apnea (see discussion of infantile apnea, p. 334). A theory that has been disproven is SIDS' association with diphtheria, tetanus, and pertussis vaccines.

Although the etiology is unknown, autopsies reveal consistent pathologic findings, such as pulmonary edema and intrathoracic hemorrhages, that confirm the diagnosis of SIDS. Consequently all infants with suspected SIDS deaths are autopsied and these findings should be shared with the parents as soon as possible after the death.

Children at Risk for SIDS

Certain groups of children are considered at increased risk from SIDS. One is the "near-miss" infant, who is defined as a child who has ceased breathing and seems to have died suddenly and unexpectedly but whose life is apparently saved by timely intervention, usually by a parent or baby-sitter. Another group includes the subsequent siblings of the infant. However, the statistics vary. Some studies report a tenfold greater risk (Brooks, 1982), while others report that the risk in the SIDS family is virtually the same as that among families of like size and maternal age (Peterson, Sabotta, and Daling, 1986). Infants with infantile apnea are also at increased risk. While they are often erroneously referred to as "near-miss SIDS," IA is not always part of the initial presentation.

Studies conducted on children considerd at risk demonstrate differences in physiologic function, especially cardiac and respiratory functions, from that of other infants. Consequently there is much concern for the survival of these children. Many of them undergo home apnea monitoring until they are past the age of vulnerability and demonstrate normal cardiac pneumograms (see discussion of home monitoring, p. 334). However, the use of pneumograms/cardiopneumograms and home monitoring on asymptomatic children at increased epidemiologic risk for SIDS, such as preterm and black infants, siblings of SIDS victims, and infants of addicted mothers, remains controversial and has not proved effective in preventing SIDS deaths (Hunt and Brouillette, 1987).

Nursing Considerations

Loss of a child from SIDS presents several crises with which the parents must cope. In addition to the grief and

TABLE 11-4

Characteristics of SIDS

Factors	Occurrence
Incidence	2:1000 live births
Peak age	2 to 4 months; 90% occur by 6 months
Sex	Higher percentage of males affected
Time of death	During sleep
Time of year	Increased incidence in winter; peak in January
Racial	Greater incidence in blacks
Socioeconomic	Increased occurrence in lower socioeconomic class
Birth	Higher incidence in: Premature infants, especially infants of low birth weight Multiple births Neonates with low Apgar scores Infants with central nervous system disturbances
Feeding habits	Not significant; breast-feeding does not prevent SIDS
Siblings	May have greater incidence
Maternal	Younger age Cigarette smoking Drug abuse, such as cocaine

mourning for the death of their child, the parents must face a tragedy that was sudden, unexpected, and unexplained. The psychologic intervention for the family must deal with these additional variables. The purpose of this discussion is to stress primarily the objectives of care for families experiencing SIDS, rather than the process of grief and mourning, which is explored in Chapter 18.

One approach toward delineating the nursing care plan for these families is to base it on the usual sequence of events that occurs after the infant is found. This approach encompasses the different areas in which nurses may be involved with the family.

Finding the infant. It is usually the mother who finds the child dead in the crib. Typically the child is in a disheveled bed, with blankets over his head, and huddled into a corner. Frothy, blood-tinged fluid fills the mouth and nostrils, and the infant may be lying face down in the secretions. The diaper is wet and full of stool, which is consistent with a cataclysmic type of death. The hands may be clutching the sheets, as if the child were in distress before he died. The initial appearance of the child combined with the shock of such an unexpected event adds to the horror and nightmare that the parents must face.

Frequently the mother is alone and must deal with her initial shock, panic, grief, questions of the other siblings, and the decision of where to find help. The first persons to arrive may be the police and ambulance attendants. Hopefully they will handle the situation by asking few questions, giving *no* indication of wrongdoing, abuse, or neglect, making sensitive judgments concerning the resuscitation efforts for the child, and comforting the members of the family as much as possible. The trend is toward public professional education about SIDS, particularly for those who arrive on the scene first. If properly informed, they should be able to recognize signs of SIDS and tell parents that their child probably died from a disease called sudden infant death syndrome, which cannot be predicted or prevented. A compassionate, sensitive approach to the family during the very first few minutes can help spare them some of the overwhelming guilt and anguish that frequently follow this type of death.

Arriving at the emergency room. The first contact that nurses have with these families is in the emergency room, when the infant is seen by a physician in order to be pronounced dead. Usually there is no attempt at resuscitation. During the time in the emergency room several aspects warrant special consideration. Parents are asked only factual questions, such as when they found the infant, how he looked, and whom they called for help. Any remarks that may suggest responsibility, such as why didn't they go in earlier, didn't they hear him cry out, was his head buried in a blanket, or were the other siblings jealous of this child, are avoided.

The events that took place when help arrived are discussed. If resuscitation was attempted, the infant may have fractured ribs, internal bleeding, and traumatic bruising, which can simulate physical abuse. If statements were made that were misguided, such as, "This looks like suffocation," they can be corrected before parents harbor them in their minds as indications of their guilt.

Another very important aspect of compassionate care toward these parents is allowing them to say good-bye to their child. A happy, beautiful, living part of themselves has suddenly been taken from them forever. Before they go into the examining room, any blood or emesis is removed from the child, he is covered partially with a sheet or blanket, and the room is put in order, especially if instruments and equipment were used. These are the parents' last moments with their child, and they should be as quiet, meaningful, peaceful, and undisturbed as possible. The child's belongings are packaged for the parents to take home if they wish. Nothing involved in the care of these grief-stricken people is complicated, difficult, or time-consuming; it only involves being human.

Returning home. When the parents return home, they should be visited by a competent, qualified professional as soon after the death as possible. A referral should also be made to the local Sudden Infant Death Foundation. Printed material that contains excellent information about SIDS (available from the national* or local chapters) should be provided.

*__National Sudden Infant Death Foundation, Inc.,__ 2 Metro Plaza, Suite 205, 8240 Professional Place, Landover, MD 20785; **Sudden Infant Death Syndrome Clearinghouse,** 8201 Greensboro Drive, Suite 600, McLean, VA 22102; **American Sudden Infant Death Syndrome Institute,** 275 Carpenter Dr., Suite 100, Atlanta, GA 30328, 1-800-232-SIDS (in Georgia, 1-800-847-SIDS); **Council of Guilds for Infant Survival,** P.O. Box 3841, Davenport, IA 52808.

During the initial visit the parents are helped to gain an intellectual understanding of the disease. The nursing objectives are to assess what the parents have been told, what they think happened, and how they have explained this to the other siblings, other family members, and friends.

Some parents are able to discuss their feelings openly and the nurse supports this coping skill. However, other families may be reluctant to express their grief and the nurse may help the parents bring their feelings out into the open.

The nurse can encourage the expression of emotions by asking about crying and feeling sad, angry, or guilty. It is an attempt to provoke a display of emotion, not just an admission of a feeling. During this session the parents should be helped to explore their usual coping mechanisms and, if these are ineffectual, to investigate new approaches. For example, one parent may refrain from discussing the death for fear of upsetting the other parent, but each may need to hear how the other feels.

The number of visits and plan for subsequent intervention need to be flexible. For example, the siblings may initially appear accepting of the explanation and well adjusted but may later refuse to go to sleep or ask questions about graves or funerals, indicating their need for further help in dealing with the death. Parents facing the question of a subsequent child will need support. Both the birth of a subsequent child and the survival of that child, especially past the age of death of the previous child, are important transitional stages for parents (Swoiskin-Schwartz, Deatrick, and Hanson, 1988).

Since the mourning process takes *at least* a year for completion of acceptance and social reorganization, nurses should call on the family periodically to evaluate their progress. Many families receive much solace and support from talking to other parents who have lost a child from SIDS. Parent groups have been formed throughout the United States and can be contacted through the national or local chapters of the Sudden Infant Death Foundation.

INFANTILE APNEA

Infantile apnea (IA) is defined as cessation of breathing for at least 20 seconds or a briefer apneic episode with bradycardia, cyanosis, or pallor. While most young infants experience periods of apnea, prolonged apnea can rarely be fatal. Although the term "near-miss SIDS" is often applied to children with IA, this is an unfortunate choice because it assumes an unproven cause-and-effect relationship between IA and SIDS. It also produces anxiety in the parents, who are now dealing with a child that they perceive may be in imminent danger of sudden death.

No universal agreement exists regarding the evaluation necessary for confirmation of the diagnosis. A number of tests may be performed to rule out specific, sometimes treatable, causes, such as seizures. The most widely used test is continuous recording of cardiorespiratory patterns (cardiopneumogram). A more sophisticated test, polysomnography ("sleep test") also records brain waves, eye and body movements, and oxygen measurements. However, none of these tests are predictive of risk. Some children with normal results may still have subsequent apneic episodes.

Treatment is also controversial but usually involves continuous home monitoring of cardiorespiratory rhythms and/or the use of respiratory stimulant drugs, such as theophylline. Shaking the child as a first-aid treatment for an apneic episode is not recommended. Guidelines for instituting home monitoring, as well as the duration of monitoring, vary. The trend is to continue monitoring only for as long as it is needed because of the family stress it generates.

Nursing Considerations

The diagnosis of IA engenders great anxiety and concern in parents, and the institution of home monitoring presents additional physical and emotional burdens. If monitoring is required, the nurse can be a major source of support to the family in terms of education about the disorder, equipment, observation of the infant's status, and immediate intervention during apneic episodes, including cardiorespiratory resuscitation (CPR). When explaining about the disorder, the nurse should avoid the term "near-miss SIDS" and clarify any misconceptions between IA and SIDS. To help the family cope with the numerous procedures they must learn, adequate preparation before discharge and written instructions are essential.*

Several types of home monitors are available and most hospitals select the model that the infant will use at home. Nurses, especially those involved in the care at home, must become familiar with the equipment, including its advantages and disadvantages. Safety is a major concern since monitors can cause electrical burns and electrocution. The following precautions are recommended (Center for Devices, 1985):

1. Remove leads from infant when not attached to monitor
2. Unplug power cord from electrical outlet when cord is not plugged into monitor
3. Use safety covers on electrical outlets to discourage children from inserting objects into a socket

Siblings should also be supervised when near the infant and taught that the monitor is not a play object. Other safety practices include informing local utility and rescue squads of the home monitoring in case of an emergency. Telephone numbers for these services should be posted near all telephones in the home.

Family support. Although IA is not a chronic illness,

*Home care instructions for apnea monitoring and CPR are available in Wong, D., and Whaley, L.: Clinical handbook of pediatric nursing, ed. 2, St. Louis, 1986, The C.V. Mosby Co. Educational materials may also be obtained from the National Sudden Infant Death Foundation and the American Sudden Infant Death Syndrome Institute.

many of the stresses observed during the monitoring period are characteristic of those of families with chronically ill children. Parents report increased stress, including marital stress, anxiety, and fatigue, especially mothers who typically have to respond 24 hours a day and feel responsible for the infant's survival (DiMaggio and Sheetz, 1983). Siblings are affected, as well as the affected child, who may be characterized as "spoiled" and have developmental delays. To deal with these potential effects nurses need to employ the same interventions as those discussed for children with chronic illness (see Chapter 18) and be aware of the need for referral when difficulties are suspected.

To lessen the continuous responsibility of monitoring, other family members such as grandparents should be taught how to manipulate the equipment, read and interpret the signals, and administer CPR. They are encouraged to stay with the infant for regular periods to allow parents respite. Support groups of other families who have successfully completed monitoring can also be of benefit. Since baby-sitters are difficult to locate, support group members or nursing students may be potential sources of qualified caregivers.

INFANTILE AUTISM

Autism is a complex, lifelong developmental disorder that is usually manifest before age 36 months and is characterized by a serious lack of social response, gross language deficit, and peculiar speech, if present. It occurs in about 4 to 5:10,000 children and is 4 times more common in males than females.

Possible Origins of Infantile Autism

The etiology of autism is still an unsolved and controversial question. Basically three theories have been proposed. The *psychogenic* or *nurture* theory proposes that the disorder has its pathology in the parent-child relationship. In the *nature-nurture* theory the infants are viewed as biologically impaired whose parents enhance the problem because of emotional inadequacies in dealing with a "vulnerable" child. The *biogenic* or *organic* theory places no blame on the parents but considers the disorder basically an expression of a biologic abnormality.

Currently there is little support for the first two theories and strong evidence for the theory that autism results from damage to the central nervous system, although the exact defect is unknown. There is also evidence for a genetic basis. Nontwin siblings have an increased incidence of autism, and many of the unaffected siblings demonstrate subnormal intellectual functioning, especially in verbal skills. A possible association also exists between fragile X syndrome and autism (Fisch and others, 1986).

Characteristics of Children with Autism

Children with autism demonstrate several peculiar and bizarre characteristics, primarily in social relations, behavior, language, and sensory-perceptual processes (see box above). Such characteristics are critical in the diagnosis of the disorder. Intellectual functioning is impaired, usually in the severe range, although some children have exceptional abilities, such as musical skills or memory. Mental functioning is an important prognostic factor, since children with IQs of 70 or above and those with useful language by age 5 have a better outcome in terms of intellectual progress and social adjustment (Connell, 1985).

Clinical Manifestations of Autism

Social Relations and Behavior
Extreme interpersonal isolation
Intense, abnormal concern for preservation of sameness
Unyielding to cuddling and holding
Do not respond to verbal stimulation
Bizarre attachment to mechanical objects
Odd repetitive behaviors, such as flicking a light switch on and off
Difficult to manage; passive or irritable
Frequent temper tantrums and/or self-destructive behavior

Development
Mental retardation, usually severe
May have advanced gross motor skills
Normal to hyperactive
May have exceptional ability, e.g., memory
Poor suck and feeding responses

Language
Echolalia or parrot speech (automatic repetition of words spoken to them)
Pronominal reversal (tendency to use "you" for "I")
Literal, concrete use of words, e.g., "in" to mean "door"

Sensory/Perceptual Processes
Sensory deficits even though vision and hearing intact
Act as if deaf, yet may be overly sensitive to sound
Hyposensitive or hypersensitive to pain
Have aversion to touch

Nursing Considerations

Therapeutic intervention for the child with autism is a specialized area, involving professionals with advanced training. While numerous therapies have been employed, the most promising results have been from highly structured and intensive behavioral modification programs. In general the objective is to increase social awareness of others, teach verbal communication, and decrease unacceptable behavior. However, the vast majority of these children need assistance and supervision throughout adulthood.

When these children are hospitalized, they usually present many management problems. Decreasing stimulation by using a private or semiprivate room, avoiding extraneous auditory and visual distraction, and encouraging parents to bring in possessions the child is attached to may lessen the disruptiveness of hospitalization. Since physical contact frequently upsets these children, minimum holding and physical care may be necessary to prevent temper tantrums. A thorough assessment of the child's usual routine and activities helps maintain an environment that is manageable and conducive to physical recovery.

A key principle in working with these children is establishing trust. They need to be introduced slowly to new situations with visits with caregivers kept short, whenever possible. Because these children have difficulty organizing their behavior and redirecting their energy, they need to be told directly what to do. Communication should be brief and concrete, such as, "sit on bed." As much as possible the parents are involved in the child's care, and effective approaches used by the family in dealing with disruptive behavior are employed.

Family support. Autism, like so many other chronic conditions, becomes a "family disease." Unfortunately the psychogenetic theory is well-known and, although unsupported by current findings, greatly multiplies the parents' guilt. Stressing what is known about the disorder from a biologic standpoint as well as how little is known can help lessen guilt and shame. Carefully questioning parents about the infant's very early behavior usually yields evidence of autistic tendencies before significant parental or environmental factors could have negatively influenced the child.

Parents need expert counseling early in the course of the disorder and should be referred to the **National Society for Autistic Children (NSAC)**.* NSAC is the most efficient clearinghouse for information about education, treatment programs and techniques, and specialized facilities, such as camps and group homes. There is also a siblings' group called SHARE (Siblings Helping Persons with Autism Through Resources and Energy).

SUMMARY

Several minor and major disorders can occur during infancy. These disorders comprise three principal categories: nutritional disturbances, feeding difficulties, and disorders of unknown etiology. The nurse's responsibilities include a thorough assessment of those factors related to the child's condition, interventions to eliminate or lessen the detrimental effects, and family support to help them cope with stresses imposed by the disorder. While some of these disorders, such as colic, are self-limiting, others, such as SIDS and autism, present numerous long-term challenges to the family.

*1234 Massachusetts Avenue, NW, Washington, DC 20005.

KEY CONCEPTS

- Common nutritional disturbances of infancy include vitamin and mineral disturbances, some types of vegetarian diets, protein and calorie malnutrition, and food intolerance.
- Malnutrition refers to poor or inadequate nutrition, and may result from undernutrition or overnutrition. Common manifestations of undernutrition in the infant include iron deficiency anemia, vitamin deficiencies, and failure to thrive. Manifestations of overnutrition are hypervitaminosis and obesity.
- Mineral disturbances may be caused by mineral-mineral interactions and mineral-diet interactions.
- Vegetarians may be classified into four groups: lacto-ovo-vegetarians, lactovegetarians, pure vegetarians, and Zen macrobiotics.
- Protein and energy malnutrition may occur as a complication of underlying disease, as a result of fad diets, from lack of parental education about infant nutrition, because of inappropriate management of food allergy, and through incorrect preparation of formula.
- Food intolerance encompasses food allergies and food sensitivities, the most serious of which are cow's milk sensitivity and lactose intolerance.
- Treatment of colic may involve change in feeding practices, correction of stressful environment, and support of parent.
- Failure to thrive may be classified as organic, resulting from some physical cause, and nonorganic resulting from psychosocial factors involving the child and caregiver (e.g., maternal deprivation), environmental causes (e.g., inadequate parental knowledge of child feeding), or unexplained causes.
- Disorders of unknown etiology include sudden infant death syndrome (SIDS), infantile apnea, and infantile autism.
- Sudden infant death syndrome is the leading cause of death in children between the ages of 1 week and 1 year. Two theories point to hypoxemia and apnea as possible causes.
- The primary nursing responsibility in care associated wih SIDS and other conditions of unknown etiology is emotional support of the family.
- Autism is a lifelong developmental disorder that is usually manifest before age 36 months. It is characterized by severe cognitive and social retardation, bizarre behavior, and gross language deficits.

STUDY QUESTIONS AND ACTIVITIES

1 Observe the eating patterns of a group of young children and compare their intake with the four food groups. Is any food group poorly represented? What vitamin or mineral deficiencies could occur?
2 Interview parents with an infant with colic. What are the stresses imposed by this child on the family? What comfort measures have the parents tried and which have been successful?
3 Observe the feeding behavior of new parents and their infant to identify possible feeding problems.
4 Compare the growth, development, feeding behavior, and interactions of a child with NFTT with a healthy child of similar age. Discuss the differences.
5 Contact the local SIDS foundation and inquire about its services to families and the community.
6 Visit a school for children with autism. List the characteristics of these children and the types of interventions used by the staff to manage the children.

REFERENCES

Altemeier, W.A., III, and others: Prospective study of antecedents for nonorganic failure to thrive, J. Pediatr. **106**(3):360-365, 1985.

Bachrach, S., Fisher, J., and Parks, J.S.: An outbreak of vitamin D deficiency rickets in a susceptible population, Pediatrics **64**(6):871-877, 1979.

Brooks, J.G.: Apnea of infancy and sudden infant death syndrome, Am. J. Dis. Child. **136:**1012-1023, 1982.

Center for Devices and Radiological Health warns of hazard with apnea monitors, Med. Devices Bull. **3**(4):1-3, 1985.

Connell, H.M.: Essentials of child psychiatry, ed. 2, Boston, 1985, Blackwell Scientific Publications.

DiMaggio, G.T., and Sheetz, A.H.: The concerns of mothers caring for an infant on an apnea monitor, MCN **8**(4):294-297, 1983.

Egan, J., Chatoor, I., and Rosen, G.: Nonorganic failure to thrive: pathogenesis and classification, Clin. Proc. Child. Hosp. DC **36**:173-182, 1980.

Fanelli, M.T., and Kuczmarski, R.J.: Food selection for vegetarians, Diet. Curr. **10**(1):1-6, 1983.

Fisch, G.S., and others: Autism and the fragile X syndrome, Am. J. Psychiatry **143:**71-73, 1986.

Hunt, C., and Brouillette, R.: Sudden infant death syndrome: 1987 perspective, J. Pediatr. **110**(5):669-678, 1987.

Oates, R.K., Peacock, A., and Forrest, D.: Long-term effects of nonorganic failure to thrive, Pediatrics **75**(1):36-40, 1985.

Olness, K.N.: Nutritional consequences of drugs used in pediatrics, Clin. Pediatr. **24**(8):417-420, 1985.

Peterson, D., Sabotta, E., and Daling, J.: Infant mortality among subsequent siblings of infants who died of sudden infant death syndrome, J. Pediatr. **108**(6):911-914, 1986.

Saal, H.M., Ratzan, S.K., and Carey, D.E.: Yogurt: contributory factor in development of nutritional rickets, Clin. Pediatr. **24:**452-454, 1985.

Swoiskin-Schwartz, S., Deatrick, J., and Hanson, D.: Parents' views about having a child after a SIDS death, J. Pediatr. Nurs. **3**(1):24-28, 1988.

Temple, W.J., and Farley, D.H.: The succussion splash as an infant "burp" sign, N. Engl. J. Med. **308**(26):1604, 1983.

BIBLIOGRAPHY

Vitamin and Mineral Disturbances

American Academy of Pediatrics, Committee on Nutrition: Vitamin and mineral supplement needs in normal children in the United States, Pediatrics **66**(6):1015-1020, 1980.

Cerrato, P.L.: Vitamin C: who needs it? and when? RN **48**(8):59-60, 1985.

Cerrato, P.L.: When to worry about vitamin overdose, RN **48**(10):69-70, 1985.

Fanelli, M.T., and Kuczmarski, R.J.: Dietetic currents, Ross Timesaver **10**(1):1-6, 1983.

Gibson, R.S.: Dietary intakes of trace elements in infants during their first year, Food Nutr. News **57**(10):1-6, 1985.

Goel, K.: Rickets: an old enemy returns, Nurs. Mirror **152**(13):16-18, 1981.

Golden, N.H.N.: Trace elements in human nutrition, Hum. Nutr. Clin. Nutr. **36C:**185-202, 1982.

Harper, A.: Recommended dietary allowances in perspective, Food Nutr. News **58**(2):7-10, 1986.

Jarvis, W.T.: Vitamin use and abuse, Contemp. Nutr. **9**(10):1-2, 1984.

Mertz, W.: The significance of trace elements for health, Nutr. Today **18**(5):26-31, 1983.

Mertz, W.: The essential elements: nutritional aspects, Nutr. Today **19**(1):22-30, 1984.

Nurses' quick guide to nutritional disorders, Nursing 83 **13**(4):56-57, 1983.

Thomas, K.: Folic acid deficiency related to the use of goat milk for infant feeding, Issues Compr. Pediatr. Nurs. **4:**37-43, 1980.

Walker, W.A., and Hendricks, K.M.: Manual of pediatric nutrition, Philadelphia, 1985, W.B. Saunders Co.

Williams, S.R.: Nutrition and diet therapy, ed. 5, St. Louis, 1985, The C.V. Mosby Co.

Vegetarian Diets

Dietz, W.H., and Dwyer, J.T.: Nutritional implications of vegetarianism for children. In Suskind, R.M., editor: Textbook of pediatric nutrition, New York, 1981, Raven Press.

Johnston, P.K.: Getting enough to grow on, Am. J. Nurs. **84**(3):336-339, 1984.

Purvis, G.A.: Vegetarian nutrition in infancy, Pediatr. Basics **34:**1, 1982.

Rudy, C.A.: Vegetarian diets for children, Pediatr. Nurs. **10**(5):329-333, 1984.

Rudy, C.A.: Teaching families about the well-balanced vegetarian diet, Child. Nurse **3**(5):1-3, 1985.

Protein and Calorie Malnutrition

Goodall, J.: Malnutrition and the family: deprivation in kwashiorkor, Proc. Nutr. Soc. **38**(1):17-27, 1979.

Karp, R.J., Scholl, T.O., and Greene, G.W.: Precursors of malnutrition in children, Public Health Curr. **25**(3):11-14, 1985.

Viteri, F.E.: Primary protein-energy malnutrition: clinical, biochemical, and metabolic changes. In Suskind, R.M., editor: Textbook of pediatric nutrition, New York, 1981, Raven Press.

Food Intolerance/Feeding Difficulties

American Academy of Pediatrics, Committee on Nutrition: The practical significance of lactose intolerance in children, Pediatrics **62**(2):240-245, 1978.

American Academy of Pediatrics, Committee on Nutrition: Soy-protein formulas: recommendations for use in infant feeding, Pediatrics **72**(3):359-363, 1983.

Carey, W.B.: "Colic" or excessive crying in young infants. In Levine, M.D., and others, editors: Developmental-behavioral pediatrics, Philadelphia, 1983, W.B. Saunders Co.

Castiglia, P.T.: Crying babies, J. Pediatr. Health Care **1**(2):110-111, 1987.

Dixie, M.: Maternal food allergy as a cause of infantile colic in the breast-fed baby, Health Visit. **54**(6):240-241, 1981.

Frappier, P., Marino, B., and Shishmanian, E.: Nursing assessment of infant feeding problems, J. Pediatr. Nurs. **2**(1):37-44, 1987.

Gillies, C.: Infant colic: is there anything new? J. Pediatr. Health Care **1**(6):305-312, 1987.

Institute of Food Technologists' Expert Panel on Food Safety and Nutrition: Food allergies and other food sensitivities, Contemp. Nutr. **10**(11):1-2, 1985.

Romanko, M.V., and Brost, B.A.: Swaddling: an effective invention for pacifying infants, Pediatr. Nurs. **8:**259-261, 1982.

Waldman, W.H., and Sarsgard, D.: Helping parents to cope with colic, Pediatr. Basics **33:**12-14, 1982.

White, J.E., and Owsley, V.B.: Helping families cope with milk, wheat, and soy allergies, MCN **8:**423-428, 1983.

Wichelow, M.J., and others: Coping with colic in the breast-fed baby, Health Visit. **53**(1):6-7, 1980.

Failure to Thrive

Ayoub, C., Pfeifer, D., and Leichtman, L.: Treatment of infants with non-organic failure to thrive, Child Abuse Negl. **3:**937-941, 1979.

Bithoney, W., and Rathbun, J.: Failure to thrive. In Levine, M.D., and others, editors: Developmental-behavioral pediatrics, Philadelphia, 1983, W.B. Saunders Co.

Castiglia, P.: Failure-to-thrive, J. Pediatr. Health Care **2**(1):50-51, 1988.

Drotar, D., and Malone, C.: Family-oriented intervention with the failure-to-thrive infant. In Klaus, M.H., and Robertson, M.O., editors: Birth, interaction and attachment, Skillman, NJ, 1982, Johnson & Johnson Baby Products Co.

Endert, C.M., and Wooldridge, N.H.: Nonorganic failure to thrive, Diet. Curr. **14**(1):1-6, 1987.

Harrison, L.: The failure-to-thrive child. In Johnson, S., editor: Nursing assessment and strategies for the family at risk, ed. 2, Philadelphia, 1986, J.B. Lippincott Co.

Hilton, A.: Approaches for feeding the young child with anorexia, J. Pediatr. Nurs. **2**(1):45-49, 1987.

Lierman, C., and others: Multidisciplinary treatment of feeding disorders in the home, Pediatr. Nurs. **13**(4):266-270, 1987.

Mira, M., and Cairns, G.: Intervention in the interaction of a mother and child with nonorganic failure to thrive, Pediatr. Nurs. **8**(2):41-46, 1981.

Showers, J., and others: Nonorganic failure to thrive: identification and intervention, J. Pediatr. Nurs. **1**(4):240-246, 1986.

Steele, S.: Nonorganic failure to thrive: a pediatric social illness, Issues Compr. Pediatr. Nurs. **9**(1):47-58, 1986.

Yoos, L.: Taking another look at failure to thrive, MCN **9**(1):32-36, 1984.

Sudden Infant Death Syndrome/Infantile Apnea

American Academy of Pediatrics, Task Force on Prolonged Infantile Apnea: Prolonged infantile apnea: 1985, Pediatrics **76**(1):129-131, 1985.

Buschbacher, V.I., and Delcampo, R.L.: Parents' response to sudden infant death syndrome, J. Pediatr. Health Care **1**(2):85-90, 1987.

Cain, L.P., Kelly, D.H., and Shannon, D.C.: Parents' perceptions of the psychological and social impact of home monitoring, Pediatrics **66**(1):37-41, 1980.

Chan, M.: Sudden infant death syndrome and families at risk, Pediatr. Nurs. **13**(3):166-168, 1987.

Cordell, A.S., and Apolito, R.: Family support in infant death, JOGNN **10**(4):281-285, 1981.

Duncan, J.A., and Webb, L.Z.: Teaching families home apnea monitoring, Pediatr. Nurs. **9**(3):171-175, 1983.

Graber, H.P., and Balas-Stevens, S.: A discharge tool for teaching parents to monitor infant apnea at home, MCN **9**(3):178, 1984.

Hartsell, M.: Selecting home monitors, J. Pediatr. Nurs. **1**(1):54-57, 1986.

Kotsubo, C.Z.: Helping families survive SIDS, Nursing 83 **13**(5):94-96, 1983.

Longo, A.: Teaching parents CPR, Pediatr. Nurs. **9**(6):445-447, 1983.

Nikolaisen, S.: The impact of sudden infant death on the family: nursing intervention, Top. Clin. Nurs. **3**(3):45-53, 1981.

Norris-Berkemeyer, S., and Hutchins, K.: Home apnea monitoring, Pediatr. Nurs. **12**(4):259-262, 304, 1986.

Price, M., and others: Maternal perceptions of sudden infant death syndrome, Child. Health Care **14**(1):22-31, 1985.

Rehm, R.S.: Teaching cardiopulmonary resuscitation to parents, MCN **8**(6):411-414, 1983.

Webb, L.Z., and Duncan, J.A.: Selecting the right home apnea monitor, Pediatr. Nurs. **9**(3):179-182, 1983.

Infantile Autism

Christian, W.P.: Childhood autism. In Levine, M., and others, editors: Developmental-behavioral pediatrics, Philadelphia, 1983, W.B. Saunders Co.

Cruz, V.K., Andron, L., and Sammons, C.: Cookie monster is autistic . . . help younger children with developmentally disabled siblings cope, Child. Today **13**(2):18-20, 1984.

DeMyer, M.K., Hingtgen, J.N., and Jackson, R.K.: Infantile autism reviewed: a decade of research, Schizophr. Bull. **7**(3):388-451, 1981.

Dudziak, D.: Parenting the autistic child, J. Psychosoc. Nurs. Ment. Health Serv. **20**(1):11-16, 1982.

Harris, M.: Understanding the autistic child, Am. J. Nurs. **78**(10):1682-1685, 1978.

Killion, S., and McCarthy, S.: Hospitalization of the autistic child, Part I—Assessment, Part II—Autistic children, intervention, MCN **5**(6):412-423, 1980.

Moss, B.K.: When autism threatens family balance, Patient Care **15:**15-33, April 1981.

Zoltak, B.: Autism: recognition and management, Pediatr. Nurs. **12**(2):90-94, 1986.

UNIT VI

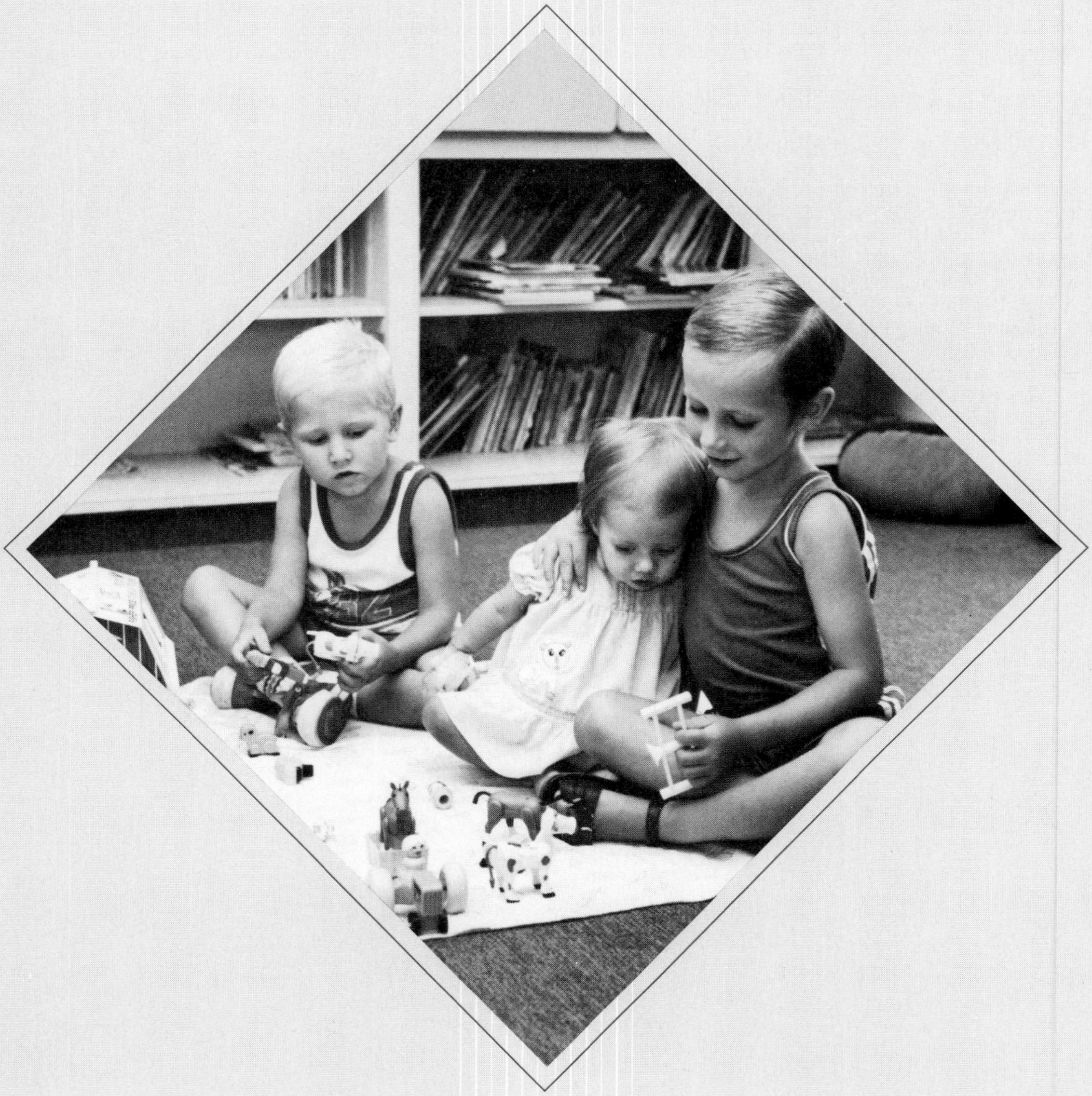

Early Childhood

Early childhood comprises the years of toddlerhood and preschool. It is primarily a period of physical development and refinement, attainment of social skills, and achievement of independent behavior. Dramatic changes occur in the child as he leaves the dependent world of infancy and readies himself for the self-sufficient life of a school-age child. Chapters 12 and 13, *Health Promotion of the Toddler and Family* and *Health Promotion of the Preschooler and Family* are concerned with the biologic growth and psychologic development of the toddler and preschooler. Emphasis is placed on promoting optimum development during each phase of early childhood, especially through anticipatory guidance regarding nutrition, achievement of self-care activities, prevention of injury, and specific parental concerns.

Chapter 14, *Health Problems of Early Childhood,* deals with health problems that commonly occur during early childhood. Although many of the disorders typical of this period are caused by infectious processes, most of the child's care is implemented in the home, necessitating nursing guidance rather than direct intervention. The other conditions discussed are results of environmental and social factors to which toddlers and preschoolers are especially vulnerable or by which they are greatly influenced. In the discussion of each of these health problems, emphasis is placed on prevention, recognition, and nursing interventions that return the child to an optimum physical and mental status.

CHAPTER 12

Health Promotion of the Toddler and Family

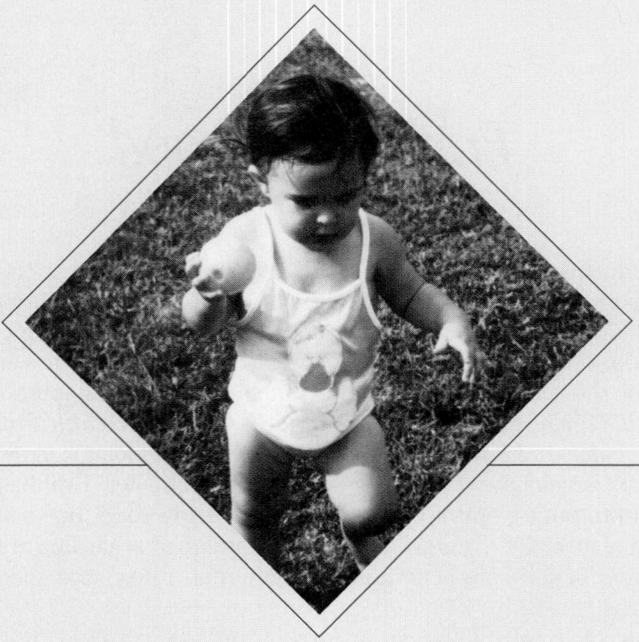

LEARNING OBJECTIVES

On completion of this chapter the reader will be able to:

- Identify the major biologic, psychosocial, cognitive, and social developments during the toddler years
- Relate separation anxiety and negativism to developmental tasks
- Recognize readiness for toilet training and offer parents guidelines
- Prepare toddlers for birth of a sibling
- Provide parents with guidelines for handling temper tantrums
- Provide parents with feeding recommendations
- Outline a preventive dental hygiene plan for toddlers
- Provide anticipatory guidance to parents regarding injury prevention based on the toddler's developmental achievements

The term *terrible twos* has often been used to describe the toddler years, a period from age 12 months to 3 years of age. It is a time of intense exploration of the environment as the child attempts to find out how things work and how to control others with temper tantrums, negativism, and obstinacy. Also, the child learns what the word "no" means. The phrase "he gets into everything" underestimates the toddler's eagerness for adventure, but the very adventure of getting into things is his means of acquiring learning and knowledge.

Although this can be a difficult time for parents and child as each learns to know the other better, it is an extremely important period for developmental achievement and intellectual growth. Successful mastery of the tasks of this age requires a strong foundation of trust during infancy and frequently necessitates guidance from others when parent and toddler face the struggles of toilet training, limit setting and discipline, and sibling rivalry. Nurses who understand the dynamics of growth and development of the toddler can help parents deal effectively with the tasks of this age.

◆ *Promoting Optimum Growth and Development*

General concepts of growth and development, such as stages and patterns of development and individual differences, are discussed in Chapter 5. This chapter is primarily concerned with biologic, psychosocial, cognitive, and social development of toddlers. It also includes a discussion of common parental concerns typical of the developmental characteristics of this age-group.

BIOLOGIC DEVELOPMENT

Biologic development and maturation of body systems is less dramatic during early childhood than during infancy. However, maturation of body systems continues, and many organs achieve mature functioning. The acquisition of fine and gross motor skills is dramatic and allows toddlers to master a wide variety of activities.

Proportional Changes

Growth slows considerably during toddlerhood. The average weight gain is 1.8 to 2.7 kg (4 to 6 pounds) per year. The average weight at 2 years is 12 kg (27 pounds). The birth weight is quadrupled by 2½ years of age. The rate of increase in height also slows. The usual increment is an addition of 7.5 cm (3 inches) per year and occurs mainly in elongation of the legs rather than the trunk. The average height of a 2-year-old is 86.6 cm (34 inches). In general, adult height is about twice the 2-year-old child's height. Accurate measurement of height and weight during the toddler years should reveal a steady growth curve that is *steplike* in nature rather than linear (straight), which is characteristic of the growth spurts during the early childhood years.

The rate of increase in head circumference slows somewhat by the end of infancy, and head circumference is usually equal to chest circumference by 1 to 2 years of age. The usual total increase in head circumference during the second year is 2.5 cm (1 inch). Then the rate of increase slows until at age 5 years the increase is less than 1.25 cm (½ inch) per year. The anterior fontanel closes between 12 and 18 months of age.

Chest circumference continues to increase in size and exceeds head circumference during the toddler years. Its shape also changes as the transverse or lateral diameter exceeds the anteroposterior diameter. After the second year the chest circumference exceeds the abdominal measurement, which, in addition to the growth of the lower extremities, gives the child a taller, leaner appearance. However, the toddler retains a squat, "pot-bellied" appearance because of the less well-developed abdominal musculature and short legs (Fig. 12-1). The legs retain a slightly bowed or curved appearance during the second year from the weight of the relatively large trunk.

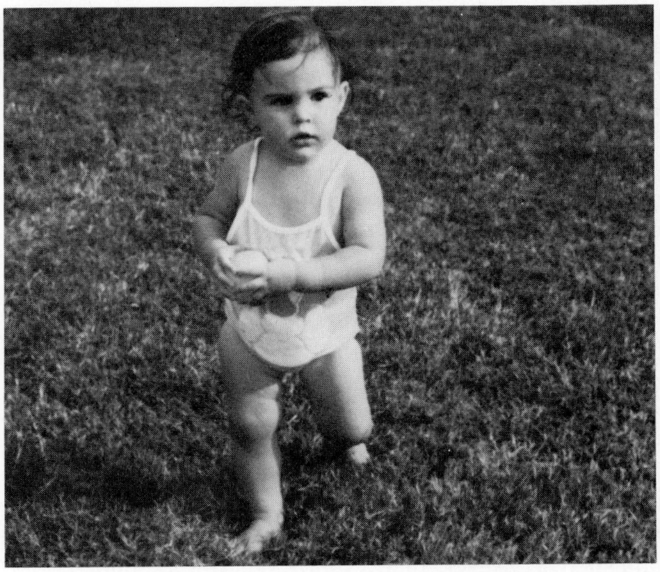

FIG. 12-1 Typical toddling gait.

Sensory Changes

Visual acuity of 20/20 is achieved during the toddler years, although 20/40 is considered acceptable. Full binocular vision is well developed by 12 months of age, and any evidence of persistent strabismus should receive professional attention as early as possible to prevent amblyopia. Depth perception continues to develop but, because of the child's lack of motor coordination, falls from heights continue to be a persistent danger.

The senses of hearing, smell, taste, and touch become increasingly well developed, coordinated with each other, and associated with other experiences. All of the senses are used to explore the environment. The toddler will visually inspect an object by turning it over; he may taste it, smell it, and touch it several times before he is satisfied with his investigation. He will shake it to see if it makes noise and vigorously test its durability. Another example of the integrated function of the senses is the toddler's development of specific taste preferences. The child is much less likely than an infant to try a new food because of its appearance or smell, not only its taste.

Maturation of Systems

Most of the physiologic systems are relatively mature by the end of toddlerhood. The volume of the respiratory tract and growth of associated structures continue to increase during early childhood, lessening some of the factors that predisposed the child to frequent and serious infections during infancy. However, the internal structures of the ear and throat continue to be short and straight, and the lymphoid tissue of the tonsils and adenoids continues to be large. As a result, otitis media, tonsillitis, and upper respiratory infections are common.

The respiratory and heart rates slow and the blood pressure increases (see inside front cover). Respirations continue to be abdominal during the toddler years. Under conditions of moderate variation in temperature, the toddler rarely has the difficulties of the young infant in maintaining body temperature. The mature functioning of the renal system serves to conserve fluid under times of stress, decreasing the risk of dehydration. The gastrointestinal tract can handle most foods consumed by adults, and the slower transit time also makes the toddler somewhat less vulnerable to dehydration from diarrhea.

The defense mechanisms of the skin and blood, particularly phagocytosis, are much more efficient in toddlers than in infants. The production of antibodies is well established. However, many young children demonstrate a sudden increase in colds and minor infections when entering nursery school or other group situations. Gradually their resistance increases, although their contact with heavily crowded areas, such as shopping centers or restaurants during holiday seasons, should be limited.

Gross and Fine Motor Development

The major gross motor skill during the toddler years is the development of locomotion. By 15 months of age toddlers walk alone, by age 18 months they try to run but fall easily, and by 2 years they walk well and run fairly well, using a wide stance for extra balance. Between 2 and 3 years refinement of the upright, biped position is evident in improved coordination and equilibrium. By 2 years toddlers can walk up and down stairs, and by age 2 1/2 years they jump, using both feet, stand on one foot for a second or two, and manage a few steps on tiptoe. By the end of the second year they can stand on one foot, walk on tiptoe, and climb stairs with alternate footing.

Fine motor development is demonstrated in increasingly skillful manual dexterity. Once the pincer grasp is achieved, usually at 9 to 10 months of age, toddlers combine this skill with other developing sensory and cognitive abilities. For example, by age 12 months they are able to grasp a very small object but are unable to release it at will. At 15 months they can drop a pellet into a narrow-necked bottle. Casting, or voluntarily throwing objects, and retrieving them become almost obsessive activities around 15 months of age. By 18 months toddlers can throw a ball overhand without losing their balance.

Mastery of gross and fine motor skills is evident in all phases of the child's activity, such as playing, dressing, language comprehension, response to discipline, social interaction, and proneness to injuries. Activities occur less in isolation and more in conjunction with other physical and mental abilities to produce a purposeful result. For example, the toddler walks to reach a new location, releases a toy to pick it up or to choose a new one, and scribbles to look at the image produced. The possibilities of the exploration, investigation, and manipulation of the environment—and its hazards—are endless.

PSYCHOSOCIAL DEVELOPMENT

The toddler is faced with the mastery of several important tasks. If the need for basic trust has been satisfied, he is ready to give up dependence for control, independence, and autonomy. Some of the specific tasks to be dealt with include (1) differentiation of self from others, particularly the mother; (2) toleration of separation from parent; (3) ability to withstand delayed gratification; (4) control over bodily functions; (5) acquisition of socially acceptable behavior; (6) verbal means of communication; and (7) ability to interact with others in a less egocentric manner. Mastery of these goals begins during late infancy and toddler years, and such tasks as developing interpersonal relationships with others may not be completed until adolescence. However, crucial foundations for successful completion of such developmental tasks are laid during these early formative years.

Developing a Sense of Autonomy (Erikson)

According to Erikson, the developmental task of toddlerhood is to acquire a sense of *autonomy* while overcoming a sense of doubt and shame. As the infant gains trust in the predictability and reliability of his parents, his environment, and his interaction with others, he begins to discover that his behavior is his own and has a predictable, reliable effect on others. However, while he realizes his will and control over others, he is confronted with the conflict of exerting his autonomy and relinquishing his much-enjoyed dependence on others. In addition, exerting his will has definite negative consequences, such as verbal disapproval or punishment, whereas retaining dependent, submissive behavior is generally rewarded with affection and approval. However, continued dependency creates in the child a sense of doubt regarding his potential capacity to control his actions. This doubt is compounded by a sense of shame for feeling this urge to revolt against others' will and a fear that he will exceed his own capacity for manipulating his environment.

Just as the infant has the social modalities of grasping and biting, the toddler has the newly gained modality of holding on and letting go. To hold on and let go is evident with the use of the hands, mouth, eyes, and, eventually, the sphincters, when toilet training is begun. These social modalities are expressed constantly in the child's play activities, such as casting or throwing objects, taking objects out of boxes, drawers, or cabinets, holding on tighter when someone says, "No, don't touch," and spitting out food as taste preferences become very strong.

Several characteristics are typical of toddlers in their quest for autonomy. Two of these, *negativism* and *ritualism,* are especially significant. As the toddler attempts to express his will, he is often contrary to everything around him. The words "no" or "me do" can be the sole vocabulary. Emotions become very strongly expressed, usually in rapid mood swings. One minute the toddler can be engrossed in an activity, and the next minute he might be violently angry because he was unable to manipulate a toy or open a door. If scolded for doing something wrong, he can have a temper tantrum and almost instantaneously pull at his mother's legs to be picked up and comforted. Often these swift changes are difficult for parents to understand and cope with. Many parents find the negativism exasperating and, instead of dealing with it, give into it, which further threatens the child in his search for learning acceptable methods of interacting with others (see also p. 353).

In contrast to negativism, which frequently disrupts the environment, ritualism becomes the needed buffer to maintain sameness and reliability. The toddler can venture out with security when he knows that familiar people, places, and routines still exist. One can easily understand why change, such as hospitalization, represents such a threat to these children. Without the comfortable rituals, there is little opportunity to exert autonomy. Consequently, dependency and regression occur (see also p. 353).

Erikson focuses on the development of the *ego* during this phase of psychosocial development. There is a struggle as the child deals with the impulses of the *id*, attempts to tolerate frustration, and learns socially acceptable ways of interacting with the environment. The ego, which may be thought of as reason or common sense, is evident as the child is able to tolerate delayed gratification.

There is also rudimentary beginning of the *superego* or conscience, which is the incorporation of the morals of society and the process of acculturation. With the development of the ego the child further differentiates himself from others and expands his sense of trust within himself. But as he begins to develop awareness of his own will and capacity to achieve, he also becomes aware of his ability to fail. This ever-present awareness of potential failure creates fear of doubt and shame. Successful mastery of the task of autonomy necessitates opportunities for self-mastery while withstanding the frustration of necessary limit setting and delayed gratification. Opportunities for self-mastery are present in appropriate play activities, toilet training, the crisis of sibling rivalry, and successful interactions with significant others.

COGNITIVE DEVELOPMENT

By the beginning of the second year it is quite clear that the toddler "thinks" and "reasons" things out. There is deliberate trial-and-error experimentation to produce certain results. The mental abstracts of time, space, and causality begin to have meaning, but the child's conception of each is different from that of the adult's. The main cognitive achievement of early childhood is the acquisition of language, which represents mental symbolism.

Sensorimotor and Preconceptual Phase (Piaget)

The period of 12 to 24 months of age is a continuation of the final two stages of the sensorimotor phase. During this time the cognitive processes develop rapidly and at times seem similar to mature thinking. However, reasoning skills are still quite primitive and need to be understood to effectively deal with the typical behaviors of this age child.

Tertiary circular reactions. In the fifth stage (from 13 to 18 months), the child uses active experimentation to achieve previously unattainable goals. Newly acquired physical skills are increasingly important for the function they serve rather than for the acts themselves. The child incorporates the old learning of secondary circular reactions to his new skills and applies the combined knowledge to new situations, with emphasis on the results of the experimentation. In this way there is the beginning of rational judgment and intellectual reasoning. During this stage there is further differentiation of oneself from objects. This is evident in the child's increasing ability to venture away from his parent and to tolerate longer periods of separation.

Awareness of a causal relationship between two events is apparent to the child. For example, as the child flips a light switch, he is aware that a reciprocal response occurs. However, he is not able to transfer that knowledge to new situations. Therefore, every time he sees what appears to be a light switch, he must reinvestigate its function. Such behavior demonstrates the beginning of categorizing data into distinct classes and subclasses. There are innumerable examples of this type of behavior in toddlers as they continuously explore the same object each time it appears in a new place.

Since classification of objects is still rudimentary, the appearance of an object denotes its function. For example, if the child's toys are stored in a paper bag or large container, that toy receptacle is no different than the garbage pail or laundry basket. If the child is allowed to turn over the toy receptacle, he will just as quickly do the same to other similar containers because, for him, there is no difference. Expecting the child to judge which receptacles are permissible to explore and which are not is inappropriate for this age-group. Instead, the forbidden object such as the garbage pail should be placed out of reach.

The discovery of objects as objects leads to the awareness of their spatial relationships. The child is able to recognize different shapes and their relationship to each other. For example, he can fit slightly smaller boxes into each other (nesting) and can place a round object into a hole, even if the board is turned around, upside down, or reversed. He is also aware of space and the relationship of his body to dimensions such as height. He will stretch, stand on a low stair or stool, and pull a string to reach an object.

Object permanence has also advanced. Although he still cannot find an object that has been invisibly displaced or moved from under one pillow to another pillow without his seeing the change, the toddler is increasingly aware of the existence of objects behind closed doors, in drawers, and under tables. Parents are usually acutely aware of this developmental achievement and find high places and locked cabinets the only places inaccessible to toddlers.

Invention of new means through mental combinations. From ages 19 to 24 months the child is in the final sensorimotor stage. During this stage the child completes the more primitive, autistic thought processes of infancy and is prepared for more complex mental operations that occur during the phase of preoperational thought. One of the most dramatic achievements of this stage is in the area of object permanence. The child will now actively search for an object in several potential hiding places. In addition, he can infer a cause when only experiencing the effect. He can infer that an object was hidden in any number of places even if he only saw the original hiding place.

Imitation displays deeper meaning and understanding. There is greater symbolization to imitation. The child is acutely aware of others' actions and attempts to copy them in gestures and in words. *Domestic mimicry* (imitating household activities) and sex-role behavior become increasingly common during this period and during the second year. Identification with the parent of the same sex becomes apparent by the second year and represents the child's intellectual ability to differentiate different models of behavior and to imitate them appropriately (Fig. 12-2).

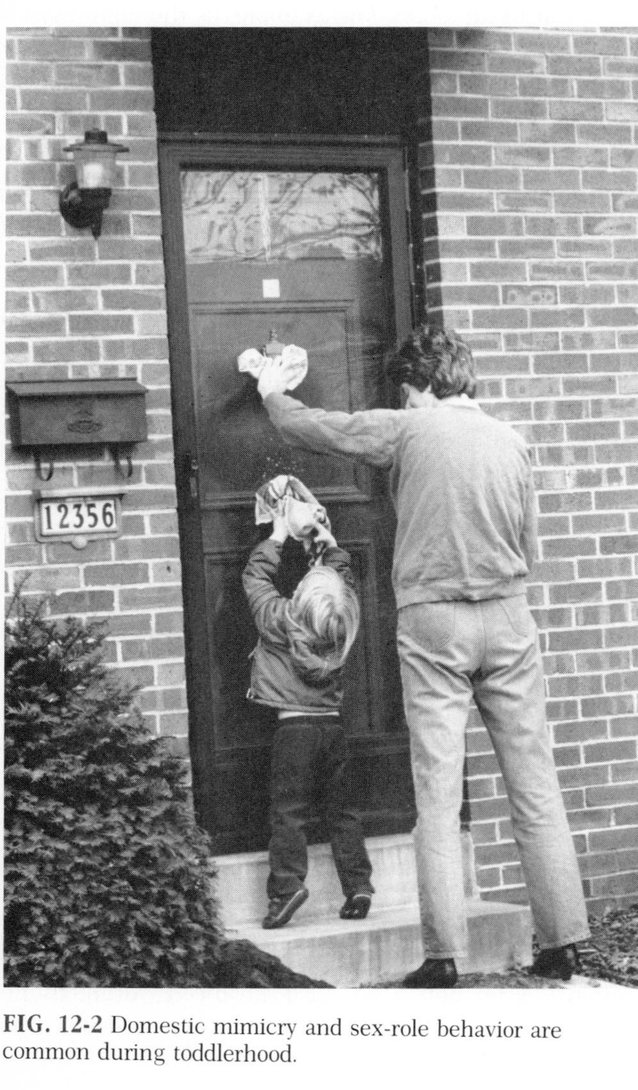

FIG. 12-2 Domestic mimicry and sex-role behavior are common during toddlerhood.

The concept of time is still embryonic, but the child has some sense of timing in terms of anticipation, memory, and the limited ability to wait. He may listen to the command, "Just a minute," and behave appropriately. However, his sense of timing is exaggerated because for him 1 minute can last an hour. The toddler's limited attention span reflects his sense of immediacy and concern for the present. His whole world is for his satisfaction and benefit. However, there is advancement from the infantile form of narcissistic behavior. This is demonstrated in the child's ability to wait, increased concern with pleasing the parent, and awareness of outside controls on this actions.

Egocentrism, or the inability to envision situations from perspectives other than one's own, is evident in all aspects of toddlers' behavior. They see, experience, and live every event in reference to themselves. For example, if a person is positioned between the toddler and another child, the toddler will explain that both children can see the middle person's face. The young child is unable to realize that the other person views the middle person from a different perspective—the back. A common example of egocentric behavior is the toddler who takes a toy away from another child. The child is concerned only with playing with the toy and is unable to conceptualize that taking the toy away will make the other child unhappy.

Preconceptual phase. At approximately 2 years of age the child enters the preconceptual phase of cognitive development, which lasts until about age 4. The preconceptual phase is a subdivision of the *preoperational phase*, which spans ages 2 to 7 years. The preconceptual phase is primarily one of transition that bridges the purely self-satisfying behavior of infancy and the rudimentary socialized behavior of latency.

Preoperational thinking implies that children cannot think in terms of "operations"—the ability to manipulate objects in relation to each other in a logical fashion. Rather, toddlers think primarily based on their perception of an event. Problem-solving is based on what they see or hear directly rather than on what they recall about objects and events. Critical to this type of thought is the concept of *centration*—the tendency to focus on one aspect rather than consider all the possible alternatives. Another aspect of their thinking relates to reasoning. Toddlers' reasoning is neither deductive (from the general to the specific) or inductive (from the specific to the general) but *transductive* (from the particular to the particular). For example, if they did not like one food on the table, they may not like any other food. This prelogic is often very difficult to understand and confusing for parents, who will respond to the previous example by stating, "What does this food have to do with that food?" As far as toddlers are concerned, the decision is logical because it is based on their frame of reference. No amount of "reasoning" will reverse this logic.

Typical of toddlers' thinking is *global organization* of thought processes, or the idea that changing any part of the whole changes the entire whole. Behaviorally this is repeatedly demonstrated in the toddler's ritualistic and rigidly traditional world. Everything must remain the same for the entire event to remain constant. Changing the smallest detail disrupts the entire experience. For example, moving the crib a few inches upsets the entire room.

Another peculiarity of preconceptual thought is the concept of *animism,* in which the child attributes lifelike qualities to inanimate objects. For example, if the child falls down the stairs, he blames the stairs for causing the accident and will frequently "scold" the stairs. Cause and effect is more related to proximity of events rather than to anything else.

Another significant cognitive characteristic is *irreversibility*—the child is unable to undo or reverse mentally the actions he initiates physically. Therefore when told to stop doing something, the child is unable to conceive of the opposite behavior. Consequently, directions should be phrased *positively,* such as "Put the toy down," rather than "Don't throw the toy."

During the second year the child increasingly uses language as symbols and is concerned with the "why" and "how" of things. For example, a pencil is "something to write with," and food is "something to eat.". Mental symbolization is closely associated with the prelogical reasoning. For instance, a needle is "something that hurts." Through the rapid acquisition of language and the ability to associate causes, the child is able to speculate and anticipate future events. If he remembers the needle as something that hurts, he will anticipate any visit to the doctor as one that causes pain. Reminding young children about other visits that did not hurt or experiences that were pleasant will usually do little to change their frame of reference regarding such events.

DEVELOPMENT OF BODY IMAGE

As in infancy, the development of body image closely parallels cognitive development. With increasing motor ability toddlers recognize the usefulness of body parts and gradually learn their respective names. They also learn that certain parts of the body have various meanings; for example, during toilet training the genitals become significant and cleanliness is emphasized. By 2 years of age there is recognition of sexual differences and reference to self by name and then by pronoun.

Once they begin preoperational thought, toddlers can use symbols to represent objects, but their thinking may lead to inaccuracies. For example, if someone who is pregnant is called "fat," they will describe all "fat" ladies as having babies. There is probably some recognition of words used to describe physical appearance, such as "pretty," "handsome," or "big boy." Such expressions eventually influence how children view their own bodies.

Although there has been little research done on body-image development in young children, it is evident that body integrity is poorly understood and that intrusive experiences are threatening. For example, during a physical assessment toddlers forcefully resist procedures such as examining the ear or mouth and taking a rectal temperature. Toddlers also have unclear body boundaries and may associate nonviable parts, such as feces, with essential body parts. This can be seen in a toddler who is upset by flushing the toilet and watching the stool disappear.

SOCIAL DEVELOPMENT

Toddlers are very social beings. As they begin to develop a sense of separateness, they are increasingly able to explore away from the parent, although anxiety related to imposed separations and strangers is at a peak. Major advances occur in language ability and personal-social behavior, although social skills, such as waiting a turn or manners, are extremely rudimentary. Play continues to be a major socializing agent and provides toddlers with invaluable opportunities to learn about the environment.

A major task of the toddler period is differentiation of self from significant others, usually the mother. The differentiation process consists of two phases: *separation,* the children's emergence from a symbiotic fusion with the mother, and *individuation,* those achievements that mark children's assumption of their individual characteristics in the environment. Although the process begins during the latter half of infancy, the major achievements occur during the toddler years.

Toddlers have an increased understanding and awareness of object permanence and some ability to withstand delayed gratification and tolerate moderate frustration. As a result, toddlers react differently to strangers than do infants. The appearance of unfamiliar persons does not represent such a significant threat to their attachment to mother. They have learned from experience that parents exist when physically absent. Repetition of events such as going to bed without mother but waking to find her there again reinforces the reliability of such brief separations. Consequently toddlers are able to venture away from their parents for brief periods of time because of the security of knowing that the parent will be there when they return.

Transitional objects, such as a favorite blanket or toy, provide security for the child, especially when he is separated from parents, dealing with a new stress, or just fatigued (Fig. 12-3). Security objects often become so important to toddlers that they refuse to have them taken away. Such behavior is normal; there is no need to discourage this tendency. During separations, such as daycare, hospitalization, or even staying overnight with a rel-

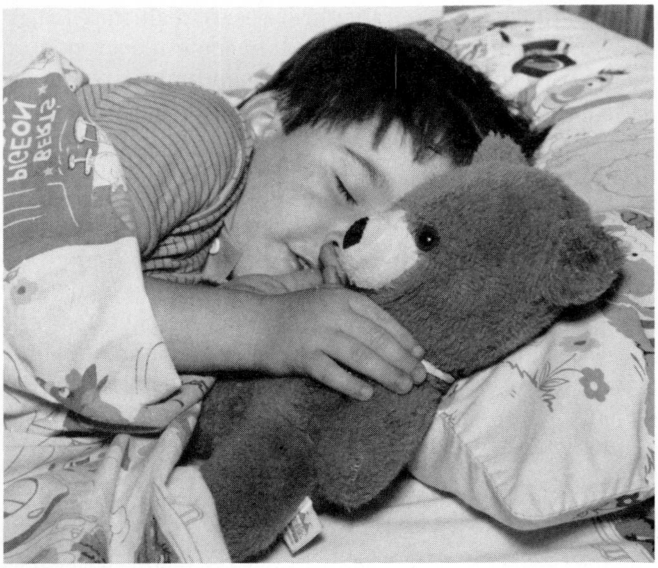

FIG. 12-3 Transitional objects, such as a warm and fuzzy stuffed animal, are sources of security to a toddler.

ative, transitional objects should be provided to minimize any feelings of fear or loneliness.

Learning to tolerate and master brief periods of separation is an important developmental task of children in this age-group. In addition, it is a necessary component of parenting, since brief periods of separation allow parents to recoup their energy and patience and to minimize directing their irritations and frustrations at the children.

Language Development

The most striking characteristic of language development during early childhood is the increasing level of comprehension. Although the number of words acquired—from about four at 1 year of age to approximately 300 at age 2 years—is notable, the ability to comprehend and understand speech is much greater than the number of words the child can say. This is particularly evident in bilingual families where the vocabulary may be delayed, but comprehension in either language is appropriate.

At age 1 year the child uses one-word sentences or holophrases. The word "up" can mean "pick me up" or "look up there." For the child the one word conveys the meaning of a sentence, but to others it may mean many things or nothing. At this age about 25% of the vocalizations are intelligible. By the age of 2 years the child uses multiword sentences by stringing together two or three words, such as the phrases, "mama go bye-bye" or "all gone," and approximately 66% of the speech is understandable.

Personal-Social Behavior

One of the most dramatic aspects of development in the toddler is his personal-social interaction. Parents frequently wonder why their manageable, docile, lovable infant has turned into a determined, strong-willed, volatile-tempered little tyrant. In addition the tyrant of the terrible twos can swiftly and unpredictably revert back to the adorable infant. All of this is part of his "growing up" and is evident in such areas as dressing, feeding, playing, and establishing self-control.

The toddler is developing skills of independence, which are evident in all areas of behavior. The 15-month-old child feeds himself, drinks well from a cup, and manages a spoon, with considerable spilling. By 24 months he uses a spoon well and may be using a fork. Between ages 2 and 3 years he eats with the family, likes to help with chores such as setting the table or removing dishes from the dishwasher, but lacks table manners and may find it difficult to sit through the family's entire meal.

In dressing, the toddler also demonstrates strides toward independence. The 15-month-old child helps his parent by putting his arm or foot out for dressing and pulls his shoes and socks off. The 18-month-old child removes his own gloves, helps with pullover shirts, and may be able to unzip. By age 2 years he removes most of his clothing and puts on his socks, shoes, and pants without regard for right or left and back or front.

Play

Play magnifies the toddler's physical and psychosocial development. Interaction with people becomes increasingly important. The solitary play of infancy progresses to *parallel* play. The toddler plays alongside, not with, other children. Although sensorimotor play is still prominent, there is much less emphasis on the exclusive use of one sensory modality. The toddler inspects the toy, talks to the toy, tests its strength and durability, and invents several uses for it. Imitation is one of the most distinguishing characteristics of play and enriches children's opportunity to engage in fantasy. With less emphasis on sex-stereotyped toys, play objects such as dolls, carriages, dollhouses, dishes, cooking utensils, child-sized furniture, trucks, and dress-up clothes are suitable for both sexes (Fig. 12-4).

Increased locomotive skills make push-pull toys, stick horses, straddle trucks or cycles, a small, low gym and slide, varied-size balls, and rocking horses appropriate for the energetic toddler. Finger paints, thick crayons, chalk, blackboard, paper, and puzzles with large simple pieces use the child's developing fine motor skills. Interlocking blocks in varied sizes and shapes provide hours of fun and, during later years, are useful objects for creative and imaginative play.

Talking is a form of play for the toddler, who enjoys musical toys such as play phonographs, "talking" dolls and animals, and play telephones. Appropriate children's television programs are excellent for children in this age-group who learn to associate words with visual images. Toddlers also enjoy "reading" stories from a picture book and imitating the sounds of animals.

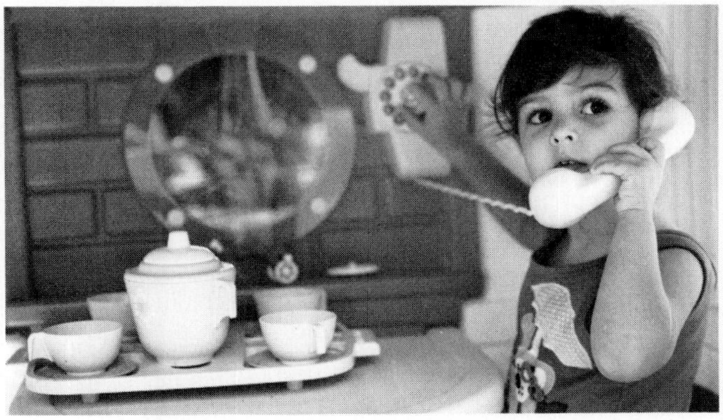

FIG. 12-4 Imitative play is common during the toddler years.

Tactile play is also important for the exploring toddler. Water toys, a sandbox with pail and shovel, finger paints, soap bubbles, and clay provide excellent opportunities for free creative and manipulative recreation. Parents sometimes forget the fascination of feeling slippery cream, catching airy bubbles, squeezing and reshaping clay, or smearing paints. These types of unstructured activities are as important as educational play to allow children freedom of expression.

Selection of appropriate toys must involve safety factors, especially in relation to size and sturdiness. The oral activity of toddlers makes them at risk for aspirating small objects. Parents need to be especially vigilant of toys played with in other children's homes or those of older siblings. Toys are a potential source of serious bodily damage to toddlers, who may have the physical strength to manipulate them but not the knowledge to appreciate their danger (see Guidelines for toy safety on p. 93).

SUMMARY OF GROWTH AND DEVELOPMENT DURING TODDLERHOOD

Developmental achievements during the toddler years occur in physical, gross and fine motor, language, and social areas. The key developmental ages are 18 and 24 months, although the chronologic ages of 15 and 30 months are also significant. Fifteen months of age is a particularly integrative period of developmental achievement since it represents the completion or fruition of many skills that were unperfected at 1 year of age. Table 12-1 presents a summary of the major features of growth and development for the age-groups of 15, 18, 24, and 30 months.

COPING WITH CONCERNS RELATED TO NORMAL GROWTH AND DEVELOPMENT

The toddler years can be trying and confusing for parents. Behaviorally the toddler can be described as untiringly energetic, insatiably inquisitive, annoyingly negative, and obstinately ritualistic. Understanding these behaviors helps parents realize their necessity and allows them to effectively deal with the developmental tasks of children in this age-group.

Toilet Training

One of the major tasks of toddlerhood is toilet training. Voluntary control of the anal and urethral sphincters is achieved sometime after the child is walking, probably between ages 18 and 24 months. However, complex psychophysiologic factors are required for readiness. The child must be able to recognize the urge to let go and hold on and be able to communicate this sensation to the mother. In addition, there is probably some necessary motivation in the desire to please mother by holding on, rather than pleasing oneself by letting go.

Usually physical and psychologic readiness is not complete until the later half of the second year. By this time the child has mastered the majority of essential gross motor skills, can communicate intelligibly, is less in conflict with self-assertion and negativism, and is aware of his ability to control his body and please his mother. One of the most important responsibilities of nurses is to help parents identify readiness in their child (Table 12-2).

Bowel training is usually accomplished before bladder training because of its greater regularity and predictability. There is a stronger sensation for defecation than urination, which can be brought to the child's attention. Nighttime bladder training may not be completed until 4 or 5 years of age. Daytime accidents are also not uncommon, particularly during periods of intense activity. Preschoolers become so engrossed in play activity that if they are not reminded they will wait until it is too late to make it to the bathroom. Boys may begin toilet training in the stand-up position or by sitting on a potty chair or toilet. Imitating father during the preschool years is a powerful motivating force.

Various helpful techniques are advocated to encourage the child's cooperation. One is the use of a free-standing potty-chair, which allows the child a feeling of security (Fig. 12-5). Another option is a portable seat attached to the regular toilet to facilitate the transition from potty-chair to regular toilet. If a potty-seat is not available, having the child sit *facing* the toilet tank provides added support. Using positive reinforcement through the use of training pants or fancy panties and encouraging imitation by watching others also works for some children. Forcing the child to sit on the potty for long periods of time, spanking him for having accidents, or other methods of negative control should be avoided.

Sibling Rivalry

The arrival of a new infant into the family represents a crisis for even the best prepared toddler, especially the firstborn, who has experienced the wonderful position of being number one. The toddler does not hate or resent the infant but the change that this additional sibling pro-

TABLE 12-1

Summary of Growth and Development during the Toddler Years

Age (months)	Physical	Gross Motor	Fine Motor
15	Steady growth in height and weight Head circumference 48 cm (19 inches) Weight 11 kg (24 pounds) Height 78.7 cm (31 inches)	Walks without help (usually since age 13 months) Creeps up stairs Kneels without support Cannot walk around corners or stop suddenly without losing balance Assumes standing position without support Cannot throw ball without falling	Constantly casting objects to floor Builds tower of two cubes Holds two cubes in one hand Releases a pellet into a narrow-necked bottle Scribbles spontaneously Uses cup well but rotates spoon
18	Physiologic anorexia from decreased growth needs Anterior fontanel closed Physiologically able to control sphincters	Runs clumsily, falls often Walks up stairs with one hand held Pulls and pushes toys Jumps in place with both feet Seats self on chair Throws ball overhand without falling	Builds tower of three to four cubes Release, prehension, and reach well developed Turns pages in a book two or three at a time In drawing, makes stroke imitatively Manages spoon without rotation
24	Head circumference 49 to 50 cm (19.5 to 20 inches) Chest circumference exceeds head circumference Lateral diameter of chest exceeds anteroposterior diameter Usual weight gain of 1.8 to 2.7 kg (4 to 6 pounds) Usual gain in height of 10 to 12.5 cm (4 to 5 inches) Adult height approximately double height at 2 years of age May have achieved readiness for beginning daytime control of bowel and bladder Primary dentition of 16 teeth	Goes up and down stairs alone with two feet on each step Runs fairly well, with wide stance Picks up object without falling Kicks ball forward without overbalancing	Builds tower of six to seven cubes Aligns two or more cubes like a train Turns pages of book one at a time In drawing, imitates vertical and circular strokes Turns doorknob, unscrews lid
30	Birth weight quadrupled Primary dentition (20 teeth) completed May have daytime bowel and bladder control	Jumps with both feet Jumps from chair or step Stands on one foot momentarily Takes a few steps on tiptoe	Builds tower of eight cubes Adds chimney to train of cubes Good hand-finger coordination; holds crayon with fingers rather than fist Moves fingers independently In drawing, imitates vertical and horizontal strokes, makes two or more strokes for cross

duces. Mother and father now share their love and attention with someone else, the usual routine is disrupted, and the toddler may lose his crib—all at a time when he thought he was in control of his world.

Preparation of a child for the birth of a sibling is quite individual, but age dictates some important considerations. Time for toddlers is a vague concept. Preparing children too soon for the birth may lessen their interest by the time the event occurs. Toddlers are aware of something when mother's belly gets large and changes have taken place within the house. A month or two in advance is ample time for preparing the child.

Toddlers also need to have a realistic idea of what newborns are like. Telling him that a new playmate will come home soon is foolish, since it is untrue and sets up unrealistic expectations. Rather, parents should stress the activities that will take place when the baby arrives home, such as diapering, bottle- or breast-feeding, bathing, and dressing. At the same time they should emphasize which routines will stay the same, such as reading stories or going to the park. If the toddler has had no contact with an infant, it is a good idea to introduce him to one, if this is feasible.

Frequently other preparations, such as introducing the toddler to a regular bed or moving him to a different room, should be made earlier. If these changes are done well in advance, they will not be associated with the infant's arrival.

Pregnancy is an abstraction for toddlers. They need concrete illustrations of how the baby is growing inside

Sensory	Language	Socialization
Able to identify geometric forms; places round object into appropriate hole Binocular vision well developed Displays an intense and prolonged interest in pictures	Uses expressive jargon Says four to six words, including names "Asks" for objects by pointing Understands simple commands May use head-shaking gesture to denote "no" Uses "no" even while agreeing to the request	Tolerates some separation from parent Less likely to fear strangers Beginning to imitate parents, such as cleaning house (sweeping, dusting), folding clothes May discard bottle Manages spoon but rotates it near mouth Kisses and hugs parents, may kiss pictures in a book Expressive of emotions, has temper tantrums
	Says 10 or more words Points to a common object, such as shoe or ball, and to two or three body parts	Great imitator ("domestic mimicry") Takes off gloves, socks, and shoes and unzips Temper tantrums may be more evident Beginning awareness of ownership ("my toy") May develop dependency on transitional objects, such as "security blanket"
Accommodation well developed In geometric discrimination, able to insert square block into oblong space	Has vocabulary of approximately 300 words Uses two- to three-word phrases Uses pronouns I, me, you Understands directional commands Gives first name; refers to self by name Verbalizes need for toileting, food, or drink Talks incessantly	Stage of parallel play Has sustained attention span Temper tantrums decreasing Pulls people to show them something Increased independence from parent Dresses self in simple clothing
	Gives first and last name Refers to self by appropriate pronoun Uses plurals Names one color	Separates more easily from parent In play, helps put things away, can carry breakable objects, pushes with good steering Begins to notice sex differences; knows own sex May attend to toilet needs without help except for wiping

TABLE 12-2

Indications of Readiness for Toilet Training

Physical Readiness	Mental Readiness	Psychological Readiness	Parental Readiness
Voluntary control of anal and urethral sphincters, usually by 18 to 24 months Ability to stay dry for 2 hours; decreased number of wet diapers; waking dry from nap Regular bowel movements Gross motor skills of sitting, walking, and squatting Fine motor skills to remove clothing	Recognizes urge to defecate or urinate Verbal or nonverbal communicative skills to indicate when wet or has urge to defecate or urinate Cognitive skills to imitate appropriate behavior and follow directions	Expresses willingness to please parent Able to sit on toilet for 5 to 10 minutes without fussing or getting off Curiosity about adults' or older sibling's toilet habits Impatience with soiled or wet diapers; desire to be changed immediately	Recognizes child's level of readiness Willing to invest the time required for toilet training Absence of family stress or change, such as a divorce, moving, new sibling, or imminent vacation

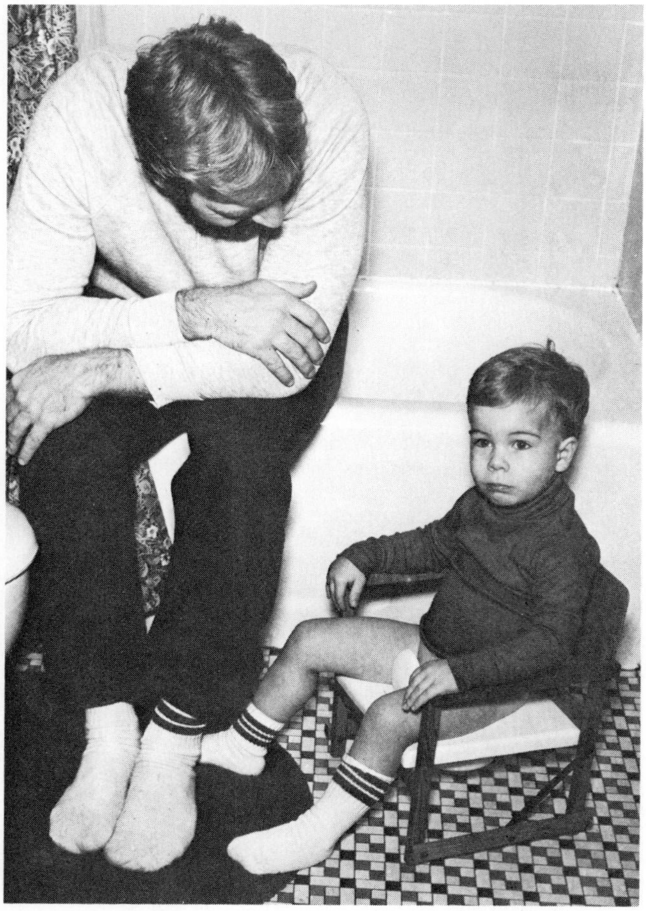

FIG. 12-5 Toddler on a free-standing potty chair.

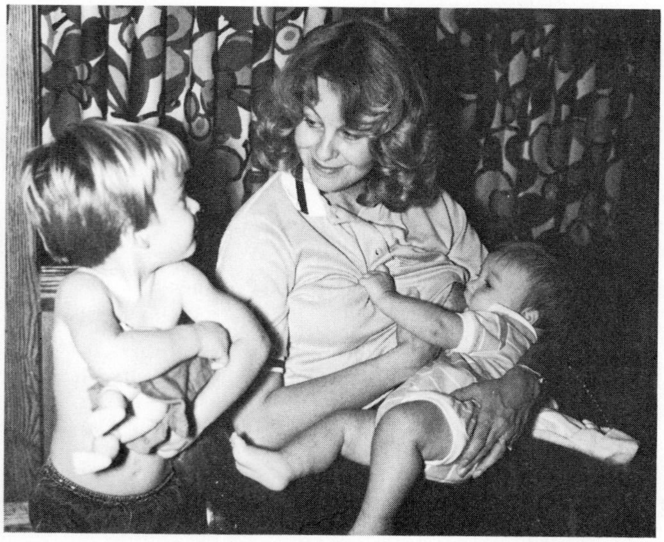

FIG. 12-6 Toddlers enjoy participating in caregiving activities for the new sibling, such as this toddler who is "breastfeeding" his doll.

the mother. It is an excellent opportunity for introducing aspects of reproduction and sexuality. Showing simple pictures of the uterus and fetus, allowing the child to feel the fetus move, and involving the child in caregiving activities after the infant is born help him feel involved in the experience (Fig. 12-6). Children also benefit from "siblings'" classes that may be part of prenatal sessions.

The way in which children exhibit jealousy is complex. Some will overtly hit the infant, push him off mother's lap, or pull the bottle or breast from his mouth. More often the expressions of hostility and resentment are much more subtle and covert. Toddlers may verbally express a wish that the infant "go back inside mommy," or they will revert to more infantile forms of behavior, such as demanding a bottle, soiling their diaper, clinging for attention, using baby talk, or aggressively acting out toward others. For this reason infants must be protected by parental supervision of the interaction between the siblings.

Discipline

Discipline becomes an important concern during the toddler years as parents are faced with the increasing need to limit and shape the child's behavior in order to protect the child and to teach socially acceptable behavior. Like all children, toddlers want and need discipline. In their striving for autonomy, unrestricted freedom is a tremendous threat to their security and safety. Through testing the limits imposed on them, they learn how far they can manipulate their environment as well as gain reassurance from knowing that others will be there to protect them from potential harm.

Numerous types of discipline may be employed during these early years and several are discussed in Chapter 4. However, one strategy that is particularly well suited to the physical needs and cognitive understanding of this age child is time out (see p. 66). At a very early age children learn that certain behaviors have undesirable consequences, such as sitting alone in a quiet room for a couple of minutes. Time out also provides young children with a safe retreat when they are unable to conform to expected behavior. For example, when a child is tired and irritable, a simple suggestion of, "Do you need to rest in your chair?", offers the child a constructive option other than continuing annoying behavior. For occasions when the child misbehaves outside the home, marking the hand with a felt pen serves as a reminder that time out will be instituted upon returning home.

Although many parents try reasoning to persuade the child to behave differently, reasoning is frequently ineffective because toddlers are egocentric. For example, explaining to a young child that "he should not hit because hitting hurts" makes little sense. Unable to take another person's perspective, the child aggressor is more concerned with the satisfaction derived from hitting than for the other child's feelings that hitting hurts. Consequently, hitting the child to demonstrate the discomfort is ineffective because the parent is modeling the very behavior he wishes to eliminate.

Temper Tantrums

Toddlers may assert their independence by violently objecting to discipline. They may lie down on the floor, kick their feet, and scream at the top of their lungs. Some have learned the effectiveness of holding their breath until the parent relents. Although holding one's breath may cause fainting from the lack of oxygen, the accumulation of carbon dioxide will stimulate the respiratory control center, resulting in no physical harm.

The best approach toward extinguishing such attention-seeking behavior is to ignore it, provided the behavior is not injuring the child, such as violently banging his head on the floor. However, the parent should remain close. When the tantrum has subsided, the child needs to feel some control and security. At this time a different toy or a favorite activity can be substituted for the ungranted request.

Frequently temper tantrums can be avoided by giving the child advance warning of a request. For example, a popular time for tantrums is before bed. Active toddlers often have trouble slowing down and when placed in bed, resist staying there. One approach is to establish limited rituals that signal readiness for bed, such as a bath or story. Parents can reinforce the pattern by stating, "After this story it is bedtime," and consistently carrying through the routine.

Negativism

One of the more difficult aspects of rearing children in this age-group is their persistent "no" response to every request. The negativism is not an expression of being fresh or insolent, but a necessary assertion of self-control. One method of dealing with the negativism is reducing the opportunities for a "no" answer. Asking the child, "Do you want to go to sleep now?" is an almost certain example of a question that will be answered with an emphatic "no." Instead, tell the child that it is time to go to sleep and proceed accordingly.

In their attempt to exert control, children like to make choices. When confronted with appropriate choices, such as, "You can have a peanut butter and jelly sandwich or chicken noodle soup for lunch," they are more likely to choose one rather than automatically say no. However, if their response is negative, parents should make the choice for the child.

Regression

Regression is the retreat from one's present pattern of functioning to past levels of behavior. It usually occurs in instances of discomfort or stress when one attempts to conserve his psychic energy by reverting to patterns of behavior that were successful in earlier stages of development. Regression is common in toddlers, because almost any additional stress hinders their ability to master present developmental tasks. Any threat to their autonomy, such as illness, hospitalization, separation, or adjustment to a sibling, represents a need to revert to earlier forms of behavior, such as increased dependency, refusal to use the potty-chair, temper tantrums, demand for the bottle, stroller, or crib, and loss of newly learned motor, language, social, and cognitive skills.

At first such regression appears acceptable and comfortable for children, but the loss of newly acquired achievements is frightening and threatening, because children are aware of their total helplessness in the recent past. Parents, too, become frightened about regressive behavior and frequently in their efforts to deal with it force the child to cope with an additional source of stress—the pressure to live up to expected standards.

When regression does occur, the best approach is to ignore it, while praising existing patterns of appropriate behavior. Regression is a child's way of saying, "I can't cope with this present stress and perfect this skill as well, but I will if given patience and understanding." For this reason it is advisable not to attempt new areas of learning when an additional crisis is present or expected, such as beginning toilet training shortly before a sibling is born or attempting new areas of learning during a brief period of hospitalization.

◆ *Promoting Optimum Health during Toddlerhood*

Physical and psychosocial changes in toddlers affect several areas of health maintenance and promotion, namely, nutrition, sleep and activity, dental health, and injury prevention. Nursing intervention, especially anticipatory guidance, can positively affect the optimal development of the child and family during this exciting, but often troublesome, period of childhood.

NUTRITION

During the period from 12 to 18 months of age, the growth rate slows, decreasing the child's need for calories, protein, and fluid. However, the protein (23 gms) and calorie (900-1800) requirements are still relatively high to meet the demands for muscle tissue growth and high activity level. Need for minerals such as iron, calcium, and phosphorus is still high, particularly when one considers the poor food habits of children in this age-group and the increased mineralization within bones. The number of servings in each food group and suggested portions are given in Table 12-3.

At approximately 18 months of age, most toddlers manifest this decreased nutritional need in a phenomenon known as *physiologic anorexia*. They become picky, fussy eaters with strong taste preferences. They may eat voraciously one day and almost nothing the next. They

TABLE 12-3

Servings per Day for Children Based on Basic Four Food Groups

Food Group	Servings per Day
Milk or equivalent ½ cup whole milk equals: ¾ ounce cheese ½ cup yogurt, milk pudding 1 cup cottage cheese ¾-1 cup ice cream	2 to 3 cups for child 4 cups for adolescent Usual serving size: Toddler and preschooler—½ to ¾ cup School-age and older—1 cup
Meat, fish, poultry, or equivalent 1 ounce meat equals: 1 egg 1 ounce cheese 2 tablespoons peanut butter ¼ cup tuna fish ½ cup cooked legumes	2 for child and adolescent Usual serving size: Toddler and preschooler—1 egg, 1 to 2 ounces meat School-age and older—1 egg, 3 ounces meat
Vegetables and fruits Citrus equivalents: 1 orange or tomato ½ cup orange or grapefruit juice ¾ cup strawberries	4 for child and adolescent 1 citrus daily 1 yellow or dark green vegetable 3 to 4 times/week Usual serving size: Toddler and preschooler—2 tablespoons to ¼ cup School-age and older—½ cup
Breads and cereals 1 slice enriched bread equals: ¾ cup dry cereal ½ cup cooked pasta, rice, or cereal ½ hamburger bun 1 small muffin or biscuit	4 for child and adolescent Usual serving size: Toddler and preschooler—½ slice bread School-age and older—1 slice bread

are increasingly aware of the nonnutritive function of food: the pleasure of eating, the social aspect of mealtime, and the control of refusing food. They are influenced by factors other than taste when choosing food. If a family member refuses to eat something, the child is likely to imitate that response. If the plate is overfilled, he is likely to push it away, overwhelmed by its size. If food does not appear or smell appetizing, he will probably not agree to try it. In essence mealtime is more closely associated with psychologic components rather than nutritional ones.

Nutritional Counseling

Eating habits established in the first 2 or 3 years of life tend to have lasting effects on subsequent years. If food is used as a reward or sign of approval, a child may overeat for nonnutritive reasons. If food is forced and mealtime is consistently unpleasant, the usual pleasure associated with eating may not develop. Mealtimes should be enjoyable rather than times for discipline or family arguments. The social aspect of mealtime may be distracting for young children; therefore, an earlier feeding hour may be appropriate. Young children are unable to sit through a long meal and become fidgety and disruptive. This is particularly common when children are brought to the table just after active play. Calling them in from play 15 minutes before mealtime allows them ample opportunity to get ready for eating while settling down their active minds and bodies.

The method of serving food also takes on more importance during this period. Toddlers need to feel control and achievement in their abilities. Giving them large, adult-size portions can overwhelm them. In general, what is eaten is much more significant than how much is consumed. Small amounts of meat and vegetables supply greater food value than a large consumption of bread or potato. Serving sizes need to be appropriate for age (see Table 12-3 and Nursing tip). Young children tend to like less spicy, bland food, although this is a culturally determined preference. Substitutions should be provided for foods that they do not enjoy.

Nursing Tip: Serving Size for Young Children

A general guide to the serving size of food is:
1 tablespoon of solid food per year of age or ¼ to ⅓ the adult portion size
Use the tablespoon guide for easily measured food such as vegetables or rice.
Use the fraction guide for bread or milk.

The ritualism of this age also dictates certain principles in feeding practices. Toddlers like the same dish, cup, or spoon every time they eat. They may reject a favorite food simply because it is served in a different utensil. If one food touches another, they often refuse to eat it. Mixed foods, such as stews or casseroles, are also rarely favorites. Since toddlers are unpredictable in their table manners, it is best to use plastic dishes and cups, both for economic and safety reasons. A regular mealtime schedule also contributes to their desire and need for predictability and ritualism.

Most children by 12 months of age are eating the same food prepared for the rest of the family. However, appetite and food preferences are sporadic. Often the interest in food parallels a growth spurt so that periods of good eating are interspersed with phases of poor eating. "Food jags" are common.

Such food fads do not ensure a well-balanced diet, but attempts to alter them are usually unsuccessful. It is preferable to accept such extremes and offer other foods in small portions. Introducing at least three items from the basic four food groups at each meal helps develop a variety of taste preferences and well-balanced eating habits.

SLEEP AND ACTIVITY

Total sleep decreases only slightly during the second year and averages about 12 hours a day. Most children take one nap a day, and by the end of the third year many relinquish this habit. The activity level of children in this age-group is high and there is rarely a problem with too little physical exercise, provided inappropriate restrictions are not instituted. With increasing numbers of young children cared for outside the home, attention to the kinds of activity provided is important. For example, children with high activity levels may benefit from an environment in which outdoor play is encouraged.

Sleep problems are common, especially going to bed and falling asleep, and are probably related to fears of separation. Bedtime rituals (same hour of sleep, snack, quiet activity) are helpful, and transitional objects, such as a favorite stuffed animal or blanket, can help ease the child's insecurity at bedtime (see Fig. 12-3).

DENTAL HEALTH

The importance of oral hygiene in preserving the teeth and maintaining healthy gums cannot be overemphasized, and the practice of oral hygiene cannot be begun too early. Nurses are in an optimum position to promote dental hygiene in their care of both healthy children and ill children during hospitalization.

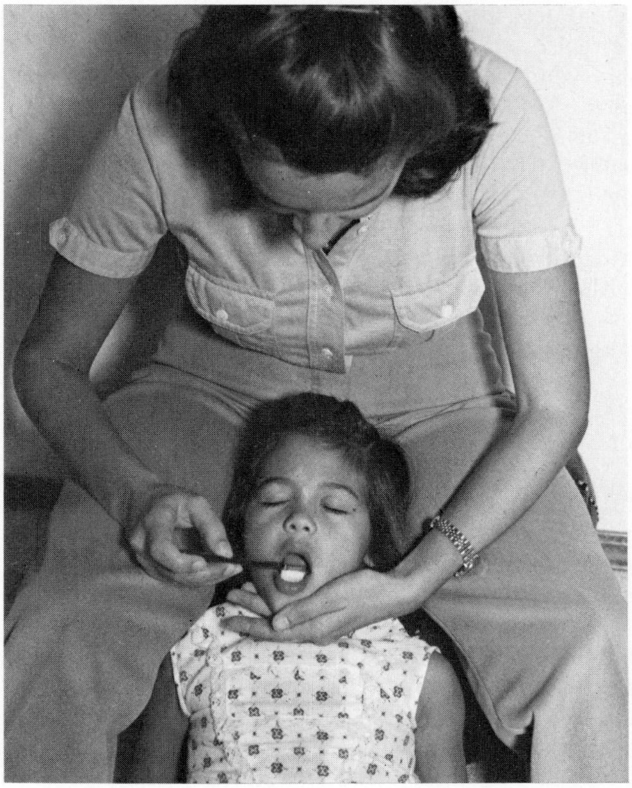

FIG. 12-7 Position that facilitates parent's brushing of child's teeth.

Regular Dental Examinations

Ideally the child should see a dentist (or pedodontist) soon after the first teeth erupt and no later than 2½ years when primary dentition is completed. Initial visits to the dentist should be nontraumatizing. Since toddlers react negatively to new and potentially frightening experiences, the initial visit can center around meeting the dentist, seeing the equipment, and sitting in the chair. If the child is cooperative, the dentist may just look at the teeth but reserve a more thorough examination for another visit. Modeling can also be effective—the child can observe procedures performed on the parent or a cooperative sibling.

Removal of Plaque

The objective of oral hygiene is removal of *plaque*, soft bacterial deposits that adhere to the teeth and cause dental caries (decay) and periodontal (gum) disease. The most effective methods for plaque removal are brushing and flossing. Several brushing techniques exist, although there is no universal agreement regarding the best method. One that is suitable for cleaning the primary teeth is the *scrub* method. The tips of the bristles are placed firmly at a 45-degree angle against the teeth and gums and moved back and forth in a vibratory motion. The ends of the bristles should be wiggling but not moving forcefully back and forth, which can damage the gums and enamel. All the surfaces of the teeth are cleaned in this manner except the lingual (inner) surfaces of the anterior teeth. To clean these surfaces, the toothbrush is placed vertical to the teeth and moved up and down. Only a few teeth are brushed at one time, using six to eight strokes for each section. A systematic approach is used so that all surfaces are thoroughly cleaned.

For young children the most effective cleaning is done by parents. Several positions can be used that facilitate access to the mouth and help stabilize the head for comfort, such as sitting on a couch or bed with the child's head in the parent's lap or sitting on a floor or stool with the child's head straddled by the parent's thighs (Fig. 12-7). The latter position is advantageous because the child can be kept amused watching television during the brushing, provided there is a receptacle for the child to spit out toothpaste. For easier access to back teeth the mouth is held partially open; fully opening the mouth causes the masseter muscle to contract, narrowing the space near the back molars.

For effective cleaning, a small toothbrush with soft, rounded, multitufted nylon bristles that are short and uniform in length is recommended. Nylon bristles dry more rapidly after use and retain their shape better than natural bristles. Children should have at least two toothbrushes, which are used alternately to allow them to dry thoroughly. Wet bristles are less resilient and consequently less effective in removing plaque. Toothbrushes are replaced as soon as the bristles are frayed or bent. With young children brushing may be more easily accomplished using only water, since many children dislike the foam from toothpaste and the foam interferes with visibilty. There is also the danger of swallowing fluoridated toothpaste (see following discussion under Fluoride). When using toothpaste, children should select the flavor they like to encourage the brushing habit.

After the teeth have been cleaned, flossing with dental floss is done to remove plaque and debris from between the teeth and below the gum margin where brushing is ineffective. Since young children do not have the dexterity to manipulate the floss, parents are taught the procedure.

A disclosing agent is helpful in identifying those areas of the teeth where plaque accumulates. It also helps motivate children to clean their teeth because plaque is difficult to see. After cleaning, the mouth is inspected to ensure that all traces of plaque have been removed.

Ideally the teeth should be cleaned after each meal and especially before bedtime, and the child should be given nothing to eat or drink after the night brushing except water. At those times when brushing is impractical, the "swish-and-swallow" method of cleaning the mouth is taught: with a mouthful of water the child rinses the mouth and swallows, repeating the procedure three or four times.

Fluoride

Several studies have documented the effectiveness of fluoride in reducing the incidence of tooth decay. Children who drink water containing 1 part per million (ppm) fluoride when their teeth are forming may have a 50% to 65% decrease in caries (Crall, 1986).

In communities where the water supply is not fluoridated, oral fluoride supplements are recommended (Table 12-4). One advantage of supplements is that the child receives a known quantity of fluoride daily. This is in contrast to fluoridated water, where the supply depends on the amount of water consumed. A major disadvantage of supplementation is compliance and cost. The supplements are considerably more expensive than community fluoridation, and adhering to a daily administration schedule for 16 years is difficult for many families.

TABLE 12-4

Supplemental Fluoride Dosage Schedule (mg/day)*

	Concentration of Fluoride in Drinking Water (ppm)		
Age	**<0.3**	**0.3-0.7**	**>0.7**
2 weeks-2 years	0.25	0	0
2-3 years	0.50	0.25	0
3-16 years	1.00	0.50	0

From American Academy of Pediatrics, Committee on Nutrition: Fluoride supplementation, Pediatrics **77**(5):758-761, 1986.
*2.2 mg sodium fluoride contains 1 mg fluoride.

Nurses have a responsibility to ensure an optimal fluoride regimen for children and to counsel families regarding correct use of supplements. The nurse should have a knowledge of the fluoride content of the community water supply and provide instruction to parents regarding correct administration of fluoride drops or tablets. Supplements should remain in the mouth 30 seconds before swallowing and taken on an empty stomach. Afterward the child should not drink or eat for 30 minutes. All fluoride products (toothpaste, supplements, and rinse) need to be stored away from young children to prevent poisoning. If the water supply is fluoridated, parents are encouraged to use water to prepare drinks and foods.

Low-Cariogenic Diet

Diet is critical to developing good teeth because the carious process depends primarily on fermentable sugars, especially sucrose. Refined table sugar is not the only concentrated sweet food that is cariogenic. Natural foods, including honey, molasses, corn syrup, and dried fruits such as raisins, are highly cariogenic.

Ideally such foods should be eliminated. However, since this is impractical, some suggestions can be helpful. First, *the frequency with which sugar is consumed is more important than the total amount eaten*. Therefore when sweets are eaten, they are less damaging if consumed immediately after a meal rather than as a snack between meals. When sweets are served as the dessert, the teeth can be cleaned afterward, decreasing the amount of time the sugar is in the mouth.

Second, the form of sugar is important. The more cariogenic foods are those that are sticky or hard, since they remain in the mouth longer. Consequently sucking on lollipops or chewing gum is more cariogenic than eating a chocolate bar.

A special form of tooth decay in children between 18 months and 3 years of age is *nursing bottle caries* (also called *bottle-mouth caries*), which occurs when the child is routinely given a bottle of milk or juice at nap or bedtime. Frequent nocturnal breast-feeding for prolonged periods also leads to extensive destruction of the teeth (Brahms and Maloney, 1983). The practice of coating pacifiers in honey can contribute to caries and may be a potential source of botulism poisoning. As the sweet liquid pools in the mouth, the teeth are bathed for several hours in this cariogenic environment. The maxillary (upper) incisors and molars are affected most, since the mandibular (lower) incisors are thought to be protected by the lower lip and tongue (Fig. 12-8).

Prevention involves eliminating the bedtime bottle completely, feeding the last bottle before bedtime, substituting a bottle of water for milk or juice, and never coating pacifiers in sweet substances. Juice in bottles, especially commercially available ready-to-use bottles, is dis-

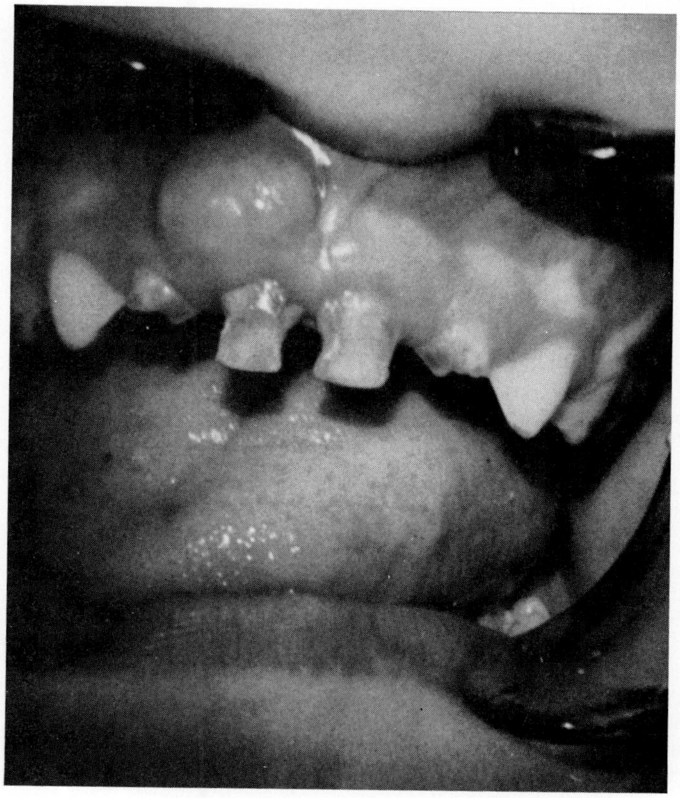

FIG. 12-8 Nursing bottle caries. Note the extensive carious involvement of maxillary primary incisors.

couraged, since the sugar in the beverage is more readily converted to acid and therefore is especially damaging. Juice should always be offered in a cup in order to avoid prolonging the bottle-feeding habit. Nurses are in an excellent position to counsel parents regarding the dangers of this habit and other aspects of dental care.*

INJURY PREVENTION

Injuries cause more deaths in children ages 1 to 4 years than in any other childhood period except adolescence. In addition, the injury death rate has remained relatively unchanged during the past decade while the corresponding rates from all other causes of death combined have declined significantly. Injury's prominence as the leading cause of death among toddlers and preschoolers underscores the need to emphasize safety awareness among parents. Child protection and parent education are key determinants in injury prevention.

*Sources of information about nursing bottle caries and other aspects of child dental health include: **National Institute of Dental Research,** Westwood Building, 5333 Westbard Ave., Bethesda, MD 20205; **American Society of Dentistry for Children,** 211 E. Chicago Ave., Suite 920, Chicago, IL 60611; and **American Dental Association,** 211 E. Chicago Ave., Chicago, IL 60611. Guidelines for children's dental care are available in Wong, D., and Whaley, L.: Clinical handbook of pediatric nursing, ed. 2, St. Louis, 1986, The C.V. Mosby Co.

A major factor in the critical increase of injuries during early childhood is the unrestricted freedom achieved through locomotion combined with an unawareness of danger within the environment. Specific categories of injuries and appropriate prevention are best understood by associating them with the major developmental achievements of young children (Table 12-5). The discussion of injuries in Chapter 10 is also relevant to safety concerns at this age.

Motor Vehicle Injuries

Motor vehicle injuries cause more accidental deaths in all pediatric age-groups after age 1 year than any other type of injury or disease and are responsible for almost half of all accidental deaths among children ages 1 to 4 years. Many of the deaths are caused by injuries within the car when restraints have not been used or have been used improperly. Approved restraints that are properly installed and applied can reduce fatalities by 71% (Ziegler, 1987).

Nurses have a responsibility to educate parents regarding the importance of car restraints and their proper use. Three basic types of federally approved restraints are available: (1) infant-only device, (2) convertible models for both infants and toddlers, and (3) toddler-only restraints. Since the infant-type restraints are discussed in Chapter 10, the other types are included here.

Toddler restraints are designed for children who can sit by themselves and are over 7.7 to 9 kg (17 to 20 pounds). Both convertible models and toddler-only models are available. The convertible type is suitable for infants in the rearward facing position and for toddlers in the forward-facing position (Fig. 12-9). Toddler-only models provide protection only in the forward-facing position and may consist of a shell or a raised booster seat. The shell restraints consist of a molded hard plastic or metal frame with energy-absorbing padding and a special harness system designed to maximize pressure over the pelvic bones rather than the more vulnerable abdomen. Booster seats are made of similar material but lack the side protection afforded by the shell (Fig. 12-10). The restraint is held in place by the car lap-belt. The shoulder strap on the seat-belt system is either placed behind the restraint or with the lap belt but never in front of the child's face or neck, which can cause strangulation in the event of a crash. If the car's shoulder/lap belt has a free-moving latch plate, a locking clip should be used to tighten the shoulder/lap belt and prevent the latch plate from sliding (see insert, Fig. 12-10). Cars with emergency locking retractor seat belts (seat belts that lock only on impact) cannot be tightened to hold a car restraint (Gunnip and others, 1987). If these are the only belts in the car, one set should be replaced with a lap belt that is used to secure the car restraint.

Some older model restraints require the use of a top anchor (tether) strap to prevent the child from pitching forward in a crash. If the tether strap is not used, up to 90% of the restraint's protection is lost. Instructions for

TABLE 12-5

Injury Prevention during Early Childhood

Major Developmental Accomplishments	Injury Prevention
Walks, runs, and climbs Able to open doors and gates Can ride tricycle Can throw ball and other objects	**Motor vehicles** Use federally-approved car restraint; if restraint is not available, use lap belt Supervise children while playing outside Do not allow to play on curb or behind a parked car Do not permit to play in pile of leaves, snow, or large cardboard container in trafficked area Supervise tricycle riding Lock fences and doors if not directly supervising children Teach children to obey pedestrian safety rules Obey traffic regulations; cross only at crosswalks and only when the traffic signal indicates it is safe to cross Stand back a step from the curb until it is time to cross Look left, right, and left again and check for turning cars before crossing the street Use sidewalks; when there is no sidewalk, walk on the left, facing the traffic Wear light colors at night, and attach fluorescent material to clothing
Able to explore if left unsupervised Has great curiosity Helpless in water; unaware of its danger; depth of water has no significance	**Drowning** Supervise closely when near *any* source of water Keep bathroom doors closed Have fence around swimming pool and lock gate Teach swimming and water safety
Able to reach heights by climbing, stretching, and standing on toes Pulls objects Explores any holes or opening Can open drawers and closets Unaware of potential sources of heat or fire Plays with mechanical objects	**Burns** Turn pot handles toward back of stove Place guard rails in front of radiators, fireplaces, or other heating elements Store matches and cigarette lighters in locked or inaccessible area Place burning candles, incense, hot foods, and cigarettes out of reach Do not let tablecloth hang within child's reach Do not let electric cord from iron or other appliance hang within child's reach Cover electrical outlets with protective plastic caps Keep electrical wires hidden or out of reach Do not allow child to play with electrical appliance Stress danger of open flames; teach what "hot" means Always check bathwater; adjust hot-water temperature to 49° C (120° F) or lower; do not allow to play with faucets
Explores by putting objects in mouth Can open drawers, closets, and most containers Climbs Cannot read labels	**Poisoning** Place all potentially toxic agents out of reach or in a locked cabinet Caution against eating nonedible items, such as plants Replace medications and poisons immediately; replace child-protector caps properly Administer medications as a drug, not as a candy Do not store large surplus of toxic agents Promptly discard empty poison containers; never reuse to store a food item or other poison Never remove labels from containers of toxic substances Have syrup of ipecac in home; use only if advised Know number and location of nearest poison control center (usually listed in front of telephone directory)
Able to open doors and some windows Goes up and down stairs Depth perception unrefined	**Falls** Keep screen in window, nail securely, and use guard rail Place gates at top and bottom of stairs Keep doors locked when there is danger of falls (stairwells, porches) Keep crib rails fully raised and mattress at lowest level Place carpeting under crib and in bathroom Keep child restrained in vehicles; never leave unattended in shopping cart Supervise at playgrounds; select safe play areas with soft ground cover Check child's shoes and trousers for possible hazards
Puts things in mouth May swallow hard or nonedible pieces of food	**Choking and suffocation** Avoid large chunks of meat, such as whole hot dogs Avoid fruit with pits, fish with bones, dried beans, hard candy, chewing gum, and nuts Choose large sturdy toys without sharp edges or small removable parts Discard old refrigerators, ovens, and so on If storing an old appliance, remove the doors Keep automatic garage door transmitter in inaccessible place Select safe toy boxes or chests without heavy, hinged lids

TABLE 12-5

Injury Prevention during Early Childhood—cont'd

Major Developmental Accomplishments	Injury Prevention
Still clumsy in many skills	**Bodily damage** Avoid giving sharp or pointed objects—such as knives, scissors, or toothpicks—especially when walking or running Do not allow lollipops or similar objects in mouth when walking or running Teach safety precautions, for example, to carry knife or scissors with pointed end away from face Store all dangerous tools, garden equipment, and firearms in locked cabinet Do not allow near machinery, such as lawnmowers Be alert to danger of unsupervised animals and household pets Have identification on child, such as plastic "shoe pocket" attached to shoelaces Use safety glass and decals on large glassed areas, especially sliding glass doors

proper installation of the tether strap and permanent bracket are included with the car restraint. If parents object to drilling holes in the car to install the bracket, they should select a model without this feature. Car restraints that do not require a top anchor strap have the lap-belt placement arched midway through the back of the car seat to hold the restraint against the back of the vehicle seat.

Children should use restraints until they have outgrown them. The "rule of fours" serves as a guide: if the child either weighs about 40 pounds (18 kg), is 40 inches (100 cm) tall, or is 4 years old, the restraint can be replaced by a lap belt. Children who outgrow the toddler shell seat may still be able to ride safely in a booster seat. If the car's restraint system is used, only the lap belt is applied until the child is tall enough for the shoulder harness to pass snugly over the shoulder, not the neck (American Academy of Pediatrics, 1987). Regardless of the child's age, the lap belt provides more protection than no restraint. The safest area of the car for children is the middle of the back seat.

When purchasing a restraint, parents should consider cost and convenience. The convertible-type seats are more expensive initially but cost less than two separate systems. Convenience is a major factor because a cumbersome restraint may be used less and improperly. Before buying a restraint, it is best to try out different models. For example, some types are too large for subcompact cars. Asking neighbors about the advantages and disadvantages of their restraints is helpful. Some service clubs

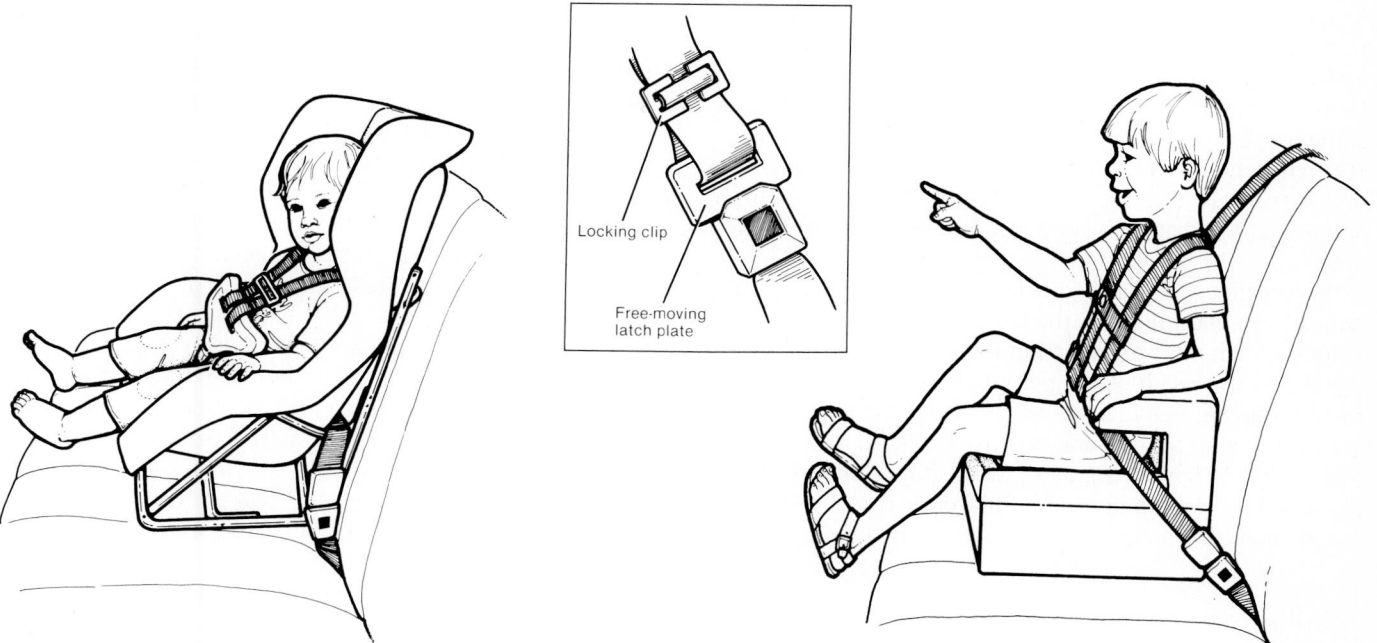

FIG. 12-9 Convertible seat in forward-facing position for older infants and children.

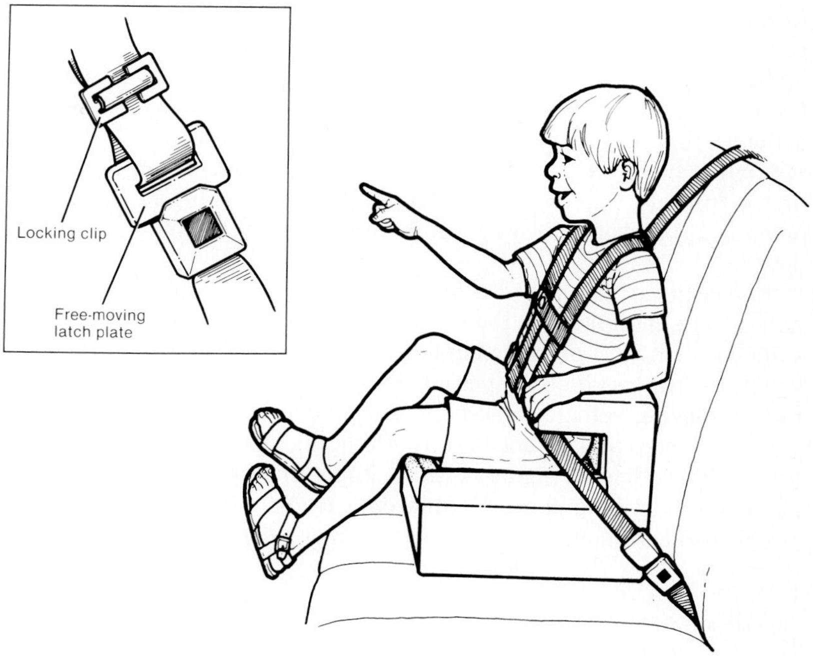

FIG. 12-10 Automobile booster seat. Model uses harness attached to auto seat belt; harness held in place by tether strap. *Inset:* use of locking clip.

and hospitals have loan programs for restraints. Information about approved models and other aspects of car restraints is available from several organizations and sources.*

For any restraint to be effective it must be used consistently and properly. Reasons for decreased compliance during the toddler years include: removal of straps by the child; inability to attach straps over heavy winter clothing; and child's crying, fussing, and boredom (Arneson and others, 1985). An advantage of restraints in addition to safety is that children riding in car seats generally behave better than children left unrestrained. To ensure compliance, these concerns and benefits must be addressed and certain "rules of riding" should be practiced:

1. Do not start the car until *everyone* is properly restrained
2. *Always* use the restraint, even for short trips
3. If the child begins to climb out or undo the harness, firmly say, "No." It may be necessary to stop the car to reinforce the expected behavior. The use of rewards, such as stars, for cooperative behavior is very effective
4. Encourage the child to help attach buckles and straps
5. Decrease boredom on long trips. Keep special toys in the car for quiet play; talk to the child; point out objects and teach the child about them. Stop periodically. If the child wishes to sleep, make sure he stays in the restraint

Children over 3 years of age are often involved in pedestrian traffic injuries, with the majority occurring between noon and 6 PM (Guyer, Talbot, and Pless, 1985). Because of their gross motor skills of walking, running, and climbing and their fine motor skills of opening doors and fence gates, they are able to leave most restricted areas when unsupervised. Unaware of danger and unable to approximate the speed of a car, they are hit by moving vehicles. Running after a ball, playing in a pile of leaves or snow or inside a cardboard box, riding a tricycle, and playing behind a parked car or near the curb are common activities that may result in a vehicular tragedy. A precaution when children are playing in driveways is attaching to the tricycle a pole with a bright flag that is high enough to be visible through an automobile's back window.

Preventing vehicular injuries involves protecting and educating children about the danger of moving or parked vehicles. Although preschool children are too young to be trusted to always obey, the parent should emphasize looking for moving vehicles before crossing the street, recognizing the stop and go colors of traffic lights, and following traffic officers' signals. Most important, what is preached must be practiced. Children learn through imitation, and consistency reinforces learning.

*__Physicians for Automotive Safety,__ 19 Church St., New Milford, CT 06776; and **American Academy of Pediatrics,** Division of Health Education, 141 Northwest Point Rd., Elk Grove, IL 60007. Guidelines for car seat safety are available in Wong, D., and Whaley, L.: Clinical handbook of pediatric nursing, ed. 2, St. Louis, 1986, The C.V. Mosby Co.

Drowning

Drowning, not including drowning from water transportation, ranks second among boys and third among girls ages 1 to 4 years as a cause of accidental death. With well-developed skills of locomotion, toddlers are able to reach potentially dangerous areas, such as bathtubs, toilets, swimming pools, hot tubs, and lakes. Their intense drive for exploration and investigation, combined with an unawareness of the danger of water and their helplessness in water, makes drowning always a viable threat. It is also one category of injuries that results in death within minutes, diminishing the chance for rescue and survival. Supervising children when near any source of water is essential, and teaching swimming and water safety can be helpful but cannot be regarded as sufficient protection.

Burns

Burns rank second to motor vehicle injuries among girls and third among boys in this age-group as a cause of accidental death. A major contributing factor to the statistical difference is that girls tend to play indoors and imitate sex-related functions, such as cooking at the stove. Their ability to climb, stretch, and reach objects above their heads makes any hot surface a potential source of danger. Scalds from children pulling pots on top of themselves are a major source of burns. As a precaution, pot handles should be turned toward the back of the stove. Ideally the knobs for controlling the range burners should be out of reach, not on the front panel where nimble fingers can turn them on and accidentally touch the hot burner. Oven doors should be closed whenever the oven is turned on or when it is cooling. The outside of doors of automatic self-cleaning ovens may become hot and, if touched, could cause a burn. Other sources of heat, such as radiators, fireplaces, accessible furnaces, kerosene heaters, or wood-burning stoves, should have guards placed in front of them. The tops of some of these heaters are designed to become hot enough to boil water to provide humidity. They are hazardous if touched or if the pan of water is spilled. Portable electric heaters must be placed in a high area, well out of reach of climbing young children.

Hot objects such as candles, incense, cigarettes, pots of tea or coffee, or irons must be placed away from children. The flame of a candle and the smoke of a cigarette invite investigation. Ashtrays with a center well are preferred to prevent the cigarette from falling off the rim and adults should try not to smoke, cook, or drink hot liquids when children are physically close. If tablecloths are used, the edges should be placed out of reach to prevent injuries from both burns and falling objects.

Flame burns represent one of the most fatal types of burns and commonly occur when children play with matches and accidentally set themselves (and the home) on fire. Butane lighters are also a hazard. Although a young child may not be able to ignite the lighter, holding the lighter at a 40 ° angle and rubbing it against fabric can cause sufficient sparks to start a fire (Meer, 1987). To prevent flame burns matches and lighters must be stored safely away from children and parents need to teach children the dangers of playing with such objects. In addition, all homes should have smoke detectors installed to alert the occupants of a fire. A safety plan for immediate escape is also essential.

Electrical burns also represent an immediate danger to children. With preschoolers' ability to manipulate small, thin objects, they are able to insert hairpins or other conductive articles into electrical sockets. Young toddlers may explore outlets and wires by mouthing them. Since water is an excellent conductor, the chance for a severe circumoral electrical burn is great. Electrical outlets should have protective guards plugged into them when not in use (Fig. 12-11) or made inaccessible by placing furniture in front of them when feasible. Children should not be allowed to play with electrical cords or appliances, which should be kept out of reach as much as possible.

An example of an appliance that interests children and can present a hazard is an electric popcorn popper. Children can become so excited by the popping that they may inadvertently pull the electric cord and popper off the table, resulting in a burn from contact with the hot oil, corn, or appliance.

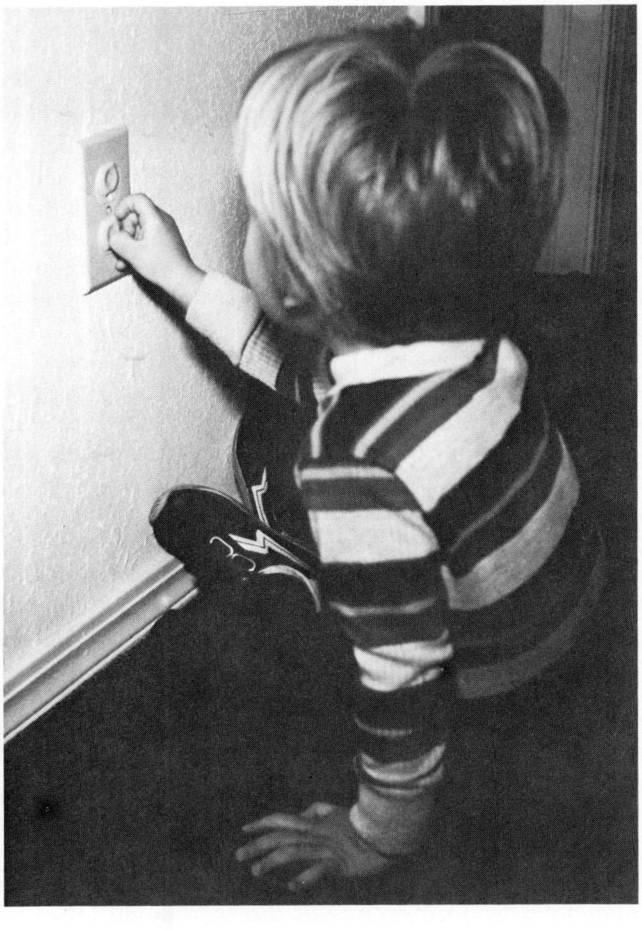

FIG. 12-11 Special plastic caps in electrical sockets prevent young fingers from exploring dangerous areas.

Scald burns are the most common type of thermal injury in children. Among young children a significant type of scalding burn is caused by high-temperature tap water, which children come in contact with either as a result of turning on the hot-water faucet, falling into a bathtub of hot water, or deliberate abuse. Besides the obvious prevention of always supervising youngsters when they are near tap water and checking bathwater temperatures, a recommended passive prevention is to limit household water temperatures to less than 49° C (120° F). At this temperature it takes 10 minutes for exposure to the water to cause a full-thickness burn. Conversely water temperatures of 54° C (130° F), the usual setting of most water heaters, expose household members to the risk of full-thickness burns within 30 seconds. Nurses can help prevent such burns by advising parents of this common household danger and recommending that they readjust the water heater to a safe temperature. A meat or candy thermometer is a convenient way to measure water temperature. An easy-to-read hot water gauge that changes color to show water temperatures between 120° to 150° is also available.* To measure bath water special "Frog Prince" or "Bath Bear" thermometers that also change color to show "hot," "cool," or "OK" water temperature are convenient for home use and can be purchased at nominal cost.*

Poisoning

Ingestion of toxic agents is common during early childhood. The highest incidence occurs in children in the 2-year-old age-group. Although in many instances poisoning does not result in mortality, it may cause significant morbidity, such as esophageal stricture from lye ingestion. Mouthing activity continues to be prevalent after 1 year of age and exploring objects by tasting them is part of children's curious investigation. Almost every nonfood substance is potentially harmful, including many house plants, and toddlers by 2 years of age are able to climb most heights, open most drawers or closets, and unscrew most lids. By trial and error younger children also manage to undo tops of bottles, plastic containers, aerosol cans, and jars. Legislature has mandated the use of child-guard tops on articles such as prescription drugs, but many young children have outwitted such "safe" caps. In addition, pharmacists often transfer drugs to regular containers for the elderly who may have difficulty with child-guard closures. Newer forms of drugs, such as transdermal patches and cough-suppressant lozenges, have created additional dangers as they are not packaged with

*Clinitemp, Inc., P.O. Box 40273, Indianapolis, IN 46240.

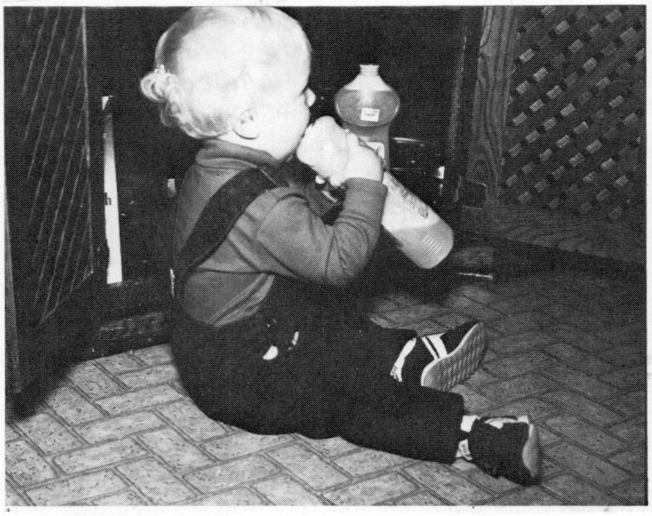

FIG. 12-12 No unlocked cabinet is safe for young children.

safety caps and the lozenges look like candy or chewing gum.

The major cause of poisoning is improper storage of toxic agents (Fig. 12-12). The guidelines suggested in Chapter 10 apply to children in this age-group as well. However, unlike the infant who was confined to certain heights and unable to unlatch inventive locks, preschoolers manage to find access to many high-level, tight-security places. Sometimes it is necessary to test a lock or high shelf by challenging the child to undo or reach it. Uncovering potential weaknesses in one's security system prevents tragedies later. Emergency measures for accidental poisoning are discussed in Chapter 14.

Falls

Falls are still a hazard to children in this age-group, although by the later part of early childhood gross and fine motor skills are well developed, decreasing the incidence of falls down stairs or from chairs. However, playground injuries are common. Children need to be taught safety at play areas, such as no horseplay on high slides or jungle gyms, *sitting* on swings, and staying away from moving swings. Passive prevention includes placement of grass, sand, or wood chips under play equipment. If loose organic material is used, it will require replacement as it pulverizes. Swing seats should be made of plastic, canvas, or rubber rather than wood and have smooth or rounded edges. Slides should not exceed an incline of 30 degress, have evenly spaced rungs for climbing, and have protective "tunnels."

The climbing and running of the typical toddler are complicated by his total neglect for and lack of appreciation of danger. Gates must be placed at both ends of stairs. Accessible windows that are left open during warm weather must be screened or guarded with a rail. Falling from open windows is a major cause of accidental death in urban, lower socioeconomic groups. Doors leading to stairwells or porches must be locked, since preschool children can easily open them. A convenient type of lock is a sliding bar or hook that can be attached to the door and frame at a level higher than the child can reach. One must be careful that inventive youngsters do not pull a chair over to unlatch the hook or bar.

Cribs and vehicles are other sources of falls. To avoid injury crib rails should be fully raised, the mattress should be kept at the lowest position, and toys or bumper pads that may be used as steps to climb out should be removed. Ideally the floor should be carpeted. Once the child reaches a height of 89 cm (35 inches) he should sleep in a bed rather than a crib. To prevent falls from vehicles, children should always be properly restrained. They should never ride in the open back of a truck; the danger of falls can be compounded by another vehicle striking the child. An unrecognized hazard is grocery shopping carts. Children left unattended can easily fall out.

Clothing can also increase the chance of falling. Slippery shoes or socks, rubber-soled shoes that "catch" on the floor and rug, and loose or cuffed pants can easily make a child fall. Simple safety measures, such as checking clothing and shoes and keeping shoelaces tied with double knots, can prevent such needless accidents.

Aspiration and Suffocation

Usually by 1 year of age children chew well, but they may have difficulty with large pieces of food, such as meat and whole hot dogs, and with hard foods, such as nuts or dried beans. Young children cannot discard pits from fruit or bones from fish as older children can. It takes practice to learn how to chew gum without swallowing it. Play objects for toddlers must still be chosen with an awareness of danger from small parts. Large, sturdy toys without sharp edges or removable parts are safest. Coins, paper clips, pins, bells, button batteries, pull-tabs on cans, thumbtacks, nails, screws, jewelry (such as label or stick pins) are household objects that can cause significant harm if swallowed. Because of the danger of aspiration, parents should be taught emergency procedures for choking (p. 733).

Another cause of death by traumatic asphyxiation is from electrically operated garage doors. Young children playing in the garage may become trapped under the door. Although the automatic doors should reverse when striking an object, they may not do so when hitting a flexible object or one that is very close to the ground. Precautions to lessen the chances of this accident occurring include placing controls where they are inaccessible to children, such as high on a wall and in a locked car, and instructing children that the transmitter is not a toy.

Suffocation is less frequent from causes seen during infancy but is an ever-present threat from old refrigerators, ovens, and other large appliances. Toddlers can climb inside these appliances and if they close the door behind them can be trapped inside. Discarding old appliances and removing all doors during storage prevent such tragic deaths. Toddlers may also suffocate when unsafe toy box lids accidently close on their head or neck. Parents should be advised of this danger and encouraged to buy storage chests with lightweight, removable covers.

Bodily Damage

Toddlers are still clumsy in many of their skills and can seriously harm themselves when walking while holding a sharp or pointed object or having food or objects, such as spoons, in their mouth. Foreseeing such potential injuries is the best approach. For the older child, teaching safety is most important. The child should be taught that when walking with a pointed object, such as a knife or scissors, the pointed end is held away from the face. Dangerous garden or workshop equipment and all firearms should be stored in a locked cabinet. Safety education should include respect for firearms and their proper use. Children should not be allowed near dangerous machinery, such as powered lawnmowers, lawn edgers, hedge trimmers, or saws, when this equipment is in use. In addition, the child should be warned of and protected against potential danger from animals, including household pets, such as dogs and cats.

Another safeguard for young children is the use of safety glass in doors and windows and the application of decals on glassed areas to lessen the likelihood of running through glass.

ANTICIPATORY GUIDANCE—CARE OF FAMILIES

Understanding toddlers is fundamental to successful childrearing, regardless of the approach used. Nurses, particularly those in ambulatory or child health centers, are in a most favorable position to assist parents in meeting the tasks and needs of children in this age-group. It seems to be an almost universal phenomenon that prevention yields better results than treatment. Anticipatory

Parental Guidance during Toddler Years

Age	Guidance
12-18 months	Prepare parents for expected behavioral changes of toddler, especially negativism and ritualism Assess present feeding habits and encourage gradual weaning from bottle and increased intake of solid foods Stress expected feeding changes of physiologic anorexia, presence of food fads and strong taste preferences, need for scheduled routine at mealtimes, inability to sit through an entire meal, and lack of table manners Assess sleep patterns at night, particularly habit of a bedtime bottle, which is a major cause of dental caries, and procrastination behaviors that delay hour of sleep Prepare parents for potential dangers of the home, particularly motor vehicular, poisoning, and falling injuries; give appropriate suggestions for safeproofing the home Discuss need for firm but gentle discipline and ways in which to deal with negativism and temper tantrums; stress positive benefits of appropriate discipline Emphasize importance for both child and parents of brief, periodic separations Discuss new toys that use developing gross and fine motor, language, cognitive, and social skills Emphasize need for dental supervision, types of basic dental hygiene at home, and food habits that predispose to caries; stress importance of supplemental fluoride
18-24 months	Stress importance of peer companionship in play Explore need for preparation for additional sibling; stress importance of preparing child for new experiences Discuss present discipline methods, their effectiveness, and parents' feelings about child's negativism; stress that negativism is important aspect of developing self-assertion and independence and is not a sign of spoiling
18-24 months	Discuss signs of readiness for toilet training; emphasize importance of waiting for physical and psychologic readiness Discuss development of fears, such as darkness or loud noises, and of habits, such as security blanket or thumb-sucking; stress normalcy of these transient behaviors Prepare parents for signs of regression in times of stress Assess child's ability to separate easily from parents for brief periods of separation under familiar circumstances Allow parents opportunity to express their feelings of weariness, frustration, and exasperation; be aware that it is often difficult to love toddlers at times when they are not asleep! Point out some of the expected changes of the next year, such as longer attention span, somewhat less negativism, and increased concern for pleasing others
24-36 months	Discuss importance of imitation and domestic mimicry and need to include child in activities Discuss approaches toward toilet training, particularly realistic expectations and attitude toward accidents Stress uniqueness of toddlers' thought processes, especially through their use of language, poor understanding of time, causal relationships in terms of proximity of events, and inability to see events from another's perspective Stress that discipline still must be quite structured and concrete and that relying solely on verbal reasoning and explanation leads to injuries, confusion, and misunderstanding Discuss investigation of nursery school or daycare center toward completion of second year

guidance in each of the areas presented in the box is paramount in order to prevent future problems.

Advice is sometimes not the only answer. Actual assistance, such as being available for home visiting or telephone consulting, should be part of nurses' flexible repertoire of interventions. Whether parents are experiencing the rearing dilemmas of a first or subsequent child, they benefit from sharing their feelings, frustrations, and satisfactions. They need adult companionship, freedom from childrearing responsibilities, and periodic separations from their children. Sometimes they lose perspective of the needs of each other in the marital relationship and fail to communicate effectively. Part of nurses' responsibility is to provide opportunities for ventilation of parents' feelings and guidance in personal areas such as marital needs, career fulfillment, and peer companionship.

SUMMARY

Toddlerhood is a period of intense developmental progress in physical, psychosocial, and cognitive skills. In the child's striving for autonomy and separation from parent, the family is faced with many childrearing challenges. Concerns related to temper tantrums, negativism, ritualism, and toileting are common. Even the experienced parent can benefit from support and guidance during the "terrible twos."

Unlike the rapid developmental changes, growth during this period is slowing and the nutritional needs are slightly less than those of infants. Nutritional counseling is concerned with providing essential nutrients as well as fostering healthy eating habits. With the completion of the primary dentition, dental care is an important area of instruction. The improved motor skills, hand-to-mouth activity, and curiosity of toddlers makes injuries a constant concern and injury prevention a matter of highest priority.

KEY CONCEPTS

- The toddler stage, extending from 12 months to 36 months, is a period of intense exploration of the environment.
- Biologic development during the toddler years is characterized by the acquistion of fine and gross motor skills that allow children to master a wide variety of activities.
- Although most of the physiologic systems are mature by the end of toddlerhood, development of certain areas of the brain is still occurring, allowing for greater intellectual capacity.
- Locomotion is the major gross motor skill acquired during toddlerhood, followed by increased eye-hand coordination.
- Specific tasks in the psychosocial development of a toddler include differentiating self from others, tolerating separation from parent, coping with delayed gratification, controlling bodily functions, acquiring socially acceptable behavior, verbally communicating, and interacting with others in a less egocentric manner.
- According to Erikson, the major developmental task of toddlerhood is acquiring a sense of autonomy while overcoming a sense of doubt and shame.
- Language is the major cognitive achievement in toddlerhood.
- In Piaget's sensorimotor and preconceptual phases of development, the toddler experiments by incorporating the old learning of secondary circular reactions with new skills and applies this knowledge to new situations. There is the beginning of a rational judgment, an understanding of causal relationships, discovery of objects as objects, imitation, and egocentrism.
- Development of body image occurs with increasing motor ability, at which point toddlers recognize the importance and capacity of body parts.
- The most striking characteristic of language development during early childhood is the increasing level of comprehension.
- Parental concerns during the toddler years include toilet training, coping with sibling rivalry, limit-setting and discipline, and dealing with temper tantrums and negativism.
- Effective discipline techniques for toddlers include reward, ignoring or extinction, and time-out.
- Nutrition is important at this stage because eating habits established in toddlerhood tend to have lasting effects on subsequent years.
- Regular dental examinations, fluoride supplementation, removal of plaque, and provision of a low-cariogenic diet promote optimum dental health.
- Because of increased locomotion, toddlers are at a high risk for sustaining injuries. Fatal injuries are primarily the result of motor vehicle mishaps, drownings, and burns.

STUDY QUESTIONS AND ACTIVITIES

1 Attend a child care center and observe the physical/cognitive abilities of children ages 1 and 2 years of age. List the observed abilities of each age-group in the areas of gross motor, fine motor, and language skills and compare these with the norms presented in Tables 10-3 and 12-1.

2 Interview at least two families who have toddlers. Have the parents describe the typical behaviors of their children that present childrearing challenges, such as temper tantrums or negativism, and their strategies to deal with the behaviors.

3 Prepare a teaching plan to help parents begin toilet training.

4 Prepare a daily menu for 2 days that meets the nutritional requirements and is appropriate for the toddler's developmental skills for self-feeding.

5 Make a home visit to a family with a toddler and assess the house for safety features and potentially dangerous areas. Instruct the family in appropriate prevention strategies to correct the hazards.

REFERENCES

American Academy of Pediatrics, Committee on Accident and Poison Prevention: Injury control for children and youth, Elk Grove, IL, 1987, the Academy.

Arneson, S., and others: Factors affecting parental use of child automobile safety restraints, Child. Health Care **13**(4):181-186, 1985.

Brahms, M., and Maloney, J.: "Nursing bottle caries" in breast-fed children, J. Pediatr. **103**(3):415-416, 1983.

Crall, J.J.: Promotion of oral health and prevention of common pediatric dental problems, Pediatr. Clin. North Am. **33**(4):887-899, 1986.

Gunnip, A., and others: Car seats: helping parents do it right! J. Pediatr. Health Care **1**(4):190-195, 1987.

Guyer, B., Talbot, A.M., and Pless, I.B.: Pedestrian injuries to children and youth, Pediatr. Clin. North Am. **32**(1):163-174, 1985.

Meer, P.A.: Safety in the home: an update, Child. Nurse **5**(4):1-4, 1987.

Ziegler, P.N.: Use of child safety seats, U.S. Department of Transportation, National Highway Traffic Safety Administration: Research Notes, March 1987.

BIBLIOGRAPHY

For additional citations relevant to toddlerhood, refer to Chapter 10.

Growth and Development

Ames, L.B., and Ilg, F.L.: Your two-year-old: terrible or tender, New York, 1979, Delacorte Press.

Griffiths, S.S.: The role of the pediatric nurse clinician in promoting the development of body image in children. In Beal, J.A., editor: Issues and advanced practice in pediatric nursing, Reston, VA, 1983, Reston Publishing Co., Inc.

Lincoln, L.M.: Fathering and the separation-individuation process, Matern. Child Nurs. J. **13**(2):103-111, 1984.

Pontious, S.L.: Practical Piaget: helping children understand, Am. J. Nurs. **82**(1):114-117, 1982.

Schuster, C.S., and Ashburn, S.S.: The process of human development: a holistic approach, ed. 2, Boston, 1986, Little, Brown & Co.

Selekman, J.: The development of body image in the child: a learned response, Top. Clin. Nurs. **5**(1):12-21, 1983.

Toilet Training

Euler, M.M., and McClellan, M.A.: Toilet training: ready or not? Pediatr. Nurs. **7**(1):15-20, 1981.

Euler-Horner, M.M.: The challenge of toilet training—bowel management for the child with psychogenic encopresis or neurogenic deficit, Pediatr. Basics **32:**4-10, 1982.

Sibling Rivalry

Bahr, J.E.: Canine and feline rivalry: another form of sibling rivalry, Pediatr. Nurs. **7** (4):14-15, 1981.

Fine, L.L., and Friedman, M.S.: The sibling experience: developmental considerations. In Children are different: behavioral development monograph series, Number 11, Columbus, OH, 1984, Ross Laboratories.

Gates, S.: Children's literature: it can help children cope with sibling rivalry, MCN **5**(5):351-352, 1979.

Honig, J.C.: Preparing preschool-aged children to be siblings, MCN **11**(1):37-43, 1986.

MacLaughlin, S.M., and Johnston, K.B.: The preparation of young children for the birth of a sibling, J. Nurse Midwife. **29**(6):371-376, 1984.

Malinowski, J.S.: Answering a child's questions about sex and a new baby, Am. J. Nurs. **79**(11):1965-1968, 1979.

Merrill, J.: Announcing the newcomer, Baby Talk **52**(3):16-20, 1987.

Sweet, P.T.: Helping children to accept and welcome a new baby, MCN **4**(2):82-83, 1979.

Swingle, M.H.: How to prepare the family for sibling rivalry, Child. Nurse **2**(2):1-3, 1984.

Wilford, B., and Andrews. C.: Sibling preparation classes for preschool children, Matern. Child Nurs. J. **15**(3):171-185, 1986.

Wright, P.: Personal view—sibling rivalry, Midwife Health Visit. Community Nurse **16**(3):100, 1980.

Limit-Setting and Discipline

American Academy of Pediatrics, Committee on Psychosocial Aspects of Child and Family Health: The pediatrician's role in discipline, Pediatrics **72**(3):373-374, 1983.

Hammer, D., and Drabman, R.S.: Child discipline: what we know and what we can recommend, Pediatr. Nurs. **7**(3):31-35, 1981.

Hirsch, D.L.O., and Russo, D.C.: Behavior management. In Levine, M.D., and others, editors: Developmental-behavioral pediatrics, Philadelphia, 1983, W.B. Saunders Co.

Kvols-Riedler, K., and Kvols-Riedler, B.: Redirecting children's misbehavior, Pediatrics: Nursing Update **1**(3), Princeton, NJ, 1985, Continuing Professional Education Center.

Melichar, M.M.: Using crisis theory to help parents cope with a child's temper tantrums, MCN **5**(3):181-185, 1980.

Nutrition

American Academy of Pediatrics, Committee on Nutrition: Pediatric nutrition handbook, ed. 2, Elk Grove Village, IL, 1985, The Academy of Pediatrics.

Brock, D.T.: Decreasing toddlers' sodium intake, Pediatr. Nurs. **11**(1):47-50, 1985.

Eden, A.N.: Toddler diet, Pediatr. Basics **39:**4-6, 1984.

Henneman, A., and Koziol, J.: Preschool feeding problems: it's not nutritious unless they eat it, Issues Compr. Pediatr. Nurs. **4:**7-12, Dec. 1980.

Lucas, B.: Nutrition in childhood. In Krause, M.V., and Mahan, L.K.: Food, nutrition, and diet therapy, ed. 7, Philadelphia, 1984, W.B. Saunders Co.

Pipes, P.: Nutrition in infancy and childhood, ed. 3, St. Louis, 1985, The C.V. Mosby Co.

Satter, E.: Child of mine: feeding with love and good sense, Palo Alto, CA, 1986, Bull Publishing Co.

Dental Health

American Academy of Pediatrics, Committee on Nutrition: Fluoride supplementation, Pediatrics **77**(5):758-761, 1986.

Current preventive concepts. In Council on Dental Therapeutics: accepted dental therapeutics, ed. 39, Chicago, 1982, American Dental Association.

Hess, C., and others: Fluoride and caries prevention, Child. Nurse **4**(2):1-4, 1986.

Hess, C.S., and others: Fluoride: too much or too little, Pediatr. Nurs. **10**(6):397-403, 1984.

Hess, C.S., and others: Preventing tooth decay in children, Baby Talk **52**(3):30-31, 1987.

Hitchens-Serota, J.A.: Assessing parent's knowledge of pediatric dental disease, Pediatr. Nurs. **12**(6):435-438, 1986.

Kilmon, F.C., and Helpin, M.L.: Update on dentistry for children, Pediatr. Nurs. **7**(5):41-44, 1981.

Kronmiller, J.E., and Nirschl, R.F.: Preventive dentistry for children, Pediatr. Nurs. **11:**446-449, 1985.

McDermott, R., and McCormack, K.: Nursing caries syndrome: implications for children's health care professionals, Child. Health Care **15**(1):49-54, 1986.

McDonald, R.E., and Avery, D.R.: Dentistry for the child and adolescent, ed. 4, St. Louis, 1983, The C.V. Mosby Co.

Nizel, A.E.: Nutritional support for optimizing children's dental health. In Suskind, R.M., editor: Textbook for pediatric nutrition, New York, 1981, Raven Press.

Injury Prevention

American Academy of Pediatrics, Committee on Accident and Poison Prevention: Automatic passenger protection systems, Pediatrics **74**(1):146-147, 1984.

D'Epiro, P.: Teaching parents about car seats, Patient Care **18**(17):166-180, 1984.

DeWitt, D.E.: Traveling with children, Pediatr. Basics **40:**10-14, 1985.

Elfert, H.: Helping preschool children learn to be safe, Can. Nurse **75:**26-29, Dec. 1979.

Killam, P., and Smith, K.: Getting kids into car seats, MCN **13**(2):124-126, 1988.

Marcus, D.F.: Child car seats: a must for safety, Pediatr. Nurs. **7**(3):13-17, 1981.

McAtee, J.M.: How to help your kids play it safe, Fam. Safety **41**(2):12-13, 1982.

Nachem, B., and Bass, R.A.: Children still aren't being buckled up, MCN **9**(5):320-323, 1984.

Questions and answers about child safety seats, Patient Care **18**(17):196-198, 1984.

Righi, F.C., and Krozy, R.E.: The child in the car: what every nurse should know about safety, Am. J. Nurs. **83**(10): 1421-1424, 1983.

Surveyer, J.A., and Halpern, J.: Age-related burn injuries and their prevention, Pediatr. Nurs. **7**(5):29-34, 1981.

CHAPTER 13

Health Promotion of the Preschooler and Family

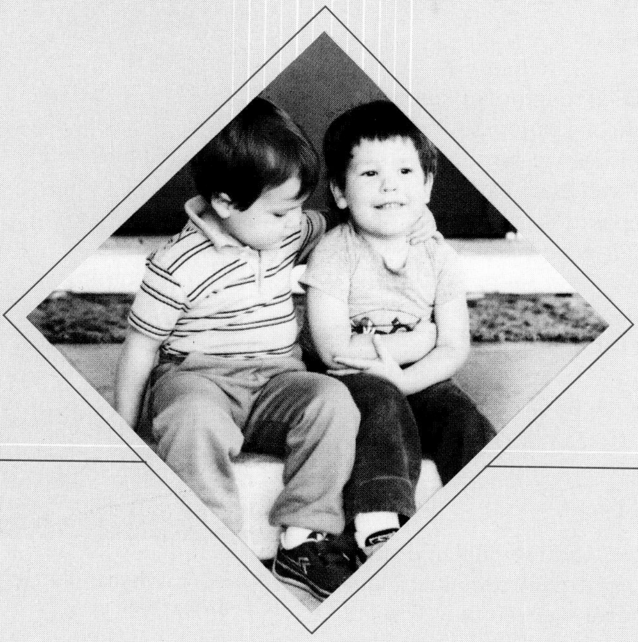

LEARNING OBJECTIVES

On completion of this chapter the reader will be able to:

- Identify the major biologic, psychosocial, cognitive, spiritual, and social developments that occur during the preschool years
- List the benefits of imaginary playmates
- Prepare preschoolers for nursery or daycare experience
- Provide parents with guidelines for sex education
- Provide parents with guidelines for dealing with a child's fears and sleep problems
- Recognize the causes of stuttering during the preschool years
- Offer parents suggestions for preventing speech problems
- Recognize feeding patterns of preschoolers
- Provide anticipatory guidance to parents regarding injury prevention based on the preschooler's developmental achievements

The preschool years, a period from 3 years of age to the completion of 5 years of age, comprise the end of early childhood. This is an age of discovery, inventiveness, curiosity, and developing sociocultural patterns of behavior. In some ways it is a period of ease and comfort for parents, particularly when many of the developmental tasks, such as toileting, independence, and self-caring abilities, have been mastered by the child. The years from birth until the child enters school are considered the most critical period for emotional and psychologic development. It is also the time of greatest parental influence on the child's development.

Once children enter school, their environment widens beyond the home. School becomes a major contributing factor, and peers, teachers, and other authority figures, as well as selected "idols" from the mass media, greatly influence their thinking and behavior. Helping families recognize and understand the adaptability and potential of young children as early as possible is an important nursing responsibility.

◆ *Promoting Optimum Growth and Development*

The combined biologic, psychosocial, cognitive, spiritual, and social achievements of preschoolers prepare them for their most significant change in life-style—entrance into school. Their control of bodily systems, experience of brief and prolonged periods of separation, ability to interact cooperatively with other children and adults, use of language for mental symbolization, and increased attention span and memory ready them for the next major period—the school years. Successful mastery of previous levels of growth and development is essential for preschoolers to refine many of the skills that were begun during the toddler years.

BIOLOGIC DEVELOPMENT

The rate of physical growth slows and stabilizes during the preschool years. Average weight gain remains about 2.3 kg (5 pounds) per year. The average weight at 3 years is 14.6 kg (32 pounds), at 4 years 16.7 kg (36.75 pounds), and at 5 years 18.7 kg (41.25 pounds).

Growth in height also remains steady at a yearly increase of 6.75 to 7.5 cm (2.5 to 3 inches) and generally occurs in elongation of the legs rather than of the trunk. The average height at 3 years is 95 cm (37.25 inches), at 4 years 103 cm (40.5 inches), and at 5 years 110 cm (43.25 inches).

Physical proportions no longer resemble those of the squat, potbellied toddler. The preschooler is slender but sturdy, graceful, agile, and posturally erect. There is little difference in physical characteristics according to sex, except as dictated by such factors as dress and hairstyle.

Most bodily systems are mature and stable and can adjust to moderate stress and change. Motor development consists mostly of increases in strength and refinement of previously learned skills, such as walking, running, and jumping. However, muscle development and bone growth are still far from mature. Excessive activity and overexertion can injure delicate tissues. Properly fitting shoes, good posture, appropriate exercise, and adequate rest are essential for optimal development of the child's musculoskeletal system.

Gross and Fine Motor Behavior

Walking, running, climbing, and jumping are well established by age 36 months. Refinement in eye-hand and muscle coordination is evident in several areas. At age 3 years a preschooler can ride a tricycle, walk on tiptoe, balance on one foot for a few seconds, and broad jump. By 4 years of age the child can skip and hop proficiently on one foot (Fig. 13-1) and catch a ball reliably. By age 5 years the child can skip on alternate feet, jump rope, and begin to skate.

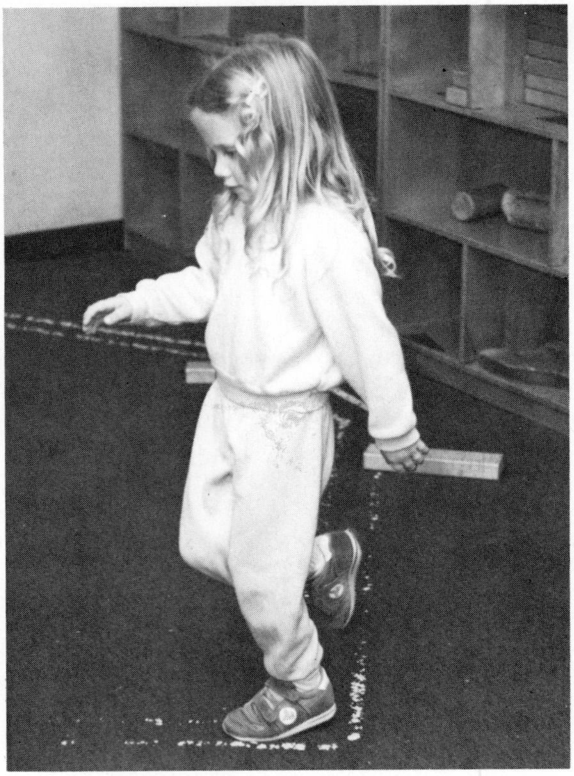

FIG. 13-1 A 4-year-old child has sufficient balance to walk or hop on one foot.

Fine motor development is evident in the child's increasingly skillful manipulation, such as in drawing and dressing. These skills provide readiness for learning and independence for entry to school.

PSYCHOSOCIAL DEVELOPMENT

By the time children reach 3 years of age their gross and fine motor abilities are sufficiently developed to enable them to pursue almost limitless activities. If they have been allowed to express their independence and negativism constructively, they are ready to direct their energy toward new learning. They learn how to interact with and relate to other children and adults; they learn appropriate sex-role functions and socially acceptable behavior; they learn right and wrong and the types of rewards or punishments associated with each. However, learning does not necessarily imply success. Without appropriate guidance and reinforcement, children can learn unacceptable behavior and, instead of feeling accomplishment, feel inadequacy, guilt, and inferiority.

Developing a Sense of Initiative (Erikson)

If preschoolers have mastered the tasks of the toddler period, they are ready to face the developmental endeavors of this stage. Erikson maintains that the chief psychosocial task of the preschool period is acquiring a sense of *initiative*. The child is in a stage of energetic learning. He plays, works, and lives to the fullest and feels a real sense of accomplishment and satisfaction in his activities. Conflict arises when the child oversteps the limits of his ability and inquiry and experiences a sense of *guilt* for not having behaved or acted appropriately. Feelings of guilt, anxiety, and fear may also result from thoughts that differ from expected behavior.

A particularly stressful thought is wishing one's parent dead. As a sense of rivalry or competition develops between the child and same-sex parent, the child may think of ways to rid himself of the interfering parent. In most situations this rivalry is resolved by strongly identifying with the same sex parent and peers during the school years. However, if that parent dies before the identification process is completed, the preschooler can be overwhelmed with feelings of guilt for having wished and, therefore, "caused" the death. Clarifying for children that wishes cannot and do not make events occur is essential in helping them overcome their guilt and anxiety.

Developing a conscience. Development of the *superego,* or *conscience,* has its beginnings toward the end of the toddler years and is a major task for preschoolers. Learning right from wrong and good from bad is the beginning of morality. Children in this age-group are generally unable to understand the reasons that something is acceptable or nonacceptable. They are aware of appropriate behavior mainly through punishment or reward and rely almost religiously on parental principles for developing their own moral judgment. However, verbal enforcement of limits is much more effective. For example, in order to avoid injuries a toddler needs to be supervised, fenced in, and told not to run into the street. A preschooler is much more aware of danger and can be relied on to listen and obey in most instances. If allowed to disagree and question, the child will develop socially acceptable behavior as well as independence in thought and action.

Developing a conscience implies *learning the sociocultural mores* of the family's heritage. Depending on the type of attitudes conveyed, the child will learn not only appropriate behaviors but also tolerant, biased, or prejudiced values concerning his ethnic, religious, and social background and that of other groups. Much of this influence may remain dormant until he associates with children or adults of a different heritage. Then, depending on the particular group, the child may be accepted or isolated for his attitudes.

COGNITIVE DEVELOPMENT

One of the tasks related to the preschool period is readiness for school and scholastic learning. Many of the thought processes of this period are crucial for achieving such readiness, and it is intentional that the child begins school between ages 5 and 6 rather than at an earlier age.

Preoperational Phase (Piaget)

Piaget's cognitive theory actually does not include a period specifically for children 3 to 5 years old. The preoperational phase comprises the age span from 2 to 7 years and is divided into two stages, the *preconceptual phase,* ages 2 to 4, and the phase of *intuitive thought*, ages 4 to 7.

One of the main transitions during these two phases is the shift from totally egocentric thought to social awareness and the ability to consider other viewpoints. This transition is closely associated with the development of the superego. The child is able to think and verbalize his mental processes without having to act out his thinking. However, he can only think of one idea at a time, a concept known as *centration*. He is unable to think of all parts in terms of the whole. Outside influences or perceptions direct his understanding of a visual concept.

The concept of *conservation,* or the idea that a mass can be changed in size, shape, volume, or length without losing or adding to the original mass, is not understood by prelogical children (below age 7 years). Preschoolers judge what they see by the immediate perceptual clues given to them. For example, if two lines of equal length are presented in such a way that one appears longer than the other, the child will state that one line is longer, even if he measures both lines with a ruler or yardstick and finds that each has the same length. The child therefore judges experiences by outside appearances and results, not by intrinsic, logical indicators.

Understanding this prelogical thinking in young children can help nurses interact with them in the most efficacious manner. One example of how manipulating matter according to the child's understanding can facilitate performing an activity concerns administration of drugs. If the child is to receive 5 ml of liquid medication, it is advisable to give it in a small medicine cup, rather than a large cup, since the child will imagine that the large vessel contains more liquid. Since he is unable to perceive the two dimensions of height and width simultaneously, the child will choose one dimension and measure the amount according to that standard. If the child refuses the medicine in the small cup, he may accept it once it is poured into a large cup because the liquid will appear to be less in a tall, wide container.

There are many everyday examples of how the young child's inability to conserve matter influences his behavior. Probably one of the most common situations involves eating and the amount of food placed on a dish. If the same amount of food is placed on a small and a large plate, the child may state that the large plate contains more food and may feel overwhelmed by the apparent large quantity. Parents are usually "taught" this by their children and "learn" ways to use this thinking. Meat that is cut thin and flat appears to be more in quantity than the same amount of meat that is cut thick, and the child will generally consume more of the thicker portion. The opposite also has its advantages. Giving a child a large, flat cookie will please and satisfy him more than giving him a small, thick one.

Language continues to develop during the preschool period. Speech remains primarily a vehicle of egocentric communication. The child assumes that everyone thinks as he does and that a brief explanation of his thinking makes his entire thought understood by others. Because of this self-referenced, egocentric verbal communication, it is frequently necessary to explore and understand the young child's thinking through other nonverbal approaches. For children in this age-group, the most enlightening and effective method is play.

Preschoolers increasingly use language without comprehending the meaning of words, particularly concepts of right or left, time, and causality. The child may use the concepts correctly but only in the circumstances he has learned them. For example, he may know how to put on his shoes by remembering that the buckle is always on the outside of the foot. However, if different shoes have no buckles, he cannot reason which shoe fits which foot. In other words he does not understand the concept of right and left.

Preschoolers believe in the power of words and accept their meaning literally. A significant example of this type of thinking is calling the child "bad" because he did something wrong. In his mind, telling him that he is bad means that he is bad. For this reason it is better to relate such words to the act, by saying, for example, "That was a bad thing to do."

Superficially, *causality* resembles logical thought. The child explains a concept as he heard it described by others, but his understanding is limited. An example is the concept of time. Since *time* is still incompletely understood, the child interprets it according to his own frame of reference, such as "A long time means until Christmas." Consequently, time is best explained in relationship to an event, such as "Your mother will visit you after you finish your lunch." Avoiding terms such as yesterday, tomorrow, next week, and Tuesday to express when an event is expected to occur and associating time with usual expected daily occurrences help children learn about temporal relationships, while increasing their trust in others' predictions.

Preschoolers' thinking is often described as *magical*. Because of their egocentrism and transductive reasoning (association of one event with a simultaneous event), they believe that thoughts are all-powerful. Such thinking places them in the vulnerable position of feeling guilty and responsible for bad thoughts, which may coincide with the occurrence of a wished event. A typical example is wishing a new sibling dead. If that sibling does die, young children think their wish caused the death. Their inability to logically reason the cause and effect of illness or an injury makes it especially difficult for them to understand such events.

DEVELOPMENT OF BODY IMAGE

The preschool years play a significant role in the development of body image. With increasing comprehension of language, preschoolers recognize that individuals have undesirable and desirable appearances. They recognize differences in skin color and racial identity and are vulnerable to learning prejudices and biases. They are aware of the meaning of words, such as *pretty* or *ugly*, and reflect the opinions of others regarding their own appearance. For example, by 5 years of age children compare their size to their peers' and can become conscious of being large or short, especially if others refer to them as "so big" or "so little" for their age.

Despite the advances in body-image development, preschoolers have poorly defined body boundaries and little knowledge of their internal anatomy. Intrusive experiences are frightening, especially those that disrupt the integrity of the skin, such as injections and surgery. There is a fear that if the skin is "broken" all their blood and "insides" can leak out. Therefore, bandages are critical to "keeping everything from coming out."

Sexual identity is developing beyond gender recognition, and children may become modest, as well as fear mutilation. There is sex-role imitation, and "dressing up" like mommy or daddy is an important activity. Attitudes and responses of others to the child's role-playing can condition him to views of himself or others. For example, comments such as "boys shouldn't play with dolls" can influence his self-concept of masculinity. Perhaps this is a time when children begin forming ideal images of how they would want to look as adults.

SPIRITUAL DEVELOPMENT

Children's knowledge of faith and religion is learned from significant others in their environment, usually from the religious practices of the parents. However, the young child's understanding of spirituality is influenced by his cognitive level. Preschoolers have a concrete conception of a God with physical characteristics who is often like an imaginary friend. They understand simple Bible stories and memorize short prayers but their understanding of the meaning of these rituals is limited. They benefit from concrete representations of religious practices, such as picture Bible books, and small statues, such as those of the Nativity scene (Shelley and others, 1982).

Development of the conscience is strongly linked to spiritual development. At this age children are learning right from wrong and behave correctly to avoid punishment. Wrongdoing provokes feelings of guilt, and preschoolers often misinterpret illness as a punishment for real or imagined transgressions. It is important that children view God as one who bestows unconditional love, rather than as a judge of good or bad behavior. Praying to God and observing religious traditions, such as prayers before meals or bedtime, can help a child through stressful periods, such as hospitalization.

SOCIAL DEVELOPMENT

Dramatic advancements in social development occur during the preschool period. The individuation-separation process is complete. Preschoolers have overcome much of the anxiety associated with strangers and the fear of separation of earlier years. They relate to unfamiliar people easily and tolerate brief separations from parents with little or no protest. However, they still need parental security, reassurance, guidance, and approval, especially when entering nursery school or elementary school. Prolonged separation, such as that imposed by illness and hospitalization, is difficult, but preschoolers respond very well to anticipatory preparation and concrete explanation. They can cope with changes in daily routine much better than toddlers; however, they may develop more imaginary fears. They gain security and comfort from familiar objects, such as toys, dolls, or photographs of family members. They are able to work through many of their unresolved fears, fantasies, and anxieties through play, especially if guided with appropriate play objects, for example, dolls or puppets, that represent family members, medical and nursing staff, and other children.

Language

Language during the preschool years is quite sophisticated and complex. It also becomes a major mode of communication and social interaction. Vocabulary increases dramatically, from 300 words at age 2 to over 2100 words at the end of 5 years. Sentence structure, grammatical usage, and intelligibility also advance to a more adult level.

Children between the ages of 3 and 4 form sentences of about three to four words and include only the most essential words to convey a meaning. Such speech is often termed *telegraphic* for its brevity in length. Three-year-old children ask many questions and use plurals, correct pronouns, and the past tense of verbs. They name familiar objects, such as animals, parts of the body, relatives, and friends. They can give and follow simple commands. They talk incessantly, regardless of whether anyone is listening or answering them. They enjoy musical or talking toys or dolls and imitate new words proficiently.

From ages 4 to 5 preschoolers use longer sentences of four to five words and use more words to convey a message, such as prepositions, adjectives, and a variety of verbs. They follow simple directional commands, such as "Put the ball on the chair," but can carry out only one request at a time. They answer questions, such as "What do you do when you are hungry?" by describing the appropriate action. The pattern of asking questions is at its peak, and children usually repeat the question until they receive an answer.

By the end of age 5 children use all parts of speech correctly, except for deviations from the rule. They can define simple words by describing their use, shape, or general category of classification, not only by stating their outward appearance. For example, they define a ball as "round, something you bounce, or a toy," rather than by its color. They can give some opposites, such as "If Mommy is a woman, Daddy is a man." By the time they are 6 years old, they can describe an object according to its composition, such as "A spoon is made of metal."

Personal-Social Behavior

The pervasive ritualism and negativism of toddlerhood gradually diminish during the preschool years. Although self-assertion is still a major theme, preschoolers demonstrate their sense of autonomy differently. They are able to verbalize their request for independence and perform independently because of their much refined physical and cognitive development. They fully care for themselves by 4 or 5 years of age, needing little if any assistance with dressing, eating, or toileting (Fig. 13-2). They can be trusted to obey warnings of danger, although 3- or 4-year-old children may exceed their boundaries at times.

They are also much more sociable and willing to please. They have internalized many of the standards and values of the family, and their conscience dictates many of their actions. By the end of early childhood they begin to question parental values and compare them to those of their peer group and other authority figures; as a result,

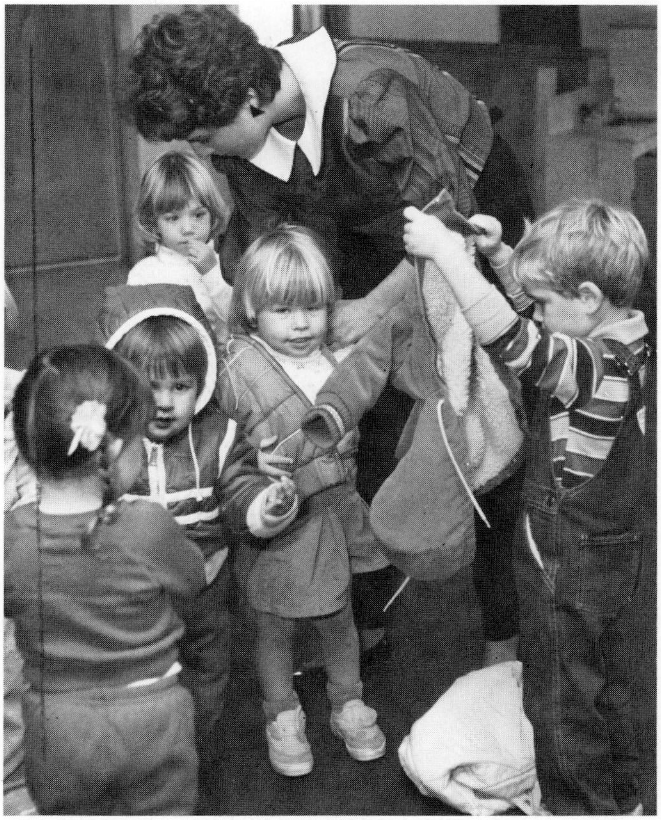

FIG. 13-2 Most preschoolers are able to dress themselves but need help with more difficult items of clothing.

they may be less willing to abide by the family's code of conduct. Preschoolers become increasingly aware of their position and role within the family. Although this is a more secure age for experiencing the addition of another sibling, relinquishing the position of first or youngest is still difficult and requires appropriate preparation (see Chapter 12).

Play

Various types of play are typical of this period, but preschoolers especially enjoy associative play—group play in similar or identical activities but without rigid organization or rules. Play should provide for physical, social, and mental development.

Play activities for physical growth and refinement of motor skills include jumping, running, and climbing. Tricycles, scooter trucks, wagons, Big wheels, gym and sports equipment, sandboxes, wading pools, and winter sleds can help develop muscles and coordination. Activities such as swimming, skating, and skiing teach safety as well as muscle development and coordination (Fig. 13-3).

Manipulative, constructive, creative, and educational toys provide for quiet activities, fine motor development, and self-expression. Easy construction sets, large blocks of various sizes and shapes, a counting frame, alphabet or number flash cards, paints, crayons, simple carpentry tools, musical toys, illustrated books, simple sewing or handicraft sets, large puzzles, and clay are suitable toys. Electronic games, such as Speak & Spell* and educational computer programs for television, are especially valuable in helping children learn basic skills, such as letters and simple words.

Probably the most characteristic and pervasive preschool activity is *imitative, imaginative,* and *dramatic play*. Dress-up clothes, dolls, housekeeping toys, dollhouses, play-store toys, telephones, farm animals and equipment, village sets, trains, trucks, cars, planes, hand puppets, and doctor and nurse kits provide hours of self-expression (Fig. 13-4). Probably at no other time is the reproduction of the behavior of significant adults so faithful and absorbing as in 4- and 5-year-old children. Toward the end of the preschool period, children are less

*Texas Instruments, Dallas, TX 75243-1108.

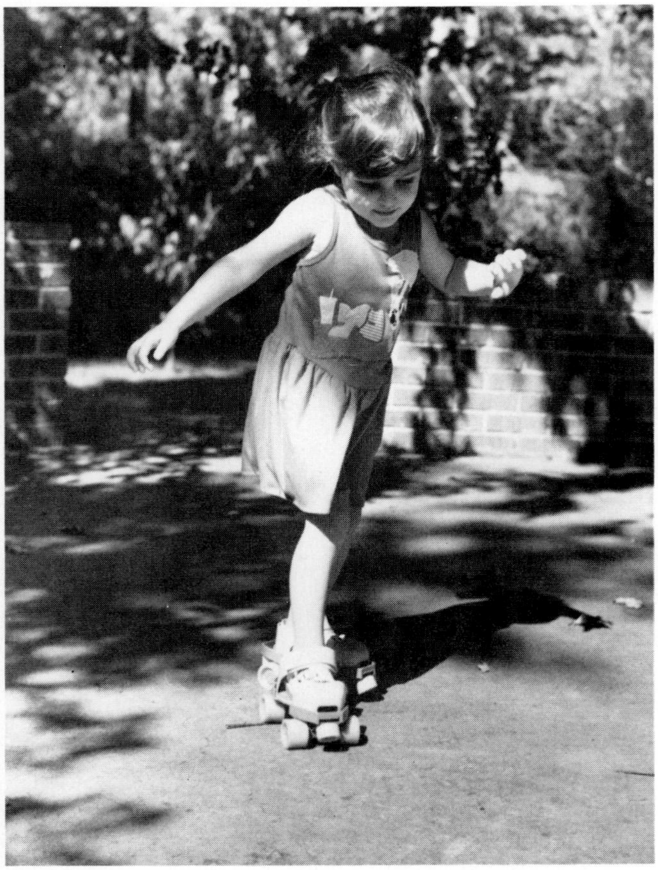

FIG. 13-3 Activities such as skating help a preschooler's muscle development and coordination.

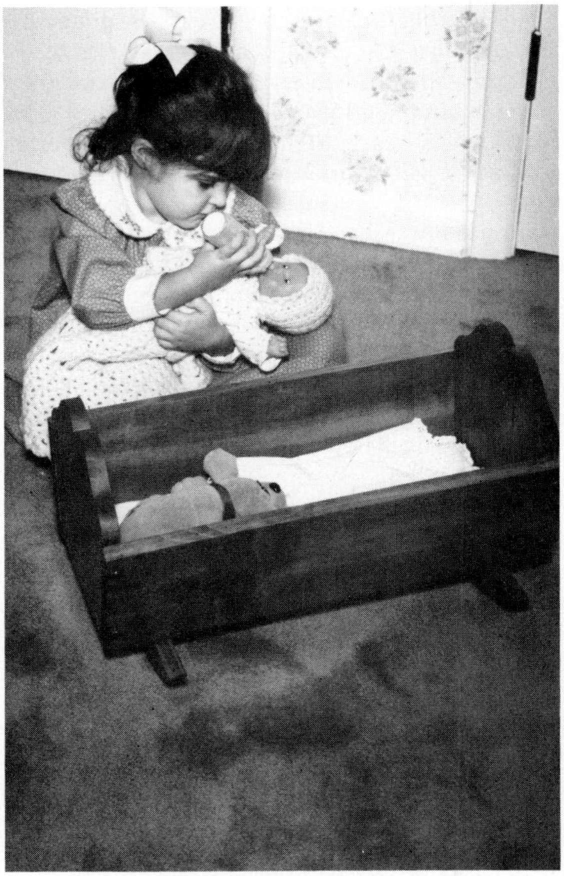

FIG. 13-4 Imaginative and dramatic play is typical of preschoolers who enjoy using fantasy.

satisfied with make believe or pretend objects and enjoy actually doing the activity, such as cooking and carpentry.

Television and video also have their places in children's play, although each should only be one part of children's total repertoire of social and recreational activities. In counseling parents regarding the effect of television on children, the nurse should explain some of the negative effects of excessive watching, such as aggressive behavior, decreased school performance, and poorer health habits (Zuckerman and Zuckerman, 1985). Parents are encouraged to supervise selection of programs, preview programs for appropriateness, and schedule hours for television viewing. Children enjoy and learn from educational children's programs, which are purposely shown before dinner or after meals to provide a quiet activity. Television can become an interactive activity when parents view programs with children and discuss program content.

Imaginary playmates. Play is so much a part of the young child's life that reality and fantasy become blurred. The make-believe is reality during play and only becomes fantasy when the toys are put away or the dress-up clothes are removed. It is no wonder that imaginary playmates are so much a part of this age period.

The appearance of imaginary companions usually occurs between the ages of 2½ to 3 years, and for the most part such playmates are relinquished when the child enters school. There seems to be a relationship between the level of intelligence and the presence of the imaginary companion (Fish and Burch, 1985). The more intelligent children tend to have the more vivid and complex pretend playmates.

Imaginary companions serve many purposes—they become friends in times of loneliness, they accomplish what the child is still attempting, and they experience what the child wants to forget or remember. It is not unusual for the "friend" to have a myriad of vices and to be blamed for wrongdoing. Sometimes the child hopes to escape punishment by saying, "My friend George broke the glass." At other times the child may fantasize that the companion misbehaved and play the role of parent. This becomes a way of assuming control and authority in a safe situation.

Parents often worry about the imaginary playmates, not realizing how normal and useful they are. They need to be reassured that children's fantasy is a sign of health that helps them differentiate between pretend and reality. Parents can acknowledge the presence of the imaginary companion by calling him by name and even agreeing to simple requests such as setting an extra place at the table, but they should not allow the child to use the playmate to avoid punishment or responsibility. For example, if the child blames the companion for messing his room, parents need to state clearly that the child is the only one they see and therefore he is responsible for cleaning up.

SUMMARY OF GROWTH AND DEVELOPMENT DURING THE PRESCHOOL YEARS

By the age of 3 the child has made tremendous strides from the dependency and callowness of infancy and the negativism and clumsiness of toddlerhood. The preschooler has excellent gross and fine motor control. He is a very social and domesticated being and cares for himself almost completely. Language is a vehicle of communication, learning, and self-expression. These and other major developmental achievements for children 3, 4, and 5 years old are summarized in Table 13-1.

COPING WITH CONCERNS RELATED TO NORMAL GROWTH AND DEVELOPMENT

In many respects the preschool years present few child-rearing problems. However, there are special situations during this period that require parental guidance. They include preschool or daycare experience, sex education, fears, and speech problems. The issue of divorce, which has a significant impact on preschoolers, is discussed in Chapter 4.

Preschool or Daycare Experience

During the preschool years many children attend some type of early childhood program, usually nursery school or a daycare center. Group care has become commonplace with the large number of mothers presently employed outside the home. The effects of early education and stimulation on children have increasingly gained recognition and importance. Since social development widens to include age-mates and other significant adults, preschool provides an excellent vehicle for expanding children's experiences with others.

In nursery school or daycare centers children are exposed to opportunities for learning group cooperation, adjusting to various sociocultural differences, and coping with frustration, dissatisfaction, and anger. If activities are tailored to provide mastery and achievement, children increasingly feel success, self-confidence, and personal competence. Whether or not structured learning is imposed is less important than the social climate, type of guidance, and attitude toward the children that is fostered by the teacher or leader. If a teacher is aware of preschoolers' developmental abilities and needs, the children will learn from any activity that is provided. Most nursery schools incorporate a similar daily schedule of quiet play, active outdoor activity, group activities such as games and projects, creative or free play, and snack and rest periods.

Nursery school is particularly beneficial for children who lack a peer-group experience, such as an only child, and for children from culturally deprived homes. Nursery school provides extensive stimulation for language, phys-

TABLE 13-1

Growth and Development during Preschool Years

Age (years)	Physical	Gross Motor	Fine Motor	Language
3	Usual weight gain of 1.8 to 2.7 kg (4 to 6 pounds) Average weight of 14.6 kg (32 pounds) Usual gain in height of 7.5 cm (3 inches) Average height of 95 cm (37.25 inches) May have achieved nighttime control of bowel and bladder	Rides tricycle Jumps off bottom step Stands on one foot for a few seconds Goes up stairs using alternate feet, may still come down using both feet on step Broad jumps May try to dance, but balance may not be adequate	Builds tower of nine or ten cubes Builds bridge with three cubes Adeptly places small pellets in narrow-necked bottle In drawing, copies a circle, imitates a cross, names what he has drawn, cannot draw stickman but may make circle with facial features	Has vocabulary of about 900 words Uses primarily "telegraphic" speech Uses complete sentences of three to four words Talks incessantly regardless of whether anyone is paying attention Repeats sentence of six syllables Constantly asks questions
4	Pulse and respiration rates decrease slightly Growth rate is similar to that of previous year Average weight of 16.7 kg (36.75 pounds) Average height of 103 cm (40.5 inches) Length at birth is doubled Maximum potential for development of amblyopia	Skips and hops on one foot Catches ball reliably Throws ball overhand Walks downstairs using alternate footing	Uses scissors successfully to cut out picture following outline Can lace shoes, but may not be able to tie bow In drawing, copies a square, traces a cross and diamond, adds three parts to stick figure	Has vocabulary of 1500 words or more Uses sentences of four to five words Questioning is at peak Tells exaggerated stories Knows simple songs May be mildly profane if he associates with older children Obeys four prepositional phrases, such as "under," "on top of," "beside," "in back of," or "in front of" Names one or more colors Comprehends analogies, such as, "If ice is cold, fire is __" Repeats four digits Uses words liberally but frequently does not comprehend meaning

Socialization	Cognition	Family Relationships
Dresses self almost completely if helped with back buttons and told which shoe is right or left Buttons/unbuttons accessible buttons Pulls on shoes Has increased attention span Feeds self completely Pours from a bottle or pitcher Can prepare simple meals, such as cold cereal and milk Can help to set table; can dry dishes without breaking any Likes to "help" entertain by passing food May have fears, especially of dark and going to bed Knows own sex and appropriate sex of others In play, parallel and associative phase Begins to learn simple games and meaning of rules, but follows them according to self-interpretation Speaks to toys, such as doll, animal, truck	Is in preconceptual phase Is egocentric in thought and behavior Has beginning understanding of time; uses many time-oriented expressions, talks about past and future as much as about present, pretends to tell time Has improved concept of space as demonstrated in understanding of prepositions and ability to follow directional command Has beginning ability to view concepts from another perspective	Attempts to please parents and conform to their expectations Is less jealous of younger sibling; may be opportune time for birth of additional sibling Is aware of family relationships and sex-role functions Boys tend to identify more with father or other male figure Has increased ability to separate easily and comfortably from parents for short periods
Very independent Tends to be selfish and impatient Aggressive physically as well as verbally Takes pride in accomplishments Has mood swings Boasts and tattles Shows off dramatically, enjoys entertaining others Tells family tales to others with no restraint Still has many fears Play is associative Imaginary playmates common Uses dramatic, imaginative, and imitative devices Works through unresolved conflicts, such as jealousy toward sibling, anger toward parent, or unconquered fear in himself. Sexual exploration and curiosity demonstrated through play, such as being "doctor" or "nurse"	Is in phase of intuitive thought Causality still related to proximity of events Understands time better, especially in terms of sequence of daily events Unable to conserve matter Judges everything according to one dimension, such as height, width, or order Immediate perceptual clues dominate judgment Can choose longer of two lines or heavier of two objects Is beginning to develop less egocentrism and more social awareness May count correctly but has poor mathematic concept of numbers Still believes that thoughts cause events Obeys because parents have set limits, not because of understanding of reason behind right or wrong	Rebels if parents expect too much, such as impeccable table manners Takes aggression and frustration out on parents or siblings Do's and don'ts become important May have rivalry with older or younger siblings, may resent older's privileges and younger's invasion of privacy and possessions May run away from home Identifies strongly with parent of opposite sex Is able to run errands outside the home

Continued.

TABLE 13-1

Growth and Development during Preschool Years—cont'd

Age (years)	Physical	Gross Motor	Fine Motor	Language
5	Pulse and respiration rates decrease slightly Systolic blood pressure increases slightly Average weight of 18.7 kg (41.25 pounds) Average height of 110 cm (43.25 inches) Eruption of permanent dentition may begin, especially if deciduous tooth eruption was early (before age 6 months) First permanent teeth to erupt are four molars, which come in behind last temporary teeth (often mistaken for temporary molars) Handedness is established (about 90% are right-handed)	Skips and hops on alternate feet Throws and catches ball well Jumps rope Skates with good balance Walks backward with heel to toe Jumps from height of 12 inches, lands on toes Balances on alternate feet with eyes closed	Ties shoelaces Uses scissors, simple tools, or pencil very well In drawing, copies a diamond and triangle, adds seven to nine parts to stickman, prints a few letters, numbers, or words, such as his first name	Has vocabulary of about 2100 words Uses sentences of six to eight words, with all parts of speech Names coins (e.g., nickel, dime) Names four or more colors Describes drawing or pictures with much comment and enumeration Asks meaning of words Asks inquisitive questions Can repeat sentence of 10 syllables or more Knows names of days of week, months, and other time-associated words Defines words using action as well as description Knows composition of articles, such as, "A shoe is made of ______" Can follow three demands in succession

ical, and social development. It also is an excellent preparation for entrance into regular school.

A major nursing responsibility is guiding parents in locating suitable facilities with a well-qualified staff.* State licensing agencies can help parents identify daycare centers that accept children of specific age-groups and are conveniently located near home and work.

State-licensed programs are supposed to abide by established standards, which represent the *minimum* requirements and safeguards. However, enforcement of the standards is sometimes inadequate. Early childhood programs may also belong to a voluntary accreditation system, the National Academy of Early Childhood Programs, which serves as a model for *optimum* care.* References from other parents are also helpful, provided the parents have investigated the center carefully and have remained involved with the agency's activities.

Other areas for parents to evaluate are the center's daily program, teacher qualifications, student-to-staff ratio, environmental safety precautions, provision of meals, sanitary conditions, adequate indoor/outdoor space per child, and fee schedule. Although fees vary considerably, it is important for the parent to realize that a program that charges a minimum fee may also be providing minimum services. In terms of an overall evaluation there is *no substitute for a personal observation of the facility.*

*A helpful booklet is *Tips on Selecting the "Right" Day Care Facility,* Elk Grove Village, IL, 1985, American Academy of Pediatrics. Single copies are $.50 and may be ordered from the Academy, P.O. Box 927, Elk Grove Village, IL 60007.

*Information about the accreditation criteria and procedures of the **National Academy of Early Childhood Programs** is available from the National Association for the Education of Young Children, 1834 Connecticut Avenue, N.W., Washington, DC 20009. These criteria are excellent guidelines for evaluating nursery or daycare centers.

Socialization	Cognition	Family Relationships

Less rebellious and quarrelsome than at age 4 years
More settled and eager to get down to business
Not as open and accessible in thoughts and behavior as in earlier years
Independent but trustworthy, not foolhardy, more responsible
Has fewer fears; relies on outer authority to control world
Eager to do things right and to please; tries to "live by the rules"
Acts "manly" or "womanly"
Has fairly consistent and polished manners
Cares for self totally, occasionally needing supervision in dress or hygiene
May complain over minor injuries but tries to be brave for major pain
Not ready for concentrated close work or small print because of slight farsightedness and still unrefined eye-hand coordination
Play is associative
  Likes rules and tries to follow them but may cheat to avoid losing
  Begins to notice group conformity and sense of belonging
Imitative play mimics the portrayed adult like a mirror image
Wants to use real objects during play, such as actual ingredients to make cookies rather than sand or mud
Very industrious, tries to accomplish a goal and feels pride and satisfaction, as well as unhappiness and discontent
May demand to watch television more now that he understands programs better
	Begins to question what parents think by comparing them to age-mates and other adults
	May notice prejudice and bias in outside world
	Is more able to view other's perspective, but tolerates differences rather than understands them
	Tends to be matter-of-fact about differences in others
	May begin to show understanding of conservation of numbers through counting objects regardless of arrangement
	Uses time-oriented words with increased understanding
	Very curious about factual information regarding world
		Gets along well with parents
		Does not try to run away from home
		May seek out parent more often than at age 4 years for reassurance and security, especially when entering school
		Is upset not to find parent, for example, when he comes home from school
		Tolerates siblings, but finds 3-year-old children a special nuisance
		Begins to question parents' thinking and principles
		Strongly identifies with parent of same sex, especially boys with their fathers
		Enjoys doing activities, such as sports, cooking, shopping with parent of same sex

Parents should arrange to meet the director and some of the employees, especially those who would be caring for the child.

One of the areas that is increasingly important in selecting child care centers is the agency's sanitary practices. Centers that care for infants and young children who are not toilet-trained can pose an increased risk of infection among children. Outbreaks of a number of organisms have been reported, including *Shigella* organisms, *Giardia lamblia,* rotavirus, cryptosporidiosis, *Campylobacter jejuni, Haemophilus influenzae* type b, cytomegalovirus, and hepatitis A (Smith, 1986).

Nurses play an important role in infection control. Not only can they advise parents regarding the evaluation of a center's sanitary practices, they can also take an active part in educating staff in measures to minimize transmission of infection by stressing the importance of (1) handwashing of children and employees (Fig. 13-5), (2) changing diapers as soon as they are soiled, (3) proper disposal of diapers, preferably placed in a plastic bag and discarded in a closed container stored away from children, (4) proper cleaning of the diaper changing surface and accessory items that may become contaminated during a diaper change, (5) not allowing staff who care for children to prepare food, and (6) excluding children who are ill from school or caring for them in a separate area.

Children need preparation for the preschool experience, whether it is a formal nursery school, organized daycare center, or casual gathering in a neighbor's home.* For young children it represents a change from their usual home environment and prolonged separation from parents.

*A recommended book to prepare young children for daycare is Rogers, F.: Going to day care, New York, 1985, G.P. Putnam's Sons.

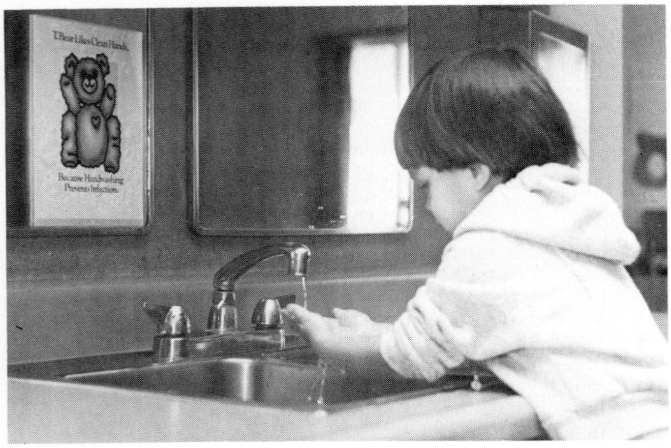

FIG. 13-5 Thorough handwashing is the single most effective method of preventing infection. Note the poster on the mirror; the T. Bear symbol is part of a national infection control campaign sponsored by the U.S. Department of Health and Human Services.

Before the child begins the school experience, the parents should present the idea as exciting and pleasurable. Talking to the child about activities such as painting, building with blocks, or enjoying swings and other outdoor equipment allows the child to fantasize about the forthcoming event in a positive manner. When the day arrives to begin school, the parents should behave confidently with no hesitancy or self-doubt about the decision, lest such feelings be transmitted to the child and influence his adjustment. Such behavior necessitates that the parents work through their own feelings regarding the nursery school or daycare center experience.

Parents should introduce their child to the teacher and familiarize him with the school. In some instances it is helpful to remain for at least some part of the first day until the child is comfortable and at ease. Other specific actions that can help lessen separation anxiety include providing the school with detailed information about the child's home environment, such as familiar routines, favorite activities, food preferences, names of siblings or pets, and personal habits. Such information helps the child feel familiar in the strange surroundings. When schools automatically request this information, the parent has a valuable clue to evaluating the quality of the program since the request represents the staff's awareness of each child's needs. Transitional objects such as a favorite toy or blanket may also help the child bridge the gap from home to school.

Sex Education and Sexual Curiosity

Preschoolers have absorbed and experienced a tremendous amount of information during their short lifetimes. Although their thinking may not be mature, they search constantly for explanations and reasons that are logical and reasonable to them. The word "why" seems to supplant the word "no," which was common in toddlerhood. It is only natural that as they learn about "me" they will also want to know "why me," and "how me." Questions such as "Where do babies come from?" are sexual in content but informational in intent. Such inquiries are as casual as "Why is the sky blue?" "What makes it rain?" or "Who is that?" It is the *way* in which questions about procreation are answered that conditions children, even the youngest, to separate these questions from others about their world.

Two rules govern answering questions about sex. The first is to *find out what the child thinks*. By investigating the theories he has conjured in his mind as a reasonable explanation, parents can not only give correct information but also help the child understand why his explanation is inaccurate. Another reason for ascertaining what the child thinks before offering any information is that the "unasked for" answer may be given. For example, 4-year-old Sally asked her father, "Where did I come from?" Both parents quickly took this inquiry as a clue for offering sex education. After a lengthy miniobstetric course, Sally exclaimed, "I don't know about all that! All I know is Mary came from New York and I want to know where I was born."

The second rule for giving information is *honesty*. It is true that much of the correct information will be forgotten or misunderstood by the preschooler, but what is more important is that the correct information can be restated until the child absorbs and comprehends the facts. Even though the correct anatomic words may be hard to pronounce or even more difficult to remember, they become foundational content for explaining other concepts later on.

Honesty does not imply revealing every fact of life or allowing children excessive permissiveness in sexual curiosity. When children ask one question, they are looking for one answer, not the entire procreation cycle. When they are ready, they will ask about the other "unfinished" parts of the story. Sooner or later they will wonder how the "sperm meets the egg" and "how the baby gets out," but it is best to wait until they ask.

Regardless of whether children are given sex education, they will engage in games of sexual curiosity and exploration. At about 3 years of age children are aware of the anatomic differences between the sexes and are very concerned with how the other "works." This is not really "sexual" curiosity, because many children are still unaware of the reproductive function of the genitals. Their curiosity is for the eliminative function of the anatomy. Little boys wonder how girls can urinate without a penis, so they watch girls go to the bathroom. Since they cannot see anything but the stream of water coming out, they want to observe further for what makes it come out. "Doctor play" is often a game invented for just such investigation. Little girls are no less curious about boys' anatomy. It is very intriguing to have a closer inspection of this "thing" that girls do not have.

One question that parents often have is how to handle

such sexual curiosity. A positive approach is neither to condone nor condemn the sexual curiosity but to express that if the child has questions he should ask his parents, and then encourage the child to engage in some other activity. In this way children can be helped to understand that there are ways other than through playing investigative games that their sexual curiosity can be satisfied. This in no way condemns the act but stresses alternate methods to seek solutions. Allowing children unrestricted permissiveness only intensifies their anxiety and concern since exploring and searching usually yield little evidence to satisfy their curiosity.

Another concern for some parents is masturbation, or self-stimulation of the genitals. This occurs at any age for a variety of reasons and, if not excessive, is normal and healthy. For preschoolers it is a part of sexual curiosity and exploration. If parents are concerned with masturbation in their children, it is essential for nurses to investigate the circumstances associated with the activity, because it may be an expression of anxiety, boredom, or unresolved conflicts. For example, a boy who repeatedly touches his penis is not masturbating for pleasure but may be reassuring himself that it is intact. Also, children who openly and publicly masturbate are inviting a reaction, such as discipline, punishment, or criticism. They may be overwhelmed by their sexual feelings and asking others to help them channel them into more constructive outlets. Since masturbation, like other forms of sex play, is a private act, parents should emphasize this to children as part of teaching them socially acceptable behavior.

Fears

The greatest number and variety of real and imagined fears are present during the preschool years and include fear of the dark, being left alone (especially at bedtime), animals (particularly large dogs and snakes), ghosts, sexual matters (castration), and objects or persons associated with pain. Parents often become perplexed about handling the fears because no amount of logical persuasion, coercion, or ridicule will send away the ghosts, boogeymen, monsters, and devils.

The best way to help children overcome their fears is by actively involving them in finding practical methods to deal with the frightening experience. This may be as simple as keeping a dim night-light on in the child's bedroom to assure him that no monsters lurk in the dark. Exposing children to the feared object in a safe situation also provides a type of conditioning or desensitization. For instance, children who are afraid of dogs should never be forced to approach or touch one, but they may be gradually introduced to the experience by watching other children play with the animal. This type of *modeling,* demonstrating fearlessness in others, can be very effective if the child is allowed to progress at his own rate.

Usually by 5 or 6 years of age children relinquish these old fears. If told about a previous fear, such as believing in ghosts, they will typically remark that they do not believe in or fear them because they have never seen one. This is quite logical and very concrete and helps explain away many of the fears of younger years. Explaining the developmental sequence of fears and their gradual disappearance may help parents feel more secure in handling preschoolers' fears.

Speech Problems

The most critical period for speech development occurs between 2 and 4 years of age. During this period the child is using his rapidly growing vocabulary to interact with the environment. However, the rate of vocabulary acquisition does not keep pace with the advancing mental ability or the degree of comprehension. Consequently, it can result in the child's stuttering or stammering as he tries to say the word he is already thinking about. This hesitancy or nonfluency in speech pattern is a *normal* characteristic of language development.

However, when parents or other significant persons place undue emphasis or stress on this pattern of dysfluency, an abnormal speech pattern may result. Chances for reversal of stuttering are good until about 7 years of age. Therefore, prevention must begin early. The nurse should discuss with parents the normal dysfluencies in children's speech. When stuttering does occur, parents are advised to use the suggestions listed in the boxed material that follows to prevent inadvertently reinforcing this pattern. If excessive concern on the part of the parent or frustration and struggling behavior from the child are noted, the child is referred for language and speech eval-

Guidelines for Parents Regarding Stuttering in Children

To Be Encouraged

- Viewing hesitancy and dysfluency as a normal part of speech development
- Giving child plenty of time and the impression of not being rushed or in a hurry
- Looking directly at child while he is talking; being patient and never ridiculing or criticizing
- Speaking clearly and articulating well but not stressing that all sounds must be perfected too early
- Identifying situations when stuttering increases and avoiding them or ignoring the hesitancy
- Capitalizing on periods of fluent speech with positive reinforcement such as singing songs or repeating nursery rhymes

To Be Avoided

- The natural tendency to "help" child by supplying word when he is having a block
- Telling him to stop or start over, to think before he speaks, or to take it easy and go slowly
- Showing great concern, embarrassment, or disapproval for hesitancy
- *Anything* that emphasizes stuttering and calls child's attention to his speech skills
- Promising reward for proper speech

uation. The critical point to remember is that the dysfluency must be arrested before the child develops an awareness or anticipation of the difficulty and begins to mistrust his speech skills.

Children who are pressured into producing sounds ahead of their developmental level may develop dyslalia (articulation problems) or revert to using infantile speech. Prevention involves discussing with parents the usual achievement of speech production during childhood. The Denver Articulation Screening Examination (DASE) is an excellent tool to assess articulation skills in the child and to explain to parents the expected progression of sounds (Appendix C).

The DASE employs the word-imitative procedure. The child repeats 22 words but pronounces 30 different sound elements. The raw score, or the number of correctly pronounced sounds, is then compared to the percentile rank for children in that age-group. The examiner must be careful to evaluate the specific sound, rather than the quality of the entire word. For beginning examiners it is helpful to validate the final score by comparing the results with a different examiner, ideally a speech therapist. The child is also scored on intelligibility, by selection of one of four possible categories: (1) easy to understand, (2) understandable half of the time, (3) not understandable, or (4) cannot evaluate. The DASE is a reliable, effective screening tool for nurses because it requires only 10 minutes to perform and it is designed to discriminate between significant delay and normal variations in the acquisition of speech sounds.

The best therapy for speech problems is prevention. One of the most essential factors involves anticipatory preparation of parents for the expected hesitation in speech during the preschool period and discussion of developmental achievements characteristic of young children.

◆ *Promoting Optimum Health during the Preschool Years*

Health promotion mainly involves guidance regarding nutrition, sleep, dental health, and injury prevention. A brief discussion of each subject is presented to emphasize the particular needs or differences of preschoolers vs toddlers. (For a more comprehensive understanding the reader is urged to also review the material presented in Chapter 12 under Promoting optimum health during the toddler years.)

NUTRITION

Nutritional requirements for preschoolers are fairly similar to those for toddlers. The requirement for calories per unit of body weight continues to decrease slightly to 85 kcal per kg for an average daily intake of 1700 calories. Fluid requirements may also decrease slightly to about 100 ml per kg daily but depend on activity level, climatic conditions, and state of health. The protein requirements are 1.5 g per kg for an average daily consumption of 30 g.

Some preschoolers still have food habits that are typical of toddlers, such as food fads and strong taste preferences. When children reach 4 years of age, they seem to enter another period of finicky eating, which is generally characteristic of the more rebellious and rowdy behavior of children in this age-group. By age 5 years children are greatly influenced by the food habits of others and are more agreeable to try new foods, especially if encouraged by an adult who allows the child to help with food preparation or experiments with a new taste or different dish (Fig. 13-6). Mealtimes can become battlegrounds if parents expect impeccable table manners. Usually the 5-year-old child is ready for the "social" side of eating, but the 3- or 4-year-old child still has difficulty sitting quietly through a long family meal.

Parents sometimes worry about the quantity of food preschoolers consume. In general, the quality is much more important than the quantity, a fact that should be stressed during nutritional counseling. Young children often consume more food than parents realize. One approach toward lessening this parental concern is advising parents to keep a weekly record of everything the child eats. In particular, the need for measuring the amount of food, such as setting aside ½ cup of vegetables, and serving the child from this premeasured amount should be

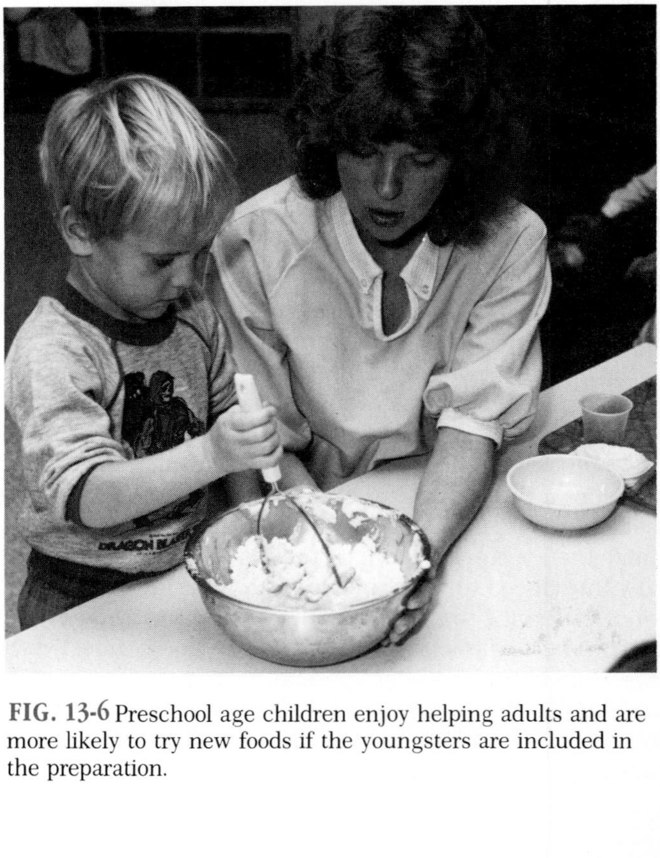

FIG. 13-6 Preschool age children enjoy helping adults and are more likely to try new foods if the youngsters are included in the preparation.

stressed. In this way there is a more accurate estimate of food intake at each meal. Usually by the end of the week, when they look at the food chart, parents are amazed at how much the child has consumed, even though at each meal the amount seemed minimum. In general, preschoolers consume only slightly more than toddlers, or about half of an adult's portion.

SLEEP AND ACTIVITY

Sleep patterns vary widely, but the average preschooler sleeps about 12 hours a night and infrequently takes daytime naps. Activity levels continue to be high, although quiet activities, such as television, are increasingly appealing and can become an unhealthy substitute for active play. Preschoolers' increased gross motor abilities and coordination provide them the opportunity to engage in many sports, if only at a novice level. Whether young children should begin formalized training in an activity at this early age is controversial. The consensus is to expose children to a wide variety of physical activities rather than concentrate on one area. However, children's interest in specific events should be respected, since early training can be advantageous.

Sleep Disturbances

The preschool years are a prime time for sleep disturbances. Young children sometimes have trouble going to sleep, especially after so much activity and stimulation during the day. Others may develop bedtime fears, wake during the night, or have nightmares. Still others may prolong the inevitable through elaborate rituals.

After a careful assessment of the events surrounding the problem, a recommended approach involves counseling parents about the importance of a consistent bedtime ritual and emphasizing the normalcy of this type of behavior in young children. Attention-seeking behavior should be ignored, and the child should not be taken into the parents' bed or allowed to stay up past a reasonable hour. If nightmares occur, the child should be comforted but left in his own bed. Sometimes the child's door must be locked in order to enforce the limits, although the safety of this procedure in case of a fire must always be considered. Other measures that may be helpful include keeping a light on in the room, providing transitional objects, such as a favorite toy, or leaving a drink of water by the bed.

Helping children slow down before bedtime also contributes to less resistance to going to bed. One approach is to establish limited rituals that signal readiness for bed, such as a bath or story. Parents can reinforce the pattern by stating, "After this story it is bedtime," and consistently carrying through the routine. If extra stimulation such as having visitors arrive at bedtime is disruptive to children's routine, it is advisable to settle children in bed beforehand.

DENTAL HEALTH

By the beginning of the preschool period, the eruption of the deciduous teeth is complete. Dental care is essential to preserve these temporary teeth and to teach good dental habits (see Chapter 12). Although preschoolers' fine motor control is improved, they still require assistance and supervision with brushing, and flossing should be done by parents. For children cared for away from home, parents are encouraged to monitor the dental care provided by others, including the diet to keep cariogenic foods to a minimum.

Injury Prevention

Because of improved gross and fine motor skill, coordination, and balance, preschoolers are less prone to falls than toddlers. They tend to be less reckless, listen more to parental rules, and are aware of potential danger, such as hot objects, sharp instruments, and dangerous heights. Putting objects in the mouth as part of exploration has all but ceased, although poisoning is still a danger. Pedestrian motor vehicle injuries increase from activities such as playing in the street, riding tricycles, running after balls, or forgetting safety regulations when crossing streets.

In general the guidelines suggested for injury prevention in Table 12-5 apply to children in this age-group as well. However, emphasis is now on *education* for safety and potential hazards, in addition to appropriate protection. Since preschoolers are great imitators, it is especially essential that parents set a good example by "practicing what they preach." Children are very quick to observe discrepancies in what they are told to do and what they see others do. Since they faithfully and unquestioningly believe in their parents' values and rules, this is an excellent opportunity for parents to practice and teach safe, cautious habits in daily living.

ANTICIPATORY GUIDANCE—CARE OF FAMILIES

Although the preschool years present fewer childrearing difficulties than earlier years, this stage of development is facilitated by appropriate anticipatory guidance in the areas already discussed. (See also the boxed material on p. 382.) There is a shift in childrearing practices from protection to education. While injury prevention previously focused on safeguarding the immediate environment with less emphasis on reasoning, now the protective guardrails or electrical outlet caps may be substituted with verbal explanations of why danger exists and how to avoid it with appropriate judgment and understanding.

During this period an emotional transition between parent and child is also occurring. Although children are still attached to their parents and accepting of all parental values and beliefs, they are nearing the period of life when they will question previous teachings and prefer

Parental Guidance during Preschool Years

Age (years)	Guidance
3	Prepare parents for child's increasing interest in widening relationships Encourage enrollment in nursery school Emphasize importance of setting limits Prepare parents to expect exaggerated tension-reduction behaviors, such as need for "security blanket" Encourage parents to offer child choices when child vacillates Expect marked changes at 3½ years when child becomes less coordinated (in motor and emotional control), becomes insecure, exhibits emotional extremes, and develops behaviors such as stuttering Prepare parents to expect extra demands on their attention as a reflection of child's emotional insecurity and fear of loss of love Warn parents that the equilibrium of the 3-year-old will change to the aggressive out-of-bounds behavior of the 4-year-old Anticipate a more stable appetite with more expansive food selection Stress needs for protection and education of child to prevent injury
4	Prepare for more aggressive behavior, including motor activity and shocking language Expect resistance to parental authority Explore parental feelings regarding child's behavior Suggest some kind of respite for primary caregiver such as placing child in nursery school for part of day Prepare for increasing sexual curiosity Emphasize importance of realistic limit-setting on behavior and appropriate discipline techniques Prepare parents for the highly imaginary 4-year-old who indulges in "tall tales" (to be differentiated from lies) and for child's acquisition of imaginary playmates Suggest swimming lessons if not begun earlier Explain Oedipus feelings and reactions Expect nightmares or an increase in them and suggest parents make certain the child is fully awakened from a frightening dream Provide reassurance that a period of calm begins at 5 years of age
5	Expect a tranquil period at 5 years Prepare and assist child through initial entrance into school environment Make certain immunizations are up-to-date before child enters school

the companionship of peers. Entry into school marks a separation from home for parents as well as for children. Parents need help in adjusting to this change, particularly if the mother has focused her daily activity primarily on home responsibilities. As preschoolers begin nursery or regular school, mothers may need to seek activities beyond the family, such as community involvement or pursuing a career. In this way all family members are adjusting to change, which is part of the process of growth and development.

SUMMARY

The preschool period is one of continued growth and refinement of developmental skills. Many of the physical, social, and cognitive changes constitute a transitional stage for readiness to enter school. In comparison to the toddler period it is a time of relative calm for parents, although concerns related to preschool or daycare experience, sex education, fears, and potential speech problems may arise.

The promotion of optimum health centers on providing good nutrition. The preschool years are an excellent time to encourage proper eating habits, introduce children to new foods, and gradually establish appropriate table manners. Since the primary teeth have completely erupted, continued dental care is essential. Although injuries are less of a risk toward the end of the preschool years, protection continues to be a priority. However, at this age children also need education in regard to safe practices.

KEY CONCEPTS

- The preschool years comprise the period from 3 to 5 years of age, a time that is considered critical for emotional and psychologic development.
- Biologic development in the preschool period is characterized by mature body systems and refinement in gross and fine motor behavior, as evidenced by participation in activities such as running, riding a bicycle, and drawing.
- According to Erikson, acquiring a sense of initiative is the chief psychosocial task of the preschooler. Development of the superego occurs during this period, and conscience begins to emerge.
- According to Piaget, the preschool age is characterized by intuitive or prelogical thinking and a move toward logical thought processes through advanced, complex learning, language, and understanding of causality.
- Social development includes further individuation-separation, more sophisticated language, greater independence, and more complex, imaginative forms of play.
- Areas of special concern to parents during the preschool period are preschool or daycare experience, sex education, fears, and speech problems.
- In selecting a daycare facility parents should inquire about daily programs, teacher qualifications, accreditation, student-to-staff ratio, safety, meals, fees, and sanitary conditions.
- Two rules that govern answering questions about sex and other sensitive issues are to find out what the child thinks and to be honest.

- Fears occur most commonly in the preschool period; examples are fear of the dark, being left alone (especially at bedtime), animals (particularly large dogs and snakes), ghosts, sexual matters (castration), and objects or persons associated with pain.
- Hesitancy or nonfluency in speech patterns is a normal characteristic of language development. Speech problems can occur when parents express excessive concern over this pattern.
- Health promotion centers on providing good nutrition, maintaining dental hygiene, and instituting appropriate safety measures to prevent injury.

STUDY QUESTIONS AND ACTIVITIES

1. Attend a child care center and observe the physical/cognitive abilities of children ages 3, 4, and 5 years. List the observed abilities of each age-group in the areas of gross motor, fine motor, and language skills and compare these with the norms presented in Table 13-1.
2. Interview the director of a daycare center and inquire about the center's policies for attending to sick children. Observe the sanitary practices of the staff, especially in regard to diapering.
3. Interview at least two families who have preschoolers. Inquire about the child's difficulties with fears, sleep, or speech and the parents' strategies in dealing with these issues.
4. Prepare two daily menus that meet the nutritional requirements and are appropriate for the preschooler's developmental skills for self-feeding.
5. Make a home visit to a family with a preschooler and assess the house for safety features and potentially dangerous areas. Identify areas of risk that require protection and those that are appropriate for education of the preschooler.

REFERENCES

Fish, L., and Burch, K.: Identifying gifted preschoolers, Pediatr. Nurs. **11**(2):125-127, 1985.

Shelly, J., and others: The spiritual needs of children, Downer's Grove, IL, 1982, Inter-Varsity Press.

Smith, D.: Common diseases children contract in day care: patterns and prevention, Pediatr. Nurs. **12**(3):175-179, 1986.

Zuckerman, D.M., and Zuckerman, B.S.: Television's impact on children, Pediatrics **75**(2):233-240, 1985.

BIBLIOGRAPHY

References specific to preschoolers are included here; additional references can be found in Chapters 10 and 12.

Growth and Development

Ames, L.B., and Ilg, F.I.: Your three-year-old: friend or enemy, New York, 1980, Delacorte Press.

Ames, L.B., and Ilg, F.I.: Your four-year-old: wild and wonderful, New York, 1981, Delacorte Press.

Ames, L.B., and Ilg, F.I.: Your five-year-old: sunny and serene, New York, 1981, Delacorte Press.

Betz, C.: Faith development in children, Pediatr. Nurs. **7**(2):22-25, 1981.

Dietz, W.H., Jr., and Gortmaker, S.L.: Do we fatten our children at the television set? Obesity and television viewing in children and adolescents, Pediatrics **75**(5):807-812, 1985.

Kay, P.: The imaginary companion: review of the literature, Matern. Child Nurs. J. **9**:8-11, 1980.

Lowrey, G.: Growth and development of children, ed. 8, Chicago, 1986, Year Book Medical Publishers.

Mitchell, S.: Imaginary companions: friend or foe? Pediatr. Nurs. **6**(6):29-30, 1980.

Murray, J.P.: Television & youth: 25 years of research & controversy, Boys Town, NE, 1980, The Boys Town Center for the Study of Youth Development.

Palumbo, F.M.: Television: effects on the development of children. In Children are different, Behavioral Development Monograph Series, No. 14, Columbus, OH, 1985, Ross Laboratories.

Rothenberg, M.B.: Role of television in shaping the attitudes of children, Child. Health Care **13**(4):148-149, 1985.

Sahler, O.J., and McAnarney, E.R.: The child from three to eighteen, St. Louis, 1981, The C.V. Mosby Co.

Schickendanz, J., and Schickendanz, D.: Toward understanding children, Boston, 1983, Little, Brown & Co., Inc.

Selekman, J.: The development of body image in the child: a learned response, Top. Clin. Nurs. **5**(1):12-21, 1983.

Shonkoff, J.P.: Preschool. In Levine, M.D., and others, editors: Developmental-behavioral pediatrics, Philadelphia, 1983, W.B. Saunders Co.

Thomas, R.M.: Comparing theories of child development, ed. 2, Belmont, CA, 1985, Wadsworth Publishing Co.

Preschool or Daycare Experience

American Academy of Pediatrics, Committee on Early Childhood, Adoption, and Dependent Care: The pediatrician's role in promoting the health of a patient in day care, Pediatrics **74**(1):157-158, 1984.

American Academy of Pediatrics, Committee on Psychosocial Aspects of Child and Family Health: The mother working outside the home, Pediatrics **73**(6):874-875, 1984.

Baker, J., and Proett, P.: One hospital's response: a child care referral service, Am. J. Nurs. **83**(4):550-551, 1983.

Ballard, P.: Selecting child care, Issues Compr. Pediatr. Nurs. **5**:219-231, 1981.

Birchfield, M.: Illnesses and children in a preschool center, Matern. Child Nurs. J. **15**(3):187-197, 1986.

Clore, E.: The working mother with young children, Child Care Newsletter **4**(1):4-6, 1985.

Seigel-Gorelick, B: The working parent's guide to child care, Boston, 1983, Little, Brown & Co., Inc.

Smith, D.: Myths about day care: fact or fantasy? Pediatr. Nurs. **10**(4):278-280, 1984.

Soderman, A., and Whiren, A.: Assessing quality day care: a checklist, Day Care Early Educ. **8**:9-12, 1980.

Summers, K.: Establishment of a hospital based children's sick room, Pediatr. Nurs. **14**(1):38-39, 1988.

Wilson, D., and Bess, C.: Establishing a community-based sick child center, Pediatr. Nurs. **12**(6):439-441, 1986.

Wong, D.: Guiding parents in selecting day-care centers, Pediatr. Nurs. **12**(3):181-187, 1986.

Sex Education

Aquilino, M.L.: Healthy sexual development in childhood, Child. Nurs. **4**(5):1-4, 1986.

Aquilino, M.L., and Ely, J.: Parents and the sexuality of preschool children, Pediatr. Nurs. **11**(1):41-46, 1985.

Bullough, V., and Bullough, B.: PNPs, patients, parents, and sexuality, Pediatr. Nurs. **8**(3):177-182, 1982.

Children's books on sex and siblings, Am. J. Nurs. **79**(11):1968, 1979.

Gallo, A.: Early childhood masturbation, Pediatr. Nurs. **5**(5):47-49, 1979.

Goldsmith, S.: Human sexuality: the family source book, St. Louis, 1986, The C.V. Mosby Co.

Malinowski, J.S.: Answering a child's questions about sex and a new baby, Am. J. Nurs. **79**(11):1965-1968, 1979.

Speech Problems

Biro, P., and Thompson, M.: Screening young children for communication disorders, MCN **9**(6):410-413, 1984.

Goldberg, R.: Identifying speech and language delays in children, Pediatr. Nurs. **15**(4):252-259, 1984.

Graham, J.M., Jr., Bashir, A.S., and Stark, R.E.: Communicative disorders. In Levine, M.D., and others, editors: Developmental-behavioral pediatrics, Philadelphia, 1983, W.B. Saunders Co.

Sleep/Fears

Edgil, A., Wood, K., and Smith, D.: Sleep problems of older infants and preschool children, Pediatr. Nurs. **11**(2):87-89, 1985.

Miller, S.R.: Children's fears: a review of the literature with implications for nursing research and practice, Nurs. Res. **28**(4):217-223, 1979.

Prescott-Day, S.: Sleep variations of the pre-school child, Health Visit. **52:**465-468, Nov. 1979.

Schumann, M.J.: A method for inducing sleep in young children, Pediatr. Nurs. **7**(5):9-13, 1981.

Siegel, F.: Eating and sleeping difficulties in young children, Consultant **22**(10):95-107, 1982.

Smith, D.: Sleep problems in children, Child Care Newsletter **5**(1):4-6, 1986.

CHAPTER 14

Health Problems of Early Childhood

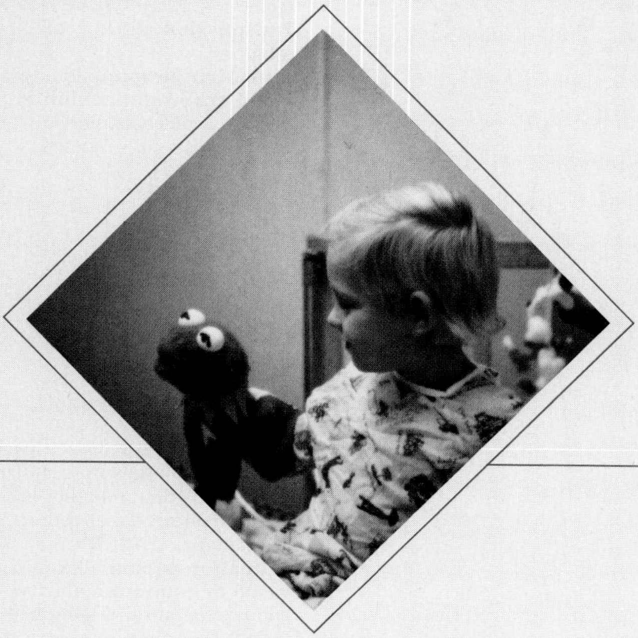

LEARNING OBJECTIVES

On completion of this chapter the reader will be able to:

- Describe the major characteristics of communicable diseases of childhood
- List three principles of nursing care of children with communicable disease
- Describe the nursing care of the child with conjunctivitis
- Outline a teaching plan designed to prevent transmission of intestinal parasites
- Identify the principles in the emergency treatment of poisoning
- Describe the nursing care of the child with lead poisoning
- State three factors thought to be associated with child abuse
- State four areas of the history that should arouse suspicion of abuse
- Describe the nursing care of the abused child

This chapter is concerned with health problems that occur most frequently during the early childhood years, such as poisoning and child abuse, and with diseases or illnesses that necessitate intervention, such as communicable disease or intestinal parasites. The influence of growth and development on each health problem is of special concern, since the cause or the treatment may be directly affected by the child's age. Optimum care includes knowledge of the pathologic, psychologic, developmental, and familial variables of the health problem in order to plan and provide individualized care to meet each child's particular needs.

Text continued on p. 392.

TABLE 14-1

Communicable Diseases of Childhood

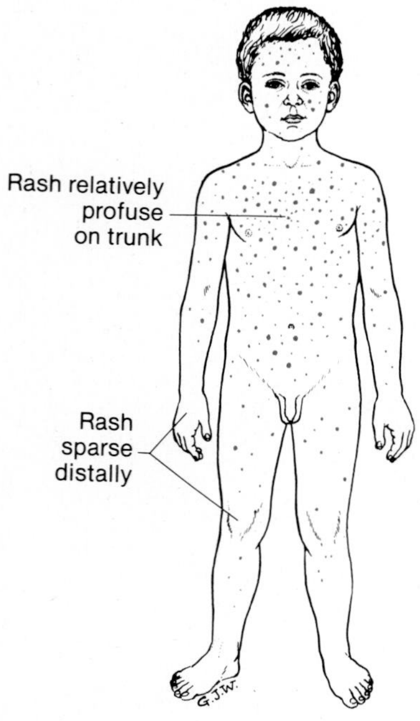

FIG. 14-1 Chickenpox.

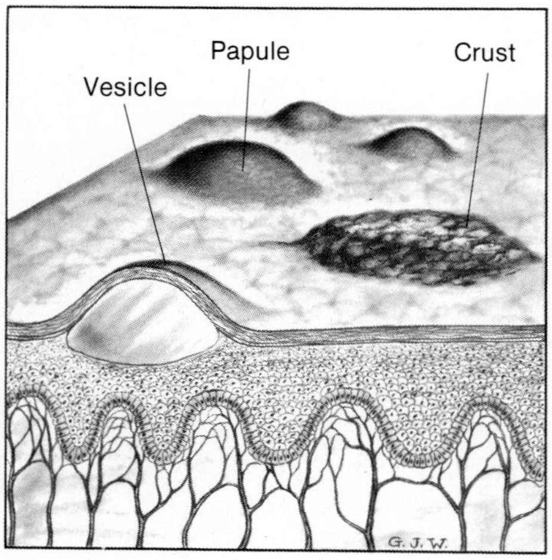

Disease

CHICKENPOX (Fig. 14-1)
Agent: varicella zoster
Source: primary secretions of respiratory tract of infected persons; to a lesser degree skin lesions (scabs not infectious)
Transmission: direct contact, droplet spread, and contaminated objects
Incubation period: 2 to 3 weeks, commonly 13 to 17 days
Period of communicability: probably 1 day before eruption of lesions (prodromal period) to 6 days after first crop of vesicles when crusts have formed

DIPHTHERIA
Agent: *Corynebacterium diphtheriae*
Source: discharges from mucous membranes of nose and nasopharynx, skin, and other lesions of infected person
Transmission: direct contact with infected person, a carrier, or contaminated articles
Incubation period: usually 2 to 5 days, possibly longer
Period of communicability: variable; until virulent bacilli are no longer present (identified by three negative cultures); usually 2 weeks but as long as 4 weeks

ERYTHEMA INFECTIOSUM (fifth disease)
Agent: parovirus
Source: infected persons
Transmission: paravirus direct contact by droplet infection
Incubation period: 6 to 14 days
Period of communicability: uncertain; most outbreaks subside in 1 to 2 months

EXANTHEMA SUBITUM (roseola)
Agent: probably virus
Source: unknown
Transmission: unknown (virtually limited to children between 6 months and 2 years of age)
Incubation period: unknown
Period of communicability: unknown

Clinical Manifestations	Therapeutic Management/Complications	Nursing Considerations
Prodromal stage: slight fever, malaise, and anorexia for first 24 hours; rash highly pruritic; begins as macule, rapidly progresses to papule and then vesicle (surrounded by erythematous base, becomes umbilicated and cloudy, breaks easily and forms crusts); all three stages (papule, vesicle, crust) present in varying degrees at one time (Fig. 14-1 and detail) **Distribution:** centripetal, spreading to face and proximal extremities but sparse on distal limbs **Constitutional signs and symptoms:** elevated temperature from lymphadenopathy, irritability from pruritus	**Specific:** none **Supportive:** Diphenhydramine hydrochloride or antihistamines to relieve itching; skin care to prevent secondary bacterial infection **Complications:** Secondary bacterial infections (abscesses, cellulitis, pneumonia, sepsis) Encephalitis Varicella pneumonia Hemorrhagic varicella (tiny hemorrhages in the vesicles and numerous petechiae in the skin) Reye syndrome (possibly related to aspirin)	Maintain *strict* isolation in hospital Isolate child in home until vesicles have dried (usually 1 week after onset of disease) and isolate high-risk children from infected children Administer skin care: give bath and change clothes and linens daily; administer topical application of calamine lotion; keep child's fingernails short and clean; apply mittens if child scratches Lessen pruritus; keep child occupied Remove loose crusts that rub and irritate skin Teach child to apply pressure to pruritic area rather than scratch it If older child, reason with him regarding danger of scar formation from scratching Avoid use of aspirin
Varies according to anatomic location of pseudomembrane **Nasal:** resembles common cold, serosanguineous mucopurulent nasal discharge without constitutional symptoms; may be frank epistaxis **Tonsillar/pharyngeal:** malaise; anorexia; sore throat; low-grade fever; pulse increased above expected for temperature within 24 hours; smooth, adherent, white or gray membrane; lymphadenitis possibly pronounced (bull's neck); in severe cases, toxemia, septic shock, and death within 6 to 10 days **Laryngeal:** fever, hoarseness, cough, with or without previous signs listed; potential airway obstruction, apprehensive, dyspneic retractions, cyanosis	Antitoxin (usually intravenously); preceded by skin or conjunctival test to rule out sensitivity to horse serum Antibiotics (pencillin or erythromycin) Complete bed rest (prevention of myocarditis) Tracheostomy for airway obstruction Treatment of infected contacts and carriers **Complications:** Myocarditis (second week) Neuritis	Maintain *strict* isolation in hospital Participate in sensitivity testing; have epinephrine available Administer antibiotics; observe for signs of sensitivity to penicillin Administer *complete* care to maintain bed rest Use suctioning as needed Regulate humidity for optimum liquefaction of secretions Observe respirations for signs of obstruction
Rash appears in three stages: *I*—erythema on face, chiefly on cheeks, "slapped face" appearance; disappears by 1 to 4 days *II*—about 1 day after rash appears on face, maculopapular red spots appear, symmetrically distributed on upper and lower extremities; rash progresses from proximal to distal surfaces and may last a week or more *III*—rash subsides but reappears if skin is irritated or traumatized (sun, heat, cold, friction)	None necessary **Complications:** Self-limited arthritis and arthralgia May be teratogenic to fetus if mother infected during pregnancy	Reassure parents regarding benign nature of condition in affected child Precautions for infected pregnant women not established
Persistent high fever for 3 to 4 days in child who appears well Precipitous drop in fever to normal with appearance of rash **Rash:** discrete rose-pink macules or maculopapules appearing first on trunk, then spreading to neck, face, and extremities; nonpruritic, fades on pressure, lasts 1 to 2 days **Associated signs and symptoms:** cervical/postauricular lymphadenopathy, injected pharynx, cough, coryza	None specific Antipyretics to control fever Anticonvulsives for child with history of febrile seizures **Complications:** Febrile seizures	Teach parents measures for lowering temperature (antipyretic drugs) If child is prone to seizures, discuss appropriate precautions Reassure parents regarding benign nature of illness

Continued.

TABLE 14-1

Communicable Diseases of Childhood—cont'd

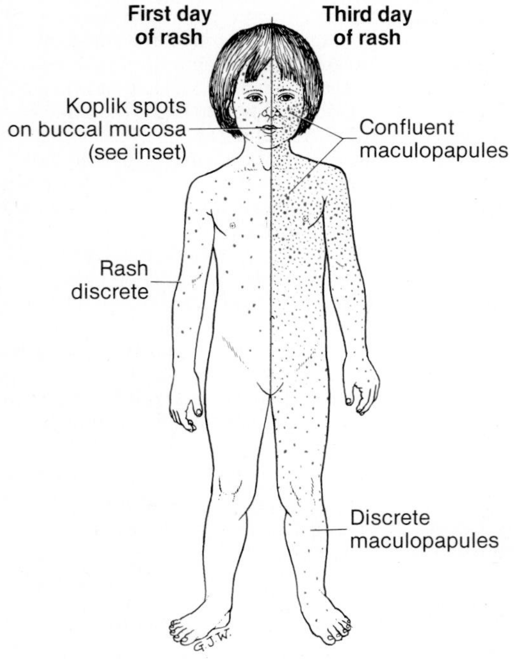

FIG. 14-2 Measles (rubeola).

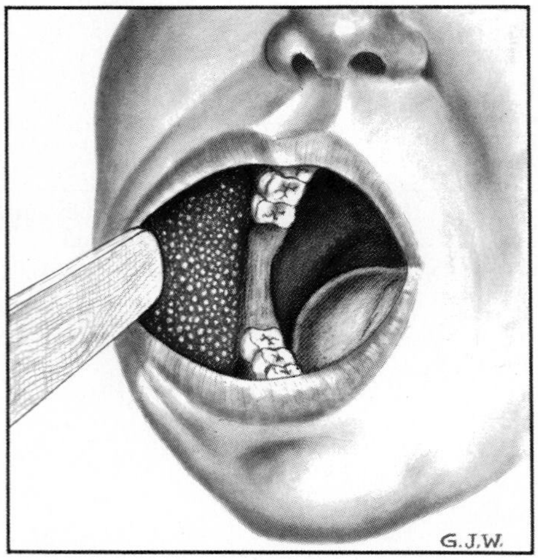

Koplik spots

Disease

MEASLES (rubeola) (Fig. 14-2)
Agent: virus
Source: respiratory tract secretions, blood, and urine of infected person
Transmission: usually by direct contact with droplets of infected person
Incubation period: 10 to 20 days
Period of communicability: from 4 days before to 5 days after rash appears but mainly during prodromal (catarrhal) stage

MUMPS
Agent: virus
Source: saliva of infected persons
Transmission: direct contact with or droplet spread from an infected person
Incubation period: 14 to 21 days
Period of communicability: most communicable immediately before and after swelling begins

PERTUSSIS (whooping cough)
Agent: *Bordetella pertussis*
Source: discharge from respiratory tract of infected persons
Transmission: direct contact or droplet spread from infected person; indirect contact with freshly contaminated articles
Incubation period: 5 to 21 days, usually 10
Period of communicability: greatest during catarrhal stage before onset of paroxysms and may extend to fourth week after onset of paroxysms

Clinical Manifestations	Therapeutic Management/Complications	Nursing Considerations
Prodromal (catarrhal) stage: fever and malaise, followed in 24 hours by coryza, cough, conjunctivitis, Koplik spots (small, irregular red spots with a minute, bluish white center first seen on the buccal mucosa opposite the molars [Fig. 14-2]) 2 days before rash; symptoms gradually increase in severity until second day after rash appears, when they begin to subside **Rash:** appears 3 to 4 days after onset of prodromal stage, begins as erythematous maculopapular eruption on face and gradually spreads downward; more severe in earlier sites (appears confluent) and less intense in later sites (appears discrete); after 3 to 4 days assumes brownish appearance, and fine desquamation occurs over areas of extensive involvement **Constitutional signs and symptoms:** anorexia, malaise, generalized lymphadenopathy	**Supportive:** bed rest during febrile period; antipyretics Antibiotics to prevent secondary bacterial infection in high-risk children **Complications:** Otitis media Pneumonia Bronchiolitis Obstructive laryngitis and laryngotracheitis Encephalitis	Isolation until fifth day of rash; if hospitalized, institute respiratory precautions Maintain bed rest during prodromal stage; provide quiet activity **Fever:** instruct parents to administer antipyretics; avoid chilling; if child is prone to seizures, institute appropriate precautions (fever spikes to 40° C [104° F] between fourth and fifth days) **Eye care:** dim lights if photophobia present; clean eyelids with warm saline solution to remove secretions or crusts; keep child from rubbing his eyes; examine cornea for signs of ulceration **Coryza/cough:** use cool mist vaporizer; protect skin around nares with layer of petrolatum; encourage fluids and soft bland foods **Skin care:** keep skin clean; use tepid baths as necessary
Prodromal stage: fever, headache, malaise, and anorexia for 24 hours, followed by "earache" that is aggravated by chewing **Parotitis:** by third day, parotid gland(s) (either unilateral or bilateral) enlarges and reaches maximum size in 1 to 3 days; accompanied by pain and tenderness **Other manifestations:** submaxillary and sublingual infection, orchitis, and meningoencephalitis	**Symptomatic and supportive:** analgesics for pain and antipyretics for fever Intravenous fluid may be necessary for child who refuses to drink or vomits because of meningoencephalitis **Complications:** Sensorineural deafness Postinfectious encephalitis Myocarditis Arthritis Hepatitis Epididymo-orchitis Sterility (extremely rare in adult males)	Isolation during period of communicability; institute respiratory precautions during hospitalization Maintain bed rest during prodromal phase until swelling subsides Give analgesics for pain; if child is unwilling to chew medication, use elixir form Encourage fluids and soft, bland foods; avoid foods requiring chewing Apply hot or cold compresses to neck, whichever is more comforting To relieve orchitis, provide warmth and local support by means of tight-fitting underpants (stretch bathing suit works well)
Catarrhal stage: begins with symptoms of upper respiratory infection, such as coryza, sneezing, lacrimation, cough, and low-grade fever; symptoms continue for 1 to 2 weeks, when dry, hacking cough becomes more severe **Paroxysmal stage:** cough that most commonly occurs at night consists of a series of short, rapid coughs followed by a sudden inspiration that is associated with a high-pitched crowing sound or "whoop"; during paroxysms cheeks become flushed or cyanotic, eyes bulge, and tongue protrudes; paroxysm may continue until a thick mucous plug is dislodged; vomiting frequently follows an attack; stage generally lasts 4 to 6 weeks, followed by convalescent stage	Antimicrobial therapy (such as erythromycin) Administration of pertussis-immune globulin **Supportive treatment:** hospitalization required for infants, children who are dehydrated, or those who have complications Bed rest Increased oxygen intake and humidity Adequate fluids Intubation possibly necessary **Complications:** Pneumonia (usual cause of death) Atelectasis Otitis media Convulsions Hemorrhage (subarachnoid, subconjunctival, epistaxis) Weight loss and dehydration Hernia Prolapsed rectum	Isolation during catarrhal stage; if hospitalized, institute respiratory precautions Maintain bed rest as long as fever is present Keep child occupied during the day (interest in play is associated with fewer paroxysms) Reassure parents during frightening episodes of whooping cough Provide restful environment and reduce factors that promote paroxysms (dust, smoke, sudden change in temperature, chilling, activity, excitement); keep room well ventilated Encourage fluids; offer small amount of fluids frequently; refeed child after vomiting Keep child in Croupette with high humidity; suction gently but often to prevent choking on secretions Observe for signs of airway obstruction (increased restlessness, apprehension, retractions, cyanosis) Involve public health nurse if child is cared for at home

Continued.

TABLE 14-1

Communicable Diseases of Childhood—cont'd

Disease

POLIOMYELITIS

Agent: enteroviruses, 3 types; type 1—most frequent cause of paralysis, both epidemic and endemic, type 2—least frequently associated with paralysis, type 3—second most frequent in association with paralysis

Source: feces and oropharyngeal secretions of infected persons, especially young children

Transmission: direct contact with persons with apparent or inapparent active infection; spread is via fecal-oral and pharyngeal-oropharyngeal routes

Incubation period: usually 7 to 14 days, with range of 5 to 35 days

Period of communicability: not exactly known; virus is present in throat and feces shortly after infection and persists for about 1 week in throat and 4 to 6 weeks in feces

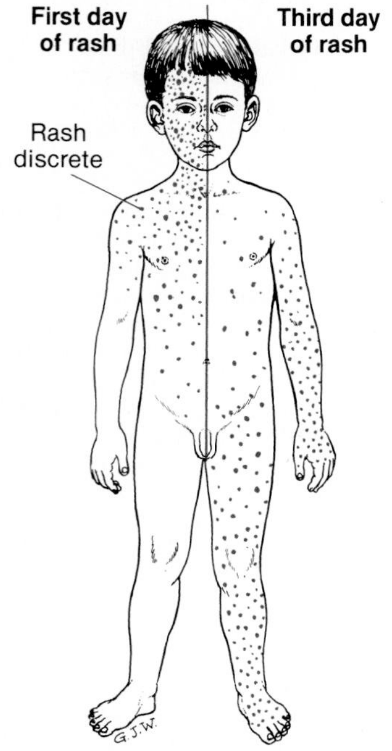

FIG. 14-3 Rubella (German measles).

RUBELLA (German measles) (Fig. 14-3)

Agent: virus

Source: primarily nasopharyngeal secretions of persons with apparent or inapparent infection; virus also present in blood, stool, and urine

Transmission: direct contact and spread via infected person; indirectly via articles freshly contaminated with nasopharyngeal secretions, feces, or urine

Incubation period: 14 to 21 days

Period of communicability: 7 days before to about 5 days after appearance of rash

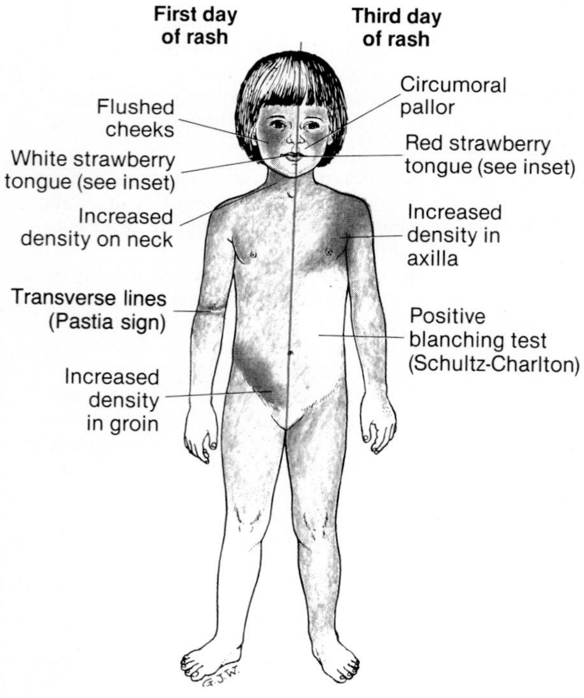

FIG. 14-4 Scarlet fever.

SCARLET FEVER (Fig. 14-4)

Agent: group A β-hemolytic streptococci

Source: usually from nasopharyngeal secretions of infected persons and carriers

Transmission: direct contact with infected person or droplet spread; indirectly by contact with contaminated articles, ingestion of contaminated milk or other food

Incubation period: 2 to 4 days, with range of 1 to 7 days

Period of communicability: during incubation period and clinical illness approximately 10 days; during first 2 weeks of carrier phase, although may persist for months

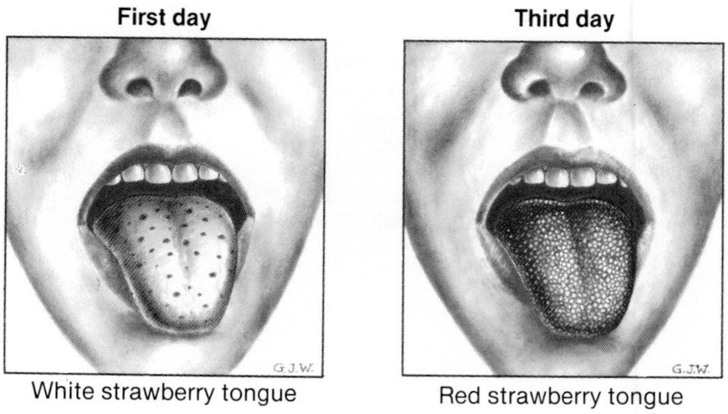

Clinical Manifestations	Therapeutic Management/Complications	Nursing Considerations
May be manifest in three different forms: **Abortive or inapparent**—fever, uneasiness, sore throat, headache, anorexia, vomiting, abdominal pain; lasts a few hours to a few days **Nonparalytic**—same manifestations as abortive but more severe, with pain and stiffness in neck, back, and legs **Paralytic**—initial course similar to nonparalytic type, followed by recovery and then signs of central nervous system paralysis	No specific treatment, including antimicrobials or gamma globulin Complete bed rest during acute phase Assisted respiratory ventilation in case of respiratory paralysis Physical therapy for muscles following acute stage **Complications:** Permanent paralysis Respiratory arrest Hypertension Kidney stones from demineralization of bone during prolonged immobility	Maintain complete bed rest Administer mild sedatives as necessary to relieve anxiety and promote rest Participate in physiotherapy procedures (use of moist hot packs and range of motion exercises) Position child to maintain body alignment and prevent contractures or decubiti; use footboard Encourage child to move; administer analgesics for maximum comfort during physical activity Observe for respiratory paralysis (difficulty in talking, ineffective cough, inability to hold breath, shallow and rapid respirations); report such signs and symptoms to physician; have tracheostomy tray at bedside
Prodromal stage: absent in children, present in adults and adolescents; consists of low-grade fever, headache, malaise, anorexia, mild conjunctivitis, coryza, sore throat, cough, and lymphadenopathy; lasts for 1 to 5 days, subsides 1 day after appearance of rash **Rash:** first appears on face and rapidly spreads downward to neck, arms, trunk, and legs; by end of first day body is covered with a discrete, pinkish red maculopapular exanthema; disappears in same order as it began and is usually gone by third day **Constitutional signs and symptoms:** occasionally low-grade fever, headache, malaise, and lymphadenopathy	No treatment necessary other than antipyretics for low-grade fever and analgesics for discomfort **Complications:** Rare (arthritis, encephalitis, or purpura); most benign of all childhood communicable diseases; greatest danger is teratogenic effect on fetus	Reassure parents of benign nature of illness Employ comfort measures as necessary Isolate child from pregnant women
Prodromal stage: abrupt high fever, pulse increased out of proportion to fever, vomiting, headache, chills, malaise, abdominal pain **Enanthema:** tonsils enlarged, edematous, reddened, and covered with patches of exudate; in severe cases appearance resembles membrane seen in diphtheria; pharynx is edematous and beefy red; during first 1 or 2 days tongue is coated and papillae become red and swollen (white strawberry tongue [Fig. 14-4]); by the fourth or fifth day white coat sloughs off, leaving prominent papillae (red strawberry tongue [Fig. 14-4]); palate is covered with erythematous punctate lesions **Exanthema:** rash appears within 12 hours after prodromal signs; red pinhead-sized punctate lesions rapidly become generalized but are absent on the face, which becomes flushed; rash is more intense in folds of joints; by end of the first week desquamation begins, which may be complete by 3 weeks or longer	Treatment of choice is a full course of penicillin (or erythromycin in penicillin-sensitive children); fever should subside 24 hours after beginning therapy Antibiotic therapy for newly diagnosed carriers (nose or throat cultures positive for streptococci) **Supportive measures:** bed rest during febrile phase, analgesics for sore throat **Complications:** Otitis media Peritonsillar abscess Sinusitis Rheumatic fever Glomerulonephritis	Institute respiratory precautions until 24 hours after initiation of treatment Ensure compliance with oral antibiotic therapy (intramuscular benzathine penicillin G [Bicillin] may be given if parents' reliability in giving oral drugs is questionable) Maintain bed rest during febrile phase; provide quiet activity during convalescent period Relieve discomfort of sore throat with analgesics, gargles, lozenges, antiseptic throat sprays (Chloraseptic), and inhalation of cool mist Encourage fluids during febrile phase; avoid irritating liquids (citrus juices) or rough foods; when child is able to eat, begin with soft diet Advise parents to consult physician if fever persists after beginning therapy Discuss procedures for preventing spread of infection

◆ *Disorders Related to Infectious Processes*

Young children are especially susceptible to infectious disease, and a number of disorders occur predominantly during these early years. At this age their resistance to infectious agents may still be low, but their exposure to such agents is beginning to increase as a result of social involvement outside the home. These disorders include the typical childhood communicable diseases, conjunctivitis, and intestinal parasitic infestations. Other common infectious diseases, such as otitis media, are discussed in those chapters devoted to specific biologic system disorders.

COMMUNICABLE DISEASES

The incidence of childhood communicable diseases has declined tremendously since the advent of immunizations. Serious complications resulting from such infections have been further reduced with the use of antibiotics and antitoxins. However, infectious diseases do occur, and nurses must be familiar with the infectious agent in order to recognize the disease and institute appropriate preventive and supportive interventions.

Nursing Considerations

The more common communicable diseases of childhood, their therapeutic management, and specific nursing care are described in Table 14-1. The following is a general discussion of nursing considerations for communicable diseases. Since most of the diseases are associated with skin manifestations, the reader is also referred to Chapter 29 for a discussion of nursing care in dermatologic conditions.

ASSESSMENT

Identification of the infectious agent is of primary importance in order to prevent exposure to susceptible individuals. Nurses in ambulatory care settings, such as emergency rooms, health maintenance centers, nursery or regular schools, and physicians' offices, are often the first persons to see signs of a communicable disease, such as a rash or sore throat. The nurse must operate under a high index of suspicion for common childhood diseases in order to identify potentially infectious cases and to recognize diseases that require medical intervention. An illustrative example is the common complaint of sore throat. Although most often a symptom of a minor viral infection, it can signal diphtheria or a streptococcal infection, such as scarlet fever. Each of these bacterial conditions requires appropriate medical treatment to prevent serious sequelae.

Assessment of the following is helpful in identifying potentially communicable diseases: (1) recent exposure to a known case, (2) prodromal symptoms or evidence of constitutional symptoms, such as a fever or rash (see Table 14-1), (3) immunization history, and (4) history of having the disease. Since immunizations are available for several of the diseases and in almost each case an attack confers life-long immunity, the possibility of many infectious agents can be eliminated based on these two criteria.

NURSING DIAGNOSES

A number of nursing diagnoses are prominent in the nursing care of the child with a communicable disease and others specific to individual cases become evident. The most common nursing diagnoses are presented in the Nursing Care Plan on pp. 393 to 394.

PLANNING

The principal nursing goals in addition to identification of the communicable disease (discussed under Assessment) are to:

1. Prevent spread of infection to others
2. Prevent complications
3. Provide comfort measures
4. Support the child and family

IMPLEMENTATION

Many of the diseases require only supportive measures until the illness runs its course. Children are usually cared for at home until the disease is no longer communicable and until they feel well enough to resume normal activity.

Prevent spread. Prevention consists of two components: prevention of the disease and control of spread of the disease to others. Primary prevention rests almost exclusively on immunization. (The nurse's role in immunization of children is discussed in Chapter 10.)

Control measures to prevent spread of the disease include appropriate techniques to reduce risk of cross-transmission of infectious organisms between patients and to protect health care workers from organisms harbored by patients. If the child is hospitalized, the institution's policies for isolation precautions are instigated (see p. 644). The most important procedure to stress is handwashing. Persons directly caring for the child or handling contaminated articles must wash their hands before beginning care of another patient. The child should be instructed to practice good handwashing technique after toileting and before eating. For those diseases spread by droplets, the nurse instructs parents in measures aimed at reducing airborne transmission. If the child is old enough, he should use a tissue to cover his face during coughing or sneezing; otherwise the parent should cover the child's mouth with a tissue and then discard it. The usual hygiene measures of not sharing eating and drinking utensils should be stressed to the family.

Prevent complications. While most youngsters recover without any difficulty, there are groups of children who

NURSING CARE PLAN

The Child with Communicable Disease

Nursing Goals	Nursing Interventions	Expected Patient/Family Outcomes
HP-HMP* Potential for infection	**Risk factors: susceptible host, infectious agents**	
Assist in identifying etiologic agent	Recognize exanthema associated with communicable diseases Operate under a high index of suspicion for children who are susceptible to infectious diseases Identify high-risk children to whom communicable disease may be fatal; in case of an outbreak, advise parents to confine child to the home Assist in performing tests used to identify the organism, such as collection of specimens for culture Be aware of significance of test results in terms of the etiologic agent and child's level of immunity	†Disease is recognized early and appropriate interventions implemented
Prevent occurrence of the disease	Participate in public education regarding prophylactic immunizations and method of spread of communicable diseases Participate in immunization programs or screening programs to identify streptococcal infections	†Disease is prevented
Prevent spread of the disease	Institute appropriate isolation procedures Make referral to public health nurse when necessary to ensure appropriate isolation procedures in the home Work with families to ensure compliance with therapeutic regimens Identify close contacts who may require prophylactic treatment (specific immune globulin or antibiotics) Report disease to local health department	Infection remains confined to original source
Prevent complications	Ensure compliance with therapeutic regimen (bed rest, antibiotics, adequate hydration) Institute seizure precautions if febrile convulsions are a possibility Monitor temperature; unexpected elevations may signal an infection Attend to good body hygiene Ensure adequate hydration with small frequent sips of water or favorite drinks and soft, bland foods (gelatin, pudding, ice cream, soups); feed again after vomiting; observe for signs of hydration	Child exhibits no evidence of complications such as infection or dehydration
N-MP Potential impaired skin integrity	**Risk factors: child's propensity to scratch**	
Prevent child from scratching the skin	Keep nails short and clean Apply mittens or elbow restraints Dress in lightweight, loose, and nonirritating clothing Cover affected areas (long sleeves, pants) Bath in cool water with no soap or apply cool compresses Apply soothing lotions Avoid exposure to heat or sun	Skin remains intact

*For an explanation of abbreviations, see p. 20.
†Nursing outcome.

Continued.

NURSING CARE PLAN

The Child with Communicable Disease—cont'd

Nursing Goals	Nursing Interventions	Expected Patient/Family Outcomes
NDx CPP Impaired social interaction **Etiology: isolation**		
Prepare child for isolation if hospitalized	Explain reason for confinement and use of any special precautions Allow child to play with gloves, mask, and gown	Child demonstrates understanding of isolation
Promote social interaction	Always introduce yourself to child and allow him to see your face before donning protective clothing Provide diversionary activity Encourage parents to remain with child during hospitalization Help child view isolation as challenging rather than solely negative experience Encourage contact with friends via telephone (in hospital can use intercom between room and nurse's station)	Child engages in suitable activities and interactions
NDx CPP Pain **Etiology: skin lesions, malaise**		
Relieve discomfort	Keep mucous membranes moist with use of cool-mist vaporizer, gargles, and lozenges Apply petrolatum to chapped lips or nares Cleanse eyes with physiologic saline solution Keep skin clean (change bedclothes and linens at least daily) Administer oral hygiene Assess need for pain or antipyretic medication Employ nonpharmacologic pain reduction techniques, such as distraction through quiet play (see also p. 598)	Skin and mucous membranes are clean and free of irritants Child exhibits minimum evidence of discomfort (specify)
NDx RRP Altered family processes **Etiology: situational crisis (child with an acute illness)**		
Provide emotional support	Reinforce family's effort to carry out plan of care Provide assistance when necessary, such as visiting nurse to help with home care Keep family aware of child's progress; stress rapidity of recovery in most cases Prepare child's peers for altered physical appearance, such as with chickenpox	Family continues to comply with expectations Peers accept child
Nursing interventions related to medical management		
Relieve discomfort Administer analgesics, antipyretics, and antipruritic medication for maximum relief of discomfort		

are at risk for serious, even fatal, complications from communicable diseases, especially those of viral etiology. Such children include those who are undergoing steroid or other immunosuppressive therapy, those who have a generalized malignancy, such as leukemia or lymphoma, or those who have an immunologic disorder. The nurse immediately refers children who have signs of a communicable disease to a physician. School nurses who are aware of such susceptible children have the responsibility of warning their parents of recent outbreaks of a communicable disease in order to prevent their exposure to known cases. In most instances the child is kept out of school until the outbreak is over. At the present time chickenpox is the most frequent disease requiring isolation of high-risk children.

Provide comfort. Many of the communicable diseases cause skin manifestations that are bothersome to the child. The chief discomfort from most of the rashes is itching, and measures such as cool baths (usually without soap) and lotions, such as calamine, are helpful. When lotions are used, they should be applied sparingly, especially over open lesions where percutaneous absorption of any active ingredients (such as diphenhydramine in Caladryl) is enhanced. To avoid overheating, which increases itching, children should wear lightweight, loose, nonirritating clothing and keep out of the sun. If the child persists in scratching, the nails are kept short and smooth; mittens and clothes with long sleeves or legs may be needed. For severe itching, antipruritic medication, such as diphenhydramine (Benadryl) or hydroxyzine (Atarax), may be required, especially when the child desires to sleep.

An elevated temperature is common, and both antipyretic medication, preferably acetaminophen, and environmental manipulation are implemented (see p. 642). Aspirin is not given if chickenpox is present because of its association with Reye syndrome. A sore throat, another frequent symptom, is managed with lozenges, saline rinses (if the child is old enough to cooperate), and analgesics. Since most children are anorectic during an illness, bland foods and increased liquids are usually preferred. During the early stages of the disease children voluntarily curtail their activity, and while bed rest is beneficial, it should not be imposed. During periods of irritability, quiet activity (e.g., reading, music, television, puzzles, and coloring) helps distract children from the discomfort.

Support the child and family. While most communicable diseases are benign, they produce a considerable degree of concern and anxiety for some parents. Often, the occurrence of a disease, such as chickenpox, is the first time the child is acutely uncomfortable. Parents need assistance to cope effectively with manifestations of the illness, such as intense itching. Sometimes, a visiting nurse may be beneficial to help the family develop a plan of care and encourage compliance with any treatments.

The family and child need reassurance that recovery from the disease is generally rapid. However, visible signs of the dermatosis may be present for some time after the child is well enough to resume usual activities. When the disease involves noticeable signs, such as the crusts of chickenpox, the child benefits from preparation before returning to school. For example, the parent can discuss the child's physical appearance with the teacher and/or school nurse and request that they explain the child's condition to classmates.

EVALUATION

The effectiveness of nursing interventions is determined by continual reassessment and evaluation of care based on the following observational guidelines and expected outcomes:

1. Observe or inquire about family members' use of control measures; observe for signs of disease in household contacts
2. Monitor vital signs, especially temperature; inquire regarding the identification of high-risk contacts and appropriate isolation of the contact; observe or inquire regarding compliance with antibiotic therapy
3. Inquire regarding effectiveness of comfort measures
4. Interview family and child regarding their feelings and concerns, especially upon child's return to school

Expected outcomes:
See Nursing Care Plan, pp. 393 to 394.

CONJUNCTIVITIS

Acute conjunctivitis, inflammation of the conjunctiva, is a common condition in children. It occurs from a variety of causes that are typically age related. In infants recurrent conjunctivitis may be a sign of nasolacrimal duct obstruction. In children the usual causes are viral, bacterial, allergic, or related to a foreign body. Bacterial infection, especially *Haemophilus influenzae,* accounts for most instances of acute conjunctivitis in children. Diagnosis is made primarily from the clinical manifestations (see box), although cultures of purulent drainage may be needed to identify the specific infecting agent.

Therapeutic Management

Treatment of conjunctivitis depends on the cause. Viral conjunctivitis is self-limiting and treatment should be limited to removal of the accumulated secretions and avoidance of topical antibiotics or steroids. Bacterial con-

Clinical Manifestations of Conjunctivitis

Bacterial Conjunctivitis ("pink eye")
Purulent drainage
Crusting of eyelids, especially upon awakening
Inflamed conjunctiva
Swollen lids
Usually both eyes infected

Viral Conjunctivitis
General:
Usually occurs with upper respiratory infection
Serous (watery) drainage
Inflamed conjunctiva
Swollen lids

Hemorrhagic:
Caused by specific virus, enterovirus 70
Severe inflammation
Subconjunctival hemorrhage
Photophobia

Allergic Conjunctivitis
Itching
Watery to viscous stringy discharge
Inflamed conjunctiva
Swollen lids

Conjunctivitis Caused by Foreign Body
Tearing
Pain
Inflamed conjunctiva
Usually only one eye affected

junctivitis is usually treated with topical antibacterial agents. Drops may be used during the day and an ointment at bedtime because the ointment preparation remains in the eye longer. Ointments are usually not used in the daytime because they blur vision.

Nursing Considerations

Nursing goals primarily include keeping the eye clean and properly administering the ophthalmic medication. Accumulated secretions are always removed by wiping from the inner canthus downward and outward, away from the opposite eye. Warm moist compresses, such as a clean washcloth wrung out with hot tap water, are helpful in removing the crusts. Compresses are *not* kept on the eye because an occlusive covering promotes bacterial growth. Medication should be instilled immediately after the eyes have been cleaned and according to correct procedure (see Chapter 21).

Prevention of infection in other family members is an important consideration with bacterial conjunctivitis. The child's washcloth and towel are kept separate from those used by others. Tissues used to clean the eye are disposed of properly. The child should refrain from rubbing his eye and is instructed in good handwashing. As with any infection, thorough handwashing by all those individuals in contact with the child is essential.

INTESTINAL PARASITIC DISEASES

Intestinal parasitic diseases, including helminths (worms) and protozoa, constitute the most frequent infections in the world. In the United States the incidence of intestinal parasitic disease, especially giardiasis, has increased among young children who are attending daycare centers.

Intestinal parasitic diseases in man are caused by a number of infecting organisms. This discussion is limited to the two most common parasitic infections among children in the United States—giardiasis and pinworms. Table 14-2 describes the outstanding features of other helminths that belong to the family of nematodes.

TABLE 14-2

Common Intestinal Parasites

Parasites/Clinical Manifestations	Comments
Ascariasis—*Ascaris lumbricoides* (common roundworm) Light infections: asymptomatic Heavy infections: anorexia, irritability, nervousness, enlarged abdomen, weight loss, fever, intestinal colic Severe infections: intestinal obstruction, appendicitis, perforation of intestine with peritonitis, obstructive jaundice, lung involvement—pneumonitis	Transferred to mouth by way of contaminated food, fingers, or toys Largest of the intestinal helminths Affects principally young children 1-4 years of age Prevalent in warm climates
Hookworm Disease—*Necator americanus* Light infections in well-nourished individuals: no problems Heavier infections: mild to severe anemia malnutrition May be itching and burning ("ground itch") followed by erythema and a papular eruption in areas to which the organism migrates	Transmitted by discharging eggs on the soil and in turn picked up infection from direct skin contact with contaminated soil Wearing shoes is recommended, although children playing in contaminated soil expose many skin surfaces
Strongyloidiasis—*Strongyloides stercoralis* (threadworm) Light infection: asymptomatic Heavy infection: respiratory signs and symptoms, abdominal pain, distention, nausea and vomiting, diarrhea—large, pale stools, often with mucus Threat to life in children with weakened immunologic defenses	Transmission is same as for hookworm except autoinfection common Older children and adults affected more often than young children Severe infections may lead to severe nutritional deficiency
Visceral Larva Migrans—*Toxocara canis* (dogs) **Intestinal Toxocariasis—*Toxocara cati* (cats)** Depends on reactivity of infected individual May be asymptomatic except for eosinophilia Specific diagnosis difficult	Transmitted by direct contamination of hands from contact with dog, cat, or objects or ingestion of soil Dogs and cats should be kept away from areas where children play; sandboxes especially important transmission areas Periodic deworming of diagnosed dogs and cats Control of dog population Continued education and laws to prevent indiscriminate canine defecation
Trichuriasis—*Trichuris trichura* (whipworm) Light infections: asymptomatic Heavy infections: abdominal pain and distention, diarrhea	Transmitted from contaminated soil, vegetables, toys, and other objects Most frequent in warm, moist climates Occurs most often in undernourished children living in unsanitary conditions

Nursing Considerations

Nursing responsibilities related to intestinal parasitic diseases are (1) identification of the parasite, (2) compliance with treatment of the infection, and (3) prevention of initial infection or reinfection. Identification of the organism is accomplished by laboratory examination of substances containing the worm, its larvae, or ova. Most are identified by examining feces smears from the stools of persons suspected of harboring the parasite. Stool specimens should be large enough to obtain an ample sampling, not merely a fecal fragment. Specimens are easily obtained from diapers, although the stool should not be contaminated with urine. For toilet-trained children, a simple procedure for collecting a specimen is described in the nursing tip (see box). Fresh specimens are best for revealing parasites or larvae; therefore collected specimens should be taken directly to the laboratory for examination. If this is not feasible, the specimen is placed in a container with a preservative.

> ***Nursing Tip: Stool Specimen***
>
> To obtain a stool specimen for identification of ova and parasites, place plastic wrap over the toilet bowl to collect the stool. Use a tongue depressor or disposable spoon or knife to collect the stool and place the specimen in a covered cup or plastic bag.

In most parasitic infections, examination of other family members, especially children, may be carried out to identify those who are similarly affected. Nurses are frequently the persons who assume the responsibility for directing and instructing the families in the collection and disposition of specimens. Parents need clear written instructions on obtaining an adequate sample and the number of samples required.

Once the diagnosis is confirmed and an appropriate treatment regimen is planned, parents need further explanation and reinforcement. Compliance in terms of drug therapy and any other measures, such as thorough handwashing, are essential for eradication of the parasite. The family needs to understand the nature of transmission and that in some cases the medication must be repeated in 2 weeks to 1 month to kill organisms hatched since initial treatment.

The nurse's most important function in relation to parasites is preventive education of children and families regarding good hygiene and health habits. Thorough handwashing before eating or handling food and after using the toilet is the most important precautionary method. Other preventive practices are listed in the box on p. 398.

GIARDIASIS

Giardiasis is caused by the protozoan *Giardia lamblia* (also called *G. intestinalis, G. duodenalis,* and *Lamblia intestinalis*). It is the most common intestinal parasitic pathogen in the United States, and its prevalence among children in daycare centers may range from 9% to 38% and even higher in some areas.

Chief modes of transmission are person-to-person; water (especially mountain lakes, streams, and pools frequented by diapered infants); food; and animals, especially puppies. In children, person-to-person transmission is the most likely cause. The potential for transmission is great since the cysts, the nonmotile stage of the protozoa, can survive in the environment for months.

Diagnostic Evaluation

Although individuals infected with giardiasis may be asymptomatic, young children, especially infants, usually manifest symptoms at any early stage (see box). Unlike most other intestinal parasites, *G. lamblia* is not easily diagnosed from stool specimens. Since *Giardia* organisms are excreted in a highly variable pattern, six or more stool specimens collected over several weeks may be necessary to identify the trophozoites (active parasites) or cysts. Other tests that appear promising for rapid and accurate diagnosis involve detecting *Giardia* antigen in the stool by counterimmunoelectrophoresis (CIE) or enzyme-linked immunosorbent assay (ELISA).

Therapeutic Management

The drugs available for treatment of giardiasis are quinacrine, furazolidone, and metronidazole. The drug of choice is furazolidone, unless cost is a factor, in which

> ***Clinical Manifestations of Giardiasis***
>
> Infants and young children
> - Diarrhea
> - Vomiting
> - Anorexia
> - Failure to thrive
>
> Children over 5 years of age
> - Abdominal cramps
> - Intermittent loose stools
> - Constipation
> - Stools may be:
>   - malodorous
>   - watery
>   - pale
>   - greasy
>
> Most infections resolve spontaneously in 4 to 6 weeks
>
> Rarely, chronic form occurs
> - Intermittent loose, foul-smelling stools
> - Possibility of:
>   - abdominal bloating
>   - flatulence
>   - sulfur-tasting belches
>   - epigastric pain
>   - vomiting
>   - headache
>   - weight loss

quinacrine is substituted. Quinacrine is less than one tenth the cost of furazolidone, and its long-term safety is established over the use of metronidazole. Unfortunately, quinacrine has the highest frequency of side effects, especially nausea and vomiting, causes temporary yellow staining of the skin, sclera, and urine, and has a very bitter taste (see Nursing tip).

Nursing Tip: Quinicrine

To decrease the side effects of quinicrine and increase its palatability:
- Administer the drug with or after meals
- Crush tablets and mix with a strong flavoring, such as jam or syrup

Nursing Considerations

The most important nursing consideration is prevention of giardiasis, especially among children and staff of daycare centers. Attention to meticulous sanitary practices, especially during diaper changes, is essential (see box and Fig. 14-5). Nurses can play an important role in educating daycare staff regarding appropriate sanitation practices.

Once children are infected, compliance with the treatment is essential. Parents often need suggestions for encouraging the child to take quinacrine (see Nursing tip).

Guidelines for Preventing Intestinal Parasitic Disease

Always wash hands and fingernails with soap and water before eating and handling food and after toileting.
Avoid placing fingers in mouth and biting nails.
Discourage children from scratching bare anal area.
Change diapers as soon as soiled and dispose of in plastic bags in closed receptable out of children's reach.
Disinfect toilet seats and diaper changing areas; use dilute household bleach (10% solution) or Lysol and wipe clean with paper towels.
Drink water that is specially treated, especially if camping.
Wash all raw fruits and vegetables or food that has fallen on the floor.
Avoid growing foods in soil fertilized with human excreta.
Teach children to defecate only in a toilet, not on the ground.
Keep dogs and cats away from playgrounds or sandboxes.
Avoid swimming in pools frequented by diapered children.
Wear shoes outside.

If other household members are infected, the nurse should inquire about any pregnant members, since treatment for giardiasis is contraindicated during pregnancy.

ENTEROBIASIS (PINWORMS)

Enterobiasis, or pinworms, caused by the nematode *Enterobius vermicularis,* is the most common helminthic

A

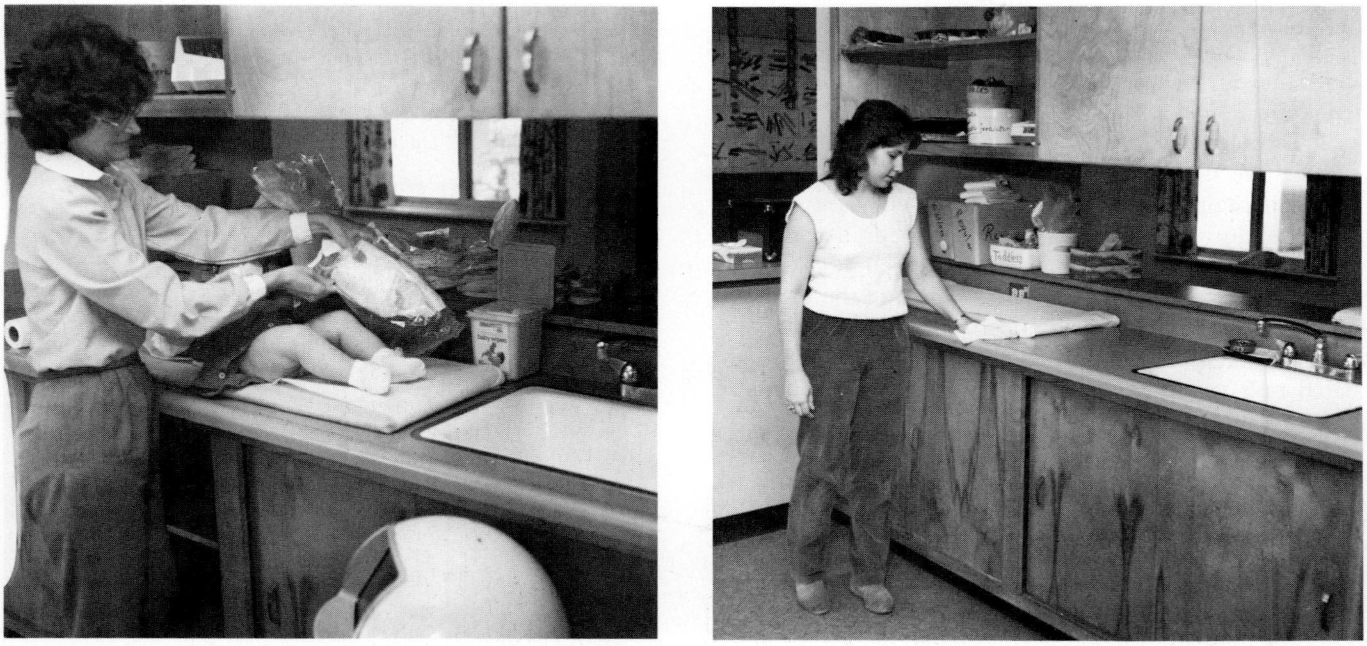

B

FIG. 14-5 Prevention of giardiasis, especially in daycare centers, requires sanitary practices during diaper changes such as **A,** wrapping diapers in plastic bags and discarding in a covered receptacle, **B,** cleaning diaper changing surfaces, and **C,** handwashing after diaper changing.

infection in the United States. It is universally present in temperate climatic zones and may infect 20% of all children at any one time. Crowded conditions, such as in classrooms and daycare centers, favor transmission.

Infection begins when the eggs are ingested or inhaled. The movement of the worms on skin and mucous membrane surfaces causes intense itching. As the child scratches, eggs are deposited on the hands and under the fingernails. The typical hand-to-mouth activity of youngsters makes them especially prone to continual reinfection. Pinworm eggs also persist in the home to contaminate anything they contact, such as toilet seats, doorknobs, bed linen, underwear, and food. Since they float in the air, they are also easily inhaled.

Clinical Manifestations of Pinworms

- Intense perianal itching (principal symptom)
  - Evidence of itching in young children includes:
    - General irritability
    - Restlessness
    - Poor sleep
    - Bed-wetting
    - Distractibility
    - Short attention span
- Perianal dermatitis and excoriation secondary to itching
- If worms migrate, possible vaginal and urethral infection

Diagnostic Evaluation

Except for the intense rectal itching associated with pinworms, the clinical manifestations (see box) are nonspecific. Diagnosis is most commonly made from the tape test (see discussion under Nursing considerations). Repeated tests to collect eggs may be necessary, and if there is a question that other family members may be infected, a tape test should be performed.

Therapeutic Management

The drugs available for treatment of pinworms include mebendazole, pyrantel pamoate, piperazine citrate, and pyrvinium pamoate. The drug of choice is mebendazole, which is safe, effective, convenient, and has few side effects. However, it is not recommended for children under 2 years of age or for pregnant women. If pyrvinium pamoate is prescribed, parents should be advised that the drug stains stool and vomitus bright red, as well as clothing or skin that comes in contact with the drug. Since pinworms are easily transmitted, all household members are treated. The drugs may be repeated in 2 weeks to prevent reinfection.

C

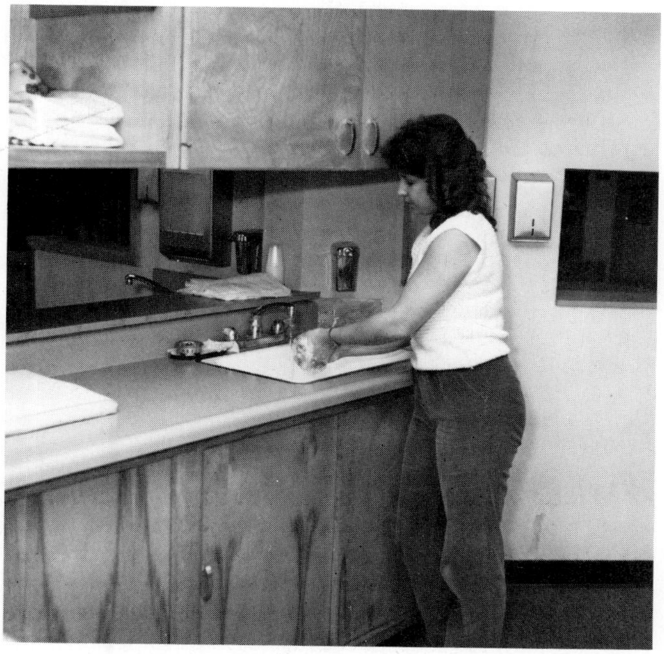

Nursing Considerations

Nursing care is directed at identifying the parasite, eradicating the organism, and preventing reinfection. Parents need clear, detailed instructions for the tape test. A loop of transparent (not "frosted" or "magic") tape, sticky side out, is placed around the end of a tongue depressor, which is then firmly pressed against the child's perianal area. A convenient commercially prepared tape is also available for this purpose. Pinworm specimens are collected in the morning as soon as the child awakens and *before* the child has a bowel movement or bathes. The procedure may need to be repeated more than once before eggs are collected. Parents are instructed to place the tongue blade in a glass jar or loosely in a plastic bag so that it can be brought in for microscopic examination. For specimens collected in the hospital, physician's office, or clinic, the tape is placed smoothly on a glass slide, sticky side down, for examination.

Compliance with the drug regime is usually excellent because the duration of treatment is typically only one dose. However, the family is reminded of the need to take a second dose in 2 weeks, if prescribed. Posting a reminder on the refrigerator door or bathroom mirror is helpful.

To prevent reinfection, certain cleaning practices, such as washing all clothes and bed linen in hot water and vacuuming the house, may be recommended. However, there is little documentation on their effectiveness, since pinworms survive on so many surfaces. Suggestions that are helpful include handwashing after toileting and before eating, keeping the child's fingernails short to minimize the chance of ova collecting under the nails, and daily showering.

◆ *Ingestion of Injurious Agents*

Children are prone to place their hands and any attractive object or substance into their mouths. Infants and young children, who explore items with their mouths, are especially at risk for ingesting toxic agents. In addition, some children practice pica, which may predispose them to certain types of poisoning, such as lead poisoning. A key nursing responsibility is education of parents regarding these common hazards to prevent their occurrence.

PICA

Pica is the Latin word for magpie, a bird of gluttonous and indiscriminate appetite. The use of the term today refers to the habitual, purposeful, and compulsive ingestion of nonfood substances, such as clay, dirt, paint chips, laundry, starch, or paper. Individuals who practice pica usually have a craving for a few particular items, which are largely determined by their availability.

In most instances pica is relatively harmless unless the substance ingested contains a harmful substance, such as lead, or the practice interferes with the ingestion of more nutritious substances. If pica persists, it should be evaluated. Certainly, if pica involves a potentially harmful substance, it should be removed from the environment or the child should be denied access to it.

POISONING

Since the passage of the Poison Prevention Packaging Act of 1970, which provides that certain potentially hazardous drugs and household products be sold in child-resistant containers, the incidence of poisonings in children has decreased dramatically. However, despite these advances, poisoning remains a significant health concern, with nearly two thirds of the cases occurring in children under 6 years of age. Children are poisoned by a variety of substances. Although the reported incidence of ingested substances varies, the most frequently ingested poisons are cleaning substances, analgesics (especially acetaminophen), plants (see box), cosmetics, cough and cold preparations, and hydrocarbons (Litovitz, Martin, and Schmitz, 1987). Over 90% of poisonings occur in the home, although a significant number take place elsewhere, such as in a grandparent's or friend's home, in a school, or in a health care facility. Most poisonings occur between 5:00 and 9:00 p.m.

The developmental characteristics of young children predispose them to poisoning by ingestion. Infants and toddlers explore their environment through oral experimentation. Since the sense of taste is less discriminatory at this age, many unpalatable substances are ingested. In addition, toddlers and preschoolers are developing autonomy and initiative, which increase their curiosity and exploration. Imitation is also a powerful motivator, especially when combined with lack of awareness of danger.

Poisonous and Nonpoisonous Plants

Poisonous Plants	Toxic Parts	Nonpoisonous Plants
Apple	Leaves, seeds	African violet
Apricot	Leaves, stem, seed pits	Aluminum plant
Azalea	Foliage and flowers	Asparagus fern
Buttercup	All parts	Begonia
Cherry (wild or cultivated)	Twigs, seeds, foliage	Boston fern
Chrysanthemum	All parts	Christmas cactus
Daffodil	Bulbs	Coleus
Dumb cane, Dieffenbachia	All parts	Gardenia
Elephant ear	All parts	Grape ivy
English ivy	All parts	Jade plant
Foxglove	Leaves, seeds, flowers	Piggyback begonia
Holly, mistletoe	Berries	Piggyback plant
Honeysuckle	All parts	Poinsettia*
Hyacinth	Bulbs	Prayer plant
Ivy	Leaves	Rubber tree
Mistletoe	Berries	Snake plant
Oak tree	Acorn, foliage	Spider plant
Philodendron	All parts	Swedish ivy
Plum	Pit	Wax plant
Poison ivy, poison oak	Leaves, fruit, stems, smoke from burning plants	Weeping fig
Pothos	All parts	Zebra plant
Rhubarb	Leaves	
Tulip	Bulbs	
Water hemlock	All parts	
Wisteria	Seeds, pods	
Yew	All parts	

*Mildly toxic if ingested in massive quantities.

This section is primarily concerned with the immediate emergency treatment of ingestion of injurious agents. Specific management of corrosive, hydrocarbon, acetaminophen, salicylate, plant, and iron poisoning are summarized in Table 14-3. Because of the importance of lead poisoning among young children, ingestion of lead is discussed separately. Appropriate suggestions for poison prevention are discussed on p. 403 and in Chapter 12.

Principles of Emergency Treatment

A poisoning may or may not require emergency intervention, but in most instances medical evaluation is necessary to initate appropriate action. Parents are advised to call the Poison Control Center (PCC) *before* initiating any intervention. The local PCC telephone number (usually listed in the front of the telephone directory; see also box on p. 403) should be posted near each phone in the house.

Based on the initial telephone assessment, the PCC counsels the parents to begin treatment at home and/or

TABLE 14-3

Selected Poisonings in Children

Poison	Clinical Manifestations	Comments/Treatment
Corrosives (strong acids or alkali) Drain, toilet or oven cleaners Electric dishwasher detergent Mildew remover Batteries Clinitest tablets Denture cleaners	Severe burning pain in mouth, throat and stomach White, swollen mucous membranes, edema of lips, tongue, and pharynx (respiratory obstruction) Violent vomiting (hemoptysis) Drooling and inability to clear secretions Signs of shock Anxiety and agitation	Household bleach is a frequently ingested corrosive but rarely causes serious damage Liquid preparations cause more damage than granular preparations **Treatment:** Inducing emesis is contraindicated (vomiting redamages the mucosa) Dilute corrosive with water, not milk (coats membranes, making assessment difficult) Provide patent airway, if needed Administer analgesics Keep NPO or place on clear liquid diet Esophageal stricture may require repeated dilations and/or surgery
Hydrocarbons Gasoline Kerosene Lamp oil Mineral seal oil (found in furniture polish) Lighter fluid Turpentine Paint thinner and remover (some types)	Gagging, choking, and coughing Nausea Vomiting Alterations in sensorium, such as lethargy Weakness Respiratory symptoms of pulmonary involvement Tachypnea Cyanosis Retractions Grunting	Immediate danger is aspiration (even small amounts can cause bronchitis and chemical pneumonia) Gasoline, kerosene, lighter fluid, mineral seal oil, and turpentine cause severe pneumonia **Treatment** (controversial): Inducing emesis is generally contraindicated Gastric lavage may be used Symptomatic treatment of chemical pneumonia includes high humidity, oxygen, hydration, and antibiotics for secondary infection
Acetaminophen	Occurs in 4 stages: 1. Initial period (2 to 4 hours after ingestion) Nausea Vomiting Sweating Pallor 2. Latent period (24 to 36 hours) Patient improves 3. Hepatic involvement (may last up to 7 days) Pain in right upper quadrant Jaundice Confusion Stupor Coagulation abnormalities 4. Patients who do not die in hepatic stage gradually recover	Most common drug poisoning in children Occurs from acute ingestion, not chronic overdose Toxic dose is uncertain **Treatment:** Emesis, lavage Antidote N-acetylcysteine is given, usually by nasogastric tube because of the antidote's offensive odor (smells like rotten eggs)
Aspirin	Acute poisoning Nausea Disorientation Vomiting Dehydration Diaphoresis Hyperpnea Hyperpyrexia Oliguria Tinnitus Coma Convulsions Chronic poisoning Same as above but subtle onset (often confused with illness being treated) Dehydration, coma, and seizures may be more severe Bleeding tendencies	May be caused by acute ingestion (severe toxicity occurs with 300 to 500 mg/kg [4 to 7 gr/kg]) May be caused by chronic ingestion (i.e., more than 100 mg/kg/day for 2 or more days); can be more serious than acute ingestion **Treatment:** Home use of ipecac for moderate toxicity Hospitalization for severe toxicity Emesis, lavage, activated charcoal, and/or cathartic Sodium bicarbonate transfusions to correct metabolic acidosis External cooling for hyperprexia Diazepam for seizures Oxygen and ventilation for respiratory depression Vitamin K for bleeding Dialysis for severest toxicity

Continued.

TABLE 14-3

Selected Poisonings in Children—cont'd

Poison	Clinical Manifestations	Comments/Treatment
Plants (see box, p. 400)	Depends on type of plant ingested May cause local irritation of oropharynx and entire gastrointestinal tract May cause respiratory, renal, and central nervous system symptoms Topical contact with plants can cause dermatitis	Some of most frequently ingested substances Rarely cause serious problems, although some plant ingestions can be fatal **Treatment:** Remove plant parts (emesis) Supportive care as needed
Iron (mineral supplement or vitamin containing iron)	Occurs in 5 stages 1. Initial period (1/2 to 6 hours after ingestion) Vomiting Hematemesis Diarrhea Hematochezia (bloody stools) Gastric pain 2. Latency (2 to 12 hours) patient improves 3. Systemic toxicity (4 to 24 hours after ingestion) Metabolic acidosis Fever Hyperglycemia Bleeding Shock Death (may occur) 4. Hepatic injury (48 to 96 hours) Seizures Coma 5. Rarely pyloric stenosis develops at 2 to 5 weeks	Factors related to frequency of iron poisoning include Widespread availability Packaging of large quantities in individual containers Lack of parental awareness of iron toxicity Resemblance of iron tablets to candy (i.e., M & Ms) **Treatment:** Emesis or lavage Chelation therapy with deferoxamine in severe intoxication

to take the child to an emergency facility. When a call is taken, the name and telephone number of the caller are recorded to reestablish contact if the connection is interrupted. Since the majority of poisonings are managed in the home, expert advice is essential in minimizing adverse effects. When the exact quantity or type of ingested toxin is not known, admission to a hospital for laboratory evaluation and surveillance for effects of the toxin (see Table 14-3) are critical during the postingestion period.

General guidelines for the emergency home treatment for poisoning are listed in the box, p. 403; selected interventions, especially those that require professional intervention, are discussed below.

Assessment. Assessment involves identifying that a poisoning has occurred and monitoring the child's condition. Identifying the poison may include searching for evidence of the ingested substance, such as an open bottle, and collecting vomitus, blood, urine, or stool samples for laboratory analysis.

Assessment must also focus on the child's physical status. Vital signs are taken and respiratory and/or circulatory support instituted as needed. The victim's condition is routinely reevaluated. The increased recovery rate from acute poisonings is largely attributable to vigorous use of supportive measures after symptoms appear. Since shock is a complication of several types of household poisons, particularly corrosives, measures to reduce the effects of shock, such as slight elevation of legs and head to promote venous drainage and provision of warmth and rest, are important. Maintenance of respiratory function may require mouth-to-mouth resuscitation or insertion of an airway and/or mechanical ventilation.

The emergency room nurse's responsibility is to be prepared for immediate intervention with any of the necessary equipment. Since time and speed are critical factors in recovery from serious poisonings, anticipation of potential problems and complications may mean the difference between life and death.

Removal of the poison. To prevent further absorption of the poison, immediate steps are taken to terminate further exposure. These steps are outlined in the Emergency treatment box. The following discussion is concerned primarily with gastric decontamination.

In general, the immediate treatment is to remove the ingested poison by inducing vomiting. The preferred method for use at home is to administer ipecac syrup, an emetic that exerts its action by direct stimulation of the vomiting center and an irritant effect on the gastric mucosa. The use of an emetic is generally contraindicated in conditions that increase the risk of aspiration and when

Nursing Guidelines for Poison Prevention

Assess possible contributing factors in occurrence of injury, such as discipline, parent-child relationship, developmental ability, environmental factors, and behavior problems
Institute anticipatory guidance for possible future injuries based on child's age and maturational level
Refer to visiting nurse agency to evaluate home environment and need for safe-proofing measures
Provide assistance with environmental manipulation when necessary, such as lead removal
Educate parents regarding safe storage of toxic substances (see Child Safety Home Inventory, p. 304)
Advise parents to take drugs out of sight of children
Advise parents to replace *immediately* all toxic substances to safe storage
Teach children the hazards of ingesting nonfood items without supervision
Advise parents against using plants for teas or medicine
Discuss problems of discipline and children's noncompliance and offer strategies for effective discipline (see p. 64)
Instruct parents regarding correct administration of drugs for therapeutic purposes and to discontinue drug if there is evidence of mild toxicity
Have syrup of ipecac available—two doses for each child in the family
Encourage grandparents or other frequent caregivers to keep syrup of ipecac in the home
Post number of local poison control center* with emergency phone list at the telephone

*Call 1-800-555-1212 to obtain number of poison control center for any state.

emesis of the poison, such as corrosives, redamages the mucosa of the esophagus and pharynx.

Proper administration of ipecac is essential (see Emergency treatment). Ipecac is available in 1-ounce (30 ml) vials. However, the label information does not include directions for a second dose. Therefore parents need clear instructions for proper use and dose. As a precaution, parents are advised to have one full dose of ipecac for *each child* in the home, to carry the emetic when traveling, and to be certain that other caregivers (baby-sitters or relatives) have the emetic available. Because children share activities, it is not uncommon for more than one child to ingest the toxic substance. In an emergency ipecac can be obtained from an all-night pharmacy, convenience store, emergency squad, or emergency department. It is inexpensive and has a shelf life of up to 16 years (Grbcich and others, 1986).

If the child is admitted to an emergency facility, gastric lavage may also be performed to empty the stomach of the toxic agent. Lavage is indicated in the following instances: young infants for whom ipecac may be contraindicated; the patient is comatose, convulsing, or requires a protected airway; or the ingested poison is one that is rapidly absorbed (strychnine or cyanide). The use of lavage in petroleum distillate poisoning is controversial because of the danger of aspiration. When lavage is performed, the largest diameter tube that can be inserted is used to facilitate passage of gastric contents.

Another method of decontaminating the stomach is the use of activated charcoal, an odorless, tasteless, fine black powder that adsorbs many compounds, creating a stable complex. It is used within 1 hour of the poisoning but *after* giving an emetic. If the charcoal is given before the emetic, it adsorbs the emetic, preventing its pharmacologic effect. It is mixed with water or saline cathartic to form a slurry. Slurries are neither gritty nor distasteful but look like black mud and are not well accepted by children (see Nursing tip, p. 404). Sorbitol, an artificial sweetener, has been used successfully as a flavoring in slurries and also acts as a cathartic. Cathartics, such as sodium or magnesium, may be administered to stimulate

EMERGENCY TREATMENT

Poisoning

1. Assess the Victim:
(a) take vital signs; re-evaluate routinely
(b) initiate cardiorespiratory support if needed
(c) treat other symptoms, such as seizures

2. Terminate Exposure:
(a) empty mouth of pills, plant parts, or other material
(b) flush thoroughly eyes and/or skin with tap water if involved
(c) remove contaminated clothing (e.g., if gasoline has spilled)
(d) bring victim of an inhalation poisoning into fresh air
(e) give water to dilute ingested poison

3. Identify the Poison:
(a) question the victim and witnesses
(b) save all evidence of poison (empty bottle, opened container, vomitus, urine)
(c) be alert to signs/symptoms of potential poisoning in absence of other evidence (see Table 14-3)
(d) call Poison Control Center or other competent emergency facility for immediate advice regarding treatment

4. Remove Poison/Prevent Absorption:
(a) induce vomiting; administer ipecac, if ordered
—9 to 12 months: 10 ml; do not repeat
—1 to 12 years: 15 ml; repeat dosage once if vomiting has not occurred within 30 minutes
—over 12 years: 30 ml; repeat dosage once if vomiting has not occurred within 30 minutes
—may administer with water or milk
(b) do not induce vomiting if:
—victim is comatose, in severe shock, or convulsing, or has lost the gag reflex
—poison is a low-viscosity hydrocarbon (mineral seal, oil) or a strong corrosive (acid or alkali)
(c) place child in side-lying, sitting, or kneeling position with head below chest to prevent aspiration
(d) administer activated charcoal (15 to 30 gm for children under 12 years and 50 to 100 g for those over 12) 30 to 60 minutes *after* inducing vomiting with ipecac, if ordered

EMERGENCY TREATMENT

> ### *Nursing Tip: Activated Charcoal*
>
> To increase the child's acceptance of activated charcoal, mix it with flavoring or a sweetener and serve through a straw and in an opaque glass with a cover, such as a disposable coffee cup and lid or an ordinary cup covered with aluminum foil or placed inside a small paper bag.

evacuation of the bowel, thus decreasing systemic absorption of the poison and aiding in removal of charcoal.

In a minority of poisonings specific antidotes are available to counteract the poison. They are highly effective and should be available in all emergency facilities. The supply of antidotes should be checked routinely and replaced as used or according to expiration dates. Among the more commonly employed antidotes are Å-acetylcysteine for acetaminophen poisoning, oxygen for carbon monoxide inhalation, naloxone for narcotic overdose, and antivenin for certain poisonous bites.

Family support. A poisoning is more than a physical emergency for the child. It usually represents an emotional crisis for the parents, particularly in terms of guilt, self-reproach, and insecurity in the parenting role. The emergency room is no place to admonish the parents for negligence, lack of appropriate supervision, or failure to safe-proof the home. Rather it is a time to calm and support the child and parents, while unaccusingly exploring the circumstances of the injury. If the nurse prematurely attempts to discuss ways of preventing such a poisoning from recurring, the parents' anxiety will block out any suggestions or offered guidance. Therefore it is preferable for the nurse to delay the discussion until the child's condition is stabilized or, if the child is discharged immediately after emergency treatment, to make a public health referral.

Prevention of recurrence. The ultimate objective is to prevent poisonings from occurring or recurring. One effective counseling method is first to discuss the difficulties of constantly watching and safeguarding young children. In this way the monumental task of raising children can lead to a discussion of injury prevention as one part of the parental role. This approach also incorporates other contributory causes for the incident, such as inadequate support systems, marital discord, discipline techniques (especially use of physical punishment), and maternal distress (Bithoney and others, 1985). A visit to the home, especially after a repeat poisoning situation, is recommended as part of the follow-up care to assess hazards, including family factors, and to evaluate appropriate safe-proofing measures. One method of identifying risk areas is to ask specific questions or to have the parent complete a questionnaire designed to isolate factors that predispose children to poisoning. Another suggestion is to encourage parents to get down to the child's eye level and survey the environment for potential hazards.

Passive measures (those that do not require active participation) have been the most successful in preventing poisoning and include child-resistant closures and limited number of tablets in one container, such as bottles of baby aspirin. However, these measures alone are not sufficient to prevent poisoning since the majority of toxic agents in the home do not have safety closures. Therefore, active measures (those that require participation) are essential. Nursing guidelines for preventing the occurrence or recurrence of a poisoning are listed in the box on p. 403.

HEAVY METAL POISONING

Heavy metal poisoning can occur from the ingestion of a variety of substances, the most common being lead. Other sources are iron from medicinal supplement preparations and mercury, most often found in excessive quantities in seafood harvested from polluted waters. Another source of mercury poisoning is the elemental form found in thermometers. Elemental mercury is nontoxic when ingested but poisonous when inhaled (vapor is produced when mercury is heated).

Heavy metals have an affinity for certain essential tissue chemicals, which must remain free for adequate cell functioning. When metals are bound to these substances, cellular enzyme systems are inactivated. Treatment involves removing the metal from the body with a chelating agent, a chemical compound that combines with the metal for rapid and safe excretion.

LEAD POISONING

Lead poisoning (plumbism) is a prevalent pediatric problem. An estimated 4%, or approximately 780,000, American preschool children have excessive amounts of lead in their blood. Black children have a six times greater prevalence than white children (Committee on Environmental Hazards, 1987). The peak age is from 2 to 3 years, and most poisoning occurs in warm weather months.

Factors Related to Lead Ingestion

Several factors influence the ingestion of lead-containing substances, and successful long-term cure and prevention of lead poisoning involves change in all the variables.

Environmental characteristics. The first contributing factor is the availability of lead in the environment. Lead enters the system either by ingestion or inhalation; the accompanying box lists potential sources of lead. Lead-based paint from dilapidated housing (especially buildings constructed before the 1950s) remains the most frequent high-dose source of lead. A chip of paint only 1 cm square in surface area may contain a thousand times the usual safe daily ingestion of lead. In addition to paint chips, another major source is small lead particles created from deleading procedures, such as sanding painted surfaces.

Other sources of lead often are related to isolated oc-

Potential Sources of Lead

Ingested
- *Lead-based paint
  - Interior: walls, window sills, floors, furniture
  - Exterior: door frames, fences, porches, siding
- Plaster, caulking
- Unglazed pottery
- Colored newsprint
- Painted food wrappers
- Cigarette butts and ashes
- Water from leaded pipes
- Foods or liquids from cans soldered with lead
- Household dust
- Soil, especially along heavily trafficked roadways
- Food grown in contaminated soil
- Urban playgrounds
- Folk remedies
- Pewter vessels or dishes
- Hobby materials, e.g., leaded paint or solder for stained glass windows

Inhaled
- *Sanding and scraping of lead-based painted surfaces
- Burning of leaded objects
  - Automobile batteries
  - Newspaper logs of colored paper
- Automobile exhaust
- Cigarette smoke
- Sniffing leaded gasoline
- Dust
  - Poorly cleaned urban housing
- Contaminated clothing and skin of household members working in smelting factories or working as urban policemen

*Most common sources.

cupations, such as lead smelter workers or urban policemen, or practices, including folk remedies that contain lead (Mexican *azarcon* or *greta* and Oriental *paylooah*—fine powders that are fed to young children as a cure for fever or rash). While these sources are much less frequent, they need to be considered when lead paint is not the cause.

Characteristics of the child. Developmentally young children are at risk for lead poisoning because of their high level of oral activity. Particularly during late infancy and toddlerhood, children explore their environment by putting objects in their mouth. This normal hand-to-mouth activity contributes to the amount of lead they ingest in dust and dirt. By virtue of their size, young children inhale air that is closer to the ground, which may be more heavily contaminated with lead, such as in areas near heavily travelled roadways. In addition, the child who ingests lead often practices *pica* (see p. 400).

Some children are more at risk than others because of nutritional deficiencies of iron, calcium, and zinc that result in increased gastrointestinal absorption of lead. Iron deficiency, even in the absence of anemia, appears to be the single most important predisposing factor for increased absorption of lead (Committee on Environmental Hazards, 1987).

Lead poisoning is not confined to the young child who ingests the substance. It can also occur in older children who habitually sniff leaded gasoline. The nurse must be aware of children experimenting with drugs or other psychotropic substances and the possibility of gasoline sniffing, which is especially prevalent among Native American children on reservations (Coulehan and others, 1983).

Parental characteristics. Parent-child interaction is another significant variable in the ingestion of lead. Children with lead poisoning generally receive less adequate child care than children without plumbism, including poor hygienic practices, insufficient feeding to promote adequate nutrition, infrequent use of medical facilities, and insufficient rest. Parents use few resources to stimulate the child, tend to be less affectionate, and have an immature attitude toward maintaining discipline. These findings are not related to differences in income, educational level, age of parents, or number of household occupants—factors commonly felt to be associated with lead poisoning (Hunt, Hepner, and Seaton, 1982).

Pathophysiology

Normally, lead is excreted very slowly via the kidneys, alimentary tract, and, to a small extent, sweat. Retained lead is stored chiefly in the bone, where it is inert. However, under conditions of chronic ingestion excess lead is deposited in the tissues and circulatory system with about 90% attached to the erythrocytes. Even when the chronic ingestion stops, it takes the body twice as long to excrete the stored lead as it did to accumulate it. As a result, several body systems continue to be affected after the environmental removal of the poison (Fig. 14-6).

Hematologic system. Lead is extremely toxic to the biosynthesis of heme, preventing the formation of hemoglobin and causing its precursors, especially erythrocyte protoporphyrin (EP), coproporphyrin, and δ-aminolevulinic acid (ALA), to increase in the body. EP is elevated in the blood when the blood-lead concentration is only minimally increased and is a sensitive, but not specific, indicator of abnormal lead levels. The latter two intermediary metabolites are excreted in the urine in excessive amounts. Reduction of the heme molecule in the red blood cell results in anemia, one of the initial, but reversible, signs of the disease.

Renal system. Lead damages the cells of the proximal tubules, resulting in abnormal excretion of glucose, protein, amino acids, and phosphate. With adequate treatment kidney damage is usually reversible.

Central nervous system. The most serious and irreversible side effects of lead intoxication are on the nervous system. Initially there is an increase in membrane permeability, with a shift of fluid into the interstitial spaces of the brain. As a result, increased intracranial pressure causes cortical atrophy and lead encephalopathy—convulsions, mental retardation, paralysis, blindness, and ultimately coma and death. Lead encephalopathy is almost always associated with a blood-lead concentration greater than 100 μg/dl.

However, before lead encephalopathy occurs, irreversible behavioral changes indicate lead toxicity (see clinical manifestations box, p. 407). Manifestations of behavioral

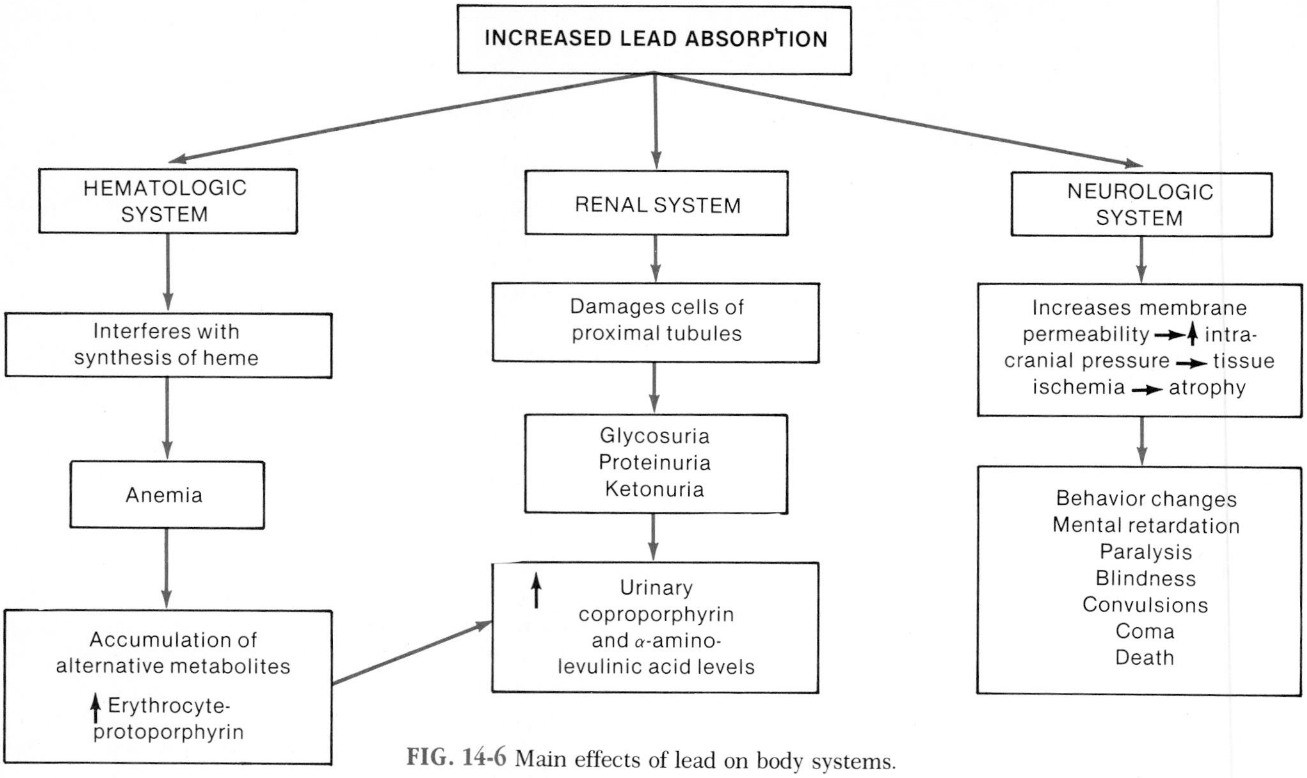

FIG. 14-6 Main effects of lead on body systems.

disturbance are important clues to the identification of children with early poisoning. Recent findings suggest that increased blood levels in fetuses adversely affect cognitive ability (Bellinger and others, 1987).

Diagnostic Evaluation

Since the clinical manifestations of lead poisoning (see box) are vague, the diagnosis is usually not made from clinical findings. For early diagnosis of asymptomatic children, screening is recommended, especially for all preschool children. When this is impractical, children at risk for lead poisoning, such as children living in older, dilapidated housing or siblings of children with known lead toxicity, should be screened.

Tests for routine screening include the blood-lead concentration and the erythrocyte-protoporphyrin (EP) level. Blood lead levels reflect absorption from recent exposure to lead, while EP determinations measure the adverse metabolic effect of lead on heme synthesis. Lead poisoning is defined as a blood lead level of 25 μg/dl and an EP level of 35 μg/dl or more.

Other tests that are helpful in determining the presence of lead in the body are (1) radiographs of the long bones for "lead lines," caused by deposition of lead, and of the abdomen for presence of recently ingested lead, (2) urinalysis for increased lead and the metabolites coproporphyrin and δ-aminolevulinic acid, (3) blood studies for evidence of anemia, and (4) lead mobilization test to help predict the amount of lead that may be removed by chelation.

Therapeutic Management

The objective of treatment is to remove lead in the body and prevent further accumulation of the metal. Therapeutic modalities include removing the source of lead, improving nutrition, and using chelation therapy. Chelation mobilizes the lead from the blood and soft tissues by enhancing its deposition in bones and its excretion in the urine. Calcium disodium edetate ($CaNa_2EDTA$) is the chelating agent of choice; it may be used in combination with the chelating drug dimercaprol, also called BAL (British anti-lewisite). A combination of the drugs is thought to result in less saturation of each (therefore fewer side effects) and better removal of lead from the brain. Because of the rapid rise in serum lead once the metal is mobilized from the bone, treatment can precipitate severe, even fatal, seizures. Success of treatment is measured by urinary excretion of lead.

The exact course of therapy depends on the severity of the child's condition and the method preferred by the physician. However, it may include a schedule of $CaNa_2EDTA$ and BAL 6 times a day for 5 days. If encephalopathy is present, fluid volume is restricted to prevent additional cerebral edema, and the drugs are administered intramuscularly. Children without encephalopathy can receive the drugs intravenously. Children with less severe lead poisoning may be treated with D-Penicillamine (Cuprimine, Depen) on an outpatient basis. D-Penicillamine is contraindicated in anyone with a history of penicillin allergy.

Symptomatic treatment involves controlling seizures,

Clinical Manifestations of Lead Poisoning

General Signs
- Anemia
- Acute crampy abdominal pain
- Vomiting
- Constipation
- Anorexia
- Headache
- Fever
- Short stature (long term)
- Decreased weight (long term)

Central Nervous System Signs (early)
- Hyperactivity
- Aggression
- Impulsiveness
- Decreased interest in play
- Lethargy
- Irritability
- Delay or reversal in verbal maturation
- Loss of newly acquired motor skills
- Clumsiness
- Deficits in sensory perception
- Learning difficulties
- Short attention span
- Distractibility

Central Nervous System Signs (late)
- Mental retardation
- Paralysis
- Blindness
- Convulsions
- Coma
- Death

Signs of Gasoline Sniffing
- Irritability
- Tremor
- Hallucinations
- Confusion
- Lack of impulse control
- Depression
- Delirium
- Chorea
- Ataxia
- Sleep disturbances

which are often severe and protracted. Hepatic and renal function is carefully monitored. Daily serum electrolyte levels should be taken. Cleansing enemas are ordered for episodes of acute lead ingestion or when lead is visible on radiologic examination in the gastrointestinal tract. Every effort is made to prevent infection and maintain adequate hydration. If nutritional deficiencies coexist, they are treated appropriately, such as administration of supplemental iron.

Nursing Considerations

The focus of nursing care depends on whether the goal is to prevent lead poisoning or to care for the child already exposed to excessive amounts of lead. Both goals are important; however, the current trend is to screen young children before lead levels become sufficiently high to cause central nervous system damage. The following discussion is concerned with nursing responsibilities for prevention and care of the lead-burdened child.

Nursing Diagnoses: Lead Poisoning

Poisoning or potential poisoning related to sources of lead in the environment
Altered parenting related to situational crises, knowledge deficit of childrearing practices and sources of lead
Fear related to pain of multiple injections

ASSESSMENT

Although screening is recommended for early identification of children with elevated lead levels, nurses should also be alert to those children who are at risk for lead poisoning. Careful history-taking is one of the most useful and valuable procedures, and the nurse should concentrate on the following areas:

1. Sources of lead in the child's environment, including home and other frequented sites, such as daycare center
2. History of pica or evidence of this behavior during the interview
3. Recent change in behavior, particularly disinterest in play
4. Developmental delay or recent loss of acquired skills, especially speech
5. Behavior problems such as aggression or hyperirritability

Parental characteristics, such as those discussed under factors related to lead ingestion, are important contributing factors to high-risk situations. The value of a home visit to evaluate the social and physical surroundings cannot be overestimated in the overall plan for diagnosis and prevention.

NURSING DIAGNOSES

A number of nursing diagnoses are prominent in the nursing care of the child with lead poisoning. The most common nursing diagnoses are presented in the box.

PLANNING

The main nursing goals for the child with lead poisoning and for prevention of plumbism include the following:

1. Prevent further exposure to lead
2. Support and encourage parents in their efforts to reduce the child's exposure to lead
3. Minimize fear and pain related to chelation therapy

IMPLEMENTATION

The most important nursing consideration is preventing the child's further exposure to lead. In most instances this involves helping the family remove lead from the child's environment. When it is not possible for the family to move to better housing or expensively refurbish their present home, some simple, inexpensive measures can be instituted. As much of the old flaking paint as possible is scraped from the walls, ceilings, and floors. However, when sanding or burning is employed, children and pregnant women must not remain in the home (day or night) until the process is completed. Since a new coating of lead-free paint does not prevent additional chips from falling away from the plaster, the walls are covered with wallpaper, contact paper, fabric, or burlap.

Other sources of lead can be minimized by meticulous housecleaning, including wet mopping; frequent handwashing, especially after outdoor play; and elimination of contaminated clothing. Workers, such as lead smelters or urban policeman, should change into clean clothing before leaving work. Members of cultures using folk remedies that contain lead must be advised of the danger and encouraged to avoid such practices.

In addition, the children must be supervised and guided toward activity other than pica. Helping parents learn methods of stimulating their children, locating preschool or daycare centers, or helping parents organize a play group are methods of improving parenting and consequently lessening those factors that contribute to plumbism. If nutritional deficiencies coexist, parents need guidance in planning meals that provide sufficient minerals or instruction regarding administration of supplements, such as iron. Consistent mealtimes should be planned with instructions that the child eat only at these times to reduce the practice of pica. As in any situational crisis, parents need support and understanding if their child is treated for plumbism. Many of the families at highest risk for lead poisoning have the fewest resources to comply with measures, such as relocation or deleading the home. Appropriate referrals are essential in locating assistance for parents.

For the child who must undergo chelation therapy, the nurse has several priorities of care, especially if the drug is injected intramuscularly, rather than given intravenously. If the intramuscular route is employed, the child may receive multiple injections. They need to be prepared for the injections and allowed to express their pain and anger. Needle play and aggressive play, such as pounding clay or throwing bean bags, provides an excellent outlet for their frustrations. Children also deserve an explanation of the need for the treatment, particularly that it is not a punishment for eating lead or paint (see Therapeutic dialogue). All the injections should be administered when the child is in an area other than his room to maintain a "safe" environment.

Since $CaNa_2EDTA$ and BAL are both viscous solutions, they must be administered deeply into a different large muscle mass. To lessen the pain during injection of the drug, a local anesthetic such as procaine may be injected simultaneously with the $CaNa_2EDTA$. For greatest

THERAPEUTIC DIALOGUE

Lead Poisoning

A 3-year old child was admitted to the pediatric unit with a diagnosis of lead poisoning and the treatment was intramuscular chelation therapy. The nurse talked with the child before initiating treatment.

NURSE: Tommy, I need to give you some medicine under the skin to make you feel better."

CHILD: What kind of medicine?

NURSE: This is a medicine that will take the paint that you ate out of your body.

CHILD: My mommy told me I was a bad boy for eating the paint.

NURSE: Eating paint is not a good thing to do. It makes you sick. But you are not a bad boy and this medicine is not a punishment. Do you understand?

CHILD: I guess so. But I still don't like to get the medicine.

NURSE: I know. After I give you the medicine I am going to bring you a doll so you can give the doll medicine too.

CHILD: OK. And I will tell the dolly that she is not bad, but she should never eat paint. It will make her sick.

SUMMARY

Following the injection, the nurse brought the child a doll and the appropriate equipment for giving an injection. The child stuck the doll several times, repeating each time, "You're not bad, but never eat paint again." Each time the child received an injection, the nurse gave the child the doll and the syringe. When the last injection was given, the nurse told the child that she would not have to give him any more medicine. The child gave the doll its injection and said, "This is the last shot. I know this hurts. You are a good dolly."

anesthetic effect, the chelating agent is drawn into the syringe, followed by the anesthetic. In this way the anesthetic is the first medication to be injected into the tissue. Injecting is performed slowly in order to allow some time for the anesthetic to exert its numbing effect. An air bubble at the top of the syringe flushes the needle of any remaining medication, thereby decreasing the chance of tracking the drug through the layers of the skin on withdrawal of the syringe. Other measures to reduce pain from the injection are summarized on p. 664.

Planning a rotation schedule for each series of injections is essential to prevent tissue damage and to ensure maximum tissue absorption. Since the peak incidence of lead poisoning is during the toddler years, the vastus lateralis, ventrogluteal, and gluteal sites are satisfactory available areas for rotation of multiple injections.

A complication of multiple injections in one site is the development of hard, painful areas of fibrotic tissue. The nodules feel firm and almost circular when palpated. It is advisable to routinely feel the muscle mass before preparing the injection site to avoid administering additional medication into the same area. A systematic approach should be used to specify the sequence of injection sites (e.g., RVL_1, right vastus lateralis, upper left corner) so that each site is used as few times as possible. Local application of warm soaks or insulated hot packs helps relieve the discomfort, although the pain may persist and be severe enough to limit movement.

Since $CaNa_2EDTA$ and lead are toxic to the kidneys, records are kept of intake and output and frequent urinalysis is performed to evaluate renal functioning. Urine and blood specimens are routinely collected to measure lead levels and assess the efficacy of treatment. Because of the risk of seizures, appropriate precautions are instituted at the bedside.

EVALUATION

The effectiveness of nursing interventions is determined by continual reassessment and evaluation of care based on the following observational guidelines and expected outcomes:

1. Inquire regarding efforts to remove lead from the environment; visit the home if possible; investigate community efforts to improve housing for families at risk
2. Interview parents regarding plans to relocate or provide activities that reduce child's tendency to practice pica; inquire regarding their compliance with therapies, such as mineral supplements
3. Observe child's reaction during chelation therapy; keep a pain assessment record; check medical record for rotation chart for injections; palpate injection sites for evidence of fibrotic tissue

Expected outcomes:

1. Sources of lead are removed from child's environment
2. Parents institute measures to prevent child's further exposure to lead and comply with prescribed treatments
3. Child demonstrates minimal fear/pain with injections

◆ *Child Maltreatment*

Child maltreatment is a broad term that includes intentional physical abuse or neglect, emotional abuse or neglect, or sexual abuse of children usually by adults. It is one of the most significant social problems affecting children. In 1985 over 1.9 million children were reported as victims of child abuse and neglect to child protective services in the United States. However, this does not represent the number of children actually maltreated. Of these reported cases, over 60% were found to be unsubstantiated and a portion of these were false reports (Highlights, 1987). It is also likely that many abuse cases are never brought to the attention of the authorities. Consequently, the best available statistics only partially reflect the true incidence of child maltreatment.

The following discussion presents an overview of the types of abuse, factors that may predispose to abuse, and nursing responsibilities related to identification of the abuse, support of the child and family, and prevention of this tragedy.

CHILD NEGLECT

Child neglect is the most common form of maltreatment. Over one half of all reported cases are related to neglect from deprivation of necessities, and the majority of deaths from maltreatment are in this group. Neglect is generally considered an omission, rather than a commission, of a direct act or behavior that has a detrimental effect on the child's psychologic development. Little is known about the etiology of neglect, although it appears that many of the risk factors identified in physical abuse apply to neglect as well (see discussion on p. 410). Ignorance of child's needs and lack of resources are important contributing factors. For example, neglectful parents often demonstrate poor parenting skills. They may be unaware that an infant needs to be fed every 3 to 4 hours, be unable to cook a meal, not know what constitutes a nutritious meal, and have insufficient funds to buy food. The most serious lack of knowledge is failure to recognize emotional nurturing as an essential need of children. Instead, emotional nurturing is viewed as spoiling the child by giving him attention. The reader is also encouraged to review the discussion of Failure to thrive (p. 327) and psychologic dwarfism (p. 473), which may be due to physical or emotional neglect.

Types of Neglect

Neglect takes many forms and can be classified broadly as physical or emotional maltreatment. *Physical neglect* involves the deprivation of necessities, such as food, clothing, shelter, supervision, medical care, and education. *Emotional neglect* generally refers to the failure to meet the child's needs for affection, attention, and emotional nurturance. It may also include lack of intervention for or fostering maladaptive behavior, such as delinquency or substance abuse. *Emotional abuse* is an even more difficult aspect of maltreatment to define but refers to the deliberate attempt to destroy or significantly impair a child's self-esteem or competence. Verbal abuse is probably the most common form and includes scapegoating, put-downs, humiliation, labeling, and unrealistic expectations.

PHYSICAL ABUSE

Physical abuse refers to the deliberate infliction of physical injury on a child, usually by the child's caregiver. Minor physical injury is responsible for about 15% of all reported cases of maltreatment. Major physical injury is infrequent, occurring in only 2.2% of abused children, but accounts for 35% of all fatalities from abuse (Highlights, 1987). Despite the importance of the problem, a universally accepted definition of what constitutes minor and major physical abuse does not exist. Rather, each state in the United States defines abuse according to its individual reporting laws.

Factors Predisposing to Physical Abuse

The exact cause of child abuse is not known. However, several theories attempt to provide an explanation for the etiology of abuse. None are proven or universally accepted, although most theories stress the importance of three factors—parental characteristics, characteristics of the child, and environmental characteristics— as influencing the potential for abuse. However, no one factor or group of factors are predictive of abuse. Rather, these factors are thought to increase the predisposition to or risk of abuse occurring in a particular family.

Parental characteristics. Extensive research has focused on parental characteristics that distinguish abusive parents from nonabusive parents. Unfortunately, the findings from most of these studies provide conflicting evidence. For example, it is commonly believed that abusive parents were abused as children. However, few studies support this relationship. While physical punishment tends to be very common in abusive parents' childhood, most of the parents were not physically abused as children. However, abusive parents who report that they were severely punished as children are much more likely to injure their own children (Kotelchuck, 1982). If the abuse was not overt physical violence, abusive parents typically recall their punishment as unfair and severe and characterize their relationship with their parents as negative. Abusive parents tend to have difficulty controlling aggressive impulses, and the free expression of violence is one of the most consistent qualities of these families (Altemeier and others, 1982).

Another finding is that abusive families are often more socially isolated and have fewer supportive relationships than nonabusive parents. With little or no available support system and the presence of concurrent stresses imposed by the child or environment, these parents are extremely vulnerable to additional crises of any nature and literally strike out at the child as a method of releasing their increasing frustration and anxiety.

Other factors that have been identified in abusing parents include low self-esteem and less adequate maternal functioning. While inadequate knowledge of childrearing is often cited as a characteristic of abusive parents, research findings do not consistently support this belief. However, this does not mean that these parents cannot benefit from learning more constructive ways of rearing their children, especially nonviolent discipline methods.

Characteristics of the child. The child also unintentionally contributes to the abusing situation. In families of two or more children it is usual to find only one child as the victim of abuse. This child's temperament, position in the family, additional physical needs if ill or disabled, or insensitivity to parental needs all in some way contribute to why he escapes or fosters physical abuse. For example, one child may not be abused if he fits into the "easy-child pattern," while another sibling with a difficult temperament may add to the parent's stress sufficiently to precipitate an abusive act. However, temperament alone is not the critical factor, but rather the "fit" or compatibility between the child's temperament and the parent's ability to deal with that behavioral style.

Occasionally, the abused child is illegitimate, unwanted, brain damaged (especially in situations where the parents cannot accept the retardation), hyperkinetic, physically disabled, or from a broken home. Sometimes the child is abused because he reminds the parent of someone the parent dislikes, for example, a younger brother or sister who received all the attention from their own parents. Premature infants may be at risk for maltreatment because of the failure of parent-child bonding during early infancy. Often a difficult pregnancy, labor, or delivery is a predisposing factor in abuse, especially when the infant is born prematurely or with congenital anomalies.

Environmental characteristics. The environment is an integral part of the potential abusive situation. Typically the environment is one of chronic stress, including problems of divorce, poverty, unemployment, poor housing, frequent relocation, and sometimes alcoholism and drug addiction. Increased exposure between children and parents, such as that which occurs in large families and in crowded living conditions, also increases the likelihood of abuse.

Although most reporting of abuse has been from lower socioeconomic populations, child abuse is by no means a problem of any one societal group. It spans all educational, social, and economic levels. Certainly stresses imposed by poverty predispose lower socioeconomic families to abusive situations, and abuse in these groups is more apt to be reported. However, concealed crises can also be present in upper class families. For example, a wealthy family experiencing major life changes, such as rehousing, the birth of an additional child, or marital discord,

Emotional N - failure to meet child need their affection, attention, emotional nurturance
lack of intervention - delinquency & substance abuse

Emotional abuse - form of Mal treatment deliberate attempt to destroy or significantly impair a child's self-esteem or competence
Verbal abuse - Most common put-downs, humiliations, labeling and unrealistic expectations

Wong 409

(Child) <u>Maltreatment</u> - intentional physical abuse or neglect, emotional sexual abuse

<u>Child</u> <u>neglect</u> is the most common form of maltreatment (or) deprivation of necessities

- neglectful parents often demonstrate poor parenting skills
- May need teaching (How to feed when) FTT, can't comprehend how to make food

* Most serious - lack of knowledge is failure to recognize emotional nurturing as an essential need of children
instead, spoiling the child c̄ lot's attention

Failure to thrive, dwarfism may be due to physical or emotional neglect

<u>Types of neglect</u> -
Many forms can be classified broadly as physical or emotional maltreatment

<u>Physical neglect</u> - deprivation of necessities, such as food clothing, shelter, supervision, medical care, education

may have sufficient environmental stressors imposed on them to produce a potentially abusive situation. Wealthy families may be so overinvolved with commitments outside the home that abuse may be inflicted by substitute caregivers. Nurses need to be aware of such factors in order to identify the less obvious examples of child abuse and neglect.

SEXUAL ABUSE

Sexual abuse is one of the most devastating types of child maltreatment, and current estimates indicate that it has increased tremendously during the past decade. This is not only because of growing public awareness but is also associated with the expansion of definitions to include extrafamilial abuse, increase in the numbers of programs to treat sexual abusers and victims, and shifts in state and local policy to increase emphasis on reporting and investigating sexual maltreatment. The number of reported occurrences was approximately 12% of all child maltreatment cases in 1985 (Highlights, 1987), but many authorities believe that this figure represents only a small percentage of the actual incidence.

As with all forms of child maltreatment, no universal definition for sexual abuse exists. The National Center on Child Abuse and Neglect (NCCAN) defines it as:

> Contacts or interactions between a child and an adult when the child is being used for the sexual stimulation of that adult or another person. Sexual abuse may also be committed by a person under age 18.

Sexual abuse includes several types of sexual maltreatment, including the following (definitions of rape are presented on p. 477) (Kempe and Kempe, 1984):

incest Any physical sexual activity between family members; blood relationship is not required and abusers can include stepparents, nonrelated siblings, grandparents, uncles, and aunts. (Does not include sexual relations between legally sanctional partners, such as spouses.)
molestation A vague term that includes "indecent liberties" such as touching, fondling, kissing, single or mutual masturbation, or oral-genital contact
exhibitionism Indecent exposure, usually exposure of the genitals by an adult male to children or female adults
child pornography Arranging and photographing in any media sexual acts including children, adults, or animals, regardless of consent by the child's legal guardian; the distribution of such material in any form with or without profit
child prostitution Involving children in sex acts for profit and usually with changing partners
pedophilia Literally means "love of child" and does not denote a type of sexual activity but the preference of an adult for prepubertal children as the means of achieving sexual excitement

Characteristics of Sexual Abuse

Anyone, including siblings and mothers, can be sexual abusers, but a typical abuser is a male that the victim knows. Offenders come from all levels of society. Some are prominent persons in the community and some, especially in the case of pedophiliacs (also called "child molesters"), are in positions, such as teaching and coaching, where they work closely with children.

Pornography and prostitution may involve strangers as well as the children's own parents. There are no typical characteristics of these offenders, although the abused children tend to be runaways—young adolescents who engage in these activities to obtain money for food, shelter, drugs, and alcohol. Incestuous relationships occur most commonly between father or stepfather and daughter and are generally prolonged. The victims are usually reluctant to report the situation because of fear of retaliation and fear that they will not be believed. Typically, incestuous relationships begin later than other forms of child abuse, and the average age of the victim is 9 years (Highlights, 1987). The eldest daughter is usually abused, but in her absence, another sister is substituted.

Boys are also victims of both intrafamilial and extrafamilial abuse. Males are much less likely to report abuse, and available research indicates that they suffer much greater emotional harm from incestuous relationships, especially between mother and son, than female victims. Boys are likely to be subjected to anal penetration and oral-genital contact, to have subtle physical findings, and to be abused by a father, stepfather, or mother's boyfriend (Spencer and Dunklee, 1986).

The cycle of sexual abuse often starts innocently, unless it involves an isolated attack, such as rape. Often offenders spend time with the victims to gain their trust before initiating any sexual contact. Most victims are then pressured into being an accessory to the sexual activity through methods such as the following:

1. The child is offered material goods, such as special favors or privileges
2. The adult misrepresents moral standards by telling the child that it is "okay to do." Children grow up believing that if an adult tells them to do something they should do it
3. Isolated and emotionally and socially impoverished children are enticed by adult males who meet their needs for warmth and human contact
4. The successful sex offender pressures the victim into secrecy regarding the activity by describing it as a "secret between us" that other people may take away if they found out
5. The offender also plays on the child's fears, including fear of punishment by the offender, fear of repercussions if the child tells, and fear of abandonment or rejection by the family

Children may not reveal the truth for fear that their parents would not believe them if they told—especially if the offender is a trusted member of the family. Some fear they will be blamed for the situation, and many young children with limited vocabulary have difficulty in describing the activity when they do have the courage or opportunity to complain.

While the reasons for incest are complicated and can occur in any number of family types, it does not occur in healthy families (Kempe and Kempe, 1984). Most relationships are directly related to sexual maladjustment and estrangement between husband and wife and begin following the cessation of sexual relationships with the usual partner. In the classic incestuous relationship, fathers experience little guilt, and the wives tolerate or deny the abuse. Consequently the home offers little protection to young victims, since abusers have easy access to their victims and the children feel they cannot reveal their secret to other family members.

However, not all incestuous relationships follow this pattern of silence. Currently, reports of father-daughter incest during child custody conflicts have become common and have raised serious concerns regarding the possibility of false accusation. Rather than tolerating or denying the child's sexual abuse, the other parent (usually the mother) is typically the chief accuser (Coleman, 1986).

NURSING CARE OF THE MALTREATED CHILD

Nursing care related to child maltreatment involves several important areas. Once an abusive act has occurred, identification and protection of the child from further abuse are essential. However, nurses also have a responsibility to prevent abuse from occurring and to minimize the wrongful accusation of abuse. The following discussion focuses on these issues for all three types of abuse.

ASSESSMENT

One of the most critical responsibilities of all health professionals is identifying abusive situations as early as possible. The characteristics that may predispose members of some families to commit abuse can serve as a framework for assessing vulnerability but are never predictive of actual abuse. Rather a thorough physical examination and a careful, detailed history are the diagnostic tools needed to identify abuse. Nurses have a very special role because they may be the first person to see the child and parent and are the consistent caregivers if the child is hospitalized.

Evidence of Maltreatment

Recognition of abuse or neglect necessitates a familiarity with both physical and behavioral signs that suggest maltreatment (Table 14-4). No one indicator is exclusively diagnostic of maltreatment; rather it is a pattern or combination of indicators that should arouse suspicion and further investigation. In addition, signs of possible abuse must be coupled with an understanding of diseases, such as bleeding disorders, osteogenesis imperfecta, or sudden infant death syndrome, or cultural practices, such as cupping or coin rubbing (see p. 42), that may mimic physical abuse.

Neglect and emotional abuse. Neglect from deprivation of necessities is easier to identify than emotional neglect or abuse because physical signs are usually evident. While emotional maltreatment may be readily suspected, it is very difficult to substantiate. Physical signs are often nonspecific, and nurses must rely on behavioral indicators, which range from depression to acting-out behavior, to help identify a possible abuse situation. Any persistent and unexplained change in the child's behavior is an important clue to possible emotional abuse.

Physical abuse. Evidence of physical abuse is not always obvious. One of the more unusual and perplexing types of physical abuse is the *Munchausen syndrome by proxy,* which refers to illness that is fabricated or induced by one person in another. In children it is usually the mother who fabricates signs and symptoms in her child, such as adding maternal blood to the child's urine to fake hematuria or sugar to the urine to simulate diabetes mellitus (Weber, 1987).

Such cases are often very difficult to confirm and require a high index of suspicion to protect the child from numerous unnecessary and painful diagnostic procedures. Warning signals of Munchausen syndrome include:

- Unexplained illnesses
- Discrepancies between clinical findings and the history
- Clinical manifestations occur primarily in mother's presence
- Mother has previous medical experience
- Mother refuses to leave child
- Child does not respond to treatment

Sexual abuse. Identifying instances of sexual abuse is particularly difficult because frequently few if any obvious physical indications of the activity may exist. Also, many individuals are hesitant to believe children and unwilling to report incidents. Even health professionals are sometimes at fault when they perform cursory physical examinations of the genitalia and ignore behavior or verbal comments that suggest abuse. When sexual abuse is suspected, other children in the family should also be evaluated, since multiple victims are not uncommon.

Unfortunately, there is no typical profile of the victim and there must be a high index of suspicion to identify these children. Physical signs vary and may include any of those listed in Table 14-4 for sexual abuse. Every effort is made to thoroughly examine children for physical clues. Most authorities agree that in any young child with a sexually transmitted disease, nonspecific vaginitis, or venereal warts (condylomata acuminata), a thorough medical and social evaluation is essential to rule out sexual abuse. However, the presence of such diseases does not automatically confirm sexual transmission.

Numerous behavioral manifestations may be exhibited by the victim, but none are specific to abuse. However, serious and unexplained manifestations, such as chronic depression, isolation from peers, apathy, and suicide attempts, should alert the health professional to consider the possibility of sexual abuse.

TABLE 14-4

Potential Signs of Child Maltreatment

I. Physical Neglect

A. 1. Failure to thrive
   2. Signs of malnutrition, such as thin extremities, abdominal distention, lack of subcutaneous fat
   3. Poor personal hygiene, especially of teeth
   4. Unclean and/or inappropriate dress
   5. Evidence of poor health care, such as nonimmunized status, untreated infections, frequent colds
   6. Frequent injuries from lack of supervision

B. Behavioral indicators
   1. Dull and inactive; excessively passive or sleepy
   2. Self-stimulatory behaviors, such as finger sucking or rocking
   3. Begging or stealing food
   4. Absenteeism from school
   5. Drug or alcohol addiction
   6. Vandalism or shoplifting
   (items 3–6: in older child)

II. Emotional Abuse and Neglect

A. Physical indicators
   1. Failure to thrive
   2. Feeding disorders, such as rumination
   3. Enuresis
   4. Sleep disorders

B. Behavioral indicators
   1. Self-stimulatory behaviors, such as biting, rocking, sucking
   2. During infancy, lack of social smile and stranger anxiety
   3. Withdrawal
   4. Unusual fearfulness
   5. Antisocial behavior, such as destructiveness, stealing, cruelty
   6. Extremes of behavior, such as overcompliant and passive or aggressive and demanding
   7. Lags in emotional and intellectual development, especially language
   8. Suicide attempts

III. Physical Abuse

A. Physical indicators
   1. Bruises and welts
      (a) On face, lips, mouth, back, buttocks, thighs, or areas of torso
      (b) Regular patterns descriptive of object used, such as belt buckle, hand, wire hanger, chain, wooden spoon, squeeze or pinch marks
      (c) May be present in various stages of healing
   2. Burns
      (a) On soles of feet, palms of hands, back, or buttocks
      (b) Patterns descriptive of object used, such as round cigar or cigarette burns, "glovelike" sharply demarcated areas from immersion in scalding water, rope burns on wrists or ankles from being bound, burns in the shape of an iron, radiator, or electric stove burner
      (c) Absence of "splash" marks and presence of symmetric burns
   3. Fractures and dislocations
      (a) Skull, nose, or facial structures
      (b) Injury may denote type of abuse, such as spiral fracture or dislocation from twisting of an extremity or whiplash from shaking the child
      (c) Multiple new or old fractures in various stages of healing
   4. Lacerations and abrasions
      (a) On backs of arms, legs, torso, face, or external genitalia
      (b) Unusual symptoms, such as abdominal swelling, pain, and vomiting from punching
      (c) Descriptive marks such as from human bites or pulling the hair out
   5. Chemical
      (a) Unexplained repeated poisoning, especially drug overdose
      (b) Unexplained sudden illness, such as hypoglycemia from insulin administration

B. Behavioral indicators
   1. Wary of physical contact with adults
   2. Apparent fear of parents or going home
   3. Lying very still while surveying environment
   4. Inappropriate reaction to injury, such as failure to cry from pain
   5. Lack of reaction to frightening events
   6. Apprehensive when hearing other children cry
   7. Indiscriminate friendliness and displays of affection
   8. Superficial relationships
   9. Acting-out behavior, such as aggression, to seek attention
   10. Withdrawal behavior

Continued.

TABLE 14-4

Potential Signs of Child Maltreatment—cont'd

IV. Sexual Abuse
- A. Physical indicators
  1. Bruises, bleeding, lacerations or irritation of external genitalia, anus, mouth, or throat
  2. Torn, stained, or bloody underclothing
  3. Pain on urination or pain, swelling, and itching of genital area
  4. Penile discharge
  5. Sexually transmitted disease, nonspecific vaginitis, or venereal warts
  6. Difficulty in walking or sitting
  7. Unusual odor in the genital area
  8. Recurrent urinary tract infections
  9. Pregnancy in young adolescent
- B. Behavioral indicators
  1. Withdrawn, excessive daydreaming
  2. Preoccupied with fantasies, especially in play
  3. Poor relationships with peers
  4. Sudden changes, such as anxiety, loss or gain of weight, clinging behavior
  5. In incestuous relationships, excessive anger at mother for not protecting daughter
  6. Regressive behavior, such as bed-wetting or thumb-sucking
  7. Sudden onset of phobias or fears, particularly fears of the dark, men, strangers, or particular settings or situations (e.g., undue fear of leaving the house or staying at the daycare center or the baby-sitter's house)
  8. Running away from home
  9. Sudden emergence of sexually-related problems, including excessive or public masturbation, age-inappropriate sexual play, promiscuity, or overtly seductive behavior
  10. Substance abuse, particularly of alcohol or mood-elevating drugs
  11. Profound and rapid personality changes, especially extreme depression, hostility, and aggression (often accompanied by social withdrawal)
  12. Rapidly declining school performance
  13. Suicidal attempts or ideation

History Pertaining to the Incident

Besides observable evidence of abuse, the type of history revealed by the parents or other caregiver, such as the baby-sitter or mother's boyfriend, is a significant factor.

Index of Suspicion of Abuse

- Physical evidence of abuse and/or neglect, including old injuries
- Conflicting stories about the "accident" or injury from the parents or others
- Cause of injury blamed on sibling or other party
- An injury inconsistent with the history, such as a concussion and broken arm from falling off a bed
- History inconsistent with child's developmental level; such as a 6-month-old turning on the hot water
- A complaint other than the one associated with signs of abuse; for example, a chief complaint of a cold when there is evidence of first- and second-degree burns
- Inappropriate parental concern for the degree of the injury, such as an exaggerated or absent emotional response
- Refusal of the parents to sign for additional tests or agree to necessary treatment
- Excessive delay in seeking treatment
- Absence of the parents for questioning
- Inappropriate response of child, such as little or no response to pain, fear of being touched, excessive or lack of separation anxiety, indiscriminate friendliness to strangers
- Previous reports of abuse in the family
- Repeated visits to emergency facilities with injuries

Those areas of the history that should arouse suspicion of abuse are summarized in the accompanying box.

Incompatibility between the history and the injury is probably the most important criterion on which to base the decision to report suspected abuse. However, maltreated children rarely betray their parents by confessing to the abuse they received. If questioned, they will repeat the same story as the parents and try to defend their parents' actions. If the interviewer directly accuses the parents of abuse, the child may accept responsibility for the act in an attempt to vindicate the parents from the accusation. Whether children respond in this way out of fear is uncertain. However, children do fear losing whatever security and love they have. Between abusive acts children may receive some measure of attention and love from the parents. If they betray the parents, they may lose this and be uncertain or fearful of the consequences, such as foster care. Preserving the present situation may be less frightening than the unknown future.

The disclosure of sexual abuse can occur in a variety of ways—the act is observed by others, resulting in a direct confrontation; the child tells someone, such as a parent of a friend; visible clues of the relationship are observed, such as an accumulation of coins, gifts, or candy; or more obvious clues are seen, such as a child coming home disheveled or becoming pregnant; and physical or behavioral signs and symptoms are observed. Children usually describe the experience in terms of whether it was unpleasant or hurt or was pleasurable (usually a response to hand-genital contact); some indicate no reaction. Young children often feel no guilt or shame because the act is pleasurable and they are unaware of its inappropriateness.

Parental Behaviors

Certain behavioral responses of the parents to their child and to the interviewer should alert the nurse to the possibility of maltreatment. Although no one pattern of behaviors is characteristic of these parents, some responses include the following. Abusive parents have difficulty in showing concern toward their child. They are unable to comfort him and give no indication of realizing how the child may feel, physically or emotionally. Instead they are critical of the child and angry with him for being injured. They maintain that the child injured himself, and, if asked any question regarding their responsibility of protecting or supervising the child, they become hostile and aggressive. They act as if the child's injury is an assault on them. Their entire perception of the incident is in terms of how it affects them, not the child, which is an indication of their preoccupation with their own needs and their inability to give any support to others.

During the child's hospitalization they may not become involved in the child's care and may show little concern for his progress, eventual discharge, or need for follow-up care. However, if they are pressured during interrogation, they immediately demand to take the child home, regardless of the child's readiness for discharge.

Families respond to sexual abuse with a wide variety of emotional reactions that may be as intense and disruptive as they are for the victim, regardless of the type of abuse. The immediate reactions range from emotional shock to near hysteria on the part of one or both of the parents, which may interfere with care of the victim. In incestuous abuse in an intact family the most common reaction is denial of the child's accusation. There may be surprising inability on the part of the parents to provide adequate emotional support to the child at this time, even when their attitude toward the child has been supportive in the past.

Parents and other family members may display the same type of emotional responses as the victim, such as inability to eat or sleep and somatic complaints of headache or backache. In the acute emotional phase, parents have a need to blame someone. The three common targets are the offender, the child, and themselves. The parents commonly express anger at the child for "stupid" behavior and may even restrict the child's privileges as punishment. When the victim is a female, the parents may question her sexual provocation of the event. Self-blaming parents assume full responsibility, believing that they have been inadequate parents or should not have allowed the child to go out. When a baby-sitter or trusted relative is involved in the assault and the child's complaint has not been believed until gross evidence is presented, the parents are often devastated by guilt.

Child Behaviors

Abused children's response to their parents or the injury may also support the suspicion of abuse. Although no one pattern is typical, extremes of behavior may be observed. Children may be very unresponsive to the parent or excessively clinging and intolerant of separation. There may be over-attachment to the abusing parent, possibly in the hope of preventing any upset that may precipitate anger and another attack. During care of the injury children may be passive and accepting of the discomfort or uncooperative and fearful of any physical contact. Some children maintain a wary watchfulness of all strangers; some shy away from strangers as if frightened; others are unusually affectionate and outgoing.

NURSING DIAGNOSES

A number of nursing diagnoses are prominent in the nursing care of the maltreated child and family, and others specific to individual cases become evident. The most common nursing diagnoses are outlined in the Nursing Care Plan on p. 419.

PLANNING

The main nursing goals related to child maltreatment are as follows:

1. Protect the child from further abuse
2. Support the child and family
3. Prevent abuse

IMPLEMENTATION

Interventions related to child maltreatment include immediate actions once a child is suspected of being abused, long-range care if the child is placed outside the home, and general strategies that may reduce the occurrence of abuse.

Protect from Further Abuse

Initially, identification of instances of suspected abuse or neglect is essential. The nurse may come in contact with abused children in an emergency room, physician's office, or school. *The priority is to remove the child from the abusive situation to prevent further injury.*

All states and provinces in North America have laws for mandatory reporting of child maltreatment. Suspected child abuse is reported to the local authorities.* Referrals usually come to the Bureau of Child Welfare and are assigned to a caseworker in an agency such as the Child Protective Services (CPS). In most states, once a referral has been made, there is an automatic court order, which gives the agency the right to keep the child in protective custody for 72 hours. This allows the caseworker suffi-

*Telephone numbers are usually listed under "Child abuse" in the business white pages of the local directory, or call the emergency child abuse hotline: 1-800-422-4453 (1-800-4-A-CHILD).

Guidelines for Assessment Data in Suspected Abuse

History of Injury
1. Date, time, and place of occurrence
2. Sequence of events with recorded times
3. Presence of witnesses, especially person caring for child at time of incident
4. Time lapse between occurrence of injury and initiation of treatment
5. Interview with child when appropriate, including verbal quotations and information from drawing or other play activities
6. Interview with parent, witnesses, or other significant persons, including verbal quotations
7. Description of parent-child interactions (verbal interactions, eye contact, touching, parental concern)
8. Name, age, and condition of other children in home (if possible)

Physical Examination
1. Location, size, shape, and color of bruises; approximate location, size, and shape on drawing of body outline
2. Distinguishing characteristics, such as a bruise in the shape of a hand; round burn (possibly caused by cigarette)
3. Symmetry or asymmetry of injury; presence of other injuries
4. Degree of pain (see p. 587); any bone tenderness
5. Evidence of old injuries; general state of health and hygiene
6. Developmental level of child; perform screening test such as Denver Developmental Screening Test (see p. 171)

cient time to investigate the report in the event of intervening holidays or weekends. If the caseworker finds no justification for the charge, the child is returned to the home. If there is evidence of abuse, further action is taken against the parents.

A court proceeding may be necessary before the child can be placed outside the home or when parental rights are to be terminated. When the courts are involved, they usually require firsthand testimony by the referring parties. Nurses' notes are often introduced as evidence in court hearings. Accurate and factual documentation is essential. A suggested outline for recording pertinent assessment data is presented in the box. Behaviors are described, not interpreted, and are recorded daily to establish a progress record. Conversations between the nurse, child, and parent should be recorded verbatim as much as possible.

Care of Child

Frequently children suspected of abuse are hospitalized for medical management of their injuries. When the sexually abused child has been physically harmed, the care is consistent with that provided a rape victim (see p. 479). Regardless of the type of abuse, their needs are the same as those of any hospitalized child. The child should be treated as a child with the usual physical needs, developmental tasks, and play interests—not as a dramatic victim of abuse. The nurse is the child's advocate in this goal. Others who want to question the child without justified reason are intercepted by the nurse, who also encourages the child in his continuing relationship with his parents. The nurse does not become a substitute parent to the exclusion of the child's natural parents. Such an intent only intensifies the parents' feelings of inadequacy, worthlessness, and isolation. It in no way helps them understand their child or promotes their trust in health professionals. The goal of the *consistent* nurse-child relationship is to provide a role model for the parents in helping them to relate positively and constructively to their child and to foster a therapeutic environment for the child in his reprieve from the abusing situation.

Sexual abuse. If nurses are involved in interviewing these children, they must use sensitivity and discretion. Every effort is made to make the child feel comfortable with appropriate introductions and to avoid duplicating the behaviors typically used by offenders, such as touching the child without permission. The interview is conducted in a quiet and private location, preferably a neutral place, such as a school playroom, or office, and not where the abuse occurred. Neutral questions are asked first, such as the child's reaction to the hospital (if appropriate), and then the conversation turns to a discussion of the incident in general terms. The interview should include such questions as "Do you know why you were brought to the hospital?" "Do you know what will happen here?" or "How do you feel about being here?" Later the question "Can you tell me what happened?" and other questions may then elicit an account of the incident. Sometimes the parents are able to help the child to describe the incident, and questions can become directed to the circumstances of the assault. Questions should progress chronologically and proceed from the nonsexual to the more sexual content. If the child shows evidence of becoming too upset, the focus can be redirected toward more neutral and less emotionally charged areas. In interviewing the victim, every effort is made to coordinate and limit the number of interviewees and to assign a primary professional to work with the child.

Children are given the opportunity to ask questions, but if they are reticent, they are never pressured into talking. Young children in particular lack the verbal skills to adequately describe body parts. These children benefit from play situations that provide opportunities for disclosure, such as drawing, using puppets or anatomically correct dolls, and doll houses. For example, the nurse can encourage the child to draw a picture "of what happened" or "of what you remember." Details of drawings, such as shading, emphasis, or deletion of body parts or persons, may reveal or lend support to the occurrence of abuse. However, drawings or anatomically correct dolls are not diagnostic tests and must be interpreted very carefully (Wong, 1987).

Discharge planning. Discharge planning should begin

as soon as the legal disposition for placement has been decided, which may be temporary foster home placement, return to the parents, or permanent termination of parental rights. The latter is the most drastic solution, but it is necessary in situations of repeated, life-threatening abuse. Whenever children are remanded to a foster home or juvenile institution, they must be allowed the opportunity to express their feelings. No matter how severe the abuse, they usually mourn the loss of their parents. They need help to understand why they must not return home and that this new home is in no way a punishment. Whenever possible, foster parents should be encouraged to visit, and the nurse should take an active role in helping these new parents understand the child. It is unfortunate that some abused children live in torment as they are sent from one foster home to another, sometimes enduring worse circumstances than those that existed in their original home. Only through constant evaluation of the placement residence and the child's adjustment to a new environment can the vicious cycle of abuse, abandonment, and neglect be stopped.

Care of Family

One of the most difficult, yet essential, components of success with abusing parents is the quality of the therapeutic relationship. It must be one of genuine concern and treatment, not one of accusation and punishment. Nurses must examine their personal feelings toward these parents, particularly when sexual abuse is present. A therapeutic approach is to view the parent as the patient and the child as the victim of abuse. Unless the nurse's attitude is positive, abusing parents will not be motivated to change, since they will not be working with a trusting person who demonstrates the kind of behavior that is being asked of them.

When parental ignorance of childrearing practices has played a part in the abuse, the nurse can educate the parent regarding children's physical and emotional needs. Because of the parents' own childrearing, they may not be aware of nonviolent methods of discipline, such as time-out or consequences. They may also need help in dealing with their frustration so that they do not vent anger on the child. Since these parents may be sensitive to criticism or domination and already possess a very low self-esteem, teaching is implemented through demonstration and example rather than through lecturing. Any competent parenting abilities they demonstrate are praised to promote their sense of parental adequacy.

Sexual abuse. Care of the family also depends on the circumstances of the sexual abuse. In the situation of a non-parent offender the family may be more able to support the child than if incest were involved. Family members are encouraged to express their feelings of anger, guilt, shame, and/or embarrassment but are also cautioned to avoid displacing such feelings on the child. For example, it is easy for parents to admonish the child with a statement, such as "We told you never to go with strangers," which makes the child feel responsible.

In cases of sexual abuse family members are advised to encourage the child to resume normal activities and to observe the child for signs of distress. Children express their feelings primarily through behavior. Parents should be alert for changes in behavior that indicate distress resulting from the incident, such as remaining in the house, refusing to go to school, changes in sleeping patterns, and frequency of dreams and nightmares. The child is encouraged to talk about these feelings and nightmares, since the more the child can talk about the experience, the more he will be able to gain control over it.

Referral. Referral to appropriate agencies is also essential. Most abusing parents tend to live in poverty, and the daily stresses imposed by their life-style are overwhelming. Resources for financial aid, improved housing, and child care should be sought. Self-help groups also provide important services. Such groups as **Parents Anonymous*** (a group for parents who have abused or fear that they may abuse their child, but only in terms of physical abuse, not sexual abuse) and **Parents United** and its adjunct, **Daughters and Sons United†** (both groups devoted to helping sexually abused families) are very accepting and nonjudgmental, because everyone has been in the same position.

Group peer pressure and commitment are important motivating factors that keep parents from reverting to previous behaviors. Parents Anonymous also provides a release mechanism because, when parents are angry, they can call a fellow member and vent their feelings over the phone rather than on the child.

Prevent Abuse

Prevention of child maltreatment has been an extremely difficult goal. Programs aimed at identifying potential abusers and instituting supportive intervention before the occurrence of an abusive act have met with variable success. However, nurses have played an important role in such programs. For example, prenatal and infancy home visiting by nurses to primiparas who were either teenagers, unmarried, or of low socioeconomic status resulted in significantly less reports of child abuse during the first two years (Olds and others, 1986). The nurses provided information on normal child growth and development and routine health care needs, served as informal support persons, and referred families to appropriate services when a need for assistance was identified.

Such programs provide models that can be used to reduce factors known to increase the risk of abuse. However, nurses in a variety of settings can implement similar activities. Nurses in prenatal clinics can prepare expectant families for the adjustment of parenthood. Nursery and postpartum nurses can foster the attachment process by encouraging parents to hold and look at their infant.

*7120 Franklin Ave., Los Angeles, CA 90046; call 1-800-421-0353.
†P.O. Box 952, San Jose, CA 95108; call 1-408-280-5055.

In neonatal intensive care units nurses can minimize the effects of separation by encouraging parents to visit and help them become comfortable in the child's care. Those in ambulatory settings can teach parents appropriate methods of bathing, feeding, toileting, disciplining, and preventing injuries, while stressing the normal needs and developmental characteristics of children. Nurses need to be sensitive to the parents' needs for attention, reassurance, and reinforcement. Nurses need to know what kinds of community services are available, including self-help groups, and make timely referrals.

Sexual abuse. Unlike preventive efforts for neglect and physical abuse, which have been aimed at the potential offender, prevention of child sexual abuse has centered on education of children to protect themselves and how to say "no." Parents have also been targets in terms of educating them on how to protect their children. Programs, such as fingerprinting of children and group discussion to help children learn the dangers of sexual exploitation, have become common, but there is little documentation of their effectiveness. The trend continues to be one of education, and the nurse is frequently in a position to discuss this topic with parents as part of health maintenance and to provide guidelines (see box). Numerous books are available to help parents prepare their child for sexual advances.* Helpful games such as "What if the baby-sitter wants to wrestle and hug but tells you to keep it a secret?" can be used to explore dangerous situations in advance and help children learn the importance of saying "no." They need reassurance that no matter what the other person says or does, the parents want to know and will not punish them. Even if the child does participate in the activity before telling the parents, he must be reassured that it was not his fault.

In addition, parents need to be made aware that "nice" people, including friends and relatives, can be offenders; parents should carefully observe how others act toward the child. A sudden change in the child's behavior and a response such as "I don't like uncle anymore" are clues to investigate the relationship. In the event of any doubt, further solitary encounters between this person and the child should be prevented. It is sometimes to the child's great misfortune that parents do not take certain comments seriously, such as "He hugs me too tight" or "I don't want to go with him." Casual parental statements such as "He just loves you" or "You do whatever adults tell you to do" can place children in jeopardy. Health professionals can alert parents to such dangers and guide them toward an appreciation of the problem, providing concrete guidelines toward child education and protection.

Guidelines for Preventing or Dealing with Sexual Abuse of Children

Sexual assault of children is much more common than most of us realize. It may be preventable if children have good preparation. *To provide protection and preparation,* as parents we can:
- Pay careful attention to who is around our children. (Unwanted touch *may* come from someone we like and trust.)
- Back up a child's right to say "No."
- Encourage communication by taking seriously what our children *say*.
- Take a second look at signals of potential danger.
- Refuse to leave our children in the company of those we do not trust.
- Include information about sexual assault when teaching about safety.
- Provide specific definitions and examples of sexual assault.
- Remind children that even "nice" people sometimes do mean things.
- Urge children to tell us about *anybody* who causes them to be uncomfortable.
- Prepare children to deal with bribes and threats, as well as possible physical force.
- Virtually eliminate secrets between us and our children.
- Teach children how to say "No," ask for help, and control who touches them and how.
- Model self-protective and limit-setting behavior for our children.

Should it ever become necessary *to help a child recover from a sexual assault,* as parents we can:
- Listen carefully and understand how children tell us.
- Support the child for telling by praise, belief, sympathy, lack of blame.
- Know local resources, and choose help carefully.
- Provide opportunities to talk about the assault.
- Provide opportunities for the entire family to go through a recovery process.

Sexual assault affects all of us, whether or not our own children are assaulted. *To help deal with this social problem,* all of us can:
- Provide sympathetic care and support to those who have been victimized.
- Recognize that offenders do not change without intervention.
- Organize neighborhood programs to support each other's efforts to protect children.
- Encourage schools to provide information about sexual assault as a problem of health and safety.
- Organize community groups to support educational, treatment, and law enforcement programs.

From Adams, C., and Fay, J.: *No more secrets: protecting your child from sexual assault*, San Luis Obispo, Calif., 1981, Impact Publishers, Inc.

Prevention of abuse must also include prevention of false allegations of abuse. Despite the fact that more than half of all reports are unsubstantiated, little attention has been directed to the problem of false accusations and its devastating consequences, such as removal of the child from the home, termination of parental rights, public ridicule of the family, loss of employment, and excessive legal fees to regain custody of the child. Nurses play a critical role in carefully documenting all evidence of abuse, giving alleged offenders the opportunity to present their

*A comprehensive listing of Child Sexual Abuse Prevention Resources is available for a fee of $2.00 from the National Committee for Prevention of Child Abuse, Publishing Dept., 332 S. Michigan Ave., Suite 950, Chicago, IL 60604-4357.

NURSING CARE PLAN

The Maltreated Child

Nursing Goals	Nursing Interventions	Expected Patient/Family Outcomes
HP-HMP* **Potential for trauma**		
Risk factors: characteristics of child, characteristics of caregiver(s), environmental characteristics		
Protect from further abuse	Perform physical assessment Assess emotional state and evaluate behaviors Implement measures to prevent abuse Report suspicions to appropriate authorities Assist in removing child from unsafe environment and establishing in a safe environment Establish protective measures for the hospitalized child as indicated Keep factual, objective records of: The child's physical condition The child's behavioral response to parents, others, and environment Interviews with family members Report suspected child abuse to local authorities	Suspected child abuse victim is removed from abusive environment
Prevent recurrence	Collaborate efforts of multidisciplinary team to continually evaluate progress of child in foster home or in return to own family Be alert for signs of continued abuse or neglect Help parents identify those circumstances that precipitate an abusive act and ways in which to deal with the release of anger in ways other than attacking child Refer for alternative placement when indicated	Signs of abuse or neglect are detected early and the child referred for appropriate intervention
Prevent abuse	Identify families at risk for potential abuse Promote parental attachment to child Emphasize childrearing practices, especially effective methods of discipline Increase parents' feeling of adequacy and self-esteem Encourage support systems that lessen stress and total responsibility for child care from one or both parents	Families exhibit evidence of positive interaction with children
SP-SCP **Anxiety**		
Etiology: interpersonal interaction and repeated abuse; powerlessness		
Provide consistent caregiver and therapeutic environment during hospitalization	Demonstrate acceptance of child while not expecting same in return Show attention while not reinforcing inappropriate behavior Plan appropriate activities for attention with nurse, other adults, and other children; use play to work through relationships Avoid displacing anger on child, such as shouting or yelling, as method of dealing with own frustration toward child's negative behavior Praise child's abilities in order to promote his self-esteem	Child exhibits minimal or no evidence of distress
Relieve anxiety in child	Treat child as one who has a specific physical problem for hospitalization, not as "abused" victim Avoid asking too many questions Use play, especially drawing or dolls, to investigate kinds of relationships perceived by child Provide one consistent person to whom child relates regarding events of abuse	Child appears calm and engages in positive relationships with caregivers

*For an explanation of abbreviations, see p. 20.

Continued.

NURSING CARE PLAN

The Maltreated Child—cont'd

Nursing Goals	Nursing Interventions	Expected Patient/Family Outcomes
NDA RRP **Altered or potential altered parenting** **Etiology: child, caregiver, or situational characteristics that precipitate abusive behavior**		
Support parents	Provide "mothering" by directing attention to parents, taking over child care responsibilities until parents feel ready to participate, and focusing on parents' needs	Parents demonstrate appropriate parenting activities
	Refer parents to Parents Anonymous (initially may need to attend with parents as their advocate) or Parents United	Parents seek group and individual support
	Help identify a support group for parents, such as extended family or nearby neighbors; help these significant others understand their important role in also preventing further abuse	
Teach parents	Teach realistic expectations of child's behavior and capabilities Emphasize alternate methods of discipline, such as reward and verbal disapproval Suggest methods of handling developmental problems or goals, such as toddler negativism, toilet training, and independence Teach through demonstration and role modeling, rather than lecture; avoid authoritarian approach	Parents demonstrate an understanding of normal expectations for their child
Lessen environmental crises	Refer to social agencies that can provide assistance in areas such as financial support, adequate housing, and employment	Parents receive assistance with problems
Promote a sense of parental adequacy during child's hospitalization	Orient parents to hospital unit and help them feel welcomed and an important part of child's care and recovery Reinforce competent child care activities Focus on the abuse as a problem that requires therapeutic intervention, not as a behavior characteristic or deficiency of the parents Emphathize with difficulties of rearing children, especially with additional life crises, while not condoning the act of abuse or neglect Foster healthy aspects of parent-child relationship	Parents demonstrate an attitude of concern for and ability to care for the child
Plan for discharge	Prepare for discharge as soon as disposition is finalized Home placement: Encourage parents to visit as much as possible during hospitalization Plan for close supervision and counseling of family	Parents demonstrate ability and desire to care for child Child is placed in appropriate environment
	Foster home placement: Encourage foster family members to visit child before discharge Stress to them child's need to regress in order to complete missed stages of development Help child grieve this loss, if parents' rights are being terminated permanently, especially if it entails separation from siblings (long-term counseling is optimum goal)	Child accepts foster parents

Nursing interventions related to medical management

Determine extent of injuries
Assist with diagnostic procedures

account of the incident, and recognizing diseases or cultural practices that may be confused with abuse (Wong, 1987). In the unfortunate event that a family is wrongly accused of abuse, they may benefit from the services of **Victims of Child Abuse Laws (VOCAL)**,* a support group for persons who have experienced false accusations.

EVALUATION

The effectiveness of nursing interventions is determined by continual reassessment and evaluation of care based on the following observational guidelines and expected outcomes:

1. Observe the child for additional physical and behavioral evidence of abuse; observe child's reactions to health professionals; if the child is hospitalized, check staffing patterns for schedule of consistent group of nurses caring for child
2. Interview parents regarding their knowledge of children's physical and development needs
3. Investigate community programs aimed at preventing child maltreatment

Expected outcomes:
See Nursing Care Plan, pp. 419 to 420.

SUMMARY

During early childhood youngsters are vulnerable to a number of communicable and infectious diseases. Their normal hand-mouth activity, inquisitiveness, and lack of awareness of danger increase the likelihood of ingesting injurious substances, such as poisons. They are also the most likely age-group for experiencing neglect or physical abuse, and a substantial number of young children are also victims of sexual abuse.

Parents are often inexperienced in caring for the sick child at home, in preventing injuries from toxic ingestions, or in coping with the numerous demands of an active toddler or preschooler. Nurses can provide valuable assistance in all of these areas and can prevent devastating consequences from repeated poisonings or maltreatment.

*P.O. Box 1135, Minneapolis, MN 55411.

KEY CONCEPTS

- Common infectious disorders during early childhood include communicable diseases, intestinal parasitic infections, and conjunctivitis.
- Nursing goals in the treatment of a communicable disease are identification, prevention of transmission, provision of comfort, and prevention of complications.
- Intestinal parasitic diseases constitute the most common infections in the world, giardiasis and enterobiasis being the most widespread parasitic infections among children in the United States.
- Although the incidence of poisoning has decreased in the last 15 years as a result of more stringent packaging regulations, childhood poisoning remains a serious health concern.
- The major principles of emergency treatment for poisoning are assessment, supportive measures, gastric decontamination, family support, and prevention of recurrence.
- The most frequently ingested poisons are cleaning substances, drugs (especially acetaminophen), plants, cosmetics, and hydrocarbons.
- Potential sources of heavy metal poisoning are lead, iron from medicinal supplements, and mercury from seafood and thermometers (only inhaled).
- Lead ingestion may be attributed to environmental factors, specific characteristics of the child, and parental characteristics. Health professionals have a major responsibility to educate parents regarding these factors.
- Child maltreatment may take the form of physical abuse or neglect, emotional abuse or neglect, and sexual abuse.
- Parental, child, and environmental characteristics are criteria that may predispose children to maltreatment.
- Identification of abuse entails securing evidence of maltreatment, taking a history pertaining to the incident, and assessing parental and child behaviors.
- The reported incidence of sexual abuse has increased in the last decade; common forms are incest, molestation, rape, exhibitionism, child pornography, child prostitution, and pedophilia.

STUDY QUESTIONS AND ACTIVITIES

1 Visit a daycare center and inquire about the types of illnesses that are most common among children 1 to 5 years of age.
2 Observe the sanitary practices in a daycare center that are likely to prevent transmission of parasites. Note any preventive measures that are not being employed.
3 Visit an old part of town and look for sources of lead in the environment. What measures could be used to delead the building?
4 Plan a schedule for rotation of injection sites for a child who must receive a total of 60 injections as part of chelation therapy.
5 Call a poison control center and inquire about the most common and the most serious poisons reported in young children. Ask if there has been a change in the pattern of poisonings over the past 5 years in this age-group.
6 Interview a hospital social worker or a caseworker in the Child Protective Services of your local welfare department regarding the types and severity of reported abuse cases. Inquire about the process of investigating these reports.
7 Attend a meeting of a local abuse support group and observe the kinds of services they provide their members.

REFERENCES

Altemeier, W.A., and others: Antecedents of child abuse, J. Pediatr. **100**(5):823-829, 1982.

Bellinger, D., and others: Longitudinal analysis of prenatal and postnatal lead exposure and early cognitive development, N. Engl. J. Med. **17:**1037-1043, 1987.

Bithoney, W.G., and others: Childhood ingestions as symptoms of family distress, Am. J. Dis. Child. **139**(3):456-459, 1985.

Coleman, L.: False allegations of child sexual abuse: have the experts been caught with their pants down?, Forum, p. 12-21, Jan./Feb. 1986.

Committee on Environmental Hazards and Committee on Accident and Poison Prevention: Statement on childhood lead poisoning, Pediatrics **79**(3):457-465, 1987.

Coulehan, J.L., and others: Gasoline sniffing and lead toxicity in Navajo adolescents, Pediatrics **71**(1):113-117, 1983.

Grbcich, P.A., and others: Expired ipecac syrup efficacy, Pediatrics **78**(6):1085-1089, 1986.

Highlights of official child neglect and abuse reporting 1985, Denver, 1987, The American Humane Association.

Hunt, T.J., Hepner, R., and Seaton, K.W.: Childhood lead poisoning and inadequate health care, Am. J. Dis. Child. **136:**538-542, 1982.

Kempe, R.S., and Kempe, C.H.: The common secret: sexual abuse of children and adolescents, New York, 1984, W.H. Freeman & Co. Publishers.

Kotelchuck, M.: Child abuse and neglect, prediction and misclassification. In Starr, R.H., editor: Child abuse prediction policy implications, Cambridge, MA, 1982, Ballinger Publishing Co.

Litovitz, T.L., Martin, T.G., and Schmitz, B.: 1986 Annual report of the American Association of Poison Control Centers National Data Collection System, Am. J. Emerg. Medicine **5**(5):405-434, 1987.

Olds, D.L., and others: Preventing child abuse and neglect: a randomized trial of nurse home visitation, Pediatrics **78**(1):65-78, 1986.

Spencer, M.J., and Dunklee, P.: Sexual abuse of boys, Pediatrics **78**(1):133-138, 1986.

Weber, S.: Munchausen syndrome by proxy, J. Pediatr. Nurs. **2**(1):50-54, 1987.

Wong, D.L.: False allegations of child abuse: the other side of the tragedy, Pediatr. Nurs. **13**(5):329-333, 1987.

BIBLIOGRAPHY

Communicable Diseases/Conjunctivitis

American Academy of Pediatrics: Report of the Committee on Infectious Diseases, ed. 20, Elk Grove Village, IL, 1986, The Academy.

Benenson, A.S., editor: Control of communicable diseases in man, ed. 14, Washington, DC, 1985, The American Public Health Association.

Fisher, M.C.: Conjunctivitis in children, Pediatr. Clin. North Am. **34**(6):1447-1456, 1987.

Fleming, J.W.: How to differentiate dermatologic conditions—often confusing and difficult—in infants and school-age children, MCN **6**(5):346-354, 1981.

Hammerschlag, M.: Conjunctivitis in infancy and childhood, Pediatr. Rev. **5**(9):285-290, 1984.

Hayman, L.L.: Varicella, Nursing 83 **13**(4):41, 1983.

Holderman, M.: Skin problems: a guide for making "rash" decisions, Nursing 84 **14**(11):22-23, 1984.

Krugman, S., and others: Infectious diseases of children, ed. 8, St. Louis, 1985, The C.V. Mosby Co.

Labson, L.H.: Doctor, I can't stand this itching! Patient Care **18**(17):89-121, 1984.

Madden, E.J.: Starting from scratch, Am. J. Nurs. **86**(7):846, 1986.

Relief for that persistent itch, Patient Care **18**(17):185, 1984.

Intestinal Parasitic Infection

Bonner, A., and Dale, R.: Giardia lamblia, Am. J. Nurs. **86**(7):818-820, 1986.

Carroll, M.J.: Routine procedures for examination of stool and blood for parasites, Pediatr. Clin. North Am. **32**(4): 1041-1046, 1985.

Getting rid of pinworms, roundworms, scabies mites, or lice, Patient Care **18**(17):189-190, 1984.

Henley, M., and Sears, J.R.: Pinworms: a persistent pediatric problem, MCN **10**(6):111-113, 1985.

Kuntz, R.E.: Parasites of children in the United States, Pediatr. Nurs. **5**(6):12-17, 1979.

Malarkay, L.M.: Ridding schoolchildren of parasites—a community approach, MCN **4:**363-366, 1979.

Sears, J.R.: To prevent reinfestation (letters to the editor), MCN **10**(6):377, 1985.

Seidel, J.S.: Treatment of parasitic infections, Pediatr. Clin. North Am. **32**(4):1077-1095, 1985.

Silverman, A., and Roy, C.: Pediatric clinical gastroenterology, ed. 3, St. Louis, 1983, The C.V. Mosby Co.

Poisoning

Arena, J.M.: Prevention of poisoning in children, Public Health Curr. **23**(1):1-4, 1983.

Barber, J.M.: Acute salicylate poisoning, Emerg. Nurs. Update Series **1**(22), Princeton, NJ, 1982, Continuing Professional Education Center.

Driggers, D.A., and Johnson, R.: Initial management of pediatric poisoning, Pediatr. Basics **35:**4-6, 1983.

Foster, S.D.: In case of an emergency: ipecac syrup, MCN **7**(4):227, 1982.

Gillies, C.: Management of pediatric poisoning, role of the nurse practitioner, Pediatr. Nurs. **6**(5):33-35, 1980.

Holbrook, M.L.: Child poisonings, Pediatr. Basics **41:**13-15, 1985.

Keim, K.A.: Preventing and treating plant poisonings in young children, MCN **8**(4):287-289, 1983.

King, R.C.: Dealing with poisonings, RN **47**(12):45-48, 1984.

Leoni, M.P.: Management of acetaminophen overdose, Crit. Care Nurse **5**(4):44-47, 1985.

Lovejoy, F.: Management of pediatric poisoning. Part I. Pediatr. Nurs. **6**(5):37-39, 1980.

Manoguerra, A.S.: Assessment and management of poisonings, Emer. Nurs. Update Series **2**(3), Princeton, NJ, 1981, Continuing Professional Education Center.

McGuigan, M.A.: Chronic salicylate poisoning: when therapy turns into intoxication, Pediatr. Consult **2**(3):1-8, 1983.

Ogzewalla, C.D., Bonfiglio, J.F., and Sigell, L.T.: Common plants and their toxicity, Pediatr. Clin. North Am. **34**(6):1557-1598, 1987.

Parks, B.R., and Fischer, R.G.: Misuse of syrup of ipecac, Pediatr. Nurs. **13**(4):261, 1987.

Shinn, A.F.: Poison control potpourri, Crit. Care Update, **10**(6):11, 1983.

Temple, A.: Management of pediatric poisoning. Part II. Pediatr. Nurs. **6**(5):40-43, 1980.

Wall, C.: The real risk of acetaminophen overdose, RN **48**(8):35-38, 1985.

Heavy Metal Poisoning

Banner, W., Jr., and Tong, T.G.: Iron poisoning, Pediatr. Clin. North Am. **33**(2):393-409, 1986.

Burdick, M.P., and Harris, V.G.: Prevention of lead poisoning in children, Public Health Curr. **24**(3):11-14, 1984.

Drummond, A.H., Jr.: Lead poisoning in children, J. Sch. Health **51**(1):43-47, 1981.

Erler, M.: Iron poisoning, J. Emerg. Nurs. **6**(2):40-42, 1980.

Galazka, S.S.: Lead poisoning in children: a multidimensional hazard, Pediatr. Basics **36:**4-6, 1983.

Langner, B., and Modrcin-McCarthy, M.A.: Lead poisoning: an ongoing pediatric nursing concern, Issues Compr. Pediatr. Nurs. **4**(3):23-36, 1980.

Miller, S.J.: Nursing care of the lead-burdened child: a problem oriented approach, Pediatr. Nurs. **7**(5):47-52, 1981.

Pearce, J., and Burg, F.D.: Lead poisoning in children, Drug Ther. **12**(5):87-102, 1982.

Robotham, J.L., and Lietman, P.S.: Acute iron poisoning: a review, Am. J. Dis. Child. **134**(9):875-879, 1980.

Rudner, N.: Children with elevated lead levels, J. Pediatr. Health Care **2**(1):46-49, 1988.

Child Maltreatment

Bergman, A.B., Larsen, R.M., and Mueller, B.A.: Changing spectrum of serious child abuse, Pediatrics **77**(1):113-116, 1986.

Besharov, D.J.: "Doing something" about child abuse: the need to narrow the grounds for state intervention, Harvard J. Law and Pub. Policy **8**(3):539-589, 1985.

Bottom, W., and Lancaster, J.: An ecological orientation toward human abuse, Fam. Community Health **4**(2):1-10, 1981.

Carley, L.: Helping the helpless: the abused child, Nursing 85 **15**(11):34-38, 1985.

Carley, L.: Reaching Julie—with a gentle touch, Nursing 87 **17**(2):39-40, 1987.

Christensen, M.L., Schommer, B.L., and Velasquez, J.: An interdisciplinary approach to preventing child abuse, MCN **9**(2):108-112, 1984.

Council on Scientific Affairs: AMA diagnostic and treatment guidelines concerning child abuse and neglect, JAMA **254** (6):796-800, 1985.

Ellerstein, N.S., editor: Child abuse and neglect: a medical reference, New York, 1981, John Wiley & Sons, Inc.

Elvik, S.L.: From disclosure to court: the facets of sexual abuse, J. Pediatr. Health Care **1**(3):136-140, 1987.

Flynn, E.M.: Preventing and diagnosing sexual abuse in children, Nurse Pract. **12**(2):47-65, 1987.

Fore, C.V., and Holmes, S.S.: Sexual abuse of children, Nurs. Clin. North Am. **19**(2):329-340, 1984.

Gelles, R.J., and Cornell, C.P.: Intimate violence in families, Beverly Hills, CA, 1985, Sage Publications, Inc.

Heindl, M.C., editor: Child abuse and neglect, Nurs. Clin. North Am. **16**(1):101-188, 1981.

Hosch, I.A.: Munchausen syndrome by proxy, MCN **12**(1):48-52, 1987.

Hurwitz, A., and Castells, S.: Misdiagnosed child abuse and metabolic disease, Pediatr. Nurs. **13**(1):33-36, 1987.

Hurwitz, S.: Child abuse: the signs may be only skin deep, Child Care Newsletter **4**(2):1-3, 1985.

Kauffman, C.K., Neill, M.K., and Thomas, J.N.: The abusive parent. In Johnson, S.J., editor: Nursing assessment and strategies for the family at risk, ed. 2, Philadelphia, 1986, J.B. Lippincott Co.

Kelley, S.J.: Drawings: critical communications for sexually abused children, Pediatr. Nurs. **11**(6):421-426, 1985.

Kelley, S.J.: Learned helplessness in the sexually abused child, Issues Compr. Pediatr. Nurs. **9:**193-207, 1986.

Kempe, C.H., and Helfer, R.E., editors: The battered child, ed. 3, Chicago, 1982, University of Chicago Press.

Ledray, L.: Victims of incest, Am. J. Nurs. **84**(8): 1010-1014, 1984.

McKittrick, C.A.: Child abuse: recognition and reporting by health professionals, Nurs. Clin. North Am. **16**(1):103-115, 1981.

Mittleman, R., Mittleman, H., and Wetli, C.: What child abuse really looks like, Am. J. Nurs. **87**(9):1185-1188, 1987.

Miller, E.L.: Interviewing the sexually abused child, MCN **10:**103-105, 1985.

Mulvihill, D.L.: Between parent and child, Can. Nurse **83**(2):12-15, 1987.

Newberger, E.H.: Understanding child abuse, Child Care Newsletter **1:**3-6, 1981.

Rhodes, A.M.: Identifying and reporting child abuse, MCN **12**(6):399, 1987.

Robertson, K.E., and Wilson-Walker, J.A.: A program for preventing sexual abuse of children, MCN **10**(2):100-102, 1985.

Ryan, M.T.: Identifying the sexually abused child, Pediatr. Nurs. **10**(6):419-421, 1984.

Schanberger, J.E.: Inflicted burns in children, Top. Emerg. Med. **3:**85-92, 1981.

Snyder, J.C., Hampton, R., and Newberger, E.H.: Family dysfunction: violence, neglect, and sexual misuse. In Levine, M.D., and others, editors: Developmental-behavioral pediatrics, Philadelphia, 1983, W.B. Saunders Co.

Sykes, M.K., and others: Nurses' knowledge of child abuse and nurses' attitudes toward parental participation in the abused child's care, J. Pediatr. Nurs. **2**(6):412-417, 1987.

Turner, R.J., and Avison, W.R.: Assessing risk factors for problem parenting: the significance of social support, J. Marriage Fam. **47**(4):881-892, 1985.

Velasquez, J., Christensen, M.L., and Schommer, B.L.: Intensive services help prevent child abuse, MCN **9**(2):113-117, 1984.

UNIT

VII

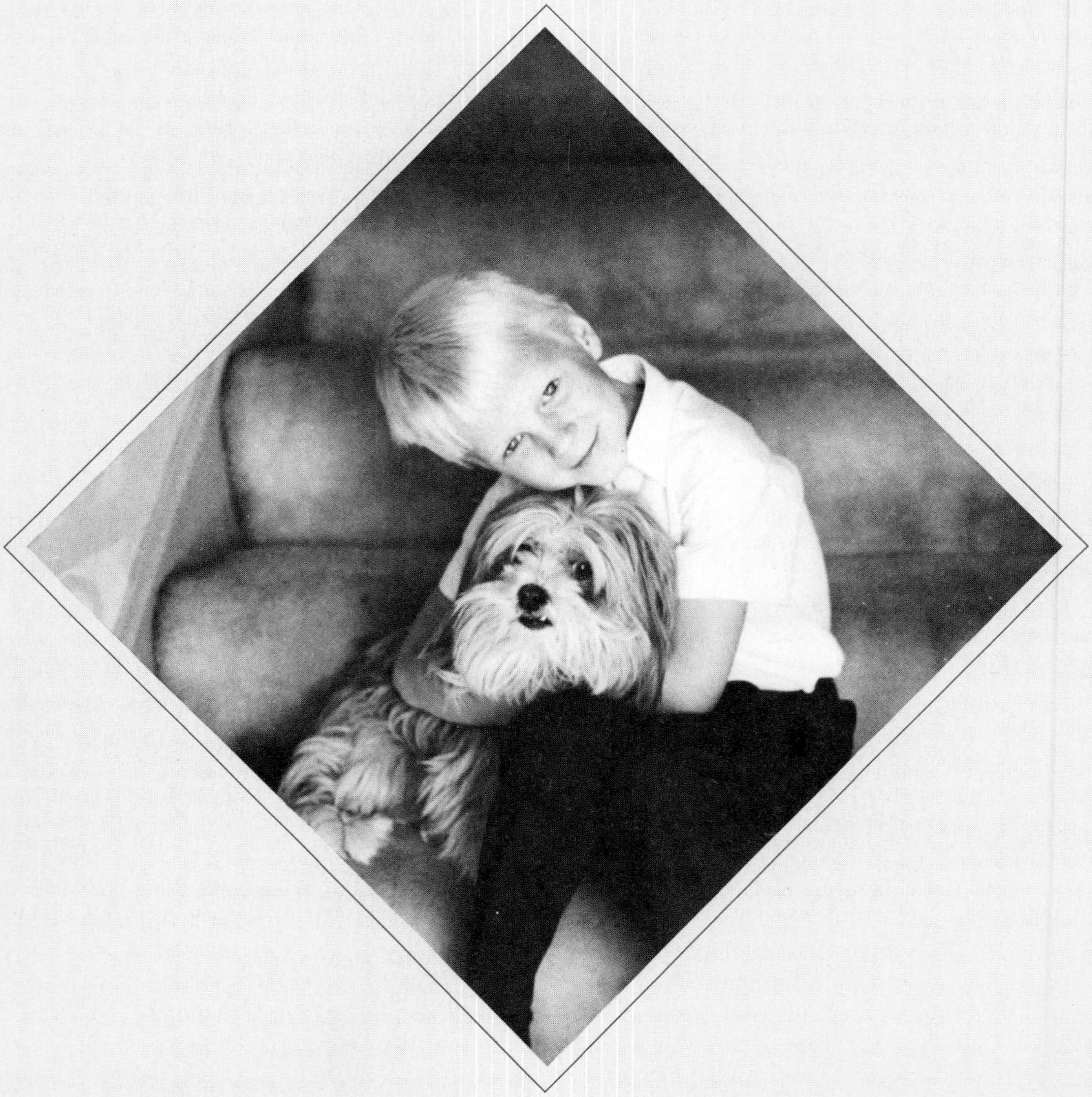

Middle Childhood and Adolescence

Children in the middle childhood years enjoy a relatively stable period of slow but steady growth and maturation with few physical or emotional stresses. It is a comfortable time of adjustment with a developmental pace sufficiently slow to meet the physical and psychologic demands placed on them. It is a period of broadening horizons when children encounter a wider sphere of influence—school, peers, and multiple opportunities for social interaction. During this time children learn the fundamental skills of their culture and develop inner resources for coping with larger social units. The emphasis is on competence in physical and mental tasks and on the equally important changes in social relationships.

Adolescence is a period of transition that is based on childhood experiences and accomplishments and that has a goal of mature, independent, and responsible functioning. This transition is a biologic, emotional, and social process, a preparatory period requiring the accomplishment of defined developmental tasks in order to attain satisfactory adjustment to adulthood. The early years of adolescence are concerned with individuation from previous dependency roles and a gradual movement toward peer-group identity. The peer group is the focus of the adolescent's world—the persons in his life who are going through the same transition and who understand the problems and frustrations he is experiencing. Later years of adolescence are centered around acquiring a personal identity, completing the separation process from family, and career-directed activity.

Chapter 15, *Health Promotion of the School-Age Child and Family,* provides a brief overview of the developmental changes that take place in middle childhood, including a lengthy summary of the major characteristics of each age within the period of middle childhood. Chapter 16, *Health Promotion of the Adolescent and Family,* provides an overview of the transitional adolescent period during which youth must adjust to rapid body changes, establish a personal identity, gain emotional and (for some) economic freedom from their parents, and evolve a set of values uniquely their own. Chapter 17, *Health Problems of Middle Childhood and Adolescence,* outlines the more common health problems encountered during these years. Few major illnesses are associated with middle childhood, although children during this time are still subject to many of the problems that characterize the earlier childhood years, and, with the wider social relationships, communicable diseases continue to be prevalent. Health problems associated with adolescence result from either the changes related to biologic maturation or the psychologic adjustments imposed by these changes and the expectations of society.

CHAPTER 15

Health Promotion of the School-Age Child and Family

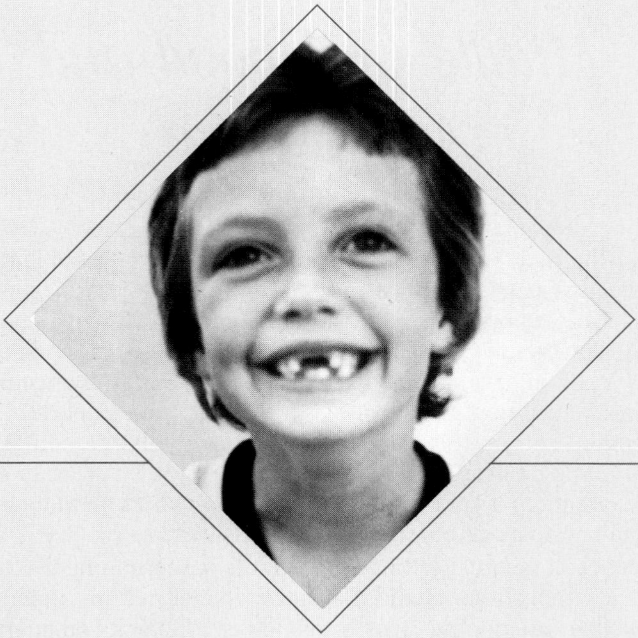

LEARNING OBJECTIVES

On completion of this chapter the reader will be able to:

- Describe the physical, cognitive, and moral changes that take place during the middle childhood years
- Describe ways to assist a child in developing a sense of accomplishment
- Demonstrate an understanding of the changing interpersonal relationships of the school-age child
- Discuss the role of the peer group in the socialization of the school-age child
- Discuss the role of schools in the development and socialization of the school-age child
- Outline an appropriate health teaching plan for the school-age child
- Plan a sex education session for a group of school-age children
- Identify the causes and discuss the preventive aspects of injury in middle childhood

The segment of the life span that extends from age 6 years to approximately age 12 years has been tagged with a variety of labels, each of which describes an important characteristic of the period. These middle years are most often referred to as *school-age* or the *school years*. This period begins with entrance into the wider sphere of influence represented by the school environment, which has a significant impact on development and relationships. The term *gang age* describes the child's affiliation with age-mates and learning the culture of childhood. With peer groups children establish the first close relationships outside the family group. From a psychoanalytic point of view, this is the period of *latency,* which has been considered to be a time of sexual tranquility between the Oedipal phase of early childhood and the eroticism of adolescence. It is during this time that children experience the intimacy of relationships with same-sex peers, following the indifference of earlier years and preceding the heterosexual fascination that accompanies the changes of puberty.

◆ *Promoting Optimum Growth and Development*

Physiologically the middle years begin with the shedding of the first deciduous tooth and end at puberty with the acquisition of the final permanent teeth (with the exception of the wisdom teeth). During the preceding 5 to 6 years, the child has progressed from a helpless infant to a sturdy, complicated individual with the capacity to communicate, conceptualize in a limited way, and become involved in complex social and motor behavior. Physical growth has been equally rapid. In contrast, the period of middle childhood, between the rapid growth of early childhood and the turmoil of the prepubescent growth spurt, is a time of gradual growth and development with steadier and more even progress in both its physical and emotional aspects. Physical health is generally good, and it is a comfortable period of physical adjustment. Physiologic processes in general have attained a stage of development that permits their maintenance at stable levels under ordinary conditions and their ready adjustment to changing needs and stresses. Under normal circumstances these children are usually well able to meet the physical and psychologic demands that are placed on them.

With a firm foundation of trust, autonomy, and initiative, the child is ready and eager for the wider world of learning and competition associated with developing a sense of industry. The child moves from the egocentricity of early childhood to the subperiod of cognitive domain described as concrete operations. Until recently middle childhood has generated the least interest and preoccupation among psychologists and others concerned with the effects of childhood experiences on later adjustments. However, it has been found that this period makes an important contribution to the child's learning the fundamental skills of his culture and the development of competence and self-esteem. It is a time of intellectual growth, investment in work, and the first real commitment to a social unit outside of and larger than the family.

BIOLOGIC DEVELOPMENT

During middle childhood growth in height and weight assumes a slower but steady pace as compared with the earlier years and the years immediately ahead. Between ages 6 and 12 years, children will grow an average of 5 cm (2 inches) per year to gain 30 to 60 cm (1 to 2 feet) in height and will almost double in weight, increasing 2 to 3 kg (4½ to 6½ pounds) per year. The average 6-year-old child is about 116 cm (45 inches) tall and weighs about 21 kg (46 pounds); the average 12-year-old child stands about 150 cm (59 inches) tall and weighs approximately 40 kg (88 pounds). During this age period girls and boys differ very little in size, although boys tend to be slightly taller and somewhat heavier than girls. Toward the end of the school-age years both boys and girls begin to increase in size, although most girls begin to surpass boys in both height and weight (to the acute discomfort of both).

Proportional Changes

School-age children are more graceful than they were as preschoolers, and they are steadier on their feet. Their body proportions take on a slimmer look, with longer legs, varying body proportion, and a lower center of gravity. Posture improves over that of the preschool period to facilitate locomotion and efficiency in using the arms and trunk. These proportions make climbing, bicycle riding, and other activities much easier. Fat gradually diminishes and its distribution patterns change, contributing to the thinner appearance of the child during the middle years.

Accompanying the skeletal lengthening and fat diminution is an increase in the percentage of body weight represented by muscle tissue. By the end of this age period, both boys and girls will double their strength and physical capabilities and their steady and relatively consistent acquisition of refined coordination will increase their poise and skill. However, this increased strength can be misleading. Although strength increases, muscles are still functionally immature when compared with those of the adolescent, and they are more readily damaged by muscular injury caused by overuse.

The most pronounced changes, and those that seem best to indicate increasing maturity in children, are a decrease in head circumference in relation to standing height, a decrease in waist circumference in relation to height, and an increase in leg length related to height. These observations often provide a clue to a child's degree of maturity that has proved useful in predicting his readiness for meeting the demands of school. There appears to be a correlation between physical indications of maturity and success in school.

Facial changes. Certain physiologic and anatomic characteristics are typical of children in the years of middle childhood. Facial proportions change as the face grows faster in relation to the remainder of the cranium. The skull and brain grow very slowly during this period and increase little in size thereafter. Since all of the primary (deciduous) teeth are lost during this age span, middle childhood is sometimes known as the *age of the loose tooth* and the early years of middle childhood as the *ugly duckling stage,* when the new secondary (permanent) teeth appear to be much too large for the face.

Maturation of Systems

Development of all body systems continues during middle childhood to become more efficient and adultlike in function. Maturity of the gastrointestinal system is reflected in fewer stomach upsets, better maintenance of blood sugar levels, and an increased stomach capacity, which permits retention of food for longer periods of time. The school-age child does not need to be fed as carefully, as promptly, or as frequently as before. Caloric needs in relation to stomach size are less than they were in the preschool years and less than they will be during the coming adolescent growth spurt.

Physical maturation is evidenced in other body tissues and organs. Bladder capacity, although differing widely among individual children, is generally greater in girls than in boys. The heart grows more slowly during the middle years and is smaller in relation to the rest of the body than at any other period of life. The heart and respiratory rates steadily decrease and the blood pressure increases during the ages from 6 to 12 years (see inside front cover).

The shape of the eye changes during growth and approaches its adult size during childhood. The normal farsightedness of the preschool child gradually changes to more nearly normal during childhood. To aid vision throughout the school years, large print is recommended for reading matter and regular vision testing should be a part of the school health program.

Bones continue to ossify throughout childhood, but, since mineralization is not completed until maturity, bones resist pressure and muscle pull less than mature bones. Consequently, care must be taken to prevent alterations in bone structure, such as providing well-fitted shoes and seeing that chairs and desks allow correct sitting posture, with the feet able to reach the floor and the hips able to fit well back in the seat. Children should have ample opportunity to move around, and they should observe appropriate caution in carrying heavy loads. For example, they should shift books from one arm to the other, and those who carry tote bags slung from the shoulders should alternate the load from one shoulder to the other to avoid developing a low shoulder or spine curvature.

There are wider differences between children at the end of middle childhood than at the beginning; such differences are sometimes striking. These differences become increasingly apparent and, if extreme or unique, may create emotional problems unless the associated characteristics of height and weight relationships, rapid or slow growth, and other important features of development are recognized and explained to children and their families. Also, physical maturity is not necessarily correlated with emotional and social maturity. The 7-year-old child who looks like a 10-year-old child will, in fact, think and act like a 7-year-old child. To expect behavior appropriate for a 10-year-old child from him is unrealistic and can be detrimental to his development of competence and self-esteem. Conversely, to treat a 10-year-old as though he were 7 years old is an equal disservice to the child.

Prepubescence

Toward the end of middle childhood the discrepancies in growth and maturation between boys and girls begin to be apparent. On the average there is a difference of approximately 2 years between girls and boys in the age of onset of pubescence. This is a period of rapid growth, especially for girls; for boys (and some girls, too) it is generally a period of steady growth in height and weight.

There is no universal age at which children assume the characteristics of preadolescence. The first physiologic signs begin to appear at about 9 years of age (particularly in girls) and are usually clearly evident in 11- to 12-year-old children. Although the preadolescent child does not want to be different, at this age the variability in physical growth and physiologic changes between children of the same sex, between the two sexes, and even within each individual child is often striking. This variability, especially in relation to the onset of secondary sexual characteristics, is of utmost concern to the preadolescent. Either early or late appearance of these characteristics is a source of embarrassment and uneasiness to both sexes.

Preadolescence is a time when there is a good deal of overlapping of developmental characteristics with elements of both middle childhood and early adolescence. However, there is a sufficient number of unique characteristics to set this period apart as an age category, even with the wide range of variability in the ages 11 and 12 years (or even 9 to 13 years in some children). Generally, the earliest age at which puberty begins is 10 years in girls and 12 years in boys, although there has been an increase in the number of girls reaching puberty at 9 years of age. The average age of puberty in girls is 12 years, and for boys it is 14 years. Boys experience little visible sexual maturation during preadolescence.

PSYCHOSOCIAL DEVELOPMENT

There is no concept more difficult to assess or more elusive than that of the personality or the "self." Personality is reflected in the way in which the child reacts to himself and others, the way in which others react to him, and the way in which he adjusts to his environment. Development of the personality involves a number of different types of development—physical, intellectual, social, emotional—all of which are profoundly influenced by the environment in which the child grows and develops.

Personality Development (Freud)

Middle childhood is the period in psychosexual development that Freud has described as the *latency period*. He maintained that this time of life involves consolidation and elaboration of previously acquired traits and skills with the assumption that no new significant conflicts or impulses will arise. Growth and development patterns follow the lines established in earlier stages. The primary personality development is that of the superego. It is a time of preparation for the important and dramatic psychosexual changes that take place during the genital stage of adolescence.

Developing a Sense of Accomplishment (Erikson)

Successful mastery of Erikson's first three stages of psychosocial development is probably the most important accomplishment in terms of development of a healthy personality (see p. 00). Successful completion of these stages implies that a child has attained confidence in an environment of loving relationships within a stable family unit that has prepared him to engage in experiences and relationships beyond this intimate group.

It has been suggested that the individual's fundamental attitude toward work is established during middle childhood. A sense of industry, for which a more descriptive term is the *stage of accomplishment,* is achieved somewhere between age 6 years and adolescence. It involves an eagerness for building skills and participating in meaningful and socially useful work. It is acquired through the process of education—formal and self-directed. Interests expand in the middle years and, with a growing sense of independence, the child wants to engage in tasks that can be carried through to completion. Children gain a great deal of satisfaction from independent behavior in exploring and manipulating their environment and from interaction with peers. Extrinsic sources of reinforcement in the form of grades, material rewards, additional privileges, and recognition provide encouragement and stimulation. Peer approval is a strong motivating power.

A sense of accomplishment also involves the ability to cooperate and to compete with others—to cope more effectively with people. Middle childhood is the time when children learn the value of doing things alongside and with others and the benefits derived from division of labor in the accomplishment of goals.

The danger inherent in this period of personality development is the imposition of situations that might result in a sense of inadequacy or inferiority. This may happen if the previous stages have not been successfully achieved or if the child is incapable of or unprepared for assuming the responsibilities associated with developing a sense of accomplishment. Feelings of inferiority or lack of worth can be derived from the child himself or from the social environment. However, no child is able to do well in everything, and children must learn that they will not be able to master each skill that they attempt. All children, even children who in most instances have positive attitudes toward work and their own capabilities, will feel some degree of inferiority in regard to a specific skill that they cannot master.

Children need and want real achievement. When they have access to tasks that need to be done, that they are able to do well despite individual differences in their innate capacities and emotional development, and for which they are suitably rewarded, children will be able to achieve a sense of industry and accomplishment (Erikson, 1963).

COGNITIVE DEVELOPMENT (PIAGET)

Somewhere around the beginning of the school years, children begin to acquire the ability to relate a series of events and actions to mental representations that can be expressed both verbally and symbolically. This is the stage in development that Piaget describes as *concrete operations,* during which the child is able to use his thought processes to experience events and actions. His rigid, egocentric outlook is replaced by thought processes that allow him to see things from the point of view of another.

During this stage the child develops an understanding and use for relationships between things and ideas. He progresses from making judgments based on what he sees (perceptual) to making judgments based on what he reasons (conceptual). He is increasingly able to master symbols and to use his memory store of past experiences in evaluating and interpreting the present.

One of the major cognitive tasks of the school-age child is mastering the concept of *conservation.* Early (about 5 to 6 years) he grasps the concept of reversibility of numbers as a basis for simple mathematic problems (for example, $2 + 4 = 6$ and $6 - 4 = 2$). He learns that certain properties of the environment are not changed simply by altering their disposition in space, and he becomes able to resist perceptual cues that suggest such alterations in the physical state of an object. For example, he recognizes that changing the shape of a substance such as a lump of clay does not alter its total mass. He no longer perceives a tall, thin glass of water as containing a greater volume than a short, wide glass; he can distinguish between the weight of items regardless of their size. He recognizes that size is not necessarily related to weight or volume. There appears to be a developmental sequence in the child's capacity to conserve matter. Conservation of mass usually is accomplished earliest (7 to 8 years), weight some time later (9 to 10 years), and volume last (11 to 12 years).

The school-age child now has the ability to classify, to place things in a sensible and logical order, to group and sort, and, in doing so, to hold a concept in his mind while he makes decisions based on that concept. It is characteristic of middle childhood that children derive a great deal of enjoyment from classifying and ordering their environment. They become occupied with numerous and varied collections of objects, such as wrappers, stamps, shells, dolls, cars, stones, and anything that is classifiable (Fig. 15-1). They even begin to order friends and relationships, such as first best friend, second best friend, and so on.

They develop the ability to understand relational terms

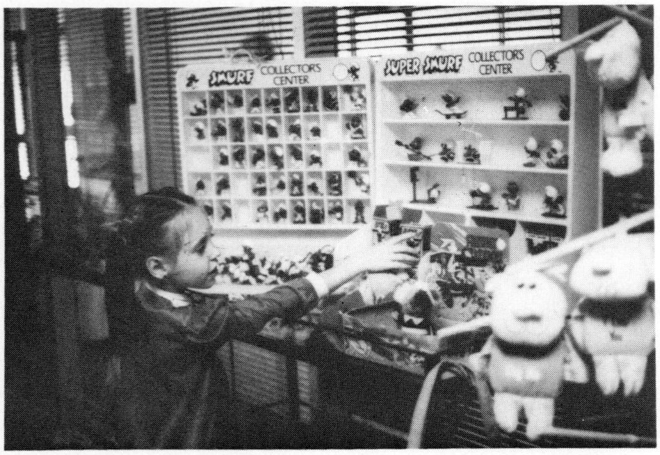

FIG. 15-1 School-age children are often avid collectors.

and concepts, such as bigger and smaller; darker and paler; heavier and lighter; to the right of and to the left of; first, last, and intermediate relationships (fourth, second, and so on); and more than and less than. They can see family relationships in terms of reciprocal roles—for example, in order to be a brother, one must have a sibling.

They learn the alphabet and the ever-widening world of symbols called words that can be arranged in terms of structure and their relationship to the alphabet. They learn to tell time, to see the relationship of events in time (history) and places in space (geography), and to combine time and space relationships (geology and astronomy).

The most significant skill, the ability to read, is acquired during the school years and becomes the most valuable tool for independent inquiry. The child's capacity for exploration, imagination, and expansion of knowledge is enhanced by the ability to read, as he progresses from the repetition and confusion of early efforts to increasing facility and comprehension.

DEVELOPING A SELF-CONCEPT

Closely associated with developing a sense of industry is developing a concept of one's value and worth. At first a child's self-concept is formed exclusively from what he perceives to be his parents' evaluation of him. During middle childhood the opinions of peers and teachers provide further input. The difficulty that children encounter in the attempt to assess their own abilities is their inclination to rely on their own expectations or on the expectations expressed by others regarding their performance. A child's self-concept is composed of his own critical self-assessment plus what he interprets as the opinions of members of his family and outside social contacts.

The significant adults in a child's life can often manage, unseen, to manipulate the child's environment so that he meets with success. Each small success increases the child's self-image a little. The more positive he feels about himself, the more confident he feels in trying again for success. Every child profits from a feeling that he is in some way special to a significant adult. A positive self-concept makes him feel likable, worthwhile, and someone with a valuable contribution to make in his world. Such feelings lead to self-respect, self-confidence, and a general feeling of happiness.

DEVELOPING A BODY IMAGE

School-age children are quite knowledgeable about the human body, and social development during this period focuses to a large extent on the body and its capabilities. As the child's social environment expands, the emphasis on peer relationships prescribes that children conform to group norms. The child continually compares his attributes and abilities with those of his peers. He is acutely conscious of the way he looks to others and is highly aware of deviations from the normal in himself and others.

At this time, physical impairments such as hearing or visual defects, ears that "stick out," or birthmarks assume greater importance. Increasing awareness of these differences, especially when accompanied by unkind comments and taunts from other children, may cause a child to feel inferior and less desirable. This is especially true if the defect interferes with his ability to participate in childhood games and activities. When children are teased or criticized about being different, the effect will be lasting.

MORAL DEVELOPMENT (KOHLBERG)

As children move from egocentrism to the more logical patterns of thought, they also move through stages in development of conscience and moral standards. Young children do not believe that standards of behavior come from within themselves but that rules are established and set down by others. They learn the standards for acceptable behavior, act according to these standards, and feel guilty when they violate the standards. Although children of 6 or 7 years of age know the rules and behaviors expected of them, they do not understand the reasons behind them. Rewards and punishment guide their judgment; a "bad act" is one that breaks a rule or does harm. Young children may believe that what other people tell them to do is right and that what they think of themselves is wrong. Consequently, children 6 or 7 years old are more likely to interpret accidents and misfortunes as punishment for misdeeds.

Older school-age children are able to judge an act by the intentions that prompted it rather than just by the consequences. Rules and judgments become less absolute and authoritarian and begin to be founded more on the needs and desires of others. For older children a rule violation is apt to be viewed in relation to the total context in which it appears; reactions are influenced by the situation as well as by the morality of the rule itself. While a younger child can judge an act only according to whether it is right or wrong, older children will take into account a different point of view to make a judgment. They are able to understand and accept the concept of treating others as they would like to be treated.

SPIRITUAL DEVELOPMENT

Children at this age think in very concrete terms but are avid learners and many have a great desire to learn about their God. They picture God as human and tend to describe him in terms of character traits such as loving and helping. He is a very important person in the lives of many children. They are fascinated by the concepts of hell and heaven and, with a developing conscience and concern about rules, they fear going to hell for misbehavior. School-age children want and expect to be punished for misbehavior and, if given the option, tend to choose a punishment that "fits the crime." Often they view illness or injury as a punishment for a real or imagined misdeed. The beliefs and ideals of family and religious personages are more influential than their peers in matters of faith.

School-age children begin to learn the difference between the natural and the supernatural but have difficulty understanding symbols. Consequently religious concepts must be presented to them in concrete terms. They are comforted by prayer or other religious rituals and, if this is a part of their daily lives, these activities can help them cope with threatening situations. Their petitions to their God in prayers tend to be for very tangible rewards and, although younger children expect their prayers to be answered, as they get older they begin to recognize that this does not always occur, and they become less concerned when prayers are not answered. They are able to discuss their feelings about their faith and how it relates to their lives (Fig. 15-2).

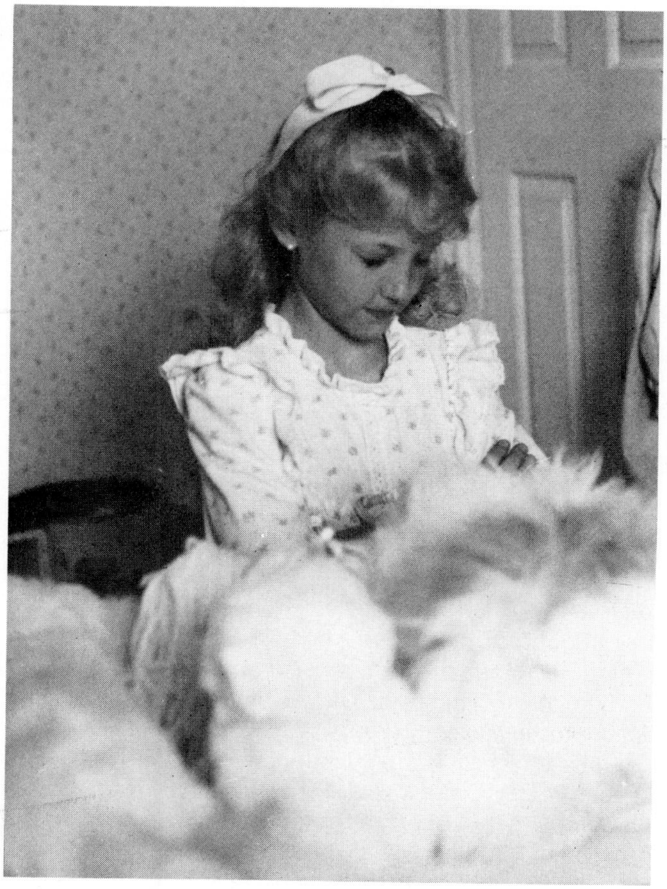

FIG. 15-2 Many children are comforted by prayer or other religious rituals.

SOCIAL DEVELOPMENT

One of the most important socializing agents in the life of the child is the peer group with whose members he explores ideas and the physical environment around him. Although it has neither the traditional authority of the parents nor the legal authority of the schools for imparting information, the peer group manages to convey a substantial amount of material to its members. Children have a culture all their own, with secrets, mores, and codes of ethics with which they promote feelings of group solidarity and detachment from adults. Through peer relationships children learn ways in which to deal with dominance and hostility and to relate to persons in positions of leadership and authority.

Identification with peers appears to be a strong influence in the child's gaining independence from parents. The aid and support of the group provide the child with enough security to risk the moderate parental rejection brought about by each small victory in his development of independence.

Much of the child's concept of the appropriate sex role is acquired through relationships with peers. During the early school years there is little difference relative to sex in play experiences of children. Games and many other activities are shared by both girls and boys. However, in the later school years the differences become marked. Boys and girls grow more intolerant of each other, especially on the surface.

Social Relationships and Cooperation

Daily relationships with age-mates provide the most important social interactions in the life of school-age children. For the first time children are able to join in group activities with unrestrained enthusiasm and steady participation when, formerly, interactions had been limited to short periods under considerable adult supervision. With increased skills and wider opportunities, children are able to become involved with one or several peer groups in which they can gain status as respected members.

There are valuable lessons to be learned from daily interaction with age-mates. First, children learn to appreciate the numerous and varied points of view that are represented in the peer group. As the child interacts with peers who see the world in ways that are somewhat different from the way he sees it, he becomes aware of the limits of his own point of view. Because age-mates are peers and are not forced to accept each other's ideas as they are expected to accept those of adults, other children have a significant influence on decreasing the egocentric outlook of the child. Consequently he learns to argue, persuade, bargain, cooperate, and compromise in order to maintain friendships.

Second, the child becomes increasingly sensitive to the social norms and pressures of the peer group. The peer group establishes standards for acceptance and rejection, and the child may be willing to modify his behavior in order to be accepted by the group. The need for peer approval becomes a powerful influence toward conformity. The child learns to dress, talk, and otherwise behave in a manner acceptable to the group. A variety of roles, such as class joker or class hero, may be assumed by individual children in order to gain approval from the group.

Third, the interaction among peers leads to the formation of intimate friendship between same-sex peers. School-age is the time when children have "best friends" with whom they share secrets, private jokes, and adventures; they come to one another's aid in times of trouble. In the course of these friendships children also fight, threaten, break up, and reunite. These dyadic relationships, in which the child experiences love and closeness for a peer, seem to be important as a foundation for heterosexual relationships in adulthood (Fig. 15-3).

Clubs and select groups. One of the outstanding characteristics of middle childhood is the formation of formalized groups, or clubs, a prominent feature of which is the rigid rules imposed on the members. There is an exclusiveness in the selection of persons who have the privilege of joining. Acceptance in the group is often determined on a pass-fail basis according to social or behavioral criteria. Conformity is the core of the group structure. There are often secret codes, shared interests, and special modes of dress, and each child must abide by a standard of behavior established by the members. Understanding of and conformity to the rules provide the child with a feeling of security and relieve him of the responsibility of making decisions. By merging his identity with that of his peers, the child is able to move from the family group to an outside group as a step toward seeking further independence. He substitutes conformity to a peer-group pattern for conformity to a family pattern while he is still too shaky and insecure to function independently.

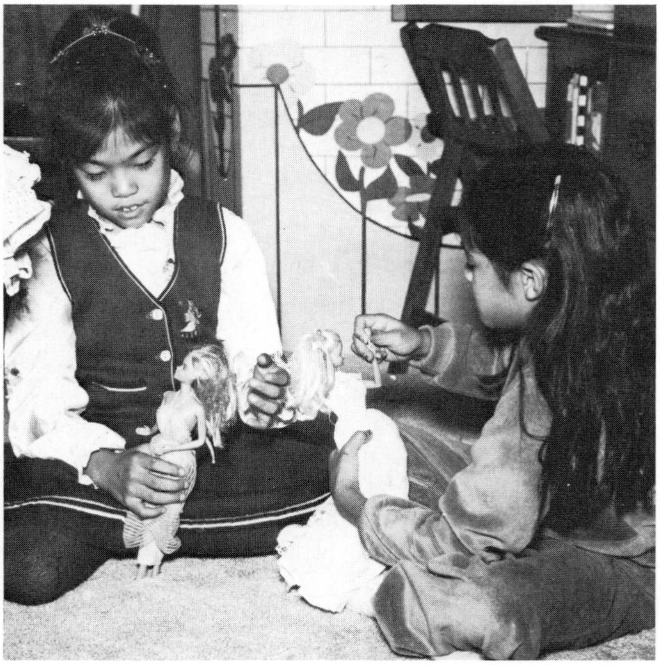

FIG. 15-3 Age-mates involved in quiet play.

During the early school years groups are rather small and loosely organized with changing membership and little formal structure and without the more prolonged cohesiveness characteristic of groups or cliques in later school years. As a rule, girls' groups are less formalized than boys', and, although there may be a mixture of both sexes in the earlier school years, the groups of later school years are composed predominantly of children of the same sex. Common interests are a frequent basis around which a group is structured.

Relationships with Families

Although the peer group is highly influential and necessary to normal child development, the parents are still the primary influence in shaping the child's personality, setting standards for behavior, and establishing a value system. It is the family values that usually predominate when parental and peer value systems come into conflict.

Peer associations seem to remain within the social class systems, and, not infrequently, there may be discrimination in membership on the basis of ethnic or racial origin.

The child will want to spend more time in the company of his peers and may seem eager to leave the house; he will often prefer activities of the peer group to family activities. This can be very disturbing to parents. The child becomes intolerant and critical of the parents and their ways when they deviate from those of the group.

Although increased independence is the goal of middle childhood, children are not yet prepared to abandon parental control. They feel more secure knowing that there is an authority greater than themselves to implement controls and restrictions. Children may complain loudly about the restrictions and try their best to break down parental barriers, but they are uneasy if they can succeed in doing so. They respect the adults on whom they can rely to prevent them from acting on each and every urge. Children sense in this behavior an expression of love and concern for their welfare.

Children also need their parents as adults, not as pals. Sometimes parents, hurt at their children's rejection, attempt to maintain their love and gratitude by assuming the role of "pals." Children need the stable, secure strength provided by mature adults to whom they can turn during troubled relationships with peers or stressful changes in their world. During a disruption in their lives, such as times of failure, periods of illness, or a move that separates them from the security of friends, children need the firm, secure anchor of parental interest and concern. With a secure base in a loving family, children are able to develop the confidence in themselves and the maturity needed to break loose from the group and stand independently.

Play

As children enter the school years, their play takes on new dimensions that reflect this new stage of development. Not only does play involve increased physical skill, intellectual skill, and fantasy, but, as children form groups and cliques, they begin to evolve a sense of belonging to a team or club. To belong to a group is of vital importance.

Rules and ritual. The need for conformity in middle childhood is strongly manifested in the activities and games that are so important in the life of school-age children. Up to this point, they have played games they have invented themselves, or they have played in the company of a friend or an adult, when rules more or less evolved with the game. Now they begin to see the need for rules, and the games they begin to play have fixed and unvarying rules that may be bizarre and extraordinarily rigid (especially those made up by the group). Clubs and secret societies become part of the culture of childhood.

Conformity and ritual permeate the play of school-age children. Not only are they present in games, but they are also evident in much of the children's behavior and language. Childhood is full of chants and taunts, such as "Eeeny, meeny, miney, mo," "Johnny's mad and I'm glad," "Last one is a rotten egg," and "Step on a crack, break your mother's back." Children derive a great deal of pleasure from such sayings, which have been handed down with few changes through generations.

Team play. A more complex form of play that evolves from group consciousness is the team games and sports that are part of the life of the early school years. The rules of a team game may even require the presence of a referee, umpire, or person of authority, in order that the rules can be followed more accurately. Through team play children learn to subordinate personal goals to goals of the group and the concept that division of labor is an effective strategy for attaining a goal. They learn about the nature of competition and the importance of winning—an attribute highly valued in the United States.

Team play can also contribute to children's social, intellectual, and skill growth. A child will work hard to develop the skills needed to become a member of a team, to improve his contribution to the group effort, and to anticipate the consequences of his behavior for the group. Team play helps stimulate cognitive growth, as children are called on to learn many complex rules, make judgments about those rules, plan strategies, and assess the strengths and weaknesses of members of their own team and the opposing team.

Quiet games and activities. Although the play of school-age children is highly active, they also enjoy many quiet and solitary activities. The middle years are the time for collections, which constitute another ritual. The early school-age child's collections are an odd assortment of unrelated objects in messy, disorganized piles. Collections of later years are more orderly and selective, and they are organized neatly in scrapbooks, on shelves, or in boxes.

School-age children become fascinated with increasingly complex board or card games, such as Monopoly and rummy, that they can play with a best friend or a group. As in all games, their adherence to rules is fanatic. There is usually much discussion and argument, but the disagreement is easily resolved through reading the appropriate rule of the game.

The newly acquired skill of reading becomes increasingly satisfying as school-age children are able to expand their knowledge of the world through books (Fig. 15-4). School-age children never tire of stories and, just like preschool children, they love to have stories read aloud. Sewing, cooking, carpentry, gardening, and creative activities such as painting are other activities that these children enjoy. Many of the creative skills, as well as athletic skills such as swimming, horseback riding, hiking, dancing, and skating, that are learned and delighted in during

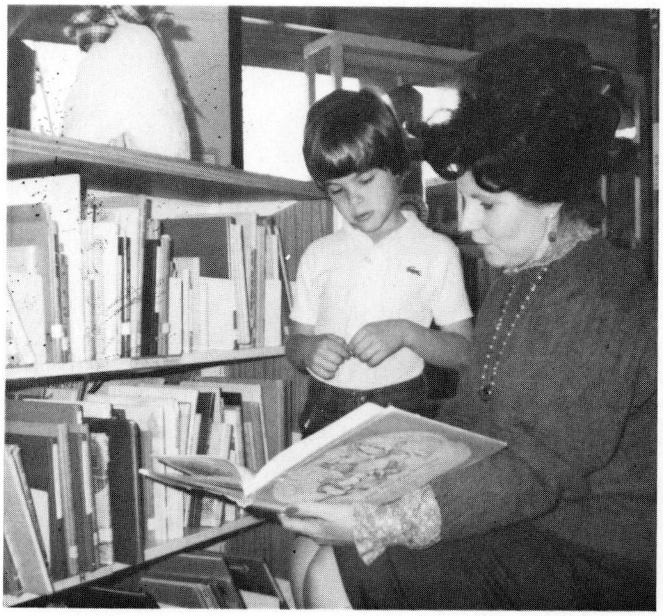

FIG. 15-4 Selecting a book with the assistance of an adult.

childhood continue to be enjoyed into adolescence and adulthood.

Ego mastery. Play also affords children the means to acquire representational mastery over themselves, their environment, and others. Through play they can feel as big, as powerful, and as skillful as their imaginations will allow, and they can attain vicarious mastery and power over whomever and whatever they choose. They need to feel in control in their play. School children still need the opportunity to use large muscles in exuberant outdoor play and the freedom to exert their newfound autonomy and initiative. They need space in which to exercise large muscles and to work off tensions, frustrations, and hostility. Physical skills practiced and mastered in play help them develop a feeling of personal competence, which contributes to a sense of accomplishment and helps provide a place of status in the peer group.

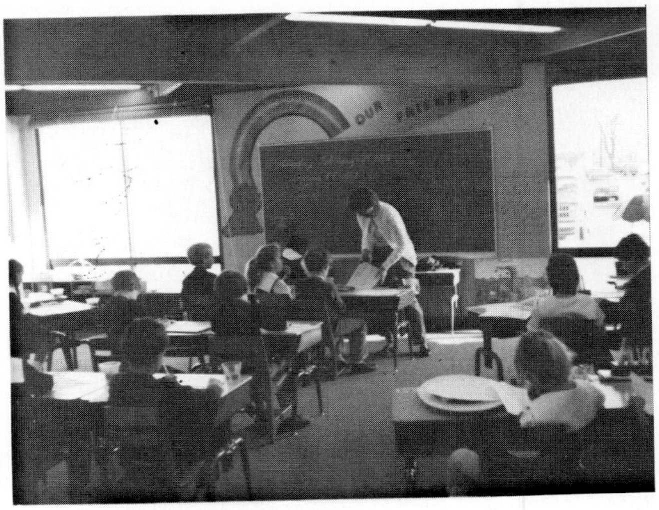

FIG. 15-5 School provides a wider range of social relationships and a new authority figure.

COPING WITH CONCERNS RELATED TO NORMAL GROWTH AND DEVELOPMENT

Middle childhood is not a period of latent development. It is a period of searching, goal-directed exploration, and increasingly complex decision-making. It is a time of preparation, trying new experiences, testing abilities, and refining performance. When difficult problems arise, most school-age children have developed sufficient coping skills to be ready to confront them and to persevere until they are solved.

School Experience

The schools serve as agents for transmitting the values of the society to each succeeding generation of children and as the setting for most of their relationships with peers. As a socializing agent second only to the family, schools exert a profound influence on the social development of children.

School entrance constitutes a sharp break in the structure of the child's world (Fig. 15-5). For many children it is their first experience in conforming to a group pattern imposed by an adult who is not a parent and who has responsibility for too many children to be constantly aware of each child as an individual. Children want to go to school and usually adapt to the new conditions with little difficulty. Successful adjustment is directly related to the physical and emotional maturity of the child and the parent's (usually the mother's) readiness to accept the separation associated with school entrance. Unfortunately some mothers express their unconscious attempts to delay the child's maturity by clinging behavior, particularly with their youngest child.

By the time they enter school, the majority of children have a fairly realistic concept of what school involves. The child receives information regarding the role of pupil from parents, playmates, and the communication media. In addition, most children have had some experience with kindergarten, and some with nursery school as well.

Although most children have had some experience with schooling before they enter first grade, the extent to which they are prepared differs. Middle-class children have fewer adjustments to make and less to learn about expected behavior, since the school tends to reflect dominant middle-class customs and values. If the child has attended a preschool program, the emphasis of the program significantly affects the child's adjustment. Some provide custodial care only, while others emphasize emotional, social, and intellectual development as well.

Classmates have a significant impact on the socialization of individual children. For the first time children become members of a large group of individuals their own age, and peer relationships become increasingly important and influential as children proceed through school. The peer group has a special impact during adolescence when it plays an important role in the transition from child to adult status. The kind of influence exerted by the peer group depends on the background, interests, and abilities of the individual child and on the degree to which the peer-group standards influence the child.

Teachers. To facilitate the transition from home to school, educators select teachers with personality characteristics that allow them to deal with potential problems of young children. As a parent surrogate, the teacher in the early grades performs many of the activities formerly assumed by the parent, such as recognizing the children's personal needs (such as a need to go to the bathroom or help with clothing) and helping to develop their social behavior (for example, manners).

Teachers, like parents, are concerned about the psychologic and emotional welfare of the child. Although the functions of teachers and parents differ, both place constraints on behavior and both are in a position to enforce standards of conduct. The teacher shares the parental influence in determining the child's attitudes and values.

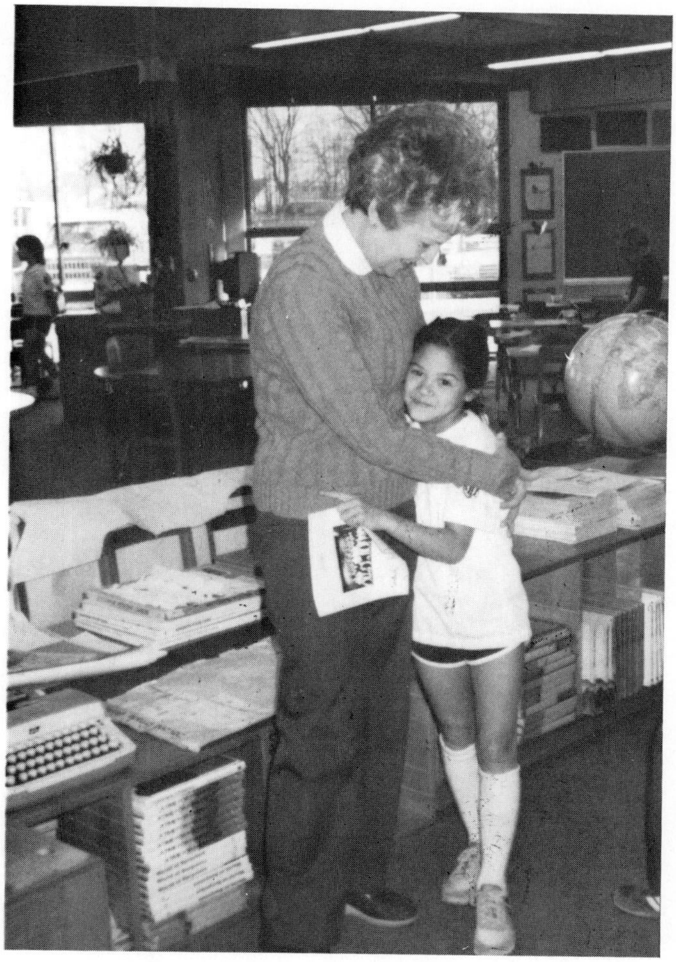

FIG. 15-6 Children develop a close relationship to their teachers.

Teachers serve as models with whom children identify and whom they try to emulate. Teacher approval is sought; teacher disapproval is avoided. The teacher is a very significant person in the life of the early school child, and hero worship of a teacher may extend into late childhood and preadolescence (Fig. 15-6).

Parents. Parents share responsibility with the schools for helping children achieve their maximum potential. There are numerous ways in which parents can supplement the school. For example, they can take an active interest in their children's schooling, send them to school every day (except when they are unwell), share information with the teacher that can help him/her to better understand the individual child, communicate with the teacher if there is a problem, provide an appropriate study area and support the children in home study, help the children learn good study habits (e.g., breaking large tasks into smaller manageable tasks spread over a longer period of time), and set goals that the children can achieve.

Latchkey Children

The term *latchkey children* is used to describe children who are left to care for themselves or whose care arrangements are so loose that they are ineffective (Long and Long, 1982). The increasing numbers of single-parent families and working mothers together with the lack of available child care has created a stress-provoking situation for a large number of school children.

The effect on these children is variable. Inadequate adult supervision after school leaves children at greater risk for injury and delinquent behavior. In some instances outside activities are curtailed and relationships with peers may be significantly diminished. Many latchkey children feel more lonely, isolated, and fearful than children who have someone to care for them. To cope with their fears and anxieties while alone, these children may devise strategies such as hiding, playing the television at loud volume, or using pets as a comfort. In other cases children benefit from the experience, becoming more responsible and secure.

Limit-Setting and Discipline

Numerous factors influence the amount and manner of discipline and limit-setting imposed on school-age children: the psychosocial maturity of the parents, childhood and childrearing experiences of the parents, temperament of the children, context of the children's misconduct, and response of the children to rewards and punishments. As children are increasingly able to see a situation from the point of view of another, they are able to understand the effects of their reactions on others and themselves.

Disciplinary techniques should help children control their own behavior. Reasoning is an effective technique for this age-group. With advancing cognitive skills they are able to benefit from more complex types of disciplinary strategies. For example, withholding privileges, requiring recompense, imposing penalties, and contracting can be used with great success. Problem-solving is the best approach to limit-setting, and children themselves can be included in the process of determining appropriate disciplinary measures.

Dishonest Behavior

During middle childhood it is not uncommon for children to engage in what is considered to be antisocial behavior. Lying, stealing, and cheating may become manifest in previously well-behaved children. It is especially disturbing to parents who may have difficulty coping with this behavior.

Lying. Preschool children often have difficulty distinguishing between fact and fantasy. By the time they reach school age they still "tell stories" but can distinguish between what is real and what is make-believe. If not, they need to be taught to distinguish between fantasy and reality. Often children will exaggerate a story or situation as a means to impress their family or friends.

TABLE 15-1

Summary of Growth and Development during School-Age Years

Age (years)	Physical and Motor	Mental	Adaptive	Personal-Social
6	Growth and weight gain slower Central mandibular incisors erupt Weight: 16-23.6 kg (35½-58 pounds); height: 106.6-123.5 cm (42-48 inches) Gradual increase in dexterity Active age; constant activity Often returns to finger feeding More aware of hand as a tool Likes to draw, print, and color	Counts 13 pennies Knows whether it is morning or afternoon Defines common objects such as fork and chair in terms of their use Obeys triple commands in succession Shows right hand and left ear Says which is pretty and which is ugly of a series of drawings of faces Describes the objects in a picture rather than simply enumerating them Period of more tension but is intellectually more stimulating Attends first grade	At table, uses knife to spread butter or jam on bread At play, cuts, folds, pastes paper toys, sews crudely if needle is threaded Enjoys making simple figures in clay Takes bath without supervision; performs bedtime activities alone Reads from memory; enjoys oral spelling game Likes table games, checkers, simple card games Giggles a lot Sometimes steals money or attractive items Has difficulty owning up to misdeeds Tries out own abilities	Can share and cooperate better Great need for children of own age Will cheat to win Often engages in rough play Often jealous of younger brother or sister Does what he sees adults doing Often has temper tantrums Is a boaster More independent, probably influence of school Has own way of doing things Increased socialization
7	Begins to grow at least 2 inches a year Maxillary central incisors and lateral mandibular incisors erupt Weight: 17.7-30 kg (39-66½ pounds); height: 111.8-129.7 cm (44-51 inches) Gross motor actions are cautious but not fearful More cautious in approaches to new performances Repeats performances to master them Posture more tense and unstable; maintains one position longer	Notices that certain parts are missing from pictures Can copy a diamond Repeats three numbers backward Reads ordinary clock or watch correctly to nearest quarter hour; uses clock for practical purposes Attends the second grade More mechanical in reading; often does not stop at the end of a sentence, skips words such as it, the, and he	Uses table knife for cutting meat; may need help with tough or difficult pieces Brushes and combs hair acceptably without help or "going over" Stealing may still be a problem Likes to help and have a choice Less resistant and stubborn	Is becoming a real member of the family group Takes part in group play Boys prefer playing with boys; girls prefer playing with girls Spends a lot of time alone; does not require a lot of companionship
8-9	Continues to grow at 5 cm (2 inches) a year Lateral incisors (maxillary) and mandibular cuspids erupt Weight: 19.6-39.6 kg (43-87 pounds); height: 117-141.8 cm (46-56 inches) Movement fluid; often graceful and poised Always on the go; jumps, chases, skips Increased smoothness and speed in fine motor control Dresses self completely Likely to overdo; hard to quiet down after recess	Gives similarities and differences between two things from memory Counts backward from 20 to 1 Repeats days of the week and months in order; knows the date Describes common objects in detail, not merely their use Makes change out of a quarter Attends third and fourth grades Greater reader; may plan to wake up early just to read Reads classic books, but also enjoys comics More aware of time; can be relied on to get to school on time	Makes use of common tools such as hammer, saw, or screwdriver Uses household and sewing utensils Helps with routine household tasks such as dusting, sweeping Assumes responsibility for share of household chores Looks after all of own needs at table Buys useful articles; exercises some choice in making purchases Runs useful errands Likes pictorial magazines Likes school; wants to answer all the questions Afraid of failing a grade; ashamed of bad grades More critical of self	Easy to get along with at home Likes the reward system Dramatizes Is more sociable Is better behaved Interested in boy-girl relationships but will not admit it Goes about home and community freely, alone or with friends Likes to compete and play games Shows preference in friends and groups Plays mostly with groups of own sex but is beginning to mix

TABLE 15-1

Summary of Growth and Development during School-Age Years—cont'd

Age (years)	Physical and Motor	Mental	Adaptive	Personal-Social
10-12	Slow growth in height and rapid weight gain; may become obese in this period Posture is more similar to an adult's; will overcome lordosis Pubescent changes may begin to appear Rest of teeth will erupt and tend toward full development (except wisdom teeth) Weight: 24.3-58 kg (54-128 pounds); height: 127.5-162.3 cm (50-64 inches) Body lines soften and round out in girls Boys like large playgrounds	Writes brief stories Produces simple paintings or drawings Attends fifth to seventh grades Writes occasional short letters to friends or relatives on own initiative Uses telephone for practical purposes Responds to magazine, radio, or other advertising by mailing coupons Reads for practical information or own enjoyment—stories or library books of adventure or romance, or animal stories	Makes useful articles or does easy repair work Cooks or sews in small way Raises pets Washes and dries own hair Is responsible for a thorough job of cleaning hair, but may need reminding to do so Is sometimes left alone at home for an hour or so Is successful in looking after own needs or those of other children left in his care	Fond of friends Chooses friends more selectively Loves conversation Beginning interest in opposite sex More diplomatic Likes his family; family really has meaning Likes mother and wants to please her in many ways Demonstrates affection Likes dad too; he is adored and idolized Respects parents Loves friends; talks about them constantly

Young children will lie to escape punishment or get out of some difficulty even when the evidence of their misbehavior is before their eyes. Older children may lie in order to meet expectations set by others to which they have been unable to measure up. However, most children are very concerned with the wrongness of lying and cheating—especially in their friends. They are quick to tell on others when they detect them in the act of cheating.

Parents need to be reassured that all children lie sometimes and that they often have difficulty separating fantasy from reality. Parents should be helped to understand the importance of their own behavior as role models and being truthful in their relationships with children.

Cheating. Cheating is most common in young children aged 5 to 6. They find it difficult to lose at a game or contest, and so they cheat in order to win. They have not yet acquired the full realization of the wrongness of this behavior and do it almost automatically. It usually disappears as they mature. However, because children model observed behaviors, parents need to be aware of their own behavior. When parents set examples of honesty, children are more likely to conform to these standards.

Stealing. Like other ethically related behavior, stealing is not an unexpected event in the younger child. Between 5 and 8 years children's sense of property rights is limited and they tend to take something simply because they are attracted to it or to take money for what it will buy. They are equally likely to give away something valuable that belongs to them. When young children are caught and punished they are penitent—"didn't mean to," and "promise never to do it again," but it is quite likely that they will repeat the performance the following day. Often they not only steal but will lie about it as well or attempt to justify the act with excuses. It is seldom helpful to trap children into admission by asking directly if they did the offensive thing. Children do not take on such responsibility until nearer the end of middle childhood.

There are several reasons why children steal: lack of a sense of property rights, trying to acquire the means with which to bribe favors from other children, a strong desire to own the coveted item, or as a means for revenge in order to "get back at someone" (usually a parent) for what they consider to be unfair treatment. Older children may steal to supplement an inadequate income from other sources. Sometimes stealing is an indication that something is seriously wrong or lacking in the child's life. For example, a child may steal to make up for love or another satisfaction that he feels is lacking.

It is difficult for many parents to cope with stealing in their children. However, in most situations it is best not to attempt to find a hidden or deep meaning to the stealing. An admonition together with an appropriate and reasonable punishment, such as having the older child pay back the money or return the stolen items, will ordinarily take care of the majority of cases. Most children can be taught to respect the property rights of others with little difficulty despite the temptations and opportunities presented to them. Some children simply need more time to learn the importance of the culture's rules regarding private property.

SUMMARY OF GROWTH AND DEVELOPMENT

The preceding stages of child development increasingly demonstrate individuality in the patterns of development. As children grow and mature, these differences become more pronounced. Although the rate generally slows during middle childhood, development continues to be uneven, with periods of acceleration in some areas followed by a leveling-off period. At the same time other areas progress normally. In addition, each child has a unique developmental pattern; therefore, any attempt to describe the typical child can only represent an average and should not be considered as absolute criteria for any given child (Table 15-1).

◆ *Promoting Optimum Health during the School Years*

Health supervision of children, begun in early childhood, is continued in middle childhood; it includes the periodic ongoing health assessment and guidance advised for children 6 to 12 years of age. Since regular health checkups and prophylactic measures such as immunizations are a routine function of health supervision, this need not be reiterated.

When school-age children enter school, they leave the relatively protected environment of home and neighborhood and experience interpersonal contacts with a larger number of children. Many childhood illnesses can be prevented by careful health supervision. For example, most of the communicable diseases, formerly a cause of high morbidity in school children, can be prevented by immunization. The body's natural defenses against illness can be supported through careful attention to diet, rest, and exercise and protection from extreme mental and physical stress.

NUTRITION

Although caloric needs are diminished in relation to body size during middle childhood, resources are being laid down for the increased growth needs of the adolescent period. It is important to impress on children and their parents the value of a diet that is balanced to promote growth. Since the child usually eats as the family does, the quality of his diet depends to a large extent on the family's pattern of eating.

Likes and dislikes established at an early age continue in middle childhood, although the propensity for single food preferences begins to end and children acquire a taste for an increasing variety of foods. However, with the influence of the mass media and the temptation of an immense variety of "junk food," it is all too easy for children to fill up on empty calories—foods that do not promote growth, such as sugars, starches, and excess fats. The easy availability of high-calorie foods, combined with the tendency toward more sedentary activities, is contributing to an increasing prevalence of childhood obesity. This problem is discussed further in Chapter 17.

Nutrition education can and should be integrated throughout the child's school years as part of classroom learning. In school the basic food groups and the elements of a wholesome diet are learned, as well as how food products are grown, processed, and prepared. The school nurse can take an active role in nutrition education by working with teachers to plan and implement units of nutrition instruction and with parents and children to give nutritional guidance.

SLEEP AND REST

The amount of sleep and rest that is required during middle childhood is a highly individual matter. There is no specific amount needed by a child at any given age. The amount depends, rather, on the child's age, the activity level, and other factors, such as his state of health. The growth rate has slowed; therefore, less energy is expended in growth than was expended during the preceding periods and than will be required during the adolescent growth spurt.

During the school years children usually do not require a nap, but they sleep an average of 11 to 12 hours nightly at age 6 years and 9 to 10 hours a night at 11 or 12 years. Although there are fewer bedtime problems with advancing years, there are still occasional difficulties associated with the necessary bedtime ritual. Usually there is little problem for children 6 and 7 years old, and the task of going to bed can be facilitated by encouraging quiet activity before bedtime, such as coloring and reading. However, most children in middle childhood must be reminded frequently to go to bed; 8- to 9-year-old children and 11-year-old children are particularly resistant. Often the child is unaware that he is tired; if he is allowed to remain up later than usual, he is fatigued the following day. Sometimes the bedtime resistance can be resolved by allowing a later bedtime in deference to his advancing age. Twelve-year-old children usually offer no difficulty in relation to bedtime. Some even retire early in order to enjoy slow preparations for bed, to read, or to listen to the radio.

EXERCISE AND ACTIVITY

The improved capabilities and adaptability of the school-age child permit greater speed and effort in motor activities, and larger, stronger muscles with greater efficiency and skill permit longer and increasingly strenuous play without exhaustion. During this age period children acquire the coordination, timing, and concentration that are required to participate in adult-type activities, even though they may be deficient in the strength, stamina, and control of the adolescent and adult. Consequently a larger amount of physical activity should be expected and encouraged during the school years. However, it must be kept in mind that, although school-age children are large and appear to be strong, they may not be prepared yet for strenuous competitive athletics.

All growing children need some regular exercise and should be afforded opportunities of various kinds that provide satisfying experiences to meet individual likes and dislikes. Appropriate activities that promote coordination and development during the school-age years include running, skipping rope, swimming, roller skating, ice skating, and bicycle riding. Positive reinforcement achieved by experiencing increasingly smooth, rhythmic, and efficient use of the body conditions the child toward regular physical activity.

Exercise is essential for developmental progress in a number of areas, including muscle development and tone, refinement of balance and coordination, gaining strength and endurance, and stimulating body functions and metabolic processes. Children need ample space in which to run, jump, skip, and climb and safe facilities and equipment to use both indoors and outdoors. Most children need little encouragement to engage in physical activity. They have so much energy that they seldom know when to stop.

Children with disabling conditions or those who hesitate to become involved in active play, such as obese children, require special assessment and help so that activities that will appeal to them, that are compatible with their limitations, and that, at the same time, meet their developmental needs can be determined.

Sports

A great deal of controversy has surrounded the trend toward earlier participation in competitive athletics and the amount and type of competitive sports that are appropriate for children in the elementary grades. The current view is that virtually every child is suited for some type of sport, and authorities do not discourage participation if the child is matched to the type of sport appropriate to his abilities and to his physical and emotional constitution. School-age children enjoy competition and, when those involved with children in this age-group understand the child's physical limitations and teach him the proper techniques and safety measures necessary to avoid injury to developing bones and muscles, a safe and appropriate sport can be found for even the most unskilled and noncompetitive child (Fig. 15-7).

Various acceptable sports activities are available to school-age children; for example, Little league, gymnastics, baseball, soccer, and swimming. However, it is important for those involved with children in this age-group to understand the child's physical limitations and to teach the proper techniques and precautions in order to avoid injury to developing bones and muscles. Equipment should be maintained in safe condition, and protective apparatus should be worn to prevent serious injury (see Sports injuries p. 464).

During the school-age years girls have the same basic body structure as boys and thus have a similar response to systematic exercise training. At puberty, when boys become larger and have more muscle mass, it is usually recommended that girls compete only against other girls. Before puberty there is no essential difference in strength and size between girls and boys, making these precautions unnecessary (Shaffer, 1980).

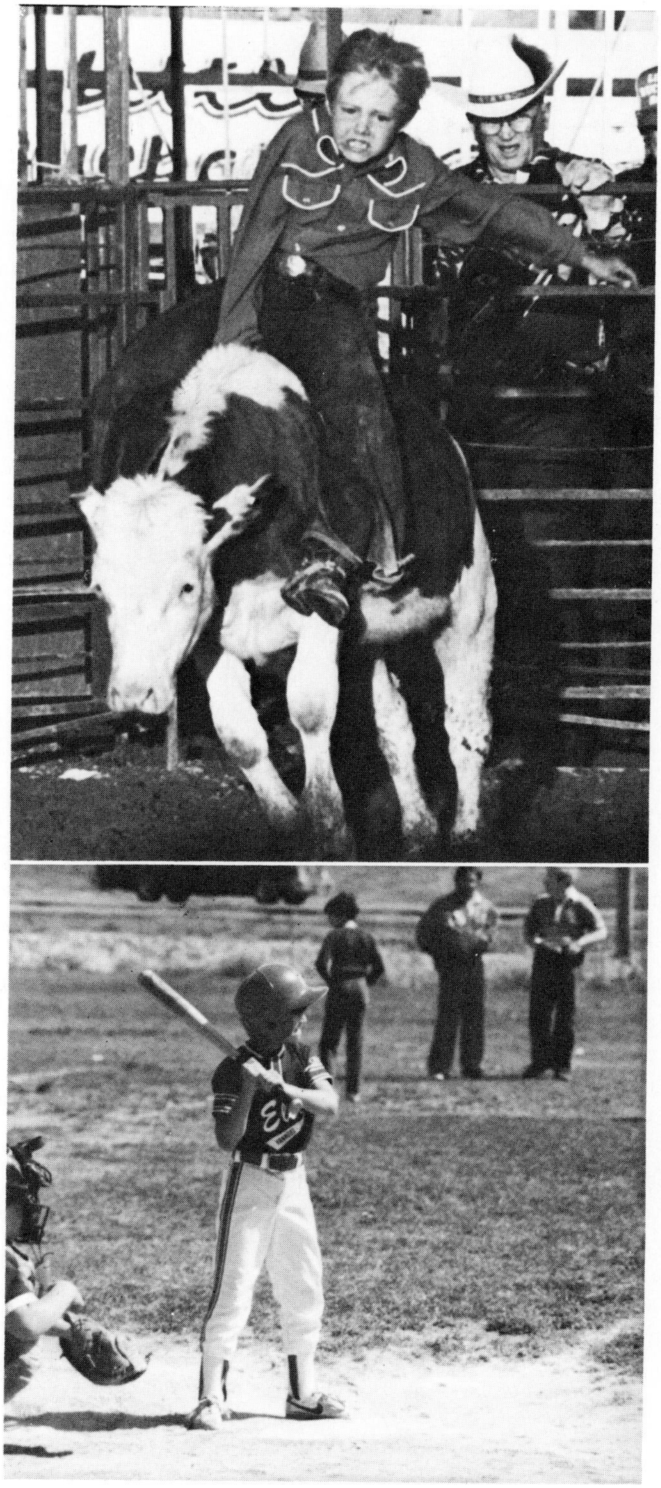

A

B

FIG. 15-7 The activities engaged in by school-age children vary according to interest and opportunity. **A,** Little Britches Rodeo competitor. **B,** Little League competitors.

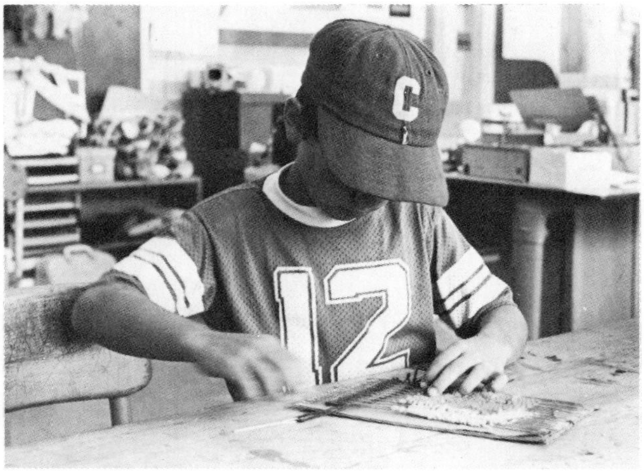

FIG. 15-8 School-age children are motivated to complete tasks working alone.

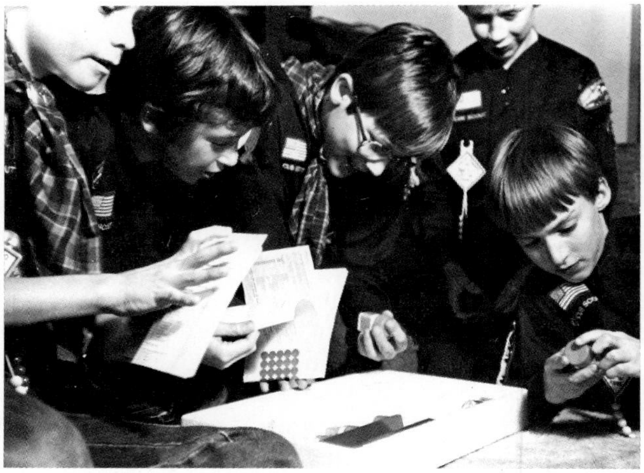

FIG. 15-9 School-age children cooperate to complete tasks working with others.

Acquisition of Skills

School-age children also demonstrate increasing capacities in fine muscle facility and complex artistic skills. Handedness is well established by the beginning of the school years, and children make great strides in writing and drawing during this age period. It is a time of energetic and vibrant creative productivity. With the tools of language and reading, children can create poems, stories, and plays. With more advanced fine motor skills, they are able to master an unlimited variety of handicrafts, such as ceramics, needlework, wood carving, and beadwork. They avidly pursue these skills in solitude (Fig. 15-8), with a friend, or in programs offered through organized groups such as boys' or girls' clubs, scouting, or special interest groups, which use crafts or other activities as a means to occupy, entertain, and educate children (Fig. 15-9).

School-age children are capable of assuming responsibility for their own needs, although their distaste for soap and water and "dress" clothes is legendary. School-age children can and want to assume their share of household tasks, which usually are related to the male and female roles that have been defined by their culture, and many assume responsibility for tasks outside the home, such as baby-sitting, mowing lawns, or paper routes.

DENTAL HEALTH

The first permanent (secondary) teeth erupt at about 6 years of age, beginning with the 6-year molar, which erupts posterior to the deciduous molars. The others appear in approximately the same order as eruption of the primary teeth (see p. 288) and follow shedding of the deciduous teeth (Fig. 15-10). With the appearance of the second permanent (12-year) molar, most of the permanent teeth are present.

Since it is during the school-age years that the permanent teeth erupt, good dental hygiene and regular attention to dental caries are vital parts of health supervision during this period. Correct brushing techniques should be taught or reinforced, and the role that fermentable carbohydrates play in production of dental caries should be emphasized. It is also important to be alert to possible malocclusion problems that may result from irregular eruption of permanent teeth and that may impair function. Regular dental supervision and continued fluo-

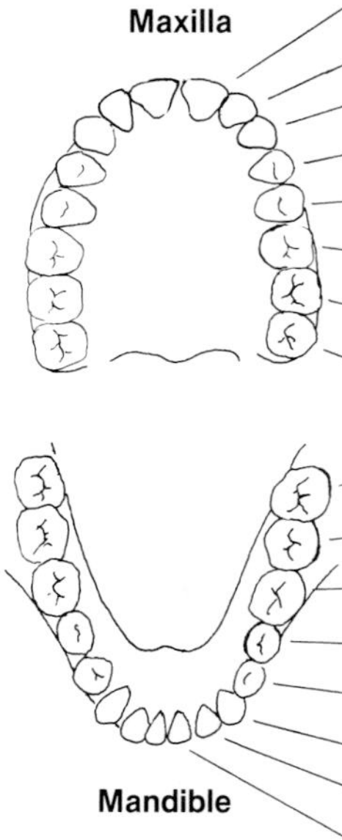

		Average age of eruption (yr)	
		BOYS	GIRLS
Maxilla	Central incisor	7.5	7.2
	Lateral incisor	8.7	8.2
	Cuspid	11.7	11.0
	First bicuspid	10.4	10.0
	Second bicuspid	11.2	10.9
	First molar	6.4	6.2
	Second molar	12.2	12.7
	Third molar	Variable 17-21	
Mandible	Third molar		
	Second molar	12.1	11.7
	First molar	6.2	5.9
	Second bicuspid	11.5	10.9
	First bicuspid	10.8	10.2
	Cuspid	10.8	9.9
	Lateral incisor	7.7	7.3
	Central incisor	6.5	6.3

FIG. 15-10 Sequence of eruption of secondary teeth.

ride supplementation are as essential as regular medical supervision and should be an integral part of the overall health maintenance program.

Brushing. One of the most effective means of preventing dental caries is a regimen of proper oral hygiene tailored to the individual child by his dentist. The child should be taught to carry out his own dental care with the supervision and guidance of the parents. Parents should learn the brushing technique along with their child, and they should inspect his efforts until he can assume full responsibility for his own care.

Teeth should be brushed after meals, after snacks, and at bedtime. Children who brush their teeth frequently and become accustomed to the feel of a clean mouth at an early age usually maintain the habit throughout life. One regimen advocated by authorities includes staining the teeth with a plaque-disclosing agent, followed by thorough brushing with plain water and flossing. After the teeth have been inspected with the aid of a mirror under adequate light, they are again cleansed, this time with a fluoridated dentifrice to freshen the mouth and provide further protection. This procedure may be carried out regularly or occasionally, according to instructions from the child's dentist.

For the school-age child with mixed and permanent dentition the best toothbrush is one of soft nylon bristles with an overall length of about 21 cm (6 inches). The design of the brush is of little importance; it is usually left to the child's preference. Numerous methods of brushing the teeth have been described and recommended for children, but there is no conclusive evidence that one method is superior over another. The thoroughness of the cleaning is more important than the specific technique used.

Dental caries. Dental caries is one of the most common chronic diseases that afflict humans at all ages; it is the principal oral problem in children and adolescents. Reducing the incidence and consequences of the disorder is of great importance in childhood because dental caries, if untreated, results in total destruction of involved teeth. The ages of greatest vulnerability are 4 to 8 years for the primary dentition and 12 to 18 years for the secondary or permanent dentition.

Dental caries is a multifactorial disease; it involves susceptible teeth, cariogenic microflora, and an appropriate oral environment. The incidence of lesions and the likelihood of progressive invasion vary considerably and depend on a number of factors being present in the right combination. Oral inspection is an integral part of the nursing assessment of the child. If there is any evidence of dental caries or other unhealthy state, the child is referred for dental services. The family may have a family dentist or a pedodontist who can provide needed care. An alarming number of children do not receive regular dental supervision, and a significant number reach adulthood without having been examined or treated by a dentist.

Malocclusion. When teeth of the upper and lower dental arches approximate in the proper relationships, the physiologic function of mastication is more effective and the cosmetic effect is more pleasing. Teeth that are uneven, crowded, or overlapping, or that otherwise interfere with their ability to meet their counterparts in the opposite jaw in the appropriate relationships, may be predisposed to disease in later years.

Orthodontic treatment is usually most successful when it is started in the later school-age years or the early teenage years, after the last primary teeth have been shed and before growth ceases. However, referral should be made as soon as malocclusion is evident, since some deformities can be corrected at an earlier age.

SEX EDUCATION

Evidence indicates that many children experience some form of sex play during or prior to preadolescence as a response to normal curiosity, not as a result of love or sexual urge. Children are experimentalists by nature, and this play is incidental and transitory. Any adverse emotional consequences or guilt feelings depend on how the behavior is managed by the parents, if it is discovered, or whether the child views his actions as wrong in the eyes of significant persons, particularly the parents.

Much of the child's attitude toward sex, which is acquired indirectly at a very early age, affects the way in which he responds to sexual information presented at a later time. Middle childhood appears to be an ideal time for formal sex education, and many authorities believe that the topic is best presented from a life-span approach. Initial curiosity about differences in body structure between boys and girls and between children and adults has arisen in the preschool years, and the next stage, adolescence, will arouse both anxiety and excitement about sexual encounters. Information about sexual maturation and the process of reproduction presented during middle childhood helps to minimize the child's uncertainty, embarrassment, and feelings of isolation that often accompany the events of puberty.

Nurse's role in sex education. No matter where nurses practice, they can provide information on human sexuality to both parents and children. Nurses can help parents by first becoming knowledgeable about human sexuality themselves, including the common myths and misconceptions associated with sex and the reproductive process. Because parents often either repress the child's sexual curiosity or avoid dealing with it, the sexual information that he receives is acquired almost entirely from his peers. When peers are the primary source of sexual information, it is transmitted and exchanged in secret, clandestine conversation and contains a large amount of misinformation. Children's questions about sex should be answered to the same extent as their questions about any other topic—honestly and at their level of understanding.

During encounters with parents, nurses can be open and available for questions and discussion. They can set an example by the language they use in discussing body

TABLE 15-2

Injury Prevention during School-Age Years

Major Developmental Accomplishments	Injury Prevention
Developing increasing independence Increased physical skills Growth in height exceeds muscular growth and coordination Needs strenuous physical activity Interested in acquiring new skills and perfecting attained skills Daring and adventurous Attempts hazardous feats Desires group loyalty; strong need for approval of friends Accompanies friends to potentially hazardous facilities Confidence often exceeds physical capacity Likely to overdo	**Motor Vehicles** Educate regarding proper use of seat belts while a passenger in a vehicle Maintain discipline while a passenger in a vehicle, for example, keep arms inside, do not lean against doors or interfere with driver Emphasize safe pedestrian behavior Teach safety and maintenance of two-wheeled vehicles, such as bicycles (see accompanying box) Insist on wearing safety apparel (e.g., helmet) where applicable, such as riding motorcycle **Drowning** Teach to swim Teach basic water safety, especially swimming with a buddy **Burns** Instruct in behavior in the areas involving contact with potential burn hazards, for example, gasoline, matches, bonfires or barbecues, firecrackers, lighters, cooking utensils, chemistry sets; avoid climbing around high-tension wires Instruct in proper behavior in the event of fire (e.g., fire drills at home or school) Teach proper behavior if clothing becomes ignited Advise regarding excessive exposure to sunlight (ultraviolet burn) **Poisoning** Educate regarding hazards of taking nonprescription drugs and chemicals, including aspirin and alcohol Keep potentially dangerous products in properly labeled receptacles—preferably out of reach **Falls** Instruct in proper use of playground equipment Instruct in proper use and care of sports equipment, especially the more hazardous devices (e.g., skateboards, trampolines, skis) Emphasize use of protective equipment when engaged in individual activities such as skateboarding and cycling and team sports such as soccer or hockey **Bodily Damage** Help provide facilities for supervised activities Encourage playing in safe places Keep firearms safely locked up except during adult supervision Teach proper care of, use of, and respect for devices with potential danger (e.g., power tools, firecrackers) Stress eye protection when using potentially hazardous objects or devices or when engaged in potentially hazardous sports Teach safety regarding use of corrective devices (glasses); if child wears contact lenses, monitor duration of wear to prevent corneal damage Stress careful selection and maintenance of sport and recreation equipment Emphasize proper conditioning for sports or other recreational activities Caution against engaging in hazardous sports, such as those involving trampolines Have identification on child, such as plastic "shoe pocket" attached to shoe laces

Bicycle Safety

Ride bicycles with traffic and away from parked cars
Ride single file
Walk bicycles through busy intersections
Give hand signals well in advance of turning or stopping
Keep as close to the curb as practical
Watch for drain grates, potholes, soft shoulders, and loose dirt or gravel
Keep both hands on handlebars, except when signaling
Never ride double on a bicycle
Do not carry packages that interfere with vision or control
Watch for and yield to pedestrians
Watch for cars backing up or pulling out of driveways
Be especially careful at intersections
Never hitch a ride on a truck or other vehicle
Learn rules of the road and respect for traffic officers
Obey all local ordinances
Wear well-fitted helmet
Wear shoes while riding
Wear light colors at night and attach fluorescent material to clothing and bicycle
Be certain the bicycle is the correct size for rider
Equip bicycle with proper lights and reflectors
Have the bicycle inspected to ensure good mechanical condition

parts and their function and by the way in which they deal with problems that have emotional overtones, such as exploratory sex play and masturbation. Parents need to be helped to understand normal behaviors and to view sexual curiosity in their children as a part of the developmental process. Assessing the parents' level of knowledge and understanding of sexuality provides cues to their need for supplemental information that will better prepare them for the increasingly complex explanations that will be needed as their children grow older.

SCHOOL HEALTH PROBLEMS

Child health maintenance is ultimately the responsibility of the parents; however, the public schools and health departments in the United States have contributed to the improvement of child health by providing a healthful school environment, health services, and health education that emphasizes sound health practices. Most of these functions constitute major components of community health services and involve large amounts of public funds and large numbers of health professionals, including nurses, on either a full-time or a part-time basis. School health programs contribute to the goals of the community for the education and development of the children.

A school health program is also involved in ongoing health maintenance through assessment, screening, and referral activities. Routine health services provided by most schools include health appraisal, emergency care and safety, communicable disease control, and counseling and follow-up care. Health education of school children is primarily directed toward providing knowledge of health and influencing habits, attitudes, and conduct in relation to health and injury prevention. The variety of topics for health instruction is endless, and eager minds are ready and willing to learn.

Traditionally, school nurses have been viewed from a limited perspective that placed them in the role of disease detector, applier of Band-Aids, and official caregiver in cases of illness and injury. Although these are still important functions and their importance is not to be minimized, this traditional role is acquiring much broader dimensions. School nurses are being prepared to provide primary health care on a broader scale that includes assessment of physical, psychomedical, psychoeducational, behavioral, and learning disorder problems and to provide comprehensive well-child care. The school nurse practitioner is also concerned with development, implementation, and evaluation of health care plans and programs.

INJURY PREVENTION

As in all age-groups, injuries are closely related to the developmental characteristics associated with normal growth and maturation. With new capabilities children are often tempted to test these abilities in activities that may not be appropriate. Because school-age children have developed more refined muscular coordination and control and can apply their cognitive capacities to a more judicious course of action, the incidence of injury is diminished in children in this age-group when compared with the incidence in early childhood.

The most common cause of severe injury and death in school-age children is motor vehicle accidents—either as pedestrian or passenger. It is imperative that nurses continue to emphasize the importance of the three automobile safety measures that have been found to reduce the severity of injuries: effective restraint systems, door-lock mechanisms, and appropriate passenger seating locations in the motor vehicle.

The school-age child's penchant for riding bicycles increases the risk of injury on streets and byways, and other serious injuries associated with moving conveyances include accidents on skateboards, roller skates, skis, and other sports equipment. All-terrain vehicles (ATVs), increasingly popular with children under 16 years of age, are unstable, difficult to handle, and responsible for an increasing number of childhood injuries (Thompson and Stroud, 1987).

The most effective means of prevention is education of the child and family regarding the hazards of risk taking and improper use of the equipment. Safety helmets are strongly recommended for children engaged in active sports, even though they may not be required equipment. For example, falls from bicycles, ATVs, and skating devices are the cause of a significant number of head injuries in school-age children.

Physically active school-age children are highly susceptible to cuts and abrasions, and the incidence of childhood fractures, strains, and sprains is noteworthy. The incidence is significantly higher in school-age boys than in school-age girls, and most occur in or near the home or school. Injuries of serious nature are discussed as appropriate elsewhere in the book—burns (p. 996), eye trauma (p. 571), near-drowning (p. 907), and head injuries (p. 902)—and need not be elaborated here. The prevalence of injuries depends on the dangers present in the environment, the protection offered by adults, and the behavior patterns of the children. See Table 15-2 for the major developmental accomplishments, suggestions for prevention, and rules for bicycle safety.

ANTICIPATORY GUIDANCE—CARE OF FAMILIES

Parents of the school-age child find themselves in the position of sharing their child's time and interests with the increasingly important peer group. It is through early peer relationships that children begin to prepare for moving from narrow, sheltered family relationships to a broader world of relationships and increased independence. Parents must learn to provide support as unobtrusively as possible without feeling rejected, hurt, or angry. The nurse can help parents of the school-age child by providing anticipatory guidance and reassurance

Parental Guidance during School Years

Age (years)	Guidance
6	Expect strong food preferences and frequent refusals of specific food items
	Expect increasingly ravenous appetite
	Prepare parents for emotionality as child experiences erratic mood changes
	Anticipate increase in susceptibility to illness and more sickness than at previous ages
	Teach injury prevention and safety, especially bicycle safety
	Respect the child's need for privacy; provide a room of his own if possible
	Prepare for increasing interests outside the home
	Encourage interaction with peers
7-10	Expect improvement in health with fewer illnesses; however, allergies may increase or become apparent
	Prepare for increase in minor injuries
	Emphasize caution in selection and maintenance of sports equipment and re-emphasize teaching safety
	Expect increased involvement with peers and interest in activities outside the home
	Encourage independence but maintain limit-setting and discipline
	Expect more demands upon mother at 8 years
	Expect increasing admiration for father at 10 years; encourage father-child activities
	Prepare for prepubescent changes in girls
11-12	Prepare child for body changes of pubescence
	Expect a growth spurt in girls
	Make certain the child's sex education is adequate with accurate information
	Expect energetic but stormy behavior at 11 to become more even-tempered at 12
	Encourage child's desire to "grow up" but allow regressive behavior when needed
	Expect an increase in masturbation
	Child may need increased amount of rest
	Educate child regarding experimentation with potentially harmful activities
	Health guidance
	Provide for regular health and dental care
	Teach and model sound health practices—including diet, rest, activity
	Encourage children to engage in appropriate physical activities
	Provide a safe physical and emotional environment
	Teach and model safety practices

throughout this period of child development and maturation (see box).

SUMMARY

There is a special quality about the school years. It is the period of childhood that the adult remembers with fond recollections, the one to which the preschooler eagerly looks ahead, and the one for which the adolescent yearns. It is a relatively healthy period of life, a period of steady growth in both body and mind, and a comfortable period of physical adjustment. Physiologic processes in general have developed to the point that they can be maintained at stable levels under ordinary conditions or can be readily adjusted to meet changing needs and stresses. Under normal circumstances children in this age-group are usually well able to meet the physical and psychologic demands that are placed on them.

Social relationships broaden, and the peer group assumes a more important role in their personality and social growth of children. As children feel the need to fit into a peer group and gain a sense of industry through individual cooperative production and performance, they move away from the close, familiar relationships of the family group.

KEY CONCEPTS

- Middle childhood, also known as the school years or the gang age, is a comfortable period of life that extends from 6 to 12 years of age.
- Although slower than previous years, there is a steady gain in height and weight with maturation of body systems; primary teeth are lost and replaced by permanent teeth.
- According to Freud, middle childhood is a period of sexual latency.
- Through the process of education school-age children develop what Erikson terms a sense of industry or accomplishment.
- School-age children, although having a limited capacity for abstract thought, are able to use their thought processes in solving more complex problems, to make judgments based on reasoning, and to see a situation from the point of view of another.
- The child develops a conscience and is able to understand and adhere to rules and standards set by others.
- Entertaining different points of view, becoming sensitive to social norms, and forming peer friendships are the most important features of social development during the school years.
- Cooperative play, team activities, and acquisition of skills are prime elements of play during the school years; rules and rituals assume greater importance.
- School-age children become proficient at many types of physical activities and are able to control various modes of locomotion.
- Typical parental concerns during middle childhood are beginning separation from the family unit, dishonest behavior, and scholastic achievement.
- Optimum nutrition is often hampered by affinity for and availability of junk foods, irregular family meals, and schedules of working parents.
- Advanced intellectual activity and reasoning make the school years an ideal time for sex education.
- School health ideally offers programs that include health appraisal, emergency care and safety, communicable disease control, counseling and guidance, and health education with adjustment to individual student needs.
- Injury prevention is directed toward safety education, providing safe play areas and equipment, and well-supervised sports activities.

STUDY QUESTIONS AND ACTIVITIES

1 Observe several school-age children of the same age. Note similarities and differences in physical development.
2 Interview an early school-age child (6 or 7 years) and an older school-age child (11 or 12 years) regarding favorite activities, a typical day's schedule, and responsibilities in the home. Compare and contrast the findings.
3 In a local eating place observe a family with school-age children. Note the type of food the child orders, parental suggestions or directives, and any disciplinary measures imposed by the parents or siblings.
4 Outline a plan for a class on injury prevention for a group of school-age children.

REFERENCES

Erikson, E.H.: Childhood and society, ed. 2, New York, 1963, W.W. Norton & Co., Inc.

Long, T.J., and Long, L.: Latchkey children: the child's view of self care, U.S. Educational Resources Information Center, ERIC Document ED 214 666, 1982.

Shaffer, T.E.: The young athlete: new guidelines in sports medicine, Pediatr. Consult. **1**(5):1-12, 1980.

Thompson, C.E., and Stroud, L.D.: The motorized tricycle: an accident waiting to happen, J. Pediatr. Nurs. **2**:120-125, 1987.

BIBLIOGRAPHY

General

Allen, M.T.: An overview of the type A behavior pattern in children and adolescents, Pediatr. Nurs. **9**:407-412, 1983.

Belkengren, R.P., and Sapala, S.: Physical fitness from infancy through adolescence, Pediatr. Nurs. **8**(4):A-I, 1982.

Betz, C.L.: Faith development in children, Pediatr. Nurs. **7**(2):22-25, 1981.

Cameron, C.O., Juszczak, L., and Wallace, N.: Using creative arts to help children cope with altered body image, Children's Health Care **12**:108-112, 1984.

Chess, S., and Thomas, A.: Temperamental differences: a critical concept in child health care, Pediatr. Nurs. **11**:167-171, 1985.

Eiden, H., Thomas, M., and Fosarelli, P.: A teaching tool for children in self-care, J. Pediatr. Health Care **1**:292-297, 1987.

Kaluger, G., and Kaluger, M.F.: Human development: the span of life, ed. 3, St. Louis, 1984, The C.V. Mosby Co.

LaMontagne, L.L.: Three coping strategies used by school-age children, Pediatr. Nurs. **10**(1):25-28, 1984.

McClellan, M.A.: On their own: latchkey children, Pediatr. Nurs. **10**:198-202, 1984.

McCown, D.E.: Moral development in children, Pediatr. Nurs. **10**:42-44, 1984.

Newman, B.M., and Newman, P.R.: Development through life: a psychosocial approach, ed. 3, Homewood, Il, 1984, The Dorsey Press.

Pipes, P.L.: Nutrition in infancy and childhood, ed. 4, St. Louis, 1989, The C.V. Mosby Co.

Reasoner, R.W.: Enhancement of self-esteem in children and adolescents, Fam. Community Health **5**(2):51-64, 1983.

Rowland, B.H., Robinson, B.E., and Coleman, M.: A survey of parents' perceptions regarding latchkey children, Pediar. Nurs. **12**:278-283, 1986.

Selekman, J.: The development of body image in the child: a learned response, Top. Clin. Nurs. **5**(1):12-21, 1983.

Shaffer, D.R.: Developmental psychology: theory, research, and applications, Monterey, CA, 1985, Brooks/Cole Publishing Co.

Stanwyck, D.J: Self-esteem through the life span, Fam. Community Health **6**(2):11-28, 1983.

Stone, L.J., and Church, J.: Childhood and adolescence, ed. 5, New York, 1983, Random House, Inc.

Health Promotion

Bausell, R.B.: A national survey assessing pediatric preventive behaviors, Pediatr. Nurs. **11**:438-444, 1985.

Bruhn, J.G., and Nader, P.R.: The school as a setting for health education, health promotion, and health care, Fam. Community Health **4**(1):57-69, 1982.

Dailey, C.P.: Teaching parents and children preventive health behaviors, Fam. Community Health **7**(1):34-43, 1985.

Denehy, J.: What do school-age children know about their bodies? Pediatr. Nurs. **10**:290-292, 1984.

Hussey, C.G., and Hirsh, A.M.: Health education for children, Top. Clin. Nurs. **5**(1):22-28, 1983.

Kaufman, D.H.: An interview guide for helping children make health-care decisions, Pediatr. Nurs. **11**:365-367, 1985.

Koster, M.K.: Self-care: health behavior for the school-age child, Top. Clin. Nurs. **5**(1):29-40, 1983.

Lasky, P.A., Gulbrandsen, M., and Scoblic, M.: Health education translated into health behavior, Issues Compr. Pediatr. Nurs. **5**:167-175, 1981.

Lewis, C.E., and Lewis, M.A.: Determinants of children's health-related beliefs and behaviors, Fam. Community Health **4**(4):85-97, 1982.

Morris, N.M.: Pediatric health promotion through risk reduction, Fam. Community Health **3**(1):63-76, 1980.

Narins, D.M., Belkengren, R.P., and Sapala, S.: Nutrition and the growing athlete, Pediatr. Nurs. **9**(3):163-168, 1983.

Otto, J.: Be prepared for camp nursing, Am. J. Nurs. **80**:906-907, 1980.

Pidgeon, V., and Olson, S.: A comparison of illness concepts of school age children and adolescents, Issues Compr. Pediatr. Nurs. **9**:209-221, 1986.

Robinson, T.: School nurse practitioners on the job, Am. J. Nurs. **81**:1674-1676, 1981.

Wood, S.P.: School aged children's perceptions of the causes of illness, Pediatr. Nurs. **9**:101-104, 1983.

Wurthman, J.J.: What do children eat? Eating styles of the preschool, elementary school, and adolescent child. In Suskind, R.M., editor: Textbook of pediatric nutrition, New York, 1981, Raven Press.

Dental Health

Babington, M.A., and Spadaro, D.C.: Cariogenic medications, Pediatr. Nurs. **8**:165-171, 1982.

Boraz, R.A.: Preventive dentistry for the pediatric patient, Issues Compr. Pediatr. Nurs. **5**:89-97, 1981.

Cormier, J.F., and Trammel, H.: Fight tooth decay: the fluoride plan, Pediatr. Nurs. **5**(3):18-22, 1979.

Heifetz, S.B., and Horowitz, H.S.: Fluorides and sealants for the prevention of dental caries, Fam. Community Health **3**(3):23-32, 1980.

Hess, C.S., and others: Fluoride: too much to too little? Pediatr. Nurs. **10**:397-403, 1984.

Jenkins, N.: Diet and dental caries, Food Nutr. News **56**:29-32, 1984.

Jolley, H.M., and Pless, I.B.: Dental health and pediatrics, Pediatr. Rev. **3**:13-22, 1981.

Josell, S.D., and Abrams, R.G.: Traumatic injuries to the dentition and its supporting structures, Pediatr. Clin. North Am. **29**:717, 1982.

Kilmon, C., and Helpin, M.L.: Update on dentistry for children, Pediatr. Nurs. **7**(5):41-44, 1981.

Kilmon, C., and Helpin, M.L.: Recognizing dental malocclusion in children, Pediatr. Nurs. **9**:204-208, 1983.

Kronmiller, K.E., and Nirschl, R.F.: Preventive dentistry for children, Pediatr. Nurs. **11**:446-449, 1985.

Starr, R.M., and Gravitz, R.F.: Pit and fissure sealants in the prevention of tooth decay, Pediatr. Nurs. **11**:289-291, 1985.

Suomi, J.D.: Methods for the prevention of periodontal diseases, Fam. Community Health **3**(3):41-49, 1980.

School Health

Andersen, A.R., and Clore, E.R.: Asbestos in schools: reducing pediatric risk factors, Pediatr. Nurs. **12:**296-321, 1986.

Hester, N.D.: Health concerns of school-age children, Issues Compr. Pediatr. Nurs. **10:**251-262, 1987.

Oda, D.: A viewpoint on school nursing, Am. J. Nurs. **81:**1677-1678, 1981.

Oda, D.S., and others: Nurse practitioners and primary care in schools, MCN **10:**127-131, 1985.

Meeker, R., and others: A comprehensive school health initiative, Image **18:**86-91, 1986.

Schor, D.P.: Temperament and the initial school experience, Child Health Care **13:**129-134, 1985.

Switzer, K.H., and Kelly, J.T.: The nurse: a member of the school team, MCN **6:**289-293, 1981.

Injury Prevention

Arenson, S., and others: Factors affecting parental use of child automobile safety restraints, Children's Health Care **13**(4):181-186, 1985.

Betz, C.L.: Bicycle safety: opportunities for family education, Pediatr. Nurs. **9:**111, 1983.

Lee, E.J.: Accident reports: survey of high school injuries, Pediatr. Nurs. **13:**151-154, 1987.

Hancock, L.A.: Safe biking—a bike helmet, J. Pediatr. Health Care **1:**334-335, 1987.

Holland, S.H.: Car safety for school children and adolescents, Children's Nurse **4**(4):1-4, 1986.

Righi, F.C., and Krozy, R.E.: The child in the car: what every nurse should know about safety, Am. J. Nurs. **83:**1421-1424, 1983.

Thomas, K.A.: Screening the child for sports participation, Issues Compr. Pediatr. Nurs. **5:**179-194, 1983.

CHAPTER 16

Health Promotion of the Adolescent and Family

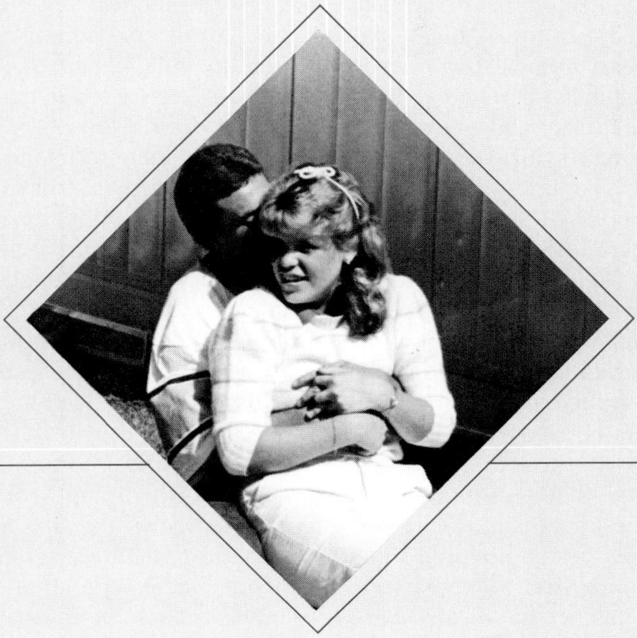

LEARNING OBJECTIVES

On completion of this chapter the reader will be able to:

- Describe the physical changes that occur at puberty in the male and the female
- Discuss the reactions of the adolescent to physical changes that take place at puberty
- Demonstrate an understanding of the processes by which the adolescent develops a sense of identity
- Discuss the significance of the changing interpersonal relationships and the role of the peer group during adolescence
- Outline a health teaching plan for adolescents
- Plan a sex education session for a group of adolescents
- Identify the causes and discuss the preventive aspects of injuries during adolescence

Adolescence is a period of transition between childhood and adulthood—a time of physical, social, and emotional maturing as the boy prepares for manhood and the girl for womanhood. The precise bounderies of adolescence are difficult to define, but this period is customarily viewed as beginning with the gradual appearance of secondary sex characteristics at about 11 or 12 years of age and ending with cessation of body growth at 18 to 20 years.

◆ *Promoting Optimum Growth and Development*

Several terms are commonly used in reference to this particular stage of growth and development. *Puberty* primarily refers to the maturational, hormonal, and growth process that occurs when the reproductive organs begin to function and the secondary sex characteristics develop. This process is sometimes divided into three stages: *pubescence,* the period of about 2 years immediately prior to puberty when the child is developing preliminary physical changes that herald sexual maturity and when he is experiencing the prepubertal growth spurt; *puberty,* the point at which sexual maturity is achieved, marked by the first menstrual flow in girls but by less obvious indications in boys; and *postpubescence,* a 1- to 2-year period following puberty during which skeletal growth is completed and reproductive functions become fairly well established. *Adolescence,* which literally means "to grow into maturity," is generally regarded as the psychologic, social, and maturational process initiated by the pubertal changes. The term *teenage years* is used synonymously with adolescence to describe ages 13 through 19.

Adolescence is a period of life that presents special problems of adjustment. With the impetus of their internal changes and the pressures of society, children must progress to emotional independence from their parents, consider prospects of economic independence, and learn the meaning of a more intimate heterosexual companionship. They learn to work with age-mates on common interests, to subordinate personal differences as they pursue a common goal, and to become responsible persons who are in control of their lives and who possess a knowledge of who they are in relation to the world.

BIOLOGIC DEVELOPMENT

The physical changes of puberty are primarily the result of hormonal activity under the influence of the central nervous system, although all aspects of physiologic functioning are mutually interacting. The very obvious physical changes are noted in increased physical growth and the appearance and development of secondary sex characteristics; less obvious are physiologic alterations and neurogonadal maturity, accompanied by the ability to procreate. Physical distinction between the sexes is determined on the basis of distinguishing characteristics: *primary sex characteristics* are the external and internal organs that carry on the reproductive functions; *secondary sex characteristics* are the characteristics that distinguish the sexes from each other but play no direct part in reproduction.

Hormonal Changes of Puberty

It is generally accepted that the events of puberty are caused by hormonal influences and controlled by the anterior pituitary (adenohypophysis) in response to a stimulus from the hypothalamus. Stimulation of the gonads has a dual function: (1) production and release of gametes—production of sperm in the male and maturation and release of ova in the female—and (2) secretion of sex-appropriate hormones—estrogen and progesterone from the ovaries (female) and testosterone from the testes (male).

Sex hormones. Sex hormones are secreted by the ovaries, testes, and adrenals, and they are produced in varying amounts by both sexes throughout the life span. The adrenal cortex is responsible for the small amounts secreted during the prepubescent years, but the sex hormone production that accompanies maturation of the gonads is responsible for the variety of biologic changes observed during pubescence and puberty.

Estrogen, the feminizing hormone, is found in low quantities during childhood; it is secreted in slowly increasing amounts until about age 11 years. In males this gradual increase continues through maturation. In females the onset of estrogen production in the ovary causes a pronounced increase that continues until about 3 years after the onset of menstruation, at which time it reaches a maximum level that continues throughout the reproductive life of the female.

Androgens, the masculinizing hormones, are also secreted in small and gradually increasing amounts up to about 7 or 9 years of age, at which time there is a more rapid increase in both sexes, especially boys, until about age 15 years. These hormones appear to be responsible for most of the rapid growth changes of early adolescence. With the onset of testicular function, the level of androgens (principally testosterone) in males increases over that in females and continues to increase until a maximum is attained at maturity.

Sexual Maturation

The visible evidence of sexual maturation is achieved in orderly sequence, and the state of maturity can be estimated on the basis of the appearance of these external manifestations. The age at which these changes are observed and the time required to progress from one stage to another may vary considerably between individual children. From the appearance of breast buds to full maturity may take from 1½ to 6 years for adolescent girls; male genitalia may take from 2 to 5 years to reach adult size. The stages of the development of secondary sex characteristics and genital development have been defined as a guide for estimating sexual maturity.

The usual sequence of appearance of maturational changes in girls is as follows: rapid increase in height and weight, breast changes, increase in pelvic girth, growth of pubic hair, appearance of axillary hair, menstruation (which usually begins 2 years after first signs), and an abrupt deceleration of linear growth.

The usual sequence of appearance of maturational changes in boys is as follows: increase in weight; enlargement of testicles; rapid increase in height; growth of pubic hair, axillary hair, hair on upper lip, hair on face and elsewhere on body (facial hair usually appears about 2 years after appearance of pubic hair); changes in the larynx and, consequently, the voice, which usually take place concurrently with growth of the penis; nocturnal emissions; and an abrupt deceleration of linear growth.

Sexual maturation in girls. Approximately 1 to 2 years before the onset of menstruation in the female, the secretion of estrogen assumes a cyclic pattern. The initial appearance of menstruation *(menarche)* occurs about 2 years after the first appearance of pubescent changes. The normal age range of menarche is usually considered to be 10 to 15 years, with the average age being 12.5 years for North American girls. Menarche has been related to a critical point in body weight (48 kg or 106 pounds) but may vary with race. During the establishment of the ovarian cycle, the menstrual periods are usually scanty and irregular and may not be accompanied by ovulation. Ovulation usually occurs 12 to 24 months after menarche.

Sexual maturation in boys. Unlike the cyclic germ cell production in the female, spermatogenesis is a continuous process that is usually well established by 17 years of age. In boys there is no sudden physical change to indicate puberty, such as menarche in girls. The overt signal in boys is the beginning of nocturnal emissions of seminal fluid, which occur spontaneously during sleep at intervals of approximately 2 weeks. Nocturnal emissions will persist into adulthood and will occur whenever there is a buildup of semen in the genital ducts. As with girls, mature germ cells may not be produced for several months. The average age range at which boys attain puberty is 12.5 to 16.5 years, with a mean of 14.5 years.

Physical Growth

A constant phenomenon associated with sexual maturation is a dramatic increase in growth. The final 20% to 25% of linear growth is achieved during puberty, and most of this growth occurs during a 24- to 36-month period—the adolescent growth spurt. This accelerated growth occurs in all children but, as in other areas of development, is highly variable in age of onset, duration, and extent. The growth spurt begins earlier in girls, usually between ages 10 and 14 years; on the average it begins between ages 12 ana 16 years in boys. During this period the average boy will gain 10 to 30 cm (4 to 12 inches) in height and 7 to 30 kg (15 to 65 pounds) in weight; the average girl, in whom the growth spurt is slower and less extensive, will gain 5 to 20 cm (2 to 8 inches) in height and 7 to 25 kg (15 to 55 pounds) in weight. Growth in height commonly ceases at 16 or 17 years in girls and 18 to 20 years in boys (Figs. 16-1 and 16-2).

This increase in size is acquired in a characteristic sequence of changes. Growth in length of extremities and neck precedes growth in other areas, and, since these parts are first to reach adult length, the hands and feet

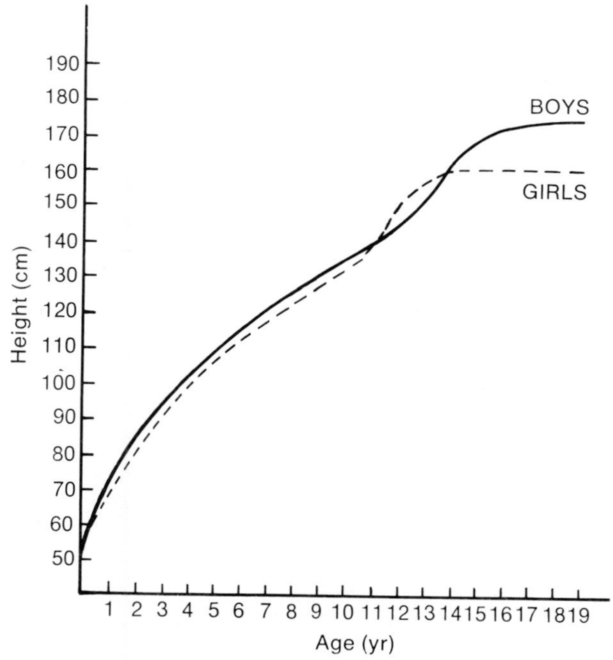

FIG. 16-1 Linear growth throughout childhood. (From Taner, J.M., Whitehouse, R.H., and Takaishi, M.: Arch. Dis. Child. **41**:454-471, 1966.)

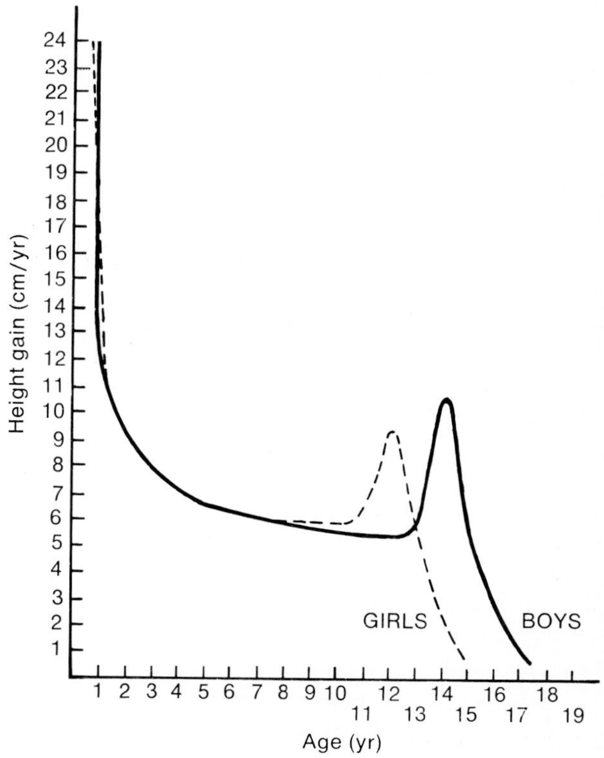

FIG. 16-2 Linear growth in centimeters per year. (From Tanner, J.M., Whitehouse, R.H., and Takaishi, M.: Arch. Dis. Child. **41**:454-471, 1966.)

appear larger than normal during adolescence. Increases in hip and chest breadth take place in a few months, followed several months later by an increase in shoulder width. These changes are followed by increases in length of the trunk and depth of the chest. It is this sequence of changes that is responsible for the characteristic long-legged, gawky appearance of the early adolescent child.

Sex differences in general growth patterns. Sex differences in general growth and distribution patterns are apparent in skeletal growth, muscle mass, adipose tissue, and skin. Skeletal growth differences between boys and girls are apparently a function of hormonal effects at puberty and are evident primarily in limb length. The earlier cessation of growth in girls is caused by epiphyseal unity under the potent effect of estrogen secretion, and the hormonal effect on female bone growth is much stronger than the similar effect of testosterone in males. In boys, the prolonged growth period prior to puberty and the less rapid epiphyseal closure are reflected in their greater overall height and longer arms and legs. Other skeletal differences are increased shoulder width in boys and broader hip development in girls.

Hypertrophy of the laryngeal mucosa and enlargement of the larynx and vocal cords occur in both boys and girls to produce voice changes. Girls' voices become slightly deeper and considerably fuller, but the effect in boys is striking. The "change of voice" in adolescent boys is one of the most noticeable traits of puberty, with the voice often shifting uncontrollably from deep to high tones in the middle of a sentence.

Growth of lean body mass, principally muscle, which tends to occur after the bone growth spurt, takes place steadily during adolescence. Lean body mass is both quantitatively and qualitatively greater in males than in females at comparable stages of pubertal development. Muscle development, under the influence of androgenic hormones, increases steadily. Muscles become remarkably well developed in boys, whereas in girls muscle mass increase is proportionate to general tissue growth.

Nonlean mass, primarily fat, is also increased but follows a less orderly pattern. There may be a transient increase in subcutaneous fat just prior to the skeletal growth spurt, especially in boys. This is followed 1 to 2 years later by a modest to marked decrease, again more marked in boys. Later, variable amounts of fat are deposited to fill out and contour the mature physique in patterns characteristic of the adolescent's sex.

Hormonal influences during puberty cause an acceleration in growth and maturation of the skin and its structural appendages. Sebaceous glands become extremely active at this time, especially those on the genitals and in the "flush areas" of the body—that is, the face, neck, shoulders, and upper back and chest. This increased activity and the structural nature of the glands are extremely important in the pathogenesis of a common problem of puberty, acne. The eccrine sweat glands, present almost everywhere on the human skin, become fully functional and respond to emotional as well as thermal stimulation. Heavy sweating appears to be more pronounced in boys than in girls. The apocrine sweat glands, nonfunctional in childhood, reach secretory capacity during puberty. Unlike the eccrine sweat glands, the apocrine glands are limited in distribution and grow in conjunction with hair follicles in the axillae, around the areola of the breast, around the umbilicus, on the external auditory canal, and in the genital and anal regions. Apocrine glands secrete a thick substance as a result of emotional stimulation that, when acted on by surface bacteria, becomes highly odoriferous.

Body hair assumes very characteristic distribution patterns and changes texture during puberty. Under the influence of gonadal and adrenal androgens, hair coarsens, darkens, and lengthens at sites related to secondary sex characteristics. Pubic and axillary hair appears in both sexes, although pubic hair is more extensive in males than in females. Beard, mustache, and body hair on the chest, upward along the linea alba, and sometimes on other areas (such as the back and shoulder) appear in males. Extremity hair appears in varying amounts in both males and females but is also more prolific in the male.

Physiologic Changes

A number of physiologic functions are altered in response to some of the pubertal changes. The size and strength of the heart, blood volume, and systolic blood pressure increase, whereas the pulse rate and basal heat production decrease (see inside front cover). Blood volume, which has increased steadily during childhood, reaches a higher value in boys than in girls, a fact that may be related to the increased muscle mass in pubertal boys. Adult values are reached for all formed elements of the blood. Respiratory rate and basal metabolic rate, decreasing steadily throughout childhood, reach the adult rate in adolescence.

Through progressive maturation of the body as it reaches adult size, the adolescent develops the ability to respond to physical stresses and strains equal to or in excess of adult competence. During this period physiologic responses to exercise change drastically—performance improves, especially in boys, and the body is able to make the physiologic adjustments needed for normal function after exercise is completed. These capabilities are a result of the increased size and strength of muscles and the increased level of cardiac, respiratory, and metabolic functioning. Adolescents enjoy physical activity, and there appears to be a positive relationship between regular exercise and physical conditioning activities and good general health, endurance, and appearance.

PSYCHOSOCIAL DEVELOPMENT

While adolescents are adjusting to physical changes that may contribute to or detract from their feelings of self-worth, they are learning how to use their developing mental capacities. Their ability to reason, to assess and evaluate, and to use divergent thinking to come up with new ideas increases during this period of life. The adolescent begins to think beyond the present and into the future. However, these capacities and the ability to make good judgments are still limited by inexperience and, as yet, insufficient knowledge from which to gain an adequate perspective for problem solving.

Personality Development (Freud)

The genital period, the longest and last of Freud's psychosexual stages, begins with puberty and extends to old age. It is the stage in which the individual arrives at full sexual potency. Throughout adolescence and young adulthood the libido is invested in activities that prepare the individual to satisfy the mature sex instinct through procreation. The activities are primarily those of forming friendships, preparing for a career, courting, and marriage.

Personality Development (Erikson)

Traditional psychosocial theory holds that the developmental crisis of adolescence leads to the formation of a sense of identity (Erikson, 1963). Throughout childhood individuals have been going through the process of identification as they concentrate on various parts of the body at specific times. During infancy the child identifies himself as separate from the mother, during early childhood he establishes a gender role identification with the appropriate-sex parent, and in later childhood he establishes who he is in relation to others. In adolescence he comes to see himself as a distinct individual, somehow unique and separate from every other individual. In the light of their observations, some authorities see the central conflict of identity vs role diffusion of adolescence as being resolved in two stages (Newman and Newman, 1984). The early period of adolescence begins with the onset of puberty and extends to relative physical and emotional stability at or near graduation from high school. During this time the adolescent is faced with the crisis of *group identity* vs alienation. In the period that follows, the individual hopes to attain autonomy from the family and develop a sense of *personal identity* as opposed to role diffusion. A sense of group identity appears to be essential as a prelude to a sense of personal identity. Young adolescents must resolve questions concerning relationships with a peer group before they are able to resolve questions about who they are in relation to family and society.

Group identity. During the early stage of adolescence the pressure to belong to a group is intensified. Teenagers find it essential to have a group to which they feel they can belong and which provides them with status. Belonging to a crowd helps adolescents to define the differences between themselves and their parents. They dress as the group dresses and wear makeup and hairstyles according to group criteria—all of which are different from those of the parental generation. Language, music, and dancing reflect a culture that is exclusive to the adolescent. When adults begin to emulate these fashions and interests, the style changes immediately. The evidence of adolescent conformity to the peer group and nonconformity to the adult group provides teenagers with a frame of reference in which they can display their own self-assertion while they reject the identity of their parents' generation.

Individual identity. The quest for personal identity is part of the ongoing identification process. As the child establishes identity within a group, he is also attempting to incorporate multiple body changes into a concept of the self. Body awareness is part of self-awareness, and for some time the adolescent will engage in assimilating the self represented by this dimension. It has been determined that the body image established during adolescence is the one that the individual retains throughout life. Much of the adolescent's search for identity takes place before a mirror as he tries to read from the reflected features just who he is and what he looks like to other people (Fig. 16-3). The adolescent practices facial expressions and postures, tries out hair arrangements, worries about a pimple, and in other ways attempts to assess the best means to achieve a maximum effect—to reveal the "true self."

In this search for identity, adolescents take into consideration the relationships that have developed between themselves and others in the past as well as the directions they hope to be able to take in the future. Significant others hold certain expectations for the behavior of the adolescent. Often these expectations or demands are persistent enough to induce certain decisions that might be made differently or not at all if the individual could be solely responsible for identity formation. It is all too easy to slip into the roles that are expected by these external influences without incorporating personal goals or questioning these decisions in relation to the developing per-

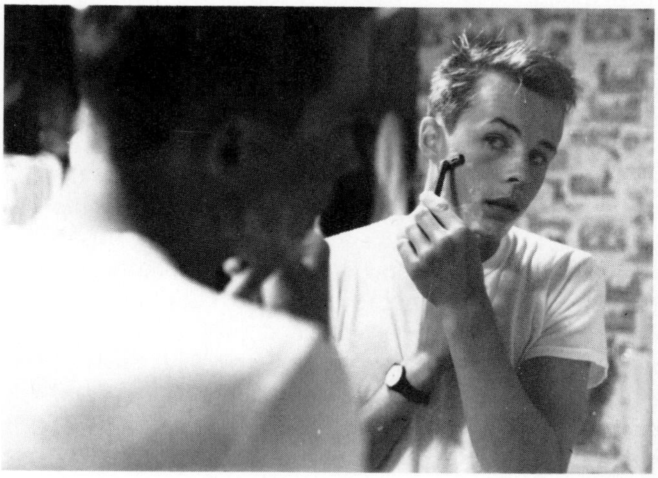

FIG. 16-3 Time spent before a mirror helps a teenager acquire a personal identity.

sonality. Thus the individual becomes what parents or others wish him to be based on these premature decisions. Also, a young person might form a negative identity when society or his culture provides him with a self-image that is contrary to the values of the community. Labels such as "juvenile delinquent," "hood," or "failure" are applied to certain adolescents, who then accept and live up to these labels with behaviors that validate and strengthen them.

The process of evolving a personal identity is time-consuming and fraught with periods of confusion, depression, and discouragement. To determine an identity and a place in the world is a critical and perilous feature of adolescence. However, as the pieces are gradually shifted and settled into place, a positive identity eventually emerges from the confusion. Role diffusion results when the individual is unable to formulate a satisfactory identity from the multiplicity of aspirations, roles, and identifications.

Sex-role identity. Adolescence is the time for consolidation of a sex-role identity. During early adolescence the peer group begins to communicate some expectations regarding heterosexual relationships, and, as development progresses, adolescents encounter expectations for mature sex-role behavior from both peers and adults. Expectations such as these vary from culture to culture, between geographic areas, and between socioeconomic groups.

COGNITIVE DEVELOPMENT (PIAGET)

Progression in the realm of cognitive thinking culminates with the capacity for abstract thinking. This stage, the period of formal operations, is Piaget's fourth and last stage. Living in the nonpresent as well as the present, adolescents are no longer concerned with and restricted to the real and actual, which was typical of the period of concrete thought, but they are also concerned with the possible. They now think beyond the present. At this time their thoughts can be influenced by more logical principles than by their own perceptions and experiences. They now become capable of scientific reasoning and formal logic. Without having to center attention on the immediate situation, they can imagine the possible—a sequence of events that might occur, such as college and occupational possibilities; how things might change in the future, such as relationships with parents; and the consequences of their actions, such as dropping out of school.

Young people are now able to think about their own thinking and the thinking of others. They wonder what opinion others have of them, and they are increasingly able to imagine the thoughts of others. With this capacity comes the ability to differentiate between others' thoughts and their own and to interpret thoughts of others more accurately. Thus they are able to see themselves and the world in a more relativistic way. As they come to know that other cultures and communities have different norms and standards from their own, it becomes easier to accept members of these other cultures and the decision to behave in their own culture in an accepted manner becomes a more conscious commitment to that culture.

MORAL DEVELOPMENT (KOHLBERG)

Late adolescence is characterized by a serious questioning of existing moral values and their relevance to society and the individual. Adolescents can easily take the role of another. They understand duty and obligation based on reciprocal rights of others, as well as the concept of justice that is founded on making amends for misdeeds and repairing or replacing what has been spoiled by wrongdoing. However, they seriously question established moral codes, often as a result of observing that adults verbally ascribe to a code but do not adhere to it.

Whereas the younger child merely accepts the decisions or point of view of adults, the adolescent, to gain autonomy from adults, must substitute his own set of morals and values. When old principles are challenged but new and independent values have not yet emerged to take their place, young people search for a moral code that preserves their personal integrity and guides their behavior, especially in the face of strong pressure to violate the old beliefs. Their decisions involving moral dilemmas must be based on an internalized set of moral principles that provides them with the resources to evaluate the demands of the situation and to plan a course of action that is consistent with their ideals.

SPIRITUAL DEVELOPMENT

As youngsters move toward independence from parents and other authorities, some begin to question the values and ideals of their families. Others cling to these values as a stable element in their lives as they struggle with the conflicts of this turbulent period. Adolescents need to work out these conflicts for themselves, but they also need support from authority figures and/or peers for their resolution. Often the peer group is more influential than parents, although values acquired during the formative years are usually maintained.

Adolescents are capable of understanding abstract concepts and of interpreting analogies and symbols. They are able to empathize, philosophize, and think logically. Most are searching for ideals and speculate about illogical statements and conflicting ideologies. Their tendency toward introspection and emotional intensity at this age often makes it difficult for others to know what they are thinking. They tend to keep their thoughts private, fearing that no one will understand these feelings that they perceive to be unique and special. It is not uncommon for them to reveal deep spiritual concerns and then become silly and deny these feelings (Shelly, 1982). They need support and encouragement in their struggle for understanding and the freedom to question without censure.

DEVELOPMENT OF A BODY IMAGE

Physical growth and maturation during adolescence occur so rapidly that these young people have difficulty in adjusting to a changing body image. Adolescence is the time when young persons' self-awareness reaches a peak and, as a result of sexual awareness, when much of their thought and concern is turned inward. The sudden growth that takes place in early adolescence creates feelings of confusion about their bodies. Teenagers are acutely aware of their appearance as they begin to acquire images of themselves as adults, but they see discrepancies between their ideal and actual skills and abilities.

Strange and unfamiliar feelings press on them as inner urges announce a sexual awakening. Sexuality is not the same for boys as it is for girls, and it has different psychic overtones that influence behavior and adaptation. Although it appears that the intensity of the sexual drive is different in adolescent boys and girls, this has not been conclusively demonstrated. Current findings indicate that the difference may be related to the physiologic nature of the sex drive rather than to its intensity. Sexual arousal in males is very direct and centered in the genitals, whereas in females it is more vague, diffuse, and closely linked to their total personality.

Boys' Responses to Puberty

The early adolescent increases in height and muscle mass are welcomed by the adolescent boy, whose growth, for several months, has lagged significantly behind that of his female age-mates. Although his more mature physique brings a highly valued increase in strength and more mature athletic skills, this rapid growth is uneven and he therefore has some trouble adjusting. When bones grow faster than muscles, muscles are taut and respond with quick, jerky movements; when muscles grow faster than bones, they become somewhat loose and sluggish. For a period of time he is awkward and uncoordinated.

The development of secondary sex characteristics, especially the growth of facial and body hair, has psychologic and social meaning to the adolescent boy. This, more than any other secondary characteristic, is associated with the masculine sex role, and the ritual act of shaving at the slightest evidence of growth is a way for the young boy to validate his identification with this role. Shaving also provides a legitimate excuse to gaze at and admire the broadening shoulders and altered features of his changing body image.

The growth of the penis and testes creates some important problems for the adolescent male. Unlike the reproductive organs in the female, the male reproductive organs are readily visible and provide the boy with concrete evidence of his masculine character. He knows by the sensations localized within these organs that he is now a man. His reproductive organs become very sensitive to sexual stimulation. Sexual feelings are directly related to the genitals, desire is urgent, and he seeks rapid relief from pressure and tension through ejaculation. Spontaneous ejaculations are frequently puzzling, troublesome, and embarrassing events. Unless he has been prepared in advance for this eventuality, the boy often finds it difficult to seek an explanation from his parents; therefore, he turns to friends or reading material to gain information, or he may puzzle about the meaning in his own mind.

The opportunity for gratification of these genital urges through heterosexual expression is often limited by Western cultural standards, early premarital sexual involvement is fraught with many problems and conflicts, and homosexual activities are generally condemned by society. As a consequence, the teenage boy resorts to masturbation, the manipulation of the genitals for the purpose of ejaculation, to relieve him of the accumulated pressures in his genital organs. It is essentially a normal activity, and almost every boy masturbates alone or in relation to sexual experimentation with others of the same sex. However, this too is often associated with guilt and anxiety. Misconceptions still dominate the feelings of many people who believe masturbation to be evil, unmanly, or "not nice" and who attribute a wide assortment of ills to the practice. Current enlightenment accepts that to engage in the practice from time to time is normal and temporarily helps provide the young man with important information about how his body works and how adult physical sexuality and reproduction are accomplished.

Girls' Responses to Puberty

As girls begin the pubertal changes, they, too, become very body conscious. Because in girls the onset of puberty is almost 2 years in advance of that in boys, their initial reaction to increased height may be embarrassment, as they find themselves towering above their male classmates. They worry about becoming too tall. Adolescent girls often slouch or adopt a hunched posture in an attempt to minimize this increased height—especially early-maturing girls, who are normally of above-average height. The increase in weight and the normal plumping of features with fat deposition are predominant concerns of the pubescent girl. They perceive these changes to be evidence of a tendency toward obesity; many attempt to avoid them by strict and rather faddish dieting. This ill-timed strategy can deprive their bodies of essential nutrients during a period of rapid body development.

The young girl is interested in her changing form and feminine curves. The average girl looks on her budding breasts with pleasure as a sign of approaching maturity and evidence of her femininity. She observes and may even measure the progress of her developing breasts and continually compares her own progress with that of her friends and classmates. She begins to wear a bra. Some girls are sensitive about their breast development and attempt to hide it, whereas others are delighted with their new figures and wear tight sweaters and clothes that accentuate their curves.

Development of some of the secondary sex characteristics may be less pleasing to girls than they are to boys, particularly the growth of body hair. A culture in which smooth-skinned females are preferred makes it necessary for the girl to shave her underarms and legs regularly to meet the standards for feminine appearance. The girl becomes increasingly conscious of the feminine ideal and, in an effort to approach this standard, experiments with a variety of cosmetics and hairstyles. Alone and together, she and her friends spend endless hours before the mirror posing, applying cosmetics, and combing their hair.

The advent of menstruation, that exclusive feature of female puberty, provides the greatest impetus toward full realization and acceptance of female sexuality. Menstruation is positive evidence of womanhood and the potential for pregnancy and childbearing. Most girls are adequately prepared for the event and take this new function in stride, looking forward to menstruation, feeling satisfaction at its onset, and seeing it as the symbol of their passage from childhood to womanhood. Others find it distressing, frightening, and difficult to accept.

Unlike the adolescent boy, strong sexual feelings in the adolescent girl are not usually centered in the genital region but are more generalized and ill defined. Her reproductive apparatus, less obvious than that of the boy, contributes in only a vague way to sexual awareness. The girl in early adolescence may experience pleasant sensations and even tingling in the genital area, but these feelings are diffuse and difficult to separate from other body sensations. Her sexual feelings are centered less on the genitals and erotic gratification with release of tension than on manipulating a pleasant state with romantic feelings about love. Sexual impulses tend to be secondary rather than primary as they are in the boy. However, with the more open, liberal views regarding female sexual responses, it is being revealed that much of the nature of the adolescent girl's sexual arousal may have a cultural rather than a biologic basis.

In the adolescent girl, the urge for self-stimulation is not as strong as it is in the male. Although many girls handle the genitals for the pleasant sensation that is evoked, not all carry the activity to a climax. Masturbation is frequently combined with fantasy.

SOCIAL DEVELOPMENT

To achieve full maturity, adolescents must free themselves from family domination and define an identity independent of parental authority. However, this process is fraught with ambivalence on the part of both teenagers and their parents. Adolescents want to grow up and to be free of parental restraints, yet they are fearful as they try to comprehend the responsibilities that are linked with independence. Part of this emancipation involves developing social relationships outside the family that help teenagers identify their role in society.

Relationships with Parents

During adolescence the parent-child relationship changes from one of protection-dependency to one of mutual affection and equality. The process of achieving independence often involves turmoil and ambiguity as both parent and adolescent learn to play new roles and work toward this end while, at the same time, resolving the often painful series of rifts essential to establishing the ultimate relationships.

Most of the behavior observed in the adolescent is related to the struggle for independence and the external restrictions and checks that are placed on this spontaneous maturation process. On the one hand, adolescents are accepted as maturing preadults. They are allowed privileges heretofore denied, and they are provided with increasing responsibilities. On the other hand, because of their unpredictability and insecurity in evaluating situations and making sound judgments, they must conform to regulations and restrictions set by adults. This state of affairs is particularly exemplified by the struggle between parents and adolescents concerning the nightly curfew.

The teenager's earliest attempts to achieve emancipation from parental controls are manifested in a period of rejection of the parents. Adolescents are critical, argumentative, and generally remote with both parents. They absent themselves from home and family activities and spend an increasing amount of time with the peer group. They are less close and confiding in relationships with parents. This rejection is not consistent, however, and varies with mood changes.

With advancing adolescence, teenagers become more competent, and with this competence comes a need for more autonomy. However, although they are psychologically better prepared for independence, they are often thwarted in their efforts by lack of money or by other parental barriers. Much conflict arises from the teenager's outside activities and the elements of privacy and trust. To gain the respect and trust of their adolescent, parents must respect his privacy and show an honest and sincere interest in what he believes and feels.

The recent trends in society in terms of equality and relaxation of previous moral standards have made the adjustments of teenagers and parents increasingly difficult. The so-called generation gap is widening in relation to a number of attitudes, values, and beliefs. Parents can no longer find guidance from their own experiences in understanding the needs of today's teenagers.

Relationships with Peers

Although parents remain the primary influence in their lives, for the majority of adolescents peers assume a more significant role in adolescence than they did during childhood. The peer group serves as a strong support to teenagers, individually and collectively, providing them with a sense of belonging and a feeling of strength and power. It forms that transitional world between dependence and autonomy.

Peer group. Adolescents have always been social, gregarious, and group minded. Except in a few small, homogeneous high schools, teenagers distribute themselves into a relatively predictable social hierarchy. The largest social division is the set. Both boys and girls are members of the crowd, but for some occasions and activities they separate into like-sex crowds. The adolescents know to which set they and others belong, although in large schools they may not all know each other.

Within the set are smaller, distinct, and rather exclusive crowds or cliques of selected close friends, based on common tastes, interests, and background, who are emotionally attached to each other. Although cliques may become formalized, most remain informal and small. But each has an identifying feature that proclaims its difference from others and its solidarity within itself, in much the same manner as the adolescent generation as a whole sets itself apart from the adult generation. Cliques are usually made up of one sex, and girls tend to be more cliquish than boys and to have a greater need for close friendships (Fig. 16-4). Within the intimacy of the group, adolescents gain support in learning about themselves, consideration for the feelings of others, and increased ego development and self-reliance.

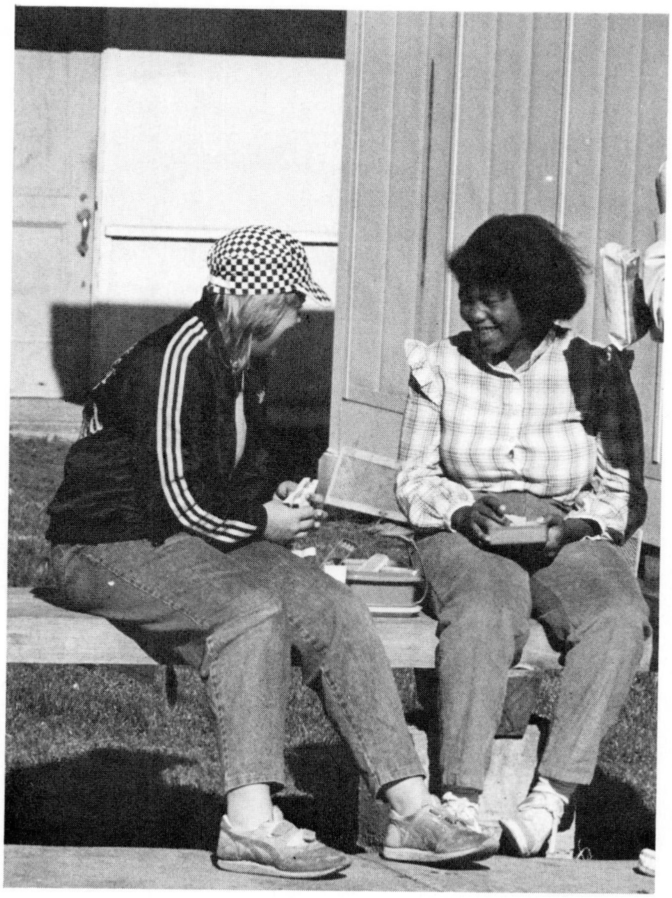

FIG. 16-4 Teenagers like to gather in small groups.

Best friends. Personal friendships of the one-to-one variety usually develop between like-sex adolescents. This relationship is closer and more stable than it is in middle childhood, and it is important in the quest for identity. A best friend is the best audience on whom to try out possible roles and identities that an adolescent wants to test. Best friends may try a role together, each providing support for the other. Each cares about what the other thinks and feels. Since a sense of intimacy grows within a permanent relationship, the stability of this like-sex friendship is an important link in the progress toward an intimate heterosexual relationship in young adulthood.

Heterosexual Relationships

During adolescence relationships with members of the opposite sex take on new importance. Although there seems to be a trend toward earlier dating, on the *average*, dating activities begin in the seventh and eighth grades and are usually "crowd" dates at organized school functions. For example, a group of girls just happens to be around a certain group of boys at most activities. By the ninth grade crowd dates are still popular, but now there is more pairing off of couples. In the tenth grade paired crowd dates, in which some boys and girls come as couples and join the crowd consisting of several couples and perhaps a few unattached friends, are the rule. Double-dating follows group dating and is the more common practice in the eleventh grade; both double-dating and single-pair dating are common by the twelfth grade. Most adolescents are dating to some degree by the time they leave high school.

The type and degree of seriousness of heterosexual relationships vary. The initial stage is usually noncommittal, extremely mobile, and seldom characterized by any deep romantic attachments. Crushes, those strong feelings of attachment to an important or well-liked adult in the youngster's life, are common in early adolescence; one of the earliest "love" attachments. With advancing adolescence and a more firm sexual identity, steady dating and boy-girl love relationships with deeper commitment become more numerous. The relationship continues until misunderstanding or boredom ends the association, and the process is often repeated with another partner.

Authorities disagree regarding the value of early opposite-sex relationships in the development of a sexual identity. Some believe that longer like-sex relationships are necessary to fully develop the characteristics of their own sex, whereas others believe that dating provides adolescents with experience in human relationships, promotes

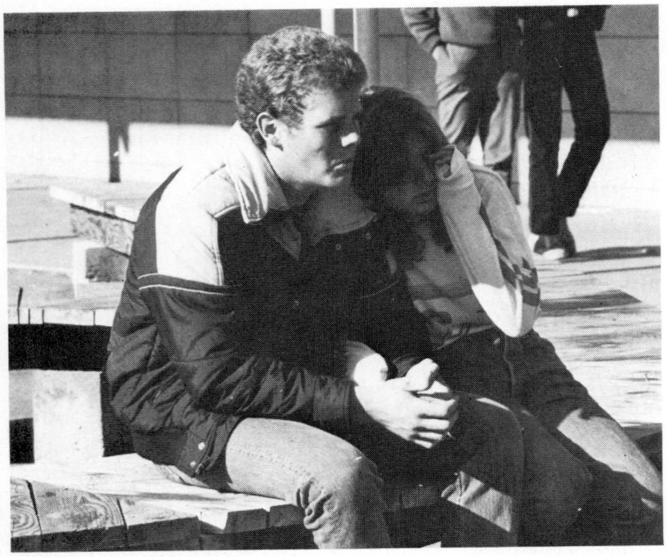

FIG. 16-5 Heterosexual friendships are characteristics of adolescence.

social skills, and enhances their ability to choose a mate wisely (Fig. 16-5).

Sexual codes. Heterosexual codes among teenage youngsters have undergone a notable change in recent years. The extent to which adolescents engage in intimate sexual relationships is not known precisely.

Some degree of permanent commitment is needed before sexual intimacy is considered appropriate. Most adolescents have indulged in petting, including transient, exploratory homosexual petting, and petting is generally more acceptable than intercourse as a form of sexual expression. However, available information indicates that at least 40% of girls and 80% to 95% of boys experience coitus by the end of adolescence. The prevalence increases with advancing age so that the largest numbers of sexually active youngsters are college students.

Adolescents engage in sexual relationships for pleasurable sensations, to satisfy sexual drives, to satisfy curiosity, as a conquest, as an expression of some degree of affection, or from inability to withstand pressures to conform. Often the urge to belong to and gain reassurance from a group and the wish to really belong to someone provoke a series of increasingly intimate physical contacts with a favored boyfriend or girlfriend, with each contact being more sexually provocative than the last. Eventually sexual intercourse becomes established as a behavior pattern and a method for ensuring social participation—or even as an end in itself.

The current trend toward greater permissiveness regarding adolescent sexual behavior will undoubtedly have an effect on the adolescent developmental experience. However, the recent concern with transmission of AIDS may influence these sexually permissive attitudes. Nonetheless, it is quite likely that young people will be accorded progressively more decision-making authority concerning control over their bodies. These alterations in the attitudes and value systems toward sex will have important implications for health professionals.

Interests and Activities

During early adolescence the interests and activities of girls and boys are in rather sharp contrast. Boys spend a great deal of time in active outdoor sports or "just going out with the guys." They enjoy hobbies and clubs, and television takes up a good part of their time. Girls and mixed-sex activities are of interest to boys but do not become prominent concerns until their development more nearly approaches that of the more rapidly maturing girls. As their bodies gain strength and size, "making the team" is a major concern for many youths, and a boy may spend an excessive amount of time in attempting to perfect athletic skills. The essential bicycle of middle childhood is replaced by the automobile, the symbol of status to the adolescent. If a car cannot be acquired, a motorcycle or motorbike is preferable to walking, riding the bus, or the humiliation of being chauffeured by a parent or sibling. Most boys avidly seek part-time employment, many because of economic necessity.

Although girls' leisure interests involve many outdoor activities, an increased interest in parties and social activities is evident. They are interested in hobbies and volunteer activities, and many seek part-time jobs through necessity or in order to purchase more clothes and other teenage "necessities." They are avid conversationalists and spend much of their time in the company of other girls, talking, listening to records, and experimenting with makeup, hairstyles, and clothes. They enjoy shopping for clothes, but there is seldom agreement between mother and daughter regarding types and styles of clothing. Many of their thoughts and feelings are confessed in a diary. Daydreaming is a prominent characteristic of the adolescent girl.

Members of both sexes enjoy movies, rock concerts, dancing, and other communal activities and entertainment, including "cruising" favorite streets in automobiles and gathering in shopping malls. Teenage horror films are attracting teenagers in large numbers, and X-rated movie theaters are crowded with adolescents. With the availability of a variety of video films adolescents are congregating in small groups to watch on home video players. However, there is little research on the types of video films teenagers watch.

Dancing has always occupied a central place in the customs of many cultures. There is delight in physical movement and a feeling of relief that comes from release of tension in activity. Dancing can also serve as a means of expressing specific sexual and aggressive urges in symbolic form and action. Many of the popular dances have decided sexual overtones and erotic movements. At

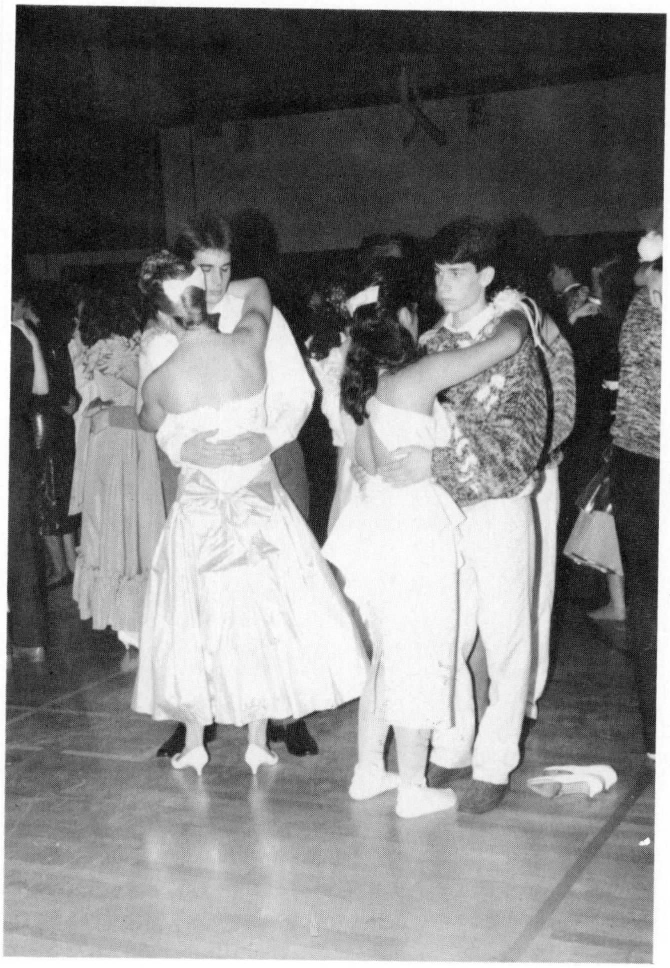

FIG. 16-6 Teenagers enjoy the activity and social aspects of dancing.

the same time the structure of the dance is such that dancers seldom touch one another. In this way the urges can be expressed without the danger of close physical contact (Fig. 16-6).

Reading is still a favorite occupation of teenagers and may serve to satisfy some of their needs for vicarious experiences. Reading is more purposeful at this stage than at earlier ages, and most adolescents prefer to read magazines rather than books.

Traditional television viewing may decline in adolescence, and many teenagers have a decided preference for the radio. Teenagers often are avidly addicted to the transistor radios that accompany many of their other activities—studying, walking, and working. Closely associated with the radio is the stereo, which assumes an important role in teenagers' lives. Much of their money is spent on recorded media, which are collected in much the same way as books.

When they are not engaged in other activities, they are probably participating in "rap sessions" or in endless telephone conversations. The telephone provides that essential link between peers when they are physically removed from one another. It is a means for fulfilling the need for flight from parents to peers without leaving the home. For boy-girl conversations, the telephone provides a way to experience closeness without the fear of complications that physical proximity may engender.

Teenage interests and activities are subject to rapid change. Each succeeding "generation" of teenagers has its own peculiar characteristics, which are evidenced in behavior, vocabulary, dress, and other external manifestations that reflect and establish a clear line of separateness, although superficial, between the peer and the adult cultures. The rapidity with which these external trappings change is often astonishing.

EMOTIONALITY

The pubertal changes in physical appearance are accompanied by changes in emotional control and response. The stability of the prepubescent period is replaced by the turmoil precipitated by the physical and psychologic alterations that teenagers experience. They are deluged with new sensations and feelings that they cannot understand. The behavior of adolescents is bewildering to others and often to the adolescents themselves. They vacillate between emotional states and between considerable maturity and childlike behavior. One minute they are exuberant and enthusiastic; the next minute they are depressed and withdrawn. Unpredictable, but essentially normal, outbursts of primitive behavior appear as the teenager loses control over instinctual drives. As the tension is relieved, emotion is brought under control and the individual retreats in order to review what has happened, to attempt to master his anger, and in the overall process to grow in his ability to control his emotions and gain from the new experience.

Teenagers begin to take hold of themselves in later adolescence. Their emotions are better controlled, they can approach problems more calmly and rationally, and, although they are still subject to periods of depression, their feelings are less vulnerable and they begin to demonstrate the more mature emotions of later adolescence. Whereas early adolescents react immediately and emotionally, older adolescents can control their emotions until socially acceptable times and places for expression present themselves. They are still subject to heightened emotion, and, when it is expressed, their behavior reflects feelings of insecurity, tension, and indecision.

SUMMARY OF GROWTH AND DEVELOPMENT

The characteristic stages described throughout the chapter are summarized as *early adolescence, middle adolescence,* and *late adolescence*. These periods represent an *average* pattern and may not necessarily apply to any single individual (Table 16-1).

TABLE 16-1

Growth and Development during Adolescence

Dimension	Early Adolescence 11–14 Years	Middle Adolescence 14–17 Years	Late Adolescence 17–20 Years
Growth	Rapidly accelerating growth Reaches peak velocity Secondary sex characteristics appear	Growth decelerating Stature reaches 95% of adult height Secondary sex characteristics well advanced	Physically mature Structure and reproductive growth almost complete
Cognition	Limited ability for abstract thinking Explores newfound ability for abstract thought Clumsy groping for new values and energies Comparison of "normality" with peers of same sex	Developing capacity for abstract thinking Enjoys intellectual powers, often in idealistic, altruistic terms Concern with philosophic, political, and social problems	Established abstract thought Can perceive and act on long-range options Able to view problems comprehensively Intellectual and functional identity established
Identity	Preoccupied with rapid body changes Trying out of various roles Measurement of attractiveness by acceptance or rejection of peers Conformity to group norms	Reestablishes body image as growth decelerates Very self-centered; increased narcissism Tendency toward inner experience and self-discovery Has a rich fantasy life Idealistic Able to perceive future implications of current behavior and decisions; variable application	Body image and gender role definition nearly secured Irreversible sexual identity Phase of consolidation of identity Stability of self-esteem Comfortable with physical growth Social roles defined and articulated
Relationships with parents	Defining independence-dependence boundaries Strong desire to remain dependent on parents while trying to detach No major conflicts over parental control	Major conflicts over independence and control Low point in parent-child relationship Greatest push for emancipation; disengagement Final and irreversible emotional detachment from parents; mourning	Emotional and physical separation from parents completed Independence from family and less conflict Emancipation nearly secured Extension of independence without conflict
Relationships with peers	Seeks peer affiliations to counter instability generated by rapid change Upsurge of close idealized friendships with members of the same sex Struggle for mastery takes place within peer group	Strong need for identity to affirm self-image Behavioral standards set by peer group Acceptance by peers extremely important—fear of rejection Exploration of ability to attract the opposite sex	Recedes in importance in favor of individual friendship Testing of male-female relationships against possibility of permanent alliance Relationships characterized by giving and sharing
Sexuality	Self-exploration and evaluation Limited dating Limited intimacy	Multiple plural relationships Decisive turn toward heterosexuality (if is homosexual, knows by this time) Exploration of "sex appeal" Feeling of "being in love" Tentative establishment of relationships	Forms stable relationships and attachment to another Growing capacity for mutuality and reciprocity Preeminence of individual as dating partner Intimacy involves commitment rather than exploration and romanticism
Emotionality	Most ambivalence Wide mood swings Intense daydreaming Anger outwardly expressed with moodiness, temper outbursts, and verbal insults and name-calling	Tendency toward inner experiences; more introspective Tendency to withdraw when upset or feelings are hurt Vascillation of emotions in time and range Feelings of inadequacy common; difficulty in asking for help	More constancy of emotion Anger more apt to be concealed

◆ *Promoting Optimum Health during Adolescence*

Adolescents are, on the whole, healthy individuals. The disease level is low during this age period, but there is heightened concern about the body. Most of the health problems and the more common illnesses are in some way related to the body changes of puberty.

Health promotion in persons in this age-group is primarily one of health teaching and guidance. Adolescents as a group are eager to learn about themselves, and nurses who are truly interested in them, who respect them as persons, and who are willing to listen to them will be able to gain their confidence and trust. Individual counseling provides adolescents with a knowledgeable adult in whom they can confide without the threat of an intimate relationship.

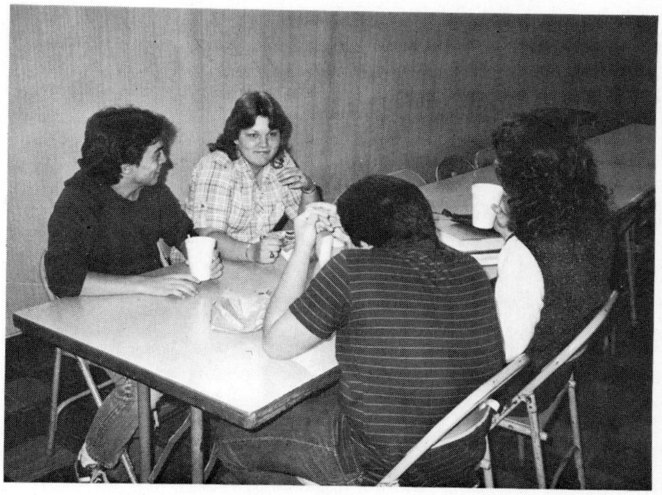

FIG. 16-7 A small group gathers for lunch.

NUTRITION

The rapid and extensive increase in height, weight, muscle mass, and sexual maturity of adolescence is accompanied by new and greater nutritional requirements. Since nutritional needs are closely related to the increase in body mass, the peak requirements occur in the year of maximum growth, during which time the body mass almost doubles. This period occurs between the tenth and twelfth years in girls and about 2 years later in boys. The calorie and protein requirements during this year are higher than at almost any other time of life. As a result of this increased anabolic need, the adolescent is highly sensitive to caloric restrictions.

Adolescents want food, their appetites soar, and their capacity to consume food is often awe-inspiring, as any parent of a teenage boy can attest. A fast-growing boy may never get filled up. His stomach may be too small to accommodate the amount of food he requires to meet his growth needs unless he eats at very frequent intervals. Not only do teenagers eat at every pause in the day's activities, but they enjoy food and the pleasures related to its consumption. Food is part of the attraction of the "hangouts" and gathering places that teenagers frequent (Fig. 16-7).

The nutritional needs of adolescents are difficult to determine, because of meager nutritional information on members of this age-group. This difficulty is further complicated by the influence of emotional and other stress factors affecting nutrient utilization and the psychologic factors that influence eating habits. In addition, the wide variations in growth rates during adolescence and the equally wide variations in ages at which these changes take place complicate any attempt to set minimum dietary standards for this age-group. Consequently the Recommended Dietary Allowances for teenagers include a safety factor that attempts to allow for these differences under average circumstances.

Protein intake remains a constant need throughout childhood and adolescence to meet continual growth needs. There is usually sufficient intake to meet these needs except in those young people who limit their food intake because of economic problems or in an attempt to lose weight.

There is a substantial increase in the need for the minerals calcium, iron, and zinc during periods of rapid growth—calcium for skeletal growth, iron for expansion of muscle mass and blood volume, and zinc for the generation of both skeletal and bone tissue. Girls may be especially susceptible to iron deficiency at menarche.

Eating Habits and Behavior

Eating and attitudes toward food are primarily family centered during early and middle childhood, and food habits are largely related to cultural and individual family preferences and patterns. With adolescence and the move toward independence, family influences on the child change. Children's interests, attitudes, and routines are altered as an increasing number of meals are eaten away from home. These changes are largely a result of the high value that teenagers place on peer acceptability and sociability; therefore, their eating habits are easily influenced by their associates.

Omitting breakfast or eating a breakfast that is nutritionally poor in quality is frequently a problem, and pressure for time and their commitments to activities adversely affect the teenager's eating habits. Snacks, usually selected on the basis of accessibility rather than nutritional merit, become more and more a part of the habitual eating pattern during adolescence. Adolescents characteristically reject or only infrequently eat a sufficient amount of fresh fruits and vegetables, especially those that are rich in ascorbic acid. Milk is usually passed over in favor of soft drinks, the appropriate social drink of the peer culture.

Overeating or undereating during adolescence presents special problems. As they experience the normal increase in weight and fat deposition of the growth spurt, teenage girls often resort to dieting. The desire for the admired slim figure and a fear of becoming "fat" prompt teenage girls to embark on nutritionally inadequate reducing regimens that sap their energy and deprive their growing bodies of essential nutrients. They resort to diets on their own or with peers in an effort to conform. Many adopt the current fad diets and are victims of food misinformation. Boys are less inclined to undereat. They are more concerned about gaining size and strength. However, they tend to eat foods high in calories but low in other essential nutrients.

Nursing Considerations

Nothing can make adolescents eat wisely. Their food habits must be considered when planning nutritional education and guidance because they reflect many influences and conditions.

In helping teenagers select a nutritious diet, it is best to begin where they are and actively involve them in the process. Teenagers dislike being talked down to or preached to, but they do respond when their independence is respected and they are given the opportunity to make their own decisions regarding food choices.

In general, adolescents are body-conscious and concerned about their appearance. When diet is associated with clear skin, firm flesh, and glossy hair, the teenager is more likely to be receptive to nutritional education. However, helping young persons arrive at a decision for change is more difficult than providing information. They respond best when the counselor provides straightforward information, talks with them and not at them, and listens to what they have to say.

SLEEP AND REST

Teenagers vary in their need for sleep and rest. Rapid physical growth, the tendency toward overexertion, and the overall increased activity of this age contribute to fatigue in adolescents. Their propensity for staying up late makes it very difficult to get out of bed in the mornings, and they sleep late at every opportunity. Adequate sleep and rest at this time are important to a total health regimen.

EXERCISE AND ACTIVITY

Adolescents probably spend more time and energy practicing and participating in sports activities than members of any other age-group. Both girls and boys participate in recreational sports and many are actively involved in competitive athletics either in conjunction with school (Fig. 16-8) or as members of amateur athletic associations.

The practice of sports and games contributes significantly to growth and development, the education process, and better health. It provides exercise for growing muscles, interactions with peers, and a socially acceptable means to enjoy stimulation and conflict. In addition, competitive activities help the teenager in the process of self-appraisal, development of self-respect, and concern for others. Nurses can encourage participation as an excellent means for health promotion and building of self-es-

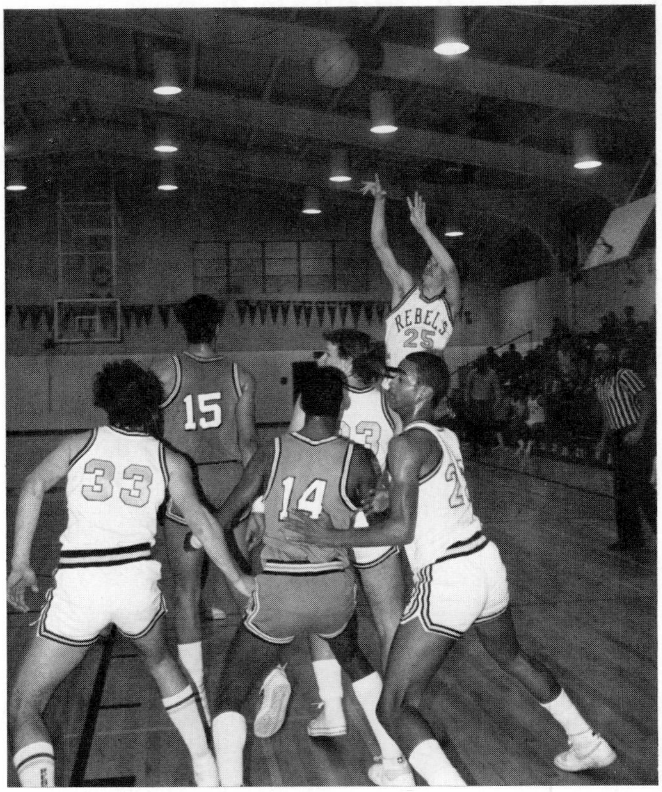

FIG. 16-8 Participation in school athletics is a primary goal of most adolescents.

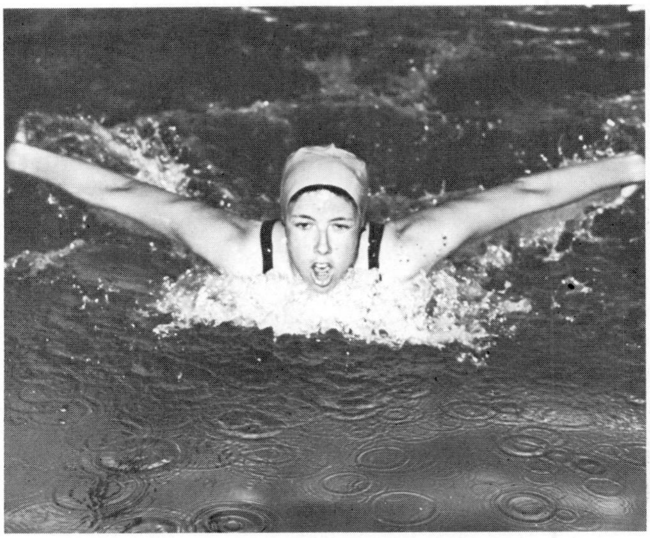

FIG. 16-9 Many sports activities can be both competitive and recreational.

teem (Fig. 16-9). However, no youngster should be encouraged to engage in physical activity that is beyond his physical or emotional capacity (see also Sports injuries, p. 464).

DENTAL HEALTH

Dental health should not be neglected during adolescence, although the rate of caries formation is not as great as it was in childhood. Early adolescence is usually the time when corrective orthodontic appliances are worn, and these are frequently a source of embarrassment and concern to the youngster. Reassurance regarding the temporary nature of the annoyance and anticipation of an improved appearance help to make the inconvenience tolerable. It is also important to reinforce the orthodontist's directions regarding use and care of the appliances and to emphasize careful attention to brushing during this time.

PERSONAL CARE

The body-conscious teenager is highly amenable to discussion and counseling about personal care and hygiene. Body changes associated with puberty bring with them special needs for cleanliness. The hyperactive sebaceous glands and newly functioning apocrine glands make the daily bath or shower imperative, and underarm deodorants assume an important place in personal care. The adolescent will find that hair requires more frequent shampooing, and girls will have questions about hair removal, use of cosmetics, and menstrual hygiene. Many group discussions center around the virtues of particular products or methods. Adolescents are continually bombarded with messages from the media regarding the best means to enhance their popularity and appeal to the opposite sex. Nurses are in a position to help them evaluate the relative merits of commercial products.

Vision

Regular vision testing is an important part of health care and supervision during adolescence. At this time the incidence of visual refractive difficulties reaches a peak that is not exceeded until the fifth decade. Adolescents may not have poorer vision than children or adults, but the increased demands of schoolwork make good vision important for academic success.

Hearing

There has been considerable concern regarding current teenage practices causing possible damage to the hearing of youngsters. Cochlear damage has been documented from relatively continuous exposure to the loud sound levels of rock music, especially from stereos and radios. The popularity of portable FM radios and stereo cassette players with lightweight earphones, both of which enable the listener to adjust the volume, are of particular concern to health care professionals (Fig. 16-10). When these units are used for extended periods, the potential for permanent hearing loss is undisputed. Appealing to individual youngsters for more judicious use is of doubtful benefit, although they should be informed of the risk. Efforts directed toward legislating legal limits to the noise exposure that can be achieved through the sets and widespread education may be possible solutions. (See p. 560 for a discussion of noise-related hearing loss.)

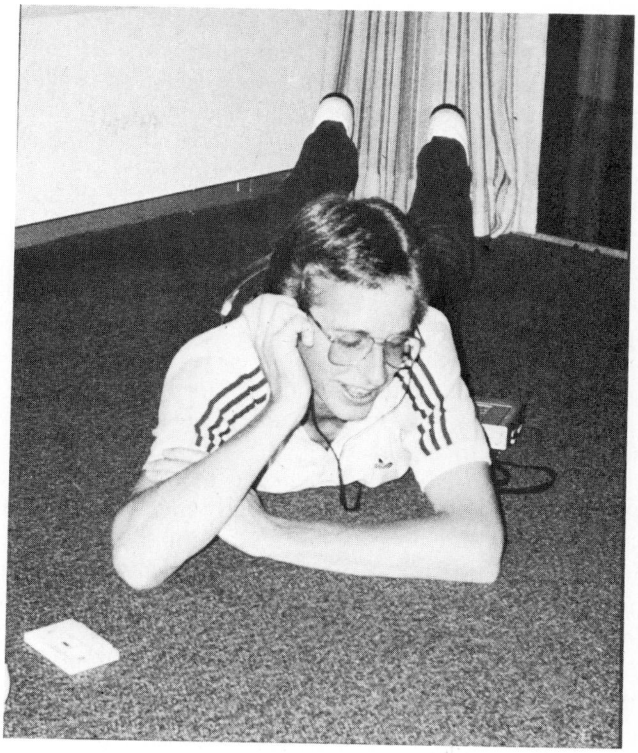

FIG. 16-10 Teenagers spend endless hours listening to music.

Posture

The process of normal development during adolescence does little to promote good posture in the teenage girl or boy. The rapid skeletal growth that is usually associated with a significant lag in muscular growth leads to weakness, easy fatigability, and awkwardness. This situation predisposes youngsters to slumping and makes them less inclined to stand or sit erectly. A relative reduction in physical activity, which often accompanies the rapid skeletal growth, aggravates the situation, especially in teenage girls. The adolescent who is routinely engaged in vigorous physical activity appears to have fewer problems with posture.

The best approach to counseling teenagers about posture is to show, not tell, them and to serve as a proper model. Good posture can be demonstrated best when the adolescent is standing before a full-length mirror. Postural defects and desired alterations can be pointed out in full view of both the young person and the nurse. A sunken chest, winged scapulas, swayback, protruberant abdomen, and drooping head and shoulders are clearly visible, and the nurse is able to demonstrate the simple corrections that can transform the youngster into a more attractive and, ultimately, healthier person. Adolescents will need reassurance that the fatigue they feel when attempting to maintain correct posture is a transient effect caused by weak muscles, especially those of the back, and that they will soon acquire the strength and endurance to maintain the desired posture. If they concentrate on assuming correct positioning several times each day, with regular practice it will eventually become a permanent aspect of their person.

Serious postural defects detected in the process of a physical assessment will require early medical intervention. Scoliosis is usually intensified during adolescence, and tight muscles often produce postural problems that need special attention. Nurses can refer a youngster to the appropriate source, such as the family physician, pediatrician, or health clinic, for evaluation and implementation of corrective therapy.

Ear Piercing

The popular trend of ear piercing may sometimes create a health problem in the uninformed teenager. It is a nursing responsibility to caution girls or boys against the practice of having their ears pierced by friends, mothers, or themselves. Although in most cases there are few if any serious side effects, there is always a danger of complications such as infection, cyst or keloid formation, bleeding, dermatitis, or metal allergy. Therefore, the procedure should be performed by a physician or qualified nurse using proper sterile technique. This is especially important if a youngster has a history of diabetes, allergies, or skin disorders. Teenagers are prone to develop keloids, particularly if there is a history of keloid formation.

Suntanning

The continuous quest for an attractive appearance leads many teenagers to excessive sunbathing and artificial means for acquiring a tan skin. However, the practice is not without risks, and the adolescent should be educated regarding the detrimental effects of sunlight on the skin (see Sunburn p. 1008). Some long-term effects include premature aging of the skin, increased risk of skin cancer, and, in susceptible individuals, phototoxic reactions.

The increasing popularity of artificial suntanning has prompted concern on the part of health professionals regarding the use of sun lamps and suntanning machines. Because the long-term effects of tanning machines (especially whole body irradiation) are unknown, most dermatologists do not recommend suntanning by this means.

SEX EDUCATION AND GUIDANCE

Contemporary adolescents are constantly exposed to sexual symbolism and erotic stimulation from the mass media. At the same time the development of primary and secondary sex characteristics and the increased sensitivity of the genitals produce thoughts and fantasies about heterosexual relationships. Although many adolescents have received sex education from parents and school throughout childhood, they are not always adequately prepared for the impact of puberty. A large portion of their knowledge is acquired from peers, provocative illustrations, and inscriptions on the walls of public restrooms. Consequently much of the sex information they accumulate is incomplete, inaccurate, riddled with cultural and moral values, and not very helpful.

Sex education should consist of instruction concerning a normal body function, and it should be presented in a straightforward manner using correct terminology. However, the questions of who is responsible for teaching and how the teaching can best be accomplished must be considered. Sex education is, and has been, assumed by parents, schools, churches, community agencies such as **Planned Parenthood Federation of America, Inc.,*** and health professionals.

The most comprehensive approach to sex education is offered by the **Sex Information and Education Council of the United States (SIECUS)**† and the **Sex Information and Education Council of Canada,**‡ interdisciplinary organizations founded to establish sexuality as a health entity and to dignify it by openness of approach, study, and scientific research. SIECUS maintains that every sex education program should present the topic from six aspects: biologic, social, health, personal adjustments and attitudes, interpersonal associations, and the establishment of values.

Whether nurses counsel young people on an individual basis, in mixed groups, or in groups segregated by sex makes little difference. Some nurses and teenagers are uneasy in mixed groups for discussions of sexuality, and no hard-and-fast rule prevails. Ideally boys and girls should be able to discuss sex objectively with one another and in groups, but this is not always possible. The difference in the rate of maturation between boys and girls and between different members of the same sex often makes it desirable to discuss certain aspects of sexuality in segregated groups. As a general rule, the need for separate discussion groups diminishes as young people progress toward maturity.

When discussing sex and sexual activities, nurses should use simple but correct language—not street language, highly scientific terminology, or evasive jargon. Once the meanings of biologic terms such as uterus, testicles, and vagina are understood, most teenagers prefer to use them in their discussions.

Both boys and girls need to know more about what is

*810 Seventh Ave., New York, NY 10019.
†Fifth Ave., Suite 801-2, New York, NY 10011.
‡41 Marchmount Road, Toronto, Ontario M6G 2A8.

going on in their bodies than they are able to see. Although most girls are adequately prepared for menstruation, they do not always understand its relationship to the total process of reproduction. Many are under the impression that the "safe" time for sexual intercourse is midway between menstrual periods. Whether they are sexually active or not, adolescents should receive accurate information about pregnancy, including when and how it occurs and ways by which it can be avoided. They need to know about sexually transmitted diseases, the manner in which they are transmitted, symptoms, and how to get treatment if they become infected.

INJURY PREVENTION

Physical injuries are the greatest single cause of death in the adolescent age-group and claim more lives than all other causes combined. The most vulnerable ages are the years 15 to 24, when accidental injuries account for 61% of deaths in boys and 39% of deaths in girls. The tragedy of this is that the figures remain fairly constant from year to year and almost all fatal injuries are preventable.

During adolescence, peak physical, sensory, and psychomotor function gives teenagers a feeling of strength and confidence that they have never experienced before and the physiologic changes of puberty give impetus to

TABLE 16-2

Injury Prevention during Adolescence

Major Developmental Accomplishments	Injury Prevention
Need for independence and freedom Testing independence Age permitted to drive a motor vehicle (varies) Propensity for risk-taking Feeling of indestructibility Need for discharging energy, often at expense of logical thinking and other control mechanisms Strong need for peer approval May attempt hazardous feats Peak incidence for practice and participation in sports Access to more complex tools, objects, and locations Can assume responsibility for own actions	**Motor vehicles** *Pedestrian*—emphasize and encourage safe pedestrian behavior *Passenger*—promote appropriate behavior while riding in a motor vehicle *Driver*—provide competent driver education; encourage judicious use of vehicle, discourage drag racing, "chicken"; maintain vehicle in proper condition (brakes, tires, etc.) Teach and promote safety and maintenance of two-wheeled vehicles Promote and encourage wearing of safety apparel such as helmet, long trousers Reinforce the danges of drugs, including alcohol, when operating a motor vehicle **Drowning** Teach to swim (if adolescent unable to do so) Teach basic rules of water safety: Judicious selection of place to swim Sufficient water depth for diving Swimming with companion **Burns** Reinforce proper behavior in areas involving contact with burn hazards (gasoline, electric wires, fires) Advise regarding excessive exposure to sunlight (ultraviolet burn) Discourage smoking Encourage use of sunscreen **Poisoning** Educate in hazards of drug use, including alcohol **Falls** Teach and encourage general safety measures in all activities **Bodily damage** Promote acquisition of proper instruction in sports and use of sports equipment Promote use of appropriate arena for sports activities Instruct in safe use of and respect for firearms and other devices with potential danger (e.g., power tools, firecrackers) Provide and encourage use of protective equipment when using potentially hazardous devices Promote access to and/or provision of safe sports and recreational facilities Be alert for signs of depression (potential suicide) Discourage use of and/or availability of hazardous sports equipment (trampoline, surfboards) Instruct regarding proper use of corrective devices such as glasses, contact lenses, hearing aids Encourage and foster judicious application of safety principles and prevention

many basic instinctual forces. One manifestation of this is an increase in energy that simply must be discharged through action, often at the expense of logical thinking and other control mechanisms. Their propensity for risk-taking behavior plus feelings of indestructibility make adolescents especially prone to injuries. Some of the developmental characteristics of teenagers and the common injuries associated with this age-group are outlined in Table 16-2.

Motor Vehicle–Related Injuries

Almost half the injuries in the adolescent age-group involve motor vehicle accidents. The adolescent's newly acquired ability to drive and the normal developmental need for independence and freedom make the automobile an attractive, if not necessary, part of an adolescent's life. Most fatal injuries involving adolescent drivers occur because of improper driving or poor judgment on the part of the driver. Many of these young people, delighted with the freedom that a driver's license affords them, are less concerned about the new responsibilities associated with this freedom.

The recent upsurge in the use of drugs, including alcohol, by adolescents has further compounded the problem of motor vehicle accidents involving youth. Overindulgence in alcohol is known to impair the ability of the best driver. The combination of inexperience, lack of defensive driving skills, and inexperience with drinking is a lethal one, and the unfortunate consequences are predictable.

Nonautomotive vehicle injuries. The increasing use of other motorized vehicles, such as motorized bicycles, all terrain vehicles (ATVs), and snowmobiles, has caused an increase in injuries, especially among youngsters below the legal age for driving automobiles, and little driver preparation and instruction are required for their use. It has been recommended that motorized bicycle use be regulated, including minimum age for driving, mandatory use of helmets, riding within prescribed limits (within 3 feet of the right side of the road), and providing safety equipment on the machine (e.g., rearview mirror, turning signals).

Firearms

Improper use of firearms continues to be one of the leading causes of accidental death in the adolescent age-group. Most of these deaths occur in or on home premises. The natural interest in gun-related activities is accelerated at this time, when almost half the victims of firearm fatalities are between the ages of 15 and 24 years. Most accidental injuries can be prevented when proper safety precautions are taken in the use and storage of firearms. For example, loaded guns should never be permitted in or around the home, and guns and ammunition must be stored where only appropriate adults have access to them.

Nonpowder firearms. Nonpowder guns (air rifles, BB guns), although viewed as toys by many, account for almost as many injuries as powder guns. The regulations regarding nonpowder guns are relaxed; they can be purchased legally by youngsters and are labeled as suitable for children as young as 8 years. Few states regulate their use. As child advocates, nurses can press for legislation to regulate the sale of these potentially dangerous "toys."

Sports Injuries

Adolescents probably spend more time and energy practicing and participating in sports activities than members of any other age-group. Because the degree of physical maturation, size, coordination, and endurance varies greatly among adolescents of the same age, sports competition between young people who differ markedly in strength and agility is unfair and hazardous. Matching candidates for sports should be done relative to physical maturity, height, weight, and physical fitness and skills, particularly in a sport involving rigorous body contact. Age is a less important consideration.

Every sport has some potential for injury—whether one participates in serious competition or is actively engaged in the activity for pure enjoyment. Serious injury is not limited to the athlete who competes in rough contact sports; a large number of severe or fatal injuries occur to persons who are not physically prepared for the activity. The increase in strength and vigor in adolescence may tempt youngsters to overextend themselves, especially boys who are egged on by teammates or are stimulated by the admiration of female observers.

Not only does the activity itself pose a hazard, but the environment and the sports or recreational equipment provide additional risks. Some of the sports that contribute to adolescent accidental injuries by their activity and equipment are bicycling, football, basketball, baseball, gymnastics, snow skiing, hockey, trampoline jumping, and water activities such as swimming, diving, and fishing. The range of injuries sustained in sports or recreational activities can involve any part of the body and extend from relatively minor cuts, bruises, and abrasions to totally incapacitating central nervous system injuries or death.

Nursing Considerations

Injury prevention is an ongoing part of nursing responsibility throughout the childhood years. Anticipatory guidance to parents regarding the expected problems and hazards related to growth and development does not end as the child nears maturity. They need the same education in basic safety precautions, encouragement to acquire proper instruction in skills required in performance of activities, handling motor vehicles and firearms, and proper maintenance of equipment. However, at adolescence health and safety education and guidance are more effective when the young people are involved directly, but

Parental Guidance during Adolescence

Accept adolescent as a human being
Respect adolescent's ideas, likes and dislikes, wishes
Provide opportunity for choosing options and accept natural consequences of these choices
Allow youngster to learn by doing, even when choices and methods differ from those of adults
Provide adolescent with clear, reasonable limits
Allow increasing independence within limitations of safety and well-being
Be available but avoid pressing youngster too far
Respect adolescent's privacy
Try to share adolescent's feelings of joy or sorrow
Respond to feelings as well as words
Be available to answer questions, give information, and provide companionship
Listen and try to be open to youngster's views, even when they disagree with parental views
Try to make communication clear
Assist adolescent in selecting appropriate career goals and preparing for adult role
Provide undemanding love

Be aware that:
Adolescent is subject to turbulent, unpredictable behavior
Adolescent is struggling for independence
Adolescent is extraordinarily sensitive to feelings and behavior that affect him or her
Message given to adolescent may not be message received
Friends are extremely important to adolescent
Adolescent has a strong need "to belong"
Adolescent sees things in black or white, good or bad

parents and health professionals can emphasize the importance of safety in the execution of activities and skills and the proper conditioning and preparation for sports.

ANTICIPATORY GUIDANCE—CARE OF FAMILIES

The parents of the adolescent are usually as confused and perplexed about the changes and behavior of this stage of development as the youngster is. Parents also need support and guidance to help them through this trying time. They need to understand the changes taking place and to understand and accept the expected behaviors that accompany the process of detachment, to be prepared to "let go," and to promote the changed relationship from one of dependence to one of mutuality. The accompanying box lists suggestions for anticipatory guidance of parents with an adolescent.

SUMMARY

Growth and development during adolescence are both physically and psychologically rapid and dramatic. Concurrent with physical changes the adolescent experiences emotional upheaval, numerous pressures to conform, and increasingly wide and varied relationships. At the end of this turbulent period young people are able to verbalize conceptually, become comfortable with their bodies, build new and meaningful relationships, seek economic and social stability, and develop a workable value system. The period culminates in severing the bonds that have tied them to their parents throughout childhood, a difficult time for both adolescent and parent.

KEY CONCEPTS

- The pubescent growth spurt that begins around age 10 in girls and 12 in boys signals the beginning of adolescence.
- Biologic development during puberty is characterized by increased activity of the pituitary gland, which results in sexual maturity and the appearance of secondary sex characteristics.
- According to Erikson, the major developmental crisis of adolescence is establishing a sense of identity.
- Cognitive development in adolescence is revealed through thinking beyond the present, logical reasoning, and a sense of idealism.
- Development of body image is closely tied to sexual awareness, as adolescents cope with sexual maturation.
- According to Kohlberg's theory of moral development, adolescents begin to question existing moral values and learn to make choices.
- Spiritual development is characterized by the questioning of family values and ideals, a move to more philosophical thinking, and emphasis on personal religion.
- Adolescent relationships with parents may be strained, while the influence of the peer group increases and heterosexual relationships assume importance.
- Teenagers demonstrate a wide variety of interests, and their increased physical and cognitive skills allow them to engage in increasingly difficult and complex activities.
- Adolescents fluctuate between periods of stability and instability.
- Nutritional needs for protein, minerals, and iron may be impaired by teenagers' eating habits, such as snacking and irregular mealtimes.
- Motor vehicle injuries constitute the primary cause of death from injury in the adolescent years.

STUDY QUESTIONS AND ACTIVITIES

1. Describe the hormonal interrelationship between the pituitary gland and the gonads.
2. Observe a group (or groups) of teenagers in a shopping mall or other gathering place. Note similarities and differences in dress, hairstyle, and general behavior.
3. Observe adolescents on or near a high school campus. Note numbers and configuration of persons within each group, loners, and interactions of individuals within groups and between groups.
4. Interview a teenager regarding a typical day's diet, eating preferences, and eating habits (where, when, and frequency).
5. Outline a plan for a sex education seminar for a group of adolescents.

REFERENCES

Erikson, E.H.: Childhood and society, ed. 2, New York, 1963, W.W. Norton & Co., Inc.

Newman, B.M., and Newman, P.R.: Development through life, a psychosocial approach, rev. ed., Homewood, IL, 1979, Dorsey Press.

Shelly, J.A.: The spiritual needs of children, Downers Grove, IL, 1982, Inter-Varsity Press.

BIBLIOGRAPHY

General

Belkengren, R.B., and Sapala, S.: Physical fitness from infancy through adolescence, Pediatr. Nurs. **8**(4):A-I, 1982.

DeMaio-Esteves, M., and Shuzman, E.: Technological society: its impact on youth, Top. Clin. Nurs. **10**:55-65, 1983.

Garrick, J.G.: The sports medicine patient, Nurs. Clin. North Am. **16**:759-766, 1981.

Kaluger, G., and Kaluger, M.F.: Human development: the span of life, ed. 3, St. Louis, 1984, The C.V. Mosby Co.

Kerrins, K.M.: Comparing the self-image of prepubescent girls before and after four sessions on body awareness, J. Sch. Health **53**:541-543, 1983.

Lowery, G.H.: Growth and development of children, ed. 8, Chicago, 1986, Year Book Medical Publishers, Inc.

Mahon, N.E.: Developmental changes and loneliness during adolescence, Top. Clin. Nurs. **5**(1):66-76, 1983.

Nelms, B.C.: What is a normal adolescent? MCN **6**:402-406, 1981.

Piaget, J.: The theory of stages in cognitive development, New York, 1969, McGraw-Hill Book Co.

Reasoner, R.W.: Enhancement of self-esteem in children and adolescents, Fam. Community Health **6**(2):51-64, 1983.

Shaffer, D.R.: Developmental psychology: theory, research, and applications, Monterey, CA, 1985, Brooks/Cole Publishing Co.

Stone, L.J., and Church, J.: Childhood and adolescence, ed. 5, New York, 1983, Random House, Inc.

Health Promotion

Adams, B.N.: Adolescent health care: needs, priorities and services, Nurs. Clin. North Am. **18**:237-248, 1983.

Anders, T.F., Carskadon, M.A., and Dement, W.C.: Sleep and sleepiness in children and adolescents, Nurs. Clin. North Am. **27**:29-43, 1980.

Bradley, J.M.: Do adolescents practice what they preach about health? Pediatr. Nurs. **10**:285-289, 1984.

Craft, M.: Rural adolescents and health care, Child. Nurse **4**(6):1-3, 1986.

Durfee, M.F., and Badger, D.W.: Adolescent health care: sharing the responsibility, Fam. Community Health **4**:43-55, 1982.

Elkind, D.: Teenage thinking: implications for health care, Pediatr. Nurs. **10**:383-385, 1984.

Jordan, D., and Kelfer, L.S.: Adolescent potential for participation in health care, Issues Compr. Pediatr. Nurs. **6**:147-156, 1983.

Keenan, T.: School-based adolescent health-care programs, Pediatr. Nurs. **12**:365-369, 1986.

Lucas, B., Rees, J.M., and Mahan, L.K.: Nutrition and the adolescent. In Pipes, P.L.: Nutrition in infancy and childhood, ed. 4, St. Louis, 1989, The C.V. Mosby Co.

Lyons, J.A.: Adolescent health and school-based clinics, Issues Compr. Pediatr. Nurs. **10**:303-314, 1987.

Mahan, L.K., and Rees, J.M.: Nutrition in adolescence, St. Louis, 1984, The C.V. Mosby Co.

Perry, C.L., and Murray, D.M.: Enhancing the transition years: the challenge of adolescent health promotion, J. Sch. Health **52**:307-311, 1982.

Sachs, B.: Cognitive screening for adolescent health education, J. Pediatr. Nurs. **2**:113-118, 1987.

Smith, K.L.D., Turner, J.G., and Jacobsen, R.B.: Health concerns of adolescents, Pediatr. Nurs. **13**:311-315, 1987.

Sex Education and Guidance

Bullough, V., and Bullough, B.: PMPs patients, parents, and sexuality, Pediatr. Nurs. **8**:A-I, 1982.

Kuhnen, K.K., and others: Barny: a computer for teaching sex education, MCN **8**:350-353, 1983.

Sapala, S., and Strokosch, G.: Adolescent sexuality: use of a questionnaire for health teaching and counseling, Pediatr. Nurs. **7**:33-34, 1981.

Sheehan, M.K., Ostwald, S.K., and Rothenberger, J.: Perceptions of sexual responsibility: do young men and women agree? Pediatr. Nurs. **12**:17-21, 1986.

Woods, N.F.: Human sexuality: in health and illness, ed. 3, St. Louis, 1984, The C.V. Mosby Co.

Injury Prevention

Bass, J.L., Gallagher, S.S., and Mehta, K.A.: Injuries to adolescents and young adults, Pediatr. Clin. North Am. **32**:31-39, 1985.

Black, R.E., and Myre, L.E.: Serious air gun injuries in children: update of injury statistics and presentation of five cases, Pediatr. Emerg. Care **3**:168-170, 1987.

Greensher, J.: Non-automotive vehicle injuries in adolescents, Pediatr. Annals **17**:116-121, 1988.

Orlowski, J.P.: Adolescent drownings: swimming, boating, diving, and scuba accidents Pediatr. Clin. North Am. **17**:126-132, 1987.

Paulson, J.A.: The epidemiology of injuries in adolescents, Pediatr. Annals Pediatr. Clin. North Am. **17**:84-96, 1988.

Rivara, F.P.: Motor vehicle injuries during adolescence, Pediatr. Annals **17**:107-113, 1988.

Schetky, D.H.: Children and handguns, Am. J. Dis. Child. **139**:229-231, 1985.

Shaffer, T.E.: New guidelines in sports medicine, Pediatr. Consult. **1**:(5):1-12, 1980.

Tanz, R., Christoffel, K.K., and Sagerman, S.: Are toy guns too dangerous? Pediatrics **75**:265-268, 1985.

CHAPTER 17

Health Problems of Middle Childhood and Adolescence

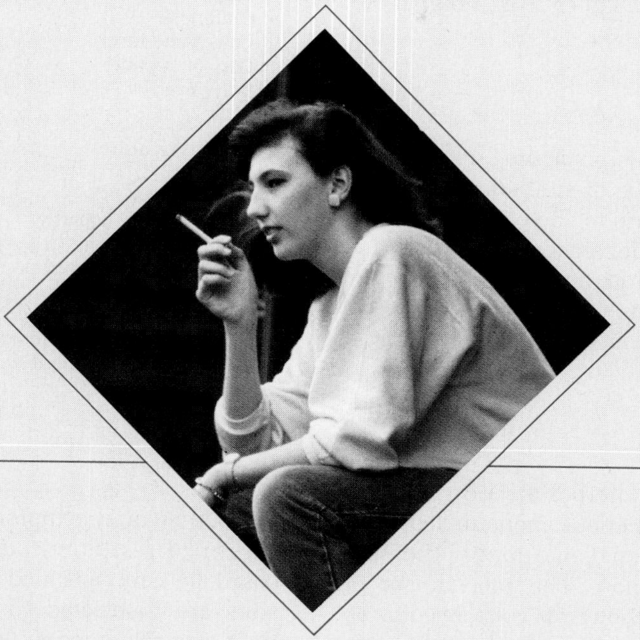

LEARNING OBJECTIVES

On completion of this chapter the reader will be able to:

- Outline a plan of care for the child or adolescent with a health problem
- Demonstrate an understanding of the types, causes, and prevention of sports injuries in middle childhood and adolescence
- Describe the most common causes of growth and/or maturation failure in later childhood
- Demonstrate an understanding of common disorders of the male and female reproductive systems
- Demonstrate an understanding of health problems related to sexuality
- Outline a plan of care for the child or adolescent with an eating disorder
- Discuss the manifestations and nursing management of selected emotional and/or behavioral problems

As a group, both school-age children and adolescents are relatively healthy individuals, especially when compared to children in infancy and early childhood. The ages 9 to 12 are the healthiest years, and this state of health continues into pubescence. Most youngsters in these age-groups have either contracted the communicable diseases of childhood or been immunized against them. Their excellent appetites, adequate rest, and sufficient physical exercise further contribute to their general good health. During the school years respiratory illnesses and gastrointestinal upsets are the most common illnesses. Most health problems of adolescents are related to the physical changes taking place in their bodies and the crucial psychosocial crisis of identity formation. Other conditions that are not uncommon are accidental injuries (see Chapters 15 and 16) and emotional or behavior disorders.

◆ *Common Health Problems*

There are a number of health problems that have their onset in middle childhood or adolescence or are more prominent at this time than at earlier ages. Most are not life-threatening but may seriously hamper physical or emotional health. Some are discussed elsewhere in the book (e.g., acne) or later in the chapter (e.g., pregnancy, attention deficit disorder).

INFECTIOUS MONONUCLEOSIS

Infectious mononucleosis (IM) is an acute, self-limiting infectious disease presumed to be of viral etiology that is common among young persons up to 25 years of age. The disease is characterized by an increase in the mononuclear elements of the blood and general symptoms of an infectious process. The course is usually mild but occasionally can be severe or, rarely, accompanied by serious complications.

Etiology and Pathophysiology

Recent evidence implicates the herpeslike EB (Epstein-Barr) virus as the cause of infectious mononucleosis. It appears in both sporadic and epidemic forms, the sporadic cases being more common. The mechanism of spread has not been proved, although it is believed to be transmitted by direct intimate contact with oral secretions. It also appears to be only mildly contagious, and the period of communicability is unknown. The incubation period following exposure is 2 to 6 weeks.

Diagnostic Tests

The onset of symptoms is anywhere from 10 days to 6 weeks following exposure and may be acute or insidious. The common presenting symptoms of infectious mononucleosis vary greatly in type, severity, and duration (see box). The leukocyte count may be normal or low, but usually lymphocyte leukocytosis develops; of these, approximately 10% are atypical lymphocytes. The heterophil antibody test determines the extent to which the patient's serum will agglutinate sheep red blood cells. In infectious mononucleosis, a titer of 1:160 is considered diagnostic, although a rising titer during the earlier stages is the best indicator.

Some rapid tests have been developed for the diagnosis of mononucleosis. These include the "spot test" (Monospot), a slide test of high specificity, and a 5-minute enzyme immunoassay test (Ventrescreen Mono Test). These can be performed in the physician's office.

Therapeutic Management

There is no specific treatment for infectious mononucleosis. Common symptoms are ordinarily relieved by simple remedies. Acetaminophen is usually sufficient to relieve the bothersome symptoms of headache, fever, and malaise. Bed rest is encouraged for fatigue but is not imposed for any specified period of time. Affected youngsters are instructed to regulate activities according to their own tolerance, unless complicating factors are present. If the spleen is enlarged, for example, activities in which they might receive a blow to the abdomen or chest should be avoided.

Oral penicillin is sometimes prescribed for sore throat, especially if β-hemolytic streptococci are present. Sore throat can be relieved by gargles, hot drinks, analgesic troches, or acetaminophen. Some physicians favor the use of corticosteroids for suppression of high fever and/or severe sore throat but usually limit its use to the period of more intense symptoms or when the youngster is severely ill.

The course of infectious mononucleosis is self-limiting and usually uncomplicated. Contrary to popular belief, mononucleosis is not necessarily a difficult, prolonged, disabling disease, and the prognosis is generally good. Acute symptoms usually disappear within 7 to 10 days, and the persistent fatigue subsides within 2 to 4 weeks. A number of affected youngsters may need to restrict activities for 2 or 3 months; the disease rarely extends for longer periods.

Nursing Considerations

Nursing responsibilities are directed toward comfort measures to relieve the symptoms and helping the affected youngster and his family determine appropriate activities according to the stage of the disease and his interests. They may need diet counseling to select foods that contain sufficient calories to meet growth and energy needs

Clinical Manifestations of Infectious Mononucleosis

Early
- Headache
- Malaise
- Fatigue
- Chilliness
- Low-grade fever
- Loss of appetite
- Puffy eyes

Full-blown Disease
- Cardinal features
  - Fever
  - Sore throat
  - Cervical adenopathy
- Common features
  - Splenomegaly (may persist for several months)
  - Palatine petechiae
  - Macular eruption (especially on trunk)
  - Exudative pharyngitis/tonsillitis
  - Hepatic involvement to some degree, often associated with jaundice

and yet are easy to swallow. Every effort should be made to prevent a secondary infection; therefore, the adolescent is counseled to limit exposure to persons outside the family, especially during the acute phase of illness.

The protracted nature of the illness and its associated weakness and fatigue frequently cause depression and resentment on the part of the usually vigorous, active teenager. It is important to spend time with the youngster to listen to his concerns and to allow him to express his feelings and vent his anger. The adolescent needs to be reassured that the limitations are only temporary, that social activities, so essential at this stage of development, can be resumed after the acute phase, and that he will have sufficient autonomy to determine the extent of his capabilities and the rate of resumption of activities.

SMOKING

The problem of smoking among teenagers is becoming increasingly serious. The habit appears to be spreading among teenagers even as the evidence of the relationship between smoking and health problems increases. Smoking is considered to be a dependence disorder and is formally included in the diagnostic nomenclature of the American Psychiatric Association (1987). Not only has smoking among teenagers increased, but the age of onset has decreased, and the proportion of girls who smoke regularly equals or surpasses the proportion of boys who smoke regularly.

The hazards of smoking at any age are undisputed; however, a preventive approach to teenage smoking is especially important. There is a high probability that regular smoking in childhood leads to a lifetime habit with concomitant increases in morbidity and mortality, since smoking has been linked to respiratory disorders in teenagers as well as adults.

Etiology

In most instances the smoking habit begins in adolescence, and there are a variety of reasons why teenagers begin smoking, such as imitation of adult behavior, peer pressure, and emulation of traits popularly attributed to smokers. Once smoking behavior is established, smoking itself is thought to produce enough reinforcement to sustain the practice without the initial pressure. The stages in the process of becoming a smoker are outlined in the accompanying box.

Stages in Becoming a Smoker

Preparation—early learning experiences provided in the environment, for example, parent or sibling smokers in the family
Initiation—trying the first cigarette; peer influences are more important than family influences in determining when cigarettes are first tried
Experimentation—learning to smoke by repeated experimentation; decision to quit or continue
Regular smoking—smokes sufficiently often to be considered a regular smoker

Smokeless Tobacco

The term *smokeless tobacco* refers to tobacco products that are placed in the mouth but not ignited, for example, snuff and chewing tobacco. This increasingly popular substitute for cigarettes is now posing a serious hazard to children and adolescents, as well as young adults. These products have been proved to be carcinogenic, and regular use has been reported to cause foul-smelling breath, periodontal disease, erosion of teeth, and tooth loss. The American Academy of Pediatrics (Committee on Environmental Hazards, 1985) states that "for the protection of the present and future health of the children of this nation, the selling and advertising of all forms of smokeless tobacco must be controlled without delay."

Nursing Considerations

Prevention of regular smoking in teenagers appears to be the most effective way to reduce the overall incidence of

Recommended Nonsmoking Strategies

Provide only a cursory mention of long-term health consequences (e.g., cardiovascular and cancer risks)
Discuss immediate physiologic consequences in some detail (e.g., changes in heart rate and blood pressure, minor respiratory symptoms, and blood carbon monoxide concentrations)
Mention alternatives to smoking for establishing a self-image that appears tough, independent, mature, or sophisticated (e.g., establishing a weight-lifting regimen, jogging and dancing, joining a Boys' Club or a Girls' Club, engaging in volunteer work for a hospital or political or religious group)
Mention the negative effects of smoking (e.g., earlier wrinkling of skin, yellow stains on teeth and fingers, tobacco odor on breath and clothing)
Mention the increasing ostracism of smokers by nonsmokers, both legal and informal, in places of work and public places
Mention the increasing evidence that second-hand smoke is injurious to the health of nonsmokers who are regularly exposed, especially small children
Acknowledge that many adults once believed that important social benefits were associated with smoking, but point out that the vast majority of adult smokers would now quit smoking if they could
Arm the cooperative adolescent with arguments for dealing with peer pressure (e.g., by not smoking, a teenager demonstrates independence and nonconformity, traits normally prized by youth)
Request posters and pamphlets from local voluntary agencies (e.g., American Cancer Society, American Heart Association, and American Lung Association) to display prominently

Modified from Wong-McCarthy, W.J., and Gritz, E.R.: Preventing regular teenage cigarette smoking, Pediatr. Ann. **11**:683-689, 1982.

smoking. A variety of methods have been employed to deal with the problem. For the most part smoking-prevention programs that focus on negative long-term effects of smoking on health have been ineffective. Those emphasizing immediate effects and youth-to-youth programs have been somewhat more effective, but primarily in improving the teenagers' attitudes toward smoking. Because smoking and smoking-related behavior function as a key social symbol, antismoking campaigns must be addressed to the norms of the potential smokers without ridicule or threat to the social norms of the group.

Two areas of focus are gaining interest among health advocates: peer-led programming emphasizing social consequences of smoking and use of media, such as videotapes and films, in smoking prevention. If a significant number of influential peers can "sell" their classmates on the idea that the habit is not popular, the followers will imitate their behavior. Short-term rather than long-term consequences are emphasized, for example, the effects of smoking on personal appearance, such as the unattractive stains on teeth and hands and the unpleasant odor that smoking gives to the breath and clothing. Several strategies are recommended for health professionals (see box).

◆ *Health Problems Related to Sports Participation*

Every sport has some potential for injury to the participant—whether the youngster engages in serious competition or participates for pure enjoyment. Serious injury can occur during rough contact sports or to persons who are not physically prepared for the activity; for example, the risk of injury is greater if the youngster's body build isn't suited to the sport, if the muscles and support systems (respiratory and cardiovascular) are insufficiently conditioned to withstand the rigors of the physical stress, or if the youngster lacks the insight and judgment to recognize when an activity is beyond his capabilities. More injuries occur during recreational sports participation than in organized athletic competition.

Not only does the activity itself pose a hazard of greater or lesser degree (Fig. 17-1), but the environment and the sports or recreational equipment present additional risks. Children participate in physical activity in a variety of environments, both indoors and outdoors, on floors, on the ground, on snow, on or beneath water surfaces, and sometimes in free air space. These activities frequently involve equipment that intensifies the risk factor.

ACUTE INJURIES

Acute overload injuries are those that occur suddenly during an activity and produce immediate symptoms. They can be caused by a blow or overstretching, twisting, or otherwise causing a sudden stress to tissues.

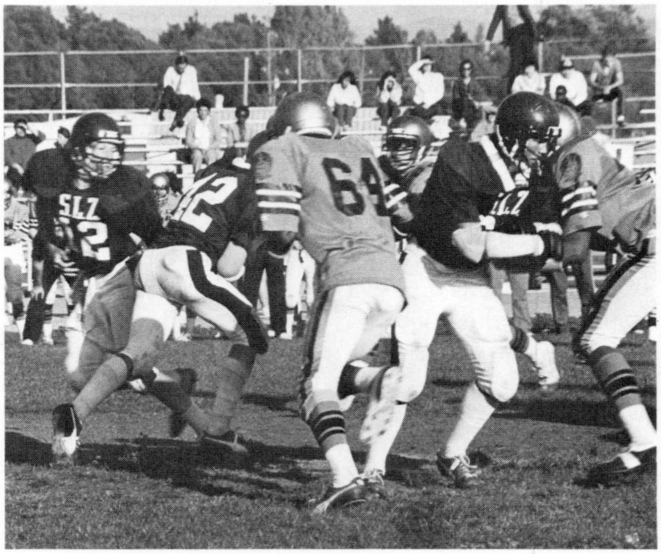

FIG. 17-1 Football is an example of a strenuous collision sport.

Contusions

Contusions are probably the most common of sports injuries and consist of damage to the soft tissue, subcutaneous structures, and muscle. The tearing of these tissues and small blood vessels and the inflammatory response lead to hemorrhage, edema, and associated pain when the youngster attempts to move the injured part. The escape of blood into the tissues will be observed as *ecchymosis*, a black and blue discoloration.

Immediate treatment consists of cold application as in the treatment of sprains described on p. 471. Return to participation is allowed when the strength and range of motion of the affected extremity are equal to those of the opposite extremity.

Dislocations

Long bones are held in approximation to one another at the joint by ligaments. Joints can be tight or loose, and loose joints are more likely to be dislocated. A dislocation occurs when the force of stress on the ligament is so great as to displace the normal position of the opposing bone ends or the bone end to its socket. The predominant symptom is pain that increases with attempted passive or active movement of the extremity. In dislocations there may be an obvious deformity and inability to move the joint. Temporary restriction of the joint, with a sling or bandage that secures the arm to the chest in a shoulder dislocation, provides sufficient comfort and immobilization until the youngster can receive medical help.

Simple dislocations should be reduced as soon as possible under sedation and often local anesthesia. An unreduced dislocation will be complicated by increased swelling, making reduction difficult and increasing the risk of neurovascular problems. Reduction is accomplished by simple traction and slight flexion followed by immobilization in a splint for 10 to 16 days or up to 3 weeks or more for healing of torn ligaments. See p. 1030 for a discussion of congenital dislocations.

Sprains

A sprain occurs when trauma to a joint is so severe that a ligament is partially or completely torn or stretched by the force created as a joint is twisted or wrenched, often accompanied by damage to associated blood vessels, muscles, tendons, and nerves. Sprains can be mild, moderate, or severe depending on the extent of damage.

The presence of laxity of the joint is the most valid indicator of the severity of a sprain. In a severe injury the athlete complains of the joint feeling "loose" or as if "something is coming apart" and may describe hearing a "snap," "pop," or "tearing." Pain is seldom the principal subjective symptom. There is a rapid onset with swelling, often diffuse, accompanied by immediate disability and appreciable reluctance to use the injured joint.

Strains

A strain is a microscopic tear to the musculotendinous unit and has features in common with sprains. The area is painful to touch and swollen. Most strains are incurred over time rather than suddenly, and the rapidity of the appearance provides clues regarding severity. In general, the more rapidly the strain occurs, the more severe the injury. When the strain involves the muscular portion, there is more bleeding, often palpable soon after injury and before edema obscures the hematoma.

Therapeutic Management

The first 6 to 12 hours constitute the most critical period for virtually all soft tissue injuries. Basic principles of managing sprains and other soft tissue injuries are summarized in the acronyms RICE or ICES:

R Rest	**I** Ice
I Ice	**C** Compression
C Compression	**E** Elevation
E Elevation	**S** Support

Soft tissue injuries should be iced immediately. This is best accomplished with crushed ice wrapped in a towel or encased in a screw-top ice bag or plastic bag (for example, a resealable storage bag). A wet elastic wrap is applied to provide compression and to keep the ice pack in place. A single layer of the wrap is placed over the injured area to protect the skin under the ice pack, and the remainder of the bandage secures the pack in place. Although the initial application remains in place only 30 minutes, the effects last up to 7 hours.

The local treatment is accompanied by appropriate exercise, depending on the severity of the injury and carried out under the direction of a competent professional experienced in care of sports injuries.

Major sprains or tears to the ligamentous tissue rarely occur in growing children. Ligaments are stronger than bone, and the epiphysis and growth plate are the weakest areas of the bone; therefore the more usual sites of injury are at the growth plate (see Fractures, Chapter 30). Torn ligaments, especially those in the knee, are usually treated by immobilization with a cast for 3 to 4 weeks or strapping of the joint with adhesive or Elastoplast bandage. Passive leg exercises, gradually increased to active ones, are begun as soon as sufficient healing has taken place.

OVERUSE SYNDROMES

To excel in sports the young athlete is forced to train longer, harder, and earlier in life than previously. The rewards are increased level of fitness, better performances, faster times, and the satisfaction of attaining a personal goal. However, the risk of overuse injury is always present. The common feature in overuse injuries is the repetitive microtrauma that occurs to a particular anatomic structure when the same movements are performed time and again, causing inflammation of the involved structure with complaints of pain, tenderness, swelling, and disability. Examples of overuse syndromes include "Little League elbow" (tendinitis and osteochondritis from repetitive throwing), "tennis elbow" (lateral epicondylitis from repetitive elbow strain), and Osgood-Schlatter disease (traction apophysitis of tibial tubercle).

Stress Fractures

Stress fractures occur as a result of repeated muscle contraction and are seen most often in repetitive weight-bearing sports such as running, gymnastics, and basketball. They occur less often in swimmers (upper extremity). The most common symptoms are a sharp, persistent, progressive pain or a deep, persistent, dull ache located over the bone. Sometimes there is pain on impact (heel strike), but the most important clinical sign is pain over the involved bony surface. Diagnosis is established on the basis of clinical observation. Occasionally a bone scan may be needed.

Therapeutic Management

Development of inflammation is common to all overuse syndromes; therefore the management is directed toward rest or alteration of activities, physical therapies, and medication. Rest is the primary therapy, usually involving reduced activity to alleviate the repetitive stress that initiated the symptoms. It is important to keep the youngster mobile, and training can be continued with alternative exercise that maintains conditioning without aggravating the injury. For example, pool running (treading water in the deep end of a pool) can use the same movements as running but without the weight-bearing.

Other modalities include cryotherapy and cold whirlpools, and sometimes taping, bracing, and splinting may be employed. Medications, such as aspirin, or nonsteroidal anti-inflammatory drugs, such as tolmetin, are sometimes prescribed for discomfort. Topical medications are of questionable value.

NURSE'S ROLE IN SPORTS FOR CHILDREN AND ADOLESCENTS

Nurses may become involved in sports activities in the areas of preparation and evaluation for activities, prevention of injury, treatment of injuries, and rehabilitation after injury. Selecting an appropriate sport for both recreation and competition is a joint effort of youngster, parents, and health professionals. The best approach to counseling children and parents regarding sports participation is to encourage activities that are most likely to provide pleasure and physical benefits throughout childhood into adulthood. Exposure to a variety of sports activities is probably better for young children than limiting them to one sport. Parents should be cautioned against overprogramming children in order that the children have ample time for other activities and associations.

When children sustain athletic injuries, nurses are often responsible for instructing the children and their parents regarding care. Instructions, such as schedule for appointments, application of ice, and any restrictions in activity, should be made clear, preferably accompanied by written directions. The importance of taking medications as prescribed is emphasized, since they may be needed for an extended period of time and compliance may be difficult.

Prevention of sports injuries is probably the most important aspect of any athletic program. The children should be suited to the activity, the environment and equipment made safe for physical activity, and the children adequately prepared for the sport, especially those requiring strenuous and/or continuous physical exertion. Nurses collaborate with coaches and athletic trainers to ensure that safety measures are carried out. Stretching exercises, warming up and cooling down activities, and an appropriate training program are only some of the requisites for safe participation. Protective measures, such as pads, taping, wrapping, or other devices, are employed for areas at risk. Nurses are also on the alert for environmental safety risks.

◆ *Altered Growth and Maturation*

The absence of physical and/or sexual maturation at a time when other children are experiencing positive evidence of sexual development and its associated spurt in growth and physical strength is a matter of concern to both the parents and their affected child. Fortunately, in most instances the delay in development is a simple physiologic or constitutional delay that merely represents one end of the normal genetically influenced variation of pubertal growth. These children will go through a delayed but normal puberty to finally catch up, in their late teens, with their more rapidly developing age-mates. Less benign causes of delayed development may be of endocrine origin or caused by chromosomal aberrations. In other situations delayed development may be a result of chronic diseases, such as malabsorption, chronic asthma, and poorly controlled diabetes mellitus, that are serious enough to retard the developmental process.

The rate of maturation is important during the school years, but at puberty it assumes gigantic proportions to the youngster and often to his parents as well. Girls or boys who lag behind their peers in physical maturation are painfully aware of their shortcomings. The adolescent girl feels out of place among her companions whose hips and bosoms are developing, feels cheated because she has not yet menstruated, and feels that she is not a part of the giggling and boy-talk of her friends. The adolescent boy feels weak and small compared with his muscular companions with whom he can no longer compete, and his high voice sounds childish in contrast to the deep tones around him. Slow-maturing youngsters need much support and reassurance that they are not abnormal and need only to be patient until the time comes when they, too, will develop the characteristics for which they yearn.

ENDOCRINE DYSFUNCTION

The child with endocrine or genetic disorders that interfere with the maturation process needs special help. The major hormones that promote physical growth are thyroid hormone, growth hormone, and sex hormones. Insulin can be said to promote growth by its effect on carbohydrate metabolism, whereas cortisol inhibits growth. Therefore, deficiencies of growth-promoting hormones or an excess of cortisol can cause growth retardation in children. Endocrine deficiencies can be the result of abnormal secretory function in the glands responsible for their production, the pituitary hormones that stimulate their secretion, or the releasing factors from the hypothalamus. (See Chapter 28 for disorders associated with endocrine dysfunction.)

Cortisol excess as a result of organic causes or of prolonged cortisone therapy also has an adverse effect on growth in children. Because of the growth-suppressing effect of cortisone in excess of minimal requirements, therapy is limited to short-term administration whenever possible.

TALL OR SHORT STATURE

Variations in height are expressions of genetic diversity among all populations. Most often the diversity is simply a manifestation of the person's genetic constitution, but it may be caused by a physiologic or emotional disorder. To the person on the extremes of height it can be a source of intense discomfort and anxiety. Boys are more distressed over short stature; girls are more likely to be disturbed by tall stature.

Tall Stature

Despite the fact that the average height of both boys and girls is steadily increasing, there is still a small group of children who, because of some organic disorder or a familial tendency, are excessively tall when compared with their contemporaries. To some it can be a source of pride or a source of intense anxiety and a severe social handicap.

When the rate of height change before puberty suggests the probability of excessive adult height, treatment with hormones may be considered, although there is a great deal of controversy regarding their use for this purpose. The selection of children for hormonal therapy is made on the basis of a careful evaluation of physical, psychologic, and social factors.

Short Stature

A small group of children suffer delay of growth or onset of adolescence because of disorders that may or may not be amenable to treatment. From a worldwide point of view, the most common cause of short stature and/or delayed development is probably inadequate nutrition; however, the major disorders that produce delayed development are chronic diseases, endocrine dysfunction, and syndromes of primary gonadal failure.

Chronic diseases can interfere with growth, but unless the illness is unduly prolonged, catch-up growth will occur. Diseases and disorders that usually cause some degree of growth delay include asthma, cystic fibrosis, gastrointestinal diseases (such as parasitic infections), malabsorption syndromes, cardiac anomalies, and chronic renal disturbances. It appears that the duration of the illness is more significant than the intensity in its effect on growth, although the precise length of time necessary to affect growth permanently has not been determined.

Skeletal disorders that affect growth in stature are principally those described as dwarfism. Most are caused by a variety of congenital defects and disorders, such as achondroplasia, and some of the inborn errors of metabolism, such as Hurler or Hunter syndromes.

Psychosocial dwarfism. *Psychosocial dwarfism, deprivation dwarfism,* and *stress-induced growth failure* are terms applied to children who are significantly retarded in growth because of environmental circumstances. The disorder affects children over 2 years of age and is associated with marked delays in physical growth and developmental skills and with immature behavior. When these children are removed from the deprived environment, their growth proceeds at a normal or increased rate. (See also nonorganic failure to thrive p. 327.)

Therapeutic Management

Management consists of continued medical observation, attention to general health and nutrition, and psychologic support. Where growth delay is accompanied by poor self-esteem and incompetence, many authorities recommend hormonal therapy. Testosterone in carefully regulated doses has proven effective in some cases. Human growth hormone, although expensive and in short supply, is capable of increasing height but is restricted to use with growth hormone deficiency. With the availability of synthetic growth hormone this treatment may become commonplace for selected children, although the potential for misuse is obvious.

Nursing Considerations

Deviation from the normal course of puberty is always of concern to the affected adolescent, and to some it assumes monumental proportions. Most of the problems of delayed development are those caused by simple constitutional delay of puberty, and in this situation the child can be assured that the normal course of events will eventually take place.

One of the difficulties related to a size that is incongruent with chronologic and mental age is the manner in which others, especially adults, relate to the child. People quite naturally respond to children with short stature as though they are younger than their age. Consequently these children often react with babyish or juvenile behavior, thus setting in motion a circular pattern of behavior and response. Conversely children who are tall or physically advanced for their age are treated as though they are more advanced than their years. They are often considered to be retarded or behaviorally immature when they actually perform according to the normal behavioral expectations for their age.

Listening to distressed adolescents and conveying to them genuine interest and concern are prerequisite to any successful intervention. Counseling and therapy are individualized to meet the needs of each youngster and his problems. Encouraging these children to accentuate the positive aspects of their bodies and personalities with sound health practices and good grooming helps foster a more positive self-image.

SEX CHROMOSOME ABNORMALITIES

Compared with most hereditary disorders, sex chromosome abnormalities are encountered with relatively high frequency. Most are caused by an alteration (usually an increase) in sex chromosome number, some of which are listed in Table 17-1. The more common of these are Turner and Klinefelter syndomes. Some general characteristics of sex chromosome abnormalites are:

1. There is a direct relationship between the male or female body type and the presence or absence of a Y chromosome. It appears that the Y chromosome is essential for development of male characteristics

TABLE 17-1

Common Sex Chromosome Abnormalities

Syndrome	Chromosomal Nomenclature	Phenotype	Incidence (live births)	Clinical Manifestations
Turner	45,X	Female	1:2500-8000 female births	Short stature; webbed neck; low posterior hairline; shield-shaped chest with widely spaced nipples; sterile
Triple X, or superfemale	47,XXX (can also be 48,XXXX or 49,XXXXX)	Female	1:850-1250 female births	Normal female characteristics; usually mentally retarded, mental deficiency in others; fertile
XYY male	47,XYY (can also be 48,XYYY or mosaic)	Male	1:840-1000 male births	Usually normal sex development; tendency to be tall with long head; poor coordination; may demonstrate aberrant behavior
Klinefelter	47,XXY (48,XXYY, 48,XXXY, 49,XXXXY, and so on, mosaics)	Male	1:500-1000 male births	Tall with long legs; hypogenitalism; sterile; male secondary sex characteristics may be deficient; may demonstrate aberrant behavior
Fragile X	46,XY or 46,XX	Predominantly male	Not established	Normocephaly or macrocephaly; prominent mandible; large ears; macroorchidism; mental retardation

2. The severity of defects is not related to the number of extra X chromosomes, except for mental retardation, which increases proportionately with each X chromosome
3. The presence of more than one Y chromosome appears to have variable but as yet not well-defined effects on an individual

Turner Syndrome

Turner syndrome is caused by absence of one of the X chromosomes. The incidence of the condition in the population has been variously estimated at 1 in 1500, 1 in 3000, and 1 in 10,000 live female births. Although this disorder is often recognized at birth, it is diagnosed most frequently at puberty because of three outstanding features: short stature, sexual infantilism, and amenorrhea (see also p. 937). Definitive diagnosis is confirmed on the basis of a negative sex chromatin test; chromosomal analysis is rarely necessary.

Therapy is always individualized for these girls and consists primarily of hormone treatment and psychologic counseling for both child and parents. Linear growth often can be increased by the administration of anabolic steroids followed by estrogen therapy to promote the development of secondary sex characteristics. Responses to estrogen therapy vary from girl to girl, but gradual feminization is accomplished to some degree in most individuals.

Klinefelter Syndrome

The most common of all chromosomal abnormalities, Klinefelter syndrome, is caused by the presence of one or more additional X chromosomes. In young boys this disorder is seldom seen before puberty, at which time varying degrees of failure of adolescent virilization occur. Some males are not detected until they appear for evaluation for infertility. All have absence of sperm in the semen (azoospermia), small testes, and defective development of secondary sex characteristics. The incidence of Klinefelter syndrome is estimated to be approximately 1 in 500 live male births. In 80% of these boys there is a chromatin-positive buccal smear, and the extra chromosome is apparent on chromosomal analysis.

The major effort in medical treatment is directed toward enhancing the masculine characteristics through the administration of male hormones, principally testosterone. Cosmetic surgery will eliminate embarrassment for the boy with gynecomastia.

Nursing Considerations

The nursing care of children with Turner or Klinefelter syndromes is primarily supportive. Nurses assist in diagnosis, explain tests and therapies to children and families, and provide support and encouragement. Since both disorders render the individual unable to reproduce, psychologic counseling will be an important aspect of care as well as modification of sex education.

PRECOCIOUS PUBERTY

Precocious puberty is the manifestation of pubertal development that appears before the expected age of onset. Although puberty is gradually appearing earlier in most societies, manifestations of sexual development before age 10 in boys or age 8½ in girls are considered precocious and should be investigated. Early sexual development can be a result of a number of causes, for example, a disorder of the gonad, the adrenal gland, or the hypothalamic-pituitary mechanism.

Precocious sexual development can be divided into two types: (1) *true,* or *complete, precocious puberty,* in which there is premature development of the gonads with secretion of sex hormones, development of secondary sex characteristics, and sometimes production of mature sperm or ova; and (2) *precocious pseudopuberty (incomplete puberty),* in which there is no maturation of the gonads, but there is appearance of secondary sex characteristics. The latter may be caused by a tumor on the adrenals or an organic brain lesion.

Psychologic management and guidance of children with true precocious puberty and their families constitute the most important aspects of treatment. Parents need a detailed explanation and reassurance of the benign nature of the condition. Dress and activities for the physically precocious child should be appropriate to the age. Heterosexual interest is not usually advanced beyond the child's chronologic age, and parents need to understand that the child's normal, overt manifestations of affection are age-appropriate and do not represent sexual advances.

GYNECOMASTIA

Some degree of bilateral or unilateral breast enlargement frequently occurs in young boys during puberty. In most instances it is a transient phenomenon that subsides spontaneously with achievement of male development. Occasionally, however, it is associated with abnormalities such as Klinefelter syndrome or endocrine dysfunction; therefore, these possibilities are ruled out by appropriate diagnostic examination.

Treatment usually consists of assurance to the boy and his parents that this is a benign and temporary situation. If the condition persists or is extensive enough to cause acute embarrassment or to produce doubts about gender identity in the young boy, plastic surgery is indicated for cosmetic and psychologic considerations. Administration of testosterone has no effect on breast development or regression and may even aggravate the condition. Since the boy is distressed about his physical integrity and masculinity, he will need reassurance regarding this apparently incongruous development.

DISORDERS OF THE MALE REPRODUCTIVE SYSTEM

It is fortunate for the male that most of the parts of the reproductive system are external and therefore visible and palpable. Therefore, most obvious anomalies, such as hypospadias, hydrocele, phimosis, and cryptorchidism, have been identified, and corrective measures can be instituted during early childhood. The most frequent problems related to the reproductive organs in later childhood are (1) infections, such as urethritis; (2) hematuria; (3) penile problems, such as nonretractable foreskin in uncircumcised males, carcinoma, and trauma; (4) scrotal conditions, such as varicocele (elongation, dilation, and tortuosity of the veins superior to the testicle); and (5) testicular torsion (a condition in which the testicle hangs free from its vascular structures, which can result in partial or complete venous occlusion with rotation). Tumors of the testes are not a common condition, but when manifested in adolescence, they are generally malignant and demand immediate evaluation.

Nursing Considerations

The adolescent male is extremely self-conscious about his changing body and often refuses a genital examination. The most successful approach is to assume a matter-of-fact attitude to the examination, explain precisely what will take place, and maintain a continuous commentary about what is being done and the findings at each phase of the examination. The adolescent male is approached as someone important as a person, with the nurse interested in his concerns. To supplement routine health assessment, every adolescent male should be taught frequent testicular self-examination (TSE) to familiarize him with his own anatomy and to ensure early detection of any abnormality.

AMENORRHEA

It is not unusual for an adolescent to skip a menstrual period or two when establishing normal menstrual and ovulatory cycles. Delay in initiation of menstruation is ordinarily a temporary problem resulting from late onset of puberty and requires no intervention. This is of little concern unless it creates undue anxiety on the part of the girl and her parents, which can ordinarily be allayed by explanation and reassurance. Careful examination will reveal any congenital defects of the genital tract (a rare cause).

Primary amenorrhea (when menarche is delayed beyond age 17 years) may be the result of absence or malformation of the female genital structures or the inability of normal structures to respond to hormonal stimulation. The most common causes of *secondary amenorrhea* (prolonged absence of menstruation for 12 months or more between periods in the first 2 years following menarche or when more than three periods have been missed after menses have become established) are emotional disturbances and pregnancy, which is accompanied by the signs and symptoms associated with this state.

Exercise-Related Menstrual Dysfunction

Delayed menarche has been associated with girls who engage in strenuous exercise. It is not clear whether exercise delays menarche, or menarcheal delay promotes athletic success. Some attribute delayed menarche and maintenance of regular ovulation to lack of development of body fat. Alterations have also been noted in menstrual bleeding patterns of girls who engage in strenuous exercise. The activities that appear to be associated with delayed or altered menstruation are ballet dancing, running, gymnastics, and swimming. This condition may cause embarrassment and concern to the youngster and her parents, which can be minimized by explanation and reassurance regarding its benign and temporary nature.

DYSMENORRHEA

A certain amount of discomfort during the first day or two of the menstrual flow is extremely common. Most girls experience cramping, abdominal pain, backache, and leg ache, but in a few the pain is intolerable and incapacitating. The term *primary dysmenorrhea* is applied to these symptoms when there is no pelvic disease to account for the cramping discomfort. When the discomfort can be attributed to endometriosis, infection, adhesions from peritonitis, or other pelvic disease, the complaint is described as *secondary dysmenorrhea*.

No specific etiology of primary dysmenorrhea is known; however, some contributory factors are recognized. In all instances of primary dysmenorrhea it is the occurrence of prior ovulation. There is also a relationship between uterine contractility and the secretion of prostaglandins. However, in some girls the discomfort may be a result of low pain tolerance.

A thorough gynecologic examination is carried out to exclude any pelvic abnormalities, and a careful history is taken regarding the type and duration of pain, its relationship to menstrual flow, and any associated symptoms. These questions not only provide information to the examiner but also serve to provide the girl with evidence that her problem is being taken seriously. An explanation of the physiology of menstruation helps to give reassurance.

Therapeutic Management

Treatment consists of administration of prostaglandin inhibitors. Aspirin has proved effective when begun a few days before the onset of the menses—approximately 11 days after ovulation. The relief appears to be the result of prostaglandin inhibitory (rather than analgesic) effect. Some relatively new prostaglandin inhibitors, such as ibuprofen, mefenamic acid, and naproxen, provide relief and can be taken at the start of menses. Simple exercises similar to those recommended for relief of prenatal discomfort, such as pelvic rocking, assuming the knee-chest position, and breathing exercises, may also be beneficial. The girl is encouraged to practice good hygiene and participate in regular activities. Sometimes cyclic estrogen therapy to prevent ovulation provides dramatic and predictable relief from pain.

Nursing Considerations

The nurse is most frequently the person to whom a young girl turns for advice regarding menstrual problems or problems related to vaginal discharge. Usually all the youngster needs is reassurance about this normal function, but this also provides an opportunity for the nurse to listen to what the adolescent is saying and to engage in health teaching concerning menstrual physiology and hygiene and the importance of a well-balanced diet, exercise, and general health maintenance. It is a time to dispel any myths the girl may have in relation to menstruation and her femininity. When assessment indicates a potential problem and need for her evaluation, the girl is referred to a physician, health service, or clinic.

One of the most difficult experiences facing the adolescent girl is the gynecologic examination. Whether it is her first experience or not, she is most likely filled with apprehension. Almost all adolescents are extremely self-conscious about their bodies and the changes taking place. She will need continuing support in the form of anticipatory guidance regarding what she can expect and suggestions of what she can do to help herself relax during the procedure. Usually the stressful experience of being placed in stirrups for the pelvic examination can be avoided. The youngster who is relaxed may be examined in the supine position with hips and knees flexed and legs abducted. If a female nurse is not the examiner, it is essential for her to remain with the patient during the examination to offer support and guidance.

◆ *Health Problems Related to Sexuality*

The child entering and progressing through the multiple physical and emotional changes of puberty is subject to some medical problems associated with these changes. The increasing incidence of adolescent pregnancy, sexually transmitted disease, and sexual trauma make it imperative that health professionals have an understanding of these disorders.

ADOLESCENT PREGNANCY

One of the consequences of adolescent experimentation, acting-out, the need to conform, impulsivity, and the search for a sexual identity is pregnancy. Although the incidence of adolescent pregnancy is influenced by the availability of contraception and abortion, pregnant teenagers present a population at risk—medically, socially, economically, and educationally.

With better facilities available for care, the mortality rates for teenage pregnancies are decreasing, but the morbidity still remains high. Teenage girls and their unborn infants are at greater risk for complications of both pregnancy and delivery. The most frequent complications are premature labor and infants of low birth weight, high neonatal mortality, toxemia of pregnancy, iron deficiency anemia, fetopelvic disproportion, and prolonged labor. There may be a greater incidence of weight gain in young mothers and, in younger girls, a competition in the nutritional needs for growth between the fetus and the teenage girl.

Nursing Considerations

The most important goal in nursing care of the pregnant teenager is to obtain medical care for her if she has not already done so. The importance of early prenatal care is well known for the welfare of both mother and infant when the girl chooses to continue the pregnancy and to facilitate a safe abortion when she elects this option. For guidelines, teaching, and general support measures during pregnancy, the reader is directed to the excellent textbooks available on nursing care throughout the maternity cycle.*

CONTRACEPTION

Family planning services in general have developed and expanded during recent years, and, with the increase in sexual activity among the teenage population, there is also an increased awareness of the need for contraceptive services as a part of the health care of adolescents.

The choice of a contraceptive method, to be safe and effective, must be suited to the individual. The choice is based on the youngster's preference and the practitioner's judgment. Although a girl may prefer to use the pill, if her menstrual pattern suggests that she is not ovulating normally, she will be guided to an alternative method. Also, the girl must be motivated to use whatever method is recommended or prescribed. No matter what method is selected, the provision of a birth control device is only part of a comprehensive sex education program.

SEXUALLY TRANSMITTED DISEASES

Sexually transmitted diseases (STDs) are among the most prevalent and dangerous of the communicable diseases and are now epidemic in the United States, with a disproportionate number occurring in adolescents and young adults. Sexually active adolescents are particularly at risk because they are often late in seeking medical attention. When a patient has one of these conditions, it is important that the history and examination should encompass the others as well.

The most prevalent STDs in the adolescent and adult populations are gonorrhea and chlamydial infections. These and other diseases that are seen less frequently are outlined in Table 17-2.

Therapeutic Management

Effective treatment of both males and females with a sexually transmitted disease is administration of the appropriate therapeutic agent. It is also suggested that all patients with gonorrhea receive a course of tetracycline therapy because of the high rate of mixed gonococcal and chlamydial infections. Treatment of sexual partners is also an essential part of therapy.

A genuine prophylaxis against infection is not yet available; therefore, preventive efforts must be directed toward finding and treating affected persons, locating and examining contacts of affected persons, educating young people regarding the facts of the disease and its spread, and encouraging the use of barriers (condoms) in sexually active young people.

Nursing Considerations

Nursing responsibilities encompass all aspects of sexually transmissible disease education, prevention, and treatment. Part of the sex education of young people should include information about these diseases, such as their symptoms and treatment, and dispelling the myths associated with their mode of transmission. It is true that most persons in the vulnerable teenage population are uninformed or misinformed about these diseases.

The major efforts of nurse counseling should be directed toward prevention, with emphasis on avoidance of sex or, when this does not seem feasible, avoidance of casual sex with multiple partners and the use of condoms. The school nurse may be involved in the controversial issue of whether or not to distribute condoms to sexually active high school students as a possible measure to control the spread of AIDS in this population.

RAPE

The adolescent girl is particularly vulnerable to sexual assault, and it is estimated that more than 50% of rape victims are between 10 and 19 years of age. In each instance the victim is potentially subject to serious physical or emotional harm or both. Males may also be assaulted (usually homosexually) and experience the same range of symptoms observed in girl victims (Brookman, 1983).

Legal definitions of rape vary from state to state but include the following categories: *completed rape*, *attempted rape*, and *statutory rape*. Most of the current definitions of rape are expanded to include all forms of sexual victimization, including anal and oral as well as genital penetration. For example, it may include intrusion of any object or body part into the genital or anal area of another person's body. Statutory rape may be charged when the victim is unable to give consent legally by virtue of age (age varies from state to state but is usually under 16 years of age), mental deficiency, psychosis, or an altered state of consciousness caused by sleep, drugs (including alcohol), or illness. Fitting the penis between the labia without disruption of the hymen or evidence of ejaculation is also considered sufficient penetration to constitute rape.

Three relationships are identified for adolescent assault: stranger (person unknown to the victim), nonstran-

*Bobak, I.M., and Jensen, M.D.: Maternity and gynecologic care: the nurse and the family, ed. 4, St. Louis, 1989, The C.V. Mosby Co.

TABLE 17-2

Selected Sexually Transmitted Diseases

Disease	Manifestations	Therapy	Nursing Considerations
Gonorrhea (*Neisseria gonorrhoeae*)	Male: urethritis—dysuria with profuse yellow discharge, frequency, urgency, nocturia Female: cervicitis (postpubertal)—may be associated with discharge, dysuria, dyspareunia; vulvovaginitis (prepubertal)	Penicillin with probenecid	Find and treat sexual contacts Educate young people regarding facts of the disease and its spread Encourage use of barrier in sexually active young people High rate of mixed disease; therefore, treat also for chlamydia (recommended)
Chlamydia (*Chlamydia trachomatis*)	Male: meatal erythema, tenderness, itching, dysuria, urethral discharge Female: mucopurulent cervical exudate with erythema, edema, congestion	Oral tetracycline	Same as above
Syphilis (*Treponema pallidum*)	Primary stage: chancre—a hard, painless, red, sharply defined lesion with indurated base, raised border, eroded surface, and scanty yellow discharge; usually located on penis, vulva, or cervix Secondary stage: systemic influenza-like symptoms and lymphadenopathy, rash; usually appears 1 to 3 weeks after healing of chancre	Penicillin	Viability of organism outside body is short Rapidly killed by oxygen, soap, common bacterial agents, and drying About 95% transmitted sexually; affected person most infectious during first year of disease
Herpes progenitalis (Herpesvirus hominis—type II)	Small (usually painful) vesicles on genital area, buttocks, and thighs; itching usually initial symptom; when vesicles break, shallow, circular, extremely painful lesions remain	No known cure Acyclovir (Zovirax) ointment decreases healing time and pain	Pregnancy should be avoided in sexually active girls Infection can be transmitted to infant during birth
Trichomoniasis (*Trichomonas vaginalis*)	Pruritus and edema of external genitalia; foul-smelling, greenish vaginal discharge; sometimes postcoital bleeding May be asymptomatic, especially in males	Oral metronidazole	May be contracted by self-infection from toilet bowls, bathtubs, or swimming pools (not total agreement on this) Patient should not consume alcohol while taking medication and for at least 48 hours following last dose
Candidiasis, or moniliasis (*Candida albicans*)	Edema and erythema of vulva and thick white, cheesy vaginal discharge May be satellite lesions on groin, thighs, and buttocks Cutaneous lesions on penis May be asymptomatic	Nystatin vaginal suppositories Miconazole vaginal cream	Possibility of predisposing factors such as oral contraceptives (which alter vaginal environment) or antibiotics Increased risk of neonatal thrush
Acquired immunodeficiency syndrome (Human immunodeficiency virus [HIV])	See p. 851	Primarily supportive	See p. 852

ger (person known to the victim), and incest (see p. 412). Although all can have serious and long-lasting effects, they are presumed to be different in a number of important ways: in the nature of the dominant, psychologic, and cognitive behavior they provoke; in the issues they raise for service providers and other potential helpers; and in the techniques that may be helpful for treating existing and new cases (Burgess, 1985).

Diagnostic Evaluation

The girl may exhibit any of a variety of reactions (see box) and the circumstances of the initial medical evaluation may also be frightening and stressful. The initial contact with the rape victim must be supportive because the interrogation and associated activities have the potential to add to the trauma of the sexual assault. First of all the victim needs to know that she (or he) is (1) all right and (2) not being blamed for the situation.

It is important to obtain a clear account of the circumstances of an alleged rape without forcing the victim to relive a very painful experience. Information includes date, time, location, and an accurate description of all types of sexual contact. The physical examination is carried out as soon as possible, since physical evidence deteriorates rapidly. The youngster is always told in advance

Clinical Manifestations of Rape Victim

- May display a variety of behaviors
  - Hysterical crying
  - Giggling
  - Agitation
  - Feelings of degradation
  - Anger and rage
  - Helplessness
  - Nervousness
  - Rapid mood swings
  - Appear calm and controlled (masking inner turmoil)
  - Confused
  - Self-blame
- Evidence of physical force
  - Roughness
  - Nonbrutal beating (slapping)
  - Brutal beating (slugging, kicking, beating repeatedly with fists)
  - Choking or gagging
- Predominant reaction is fear—of the rape and of injury
- Medical examination provides evidence of:
  - Penetration
  - Ejaculation
  - Use of force (when possible)

in understandable terms exactly what to expect in the way of tests and procedures, and the explanation is accompanied by strong emotional support. The victim is examined thoroughly, including nongenital areas, for evidence of injury that might substantiate the use of force.

Specimens are obtained for examination, including vaginal secretions for evidence of sperm and blood for serology, and a gonococcal culture is obtained to prove that the victim did not have any preexisting infection. The child is reexamined at appropriate intervals (4 to 6 weeks for syphilis; 2 to 3 days for gonorrhea) to determine if the child acquired disease from the assailant. At present testing for AIDS is not a routine procedure. However, if the family requests it, testing is carried out after a 2-month period.

Therapeutic Management

Adolescents who have been raped arrive at the emergency room or physician's office under a variety of circumstances. They are usually brought in by parents, friends, or police officers, but some may seek medical help on their own. It is advisable to obtain parental consent for examination, but the examination may be performed without consent if the adolescent is mature and the parents are unavailable. A female nurse should be present during the history and examination of female victims. Whether a parent should be present during the examination is determined on an individual basis. The parent's presence is usually encouraged but only *if the parent is supportive*.

Any injuries sustained by the victim that require surgical treatment are repaired. Lacerations of the vagina are not uncommon. Most physicians prescribe, and many of the victims and/or their parents prefer the youngster to receive, prophylactic administration of penicillin at the time of initial examination. Pregnancy prophylaxis, usually diethylstilbestrol, is offered to the victim who is not using oral contraceptives, pregnant, or menstruating. Follow-up care is needed to observe the youngster for possible development of pelvic inflammatory disease or other sexually transmitted disease.

Rape Trauma Syndrome

Through observations of victims the term *rape trauma syndrome* has been applied to the reaction to a sexual assault. The syndrome involves two phases: (1) the acute phase of disorganization of life-style, and (2) a long-term process of reorganization. These phases encompass behavioral, somatic, and psychologic reactions to the stressful event.

Acute phase of disorganization. During the acute phase victims exhibit either an expressed style or a controlled style of demonstrating emotional reactions in coping with the stress of the experience. Those with the expressed style are able to express their feelings of fear, anger, and/or anxiety. Those with the controlled style hide or mask their feelings and display a calm, subdued affect. However, the controlled victim is equally as upset as the victim who expresses feelings. Other acute reactions include physical reactions such as body soreness, disturbances in sleep patterns, and alterations in eating patterns. Feelings of embarrassment are prominent in adolescents. Many concerns of youngsters focus on how the event will affect them at school.

Long-term reorganization process. Changes in life-style are often observed during the reorganization phase. Victims may continue previous activities such as attending school but achieve only a minimum level of functioning. A teenager may attend school but be apprehensive that other students know about the incident and are talking about her. Most children experience nightmares, phobias about being left alone, and panic reactions on seeing the assailant, the scene of the crime, or a symbolic reminder of the assault. Sexual fears are prominent and difficult for the victim to discuss.

Feelings of helplessness and powerlessness are experienced as the victim feels that events are totally beyond her control. Victims are concerned about the potential effects that the assault will have on their relationships with others, particularly regarding the extent to which persons close to them will blame them for the assault. There are concerns about whom to tell about the event and how to go about telling them.

Nursing Considerations

Many of the approaches that have been described for the sexually abused child (p. 415) are applicable to the adolescent. Sexual assault is a devastating experience with long-lasting effects. The primary goal of nursing care is to avoid inflicting further stress on the youngster who is often angry, confused, frightened, embarrassed, and filled with self-blame. The nurse must do everything possible to reduce the stress of the interrogation and examination. Although most health professionals and law enforcement officers are sensitive to the needs of the youngster and attempt to make the process as nonstressful as possible, the nurse should be alert to cues that indicate the victim is being overstressed.

Follow-up care of the rape victim is essential and extends over a long period of time. Aside from the universal need for emotional support, there are no firm guidelines for meeting the needs of rape victims. Their needs vary widely and depend on the nature of the incident, when it took place, the physical and emotional injuries sustained by the victim, the actions being considered as a result, the resources available for informal support, and the anticipated reactions of persons in the informal support network (Burgess, 1985).

Family support. In addition to the needs of the adolescent rape victim, the nurse is also sensitive to the needs and reactions of the youngster's parents. Some will be angry and blame the adolescent; others will be guilt-ridden. Many reactions can be expected at the time of the incident, ranging from despair to extreme agitation. Frequently the parents require as much support and reassurance as the victim. Agitated, angry, or incapacitated parents are unable to provide support for their youngster. Meeting their needs can facilitate their ability to support the teenager during the crisis.

◆ *Eating Disorders*

Eating disorders are among the most frequently encountered health problems in childhood and adolescence. Overeating often begins in infancy and continues throughout childhood; undereating usually does not become apparent until later childhood or adolescence. Either overeating or undereating can have a detrimental effect on health and well-being and, especially in the case of undereating, can be a decided threat to life.

OBESITY

There is probably no problem related to childhood and adolescence that is so obvious to others, is so difficult to treat, and has such long-term effects on psychologic and physical health status as obesity. It is the most common nutritional disturbance of children and one of the most challenging contemporary health problems at all ages.

Obesity is an increase in body weight resulting from an excessive accumulation of fat or simply the state of being too fat. *Overweight* refers to the state of weighing more than average for one's height and body build, which may or may not include an increased amount of fat. It is possible for two children to have the same height and weight and for one to be obese whereas the other is not.

Etiology/Pathophysiology

Obesity results from a caloric intake that consistently exceeds calorie requirements and expenditure. The causes that produce this disequilibrium are complex and may involve a variety of influences, including metabolic, hypothalamic, hereditary, social, cultural, and psychologic factors (Fig. 17-2).

In a very small percentage of children childhood obesity can be attributed to an underlying disease such as hypothyroidism, adrenal hypercorticoidism, hyperinsulinism, and dysfunction of or damage to the central nervous system.

It is known that the metabolism of glucose plays an important role in the regulation of fat deposition, since excess calories from carbohydrates are stored as fat and a lack of glucose prompts the release of fat as a source of energy. It appears that the obese are able to store fat easily but are unable to release this fat or burn it for energy. Obese persons also appear to be more efficient in fat storage and have less heat-producing brown fat than nonobese persons.

Heredity has been demonstrated to be an important factor in the development of obesity. For example, identical twins reared apart tend to resemble their natural parents to a greater extent than they do their adoptive

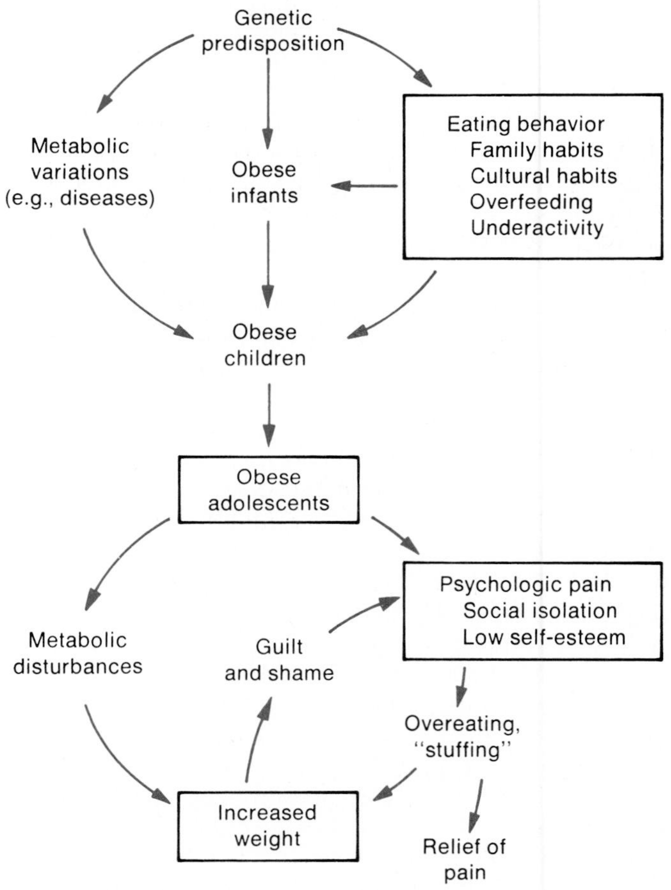

FIG. 17-2 Complex relationships in adolescent obesity.

parents. Children who are inclined toward a rounded body build with soft body contours and larger amounts of subcutaneous fat are somewhat predisposed to the accumulation of fat. However, it is almost impossible to distinguish between hereditary and environmental factors, since both may be operating in any situation when other family members are obese.

Obese children are less active than lean children although it is uncertain whether the inactivity creates the obesity or if the obesity is responsible for the inactivity. Obese persons also demonstrate an overwhelming appetite and often overeat when they are not hungry or have no appetite. They eat more rapidly and tend to ingest more calories at one meal rather than over a period of time. Obese adolescents are characteristically night eaters and often skip meals, particularly breakfast.

Recent theories that attempt to explain the development of obesity are:

Adipose cell theory—The number of cells in adipose tissue is increased, the size of the fat cells is increased, or a combination of these. It is believed that there are sensitive periods in development when cell numbers increase. Obese children have larger cells that stay the same size once they reach a maximum, and their fat cells appear to increase in number during childhood.

Set point theory—Individuals have a predetermined level for body weight that remains relatively stable during adulthood. With increased caloric intake the metabolic rate increases to burn the excess; when intake is reduced, metabolism decreases to conserve energy.

Sociocultural factors play an important role in weight gain. Patterns of eating are culturally and socially based in most instances, and in some the food preferences of the culture contribute to the development of obesity. Many cultures consider plump children to be a sign of health, and some look on obesity as evidence of well-being and foster weight gain as a desirable feature.

Psychologic factors may provide a basis for eating patterns in childhood. In infancy the child first experiences relief from discomfort through feeding and learns to associate eating with feelings of well-being, security, and the comforting presence of the mothering person. Soon eating is deeply associated with the feeling of being loved. Many parents use food, such as candy and other "treats," as a positive reinforcer for desired behavior or as a way to compensate for their own feelings of guilt, especially if the child was unwanted or overvalued because of loss of a previous child. This practice soon acquires symbolic significance to the extent that the child continues to use food as a reward, a comfort, and a means by which to deal with feelings of depression or hostility.

Diagnostic Evaluation

An obese child looks "too fat." Several tests, both scientific and unscientific, can be employed to assess obesity (see box and p. 134). Appropriate diagnostic tests rule out suspected metabolic and endocrine disorders.

Clinical Manifestations of Obesity

Child appears overweight
Weight over established standards
Skin fold thickness greater than established standard
Body fat increased above established standards as determined by densimetric, hydrometric, and radiopotassium measurements

Nursing Considerations

Medical and nursing management are considered together since nearly all successful weight-reduction programs involve nurses. Few physicians are able or inclined to devote the time to the long-term supportive care needed to maintain the motivation of obese youngsters.

ASSESSMENT

The presence of obesity is obvious from appearance alone, and a gross determination can be made by a rough comparison of height and weight with standard growth charts. Children who are 20% over the normal for their height and weight should be further evaluated. Evaluation includes height and weight history of the child, parents, and siblings, as well as eating habits, appetite and hunger patterns, and physical activities engaged in. It is useful to have an estimation of the degree of fatness in order to have some idea of the component of body weight that can be modified.

NURSING DIAGNOSES

Based on a thorough assessment of the obese child or adolescent, nursing diagnoses become apparent. Although the diagnoses vary according to the needs of each individual child, some of the more prominent are outlined in the Nursing Care Plan on pp. 484-485.

PLANNING

The goals of a weight-loss program include the following:

1. Modify diet to provide loss of fat content without interfering with growth, normal activity, and psychologic well-being.
2. Implement a regular exercise program.
3. Modify eating behavior.
4. Provide psychologic support.

IMPLEMENTATION

Motivation to lose weight is the key to success. The reasons behind the teenager's desire to lose weight need to be explored with him, but success is rarely achieved unless the youngster is motivated to lose weight and takes personal responsibility for his dietary habits and exercise

TABLE 17-3

Caloric Values for Selected Fast Food

Food	Caloric Value
Burger King	
Cheeseburger	317
Hamburger	275
Whopper, regular	640
w/cheese	723
Double beef, plain	850
w/cheese	950
French fries, regular	227
Onion rings, regular	274
Chocolate shake	320
McDonald's	
Big Mac	570
Hamburger	263
Cheeseburger	328
Chicken McNuggets (6 pieces)	323
Quarter Pounder	427
w/cheese	525
Egg McMuffin	340
French fries, regular	220
Filet-O-Fish	435
Milk shake, vanilla	352
chocolate	383
Wendy's	
Hamburger, single	350
Hamburger, double	570
Chicken sandwich	320
French fries	280
Frosty	400
Long John Silver's	
Fish, 2 pieces & fries	651
3 pieces & fries	853
Fish sandwich	337
Cole slaw	180
Hushpuppies (3)	145
Taco Bell	
Beef Burrito	466
Burrito Supreme	457
Beefy Tostada	291
Dairy Queen	
Super Hot Dog/chili	570
Super Hot Dog w/cheese	580
Fries, small	200
Pizza Hut	
Thin 'n Crispy (¼ medium)	
Standard cheese	340
Superstyle cheese	410
Standard pepperoni	370
Superstyle pepperoni	430
Thick 'n Chewy (¼ medium)	
Standard cheese	390
Superstyle cheese	450
Standard pepperoni	450
Superstyle pepperoni	490
Supreme	480
Super Supreme	590
Fruit	
Apple w/skin, 2½ in. diameter	66
Banana, medium	100
Peach w/skin, 2 in. diameter	38
Cookies and cakes	
Hostess, 1 cup cake	
orange	151
chocolate	166
Hostess Twinkie, 1	147
Oreo, each	50
Chocolate chip	50-80

Food	Caloric Value
Cookies and cakes—cont'd	
Brownie	200
Fig Newton, 1	60
Doughnut, regular, 1 oz	113
old fashioned, 1 oz	151
powdered, 1 oz	117
Crackers	
Cheese balls & curls, 1 oz	160
Corn chips, 1 oz	150-160
Graham crackers, 1 piece	30
Pretzels, 1 oz	110-116
Rye Krisp, 1 triple	25
Saltine, 1 piece	12-18
Tortilla chips, 1 oz	130-140
Trisket, 1 piece	20
Wheat Thins, 1 piece	9
Candy	
Heath, 2½ oz	334
Hershey's, 1.2 oz bar	187
Nestle's, 1.1 oz bar	159
Hershey's Kisses, 1 piece	27
Krackle bar, .35 oz	52
Life Savers, 1 piece	10
Milk Duds, ¾ oz box	89
1¼ oz box	148
M & Ms, peanut, 1½ oz	219
plain, 1½ oz	202
Mr. Goodbar, 1½ oz	233
Snickers, 1.8 oz	247
Crackerjack, ¾ oz	90
Chewing gum	
Any brand, 1 stick	10
Dentyne, 1 stick	4
Chiclets, Beechies, 1 piece	6
Miscellaneous snacks	
Potato chips, 1 oz	150-160
Pringles, 1 oz	172
Yogurt, plain, 8 oz	150-160
fruit, 8 oz	230-262
Popcorn, plain, 1 cup	54
Nuts	
Almonds, 1 oz	170-178
Peanuts, dry roasted, 1 oz	160-173
oil roasted, 1 oz	179
Pecans, 1 oz	190-220
Pistachios, 1 oz	174
Pumpkin seeds, unshelled, 1 oz	116
Sunflower seeds, shelled, 1 oz	164
unshelled, 1 oz	86
Dessert snacks	
Popsicle, 1 twin pop	70
Turnover	310-340
Pop Tart	200-220
Baskin-Robbins	
Ice cream, 1 scoop	
vanilla	147
French vanilla	181
chocolate	165
chocolate fudge	178
Sherbet, 1 scoop	99-139
Beverages	
Chocolate milk, 8 oz	213
Skim milk, 8 oz	88
Whole milk, 8 oz	159
Coca Cola, 8 oz	96
Sprite, 8 oz	95

Essentials of a Good Dietary Regimen for Children and Adolescents

The diet should provide for:
- Rapid weight loss
- Lack of metabolic complications
- Lack of hunger
- Preservation of lean body mass
- Absence of psychiatric reactions
- Normal activity
- Growth

After Merritt, R.J.: Obesity in paediatric patients, Compr. Ther. **5**:26-34, 1979.

program. Teenagers who are forced by parents to seek help are seldom sufficiently motivated, become rebellious of parental nagging, and are unwilling to control dietary intake. A rigid approach and one that is based on parental enforcement of the regimen is usually doomed from the start.

Diet. Planning caloric restriction for the adolescent during the rapid growth period requires a careful design (see box). Since obesity is usually a lifelong problem, it is best to provide the individual with a diet that can be maintained throughout life with the emphasis on restricting calories. The most successful diets are those that use ordinary foods in controlled portions rather than diets that require the avoidance of any specific food. The youngster is taught how to incorporate favorite foods into the diet and how to select substitutes that are also satisfying. The dieting youngster should eat what the rest of the family eats, but less of it, and should not be deprived of favorite foods. These can be allowed—in small amounts. There are a multitude of restricted calorie diets available from a number of sources, such as the American Dietetic Association, and the caloric values for a wide variety of commercial foods are available to facilitate meal planning.

For children, especially teenagers, snacking is an integral part of the daily routine, which makes dieting particularly difficult for obese children. They have little concept of the caloric content of even the most commonplace snack foods. Vending machines are usually stocked with high-calorie, low-nutrient temptations, they are readily accessible, and the children have ample pocket money with which to purchase these items. Following pressures from concerned parents and nutritionists, many school cafeterias are providing more wholesome "treats," such as fruit, juices, and raw vegetables, in vending machines in school cafeterias. However, the favorite gathering places for children and teens are the fast-food establishments, which are often located curiously near to large schools. See Table 17-3 for the caloric values for some of the fast-food items and snack foods.

No child or adolescent should be encouraged to initiate a reduction diet without a health assessment, evaluation, and counseling. It is also important to emphasize the undesirable nature of the fad diets and crash programs that continually appear in various publications. Although some success has been achieved with low-carbohydrate, high-fat diets, their unpalatability and dietary boredom contribute to a high failure rate. Exotic diets have not been successful, and their unbalanced nature makes them potentially dangerous for growing children or adolescents. To be successful from all aspects, a dietary program should be nutritionally sound with sufficient satiety value, produce the desired weight loss, and be accompanied by nutrition education and continued support.

Exercise. Since weight loss will occur only when caloric expenditure is greater than caloric intake, physical activity in the form of regularly scheduled exercise, progressively increased over the child's usual activity, is an integral part of a weight-reduction program. Activities should be those that stress self-improvement rather than competition, and teenagers need continued psycholgic support and encouragement to prevent the beginning of the destructive cycle of passivity, withdrawal, and rejection.

Behavioral therapy. Probably the most successful method for treating obesity is diet combined with behavior modification, which emphasizes identification and elimination of inappropriate eating habits. Although the long-term effects of this method are still in need of evaluation, it appears to hold promise for the treatment of obesity in adolescents. Some of the techniques used in this approach are listed in the Nursing Care Plan on p. 484.

Group involvement. Some persons on weight-reduction programs find that support and mutual reinforcement provided by a group of persons with a similar problem help them to adjust to the changes needed for successful accomplishment of their goals, including weight loss. Commercial groups, such as Weight Watchers, TOPS, or diet workshops, composed primarily of adults may be helpful to a few, but, for teenagers, a group composed of persons their own age is more acceptable. Some types of teenage groups include summer camps designed for obese youngsters and conducted by health professionals, school groups organized and led by the school nurse, and groups associated with special clinics.

The group is concerned not only with weight loss but also emphasizes the development of a positive self-image. Nutrition education and diet planning are essential elements of the group function, but equally important are discussions centered around better grooming and improvement of social skills. Improvement is measured by positive changes in all aspects of endeavor. Group support and reinforcement are basic to success.

Medical therapies. A variety of preparations have been introduced as a means for achieving weight loss, ostensibly to decrease appetite to help the individual follow a reduction diet or to use energy more effectively and to a greater degree. Most authorities agree that drugs have limited value in achieving permanent weight loss and are transient in action, useless, or actually harmful.

NURSING CARE PLAN

The Obese Child

Nursing Goals	Nursing Interventions	Expected Patient/Family Outcomes
N-MR* **Altered nutrition: more than body requirements** **Etiology: dysfunctional eating patterns, hereditary factors**		
Identify eating patterns and behaviors	Instruct child and family to: Keep a record of everything eaten, including Time eaten Amount eaten Where food was consumed Activity engaged in while eating With whom the food was eaten or if it was eaten alone Feelings at the time food was eaten, for example, angry, depressed, lonely, elated Identify food stimuli Feelings of hunger Television commercials Smell or sight of food Assess eating environments Where food is eaten With whom food is eaten, or eaten alone Feelings at time of food consumption Activity in which engaged while eating Analyze preceding data for patterns of eating and relationships of other factors as a basis for making adjustments	Child's eating patterns become apparent
Control food stimuli	Encourage child to: Separate eating from other activities Minimize food cues Get rid of "junk" food Prepare and serve only amounts to be eaten Put snacks out of sight Avoid purchase of problem foods Serve food from stove or other place out of reach of the established eating place	Child demonstrates an understanding of eating patterns and endeavors to alter destructive patterns
Change eating patterns	Encourage child to: Eat at a specific place reserved just for eating Eat orderly meals at regular hours Use smaller plates to make amounts of food appear larger Eat at slow pace Leave a small amount of food on plate Eliminate eating during television viewing Substitute raw vegetables for "junk" food snacks	Child alters eating behaviors
Use activities other than eating to deal with emotional stress, boredom, and fatigue	Encourage child to: Engage in hobby activity, take a walk, straighten up room Become involved in activities away from food	Child engages in suitable activities according to age and interest
Eat the prescribed diet	Assist the child with meal planning Employ strategies outlined above	Child conforms to prescribed diet plan Child evidences a steady weight loss (or weight maintenance in a growing child)
A-EP **Activity intolerance** **Etiology: sedentary life-style, physical bulk**		
Increase physical activity	Arrange programmed activity such as running, swimming, cycling Encourage routine activity such as walking, climbing stairs	Child engages in preferred exercise and activities regularly (specify)

*For an explanation of abbreviations, see p. 20.

NURSING CARE PLAN

The Obese Child

Nursing Goals	Nursing Interventions	Expected Patient/Family Outcomes
SP-SCP Body image or self-esteem disturbance Etiology: perceived physical appearance, internalization of negative feedback from others		
Reinforce accomplishments	Provide a system of rewards for changes in eating behavior, exercise, and weight loss Point system Tangible rewards such as a trip, a new record, a concert Have a family member serve as a monitor at home to help in progress toward goals and to encourage child with positive statements daily	Child expresses feelings and concerns regarding problems
Maximize positive aspects of appearance	Encourage good grooming, hygiene, and posture Assist with exploring positive aspects of appearance and ways to enhance these aspects	Child makes measurable efforts to improve appearance (specify)
Improve self-esteem	Relate to child as an important, worthwhile individual Encourage to set small, attainable goals for self Encourage and support positive thinking (overweight persons are negative thinkers) Encourage in activities to relieve boredom Encourage interaction with peers	Child sets realistic short-term goals for self-improvement (specify) Child voices positive attitudes toward self Child engages in appropriate activities and interaction with peers (specify)
CSTP Ineffective individual coping Etiology: little or no exercise, poor nutrition, personal vulnerability		
Involve family in child's weight-loss program	Educate family regarding weight-loss program, including nutrition, relationship of food intake and exercise, psychologic support Encourage family to: Use appropriate reinforcement Alter food and eating environment Maintain proper attitudes regarding program Assist in monitoring eating behavior, food intake, physical activity, weight change Eliminate food as a reward Encourage youngster with positive statements only	Family becomes actively involved in child's weight-loss program
Implement a school weight-loss program	Employ a buddy system Use peers as sponsors and positive reinforcers Employ frequent weigh-ins conducted by involved adult, nurse, teacher, physical education instructor Provide reinforcement for weight change Social—praise Tangible—contract that earns simple rewards Graph positive weight changes and display where others in the program can see it Provide nutrition education	Child engages in school-based program (specify)
Promote goal attainment	Encourage child to discuss his or her feelings and concerns	Child maintains a positive attitude toward the weight-loss program

Surgical techniques are available that bypass a substantial portion of the intestine or occlude a large segment of the stomach to produce a marked diet restriction and, hence, weight loss. These shunting techniques are hazardous surgical procedures with many metabolic complications. Most authorities believe that the complex metabolic effects need clarification and that certainly this procedure should be restricted to those massively obese youngsters in whom other therapies have failed and whose obesity is life-threatening in disease states that demand weight loss for effective management.

EVALUATION

The effectiveness of nursing interventions is determined by continual reassessment and evaluation of care based

on the following observational guidelines and expected outcomes:

1. Assess weight at regular intervals (usually weekly); discuss with the youngster his/her feelings, reactions, and concerns; analyze daily recordings (log) of activities (eating, behavior, exercise) and feelings.
2. Review exercise program with the youngster.
3. Review log of eating behaviors; discuss the observations with the youngster.
4. Interview the youngster about the plan of care and progress toward short-term and long-term goals.

Expected outcomes:
See Nursing Care Plan, pp. 484-485.

Clinical Manifestations of Anorexia Nervosa

Severe and profound weight loss
Signs of altered metabolic activity:
- Secondary amenorrhea (if menarche attained)
- Primary amenorrhea (if menarche not attained)
- Bradycardia
- Lowered body temperature
- Decreased blood pressure
- Cold intolerance
- Dry skin and brittle nails
- Appearance of lanugo hair

ANOREXIA NERVOSA

Anorexia nervosa (AN) is the term applied to a long-recognized disorder characterized by severe weight loss in the absence of obvious physical cause. The term "anorexia nervosa" inaccurately describes the disorder in which emaciation occurs as a result of self-inflicted starvation. AN occurs predominantly in adolescent and young adult females, and the incidence appears to be increasing significantly.

The onset of AN generally takes place at or near menarche, but it may begin in preadolescence or in adulthood. The peak ages are 12 and 13 years, with another peak occurring around ages 19 to 20 years or in the mid-20s. Young women who have this disorder are most frequently from the upper or middle socioeconomic groups, often described as "good children," academically high achievers, conforming, conscientious, and have a high energy level, even with marked emaciation. These girls are usually strongly dependent on their parents, and frequently an ambivalent mother-daughter relationship is present.

Etiology/Pathophysiology

The etiology of the disorder remains unclear. There is a distinct psychologic component, and the diagnosis is based primarily on psychologic and behavioral criteria. Nevertheless, the physical manifestations of anorexia lend support to possible organic factors in the etiology.

Dominating the psychologic aspects of anorexia nervosa are a relentless pursuit of thinness and a fear of fatness, usually preceded by a period of a year or two of mood disturbances and behavior changes. The weight loss is usually triggered by a typical adolescent crisis such as the onset of menstruation or traumatic interpersonal incidents that precipitate serious dieting that continues out of control.

Frequently there is an exaggerated misinterpretation of the normal fat deposition characteristic of the early adolescent period, or someone may comment that the adolescent girl is putting on weight. The weight loss may be a response to teasing, some change in her life (such as changing schools or going off to college), or an incident that requires an independent decision that she is unprepared to make (such as a career choice). The current emphasis on slimness is a significant factor. For example, the standard for beauty is one exemplified by the models chosen for advertising clothing. Youngsters entering the growth phase of puberty when biologic fat accumulation is normal are particularly vulnerable.

Diagnostic Evaluation

Diagnosis is made on the basis of clinical manifestations (see box) and conformity to the criteria established by the American Psychiatric Association (1987) (see box).

Therapeutic Management

The initial goal is to treat the life-threatening malnutrition with strict adherence to dietary requirements, which sometimes necessitates intravenous and tube feedings. The most successful approach uses simple operant conditioning that emphasizes positive reinforcement for

Diagnostic Criteria for Anorexia Nervosa

A. Refusal to maintain body weight over a minimal normal weight for age and height, e.g., weight loss leading to maintenance of body weight 15% below that expected; or failure to make expected weight gain during period of growth, leading to body weight 15% below that expected
B. Intense fear of gaining weight or becoming fat, even though underweight
C. Disturbance in the way in which one's body weight, size, or shape is experienced, e.g., the person claims to "feel fat" even when emaciated, believes that one area of the body is "too fat" even when obviously underweight
D. In females, absence of at least three consecutive menstrual cycles when otherwise expected to occur (primary or secondary amenorrhea). (A woman is considered to have amenorrhea if her periods occur only following hormone, e.g., estrogen, administration.)

From Diagnostic and statistical manual of mental disorders, ed. 3-revised (DSM-III-R), Washington, DC, 1987, American Psychiatric Association.

weight gain. A clearly defined behavior modification plan is communicated to the child and maintained through a unified team approach by all persons involved in her care. Children whose disorder can be clearly related to a dysfunctional family situation respond to therapy best when separated from the family. Many of those whose therapy plan is implemented in the hospital need a continued behavior modification program after discharge in order to maintain the desired weight.

Family therapy seems to be effective when begun soon after the onset of illness, but it is less successful when the condition has existed for some time. Therapy is directed toward disengagement and redirection of malfunctioning processes in the family. Individual psychotherapy is aimed at helping the child resolve the adolescent identity crisis, particularly as it relates to a distorted body image.

Nursing Considerations

The management of anorexia nervosa is directed toward correction of the severe state of malnutrition and resolution of the psychologic disorganization. Because of the psychogenic nature of the disorder, treatment is difficult and requires long-term management. All of those involved in therapy must keep in mind the adolescent's distorted sense of body image and self-awareness and her feelings of self-doubt, ineffectiveness, and helplessness that prompt such bizarre behavior in order to feel in control of her own body functions.

Nurses need to adopt and maintain a kind, supporting, yet firm manner in managing the care of an anorectic child. The child requires the sustained support and reassurance as she copes with ambivalent feelings related to her own body concept and the desire to see herself as cooperative, reliable, and worthy of the kindness she receives. Encouraging the child with education and activities that strengthen her self-esteem facilitates her resocialization process and social acceptance among her peers.

One approach that has met with varied degrees of success is behavior modification. This requires team involvement with the following essential aspects:

1. The health team determines an approach and adheres to it consistently.
2. All team members are involved.
3. There is continuity of caregivers (team members).
4. There is clear communication among team members and with the patient so that she understands precisely what is expected.
5. The patient is supported in her efforts, e.g., positive feedback for accomplishments.

It is important for nurses to be aware of some of the physical side effects of AN. Patients with anorexia nervosa often limit their fluid intake, leading to urinary tract problems, and ketones and protein may be detected in the urine as a result of breakdown of fat and protein. Vital sign instability can be severe (including orthostatic hypotension). The pulse becomes irregular and the rate decreases markedly. The bradycardia and hypothermia can result in cardiac arrest.

Health professionals, patients, and families can find assistance and information from any of the following organizations: The **National Anorectic Aid Society, Inc.,*** the **National Association of Anorexia Nervosa and Associated Disorders, Inc.,**† and the **American Anorexia/Bulimia Association, Inc.**‡

BULIMIA

Bulimia is the term applied to an eating disorder that is characterized by binge eating. The binge behavior consists of secretive, frenzied consumption of large amounts of high-calorie (or "forbidden") foods during a brief period of time (usually less than 2 hours). The binge is counteracted by a variety of weight-control methods (purging), including self-induced vomiting, diuretic and laxative abuse, and rigorous exercise. These binge/purge cycles are followed by self-deprecating thoughts, depressed mood, and an awareness that the eating pattern is abnormal.

The disorder is observed more frequently in older adolescent girls and young women. Characteristically bulimic persons are those who have been unsuccessful dieters, have low impulse control, and may have been self-conscious about being overweight in childhood. They fall into two categories: (1) those who consume vast quantities of food followed by purging but who, if unable to purge, still consume large amounts, and (2) those who restrict their caloric intake, especially when unable to purge. Some bulimic women are of normal or (more often) slightly above normal weight; others become as underweight as anorectic individuals—*bulimarexia.*

Diagnostic Evaluation

The diagnosis may be first suspected from the presence of complications, including fluid and electrolyte disturbances from gastrointestinal losses, abdominal complaints from laxative abuse, erosion of tooth enamel and increased dental caries from vomited gastric acid, and throat complaints. The diagnosis is established on the basis of criteria established by the American Psychiatric Association (1987) (see box).

Therapeutic Management

Therapy is similar to management of anorexia nervosa. Hospitalization may be required, especially for complications such as potassium depletion and esophageal damage. Intravenous fluids and potassium replacement are essential elements of care, and cardiac monitoring is indicated.

*550 S. Cleveland Ave., Suite F, Westerville, OH 43081.
†Box 7, Highland Park, IL 60035.
‡133 Cedar Lane, Teaneck, NJ 07666.

Diagnostic Criteria for Bulimia

A. Recurrent episodes of binge eating (rapid consumption of a large amount of food in a discrete period of time)
B. A feeling of lack of control over eating behavior during the eating binges
C. The person regularly engages in either self-induced vomiting, use of laxatives or diuretics, strict dieting or fasting, or vigorous exercise in order to prevent weight gain
D. A minimum average of two binge eating episodes a week for at least 3 months
E. Persistent overconcern with body shape and weight

From Diagnostic and statistical manual of mental disorders, ed. 3-revised (DSM-III-R), Washington, DC, 1987, American Psychiatric Association.

Nursing Considerations

Nursing care is similar to care of the patient with anorexia nervosa. Acute care also involves careful monitoring of fluid and electrolyte alterations and observation for signs of cardiac complications.

◆ *Behavior Disorders in School-Age Children*

A number of classification systems have been employed to outline the various problems of middle childhood that interfere with development, learning, and social relationships. Although there is no universal categorization, most authorities seem to broadly classify behavioral disorders in some manner that identifies mental subnormality, learning disabilities, neuroses, psychoses, and antisocial behavior. Some are seen almost exclusively in children of school age, others are primarily problems of adolescence, but many extend throughout the course of childhood. Many disorders have a major organic or developmental component. Very often a change in behavior is one of the manifestations of an organic disease; at other times emotional problems produce somatic symptoms of greater or lesser seriousness.

ATTENTION DEFICIT DISORDER

Attention deficit disorder (ADD) is the term applied to various behavior problems that in some way impair the child's capacity to profit from new experiences. ADD is further delineated into two subtypes: (1) *ADD with hyperactivity* and (2) *ADD without hyperactivity*. The term *specific learning disabilities* refers to the behavioral outcomes of impaired functioning in central processing, such as dyslexia, dysphasia, and inability to calculate or draw. It is primarily an educational concern and mentioned briefly at the conclusion of this segment.

Early identification of affected children is needed since the characteristics of the disorder significantly interfere with the normal course of emotional and psychologic development. Many of these children, in the attempt to cope with cerebral dysfunction, develop maladaptive behavior patterns that are a deterrent to psychosocial adjustment. Their behavior evokes negative responses from others, and repeated exposure to negative feedback adversely affects the child's self-concept.

Diagnostic Criteria for Attention Deficit/Hyperactivity Disorder

Note: Consider a criterion met only if the behavior is considerably more frequent than that of most people of the same mental age.

A. A disturbance of a least 6 months during which at least eight of the following are present:
(1) Often fidgets with hands or feet or squirms in seat (in adolescents, may be limited to subjective feelings of restlessness)
(2) Has difficulty remaining seated when required to do so
(3) Is easily distracted by extraneous stimuli
(4) Has difficulty awaiting turn in games or group situations
(5) Often blurts out answers to questions before they have been completed
(6) Has difficulty following through on instructions from others (not due to oppositional behavior or failure of comprehension), e.g., fails to finish chores
(7) Has difficulty sustaining attention in tasks or play activities
(8) Often shifts from one uncompleted activity to another
(9) Has difficulty playing quietly
(10) Often talks excessively
(11) Often interrupts or intrudes on others, e.g., butts into other children's games
(12) Often does not seem to listen to what is being said to him or her
(13) Often loses things necessary for tasks or activities at school or at home (e.g., toys, pencils, books, assignments)
(14) Often engages in physically dangerous activities without considering possible consequences (not for the purpose of thrill-seeking), e.g., runs into street without looking

Note: The above items are listed in descending order of discriminating power based on data from a national field trial of the DSM-III-R criteria for Disruptive Behavior Disorders.

B. Onset before the age of seven.
C. Does not meet the criteria for a Pervasive Developmental Disorder.

Criteria for severity of attention deficit/hyperactivity disorder:
Mild: Few, if any symptoms in excess of those required to make the diagnosis and only minimal or no impairment in school and social functioning.
Moderate: Symptoms or functional impairment intermediate between "mild" and "severe."
Severe: Many symptoms in excess of those required to make the diagnosis and significant and pervasive impairment in functioning at home and school and with peers.

From Diagnostic and statistical manual of mental disorders, ed. 3-revised (DSM-III-R), Washington, DC, 1987, American Psychiatric Association.

Diagnostic Evaluation

The behaviors exhibited by the child with ADD are not unusual aspects of child behavior. The difference lies in the quality of motor activity and developmentally inappropriate inattention, impulsivity, and hyperactivity the child displays. The manifestations may be numerous or few, mild or severe, and will vary with the developmental level of the child. Any given child will not have every manifestation that is characteristic of a syndrome, and the degree of severity is highly variable. The diagnostic criteria established by the American Psychiatric Association (1987) for identifying the child with ADD are outlined in the box.

Therapeutic Management

Management of the child with ADD usually involves a multiple approach that includes family education and counseling, medication, remedial education, environmental manipulation, and sometimes psychotherapy for the child. Diet modification has proved effective for some children but is not considered a standard therapy.

Medication. Extensive experience with central nervous stimulants has demonstrated them to be highly effective in reducing many of the symptoms in children with ADD. The most frequently prescribed medications are dextroamphetamine (Dexedrine) or methylphenidate (Ritalin). However, not all children benefit from medications. Those who do may respond to only one medication or to a combination of two medications, and the effective dosage varies from child to child.

Environmental manipulation. The child's environment is simplified by decreasing external stimuli, reducing alternatives, encouraging desired patterns of behavior, and, sometimes, controlling his diet. The child needs an environment in which distractions and external stimuli are reduced to a minimum. Also, the more the environment is controlled, the less medication is required.

Remedial education. Special training activities in the schools are designed to offer a direct attack on such areas of deficit as visual perception, auditory perception, and other areas involving integration and coordination. The purpose of programs for children with special learning disabilities is to assist them toward more successful achievement, personal adjustment, and eventual retention in the regular classroom.

Nursing Considerations

Nurses are active participants in all aspects of management of the child with ADD. Nurses in the community setting work with families in the home on a long-term basis to help plan and implement therapeutic regimens and to evaluate the effectiveness of therapy.

ENURESIS

Enuresis is a common and troublesome disorder that is difficult to define because of the variable ages at which children achieve bladder control. In a broad sense enuresis can be defined as repeated involuntary urination (usually nocturnal) in children who are beyond the age when voluntary bladder control should normally have been acquired. Some authorities place 4 years as an arbitrary age by which diurnal and nocturnal bladder control is normally accomplished, although 5 years of age is probably more accurate. The incidence is approximately 5% to 17% in otherwise normal children between 3 and 15 years of age. Enuresis is more common in boys than in girls.

Organic causes that may be related to enuresis should be ruled out before psychogenic factors are considered. These include structural disorders of the urinary tract, urinary tract infection, major neurologic deficits, nocturnal epilepsy, disorders such as diabetes mellitus and diabetes insipidus that increase the normal output of urine, and disorders such as chronic renal failure or sickle cell disease that impair the concentrating ability of the kidneys. In other cases the enuresis is influenced by emotional factors, although it is doubtful that they are causative factors.

In most enuretic children nocturnal bed-wetting is a primary maturational problem and usually ceases between 6 and 8 years of age, although it sometimes continues into adolescence. The predominant symptom is urgency that is immediate and accompanied by acute discomfort, restlessness, and sometimes urinary frequency. Nocturnal enuresis is most common and is occasionally accompanied by diurnal wetting; diurnal wetting without nocturnal bed-wetting is unusual.

Various therapeutic techniques are employed in the management of enuresis. These include anticholinergic drugs, bladder training, restriction or elimination of fluids after the evening meal, interruption of sleep to void, and some type of electrical device designed to establish a conditioned reflex response to waken the child at the initiation of micturition.

Nursing Considerations

No matter what techniques are employed, the nurse can help both child and parents to understand the problem of enuresis, the treatment plan, and the probable difficulties they may encounter in the process. More important, the nurse can provide consistent support and encouragement to help sustain them through the inconsistent and unpredictable treatment process. The child needs to believe that he is helping himself and to sustain feelings of confidence and hope.

ENCOPRESIS

Encopresis is the repeated voluntary or involuntary passage of feces of normal or near-normal consistency into places not appropriate for that purpose according to the individual's own sociocultural setting; it is not the result of any physical disorder. The disorder is less common than enuresis, but the two may coexist. It is seldom an isolated symptom and is commonly clustered with other somatic symptoms—social withdrawal, antisocial-aggressive behaviors, affective-dependent behaviors, and somatic manifestations.

Primary encopresis is identified by age 4 when the

child has not achieved fecal continence for at least a year. Secondary encopresis is fecal incontinence occurring between ages 4 and 8 that has been preceded by a period of fecal continence. Predisposing factors seem to be inadequate, inconsistent toilet training and psychosocial stress, such as entering school or the birth of a sibling. The disorder is more common in males than in females. When incontinence is involuntary, it frequently occurs secondary to constipation, impaction, or retention of feces with subsequent overflow. It is not unusual for soiling to take place after bathing because of reflex stimulation.

School performance and attendance is affected as the child's offensive odor becomes a target for scorn and derision from classmates. This causes further withdrawal and other behavioral manifestations. Therapeutic management consists of determining the cause of the soiling and application of appropriate interventions to correct the problem. It may involve dietary changes, relief of a fecal impaction, and/or behavioral therapy. Frequently psychotherapeutic intervention with the child and the family becomes necessary.

Nursing Considerations

The nursing care of the child with encopresis involves primarily education and support of the family. Families are taught the physiology of normal defecation, toilet training as a developmental process, and the treatment outlined for the particular family. Family counseling is directed toward reassurance that most problems resolve successfully. Parents are relieved to know that other parents share this problem and are surprised to learn that functional changes that take place as the condition develops make control of seepage impossible.

SCHOOL PHOBIA

School phobia is a term used to describe children, other than beginning students, who resist going to school because of dread of the school situation, concerns with leaving home, or both. Anxiety—especially anxiety over separation from the mother—that frequently verges on panic is a constant manifestation. Some children are afraid the mother will not be home when they get there. Simple reassurance is often sufficient for these children.

Physical symptoms are prominent and may affect any part of the body—anorexia, nausea, vomiting, diarrhea, dizziness, headache, leg pains, or abdominal pains, to name a few. There may even be a low-grade fever. A striking feature of school phobia is the prompt subsiding of symptoms when it is evident that the child can remain at home. Another significant observation is absence of symptoms on weekends and holidays unless they are related to other places such as Sunday school or parties. Occasional mild reluctance is not uncommon among schoolchildren, but if the fear continues for longer than a few days it must be considered as a serious problem—a warning of an important personality problem.

Nursing Considerations

The primary goal for the child with school phobia is to keep the child in school. The longer a child is permitted to stay out of school, the more difficult it is to reenter. Parents must be convinced gently but firmly that *immediate* return is essential and that it is their responsibility to insist upon school attendance.

The child with severe symptoms may require modified school attendance, such as part-time class attendance and spending time in the counselor's office or nurse's office, then getting homework from the teacher after class. It may be necessary for a parent to attend class with the child. If the problem persists, professional help is recommended.

RECURRENT ABDOMINAL PAIN

Recurrent abdominal pain is one of the somatic complaints of childhood that is almost always attributed to a psychogenic etiology, although it can be a symptom of either psychosomatic or organic disease.

The characteristic feature of the disorder is abdominal pain that the child usually locates in the periumbilical area. However, on palpation the pain is more likely to be experienced in the epigastric area or in the lower right or left quadrant and is accompanied by vague tenderness without muscle guarding. The pain is irregular in time, duration, and intensity and is associated with either loose or pellet-formed stools. Other symptoms that may accompany the abdominal pain are headache, pallor, dizziness, and dysuria.

Support for the psychologic aspects of this disorder is based on observations of aggravation of symptoms during times of tension or stress. Children with recurrent abdominal pain tend to be highly sensitive, have a poor self-image, and are uncomfortable with expressions of anger or argument, especially in those persons who are significant in their life. School attendance is adversely affected, and these children generally exhibit poor learning performance. It is not uncommon for symptoms to be aggravated during school days.

Treatment is difficult. Hospitalization may be necessary, and the child frequently shows improvement in the hospital environment. Initial efforts are directed toward ruling out organic causes of the pain, relieving discomfort, and attempting to determine the situations that precipitate attacks. When simple measures are ineffective, an antispasmodic drug such as propantheline bromide may be prescribed to relieve the muscle spasm.

Nursing Considerations

Once the diagnosis has been established, the parents and the child need an explanation of the pain, which can be compared to a skeletal muscle cramp or "charley horse" for easier comprehension. Reassurance that the symptoms are not unique to their child and that the pain can be expected to subside is helpful in relieving parental fears and anxieties. When parents are reassured that there is no organic cause of the pain, they will need some guidance regarding what they can do during a pain episode. All too often they feel helpless and anxious, which tends to compound the child's distress.

The simple expedient of putting the child at rest by having him lie down in a peaceful, quiet environment and providing comfort will often relieve the symptoms in a short time. A heating pad may also help ease the discomfort. If pain is not relieved by these simple measures, the parents are taught how to administer antispasmodics, if prescribed. For example, if pain is precipitated by meals, having the child take the medication 20 to 30 minutes before mealtime may prevent an episode.

The most valuable measures that the nurse can provide are support and reassurance to the family. When open communication is established and families are able to see a relationship between stress-provoking situations and the child's symptoms, the chance for remedial action is enhanced. Follow-up care and continued support are essential, because the symptoms tend to remit and exacerbate; therefore, the availability of a supportive health professional can be a source of comfort to the child and family.

CONVERSION REACTION

Conversion reaction, also known as hysteria, hysterical conversion reaction, and childhood hysteria, is a psychophysiologic disorder with a sudden onset that can usually be traced to a precipitating environmental event. The manifestations involve primarily the voluntary musculature and special senses and include abdominal pain, fainting, pseudoseizures, paralysis, headaches, and visual field restriction. The most commonly observed symptom is seizure activity, which can be differentiated from those of neurogenic origin by formal tests, the most useful of which is the finding of a normal electroencephalogram.

It has been observed that nearly all children with conversion reaction have experienced a major family crisis before the onset of symptoms, such as loss of a parent or other significant person through death, divorce, or moving.

Nursing Considerations

Nursing care is similar to that for the child with recurrent abdominal pain.

CHILDHOOD DEPRESSION

Depression in childhood is often difficult to detect. Children may be unable to express their feelings and tend to act out their problems and concerns. Some states of depression are of a temporary nature, for example, acute depression precipitated by a traumatic event. This might include a period of hospitalization, loss of a parent through death or separation, or loss of a significant relationship with something (a pet), someone (a friend or family member), or a place (move from a familiar home, neighborhood, or city). The easily identified manifestations are outlined in the accompanying box. The child tends to spend more time in solitary activities, especially television viewing, and schoolwork is impaired. Some children become more dependent and clinging; others become more aggressive and disruptive. The manifestations may last a few days or weeks, usually resolving spontaneously.

More serious and less common are depressive responses to more chronic stress and loss; these are frequently observed in children with chronic illness or disability. There is no apparent precipitating event, but there is often a history of frequent disruptions in important relationships. Manifestations are as varied as those observed in acute depression but occur more frequently and extend over a longer period of time.

Primary and Associated Symptoms of Depression in Children

Primary symptoms
- Depressed affect (dysphoric mood)
- Anhedonia (loss of pleasure)
- Self-deprecatory ideation
- Tearfulness
- Low sense of self-worth/self-esteem
- Social withdrawal
- Impairment of schoolwork
- Psychomotor retardation
- Difficulty with biologic functions (sleeping, eating)
- Morbid ideation/suicide attempts

Associated symptoms
- Irritability
- Moodiness
- Social interactive difficulties
- Pathologic guilt
- Fatigue
- Somatic complaints
- Anxiety, decreased concentration
- Obsessive rumination and thoughts
- Attention deficit
- Feelings of helplessness/hopelessness
- Enuresis/encopresis
- Aggressive and explosive behaviors

From Aylward, G.P.: Understanding and treatment of childhood depression, J. Pediatr. **107**:1-9, 1985.

Nursing Considerations

The management of childhood depression is usually psychotheraputic and highly individualized. Nurses should be aware that depression is a problem that can easily be overlooked in the school-age child and one that can interrupt normal growth and development. Recognizing depression and making appropriate referrals is an important nursing function. Identification of the depressed child requires a careful history (health, growth and development, social, and family health), interviews with the child, and observations by the nurse, parents, and teachers. See also Suicide, p. 494.

CHILDHOOD SCHIZOPHRENIA

Childhood schizophrenia is a term used to describe severe deviations in ego functioning and is generally reserved for psychotic disorders that appear after the first 4 or 5 years of life. Schizophrenia in adults occurs with relative frequency, and, although childhood psychosis is not as common, it is by no means rare.

Childhood schizophrenia is characterized by a gradual onset of neurotic symptoms that show wide variation according to each affected child's developmental level, the age of onset, the nature of early childhood experiences, and the type of defense mechanisms used. However, the basic core disturbance is a lack of contact with reality and the subsequent development of a world of the child's own. Secondary characteristics represent impairment in a wide number of areas of development including cognition, perception, emotion, language, and physical motor control. The most common manifestations involve language disturbances, impaired interpersonal relationships, and inappropriate affect (outward expression of emotion).

Nursing Considerations

Nursing of psychotic children is a highly specialized area, but since these problems are being recognized with increasing frequency, nurses should be alert to the possibility. A child who consistently demonstrates abnormal behavior should be referred for evaluation.

◆ *Serious Health Problems of Later Childhood and Adolescence*

The transition to adulthood with its prescribed developmental tasks produces a sense of diffuse discomfort within some adolescents, who respond with faulty problem solving in their search for relief from the discomfort and stress of this transitional period of life. Some of the more serious health problems may arise during this time of developmental stress, although there is an increased incidence of suicide and substance abuse among school-age children.

SUBSTANCE ABUSE

The use of drugs and other substances by children and adolescents to produce an altered state of consciousness is widespread and is believed to reflect the variety of changes taking place in their lives and the stresses engendered by these changes. Drug abuse is the regular use of drugs for other than the accepted medical purposes and to the extent that it results in physical or psychologic harm to the user and/or is used in a way that is detrimental to society.

Most drugs to which young people turn induce changes in perception, a feeling of well-being, and a sense of closeness. To most, they provide a feeling of happiness. With the exception of some stimulant drugs used for practical purposes, such as working better, studying, or increasing cognitive effectiveness, the drugs used are simply pleasure-promoting chemicals used in the hope for altered consciousness or the attainment of a different level of functioning. In the majority of cases drug use begins with experimentation. The individual may try a drug only once, it may be used occasionally, or it may become an integral part of a drug-centered life-style.

Motivation

There are several common motives for drug use. Children and adolescents try drugs out of curiosity, for kicks. Drugs produce for some persons a dreamy state of altered consciousness and a feeling of power, excitement, heightened acuity, or confidence. Others seek visual hallucinatory experiences and sexual sensation. Many youngsters use drugs not only for the perceptual and sensory experiences but also for the social aspects. They use drugs because others use them, and because they want to "turn on" or "tune in" to the drug culture. Teenagers are highly influenced by fads and fashions within their society, and they are, developmentally, sensation-hungry risk takers. It is characteristic that they are eager to test their mental and physical capabilities to the utmost.

Types of Drugs Abused

Any drug can be abused, and most are potentially harmful to youngsters still going through formative life experiences. Although rarely conceived of as drugs by society, the chemically active substances most frequently abused are the xanthines and theobromines contained in chocolate and in common beverages such as tea, coffee, and colas. Common analgesics such as aspirin, propoxyphene hydrochloride (Darvon compound), and butalbital (Fiorinal); ethyl alcohol; and nicotine are others that, although recognized as drugs, are sanctioned by society. Any of these can produce mild to moderate euphoric and/or stimulant effects and can lead to physical and psychic dependence.

Drugs with mind-altering capacity that are available on the black market and that are of medical and legal concern are the hallucinogenic, narcotic, hypnotic, and stimulant drugs. In addition, those of concern to the health professionals are alcohol and various volatile substances, such as antifreeze, plastic model airplane cement, typewriter correction fluid, and organic solvents, which are inhaled to achieve altered sensation in the user. Drugs available on the street are often mixed with other compounds and fillers so that the purity of the drug, its strength, and the nature of additives are highly variable.

Alcohol. Acute or chronic abuse of ethanol, a socially accepted depressant, is responsible for many acts of violence, suicide, and accidental injury and death. It is the most widely accepted drug, can be purchased legally by adults, is relatively inexpensive, is often used as a part of a meal (wine and beer), and is approved by adults throughout the world when used in moderation. Youngsters may be afraid of hard drugs but feel comfortable with alcohol.

The most noticeable effects of alcohol are on the central nervous system—incoordination, emotional lability, and impaired judgment, memory, and perception. Youthful alcoholics enjoy the effect of the alcohol and look forward to becoming intoxicated. They drink rapidly to obtain a "high" emotional state, often drink alone, cannot predictably control their use of alcohol, and protect their supply, afraid that they will be caught without anything to drink. Not all of these characteristics are observed in the alcoholic but if several of the signs are evident, the youngsters should be considered at risk and detoxification therapy initiated to assure safe and complete withdrawal from the drug.

Cocaine. The use of cocaine by adolescents is increasing more rapidly than any other form of substance abuse. Cocaine is available in two forms: water-soluble cocaine hydrochloride administered by insufflation or "snorting" and a nonsoluble alkaloid (freebase) used primarily for smoking. "Crack" or "rock" is a new, purer, and more menacing form of the drug; it can be produced cheaply and smoked in either water pipes or mentholated cigarettes. The increased use of cocaine is related to its availability and affordability, the false perception of safety in its use, association with persons in glamorous occupations, snob appeal, a reputation as a sexually enhancing drug, and peer pressure (Tarr and Macklin, 1987).

The drug creates a sense of euphoria, or an indefinable high. Withdrawal does not produce the dramatic symptoms observed in withdrawal from other substances. The effects are those more commonly seen in depression, including lack of energy and motivation, irritability, appetite changes, psychomotor retardation, and irregular sleep patterns. More serious symptoms include cardiovascular manifestations and seizures. Withdrawal is not to be confused with the so-called crash after a cocaine high, which consists of a long period of sleep. Answers to questions about health risks of cocaine can be obtained by calling the **National Cocaine Hotline.*** It also provides referrals to support groups and treatment centers.

Narcotics. Narcotic drugs include opiates such as heroin, morphine, meperidine hydrochloride (Demerol), and codeine. They produce a state of euphoria by removing painful feelings and creating a pleasurable experience of specific quality and a sense of success accompanied by clouding of consciousness and a dreamlike state. Physical signs of narcotic abuse include constricted pupils, respiratory depression, and, often, cyanosis. Needle marks may be visible on arms or legs in chronic users. Withdrawal from opiates is extremely unpleasant unless controlled with supervised substitution of methadone.

Central nervous system depressants. A variety of hypnotic drugs that produce physical dependence and withdrawal symptoms on abrupt discontinuation may be used by adolescents. They create a feeling of relaxation and sleepiness but impair general functioning. Drugs in this category include both barbiturates and nonbarbiturates (such as methaqualone [Quaalude]) as well as alcohol. Barbiturates combined with alcohol produce a profound depressant effect.

Central nervous system stimulants. Amphetamines and cocaine do not produce strong physical dependence and can be withdrawn without much danger. However, psychologic dependence is strong, and acute intoxication can lead to violent aggressive behavior or psychotic episodes manifest by paranoia, uncontrollable agitation, and restlessness. When combined with barbiturates, the euphoric effects are particularly addictive.

Mind-altering drugs. Hallucinogens (psychedelic, psychotomimetic, psychotropic, or illusionogenic) are drugs that produce vivid hallucinations and euphoria. These drugs do not produce physical dependence, since they can be abruptly withdrawn without ill effect. However, acute and long-term effects are variable, and in some individuals the dissociative behavior may be unduly protracted. This category includes cannabis (marijuana, hashish) and lysergic acid diethylamide (LSD).

Hydrocarbons and fluorocarbons. Glue "sniffing," the inhalation of plastic cement, and inhalation of other volatile substances that youngsters breathe and rebreathe in paper or plastic bags produce euphoria and altered consciousness. They are extremely hazardous to the individual, causing rapid loss of consciousness and respiratory arrest. Many persons taking these drugs do not have time to remove the bag from their heads and quickly become asphyxiated.

Nursing Considerations Related to Therapeutic Management

Nurses in almost every setting are increasingly likely to have contact with youthful drug abusers or to be in a position to serve as educator and patient advocate. The nurse most often encounters youthful drug abusers when they are (1) experiencing overdose symptoms, (2) experiencing withdrawal symptoms, (3) manifesting bizarre behavior or confusion secondary to drug ingestion, or (4) worried that they are becoming or will become addicted.

Drug use may be encountered in relation to other health problems; therefore, nurses caring for adolescents who are in the hospital or under treatment for other illnesses need to know if the youngsters use drugs compulsively, since withdrawal phenomena can seriously complicate the illness. Nurses should be able to recognize physical or behavioral clues that indicate the onset of withdrawal or the effects of drugs that might have been

*800-COCAINE.

brought to the youngster secretly by well-meaning relatives or friends.

Acute care. Adolescents experiencing toxic drug effects or withdrawal symptoms are frequently seen as emergencies. Experienced emergency room personnel are familiar with the management of acute drug toxicosis; the signs, symptoms, and behavioral characteristics of a variety of substances; and differences and similarities among them. When the drug is questionable or unknown, knowledge of these factors facilitates handling of the youngster and implementation of a treatment regimen. Often observation of or description of the behavior is of more value than a report by patients or their friends as to the chemical agent taken.

The treatment for drug toxicity or withdrawal varies according to the drug and the method used. Every effort should be made to determine the type and amount of drug taken, the time it was taken, the mode of administration, and factors related to the onset of presenting symptoms. It is helpful to know that patient's pattern of use. For example, if two types of drugs are involved, they may require different treatments. Gastric lavage may be employed when the drug has been ingested recently and the cough reflex is intact, but it would be of little value when the drug has been administered by the intravenous ("mainlined") or intranasal ("sniffed") route. Since the actual content of most street drugs is highly questionable, other pharmaceutical agents are administered with caution, except perhaps the narcotic antagonists in cases of suspected opiate overdose. It is necessary to assess for possible trauma that might have been sustained while under the influence of the drug.

Long-term management. A major factor in the treatment and rehabilitation of the young drug user is careful assessment, in the nonacute stage, to determine the function that the drug plays in the youngster's life. The adolescent needs help to identify the problem that motivated him to resort to drugs and to recognize his own role in self-destructive, inappropriate drug-abuse behavior before he can embark on a rehabilitation program.

Rehabilitation begins when a youngster has decided that, with the help of concerned and supportive adults, he can and is willing to change. Rehabilitation implies not only environmental manipulation and involvement therapy but also commitment on the part of the patient to substitute dependency on people for his dependency on drugs and to explore alternative mechanisms for problem solving and coping with stress. Persons working with troubled youth must be prepared for recidivism, or the tendency to relapse, and maintain a plan for reentry into the treatment process.

Family support. Organizations that have achieved success in helping others cope with problems of drug abuse are excellent sources for both youngsters and their families. The **Tough Love*** philosophy first employed by Alcoholics Anonymous and Al-Anon is based on the conviction that parents have the right and responsibility to be the policymakers in the family, set limits on the behavior of their children, and take control of the household from out-of-control youngsters. The premise is that allowing teenagers to experience the negative consequences of their behavior will bring them closer to accepting help and/or changing their behavior (Newton, 1985).

*Community Service Foundation, P.O. Box 70, Sellersville, PA 18960.

Other groups that provide support and counseling for families experiencing crises with their children include **Parents Anonymous*** and **Parental Stress, Inc.,†** both of which maintain crisis counseling on a 24-hour basis.

Prevention. Drug abuse in adolescence is both an individual and a community problem, and nurses play an important role in education and legislation, as well as in individual observation, assessment, and therapy. In this drug-oriented society, patterns of drug use may be established through parental models and the influence of the media as an effective means to make the user "feel better." Impressionable youth need to be educated regarding appropriate use of chemicals. More important, those associated with adolescents should listen to what they are saying, determine what is bothering them, and try to help them meet these needs through alternative methods before they resort to drugs.

Peer pressure is a powerful tool and can be used effectively in prevention. A group that has had some success in reducing injury from drunk driving is **Students Against Driving Drunk (SADD),‡** an organization designed to help eliminate drunk driving in teenagers. Some of the techniques used by the group include peer counseling, parental guidelines for teenage parties, and community awareness. Nurses can encourage the formation of chapters of SADD in the high schools in their communities.

SUICIDE

Suicide is defined as the deliberate act of self-injury with the intent that the injury should kill. It is the second leading cause of death during the teenage years, surpassed only by death from injury (see pp. 4-5). A striking feature is the rise among persons in the younger age-groups. During the years 1950 to 1981 the suicide rate tripled in people between the ages of 15 and 24 (Raley, 1985).

Most authorities distinguish between a suicidal gesture and an attempt, and both must be acknowledged. A *gesture* is made without any real attempt to cause either serious injury or death but rather to send out a signal that

*22330 Hawthorne Blvd., #208, Torrance, CA 90505, 800-352-0386 (California) and 800-421-0353 (elsewhere).

†617-742-7535 (Massachusetts) and 800-632-8188 (elsewhere). Other sources of information include: **National Clearinghouse for Alcohol Information,** P.O. Box 416, Kensington, MD 20795; **National Federation of Parents for Drug-Free Youth,** 800-554-KIDS or 301-585-5437 (Maryland); **National Institute on Drug Abuse Prevention Branch,** 800-638-2045 or 301-443-2450 (Maryland).

‡110 Pleasant St., Corbin Plaza, Marborum, MA 01752.

something is wrong. An *attempt*, unlike a gesture, is intended to cause injury or death. Teenagers sometimes make a number of gestures to draw attention to the fact that they are unable to cope. If the signals are not detected and responded to promptly, they may escalate in seriousness until they become serious attempts or completed acts.

Etiology

Adolescence has always been characterized by turmoil, heightened emotionality, and wide variations in mood. With limited capacities for problem solving and with fewer and less sophisticated resources for resolving difficulties, some teenagers have difficulty coping well with critical events, especially a situation that is forced upon them, such as death of a friend, parent, or sibling. Most adolescents are able to function quite well, but when health professionals see those who do not, further investigation is indicated.

Suicidal youngsters almost invariably come from a disturbed family situation, such as economic stresses, family disintegration, medical problems, or psychiatric illness. Broken homes, divorce, separation, abandonment, alcoholism, and death are highly significant factors and are frequently noted in the histories of suicidal youth. History of suicide by another family member is a common finding.

Suicidal Methods

The outcome of suicide behavior is influenced to some extent by the method used. Violent methods of destruction used by adults, such as jumping from heights or in front of trains, are less frequently employed by younger persons. Overdose of drugs is the method of choice for most adolescents who attempt suicide, and these are usually medications prescribed for parents (such as barbiturates and antidepressants), those intended for household use (aspirin), or solvents. Ingestion of medications and wrist lacerations are the favored methods of females; males tend to use more lethal methods such as knives, guns, and automobiles. Younger children (under 13½) are more likely to resort to hanging (Garfinkel and others, 1982).

Motivation

Most suicidal gestures are impulsive acts committed to force parents or other significant persons in youngsters' lives to pay attention to the need for help. The attempt usually is the culmination of a behavioral pattern. These youngsters often have a history of attention-getting behaviors that range from minor acts to increasingly dramatic ones. With the ultimate act of attempted suicide, the child finally makes himself heard. He seldom actually plans a suicidal act because he really wants to die; successful suicides are committed either impulsively or accidentally.

Occasionally there are adolescents who are so severely depressed that suicide appears to them to be the only means of release from their despair. These youngsters rarely give evidence of their intent, concealing their suicidal thoughts for fear of outside intervention. Sometimes this self-destructive behavior on the part of adolescents is a desire to punish themselves for guilt-filled actions, such as masturbation or, more often, thoughts. Peer pressure, too, has convinced many young persons that there is something wrong with them if they feel lonely or depressed; therefore, they direct these feelings inward to avoid the risk of rejection. Social isolation is seen in many suicidal adolescents, but it appears to be the most significant factor in distinguishing those who will kill themselves from those who will not. It is more characteristic

Clinical Manifestations of Suicidal Youth

Mood/Affect

- Marked persistent depression
- Feelings of hopelessness, helplessness, isolation
- Deteriorating schoolwork
- Remains distant, sad, remote
- Flat affect—has "frozen" facial expression
- Persistently looks or sounds sad and unhappy
- Describes self as worthless
- Feelings of self-hatred or excessive guilt
- Feelings of humiliation, often brought on by inadequate performance at school
- Sudden cheerfulness following deep depression
- Wish to be punished

Behavior

- Changes in physical appearance—a child previously neat and well-groomed will stop bathing and begin to look slovenly
- Loss of function due to illness or trauma
- Loss of energy—loss of interest, listlessness, exhaustion without obvious cause
- Sleep disturbances—difficulty going to sleep or sleeping excessively, takes voluntary naps during afternoon or evening
- Increased irritability, argumentativeness, or stubbornness
- Physical complaints—recurrent stomachaches, headaches
- Repeated visits to doctor's office or emergency room for treatment of injuries
- Antisocial behavior—engages in drinking, uses drugs, fights, commits acts of vandalism, runs away from home, becomes sexually promiscuous
- *Preoccupation with death—focuses on morbid thoughts; speaks repeatedly about people getting killed
- May begin referring to own death

School and Interpersonal Relationships

- Resists or refuses to go to school
- May become truant, cuts classes, does not complete assignments
- Social withdrawal from friends, activities, interests that were previously enjoyed
- *Wants to give away cherished possessions
- Lacks an effective social support system

Coping Skills

- Loses reality boundaries
- Withdraws and isolates self
- No use of support systems
- Sees self as totally helpless, a victim of fate

*Absolute red flags.

of those who complete suicide than of those who make attempts or threats.

A cluster phenomenon, known as "contagion," has also been observed. Sometimes referred to as a teenage "epidemic," this situation occurs when one suicide appears to trigger several other suicides in a group such as a school or community. Suicide of a public figure sometimes prompts a number of suicides.

Diagnostic Evaluation

Depression is a symptom common to all human beings. It is characterized by both subjective symptoms and objective signs that reflect the adolescent's grief. Depressed persons describe feelings of sadness, despair, helplessness, hopelessness, boredom, loss of interest, and isolation. They may also feel self-reproach, self-deprecation, and guilt. These subjective symptoms are evidenced by changes in behavior (see box).

Therapeutic Management

Suicidal threats should be taken very seriously. There has been a general tendency to dismiss a suicide attempt as an impulsive act resulting from a temporary crisis or depression. If this drastic move to gain attention fails to draw attention to their problems or makes them worse, adolescents may conclude that taking their lives is their only means to solve these escalating, unsolvable, and unbearable problems.

Children need to know that someone cares and must be provided with swift and efficient crisis intervention. Although an acute depressive reaction can be managed without difficulty by ordinary practitioners, the youngster who has made a serious attempt or has made a plan for suicide should receive competent psychiatric care.

Nursing Considerations

Care of the suicidal adolescent includes early recognition, management, and prevention. Probably the most important aspect of management is the recognition of prodromal signs that indicate that a youngster is troubled and might attempt to take his life. Health professionals need to be alert to the signs of adolescent depression, and any youngster who exhibits such behavior, subtle or overt, should be referred for thorough psychologic assessment. Depression can be manifest in two ways: youngsters who feel depressed may talk about suicide and feelings of worthlessness, or they may build themselves a solid defense against such intolerable feelings of depression with behavioral or psychosomatic disturbances. A sudden change in behavior from depression to cheerfulness can be mistaken for apparent adjustment but should be investigated. It frequently indicates that the child has reached the decision to take his life.

Too often suicidal threats or minor attempts are confused with bids for attention. No threat of suicide should be ignored or challenged in any way. The child needs to know that someone cares and must be provided with swift and efficient crisis intervention. Most larger communities have 24-hour service in the form of "hot lines"—telephone communication that is within reach of troubled youngsters or their families where they can make ready contact with someone to listen to them. The function of the hot line is to help them through the immediate crisis. Through skillful questioning, but without imposing a solution on the caller, the listener helps the caller arrive at a course of action that will contribute to a solution for his problem.

Some schools have instituted suicide prevention programs designed primarily for high school–age youth. However, many are attempting to reach children in middle and elementary schools. Those with programs in operation offer services such as drop-in counseling and a peer counseling telephone line. Information can be obtained from the **American Association of Suicidology.***

SUMMARY

Although the school-age and adolescent years are relatively healthy periods of development from a biologic perspective, injuries continue to be a significant source of health problems during middle and late childhood. Emotional problems that become more apparent during middle childhood include hyperactivity, learning disorders, and problems of elimination. Many adolescent health problems are a consequence of certain behaviors related to these turbulent years, including sexual experimentation, indiscriminate drug and alcohol use, indiscriminate automobile driving, and competitive athletics. Problems related to growth and maturation become increasingly evident and distressful to affected children and their families. Intense body image concerns that stem from preoccupation with pubertal changes render the adolescent singularly vulnerable to psychologic complications related to real or perceived alterations in appearance.

*2459 Ash, Denver, CO 80222, 303-692-0985.

KEY CONCEPTS

- Middle childhood is a relatively healthy period, and most problems encountered are not considered serious.
- The change, growth, and stress accompanying the transition to adulthood may predispose adolescents to faulty problem solving.
- Smoking is a widespread problem among teenagers; reasons for smoking include social pressures, mass media influence, and a need to develop a self-concept.
- Participation in sports predisposes children and adolescents to both acute injuries and overuse syndromes.
- Alterations in growth and maturation may be manifest in short stature, tall stature, precocious puberty, and delayed sexual development.
- Tools for assessment of growth include a family history, previous growth patterns, physical examination, bone age determination, and endocrine studies.
- The most frequent health problems related to the female reproductive system involve menstrual dysfunction.
- Health problems related to sexuality are pregnancy, rape, and sexually transmitted diseases.
- Eating disorders observed in middle and late childhood are obesity, anorexia nervosa, and bulimia.
- Effective therapy for attention deficit disorder usually involves a multiple approach: family education and counseling, medication, remedial education, environmental manipulation, and psychotherapy.
- Behavior problems in middle childhood include attention deficit disorder, enuresis, encopresis, school phobia, recurrent abdominal pain, childhood depression, conversion reaction, and childhood schizophrenia.
- The substances abused by children and adolescents are alcohol, narcotics, central nervous system depressants, central nervous system stimulants, hydrocarbons and fluorocarbons, and mind-altering drugs.
- Suicide, the deliberate act of self-injury with the intent to kill, may occur because of difficulties coping with stress, disturbed family environment, and psychoses.

STUDY QUESTIONS AND ACTIVITIES

1 Analyze 5 different cigarette advertisements. What aspects of the advertisement would be likely to entice a teenager to smoke?

2 Interview a school nurse to determine the types of sports injuries sustained by children and/or adolescents at school and the role of the school nurse in injury management and prevention.

3 Investigate the philosophy and general plan of two weight-loss programs (commercial or noncommercial) in the community.

4 Design a teaching plan for an adolescent on one of the following topics:
   Contraception
   Sexually transmitted disease
   Pregnancy

5 Interview a school-age child and an adolescent to determine his/her understanding of chemical substances frequently abused. Determine their concept of the substance's effect on an individual, availability, and adverse consequences of its use.

REFERENCES

American Psychiatric Association: Diagnostic and statistical manual of mental disorders, ed. 3-revised (DSM-III-R), Washington, DC, 1987, The Association.

Brookman, R.R.: Adolescent sexuality and related health problems. In Hofmann, A.D., editor: Adolescent medicine, Menlo Park, CA, 1983, Addison-Wesley Publishing Co.

Burgess, A.W.: The sexual victimization of adolescents, Washington, DC, 1985, U.S. Government Printing Office, DHHS Publication No. (ADM) 858-1382.

Committee on Environmental Hazards: Smokeless tobacco—a carcinogenic hazard, Pediatrics **76:**1009-1011, 1985.

Garfinkel, B.D., and others: Suicide attempts in children and adolescents, Am. J. Psychiatry **129:**1257-1261, 1982.

Newton, B.: Tough Love: help for parents with troubled teenagers—reorganizing the hierarchy in disorganized families, Pediatrics **76:**691-694, 1985.

Raley, G.: Youth suicide: the federal response, Soc. Legis. Bull. **29:**65-68, 1985.

Tarr, J.E., and Macklin, M.: Cocaine, Pediatr. Clin. North Am. **34:**319-331, 1987.

BIBLIOGRAPHY

General

Hofmann, A.D., editor: Adolescent medicine, Menlo Park, CA, 1983, Addison-Wesley Publishing Co.

Howe, J.: Nursing care of adolescents, New York, 1980, McGraw-Hill Book Co.

Mahan, L.K., and Rees, J.M.: Nutrition in adolescence, St. Louis, 1984, Times Mirror/Mosby College Publishing.

Pipes, P.L.: Nutrition in infancy and childhood, ed. 4, St. Louis, 1989, The C.V. Mosby Co.

Smoking

Coe, R.M., and others: Patterns of change in adolescent smoking behavior and results of a one year follow-up of a smoking prevention program, J. Sch. Health **52:**348-353, 1982.

Demuth, P.J.: Clove cigarettes: a hazardous fad, Am. J. Nurs. **85:**950-951, 1985.

Flay, B.R., and others: Cigarette smoking: why young people do it and ways of preventing it. In McGrath, P.J., and Firestone, P.: Pediatric and adolescent behavioral medicine. Issues in treatment, New York, 1983, Springer Publishing Co.

Masironi, R., and Roy, L.: Smoking and youth: a special report, World Smoking and Health **8**(1):27-31, 1983.

McCaul, K.D., and others: Predicting adolescent smoking, J. Sch. Health **52:**342-346, 1982.

Murray, M., Kiryluk, S., and Swan, A.V.: School characteristics and adolescent smoking. Results from the MRC/Derbyshire smoking study 1974-8 and from a follow-up in 1981, J. Epidemiol. Community Health **38:**167-172, 1984.

Young, T.L., and Rogers, K.D.: School performance characteristics preceding onset of smoking in high school students, Am. J. Dis. Child. **140:**257-259, 1985.

Disorders Related to Sports

Carey, R.J., and Shute, R.E.: Sports trauma management and the high school nurse, J. Sch. Health **52:**156-158, 1982.

Cook, D.E., and Gustafson, P.R.G.: Sports health care for children and adolescents, Nurs. Update **1**(15):1-8, 1986.

Frisch, R.E., Wyshak, G., and Vincent, L.: Delayed menarche and amenorrhea in ballet dancers, N. Engl. J. Med. **303:**17-19, 1980.

Goldberg, B.: Pediatric sports medicine. In Scott, W.N., Nisonson, B., and Nicholas, J.A., editors: Principles of sports medicine, Baltimore, 1984, Williams & Wilkins.

Kris-Etherton, P.M.: Nutrition, exercise and athletic performance, Food Nutr. **57**(3):13-15, 1985.

Latinis, B.: Frequent sports injuries of children: etiology, treatment, and prevention, Issues Compr. Pediatr. Nurs. **6:**167-178, 1983.

Macvicar, M.G., Harlan, J.D., and Ouellette, M.: What do we know about the effects of sports training on the menstrual cycle? MCN **7:**55-58, 1982.

Narins, D.M., Belkengren, R.P., and Sapala, S.: Nutrition and the growing athlete, Pediatr. Nurs. **9:**163-168, 1983.

Osguthorpe, N.C., and Osguthorpe, J.D.: Scuba diving hazards: emergency management, Am. J. Nurs. **81:**1456-1458, 1981.

Thomas, K.A.: Screening the child for sports participation, Issues Compr. Pediatr. Nurs. **6:**179-194, 1983.

Thompson, C.E., and Stroud, S.D.: The motorized tricycle: an accident waiting to happen, J. Pediatr. Nurs. **2:**120-125, 1987.

Thorne, B.P.: A nurse helps prevent sports injuries, MCN **7:**236-239, 1982.

Wilson, M.C., and Fischer, R.G.: Drug use in sports, Pediatr. Nurs. **12:**452, 464, 1986.

Altered Growth and/or Maturation

Cohen, F.L., and Durham, J.D.: Update your knowledge of Klinefelter syndrome, J. Psychosocial Nurs. **23:**19-25, 1985.
Cohen, F.L., and Durham, J.D.: Sex chromosome variations in school-aged children, J. Sch. Health **55:**99-102, 1985.
Holmes, C.S., Hayford, J.T., and Thompson, R.G.: Personality and behavior differences in groups of boys with short stature, Child Health Care **11:**61-64, 1982.
Solomon, S.B.: Children with short stature, J. Pediatr. Nurs. **1:**80-89, 1986.
Stern, N., and Zaiken, H.: Assessing the child with short stature, Pediatr. Nurs. **11:**106-110, 1985.

Disorders of the Reproductive System

Brown, M.A., and Zimmer, P.A.: Personal and family impact of premenstrual symptoms, JOGNN **15:**31-38, 1986.
Coyne, C.M., Woods, N.F., and Mitchell, E.S.: Premenstrual tension syndrome, JOGNN **14:**446-454, 1985.
Frank, E.P.: What are nurses doing to help PMS patients?, Am. J. Nurs. **86:**137-140, 1986.
Gault-Catarrinho, P.L.: Testicular cancer, Crit. Care Update **10**(2):32-35, 1983.
Gever, L.N.: From arthritis pain to dysmenorrhea, a new indication for prostaglandin inhibitors, Nursing 80 **10:**81, 1980.
Lauver, D.: Irregular bleeding in women: causes and nursing intervention, Am. J. Nurs. **83:**396-401, 1983.
Meyer, M.R.: Adolescent gynecology: problems and ponderings, Pediatr. Nurs. **4**(4):43-47, 1978.
Mitchell, J.R.: Male adolescents' concern about a physical examination conducted by a female, Nurs. Res. **29:**165-169, 1980.
Muscari, M.E.: Obtaining the adolescent sexual history, Pediatr. Nurs. **13:**307-310, 1987.
Peach, E.H.: Counseling sexually active very young adolescent girls, MCN **5:**191-195, 1980.
Primrose, R.B.: Taking the tension out of pelvic exams, Am. J. Nurs. **84:**72-74, 1984.
Rx drugs switched to OTC, FDA Drug Bulletin **13**(3):29-30, 1984.
Sasso, S.C.: Prostaglandin inhibitors for primary dysmenorrhea, MCN **9:**177, 1984.
Wawrzyniak, M.N.: The painless pelvic, MCN **11:**178-179, 1986.
Williams, A.W.: Screening for testicular cancer, Pediatr. Nurs. **7**(5):38-40, 1981.

Adolescent Pregnancy

Abbott, M.I.: Parenting group for teen-agers fails, Pediatr. Nurs. **6**(5):54-65, 1980.
Abrams, B.: Helping pregnant teenagers eat right, Nursing 81 **11**(3):46-47, 1981.
Admire, G., and Byers, L.: Counseling the pregnant teenager, Nursing 81 **11**(4):62-63, 1981.
Berland, A.: Young father's support group, Pediatr. Nurs. **13:**255-256, 278, 1987.
Bobak, I.M., and Jensen, M.D.: Maternity and gynecologic care: the nurse and the family, ed. 4, St. Louis, 1989, The C.V. Mosby Co.
Burke, P.J.: A community health model for pregnant teens, MCN **8:**340-344, 1983.
Clarke, B.A.: Improving adolescent parenting through participant modeling and self-evaluation, Nurs. Clin. North Am. **18:**303-311, 1983.
Cusson, R.M.: Attitudes toward breast-feeding among female high-school students, Pediatr. Nurs. **11:**189-191, 1985.
Daniels, M.B., and Manning, D.: A clinic for pregnant teens, Am. J. Nurs. **83:**68-71, 1983.
Dibble, J.C.: ABC for teens: parent education after the baby comes, Pediatr. Nurs. **7**(4):21-23, 1981.
Donlen, J., and Lynch, P.: Teenage mother: high-risk baby, Nursing 81 **11**(5):51-56, 1981.
Howard, J.S., and Sater, J.: Adolescent mothers: self-perceived health education needs, JOGNN **14:**399-404, 1985.
Mercer, R.: Assessing and counseling teenage mothers during the perinatal period, Nurs. Clin. North Am. **18:**293-301, 1983.
Mercer, R.T.: Teenage motherhood: the first year, JOGNN **9:**16-27, 1980.
Moore, D.S., Erickson, P.I., and Wurgel, M.: Adolescent pregnancy and parenting: the role of the nurse, Top. Clin. Nurs. **6**(3):72-78, 1984.
Morgan, B.S., and Barden, M.E.: Unwed and pregnant: nurses' attitudes toward unmarried mothers, MCN **10:**114-117, 1985.
Poole, C.J., and Hofmann, M.: Mothers of adolescent mothers: how do they cope? Pediatr. Nurs. **7**(1):28-31, 1981.
Sewall, K.S.: Peer-group reality therapy for the pregnant adolescent, MCN **8:**67-69, 1983.
Smith, D.L.: Meeting the psychosocial needs of teen-age mothers and fathers, Nurs. Clin. North Am. **19:**369-379, 1984.
Taylor, B., Wadsworth, J., and Butler, N.R.: Teenage mothering, admission to hospital, and accidents during the first 5 years, Arch. Dis. Child. **58:**6-11, 1983.
Teenage pregnancy: the problem that hasn't gone away, New York, 1981, Alan Guttmacher Institute.
Vukelich, C., and Kliman, D.S.: Mature and teenage mothers' infant growth expectations and use of child development information sources, Fam. Rel. **34:**189-196, 1985.
Winkelstein, M.L., and Carson, V.J.: Adolescents and rooming-in, Matern. Child Nurs. J. **16**(1):75-88, 1987.

Contraception

Babington, M.A.: Adolescent use of oral contraceptives, Pediatr. Nurs. **10:**111-114, 1984.
Gara, E.: Nursing protocol to improve the effectiveness of the contraceptive diaphragm, MCN **6:**41-45, 1981.
Hewson, P.M.: Research on adolescent male attitudes about contraceptives, Pediatr. Nurs. **12:**114-116, 1986.
Peach, E.H.: Counseling sexually active very young adolescents, MCN **5:**191-195, 1980.
Reis, J., and Herz, L.: Young adolescents' contraceptive knowledge and attitudes: implications for anticipatory guidance, J. Pediatr. Health Care **1:**247-254, 1987.
Tauer, K.M.: Promoting effective decision-making in sexually active adolescents, Nurs. Clin. North Am. **18:**275-292, 1983.
White, J.E.: Influence of parents, peers, and problem-solving on contraceptive use, Pediatr. Nurs. **13:**317-321, 360, 1987.
White, J.E.: Initiating contraceptive use: how do young women decide? Pediatr. Nurs. **10:**347-352, 1984.
Yoos, L.: Adolescent cognitive and contraceptive behaviors, Pediatr. Nurs. **13:**247-250, 1987.

Sexually Transmitted Diseases

Bettoli, E.J.: Herpes: facts and fallacies, Am. J. Nurs. **82:**111-114, 1982.
Campbell, C.E., and Herten, R.J.: VD to STD: redefining venereal disease, Am. J. Nurs. **81:**1629, 16-35, 1981.
DiClemente, R.J., Zorn, J., and Temoshok, L.: Adolescents and AIDS: a survey of knowledge, attitudes, and beliefs about AIDS in San Francisco, Am. J. Public Health **76:**1443-1445, 1986.
Hamm, P., and Jemison-Smith, P.: Chlamydia, Crit. Care Update **8**(3):34-36, 1981.
Hamm, P., and Jemison-Smith, P.: Herpesvirus hominus, Crit. Care Update **8**(8):34-37, 1981.
Helgerson, S.D., Peterson, L.R., and the AIDS Education Study Group: acquired immunodeficiency syndrome and secondary school students: their knowledge is limited and they want to know more, Pediatrics **81:**350-355, 1988.
Larson, E.: Intransigent genital infection? Suspect chlamydiae, RN **46**(1):42-43, 1984.
Lucey, J., and Baron, M.: Herpetic whitlow, Am. J. Nurs. **84:**60-61, 1984.
Perley, N.Z., and Bills, B.J.: Herpes genitalis and the childbearing cycle, MCN **8:**213-217, 1983.
Price, J.H., Desmond, S., and Kukulka, G.: High school students' perceptions and misperceptions of AIDS, J. Sch. Health **55:**107-109, 1985.

Rape

Burgess, A.W., and Brodsky, S.L.: Applying flight education principles to rape prevention, Fam. Community Health **4**(2):45-51, 1981.

Cline, F.: Dealing with sexual abuse of children, Nurse Pract., pp. 52-54, May/June 1980.

Foley, T.S., and Davies, M.A.: Rape: nursing care of victims, St. Louis, 1983, The C.V. Mosby Co.

Platt, C.R., Hicks, D.J., and Mori, D.M.: Medical care for the rape victim. In Reinhardt, A.M., and Quinn, M.D., editors: Family-centered community nursing, vol. 2, St. Louis, 1981, The C.V. Mosby Co.

Resisting rape without getting killed, Am. J. Nurs. **85:**947-948, 1985.

Sisney, K.F.: Breaking the link: nursing intervention in the incestuous family, Issues Compr. Pediatr. Nurs. **4**(4):51-59, 1980.

Warner, C.G.: Comforting and caring for the rape victim using crisis intervention wisely, Nursing Skillbooks, 1979, Nursing 79 Books.

Obesity

Brownell, K.D., and others: School-based behavior modification, nutrition education and physical education program for obese children, Am. J. Clin. Nutr. **35:**277-281, 1982.

Castiglia, P.T.: Obesity in infants and toddlers, J. Pediatr. Nurs. **1:**218-220, 1987.

Cecere, M.C.: PIP (Positive Image Program): a group approach for obese adolescents, Nurs. Clin. North Am. **18:**249-256, 1983.

Clark, M.K.: The risks of repeated dieting, Child. Nurse **2:**1, 3-4, 1984.

Dietz, W.H., Jr., and Gortmaker, S.L.: Factors within the physical environment associated with childhood obesity, Am. J. Clin. Nutr. **39:**619-624, 1984.

Hagenbuch, V.E.G.: Obesity and the school-age child, Nurs. Clin. North Am. **17:**207-216, 1982.

Hataway, H., Raines, J.L., and Weinsier, R.L.: Nutrition: its ever-increasing role, Fam. Community Health **7:**22-37, 1984.

Hoerr, S.M.: An overlooked factor in adolescent obesity, Food Nutr. News **57:**17-19, 1985.

Hoover, M.L.: The self-image of overweight adolescent females: a review of the literature, MCN **13:**125-137, 1984.

Jessor, R.: Problem behavior and developmental transition in adolescence, J. Sch. Health **52:**295-300, 1982.

Jonides, L.: Childhood obesity: a treatment approach for private practices, Pediatr. Nurs. **8:**320-322, 1982.

Kahn, A.N.: Group education for the overweight, Am. J. Nurs. **78:**254, 1978.

Lasky, P.A.: Implications, considerations, and nursing interventions of obesity in neonatal and preschool patients, Nurs. Clin. North Am. **17:**199-205, 1982.

Mogan, J.: Prevention of childhood obesity, Issues Compr. Pediatr. Nurs. **9:**33-38, 1986.

Mowrey, B.D.: Family oriented approach to childhood obesity, Pediatr. Nurs. **6**(2):40-44, 1980.

Overfield, T.: Obesity: prevention is easier than cure, Nurse Pract. **5:**25, Sept./Oct. 1980.

Rowe, N.R.: Childhood obesity: growth charts vs. calipers, Pediatr. Nurs. **6**(2):24-27, 1980.

Simonson, M.: An overview: advances in research and treatment of obesity, Food Nutr. News **53:**1-4, 1982.

Taitz, L.S.: The obese child, Boston, 1983, Blackwell Scientific Publications.

White, J.H.: An overview of obesity: its significance to nursing, Nurs. Clin. North Am. **17:**191-198, 1982.

Anorexia Nervosa/Bulimia

Bhanji, S.: Anorexia nervosa: two schools of thought, Nurs. Time. **76**(1):324-325, 1980.

Block, P.J.: Working with anorexic and bulimic adolescents, Food Nutr. News **56:**33-34, 1984.

Carino, C.M., and Chmelko, P.: Disorders of eating in adolescence: anorexia nervosa and bulimia, Nurs. Clin. North Am. **18:**343-352, 1983.

Ciseaux, A.: Anorexia nervosa: a view from the mirror, Am. J. Nurs. **80:**1468-1470, 1980.

Claggett, M.S.: Anorexia nervosa: a behavioral approach, Am. J. Nurs. **80:**1471-1472, 1980.

Dexter, J.M.: Anorexia nervosa, Nurs. Time. **76:**325-327, 1980.

Doyen, L.: Primary anorexia nervosa: a review and critique of selected papers, J. Psychosoc. Nurs. Ment. Health Serv. **20**(6):12-18, 1982.

Goodwin, R.A., and Mickalide, A.D.: Parent-to-parent support in anorexia nervosa and bulimia, Child. Health Care **14:**32-37, 1985.

Harding, S.E.: Anorexia nervosa, Pediatr. Nurs. **11:**275-277, 1985.

Marks, R.G.: Anorexia and bulimia: eating habits that can kill, RN **46**(1):44-47, 1984.

McNab, W.L.: Anorexia and the adolescent, J. Sch. Health **53:**427-430, 1983.

Misik, I.M.: When the anorectic patient challenges you, Nursing 81 **11**(12):46-49, 1981.

Muscari, M.E.: Identification and management of the early anorectic child. J. Pediatr. Health Care **1:**196-203, 1987.

Potts, N.: The secret pattern of binge/purge, Am. J. Nurs. **84:**32-35, 1984.

Rees, J.M.: Eating disorders. In Mahan, L.K., and Rees, J.M.: Nutrition in adolescence, St. Louis, 1984, The C.V. Mosby Co.

Richardson, T.F.: Anorexia nervosa: an overview, Am. J. Nurs. **80:**1470-1471, 1980.

Sanger, E., and Cassino, T.: Eating disorders—avoiding the power struggle, Am. J. Nurs. **84:**31-35, 1984.

Attention Deficit Disorder

Bassett, L.B., Gudas, L.J., and McAnulty, E.H.: The learning disabled child: recognition, evaluation, and management, Pediatr. Nurs. **8**(5):323-330, 1982.

Brown, R.T., and Wynne, M.E.: Sustained attention in boys with attention deficit disorder and the effect of methylphenidate, Pediatr. Nurs. **10:**35-39, 1984.

Cantwell, D.P.: Recognition, evaluation and management of the hyperactive child, Pediatr. Nurs. **5**(5):11-22, 1979.

Erb, L., and Andresen, B.D.: Hyperactivity: a possible consequence of maternal alcohol consumption, Pediatr. Nurs. **7**(4):30-33, 1981.

Huber, C.J., and Dalldorf, J.S.: Minimal brain dysfunction syndrome, Nurs. Clin. North Am. **15:**551-569, 1980.

Robinson, L.A.: Food allergies, food additives, and Feingold diet, Pediatr. Nurs. **6**(6):38-39, 1980.

Silverstein, R.A.: Learning problems as a symptom of family dysfunction, J. Assoc. Care Child Health **9**(4):122-125, 1981.

Varley, C.K.: A clinical nurse specialist's role in the comprehensive management of attention deficit disorder, Child. Health Care **13:**139-142, 1985.

White, J.E.: Special nursing needs of hospitalized children with learning disabilities, MCN **8:**209-212, 1983.

Enuresis/Encopresis

Ack, M., Norman, M.E., and Schmitt, B.D. (in discussion): Enuresis: the role of alarms and drugs, Patient Care **19:**75-90, 1985.
Castiglia, P.T.: Nocturnal enuresis, J. Pediatr. Health Care **1:**280-282, 1987.
Crowley, A.A.: A comprehensive strategy for managing encopresis, MCN **9:**395-400, 1984.
Hague, M., and others: Parental perceptions of enuresis, Am. J. Dis. Child. **135:**809-811, 1981.
Johns, C.: Encopresis, Am. J. Nurs. **85:**153-156, 1985.
Levine, M.D.: Encopresis: its potentiation, evaluation, and alleviation, Pediatr. Clin. North Am. **29:**315-330, 1982.
Levine, M.D., Mazonson, P., and Bakow, H.: Behavioral symptom substitution in children cured of encopresis, Am. J. Dis. Child. **134:**663-667, 1980.
Olness, K., McParland, F.A., and Piper, J.: Biofeedback: a new modality in the management of children with fecal soiling, J. Pediatr. **96:**505-509, 1980.
O'Regan, S., and others: Constipation: a commonly unrecognized cause of enuresis, Am. J. Dis. Child. **140:**260-261, 1986.
Ruble, J.A.: Childhood nocturnal enuresis, MCN **6:**26-31, 1981.
Schmitt, B.D.: Encopresis, Primary Care **11:**497-511, 1984.
Schmitt, B.D.: Nocturnal enuresis: an update on treatment, Pediatr. Clin. North Am. **29:**21-35, 1982.
Shapiro, S.R.: Enuresis: treatment and overtreatment, Pediatr. Nurs. **11**(3):203-207, 1985.
Younger, J.B., and Hughes, L.S.: No-fault management of encopresis, Pediatr. Nurs. **9:**185-187, 1983.

Behavior Disorders in School-Age Children

Brady, M.A., and others: Childhood depression: development of a screening tool, Pediatr. Nurs. **10:**222-227, 1984.
Bumbalo, J.A., and Siemon, M.K.: Nursing assessment and diagnosis: mental health problems of children, Top. Clin. Nurs. **5**(1):41-54, 1983.
Child, A.A., Murphy, C.M., and Rhyne, M.C.: Depression in children: reasons and risks, Pediatr. Nurs. **6**(4):9-13, 1980.
Fond, K., and Brosnan, J.: School phobia: the school anxiety syndrome, Pediatr. Nurs. **6**(5):9-13, 1980.
McConville, B.J.: The causes and treatment of depression in young children, J. Child. Contemp. Soc. **15**(6):61-68, 1982.
Nelms, B.C.: Assessing childhood depression: do parents and children agree? Pediatr. Nurs. **12:**23-26, 1986.
Nelms, B.C., and Brady, M.A.: Assessment and intervention: the depressed school-age child, Pediatr. Nurs. **6**(4):15-19, 1980.
Ryan, N.M.: Recurrent abdominal pain among school-age children, MCN **11:**102-106, 1986.

Substance Abuse

Burton, J.: Intoxication by centrally acting substances, Crit. Care Update **10:**34-35, 1983.
Cuddy, P.G.: Management of acute opioid intoxication, Crit. Care Q. **4**(4):65-74, 1982.
Fields, B.L.: Adolescent alcoholism: treatment and rehabilitation, Fam. Community Health **2**(1):61-90, 1979.
Hahn, A.B., Oestreich, S.J.K., and Barkin, R.L.: Mosby's pharmacology in nursing, ed. 16, St. Louis, 1986, The C.V. Mosby Co.
Lukwikowski, K.L.K.: PPA: an innocent over-the-counter drug? Pediatr. Nurs. **10:**387-390, 1984.
Pallikkathayil, L., and Tweed, S.: Substance abuse: alcohol and drugs during adolescence, Nurs. Clin. North Am. **18:**313-321, 1983.
Palmer-Erbs, V.K., and DeForge, V.M.: Interventions with the adolescent drug user and the family, Issues Compr. Pediatr. Nurs. **3**(5):15-24, 1979.
Rehrig, M.: Cocaine look-alikes, Crit. Care Update **10:**47-49, 1983.
Rice, M.A., and Kibbee, P.E.: Review: identifying the adolescent substance abuser, MCN **8:**139-142, 1983.
Tennant, F.S., Jr., and LaCour, J.: Children at risk for addiction and alcoholism: identification and intervention, Pediatr. Nurs. **6**(1):26-27, 1980.
Woolf, D.S., Vourakis, C., and Bennett, G.: Guidelines for management of acute phencyclidine intoxication, Crit. Care Update **7**(6):17-24, 1980.
Wright, L.S.: High school polydrug users and abusers, Adolescence **20:**853-861, 1985.

Suicide

Carmack, B.J.: Suspect a suicide? RN **46**(44):43-45, 90, 1983.
Hafen, B.Q.: and Peterson, B: Preventing adolescent suicide, Nursing 83 **13**(9):47-48, 1983.
Hart, N.A., and Prophit, P., Sr.: Adolescent suicide, Pediatr. Nurs. **5**(6):22-28, 1979.
Hoff, L.A., and Resing, M.: Was this suicide preventable? Am. J. Nurs. **82:**1107-1111, 1982.
Keidel, G.C.: Adolescent suicide, Nurs. Clin. North Am. **18:**323-332, 1983.
Lewis, L., McDowell, W.A., and Gregory, R.J.: Saving the suicidal patient from himself, RN **49**(12):26-28, 1986.
Litt, I.F., Cuskey, W.R., and Rudd, S.: Emergency room evaluation of the adolescent who attempts suicide: compliance with follow-up, J. Adolesc. Health Care **4:**106-109, 1983.
Mitchell, K.: Suicide: a preventable tragedy, Pediatr. Nurs. **11:**165, 1985.
Nursing Grand Rounds: Nursing care of a suicidal adolescent, Nursing 80 **10**(4):56-59, 1980.
Tishler, C.L.: Adolescent suicide: prevention, practice, and treatment, Feelings Med. Significance **23:**23-26, 1981; **24:**1-4, 1982.
Tishler, C.L.: Depression in children and adolescents: identification and intervention, Public Health Curr. **24:**1-3, 1984.
Tishler, C.L.: Intentional self-destructive behavior in children under age ten, Clin. Pediatr. **19:**451-453, 1980.
Valente, S.: The suicidal teenager, Nursing 85 **15:**47-49, 1985.
Valente, S.: Suicide in school-aged children: theory and assessment, Pediatr. Nurs. **9:**25-29, 1983.

UNIT

VIII

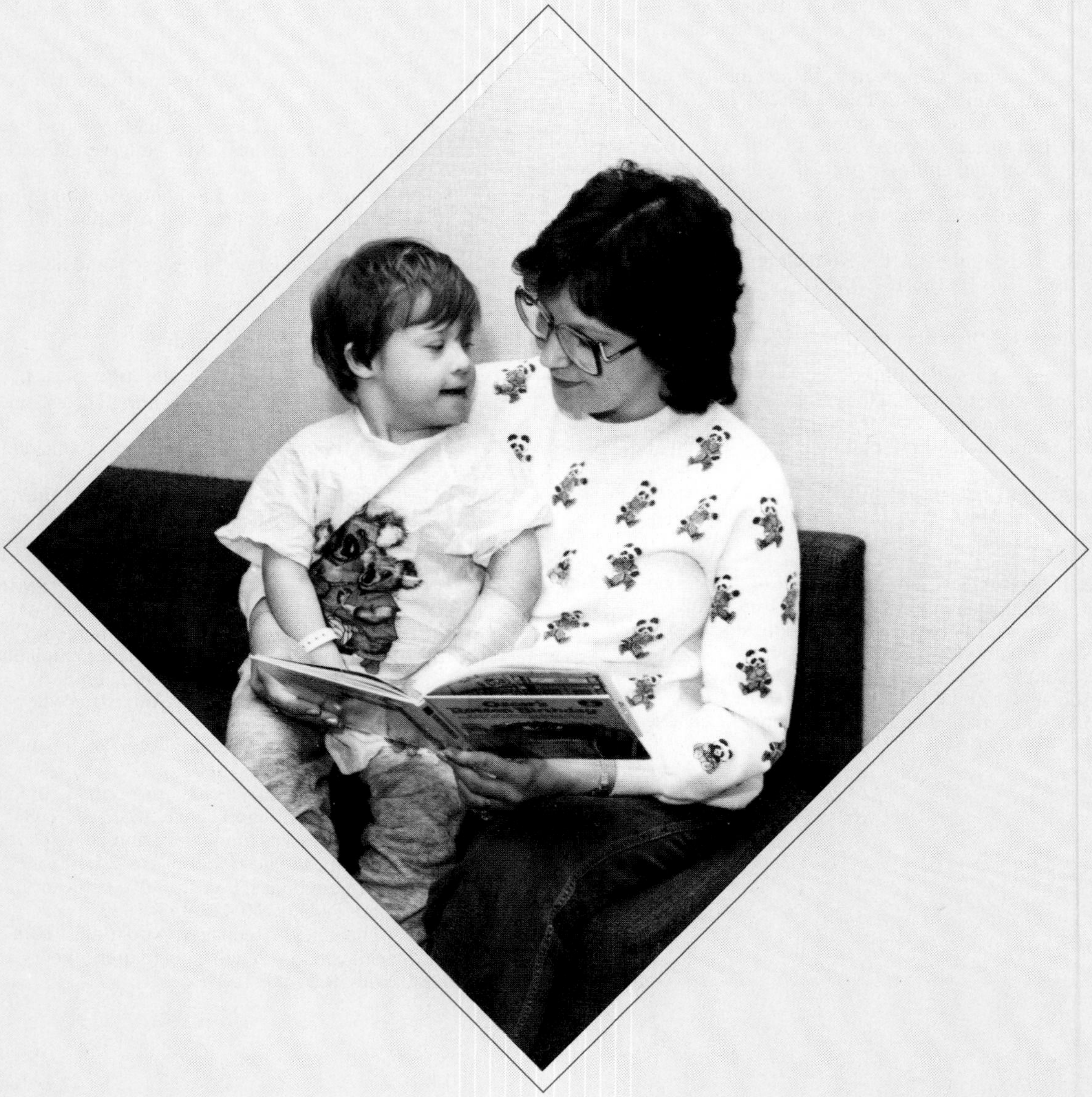

The Child and Family with Special Needs

Units IV through VII have focused on the growth and development of the well child. Most of the health problems discussed for each age-group were those that temporarily incapacitated the child. Unit Eight is concerned with the child who has special needs imposed by a permanent or chronic physical and/or developmental disability. These children need to master the same developmental achievements as well children, in accordance with their potential abilities and despite the limitations of their condition. Families of these children are faced with exceptional challenges for which there is little guidance or few role models. As a result, the entire family unit is highly vulnerable to psychologic and sometimes physical problems that arise from unsuccessful attempts to deal with the child's special needs.

Chapter 18, *Impact of Chronic Illness, Disability, or Death on the Child and Family,* is an overview of the child's and family's reactions to the disorder and nursing interventions that assist each member in adjusting to the condition and developing to their fullest despite the disability. This chapter serves as a basis for understanding the stresses and needs of families when the child is chronically ill, fatally ill, physically disabled, mentally retarded, or sensory impaired. Chapter 19, *Impact of Cognitive or Sensory Impairment on the Child and Family,* discusses the classification of mental retardation, causes of cognitive, auditory, and visual impairments, and the nursing interventions required to help the child become independent. Emphasis is placed on the effect of the impairment on development, detection of the disorder, and nursing interventions that promote rehabilitation.

CHAPTER 18

Impact of Chronic Illness, Disability, or Death on the Child and Family

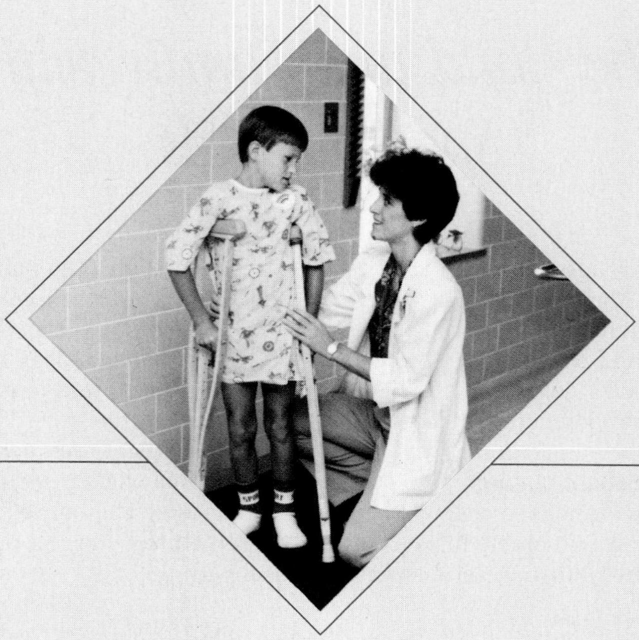

LEARNING OBJECTIVES

On completion of this chapter the reader will be able to:

- Identify the scope of and changing trends in care of children with special needs
- Define the stages of adjustment to the diagnosis of a chronic condition
- Define the stages of grief for the anticipated or actual loss of a child
- Identify the major reactions of and effects on the family with a child with a special need
- Recognize the impact of the illness or disability on the developmental stages of childhood
- Outline nursing interventions that promote the family's optimal adjustment to the child's chronic disorder
- Outline nursing interventions that support the family at the time of death

With advances in early diagnosis and treatment of many chronic illnesses and with improved technology for people with physical impairments, a growing number of children with these conditions are surviving and need care. Because nurses are intimately involved in nearly every type of health deviation, they will inevitably be responsible for some phase of care with these families. This chapter is primarily concerned with the child's and the family's responses to the disorder, the effects of chronic or fatal illness or disability on the child and family unit, and nursing interventions that promote the optimum adjustment of each family member and acceptance of the child as a unique individual with special attributes as well as needs.

◆ *Perspectives in the Care of Children with Special Needs*

Children with special needs related to their physical or mental health status comprise an increasingly important group of children who require both routine and specialized health care. The following discussion is an overview of the incidence of chronic illness, life-threatening illness, and disability in children and the current trends in caring for these children.

SCOPE OF THE PROBLEM

Despite the interest and concern for these children, exact definitions and incidence rates of chronic illness, disability, and terminal illness do not exist. For the purposes of this chapter, the following definitions are used and collectively refer to *special needs*:

chronic illness A condition that interferes with daily functioning for more than 3 months in a year, causes hospitalization of more than 1 month in a year, or (at time of diagnosis) is likely to do either of these (Hobbs and Perrin, 1985).
disability Broadly, refers to a loss of function (Reynolds, 1984).
developmental disability Any severe, chronic disability that is attributable to a mental (cognitive) and/or physical impairment, is manifested before age 22 years, is likely to continue indefinitely, results in substantial limitation of function, and requires special services (Golden, 1984).
terminal illness Any illness, of long or short duration, with a life-threatening outcome.

Individuals with chronic illnesses or disabilities are not necessarily handicapped. A *handicap* refers to environmental barriers preventing or making it difficult for full participation or integration, such as curbs or steps for a person in a wheelchair. Consequently, the term *disabled*, rather than the term *handicapped,* is preferred when describing these individuals.

Statistics regarding chronic illness and disability are at best only estimates of the true incidence of the problem. Overall rates of children with any chronic disorder range from 10% to 15%; approximately 1% to 2% of the total population (1 to 2 million children) have a severe chronic illness (Hobbs and Perrin, 1985). Two thirds of all cases of chronic illness in children are attributable to asthma and congenital heart defects; however, in terms of mortality, congenital heart defects, spina bifida, and leukemia are the most lethal.

Broadly expanding chronic conditions to include speech, learning, emotional, sensory, and cognitive disorders yields an estimated 40% of children from kindergarten through sixth grade who have a significant long-term condition (Reynolds, 1984). Terminal illness also significantly adds to the number of children with special needs. Cancer, the leading cause of death from disease in children ages 3 through 14 years, claims the lives of approximately 1800 children each year (Cancer Facts & Figures, 1988). However, because of advances in the treatment of several types of cancer, many children survive for long periods and experience problems commonly associated with chronic illness or physical disability. In addition to death from diseases such as cancer, a much larger number of children die unexpectedly from injuries (see Chapter 1). Considering also those who care deeply about the child, the number of individuals intimately affected by these children's illnesses and disabilities is staggering.

CHANGING TRENDS IN CARE

Several changes have occurred in providing services to children with special needs. One is the focus on the child's *developmental* age rather than chronologic age or diagnosis. Using the developmental approach emphasizes the child's abilities and strengths rather than disabilities. Nurses often are in vital positions to redirect attention from the pathologic model to the developmental model to meet the unique needs of the child and family.

Another principle that is increasingly employed is that of *normalization,* which refers to establishing a normal pattern of living (see also p. 524). By applying the principles of normalization, the environment for the child is "normalized" and "humanized." Concurrent with the trend toward normalization has been the earlier discharge of children from acute or chronic care facilities to the family and community. *Home care* represents the return to a system and set of priorities in which family values are as important to the care of a child with a chronic health problem as they are in the care of the well child. Home care seeks to achieve goals that are consistent with the developmental model (Stein, 1985):

1. Normalize the life of a child with special needs, including those with technologically complex care, in a family and community context and setting.
2. Minimize the disruptive impact of the child's condition on the family.
3. Foster the child's maximum growth and development.

Throughout the text home care is discussed as appropriate for specific conditions, and the process of transition from hospital to home is elaborated in Chapter 20.

Paralleling normalization and home care, there also has been a trend toward *mainstreaming,* or integrating children with special needs into regular classrooms. Just as the home is the natural environment for children, so school must also be included as an essential component of the children's overall physical, intellectual, and social development. Children who attend school have the advantages of learning and socializing with a wide group of peers. There is an increased focus on individualization as the academic needs of these children are planned along with those of the rest of the students. A variety of supplemental programs have been designed in the school system to accommodate special needs, thus providing these children with an equal educational opportunity. This change has largely been a result of the passage of Public

Law 94-142, the Education for All Handicapped Children Act of 1975, and Public Law 99-457, the Education of the Handicapped Act Amendments of 1986 (see also p. 10).

◆ *The Family of the Child with Special Needs*

Families of children with special needs are faced with the crisis of losing a perfect child and the task of adjusting to and accepting the child and his condition. Many of the responses of parents to the birth of a child with a congenital anomaly are similar to those observed when the diagnosis of a problem is made later in a child's life. When a child dies, the family experiences the grief process, which in many respects is similar to the reactions that occur at the time of diagnosis. Nurses who understand the responses to the diagnosis and the usual effects the diagnosis has upon each family member are able to emotionally support the family, anticipate and prevent potential problems, and foster growth despite the disorder.

REACTIONS OF FAMILIES TO A CHRONIC ILLNESS OR DISABILITY

When the diagnosis of a disability or chronic illness is made, the family progresses through a fairly predictable sequence of stages, regardless of the nature of the condition. The following discussion focuses on stages that are common to most families, with the exception of the freezing-out stage. Not all families experience this process, and the time needed to progress through any of the stages varies widely with each family member.

Shock and Denial

The initial stage is a period of intense emotion and is characterized by shock, disbelief, and sometimes denial, especially if the disorder is not obvious, such as in chronic illness. Denial as a defense mechanism is a necessary cushion to prevent disintegration and is a normal response to grieving in any type of loss. All family members experience various degrees of adaptive denial as they learn of the impact that the diagnosis has on their lives. Denial becomes maladaptive when it prevents recognition of treatment or rehabilitative goals necessary for the child's optimum survival or development. For example, protracted denial may be seen in the response of a family to mental retardation; as long as the family can maintain a semblance of normality and handle the deviance within the present familial roles and values, no recognition of the diagnosis may exist. Instead the family may explain the problem as slow maturation or an easily remedied disorder. Not infrequently this ability to rationalize delayed development is successful until the child enters school, when his differences are compared to other children and become very evident. At this point the family may begin to recognize the diagnosis as a crisis and react with shock and disbelief.

Shock and denial can last from days to months, sometimes even longer. Examples of denial that may be exhibited at the time of diagnosis include: (1) physician shopping, (2) attributing the symptoms of the actual illness to a minor condition, (3) refusing to believe the diagnostic tests, (4) delaying treatment, (5) acting very happy and optimistic despite the revealed diagnosis, (6) refusing to tell or talk to anyone about the condition, (7) insisting that no one is telling the truth regardless of others' attempts to do so, (8) denying the reason for admission, and (9) asking no questions about the diagnosis, treatment, or prognosis. Each of these mechanisms allows individuals to distance themselves from the onslaught of a tremendous emotional impact and to collect and mobilize their energies toward goal-directed, problem-solving behaviors.

Partial denial, such as seeking additional professional consultations or occasionally acting as if nothing were wrong, is used by most people throughout the dying process. Without such a temporary protective mechanism, few people could survive the constant emotional drain of anticipating their own death or the death of a family member. Particularly with parents, anticipating the death of the child is the same as losing part of one's personal hope for achievement, prestige, and accomplishment. There is no comfort or justice in the loss of youth because death occurs before self-fulfillment.

Denial is probably the least understood and most poorly dealt with reaction. Nurses and physicians typically label denial as "maladaptive" and actively attempt to strip it away by repeated and sometimes blunt explanations of prognosis. In children, the importance of denial has repeatedly been demonstrated as a factor in their positive coping with the diagnosis. Children who use denial to cope with illness are often better able to deal with anxiety and have a more productive attitude about life (O'Malley and others, 1979). Denial allows an individual to maintain hope in the face of overwhelming odds. Like hope, denial may be an adaptive mechanism for dealing with loss that persists until a family or patient is ready to progress beyond this behavior.

Adjustment

Adjustment gradually follows shock and is usually characterized by an open admission that the condition exists. This stage is one of "chronic sorrow" and only partial acceptance and is manifest by several responses, probably the most universal of which are *guilt* and *anger*. Guilt arises from a human need to find rational causes for events. The concept of cause and effect implies an ability to change future events. It is often greatest when the cause of the disorder is directly traceable to the parent, such as in genetic diseases or from accidental injury. However, it occurs even without any scientific or realistic basis for parental responsibility. Frequently the guilt stems from a fallacious assumption that the disability is a result of personal failing or wrongdoing, such as drinking, smoking, not eating correctly, having sex or an affair, exercising, or not doing something correctly during pregnancy or the birth (Childs, 1985). Guilt may also be related to thoughts of wishing the child dead, especially when the demands of care seem overwhelming and unrelenting, and may be associated with religious beliefs, either as a punishment or as a test of faith.

Children, too, may interpret their serious illness as retribution for past misbehavior. The nurse should be particularly sensitive to the child who passively accepts all painful procedures. This child may believe that such acts are inflicted as punishment that he deserves. It is always vital to assure children that what happens to them during diagnosis or treatment is to make them well.

Another common reaction in family members is anger. Anger directed inwardly may be evident as self-reproaching or punitive behavior, such as neglecting one's health and verbally degrading oneself. Anger directed outwardly may be manifest in open arguments or withdrawal from communication and may be evident in the person's relationship with any number of individuals, such as the spouse, the child, and siblings. Passive anger toward the ill child may be evident in decreased visiting, refusal to believe how sick he is, or inability to comfort him. One of the most common targets for parental anger is the staff member.

Children, including the sick or disabled child and his siblings, are apt to respond with anger. Affected children are aware of the loss engendered by the illness or disability and may react angrily to the imposed restrictions or the feelings of being different. Siblings also feel anger and resentment toward the ill child and parents for the loss of a routine and of parental attention. It is difficult for older children and almost impossible for younger children to comprehend the plight of the affected child. Their perception is of a brother or sister who has the undivided attention of their parents, is showered with cards and gifts, and is the focus of everyone's concern.

A number of other reactions among family members are typical and include:

1. **Lowered self-esteem,** in which parents perceive a defect in their child as a defect in themselves; their life goals may be abruptly and dramatically altered, and they lose the fantasy of immortality through their child
2. **Shame,** in which family members anticipate social rejection, pity, or ridicule and related loss of social prestige and may experience social withdrawal
3. **Ambivalence,** in which the simultaneous experience of love and hatred normally experienced by parents toward their children is likely to be greatly intensified
4. **Self-sacrifice,** in which parents become acutely sensitive to implied criticism of their child and may react with resentment and belligerence, or they may deny the existence of the problem and seek professional opinions to substantiate their own belief that "there is really nothing wrong with him"

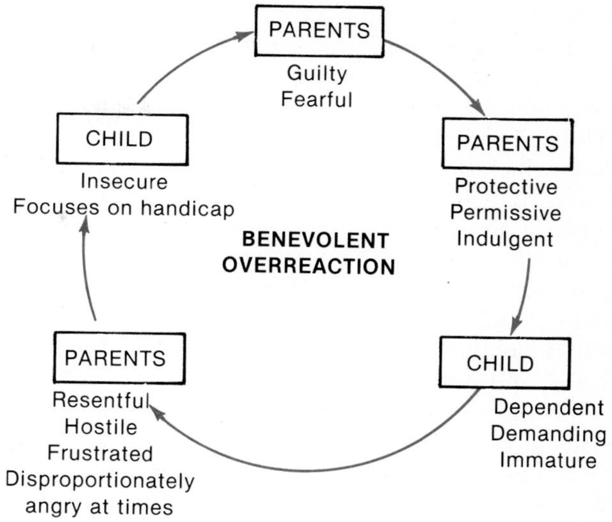

FIG. 18-1 Common cyclical response between parents and child. (From Boone, D.R., and Hartman, B.H.: The benevolent over-reaction, Clin. Pediatr. **11**(5):268-271, 1972.)

During the period of adjustment, four types of parental reactions to the child may occur that influence the child's eventual response to the disorder (see p. 515):

1. **Overprotection,** in which the parents fear letting the child achieve any new skill, avoid all discipline, and cater to the child's every desire so as to prevent frustration
2. **Rejection,** in which the parents detach themselves emotionally from the child but usually provide adequate physical care or constantly nag and scold the child
3. **Denial,** in which parents act is if the disorder does not exist or attempt to have the child overcompensate for it
4. **Gradual acceptance,** in which parents place necessary and realistic restrictions on the child, encourage self-care activities, and promote reasonable physical and social abilities

The most common initial response, especially among mothers, is *benevolent overreaction*. This is usually a consequence of unresolved guilt or fear, such as ambivalent feelings or not wanting the child during pregnancy, feeling responsible for the disorder, believing that the child would die at the time of birth or diagnosis, or reactivated feelings about a previous death of a loved one. The benevolent overreaction results in a vicious cycle of overprotective, permissive parent and dependent, demanding child (Fig. 18-1). It prevents the child from developing self-control, independence, initiative, and self-esteem. The reaction responds to early intervention and prevention but is resistant to change once firmly established.

Reintegration and Acceptance

For many families the last stage is characterized by realistic expectations for the child and reintegration of family life with the illness or disability in proper perspective. Since a large portion of the adjustment phase is one of grief for a loss, total resolution is not possible until the child dies or leaves home as an independent adult. Therefore one can regard adjustment to chronic sorrow as "increased comfortableness" with everyday living.

This adjustment phase also involves social reintegration, in which the family broadens its activities to include relationships outside of the home, with the child as an acceptable and participating member of the group. This last criterion often differentiates gradual acceptance during the adjustment period from total acceptance.

One of the most important aspects of acceptance for health professionals to understand is that it is not an "all-or-none" phenomenon. Rather, acceptance is interspersed with periods of intensified sorrow for the loss, especially at certain landmarks of the child's development, such as entry into school and the onset of puberty. Consequently even families who have achieved a high level of adjustment and acceptance are, at predictable times, in need of professional support.

Freezing-Out Phase

If strategies of coping cannot be employed to minimize the stress and disorganization of maintaining the child within the home to tolerable levels, the affected child may be permanently placed outside the home in a residential setting. Evolution of this phase is directly related to the degree of physical and mental disability.

This phase is not necessarily one of maladjustment. Placement may be the only option that will preserve the integrity of the family. Aging parents may be forced to accept this alternative from progressive inability to meet the demands of a severely disabled offspring. Relinquishing the role of primary caregiver is followed by an initial sense of loss, relief, guilt, and ambivalence, a pattern of reactions not unlike that seen following the death of a terminally ill child (see p. 512).

IMPACT OF CHILD'S CHRONIC ILLNESS OR DISABILITY ON FAMILY MEMBERS

Each family who has a child with special needs is affected by the experience. The effects on the parents and their responses are so critical that there is a direct influence on the other members' reactions. In addition, members of the extended family are affected, and their response, as well as the community's acceptance of the child, can further assist or hinder the family's coping with the stresses imposed by caring for their child.

Parents

All parents wish for the birth of a perfect child and hope that no serious illness or disability occurs at any time in the child's life. Unfortunately, the child may be born with a problem or develop one after birth. While the responses of the parents are similar regardless of the timing of the diagnosis, some important differences do exist.

Parental responses at the time of birth. When a child is born with a congenital anomaly, parents must mourn the loss of the anticipated "perfect" child and accept a child who has an imperfection. Normally every parent wishes for a perfect child but, at the same time, fears that the infant will be abnormal. This fear is often expressed by parents who state that their concern is not whether the child is to be a girl or a boy, just that the infant is healthy. One of the first things parents want confirmed at the time of birth is, "Is our baby all right?"

In most instances there is some discrepancy between the parent's idealized child and the newborn—for example, the birth of a boy when a girl was hoped for. Resolution of this discrepancy is a developmental task of parenthood, and it is essential to the establishment of a healthy parent-child relationship. If the discrepancy is too great, as in the birth of an infant with a serious problem, the resulting emotional stress may be overwhelming.

The birth of a child with a serious disorder abruptly ends the psychologic attachment the parents have formed for the child they idealized during pregnancy. They must now deal with loss of this wished-for, healthy child. Their fears have been realized, and they are faced with meeting the demands of this child for care and affection. The parents' grief places overwhelming demands on them, especially when their own psychologic and physiologic resources have been depleted by the birth experience.

Most parents are able to deal with the impact of the loss, even though most require considerable time to resolve their grief. When parents are unable to face the reality of the infant's condition, they may withdraw from the situation either physically or emotionally. Parents often extend this avoidance behavior to include the infant. They are unable to face the infant and do not visit the child in the nursery or the pediatric unit. Sometimes it takes time for the parents to master their own feelings before they are able to deal constructively with the situation. A more subtle form of isolation is seen in parents who are very objective in their behavior toward the infant and his defect. They are intellectually concerned with their infant's medical care, but they display no emotional involvement. Their attention is focused on the abnormality, not on the infant.

Parental reactions depend to a large extent on the type and severity of the defect. A gross, visible anomaly, especially one involving the face, elicits a more intense emotional response than one that is less apparent, such as a heart defect. The extent of the impairment cannot be used as a criterion to determine the degree of parental depressive reactions. Also, because of their limited contact with congenital defects, the parents' perceptions of the situation may be distorted; much depends on feelings they may have experienced with a similar abnormality. Therefore, their reactions may seem out of proportion to the actual extent and severity of the impairment as viewed by health professionals.

Parental responses after the birth or after discovery of the diagnosis. Besides grieving for the loss of a perfect child, parents are faced with many practical difficulties. They may have excessive demands placed on their time, energy, and financial resources. Depending on the roles assumed by each spouse, the wife often receives the brunt of the time and energy demands and the husband, the financial responsibilities. However, with changing sex roles these responsibilities may be shared or shifted more heavily to one member. For example, the working mother may feel the need to continue employment to help defray the expenses, but this also incurs the added burden of additional child/home responsibilities.

The result can eventually be marital conflicts as one partner views his or her share as unequal. In addition, the partner who is not included in the caregiving activities may feel neglected, since all the attention is directed toward the child, and resentful that he or she is not sufficiently informed to be competent in the care. Without active participation in the care of the child, the parent has little appreciation of the time and energy involved in performing those activities. When the less competent partner does attempt to participate, the other parent frequently criticizes the less skillful efforts. As a result, communication breaks down and neither is able to support the other. Unfortunately, the problems are seldom recognized until they are well established rather than early, when intervention can be most effective.

Although increased marital discord is common among the partners, studies show that the divorce rate is no higher than that for the general population (Kalnins, 1983; Sabbeth and Leventhal, 1984). The stresses often cited as having an impact on the marriage are (1) the home care program with the burden of care assumed by primarily one parent; (2) the financial burden; (3) the fear of the child dying; (4) pressure from relatives; (5) the hereditary nature of the disease (if applicable); (6) fear of pregnancy; and (7) the inconveniences associated with care, such as long waiting for appointments, lack of parking near care facilities, or lack of overnight accommodations. Certainly, these latter stressors are within health professionals' domain to minimize, if not eliminate.

These parents are less likely than most parents to receive positive feedback from transactions with their child. Parenting such children may be a series of unrewarding experiences, which continually support the parents' feelings of inadequacy and failure. These responses may be most evident in parents who are responsible for the child's care. For example, they may become preoccupied with their ability to carry out certain procedures, overlooking the child's personal comfort and satisfaction or failing to praise him for anything less than perfect cooperation or performance. They often pursue a frustrating activity until they achieve "success"—long after the child has become irritable and uncooperative. They may unrealistically withhold privileges until the child completes a certain task or exercise. As a result, the parent becomes caught in a pattern of interaction that is mutually unrewarding and minimally productive. For these parents it may be beneficial to reduce the quantity of time spent with the child to increase the quality of the relationship.

Communication tends to be centered on the affected child, with mothers typically assuming the role of interpreter between the child and other family members. This, combined with mothers' heavy investment in the caregiving role, leads to a very close relationship between the child and parent, usually the mother. However, problems frequently arise because the mother interferes with the child's functioning at maximum potential (Cleveland, 1980). Levels of stress appear to be related to the ease with which mothers can relate to their children and the demands their children make on them. Feelings of restriction and social isolation add further stress.

Compared to mothers, fathers generally have fewer opportunities to do something directly helpful for the child, such as taking the child to the physician, the drugstore, the physical therapist, the special school, or other special health services. Organizations for parents of children with special needs tend to offer fewer services to fathers. Fathers are less adequately provided for than are mothers by supportive mental health services. As a result, they have fewer opportunities available to them to mourn the loss of the perfect child and to deal with lowered self-esteem often associated with fathering a child with special needs. Their needs to adjust to the loss of a perfect male child may be even greater than the mother's when the expectations of immortality through a son can no longer be realized.

The main concerns of fathers of children with chronic illness often involve the child's future and the unpredictable nature of the illness (McKeever, 1981). Although fathers speak of intense feelings at the time of diagnosis, many believe it is their responsibility to support the wife during the crisis. Many fathers believe their marital relationship has been affected by the child's illness, a major change being less time to enjoy leisure activities together. A significant finding for health professionals is paternal use of denial in coping with the diagnosis and fathers' hesitancy to associate with support groups.

Siblings

Siblings are deeply affected by the special child's membership in the family. Younger siblings in particular may be affected because they are uprooted and displaced more than older children. For example, if the child with cognitive impairment is firstborn, he becomes the "youngest" by virtue of his developmental age. Conversely, the child born second becomes the oldest, often shouldering adult-like responsibilities. These children are often pressed into parental roles that they are unprepared to fulfill and that force them too rapidly through the developmental stages so necessary for normal growth (Seligman, 1987).

Siblings are likely to show symptoms of irritability and social withdrawal and to fear for their own health. Healthy siblings may have a wide variety of physical complaints, such as headache, abdominal pain, or symptoms mimicking those of the affected child, as a reflection of their anxiety and fear. Their reactions to the child often do not parallel the severity of the condition. For example, siblings of children with obvious but less serious physical problems may have more adjustment difficulties than siblings of children with less visible but more life-threatening illnesses (Lavigne and Ryan, 1979). However, other findings indicate that the degree of the child's disability has no significant effect on the siblings' adjustment (Breslau, Weitzman, and Messenger, 1981).

Most parents can identify specific behaviors in the well children that have a negative effect on the family, such as jealousy, increased competition and fighting among siblings, anger, hostility, social withdrawal, attention-seeking behavior, and a decline in school performance. However, positive behaviors are also cited, such as increased nurturing, cooperation, sensitivity, compassion, and mastery of new skills. A common pattern among the siblings is periods of good adjustment alternating with times of poorer adjustment (Taylor, 1980). As siblings reach adulthood, they may develop increased altruism and tolerance and an orientation to humanitarian interests (Siemon, 1984).

Siblings may reveal feelings of isolation, deprivation, inferiority, and inadequate knowledge about the child's condition. Their lives are most affected in terms of the parent-child relationship, the medical care and treatment, and play and socialization. For example, the greatest effect of the ill child on the well siblings is a feeling of isolation and of being outside the parent(s)/sick child dyad. This is often increased by social restriction in peer relationships because of additional responsibilities in the home. Many siblings report receiving rewards in terms of "bribes" to overlook shortcomings in their parent-child relationship, but few receive any reward in the form of praise, personal attention, or tangible items. They often feel left out and uninvolved in the child's care, especially when the child is treated away from home. In particular they report feeling ignored by health care members, a finding that stresses the need for nurses to include the siblings as much as possible in what is happening to the affected child.

Extended Family Members and Society

Two other groups of people may experience the effects of the child with special needs: (1) significant nonnuclear family members or friends and (2) society as a whole. Although extended family relationships are often helpful to parents in rearing a child with special needs, they may also be sources of stress. Grandparents may have more difficulty in accepting the diagnosis than the parents themselves have, and parents may have concerns about the best way in which to respond to the grandparents' anger over the diagnosis or to their criticism regarding parental care. For example, grandparents or other well-meaning relatives may attempt to reassure the parents that the child "will grow out of" his slowness at a time when parents are struggling to accept reality.

Although society's views of individuals with chronic illness or disability are changing toward a more accepting, nonjudgmental, and open attitude, parents, siblings, and the affected child frequently are victims of prejudice, ostracism, or criticism. A great deal of this stems from public ignorance and fear, and this remains a crucial area for intervention by health professionals.

REACTIONS OF FAMILIES TO CHILDHOOD DEATH: THE GRIEF PROCESS

Although the existence of a chronic illness or disability is stressful for families, no event is more devastating than the threatened or actual loss of a child. Families, especially parents, are deprived of the joy and fulfillment of watching a child grow. All family members are affected by the loss, and their needs must be recognized for the family unit to resolve the grief. Nurses require a basic understanding of the grief process before (if the death is anticipated), at the time of, and after the death to provide guidance and emotional support to the survivors.

Anticipatory Grief

When death is the expected or possible outcome of a disorder, the child and family members experience behavioral reactions of anticipatory grief. Although the grieving behaviors vary and are experienced in varying intensities by different people, five stages are described (Kübler-Ross, 1969). These stages represent a set of *ever-changing behaviors* that surface as the need for them arises within the individual's attempts to cope with expected loss. They are not sequential stages that persons progress through, and the helping person's role is not to move the person from one stage to another, but to support the person in the stage at which he or she has arrived.

Denial. Just as a person responds with shock and denial to any serious loss (see p. 506), the first stage of anticipatory grief is also denial and disbelief. The "No, not me" reaction occurs regardless of whether the person is explicitly told the diagnosis. The duration of the denial depends on the coping mechanisms used by the person in previous crises, the support systems available to the person to help him give up the denial, and the reactions of others, especially physicians and nurses, to the resistance that is demonstrated. Unfortunately the need of others to deny the reality of the situation may be so great that it supports and fosters the patient's own denial and retards progress toward other stages.

Anger. The second stage in the dying process is anger. Although it usually follows denial, it may occur and recur at any time during the dying process. When the denial fails and the reality of the situation penetrates consciousness, the person's reaction is, "Why me?" The anger, rage, hostility, envy, or resentment may be directed at oneself or at others, notably members of the medical and nursing staff. However, unlike denial, anger is not socially approved or condoned. As a result, the person is often harshly judged for his angry refusal to accept mortality and may be further isolated in his struggle for life, and death.

To think about why the dying person or the parents of a dying child become enraged and resentful is only to begin to imagine the tremendous consequences of loss. Everything in life that the person dreamed of, hoped for, and expected to achieve is now only painful memories. He is angry toward those who are physically strong, who can make the dreams reality, and who live without pain or suffering. He is not angry at these people but at the things they represent, which for the dying person are no longer possible.

Bargaining. The next stage, and one that is often difficult to identify, is bargaining. It is the person's attempt to postpone the inevitable. The bargaining for additional time may be with God, with oneself, or with the most significant other person. Bargaining also occurs in children. The dying child may wish for additional time for himself, or the child who is facing the loss of a parent may hope for a delay of that person's death. One must listen very carefully to children to understand their symbolic language. One child who had recently been told that his leukemia had relapsed casually said to his mother, "Do you know what I wished for on my last birthday? Another birthday."

Depression. Without the denial to protect the person from realizing the seriousness of his condition, the anger to displace the emotional anxiety, and the bargaining to postpone the inevitable, the person eventually experiences depression. Generally there are two types of depression: for past losses and for anticipated or impending losses.

In a chronic terminal illness there are many reasons for the first kind of depression, such as loss of hair from therapy, loss of a body part or function, restricted physical ability, and change in life-style. The second kind of depression signals the person's preparation for the impending loss of all love objects. It is a difficult time for the dying person because he realizes the enormity of his loss. Unlike the survivors who are saying good-bye to one person, the dying person is saying good-bye to everyone and everything he ever loved.

Acceptance. The final stage of dying is acceptance. The person is no longer angry or depressed. If bargaining occurs, it is usually for a peaceful, painless death rather than for prolongation of life. It is not a happy time but one of inner peace and resolution that death is a certainty. The person may signal his acceptance by being disinterested in present or future events and preoccupied with past events, preferring few visitors and wanting quiet and solitude.

Such behavior may be very upsetting to others close to him, including health team members who have not reached the same level of acceptance. One critical nursing objective is to recognize the behaviors of acceptance in the patient and help others understand their relevance. Often the medical plan for continued treatment does not allow the patient the opportunity to accept the inevitable end. Nurses can be instrumental in planning care with all members of the health team, with fulfilling the patient's and family's wishes as the priority. This may involve the willingness to terminate extraordinary or lifesaving measures when death is imminent.

Acute Grief

When death occurs, whether it is expected or unexpected, acute grief develops within hours to days. Acute grief is a definite syndrome with psychologic and somatic symptoms that cause intense distress (see box). Reactions such as hearing the dead person's voice, feeling distant from others who want to help, or feeling overwhelming guilt for failing to prevent the death may make grieving persons fear that they are approaching a mental breakdown or insanity. On the contrary, these symptoms are normal, necessary, and expected responses. They signify that the survivor is working through the acute grief and will probably satisfactorily resolve the loss and resume or restructure a meaningful role in his social environment.

Although grief symptoms should appear immediately after a crisis, they may be delayed, be exaggerated, or be apparently absent. In the place of normal grief responses, distorted reactions, such as excessive hostility, depression with signs of suicide, or overactivity without a sense of loss, may occur. Such distorted reactions can be trans-

Characteristics of Normal Grief Reaction

Sensations of Somatic Distress
- Feeling of tightness in the throat
- Choking, with shortness of breath
- Marked tendency toward sighing
- Empty feeling in abdomen
- Lack of muscular power
- Intense subjective distress described as tension or mental pain

Preoccupation with Image of the Deceased
- Hears, sees, or imagines that the dead person is present
- Slight sense of unreality
- Feeling of emotional distance from others
- May believe that he is approaching insanity

Feelings of Guilt
- Searches for evidence of failure in preventing the death
- Accuses himself of negligence or exaggerates minor omissions

Feelings of Hostility
- Loss of warmth toward others
- Tendency toward irritability and anger
- Wish not to be bothered by friends or relatives

Loss of Usual Pattern of Conduct
- Restlessness, inability to sit still, aimless moving about
- Continual searching for something to do or what he thinks he ought to do
- Lack of capacity to initiate and maintain organized patterns of activity

Modified from Lindemann, E.: Symptomatology and management of acute grief, Am. J. Psychiatry **101:**141-143, 1944. Copyright 1944 American Psychiatric Association.

formed into normal grief with appropriate intervention, such as by a grief counselor. Nurses working with grieving families should be aware of the symptomatology of normal grief to recognize morbid grief reactions.

Mourning

After the death the lengthy process of grief work or mourning begins and extends into a period of adjustment to the loss, with attachment to new people and the development of new interests. Contrary to the common belief that mourning is completed in a year, data from clinical studies indicate that resolution of grief may take years and that there may be an *intensification* of grief during the third year (Rando, 1983).

Shock and disbelief. Shock, numbness, and disbelief are seen during the immediate phase of grief. As one parent described, "We were as prepared for our son's death as anyone could be, but it was a shock when in a moment his life was finished. I just can't get over the rapidity with which life ends." This temporary numbness protects the survivors from the overwhelming pain associated with grief. Often decisions are made automatically and only certain details are remembered.

Expression of grief. When the numbness fades there begins a period of intense grief characterized by a yearning and loneliness for the deceased. During this stage many of the signs of acute grief are evident, and physical complaints such as inability to sleep and appetite changes are common. There is a tendency to review the events of the deceased's life and to evaluate the relationship with the loved one. At this time feelings of guilt and anger are common.

Disorganization and despair. During this stage the pain of the loss is replaced primarily by emptiness, apathy, and deep depression. There is a feeling that life has no meaning and that the pain will never end. This is particularly relevant for parents. For example, mothers often comment that they feel they have suffered a double loss—loss of their child and loss of the mothering role (Wong, 1980). Feelings of estrangement from other loved ones are common, and social isolation may foster the depression.

Reorganization. Reorganization refers to recovery from the loss. It is a very gradual process in which the survivors again find meaning in living, readjust to life without the deceased, develop new or renewed relationships, and learn to live with the memory of the deceased with much less pain. It never means that the loved one is forgotten and the pain is gone. There always remains a deep ache that is never totally replaced with happiness and one that returns more intensely, for example, on holidays or anniversaries.

◆ *The Child with Special Needs*

Children with special needs are in many ways no different from any other children—they have the same requirement for love, security, and self-esteem. But in addition to dealing with all the normal developmental tasks of childhood, they must also cope with the challenges imposed by their illness or disability. While the family's responses are critical to the child's adjustment, other factors, such as the child's age, are important in planning individualized care.

IMPACT OF CHRONIC ILLNESS OR DISABILITY ON THE CHILD

The child's reaction to chronic illness or disability depends to a great extent on his developmental level, available coping mechanisms, and the reactions of significant others to him, and to a lesser extent on the condition itself. Knowledge of these variables is essential in providing the kind of support needed by these children to cope with a sometimes overwhelming situation.

Developmental Aspects

The impact of a chronic illness or disability is influenced by the age at onset. Chronic illness affects children of all ages, but the developmental aspects of each age-group dictate particular stresses and risks for the child. The following discussion presents the major stresses that these conditions can impose on children at each developmental stage. Children's developmental concepts of illness are discussed on p. 582. An understanding of these developmental factors facilitates planning care to support the child and minimize the risks.

Infancy. During infancy the child is engaged in the task of developing trust, which necessitates a reciprocal satisfying relationship between child and parent. When illness or disability occurs, this relationship is potentially affected. For example, a visible defect can retard parent bonding as the parent mourns the loss of the perfect child. In addition, prolonged illness may impose separations that prevent the child and parent from normal attachment and deprive the infant of the nurturing relationship.

The illness itself affects the infant, especially since sensorimotor experiences are critical at this age. Illness and/or disability often impairs the child's motor abilities by confining the child to a crib and lessening contact with the environment. Certainly the messages transmitted to infants about their bodies are influenced by the amount of pain and discomfort they experience. This lack of pleasurable sensations can lead to an irritable and unhappy child. Consequently, parents may interpret the behaviors as evidence that they are not adequately meeting the child's physical and emotional needs, which further affects the parent-child relationship and the acquisition of trust.

To compensate for some of these feelings, parents, especially the mother, may become overly involved with the infant and promote increased dependency. This is significant during infancy when one of the tasks is separation and individuation from the parent. Such a response hinders the child's future self-development and often leads to the pattern of marked dependency, fearfulness, and passivity. One of the critical aspects of this pattern is that it is amenable to change if intervention is begun *early*.

Toddler. The toddler is in the stage of autonomy; the need for mastery of locomotor and language skills is paramount. As the child learns to walk and talk he progresses toward becoming a separate person, both physically and psychologically. However, illness or disability can hinder mobility and deprive the child of mastery. In addition, overprotective parents can magnify the problem by setting limits on the child's exploration and experimentation for fear that the child will hurt or overexert himself. Even the most basic self-help skills, such as feeding and dressing, may be done for the child. Age-appropriate tasks such as toilet training may be delayed. With such limited opportunities for testing mastery the child soon fears to venture on his own and develops little confidence in his ability. Over time the child may feel defeated and become apathetic, passive, and clinging (Perrin and Gerrity, 1984).

Illness can impose separations that are detrimental to the toddler, for whom, like the infant, separation is the most anxiety-producing event. A chronic illness or disability can necessitate repeated hospitalizations and painful procedures. If the need to preserve the parent-child relationship is not appreciated, the child may become depressed and eventually detach from the parent. Children seem to have a tremendous capacity to withstand stress, provided their attachment to the parent is preserved.

Preschooler. The preschooler is in the stage of initiative; numerous tasks are achieved during this age that can be severely hampered by chronic illness and disability. Impairment can limit the preschooler's learning about the environment, especially in terms of social development. Rather than being encouraged to play with peers and participate in nursery school activities, the preschooler may be confined to the home, where socialization is limited to the secure and tolerant family. He may be allowed immature behavior because age-appropriate standards and discipline are not enforced. Consequently, when paired with children his own age or placed in school, he may not know how to act and can easily be criticized by peers who view him as a "baby." In fact, his illness or disability may provoke much less criticism than his inappropriate behavior. Faced with such reactions from others, in contrast to the security of the home, the child may gradually choose a life of social isolation and loneliness, especially during the school-age years.

One of the major tasks of this period is establishing sexual identity, and one of the principal methods is through imitation of sex-related activities. However, the sick child may have fewer opportunities to engage in such activity and may view the parent predominantly in the caregiving role, since this may be the focus of their relationship. In some families it is expected that the mother assume the care of the child while the father provides the financial base by working outside the home. This can limit the child's identification with the male role.

In addition to sexual identity, the child's image of his body is forming. The child's knowledge of his body is limited to what he sees, feels, and uses. If the child is chronically ill, his awareness of his body is focused on the pain and anxiety it causes him. For example, the young child may lose control over certain bodily functions, such as newly acquired bowel and bladder function, and feel embarrassed and inferior. The child with a disability may have difficulty forming a mental image of impaired body parts, such as paralyzed extremities. This poorly developed sense of body integrity makes children especially fearful of intrusive or mutilating experiences, which can be frequent during prolonged illness.

One of the more critical influences of chronic illness or disability on the preschooler is the feeling of guilt that he "caused" the condition by a real or imagined misdeed. This is probably less a factor if the child is born with the disorder than if it occurs during the preschool years. Such guilt can greatly affect the child's developing but fragile self-esteem. Unlike the child with a temporary physical impairment who has additional opportunities for achieving mastery and thus overcoming feelings of guilt and inferiority, the child with a chronic illness or disability experiences continual insults. Unless situations are structured for him to succeed, life can become a series of failures—of never being strong enough or good enough to compete with peers.

School-age child. The child of school age is striving to achieve a sense of accomplishment while overcoming a sense of inferiority. Successful mastery of this task depends on the child's ability to cooperate and compete with others. Consequently, physical impairments can greatly affect the ability to achieve and compete. For example, physical disability may hinder participation in sports, and repeated absences from school caused by illness can place the child at an academic disadvantage. To repeat a grade can saddle the child with feelings of shame, inadequacy, and inferiority. However, the decision to remain in the same grade can also enhance feelings of success because the work requirements may be easier and new classmates provide a second chance for forming friendships.

During this age there is a transition from relationships with family members to strong identification with peers. Peers increasingly influence the school-age child's view of himself and the child's self-esteem. Anything that labels the child as "different" can affect his sense of belonging to the group. Many children cope with their "differentness" by retreating from socialization. As they withdraw farther from the group, their sense of belonging diminishes and intense loneliness and isolation dominate. However, if they are helped to deal with their feelings of being different and to recognize their unique abilities, these children can cope very well. It is to be expected that all children will be unable to master some tasks and that they will feel some degree of inferiority. If this is stressed to children with physical impairment, the burden to achieve is lessened.

As school-age children identify more with the peer group and authority figures outside the home, there is a concurrent striving for independence from the family. However, the ill child may be forced into an extended period of dependency either from the disorder or from parental overprotectiveness. Attempts to demonstrate independence may be manifest as resentment toward the parents, refusal to comply with treatment, or risk-taking behavior, such as cheating on the special diet. If parents can understand that these behaviors represent a normal phase of development, they may be more tolerant and able to find appropriate outlets for independence (e.g., increasing the child's responsibility for home care).

Adolescence. The major task of the adolescent is to establish an identity of his own. Pubertal changes must be integrated into the self-image while the teenager is gaining control and mastery over his increased physical capabilities and sexuality. During early adolescence this takes place primarily within the peer group. Illness or injury at this time interferes with the teenager's sense of mastery and control over his changing body. He is different at a stage of development when being different is unacceptable to the peer group, who may view a disability in one member as a threat to the established uniformity by which all are measured. At no time of life is an individual so vulnerable to the emotional stress of biologic impairment (Hofmann, 1980). Appearance, skills, and abilities are highly valued by peers (Fig. 18-2); a teenager who is limited in any of these qualities is subject to rejection by this important group. This is especially marked when a physical disability interferes with sexual attractiveness.

Teenagers with special needs are faced with the task of incorporating their disabilities into the changing self-concept. The youngster who develops the illness or acquires the disability during the crucial adolescent years has more difficulty accomplishing this task than has the teenager who has been affected since childhood. It appears that the earlier the onset of a limiting condition, the better the individual is able to adapt to it. The youngster with a newly acquired disorder will have the additional task of grieving for his lost "perfection" while adjusting to the changes taking place as a natural course of events. He often feels rejected because of his appearance or his inability to engage in activities expected of a healthy adolescent. The threat is greatest during middle adolescence, when the teenager has less available energy to cope with illness, since his emotional resources are being used to meet the normal demands of this developmental phase.

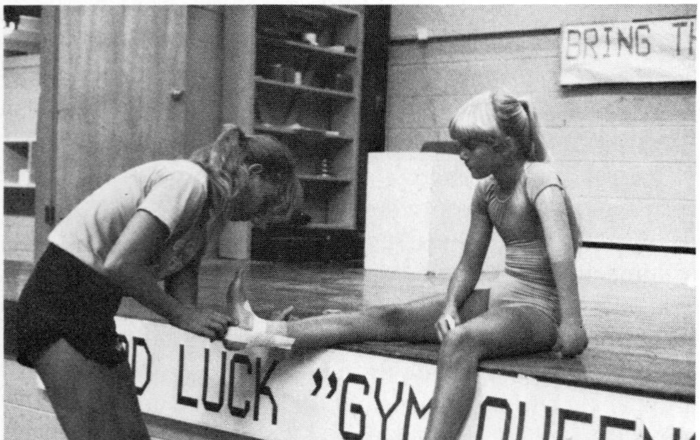

FIG. 18-2 Children with any type of impairment should have the opportunity to develop their skills. Despite her prosthetic left arm, this youngster excels in competitive sports.

Adolescence is a time for achieving independence from the family and planning for future goals and responsibilities. Adolescents with long-term chronic illness tend to be less future directed and less independent than well peers (Orr and others, 1984). Enforced dependency caused by physical impairment can exacerbate the parent-child conflicts surrounding independence. Lack of understanding from both parties can result in bitter feelings and intrafamilial turmoil. The tendency toward rebellion may be directed at the disorder and reflected in decreased compliance with treatment, denial of the disorder to preserve a sense of normalcy with peers, and risk-taking behavior that can place the teenager in jeopardy, such as driving a car despite a disorder that increases the chance of an injury. Such behaviors can further strain an already tense parent-child relationship.

Coping Mechanisms

Children's innate and learned coping mechanisms are very important in their ability to deal with their disorder. A number of individual factors influence the ability to cope with stress. Children who have poorer coping skills and therefore are more vulnerable to stress include (1) males; (2) children between ages 6 months and 4 years; (3) children with a "difficult temperament"; and (4) children with below-average intelligence (Rutter, 1983). In addition to these variables, the child's inborn traits and the social support available to the child influence the overall ability to adapt. Therefore the better the family copes, the better the child is able to deal with the stressors imposed by the illness or disability.

Because it is often easier to recognize the child who copes poorly with the illness or disability, it is helpful to describe those behaviors typical of the well-adjusted child. The well-adapted child slowly learns to accept his physical limitations but finds achievement in a variety of compensatory motor and intellectual pursuits. He functions well at home, at school, and with peers. He has an understanding of his disorder that allows him to accept his limitations, assume responsibility for care, and assist in treatment and rehabilitation regimens.

He expresses appropriate emotions, such as sadness,

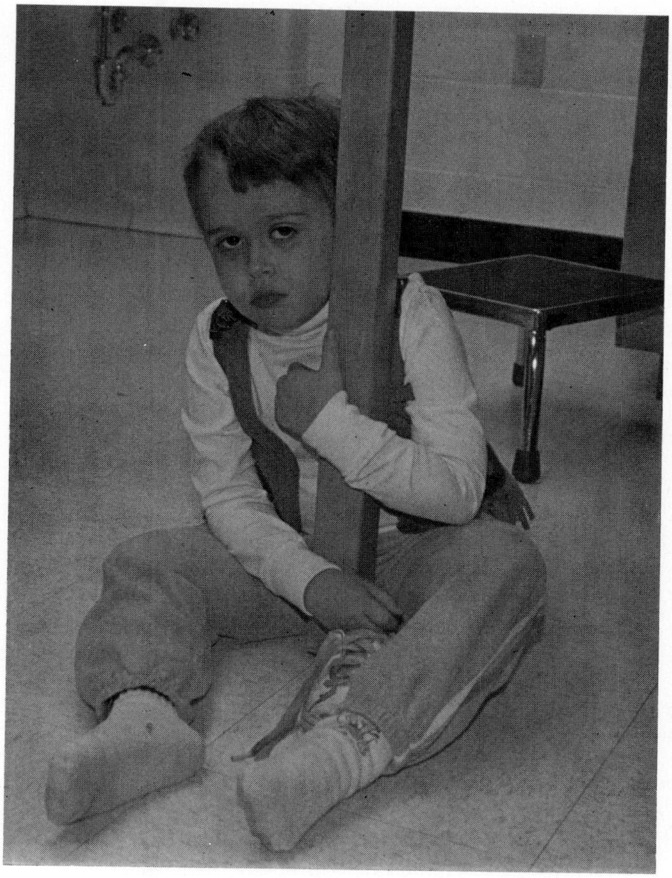

FIG. 18-3 Periods of sadness and anger are appropriate in the child's adjustment to a chronic illness or disability, especially during exacerbations of the disorder.

anxiety, and anger at times of exacerbations but confidence and guarded optimism during periods of clinical stability (Fig. 18-3). He is able to identify with other similarly affected individuals, promoting positive self-images and displaying pride and self-confidence in his ability to master a productive, successful life despite the disability.

Responses to Parental Behavior

The parents' behavior toward the child, especially in terms of childrearing, is one of the most important influencing factors in the child's adjustment. For example, children whose parents are overprotective tend to have marked dependency (especially on the mother), fearfulness, inactivity, and lack of outside interests. Children who are raised by overly solicitous and guilt-ridden parents are often overly independent, defiant, and risk takers. Children who are reared by parents who emphasize their deficits and tend to "hide" or isolate them appear as shy and lonely individuals who harbor resentful and hostile attitudes toward unaffected persons. In contrast children who are reared by parents who establish reasonable limits tend to develop independence that is appropriate for their age and achievement commensurate with their limitations. They often display pride and confidence in their ability to cope successfully with the challenges imposed by their disorder.

Type of Illness or Disability

The type of illness or disability also influences the child's emotional response. Interestingly, children with *more severe* disorders often cope better than those with milder conditions (Pless, 1984). Considering children's cognitive ability and their delay in achieving abstract thinking until adolescence, it is likely that an obvious condition is easier to accept because its limitations are concrete. For example, the child who is blind or crippled is constantly reminded of his inability to run. However, not only must the child with hemophilia live by rules he does not understand, but he also only vaguely and occasionally senses his illness, such as when he runs and accidentally initiates a bleeding episode. Therefore some chronic illnesses pose special threats to the child.

Diseases transmitted by hereditary factors may cause strain in the parent-child relationship once children discover the cause of the disorder. There may be considerable concern for their potential to transmit the disorder to their offspring. With improved survival among many of these young people, this is an increasingly important issue.

The severity, type, and visibility of the illness also influence the adjustment process and appear to be sex related. Boys seem to be more concerned about diseases or therapies that interfere with their ability to function independently and to achieve vocational and academic goals. Consequently, they may tolerate wearing a visible device or having a somewhat altered appearance as long as their physical and academic goals are not affected; for them confinement and restricted independence are less tolerable. Girls are more upset by conditions that they perceive to interfere with their ability to attract important others and maintain relationships. Thus they are more likely to tolerate restriction of movement and confinement provided they continue to look attractive; however, disorders or treatments that affect their appearance are devastating (Coupey and Cohen, 1984).

IMPACT OF IMPENDING DEATH ON THE CHILD

Children with life-threatening conditions must face the possibility of death, a realization that can have a profound effect upon their lives. However, the impact of impending death is greatly influenced by a number of factors. Two of these factors are the child's developmental age and the child's experience with his diagnosis.

Developmental Concepts of Death

Children's understanding of death parallels their cognitive and psychosocial development. Death has the least

TABLE 18-1

Children's Understanding of and Reactions to Death

Concepts of Death	Reactions to Death	Interventions
Infants and Toddlers Death has least significance to children under 6 months. After parent-child attachment and the development of trust is established, the loss, even temporary, of the significant person is profound. Prolonged separation during the first several years is thought to be more significant in terms of future physical, social, and emotional growth than at any subsequent age. Toddlers are egocentric and can only think about events in terms of their own frame of reference—living. Their egocentricity and vague separation of fact and fantasy make it impossible for them to comprehend absence of life. Instead of understanding death, this age-group is affected more by any change in life-style.	In the death of someone else, they may continue to act as though the person is alive. As the child grows older, he will be increasingly able and willing to let go of the dead person. Ritualism is important; a change in life-style could be anxiety producing. This age-group reacts more to the pain and discomfort of a serious illness than to the probable fatal prognosis.	Help parents deal with their feelings, allowing them more emotional reserve to meet the needs of their children. Encourage the parents to remain as near to the child as possible, yet be sensitive to the parents' needs. Maintain as normal an environment as possible to retain ritualism. If a parent has died, encourage a consistent caregiver for the child. If parents are unable to visit frequently, assign a primary nurse.
Preschool Children Believe their thoughts are sufficient to cause death; the consequence is the burden of guilt, shame, and punishment. Their egocentricity implies a tremendous sense of self-power and omnipotence. Usually have some connotation of its meaning. Seen as a departure, a kind of sleep. May recognize the fact of physical death but do not separate it from living abilities. Seen as temporary and gradual; life and death can change places with one another. No understanding of the universality and inevitability of death.	If they become seriously ill, they conceive of the illness as a punishment for their thoughts or actions. May feel guilty and responsible for a death of a sibling. Greatest fear concerning death is separation from parents. May engage in activities that seem strange or abnormal to adults. Because of their fewer defense mechanisms to deal with loss, young children may react to a less significant loss with more outward grief than to the loss of a very significant person. The loss is so deep, painful, and threatening that the child must deny it for the present in order to survive its overwhelming impact. Behavior reactions such as giggling, joking, attracting attention, or regressing to earlier developmental skills indicate the child's need to distance himself from tremendous loss.	Help parents deal with their feelings, allowing them more emotional reserve to meet the needs of their children. Help parents to understand behavioral reactions of their children. Encourage the parents to remain near the child as much as possible, to minimize his great fear of separation from parents. If a parent has died, encourage a consistent caregiver for the child. If parents are unable to visit frequently, assign a primary nurse.
School-Age Children Still associate misdeeds or bad thoughts with causing death and feel intense guilt and responsibility for the event. Because of their higher cognitive abilities, they respond well to logical explanations and comprehend the figurative meaning of words. Have a deeper understanding of death in a concrete sense. Particularly fear the mutilation and punishment they associate with death. Personify death as devil, monster, or bogeyman. May have naturalistic/physiologic explanations of death. By 9 or 10, children have an adult concept of death, realizing that it is inevitable, universal, and irreversible.	Because of their increased ability to comprehend, they may have more fears, for example: —the reason for the illness —communicability of the disease to themselves or others —consequences of the disease —the process of dying and death itself Their fear of the unknown is greater than the known. The realization of impending death is a tremendous threat to their sense of security and ego strength. Likely to exhibit fear through verbal uncooperativeness rather than actual physical aggression. Very interested in postdeath services. May be inquisitive about what happens to the body.	Help parents deal with their feelings, allowing them more emotional reserve to meet the needs of their children. Encourage the parents to remain near the child as much as possible, yet be sensitive to the parents' needs. Because of children's fear of the unknown, anticipatory preparation is very important. Since the developmental task of this age is industry, helping children maintain control over their bodies and increasing their understanding allows them to achieve independence, self-worth, and self-esteem and avoids a sense of inferiority. Encourage children to talk about their feelings and provide aggressive outlets. Encourage parents to honestly answer questions about dying rather than avoiding or fabricating euphemisms. Encourage parents to share their moments of sorrow with their children. Provide preparation for postdeath services.

TABLE 18-1

Children's Understanding of and Reactions to Death—cont'd

Concepts of Death	Reactions to Death	Interventions
Adolescents		
Have a mature understanding of death. Still very much influenced by "remnants" of magical thinking and are subject to guilt and shame. Likely to see deviations from accepted behavior as reasons for their illness.	Straddle transition from childhood to adulthood. Have the most difficulty in coping with death. Least likely to accept cessation of life, particularly if it is their own. Concern is for the present much more than for the past or the future. May consider themselves alienated from their peers and unable to communicate with their parents for emotional support—feeling alone in their struggle. Adolescents' orientation to the present compels them to worry about physical changes even more than the prognosis. Because of their idealistic view of the world, they may criticize funeral rites as barbaric, money-making, and unnecessary.	Help parents deal with their feelings, allowing them more emotional reserve to meet the needs of their children. Avoid alliances with either parent or child. Structure the hospital admission to allow for maximum self-control and independence. Answer adolescents' questions honestly, treating them as mature individuals, and respecting their needs for privacy, solitude, and personal expressions of emotions. Help parents understand their child's reactions to death/dying, especially that concern for present crises, such as loss of hair, may be much greater than for future ones, including possible death.

significance to infants younger than 6 months of age. However, once parent-child attachment and the development of trust have been well established, the loss, even temporarily, of that significant person elicits profound resistance from the child. Therefore, separation is the major fear associated with death.

Children between 3 and 5 years of age usually have heard the word *death,* and they have some idea of its meaning. They see death as a departure, possibly as a kind of sleep. They may recognize the fact of physical death, but they do not see that it involves the loss of the abilities a person has in life. The dead person in the coffin still breathes, eats, and sleeps. Death is temporary and gradual; life and death can change places with one another. Because of their immature concept of time, there is no real understanding of the universality and inevitability of death. Words such as *forever* and *everyone* have meaning only in the child's egocentric thinking.

Much of what pertains to the preschool period regarding the understanding of death also relates to school-age children, particularly those near 6 or 7 years of age. However, these children have a deeper understanding of death in the concrete sense. They may attempt to ascribe a more comprehensible meaning to the event by personifying death as a devil, God, a ghost, or a bogeyman. As some of these names imply, children attach a destructive connotation to death that is often associated with fear of mutilation and punishment. Naturalistic and physiologic explanations of death, such as "When you die, your body decays in the ground," are also common.

By 9 or 10 years of age most children have an adult concept of death. They realize that it is inevitable, universal, and irreversible. Their attitudes toward death are greatly influenced by the reactions and attitudes of others, particularly their parents.

Table 18-1 summarizes children's concepts of and reactions to death and outlines supportive interventions for each developmental stage.

Influence of Experience

Although children's concept of death is limited by their cognitive abilities, children develop an appreciation for what is happening to them through their experience with life-threatening illness. Studies conducted on these children have found that terminally ill children have some level of comprehension about their prognosis, even if they have been protected from the truth (Waechter, 1985). As these children acquire information about their situation, they develop different conceptions of themselves, a process that occurs in five stages (Bluebond-Langner, 1978):

Stage 1 Disease is a serious illness. New identity of "sick" child.

Stage 2 Discovery of the relationship of medication and recovery. Learns the taboos of disease and death.

Stage 3 Marked by an understanding of the purposes and implications of special procedures. Sense of well-being begins to fade and perceives self as different from other children.

Stage 4 Illness is viewed as a permanent condition. Sense of always being sick and never getting better.

Stage 5 Realization that there is only a finite number of medications. Awareness (directly or indirectly) of the fatal prognosis.

Time lapse between stages tends to be the same for all children regardless of age. Passage from the first stage to the second stage occurs rapidly on relapse. Passage through the second, third, and fourth stages takes somewhat longer, but passage to the fifth stage may take place as soon as the child learns of the death of another, and all knowledge from previous stages is quickly synthesized into a new self-awareness. Since experience, not age or intellectual ability, is the critical factor in passing through these stages, young children who have undergone treatment for several months may know more about their prognosis than adolescents whose disease is newly diagnosed.

◆ *The Nurse, the Child, and the Family*

Throughout the long process of caring for a child with special needs, family members become expert in management of their child's care. Nurses working with these families must become partners in the process. A supportive relationship includes coordination of care with family members, respect for their knowledge, and willingness to include their suggestions and recommendations whenever possible.

NURSING CARE OF THE FAMILY AND CHILD WITH SPECIAL NEEDS

The major nursing objective in caring for these families is to help the family remain healthy and functioning at maximum levels throughout the child's life or beyond if the child dies. The most effective approach is to use the *mutual participation model*, which invites the parents' early input, encourages them to be more accountable and responsible for the child's care, and reinforces the fact that it is not so much the condition itself that affects the child's progress but the family's ability to cope successfully with the child's problems.

ASSESSMENT

Since the nurse may meet a family during any phase of the adjustment process, several assessment areas are important. Knowledge of the family's available support system is essential and may include the marital relationship, nonmarital partners, extended family, friends, and professionals. The family's perception of the illness or disability is also an area that influences family adjustment. Assessment questions should focus on members' general knowledge of the condition even before the child's diagnosis was made, influence of religion on their thinking, imagined causes of the condition, and the effects of the child's disorder on the family.

Since the family's ability to cope with previous stresses influences the current situation, answers to questions about their usual coping skills are enlightening. Knowledge of concurrent stresses, such as financial, marital, career, or unemployment, helps identify families who may have fewer resources to cope with the child's needs. Finally, awareness of the family members' reactions to the child is important and can uncover the type of childrearing or attitudes that may hamper the child's optimum development. Sample questions designed to elicit information for evaluating the family in these areas are listed

TABLE 18-2

Assessment of Factors Affecting Family Adjustment

Factors Affecting Adjustment	Assessment Questions
Available Support System	
Status of marital relationship Alternate support systems Ability to communicate	Whom do you talk to when you have something on your mind? (If answer is not the spouse, ask for the reason.) When something is worrying you, what do you do? What helps you most when you are upset? Does talking seem to help when you feel upset?
Perception of the Illness/ Disability	
Previous knowledge of disorder Influence of religion Imagined cause of disorder Effects of illness or disability on family	Have you ever heard the word (name of diagnosis) before? Tell me about it (if answer is yes). Has your religion or faith been of help to you? Tell me how (if answer is yes). I know the doctors said there is no known cause of this disorder, but what do you think *really* caused it? How has your child's illness or disability affected you and your family?
Coping Mechanisms	
Reactions to previous crises Concurrent stresses	Tell me one time you've had another crisis (problem, bad time) in your family. How did you solve that problem? What other problems are you facing now? (Be specific—ask about financial, marital, and sibling concerns).
Reactions to the Child	
Childrearing practices Attitudes	Do you find yourself being a little more cautious with this child than with your other children? Do you feel as comfortable disciplining this child as compared to your other children? How is this child different from his siblings or other children his age? Describe your child's personality. When you think of your child's future, what thoughts come to mind?

in Table 18-2. Because the family's response in terms of support systems, perception of events, coping mechanisms, and reactions to the child may change at any point during the illness, assessment must be a continuous process.

Special challenges exist in assessing the child's feelings about having a disability. Chapter 6 presents several approaches to encourage a child to discuss feelings about the condition. The nurse should use a variety of communication techniques, such as drawing and play, as assessment tools rather than rely solely on parental reports. Often the child is a neglected partner in his care, and his unique needs are not identified.

The needs of fathers and siblings also need to be assessed, a goal that requires flexibility in scheduling appointments to include these important family members. When fathers know that their input is valuable, they will often change their work schedule to meet with a health professional. Since siblings can be of any age, the use of appropriate communication strategies for assessment must be considered. Nonverbal techniques such as those discussed in Chapter 6 should be considered for these children.

NURSING DIAGNOSES

A number of nursing diagnoses are prominent in the nursing care of the family and child with special needs. Others specific to individual cases become evident, especially when the child's actual disorder is considered. The most common nursing diagnoses are outlined in the Nursing Care Plan on pp. 531-537.

PLANNING

The nursing plan depends to a large extent on the child's actual illness or disability. However, the following are basic goals for all families and children with special needs:

1. Provide support at the time of diagnosis
2. Educate the family about the child's condition
3. Accept the family's emotional reactions
4. Help the family cope
5. Promote normal development
6. Provide support at the time of death

IMPLEMENTATION

The main objective in caring for the family is to help them cope effectively with those stresses imposed by the child's special needs. To achieve this goal the entire family unit must be viewed as the patient and included in every aspect of the implementation process.

Provide Support at Time of Diagnosis

The impact of the crisis usually occurs at the time of diagnosis, which may be at the time of birth, following a long period of physical and/or psychologic testing, or immediately after a tragic injury. It is a critical time for parents. Although they may not hear or remember all that is said to them, they frequently sense a certain attitude of acceptance, rejection, hope, or despair that may influence their ability to absorb the shock and to begin adapting to the family's altered future (Halpern, 1984). Although it is usually the physician's responsibility to inform the family of the diagnosis, nurses need guidelines to follow during the informing interview to provide the family with support during this critical time.

Parents are encouraged to be together when they are informed of their child's condition, thus avoiding the problem of one parent having to interpret complex findings and deal with the initial emotional reaction of the other (Fig. 18-4). Being together also provides an opportunity for the nurse to observe the interaction between the parents as they are confronted with the tragedy of discovering a serious problem in their child. Their emotional needs are acknowledged by showing acceptance of such expressions as crying, sadness, anger, and disappointment. Emotional support is offered by having tissues available if a family member cries and demonstrating through facial and body language that indeed this is a difficult and painful period. Although touching is a powerful expression of empathy, it must be used wisely. For example, touching can prematurely terminate free expression of feelings, especially when combined with statements such as "Everything will be all right."

Last, the informing conference should not end with presentation of devastating news. Instead the strengths of the child, his appealing behaviors, his potential for development, and available rehabilitation efforts or treatment are stressed. Parents are encouraged to view life with their child as very similar to life with other children. Their experiences should be thought of as a series of problem-solving processes that they are capable of handling, particularly with available professional feedback.

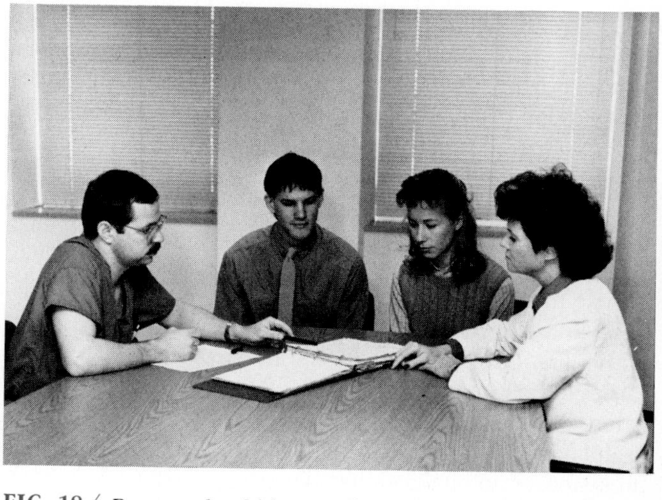

FIG. 18-4 Parents should be together when information about their child is given, especially during the informing conference.

The parents are assured that the nurse or another health professional will be available to answer questions and to provide further assistance as it is needed in the future.

The preceding discussion presented general guidelines; however, some situations require consideration of special problems, which are discussed briefly below.

Congenital anomaly. The first indication that all is not well occurs at the time of delivery. The atmosphere of happy anticipation suddenly changes to one laden with anxiety. Even when parents are unable to see the infant, they sense with terrified awareness the heightened and prolonged tension in the room, which conveys that something is seriously wrong. Personnel unprepared for this disturbing experience find it difficult to cope with their own feelings and react with feelings of frustration and resentment toward a situation that they are powerless to change. As a result they may forget about or retreat from the parents, who, at this moment, are suffering the most.

Most physicians believe that it is their responsibility to inform the parents of a congenital anomaly. Nurses and physicians need to clarify their roles in regard to revealing information, so that parents will be supported immediately after the birth of their child. For example, at the time of delivery, unless a pediatrician is in attendance, communication with the mother is delayed while the physician is involved with the mother's care. During this period the mother, unable to see her child and feeling the tense atmosphere, will believe either that the child is normal but that others do not share her enthusiasm or that the condition of the child is so terrible that the professional people in the room are unable to talk about it. A nurse, the person who is most likely to be free to support the mother and who is familiar with most common congenital anomalies, should have the freedom to make truthful statements about the defect.

The manner in which the infant is presented to the parents may well set the tone for the early parent-child relationship. It is best to explain briefly to them in simple language what the defect is and something concerning the immediate prognosis before the infant is shown to them, when they are more apt to "hear" what is said. Parents attach a great deal of meaning to the behavior of others during this critical period and watch the facial expressions of others closely for signs of revulsion or rejection. Presenting the infant as something precious, although incomplete, and emphasizing the well-formed aspects of the infant's body provide some reassurance to parents in this crisis period. It is important to allow time and opportunity for the parents to express their initial response to the situation. They are encouraged to ask questions and should receive honest, straightforward answers without undue optimism or pessimism.

Cognitive impairment. Unless cognitive impairment (mental retardation) is associated with other physical problems, it is often easy for parents to miss clues to its presence or to make defensive excuses regarding diagnosis. Since the impact of a diagnosis is associated with the reactions of shock and denial, parents may need help to develop self-awareness of the condition. The best approach lies not so much in careful preparation of how to relay the diagnosis but in planning situations that help them become aware of the problem. This may deliberately involve a prolonged period of evaluation to help the parents gain an appreciation of the child's strengths and weaknesses.

The nurse can encourage parents to discuss their observations of the child but must withhold diagnostic opinions. For example, the parents may be asked how this child's development compares with that of other siblings or peers, how he is doing in school, if they have any concerns about his progress, or what they have been told by others. By focusing on what the child can do and appropriate interventions to help him progress, such as infant stimulation programs, the nurse can involve parents in their child's care while helping them gain an awareness of his disability.

Physical disability. If loss of a motor or sensory ability occurs during childhood, there is usually little difficulty in revealing the diagnosis because it is readily apparent. The challenge lies in helping the child and parents over the period of shock and grief and toward the phase of acceptance and reintegration. One of the most helpful interventions is to institute early rehabilitation, such as using a prosthetic limb, learning to read braille, or learning to read lips. However, physical rehabilitation usually precedes psychologic adjustment. Therefore persons working with these children must be aware that even though the child is proficient in compensatory skills, he may still be grieving for his loss and in great need of emotional support.

A special dilemma exists when the cause of the disability is accidental, since parental and child guilt can be overwhelming. It is imperative at the time of diagnosis to avoid implying that the parents or child was responsible for the injury. However, at the same time the nurse should allow the parents and child the opportunity to discuss feelings of blame. The third-person technique (see p. 110) can be used to encourage parents to express their feelings by stating, "Sometimes it is so difficult for a parent to anticipate hidden dangers in a child's life," or "Parents often feel responsible for things that happen to their child even if there was no way they could have prevented it."

Statements directed at eliciting the child's feelings are, "Sometimes when tragic things happen, people often wonder what they did to deserve them," or "When people are warned not to do things, those warnings are easy to forget because the actual dangers may not be apparent, but then when something happens, they feel responsible." The nurse can either wait for a response with silence or encourage a reply with a statement such as, "Did you ever feel that way?"

Chronic illness. Realization of the true impact of a diagnosis of chronic illness may take months or years. Conflict over parents' vs the child's concerns may result in serious problems. For example, whereas parents worry about preventing bleeding episodes and joint deformity, the child with hemophilia may only focus on the activity restriction. Unless each member is able to gain an appreciation of the other's concerns, it is likely that no one's needs will be met.

A special dilemma arises when the illness is inherited, since parents may blame themselves and/or the child may blame the parents. This aspect should be discussed with parents at the time of diagnosis to lessen guilt and accusatory feelings on any person's part. The child should be allowed to express his feelings. Using the third-person technique helps open discussion in this area. For example, the nurse may comment, "Sometimes when a person has an illness that was passed on by the parents, that person feels angry or bitter toward them."

Multiple disabilities. The child with multiple disabilities may present special challenges because the child or parent may require additional time for the shock phase. The child or parent may only be able to attend to one diagnosis before hearing significant information regarding the other disorder. When an obvious and a more hidden disability coexist, such as cerebral palsy and mental retardation, the nurse must be careful to acknowledge parents' understanding and acceptance of both diagnoses. Not infrequently the parents intellectualize that any retarded development is the result of the physical impairment and resist accepting the intellectual deficit.

The nurse must also appreciate the devastating consequences of two disabilities to a child, especially if they interfere with expressive-receptive abilities. The overwhelming example is the child who is blind and deaf. Although both these defects may be present at birth, they may also have different onsets, such as partial deafness at birth with progressive loss of vision. In this situation the child's experiences with the outside world are severely limited.

Terminal illness. A particular dilemma arises when the diagnosis indicates a potentially life-threatening disorder. Not only do parents require much support to deal with their own feelings, but they also need guidance in how to tell the child the diagnosis. Sometimes parents wish to conceal the diagnosis from the child. They may believe that the child is too young to know, that he will not be able to cope with the information, or that he will lose hope and his will to live. A decision not to tell the child has several disadvantages. It deprives the child of the opportunity to openly discuss his feelings and ask questions, it incurs the risk of the child's learning the truth from outside and sometimes less tactful sources, and it may lessen the child's trust and confidence in his parents once he learns the truth.

While the decision to "tell or not to tell" ultimately belongs to the parents, they can be guided to see the potential problems involved in fostering a conspiracy. One way of approaching the subject is by asking, "*How* will you tell your child about the diagnosis?" rather than "What will you tell him?" The former question implies that the child should be informed of the diagnosis.

Exactly how and what to tell children about their disease or the possibility of death is a very individual matter. However, certain guidelines can be offered.: (1) the explanation should be tailored to the child's cognitive ability, (2) it should be based on knowledge that the child already has, and (3) it should be honest. Children's developmental concept of death is discussed on p. 516 and serves as a basis for the kind of explanation a child can understand. Finding out what the child already knows or what he is thinking before answering a question offers

THERAPEUTIC DIALOGUE

Questions on Death

Shortly after learning of the diagnosis of cancer and beginning chemotherapy, a school-age child has the following conversion with the nurse.

CHILD: What is happening to me?
NURSE: What do you mean?
CHILD: I feel so awful. I hate the throwing up after those drugs. Sometimes I think I may die.
NURSE: What do you think about dying?
CHILD: I get very scared. I don't know how it would be or if anyone would be there to help me. (Starts to cry; nurse comforts child in her arms.) Am I going to die?
NURSE: I don't know. You have a serious illness, but we hope these medications will make it go away. But no matter what happens, you won't be alone. People who care for you, like your parents and I, will be here.
CHILD: I'm glad. Being by myself scares me.

SUMMARY

Nurse remains silent to allow the child to continue with the conversation but stays with him for a short time to reinforce the promise that he won't be left alone.

important clues to the kind of answer the child is seeking. Honesty must be tempered with concern for the child's feelings. There is a difference between "cruel" truth and "gentle" truth. To tell someone that he has a potentially fatal disease and that he is probably going to die is cruel. However, telling a child the name of the illness and the reason for treatment instills hope, provides support from others, and serves as a foundation for explaining and understanding subsequent events. However, being honest is not always easy because the truth may prompt children to ask other distressing questions, such as "Am I going to die?" However, even this difficult question must be answered (see Therapeutic dialogue, p. 521).

Educate the Family

Educating the family about the disorder is actually an extension of revealing the diagnosis. Education involves not only supplying technical information but also discussing how the condition will affect the child. For example, it is of little benefit to discuss mental retardation in terms of numbers. Rather, parents need to understand what the child can do in terms of self-help, academic learning, and independence. Similarly the child who has lost a limb needs more than an explanation of the prosthetic leg. He must know the limitations it places on his activity as well as the opportunities available to him.

Parents also need guidance in how the condition may interfere with or alter activities of daily living. One area frequently affected is nutrition. Common problems are undernutrition as a result of food being inappropriately restricted, loss of appetite, or motor deficits that interfere with feeding and overnutrition usually caused by a caloric intake in excess of energy expenditure or boredom and lack of stimulation in other areas. Although the child requires the same basic nutrients as other children, the daily requirements may differ.

Another area that is part of all children's lives, but only recently has received attention in terms of children with special needs, is car safety. Children who need ventilators, who cannot sit upright, or who are in casts or other appliances often need adaptations of federally approved car restraints to receive the maximum crash protection.* These considerations, as well as other aspects of care that are affected by the diagnosis, are discussed as appropriate throughout the text.

Parents also need to be aware of the importance of communicating the child's condition in the event of a medical emergency. Young children are unable to give information about their disorder, and although older children may be reliable sources, after an accident they may be physically unable to speak. Therefore all children with any type of chronic condition that may affect medical care should wear some type of identification, such as a Medic Alert bracelet,* which lists the medical condition and a collect phone number for emergency medical records and other personal information, or a MediScope,† a cylinder-shaped pendant that contains a microfilm medical record and a magnifying lens. Other types of identification usually employ plastic-laminated cards, which are less convenient for young children.‡

Children need information about their condition, the therapeutic plan, and how the disease or the therapy might affect their particular situation. Children nearing puberty also need to understand the maturation process and how their disability may alter this event. For example, the youngster with Crohn disease should understand that this disorder is associated with growth failure and delayed puberty; the child with diabetes needs to know that hormonal changes and increased growth needs will alter food and insulin requirements at this time; and the sexually active girl with sickle cell anemia or systemic lupus erythematosus needs to be aware of the hazards of pregnancy. The information should not be given all at once but timed appropriately to meet the changing needs of the youngsters, and it should be described and repeated as often as the situation demands.

The subject of sexuality as it relates to the effects of the disorder is a prominent concern of adolescents, but they rarely initiate a discussion of this sensitive topic. Any probable interference in sexual function because of the disability should be discussed openly and candidly with the teenager. Adults often underestimate the degree to which adolescents engage in unrealistic fantasies regarding sexual activities and related matters. The health professional must be alert to cues that signal when the teenager is ready for more detailed and prognostic information about his condition relative to sexuality and reproduction.

Accept the Family's Emotional Reactions

One of the most supportive interventions is to accept the family's emotional reactions to the child's condition in as nonjudgmental a manner as possible. Although all families respond differently and in varying degrees of intensity, three responses are so common and often so poorly handled that they deserve special consideration.

Denial. The nurse's response to denial is a critical component of the individual's continuing need for this defense mechanism. The most effective method of support is active listening. Silence neither reinforces nor rejects denial (or any other emotional reaction) but implies a willingness and acceptance of the person's need for this behavior. However, silence alone can be misinterpreted. For example, if the person demonstrates denial, such as

*Information on safe transportation of children with special needs is available from the Automotive Safety for Children Program, James Whitcomb Riley Hospital for Children, 702 Barnhill Dr., Indianapolis, IN 46223.

*Medic Alert Foundation International, Turlock, CA 95381-1009. 1(800)ID-ALERT.

†**MicroDesign Systems,** P.O. Box 188, Arverne, NY 11692.

‡**National Safety Council Medical Information Card,** National Health & Safety Awareness Center, Dept. FP, 333 North Michigan Ave., Chicago, IL 60601.

by saying, "I am sure the doctors made a mistake," and the nurse responds silently and leaves, the person may infer disapproval, agreement, avoidance, or rejection from this behavior.

To be effective, silence and listening must be accompanied by physical and mental concentration and use of body language to communicate interest and concern. Direct eye contact, touch, physical geographic closeness, and body posture, such as sitting and leaning slightly forward, demonstrate silent but effective communication. (See also the discussion on p. 103.)

Guilt. Since guilt is such a common response and can cause family members tremendous anxiety, they should be told directly that there is no known cause of the disorder (when appropriate) and that they are not to be blamed. Using the third-person technique (see p. 110) is valuable in eliciting thoughts of guilt. For example, with children an appropriate statement may be, "When people get sick they often wonder if they did anything to make themselves sick." This allows children an opportunity to explore any feelings of responsibility they harbor.

If family members are expressing feelings of guilt, it is important to allow them to talk about their feelings rather than quickly trying to dispel them with long "scientific" explanations. An effective method in lessening guilt is to *encourage the irrationality of thought*. For example, one mother stated that her son probably developed cancer by sitting too close to the television, which she could have prevented by being more strict. By following her reasoning and talking about how *many* children sit close to the television and how *few* of them ever have cancer, the nurse was able to help the mother realize that this activity was not a cause.

Anger. Anger is one of the more difficult reactions to accept and deal with therapeutically. The responses to anger may be reciprocal anger, fear, acceptance, and/or encouragement. The first two reactions close off communication and express disapproval and rejection of the person. They most commonly occur when the listener views the anger as a personal assault. The last two responses allow the individual to ventilate his feelings in an atmosphere of nonjudgmental acceptance. Two basic rules for dealing with the angry person is to avoid losing one's temper and to encourage the person to talk. The following steps encourage expression of emotions, such as anger:

1. Describe the behavior: "You seem angry at everyone."
2. Give evidence of understanding: "Being angry is only natural."
3. Give evidence of caring: "It must be difficult to endure so many painful procedures."
4. Help focus on feelings: "Maybe you wonder why this happened to your child."

One essential element to the successful implementation of this process is to wait for the person to respond to a statement before proceeding to the next step. Since the objective of each statement is for the person to speak freely, the responses should avoid "yes" or "no" type of answers. For example, the behavior can be described as above or the nurse can ask directly, "Are you angry?" The latter question, however, may hinder further expressive communication and places the burden of subsequent conversation on the nurse, who should be the listener.

Help the Family Cope

In order for the family to meet the stresses of optimally adjusting to the child's condition, each member must be individually supported so that the family system is healthy. Although the family unit can indefinitely support a member who is in need of assistance, its greatest strength lies in every member supporting each other. The nurse should bear in mind that the "member in need" is not necessarily the affected child but may be a parent or sibling who is dealing with stresses that require intervention.

Parents. The nurse can provide support by being attentive to the family's responses to the child. Mothers and fathers need to experience success, joy, and pride in their child to give him the support he needs from them. Since parents of children with special needs have few role models to imitate, they need support to help them adjust. Above all, the nurse should ensure that the parents and siblings learn to perceive the child as a child first with unique and individual needs. The nurse needs to convey a humanistic, accepting approach of the child so that the parents can observe this acceptance. The way the nurse interacts with, approaches, touches, or holds the child makes this obvious. Any signs of rejection of the child, though subtle in nature, are readily interpreted by parents. This attitude of liking, concern for, and acceptance of the child should begin in early infancy and continue throughout the child's life.

Parents are asked for suggestions on care planning, implementation, and evaluation, as in the mutual participation model. The nurse can play a valuable role in ensuring that the child learns about his disorder and in fostering communication between child and parents so that the child shares his concerns with them. The parents are helped to realize the child's level of maturity and understanding and that his need for information changes as his development progresses.

Communication among all family members is encouraged. Parent group sessions are helpful in assisting parents to verbalize thoughts and feelings to each other but often do not take into account siblings' or the child's viewpoint. Therefore the nurse may need to set up a family session, such as during a home or clinic visit. Although the ideal situation is to have all the members present at once, this is often not possible within the confines of traditional nursing practice. However, inviting members to participate at various visits is an appropriate alternative.

Parents are encouraged to discuss their feelings toward the child, the impact of this event on their marriage, and associated stresses, such as financial burdens. For most families, regardless of their income or insurance coverage, financial concerns exist. The costs of caring for a child with special needs can be overwhelming. In addition, the family wage earner may have to sacrifice job opportunities to remain close to a medical facility or to avoid losing insurance benefits.

Fathers are encouraged to express their expectations for the child now and in the future. Because fathers tend to repress their feelings and feel less competent, the nurse acknowledges their difficulties and strengths, such as parenting skills and problem-solving abilities. Fathers are also encouraged to be involved with the child's care; maximizing their involvement while minimizing the mother's participation is effective in strengthening family relationships and preventing overdependency between the child and mother (Cleveland, 1980).

Numerous volunteer and community resources are available that provide assistance, rehabilitation, equipment, and funding for a variety of health problems.* National and local disease-oriented organizations may provide needed assistance and support to families that qualify. Many of these are discussed elsewhere in the text under the condition. State and federal departments of health, mental health, social service, and labor may be able to help locate appropriate regional resources. For example, state **Crippled Children's Services** provide financial assistance for children with many disabling conditions. Parents' organizations are especially helpful in providing information and support. Nurses should become acquainted with those in their communities and with vocational programs for special groups.

The child. The child, too, requires support for his interactions, adjustments, and efforts. Through ongoing contacts with the child, the nurse (1) observes his responses to the disorder, ability to function, and adaptive behaviors within the environment and with significant others, (2) explores the child's understanding of the nature of his condition, and (3) supports him while he learns to cope with his feelings. He is encouraged to express his concerns rather than to allow others to express them for him, since open discussions may reduce anxiety.

One of the most important interventions in helping the child to cope with a deviation from his peers is alleviating the child's feeling of being different and normalizing his life as much as possible. The principles in the accompanying box are fundamental in implementing the normalizing process (Krulik, 1980). Whenever possible the nurse should assess the child's daily routine for indications of lack of normalizing practices. The child who remains in a bedroom all day is in need of a restructured daily routine to provide activities in different parts of the house, such as eating in the kitchen with the family. Such children may also be deprived of social, recreational, and academic activities. For example, home and out-of-home treatments should be planned at times that interfere least with normal daily activities (Fig. 18-5).

Principles of Normalization

1. **Preparation.** Prepare the child in advance for changes that may occur from the illness or disability; for example, the child is told in advance of the possible side effects of drug therapy.
2. **Participation.** Include the child in as many decisions as possible, especially those relating to his care regimen; for example, the child is responsible for taking his medications or scheduling his home treatments.
3. **Sharing.** Allow both family members and the child's peers to be a part of the care regimen whenever possible; for example, the child is given his medication when the other siblings receive their vitamins; mother cooks the same menu for the whole family; and if the child is invited to another's home, the mother advises the family of the child's dietary restrictions.
4. **Control.** Identify areas where the child can be in control so that feelings of uncertainty, passivity, and helplessness are decreased; for example, the child identifies activities that are appropriate to his energy level and chooses to rest when he is fatigued.

Children who are concerned that their condition detracts from their physical attractiveness need attention focused on the normal aspects of appearance and capabilities. Health professionals must help strengthen and consolidate the self-image by emphasizing the normal, while at the same time allowing children to express anger, isolation, fear of rejection, feelings of sadness, and loneliness. They need positive reinforcement for compliance and any evidence of improvement. Anything that might improve attractiveness and contribute to a positive self-image is employed, such as makeup for a teenager with a scar; clothing that disguises a prosthesis; or a hairstyle or wig to cover a deformity or lost hair.

Siblings. As pointed out, the presence of a child with special needs in a family may result in parents paying less attention to the other children or expecting older siblings to take on greater responsibility for the care of the child. The siblings may respond by developing negative attitudes toward the child or by expressing anger in different forms. The nurse can help by using "anticipatory guidance," questioning the parents about what they believe is the best way to have siblings respond to the child and whether they have any concerns regarding the way in which they are assigning responsibility to older sib-

*General sources of information are **Clearinghouse on the Handicapped,** Office of Special Education and Rehabilitative Services, Room 3132, Switzer Building, C St. SW, Washington, DC 20202, (202) 732-1250; and **National Information Center for Handicapped Children and Youth,** P.O. Box 1492, Washington, DC 20013, (703) 522-3332. A comprehensive list of books and pamphlets for parents and teachers of children with disabilities is available from **The National Easter Seal Society,** 2023 W. Ogden Ave., Chicago, IL 60612, (312) 243-8400. In Canada: **Coalition of Provincial Organizations of the Handicapped,** 929 294 Portage Ave., Winnipeg, Manitoba R3C 0B9, (204) 947-0303; **Canadian Rehabilitation Council for Disabled,** Suite 2110, 1 Yonge St., Toronto, Ontario M5E 1E5, (416) 862-0340.

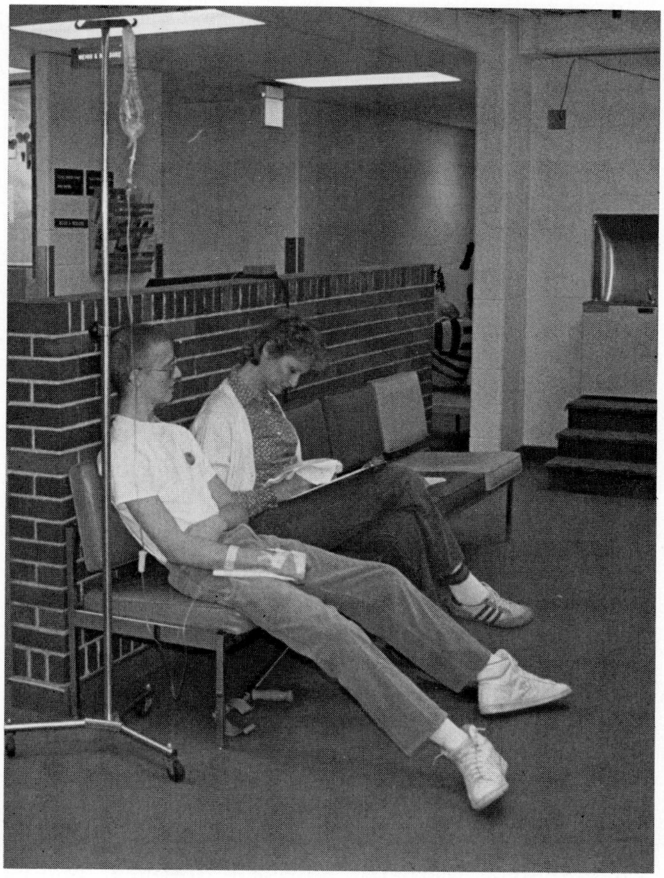

FIG. 18-5 Treatment often involves long periods of outpatient visits that should be scheduled at times that least interfere with the youngster's daily routine.

lings. This questioning should take place before serious negative effects occur.

Siblings may also experience embarrassment associated with the stigma of a disorder such as mental retardation. Parents are then faced with the difficulty of responding to this embarrassment in an understanding and appropriate manner without punishing the siblings for feeling the way they do. Parents should talk with the siblings about how they view their affected sibling. For example, when the child is mentally retarded, siblings may express fears of their ability to bear children with normal intelligence. Adolescents in particular may not be able to discuss these vital issues with their parents and may prefer to consult with the nurse. Many siblings benefit from sharing their concerns with other young people who are experiencing a similar situation.

The nurse must be sensitive to the reactions of siblings and whenever possible intervene to promote more positive adjustments. For example, siblings often mention that they are expected to take on additional responsibilities to help the parents care for the child. It is not unusual for them to express a positive reaction to assuming the extra duties but a negative response to feeling unappreciated for doing so. Such feelings can often be minimized by encouraging the siblings to discuss this with the parents and by suggesting to parents ways of showing gratitude, such as an increase in allowance, special privileges, and most significantly verbal praise.

Extended family members and society. The nurse must also be sensitive to the family's cues regarding sources of stress from extended members, such as grandparents. For example, the nurse may encourage the parents to invite the grandparents to be present during one of the child's visits to a clinic, during the diagnostic workup, or at a parent conference or to provide appropriate literature. Including grandparents in a discussion in which they can share their concerns may help them deal with their feelings, thus reducing stress on the entire family. Grandparents' feelings of blame and anger as well as any "cure fantasies" they harbor can be brought out in the open and discussed if necessary. Grandparents can be helped to understand the effects of their behavior on the family with an appropriate statement, such as, "Your daughter is currently experiencing a great deal of pain and anguish. We realize that this is difficult for you as well as your daughter; however, you can be of tremendous help by being supportive toward her."

Considerable stress can also arise from nonfamilial sources, such as friends, neighbors, or strangers. Inability to cope with comments about the disorder or curious stares by others may foster the tendency to isolate and protect the child within the home. The family needs guidance in preparing for these inevitable experiences. One approach is encouraging parents to dress the child as much as possible like other children. Good grooming is very important in minimizing differences in appearance. Through role playing parents can practice responses to comments such as, "Is your child retarded?" or "Has he always been crippled?" Through parent groups family members can share experiences and learn from each other how to successfully deal with probing questions or unkind remarks. Such interventions must include the siblings and the affected child, who also must face and deal with these events. Nurses can be instrumental in teaching young healthy children about disabilities to familiarize them with the special needs and abilities of these individuals.

Promote Normal Development

Aside from knowledge of the condition and its effect on the child's abilities, the family must be guided toward fostering appropriate development in their child. With appropriate planning and knowledge of strategies to improve the child's functional abilities, most children can live fulfilling and productive lives.

Early childhood. During infancy the child is achieving basic *trust* through a satisfying, intimate, consistent relationship with his parents. However, the affected child's early existence may be stressful, chaotic, and unsatisfying. Consequently he may need more parental support and expressions of affection to achieve trust. Likewise the parents require assistance in finding ways to meet the infant's needs, such as how to hold a rigid or flaccid infant, how to feed a child with tongue thrust or episodes of dyspnea, and how to stimulate a child who seems incapable of achieving any skills. If hospitalizations are frequent or prolonged, every effort is made to preserve the parent-child relationship (see also Chapter 20).

During early childhood the goal is to achieve separation from parents, autonomy, and initiative. However, the natural parental response to having a sick child is overprotection. Parents need help in realizing the importance of brief separations from the child and from others involved in the child's care and of providing social experiences outside the home whenever possible. Respite care, which provides temporary relief for family members, is essential in allowing caregivers time away from the daily burdens.

Young children also need the opportunity to develop independence. Frequently the child is able to learn self-help skills, such as holding the bottle, finger feeding, and removing simple articles of clothing, but the parent continues to perform the act. Therefore the nurse must guide parents to the usual milestones expected from the child.

When a child is unable to perform a skill independently, functional aids should be used (see p. 547 for feeding aids). With innovation many adaptations can be implemented in children's environments to increase their mobility and independence and allow them to play like other children their age. For example, with slight modifications, a child with physical limitations may be able to ride a tricycle* (Fig. 18-6).

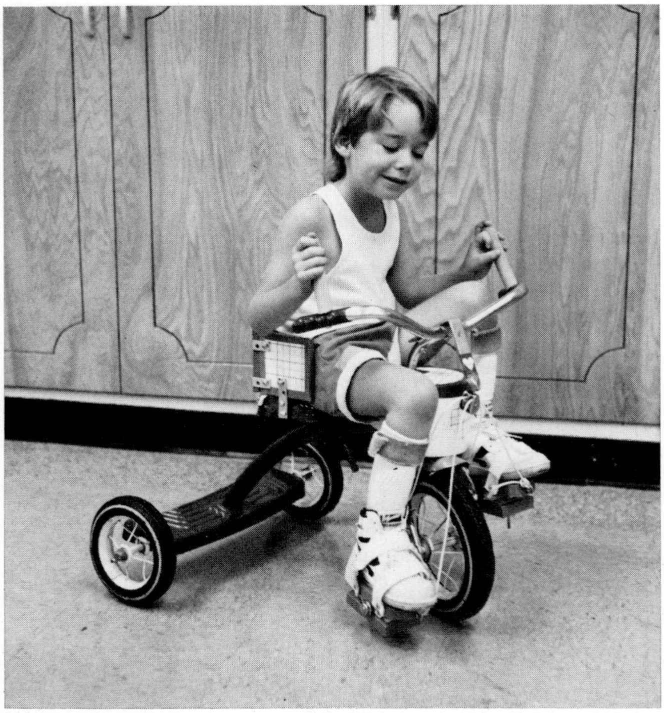

FIG. 18-6 A modified tricycle with block peddles, Velcro straps for support, and modified seat and handle bars can help a child with disabilities gain mobility.

Another critical component for normal child development is discipline. Unfortunately this is one of the child-rearing practices eliminated earliest when parents react with "overbenevolence." Not only does lack of discipline destroy the child's security because he has no boundaries on which to test out his behavior, it also fails to teach the child socially acceptable behavior and creates resentment and hostility among the siblings if different standards are applied to each child. The nurse's responsibility is to help parents learn successful methods of controlling behaviors before they become problems (see Chapter 4).

School age. For school-age children, the major tasks are entry into school and achieving a sense of industry. While the importance of school in the life of all children is well known, school absences are significantly higher among children with chronic illness than among their healthy peers (Weitzman, Walker, and Gortmaker, 1986). The more school absences the child experiences, the more difficult it is to resume attendance and "school phobia" may result. To prevent school phobia the child should return to school as soon as possible following diagnosis or treatments.

Preparation for entry into or resumption of school is best accomplished through a team approach with the parents, child, school teacher, school nurse, and primary nurse in the hospital. Ideally this planning should begin before hospital discharge, provided the child is well enough to resume usual activities. A structured plan should be developed, with attention to those aspects of care that must be continued during school hours, such as administration of medication or other treatments.

Children also need preparation before entering or resuming school. Having a tutor in the hospital or home as soon as children are physically able helps them realize that school will continue and gives them time to consider this prospect (Fig. 18-7). They need to investigate possible answers to the many questions others will ask. One method of anticipatory preparation is to role play, with the child as the "returned pupil" and the nurse or parent as "other schoolmates." If the child returns to school with some obvious physical change, such as hair loss, amputation, or visible scar, the nurse might also ask questions about these alterations to prompt preparatory responses from the child.

Classroom peers also need preparation, and a joint plan of the school teacher, nurse, and child is best. At a minimum the classmates should be given a description of the child's condition, prepared for any visible changes in the child, and allowed an opportunity to ask questions. The child should have the option of attending this session. As the child's condition changes, particularly if the illness is potentially fatal, school personnel, including the

*For information about the HOT (Hand Operated Tricycle) Project, contact Telephone Pioneers of America—AT-39, Rolling Meadows—Chapter 93, 3800 Gold Road, Rolling Meadows, IL 60008.

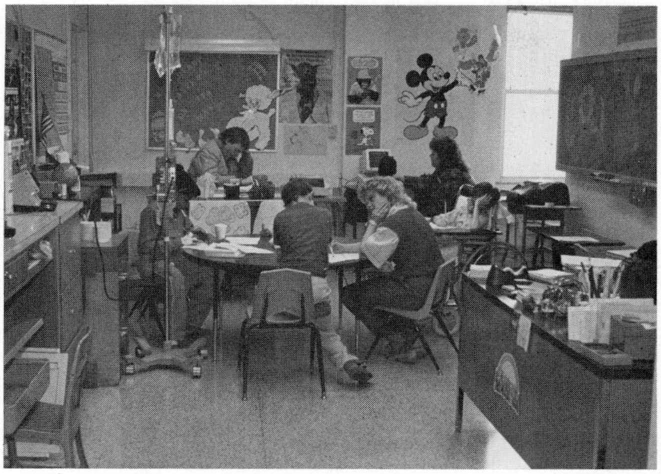

FIG. 18-7 Children with special needs should continue their schooling as soon as their condition permits.

students, need periodic appraisal of the child's status and preparation for what to expect.

Children with special needs are encouraged to maintain or reestablish relationships with peers and to participate according to their capabilities in any age-appropriate activities. Alternative activities may be substituted for those that are impossible or that place a strain on the child's condition. It is important for these children to have the opportunity to interact with healthy peers as well as to engage in activities with groups or clubs composed of similarly affected age-mates. Such organizations as ostomy clubs, diabetes clubs, and cerebral palsy groups share information and provide support related to the special problems the members face.

Adolescence. Adolescence can be a particularly difficult period for the teenager and family. All the needs already discussed apply to this age-group as well; however, fostering independence and autonomy is particularly important at this time. This can be accomplished by encouraging the teenager to assume responsibility for making and keeping appointments (ideally alone), by encouraging self-management of the disease, and by helping him make decisions regarding his life whenever possible. Age-appropriate pursuits are encouraged, such as driving a car, making plans for college, or securing a job. Planning for the future is a prominent concern.

Establish Realistic Future Goals

One of the most difficult adjustments is setting realistic future goals for the child and for those involved in his continued care. Sometimes the impact of this decision does not surface until the child finishes school or the parents near retirement, when a crisis can arise because all the family roles and relationships that maintained stability are now disrupted.

Planning for the future should be a gradual process. All along the parents should cultivate realistic vocations for the child. For example, if the child has a physical disability, he is directed to intellectual, artistic, or musical pursuits. If the child is developmentally disabled, he is taught a skill that can be performed in a special workshop. In this way the child's development proceeds in the direction of self-support through gainful employment.

With prolonged survival young people with chronic illnesses must deal with new decisions and problems, such as marriage, employment, and insurance coverage. Many of these individuals are capable of gainful employment and may choose to marry and raise a family. For those whose conditions are genetic, there is the need for counseling regarding future offspring. Prospective spouses often benefit from an opportunity to discuss their feelings regarding marriage to an individual with continued health needs and possibly a limited life span. Health insurance coverage is a critical issue because some private carriers may no longer insure a young person who leaves home or may be unwilling to reinsure the person who is independent. Life insurance is another dilemma, especially when children have serious defects, such as congenital heart anomalies. These issues are only beginning to receive attention but will become increasingly prominent as the number of survivors increases.

Unfortunately vocational pursuits and independence are not realistic goals for all persons. Persons with multiple or severe disabilities may require lifelong care and assistance. In these situations parents must look to the time when they will no longer be able to care for their child. Residential placement may be very difficult unless the family mutually participates in the decision-making and planning process. Placement outside the home should not be viewed as abandonment. Not infrequently it is the only way to preserve the family unit. The nurse should help the family investigate suitable placements, discuss their feelings regarding this decision, and explore measures to maintain meaningful communication with the member who has a disability.

Provide Support at the Time of Death

For some families no options for their child's future exist because the child dies. These families require compassionate, competent nursing care during the child's terminal phase, at the death, and during the bereavement (postdeath) period. Guidelines for supporting grieving family members are given in the box (p. 528) and Table 18-1.

Terminal phase. When death is anticipated, a terminal phase, the time of dying before the actual death, presents the opportunity for the family to decide the kind of care they wish for their child. As the group of health professionals who are most involved with families, nurses are in a excellent position to ensure that families are given the options available to them at the time of death. The nurse's first responsibility is to explore the family's wishes. This is best done in concert with the physician but at times may need to be initiated by the nurse. Statements such as, "Tell me about your thoughts for the kind

*Nursing Guidelines for Supporting Grieving Families**

General

- Stay with the family; sit quietly if they prefer not to talk; cry with them if desired
- Accept the family's grief reactions; avoid judgmental statements, e.g., "You should be feeling better by now"
- Avoid offering rationalizations for the child's death, e.g., "You should be glad your child isn't suffering anymore"
- Avoid artificial consolation, e.g., "I know how you feel" or "You are still young enough to have another baby"
- Deal openly with feelings such as guilt, anger, and loss of self-esteem
- Focus on feelings by using a feeling word in the statement, e.g., "You're still feeling all the pain of losing a child"; see also Facilitative responding, p. 110
- Refer the family to an appropriate self-help group or for professional help if needed

At the Time of Death

- Reassure the family that everything possible is being done for the child, if they wish lifesaving interventions
- Do everything possible to ensure the child's comfort, especially relieving pain
- Provide the child and family the opportunity to review special experiences or memories in their lives
- Express personal feelings of loss and/or frustrations, e.g., "We will miss him so much" or "We tried everything; we feel so sorry that we couldn't save him"
- Provide information that the family requests and be honest
- Respect the emotional needs of family members, such as siblings, who may need brief respites from the dying child
- Make every effort to arrange for family members, especially parents, to be with the child at the moment of death, if they wish to be present
- Allow the family to stay with the dead child for as long as they wish and to rock, hold, or bathe the child
- Provide practical help when possible, such as collecting the child's belongings
- Arrange for spiritual support, such as clergy; pray with the family if no one else can stay with them

After the Death

- Attend the funeral or visitation if there was a special closeness with the family
- Initiate and maintain contact, e.g., sending cards, telephoning, inviting them back to the unit, or making a home visit
- Refer to the dead child by name; discuss shared memories with the family
- Discourage the use of drugs or alcohol as a method of escaping grief
- Encourage all family members to communicate their feelings rather than to remain silent to avoid upsetting another member
- Emphasize that grieving is a painful process that often takes *years* to resolve

*The *family* refers to all significant persons involved in the child's life, such as the parents, siblings, grandparents, or other close relatives or friends.

of care you want your child to receive when he is dying" or "Have you considered the kinds of interventions you would like us to use when your child is near death?" can begin discussion of this sensitive but critical aspect of terminal care.

One of the issues the family should discuss is the extensiveness of lifesaving measures as death approaches. To make an informed decision, the family needs an honest appraisal of the child's prognosis, especially if the condition is a sudden illness or injury. If parents choose "no code," they are assured that this does not mean "no care" and that everything possible will be done to make the child comfortable. Once a decision to not resuscitate is made, it must be communicated to all members of the health team, including a *written* medical order that specifies the exact nature of the treatments that are to be withheld. Do not resuscitate (DNR) orders should be reviewed on a regular basis (Olson and Hooke, 1988).

Another important option for the family should be the choice of hospice* or hospital care for the terminal stage of illness. Hospital care refers to the traditional practices of caring for dying patients in an acute care facility; hospice is a concept, not necessarily a facility, that is intended to maximize the present quality of life whenever there is no reasonable expectation of cure (Corr and Corr, 1985). The three basic ways of providing hospice care are in a hospice, in a facility that employs the hospice concept, or in the child's home. If the home is chosen, the goal is to enable the child and family to enjoy the best possible quality of life until the time of death. The child may or may not die in the home.

Regardless of where the child is cared for during the terminal stage, both the child and family commonly experience the following fears: (1) fear of what the actual death will be like, (2) fear of dying alone or not being present when the child dies, and (3) fear of pain. Nurses play a major role in managing care so that each of these fears is lessened. Although no one can predict exactly what the child's death will be like, the nurse can explore the family's expectations, clarify misconceptions, and supply information based on how the death is most likely to occur. Since the child and family have fears of isolation and loneliness, their wishes to be together must be respected (Fig. 18-8). If the family members temporarily leave the child's room, they need reassurance that they will be summoned if the child's condition worsens (see Table 18-3 for signs of approaching death.)

Every parent's wish is for his child to die a comfortable death and no nursing intervention is more important than control of pain. Ideally pain should be managed throughout the terminal phase on a *preventive schedule*, with adjustments made as needed to provide maximum comfort. Optimum pain relief requires using narcotic analgesics such as morphine, increasing doses of narcotics beyond

*Information can be obtained from **Children's Hospice International**, 101 King St., Suite 131, Alexandria, VA 22314.

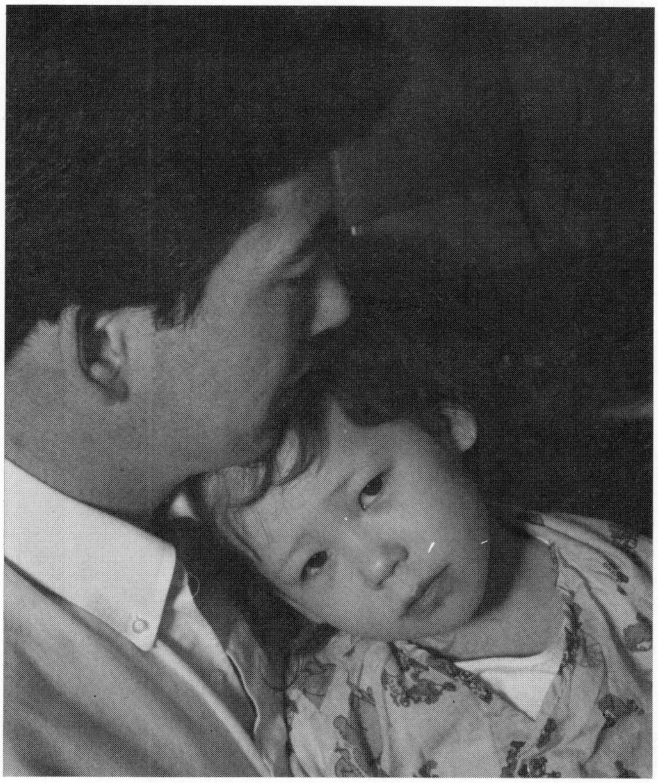

FIG. 18-8 For the dying child there is no greater comfort than the security and closeness of a parent.

those normally recommended, decreasing the duration between doses, and changing routes of administration to comply with the child's needs and wishes. Whenever possible the oral route is preferred, but when no longer possible, continuous intravenous infusion or rectal administration may provide the greatest benefit. Any nonpharmacologic measures that may augment pain relief and promote relaxation are employed, such as cutaneous stimulation (for example, rocking or stroking the skin) or diversion (for example, reading to the child or playing music). (See also p. 587 for an extensive discussion of pain assessment and management.)

At the time of death. As death approaches, the nurse should recognize the physical signs and institute appropriate care to make the death as peaceful as possible (Table 18-3). The nurse should explain everything she is doing to make the child comfortable, even if the child does not appear to be coherent. The nurse can offer support to the family by visiting frequently, sitting quietly with them, and attending to their needs, such as bringing them some nourishment. Immediately after the death the family should be allowed to stay with the child as long as they wish. Many parents want to hold or rock the child one last time.

Although most institutions recognize the need for the family to spend time with the dead child, a dilemma may arise when the body is mutilated, as may occur in an accident or from a criminal act. Although the memory of the child's disfigurement can be extremely upsetting and generate concern for how much the child suffered, not seeing the body leaves the parents with imagined ideas of how their child looked, which can be worse than the reality and can delay the acceptance of the death (Miles and Perry, 1985). However, family members need preparation for this upsetting experience. They should be told what to expect and why certain parts of the body are covered or bandaged. They should be allowed to visit in a private room. Some people appreciate the presence of a nurse in the room with them; others prefer to be alone. Regardless of how badly the body is harmed, parents may want to hold the child. Such options are offered and respected. Family members should be given as much time as they need to say good-bye.

A topic that should be discussed when a child dies is tissue donation. For some families this may be a meaningful act—one that benefits another human being despite the loss of their child. Some states have "required request" laws that mandate that the hospital make a request for tissue donation from the family of the deceased, especially if the patient has been pronounced brain dead. The request should be made in a private and quiet area of the hospital and should be simple and direct, with questions such as "Are you a donor family?" or "Have you ever considered organ donation?" (Weber, 1985). The family should know that tissue donation incurs no cost to the donor family and does not mutilate the body or delay the burial.

At some point the nurse should discuss if the family has made preparations for the burial service and if the staff can help in any way. Parents often have concerns about the funeral, such as siblings' involvement in the death rituals. Although no absolute answers exist regarding the question of siblings attending the funeral or burial services, the general consensus is that the surviving children benefit from being involved in these events. However, children need preparation for postdeath services. They should be told what to expect, particularly how the deceased person will look if the coffin is open, allowed their private time to say good-bye, and permitted to stay as long as they wish. Ideally the parent should prepare the siblings. If the parent's grief prevents this communication, a significant family member or friend should substitute.

Postdeath. The crisis of loss does not end with the child's death. In many ways it only begins. Unfortunately, the child's death often marks the close of the family's contacts with health professionals involved in the care. Consequently, many of these families never receive the support and guidance that could assist them in resolving the loss. Fortunately, hospice programs recognize this need and provide regular follow-up after the death. In addition, self-help groups are present in many communities, such as **The Compassionate Friends,*** an international organization for bereaved parents and sib-

*P.O. Box 3696, Oak Brook, IL 60522-3696.

TABLE 18-3

Physical Signs of Approaching Death and Related Nursing Care

Signs	Interventions
Loss of sensation and movement in the lower extremities, progressing toward the upper body Sensation of heat, although body feels cool	Keep bedsheets untucked Keep child uncovered if sheets are bothersome Apply loose, cool clothing Keep fresh air circulating in room (open window, use small fan) Change child's position only as tolerated Give cool sponge baths Preserve physical closeness with family members (e.g., parent may want to rock child in chair or lie next to child in bed)
Loss of senses Tactile sensation decreases Sensitive to light Hearing is last sense to fail	Limit care to essentials May need to forego usual hygienic measures such as bath or clothing change but provide comfort measures (e.g. mouth care, wiping forehead, gentle back rub) Avoid bright, direct light, but do not keep room too dim Sit at head of bed where child can easily see face Talk to child in clear, distinct voice, not whispers Avoid conversation about the child in his presence
Confusion, loss of consciousness, slurred speech	Talk to child even though may not appear awake Play favorite music; may soothe child Offer calm reassurance and orient child to surroundings when awake Phrase questions for yes or no answers
Muscle weakness	Use pillows or other supports to prop child in comfortable position Carry (if possible) to other areas for diversion if desired
Loss of bowel and bladder control	Place absorbent pads under hips Help child to toilet if he desires
Decreased appetite/thirst Difficulty swallowing	Offer any foods child desires Avoid excessive encouragement to eat or drink Avoid foods with strong odors Serve foods that require the least energy to eat (soups, shakes) Feed slowly Provide mouth care before and after eating; lubricate lips with petrolatum
Change in respiratory pattern Cheyne-Stokes respirations (waxing and waning of depth of breathing with regular periods of apnea) "Death rattle" (noisy chest sounds from accumulation of pulmonary and pharyngeal secretions)	Administer anticholinergic drugs (atropine or scopolamine) to reduce secretions (lessens "death rattle," which can be distressing to family) Position with head slightly elevated or in well-supported sitting position if tolerated
Weak, slow pulse; decreased blood pressure	No intervention other than reassurance of family Do not disturb child with repeated measurements of vital signs

lings, and specialty groups such as **Parents of Murdered Children.***

Follow-up can help the family understand the process of mourning, particularly its duration and pain, and can provide assistance in making decisions that involve the loss. One especially difficult dilemma faced by many parents is the decision to have additional children. The advisability of having another child soon after the death is controversial. Consequently, the nurse's role cannot be one of giving answers but of assessing readiness for another pregnancy through knowledge of the parents' progress through grief and their motivations for conceiving.

At times family members may need assistance in their grieving. Mothers, in particular, often feel a great sense of loneliness and emptiness, and part of their resolving the grief is finding a substitute role that is fulfilling and rewarding. Nurses can be instrumental in this process by (1) preparing the mother for anticipating the *normal* feelings of emptiness, loneliness, and sometimes even failure, (2) helping her reevaluate her role as parent and spouse, stressing that giving up the lost child must occur before she can reestablish emotional relationships, (3) encouraging her to explore fulfilling activities that utilize her special interests, talents, and qualifications, and (4) supporting her as her role changes, particularly assisting with communication between affected family members (Wong, 1980).

Nurses should also be aware of behaviors that indicate siblings' difficulty with resolving their grief, such as persistent blame and guilt, patterns of overactivity with ag-

Text continued on p. 538.

*100 E. 8th St., Rm. B41, Cincinnati, OH 45202.

NURSING CARE PLAN

The Child with Chronic or Terminal Illness or Disability

Nursing Goals	Nursing Interventions	Expected Patient/Family Outcomes
HP-HMP Potential for injury Etiology: specify		
Decrease risk of injury	Assess environment for hazards if indicated Teach safety precautions Encourage activities that are compatible with the disease or disability	Child remains free of injury and complications
Help child adjust to restricted activities	Help devise alternatives for restricted activities and help child cope with physical limitations	Child demonstrates appropriate adaptation to limitations (specify)
Prevent complications	Stress importance of sound health practices and frequent health supervision Make certain child and family understand the therapeutic measures prescribed Encourage older child to choose activities but take responsibility for his own safety Plan with allied personnel (e.g., teachers, coaches, counselors) appropriate activities Confer with school nurse (or other person) regarding any special needs of the child Discuss with parents any indicated limit-setting	Child maintains optimum health
HP-HMP Noncompliance (specify) Etiology: specify		
Promote positive adjustment to the disease or disability	Anticipate problems associated with each of the child's developmental stages Assist child and family to devise strategies for coping with anticipated problems Encourage child to maintain normal activities and relationships Be available for consultation when needed Be alert to signs that child may be using his symptoms to manipulate his interpersonal relationships	Child and/or family demonstrates an understanding of his disease and complies with therapies
Promote compliance	Establish communication with child and family Assess understanding of plan of care Help child and family set realistic goals Help plan therapies and medical care so they do not interfere with child's or family's regular activities and social interaction Help child or family devise cues or reminders to encourage compliance Provide praise and encouragement for compliance and innovation; tangible reward for positive behavior Provide assistance and encouragement when needed Arrange appointments with family's input Assist family with transportation to appointments	Child and/or family demonstrates an understanding of the therapeutic plan (specify) Family participates in scheduling therapies and evaluations

	Contract with child or family if appropriate
	  Identify goals, activities needed to reach goals, and method for keeping records
	  Explore possible deterrents to goal achievement
	  Select meaningful reward for achievement, penalty for noncompliance
	Emphasize positive aspects of compliance
		Child and/or family plans in terms of realistic long-range goals as well as short-range ones

Carry out ongoing evaluation	Assess psychologic responses to the disorder and its therapies Carry out frequent assessments with particular attention to identified problem Take history for new or increasing symptoms Investigate any complaints of discomfort (especially in relation to equipment or appliances) Encourage child and family to discuss feelings about therapy Be alert to signs that may indicate rebellion against the disorder, such as acting out behavior	†Problems or incipient problems are identified and appropriate interventions implemented

†Nursing outcome.

Continued.

NURSING CARE PLAN

The Child with Chronic or Terminal Illness or Disability—cont'd

Nursing Goals	Nursing Interventions	Expected Patient/Family Outcomes
A-EP* **Altered growth and development** **Etiology: chronic illness, terminal illness, disability, parental reactions such as overbenevolence, repeated hospitalizations**		
Promote age-appropriate developmental tasks:		
Infancy		
Develop a sense of trust	Encourage consistent caregivers in hospital or other care settings Encourage parents to visit frequently or "room in" during hospitalization Encourage parents to participate in care	†Consistent caregivers are assigned to infant Parents visit frequently and participate in care
Bond/attach to parent	Emphasize healthy, perfect qualities of infant; see also p. 210 Help parents learn special care needs of infant for them to feel competent	Parents and infant demonstrate attachment behaviors Parents learn to care for infant
Learn through sensorimotor experiences	Expose infant to pleasureable experiences through all senses (touch, hearing, sight, taste, movement) Encourage age-appropriate developmental skills (i.e., sitting unsupported, holding bottle, finger feeding, crawling)	Infant engages in appropriate sensorimotor experiences Infant learns age-appropriate skills (specify)
Begin to develop sense of separateness from parent (older infant)	Encourage family members to participate in care Encourage parents to take periodic respites from burdens of care	Infant has opportunities to separate from parent
Toddlerhood		
Develop autonomy	Encourage independence in as many areas as possible (i.e., toileting, dressing, feeding) Offer choices to allow opportunities for control	Child achieves independence as expected for age (specify)
	Recognize that negative and ritualistic behavior are normal and expected	Parents demonstrate an understanding of typical toddler behavior
	Institute age-appropriate discipline and limit-setting	Appropriate discipline strategies are implemented
Master locomotor and language skills	Provide gross motor skill activity and modification of toys or equipment	Child achieves appropriate motor and language skills
Learn through sensorimotor experience, beginning preoperational thought	Provide a variety of play experiences, especially sensory play Use simple explanations to explain aspects of child's condition	Child engages in appropriate play experiences Child has beginning understanding of condition
Preschool		
Develop initiative and purpose	Encourage mastery of self-help skills Provide devices that make task easier (i.e., self-dressing or feeding)	Child achieves independence as expected for age (specify)
Begin to develop social relationships with peers	Encourage socialization, such as inviting friends to play, daycare experience Provide age-appropriate play, especially cooperative play opportunities	Child forms relationships with peers
	Help child deal with criticisms; realize that too much protection prevents child from realities of world and may foster social isolation	Child demonstrates beginning ability to deal with criticism
Develop sense of body image and sexual identity	Emphasize child's abilities; dress appropriately to enhance desirable appearance Encourage relationships with same-sex and opposite-sex peers and adults	Child demonstrates a positive body image
Learn through preoperational thought (magical thinking)	Clarify that cause of child's illness or disability is not his fault or a punishment	Child has beginning understanding of condition without self-blame

*For an explanation of abbreviations, see p. 20.
†Nursing outcome.

NURSING CARE PLAN

The Child with Chronic or Terminal Illness or Disability—cont'd

Nursing Goals	Nursing Interventions	Expected Patient/Family Outcomes
School-age		
Develop a sense of accomplishment	Encourage school attendance Schedule medical visits at times other than school Provide opportunity to make up missed work Educate teachers and classmates about child's condition, abilities, and special needs	Child attends school and has opportunity to achieve within his abilities
Form peer relationships	Encourage sports activities (i.e., Special Olympics) Encourage socialization (i.e., Girl Scouts, Campfire Girls, having a best friend or a club)	Child forms relationships with peers
Learn through concrete operations	Provide child with knowledge about his condition	Child demonstrates an understanding of his condition
Adolescence		
Develop personal and sexual identity	Realize that many of the difficulties the teenager is experiencing are part of normal adolescence (i.e., rebelliousness, risk-taking, lack of cooperation)	Parents demonstrate an understanding of typical adolescent behavior
Form heterosexual relationships	Encourage socialization with peers, including peers with special needs and those without special needs Encourage activities appropriate for age, such as attending mixed-sex parties, sports activities, driving a car (when possible)	Adolescent forms relationships with same-sex and opposite-sex peers
	Emphasize good appearance and wearing stylish clothes, use of make-up	Adolescent is well groomed and stylish
	Help parents understand that adolescent has same sexual needs and concerns as any other teenager	Parents demonstrate an understanding of adolescent sexual needs and concerns
Achieve independence from family	Involve adolescent and family in discussion regarding teenager's potential for independence outside the home	Adolescent achieves independence in accordance with his potential
	Explore appropriate educational/vocational pursuits	Adolescent engages in suitable educational/vocational activities
Learn through abstract thinking	Realize that adolescent may be concerned about future issues (e.g., employment, marriage, financial support) Discuss planning for future and how condition can affect choices (i.e., inheritance of disease and childbearing)	Adolescent demonstrates an understanding of his condition and how it affects future choices
NDx A-EP Diversional activity deficit **Etiology: environmental lack of diversion, physical limitations (specify), hospitalization**		
Provide diversion	Provide appropriate stimulation Encourage activities appropriate to age, interests, and capabilities of child Encourage physical exercise that does not overtax the child (if indicated) Incorporate therapeutic needs in play activities as appropriate Supervise and encourage activities of daily living Encourage child's natural tendency to be active	Child engages in age-appropriate activities within the limits of his capabilities
	Encourage interaction with family and peers Include child in planning and scheduling care	Child accepts efforts of family and caregivers
Discourage sedentary habits	Encourage child to participate in normal childhood activities commensurate with his interests and capabilities Encourage and reinforce age-appropriate behaviors, experiences, and socialization with peers Discourage physical inactivity	Child engages in nonsedentary activities within the limits of his condition

†Nursing outcome.

Continued.

NURSING CARE PLAN

The Child with Chronic or Terminal Illness or Disability—cont'd

Nursing Goals	Nursing Interventions	Expected Patient/Family Outcomes
NDx A-EP (Specify) self-care deficit Etiology: specify impairment		
Promote self-help (self-care)	Teach child about the disease and therapies Encourage child to assist in his care as age and capabilities permit Provide and/or help devise methods to facilitate maximum functioning Incorporate play that encourages desired behavior Select toys and activities that allow maximum participation by the child Modify environment if needed (specify) Assist with self-care activities where needed (specify) Avoid undue persistence to accomplish a goal Provide incentives to achieve desired behavior Instruct when to seek assistance from family or health care providers	Child engages in self-help activities commensurate with his capabilities (specify activities and extent of involvement)
Enhance child's sense of competence and mastery	Capitalize on child's assets; help him compensate for liabilities Praise child for accomplishments and "near" accomplishments, such as partial completion of a task Ensure adequate rest before attemptimg energy-expending activities Emphasize the child's abilities and focus on realistic endeavors Emphasize positive coping behaviors Discourage activities that are beyond the child's capabilities; promote and reinforce successful endeavors Encourage participation in own care to the extent that he is able Teach and encourage responsibility for use of equipment, appliances, testing, medication (specify) Help child become adept at self-management to his maximum capabilities	Child takes responsibility for self-care according to age and capabilities (specify) Child engages in appropriate activities with undue fatigue
NDx SP-SCP Anxiety/fear Etiology: Specify		
Prepare for tests and procedures Prepare for hospitalization Provide support and reassurance	See Nursing care of the hospitalized child, p. 603	
NDx SP-SCP Body image or self-esteem disturbance Etiology: perception of disability (self and others), feeling of differentness, inability to participate in specific activities (specify)		
Meet child's emotional needs	Convey an attitude of understanding, caring, and acceptance Avoid conveying an attitude of intrusion Maintain open communications with child Relate to the child on his cognitive level Serve as a role model for others	Child maintains a positive attitude (specify behaviors)
Determine extent of disturbance	Encourage verbalization of feelings and perceptions, especially feelings of "differentness" Explore feelings concerning disease or disability and its implications: stress of being "different," physical limitations, difficulty competing, relationships with peers, self-image Encourage child to discuss his feelings about how he thinks others feel about his disorder	Child openly discusses feelings and concerns about his condition, therapies, and perceived reactions of others

†Nursing outcome.

NURSING CARE PLAN

The Child with Chronic or Terminal Illness or Disability—cont'd

Nursing Goals	Nursing Interventions	Expected Patient/Family Outcomes
Help child cope with actual and perceived differentness	Acknowledge feelings and facilitate sharing feelings with family and other health professionals Clarify misconceptions child may have acquired Assist child to identify positive aspects of situation	Child discusses his disorder and his feelings regarding his limitations
Assist child to adjust to the disorder and its effects	Help child assess his strengths and assets; emphasize strengths Identify coping behaviors Support positive coping mechanisms and extinguish negative ones Help child set realistic goals	Child identifies his assets and strengths realistically
	Encourage as much independence as condition allows Introduce child to other children who have adjusted well to this or a similar disorder	Child verbalizes positive suggestions for adjusting to his disability
	Suggests involvement with special groups and facilities for children with similar problems	Child becomes involved with special group activities
Help child build self-esteem and a positive self-concept	Encourage an appealing physical appearance: good body hygiene, clean straight teeth, good grooming, stylish clothing, makeup for teenage girls	Child demonstrates a positive appearance and attitude (specify)
	Assist with improving appearance and grooming Point out positive aspects of his coping, appearance, and other capabilities Promote constructive thinking in child; encourage to maximize strengths Reinforce positive behaviors	Child appears clean, well groomed, and attractively dressed
	Assist child to determine and engage in activities that foster self-esteem Promote independence	Child exhibits behaviors that indicate elevated self-esteem (specify)
Provide child with appropriate feeling of control	Channel need for control and feeling of effectiveness in appropriate directions Encourage child to monitor own care as appropriate Provide opportunities for child to make choices and participate in care when appropriate Assist the child with vocational planning when appropriate	Child becomes actively involved in own care and management
Help prepare hospitalized child for discharge	Begin early in hospitalization to discuss "going home" Help child develop independence and self-help capabilities Encourage visits from friends to help child assess the impact of any change in appearance or behavior that might interfere with returning to previous environments	Child verbalizes and otherwise demonstrates interest in going home
NDx RRP Altered family processes **Etiology: situational crisis (child with a chronic disease or disability)**		
Help family adjust to the diagnosis	Provide opportunity for family to adjust to discovery of diagnosis Anticipate the usual grief reaction to loss of "perfect" child Explore family's feelings regarding the child and their ability to cope with his disorder Serve as a role model regarding attitudes and behavior toward the child	Parents verbalize feelings and concerns regarding implications of the disease
Increase family's understanding of the disorder	Assist family to understand the disorder, its therapies, and implications Reinforce information given by others Clarify misconceptions Provide accurate information at a rate family can absorb Discuss advantages and limitations of therapeutic plan Encourage family to ask questions and express concerns	Family expresses feelings and concerns regarding child, his condition, and ability to care for him

†Nursing outcome.

NURSING CARE PLAN

The Child with Chronic or Terminal Illness or Disability—cont'd

Nursing Goals	Nursing Interventions	Expected Patient/Family Outcomes
Promote positive adaptation to the child	Explore family's reaction to the child and his disorder Assess family's coping skills, abilities, and resources Help family to achieve a realistic view of the child and his capabilities and limitations Foster positive family relationships Assess interpersonal relationships within the family, especially behaviors that reflect family attitudes toward the affected child Intervene appropriately if there is evidence of maladaptation Encourage parents in their attempts to promote child's development Emphasize positive aspects of the child's abilities or attributes	Family verbalizes feelings and concerns regarding the special needs of the child and their effect on the family process
	Help family gain confidence in their ability to cope with the child, the disorder, and its impact on other family members	Family members demonstrate an attitude of confidence in their ability to cope
Promote family's ability to provide child's care	Help family develop a thorough plan of care Teach skills needed to provide optimum care Interpret child's behavior to parents (e.g., anger, depression, regression, physical modifications as a result of disorder) Help family plan for the future	Family sets realistic goals for selves, child, and others
Rally support systems	Identify family support systems (immediate family, extended family, friends, health service providers) Assess systematically the number, affiliation, and interrelationships (if any) of persons the family sees as important Assist family to assign specific tasks to specific people	Family avails itself of support
Provide support	Be available to the family Listen to family members—singly or collectively Allow for expression of feelings including feelings of guilt, helplessness, and their perception of the impact that the condition may have (or does have) on the family Refer to community agencies or special organizations providing assistance—financial, social, and support Refer for genetic counseling if appropriate Help family learn to expect feelings of frustration and anger toward the child; reassure that it is not a reflection on their parenting	Family maintains contact with health providers Family demonstrates an understanding of the needs of the child and the impact his condition will have on them
	Assist family in problem solving Encourage interaction with other families who have a similarly affected child Introduce to families Provide information regarding support groups Help families learn when to accept and when to "fight"	Problems are dealt with early Family becomes involved with local agencies and support groups
Prepare family for hospitalized child's discharge	Teach skills needed for home care Assess home situation, including family's strengths, weaknesses, and support systems Help devise an individualized plan of care based on assessment of family's needs and resources Encourage family involvement in care while still in the hospital Encourage family to ask questions regarding posthospital care Explore family's attitudes toward the child's entry (or reentry) into the home	Family demonstrates an understanding of needed skills (specify skills and method of demonstration)
	Help family acquire needed drugs, supplies, and equipment Refer to special agencies based on need assessment Arrange for regular follow-up care to reassess effectiveness of home management	Family members avail themselves of resources within their community (specify) Family complies with home care program

NURSING CARE PLAN

The Child with Chronic or Terminal Illness or Disability—cont'd

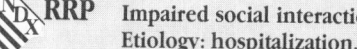

Nursing Goals	Nursing Interventions	Expected Patient/Family Outcomes
Continue ongoing evaluation	Participate in follow-up care Coordinate team management of child and family Be alert to comments by child or family members that indicate possible problems Assess interpersonal relationships within the family, especially behaviors that reflect family attitudes toward the child	Family participates in follow-up care
	Be alert for cues that signal undue anxiety and guilt: preoccupation with causative factors, constant analysis of effects of therapies, experimentation with diets and folk remedies, seeking magical cures Be alert for overprotective behaviors such as assuming self-care activities for child, restricting child's activities or interaction with peers	†Signs that may indicate family's difficulty in adjusting to the child's condition are identified early
	Allow family to express discouragement at interference with activities and what appears to be slow progress	Family expresses discouragement and concerns related to child's progress
Support siblings of affected child	Assess siblings to identify areas of concern Communicate honestly with siblings about the child's disease or disability Provide opportunity for siblings to ask questions and express feelings but avoid lengthy explanations before they ask	Siblings verbalize or otherwise demonstrate their feelings and concerns
	Help parents talk to siblings about the child's condition and interpret the siblings' needs and questions	Parents include siblings in discussions of the disabled child
	Encourage parents to spend special time and demonstrate gratitude to the siblings Help siblings and family understand that it is normal for them to have negative feelings about the child	Parents make an effort to spend time with their other children and express appreciation for cooperation
	Prepare siblings in advance for any household changes	Siblings exhibit an understanding of household changes
	Allow sibling(s) to participate in the child's care and therapy as appropriate Help siblings learn how to explain the child's condition to their peers and others Acknowledge siblings' strengths and abilities to cope	Siblings assist with affected child's care (specify)
	Refer to sibling groups and networks composed of siblings of children with the same or similar conditions Assess siblings periodically to determine their adjustment to the family situation	Siblings become involved in support groups (specify)
RRP Anticipatory grieving **Etiology: child with a life-threatening disorder**		
Help family face the possibility of the child's death	Maintain contact with the family Clarify, refocus, and supply information as needed	Family verbalizes concerns and plans
	Arrange for spiritual support according to family's beliefs and/or affiliations	Family receives appropriate religious representative (specify)
	Help family plan care of the child, especially at terminal stage (hospice care, extent of extraordinary life-saving measures)	†Family's wishes for terminal care are implemented
RRP Impaired social interaction **Etiology: hospitalization, confinement to home, frequent illness, activity intolerance, fatigue (specify)**		
Promote interpersonal relationships	Encourage to maintain usual activities	Child engages in appropriate activities
	Arrange for continued interpersonal contacts while hospitalized or otherwise confined Provide opportunities for interaction with others, especially peers	Child associated with peers and family
	Encourage regular school attendance (including daycare, beginning school, return to school) Arrange for rest periods at school if needed Promote peer contact wherever possible Encourage recreational outlets and after-school activities appropriate to the child's interests and capabilities Discourage activities that increase isolation from others	Child attends school with reasonable regularity

†Nursing outcome.

gressive and destructive outbursts, compulsive caregiving, persistent anxieties (such as fear of another family death or of their own), excessive clinging to the parent, difficulty with forming new relationships, problems at school, or delinquency (such as stealing) (Krupnick, 1984). In these situations professional assistance may be required, and the nurse can provide appropriate referral.

Communication with the bereaved family is essential, but often there is a feeling of not knowing what to say and of helplessness in offering words of comfort. The most supportive approach is to avoid judging the family's reactions or offering advice or rationalizations and to focus on feelings. Families understand that no words will relieve their pain; all they want is acceptance, understanding, and respect for their grief.

EVALUATION

The effectiveness of nursing interventions is determined by continual reassessment and evaluation of care based on the following observational guidelines and expected outcomes:

1. Observe family members' response to the diagnosis and the type of questions or concerns that they have
2. Interview the family regarding their knowledge and understanding of the child's condition; observe if they have instituted suggestions, such as the use of identification devices for children with certain conditions
3. Observe the response of professionals to reactions such as denial, guilt, and anger and whether supportive interventions are used with the family
4. Observe the family's communication patterns with each other and their ability to discuss feelings about issues such as the impact of the child's condition on the marriage or additional care responsibilities; investigate the family's use of services, such as self-help groups or other community resources
5. Perform a developmental screening test on young children and compare the results to expected milestones for the child's abilities; investigate the use of functional aids to assist children to develop to their potential; question the family about the child's attendance at school and interaction with peers
6. Review the child's nursing record for evidence of adequate physical care, especially pain relief measures, before and at the time of death; observe the family's grief reactions and compare them to behaviors expected in acute grief; investigate the family's use of bereavement support, such as self-help groups

Expected outcomes:

See Nursing Care Plan, pp. 531 to 537.

SUMMARY

Caring for children with chronic illness or disability or at the time of their death presents immense challenges to their families, as well as to nurses. To meet the needs of this group of people, nurses need knowledge of families' and children's reactions to chronic illness, disability, and death, especially the grief process. They must be aware of the impact that these conditions have on family members, both from a theoretic basis and from assessment of the family's actual responses.

In planning care nurses must consider the needs of the child and the other family members. The goals of care focus on providing support to the family at the time of diagnosis and throughout the child's course, including those instances in which the child dies. Nurses are involved in educating the family about those aspects of the disorder that affect the child's immediate and long-term adjustment. They need to be aware of the child's normal developmental needs and to assist the family in promoting age-appropriate skills and tasks. The approach with the family needs to convey acceptance of the family's response to the child's condition in a manner that supports appropriate behaviors but sensitively guides the family to recognize areas that need improvement. By taking an active role in implementing these goals, nurses can influence the quality of life for families and children with special needs.

KEY CONCEPTS

- Trends in the treatment of children with chronic illness or disability have focused on developmental age, the child's strengths and uniqueness, family relationships, establishment of normalization, early discharge, home care, and mainstreaming.
- Families' reactions to disability or chronic illness are manifested in the following stages: shock and denial, adjustment, reintegration and acceptance, and freezing out.
- The family's reactions to impending or actual death include anticipatory grief, acute grief, and mourning.
- The stages of anticipatory grief are denial, anger, bargaining, depression, and acceptance.
- Acute grief is a syndrome with intense and distressing psychologic and somatic symptoms that appear at the time of death.
- Mourning is a prolonged, painful process that consists of four phases: shock and disbelief, expression of grief, disorganization and despair, and reorganization.
- In response to the child with chronic illness or disability, parents may be affected by feelings of inadequacy and failure; excessive demands on time, energy, and financial resources; and strain on the marital relationship.
- Effects of chronic illness on siblings include changes in role status, irritability and physical complaints, jealousy, competition, anger, hostility, attention-seeking behavior, social withdrawal, and decline in school performance.
- The child's reaction to illness or disability depends on developmental level, coping mechanisms, others' reactions, and the illness itself.
- Children's concept of death is determined by their cognitive ability and their experience with life-threatening illness.
- Young children see death as temporary and reversible and mainly fear separation.
- School-age children view death as irreversible but not necessarily inevitable and may fear mutilation.
- Children beyond 9 to 10 years realize death is irreversible, universal, and inevitable but may resist the thought of their own death.
- Assessment of the family's adjustment to a child's chronic illness, disability, or death includes the availability of a

support system, their perception of the event, their coping mechanisms, and response to the child.

- To help parents cope with their child's chronic illness or disability, nurses must offer attentiveness, humanistic support, solicitation of suggestions for care, facilitation of communication, verbalization of feelings, and referral to volunteer and community agencies.
- Supporting the child involves encouraging self-expression, alleviating feelings of being different, and strengthening self-image.
- Fostering reality adjustment entails supplying information about the disorder, promoting normal development, and establishing realistic future goals.
- At the time of dying and death important decisions for the family may include the extensiveness of lifesaving interventions, the choice of hospital or hospice care, viewing the body (particularly following a traumatic death), tissue donation, and the siblings' attendance at the funeral.

STUDY QUESTIONS AND ACTIVITIES

1 Select three chronic illnesses, read the description given in the text, and compare the impact that these disorders can have on the child and family. Consider the amount of home care involved, the educational needs of the family to care for the child, and the effect of the illness on the child's overall health.
2 Interview a school nurse, a pediatric clinical nurse specialist, or a pediatrician who cares for children with chronic illness and/or disability. Have they identified any trends in children's adjustment based on the diagnosis, such as children with less obvious problems having a more difficult adjustment than children with highly visible conditions?
3 Outline a plan of care for a child with a chronic illness that is designed to meet the development tasks of each age-group.
4 Visit a rehabilitation center for children with physical disabilities and observe the type of functional aids that children use to maximize their motor abilities.
5 Attend a meeting of bereaved parents and observe the kinds of services that the group provides. Interview one parent and ask him or her to identify those interventions by those caring for the child that were helpful at the time of the child's death and those that were harmful.

REFERENCES

Bluebond-Langner, M.: The private worlds of dying children, Princeton, NJ, 1978, Princeton University Press.

Breslau, N., Weitzman, M., and Messenger, K.: Psychologic functioning of siblings of disabled children, Pediatrics **67**(3):344-353, 1981.

Cancer facts & figures—1988, New York, 1988, American Cancer Society, Inc.

Childs, R.: Maternal psychological conflicts associated with the birth of a retarded child, MCN **14**(3):175-182, 1985.

Cleveland, M.: Family adaptation to traumatic spinal cord injury: response to crisis, Fam. Relations **29:**558-565, 1980.

Corr, C.A., and Corr, D.M.: Pediatric hospice care, Pediatrics **76**(5):774-780, 1985.

Coupey, S.M., and Cohen, M.I.: Special considerations for the health care of adolescents with chronic illnesses, Pediatr. Clin. North Am. **31**(1):211-219, 1984.

Golden, G.S.: The developmentally disabled child: detection, assessment, referral and treatment, Child Care Newsletter **3**(1):8-11, 1984.

Halpern, R.: Physician-parent communication in the diagnosis of child handicap: a brief review, Child. Health Care **12**(4):170-173, 1984.

Hobbs, N., and Perrin, J.M., editors: Issues in the care of children with chronic illness, San Francisco, 1985, Jossey-Bass Inc.

Hofmann, A.D.: Managing handicapped adolescents with impaired body image, Feelings Med. Signif. **22**(4):13-18, 1980.

Kalnins, I.: Cross-illness comparisons of separation and divorce among parents having a child with a life-threatening illness, Child. Health Care **12**(2):72-77, 1983.

Krulik, T.: Successful "normalizing" tactics of parents of chronically ill children, J. Adv. Nurs. **5**(6):573-578, 1980.

Krupnick, J.: Bereavement during childhood and adolescence. In Osterweis, M., Solomon, F., and Green, M., editors: Bereavement: reactions, consequences, and care, Washington, DC, 1984, National Academy Press.

Kübler-Ross, E.: On death and dying, New York, 1969, Macmillan, Inc.

Lavigne, J.V., and Ryan, M.: Psychologic adjustment of siblings of children with chronic illness, Pediatrics **63**(4):616- 627, 1979.

McKeever, P.T.: Fathering the chronically ill child, MCN **6**(2):124-128, 1981.

Miles, M.S., and Perry, K.: Parental responses to sudden accidental death of a child, Crit. Care Q. **8**(1):73-84, 1985.

Olsen, V., and Hooke, M.: The complexities of do not resuscitate orders, MCN **13**(3):157–162, 1988.

O'Malley, J.E., and others: Psychiatric sequelae of surviving childhood cancer, Am. J. Orthopsychiatry **49**(4):608-616, 1979.

Orr, D.P., and others: Psychosocial implications of chronic illness in adolescence, J. Pediatr. **104**(1):152-157, 1984.

Perrin, E.C., and Gerrity, P.S.: Development of children with a chronic illness, Pediatr. Clin. North Am. **31**(1):19-31, 1984.

Pless, I.B.: Clinical assessment: physical and psychological functioning, Pediatr. Clin. North Am. **31**(1):33-45, 1984.

Rando, T.: An investigation of grief and adaptation in parents whose children have died from cancer, J. Pediatr. Psychiatry **8**(1):3-20, 1983.

Reynolds, M.C.: The educational needs of disabled children and youths. In Blum, R., editor: Chronic illness and disabilities in childhood and adolescence, New York, 1984, Grune & Stratton, Inc.

Rutter, M.: Stress, coping, and development: some issues and some questions. In Garmezy, N., and Rutter, M., editors: Stress, coping, and development in children, New York, 1983, McGraw-Hill Book Co.

Sabbeth, B.F., and Leventhal, J.M.: Marital adjustment to chronic childhood illness: a critique of the literature, Pediatrics **73**(6):762-768, 1984.

Seligman, M.: Adaptation of children to a chronically ill or mentally handicapped sibling, Can. Med. Assoc. J. **136**(12):1249-1252, 1987.

Siemon, M.: Siblings of the chronically ill or disabled child: meeting their needs, Nurs. Clin. North Am. **19**(2):295-307, 1984.

Stein, R.: A home care program for children with chronic illness, Child. Health Care **12**(2):90-92, 1983.

Stein, R.E.K.: Home care: a challenging opportunity, Child. Health Care **14**(2):90-95, 1985.

Taylor, S.C.: The effects of chronic childhood illnesses upon well siblings, MCN **9**(2):109-116, 1980.

Waechter, E.: Dying children: patterns of coping, Issues Compr. Pediatr. Nurs. **8**(1-6):51-68, 1985.

Weber, P.: The human connection: the role of the nurse in organ donation, J. Neurosurg. Nurs. **17**(2):119-122, 1985.

Weitzman, M., Walker, D.K., and Gortmaker, S.: Chronic illness, psychosocial problems, and school absences, Clin. Pediatr. **25**(3):137-141, 1986.

Wong, D.: Bereavement: the empty-mother syndrome, MCN **5**(6):385-389, 1980.

BIBLIOGRAPHY

Congential Anomalies

Hall, L.F., and Stoops, P.M.: Acquainting a new mother with her less-than-perfect baby, MCN **9:**136, 1984.

Horan, M.L.: Parental reaction to the birth of an infant with a defect: an attributional approach, Adv. Nurs. Sci. **4**(1):57-68, 1982.

Irvin, N.A., Kennell, J.H., and Klaus, M.H.: Caring for the parents of an infant with a congenital malformation. In Klaus M.H., and Kennell, J.H., editors: Parent-infant bonding, ed. 2, St. Louis, 1982, The C.V. Mosby Co.

Jackson, P.L.: When the baby isn't "perfect," Am. J. Nurs. **85:**396-399, 1985.

Kikuchi, J.: Assimilative and accommodative responses of mothers to their newborn infants with congenital defects, Matern. Child Nurs. J. **9:**141-219, 1980.

Lemons, P.M., and others: Beyond the birth of a defective child, Neonatal Network **5**(3):13-20, 1986.

Romney, M.C.: Congenital defects: implications on family development and parenting, Issues Compr. Pediatr. Nurs. **7:**1-15, 1984.

Chronic Illness/Disability

American Academy of Pediatrics, Ad Hoc Task Forces on Home Care of Chronically Ill Infants and Children: Guidelines for home care of infants, children and adolescents with chronic disease, Pediatrics **74**(3):434-436, 1984.

Bakke, K.: Ethical dilemmas: institutionalizing a severely disabled child, Pediatr. Nurs. **7**(6):27-29, 1981.

Baskin, C.H., and others: Helping teachers help children with cancer: a workshop for school personnel, Child. Health Care **12**(2):78-83, 1983.

Bernard, B., and others: Exercise for children with physical disabilities, Issues Compr. Pediatr. Nurs. **5:**99-107, 1981.

Bernardo, M.L.: A conceptual model of children's cognitive adaptation to physical disability, J. Adv. Nurs. **7:**595-601, 1982.

Blum, R.: Chronic illness and disabilities in childhood and adolescence, New York, 1984, Grune & Stratton.

Bock, R.H., and others: There's no place like home, Child. Health Care **12**(2):93-96, 1983.

Boren, H.A., and Meell, H.: Adolescent amputee ski rehabilitation program, J. Assoc. Pediatr. Oncol. Nurses **2**(1):16-23, 1985.

Brandt, P.A.: Clinical assessment of the social support of families with handicapped children, Issues Compr. Pediatr. Nurs. **7:**187-201, 1984.

Brewster, A.B.: Chronically ill hospitalized children's concepts of their illness, Pediatrics **69**(3):355-362, 1982.

Chekryn, J., Deegan, M., and Reid, J.: Impact on teachers when a child with cancer returns to school, Child. Health Care **15**(3):161-165, 1987.

Crummette, B.: Assessing the impact of illness upon an adolescent and family, MCN **12**(3):155-167, 1983.

Deatrick, J.A.: It's their decision now: perspectives of chronically disabled adolescents concerning surgery, Issues Compr. Pediatr. Nurs. **7:**17-31, 1984.

Eiser, C., and Town, C.: Teachers' concerns about chronically sick children: implications for paediatricians, Dev. Med. Child Neurol. **29**(1):56-63, 1987.

Feller, N., and others: A multidisciplinary approach to developing safe transportation for children with special needs, Orthopaedic Nurs. **5**(5):25-27, 1986.

Ferrari, M.: Perceptions of social support by parents of chronically ill versus healthy children, Child. Health Care **15**(1):26-31, 1986.

Frauman, A.C., and Sypert, N.S.: Sexuality in adolescents with chronic illness, MCN **4**(6):371-375, 1979.

Gallo, A.M.: The special sibling relationship in chronic illness and disability: parental communication with well siblings, Holistic Nurs. Pract. **2**(2):28-37, 1988.

Goldfarb, L.A., and others: Meeting the challenge of disability or chronic illness—a family guide, Baltimore, 1985, Brookes Publishing Co.

Goodell, A.: Peer education in schools for children with cancer, Issues Compr. Pediatr. Nurs. **7:**101-106, 1984.

Grindley, J.F.: The handicapped child in school: considerations for health care, Holistic Nurs. Pract. **2**(2):11-19, 1988.

Hingsburger, D.: Stranger in a strange bed, Can. Nurse **83**(7):21-22, 1987.

Holaday, B.: Challenges of rearing a chronically ill child, Nurs. Clin. North Am. **19:**361-368, 1984.

Holaday, B.: Patterns of interaction between mothers and their chronically ill infants, MCN **16**(1):29-45, 1987.

Holaday, B., and Turner-Henson, A.: Chronically ill school-age children's use of time, Pediatr. Nurs. **13**(6):410-414, 1987.

Horner, M.M., Rawlins, P., and Giles, K.: How parents of children with chronic conditions perceive their own needs, MCN **12**(1):40-43, 1987.

Iscoe, L., and Bordelon, K.: Pilot parents: peer support for parents of handicapped children, Child. Health Care **14**(2):103, 1985.

Kegel, B.: Sports and recreation for those with lower limb amputation or impairment, J. Rehabil. Res. Dev., Clinical Supplement No. 1, 1985.

Kinrade, L.C.: Preventive group intervention with siblings of oncology patients, Child. Health Care **14**(2):110, 1985.

Knowles, R.D.: Handling anger: responding vs. reacting, Am. J. Nurs. **81**(12):2196, 1981.

Knox, J.E., and Hayes, V.E.: Hospitalization of a chronically ill child: a stressful time for parents, Issues Compr. Pediatr. Nurs. **6:**217-226, 1983.

Lansky, S.B.: Management of stressful periods in childhood cancer, Pediatr. Clin. North Am. **32**(3):62-63, 1985.

Menke, E.M.: The impact of a child's chronic illness on school-aged siblings, Child. Health Care **15**(3):132-140, 1987.

Miller, M., and Diao, J.: Family friends: new resources for psychosocial care of chronically ill children in families, Child. Health Care **15**(4):259-264, 1987.

Monsen, R.: Phases in the caring relationship: from adversary to ally to coordinator, MCN **11**(5):316-318, 1986.

Morrow, G.: Helping chronically ill children in school, New York, 1985, Parker Publishing Co., Inc.

Oremland, E.: Communicating over chronic illness: dilemmas of affected school-aged children, Child. Health Care **14**(4):218-223, 1986.

Patton, A.C., Ventura, J.N., and Savedra, M.: Stress and coping responses of adolescents with cystic fibrosis, Child. Health Care **14**(3):153-156, 1986.

Pipes, P.L., and Pritkin, R.: Nutrition and feeding of children with developmental delays and related problems. In Pipes, P.L., editor: Nutrition in infancy and childhood, ed. 3, St. Louis, 1985, The C.V. Mosby Co.

Pollard, A., and others: School and the child with cancer: a program to assist school personnel, J. Assoc. Pediatr. Oncol. Nurses **2**(3):7-10, 1985.

Rawlins, P.S., and Horner, M.M.: Does membership in a support group alter needs of parents of chronically ill children? Pediatr. Nurs. **14**(1):70-72, 1988.

Robinson, C.: Double bind: a dilemma for parents of chronically ill children, Pediatr. Nurs. **11**(2):112-115, 1985.

Rollins, J.A.: Self-help groups for parents, Pediatr. Nurs. **13**(6):403-409, 1987.

Rose, M.H.: The concepts of coping and vulnerability as applied to children with chronic conditions, Issues Compr. Pediatr. Nurs. **7:**177-186, 1984.

Sahin, S.: The physically disabled child. In Johnson, S., editor: Nursing assessment and strategies for the family at risk, ed. 2, Philadelphia, 1986, J.B. Lippincott Co.

Strauss, S.S., and Munton, M.: Common concerns of parents with disabled children, Pediatr. Nurs. **11**(5):371-375, 1985.

Tamlyn, D., and Arklie, M.M.: A theoretical framework for standard care plans: a nursing approach for working with chronically ill children and their families, Issues Compr. Pediatr. Nurs. **9**(1):39-45, 1986.

Thomas, R.B.: Nursing assessment of childhood chronic conditions, Issues Compr. Pediatr. Nurs. **7:**165-176, 1984.

Yoos, L.: Chronic childhood illnesses: developmental issues, Pediatr. Nurs. **13**(1):25-28, 1987.

Terminal Illness/Death

Adams, D.W.: Helping the dying child: practical approaches for nonphysicians, Issues Compr. Pediatr. Nurs. **8**(1-6):95-112, 1985.

Balk, D.: Effects of sibling death on teenagers, J. Sch. Health **53**(1):14-18, 1983.

Carlson, P., and others: Helping parents cope: a model home-care program for the dying child, Issues Compr. Pediatr. Nurs. **8**(1-6):113-128, 1985.

Coleman, F.W., and Coleman, W.S.: Helping siblings and other peers cope with dying, Issues Compr. Pediatr. Nurs. **8**(1- 6):129-150, 1985.

Conrad, N.L.: Spiritual support for the dying, Nurs. Clin. North Am. **20**(2):415-426, 1985.

Coolican, M.B.: Katie's legacy: organ donation helped this family begin to resolve the tragedy, Am. J. Nurs. **87**(4):483-485, 1987.

Corr, C.A., and Corr, D.M., editors: Hospice approaches to pediatric care, New York, 1985, Springer Publishing Co.

Davidhizar, R.M., and Monhaut, N.: Guidelines for giving bad news by phone, Nursing 85 **15**(4):58-60, 1985.

Davidowitz, M., and Myrick, R.: Responding to the bereaved: an analysis of "helping" statements, Death Education **8:**1-10, 1984.

Davis, A.J.: Breaking the news...to inform relatives of a family member's death, Am. J. Nurs. **83**(10):1457-1478, 1983.

Edwardson, S.R.: The choice between hospital and home care for terminally ill children, Nurs. Res. **32**(1):29-34, 1983.

Foley, G.V.: Facilitating death discussions with children, Pediatrics: nursing update, lesson 19, Princeton, NJ, 1986, Continuing Professional Educational Corp.

Gaffney, D.A.: Death in the classroom: a lesson in life, Holistic Nurs. Pract. **2**(2):20-27, 1988.

Hall, M., Hardin, K., and Conatser, C.: The challenges of psychological care. In Fochtman, D., and Foley, G.V., editors: Nursing care of the child with cancer, Boston, 1982, Little, Brown & Co.

Hazinski, M.F.: Organ donation: what the new "required request" law means to you, Pediatr. Nurs. **13**(6):415-439, 1987.

Johnson, S.: Giving emotional support to families after a patient dies, Nurs. Life **3**(1):34-39, 1983.

Johnson-Soderberg, S.: The development of a child's concept of death, Oncol. Nurs. Forum **8**(1):23-26, 1981.

Kübler-Ross, E.: On children and death, New York, 1983, Macmillan Publishing Co.

Lauer, M.E., and others: Children's perceptions of their sibling's death at home or hospital: the precursors of differential adjustment, Cancer Nurs. **8**(1):21-27, 1985.

Martinson, I.M.: Symposium on child psychiatric nursing: caring for the dying child, Nurs. Clin. North Am. **14:**467-474, Sept. 1979.

Martinson, I.M., Davies, E.B., and McClowry, S.G.: The long-term effects of sibling death on self-concept, J. Pediatr. Nurs. **2**(4):227-235, 1987.

Martinson, I.M., and others: Home care for children dying of cancer, Res. Nurs. Health **9**(1):11-16, 1986.

Martocchio, B.C., and Dufault, K., editors: Symposia on hospice and compassionate care and the dying experience, Nurs. Clin. North Am. **20**(2):267-466, 1985.

McCown, D.E.: When children face death in a family, J. Pediatr. Health Care **2**(1):14-19, 1988.

Miles, M.S.: Emotional symptoms and physical health in bereaved parents, Nurs. Res. **34**(2):76-81, 1985.

Miles, M.S.: Helping adults mourn the death of a child, Issues Compr. Pediatr. Nurs. **8**(1-6):219-241, 1985.

Miles, M.S., and Perry, K.: Parental responses to sudden accidental death of a child, Crit. Care Q. **8**(1):73-84, 1985.

Moore, I., Gilliss, C., and Martinson, I.: Psychosomatic symptoms in parents 2 years after the death of a child with cancer, Nurs. Res. **37**(2):104-107, 1988.

Osterweis, M., Solomon, F., and Green, M., editors: Bereavement: reactions, consequences, and care, Washington, DC, 1984, National Academy Press.

Parkes, C., and Weiss, R.: Recovery from bereavement, New York, 1983, Basic Books, Inc.

Petix, M.: Explaining death to school-age children, Pediatr. Nurs.**13**(6):394-396, 1987.

Ross-Alaolmolki, K.: Supportive care for families of dying children, Nurs. Clin. North Am. **20**(2):457-466, 1985.

Schultz, C.A.: Grief at sudden death ... you can help, Crit. Care Update **10**(2):9-15, 1983.

Walker, K.L.: Easing the pain of bereaved parents, Nursing 86 **16**(4):49-50, 1986.

Wass, H., and Corr, L., editors: Special issue on childhood and death, Issues Compr. Pediatr. Nurs. **8**(1-6):3-383, 1985.

Weber, J.A., and Fournier, D.G.: Family support and a child's adjustment to death, Fam. Relat. **34**(1):43-49, 1985.

Williams, H.A., Frederick, P.R., and Rothenberg, M.B.: The child is dying: who helps the family? MCN **6**(4):261, 1981.

Williams, L.: Organ procurement: what nurses need to know, Crit. Care Q. **8**(1):27-30, 1985.

Wong, D.: The terminally ill child. In Johnson, S., editor: Nursing assessment and strategies for the family at risk, ed. 2, Philadelphia, 1986, J.B. Lippincott Co.

CHAPTER 19

Impact of Cognitive or Sensory Impairment on the Child and Family

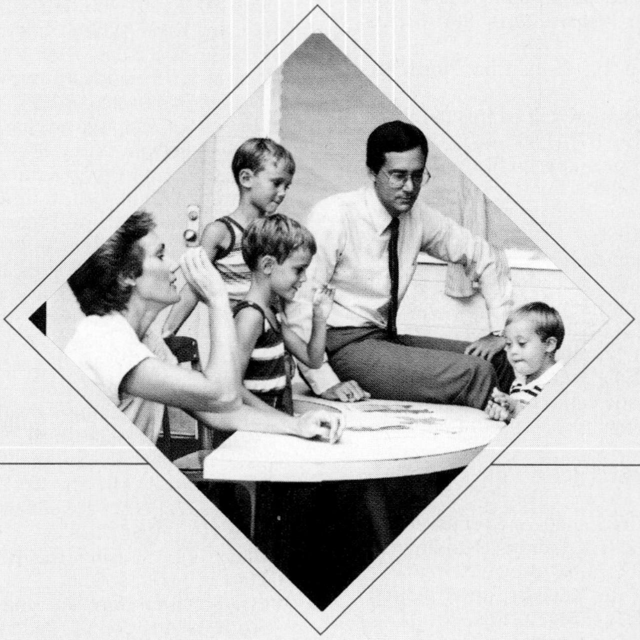

LEARNING OBJECTIVES

On completion of this chapter the reader will be able to:

- Define the classifications of mental retardation
- Outline nursing interventions for the child with cognitive impairment that promote optimum development, including during hospitalization
- Identify the major biologic and cognitive characteristics of the child with Down syndrome
- Outline nursing interventions for the child with Down syndrome
- Identify the major characteristics associated with fragile X syndrome
- List the general classifications of hearing impairment and the effect on speech
- Outline nursing interventions for the child with hearing impairment, including during hospitalization
- List the common types of visual disorders in children
- Outline nursing interventions for the child with visual impairment, including during hospitalization
- Outline nursing interventions for the child with retinoblastoma

*T*his chapter is concerned with the complex problems often associated with cognitive and sensory impairments. Throughout the chapter the term cognitive impairment is used to refer to mental retardation. In addition to the general concepts related to mental retardation, two syndromes associated with cognitive impairment are discussed, Down syndrome and fragile X syndrome, a recently recognized disorder. The term sensory impairment focuses on the problems of hearing and vision loss. Each type of impairment poses special threats to a child's developmental potential. Without assistance in dealing with the impairments, these children are vulnerable to lifelong disadvantages. While the needs and concerns of the child and family are a primary focus throughout the chapter, the reader is encouraged to review Chapter 18, which details the family members' adjustment to disabilities in general.

◆ *Cognitive Impairment*

Mental retardation is the most common developmental disability in the United States, affecting some 3% of the population. In recent years, major changes have occurred in the philosophy of care toward people with cognitive impairment. Children with mental retardation are no longer automatically admitted into institutional settings but often remain at home. Therefore parents need role models and adequate preparation to effectively teach the child to function at optimum level within the environment. Nurses are in a strategic position to assume a vital role in assisting these parents with observation, problem solving, and decision making.

GENERAL CONCEPTS

The American Association on Mental Retardation (AAMR) defines mental retardation as "significantly subaverage general intellectual functioning existing concurrently with deficits in adaptive behavior and manifested during the developmental period" (Grossman, 1983). *General intellectual functioning* refers to the results of various individually administered general intelligence tests. *Significantly subaverage intellectual functioning* is defined as an intelligence quotient (IQ) of approximately 70 or below. *Adaptive behavior* is the effectiveness or degree with which individuals meet the standards of personal independence and social responsibility expected for age and cultural group. It is a critical component of the definition, since it implies that intelligence alone is not the criterion for mental retardation. For example, individuals with IQ scores near 70 may not be classified as retarded based on their ability to adapt to the environment. *Developmental period* comprises the period between conception and the eighteenth birthday. Consequently, if cognitive impairment occurs after this time, such as from injury or disease, the person is not considered retarded.

Diagnosis and Classification

The diagnosis of cognitive impairment is usually made after a period of suspicion, by professionals and/or the family, that the child's developmental progress is delayed. In some cases it is confirmed at birth because of recognition of distinct syndromes, such as Down syndrome. At the other extreme, it is determined after the child begins school, when problems such as speech delays arouse concern when compared to peer achievement. In all cases a high index of suspicion for developmental delay and behavioral signs (see accompanying box) is necessary for early diagnosis, and the importance of routine developmental screening with such instruments as the Denver Developmental Screening Test (DDST) (see p. 171) cannot be overemphasized. Delays are commonly seen in gross and fine motor and speech development, although the latter is most predictive.

Early Behavioral Signs Suggestive of Cognitive Impairment

Nonresponsiveness to contact
Poor eye contact during feeding
Diminished spontaneous activity
Decreased alertness to voice or movement
Irritability
Slow feeding

From Crocker, A., and Nelson, R.: Mental retardation. In Levine, M., and others: Developmental-behavioral pediatrics, Philadelphia, 1983, W.B. Saunders Co., p. 760.

The diagnosis and classification of mental retardation are based on standard intelligence tests, such as the Stanford-Binet Test and Wechsler Intelligence Scale for Children (WISC). Tests for assessing adaptive behaviors include the Vineland Social Maturity Scale and the AAMR Adaptive Behavior Scale. Informal appraisal of adaptive behavior may be made by those fully acquainted with the child (e.g., teachers, parents, or other care providers). Frequently these observations lead parents to seek evaluation of the child's development.

The severity of retardation is based on the IQ scores, which represent mild, moderate, severe, and profound levels of deficit (Table 19-1). A more useful approach for clinical application is classification based on educational potential or symptom severity. For educational purposes the terms *educable mentally retarded (EMR)* or *trainable mentally retarded (TMR)* may be used. EMR corresponds to the mildly retarded group and TMR primarily to children with moderate levels of cognitive impairment. Mild mental retardation is about six times more common than moderate or severe retardation (Coplan, 1982). While nurses should be familiar with the approximate range of IQ for classifying severity, they should refrain from using numbers as the criterion for assessing or evaluating the child's abilities, since numbers are of little value in counseling parents or training these children.

Etiology

The causes of severe mental retardation are primarily genetic, biochemical, viral, and developmental. Although the etiology is unknown in the majority of cases, general categories of events that may lead to retardation include (Grossman, 1983):

1. Infection and intoxication, such as congenital rubella, syphilis, maternal drug consumption (such as excessive alcohol), chronic lead ingestion, or kernicterus

TABLE 19-1

Classification of Mental Retardation

Level (IQ)*	Preschool (birth-5 years)—Maturation and Development	School Age (6-21 years)—Training and Education	Adult (21 years and older)—Social and Vocational Adequacy
Mild—50-55 to approximately 70	Often not noticed as retarded by casual observer but is slower to walk, feed self, and talk than most children; follows same sequence in development as normal children	Can acquire practical skills and useful reading and arithmetic to a third- to sixth-grade level with special education; can be guided toward social conformity; achieves mental age of 8 to 12 years	Can usually achieve social and vocational skills adequate to self-maintenance; may need occasional guidance and support when under unusual social or economic stress; can adjust to marriage but not childrearing
Moderate—35-40 to 50-55	Noticeable delays in motor development, especially in speech; responds to training in various self-help activities	Can learn simple communication, elementary health and safety habits, and simple manual skills; does not progress in functional reading or arithmetic; achieves mental age of 3 to 7 years	Can perform simple tasks under sheltered condition; participates in simple recreation; travels alone in familiar places; usually incapable of self-maintenance
Severe—20-25 to 35-40	Marked delay in motor development; little or no communication skills; may respond to training in elementary self-help, for example, self-feeding	Usually walks, barring specific disability; has some understanding of speech and some response; can profit from systematic habit training; achieves mental age of toddler	Can conform to daily routines and repetitive activities; needs continuing direction and supervision in protective environment
Profound—below 20-25	Gross retardation; minimal capacity for functioning in sensorimotor areas; needs total care	Obvious delays in all areas of development; shows basic emotional responses; may respond to skillful training in use of legs, hands, and jaws; needs close supervision; achieves mental age of young infant	May walk; needs complete custodial care; has primitive speech; usually benefits from regular physical activity

*Based on classification from American Association on Mental Deficiency.

2. Trauma or physical agent, namely injury to the brain suffered during the prenatal, perinatal, or postnatal period
3. Inadequate nutrition and metabolic disorders, such as phenylketonuria
4. Gross postnatal brain disease, such as neurofibromatosis and tuberous sclerosis
5. Unknown prenatal influence, including cerebral and cranial malformations, such as microcephaly and hydrocephalus
6. Gestational disorders, including prematurity, low birth weight, and postmaturity
7. Psychiatric disorders that have their onset during the child's developmental period up to age 18 years, such as autism
8. Environmental influences, including evidence of a deprived environment associated with a history of mental retardation among parents and siblings
9. Chromosomal abnormalities, such as Down syndrome and fragile X syndrome

Nursing Considerations

The goal of caring for children with mental retardation is to promote their optimum development as individuals within a family and community. Since the general guidelines for coping with and adjusting to the child with special needs are discussed extensively in Chapter 18, the following discussion focuses on principles specific to children with mental disability and their families. Prevention is also discussed, since nurses should be concerned with measures that may prevent mental retardation.

ASSESSMENT

Nurses play a major role in identifying children with cognitive impairment. In the newborn and early infancy period few signs are present, with the exception of Down syndrome (see p. 550). However, after this age delayed developmental milestones are the major clues to mental retardation. In addition, nurses must have a high index of suspicion for early behavior patterns that may suggest cognitive impairment (see box, p. 543) and be aware of stereotypes that may delay diagnosis, such as "retarded children have to look dumb." Parental concerns, such as delayed development compared to siblings, need to be taken seriously. All children should receive regular developmental assessment, and the nurse is often the person responsible for performing such assessments using the Denver Developmental Screening Test (see p. 171). When delays are found, the nurse must use sensitivity and discretion in revealing this finding to parents (see Therapeutic dialogue).

NURSING DIAGNOSES

A number of nursing diagnoses are prominent in the nursing care of the child with cognitive impairment and

THERAPEUTIC DIALOGUE

Developmental Delay

During a well child visit the nurse performs a Denver Developmental Screening Test on a 13 month-old child. The child has delays in each of the 4 sectors. However, the mother has not expressed any concern for the child's delayed development.

NURSE: Mrs. M., when I was seeing what Carey is able to do, was his performance typical?

MOTHER: Yes, I would say so.

NURSE: How do you think Carey is developing?

MOTHER: I think he is a little slow, but he was born 2 weeks early and I have read that premature babies can take longer to catch up.

NURSE: Were you told that the baby was premature?

MOTHER: No, but the baby was early and I thought that meant he was premature.

NURSE: Usually if babies are two weeks early or late they are still considered born at the correct time. I wouldn't expect Carey to have any slower development because of his birth date.

MOTHER: Do you think he is behind? What did that Denver test show?

NURSE: The Denver Developmental Screening Test is only a way to screen children to see how they are developing. It isn't a diagnostic test, but it does show that Carey is behind in these areas. (Nurse explains the results and what delays mean.)

MOTHER: It doesn't seem like very good news. I don't have any other children to compare with Carey, but I thought he should be sitting up by now and talking a little. Anytime I mentioned my concern to my family, they always told me not to worry. They said that Carey is so cute and lovable that he had to be normal.

NURSE: Unfortunately, cute and lovable children can have problems also. At your next visit I will do the Denver again, and I will talk with Carey's doctor. I believe your concerns are correct. Carey should be sitting up by himself and imitating some speech sounds.

MOTHER: I wish what you are saying weren't true, but if it is, I want to find out right away so that we can get the help we need.

NURSE: I can understand that this is difficult news. Once we know more, I can discuss with you what community programs are available. Starting early is very important.

the child's family; other diagnoses specific to individual cases become evident. The most common nursing diagnoses are outlined in the Nursing Care Plan for the child with Down syndrome on p. 553.

PLANNING

The goals of nursing care for the child with mental retardation and family are:

1. Educate the child using effective teaching strategies
2. Teach the child self-care skills
3. Promote the child's optimum development
4. Help the family adjust to future care
5. Care for the child during hospitalization
6. Assist in measures to prevent mental retardation

IMPLEMENTATION

Once the goals are identified, specific interventions are carried out. The following discussion presents general interventions for most children with mental disability. Modifications are needed in specific situations and in accordance with the child's educability.

Educate the child. In order to teach children with subaverage intelligence, it is necessary to know their learning abilities and deficits. This is important for the nurse who may be involved in a home care type of program or who may be caring for the child in a health care setting. The nurse who understands how these children learn can effectively teach them basic skills or prepare them for various health-related procedures.

Children with cognitive impairment have a marked deficit in their ability to discriminate between two or more stimuli because of difficulty in paying attention to relevant cues. However, these children can learn to discriminate if the cues are presented in an exaggerated concrete form and all extraneous stimuli are eliminated. For example, the use of colors to emphasize visual cues or the use of singing or rhymes to stress auditory cues can help them learn. Their deficit in discrimination also implies that concrete ideas are learned much more effectively than abstract ideas. Therefore, demonstration is preferable to verbal explanation, and learning should be directed toward mastering a skill rather than understanding the scientific principles underlying a procedure.

Another cognitive deficit is in short-term memory. Whereas children of average intelligence can remember several words, numbers, or directions at one time, these

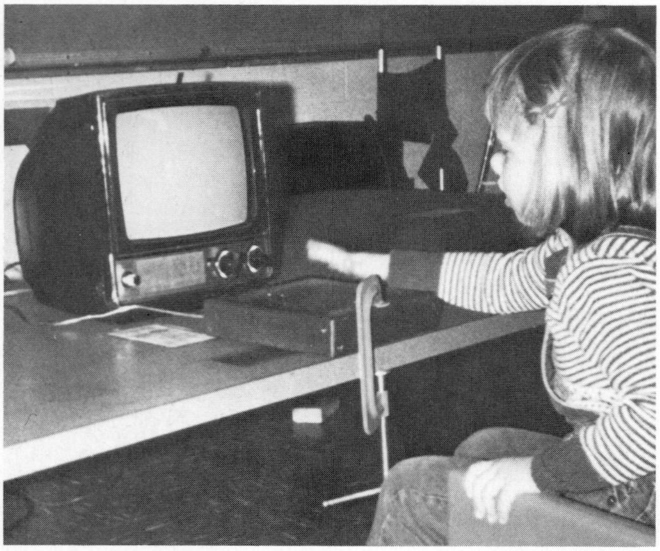

FIG. 19-1 A single push panel allows a child with mental retardation to turn a television on and off.

children are less able to do so. Therefore, they need simple one-step directions. Learning through a step-by-step process requires a *task analysis,* in which each task is separated into its necessary components and each step is taught completely before proceeding to the next activity.

One critical area of learning that has had a tremendous impact on education for cognitively impaired individuals is motivation. Programs based on the motivational principles of behavior modification, employing positive reinforcement for specific tasks or behaviors, have demonstrated marked improvement in children's ability to learn. Advances in technology have greatly aided in providing reinforcement, especially in children who are severely retarded and may have physical disabilities that limit their range of capabilities. For example, with the use of specially designed switches children are given control of some event in the environment, such as turning on the television (Fig. 19-1). The television picture becomes reinforcement for activating the switch. Repetitive use of these switches provides an early, simplistic association with a technical device that may progress to increasingly more complex aids.

Early intervention or stimulation programs have been widely promoted for children with mental disabilities, and there is considerable evidence that early intervention programs are valuable for cognitively impaired children. Nurses working with these families need to be aware of the types of programs in their community. Under Public Law 99-457, the Education of the Handicapped Act Amendments of 1986, federal funds are available to states to develop early intervention services for infants and young children. This act expanded earlier legislation that required states to provide educational programs for children from 3 years of age. Programs may be provided under state **Crippled Children's Program** or by private organizations such as **The National Easter Seal Society*** and **Association of Retarded Citizens.†** Parents should inquire about these programs by contacting the appropriate agencies as soon as possible.

Promote independent self-help skills. When a child with cognitive impairment is born, parents need assistance in promoting normal developmental skills that are almost automatically learned by other children. These include self-help skills such as feeding, toileting, dressing, and grooming. Teaching these skills requires a basic knowledge of the developmental sequence in learning the skills demonstrated by children of average intelligence. For example, a child with subaverage intelligence would not be expected to dress himself as early as an unaffected youngster.

Teaching self-help skills also necessitates a working knowledge of the individual steps needed to master a skill. For example, before beginning a self-feeding program, a task analysis is performed. Following a task analysis, the child is observed in a particular situation, such as eating, to determine what skills he possesses and his developmental readiness to learn the task. Family members are included in this process because their "readiness" is as important as the child's. Numerous self-help aids are available to facilitate independence and can be most helpful in eliminating some of the difficulties of learning, such as using a plate with suction cups to prevent accidental spills (Fig. 19-2).‡

Specific stimulation programs for learning self-help skills and gross motor development are described in *Nursing Care of Infants and Children,* Chapter 24 (Whaley and Wong, 1987), and other texts devoted to the care of developmentally disabled children. The reader is encouraged to review these sources for a more in-depth discussion of the subject.

Promote optimum development. Optimum development involves more than achieving independence. It requires appropriate guidance for establishing acceptable social behavior and personal feelings of self-esteem, worth, and security. These attributes are not simply learned through a stimulation program. Rather they must arise from the genuine love and caring that exist among family members. However, parents need guidance in providing an environment that fosters optimum development. Often it is the nurse who can provide assistance in these areas of childrearing.

Another important area for promoting optimum development and self-esteem is ensuring the child's physical well-being. Any congenital defects should be repaired, such as cardiac, gastrointestinal, or orthopedic anomalies.

*2023 W. Odgen Ave., Chicago, IL 60612.

†2501 Avenue J, Arlington, TX 76006.

Information on early intervention programs in each state is available from the **National Down Syndrome Society,** 141 Fifth Ave., New York, NY 10010.

‡A resource for a wide variety of equipment, including self-help devices, is available from J.A. Preston, Catalog: Equipment for rehabilitation and special education, 60 Page Rd., Clifton, NJ 07012.

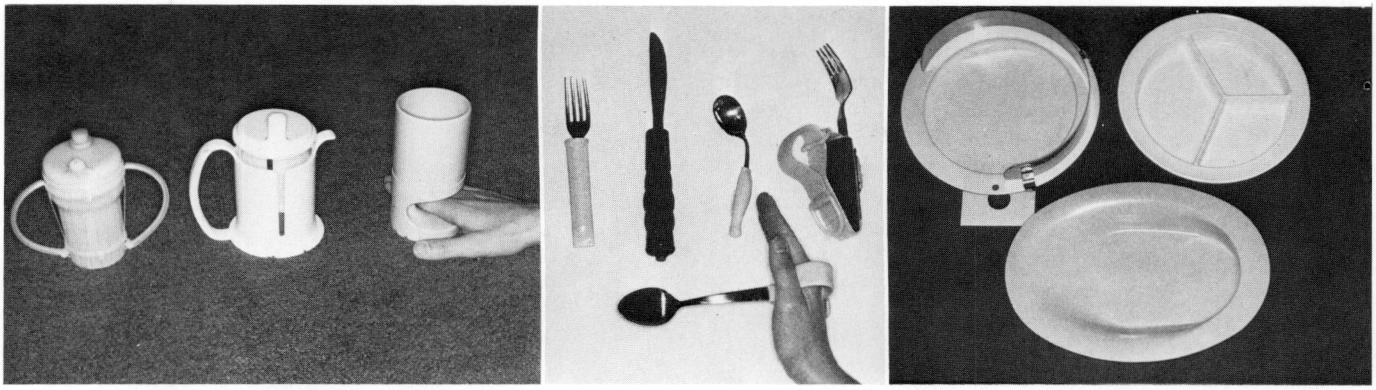

A B C

FIG. 19-2 Self-help aids for feeding: **A** *(left to right)*: modified drinking cup, glass with holder and lid, pedestal cup; **B** *(left to right)*: soft build-up handle utensil, weighted knife, child's bent spoon, quad-quip utensil holder (holds most household utensils) and *(bottom)* vertical palm self-handle utensil; **C** *(left to right, top)*: plastic plate with suction feet and optional metal food guard, partitioned scoop dish, and *(bottom)* scoop dish.

Plastic surgery should be considered in situations where the child's appearance may be substantially improved. Dental health is very significant, and orthodontic and restorative procedures can immensely improve facial appearance.

Play/exercise. The child with mental retardation has the same needs for recreation and exercise as any other child. However, because of his slower development, parents may be less aware of the need to provide such activities. Therefore, the nurse guides parents toward selection of suitable play and exercise activities. Since play has been discussed for children in each age-group in earlier chapters, only the exceptions are presented here.

The type of play is based on the child's developmental age, although the need for sensorimotor play may be prolonged for several years. Parents should use every opportunity to expose the child to as many different sounds, sights, and sensations as possible. Appropriate play includes musical mobiles, stuffed toys, water play, floating toys, rocking chair or horse, swing, bells, and rattles. The child should be taken on outings, such as trips to the grocery store or shopping center; other people should be encouraged to visit in the home; and the child should be related to directly, such as by cuddling, holding, rocking, talking to him in the *en face* (face to face) position, and giving him "rides" on the parents' shoulders.

Toys are selected for their recreational and educational value. For example, a large inflatable beach ball is a good water toy, encourages interactive play, and can be used to learn motor skills, such as balance, rocking, kicking, and throwing. A doll with removable clothes and different types of closures can help the child learn dressing skills. Musical toys that mimic animal sounds or respond with social phrases are excellent ways of encouraging speech. Toys should be simple in design so that the child can learn to manipulate them without help. For children with severe cognitive and physical impairment, electronic switches can be used to allow them to operate toys (Fig. 19-3).

Suitable activities for physical activity are based on the child's size, coordination, physical fitness and maturity, motivation, and health. Some children may have physical problems that prevent certain sports, such as atlantoaxial instabililty in children with Down syndrome (see p. 551). These children often have greater success in individual and dual sports than in team sports and enjoy themselves most with children of the same developmental level (American Academy of Pediatrics, 1987). The **Special**

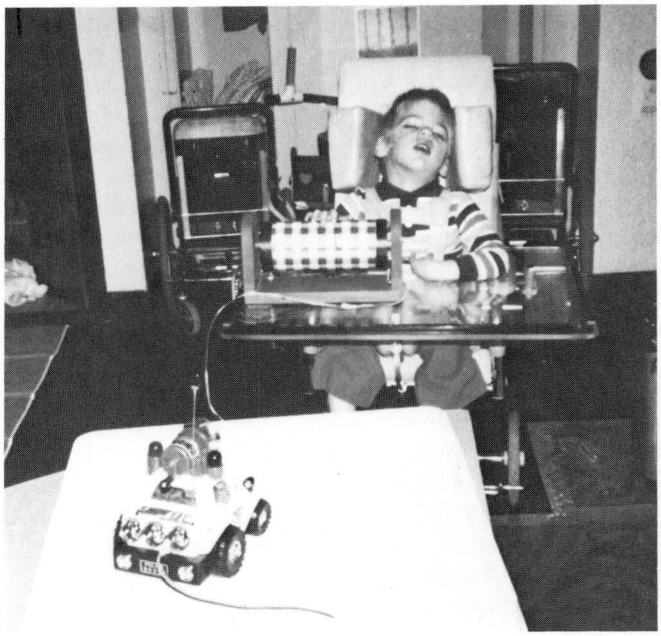

FIG. 19-3 A barrel switch allows a child with mental retardation to play with a battery-operated truck.

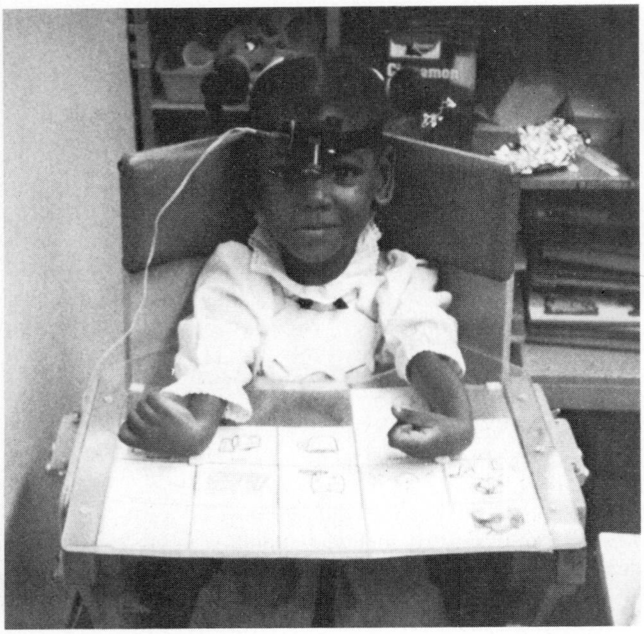

FIG. 19-4 A child with cognitive and physical impairments can use a communication board by pointing with an optical head pointer.

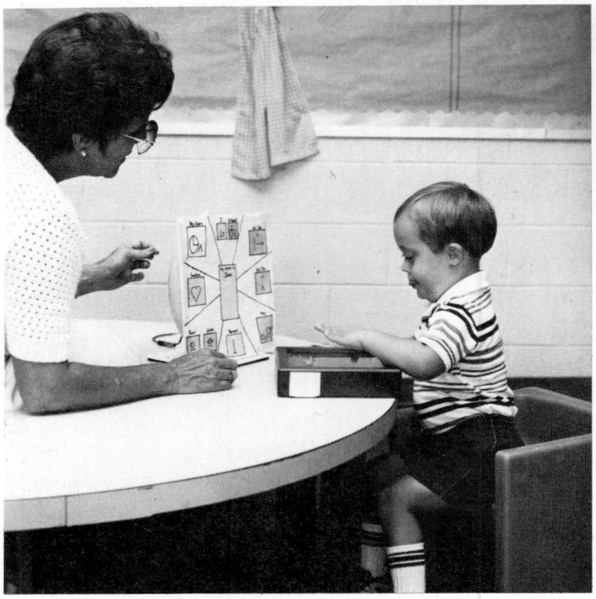

FIG. 19-5 Blissymbols can help a young child communicate nonverbally. This device uses a light behind each symbol; the child rotates the light around the board by pressing the push panel.

Olympics Program* provides these children with a unique competitive opportunity.

Safety is a major consideration in selecting recreational and exercise activities. For example, toys that may be appropriate developmentally may present dangers to a child who is strong enough to break them or use them incorrectly.

Communication. Verbal skills are typically delayed more than other physical skills. Speech requires hearing and interpretation (receptive skills) and facial muscle coordination (expressive skills). Since both types of skills may be impaired, these children need frequent audiometric testing and should be fitted with hearing aids if this is indicated. In addition, they may need help in learning to control their facial muscles. For example, some children may need tongue exercises to correct the tongue thrust or gentle reminders to keep the lips closed.

Nonverbal communication may be appropriate for some of these children and various devices are available. For the child without associated physical disabilities, a talking picture board is helpful. For children with physical limitations a number of adaptations or types of communication devices are available to facilitate selection of the appropriate picture or word (Fig. 19-4). Some children may be taught sign language or *Blissymbols*. Blissymbols is a highly stylized system of graphic symbols that represent words, ideas, and concepts. Although they require education to learn their meaning, no reading skill is needed. The symbols are usually arranged on a board and the person points or uses some type of selector to convey a message (Fig. 19-5).

Discipline. Discipline must begin early. Limit-setting measures need to be simple, consistently applied, and appropriate for the child's mental age. Control measures are based primarily on teaching a specific behavior rather than on understanding the reasons behind it. Stressing moral lessons are of little value to a child who lacks the cognitive skills to learn from self-criticism or from a lesson based on previous wrongdoing. Behavior modification, especially reinforcement of desired actions, and time-out are appropriate forms of behavior control (see Chapter 4).

Socialization. Acquiring social skills is a complex task, as is learning self-care procedures. Active rehearsal with role playing and practice sessions and positive reinforcement for desired behavior have been the most successful approaches. Parents should be encouraged early to teach their child socially acceptable behavior—waving goodbye, saying hello and thank you, responding to his name, greeting visitors but not being overly affectionate, and sitting modestly. The teaching of socially acceptable sexual behavior is especially important to minimize sexual exploitation (Williams, 1983). Parents also need to expose the child to strangers so he can practice manners, since there is no automatic transfer of learning from one situation to another.

Dressing and grooming are also important aspects of socialization. A child who is dressed in appropriate-age clothing and is well-groomed is much more likely to be

*1350 New York Ave., NW, Suite 500, Washington, DC 20005-1518; **Canadian Special Olympics, Inc.,** 40 St. Clair Ave. West, Suite 209, Toronto, Ontario M4V 1M6.

accepted and to develop good self-esteem. Clothes should be clean, up-to-date, and well-fitted. Many attractive outfits can be adapted with Velcro fasteners and elastic openings to facilitate self-dressing.*

Children of all ages need peer relationships, and these children are no exception. As soon as possible parents should enroll the child in appropriate preschool programs. Not only do these programs provide education and training, they also offer an opportunity for social experiences among the children.

As the child grows older, he should have peer experiences similar to those of normal children, including group outings, sports, and organized activity, such as Boy Scouts, Girl Scouts, or Special Olympics. He should be encouraged to form a close relationship with a best friend.

Adolescence may be a particularly difficult time for parents, especially in terms of the child's sexual behavior, possibility of pregnancy, future plans to marry, and ability to be independent. Frequently little anticipatory guidance has been offered parents to prepare the child for physical and sexual maturation. The nurse can help in this area by providing parents with information about sex education that is geared to the child's developmental level. For example, the adolescent female needs a *simple* explanation of menstruation and instructions on personal hygiene during the menstrual cycle.

The question of contraceptive protection for female retarded adolescents is often a parental concern. Of the available methods, medroxyprogesterone, the intrauterine device (IUD), or birth control pills are most commonly used. However, each has its disadvantages. Medroxyprogesterone (Depo-Provera) requires intramuscular injections every 3 months and initially is associated with heavy breakthrough bleeding. The IUD requires regular checking of the string's placement and can cause menorrhagia. Birth control pills must be used regularly; their effectiveness can be maximized by devising reminder charts or by using dated pill dispensers. Sterilization as a form of contraception is a special dilemma because of moral and ethical questions as well as psychologic effects on the adolescent. The decision regarding sterilization of minors and incompetent adults is a legal one; if parents consider permanent sterilization for their daughter, she should be included in the decision according to her level of understanding.

Because of the embarrassment some parents feel regarding sexual information, many concerns may go unvoiced. The nurse can be instrumental in discussing topics such as contraception or advisability of marriage with the parents and the adolescent. In this way plans can be made early and potential problems avoided.

Help families adjust to future care. Not all families are able to cope with home care of their affected child, especially one who is severely or profoundly retarded and/or multidisabled. Older parents may not be able to assume care responsibilities once they reach retirement or old age. For these parents, the decision regarding residential placement is a difficult one.

A number of alternatives exist regarding out-of-home care, but the availability of these facilities varies widely depending on the community's resources. Basically, care options range from the least to the most restrictive types of environments—foster homes, semi-independent living programs, group residence homes, and institutions. The nurse working with a family should help them investigate and evaluate various programs, in addition to assisting them in their adjustment to the decision for placement.

Care for the child during hospitalization. Caring for the child during hospitalization is a special challenge. Frequently nurses are unfamiliar with children who are retarded, and so they cope with their feelings of insecurity and fear by ignoring or isolating the child. Not only is this approach nonsupportive, it may also be destructive for the child's sense of self-esteem and optimum development and hamper the parents' ability to cope with the stress of the experience. One method that successfully avoids this nontherapeutic approach is the use of the mutual participation model in planning the child's care. Parents should be encouraged to room with their child but should not be made to feel as if the responsibility is totally theirs.

When the child is admitted, a detailed history is taken (see Chapter 20), especially in terms of all self-help activity. During the interview the child's developmental age is assessed. It is best to avoid directly asking about IQ levels, since this may make the parents uncomfortable and often tells little about the child's actual abilities. Questions are approached positively. For example, rather than asking, "Is he toilet trained yet?" the nurse may state, "Tell me about his toileting habits." The assessment should also focus on any special devices the child uses, effective measures of limit setting, unusual or favorite routines, and any behaviors that may require intervention. For example, if the parent states that the child engages in self-stimulatory activities, the nurse inquires about events that precipitate them and techniques that the parents use to manage them.

The child's functional level of eating and playing, his ability to express his needs verbally, his progress in toilet training, and his relationship with objects, toys, and other children are also assessed. He is encouraged to be as independent as possible, even though he is in a hospital setting.

Realizing that the child may be lonely in the hospital, the nurse makes certain that he has toys and other activities to entertain him, includes him in group activities on the unit, and sets time aside each day to talk to or play with him. The child is placed in a room with other children of approximate developmental age, preferably a room with two beds, to avoid overstimulation. The nurse discusses with the other parents the child's abilities and introduces the parents and children to each other. By the nurse's example of treating the child with dignity and respect, others who may be fearful of what they

*A helpful book is Hotte, E: *Self-Help Clothing,* available from The National Easter Seal Society, 2023 W. Odgen Avenue, Chicago, IL 60612.

do not understand are encouraged to accept the child.

Procedures are explained to the child through methods of communication that are at his cognitive level. Generally explanations should be simple, short, and concrete, emphasizing what the child will experience *physically*. Demonstration either through actual practice or with visual aids is always preferable to verbal explanation. The nurse repeats instructions often and evaluates the child's understanding by asking questions such as, "What did I say it will feel like?" "What will the doctor look like?" "Show me how you must lie." or "Where will the dressing be?" Parents are included in preprocedural teaching for their own learning and to help the nurse learn effective methods of communicating with the child.

During hospitalization the nurse should also focus on growth-promoting experiences for the child. For example, hospitalization may be an excellent opportunity to emphasize to parents abilities that the child does have but has not had the opportunity to practice, such as self-dressing. It may also be an opportunity for social experiences with peers, group play, or new educational/recreational activities. For example, one child who had the habit of screaming and kicking demonstrated a definite decrease in those behaviors after he learned to pound pegs and use a punching bag. Through social services the parents may become aware of specialized programs for the child. Nutritional counseling is available if the child is overweight or has evidence of specific deficiencies, such as iron deficiency. Hospitalization may also offer parents a respite from everyday care responsibilities and an opportunity to discuss their feelings with a concerned professional.

Assist in measures to prevent retardation. Not only do nurses have a responsibility to families with a child with cognitive retardation; they also need to be involved in programs aimed at preventing mental retardation. Many of the familial, social, and environmental factors known to cause mild retardation are preventable. Counseling and education can reduce or eliminate such factors, for example, poor nutrition, cigarette smoking, and chemical abuse, which increase the risk of prematurity and intrauterine growth retardation. Consequently, the major interventions are directed at improving maternal health and educating women regarding the dangers of chemicals used during pregnancy. Other preventive strategies that play an important role include optimal medical care for high-risk newborns; rubella immunization; genetic counseling and amniocentesis, especially in terms of Down or fragile X syndrome; newborn screening for treatable inborn errors of metabolism, such as congenital hypothyroidism, phenylketonuria, and galactosemia; and early appropriate therapies and rehabilitation services for children with developmental disabilities.

EVALUATION

The effectiveness of nursing interventions is determined by continual reassessment and evaluation of care based on the following observational guidelines and expected outcomes:

1. Observe the techniques used to teach the child and their success in accomplishing education; inquire if child is enrolled in early stimulation program
2. Observe those activities of daily living that the child can completely or partially perform
3. Interview the family regarding the provision of appropriate play, socialization, and discipline for the child; observe the child's ability to communicate with others; interview the child regarding feelings of self-worth if possible
4. Interview the family regarding any plans for future care and their awareness of community services
5. Check medical record or Kardex for evidence of nursing admission history, especially for self-help activities; observe parent's involvement in child's care; observe social interaction of child and family with other patients
6. Investigate community programs aimed at preventing retardation and inquire as to nursing involvement in these efforts

Expected outcomes:

1. Child is enrolled in early stimulation program; family members use appropriate education techniques
2. Child participates in self-care to his maximum capabilities
3. Child develops to maximum potential
4. Family identifies realistic goals for future care of child
5. Child receives appropriate care during hospitalization
6. Nurses participate in measures to prevent mental retardation

DOWN SYNDROME

Down syndrome is the most common chromosomal abnormality, occurring once in every 650 to 1000 live births. It owes its once common but unacceptable name, *mongolism*, to the particular facial characteristics, which resemble those of the Mongol race.

Etiology

The cause of Down syndrome is not known, but evidence from cytogenetic and epidemiologic studies supports the concept of multiple causality. Although the etiology is unclear, the cytogenetics of the disorder are well established. Approximately 92% to 95% of all cases of Down syndrome are attributable to an extra chromosome 21 (group G), hence the name *trisomy 21*. Although children with trisomy 21 are born to parents of all ages, there is a statistically greater risk in older women, particularly those over 35 years. For example, in women less than 30 years of age the incidence of Down syndrome is less than 1 in 1000 live births, but in women age 40 it is about 1 in 100. Paternal age is also a factor, especially in males 55 years and over.

About 4% to 6% of the cases may be caused by *translocation* of chromosomes 15 and 21 or 22. This type of genetic aberration is usually hereditary and is not associated with advanced parental age. From 1% to 3% of affected persons demonstrate *mosaicism*, which refers to

Clinical Manifestations in Down Syndrome

Physical Characteristics (most frequently observed)
Small rounded skull with a flat occiput
Inner epicanthal folds and oblique palpebral fissures (upward, outward slant of the eyes)
Small nose with a depressed bridge (saddle nose)
Protruding, sometimes fissured, tongue
Hypoplastic mandible (makes tongue appear large)
High-arched palate
Short, thick neck
Hypotonic musculature (protruding abdomen, umbilical hernia)
Hyperflexible and lax joints
Simian line (transverse crease on the palmar side of the hand; see Fig. 7-9, *B*)
Broad, short, and stubby hands and feet

Intelligence
Varies from severely retarded to low normal intelligence
Generally within mild to moderate range

Social Development
May be 2 to 3 years beyond mental age, especially during early childhood

Congenital Anomalies (increased incidence)
Most common is congenital heart disease
Other defects include:
- Renal agenesis
- Duodenal atresia
- Hirschsprung disease
- Tracheoesophageal fistula
- Hip subluxation
- Instability of the first and second cervical vertebrae (atlantoaxial instability)

Sensory Problems (frequently associated)
May include:
- Conductive hearing loss (very common)
- Strabismus
- Myopia
- Nystagmus
- Cataracts
- Conjunctivitis

Growth and Sexual Development
Growth in both height and weight reduced; obesity common
Sexual development delayed, incomplete, or both
Males infertile; females can be fertile
Premature aging common; lowered life expectancy

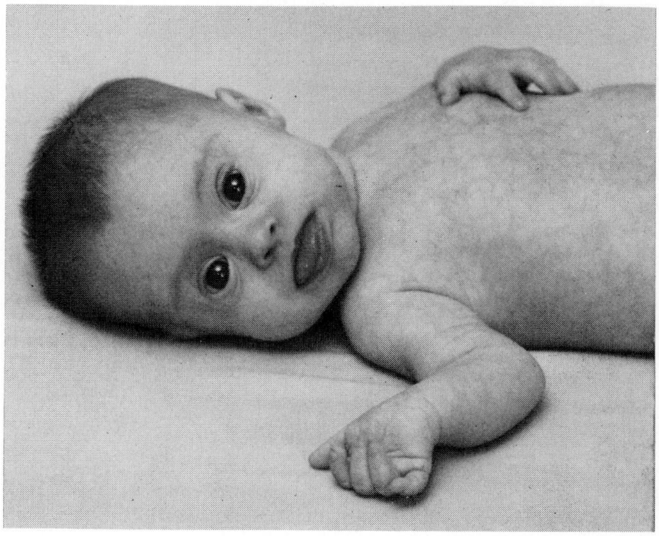

FIG. 19-6 Down syndrome in infant. Note small square head with mongoloid slant to the eyes, flat nasal bridge, protruding tongue, mottled skin, and hypotonia.

cells with both normal and abnormal chromosomes. The degree of physical and cognitive impairment is related to the percentage of cells with the abnormal chromosome makeup.

Diagnostic Evaluation

Down syndrome can usually be diagnosed by the clinical manifestations alone (see box and Fig. 19-6), but a chromosomal analysis should be done to confirm the genetic abnormality if the parents are young or if the diagnosis is doubtful, as in mosaicism.

Several physical problems are associated with Down syndrome. Many of these children have congenital heart malformations, the most common being septal defects. Respiratory infections are very prevalent, and when combined with cardiac anomalies, they are the chief cause of death, particularly during the first year of life. Hypotonicity of chest and abdominal muscles probably predisposes to the development of respiratory infection. Other physical problems include thyroid dysfunction, especially congenital hypothyroidism, and an increased incidence of leukemia.

Therapeutic Management

Although there is no cure for Down syndrome, a number of therapies are advocated, such as surgery to correct serious congenital anomalies and possibly the physical stigmata, although the latter is controversial. These children also benefit from regular medical care. Evaluation of sight and hearing is essential, and treatment of otitis media is required to prevent auditory loss, which can influence cognitive function. Periodic testing of thyroid function is recommended, especially if growth is severely delayed. Children participating in sports that may involve stress on the head and neck, such as gymnastics, diving, butterfly stroke in swimming, high jump and soccer, should be evaluated for atlantoaxial instability. Symptoms of the disorder, such as neck pain, weakness, and torticollis, require prompt attention.

Nursing Considerations

Caring for the child with Down syndrome involves several short- and long-term goals. Support for parents from health professionals, especially nurses, is increasingly important with the present trend to rear these children at home. Prevention is also discussed since nurses should be concerned with measures that may prevent Down syndrome.

ASSESSMENT

Assessment of the child with Down syndrome usually presents little difficulty because of the obvious physical characteristics (see box, p. 551). However, the nurse needs to be aware of newborns who manifest these stigmata in order to ensure early diagnosis and support for the family.

NURSING DIAGNOSES

A number of nursing diagnoses are prominent in the nursing care of the child with Down syndrome and the child's family; other diagnoses specific to individual cases become evident. The most common nursing diagnoses are outlined in the Nursing Care Plan on p. 553.

PLANNING

The goals of nursing care for the child with Down syndrome and family are:

1. Support the family at time of diagnosis
2. Assist the family in preventing physical problems
3. Assist with measures to prevent Down syndrome

IMPLEMENTATION

Once the goals are identified, specific interventions are carried out. The following discussion presents general interventions for most children with Down syndrome. Long-term interventions for the child with mental retardation have been discussed earlier in this chapter.

Support the family at time of diagnosis. Because of the unique physical characteristics, the infant with Down syndrome is usually diagnosed at birth. However, parents are not always informed of the diagnosis at this time. This presents special difficulties for those caring for the postpartal mother, since she or the father may notice differences in the child and question others about their concern.

Generally parents wish to know the diagnosis as soon as possible. This approach prevents such dilemmas as telling others that the child has Down syndrome after indicating that he was fine and experiencing unconfirmed doubt over the child's development. Most parents prefer that both of them be present during the informing interview because it is a problem that both of them will have to face, they can emotionally support one another, and it eliminates the difficult task of revealing the diagnosis to the other partner. They appreciate receiving reading material about the syndrome* and being referred to others for help or advice, such as parent groups or professional counseling.

Once parents are aware of the diagnosis, they are confronted with the crisis of losing a perfect or dream child and grieving for and accepting their reality child. Consequently, the parents' responses to the child may greatly influence decisions regarding future care. Whereas some families willingly wish to take the child home, others consider immediate residential placement. The nurse must carefully answer questions regarding developmental potential and out-of-home placement, since the responses may influence the parents' decision. It is important to stress to parents that a decision regarding placement will affect all of their lives and need not be made at the time of diagnosis.

Assist the family in preventing physical problems. Many of the physical characteristics of Down syndrome present nursing problems. The hypotonicity of muscles and hyperextensibility of joints complicate positioning. The limp, flaccid extremities resemble the posture of a rag doll; as a result, holding the infant is difficult and cumbersome. Sometimes parents perceive this lack of molding to their bodies as evidence of inadequate parenting. The extended body position promotes heat loss because more surface area is exposed to the environment. Parents are encouraged to swaddle or wrap the infant tightly in a blanket before picking him up to provide security and warmth. The nurse also discusses with parents their feelings concerning attachment to the child, emphasizing that the child's lack of clinging or molding is a physical characteristic, not a sign of detachment or rejection.

Decreased muscle tone compromises respiratory expansion. In addition, the underdeveloped nasal bone causes a chronic problem of inadequate drainage of mucus. The constant stuffy nose forces the child to breathe by mouth, which dries the oropharyngeal membranes, increasing the susceptibility to upper respiratory infections. Measures to lessen these problems include clearing the nose with a bulb-type syringe, rinsing the mouth with water after feedings, using a cool-mist vaporizer to keep the mucous membranes moist and the secretions liquefied, changing the child's position frequently, and performing postural drainage and percussion. If antibiotics are ordered, the importance of completing the full course of therapy for successful eradication of the infection and prevention of growth of resistant organisms is stressed.

Inadequate drainage and pooling of mucus in the nose also interfere with feeding. Because the child breathes by mouth, he is unable to suck for any length of time as a result of his need for air. When eating solids, he may gag on the food because of mucus in the oropharynx. Parents are advised to clear the nose before each feeding, give small, frequent feedings, and allow opportunities for rest at mealtime.

The protruding tongue also interferes with feeding, especially solid foods. Parents need to know that the tongue thrust is not an indication of refusal to feed, but a physiologic response. Parents are advised to use a small but long, straight-handled spoon to push the food toward the back and side of the mouth. If food is thrust out, it is refed.

Dietary intake needs supervision. Decreased muscle tone affects gastric motility, predisposing the child to con-

*Information is available from the **National Down Syndrome Society,** 141 Fifth Ave., New York, NY 10010 (1-800-221-4602); **Down Syndrome Congress,** 1800 Dempster, Park Ridge, IL 60068 (1-800-232-6372.)

NURSING CARE PLAN

The Child with Down Syndrome

Nursing Goals	Nursing Interventions	Expected Patient/Family Outcomes
NDx HP-HMP* Potential for infection **Risk factors: hypotonia, increased susceptibility to infection**		
Prevent respiratory infection	Teach the parents postural drainage and percussion Stress importance of changing child's position frequently, especially sitting posture Encourage use of cool-mist vaporizer Teach suctioning of nares Stress importance of good mouth care (follow feedings with clear water)	Child exhibits no evidence of infection or respiratory distress
NDx HP-HMP Potential for abnormal development **Risk factors: parental age**		
Prevent Down syndrome	Discuss with high-risk women risks of giving birth to child with Down syndrome Encourage all pregnant women at risk (over age 35, family history of Down syndrome, or previous birth of child with Down syndrome) to consider amniocentesis during twelfth to sixteenth week of pregnancy to rule out Down syndrome in fetus Discuss option of elective abortion with women who are carrying an affected fetus Discuss with parents of adolescent children with Down syndrome the possibility of conception in a female and the need for contraceptive methods	Pregnant women at risk seek evaluation for Down syndrome Families demonstrate an understanding of options available to them Families of an affected female child seek contraceptive advice
NDx N-MP Potential impaired skin integrity **Risk factors: hypotonia, increased susceptibility to infection**		
Prevent skin breakdown	Keep skin well lubricated with topical creams or lotions Use soap sparingly Apply lip balm when the child is outdoors	Skin remains clean and intact with no evidence of inflammation
NDx A-EP Feeding, bathing/hygiene, dressing/grooming, toileting (specify level) self-care deficit **Etiology: mental retardation**		
Facilitate self-care†	Enroll child in stimulation program Reinforce self-care activities	Child participates in self-care to his maximum capabilities
Minimize feeding difficulties in infancy	Suction nares before each feeding, if needed Schedule small, frequent feedings; allow child to rest during feedings Feed solid food by pushing it to back and side of mouth; use long, straight-handled infant spoon Point out to family that tongue thrust does not indicate refusal of food Calculate caloric needs to meet energy requirements; base intake on height and weight, not chronologic age Monitor height and weight at regular intervals Provide sufficient fiber and fluids to prevent constipation	Infant consumes an adequate amount of food for age and size (specify) Family reports satisfactory feeding Infant gains weight in accordance with standard weight tables
NDx CPP Altered growth and development **Etiology: mental retardation**		
Promote optimum development†	Involve child and family in an early infant stimulation program Assess child's developmental progress at regular intervals; keep detailed records to distinguish subtle changes in functioning Help family set realistic goals for child	Child and family are actively involved in infant stimulation program Family applies concepts and continues activities in home care of child

*For an explanation of abbreviations, see p. 20.
†Applicable to any child with mental retardation.

Continued.

NURSING CARE PLAN

The Child with Down Syndrome—cont'd

Nursing Goals	Nursing Interventions	Expected Patient/Family Outcomes
	Encourage learning of self-care skills as soon as child achieves readiness	Child performs activities of daily living at his optimum capacity
	Encourage family to investigate special day-care programs and educational classes as soon as possible	Family investigates educational programs
	Emphasize that child has same needs as other children Play Discipline Social interaction	Appropriate limit setting, recreation, and social opportunities are provided
	Prior to adolescence, counsel child and parents regarding physical maturation, sexual behavior, marriage, and family Encourage optimum vocational training	Adolescent issues are explored and implemented as appropriate
NDx RRP Altered family processes **Etiology: birth of a child with mental deficiency**		
Support family at time of diagnosis*	Inform family as soon as possible after birth Have both parents present at informing conference Give family written information about syndrome Discuss with family members benefits of home care vs foster care or adoption; allow them opportunities to investigate all residential alternatives before making a decision Encourage family to meet other families with Down children Refrain from giving definitive answers about the degree of retardation; stress the potential learning abilities of their children, especially with early stimulation	Family expresses feelings and concerns regarding the birth of child with mental retardation and its implications Family members make realistic decisions based on their needs and capabilities
	Demonstrate acceptance of infant through own behavior Emphasize normal characteristics of child Encourage family members to express their feelings and concerns	Family members demonstrate acceptance of child
Help family prepare for future care of child	As child grows older, discuss with parents alternatives to home care, especially as parents near retirement or old age Help family investigate residential settings Encourage family to include affected member in planning and to continue meaningful relationships with him after placement	Family identifies realistic goals for future care of child
	Refer to agencies that provide support and assistance	Family avails themselves of supportive services

*Applicable to any child with mental retardation.

stipation. Dietary measures such as increased fiber and fluid promote evacuation. The child's eating habits may need careful scrutiny to prevent obesity. Height and weight measurements should be obtained on a serial basis, especially during infancy, since excessive weight gain can impede motor development. The child should receive calories in accordance with his height and weight, not his chronologic age.

During infancy the child's skin is pliable and soft. However, it gradually becomes rough and dry and is prone to cracking and infection. Skin care involves the use of minimum soap and application of lubricants. Lip balm is applied to the lips, especially when the child is outdoors, to prevent excessive chapping.

Assist with prenatal diagnosis Down syndrome. There is no cure for Down syndrome. However, through amniocentesis, chromosomal analysis of fetal cells can detect the presence of trisomy or translocation. The nurse has a role in genetic counseling of those parents of advanced age or who have a family history of the disorder to discuss the possibility of amniocentesis. If the fetus is affected, the nurse must allow the parents to express their feelings concerning elective abortion and support their decision either to terminate or proceed with the pregnancy.

EVALUATION

The effectiveness of nursing interventions is determined by continual reassessment and evaluation of care based on the following observational guidelines:

1. Observe the parents' response to the newborn; interview family regarding plans for home care or residential placement

2. Observe the parents' ability to care for child; monitor weight and height; observe condition of the skin
3. Interview parents regarding their beliefs on abortion if result of amniocentesis is positive; check follow-up if family is referred for genetic counseling

Expected outcomes:
See Nursing Care Plan, pp. 553 to 554.

FRAGILE X SYNDROME

Fragile X syndrome is a recently described chromosomal condition characterized by a marker found on the X chromosome when the chromosome is placed in a special culture medium. The fragile X syndrome affects approximately 30% to 50% of families with X-linked mental retardation, making it the second most common specific cause of mental retardation after Down syndrome (Cohen, 1984). Identification of this marker allows for genetic counseling that was not possible previously for families of an affected individual.

In some males with the fragile X chromosome there is a reçognizable clinical phenotype and associated developmental characteristics (see box). However, none of these features is specific to individuals with the fragile X site and in females the clinical manifestations are extremely varied. Both affected sexes are fertile and therefore capable of transmitting the fragile X disorder.

Nursing Considerations

Since cognitive impairment is a fairly consistent finding in individuals with fragile X syndrome, the care afforded to these families is the same as for any child with mental retardation. Because the disorder is hereditary, genetic counseling is necessary to inform parents of the risks of transmission; a woman who carries a fragile X chromosome has a 25% recurrence risk for transmission to her offspring, regardless of their sex (Cohen, 1984). In addition, any male or female with unexplained or nonspecific mental impairment should be referred for chromosomal analysis and appropriate genetic counseling (Brady, 1984).

Clinical Manifestations Associated with Fragile X Syndrome

Short stature
Normal to increased head size
"Long face" with prominent jaw
Large nose with broad nasal bridge
Large or prominent ears
Large testicles (macroorchidism or macrotestes)
Mild to severe mental retardation
Speech or language abnormality
Hyperactivity
Visual motor incoordination
Autistic tendencies

◆ *Sensory Impairments*

Sensory impairments pose special threats to a child's developmental potential. Deprived of visual or auditory cues, the child must rely more heavily on other sensory experiences to learn about and relate to the environment. Without assistance and rehabilitation, these children are vulnerable to the lifelong disadvantages of their disability. However, with assistance they can lead essentially normal and productive lives.

HEARING IMPAIRMENT

Hearing impairment is one of the most common disabilities in the United States. The exact prevalence of hearing loss is not known, especially in young children with unilateral impairment. However, national data indicate that about 11 of 1000 children 6 to 17 years of age have a hearing impairment (Gortmaker and Sappenfield, 1984). With improved neonatal detection methods, the incidence of moderate to profound hearing loss in high-risk infants is 2.5% to 5% (American Academy of Pediatrics, 1982).

Definition and Classification

Hearing impairment is a general term indicating disability that may range in severity from mild to profound and includes the subsets of deaf and hard-of-hearing. *Deaf* refers to a person whose hearing disability precludes successful processing of linguistic information through audition, with or without a hearing aid. *Hard-of-hearing* refers to a person who, generally with the use of a hearing aid, has residual hearing sufficient to enable successful processing of linguistic information through audition. Other terms, such as deaf and dumb, mute, or deaf-mute, are unacceptable. Hearing-impaired persons are not dumb and, if mute, have no physical speech defect other than that caused by the inability to hear.

Hearing defects may be classified according to etiology, pathology, or symptom severity. Each is important in terms of treatment, possible prevention, and rehabilitation.

Etiology. Hearing loss may be caused by a number of prenatal and postnatal conditions. These include a family history of childhood hearing impairment, anatomic malformations of the head or neck, low birth weight, severe perinatal asphyxia, perinatal infection (cytomegalovirus, rubella, herpes, syphilis, toxoplasmosis, and bacterial meningitis), chronic ear infection, cerebral palsy, Down syndrome, or administration of ototoxic drugs.

Another significant potential cause is excessive exposure to high noise levels. This may occur from urban living, loud rock music, model airplanes, snowmobiles, sport shooting, motorcycle and sport racing, or heavy machinery.

In addition, high-risk neonates who are surviving formerly fatal prenatal or perinatal conditions may be susceptible to hearing loss from the disorder or its treatment.

For example, sensorineural hearing loss may be the result of continuous humming noises or high noise levels associated with incubators, oxygen hoods, or intensive care units, especially when combined with the use of potentially ototoxic antibiotics.

Pathology. Disorders of hearing are divided according to location of the defect. *Conductive* or middle-ear hearing loss results from interference of transmission of sound to the middle ear. It is the most common of all types of hearing loss and most frequently is a result of recurrent serous otitis media. Conductive hearing impairment mainly involves interference with loudness of sound.

Sensorineural hearing loss, also called perceptive or nerve deafness, involves damage to the inner ear structures and/or the auditory nerve. The most common causes are congenital defects of inner ear structures or consequences of acquired conditions, such as kernicterus, infection, administration of ototoxic drugs, or exposure to excessive noise. Sensorineural hearing loss results in distortion of sound and problems in discrimination. Although the child hears some of everything going on around him, the sounds are distorted, severely affecting discrimination and comprehension.

Mixed conductive-sensorineural hearing loss results from interference with transmission of sound in the middle ear and along neural pathways. It frequently results from recurrent otitis media and its complications.

Central auditory imperception includes all hearing losses that do not demonstrate defects in the conductive or sensorineural structures. They are usually divided into organic or functional losses. In the organic type of central auditory imperception, the defect involves the reception of auditory stimuli along the central pathways and the expression of the message into meaningful communication. Examples are *aphasia,* an inability to express ideas in any form, either written or verbally; *agnosia,* the inability to interpret sound correctly; and *dysacusis,* difficulty in processing details or discrimination among sounds.

In the functional type there is no organic lesion to explain a central auditory loss. Examples of functional hearing loss are conversion hysteria (an unconscious withdrawal from hearing to block remembrance of a traumatic event), infantile autism, and childhood schizophrenia.

Symptom severity. Hearing impairment is expressed in terms of a decibel (dB), a unit of loudness (Table 19-2). Hearing impairment can be classified according to hearing-threshold level (the measurement of an individual's hearing threshold by means of an audiometer) and the degree of symptom severity as it affects speech (Table 19-3). These classifications offer only general guidelines regarding the effect of the impairment on any individual child, since children differ greatly in their ability to use residual hearing.

Therapeutic Management

Treatment of hearing loss depends on the cause and type of hearing impairment. Many conductive hearing defects are amenable to medical or surgical treatment, such as antibiotic therapy for acute otitis media or insertion of tympanostomy tubes for chronic otitis media. When the conductive loss is permanent, hearing can be improved with the use of a hearing aid to amplify sound.

Treatment for sensorineural hearing loss is much less

TABLE 19-2

Intensity of Sounds Expressed in Decibels

Decibels (dB)	Representative Sound
0	Softest sound normal ear can hear
10	Heartbeat, rustling of leaves
20	Whisper at 1.8 m (5 feet)
30-45	Normal conversation
60	Noise in average restaurant
70-80	Street noises
80	Loud radio in home
90-100	Train
120	Thunder, rock music
140	Jet airplane during departure
>140	Pain threshold

TABLE 19-3

Classification of Hearing Loss Based on Symptom Severity

Hearing Level (dB)	Effect
Slight—<30 (hard of hearing)	Has difficulty in hearing faint or distant speech Usually is unaware of hearing difficulty Likely to achieve in school but may have problems No speech defects
Mild to moderate—30-55 (hard of hearing)	Understands conversational speech at 3 to 5 feet but has difficulty if speech faint or not facing speaker May have speech difficulties
Marked—55-70 (hard of hearing)	Unable to understand conversational speech unless loud Considerable difficulty with group or classroom discussion Requires special speech training
Severe—70-90 (deaf)	May hear a loud voice if nearby May be able to identify loud environmental noises Can distinguish vowels but not most consonants Requires speech training
Profound—>90 (deaf)	May hear only loud sounds Requires extensive speech training

satisfactory. Since the defect is not one of intensity of sound, hearing aids are of less value in this type of defect. The use of cochlear implants (a surgically implanted prosthetic device) may provide hope for some affected children in the future.

Disorders of central auditory imperception depend on the cause. Functional types, such as conversion hysteria, may require psychologic intervention, but others, such as autism, may not respond to any therapy.

Nursing Considerations

Nursing care of hearing-impaired children is often a specialized area, requiring additional training in auditory testing and rehabilitation. However, general nursing goals that focus on assessment, prevention, and rehabilitation of the child with a hearing impairment are every nurse's responsibility. In addition, nurses may have to care for a hearing-impaired child who is hospitalized and must know how to best meet the child's and family's special needs.

ASSESSMENT

Assessment of children for hearing impairment is a critical nursing responsibility. Discovery of a hearing impairment within the first 6 to 12 months of life is essential to prevent social, physical, and psychologic damage to the child. Assessment involves (1) identifying those children who by virtue of their history are at risk, (2) observing for behaviors that indicate a hearing loss, and (3) screening all children for auditory function. This discussion focuses on developmental/behavioral indices associated with hearing impairment. Tests for assessing hearing are included in Chapter 7.

Infancy. At birth the nurse can observe the neonate's response to auditory stimuli as evidenced by the startle reflex, head turning, eye blinking, and cessation of body movement. The infant may vary in the intensity of the response, depending on the state of alertness. However, a consistent absence of a reaction should lead to suspicion of hearing loss. Other clinical manifestations of hearing impairment in the infant are summarized in the box.

Childhood. The profoundly deaf child is much more likely to be diagnosed during infancy than the less severely affected one. If the defect is not detected during early childhood, the likelihood is that it will surface during entry to school, when the child has difficulty in learning. Unfortunately some of these children are erroneously placed in special classes for students with learning disabilities or mental retardation. Therefore it is essential that the nurse suspect a hearing impairment in any child who demonstrates the behaviors listed in the box.

Of primary importance is the effect of hearing impairment on speech development. A child with a mild conductive hearing loss may speak fairly clearly but in a loud, monotone voice. A child with a sensorineural defect usually has difficulty in articulation. For example, inability to hear higher frequencies may result in the word *spoon* being pronounced *poon*. Children with articulation problems need to have their hearing tested.

Clinical Manifestations of Hearing Impairment

Infants

Lack of startle or blink reflex to a loud sound
Failure to be awakened by loud environmental noises
Failure to localize a source of sound by 6 months of age
Absence of babble or inflections in voice by age 7 months
General indifference to sound
Lack of response to the spoken word; failure to follow verbal directions
Response to loud noises as opposed to the voice

Children

Use of gestures rather than verbalization to express desires, especially after age 15 months
Failure to develop intelligible speech by age 24 months
Monotone quality, unintelligible speech, lessened laughter
Vocal play, head banging, or foot stamping for vibratory sensation
Yelling or screeching to express pleasure, annoyance (tantrums), or need
Asking to have statements repeated or answering them incorrectly
Responding more to facial expression and gestures than verbal explanation
Avoidance of social interaction; often puzzled and unhappy in such situations, prefers to play alone
Inquiring, sometimes confused facial expression
Suspicious alertness, sometimes interpreted as paranoia, alternating with cooperation
Frequently stubborn because of lack of comprehension
Irritable at not making himself understood
Shy, timid, and withdrawn
Often appears "dreamy," "in a world of his own," or markedly inattentive

NURSING DIAGNOSES

A number of nursing diagnoses are prominent in the nursing care of the child with hearing impairment and the child's family; other diagnoses specific to individual cases become evident. The most common nursing diagnoses are outlined in the Nursing Care Plan on pp. 561-562.

PLANNING

The goals of nursing care for the child with hearing impairment and family are:

1. Promote the child's optimum development through enhancing the communication process and socialization
2. Support the child and family
3. Care for the child during hospitalization
4. Assist in measures to prevent hearing impairment

IMPLEMENTATION

Once the goals are identified, specific interventions are carried out. The following discussion presents general in-

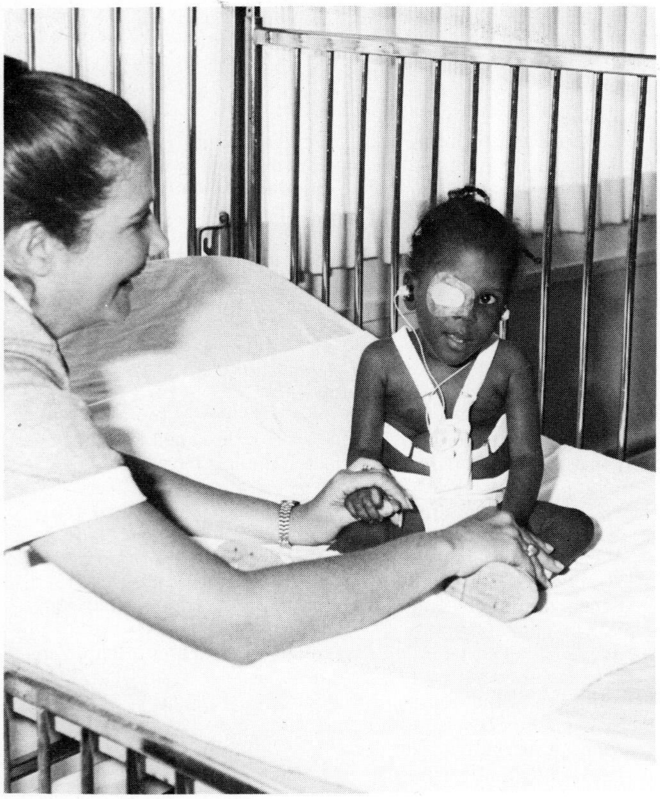

FIG. 19-7 On-the-body hearing aids are convenient for young children, such as this child with severe bilateral hearing loss. Note the eye patching for strabismus.

terventions for most children with hearing impairment. Modifications are needed in specific situations, particularly if other physical or mental disabilities coexist.

Promote communication process. The nurse's initial role in rehabilitation is to encourage the family to participate in an auditory training program.* Rehabilitation training consists of using a hearing aid and learning lipreading (speech reading), sign language, and verbal communication.

Hearing aids. The nurse should be familiar with the types, basic care, and handling of hearing aids, especially when the child is hospitalized.† Types of aids include those worn in or behind the ear, models incorporated into an eyeglass frame, or types worn on the body with a wire connection to the ear (Fig. 19-7). One of the most common problems with a hearing aid is *acoustic feedback*, an annoying whistling sound usually caused by improper fit of the ear mold. Sometimes the whistling may be at a frequency that the child cannot hear but that is annoying to others. In this case, the child should be told of the noise and asked to readjust the aid (see also Nursing tip).

Nursing Tip: Hearing Aid

To reduce or eliminate whistling from a hearing aid, try reinserting the aid, making certain that no hair is caught between the ear mold and canal, cleaning the ear mold or ear, or lowering the volume of the aid.

As the child grows older, he may be self-conscious about the device. Every effort should be made to make the aid inconspicuous, such as an appropriate hairstyle to cover behind-the-ear or in-the-ear models, attractive frames for glasses, and placement of the on-the-body type where it is not seen, such as under a blouse or sweater. The child is given responsibility for the care of his device as soon as he is able, since fostering independence is a primary goal of rehabilitation.

Lipreading. Even though the child may become expert at lipreading, only about 40% of the spoken word is understood, and less if the speaker has an accent, mustache, or beard. Exaggerating pronunciation or speaking in an altered rhythm further lessens comprehension. Parents can help the child understand the spoken word by using the suggestions in the box below. The child learns to supplement the spoken word with sensitivity to visual cues, primarily body language and facial expression (e.g., tightening the lips, muscle tension, and eye contact).

Sign language. Sign language, such as the American Sign Language (ASL) or British Sign Language (BSL), is a visual-gestural language that uses hand signals that roughly correspond to specific words and concepts in the

Guidelines for Facilitating Lipreading

Attract child's attention before speaking; use light touch to signal speaker's presence
Stand close to child
Face child directly or move to a 45-degree angle
Stand still; do not walk back and forth or turn away to point or look elsewhere
Establish eye contact and show interest
Speak at eye level and with good lighting on speaker's face
Be certain nothing interferes with speech patterns, such as chewing food or gum
Speak clearly and with a slow and even rate
Use facial expression to assist in conveying messages
Keep sentences short
Do not repeat if child does not understand the words; rephrase message

*Home training correspondence programs are sponsored by the **John T. Tracy Clinic,** 806 West Adams Blvd., Los Angeles, CA 90007. Other sources of information on several aspects of hearing loss and on the International Parents' Organization are the **Alexander Graham Bell Association for the Deaf,** 3417 Volta Place, NW, Washington, DC 20007, and **Canadian Hearing Society,** 271 Spadina Rd., Toronto, Ontario M5R 2V3.

†Information about hearing aids is available from the **National Hearing Aid Society,** 20361 Middlebelt Rd., Livonia, MI 48152; 1-800-521-5247 (in Michigan, 1-313-478-2610).

English language. Family members are encouraged to learn signing because using or watching hands require much less concentration than lipreading or talking. Also a symbol method enables some deaf children to learn more and to learn faster.

Speech therapy. The most formidable task in the education of a deaf child is learning to speak. Speech is learned through a multisensory approach, using visual, tactile, kinesthetic, and auditory stimulation. Since the usual mechanism for learning language (imitation and reinforcement) is not available to the deaf child, systematic formal education is required. Parents are encouraged to participate fully in the learning process.

Additional aids. Everyday activities present problems to the older child. For example, he may not be able to hear the telephone, doorbell, or alarm clock. Several commercial devices are available to help the deaf person adjust to these dilemmas. Flashing lights can be attached to a telephone or doorbell to signal its ringing. Trained hearing ear dogs can provide great assistance to deaf individuals because they alert the person to sounds, such as someone approaching, a moving car, a signal to wake up, and a child's cry. Special teletypewriters (TYY) or telecommunications devices for the deaf (TDD) help deaf people communicate with each other over the telephone; the typed message is conveyed via the telephone lines and displayed on a small screen.

Any audiovisual medium presents dilemmas to the child because, although he can see the picture, he cannot hear the message. However, *closed captioning* offers a solution. Through a special decoding device attached to a television, the audio portion of a program is translated into subtitles that appear on the screen.*

As the deaf child learns to compensate for his lack of hearing, he becomes extremely perceptive to visual and vibratory changes. He often knows when another person wishes to talk to him because the person will walk close by him but not pass. He learns to be alert to other people approaching him by seeing their shadows or feeling the vibrations of their footsteps. He is acutely aware of facial expressions and may comprehend the unspoken word more quickly than the spoken word.

Socialization. Since socialization is extremely important to the child's development, the nurse discusses with the family methods of fostering social contact. If the child attends a special school for the deaf, he is able to socialize with peers in that setting. Classmates become a potential source of close friendships because they communicate more easily among themselves. Parents are encouraged to promote these relationships whenever possible.

The child with a hearing impairment may need special help in school or social activities. For those children wearing hearing aids, background noise should be kept to a minimum. Since many of these children are able to attend regular classes, the teacher may need assistance in adapting methods of teaching for the child's benefit. The school nurse is often in an optimum position to emphasize methods of facilitated communication, such as lipreading (see box). Since group projects and audiovisual teaching aids may hinder the deaf child's learning, these educational methods should be carefully evaluated.

When the child is in a group setting, it is helpful for the other members to sit in a semicircle in front of him so that he can see their faces. Since one of the difficulties in following a group discussion is that the deaf child is unaware of who will speak next, it helps to have someone point out each speaker. This can be accomplished by giving each speaker a number or using his name and marking this down as that person talks. If one person writes down the main topic of the discussion, the child is able to follow lipreading more closely. Such suggestions can increase the child's ability to participate in sports, clubs such as Boy Scouts or Girl Scouts, and group projects.

Support the child and family. Once the diagnosis of hearing impairment is made, parents need extensive support to adjust to the shock of learning about their child's disability and an opportunity to realize the extent of the hearing loss. If the hearing loss occurs during childhood, the child also requires sensitive, supportive care during the long, and often difficult adjustment, to this sensory loss. Early rehabilitation is one of the best strategies for fostering adjustment. However, progress in learning communication may not always coincide with emotional adjustment. Depression or anger is common and such feelings are a normal part of the grieving process. (See also Chapter 18 for an extensive discussion of the emotional support of the child and family.)

Care for the child during hospitalization. The needs of the hospitalized deaf child are the same as those of any other child, but his disability presents special challenges to the nurse. For example, verbal explanations as the primary method of preparation for admission or procedures must be supplemented with tactile and visual aids, such as books or actual demonstration and practice. The child's understanding of the explanation needs to be constantly reassessed. If the child's verbal skills are poorly developed, he can answer questions through drawing, writing, or gesturing. For example, if the nurse is attempting to clarify where a spinal tap is done, the child is asked to point to where the doctor will insert the needle. Since deaf children often need more time to grasp the full meaning of an explanation, the nurse is careful not to judge the slowness as a sign of retardation and to allow ample time for understanding.

When communicating with the child, the nurse should use the same principles as those that are outlined for facilitating lipreading. Ideally, nurses without foreign accents should be assigned to the child. The child's hearing aid is checked to ensure that it is working properly. If it is necessary to awaken the child at night, the nurse gently shakes him to signal his or her presence or turns on the hearing aid before arousing the child and always makes sure that the child can see him or her before any

*Additional information is available from the **National Captioning Institute, Inc.,** 5203 Leesburg Pike, Falls Church, VA 22041.

procedures, even routine ones such as changing a diaper or regulating an infusion, are performed. It is important to remember that the child may not be aware of one's presence until alerted through visual or tactile cues.

Ideally parents are encouraged to room with the child. However, it must be conveyed to them that this is not to serve as a convenience to the nurse but as a benefit to the child. Although the parents' aid can be enlisted in familiarizing the child with the hospital and explaining procedures, the nurse also talks directly to him, encouraging expression of his feelings about the experience. If there is difficulty in understanding the child's speech, an effort is made to become familiar with his pronunciation of words. Parents often can be helpful by explaining the child's usual speech habits.

The nurse honestly admits if the child cannot be understood, and encourages him to write his statements. However, at no time is it implied that the child's speech is imperfect. Rather the nurse lets the child know that it will take some time to become familiar with his words and that in the meantime he can help by using gestures or written messages. Expressing an interest in learning sign language, especially useful words, such as yes, no, water, and toilet, not only improves communication efforts but greatly strengthens the nurse-child-parent relationship. Nonvocal communication devices that employ pictures or words that the child can point to are also available (see p. 548). Such boards can also be made up by drawing pictures or writing the words of common needs on cardboard, such as parent, food, water, or toilet.

The nurse has a special role as child advocate with the deaf and is in a strategic position to alert other health team members and other patients to the child's special needs regarding communication. For example, the nurse should accompany the physician on visits to the child's room to ensure that the physician speaks to the child and that the child understands what is said. Not infrequently caregivers forget that the child has the abilities to perceive and learn despite a hearing loss and consequently communicate only with the parents. As a result, the child's needs and feelings remain unrecognized and unmet.

Since deaf children often have difficulty in forming social relationships with other children, the child is introduced to his roommates and encouraged to engage in play activities. The hospital setting can provide growth-promoting opportunities for social relationships. With the assistance of a child-life specialist, the child can learn new recreational activities, experiment with group games, and engage in therapeutic play. The use of puppets, dollhouses, role playing with dress-up clothes, building with a hammer and nails, finger painting, needle play, and water play can help the child express feelings that previously were suppressed.

Assist in measures to prevent hearing impairment. A primary nursing role is prevention of hearing loss. Since the most common cause of impaired hearing is chronic otitis media, it is essential that appropriate measures be instituted to treat existing infections and prevent recurrences (see Chapter 22). Children with histories of ear or respiratory infections or any other condition known to increase the risk of hearing impairment should receive periodic auditory testing.

To prevent the causes of hearing loss that begin prenatally and perinatally, pregnant women need counseling regarding the necessity of early prenatal care, including genetic counseling for known familial disorders; avoidance of all ototoxic drugs, especially during the first trimester; tests to rule out syphilis, rubella, or blood incompatibility; medical management of maternal diabetes; control of alcoholism; and adequate dietary intake. During childhood, the necessity of routine immunization to eliminate the possibility of acquired sensorineural loss from rubella, mumps, and measles (encephalitis) is stressed.

Exposure to excessive noise pollution is a well-established cause of sensorineural hearing loss. The nurse should routinely assess the possibility of environmental noise pollution and advise children and parents of the potential danger. Signals suggesting exposure to excessive noise are ringing or buzzing in the ears and/or perceiving sounds as muffled or dull after leaving the source of the noise. When individuals engage in activities associated with high-intensity noise, such as flying model airplanes, target shooting, or snowmobiling, they should wear ear protection such as earmuffs or earplugs (not ordinary dry cotton). However, any protection is better than none. Even common household equipment can be hazardous, such as lawn mowers, power vacuum cleaners, and cordless telephones.

EVALUATION

The effectiveness of nursing interventions is determined by continual reassessment and evaluation of care based on the following observational guidelines and expected outcomes:

1. Observe the techniques used to communicate with the child; inquire if child is enrolled in auditory training program; inquire about socialization opportunities for the child (i.e., who are child's friends, what are his extracurricular activities)
2. Interview the family regarding their adjustment to the sensory impairment; observe the family members' relationship with the child; interview the child regarding feelings about the sensory impairment and its effect on activities of daily living (especially important if a recent impairment)
3. Observe types of preparation/communication used to prepare child for hospitalization or procedures; observe parents' involvement in child's care; observe interaction of child and family with other patients
4. Investigate community programs aimed at preventing or detecting hearing loss and inquire as to nursing involvement in these efforts

Expected outcomes:
See Nursing Care Plan, pp. 561 to 562.

NURSING CARE PLAN

The Child with Hearing Impairment

Nursing Goals	Nursing Interventions	Expected Patient/Family Outcomes
ND HP-HMP* **Potential for tissue damage**	**Risk factors: developmental (maternal infection), chemical (drugs), biologic (genetic), environmental**	
Detect hearing impairment		
Infancy	Assess neonate's response to a loud noise Observe for signs associated with congenital deafness	†Child's hearing impairment is detected early and appropriate management strategies are implemented
Childhood	Listen carefully to family's concerns regarding hearing loss Take a thorough history regarding factors that support an auditory impairment Evaluate speech development carefully Observe for behaviors that may suggest a hearing impairment (p. 557) Administer hearing tests and refer for audiometry	Family expresses fears and concerns †Family's concerns are recognized Child is referred for testing
Prevent hearing loss		
Infancy	Encourage immunization at appropriate age Prevent ear infection; detect early	Infant does not develop hearing loss Children are properly immunized
Childhood	Assess hearing ability of children who are receiving ototoxic antibiotics Promote compliance with treatment regimens for otitis media Discuss with parents measures to prevent otitis media Evaluate auditory ability of children prone to chronic ear or respiratory problems	Child does not develop hearing loss
	Assess sources of excessive noise in child's environment Institute appropriate measures to decrease sound levels (turn music lower, use ear protection)	Child is not exposed to excess noise levels
ND CPP **Altered growth and development**	**Etiology: Sensory-perceptual alteration: auditory**	
Promote communication process	Encourage family to attend rehabilitation program in order to continue learning in home; encourage them to learn sign language, finger spelling Teach language that serves a useful purpose Encourage use of language and books in home Encourage spontaneous language but correct speech impairments	Family continues communication practices in home environment Family provides stimulation to child
Facilitate lipreading	Test child for visual problems that may interfere with learning to lipread or use sign language Teach family and others involved with child (e.g., teacher) behaviors that facilitate lipreading (see box, p. 558)	Child communicates with others in manner taught (specify) Persons communicating with child use good communication techniques
Maximize residual hearing	Help family investigate reliable hearing aid dealers Discuss types of hearing aids and their proper care Teach child how to regulate hearing aid for maximum benefit Help child focus on all sounds in environment and talk to him about them For older child, discuss methods of camouflaging aid to make it less conspicuous	Child acquires and uses hearing aid
Provide opportunities for play/socialization	Guide family in selection of toys that maximize visual and tactile senses, as well as residual hearing Encourage child to participate in group activities Help him follow group discussion by pointing out speaker and arranging group in semicircle Help child develop friendships among hearing and deaf peers Help child achieve a sense of security in his ability to compete with peers	Child engages in activities appropriate to his developmental level

*For an explanation of abbreviations, see p. 20.
†Nursing outcome.

Continued.

NURSING CARE PLAN

The Child with Hearing Impairment—cont'd

Nursing Goals	Nursing Interventions	Expected Patient/Family Outcomes
Encourage education within a regular classroom	Discuss with teacher ways of communicating effectively with child (such as through facilitating lipreading) Promote socialization with classmates	Child attends school regularly
Promote independence and development	Help family transfer normal childrearing practices to this child Emphasize importance of attaining independence in self-care Provide child with devices that foster independence (hearing ear dog, special signaling aids for telephone or door bell) Discuss importance of discipline and limit setting	Child performs activities of daily living appropriate to level of development
NDx RRP Altered family processes **Etiology: situational crisis (diagnosis of deafness in a child)**		
Assist family in adjusting to child's loss of hearing	Anticipate usual grief reaction to loss Help family deal with any guilt feelings regarding previous responses to child when true nature of problem was unknown Help family realize extent of child's disability and its tremendous influence on speech and language development Discuss advantages and limitations of amplifying devices with different types of hearing loss Encourage formal rehabilitation as soon as possible	Family expresses feelings and concerns regarding child's loss of hearing Family demonstrates an understanding of implications of hearing loss Family becomes involved in programs
Provide emotional support	Be available to family for assistance Encourage family members to discuss their feelings regarding disability Stress child's abilities rather than disability Become familiar with techniques used for communication if following family on a long-term basis Refer family to appropriate community agencies for medical, psychiatric, educational, vocational, or financial assistance Involve parents in local parent groups for hearing impaired children	Family expresses feelings and concerns about disability and its ramifications Family members avail themselves of available resources
Promote parent-child attachment	Help family identify clues other than verbal ones that signify infant's communication with them Encourage family to stimulate child with visual and tactile cues Stress importance of continuing to talk to child even though he may not hear their voices Encourage parents to discuss their feelings regarding attachment process	Parents and child demonstrate a positive relationship

VISUAL IMPAIRMENT

Visual impairments are a common problem during childhood; prevalence rates for some degree of visual impairment even with corrective glasses is approximately 20 to 35 per 1000 children. Of this group 0.5 to 1.0 per 1000 are considered legally blind (Gortmaker and Sappenfield, 1984). Nearly 50% of blind children under 5 years of age have no useful vision, and for the remainder the visual acuity is unknown (Vision problems in the United States, 1980). The nurse's role is clearly one of assessment, prevention, referral, and in some instances rehabilitation.

Definition and Classification

Vision impairment is a general term that refers to visual loss that cannot be corrected with regular prescription lenses. However, more useful definitions for classifying visual impairments include the following. *School vision* (also known as partially sighted) refers to visual acuity between 20/70 and 20/200. The child should be able to obtain an education in the usual public school system with the use of normal-sized print. Near vision is almost always better than distance vision. *Legal blindness* is visual acuity of 20/200 or less and/or a visual field of 20 degrees or less in the better eye. This is useful only as a

Table 19-4

Types of Visual Problems

Defect	Description	Pathophysiology	Treatment
Refractive errors			
Myopia (near-sightedness)	Ability to see objects clearly at close range but not at a distance	Results from eyeball that is too long, causing image to fall in front of retina	Corrected with biconcave lenses that focus rays on retina
Hyperopia (hypermetropia or farsightedness)	Ability to see objects clearly at a distance Because of accommodative ability, child can usually see objects at all ranges Most children normally hyperopic until about 7 years of age	Results from eyeball that is too short, causing image to focus beyond retina	If correction is required, use convex lenses to focus rays on retina
Astigmatism	Unequal curvatures in refractive apparatus	Results from unequal curvatures in cornea or lens that cause light rays to bend in different directions	Corrected with special lenses that compensate for refractive errors
Anisometropia	Different refractive strengths in each eye	May develop amblyopia as weaker eye is used less	Treated with corrective lenses, preferably contact lenses, to improve vision in each eye so they work as a unit
Amblyopia (lazy eye)	Reduced visual acuity in one eye	Results when one eye does not receive sufficient visual stimulation Each retina receives different images, resulting in diplopia (double vision) Brain accommodates by suppressing less intense image Visual cortex eventually does not respond to visual stimulation with loss of vision in that eye	Preventable if primary visual defect, such as anisometropia or strabismus, begins before 6 years of age
Strabismus (squint or crosseye)	Malalignment of eyes Esotropia-inward deviation of eye (Fig. 19-8) Exotropia-outward deviation of eye	May result from muscle imbalance or paralysis, poor vision, or as congenital defect Since visual axes not parallel, brain receives two images, and amblyopia can result	Treatment depends on cause of strabismus May involve occlusion therapy (patching stronger eye) to increase visual stimulation to weaker eye Early diagnosis essential to prevent vision loss
Cataracts	Opacity of crystalline lens	Prevents light rays from entering eye and refracting them on retina	Requires surgery to remove cloudy lens and replacement of lens (contact or prescription glasses) Must be treated early to prevent blindness from amblyopia
Glaucoma	Increased intraocular pressure	Congential type results from defective development of some component related to flow of aqueous humor Increased pressure on optic nerve causes eventual atrophy and blindness	Requires surgical treatment (goniotomy) to open outflow tracts May need more than one operation

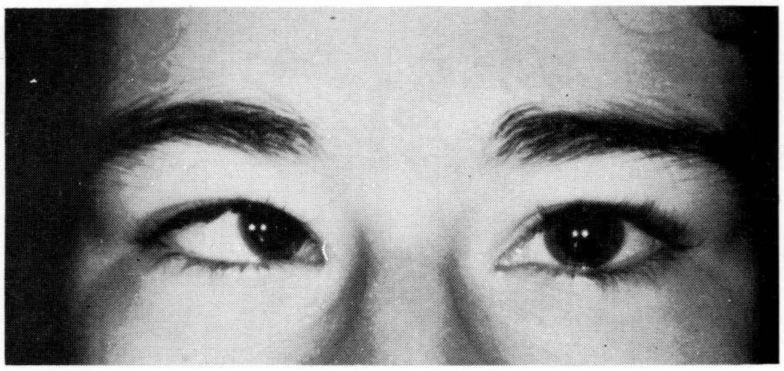

FIG. 19-8 Strabismus (esotropia). Note obvious malalignment of eyes. The light reflections are centered in the left cornea but to side of the right cornea. (From Havener, W.H., Saunders, W.H., Keith, C.F., and Prescott, A.W.: Nursing care in eye, ear, nose, and throat disorders, ed. 3, St. Louis, 1974, The C.V. Mosby Co.)

legal definition, not as a medical diagnosis. It allows special considerations with regard to taxes, entrance into special schools, eligibility for aid, and other benefits.

Etiology

Visual impairment can be caused by a number of genetic and prenatal or postnatal conditions. These include Tay-Sachs disease, perinatal infections (herpes, chlamydia, gonococci, rubella, syphilis, or toxoplasmosis), retinopathy of prematurity, trauma, postnatal infections (meningitis), and disorders such as sickle cell disease, juvenile rheumatoid arthritis, and retinoblastoma. In many instances, such as with refractive errors, the cause of the defect is unknown.

Refractive errors are the most common types of visual disorders in children. The term *refraction* means bending and refers to the bending of light rays as they pass through the lens of the eye. Normally light rays enter the lens and fall directly on the retina. However, in refractive disorders the light rays either fall in front of the retina (myopia) or beyond it (hyperopia). Other eye problems, such as strabismus, may or may not include refractive errors, but they are very important because, if untreated, they result in blindness from amblyopia. These along with other less frequent visual disorders are summarized in Table 19-4. Their clinical manifestations are listed in Table 19-5. In addition to these disorders, other visual problems can be the result of infection or trauma.

Trauma. Trauma is a common cause of blindness in children. Injuries to the eyeball and adnexa (supporting or accessory structures, such as eyelids, conjunctiva, and lacrimal glands) can be classified as penetrating or nonpenetrating. *Penetrating wounds* are most often the result of sharp instruments, such as knives or scissors; propulsive objects, such as firecrackers, guns, bows and arrows, or slingshots; and a powerful contusion by a blunt object, which may occur during a fight or from a serious car accident. *Nonpenetrating injuries* may be the result of foreign objects in the eyes, lacerations, a blow from a blunt object such as a fist, and thermal or chemical burns.

Treatment is aimed at preventing further ocular damage and is primarily the responsibility of the ophthalmologist. It involves adequate examination of the injured eye (with the child sedated or anesthetized in severe injuries), appropriate immediate intervention such as removal of the foreign body or suturing of the laceration, and prevention of complications, such as administration of antibiotics or steroids and complete bed rest to allow the eye to heal and blood to reabsorb. Prognosis varies according to the type of injury. It is usually guarded in all cases of penetrating wounds because of the high risk of serious complications.

Infections. Infections of the adnexa and the structures of the eyeball or globe are not infrequent in children. The most common eye infection is conjunctivitis (see Chapter 14). Treatment is usually ophthalmic antibiotics. Severe infections may require systemic antibiotic therapy. Steroids are used cautiously because they exacerbate viral infections such as herpes simplex, increasing the risk of damage to the involved structures.

Nursing Considerations

Nursing care of visually impaired children is often a specialized area, requiring additional training in vision testing and rehabilitation. However, general nursing goals that focus on assessment, prevention, and rehabilitation of the child with a vision impairment are every nurse's responsibility. In addition, nurses may have to care for a vision-impaired child who is hospitalized and must know how to best meet the child's and family's special needs.

ASSESSMENT

Assessment of children for vision impairment is a critical nursing responsibility. Discovery of a vision impairment as early as possible is essential to prevent social, physical, and psychologic damage to the child. Assessment involves (1) identifying those children who by virtue of their history are at risk, (2) observing for behaviors that indicate a vision loss, and (3) screening all children for visual acuity and signs of other ocular disorders, such as strabismus. This discussion focuses on clinical manifestation of various types of visual problems (Table 19-5). Vision testing is discussed in Chapter 7.

Infancy. At birth the nurse should observe the neonate's response to visual stimuli, such as following a light or object and cessation of body movement. The infant may vary in the intensity of the response, depending on the state of alertness. However, a consistent absence of a reaction should lead to suspicion of vision loss.

Of special importance in detecting visual impairment during infancy are the parents' concerns regarding visual responsiveness in their child. Their concerns must be taken seriously, such as lack of eye-to-eye contact from the infant. During infancy the child should be tested for strabismus. Lack of binocularity after 4 months of age is

TABLE 19-5

Clinical Manifestations of Visual Impairment

Cause	Behavioral Manifestations	Signs/Symptoms
Congenital blindness	Does not follow a moving light No orientation response to visual stimuli Does not initiate eye-to-eye contact with caregiver	Constant nystagmus Fixed pupils Marked strabismus Slow lateral movements
Refractive errors	Rubs eyes excessively Tilts head or thrusts head forward Has difficulty in reading or other close work Holds books close to eyes Writes or colors with head close to table Clumsy; walks into objects Blinks more than usual or is irritable when doing close work Is unable to see objects clearly Does poorly in school, especially in subjects that require demonstration, such as arithmetic	Dizziness Headache Nausea following close work
Strabismus	Squints eyelids together or frowns Has difficulty in focusing from one distance to another Inaccurate judgment in picking up objects Unable to see print or moving objects clearly Closes one eye to see Tilts head to one side If combined with refractive errors, may see any of above	Diplopia Photophobia Dizziness Headache Cross-eye
Glaucoma	Mostly seen in acquired types—loses peripheral vision May bump into objects that are not directly in front of him Sees halos around objects May complain of mild pain or discomfort (severe pain, nausea, vomiting if sudden rise in pressure)	Redness Excessive tearing (epiphora) Photophobia Spasmodic winking (blepharospasm) Corneal haziness Enlargement of eyeball (buphthalmos)
Cataract	Gradually less able to see objects clearly May lose peripheral vision	Nystagmus (with complete blindness) Gray opacities of lens Strabismus Absence of red reflex

considered abnormal and must be treated to prevent amblyopia.

Childhood. Since the most common visual impairment during childhood is refractive errors, testing for visual acuity is essential. The school nurse usually assumes major responsibility for vision testing in school children. Besides refractive errors, the nurse should be aware of signs and symptoms that indicate other ocular problems. If a referral is made to the family requesting further eye testing, the nurse is responsible for follow-up concerning the recommendation.

NURSING DIAGNOSES

A number of nursing diagnoses are prominent in the nursing care of the child with visual impairment and the child's family; other diagnoses specific to individual cases become evident. The most common nursing diagnoses are outlined in the Nursing Care Plan on pp. 568-570.

PLANNING

The goals of nursing care for the child with visual impairment and family are:

1. Support the child and family
2. Promote parent-child attachment
3. Promote the child's optimum development
4. Care for the child during hospitalization
5. Assist in measures to prevent vision impairment

IMPLEMENTATION

Once the goals are identified, specific interventions are carried out. The following discussion presents general interventions for most children with vision impairment, especially blindness. Modifications are needed in specific situations, particularly if other physical or mental disabilities coexist.

Support the child and family. The shock of learning that their child is blind or partially sighted is an immense crisis for families. Of all types of disabilities, many people fear loss of sight the most. Certainly it is one of the senses that is involved in almost every activity of daily living. Parents need support during the initial phase of learning about the diagnosis and help to gain a realistic understanding of their child's abilities. The family is encouraged to investigate appropriate stimulation and educational programs for their child as soon as possible.

Sources of information include state **Commissions for the Blind,** local schools for the blind, the **American Foundation for the Blind,*** **National Federation of the Blind,†** **National Association for Parents of the Visually Impaired, Inc.,‡** **National Association for Visually Handicapped,§** and **American Council of the Blind.‖**

When blindness is not congenital but acquired, the newly blind child needs a great deal of support to help him adjust to the disability. He is usually frightened and confused by the sudden or progressive loss of sight and benefits from an environment that provides security and familiarity. This is especially important to remember when he is hospitalized.

Promote parent-child attachment. A crucial time in the life of the blind infant is when he and his parents are getting acquainted with each other. Pleasurable patterns of interaction between the infant and his parents may be lacking if there is not enough reciprocity. For example, if the parent gazes fondly at the infant's face and seeks eye contact but the infant fails to respond because he cannot see the parent, a troubled cycle of responses may occur. The nurse can help parents learn to look for other cues that indicate the infant is responding to them, such as if his eyelids blink, whether his activity level accelerates or slows, if respiratory patterns change, such as if he breathes faster or slower when they come near, and whether the infant makes throaty sounds when they speak to him. In time parents learn that the infant has unique ways of relating to them. They are encouraged to show affection using nonvisual methods, such as talking or reading, cuddling, and walking the child.

Promote the child's optimum development. Promoting the child's optimum development requires rehabilitation in a number of important areas. These include learning self-help skills and appropriate communication techniques to become independent. Although nurses may not be directly involved in such programs, they can provide direction and guidance to families regarding the availability of programs and the need to promote these activities in their child.

Development and independence. Motor development is almost as dependent on sight as verbal communication is on hearing. From earliest infancy parents are encouraged to expose the infant to as many visual-motor experiences as possible, such as sitting supported in an infant seat or swing and being given opportunities for holding up his head, sitting unsupported, reaching for objects, and crawling. Ideally the child should be enrolled in an educational stimulation program for blind infants to develop age-appropriate motor skills.

Despite visual impairment the child can become independent in all aspects of self-care. The same principles used for promoting independence in sighted children apply with additional emphasis on nonvisual cues. For example, the child may need help in dressing, such as special arrangement of clothing for style coordination and braille tags to distinguish colors and prints.

The blind child also must learn to become independent in navigational skills. The two main techniques are the *tapping method* (use of a cane to survey the environment for direction and to avoid obstacles) and *guides*, such as a human sighted guide or a dog guide, such as a Seeing Eye dog. Partially sighted children may benefit from ocular aids, such as a monocular telescope.

Play and socialization. The blind child does not learn to play automatically. Because he cannot imitate others or actively explore his environment as sighted children do, he depends much more on others to stimulate and teach him how to play. Parents need help in selecting appropriate play material, especially those that encourage fine and gross motor development and stimulate the senses of hearing, touch, and smell. Toys with educational value are especially useful, such as dolls with various clothing closures.

The blind child has the same needs for socialization as sighted children. Since he has little difficulty in learning verbal skills, he is able to communicate with age-mates and participate in suitable activities. The nurse discusses with parents opportunities for socialization outside of the home, especially regular nursery schools. The trend is to include these children with sighted children to help them adjust to the outside world for eventual independence.

To compensate for inadequate stimulation, these children may develop *blindisms,* such as body rocking, finger flicking, or arm twirling. Such habits retard the child's social acceptance and should be discouraged. Behavior modification is often successful in reducing or eliminating blindisms.

Education. The main obstacle to learning is the child's total dependence on nonvisual cues. Although the child can learn via verbal lecturing, he is unable to read the written word or to write without special education. Therefore, he must rely on *braille,* a system that uses raised dots to represent letters and numbers. The child can then read the braille with his fingers and can write a message using a braille writer. However, unless others read braille this type of communication is not useful for communicating with others. A more portable system for written communication is the use of a braille slate and stylus (Fig. 19-9) or a microcassette tape recorder. A recorder is especially helpful for leaving messages for others and for note-taking during classroom lecturing. Both the braille slate and stylus and the tape recorder are as important to a blind person as paper and pencil are to a sighted indi-

*15 W. 16th St., New York, NY 10011.
†1800 Johnson St., Baltimore, MD 21230.
‡ P.O. Box 180806, Austin, TX 78718.
§22 West 21th St., New York, NY 10010.
‖ 1010 Vermont Ave., NW, Washington, DC 20005.
Sources of information in Canada include the **Canadian National Institute for the Blind,** 1931 Bayview Ave., Toronto, Ontario M4G 4C8; **Low Vision Association of Canada,** 145 Adelaide St. West, Toronto, Ontario M5H 3H4; and **Blind Organization of Ontario,** 597 Parliament St., Suite B-3, Toronto, Ontario M4X 1W3.

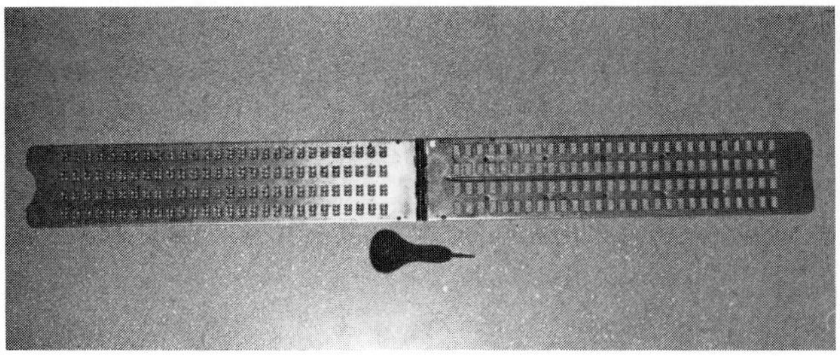

FIG. 19-9 Braille slate and stylus. The hinged slate consists of a series of open rectangles on one side and standard braille cells on the other. The paper is clamped or sandwiched between these two metal bars and the appropriate dots are punched with the stylus.

vidual. For mathematical calculations portable calculators with voice synthesizers are available.*

Records and tapes are significant sources of reading material other than braille books, which are large and cumbersome. The **Library of Congress**† has talking books, braille books, and a special records program, which are available at many local libraries, state libraries, and directly from the Library of Congress. The talking book machine and tape player are provided at no cost to families and there is no postage fee for returning the materials. **Recording for the Blind, Inc.**‡ also provides texts and tapes of books, which are very helpful for secondary and college students who are blind.

Learning to use a regular typewriter is another form of writing but has the disadvantage of the blind person being unable to check the accuracy of the typing. Recent developments with computers have eliminated this drawback. A home computer with a voice synthesizer can be adapted to speak each letter or word that has been typed.

The partially sighted child benefits from specialized visual aids, which produce a magnified retinal image. The basic devices are accommodation, such as bringing the object closer, special plus lenses, hand-held and stand magnifiers, telescopes, video projection systems, and large print. Special equipment is available to enlarge print. Information about services for the partially sighted is available from the **National Association for Visually Handicapped** and **American Foundation for the Blind.** Children with diminished vision often prefer to do close work without their glasses and compensate by bringing the object very near to their eyes. This should be allowed. The exception is the child with vision in only one eye, who should always wear glasses for protection.

Care for the child during hospitalization. Because nurses are more likely to care for children who are hospitalized for procedures that involve temporary loss of vision than for children who are blind, the following discussion concentrates primarily on the needs of such children. The nursing care objectives in either situation are to (1) reassure the child and family throughout every phase of treatment, (2) orient the child to his surroundings, (3) provide a safe environment, and (4) encourage independence. Whenever possible the same nurse should care for the child to ensure consistency in the approach. These same principles also apply to a blind child who requires hospitalization.

When a sighted child temporarily loses his vision, almost every aspect of his environment becomes bewildering and frightening. He is forced to rely on nonvisual senses for help in adjusting to the blindness without the benefit of any special training. Nurses have a major role in minimizing the effects of temporary loss of vision. They need to talk to the child about everything they are doing, emphasizing aspects of procedures that are felt or heard. They should approach the child by always identifying themselves as soon as they enter the room. Since unfamiliar sounds are especially frightening to the child, these are explained. Parents are encouraged to room with him and participate in his care. Familiar objects, such as a teddy bear or doll, should be brought from home to help lessen the strangeness of the hospital. As soon as the child is able to be out of bed, he is oriented to his immediate surroundings. If the child is able to see on admission, this opportunity is taken to point out significant aspects of his room, and he is encouraged to practice ambulating with his eyes closed to accustom him to this experience.

The room is arranged with safety in mind. For example, a stool or chair is placed next to the bed to help the child climb in and out of bed. The furniture is always placed in the same position to prevent accidental collisions. Cleaning personnel are reminded of the need to keep the room in order. If the child has difficulty navigating by feeling the walls, a rope can be attached from the bed to the point of destination, such as the bathroom. Attention to details such as well-fitting slippers or robes that do not hang on the floor is important in preventing tripping. Unlike the child who is blind, these children are not familiar with navigating with a cane.

The child is encouraged to be independent in self-care activities, especially if the visual loss may be prolonged or potentially permanent. For example, during bathing the nurse sets up all the equipment and encourages the child to participate. At mealtime the nurse explains where each food item is on the tray, opens any special containers, prepares cereal or toast, but encourages the child to feed himself. Favorite finger foods, such as sandwiches, hamburgers, hot dogs, or pizza, may be good selections. The child is praised for efforts at being cooperative and independent, and any improvements he makes in self-care, no matter how small, are stressed.

Appropriate recreational activities are provided for the child. If a child life specialist is available, such planning is done jointly. Since the child with temporary blindness has a wide variety of play experiences to draw on, he is encouraged to select activities. For example, if he liked to

*A catalog of numerous products for people with vision problems is available from the American Foundation for the Blind.

†**Division for the Blind and Visually Handicapped,** 1291 Taylor St., NW, Washington, DC 20542.

‡20 Roszel Rd., Princeton, NJ 08540.

NURSING CARE PLAN

The Child with Visual Impairment

Nursing Goals	Nursing Interventions	Expected Patient/Family Outcomes
NDx HP-HMP* **Potential for tissue damage** **Risk factors: environmental hazards**		
Detect eye problems Infancy	At birth assess neonate's response to a bright, shiny object; observe for signs associated with congenital blindness Check for strabismus (lack of binocularity); refer to ophthalmologist for evaluation if malalignment persists past 2 to 3 months of age	†Evidence of visual problems is detected early and appropriate action initiated
Childhood	Test for visual acuity as soon as child is cooperative (sometimes by age 2 years) Advise parents of Home Eye Test for Preschoolers, which is available from National Society for the Prevention of Blindness Observe for signs or behaviors that indicate eye problems (see Table 19-5); include questions regarding behavioral indications of vision impairment in health histories Assume responsibility as school nurse for follow-up care of children who require corrective lenses or other types of treatments, such as patching Stress to parents importance of continued periodic eye examinations, since child's eyesight may change significantly in a short period of time	
Prevent defects of vision	Provide prophylactic eye care at birth Administer oxygen cautiously to premature infant Periodically screen all children from birth through adolescence for visual impairment Participate in immunization programs for children Teach safety regarding common causes of eye injuries Stress importance of good eye care—use of proper lighting, avoidance of excessive close work, proper rest and nutrition, and yearly eye examinations	Infant receives prophylactic eye care †Screening and immunization programs are conducted and education programs implemented Healthy child does not acquire visual defect
Infections	Teach family correct procedure for instilling ophthalmic preparations (always in conjunctival cul-de-sac) Ensure proper dosage by holding dropper vertically, slowly closing lids, and having child rotate eyeball for even distribution Wipe excess medication for inner canthus outward to prevent contamination of contralateral eye Emphasize regular administration of drug for entire term of therapy to completely eradicate infection	Family complies with instructions and performs procedures correctly (specify)
Trauma	Prevent further injury by instituting appropriate emergency care (see box, p. 571) Obtain history of incident; avoid any implication of guilt Reassure parent and child; avoid giving false reassurance; appraise them of each step of treatment, especially if therapy interferes with vision (patching eyes)	Child does not develop complications
Prevent complications of eye defects	Encourage compliance with corrective therapies	Child and family comply with therapy and perform procedures correctly
Strabismus	Discuss with school-age child necessity of patch in preserving vision; allow him to verbalize feelings regarding altered facial appearance Stress importance of wearing corrective lenses, if prescribed Teach parents correct procedures for instilling anticholinesterase drugs, if ordered	

*For an explanation of abbreviations, see p. 20.
†Nursing outcome.

NURSING CARE PLAN

The Child with Visual Impairment—cont'd

Nursing Goals	Nursing Interventions	Expected Patient/Family Outcomes
Refractive errors	For secure fit of glasses, use ones with rounded temporal pieces or attach elastic strap to handles and around back of head Include older child in selection of frames Encourage parents to compare value of more expensive attractive frames and inducement for wearing them against cost If glasses are recommended for continuous wearing, discuss possibility of temporary removal for special occasions Encourage use of protective shields during contact sports Stress improvement in visual acuity as reason for wearing glasses Discuss feasibility of contact lenses with selected families Know procedures for care, insertion, and removal of lens; teach to parents and older children	Child wears corrective lenses and cares for equipment correctly
NDx CPP Altered growth and development **Etiology: Sensory-perceptual alteration: visual**		
Provide opportunities for play/socialization	Talk to child about environment Guide family to selection of play material that encourages motor development and stimulates senses of hearing and touch Discuss with family how play for blind children differs from that of sighted children Encourage family to initiate play activities and teach child how to use toys	Parents engage in appropriate activities with blind child and have realistic expectations for child
	Assess adequacy of environmental stimulation if blindisms are present Use behavior modification to discourage blindisms Discuss importance of consistent limit-setting in helping child learn acceptable behavior and tolerate frustration	Blindisms are minimized or eliminated
Promote development and independence	Provide visual-motor activities for infant (e.g., sitting in chair or swing, holding head up, standing, crawling, grasping for objects) Provide an environment that fosters familiarity and security; arrange furniture to allow safe ambulation; place identifying markets to denote steps or other dangerous areas Enroll child in special programs for the blind as soon as possible to learn independent skills, braille reading and writing, and navigational skills (cane method, sighted guide, guide dog) Encourage participation in active play Discuss need for experimenting with active play in safe environment and with other children	Infant or child engages in appropriate activities for level of development (specify) Child demonstrates an attitude of security in his environment
NDx RRP Altered family processes **Etiology: situational crisis (birth of a blind child; diagnosis of blindness of a child)**		
Assist family in adjusting to child's loss of sight	Anticipate usual grief reactions to loss Stress to family (and older child) that such feelings are normal and that grief takes time to resolve Help family gain a realistic concept of child's impairment and abilities Encourage formal rehabilitation as soon as realistically feasible Assist family in orienting newly blind child to environment and in making immediate surroundings safe to encourage ambulation Listen to family's concerns of child's visual loss	Parents express their feelings and concerns regarding loss of sight Parents demonstrate an understanding of the child's impairment and its implications

NURSING CARE PLAN

The Child with Visual Impairment—cont'd

Nursing Goals	Nursing Interventions	Expected Patient/Family Outcomes
Provide emotional support	Be available to family for assistance Encourage child, parents, and siblings to discuss their feelings regarding disability Stress child's abilities rather than disability Refer families to appropriate community agencies for medical, psychiatric, vocational, or financial assistance	Parents express their feelings and concerns regarding child and his special needs Child expresses his feelings and concerns Family members avail themselves of supportive services
Promote parent-child attachment	Help parents identify clues other than eye contact from infant that signify communication with them Encourage parents to discuss their feelings regarding lack of visual contact or smiling from child Stress that lack of such responses is not an indication of child's rejection or dislike of parents Demonstrate by own example acceptance of child Emphasize positive abilities or attributes Encourage parents in their attempts to promote child's development	Parents and child exhibit a positive relationship

read, he may enjoy being read to. If he preferred manual activity, he may appreciate playing with clay or building blocks or feeling different textures and naming them. If he needs an outlet for aggression, activities such as pounding or banging on a drum can be helpful. Simple board and card games can be played if the child has a "seeing partner" or if the opponent helps him with the game. He should have familiar toys from home to play with, since they are more easily manipulated than new ones. If parents wish to bring him presents, they should be things that stimulate hearing and touch, such as a radio, music box, or stuffed animal.

Occasionally children who are blind come to the hospital for procedures to restore their vision. Although this is an extremely happy time, it also requires intervention to help the child adjust to sight. The child needs an opportunity to take in all that he sees. He should not be bombarded with visual stimuli. He may need to concentrate on people's faces or his own to accustom himself to this experience. He often has the need to talk about what he sees and to compare the visual image with his mental one. The child may also go through a period of depression as he begins to realize all that he had lost. This depression must be respected and supported. The nurse or parents should refrain from statements, such as, "How can you be so sad when you can see again?" Instead the child should be encouraged to discuss how it feels to see, especially in terms of seeing himself.

The child also needs time in adjusting to his ability to engage in activities that were impossible before. For example, he may prefer to use braille to read, rather than learning a new "visual approach" because of his familiarity with the touch system. Eventually, as he learns to recognize letters and numbers, he will integrate these new skills into reading and writing. However, parents and teachers must be careful not to push the child before he is ready. This applies to social relationships and physical activities as well as learning situations.

Assist in measures to prevent vision impairment. An essential nursing goal is to prevent visual impairment. This involves many of the same interventions discussed under hearing impairments, namely (1) prenatal screening for pregnant women at risk, such as those with rubella or syphilis infection and family histories of genetic disorders associated with visual loss, (2) adequate prenatal and perinatal care to prevent prematurity and iatrogenic damage from excessive administration of oxygen, (3) periodic screening of all children, especially newborns through preschoolers, for congenital blindness and visual impairments caused by refractive errors, strabismus, and so on, (4) rubella immunization of all children, and (5) safety counseling regarding the common causes of ocular trauma.

Following detection of eye problems, the nurse has a responsibility to prevent further ocular damage by ensuring that corrective treatment is employed. For the child with strabismus, this often necessitates occlusion patching of the stronger eye. Compliance with the procedure is greatest during the early preschool years. It is more difficult to encourage school-age children to wear the occlusive patch because the poor visual acuity of the uncovered weaker eye interferes with schoolwork and the patch sets them apart from their peers. In school they benefit from being positioned favorably (closer to the blackboard) and allowed extra time to read or complete an assignment. If treatment of the eye disorder requires instillation of ophthalmic medication, the family is taught the correct procedure (see Chapter 21).

For the child with refractive errors, the nurse helps the child adjust to wearing glasses. Young children who often pull glasses off benefit from temporal pieces that wrap around the ears or an elastic strap attached to the frames and around the back of the head to hold them on securely. Once a child appreciates the value of clear vision, he is more likely to wear the corrective lenses.

Glasses should not interfere with any activity. Special protective guards are available during contact sports to prevent accidental injury and all corrective lenses should be made from safety glass, which is shatterproof. Often corrective lenses improve visual acuity so dramatically that children are able to compete more effectively in sports. This in itself is a tremendous inducement to continue wearing glasses.

Contact lenses are a popular alternative, especially for adolescents. Several types are available, such as hard lenses, including gas permeable ones, and soft lenses, which may be designed for daily or extended wear. Contact lenses offer several advantages over glasses, such as greater visual acuity, total corrected field of vision, convenience (especially with the extended wear type), and optimum cosmetic benefit. Unfortunately they are more expensive and require much more care than glasses, including considerable practice to learn techniques for insertion and removal. If they are prescribed, the nurse can be very helpful in teaching parents or older children how to care for the lenses.

Since trauma is the leading cause of blindness, the nurse has the major responsibility of preventing further eye injury until the specific treatment is instituted. The major principles to follow when caring for an eye injury are outlined in the emergency treatment box. Since patients with a serious eye injury fear blindness, the nurse should stay with the child and family to provide support and reassurance.

EVALUATION

The effectiveness of nursing interventions is determined by continual reassessment and evaluation of care based on the following observational guidelines and expected outcomes:

1. Interview the family regarding their adjustment to the sensory impairment; observe the family members' relationship with the child; interview the child regarding feelings about the sensory impairment and its effect on activities of daily living (especially important if a visual loss)
2. Have parents identify those cues that indicate the infant is responding to them; observe nonvisual behaviors of parents as they respond to infant
3. Observe the techniques the child uses to read and navigate; inquire if child is enrolled in visual training program; inquire about socialization opportunities for the child (i.e., who are child's friends, what are his extracurricular activities)
4. Observe preparation of room and self-care activities that provide for safety and independence during hospitalization
5. Investigate community programs aimed at preventing or detecting vision loss and inquire as to nursing involvement in these efforts.

Expected outcomes:

See Nursing Care Plan, pp. 568 to 570.

EMERGENCY TREATMENT

Eye Injuries

Foreign Object

Examine eye for presence of a foreign body (evert upper lid to examine upper eye)
Remove a freely movable object with pointed corner of gauze pad lightly moistened with water
Do not irrigate eye or attempt to remove a penetrating object (see below)
Caution child against rubbing eye

Chemical Burns

Irrigate eye copiously with tap water for 20 minutes
Evert upper lid to flush thoroughly
Hold child's head with eye under tap of running lukewarm water
Allow child to rest with eyes closed
Keep room darkened
Refer to an ophthalmologist

Ultraviolet Burns

If skin is burned, patch both eyes (make sure lids are completely closed); secure dressing with Kling bandages wrapped around head rather than tape
Allow child to rest with eyes closed
Refer to an ophthalmologist

Hematoma ("black eye")

Use a flashlight to check for gross hyphema (visible fluid meniscus across iris; more easily seen in light-colored than in brown eyes)
Apply ice for first 24 hours to reduce swelling if no hyphema is present
Refer to an ophthalmologist if hyphema is present

Penetrating Injuries

Never remove an object that has penetrated eye
Follow strict aseptic technique in examining eye
Observe for:
- Aqueous or vitreous leaks (fluid leaking from point of penetration)
- Hyphema
- Shape and equality of pupils, reaction to light
- Prolapsed iris (not perfectly circular)

Apply a Fox shield if available (not a regular eye patch)
Maintain bed rest with child in 30-degree Fowler position
Apply patch over unaffected eye to prevent bilateral movement
Caution child against rubbing eye
Refer to ophthalmologist

DEAF-BLIND CHILDREN

The most traumatic sensory impairment is loss of sight and hearing. Obviously, auditory and visual disabilities have profound effects on the child's development. They interfere with the normal sequence of physical, intellectual, and psychosocial growth. Although the child often achieves the usual motor milestones, he is more slowly developed. Children only learn communication with specialized training. Some deaf-blind children, especially those with residual hearing or sight, can learn to speak. Whenever possible, speech is encouraged, since it allows communication with other individuals.

The future prospects for deaf-blind children are at best unpredictable. Not infrequently congenital blindness and/or deafness is accompanied by other physical or neurologic problems, which further lessen the child's learning potential. The most favorable prognosis is for children who have acquired deaf blindness and have few, if any, associated disabilities. Their learning capacity is greatly potentiated by their previous developmental progress prior to the sensory impairments. Although total independence, including gainful vocational training, is the goal, some deaf-blind children are unable to develop to this level. They may require lifelong parental or residential care. The nurse working with such families helps them deal with future goals for the child, including possible alternatives to home care during the parents' advancing years.

RETINOBLASTOMA

Retinoblastoma is a rare congenital malignant tumor arising from the retina. It may be present at birth or may arise in the retina during the first 2 years of life. Retinoblastoma may be hereditary or nonhereditary and unilateral or bilateral. Hereditary retinoblastomas are transmitted as an autosomal-dominant trait with incomplete penetrance.

Diagnostic Evaluation

Retinoblastoma has few grossly obvious signs (see clinical manifestations box). Typically it is the parent who first observes a whitish "glow" in the pupil. The white reflex or white pupil (leukokoria) known as the *cat's eye reflex* represents visualization of the tumor as the light momentarily falls on the mass (Fig. 19-10).

The first step in diagnosis is carefully listening to and recognizing the significance of reports from family members regarding suspected abnormalities within the eye. Since the cat's eye reflex is a momentary sign visualized

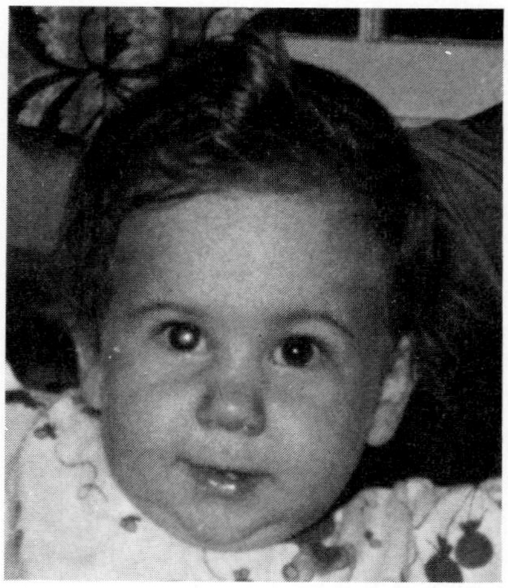

FIG. 19-10 Cat's eye reflex. Whitish appearance of lens is produced as light falls on tumor mass in right eye.

Clinical Manifestations of Retinoblastoma

Cat's eye reflex (most common sign)
Strabismus (second most common sign)
Red, painful eye, often with glaucoma
Blindness (late sign)

only under specific conditions, the physician or nurse must attempt to duplicate those conditions necessary to observe the tumor. Children suspected of having this disorder are referred to an ophthalmologist. Definitive diagnosis is usually based on indirect ophthalmoscopy, which is performed under general anesthesia with maximum dilation of the pupils.

Therapeutic Management

Treatment of retinoblastoma depends chiefly on the stage of the tumor at diagnosis. Staging includes five groups; group I refers to a small localized tumor(s), whereas group V is reserved to tumors involving more than half the retina and vitreous seeding. In general, early stage unilateral retinoblastomas are treated with irradiation or other techniques, such as cryotherapy, which freezes the tumor. Treatments other than radiotherapy are preferred to minimize the risk of radiation-induced malignancies, especially osteogenic sarcoma, later in life. The aim of therapy is to preserve useful vision in the affected eye and eradicate the tumor.

With advanced tumor growth, especially optic nerve involvement, enucleation of the affected eye is the treatment of choice. The use of chemotherapy in advanced disease is controversial but, if employed, may include the drugs vincristine, cyclophosphamide, and adriamycin.

With bilateral disease, every attempt is made to preserve useful vision in the least affected eye with enucleation of the severely diseased eye. When bilateral tumors are found early, radiotherapy or other treatments to both eyes may prevent the need for enucleation.

The overall prognosis for retinoblastoma is very favorable, with a survival rate of nearly 90% for both unilateral and bilateral tumors. Retinoblastoma is one of the tumors that may spontaneously regress.

Nursing Considerations

One of the most important nursing goals is to have a high index of suspicion for this rare malignancy. If parents report noticing a strange light in the eye or expression, these concerns must be taken seriously. Families with a history of retinoblastoma require follow-up and the nurse can be instrumental in reminding parents of appointments.

Since the tumor is usually diagnosed in infants or very young children, most of the preparation for diagnostic tests and treatment involves parents. After indirect ophthalmoscopy, the child may not see very clearly or his eyes may be sensitive to light because of pupillary dilation. Parents are made aware of these normal reactions prior to the procedure. They also are informed that a battery of screening tests, such as bone surveys and bone marrow aspiration, may be performed to detect metastasis.

Once the disease is staged, the physician confers with the parents regarding treatment. Unless the diagnosis is made very early, an enucleation is performed. Parents are told about the procedure as well as about the positive benefits of a prosthesis. Showing them pictures of another child with an artificial eye may be very helpful in their adjusting to the thought of disfigurement (Fig. 19-11). Although the idea of blindness is a very distressing one, most parents seem to realize that there is no alternative. The fact that the unaffected eye retains normal vision is particularly helpful in their accepting the loss and should be emphasized.

After surgery the parents are prepared for the child's facial appearance. An eye patch is in place, and the child's face may be edematous or ecchymotic. Parents often fear seeing the surgical site because they imagine a cavity in the skull. On the contrary, the lids are usually closed and the area does not appear sunken because a surgically implanted sphere maintains the shape of the eyeball. The implant is covered with conjunctiva, and when the lids are open the exposed area resembles the mucosal lining of the mouth. Once the child is fitted for a prosthesis, usually within 3 weeks, the facial appearance returns to normal. Initial instructions for care of the prosthesis are given by the ocularist, who fits and manufactures the device.

Care of the socket is minimal and easily accomplished. The wound itself is clean and has little or no drainage. If an antibiotic ointment is prescribed, it is applied in a thin line on the surface of the tissues of the socket. To cleanse the site, an irrigating solution may be ordered and is instilled daily or more frequently if necessary, *before* application of the antibiotic ointment. The dressing consists of an eye pad taped over the surgical site with nonirritating tape; it is changed daily. Once the socket has healed completely, a dressing is no longer necessary, although it is a preventive measure against infection.

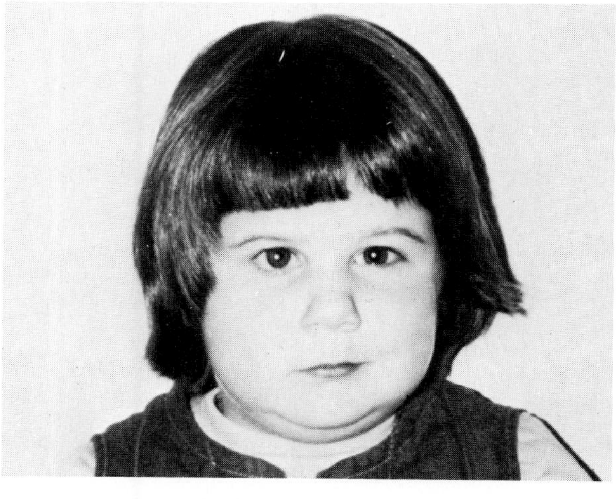

FIG. 19-11 Preschooler with right prosthetic eye.

A long-term consideration is the survivor's ability to transmit the defective gene to his offspring. Parents are encouraged to seek genetic counseling for themselves and for the child after he reaches puberty.

Family support. Families with a history of the disorder may feel great guilt for transmitting the defect to their offspring. In families with no history of retinoblastoma, the discovery of the diagnosis is a shock, frequently complicated by guilt for not having found it sooner. Since parents frequently are the first to observe the cat's eye reflex, they may feel angry at themselves or others, especially health professionals, for delaying a more thorough examination. The nurse assesses each of these variables in planning care based on understanding the family's emotional reactions and adjustment (see Chapter 18).

SUMMARY

Cognitive and sensory impairments constitute some of the most devastating disabilities for the child and the family. The impairments are usually life-long and require special training and education for children to develop to their optimum potential. Parents are unprepared for the special needs of rearing these children and benefit from the guidance and support of health professionals. Although nurses may not be involved in the direct rehabilitation of such children, they have important responsibilities in the areas of early detection of cognitive and sensory problems and involvement in preventive efforts. Nurses may also provide direct care to these children during hospitalization or follow-up in the home. School nurses are playing an increasingly important role as many children with special needs are mainstreamed into the regular classroom.

KEY CONCEPTS

- Mental retardation is the most common developmental disability in the United States, affecting about 3% of the population.
- According to the American Association of Mental Deficiencies, mental retardation is a "significantly subaverage general intellectual functioning existing concurrently with deficits in adaptive behavior and manifested during the developmental period."
- Causes of severe mental retardation are primarily genetic, biochemical, viral, and developmental. Mild retardation is associated primarily with familial, social, and environmental causes, whereas severe retardation is more likely associated with specific syndromes.
- Education of children with cognitive impairment emphasizes sensory and verbal discrimination, improvement of short-term memory, motivation, and technologic support.
- Promoting optimum development may be achieved through family guidance regarding play, communication, discipline, socialization, and sexuality.

- Prevention efforts regarding mental retardation focus on support for the premature neonate and other high-risk newborns, rubella immunization, genetic counseling, and maternal education regarding the risks of chemical use and the importance of adequate nutrition.
- Down syndrome, a chromosomal abnormality, is characterized by retarded intelligence, slowed social development, congenital anomalies, sensory problems, and diminished growth and sexual development.
- Fragile X syndrome is a recently recognized clinical entity characterized by mental retardation and phenotypic findings in some affected males. It is considered the second leading cause of mental retardation after Down syndrome.
- Hearing disorders may be classified according to the location of the defect: conductive, sensorineural, mixed conductive-sensorineural, and central auditory imperception.
- Rehabilitation for hearing loss involves parent education and support, hearing aids, lipreading, sign language, speech therapy, and promotion of socialization.
- Prevention of hearing loss includes treatment of infection, auditory testing, immunization, pregnancy and genetic counseling, and reduction of noise pollution.
- Visual impairments in childhood include refractive errors, amblyopia, strabismus, cataracts, glaucoma, trauma, and infections.
- Nursing goals in visual rehabilitation are helping the family and child adjust to the child's visual impairment, promoting parent-child attachment, fostering optimum development and independence, providing for play and socialization, and being aware of educational facilities.
- For the child undergoing ocular surgery, nursing care is aimed at reassuring the child and family throughout treatment, orienting the child to his surroundings, providing a safe environment, and encouraging independence.
- Prevention of visual impairment focuses on prenatal screening, prenatal and perinatal care, and periodic vision screening of all children, immunization, and safety counseling.
- Retinoblastoma is a rare congenital malignant tumor; its most common clinical manifestations are cat's eye reflex (white pupil) and strabismus.

STUDY QUESTIONS AND ACTIVITIES

1 Visit a long-term facility for children with mental retardation and ask about the training strategies used to teach the residents.
2 Interview a family who has chosen to rear a child with Down syndrome at home. What were the reasons for the parents' choosing home care? What have been the difficulties and rewards of the child's membership in the family?
3 Visit an audiologist and inquire about the different types of hearing aids and their care.
4 Visit a school for the deaf and observe the types of communication training that are taught to the child and family.
5 Visit a school for the blind and observe the types of reading training and activities of daily living that are taught to the child and family.

REFERENCES

American Academy of Pediatrics, Committee on Sports Medicine, Committee on Children with Disabilities: Exercise for children who are mentally retarded, Pediatrics **80**(3):447-448, 1987.
American Academy of Pediatrics, Joint Committee on Infant Hearing: Position statement 1982, Pediatrics **70**(3):496-497, 1982.
Brady, M.A.: Fragile-X syndrome: an overview, Pediatr. Nurs. **10**(3):210-211, 1984.
Cohen, F.: Clinical genetics in nursing practice, Philadelphia, 1984, J.B. Lippincott Co.
Coplan, J.: Three pitfalls in the early diagnosis of mental retardation, Clin. Pediatr. **21**(5):308-310, 1982.
Gortmaker, S.L., and Sappenfield, W.: Chronic childhood disorders: prevalence and impact, Pediatr. Clin. North Am. **31**(1):3-18, 1984.
Grossman, H.J., editor: Classification in mental retardation, Washington, DC, 1983, American Association on Mental Retardation.
Vision problems in the United States, New York, 1980, National Society to Prevent Blindness.
Whaley, L., and Wong, D.: Nursing care of infants and children, ed. 3, St. Louis, 1987, The C.V. Mosby Co.
Williams, J.K.: Reproductive decisions: adolescents with Down syndrome, Pediatr. Nurs. **9**(1):43-44, 1983.

BIBLIOGRAPHY

Cognitive Impairment

Bernardo, M.L.: Premarital counseling and the couple with disabilities: a review and recommendations, Rehabil. Lit. **42**(7-8):213-216, 1981.
Blackwell, M.W., and Roy, S.A.: Surgical "routines" for profoundly retarded patients, Am. J. Nurs. **78**(3):402-404, 1978.
Bowness, S., and Zadik, T.D.: Implementing the nursing process at a unit for mentally handicapped children, Nurs. Times **77**(16):695-696, 1981.
Brinkworth, R.: Helping the child with Down's syndrome, Midwife Health Visit. Community Nurse **19**:93-96, 1983.
Carpenter, N.J., Leichtman, L.G., and Say, B.: Fragile X–linked mental retardation, Am. J. Dis. Child. **136**:392-398, 1982.
Chatterjee, M.S.: Paternal age and Down's syndrome, Contemp. OB/GYN **21**(5):171-174, 1983.
Chudley, A.E., and Hagerman, R.J.: Fragile X syndrome, J. Pediatr. **110**(6):821-831, 1987.
Davies, R.R., and Rogers, E.S.: Social skills training with persons who are mentally retarded, Ment. Retard. **23**(4):186-196, 1985.
de la Cruz, F.F., and Muller, J.Z.: Facts about Down syndrome, Child. Today **12**(6):2-7, 1983.
Erickson, M.L.: Care approaches to the child with mental retardation in a hospital setting, Clin. Pediatr. **17** (7):539-547, 1978.
Fryns, J.: Fragile X syndrome: a study of 83 families, Clin. Genet. **26**(6):497-528, 1984.
Hogge, W.A., and others: Prenatal diagnosis of fragile "X" syndrome, Obstet. Gynecol. **63**(3)[suppl.]:19S-21S, 1984.
Kihlstrom, A.: A very special boy, Child. Today **12**(6): 8-11, 1983.
Koch, R.: Down's syndrome: pediatric care, Feelings Med. Signif. **22**(1):1-6, 1980.
McKerrow, K: Minimal hearing loss may not be benign, Am. J. Nurs. **87**(7):904-905, 1987.
Miola, E.S.: Down syndrome: update for practitioners, Pediatr. Nurs. **13**(4):233-237, 1987.
Pipes, P.L., and Pritkin, R.: Nutrition and feeding of children with developmental delays and related problems. In Pipes, P.L., editor: Nutrition in infancy and childhood, ed. 3, St. Louis, 1985, The C.V. Mosby Co.
Pueschel, S.M.: The child with Down syndrome. In Levine, M.D., and others, editors: Developmental-behavioral pediatrics, Philadelphia, 1983, W.B. Saunders Co.
Roberts, M.J., and Canfield, M.: Behavior modification with a mentally retarded child, Am. J. Nurs. **80**(4):679, 1980.
Roberts, S.E., Coffin, G., and Dunn, M.J.: Feeding techniques for the physically impaired child, Pediatr. Basics **21**:4-7, 1978.

Silva, M.C.: Assessing competency for informed consent with mentally retarded minors, Pediatr. Nurs. **10**(4): 261-265, 306, 1984.
Steele, S.: Assessment of functional wellness behaviors in adolescents who are mentally retarded, Issues Compr. Pediatr. Nurs. **9:**331-340, 1986.
Task Force on Joint Assessment of Prenatal and Perinatal Factors Associated with Brain Disorders: National Institutes of Health report on causes of mental retardation and cerebral palsy, Pediatrics **76**(3):457-458, 1985.
Tudor, M.: Nursing intervention with developmentally disabled children, MCN **3**(1):25-31, 1978.
Veach, S.A.: Down's syndrome: helping the special parents of a special infant, Nursing 83 **13**(9):42-43, 1983.
Vessey, J.A.: Care of the hospitalized child with a cognitive developmental delay, Holistic Nurs. Pract. **2**(2):48-54, 1988.
Wasch, S.W.: Hospitalization of profoundly and severely mentally retarded children, Child Health Care **9:**126-131, 1981.
Williams, J.K.: Down syndrome update, Child. Nurse **3**(5):1-4, 1985.
Williams, R.: A community nursing service for mentally handicapped children, Nurs. Times **76:**2011-2012, Nov. 1980.
Wilson, B.: Toilet training the mentally handicapped child, Dev. Med. Child Neurol. **22**(2):225-229, 1980.

Hearing Impairment

Anagnostakis, D., and others: Hearing loss in low-birth-weight infants, Am. J. Dis. Child. **136**(7):602-604, 1982.
Bergstrom, L.: Causes of severe hearing loss in early childhood, Pediatr. Ann. **9**(1):23-30, 1980.
Boffman, J.H., and Boffman, R.T.: Early detection of hearing impairment, Issues Compr. Pediatr. Nurs. **5**(1):11-20, 1981.
Campbell, S.L.: Some sound advice from managing a hearing-impaired patient, Nursing 84 **14**(12):46, 1984.
Gibbons, C.L.: Deaf children's perception of internal body parts, Matern. Child Nurs. J. **14**(1):37-46, 1985.
Hanawalt, A., and Troutman, K.: If your patient has a hearing aid, Am. J. Nurs. **84**(7):900-901, 1984.
Holder, L.: Hearing aids: handle with care, Nursing 82 **12**(4):64-67, 1982.
Holm, C.: Deafness: common misunderstandings, Am. J. Nurs. **78**(11):1910-1912, 1978.
Kaufman, D.H., Grothe, G., and Brasser, B.: Early identification of ear infection and hearing loss in an early childhood population, School Nurse **3**(1):18-21, 1987.
Matkin, N.D.: Early recognition and referral of hearing-impaired children, Pediatr. Rev. **6**(5):151-156, 1984.
McFarland, W.H., and Simmons, F.B.: The importance of early intervention with severe childhood deafness, Pediatr. Ann. **9**(1):13-19, 1980.
McRae, M.J.: Bonding in a sea of silence, MCN **4**(1):29-34, 1979.
Morgan, R.H.: Breaking through the sound barrier, Nursing 83 **13**(2):112-113, 1983.
Northern, J., and Downs, M.: Hearing in children, ed. 4, Baltimore, 1984, The Williams & Wilkins Co.
Robinson, T.: Early identification of vision and hearing problems. In Pediatrics: nursing update, vol. 1, no. 12, Princeton, NJ, 1986, Continuing Professional Education Center, Inc.
Sataloff, R.: Pediatric hearing loss, Pediatr. Nurs. **6**(5):16-18, 1980.
Smith, M.P., and Cloonan, P.A.: Meeting the special needs of the hearing-impaired child, Issues Compr. Pediatr. Nurs. **3**(6):21-34, 1979.

Vision Impairment

Als, H.: Reciprocity and autonomy: parenting a blind infant, Zero to Three **5**(5):8-10, 1985.
Bischoff, R.W.: Early childhood development of the visually handicapped, Issues Compr. Pediatr. Nurs. **3**(6):35-49, 1979.
Carden, R.G.: The ins and outs of contact lenses, RN **48** (2):48-50, 1985.
Fenwick, A., and others: Traumatic blindness: a flexible approach for helping a blind adolescent, Nursing 79 **9**(1):36-41, 1979.
Grin, T.R., Nelson, L.B., and Jeffers, J.B.: Eye injuries in childhood, Pediatrics **80**(1):13-17, 1987.
Helveston, E., and Ellis, F.: Pediatric ophthalmology practice, ed. 2, St. Louis, 1984, The C.V. Mosby Co.
Herget, M.: For visually impaired diabetics, Am. J. Nurs. **83**(11):1557-1560, 1983.
Kovalesky, A.: Nurses' guide to children's eyes, New York, 1985, Grune & Stratton, Inc.
McNeer, K.W.: Pediatric ophthalmology, Pediatr. Nurs. **5**(6):47-49, 1979.
Nelson, L.B.: The visually handicapped child, Pediatr. Rev. **6**(6):173-182, 1984.
Osguthorpe, N.C.: If your patient has contact lenses, Am. J. Nurs. **84**(10):1255-1256, 1984.
Pugh, R.: Effects of visual impairment on children: development in sight, Nurs. Mirror **150**(21):30-32, 1980.
Severtsen, B.M.: Sensory impairment: its effect on the family. In Hymovich, D.P., and Barnard, M.U., editors: Family health care, New York, 1979, McGraw-Hill Book Co.
Steffe, D.R., Suty, K.A., and Delcalzo, P.V.: More than a touch: communicating with a blind and deaf patient, Nursing 85 **15**(8):36-39, 1985.
Tumulty, G., and Resler, M.M.: Eye trauma, Am. J. Nurs. **84**(6):740-744, 1984.
Wassenberg, C.: Common visual disorders in children, Nurs. Clin. North Am. **16**(3):479-485, 1981.
Wong, D.L., and Dorman, L.R.: Nursing care in childhood cancer: retinoblastoma, Am. J. Nurs. **82**(3):425-431, 1982.

UNIT

IX

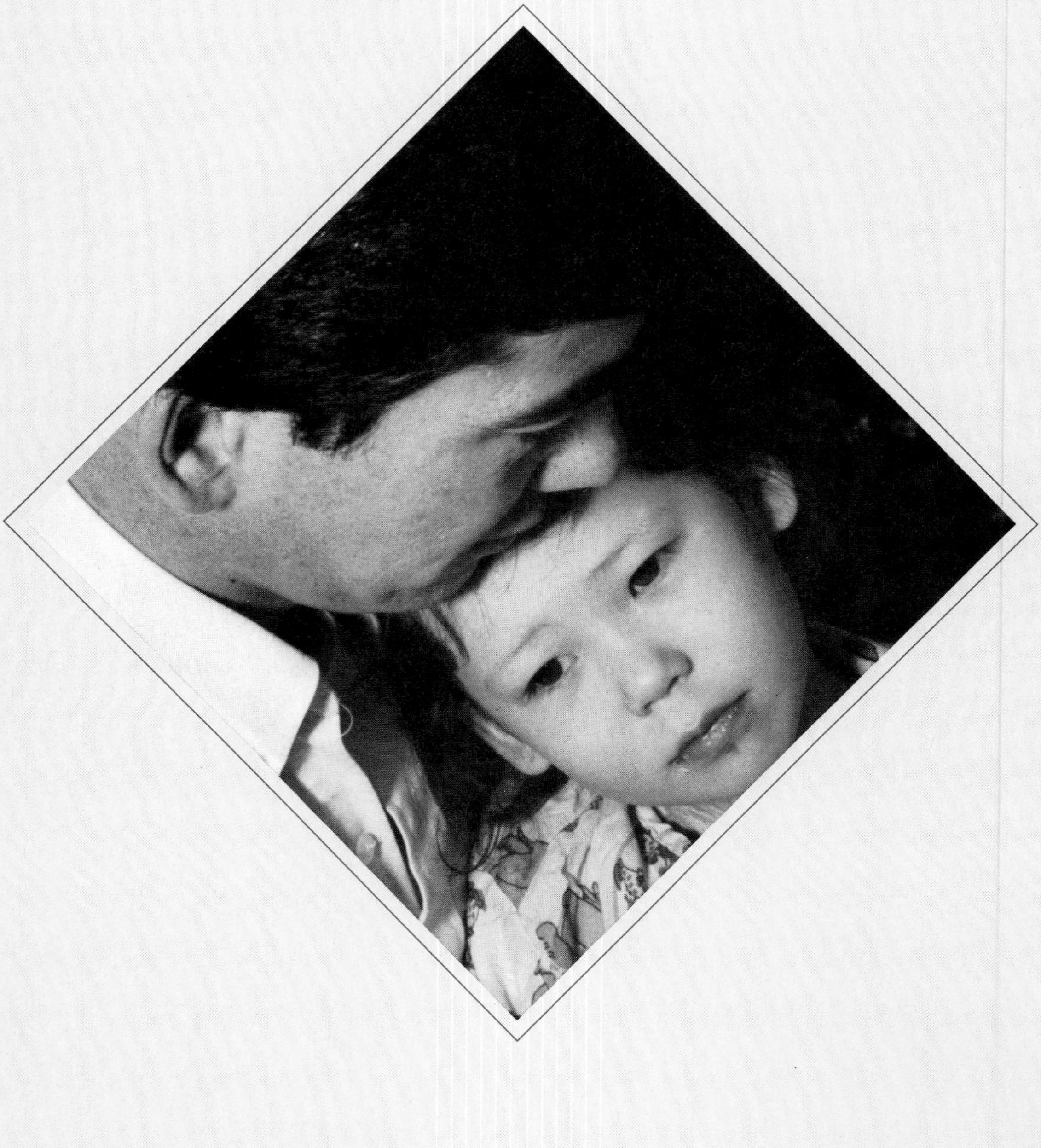

Impact of Hospitalization on the Child and Family

Putting a sick child in the hospital creates a crisis for both the child and the family. The child faces separation from familiar caregivers and surroundings, loss of independence, exposure to painful experiences, and disruption of nearly every aspect of his usual life-style. Often the reason for the hospitalization is of much less concern to the child than the consequences of confinement. Emergency and intensive care admissions pose an even greater threat because of the lack of time to prepare the child and the seriousness of the child's condition. In addition, treatments are often painful and frightening.

Chapter 20, *Reaction of Child and Family to Illness and Hospitalization,* is concerned with the child's age-related reactions to illness and hospitalization and with interventions that lessen the psychologic trauma of the experience, particularly parent participation and preparation of the child for admission to the hospital. The effects of the child's hospitalization on the family are discussed, making the point that care must be extended to these important individuals as well. The needs of the child and family during special hospital admissions are explored. The chapter concludes with a discussion of discharge planning and home care.

Chapter 21, *Pediatric Variations of Nursing Interventions,* deals with pediatric variations of nursing procedures and psychologic and physical preparation of the child for various procedures. The chapter is not designed to present a detailed description of how to perform specific procedures, but rather to show how to safely implement those procedures with children.

CHAPTER 20

Reaction of Child and Family to Illness and Hospitalization

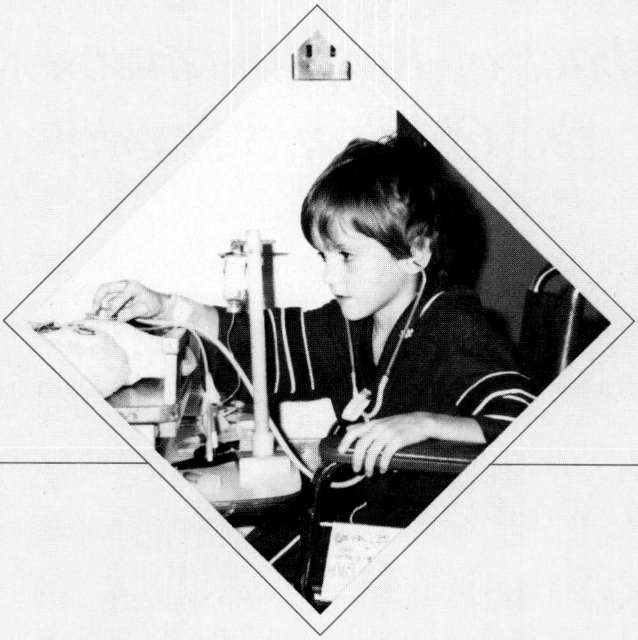

LEARNING OBJECTIVES

On completion of this chapter the reader will be able to:

- Identify the stressors of illness and hospitalization for children during each developmental stage
- Outline nursing interventions that prevent or minimize the stress of separation during hospitalization
- List the admission procedures for a child on admission to the hospital
- Outline nursing interventions that minimize the stress of loss of control during hospitalization
- Outline nursing interventions that minimize the fear of bodily injury during hospitalization
- Describe methods of assessing and managing pain in children
- Outline nursing interventions that support parents and siblings during a child's illness and hospitalization
- Describe nursing interventions needed when children are admitted to special units

For children and their families illness and hospitalization create a stressful experience. Often these two crises are the first ones children must deal with. Children, especially during the early years, are particularly vulnerable to the crises of illness and hospitalization because (1) stress represents a change from the usual state of health and environmental routine, and (2) children have a limited number of coping mechanisms to resolve the stressful events. Children's reactions to these crises are influenced by their developmental age; previous experience with illness, separation, or hospitalization; innate and acquired coping skills; the seriousness of the diagnosis; and the support system available. This chapter focuses on the various aspects of pediatric illness and hospitalization to help nurses provide the quality of care that promotes optimum resolution of the crises and positive growth from the experience for the entire family unit.

◆ *Stressors and Reactions Related to Developmental Stage*

Children's understanding of, reaction to, and method of coping with illness or hospitalization are influenced by the significance of individual *stressors* (those events that produce stress) during each developmental phase. Although the major stressors of separation, loss of control, and bodily injury and their behavioral reactions are discussed in the following section, a review of the previous chapters on normal growth and development will facilitate a more thorough understanding of children's physical, psychosocial, and cognitive abilities and limitations. In addition, Chapter 18 presents an in-depth discussion of children's and family members' reactions to a disability or chronic or life-threatening illness.

Manifestations of Separation Anxiety in Young Children

Phase of Protest

Observed behaviors during later infancy
- Cries
- Screams
- Searches for parent with eyes
- Clings to parent
- Avoids and rejects contact with strangers

Additional behaviors observed during toddlerhood
- Verbally attacks strangers, i.e., "go away"
- Physically attacks strangers, i.e., kicks, bites, hits, pinches
- Attempts to escape to find parent
- Attempts to physically force parent to stay

Behaviors may last from hours to days

Protest, such as crying, may be continuous, ceasing only with physical exhaustion

Approach of stranger may precipitate increased protest

Phase of Despair

Observed behaviors
- Inactive
- Withdraws from others
- Depressed, sad
- Uninterested in environment
- Uncommunicative
- Regresses to earlier behavior, i.e., thumb sucking, bed-wetting, use of pacifier, use of bottle

Behaviors may last for variable length of time

Child's physical condition may deteriorate from refusal to eat, drink, or move

Phase of Detachment

Observed behaviors
- Shows increased interest in surroundings
- Interacts with strangers or familiar caregivers
- Forms new but superficial relationships
- Appears happy

Detachment usually occurs after prolonged separation from parent; rarely seen in hospitalized children

Behaviors represent a superficial adjustment to loss

SEPARATION ANXIETY

The major stress from middle infancy throughout the preschool years, especially for children ages 15 to 30 months, is separation anxiety (also called *anaclitic depression*). The principal behavioral responses to each stressor during early childhood are summarized in the box.

During the phase of *protest,* the child reacts aggressively to the separation from the parent. The child cries and screams for his parents, refuses the attention of anyone else, and is inconsolable in his grief (Fig. 20-1). During the phase of *despair,* the crying stops, and depression is evident. The child is much less active, is uninterested in play or food, and withdraws from others (Fig. 20-2).

The third stage is *detachment,* which is sometimes also called *denial.* Superficially it appears that the child has finally adjusted to the loss. He becomes more interested in his surroundings, plays with others, and seems to form new relationships. However, this behavior is the result of resignation and is not a sign of contentment. The child detaches from the parent in an effort to escape the emotional pain of desiring the parent's presence and copes by forming shallow relationships with others, becoming increasingly self-centered, and attaching primary importance to material objects. This is the most serious stage in that reversal of the potential adverse effects is

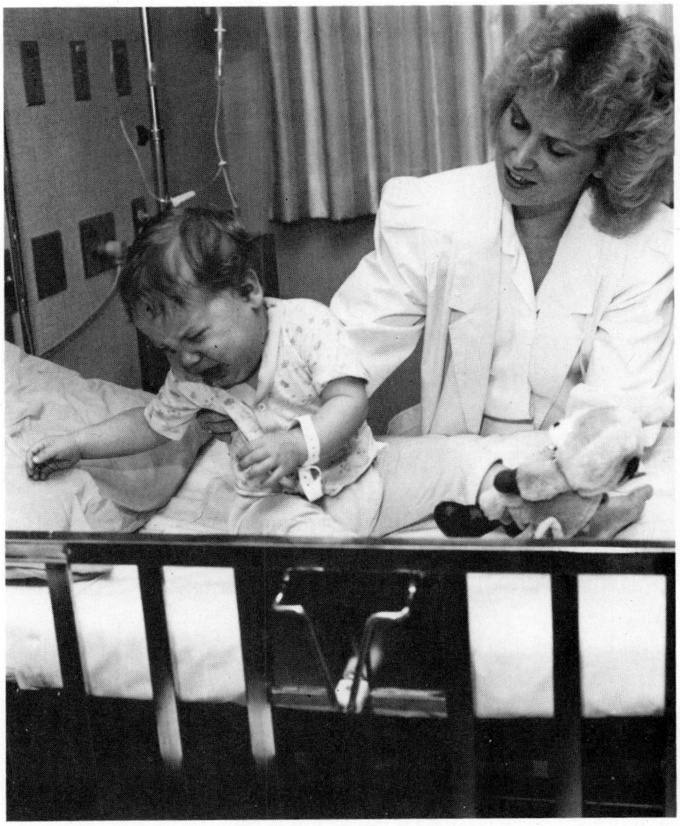

FIG. 20-1 During the phase of protest, the child cries loudly, rejects the nurse, and grieves inconsolably for the parents.

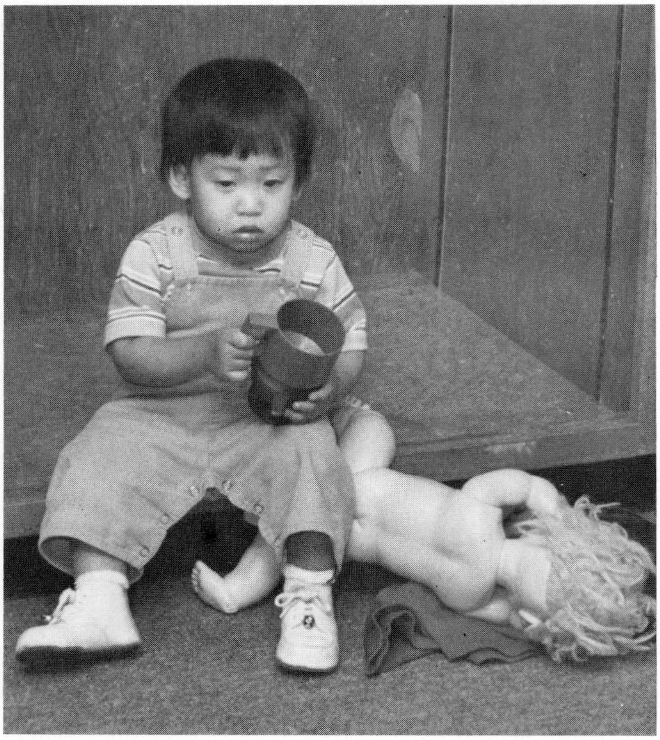

FIG. 20-2 During the phase of despair, the child is sad, lonely, and uninterested in play or food.

less likely to occur once detachment is established. However, in most situations the temporary separations imposed by hospitalization do not cause such prolonged parental absences that the child enters into detachment. In addition, there is considerable evidence to suggest that, even with stresses such as separation, children are remarkably adaptable and permanent ill effects are rare.

While progression to the stage of detachment is uncommon, the initial stages are frequently observed even with very brief separations from either parent. Unless health team members understand the meaning of each stage of behavior, they may erroneously label the behaviors as positive or negative. For example, they may see the loud crying of the protest phase as "bad" behavior. Since the protesting increases when a stranger approaches the child, they may interpret that reaction as meaning they should stay away. During the quiet, withdrawn phase of despair, health team members may think the child is finally "settling in" to his new surroundings, and they may see the detachment behaviors as proof of a "good adjustment." The faster this stage is reached, the more likely the child will be regarded as the "ideal patient."

Since children seem to react "negatively" to visits by their parents, uninformed observers feel justified in restricting parental visiting privileges. For example, during the protest stage, children outwardly do not appear happy to see their parents. In fact, they may even cry louder. If they are depressed, they may reject their parents or begin to protest once more. Often they cling to their parents in an effort to ensure their continued presence. Consequently, such reactions may be regarded as "disturbing" the child's adjustment to the new surroundings. If the separation has progressed to the phase of detachment, children will respond no differently to their parents than to any other strange or familiar person.

Such reactions are equally distressing to parents, who are unaware of their meaning. If parents are regarded as intruders, they will see their absence as "beneficial" to the child's adjustment and recovery. They may respond to the child's behavior by staying for only short periods of time, visiting less frequently, or deceiving the child when it is time to leave. The result is a *destructive* cycle of misunderstanding and unmet needs.

Early Childhood

Separation anxiety is most evident during the ages of 6 to 30 months and is the greatest stress imposed by hospitalization. If separation is avoided, young children have a tremendous capacity to withstand any other stress. During this time the typical reactions previously described are seen. However, children in the toddler stage demonstrate more goal-directed behaviors. For example, they may plead with the parents to stay and physically try to keep the parents with them or try to find parents who have left. They may demonstrate displeasure on the parents' return or departure by having temper tantrums; refusing to comply with the usual routines of mealtime, bedtime, or toileting; or regressing to more primitive levels of development.

Since preschoolers are more secure interpersonally than toddlers, they can tolerate brief periods of separation from their parents and are more inclined to develop substitute trust in other significant adults. However, the stress of illness usually renders preschoolers less able to cope with separation; as a result, they manifest many of the stage behaviors of separation anxiety, although in general the protest behaviors are more subtle and passive than those seen in younger children. Preschoolers may demonstrate separation anxiety through refusing to eat, difficulty in sleeping, crying quietly for their parents, continually asking when the parents will visit, or withdrawing from others. They may express anger indirectly by breaking their toys, hitting other children, or refusing to cooperate during usual self-care activities. Nurses need to be sensitive to these less obvious signs of separation anxiety in order to intervene appropriately.

Later Childhood and Adolescence

Although school-age children are better able to cope with separation in general, the stress imposed by illness or hospitalization may increase their need for parental security and guidance. This is particularly true for young school-age children who have only recently left the safety of the home and are struggling with the crisis of school adjustment. Middle and late school-age children may react more to the separation from their usual activities and peers than to the absence of their parents. These children have a high level of physical and mental activity that frequently finds no suitable outlets in the hospital environment, and even when they dislike school, they admit to missing its routine and worry that they will not be able to compete with their classmates when they return to school. Feelings of loneliness, boredom, isolation, and depression are common. It is important to recognize that such reactions may occur more as a result of separation than from concern over the illness, treatment, or hospital setting.

School-age children may need and desire parental guidance or support from other adult figures but be unable or unwilling to ask for it. Because the goal of attaining independence is so important to them, they are reluctant to seek help directly for fear that they will appear weak, childish, or dependent. Cultural expectations to "act like a man" or to "be brave and strong" bear heavily on these children, especially boys, who tend to react to stress with stoicism, withdrawal, or passive acceptance. Often the need to express hostile, angry, or other negative feelings finds outlets in alternate ways, such as irritability and aggression toward parents, withdrawal from hospital personnel, inability to relate to peers, rejection of siblings, or subsequent behavioral problems in school.

For adolescents separation from home and parents may be a welcomed and appreciated event. However, loss of peer-group contact may pose a severe emotional threat because of loss of group status, inability to exert group control or leadership, and loss of group acceptance. Deviations within peer groups are poorly tolerated, and, although group members may express concern for the adolescent's illness or need for hospitalization, they continue their group activities, quickly filling the gap of the absent member. During the temporary separation from their usual group, ill adolescents may benefit from group associations with other hospitalized age-mates.

LOSS OF CONTROL

One of the factors influencing the amount of stress imposed by hospitalization is the amount of control people feel they have. Lack of control increases the perception of threat and can affect children's coping skills. In the hospital numerous situations exist that decrease the amount of control a child feels. The major areas of loss of control in terms of physical restriction, altered routine or rituals, and dependency are discussed for each age-group.

Toddlers

Toddlers are striving for autonomy, and this goal is evident in most of their behaviors—motor skills, play, interpersonal relationships, activities of daily living, and communication. When their egocentric pleasures meet with obstacles, toddlers react with negativism, especially temper tantrums. Any restriction or limitation of movement, such as the simple act of making toddlers lie down, can cause forceful resistance and noncompliance.

Loss of control also results from altered routines and rituals. Toddlers rely on the consistency and familiarity of daily rituals to provide a measure of stability and control in their complex world of growing and developing. The experience of hospitalization or illness severely limits their sense of expectation and predictability, since practically every detail of the hospital environment differs from that of the home.

Toddlers' main areas for rituals include eating, sleeping, bathing, toileting, and play. When the routines are disrupted, difficulties can occur in any or all of these areas. The principal reaction to such change is regression. For example, when mealtime and food choices differ from those at home, toddlers often refuse to eat, demand a bottle, or ask others to feed them. Although regression to earlier forms of behavior may seem to increase toddlers' security and comfort, in reality it is very threatening for them to relinquish their most recently acquired achievements.

Enforced dependency is a chief characteristic of the sick role and accounts for the numerous instances of toddler negativism. For example, rigid schedules, altered caregiving activities, unfamiliar surroundings, separation from parents, and medical procedures usurp toddlers' control over their world. Although most toddlers initially react negatively and aggressively to such dependency, prolonged loss of autonomy may result in passive withdrawal from interpersonal relationships and regression in all areas of development. Therefore the effects of the sick role are most severe in instances of chronic, long-term illnesses or in those families in which the sick role is fostered despite the child's improved state of health.

Preschoolers

Preschoolers also suffer from loss of control caused by physical restriction, altered routines, and enforced dependency. However, their specific cognitive abilities, which make them feel omnipotent and all-powerful, also make them feel out of control. This loss of control in the context of their sense of self-power is a critical influencing factor in their perception of and reaction to separation, pain, illness, and hospitalization.

Preschoolers' egocentric and magical thinking limits their ability to understand events because they view all experiences from their own self-referenced (egocentric) perspective. Without adequate preparation for unfamiliar settings or experiences, preschoolers' fantasy explanations for such events are usually more exaggerated, bizarre, and frightening than the actual facts. One typical fantasy to explain the reason for illness or hospitalization is that it represents punishment for real or imagined misdeeds. In response to such thinking the child usually feels shame, guilt, and fear.

School-Age Children

Because of their striving for independence and productivity, school-age children are particularly vulnerable to events that may lessen their feeling of control and power. In particular, altered family roles; physical disability; fears of death, abandonment, or permanent injury; loss of peer acceptance; lack of productivity; and inability to cope with stress according to perceived cultural expectation may result in loss of control.

Because of the nature of the patient role, many routine hospital activities usurp individual power and identity. For school-age children, dependent activities such as enforced bed rest, use of a bedpan, inability to choose a menu, lack of privacy, help with a bed bath, or transport by use of a wheelchair or stretcher can be a direct threat to their security. Although all of these usual hospital procedures seem routine and inconsequential, to children who want to "act grown-up" they allow no freedom of choice. However, when children are allowed to exert a measure of control, regardless of how limited it may be, they generally respond very well to any procedure. For example, some of the most cooperative, satisfied, and contented patients are those school-age children who help make their beds, choose their schedule of activities, assist in procedures, and help the nurses care for the younger children. An increased sense of control is usually an outcome of a feeling of usefulness and productivity.

Besides the hospital environment, illness also may cause a feeling of loss of control. One of the most significant problems of children in this age-group centers on boredom. When physical or enforced limitations curtail their usual abilities to care for themselves or to engage in favorite activities, school-age children generally respond with depression, hostility, or frustration. Keeping a normally active child on bed rest is no small challenge. However, by emphasizing areas of control for the child and capitalizing on quiet activities, particularly hobbies such as building models or collecting specific objects, nurses can promote school-age children's adjustment to physical restriction. Nursing judgment regarding selection of a roommate is one of the most important contributing factors to the overall adjustment of children in this age-group to illness and hospitalization.

Adolescents

Adolescents' struggle for independence, self-assertion, and liberation centers on the quest for personal identity. Anything that interferes with this poses a threat to their sense of identity and results in a loss of control. Illness, which limits their physical abilities, and hospitalization, which separates them from usual support systems, constitute major situational crises.

The patient role fosters dependency and depersonali-

TABLE 20-1

Children's Developmental Concepts of Illness and Pain

Cognitive Stage (age)	Concept of Illness*	Concept of Pain†
Preoperational thought (2 to 7 years)	*Phenomenism:* Perceives an external, unrelated, concrete phenomenon as the cause of illness; e.g., "being sick because you don't feel well" *Contagion:* Perceives cause of illness as proximity between two events that occurs by "magic"; e.g., "getting a cold because you are near someone who has a cold"	Related to pain primarily as physical, concrete experience Thinks in terms of magical disappearance of pain May view pain as punishment for wrongdoing Tends to hold someone accountable for own pain and may strike out at person
Concrete operational thought (7 to 10+ years)	*Contamination:* Perceives cause as a person, object, or action external to the child that is "bad" or "harmful" to the body; i.e., "getting a cold because you didn't wear a hat" *Internalization:* Perceives illness as having an external cause but as being located inside the body; i.e., "getting a cold by breathing in air and bacteria"	Relate to pain physically; i.e., headache, stomachache Able to perceive of psychologic pain, such as someone dying Fears bodily harm and annihilation (body destruction and death) May view pain as punishment for wrongdoing
Formal operational thought (13 years and older)	*Physiologic:* Perceives cause as malfunctioning or nonfunctioning organ or process; can explain illness in sequence of events *Psychophysiologic:* Realizes that psychologic actions and attitudes affect health and illness	Able to give reason for pain; i.e., fell and hit nerve Perceives several types of psychologic pain Has limited life experiences to cope with pain as adult might cope despite mature understanding of pain Fears losing control during painful experience

*From Bibace, R., and Walsh, M.E.: Development of children's concepts of illness, Pediatrics **66**(6):912-917, 1980.
†From Hurley, A., and Whelan, E.G.: Cognitive development and children's perception of pain, Pediatr. Nurs. **14**(1):21-24, 1988.

zation. Adolescents may react to dependency with rejection, uncooperativeness, or withdrawal. They may respond to depersonalization with self-assertion, anger, or frustration. Regardless of which response they manifest, hospital personnel generally tend to regard them as difficult, unmanageable patients. Parents may not be a source of help because these behaviors serve to further isolate them from understanding the adolescent. Although peers may visit, they may not be able to offer the kind of support and guidance needed. Sick adolescents often voluntarily isolate themselves from age-mates until they feel they can compete on an equal basis and meet group expectations.

Loss of control also occurs for many of the reasons discussed for school-age children. However, adolescents are more sensitive to potential instances of loss of control and dependency than younger children. For example, both groups seek information about their physical status and rely heavily on anticipatory preparation to decrease fear and anxiety. However, adolescents react not only to the kinds of information supplied them but also to the means by which it is conveyed. They may feel very threatened by others who relate facts in a derogatory manner. Adolescents want to know that others can relate to them on their own level. This necessitates a careful assessment of their intellectual abilities, previous knowledge, and present needs.

BODILY INJURY AND PAIN

Fears of bodily injury and pain are prevalent among children and recent research documents that young children, including newborns, react to painful stimuli. In caring for children, nurses must have an appreciation of a child's concerns about bodily harm and the reactions to pain at different developmental periods. Developmental considerations related to children's understanding of illness and pain are summarized in Table 20-1. Developmental characteristics of children's reactions to pain are summarized in the box.

Infants

In the research exploring children's development of illness concepts and how their understanding of illness relates to fears of bodily injury, no findings are available for preverbal children. Consequently, the following discussion is limited to infants' reactions to pain.

Neonates' reaction to painful stimuli is generalized body movement associated with brief, loud crying and facial expressions of pain. Physiologic indications of pain may include palm sweating, increased heart rate and blood pressure, and decreased blood oxygenation. However, these changes may be less apparent in premature infants; for example, during heelstick procedures these infants may not demonstrate decreased oxygenation but may be more responsive physiologically to procedures such as suctioning and position changes (Norris, Campbell, and Brenkert, 1982).

Infants' response to pain after the neonatal period is quite similar to earlier reactions, although there is marked variability in measures of distress, especially initial cry and heart rate, which may decrease in some infants (Dale, 1986). The most consistent indicator of distress is a facial expression of discomfort (Fig. 20-3). Body movements consist initially of rigidity of the extremities

Developmental Characteristics of Children's Responses to Pain

Young Infants

Generalized body response of rigidity or thrashing, possibly with local reflex withdrawal of stimulated area
Loud crying
Facial expression of pain (brows lowered and drawn together, eyes tightly closed, and mouth open and squarish) (Fig. 20-3)
Demonstrates no association between approaching stimulus and subsequent pain

Older Infants

Localized body response with deliberate withdrawal of stimulated area
Loud crying
Facial expression of pain and/or anger (same facial characteristics as pain but eyes are open)
Physical resistance, especially pushing the stimulus away *after* it is applied

Young Child

Loud crying, screaming
Verbal expressions of "Ow," "Ouch," "It hurts"
Thrashing of arms and legs
Attempts to push stimulus away *before* it is applied
Uncooperative; needs physical restraint
Requests termination of procedure
Clings to parent, nurse, or other significant person
Requests emotional support, such as hugs or other forms of physical comfort
May become restless and irritable with continuing pain
All of these behaviors may be seen in anticipation of actual painful procedure

School-Age Child

May see all behaviors of young child, especially *during* actual painful procedure but less in anticipatory period
Stalling behavior, such as "Wait a minute" or "I'm not ready"
Muscular rigidity, such as clenched fists, white knuckles, gritted teeth, contracted limbs, body stiffness, closed eyes, wrinkled forehead

Adolescent

Less vocal protest
Less motor activity
More verbal expressions, such as "It hurts" or "You're hurting me"
Increased muscle tension and body control

Principle references: Craig, K.D., and others: Developmental changes in infant pain expression during immunization injections, Soc. Sci. Med. **19**(12):1331-1337, 1984; Katz, E.R., Kellerman, J., and Siegel, S.E.: Behavioral distress in children with cancer undergoing medical procedures: developmental considerations, J. Consult. Clin. Psychol. **48**(3)356-365, 1980.

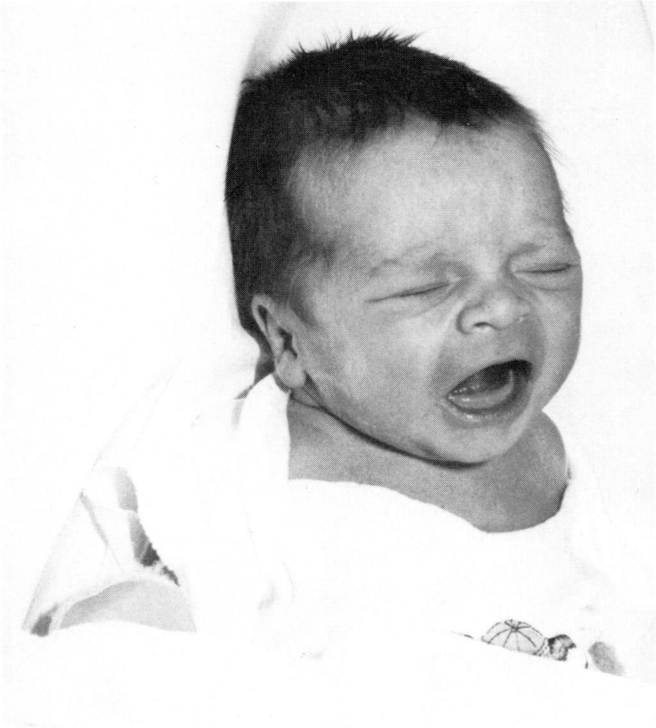

FIG. 20-3 Facial expression of physical distress is the most consistent behavioral indicator of pain in infants.

followed by thrashing and deliberate withdrawal of the stimulated body part.

Toddlers

Toddlers' concept of body image, particularly the definition of body boundaries, is very poorly developed. Intrusive experiences, such as examining the ears or mouth or taking a rectal temperature, are very anxiety producing. Toddlers may react to such painless procedures as intensely as they do to painful ones.

Toddlers' reactions to pain are similar to those seen during infancy, except that the combination of variables influencing the individual response is highly complex. Memory of previous experiences, physical restraint, separation from parents, emotional reactions of others, and lack of preparation partially determine the intensity of the behavioral response. In general children in this age-group continue to react with intense emotional upset and physical resistance to any actual or perceived painful experience. Unlike adults who usually decrease their activity when in pain, young children typically become restless and overly active; frequently this response is not recognized as a consequence of pain.

By the end of this age period, toddlers usually are able to communicate about their pain. Although they have not developed the ability to describe the type or intensity of the pain, they usually are able to localize it by pointing to a specific area.

Preschoolers

Concepts of illness begin during the preschool period and are influenced by the cognitive abilities of the preoperational stage. Preschoolers differentiate poorly between themselves and the external world. Their thinking is focused on externally perceived events, and causality is based on the proximity of two events. Consequently, a child defines illness according to when he is told he is sick or is given external evidence of illness, such as, "You are sick because you have a fever." The cause of illness is seen as a concrete action the child does or fails to do and often implies a degree of responsibility and self-blame. Another explanation may be based on contagion, that the proximity of two objects or persons causes the illness.

The psychosexual conflicts of children in this age-group make them very vulnerable to threats of bodily injury. Intrusive procedures, whether painful or painless, are threatening to preschoolers, whose concept of body integrity is still poorly developed. It is not uncommon for preschoolers to react to an injection with as much concern for withdrawal of the needle as for the actual pain. They fear that the intrusion or puncture will not close and that their "insides" will leak out.

Concerns of mutilation are paramount during this age period. Loss of any body part is threatening, but preschool boys' fears of castration complicate their understanding of surgical or medical procedures associated with the genital area, such as circumcision, repair of hypospadias or epispadias, cystoscopy, or catheterization. Their limited comprehension of body functioning also increases their difficulty in understanding how or why body parts are "fixed." For example, telling preschoolers that their tonsils are to be removed may be interpreted as "taking out their voice," or having the penis "fixed" may be understood as cutting it off. Words such as "dye," "cut off," "take out," or "draw" (e.g., "draw some blood") are interpreted literally and can lead to confusion and fear.

Reactions to pain tend to be similar to those seen during toddlerhood although some differences become apparent. For example, preschoolers respond more favorably to preparatory interventions, such as explanation and distraction, than younger children. Physical and verbal aggression are more specific and goal directed. Instead of showing total body resistance, preschoolers may push the offending person away, try to secure the equipment, or attempt to lock themselves in a safe place. Much more thought is evident in their plan of attack or escape.

Verbal expression in particular demonstrates their advanced development in response to stress. They may verbally abuse the attacker by stating, "Get out of here" or "I hate you." They may also use the more cunning approach of trying to persuade the person to give up the intended activity. A common plea is, "Please don't give me a shot; I'll be good." Some statements are not only attempts to avoid the event but also evidence of children's perceptions about the experience.

Attempts to secure comforting may also be evident and may be expressed through behaviors such as clinging to a parent, wanting to be held, or refusing to be left alone. A common expression denoting the need for dependency is, "Help me." It is important to recognize such requests as the need for support from others during a time of stress. Admonishing children to act grown-up or encouraging them to do things by stating, "I know you can do it yourself," deprives them of the support they are requesting and increases their own feelings of guilt and shame.

School-Age Children

Fears of the physical nature of the illness surface at this time. There may be less concern with actual pain than there is for disability, uncertain recovery, or possible death. Girls tend to express more and stronger fears than boys, and previous hospitalizations may have no effect on the frequency or intensity of these fears (Aho and Erickson, 1985). Because of their developing cognitive abilities, school-age children are aware of the significance of different illnesses, the indispensability of certain body parts, potential hazards in treatments, lifelong consequences of permanent injury or loss of function, and the meaning of death. A paramount concern of hospitalized school-age children is their fear of not being well again.

The school-age child defines illness by a set of multiple, concrete symptoms, such as signs of a cold, and sees the cause as primarily germs or bacteria. The germs have a powerful, almost magical quality, so that in the child's mind, illness can be prevented by avoiding people with the germs. Also, the school-age child's idea of contamination is similar to that of the younger age-group; for example, the illness occurs because of physical contact or because the child engaged in a harmful action and became contaminated. Consequently, feelings of self-blame and guilt may be associated with the reason for becoming ill.

School-age children begin to show concern for the potential beneficial and hazardous effects of procedures. Besides wanting to know if a procedure will hurt, they want to know what it is for, how it will make them better, and what injury or harm could result. For example, these children fear the actual procedure of anesthesia. Unlike preschoolers, who fear the mask and the strange surroundings, school-age children fear what may happen while they are asleep. They wonder if they will wake up and if they might die. Preadolescents also worry about the operation itself, particularly one that will result in visible changes in body image.

Intrusive procedures of a nonsexual nature, such as routine physical examination of the ears, nose, mouth, and throat, are generally well tolerated. However, concerns for privacy become evident and increasingly significant. Although school-age children may be cooperative during examination of the genitals or during procedures performed in that area, such situations are usually very stressful for them, especially for preadolescents who are beginning pubertal changes.

Young school-age children react to painful procedures with many of the same behaviors exhibited by younger children, although the school-age child tends to be able to maintain control up to, but not including, the actual infliction of pain. By the age of 9 or 10, most school-age children show less fright or overt resistance to pain than younger children. They generally have learned passive methods of dealing with discomfort, such as holding rigidly still, clenching their fists or teeth, or trying to act brave by the "grin-and-bear-it" routine.

School-age children verbally communicate about their pain in respect to its location, intensity, and description. Unlike younger children, who have difficulty choosing words to describe pain, children 9 years or older use a wide variety of words and phrases, such as throbbing, piercing, bad, terrible, awful, or "like a torture treatment" (Savedra and others, 1982).

School-age children also use words as a means of controlling their reactions to pain. For example, these children may ask the nurse to talk to them during a procedure. Some prefer to participate in a procedure, whereas others choose to distance themselves by not looking at what is happening. Most appreciate an explanation of the procedure and seem less fearful when they know what to expect. Others try to gain control through stalling techniques, such as, "Give me the shot when I am finished with this." Although the ability to make decisions does increase the procrastinator's sense of control, unlimited procrastination results in heightened anxiety. When choices are allowed, such as selection of the injection site, it is best to structure the number of possible sites and to limit the number of "procrastination" techniques.

Similar to school-age children's more passive acceptance of pain is their indirect way of asking for support or help. School-age children will rarely initiate a conversation about their feelings or ask someone to stay with them during a lonely or stressful period. In fact, their visible composure, calmness, and acceptance often belie their inner longing for support. It is especially important to be aware of nonverbal clues, such as a serious facial expression, a halfhearted reply of "I am fine," silence, lack of activity, or social isolation, as signs of the need for help. Usually when someone identifies the unspoken messages and offers support, school-age children readily accept it.

Adolescents

Although the development of body image begins at birth, its relevance is paramount during adolescence. Injury, pain, disability, and death are viewed primarily in terms of how each affects the adolescent's view of himself in the present. Any change that differentiates adolescents from their peers is regarded as a major tragedy. For example, diseases such as diabetes mellitus often present a more difficult adjustment period for children in this age-group than for younger children because of the necessary changes in the adolescent's life-style. Conversely, serious, even life-threatening illnesses that entail no visible body changes or physical restrictions may have less immediate significance for the adolescent. Therefore the nature of bodily injury may be more important in terms of the adolescent's perception of the illness than the disorder's actual degree of severity.

Adolescents' rapidly changing body image during pubertal development often makes them feel insecure about their bodies. Illness, medical or surgical intervention, and hospitalization increase their existing concerns for normalcy. They may respond to such events by asking numerous questions, withdrawing, rejecting others, or questioning the adequacy of care. Frequently their fear of loss of control and body image change is demonstrated as overconfidence, conceit, or a "know-it-all" attitude.

Because of sexual changes, adolescents are very concerned about privacy. Lack of respect for this need can cause greater stress than physical pain. In addition, adolescents look for signs that indicate that they are developing normally and according to acceptable standards. When illness occurs, they fear that growth may be retarded, leaving them behind their peers. Although they may not voice this concern, they may demonstrate it by carefully observing others' reactions to them during physical examinations or procedures.

Adolescents react to pain with much self-control. Physical resistance and aggression are unusual at this age, unless the adolescent is totally unprepared for a procedure. Like older school-age children, adolescents are very concerned with remaining composed and feel embarrassed and ashamed if they lose control. They are able to describe their pain experience and to use any of the pain assessment tools developed for adults. However, they may be reluctant to disclose their pain unless the nurse is willing to listen closely and observe physical indications, such as limited movement, excessive quiet, or irritability.

EFFECTS OF HOSPITALIZATION ON THE CHILD

Admission is not the only time when children react to the stresses of illness and hospitalization; many children demonstrate temporary behavioral changes following discharge, especially children under 4 years of age (see box). These changes are a result of (1) separation from significant people, (2) a lack of opportunity to form new attachments, and (3) a strange environment. In addition, the development of subsequent long-term emotional disturbance may be related to the *length* and *number* of hospital admissions and the type of hospital practices. A single hospitalization of 4 weeks or more and repeated hospital admissions have been associated with later disturbances. However, supportive practices, such as frequent family visiting, may lessen the detrimental effects of such admissions.

While hospitalization can be and usually is stressful for children, it can also be beneficial. The most obvious benefit is the recovery from illness, but hospitalization also can present an opportunity for children to master stress and feel competent in their coping abilities. The hospital environment can provide children with new socialization experiences that can broaden their interpersonal relationships. The psychologic benefits need to be considered and maximized during any hospitalization. Appropriate nursing strategies to achieve this goal are presented on p. 601.

Posthospital Behaviors in Children

Young Children

Some initial aloofness toward parents; may last from a few minutes (most common) to a few days
Frequently followed by dependency behaviors:
- Tendency to cling to parents
- Demand parents' attention
- Vigorously oppose any separation, e.g., staying at nursery school or with a baby-sitter

Other negative behaviors include:
- New fears, e.g., nightmares
- Resistance to going to bed, night waking
- Withdrawal and shyness
- Hyperactivity
- Temper tantrums
- Food finickiness
- Attachment to blanket or toy
- Regression in newly learned skills, e.g., self-toileting

Older Children

Negative behaviors include:
- Emotional coldness, followed by intense, demanding dependence on parents
- Anger toward parents
- Jealousy toward others, i.e., siblings

NURSING CARE OF THE HOSPITALIZED CHILD

Children require competent and sensitive care to minimize the potential negative effects of hospitalization and also to promote positive effects from the experience. From the initial preparation for the hospital admission to planning for discharge, nursing care should be based on an understanding of the child's developmental and physical needs.

ASSESSMENT

A number of important areas must be assessed to identify nursing diagnosis and plan care for an individual child. In some instances, such as elective admission, assessment begins even before the child is hospitalized so that appropriate preadmission preparation can be instituted. At other times assessment occurs at the time of admission and should be integrated into other admission procedures so that the child's specific needs are recognized *early* in the hospitalization. Another critical area is assessment of pain for implementing appropriate relief of discomfort. While assessment is discussed under nursing care of the hospitalized child, a comprehensive approach must involve the child's parents or other caregivers.

Admission Assessment

Whenever a child is admitted to a hospital, a nursing admission history should be taken. The nursing admission history refers to a systematic collection of data about the child and family that allows the nurse to plan individualized care. The nursing admission history presented in the box is organized according to the Functional Health Patterns outlined by Gordon (1987) (see p. 19) to facilitate the formulation of nursing diagnoses.

One of the main purposes of the history is to assess the child's usual health habits at home to promote a more normal environment in the hospital. Therefore questions related to activities of daily living in the nutritional-metabolic, elimination, sleep-rest, and activity-exercise patterns are a major part of the assessment.

The questions found under the health-perception–health-management pattern are directed toward evaluation of the child's preparation for hospitalization and are key factors in determining if additional preparation is needed. The questions included in the self-perception–self-concept and role-relationship patterns offer insight into the child's potential reaction to hospitalization, especially in terms of separation.

Once the data is collected, it must be applied to the nursing process and communicated to other staff. It makes little sense to assess a child's home routine if none of this knowledge is integrated into the plan of care. Most nursing units have provisions for care plans in which specific information about the child's habits and needs are recorded and incorporated in the hospital routine.

Besides taking the nursing admission history, nurses should also perform a physical assessment (see Chapter 7) or obtain the information from the medical examination before planning care. At the very least the nurse's physical assessment of the child should include observation of the body for any bruises, rash, signs of neglect, deformities, or physical limitations. The nurse should also listen to the heart and lungs to assess overall physical status. For example, it is impossible to evaluate improvement in respiratory function in a child admitted with pulmonary disease unless there is baseline data with which to compare subsequent findings.

Pain Assessment

Pain assessment is a critical component of the nursing process. Unfortunately, health professionals, including nurses, tend to underestimate the existence of pain in children. Several studies have documented the enormous disparity between medication practices with children and adults. For example, one study found that hospitalized adults received almost 30 times more doses of analgesics than a matched group of children. One of the most disturbing finding was that more than twice as many children had pain medication ordered as received it (Eland and Anderson, 1977). This lack of response to the need for pain medication directly relates to the nurses who failed to administer the analgesic.

TABLE 20-2

Myths about Children and Pain

Myth	Facts
Infants do not feel pain	Infants demonstrate behavioral, physiologic, and hormonal indicators of pain (Johnston and Strada, 1986; Anand, Sippell, and Aynsley-Green, 1987)
Children tolerate pain better than adults	Children's tolerance to pain actually *increases* with age (Haslam, 1969)
Children cannot tell where they hurt	Children beyond infancy can accurately point to the body area or mark the site on a drawing (Eland and Anderson, 1977)
Children always tell the truth about pain	Children may not admit feeling pain to avoid an injection; because of constant pain they may not realize how much they are hurting (Eland, 1985)
Children become accustomed to pain or painful procedures	Children do not demonstrate decreased behavioral signs of discomfort with repeated painful procedures (Katz, Kellerman, and Siegel, 1980)
Active children are not in pain	Increased activity is frequently a sign of pain (Eland, 1985), although children with more severe pain may be less active (Hester, 1979)
Narcotics are dangerous drugs for children and cause addiction	Narcotics are no more dangerous for children than adults; addiction is extremely rare (Porter and Jick, 1980)

One of the reasons for inadequate management of pain is a lack of understanding of what pain is—a personal phenomenon that *cannot* be experienced by any other individual. Therefore defining what pain is in terms of another's perceptions is inappropriate and inaccurate. McCaffery (1979) offers an operational definition that is useful in clinical practice: *pain is whatever the experiencing person says it is, existing whenever he says it does.* This definition implies a very important attitude toward the patient—*that he is believed.* It is meant to encompass both verbal and nonverbal expressions of pain. Pain in children also is misunderstood because numerous myths erroneously influence nurses' assessment and management of pain (Table 20-2).

A comprehensive assessment of pain must include a variety of factors. One approach to assessment is QUEST, a process that consists of five components (Baker and Wong, 1987):

Question the child
Use pain rating scales
Evaluate behavior
Secure parents' involvement
Take action

*Nursing Admission History According to Functional Health Patterns**

HEALTH-PERCEPTION–HEALTH-MANAGEMENT PATTERN

1. Why has your child been admitted?
2. How has your child's general health been?
3. What does your child know about this hospitalization?
   a. Ask the child why he came to the hospital.
   b. If answer is "For an operation or for tests," ask the child to tell you about what will happen before, during, and after the operation or tests.
4. Has your child ever been in the hospital before?
   a. How was that hospital experience?
   b. What things were important to you and your child during that hospitalization? How can we be most helpful now?
5. What medications does your child take at home?
   a. Why are they given?
   b. When are they given?
   c. How are they given (if a liquid, with a spoon; if a tablet, swallowed with water, or other)?
   d. Does your child have any trouble taking medication? If so, what helps?
   e. Is your child allergic to any medications?

NUTRITIONAL-METABOLIC PATTERN

1. What are the family's usual mealtimes?
2. Do family members eat together or at separate times?
3. What are your child's favorite foods, beverages, and snacks?
   a. Average amounts consumed or usual size portions
   b. Special cultural practices, such as family eats only ethnic food
4. What foods and beverages does your child dislike?
5. What are your child's feeding habits (bottle, cup, spoon, eats by self, needs assistance, any special devices)?
6. How does he like his food served (warmed, cold, one item at a time)?
7. How would you describe your child's usual appetite (hearty eater, picky eater)?
   a. Has being sick affected your child's appetite?
8. Are there any known or suspected food allergies; is your child on a special diet?
9. Are there any feeding problems (excessive fussiness, spitting up, colic); any dental or gum problems that affect feeding?
10. What do you do for these problems?

ELIMINATION PATTERN

1. What are your child's toilet habits (diaper, toilet trained—day only or day and night, use of word to communicate urination or defecation, potty chair, regular toilet, other routines)?
2. What is your child's usual pattern of elimination (bowel movements)?
3. Do you have any concerns about elimination (bed-wetting, constipation, diarrhea)?
4. What do you do for these problems?
5. Have you ever noticed that your child sweats a lot?

SLEEP-REST PATTERN

1. What is your child's usual hour of sleep and awakening?
2. What is your child's schedule for naps; length of naps?
3. Is there a special routine before sleeping (bottle, drink of water, bedtime story, nightlight, favorite blanket or toy, prayers)?
4. Is there a special routine during sleep time, such as waking to go to the bathroom?
5. What type of bed does your child sleep in?
6. Does your child have his own room or share a room; if shares, with whom?
7. What are the home sleeping arrangements (alone or with others, such as sibling, parent, or other person)?
8. What is your child's favorite sleeping position?
9. Are there any sleeping problems (falling asleep, waking during night, nightmares, sleep walking)?
10. Are there any problems awakening and getting ready in the morning?
11. What do you do for these problems?

ACTIVITY-EXERCISE PATTERN

1. What is your child's schedule during the day (nursery school, daycare center, regular school, extracurricular activities)?
2. What are your child's favorite activities or toys (both active and quiet interests)?
3. What is your child's usual television viewing schedule at home?
   a. What are your child's favorite programs?
   b. Are there any TV restrictions?
4. Does your child have any illness or disabilities that limit activity? If so, how?
5. What are your child's usual habits and schedule for bathing (bath in tub or shower, sponge bath, shampoo)?
6. What are your child's dental habits (brushing, flossing, fluoride supplements or rinses, favorite toothpaste); schedule of daily dental care?
7. Does your child need help with dressing or grooming, such as hair combing?
8. Are there any problems with the above (dislike of or refusal to bathe, shampoo hair, or brush teeth)?
9. What do you do for these problems?
10. Are there special devices that your child requires help in managing (eyeglasses, contact lenses, hearing aid, orthodontic appliances, artificial elimination appliances, orthopedic devices)?

NOTE: Use the following code to assess functional self-care level for feeding, bathing/hygiene, dressing/grooming, toileting:

- **O:** Full self-care
- **I:** Requires use of equipment or device
- **II:** Requires assistance or supervision from another person
- **III:** Requires assistance or supervision from another person and equipment or device
- **IV:** Is dependent and does not participate

*The focus of the admission history is the child's psychosocial environment. For an assessment of physical aspects, see Chapter 7. Most of the questions are worded in terms of parental responses. Depending on the child's age, they should be addressed directly to the child when appropriate.

Nursing Admission History According to Functional Health Patterns—cont'd

COGNITIVE-PERCEPTUAL PATTERN

1. Does your child have any hearing difficulty?
   a. Does the child use a hearing aid?
   b. Have "tubes" been placed in your child's ears?
2. Does your child have any vision problems?
   a. Does the child wear glasses or contact lenses?
3. Does your child have any learning difficulties?
   a. What is the child's grade in school?
4. For information on pain, see Table 20-3.

SELF-PERCEPTION–SELF-CONCEPT PATTERN

1. How would you describe your child (e.g., takes time to adjust, settles in easily, shy, friendly, quiet, talkative, serious, playful, stubborn, easygoing)?
2. What kinds of things make your child angry, annoyed, anxious, or sad? What helps?
3. How does your child act when annoyed or upset?
4. What have been your child's experiences with and reactions to temporary separation from you (parent)?
5. Does your child have any fears (places, objects, animals, people, situations)? How do you handle them?
6. Do you think your child's illness has changed the way he thinks about himself (e.g., more shy, embarrassed about appearance, less competitive with friends, stays at home more)?

ROLE-RELATIONSHIP PATTERN

1. Does your child have a favorite nickname?
2. What are the names of other family members or others who live in the home (relatives, friends, pets)?
3. Who usually takes care of your child during the day/night (especially if other than parent, such as baby-sitter, relative)?
4. What are the parents' occupations and work schedules?
5. Are there any special family considerations (adoption, foster child, stepparent, divorce, single parent)?
6. Have any major changes in the family occurred lately (death, divorce, separation, birth of a sibling, loss of a job, financial strain, mother beginning a career, other)? Describe child's reaction.
7. Who are your child's play companions or social group (peers, younger or older children, adults, prefers to be alone)?
8. Do things generally go well for your child in school or with friends?
9. Does your child have "security" objects at home (pacifier, thumb, bottle, blanket, stuffed animal or doll)? Did you bring any of these to the hospital?
10. How do you handle discipline problems at home? Are these methods always effective?
11. Does your child have any speech or hearing problems? If so, what are your suggestions for communicating with him?
12. Will your child's hospitalization affect the family's financial support or care of other family members, such as other children?
13. What concerns do you have about your child's illness and hospitalization?
14. Who will be staying with your child while he is in the hospital?
15. How can we contact you or another close family member outside of the hospital?

SEXUALITY-REPRODUCTIVE PATTERN

(Answer questions that apply to your child's age-group.)

1. Has your child begun puberty (developing physical sexual characteristics, menstruation)? Have you or your child had any concerns?
2. Does your daughter know how to do breast self-examination?
3. Does your son know how to do testicular self-examination?
4. How have you approached topics of sexuality with your child? Do you feel you might need some help with some topics?
5. Has your child's illness affected the way he or she feels about being a boy or a girl? If so, how?
6. Do you have any concerns with behaviors in your child, such as masturbation, asking many questions or talking about sex, not respecting others' privacy or wanting too much privacy?
7. Initiate a conversation about adolescent's sexual concerns with open-ended to more direct questions and using the terms "friends" or "partners" rather than "girlfriend" or "boyfriend":
   a. Tell me about your social life.
   b. Who are your closest friends? (If one friend is identified, could ask more about that relationship, such as how much time they spend together, how serious they are about each other, if the relationship is going the way the teenager hoped it would)
   c. Might ask about dating and sexual issues, such as the teenager's views on sex education, "going steady," "living together," or premarital sex.
   d. Which friends would you like to have visit in the hospital?

COPING-STRESS TOLERANCE PATTERN

(Answer questions that apply to your child's age-group.)

1. What does your child do when tired or upset?
   a. If upset, does your child want a special person or object? If so, explain.
2. If your child has temper tantrums, what causes them and how do you handle them?
3. Whom does your child talk to when worried about something?
4. How does your child usually handle problems or disappointments?
5. Have there been any big changes or problems in your family recently? How did you handle them?
6. Has your child ever had a problem with drugs or alcohol or tried suicide?
7. Do you think your child is "accident prone?" If so, explain.

VALUE-BELIEF PATTERN

1. What is your religion?
2. How is religion or faith important in your child's life?
3. What religious practices would you like continued in the hospital, such as prayers before meals/bedtime; visit by minister, priest, or rabbi, prayer group?

TABLE 20-3

Pain Experience Inventory

Questions for Parents	Questions for Child
Describe any pain your child has had before. How does your child usually react to pain? Does your child tell you or others when he is hurting? How do you know when your child is in pain? What do you do for your child when he is hurting? What does your child do for himself when he is hurting? Which of these actions work best to decrease or take away your child's pain? Is there anything special that you would like me to know about your child and pain? (If yes, have parent[s] describe.)	Tell me what pain is. Tell me about the hurt you have had before. What do you do when you hurt? Do you tell others when you hurt? What do you want others to do for you when you hurt? What don't you want others to do for you when you hurt? What helps the most to take away your hurt? Is there anything special that you want me to know about you when you hurt? (If yes, have child describe.)

From Hester, N., and Barcus, C.: Assessment and management of pain in children. In Pediatrics: nursing update **1**(14):3, Princeton, NJ, 1986, Continuing Professional Education Center, Inc.

Question the child. Children can be excellent sources of information about pain and a pain history can be invaluable in providing basic information about the child's understanding and previous response to pain (Table 20-3). Although verbal indications are much less common in children than in adults, children can describe pain if asked appropriate questions. Children, even those up to preadolescence, do not necessarily understand the meaning of terms like "pain" and "discomfort" and have very limited use of descriptive words, such as "burning," "cramping," "severe," or "excruciating." Children may globally describe pain as, "I hurt," or "I don't feel good." Using a variety of words that may be associated with pain, such as "owie," "funny," "booboo," "hot," "pushing," or "banging," may help children describe the sensation. Asking children to locate the pain is also helpful and play can provide other means for helping children to reveal discomfort (see Nursing tip).

Nursing Tip: Helping Children Locate Pain

- Ask child to point to where it hurts or to "where mommy would put a Band-Aid."
- Have child mark or color the painful area on a drawing of a human figure (see Fig. 21-1, p. 627).
- Ask child to tell how a puppet, doll, or stuffed animal is feeling or to point out areas on these models that "hurt" or "don't feel good."

Several factors may influence children's truthfulness about pain. For example, some children may see pain as a punishment for wrongdoing and may believe that they deserve to suffer. Others may fear that admitting they hurt will result in a "shot"—a second pain. To minimize these fears nurses should clarify that the child did nothing wrong to deserve to suffer and that the brief discomfort of an injection will take away the more severe, continuous pain (see also discussion of pain management on p. 598).

Children often may not tell strangers how they feel but will confide in their parents, who are safe and trusted persons. It is not unusual for a child who has been quiet to start crying when the parents visit and to complain, "I hurt." Nurses sometimes erroneously judge this behavior as seeking attention, when it represents the child's true feelings. The best intervention is to talk with the parent and child and to *believe* that the child hurts.

Use pain rating scales. Several pain rating scales have been developed that provide a quantitative, subjective measurement of a person's pain. Most of the scales were designed for use with adults, but some have been constructed for and tested with children as young as 3 years of age. Scales that are available and appropriate for children of different ages are presented in Table 20-4. If the pain rating scales are to be used effectively, they should be explained to the child *before* they are needed, such as during the admission process or preoperative teaching.

Pain rating scales also are useful after the initial assessment of pain. They should be used to continually evaluate the effectiveness of pain management. A pain assessment record provides documentation of pain relief at regular intervals and can be instrumental in persuading other health professionals of the child's need for analgesics (Fig. 20-5).

Evaluate behavior. A valuable tool in assessing pain is observing behavioral changes and physiologic responses. *Behavioral changes* are common indicators of pain in children, particularly in preverbal youngsters and those with mental retardation or sensory/communication deficits. Such changes include irritability, lethargy, loss of appetite, unusual quietness, disturbed sleep patterns, voluntary resting, increased restless movement or rigid posturing, flat affect, or anger. Specific reactions often indicate discomfort in localized body regions—such as rolling the head from side to side or pulling the ears for an earache, lying on the side with legs flexed on the abdomen for abdominal pain, or favoring a body part during usual activity. However, behavioral manifestations of pain vary

TABLE 20-4

Pain Rating Scales for Children

Pain Scale	Description	Comments
Faces scale*	Consists of series of drawn faces ranging from very happy, smiling face for "no pain" to sad, tearful face for "worst pain." Child chooses face that most nearly describes his pain (Fig. 20-4)	Can be used with children as young as 3 years
Color scale	Uses crayons in various colors; child creates own scale by choosing color that is like "worst or most hurt," then another color that is like "little less pain," until last color represents "no hurt." Child chooses color that most nearly describes his pain (Eland, 1985)	Recommended for children as young as 4 years provided children know their colors and are not color blind
Chips scale	Uses plastic chips that are compared to pieces of hurt: one chip is "little hurt" and all chips are "most hurt," with other chips representing intermediate amounts of hurt. Child chooses number of chips that most nearly describes his pain (Hester, 1979)	Recommended for children as young as 4 years although children who cannot count may have difficulty with the concept
Glasses scale	Consists of drawing of six cylinders or "glasses," five of which are filled with increasing amounts of "pain." First glass is empty and represents "no pain." Completely filled glass is for "worst pain." Glasses in between have from very little to a whole lot of pain. Child chooses glass that best describes his pain	Can be used with children as young as 3 years
Numeric scale	Uses a straight line with end points identified as "no pain" and "worst pain" and divisions along the line marked in units from 0 to 10 (high number may vary). Child chooses number that best describes his pain	May be appropriate for children as young as 5 years although children who cannot count may have difficulty with the concept
Simple descriptive scale	Uses descriptive words (no pain, mild, moderate, quite a lot, very bad, and worst pain) to denote varying intensities of pain. Child chooses word that most nearly describes his pain	May be appropriate for children as young as 5 years although words may need explanation
Oucher scale	Consists of six photographs of a child's face representing "no hurt" to "biggest hurt you could ever have." Child chooses face that most nearly describes his pain. Also consists of vertical numeric scale with numbers from 0 to 100. Child chooses number that best describes his pain (Beyer, 1984)	Recommended for children approximately 3 to 15 years; if children can count to 100, they can use numerical scale; otherwise they should use photographic scale

*Scales (with exception of Oucher) are listed in order of children's preference for using them (Wong and Baker, 1988).

FIG. 20-4 Faces pain rating scale.

Date	Time[1]	Drug administered	Reason for drug administration[2]	Pain rating[3]	Respirations	Signature

[1]Record time of administering drug and assess analgesic effect 30 minutes later and then hourly.
[2]State reason in behavioral terms.
[3]Use pain rating scale.

FIG. 20-5 Pain assessment record.

widely, and some children with more severe pain may show fewer facial and body movements than those with less pain (Hester, 1979).

The child's response to medication is another valuable indicator of pain. For example, in preverbal children, who communicate a wide variety of emotions through behavior, obvious change in behavior following administration of an analgesic is evidence that the child was in pain. This knowledge can help in determining the cause of behaviors suggestive of pain, such as crying or restlessness. If after administering one dose of an analgesic the child's behavior improves, it is likely that the cause was pain, which requires further relief.

Recognition of the existence of pain and evaluation of its severity are facilitated by an understanding of the developmental response to pain of children in each age-group (see box on p. 583), as well as the influence of factors such as cultural or ethnic background. While studies of cultural components of pain demonstrate some differences in children's descriptions of pain and comfort measures, the differences are slight and should not be overemphasized (Abu-Saad, 1984). Individual differences related to temperament also play a role in children's responses to pain. Some children may cry loudly following a procedure, whereas others are easily calmed by a gentle hug. It is important to recognize and respect such signs of individuality and to realize that children who react less intensely may still be experiencing significant discomfort (Chess and Thomas, 1985).

Physiologic responses indicating pain include flushing of the skin; increases in sweating, blood pressure, pulse, and respiration; restlessness; and dilation of the pupils. However, these signs vary considerably—for example, heart rate may actually decrease (Dale, 1986)—and they may be produced by emotions, such as fear, anger, or anxiety. They occur primarily in acute pain from stimulation of the sympathetic nervous system. If pain persists, the body begins to adapt and there is a decrease or stabilization of these responses. Consequently, if nurses rely primarily on observing these physiologic indications before believing that pain exists, many instances of pain will go unrecognized.

Secure parents' involvement. Parents know their child and are sensitive to changes in behavior. However, there is no documentation of exactly how astute parents are in recognizing pain in their children. Some parents may never have seen their child in severe pain. However, others are aware that certain behaviors signal pain because the child has acted similarly during previous painful events. To better assess the child's pain, the nurse can interview the parents about their child's previous pain experiences (see Table 20-3). Ideally this questioning should occur before the child is in pain, such as on admission to the hospital. Parents need to know that their knowledge of their child is important in providing care. Parents sometimes tend to leave the assessment of pain up to the nurse because "nurses are more experienced." While this may be true, the best care is provided with joint assessment and planning.

Take action. The reason for assessing pain is to relieve it. Consequently, nurses must be knowledgeable about pain reduction strategies and implement them as appropriate. Pain management is discussed on p. 597.

NURSING DIAGNOSES

A number of nursing diagnoses are prominent in the nursing care of the ill and/or hospitalized children. Other nursing diagnoses specific to individual cases may become evident in addition to those outlined in the Nursing Care Plan on pp. 603-605.

PLANNING

The main nursing goals for the ill and/or hospitalized child are:

1. Prepare the child for hospitalization
2. Prevent or minimize separation
3. Minimize loss of control
4. Prevent or minimize bodily injury and pain
5. Use play to minimize stress
6. Maximize potential benefits of hospitalization

IMPLEMENTATION

Implementing the plan of care may begin even before the child is hospitalized, such as during a preadmission visit. While the goal is to prevent predictable stresses during hospitalization, often prevention is not possible and the objective becomes one of minimizing stress and helping the child cope with the experience.

Prepare Child for Hospitalization

The rationale for preparing children for the hospital experience and related procedures is based on the principle that fear of the unknown (fantasy) exceeds fear of the known. Therefore decreasing the elements of the unknown results in less fear. When children do not have paralyzing fear to cope with, they are able to direct their energies toward dealing with the other unavoidable stresses of hospitalization and to benefit optimally from the growth potential of the experience.

Children may be prepared before or the day of admission. The preparation process may be elaborate, with tours, puppet shows, and playtime with miniature hospital equipment; it may involve the use of books (see p. 620 and/or films; or it may be limited to a brief description of the major aspects of any hospital stay. Regardless of the specific type of program, all children, even those who have been hospitalized before, benefit from an introduction to the environment and routine of the unit.

Hospital admission. The preparation that children require on the day of admission depends on the kind of prehospital counseling they have received. If they have been prepared in a formalized program, they will usually know what to expect in terms of initial medical procedures, inpatient facilities, and nursing staff. However, prehospital

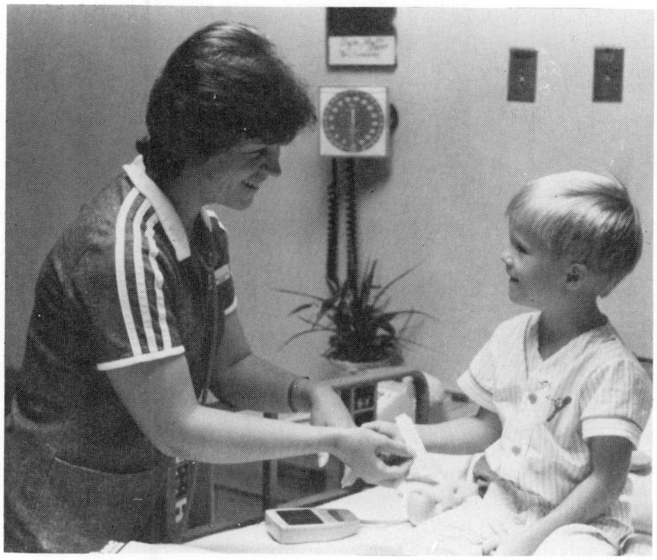

FIG. 20-6 The initial admission procedures give the nurse an opportunity to get to know the child and to assess the child's understanding of the hospital experience.

Guidelines for Admission

Preadmission

Assign a room based on developmental age, seriousness of diagnosis, communicability of illness, and projected length of stay

Prepare roommate(s) for the arrival of a new patient; when children are too young to benefit from this consideration, prepare parents

Prepare room for child and family, with admission forms and equipment nearby to eliminate need to leave child

Admission

Introduce primary nurse to child and family

Orient child and family to inpatient facilities, especially to assigned room and unit; emphasize positive areas of pediatric unit

- Room: explain call light, bed controls, television, etc.; direct to bathroom, telephone, etc.
- Unit: Direct to playroom, desk, dining area, or other areas

Introduce family to roommate and his or her parents

Apply identification band to child's wrist, ankle, or both (if not done)

Explain hospital regulations and schedules (e.g., visiting hours, mealtimes, bedtime, limitations [give written information if available])

Perform nursing history

Take vital signs, blood pressure, height, and weight

Obtain specimens as needed and order needed laboratory work

Support child and assist physician with physical examination (for purposes of nursing assessment)

counseling does not preclude the need for support during procedures such as obtaining blood specimens, x-ray tests, or physical examination. For example, undressing young children before they feel comfortable in their new surroundings can be very upsetting. Causing needless anxiety and fear during admission may adversely affect the nurse's establishment of trust with these children. Therefore nursing assistance during the admission procedure is vital, regardless of how well prepared any child is for the experience of hospitalization. In addition, spending this time with the child gives the nurse an opportunity to evaluate the child's understanding of subsequent procedures (Fig. 20-6). Ideally a primary nurse is assigned whenever possible to allow for individualized care and to provide a substitute support person for the child.

When a child is admitted, nurses follow several fairly universal admission procedures, which are outlined in the box. One particularly important decision is room assignment. The minimum considerations for room assignment are age, sex, and nature of the illness. Ideally, however, room selection should be based on a variety of developmental and psychobiologic needs. Determining compatible roommates, both for the children and for rooming-in parents, greatly influences the growth potential from the hospital experience.

No absolute rules govern room selection, but in general, placing children of the same age-group and with similar types of illness in the same room is both psychologically and medically advantageous. However, there are many exceptions. For example, a school-age child may thrive on the responsibility of caring for a younger child. A child in traction may be very therapeutic for another child confined to bed because of a serious illness. A child who is very independent despite physical disabilities may help another child with similar or different limitations and the parents of the child with disabilities may achieve deeper insight and acceptance of their child's disorder.

Prevent or Minimize Separation

The primary nursing goal is to prevent separation, particularly in children under 5 years of age. Unrestricted visiting hours and facilities such as a chair or bed for at least one person per child provide a welcoming atmosphere for parents. However, not all hospitals provide such an invitation, and parents' own schedules may prevent rooming-in. In such instances, strategies to minimize the effects of separation must be implemented.

Ideally a primary nurse is assigned to meet the child's needs. Becoming a surrogate parent requires a thorough, detailed nursing history (see p. 588) that specifically identifies the child's established daily routine. Usual daily activities such as food preparation and method of feeding help establish a complementary schedule of caregiving practices. Incorporating these normal activities also helps the parents feel that they are participating in the child's care, even if through another person.

The nurse caring for the child must have an appreciation of the child's separation behaviors. As discussed earlier, the phases of protest and despair are normal. The child is allowed to cry. Even if he rejects strangers, the nurse provides support through physical presence in the room. Saying to the child, "I know you are unhappy because you miss your mommy and daddy. It's all right to cry. I will sit here for a while so you are not alone," reinforces for the child that the nurse is aware of his feelings and will not abandon him. If behaviors of detachment are evident, the child's contact with the parents is maintained by frequently talking about them, encouraging the child to remember them, and stressing the significance of their visits, telephone calls, or letters.

Separation may be equally as difficult for parents, especially when they do not understand the behaviors of separation anxiety. To avoid the immediate protest, parents may sneak out or lie to the child about leaving. As a result, the child learns not that absence is associated with a guaranteed return, but that absence means loss of parents. Helping parents recognize that separation behaviors are normal and expected can decrease the parents' anxiety and may ease their fears about leaving the child without telling him. Explaining to parents how the child reacts after they leave may also be helpful. Many parents imagine that the child cries for hours after they leave, whereas in reality the child may cry for a few minutes but settle down when comforted by someone else.

Toddlers and preschoolers have a very limited concept of time. The young child's question, "Will my mommy come yesterday?" symbolizes a lack of understanding for usual measurements of time, such as days, hours, and weeks. Time is measured in associations, such as eating dinner "when daddy comes home." Therefore, when helping parents with their fears of separation, nurses need to suggest ways of explaining leaving and returning. For example, if parents must leave to go to work or to make meals for the other family members, they should tell the hospitalized child the reason for leaving. They also need to convey the expected time of return in terms of anticipated events. For example, if the parents will return in the morning, they can say to the child, "We'll see you after the sun comes up" or "We'll come back when (a favorite program) is on television."

The young child's ability to tolerate parental absence is very limited. Therefore parental visits should be frequent. For example, it is better for parents to visit three times a day for short periods than once a day for an extended time. This may necessitate that each parent visit at different times to lessen the length of separation. When parents cannot visit, the presence of other significant people can be most comforting for the child (Fig. 20-7).

If parents leave after the child is asleep, they still need to communicate their absence. The parents of a 5-year-old boy solved this problem by devising a sign; on one side they drew a picture of a telephone, and on the other they drew a hamburger. Before they left, they turned the sign to the apppropriate side to tell the child when he awoke that they were out using the telephone or eating.

Older children who know how to tell time may find it helpful to have a clock or watch. However, these children also need honesty from their parents regarding visiting schedules. Because their peer groups are important, adolescents often appreciate planning visiting hours with their parents to ensure that the patient has some private time for friends.

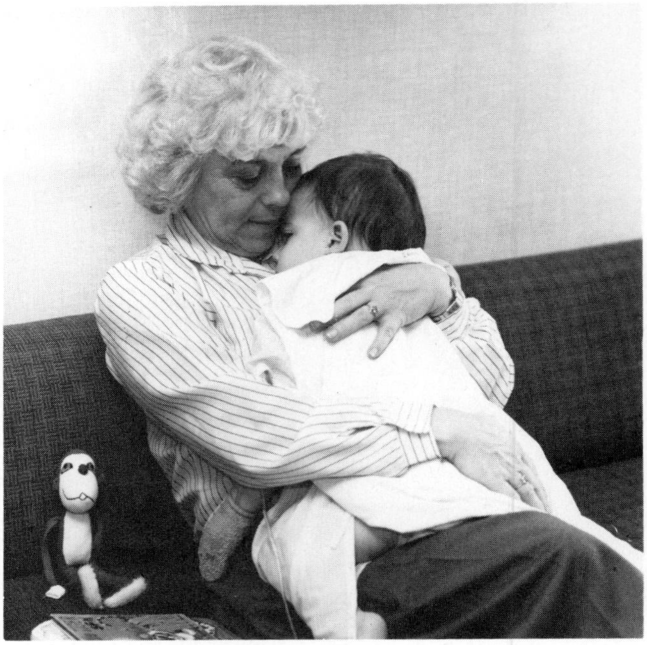

FIG. 20-7 When parents cannot visit, other significant persons, such as a grandparent, can provide comfort to the hospitalized child.

Familiar surroundings also increase the child's adjustment to separation. If parents cannot room-in, they should leave favorite home articles with the child, such as a blanket, toy, bottle, feeding utensil, or article of clothing (Fig. 20-8). Since young children associate such inanimate objects with significant people, they gain comfort and reassurance from these possessions. They make the association that if the parents left this, the parents will surely return. Placing an identification band on the toy lessens the chances of its being misplaced and provides a symbol that the toy is experiencing the same needs as the child. Other mementos of home include photographs and tape recordings of family members reading a story, singing a song, saying prayers before bedtime, relating events at home, or taking a "talking walk" through the home. The tapes can be played at lonely times, such as on awakening or before sleeping (McCain, 1982). Some units allow pets to visit, which can be a special event for a child and can have therapeutic benefits (Davis, 1985).

Older children also appreciate familiar articles from home, particularly photographs, a radio, a favorite toy or game, and the usual pajamas. Often the importance of treasured objects to school-age children is overlooked or criticized. However, it is reported that about half of school-age children have a special object to which they formed an attachment in early childhood and that this is a normal and healthy phenomenon (Sherman and others, 1981). Therefore such treasured or transitional objects

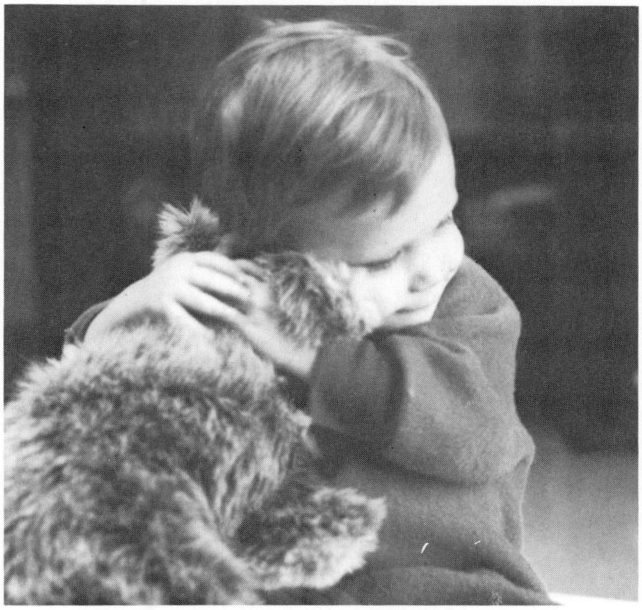

FIG. 20-8 A favorite "friend" can help a child feel more secure in the strange environment of the hospital.

can help even older children feel more comfortable in a strange environment.

Helping children maintain their usual contacts outside the home by continuing school lessons during the period of illness and confinement, visiting with friends either directly or through letter writing or telephone calls, and participating in extracurricular projects whenever possible also minimizes the effects of separation imposed by hospitalization.

Minimize Loss of Control

Feelings of loss of control result from separation, physical restriction, changed routines, and enforced dependency. Although some of these, such as separation from parents, can sometimes be prevented, most of them can be minimized through individualized planning of nursing care.

Physical restriction. Younger children react most strenuously to any type of physical restriction or immobilization. Although some restraint, such as immobilizing an extremity for maintenance of an intravenous line, is frequently necessary, most physical restriction can be prevented if the nurse gains the child's cooperation.

For young children, particularly infants and toddlers, preserving parent-child contact is the best means of decreasing the need for or stress of restraint. For example, almost the entire physical examination can be done in a parent's lap, with the parent hugging the child for procedures such as otoscopy. For painful procedures the parents' preferences for assisting, observing, or waiting outside the room are assessed (see also discussion on p. 624). Older children may or may not want their parents present, particularly if privacy is a concern.

Most children feel more in control when they know what to expect because the element of fear is reduced. Anticipatory preparation and information-giving is a significant method of lessening stress and often results in little need for physical restraint (see p. 624 on Preparing for procedures).

Environmental factors also influence the need for physical restraint. Keeping children in cribs or playpens may not represent immobilization in a concrete sense, but it certainly limits sensory stimulation. Increasing mobility by transporting children in carriages, wheelchairs, carts, wagons, or on stretchers or beds provides them with mechanical freedom.

In some cases physical restraint or isolation is necessary for recovery. Whenever possible, restraints should be removed to allow the child some period of supervised freedom, such as during the bath or when parents visit. In those instances when restraints or isolation cannot be discontinued, such as in severe burns, the environment can be manipulated to increase sensory freedom. For example, moving the bed toward the door or window; opening window shades; providing musical, visual, or tactile toys; and increasing interpersonal contact can substitute mental mobility for the limitations of physical movement.

Altered routines. Altered daily schedules and loss of rituals are particularly stressful for toddlers and early preschoolers and may increase the stress of separation. As discussed previously, the nursing admission history provides a baseline for planning care around the child's usual home activities.

Children's response to loss of routine and ritualism is often demonstrated in problems with activities such as feeding, sleeping, dressing, bathing, toileting, and social interaction. Although some regression is to be expected in all of these areas, sensitivity to the special needs of children can minimize the negative effects. For example, loss of appetite and marked food preferences are common in ill or hospitalized children. In addition, the food selections on hospital menus may differ greatly from preferred cultural or ethnic food preparation. Encouraging the child to eat while avoiding a battle is often a challenge, yet it is an essential nursing responsibility. Suggestions for feeding hospitalized children are discussed on p. 641.

Although regression is expected and normal, nurses also have the responsibility of fostering children's optimum growth and development. There are instances when hospitalization becomes a significant opportunity for learning and advancing. For example, extended hospitalization for long-term chronic illness or situations of failure to thrive, abuse, or neglect represent instances in which regression must be seen as an adjustment period, to be followed by plans for promoting appropriate developmental skills.

One of the aspects of altered routines that is frequently neglected is the change in the child's daily activities. A nonhospitalized child's day, especially during the school years, is structured with specific times for eating, dressing, going to school, playing, and sleeping. However, this time structure vanishes when the child is hospitalized. Although the nurses have a set schedule, the child is frequently unaware of it; new schedules are imposed that may be rigid or flexible. For example, some units have uniform nap and bedtimes for all children, while other units allow children to stay up very late. Many children get significantly less sleep in the hospital than at home; the primary causes are delay in sleep onset and early termination of sleep because of hospital routines. Not only are hours of sleep disrupted, but waking hours are spent in passive activities. For example, few institutions impose any regulation on the amount of time the child spends watching television. Studies show that children spend an average of 8 hours a day watching television in the hospital, considerably more time than they spend watching television at home (McCain and Bies, 1983).

One technique that can minimize the disruption in the child's routine is *time structuring* (Volz, 1981). This approach is most suitable for the school-age or adolescent child who is not critically ill and who has mastered the concept of time. The technique involves scheduling the child's day to include all those activities that are important to the nurse and child, such as treatment procedures, schoolwork, exercise, television, playroom, and hobbies. Together the nurse, parents, and child then plan a daily schedule, which has each activity and its time written down (Fig. 20-9). This schedule is left in the child's room, and the child is given a clock or watch to keep track of the activities. Whenever possible, a calendar is also constructed with special events marked, such as favorite television programs, visits by friends or relatives, events in the playroom, and holidays or birthdays. If specific changes in treatment are expected ("beginning physical therapy in 2 days"), these are added.

Enforced dependency. The dependent role of the hospitalized patient imposes tremendous feelings of loss on older children. Principal interventions should focus on respect for individuality and the opportunity for decision

ERIC'S DAILY SCHEDULE:

7:00 AM	Breakfast, Watch TV, Brush Teeth, Wash up	3:00 PM	Tutor (M,W,F) Study Time (T,Th)
9:00	Tub Room, Dressing Change	4:00	Physical Therapy
		5:00	Dinner
10:00	Rest, TV, Snack	6:30	Dressing Change
11:00	Physical Therapy	7:00 to 9:00	TV, Reading, Snack, Friends Visit
12:00 PM	Lunch		
1:00	Playroom, Quiet Play, Rest, Friends Visit	9:00	Brush Teeth, Wash up
		9:15	Bedtime

FIG. 20-9 Time structuring is an effective strategy for normalizing the hospital environment and increasing the child's sense of control.

making. Although these sound simple, their efficacy lies with nurses who are flexible, tolerant, and personally secure. The last is particularly important because when decision making is geared toward the patient, nurses can feel threatened by a sense of lessened control.

Promoting children's control involves maintaining independence, and the concept of *self-care* can be most beneficial. Self-care refers to the practice of activities that individuals personally initiate and perform on their own behalf in maintaining life, health, and well-being (Orem, 1985). While self-care is limited by the child's age and physical condition, most children beyond infancy can perform some activities with little or no help. Whenever possible, these activities are encouraged in the hospital. Other approaches include jointly planning care; time structuring; wearing street clothes; making choices in food selections and bedtime; continuing school activities; and rooming with an appropriate age-mate. For example, although school-age children may enjoy the responsibility of caring for a toddler or preschooler in their room, adolescents generally prefer quarters separate from the pediatric unit.

Prevent or Minimize Bodily Illness and Pain

Beyond early infancy all children fear bodily injury either from mutilation, bodily intrusion, body image change, disability, or death. In general, preparation of children for painful procedures decreases their fears. Manipulating procedural techniques for children in each age-group also minimizes fear of bodily injury. For example, since toddlers and young preschoolers are traumatized by insertion of a rectal thermometer, axillary temperatures or electronic temperature probes can effectively be substituted. Whenever procedures are performed on young children, the most supportive intervention is to do the procedure as quickly as possible while maintaining parent-child contact.

Children also need permission to express pain. Telling young children that the procedure may be uncomfortable but that it is all right to say "ouch," scream, or cry allows them to express their feelings in an atmosphere of support and acceptance.

Because of young children's poorly defined body boundaries, the use of bandages may be particularly helpful. For example, telling children that the bleeding will stop after the needle is removed does little to relieve their fears, whereas applying a small Band-Aid usually provides much reassurance. The size of bandages is also significant to children in this age-group; the larger the bandage, the more importance is attached to the wound. Watching their surgical dressings get successively smaller is one way young children can measure healing and improvement. Prematurely removing a dressing may cause these children considerable concern for their well-being.

For children who fear mutilation of body parts, it is essential that the nurse repeatedly stress the reason for a procedure and evaluate the child's understanding. For example, explaining cast removal to preschoolers may seem simple enough, but the children's comprehension of the details may vary considerably from the explanation. Asking them to draw a picture of what they think will happen presents substantial evidence of the perceived events.

Children may fear bodily injury from a great variety of sources. X-ray machines, use of strange equipment for examination, unfamiliar rooms, or awkward positions can be perceived as potentially hazardous. In addition, thoughts and actions can be imagined sources of bodily damage. For older children masturbation or sex play may be perceived as powerful weapons of potential destruction. Therefore it is important to investigate imagined reasons, particularly of a sexual nature, for illness. Since children may fear revealing such thoughts, using projective techniques such as drawing or doll play may elicit previously undisclosed misconceptions.

Older children fear bodily injury of both internal and external origins. For example, school-age children are aware of the significance of the heart and may fear the actual operation as much as the pain, the stitches, and the possible scar. Adolescents may express concern about the actual procedure but be much more anxious over the resulting scar. An appreciation of each child's special concerns helps nurses focus on critical areas during preparation for procedures or when giving explanations of the disease processes.

Children can grasp information only if it is presented on or close to their level of cognitive development. When a child is upset about his illness, his perception can be changed by (1) providing a somewhat different and less negative account of the disease or (2) by offering an explanation that is characteristic of the next stage of cognitive development (Bibace and Walsh, 1980). An example of the first strategy is reassuring a preschool child who fears that after a tonsillectomy, another sore throat means a second operation. Explaining that once tonsils are "fixed" they do not need fixing again can help relieve the fear. An example of the latter strategy is to explain that germs made the tonsils sick and even though germs can cause another sore throat, they cannot cause the tonsils to ever be sick again. This higher-level explanation is based on the school-age child's concept of germs as a cause of disease.

Pain management. Relief of pain is a basic need and right of all children, yet physicians and nurses are often reluctant to order and administer analgesics for children. The reason cited most often for withholding analgesics is that narcotics are dangerous—they depress respirations and cause addiction. In reality, narcotics given in safe dosages rarely cause respiratory depression because pain is a physiologic antidote to side effects, such as respiratory depression. In addition, as tolerance to the narcotic occurs, it also develops against side effects, such as respiratory depression and sedation (but not constipation). Fears of addiction typically stem from confusion between what addiction is and what occurs physiologically when patients take narcotics for extended periods. Addiction is a *voluntary psychologic dependence* on drugs. Studies on hundreds of terminally ill patients receiving narcotics daily for long periods show that psychologic dependence is virtually nonexistent. Although drug tolerance (need for increased dosage) and physical dependence (withdrawal when the drug is discontinued) may occur, these are *involuntary physiologic events* and in no way are synonymous with addiction. Even when patients require a considerably greater amount of a drug than its recommended dosage, there are relatively few side effects and a dose remains that can continue to relieve pain.

Effective pain management requires that health professionals be willing to try a number of interventions. Basically, methods to relieve pain can be grouped into two categories: nonpharmacologic and pharmacologic. Whenever possible, both of these should be used; however, nonpharmacologic measures should not be considered substitutes for analgesics.

Nonpharmacologic management. A number of nonpharmacologic techniques exist for lessening the perception of pain. These include (1) distraction, (2) relaxation, (3) guided imagery, (4) thought-stopping, (5) cutaneous stimulation, and (6) behavioral contracting (see box, p. 598). These techniques can lessen the perception of pain, and, when used with analgesics, can enhance the analgesic's effectiveness. Virtually no risks exist when these procedures are used, and nurses can implement them as an independent nursing function.

Pharmacologic management. Numerous nonnarcotic and narcotic analgesics exist; however, the purpose of this discussion is not to describe individual drugs but to present general guidelines in selecting and administering analgesics. Two basic principles govern successful pharmacologic pain control:

1. Schedule the medication for *prevention* of pain
2. Titrate the dosage for maximum comfort

If pain is continuous, which is often the case postoperatively and in illnesses such as cancer, the goal is pain relief with maximum mental functioning. Administration of medications as needed (PRN) is not conducive to meeting this goal. Rather, scheduled medication times around the clock (ATC) are necessary. The nurse plans such a schedule by anticipating that pain will be continuous, such as after certain procedures, or by recording for at least one 24-hour period the times of day when the child needs pain medication. Based on these findings, a *preventive* schedule of drug administration is outlined. For example, if the child complains of pain at 4- to 6-hour intervals, pain medication is given every 3½ hours. One approach to preventive pain management is patient-controlled analgesia (PCA). With this system, the patient self-administers small intravaneous bolus doses of a narcotic analgesic using a programmable infusion pump.

Dosage is increased or decreased as necessary to provide maximum relief. For example, if a prescribed dose fails to relieve pain, the dosage is increased until analgesia is achieved. Conversely, if the dosage causes excessive sleepiness, it is decreased gradually until the dose

Guidelines for Nonpharmacologic Pain Management in Children

General Strategies

Prepare the child before potentially painful procedures but avoid "planting" the idea of pain. For example, instead of saying "This is going to (or may) hurt," say "Sometimes this feels like pushing, sticking, or pinching and sometimes it doesn't bother people. You tell me what it feels like to you." This allows for variation in sensory perception, avoids suggesting pain, and gives the child control in describing reactions.

Avoid evaluative statements or descriptions, such as "This is a terrible procedure" or "It really will hurt a lot."

Stay with the child during a painful procedure; parents are often a neglected source of support for the child and can be involved in distracting him.

Use the power of positive suggestion by saying "I am giving you a medicine that *will* take the hurt away."

Reinforce the effect of the analgesic by telling the child he will begin to feel better in Å amount of time (according to drug use); use a clock or timer to measure onset of relief with the child; reinforce the cause and effect of pain—analgesic, so the child becomes conditioned to *expecting* relief.

Avoid saying "I am going to give you an injection for pain," since this is another pain in addition to the existing pain; if the child refuses an injection, explain that the little hurt from the needle will take away the bigger hurt for a long time.

Give the child control whenever possible (e.g., choosing which leg for an injection, taking bandages off, holding the tape or other equipment).

Educate the child about the pain, especially when explanation may lessen anxiety (e.g., that the pain the child is experiencing is expected after surgery and does not indicate that something is wrong; reassure the child that he is not responsible for the pain).

For long-term pain control give the child a doll that becomes "his patient" and allow him to do everything to the doll that is done to him; pain control can be emphasized through the doll by stating, "Dolly feels better after her medicine."

Specific Strategies

Distraction

Involve parent and child in identifying strong distractors.

Involve child in play; use radio, tape recorder, record player; have him sing or use rhythmic breathing.

Have the child concentrate on yelling or saying "ouch" by focusing on "yelling loud or soft as you feel it hurt; that way I know what's happening."

Relaxation

With an infant or young child:

- Hold in a comfortable, well-supported position, such as vertically against the chest and shoulder.
- Rock in a wide, rhythmic arc in a rocking chair or sway back and forth, rather than bouncing the child.
- Repeat one or two words softly, such as "Mommy's here."

With a slightly older child:

- Ask the child to take a deep breath and "go limp as a rag doll" while exhaling slowly, then ask the child to yawn (demonstrate if needed).
- Help the child assume a comfortable position (e.g., pillow under neck and knees).
- Begin progressive relaxation: starting with the toes, systematically instruct the child to let each body part "go limp" or "feel heavy"; if the child has difficulty with relaxing, instruct him to tense or tighten each body part and then relax it.

Guided Imagery

Have the child identify some highly pleasurable experience.

Have the child describe the details of the event, write down the script, or record it.

Encourage the child to concentrate only on the pleasurable event during the painful time and/or enhance the image by recalling specific details, such as reading the script or playing the record.

Combine with relaxation.

Thought-Stopping

Identify positive facts about the painful event, such as "It does not last long."

Identify reassuring information, such as, "If I think about something else, it does not hurt as much."

Condense positive and reassuring facts into a set of brief statements and have the child memorize them.

Have the child repeat the memorized statements whenever thinking about or experiencing the painful event.

Cutaneous Stimulation

Includes simple rhythmic rubbing; use of pressure; electric vibrator; massage with hand lotion, powder, or menthol cream; application of heat or cold, such as an ice cube on the site before giving injection or application of ice to the site opposite the painful area (e.g., if right knee hurts, place ice on left knee).

Most effective if rhythmic or constant and moderate in intensity.

Behavioral Contracting

May be used informally with children as young as 4 or 5; use stars or tokens as rewards. For example, if the child is uncooperative and procrastinates during a procedure, give a limited amount of time (measured by a visible timer) to complete the procedure, and if the child is unable to comply, proceed as needed; if the procedure is accomplished within the set time, reinforce cooperation with a reward. With older children a written contract may be used (see p. 66).

---

provides analgesia with minimal sedation. Successful manipulation of pain medication requires use of a pain assessment record (see Fig. 20-5) that records the time the medication was administered, the medication given, and an assessment or rating of pain at the time the drug was given and every hour thereafter until the next dose of analgesic. This documentation provides evidence of the drug's effectiveness and facilitates collaboration with the physician regarding changes in medication orders.

Whenever possible, the oral form of the safest drug is used. For example, the effective use of oral nonnarcotic analgesics may eliminate the need for injectable narcotics. When pain is more severe, a very effective approach is the combination of a narcotic with a nonnarcotic analgesic. The rationale for combining the two is that pain is attacked at different physiologic levels—the central nervous system (narcotics) and the peripheral nervous system (nonnarcotics). By adding a nonnarcotic, analgesia may be significantly increased without increasing the narcotic dose.

When combining narcotics and nonnarcotics, it is important to take maximum advantage of the nonnarcotic. For example, Tylenol (acetaminophen) with codeine is available in several preparations, each with a constant

TABLE 20-5

Pediatric and Equianalgesic Dosages of Selected Narcotics

Drug	Dosage (IM)*	Equianalgesia IM (MG)	Equianalgesia PO (MG)
Codeine	Newborn—not established Infants and children—0.5 mg per kg q 4 to 6 hr	130	200
Meperidine (Demerol)	1.1 to 1.6 mg per kg q 2 to 4 hr	75	300
Methadone	Children under 6 yrs—0.1 to .7 mg/24 hr Children over 6 yrs—2.5 mg/24 hr†	10	20
Morphine	0.1 to 0.2 mg per kg q 4 to 6 hr Rectal suppositories—dose not established but 5 mg suppository approximately equal in analgesia to 5 mg morphine IM	10	60‡

*IV dose is half IM dose, given very slowly.
†In clinical practice a higher dose than that recommended has been found necessary to achieve analgesia. The dose ranged from 2.5 to 40 mg q 4 to 12 hours with a "typical dose" being 5 to 10 mg q 6 to 8 hours. (Martinson, I., and others: Nursing care in childhood cancer: methadone, AJN, **82**(3):432-435, 1982.)
‡For relief of chronic pain, the parenteral-oral ratio may decrease to 1:2 or 1:3, although this is controversial (Kaiko, A.: Controversy in the management of chronic cancer pain: therapeutic equivalents of IM and PO morphine, J. Pain Sympt. Manag. **1**:42-45, 1986.)
NOTE: Research has not proven that the above recommended doses are effective in relieving pain. Rather, clinical experience has shown that these doses are safe for most children. Children metabolize narcotics faster than adults. Therefore doses need to be given more frequently for optimum pain control. Long-acting drugs such as methadone or sustained-release morphine are preferable in treating prolonged pain.

dosage of Tylenol and varying amounts of codeine. If inadequate pain relief is achieved, it is preferable to add additional plain Tylenol before doubling the Tylenol with codeine dosage.

Morphine is the narcotic of choice for severe pain. It is available for parenteral, oral (immediate release and sustained release), or rectal administration. The oral form and to a lesser extent the suppository form (Numorphan) are especially useful with children because they provide maximum pain relief without the trauma of an injection. When large doses of morphine are required for intractable pain, continuous morphine infusion is effective.

Meperidine (Demerol), a widely used narcotic, is not recommended for severe or continuous pain. Meperidine has a short duration (2 to 4 hours) and, when given repetitively, can result in central nervous system stimulation, such as anxiety, tremors, myoclonus, and generalized seizures (American Pain Society, 1987).

When parenteral narcotics are required, every effort is made to avoid intramuscular or subcutaneous injections. If the child has an existing intravenous line, such as after surgery, narcotic analgesics can be given safely by this route. The intravenous dosage is usually half of the recommended intramuscular dosage. When converting from parenteral to oral medication, the equianalgesic doses for the oral drug *must* be used. For example, a child receiving 5 mg of parenteral morphine must receive 30 mg of oral morphine to achieve the same amount of analgesia. Table 20-5 lists common narcotics and their equianalgesic doses.

Use Play to Minimize Stress

Play is one of the most important aspects of a child's life and one of the most effective tools for managing stress. Since illness and hospitalization constitute crises in the life of a child, and since these situations are often fraught with overwhelming stresses, children need to play out their fears and anxieties as a means of coping with these stresses.

Play is the "work" of children. It is essential to their mental, emotional, and social well-being, and, like their developmental needs, the need for play does not stop when children are ill or in the hospital. On the contrary, play in the hospital serves many functions:

1. Provides diversion and brings about relaxation.
2. Helps the child feel more secure in a strange environment.
3. Helps to lessen the stress of separation and the feelings of homesickness.
4. Provides a means for release of tension and expression of feelings.
5. Encourages interaction and development of positive attitudes toward others.
6. Provides an expressive outlet for creative ideas and interests.
7. Provides a means for accomplishing therapeutic goals (see box, p. 637).

Of all hospital facilities, probably no room does more to alleviate the stressors of hospitalization than the playroom. In this room children temporarily distance themselves from the fears of separation, loss of control, and bodily injury. They can work through their feelings in a nonthreatening, comfortable atmosphere and in the manner that is most natural for them. They also know that the boundaries of this room are safe from intrusive or painful procedures, strange faces, and probing questions. The playroom becomes a sanctuary of peace and safety in an otherwise frightening environment.

Diversional activities. Almost any form of play can be used for diversion and recreation, but the activity should

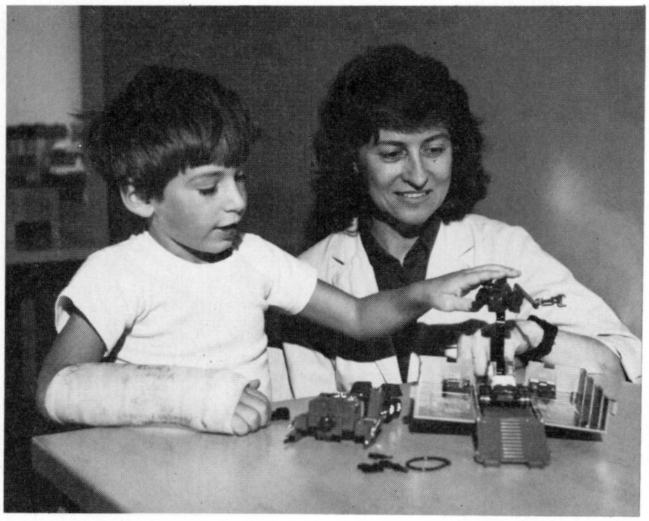

FIG. 20-10 Play materials for hospitalized children need to be appropriate for their age, interests, and limitations.

be selected on the basis of the child's age, interests, and limitations (Fig. 20-10). Children do not necessarily need special direction for using play materials. All they require is the raw materials with which to work and adult approval and supervision to help keep their natural enthusiasm or expression of feelings from getting out of control. Small children enjoy a variety of small, colorful toys that they can play with in bed or in their room, or more elaborate play equipment, such as playhouses, sandboxes, rhythm instruments, or large boxes and blocks, that may be a part of the hospital playroom.

Games that can be played alone or with another child or an adult are popular with older children, as are puzzles; reading material; quiet individual activities, such as sewing, stringing beads, and weaving; and Tinker-Toys, Lego blocks, and other building materials. Assembling models is an excellent past time, but it is a good idea to make certain that all pieces and necessary materials are included in the package. It is disappointing to the child to be ready to begin a project only to find that an essential item, such as glue, is missing from the set.

Well-selected books are of infinite value to the child. Children never tire of stories; having someone read aloud gives them endless hours of pleasure and is of special value to the child who has limited energy to expend in play. A radio and/or television set, included among most hospital room equipment, is a useful tool for entertaining a child, but parents and nurses should monitor program selection, and the television or radio should not be used as a substitute for social interaction or therapeutic play.

When supervising play for ill or convalescent children, it is best to select activities that are simpler than would normally be chosen according to the specific developmental level of the child. These children usually do not have the energy to cope with more challenging activities. Other limitations also influence the type of activities. Special consideration must be given to the child who is confined in terms of movement, has a restricted extremity, or is isolated. Toys for isolated children may need to be disposed of or disinfected after use.

Toys. Parents of hospitalized children often ask nurses about the types of toys that would be best to bring for their child. Most parents want to bring new ones to cheer and comfort the child and assuage their own guilt feelings regarding the child's need for hospitalization. It is wise to assure the parents that, although it is natural to want to provide these things for their child, it is often better to wait awhile to bring new things, especially in the case of younger children. Small children need the comfort and reassurance of familiar things, such as the stuffed animal the child hugs for comfort and takes to bed at night. These familiar items are a link with home and the world outside the hospital.

Large numbers of toys often confuse and frustrate a small child. A few small, well-chosen toys are usually preferred to one large, expensive one. Children who are hospitalized for an extended time benefit from changes. Rather than a confusing accumulation of toys, older toys should be replaced periodically as interest wanes. A helpful suggestion is to have parents provide the child with a shoe box, a child's small suitcase, or knapsack to attach to the bed for an easy storage receptacle to prevent small items from becoming lost in the sheets or under the bed. Children love putting things in and taking things out of a larger container. Many simple items, such as a small magnifying glass, a magnet, grooming aids, a small mirror, crayons and coloring books, colorful paper with scissors and paste, a magic slate, small dolls or toy soldiers, small cars, and beads to string, afford endless hours of amusement. It is the responsibility of the nurse to assess the safety of the toys brought to the child.

A highly successful diversion for a child who is hospitalized for a length of time and whose parents are unable to visit frequently is having the parents bring a box with seven small, inexpensive, brightly wrapped items with a different day of the week printed on the outside of each package. The child will eagerly anticipate the time for opening each one. When the parents know when their next visit will be, they can provide the number of packages that corresponds to the days between visits. In this way the child knows that the diminishing packages also represent the anticipated visit from the parent.

Expressive activities. Play provides one of the best opportunities for encouraging emotional expression, including the safe release of anger and hostility. Nondirective play that allows children freedom for expression can be tremendously therapeutic. Therapeutic play, however, should not be confused with the psychologic technique of play therapy. *Play therapy* is reserved for use by trained and qualified therapists who use the technique as an interpretative method with emotionally disturbed children. *Therapeutic play,* on the other hand, is a very effective, nondirective modality for helping children deal with their concerns and fears, whereas at the same time it often helps the nurse to gain insights into their needs and feelings.

Tension release can be facilitated through almost any activity and, with younger ambulatory children, large-muscle activity such as use of tricycles and wagons is especially beneficial. A great deal of aggression can be safely directed into pounding and throwing games and activities. Bean bags are often thrown at a target or open receptable with surprising vigor and hostility. A pounding board is employed with enthusiasm by young children; clay and Play Doh are marvelous media for use at any age. It is not uncommon to see an angry child of 9 or 10 years of age attacking a mound of clay with the same intensity that is observed in a 3- or 4-year-old counterpart.

Creative expression. Drawing and painting are excellent media for expression. The child needs only to be supplied with the raw materials, such as crayons and paper; plots of bright poster color, large brushes, and an ample supply of newsprint supported on easels; or materials for finger painting. Children usually require little direction for self-expression; however, older children may be given some direction in what to paint or draw. For example, they may be asked to draw the hospital room, draw what they like about the hospital, or draw what they do not like about the hospital. Groups of children can enjoy this creative activity either working individually or, with older children, collaborating on a group project, such as a mural painted on a long piece of paper. For children confined to bed, an old sheet (acquired from the laundry) spread over the bed and a large gown that extends down over the bedclothes to cover the child's own gown provide protection for clean linen.

Holidays provide stimulus and direction for unlimited creative projects. The children can participate in decorating the pediatric unit, and making pictures and decorations for their rooms gives the children a sense of pride and accomplishment. This is especially beneficial for immobilized and isolated children. Making gifts for someone at home helps to maintain interpersonal ties.

Dramatic play. Dramatic play is a well-recognized technique for emotional release, allowing children to reenact frightening or puzzling hospital experiences. Through use of puppets, replicas of hospital equipment, or some actual hospital equipment, children can play out the situations that are a part of their hospital experience. Dramatic play enables children to learn about procedures and events that will concern them and to assume the roles of the adults in the hospital environment.

Puppets are universally effective for communicating with children. Most children see them as peers and readily communicate with them. Children will relate to the puppet feelings that they hesitate to express to adults. Puppets can share children's own experiences and help them to find solutions to their problems. Puppets dressed to represent figures in the child's environment—for example, a physician, nurse, child patient, therapist, and members of the child's own family—are especially useful

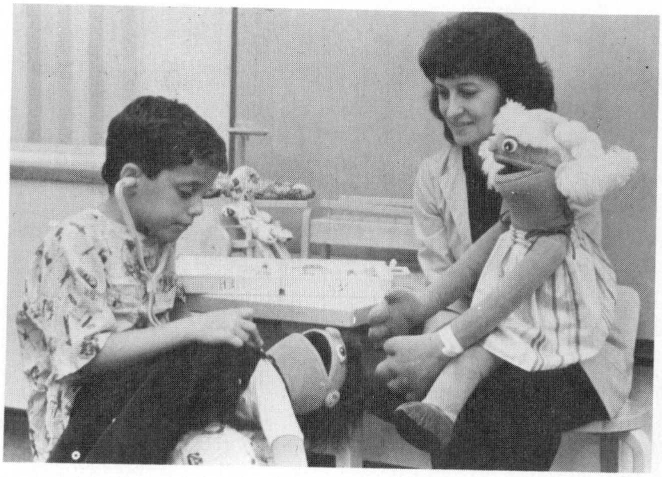

FIG. 20-11 Playing with miniature hospital equipment and puppets allows children to safely explore feelings and concerns.

(Fig. 20-11). Small, appropriately attired dolls are equally effective in encouraging the child to play out situations, although puppets are usually best for direct conversation.

In planning any play activities for the hospitalized child, the nurse must not lose sight of the fact that the reason for the child's hospitalization always takes precedence over other considerations, including the need for play. Play must be scheduled around medical needs and any limitations imposed by the child's condition. For example, it is not uncommon for small children to eat paste and other creative media; therefore, a child who is allergic to wheat should not be given finger paint made from wallpaper paste or play dough made with flour. A child on a restricted salt intake should not play with modeling dough, since salt is one of its major constituents. Treatment schedules and the rules and policies of the institution must be considered also. At home the play program should be planned around the therapy regimen. However, play can be satisfactorily incorporated into the child's care if the nurse and others involved allow some flexibility and use creativity in planning for play.

Maximize Potential Benefits of Hospitalization

While hospitalization generally represents a stressful time for children and families, it also presents an opportunity for facilitating positive change within the child and among family members. Therefore nursing interventions must also focus on maximizing the potential benefits of the experience.

Foster parent-child relationships. The crisis of illness and/or hospitalization can mobilize parents into more acute awareness of the needs of their children. For example, one school-age child who was diagnosed with a serious physical condition commented to the nurse that he "enjoyed" the hospital because it was the first time that he had seen so much of his parents. He expressed concern over discharge because he anticipated the loss of the intensified love and attention. The nurse was able to discuss these feelings with the parents and to increase their awareness of their child's need for them.

Hospitalization provides opportunities for parents to learn more about their children's growth and development. When parents are helped to understand children's usual reactions to stress, such as regression or aggression, they are not only better able to support the child through the hospital experience but also may extend their insights into childrearing practices following discharge.

Difficulties in parent-child relationships that may result in feeding problems, negative behavior, and enuresis may decrease during hospitalization. The temporary cessation of such problems sometimes alerts parents to the role they may be playing in propagating the negative behavior. With assistance from health professionals, parents can restructure ways of relating to their children to foster more positive behavior.

Hospitalization may also represent a temporary reprieve or refuge from a disturbed home. Typically abused or neglected children's dramatic physical and social improvement during hospitalization is proof of the growth potential of this experience. Hospitalized children temporarily are able to seek support, reassurance, and security from new relationships, particularly with nurses and hospitalized peers.

Provide educational opportunities. Illness and hospitalization represent excellent opportunities for children and other family members to learn more about their bodies, each other, and the health professions. For example, during a hospital admission for a diabetic crisis, the child may learn about the disease, the parents may learn about the child's needs for independence, normalcy, and appropriate limits, and each of them may find a new support system in the hospital staff.

During extended hospitalization, special tutoring can help children advance their studies and concentrate on subjects that were difficult. The child's relationship with a tutor can foster a more positive attitude toward school and learning.

Illness or hospitalization can also help older children in choosing a vocational career. Frequently children have impressions of physicians or nurses that are disproportionately glorified or horrified. Actual experience with different health professionals can influence their attitude about health professionals and even a decision for or against a health career.

Promote self-mastery. The experience of facing a crisis such as illness or hospitalization, coping successfully with it, and maturing as a result of it constitutes an opportunity for self-mastery. Younger children have the chance to test fantasy vs reality fears. They realize that they were not abandoned, mutilated, castrated, or punished. In fact, they were loved, cared for, and treated with respect for their individual concerns. It is not unusual for children who have undergone hospitalization or surgery to tell others that "it was nothing" or to proudly display their scars or bandages. For older children hospitalization may represent an opportunity for decision making, independence, and self-reliance. They are proud of having survived the experience and may feel a genuine self-respect for their achievements. Nurses can facilitate such feelings of self-mastery by emphasizing aspects of personal competence in the child and avoiding paying attention to uncooperative or negative behavior.

Provide socialization. Hospitalization may offer children a special opportunity for social acceptance. Lonely, asocial, sometimes delinquent children find a sympathetic environment in the hospital. Children who are physically deformed or in some other way "different" from their agemates may find an accepting social peer group (Fig. 20-12). Although this does not always spontaneously occur, nurses can structure the environment to foster a supportive child group. For example, judicious selection of a roommate can help a child gain a new friend and learn more about himself. Forming relationships with significant members of the health care team, such as the physician, nurse, child life specialist, or minister, can greatly enhance the child's adjustment in many areas of life.

Parents may also encounter a new social group in other parents who have similar problems. The waiting room or hallway "self-help" groups are inherent to every institution. Nurses can capitalize on this informal gathering by encouraging parents to collectively discuss their concerns and feelings. Nurses can also refer parents to organized parent groups or can use the help and support of recovered hospitalized patients.

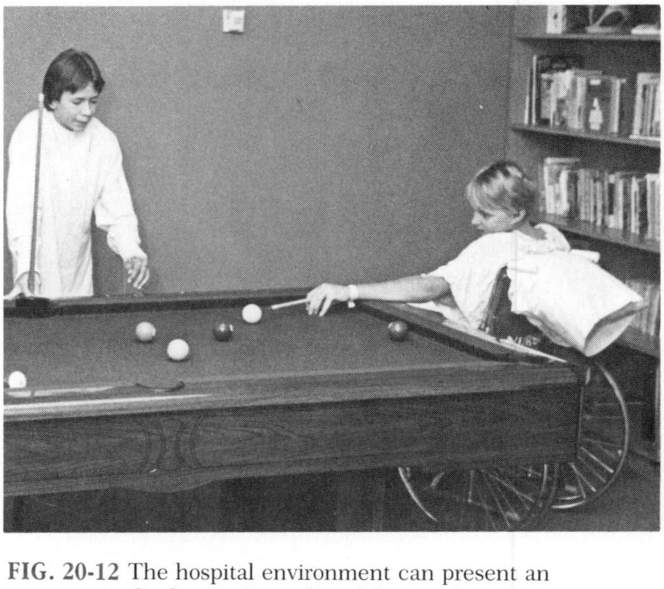

FIG. 20-12 The hospital environment can present an opportunity for forming new friendships and an accepting peer group for children.

NURSING CARE PLAN

The Hospitalized Child

Nursing Goals	Nursing Interventions	Expected Patient/Family Outcomes
A-EP* **Diversional activity deficit** **Etiology: hospitalization, effects of illness**		
Provide opportunity for play	Allow ample time for play Make play materials available to the child Encourage play activities and diversions appropriate to the child's age, condition, and capabilities Use play as a teaching strategy and an anxiety-reducing technique Provide diversional activities or consult with a child-life specialist Encourage interaction with other children Choose a roommate compatible in age, sex, and physical abilities Monitor time spent watching television versus interactive or creative activities	Child engages in age-appropriate diversional activities (specify)
CPP **Pain** **Etiology: discomfort/pain related to illness or therapies**		

Modify procedures to minimize discomfort	Avoid intrusive procedures
	  Take axillary temperatures
	  Administer medications orally or through an existing intravenous route
	Use restraints only when necessary
	Allow the child to sit rather than lie down, if feasible, during procedures
	Maintain the child's contact with parent
	Keep strange and potentially frightening equipment out of view
	Use correct technique (for intramuscular injections, see p. 660)
		Child displays evidence of no, or only minimum, discomfort

Increase control during procedures	Warn the child before implementing a procedure
	  Wake a sleeping child
	Offer choices only when they exist
	Avoid undue delay during a procedure
	Apply a small bandage after injections in young children
	Allow expression of feelings, such as crying, saying "ouch"
	Praise for cooperation
	  Give a small reward, such as a star, sticker, badge
	See also guidelines for preparing children for procedures, (p. 624)
		Child expresses discomfort but maintains some degree of control

Assess pain	See suggestions (p. 587)	
Manage pain	Implement both nonpharmacologic and pharmacologic techniques (p. 597)	Same as above
SP-SCP **Anxiety** **Etiology: separation from support system; unfamiliar environment**		
Prepare for hospitalization	Assess type of preparation the child has received Prepare the child as needed Select appropriate preparatory materials Involve the parents Modify preparation in special situations, e.g. day hospital, emergency admission, or ICU	Child is prepared for hospital experience
Prevent or minimize separation	Provide consistency of nursing personnel as much as possible; assign a primary nurse Arrange workload and schedule to allow personal contact with the child	Child has consistent caregivers

*For an explanation of abbreviations, see p. 20.

Continued.

NURSING CARE PLAN

The Hospitalized Child—cont'd

Nursing Goals	Nursing Interventions	Expected Patient/Family Outcomes
Prevent or minimize separation—cont'd	Encourage parents to room-in whenever possible	Parents visit as much as possible
	Provide an atmosphere of warmth and acceptance for both child and parents	
	Encourage parents and others to cuddle, fondle, and otherwise demonstrate affection for the child	Parents cooperate in care (specify)
	Recognize the child's separation behaviors as normal	
	Allow the child to cry	
	Provide support through physical presence	
	Maintain the child's contact with parents and siblings	Child discusses the family, including pets
	Talk about the child's parents frequently	
	Encourage the child to talk about and remember parents	
	Stress the significance of the parents' visits, telephone calls, or letters	
	Help the parents understand the behaviors of separation anxiety and suggest ways of supporting the child	Parents demonstrate an understanding of separation behaviors
	Explain to the child when they leave and when the parents will return	
	Tell the hospitalized child the reason for leaving	
	Convey the expected time of return in terms of anticipated events. For example, if the parents will return in the morning, they can say they will see the child, "After the sun comes up," or, "When (a favorite program) is on television"	
	Use a clock or calendar for an older child	
	Visit for short but frequent times rather than one long time; encourage parents and relatives to take turns visiting	
	Allow siblings to visit	Siblings visit as much as possible
	Leave favorite home articles, such as a blanket, toy, bottle, feeding utensil, or article of clothing, with the child	Family provides the child with familiar and/or cherished articles from home
	Respect treasured objects of older children, such as a stuffed animal	
	Encourage the family to provide photographs of family members and tape recordings of the parents' voices, such as reading a story, singing a song, saying prayers before bedtime, or relating events at home	
	Play tape recordings at lonely times, such as before sleep	
	Encourage the child to talk about family members	
	Suggest that the family leave small gifts for the child to open each day; if the parents know when their next visit will be, have them leave the number of packages that correspond to the days between visits	
	Assign a "foster grandparent" or consistent volunteer to be with the child if available	*Assigned person spends time with the child (specify amount of time)
Establish a trusting relationship with the child	Be positive in approach to the child	Child develops rapport with primary nurse
	Be honest with the child	
	Convey to the child the behaviors expected of him	
	Be consistent in expectations and in relationships with the child	
	Treat the child fairly and help him feel that he is being treated fairly	
	Encourage parents to maintain a truthful relationship with the child	Child maintains trust of family

*Nursing outcome.

NURSING CARE PLAN

The Hospitalized Child—cont'd

Nursing Goals	Nursing Interventions	Expected Patient/Family Outcomes
Allow expression of feelings	Accept expression of feelings Provide an atmosphere that encourages free expression of feelings Provide opportunities for the child to verbalize, "play out," or otherwise express feelings without fear of punishment	Child verbalizes or plays out feelings or concerns
Help the child to feel he is cared for as a person	Maintain the child's identity Address the child by name or usual nickname Avoid assigning a nickname to the child or converting a given name to its counterpart in another language, such as using Joe instead of José Avoid communicating any signals of rejection, distaste, or other negative feelings to the child Criticize or communicate disapproval of unacceptable *behavior* not disapproval of the *child* Communicate (verbally and nonverbally) that the child is a valued person	Child interacts with staff *Staff demonstrates respect for the child
Allow for regression during periods of illness	Recognize that regressive behavior is a feature of illness Accept regressive behavior and help the child with dependency Assist the child in reconquering the negative counterpart of the psychosocial stage to which he has regressed, (e.g., overcome mistrust; facilitate development of trust)	*Staff and parents exhibit an attitude of acceptance of regressive behaviors
Reduce or alleviate fear of the unknown	Explain routines, items, procedures, and events in a language appropriate to the child's developmental level; use simple language Reassure the child and repeat reassurance as necessary Absolve the child from any guilt about being hospitalized Allow the parent(s) to participate in the child's care Allow the child to handle items that may seem strange or threatening	Child exhibits understanding of information presented (specify information and means of demonstration)
NDx SP-SCP Powerlessness **Etiology: health care environment**		
Modify the hospital environment to resemble home	Determine from the parents or other caregiver the child's customary routine and manner of handling (see nursing admission history, p. 588) Maintain a routine similar to the one the child is accustomed to at home Minimize a hospital-like environment as much as possible; allow the child to sit at a table to eat meals, wear own pajamas or street clothes Use terms familiar to the child, such as those for body functions	Child's routines and environment are similar to those at home (specify)
Provide opportunities for acceptable control	Allow the child choices whenever possible, such as food selection, clothing, options for time of basic care (bath, play, bedtime), selection of television channels Use time structuring with an older child, a jointly planned and written schedule of daily activities	Child participates in planning care (specify)
	Permit freedom on the unit within defined and enforced limitations Limit use of restraints	Child moves about the unit but respects limits
	Encourage self-care according to the child's abilities	Child participates in care activities (specify activities)
	Assign tasks to an older child, especially in extended hospitalization—such as making the bed, supervising younger children, distributing menus, collating charts Respect the child's need for privacy	Child assumes responsibility for tasks (specify)

*Nursing outcome.

EVALUATION

The effectiveness of nursing interventions is determined by continual reassessment and evaluation of care based on the following observational guidelines and expected outcomes:

1. Interview the child and parents regarding the type of preparation for hospitalization the child received.
2. Review the medical record for evidence of parental visitation; interview parents and child regarding strategies used to minimize separation.
3. Observe child's hospital schedule and compare it to the schedule the child typically follows at home; interview child and family for examples of when they were allowed choices in the child's care.
4. Review the medical record for evidence of pain assessment and administration of analgesics or nonpharmacologic pain reducers. Compare the child's behavior and pain scores before and after administration of pain reducers for evidence of pain relief.
5. Interview child regarding the types of play that were introduced to him by the nurses or child life specialist and the times he visited the playroom. For preverbal child, observe the child's use of play materials.
6. Interview the child and parents regarding their perception of any beneficial aspects of the hospitalization. Observe behaviors that indicate benefits, such as formation of new friendships.

Expected outcomes:
See Nursing Care Plan, pp. 603 to 605.

◆ *Stressors and Reactions in the Family of a Hospitalized Child*

The crises of childhood illness and hospitalization affect every member of the nuclear family and, to varying degrees, members of the extended family. The stressors and reactions of families have been discussed in detail in Chapter 18 in relation to chronic illness, disability, and life-threatening illness. In many respects these stressors and reactions differ little regardless of the diagnosis except for their intensity and persistence, which are proportional to the degree of severity of the illness. Consequently, when a child is admitted to an intensive care facility, the family members' reactions and needs are typically greater than when a child is admitted with a less serious condition to the regular pediatric unit. The following discussion briefly reviews the common reactions of the family; specific reactions during intensive care admissions are discussed on p. 616.

PARENTAL REACTIONS

Parents' reactions to illness in their child depend on a variety of influencing factors, but in many instances they are quite similar. Initially parents may react with *disbelief,* especially if the illness is sudden and serious. Following the realization of illness, parents react with *anger, guilt,* or both. There is a tendency to search for self-blame regarding why the child became ill or to project anger at others for some wrongdoing. Even in the mildest of illnesses, parents question their adequacy as caregivers and review any actions or omissions that could have prevented or caused the illness. When hospitalization is indicated, parental guilt is intensified because they feel helpless to alleviate the child's physical and emotional pain.

Fear, anxiety, and *frustration* are common feelings expressed by parents. Fear and anxiety may be related to the seriousness of the illness and the type of medical procedures involved. Often a great deal of anxiety is related to the trauma and pain inflicted on the child because of the various procedures. Feelings of frustration are often related to lack of information about procedures and treatments, unfamiliarity with hospital rules and regulations, a sense of unwelcomeness from the staff, or fear of asking questions. Much frustration can be alleviated if parents are encouraged to participate in their child's care and are regarded as the most significant contributors to the child's total health.

Parents eventually may react with some degree of *depression.* The depression usually occurs when the acute crisis is over, such as following hospital discharge or complete recovery. Mothers often comment on their feeling of physical and mental exhaustion after all the other family members have adapted to the crisis. Other reasons for anxiety and depression are related to concerns for the child's future well-being, including negative effects produced by the hospitalization and any subsequent financial burden incurred from the hospitalization.

SIBLING REACTIONS

Siblings' reactions to a sister's or brother's illness or hospitalization are discussed in Chapter 18 and differ little from instances when a child becomes temporarily ill. Siblings' main reactions are anger, resentment, jealousy, and guilt. A number of factors have been identified that influence the effects of the child's hospitalization on siblings, and although these factors are similar to those seen when a child has a chronic illness, the following are related specifically to the hospital experience and were found to *increase* the negative effects on the siblings (Craft, Wyatt, and Sandell, 1985):

1. Fear of contracting the illness
2. Younger age
3. Close relationship to sick sibling
4. Living away from home while sick sibling is hospitalized
5. Minimal explanation of the sick child's illness
6. Perceived changes in parenting, such as increased parental anger

Parents often are unaware of the number of effects that siblings experience during the sick child's hospitalization and of the benefit of simple interventions to minimize such effects, such as explicit explanations about the illness and provisions for the siblings to remain at home. Sibling visitation helps the well children gain a more realistic perspective of the ill child's hospital experience. Ideally sibling visiting can provide nurses with the opportunity to see the family interact and to directly intervene to supply information or listen to the siblings' concerns.

NURSING CARE OF THE FAMILY

The family of the ill or hospitalized child requires sensitive care that relieves or minimizes the stresses imposed by the temporary crisis. Although the needs of the family are discussed below and are summarized in the Nursing Care Plan on p. 610, the family benefits from all those interventions directed toward the child's recovery. Consequently, comprehensive care requires attention to the needs of all family members.

ASSESSMENT

Assessment involves those factors that are most likely to influence the family's responses to the child's illness and/or hospitalization. While it is not possible to predict exactly which factors are most likely to have an effect on the family's reactions, the areas discussed on p. 518 and in Table 18-2 should be included in the assessment process. Other important variables are (1) the seriousness of the child's illness, (2) the family's previous experience with hospitalization, and (3) the medical procedures involved in the diagnosis and treatment. Important information is also obtained in the nursing admission history (see p. 588).

Discharge Assessment

Throughout the hospitalization the nurse should be aware of the need for discharge planning and those assessment factors that affect the family's ability to provide home care. Ideally discharge planning begins early in the hospital admission to permit sufficient time to assess the family's ability to perform care at home and to institute needed teaching. With the current concern for cost containment and recognition of children's emotional needs, home care for children with technologically complex care, such as youngsters on ventilators, has become increasingly common.

In terms of home care for children with complex care, a thorough assessment of the family and home environment should be performed to ensure that the family's emotional and physical resources are sufficient to manage the tasks of home care (for a discussion of family and home assessment strategies, see Chapter 6). In addition to adequate family resources, an investigation of community services, including respite care, is needed to ensure that appropriate support agencies are available, such as emergency facilities, home health agencies, and equipment vendors. To coordinate the immense task of assessment and plan implementation, a case coordinator should be appointed early in the discharge program.

Discharge planning is also concerned with those skills that parents or children are expected to continue at home. Assessment for planning appropriate teaching includes knowledge of (1) the actual and perceived complexity of the skill, (2) the parents' or child's ability to learn the skill, and (3) the parents' or child's previous or present experience with such procedures.

NURSING DIAGNOSES

A number of nursing diagnoses are prominent in the nursing care of the family of the hospitalized child, and others specific to individual cases become evident. The most common nursing diagnoses are outlined in the Nursing Care Plan on pp. 610-613.

PLANNING

The main nursing goals for the family are:

1. Encourage parents to participate
2. Provide support
3. Supply information
4. Prepare for discharge and home care

IMPLEMENTATION

As soon as the child is admitted to the hospital, or if the care is given in the home, nurses need to begin providing care that incorporates the suggestions and needs of the family. The most effective approach is the mutual participation model (see p. 518) in which the family and health care professionals become partners in the child's care.

Encourage Parent Participation

As discussed previously, preventing or minimizing separation is a key nursing goal with the hospitalized child, but maintaining parent-child contact is also beneficial for the family. One of the best approaches is encouraging parents to stay with their child and to participate in the care whenever possible. Although some health facilities provide special accommodations for parents, the concept of "rooming-in" can be instituted anywhere. The first requirement is the staff's positive attitude toward parents. When hospital staff genuinely appreciate the importance of continued parent-child attachment, they foster an environment that encourages parents to stay. When parents are included in the care planning and made to feel as if they are a contributing factor to the child's recovery, they are more inclined to remain with their child and have more emotional reserves to support themselves and the child through the crisis.

Since the mother tends to be the usual family caregiver, she usually spends more time in the hospital than the father. However, not all mothers feel equally comfortable in assuming responsibility for their child's care. Some may be under such great emotional stress that they need a temporary reprieve from total participation in care-

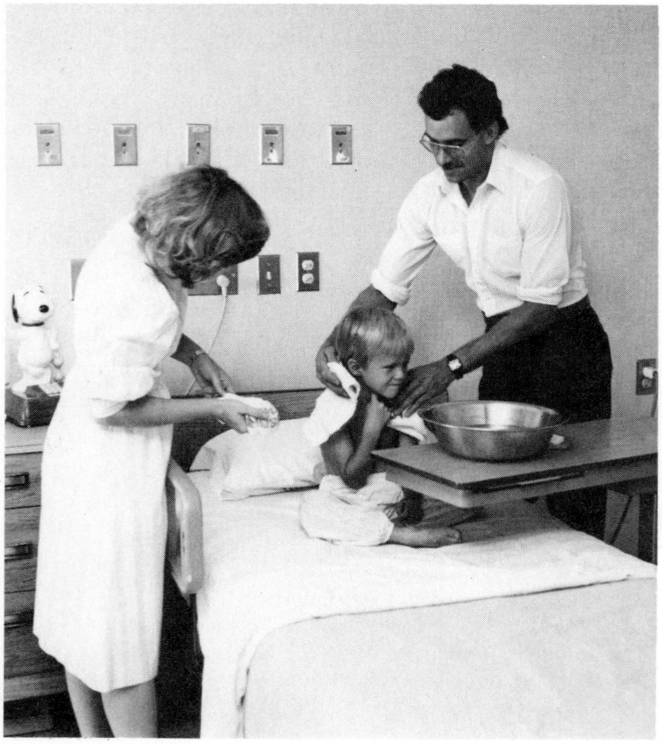

FIG. 20-13 Parents are encouraged to participate in their child's care to the extent that they feel comfortable.

giving activities. Others may feel insecure in participating in specialized areas of care, such as bathing the child after surgery. Individual assessment of each parent's preferred involvement is necessary in order to prevent the effects of separation while supporting parents in their needs as well. Both under and overinvolvement of parents' in the child's care can be detrimental; therefore every effort is extended to help parents identify moderate amounts of visiting and participation (Fig. 20-13).

With life-styles and sex roles changing, fathers may assume all or some of the usual mothering roles in the household. In this case it may be the father-child relationship that requires preservation. Fathers need to be included in the plan of care and respected for their parental role. For some fathers the child's hospitalization may represent an opportunity to alter their usual caregiving role and increase their involvement. In single-parent families, the caregiver may not be a parent but an extended family member, such as a grandparent or aunt.

One of the potential problems with continuous parent visiting is neglect of the parent's need for sleep, nutrition, and relaxation. Often the sleeping accommodations are limited to a chair, and sleep is disrupted by nursing procedures. After a few days parents can become exhausted but feel obligated to stay. Encouraging them to leave for brief periods, arranging for sleeping quarters on the unit but outside the child's room, and planning a schedule of alternating visiting with the other parent or with a family member can minimize the stresses for the parent.

All too often nurses respond to parent participation by abandoning their patient responsibilities. Nurses need to restructure their roles to complement and augment the caregiving functions of parents. Even in units structured to provide care by parents, parents frequently feel anxiety in their caregiving responsibilities; those more involved in direct care may feel more anxiety than those less involved in direct care. Therefore 24-hour responsibility may be too much for some parents. Assistance and relief by nursing personnel should always be available to these families.

Support Family Members

The term *family-centered care* defines the focus of pediatric care, because nursing of children cannot be optimally performed unless each family member is designated the "patient" or "client." Support involves the willingness to stay and listen to parents' verbal and nonverbal messages. Sometimes the nurse does not give this support directly. For example, the nurse may offer to stay with the child to allow the parents time alone or may discuss with other family members the parents' need for extra relief. Often relatives and friends want to help but do not know how. Suggesting ways, such as baby-sitting, preparing meals, tending the garden or home, doing laundry, or transporting the siblings to school, can prompt others to help lessen the responsibilities that burden parents.

Support may also be provided through the clergy. Parents with deep religious beliefs may appreciate the counsel of a clergy member, but because of their stress they may not have sufficient energy to initiate the contact. Nurses can be supportive by arranging for clergy to visit, upholding parents' religious beliefs, and respecting those beliefs' individual meaning and significance.

Support involves an acceptance of cultural, socioeconomic, and ethnic values. For example, health and illness are defined differently by various ethnic groups. For some, a disorder that has few outward manifestations of illness, such as diabetes, hypertension, or cardiac problems, is not a sickness. Consequently, following a prescribed treatment may be seen as unnecessary. Nurses who appreciate the influences of culture are more likely to intervene therapeutically (see also Chapter 3 for an extensive discussion of cultural and religious influences on health care).

Parents need help in accepting their own feelings toward the ill child. If given the opportunity, parents often disclose their feelings of loss of control, anger, and guilt. They often resist admitting to such feelings because they expect others to disapprove of behavior that is less than perfect. Unfortunately health personnel, including nurses, sometimes do exercise little tolerance for deviation from the expected norm. This only increases the psychologic impact of a child's illness on family members. Helping parents identify the specific reason for such feelings and emphasizing that each is a normal, expected, and healthy response to stress provides the parents with an opportunity to lessen their emotional burden.

Provide Information

One of the most important nursing interventions is providing information about (1) the disease, its treatment, and prognosis; (2) the child's emotional, as well as physical, reaction to illness and hospitalization; and (3) the probable emotional reactions of family members to the crisis.

For many families the child's illness is the first contact they have with the hospital experience. Often parents are not prepared for the child's behavioral reactions to hospitalization, such as separation behaviors, regression, aggression, and hostility. Providing the parents with information about these normal and expected behavioral responses can lessen the parents' anxiety during the hospital admission (Vulcan and Nikulich-Barrett, 1988). The family is equally unfamiliar with hospital rules, which often adds to feelings of confusion and anxiety. Therefore the family needs clear explanations about what to expect and what is expected of them.

Parents also need to be aware of the effects of illness on the family and strategies that prevent negative changes. Specifically, parents should keep the family well informed and communicating as much as possible. They should treat all the children as equally and as normally as before the illness occurred. Discipline, which initially may be lessened for the ill child, should be continued to provide a measure of security and predictability. When ill children know that their parents expect certain standards of conduct from them, they feel certain that they will recover. Conversely, when all limits are removed, they fear that something catastrophic will happen.

Nurses should help parents understand and accept the meaning of posthospitalization behaviors in the sick child so the parents can tolerate and support such behaviors. Consequently, parents should be forewarned of the usual continuance of such reactions following discharge (see box, p. 586). Parents who do not expect such reactions may misinterpret them as evidence of the child's "being spoiled" and demand perfect behavior at a time when the child is still reacting to the stress of illness and hospitalization. If the behaviors, especially the demand for attention, are dealt with in a supportive manner, most children are able to relinquish them and assume precrisis levels of functioning.

Nurses should also forewarn parents of the reactions of siblings to the ill child—particularly anger, jealousy, and resentment. Older siblings may deny such reactions because they provoke feelings of guilt. However, everyone needs outlets for emotions, and the repressed feelings may surface as problems in school, with age-mates, as psychosomatic illnesses, or in delinquent behavior.

Probably one of the most neglected areas involves giving information to siblings. Frequently age becomes the only factor that leads to an awareness of this problem, because older children may begin to ask questions or request explanations. However, even in this situation the information may be seriously inadequate. Children in every age-group deserve some explanation of the child's illness or hospitalization. Although the exact wording may differ, the explanation should focus on the following concerns: (1) "Will I get sick and have to go to the hospital?" (2) "Did I cause the illness?" (for actual or imagined reasons), and (3) "Will my parents abandon me if my brother or sister doesn't recover?" If parents or nurses address the explanations to these three questions, the siblings' own fears of illness, guilt, and abandonment are minimized.

Prepare for Discharge and Home Care

Most hospitalizations necessitate some type of discharge preparation. Often this involves education of the family for continued care and follow-up in the home. Depending on the diagnosis, this may be relatively simple or highly complex. Preparing the family for home care demands a high degree of competence in planning and implementing discharge instructions. Although this is usually a team effort, nurses are often key individuals in initiating the process and collaborating with others in the planning and implementing stages.

Nurses frequently are responsible for all or some of the teaching as well. The teaching plan should incorporate levels of learning, such as observing, participating with assistance, and, finally, acting without help or guidance. The skill should be divided into discrete steps and each step taught to the family member until it is learned. Return demonstration of the skill should be requested before new skills are introduced. A record of teaching and performance provides an efficient checklist for evaluation. All families should receive detailed *written* instructions about home care, with telephone numbers for assistance,* before they leave the hospital.

Once the family is competent in performing the skill, they should be given responsibility for the care. Whenever possible, the family should have a transition or trial period to assume care with minimum supervision. This may be arranged on the unit, during a home pass, or in a facility, such as a motel, near the hospital. Some programs incorporate a hospital trial into their discharge criteria, necessitating that the family successfully manage this phase before discharge to home (Steel and Harrison, 1986). Such transitions provide a safe practice period for the family with assistance readily available when needed, and are especially valuable when the family lives at a distance from the treating center.

In most instances parents need only simple instructions and understanding of follow-up care. However, the often overwhelming care assumed by some families ne-

*Home care instructions for a wide variety of technical skills are available in Wong, D., and Whaley, L., *Clinical Handbook of Pediatric Nursing*, ed. 2, St. Louis, 1986, The C.V. Mosby Co.

Text continued on p. 614.

NURSING CARE PLAN

The Family of the Hospitalized Child

Nursing Goals	Nursing Interventions	Expected Patient/Family Outcomes
NDx SP-SCP*	**Anxiety** **Etiology: situational crisis, threat to role functioning, change in environment**	
Help family adjust to the hospital	Introduce family to significant staff members Describe hospital routine that affects the child Acclimate family to the new and strange surroundings Physical layout of unit including playroom, unit kitchen, toilet, telephone, where they can stay Direct family to areas they may need to use outside the unit, (e.g., dining room, chapel)	Family demonstrates familiarity with hospital environment
	Provide an atmosphere that promotes questioning, expression of doubts and feelings Be available to family Be alert to signs of tension in family members Provide for privacy	Family members ask questions
Make family feel important as members of the health team	Employ a polite approach and demeanor Greet family by name when they arrive on the unit Encourage frequent visiting Include family in planning patient care Encourage family to select and assume specific roles in the child's care Offer encouragement for their efforts Ask family to share with the staff what they know about the child's care and needs Convey an attitude of collegiality with family—not competition	Family becomes involved in planning and carrying out care for the child
Reduce apprehension	Allow for expression of feelings about the child's hospitalization and illness	Family members verbalize feelings and concerns
	Provide needed information Prepare family for what to expect (e.g., procedures, behaviors) Explore family's concerns and feelings of irritation, guilt, anger, disappointment, inadequacy Explore family's fears and anxieties regarding the child's status and expectations of results of procedures or therapy	Family demonstrates an understanding of procedures and behaviors (specify manner of demonstration and learning)
	Introduce parents to other families who have a child in the hospital—especially a child who is similarly affected	Family interacts with other families
	Provide something legitimate for family to focus on (e.g., a small task such as assuring a specified amount of fluid, collecting a specimen)	Family complies with directions (specify)
Prepare family for special procedures (x-ray, diagnostic tests, surgery)	Assess family's understanding of the procedure and its purpose Provide needed information, clarify misconceptions Explain special preparation needed (e.g., NPO, shaving, preprocedure medication or equipment) Describe Where the child will be during the procedure Whether the family can be with the child Where the family can wait Approximate length of time procedure requires Reassure family that they will be notified regarding progress of the procedure	Family demonstrates an understanding of procedures and tests (specify)
Support the family during child's absence	Provide a comfortable place for the family to wait Suggest activities to help reduce anxiety (e.g., go to the coffee shop or dining room, take a short walk [specify activity]) Be available to family Make contact with family at frequent intervals to relay information, provide comforts	Family takes advantage of suggestions (specify)

*For an explanation of abbreviations, see p. 20.

NURSING CARE PLAN

The Family of the Hospitalized Child—cont'd

Nursing Goals	Nursing Interventions	Expected Patient/Family Outcomes
Help family adjust to the child's appearance and behavior following procedure(s) or in special care unit	Remain calm Describe the environment, if appropriate (e.g., ICU) Apply principles of learning to explanations Begin with small amounts of information Begin with very general information Allow ample time for family to absorb information and to ask questions Explain how the child will look and the reasons for his appearance and equipment Explain what the child is experiencing Prepare the child and surroundings to lessen the impact of first impression Tidy the bed Personalize the bed and bedside with a toy or other item(s) Provide chairs for the family Be prepared for possible adverse reaction (e.g., fainting) Convey an attitude of caring *about* as well as *for* the child Accompany the family to the child's bedside	Family comes to child's bedside without evidence of distress
NDx SP-SCP Fear **Etiology: knowledge deficit, environmental stimuli**		
Alleviate fears	Help family distinguish between realistic and unfounded fears Help eliminate unfounded fears Discuss with family their fears regarding Child's signs and symptoms Child's anxiety Dire consequences of disease or therapy Deterioration of child's condition Tests and procedures Death Answer questions	Family members verbalize fears and explore nature and ramifications of these fears
NDx SP-SCP Powerlessness **Etiology: health care environment**		
Provide a sense of control	Encourage family visiting at times convenient for them (there will be cultural variations in the amount and type of visiting)	Family schedules visiting times
	Allow expression of concerns regarding the child's care and progress Explore the family's feelings regarding prescribed therapies	Family readily discusses feelings and concerns
	Permit the family as much control as possible in the child's management Encourage participation in the child's care Include family in setting goals for care Involve family in scheduling and other aspects of care Explain what family can do for the child and how to handle him to maintain therapy, (e.g., how to pick up the child with an IV)	Family contributes to care and management of the child
	Employ family's suggestions regarding the child's care whenever possible	*Family's suggestions are incorporated into plan of care

*Nursing outcome.

Continued.

NURSING CARE PLAN

The Family of the Hospitalized Child—cont'd

NDx RRP Altered family processes
Etiology: situational crisis (threat to role functioning, hospitalization of a child)

Nursing Goals	Nursing Interventions	Expected Patient/Family Outcomes
Help family understand the child's illness	Recognize family concern and need for information and support Assess family's understanding of the diagnosis and the plan of care Reinforce and clarify physician's explanation of the child's condition, suggested procedures and therapies, and the prognosis Use every opportunity to increase the family's understanding of the disease and its therapies Repeat information as often as necessary Interpret technical information Help family interpret the infant's or child's behaviors and responses Do not appear rushed—if time is inappropriate, set a date for discussion as soon as feasible Keep appointment meticulously	Family demonstrates an understanding of the disease and its therapies (specify knowledge)
Help alleviate guilt feelings	Provide accurate and specific information regarding the causes of the illness Clarify misconceptions and false assumptions	Family verbalizes their understanding of the cause of the illness (specify)
Support family	Respect parental rights Convey an attitude of respectful caring for both the child and the family Support and emphasize the strengths and abilities of the family Provide feedback and praise for compliance Refer to other professionals for additional interpersonal and concrete support (e.g., social service, clergy)	Family exhibits behaviors that indicate a feeling of self-respect Family avails itself of supportive services
Help family cope with the child's behavior	Determine family's understanding of the normal childhood responses to stress of illness and hospitalization Explain child's regression, magical thinking, egocentricity, separation anxiety, fears Explain behavioral reactions generally expected of the child (specify according to age and developmental level) Explain what the child is (family are) permitted to do in coping with the child's behavior Reinforce family's endeavors	Family demonstrates an understanding of the child's unfamiliar behaviors (specify manner of demonstration—verbalization, physical attitude, behaviors with child)
Help family to assist the child to cope with his hospitalization	Help parents determine the best way to prepare the child for hospitalization, procedures Provide family with precise information about what will take place so they know what the child is likely to experience Encourage family to trust the child's capacity to cope Impress upon family the need for honesty in relating to the child Encourage family to use play as a coping strategy Suggest appropriate items to bring to the child (e.g., pajamas, favorite toys) See also The hospitalized child, p. 603	Family helps in planning strategies Family is honest with the child and staff Family uses play as a tool for relating with the child
Promote and foster positive family relationships	Recognize that family members know the child best and are "cued in" to the child's needs Allow unlimited visiting times Encourage family to bring other significant family members to visit (e.g., siblings, grandparents, and [where permitted] pets) Encourage family to provide the child with significant, but manageable, items from home	Child and family exhibit behaviors that indicate positive coping Family visits child at appropriate times and in appropriate numbers Child demonstrates an attitude of security with familiar persons and things

NURSING CARE PLAN

The Family of the Hospitalized Child—cont'd

Nursing Goals	Nursing Interventions	Expected Patient/Family Outcomes
Promote family health	Stress the importance of maintaining family members' health during the child's illness and hospitalization Encourage adequate rest Provide sleeping facilities where possible Encourage members to alternate visiting with the child to allow some time at home Explore means for respite care of dependent family members Convey to family the assurance that the child will receive optimum care in their absence Provide relief for family from direct care of child as needed	Family shows no evidence of illness Family members appear well rested
	Promote adequate nutrition Provide meals for parents if possible Direct family to nutritious resources for meals Encourage regular mealtimes away from unit	Family members eat regularly
Promote a smooth transition from hospital to home	Assess the learning needs of the family Outline and carry out a teaching plan Determine services needed and make necessary referrals Include family in planning and problem solving Maintain open communication between family and health care providers	Child and family demonstrate the ability to provide needed care in the home
Prepare for discharge	Assess the family's knowledge Teach family the skills needed to carry out the therapeutic program (specify) Allow ample time for preparation Teach necessary techniques and observations Help family by demonstration Distribute appropriate Home Care Instructions or other educational materials or both Encourage questions and expression of feelings and concerns Allow sufficient time for family to perform procedures under supervision Inform parents of Signs of progress to observe for Any unfavorable signs to be alert for Problems that can be anticipated (e.g., care of equipment or devices) Behaviors that indicate special needs (e.g., pain medication, imminent seizures) A course of action to follow (e.g., seizure care, CPR)	Family demonstrates the procedures needed to care for the child in the home (specify learning and method of demonstration)
	Make certain family knows how to contact appropriate persons if or when needed Prepare family for possible posthospital behaviors of the child Ensure family's comprehension of the child's needs before discharge	Family is aware of how to seek help
Maintain continuity of care	Inform family of community resources available Refer to agencies as appropriate (specify) Help identify support group(s) for family Be available to family by telephone or other means	Family seeks appropriate assistance
	Schedule follow-up appointments as needed	Family keeps appointments

cessitates continued professional support after discharge. Appropriate referrals and resources may include visiting nurse or home health agencies, private nurse services, the school system, physical therapist, mental health counselor, social worker, or any number of community agencies, including special organizations, such as SKIP.* Sharing the important issues surrounding the child's and family's needs is essential. Referral summaries should be concise, specific, and factual. When numerous support services are involved, periodic collaboration among the professionals involved and the family is an excellent strategy to ensure efficient usage and comprehensive delivery of services.

EVALUATION

The effectiveness of nursing interventions is determined by continual reassessment and evaluation of care based on the following observational guidelines and expected outcomes:

1. Observe parents' visiting schedule and amount of participation in child's care; observe their willingness and ability to take care of their own needs, such as regular breaks to eat, sleep, and care for the family's needs at home.
2. Interview family regarding their concerns; observe support offered by others, such as relatives, friends, and clergy; observe if special cultural practices (if applicable) are respected in the hospital.
3. Interview the family regarding their knowledge of the child's illness, the child's expected reactions to the hospitalization experience, and the emotional needs of the other family members, especially siblings. Observe frequency of siblings' visits and interview siblings regarding their understanding of the ill child's condition.
4. Observe the family's performance of skills and determine their understanding of other aspects of home care before discharge; interview family and/or resource persons regarding the family's use of appropriate referral services.

Expected outcomes:
See Nursing Care Plan, pp. 610 to 613.

◆ *Care of the Child and Family in Special Hospital Situations*

Children may sometimes be admitted to special facilities in the hospital, such as a day hospital, an isolation room, or an intensive care unit. Some admissions are unexpected and frequently constitute medical emergencies. Such situations require special preparation of the child and family and nursing care interventions based on an awareness of the child's needs and the unique stressors associated with these hospital facilities.

*SKIP (Sick Kids need Involved People) serves as an educational, support, and resource agency that provides assistance to families who have chosen home care for their hospitalized child. The address of the national headquarters is 216 Newport Drive, Severna Park, MD 21146.

DAY HOSPITAL

A day hospital is intended to provide needed medical services for the child while eliminating the necessity of overnight admission. Among the benefits of a day hospital are (1) minimization of the stressors of hospitalization, especially separation from the family, (2) reduced chance of infection, and (3) economic saving. Typically, a child is admitted to the day hospital for operative or diagnostic procedures, such as insertion of tympanostomy tubes, removal of tonsils, hernia repair, cystoscopy, or bronchoscopy.

Because of the limited contact with the child, nursing admission procedures are extremely important. Ideally each child and family should receive preadmission counseling, including a tour of the facility and a review of the expected day's procedures. However, when that is not possible, surgery should be scheduled to allow some time for children to get acquainted with their surroundings and nurses to assess, plan, and complement appropriate teaching.

ISOLATION

Admission to an isolation room increases all the stressors typically associated with hospitalization. There is further separation from familiar persons, additional loss of control, and added environmental changes such as sensory deprivation and the strange appearance of visitors. These stressors are compounded by children's limited understanding of isolation. Preschool children have difficulty understanding the rationale for isolation because they are unable to comprehend the cause-and-effect relationship between germs and illness. These children are likely to consider isolation as punishment. Older children understand the causality better but still require factual information to decrease fantasizing or misinterpretation (Broeder, 1985).

When a child is to be placed in isolation, preparation is essential so that the child will feel in control. With young children the best approach is a simple explanation, such as, "You need to be in this room to help you get better." With older children and parents the explanation can be based more on the cause-and-effect relationship, including how germs enter another's body, such as "by breathing them in." Family members are more likely to practice precautions such as good handwashing and toileting hygiene if they are aware of the value of these measures.

All children, but especially younger ones, need preparation in terms of what they will see, hear, or feel in isolation. Therefore they are shown the mask, gloves, and gown and are encouraged to "dress up" in them. Playing with the strange apparel lessens the fear of seeing "ghost-like" people walk into the room. Before entering the room, nurses and other health personnel should introduce themselves and let the child see their face before donning a mask. In this way the child associates them with significant experiences and gains a sense of familiarity in an otherwise strange and lonely environment.

When the child's condition improves, appropriate play activities are provided to minimize boredom. Rather than dwelling on the negative aspects of isolation, the child can be encouraged to see this experience as challenging and positive. For example, the nurse can help the child look at isolation as a method of keeping others out and letting only special people in. Children often think of intriguing signs for their doors, such as "Enter at your own risk" or "Many have entered but few have left." These posterlike signs also encourage people "on the outside" to enter and talk with the child about the ominous greetings.

EMERGENCY ADMISSION

One of the most traumatic hospital experiences for the child and parents is an emergency admission. The sudden onset of an illness or the occurrence of an injury leaves little time for preparation and explanation. Sometimes the emergency admission is compounded by admission to an intensive care unit or the need for immediate surgery. However, even in those instances requiring outpatient treatment, the child is exposed to a strange, frightening environment and to people who often inflict pain. Therefore every medical emergency requires psychologic intervention to reduce the fear and anxiety so frequently associated with the experience.

Lengthy preparatory admission procedures are often impossible and inappropriate for emergency situations. In such instances nurses must focus their nursing interventions on the essential components of admission counseling, which include the following:

1. Appropriate introduction to the family
2. Use of child's name, not terms such as "honey" or "dear"
3. Determination of child's age and some judgment made about developmental age (if the child is of school age, asking about the grade level will offer some evidence for concurrent intellectual ability)
4. Information about child's general state of health, any problems that may interfere with medical treatment, such as sensitivity to medication, and previous experience with hospital facilities
5. Information about the chief complaint from both the parents and the child

Unless an emergency is life threatening, children need to participate in their care to maintain a sense of control. Because emergency rooms are frequently hectic, there is a tendency to rush through procedures in order to save time. However, when possible, the extra few minutes needed to allow children to participate may save many more minutes of useless resistance and uncooperative-

THERAPEUTIC DIALOGUE

"Postvention" Counseling

A child admitted to the hospital for an emergency appendectomy described the usual admission and preoperative procedures correctly but had no understanding of why they were done. His most prominent recollection focused on all the "shots" he had received (blood tests, intravenous fluid, sedation).

NURSE: Tell me about all these shots.
CHILD: I got millions of shots!
NURSE: Tell me what they were for.
CHILD: To make me better.
NURSE: Why wouldn't one shot have been enough?
CHILD: I guess because I didn't tell my mommy about my stomachache soon enough.
NURSE: I'm not sure about that. Let's count how many shots you got and why you got them. (The nurse reviewed with the child the entire admission, preoperative procedure, and postoperative care and the reason for each injection and venipuncture.) Now, how many shots did we count?
CHILD: Six.
NURSE: Is that a little less than a million?
CHILD: Yes, but they still feel like a million shots when you get them!
NURSE: I can understand that, but do you understand why you got them?
CHILD: I guess so.
NURSE: Do you still think you got extra shots because you didn't tell your mom about your stomachache?
CHILD: Well, you told me everybody gets these same shots when they have their appendix taken out, so I don't think so. My stomach didn't hurt that bad in the beginning, so I didn't say anything until it hurt a lot.
NURSE: That's right. There were reasons for all the shots, and you didn't do anything wrong. In fact, you should feel proud of yourself for having the operation and doing so well.
CHILD: Thanks. I'm going to tell my friends about my operation and how brave I was to get so many shots.

ness during subsequent procedures. Other supportive measures include ensuring privacy, accepting various emotional responses to fear or pain, preserving parent-child contact, explaining all events before or as they occur, and personally remaining calm.

There are occasions when, because of the child's physical condition, little or no preparatory counseling for emergency hospitalization can be done. In such situations the implementation of "postvention," or counseling subsequent to the event, has therapeutic value. The process of postvention involves evaluating children's thoughts regarding admission and related procedures. It is similar to precounseling techniques; however, instead of supplying information, the nurse listens to the explanations offered by the child. Projective techniques, such as drawing, doll play, or storytelling, are especially effective. The nurse then bases additional information on what has already been revealed (see Therapeutic Dialogue).

INTENSIVE CARE UNIT

Admission to an intensive care unit (ICU) can be a particularly traumatic event for both the child and the parents (Fig. 20-14). The nature and severity of the illness and the circumstances surrounding the admission are major factors, especially for parents. Parents experience significantly more stress when the admission is unexpected than expected (Eberly and others, 1985). Stressors that have been identified for the child and parent are (Tichy and others, 1988):

physical stressors, such as pain and discomfort, restraint, inability to eat or drink, changes in elimination habits, and sleep deprivation

environmental stressors, such as unfamiliar surroundings, monitors, ventilators, constant lights, noise, physicians, other staff, and other patients

psychologic stressors, such as lack of privacy, inability to communicate, inadequate knowledge and understanding of the situation, parental behavior, and severity of illness

social stressors, such as disruption of relationship with others, disruption of school attendance, and play deprivation

The emotional needs of the family are paramount when a child is admitted to an ICU. While the same interventions that were discussed earlier for the stressors of separation, loss of control, and bodily injury and pain apply here, additional interventions may also benefit the family and child (see box).

Despite the stresses normally associated with ICU admission, a special security develops from being carefully monitored and receiving individualized care. Therefore planning for transition to the regular unit is essential and should include (1) assignment of a primary nurse on the

Nursing Guidelines for Providing Support during ICU Admission

- Prepare child and parents for elective ICU admission, such as for postoperative care after cardiac surgery
- Prepare child and parents for unanticipated ICU admission by focusing primarily on the sensory aspects of the experience and on usual family concerns, e.g., persons in charge of child's care, schedule for visiting, area where family can wait
- Prepare parents regarding child's appearance and behavior when they first visit child in ICU
- Accompany family to bedside to provide emotional support and answer questions
- Prepare siblings for their visit; plan length of time for sibling visitation; monitor siblings' reactions during visit to prevent them from becoming overwhelmed
- Encourage parents to stay with their child:
  - If visiting hours are limited, allow flexibility in schedule to accommodate parental needs
  - Give family members a written schedule of visiting times
  - If visiting hours are liberal, be aware of family members' needs and suggest periodic respites
  - Assure family they can call the unit at any time
- Prepare parents for expected role changes and identify ways for parents to participate in child's care without overwhelming them with responsibilities:
  - Help with bath or feeding
  - Touch and talk to child
  - Help with procedures
- Provide information about child's condition in understandable language:
  - Repeat information often
  - Seek clarification of understanding
  - Avoid medical discussions among health professionals at bedside or where family and child can overhear
  - If bedside conferences are necessary, interpret information for family members and child or, if appropriate, ask family to leave area during report
- Prepare child for procedures, even if this involves explanation while procedure is performed
- Assess and manage pain; recognize that a child who cannot talk, such as an infant or child in a coma or on a ventilator, can be in pain
- Establish a routine that maintains some similarity to daily events in child's life whenever possible:
  - Organize care during normal waking hours
  - Keep regular bedtime schedules, including quiet times when television/radio is lowered or turned off
  - Close and open drapes and dim lights to allow for day/night
  - Place curtain around bed for privacy
  - Orient child to day and time; have clocks or calendars in easy view for older children
- Schedule a time when child is left undisturbed, e.g. during naps, visit with family, or favorite televised program
- Reduce stimulation in environment:
  - Refrain from loud talking or laughing
  - Keep equipment noise to a minimum:
    - Turn alarms as low as safely possible
    - Perform treatments requiring equipment at one time
    - Turn off bedside equipment that is not in use, such as suction and oxygen
    - Avoid loud, abrupt noises, such as clattering bedpans or toilet flushing

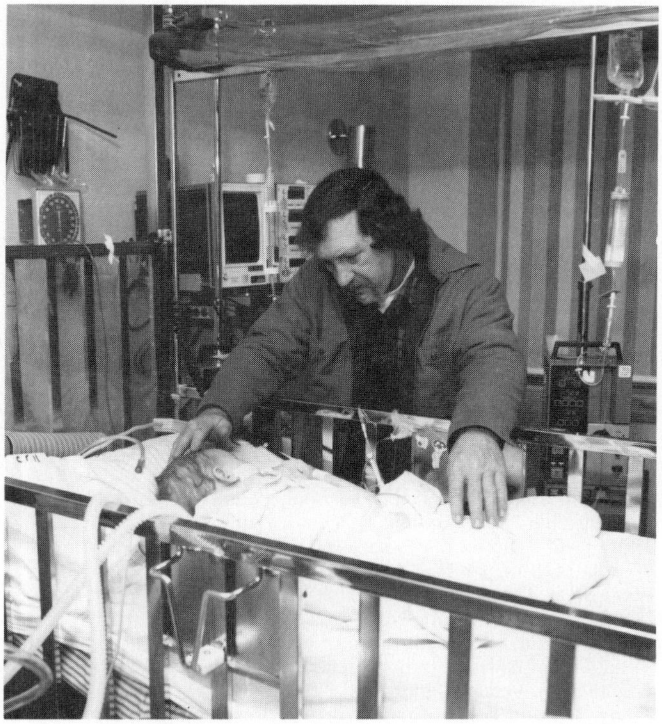

FIG. 20-14 Parents can be overwhelmed when their child is critically ill and requires care in an ICU.

regular unit who visits before the transfer, (2) continued visits by the ICU staff to assess the child's and parents' adjustment and to act as a temporary liaison with the nursing staff, (3) explanation of the differences between the two units and the rationale for the change to less intense monitoring of the child's physical condition, and (4) selection of an appropriate room, such as one that is close to the nursing station, and a compatible roommate.

SUMMARY

Illness and hospitalization represent two of the most significant stresses a child and family may experience. Children are especially vulnerable to the stresses of separation from parents, loss of control in a new and strange environment, and fear of bodily injury and pain. Family members, particularly parents, share many of these same stresses. Even though parents may not feel the physical pain, they hurt for the child. In addition to the child's illness and/or hospitalization, parents are responsible for the care of siblings, who are also affected by the unique stresses imposed by the crisis.

Because nurses spend more time with hospitalized patients than any other group of health professionals, they play a critical role in preventing or minimizing the stresses for the hospitalized child and the family. To provide effective care, nurses must understand the age-related stresses of illness and hospitalization for the child, the reactions of the other family members, and appropriate nursing interventions to deal with the needs of the family.

KEY CONCEPTS

- Children are particularly vulnerable to the stresses of illness and hospitalization because stress represents a change from the usual state of health and routine and because they possess limited coping mechanisms.
- The three phases of separation anxiety are protest, despair, and detachment.
- Feelings of loss of control are caused by unfamiliar environmental stimuli, physical restriction, altered routine, and dependency.
- Fear of bodily pain may be manifested in the following ways: infants—facial expressions, body movements; toddlers—intense emotional upset, physical resistance; preschoolers—aggression, verbal expression, dependency; school-age children—precise verbalization of pain, passive requests for support or help, procrastination technique; adolescents—self-control, limited movement.
- Because of their separation from significant people, hospitalized children may lack the opportunity to form new attachments in the strange environment of the hospital and exhibit negative behaviors after discharge.
- Nursing care of the hospitalized child is aimed at preventing or minimizing separation, decreasing loss of control, minimizing bodily injury and pain, using play to lessen stress, and maximizing the potential benefits of hospitalization.
- Pain assessment includes questioning the child, using pain rating scales, evaluating behavior, securing parents' involvement, and taking action. Pain management should incorporate both pharmacologic and nonpharmacologic methods.
- Diversional or expressive play is an effective tool in minimizing stress.
- The nurse can maximize potential benefits of hospitalization by fostering parent-child relations, providing educational opportunities, promoting self-mastery, and encouraging socialization.
- Family reactions are influenced by the seriousness of illness; experience with illness or hospitalization and diagnostic or therapeutic procedures; available support systems; personal ego strengths; coping abilities; presence of additional stresses; cultural and religious beliefs; and family communication patterns.
- Fear of contracting illness, their younger age, a close relationship with the ill sibling, substitute child care, minimum explanation of the illness, and perceived changes in parenting all increase the deleterious effects of a brother's or sister's illness/hospitalization on siblings.
- Nursing care of the family involves listening to parents' verbal and nonverbal messages, providing clergy support, accepting cultural, socioeconomic, and ethnic values, giving information to families and siblings, and preparing for discharge and home care.
- Emergency admission, or admission to day hospital, isolation room, or intensive care unit requires additional intervention strategies to meet the child's and family's needs.

STUDY QUESTIONS AND ACTIVITIES

1 Attend a preadmission hospital tour for children or read two books written about children and hospitalization and list the various approaches used to familiarize children with the hospital environment and routine.
2 Observe the reactions of a toddler who has been recently admitted to a hospital when the parent leaves or a stranger approaches the child. Compare the behaviors with those listed in the box on p. 579.
3 Complete a nursing admission history for a hospitalized child using the form on pp. 588-589.
4 Care for a child who is in pain, such as a postoperative patient, and assess the child using the QUEST process.
5 Interview a parent whose child has been recently discharged from the hospital and inquire about the presence of posthospital behaviors in the child. Compare the behaviors with those listed in the box on p. 586. If no posthospital changes in behavior were evident, consider the child's age, length of admission, any separation from parents, and reason for hospitalization as possible factors.

REFERENCES

Abu-Saad, H.: Cultural group indicators of pain in children, Matern. Child Nurs. J. **13**(3):187-196, 1984.
Aho, A.C., and Erickson, M.T.: Effects of grade, gender, and hospitalization on children's medical fears, Dev. Behav. Pediatr. **6**(3):146-153, 1985.
American Pain Society: Principles of analgesic use in the treatment of acute pain or chronic cancer pain, Clin. Pharm. **6**(7):523-532, 1987.
Anand, K., Sippell, W., and Aynsley-Green, A.: Randomised trial of fentanyl anaesthesia in preterm babies undergoing surgery: effects on the stress response, Lancet **1**(8525):62-66, 1987.
Baker, C., and Wong, D.: Q.U.E.S.T.: a process of pain assessment in children, Orthop. Nurs. **6**(1):11-21, 1987.
Beyer, J.: The Oucher: a user's manual and technical report, Evanston, IL, 1984, The Hospital Play Equipment Co.
Bibace, R., and Walsh, M.E.: Development of children's concepts of illness, Pediatrics **66**(6):912-917, 1980.
Broeder, J.L.: School-age children's perceptions of isolation after hospital discharge, Matern. Child Nurs. J. **14**(3):153-174, 1985.
Chess, S., and Thomas, A.: Temperamental differences: a critical concept in child health care, Pediatr. Nurs. **11**(3):167-171, 1985.
Craft, M., Wyatt, N., and Sandell, B: Behavior and feeling changes in siblings of hospitalized children, Clin Pediatr. **24**(7):374-378, 1985.
Dale, J.C.: A multidimensional study of infants' responses to painful stimuli, Pediatr. Nurs. **12**(1):27-31, 1986.
Davis, J.H.: Children and pets: a therapeutic connection, Pediatr. Nurs. **11**(5):377-379, 1985.
Eberly, T.W., and others: Parental stress after the unexpected admission of a child to the intensive care unit, Crit. Care Q. **8**(1):57-65, 1985.
Eland, J.M.: The child who is hurting, Semin. Oncol. Nurs. **1**(2):116-122, 1985.
Eland, J.M., and Anderson, J.E.: The experience of pain in children. In Jacox, A., editor: Pain: a source book for nurses and other health professionals, Boston, 1977, Little, Brown & Co.
Gordon, M.: Nursing diagnosis: process and application, ed. 2, New York, 1987, McGraw-Hill Book Co.
Haslam, D.R.: Age and the perception of pain, Psychonom. Sci. **15:**86, 1969.
Hester, N.: The preoperational child's reaction to immunization, Nurs. Res. **28**(4):250-255, 1979.
Johnston, C.C., and Strada, M.E.: Acute pain response in infants: a multidimensional description, Pain **24**(3):373-382, 1986.
Katz, E.R., Kellerman, J., and Siegel, S.: Behavioral distress in children with cancer undergoing medical procedures: developmental considerations, J. Consult. Clin. Psychol. **48**(3):356-365, 1980.
McCaffery, M.: Nursing management of the patient with pain, ed. 2, Philadelphia, 1979, J.B. Lippincott Co.
McCain, G.C.: Parent-created tape recordings for hospitalized children, Child. Health Care **10**(3):104-105, 1982.
McCain, G.C., and Bies, D.C.: Television viewing and the hospitalized child, Pediatr. Nurs. **9**(1):33-35, 1983.
Norris, S., Campbell, L.A., and Brenkert, S.: Nursing procedures and alterations in transcutaneous oxygen tension in premature infants, Nurs. Res. **31**(6):330-336, 1982.
Orem, D.: Nursing: concepts of practice, ed. 3, New York, 1985, McGraw-Hill Inc.
Porter, J., and Jick, H.: Addiction rare in patients treated with narcotics, New Engl. J. Med. **302**(2):123, 1980.
Savedra, M., and others: How do children describe pain? a tentative assessment, Pain **14:**95-104, 1982.
Sherman, M., and others: Treasured objects in school-aged children, Pediatrics **68**(3):379-386, 1981.
Steele, N., and Harrison, B.: Technology-assisted children: assessing discharge preparation, J. Pediatr. Nurs. **1**(3):150-158, 1986.
Tichy, A.M., and others: Stressors in pediatric intensive care units, Pediatr. Nurs. **14**(1):40-42, 1988.
Volz, D.D.: Time structuring for hospitalized school-aged children, Issues Compr. Pediatr. Nurs. **5:**205-210, 1981.
Vulcan, B., and Nikulich-Barrett, M.: The effect of selected information on mothers' anxiety levels during their children's hospitalizations, J. Pediatr. Nurs. **3**(2):97-102, 1988.
Wong, D., and Baker, C.: Pain in children: comparison of assessment scales, Pediatr. Nurs. **14**(1):9-17, 1988.

BIBLIOGRAPHY

Hospitalization: The Child and Family

Alexander, D., White, M., and Powell, G.: Anxiety of non-rooming-in parents of hospitalized children, Child. Health Care **15**(1):14-20, 1986.
Azarnoff, P.: Preparing children for hospitalization. In Preparing children and families for health care encounters, Washington, DC, 1980, Association for the Care of Children's Health.
Bates, T.A., and Broome, M.: Preparation of children for hospitalization and surgery: a review of the literature, J. Pediatr. Nurs. **1**(4):230-239, 1986.
Betz, C.L., and Poster, E.C.: Incorporating play into the care of the hospitalized child, Issues Compr. Pediatr. Nurs. **7:**343-355, 1984.
Birchfield, M.E.: Nursing care for hospitalized children based on different stages of illness, MCN **6**(1):46-52, 1981.
Bordeaux, B.R.: Television viewing patterns of hospitalized school-aged children and adolescents, Child. Health Care **15**(2):70-75, 1986.
Cave, N.: What a little care can do, Can. Nurse **75**(11):38-40, 1979.
Clatworthy, S.: Therapeutic play: effects on hospitalized children, Child. Health Care **9**(4):108-113, 1981.
Coucouvanis, J.A., and Solomons, H.C.: Handling complicated visitation problems of hospitalized children, MCN **8**(2):131, 1983.
Craft, M.J.: Validation of responses reported by school-aged siblings of hospitalized children, Child. Health Care **15**(1):6-13, 1986.
Craft, M.J., and Wyatt, N.: Effect of visitation upon siblings of hospitalized children, Matern. Child Nurs. J. **15**(1):47-59, 1986.
Curry, N.E.: Enhancing dramatic play potential in hospitalized children, Child. Health Care **16**(3):142-149, 1988.
Denehy, J.: What do school-age children know about their bodies? Pediatr. Nurs. **10**(4):290-292, 1984.
Denholm, C.J.: The adolescent patient at discharge and in the post-hospitalization environment: a review, Matern. Child Nurs. J. **16**(2):95-102, 1987.
Denholm, C.J.: Hospitalization and the adolescent patient: a review and some critical questions, Child. Health Care **13**(3):109-116, 1985.

Denholm, C.J., and Ferguson, R.V.: Strategies to promote the developmental needs of hospitalized adolescents, Child. Health Care **15**(3):183-187, 1987.
Dorn, L.D.: Children's concepts of illness: clinical applications, Pediatr. Nurs. **10**(5):325-327, 1984.
Elfert, H., and Anderson, J.M.: More than just luck, Can. Nurse **83**(4):14-17, 1987.
Ferraro, A.R., and Longo, D.C.: Nursing care of the family with a chronically ill, hospitalized child: an alternative approach, Image: Journal of Nursing Scholarship **17**(3):77-81, 1985.
Fletcher, B.: Psychological upset in posthospitalized children: a review of the literature, Matern. Child Nurs. J. **10**(3):185-195, 1981.
Fore, C.V., and Holmes, S.S.: A care-by-parent unit revisited, MCN **8**(6):408-410, 1983.
Fosson, A., and deQuan, M.M.: Reassuring and talking with hospitalized children, Child. Health Care **13**(1):37-44, 1984.
Garot, P.A.: Therapeutic play: work of both child and nurse, J. Pediatr. Nurs. **1**(2):111-116, 1986.
Giesy, J.: Teaching discharge management, J. Pediatr. Nurs. **2**(5):353-354, 1987.
Goldberger, J.: Issue-specific play with infants and toddlers in hospitals: rationale and intervention, Child. Health Care **16**(3):134-141, 1988.
Gratz, R.R., and Piliavin, J.A.: What makes kids sick: children's beliefs about the causative factors of illness, Child. Health Care **12**(4):156-162, 1984.
Hagemann, V.: Night sleep of children in a hospital. Part 1. Sleep duration, Matern. Child Nurs. J. **10:**1-13, 1981a.
Hagemann, V.: Night sleep of children in a hospital. Part 2. Sleep disruption, Matern. Child Nurs. J. **10:**127-142, 1981b.
Hester, N.O.: Health perceptions of school-age children, Issues Compr. Pediatr. Nurs. **10:**137-147, 1987.
Hudson, C., and others: Storytelling: a measure of anxiety in hospitalized children, Child. Health Care **16**(2):118-122, 1987.
Knafl, K.A., Cavallari, K.A., and Dixon, D.M.: Pediatric hospitalization: family and nurse perspectives, Boston, 1988, Scott, Foresman & Co.
Kruger, S.F., and Rawlins, P.: Pediatric dismissal protocol to aid the transition from hospital care to home care, Image **16:**120, 1984.
Lamb, J.M., and Rodgers, D.R.: Assisting the hostile, hospitalized child, MCN **8**(5):336-339, 1983.
LaMontagne, L.L.: Three coping strategies used by school-age children, Pediatr. Nurs. **10**(1):25-28, 1984.
Maheady, D.C.: Health concepts of preschool children, Pediatr. Nurs. **12**(3):195-197, 1986.
Marchant, R.: Caring for hospitalized inner-city children, Pediatr. Nurs. **11**(2):129-131, 1985.
McCue, K.: Medical play: an expanded perspective, Child. Health Care **16**(3):157-161, 1988.
Miller, S.A.: Promoting self-esteem in the hospitalized adolescent: clinical interventions, Issues Compr. Pediatr. Nurs. **10:**187-194, 1987.
Mishel, M.H.: Parents' perception of uncertainty concerning their hospitalized child, Nurs. Res. **32**(6):324-330, 1983.
O'Mears, K., and others: Preadmission programs: development, implementation, and evaluation, Child. Health Care **11**(4):137-141, 1983.
Oremland, E.K.: Mastering developmental and critical experiences through play and other expressive behaviors in childhood, Child. Health Care **16**(3):150-156, 1988.
Pass, M.D., and Pass, C.M.: Anticipatory guidance for parents of hospitalized children, J. Pediatr. Nurs. **2**(4):250-258, 1987.
Pazola, K.J., and Gerberg, A.K.: Teen group: a forum for the hospitalized adolescent, MCN **10**(4):265-269, 1985.
Perrin, E.C., and Gerrity, P.S.: There's a demon in your belly: children's understanding of illness, Pediatrics **67**(6):841-849, 1981.
Petrillo, M., and Sanger, S.: Emotional care of hospitalized children, ed. 2, Philadelphia, 1980, J.B. Lippincott Co.
Pidgeon, V.: Children's concepts of illness: implications for health teaching, Matern. Child Nurs. J. **14**(1):23-35, 1985.
Poster, E.C.: Stress immunization: techniques to help children cope with hospitalization, Matern. Child Nurs. J. **12**(2):119-134, 1983.
Poster, E.C., and Betz, C.L.: Allaying the anxiety of hospitalized children using stress immunization techniques, Issues Compr. Pediatr. Nurs. **67:**227-233, 1983.
Powell, G.M., and others: Maternal anxiety and the nature of sleep onset latency in hospitalized children, Pediatr. Nurs. **13**(6):397-401, 1987.
Reynolds, E.A., and Ramenofsky, M.L.: The emotional impact of trauma on toddlers, MCN **13**(2):106-109, 1988.
Robinson, C.A.: Preschool children's conceptualizations of health and illness, Child. Health Care **16**(2):89-95, 1987.
Ruddy-Wallace, M.: Temperament: assessing individual differences in hospitalized children, J. Pediatr. Nurs. **2**(1):30-36, 1987.
Sanborn, C.W., and Blount, M.: Standard plans for care and discharge, Am. J. Nurs. **84**(11):1394-1396, 1984.
Savedra, M., Tesler, M., and Ritchie, J.: Parents' waiting: is it an inevitable part of the hospital experience? J. Pediatr. Nurs. **2**(5):328-332, 1987.
Stevens, M.: Adolescents' perception of stressful events during hospitalization, J. Pediatr. Nurs. **1**(5):303-313, 1986.
Stevens, M.S.: Which adolescents breeze through surgery? Am. J. Nurs. **87**(12):1564-1565, 1987.
Strickland, M.P.: Children's adjustment to the hospital: a rural/urban comparison, Matern. Child Nurs. J. **16**(3):251-260, 1987.
Terry, D.G.: The needs of parents of hospitalized children, Child. Health Care **16**(1):18-20, 1987.
Thompson, R.H.: Psychosocial research on pediatric hospitalization and health care: a review of the literature, Springfield, IL, 1985, Charles C Thomas, Publisher.
White, J.E.: Special nursing needs of hospitalized children with learning disabilities, MCN **8**:209-212, 1983.
Wilson, C.J.: Comparison of two methods of preparation for hospitalization, Child. Health Care **16**(1):24-27, 1987.
Winkelstein, M.L., and Carson, V.J.: Adolescents and rooming-in, Matern. Child Nurs. J. **16**(1):75-88, 1987.
Wolfer, J., and Visintainer, M.: Prehospital psychological preparation for tonsillectomy patients: effects on child's and parents' adjustment, Pediatrics **64:**646-655, 1979.
Wood, S.P.: School-aged children's perceptions of the causes of illness, Pediatr. Nurs. **9**(2):101-104, 1983.
Zweig, C.D.: Reducing stress when a child is admitted to the hospital, MCN **11**(1):24-26, 1986.

Pain Assessment and Management

Abu-Saad, H., and Holzemer, W.L.: Measuring children's self-assessment of pain, Issues Compr. Pediatr. Nurs. **5:**337-349, 1981.
Aradine, C.R., Beyer, J.E., and Tompkins, J.M.: Children's pain perception before and after analgesia: a study of instrument construct validity and related issues, J. Pediatr. Nurs. **3**(1):11-23, 1988.
Beyer, J.E., and Aradine, C.R.: Content validity of an instrument to measure young children's perceptions of the intensity of their pain, J. Pediatr. Nurs. **1**(6):386-395, 1986.
Beyer, J.E., and Byers, M.L.: Knowledge of pediatric pain: the state of the art, Child. Health Care **13**(4):150-159, 1985.
Beyer, J.E., and Levin, C.R.: Issues and advances in pain control in children, Nurs. Clin. North Am. **22**(3):661-676, 1987.
Beyer, J.E., and others: Patterns of postoperative analgesic use with adults and children following cardiac surgery, Pain **17:**71-81, 1983.
Bradshaw, C., and Zeanah, P.D.: Pediatric nurses' assessments of pain in children, J. Pediatr. Nurs. **1**(5):314-322, 1986.
Broome, M.E.: The child in pain: a model for assessment and intervention, Crit. Care Q. **8**(1):47-56, 1985.
Craig, K.D., and others: Developmental changes in infant pain expression during immunization injections, Soc. Sci. Med. **19**(12):1331-1337, 1984.
D'Apolito, K.: The neonate's response to pain, MCN **9**(4):256-257, 1984.
Gaffney, A., and Dunne, E.A.: Developmental aspects of children's definitions of pain, Pain **26:**105-117, 1986.
Hawley, D.D.: Postoperative pain in children: misconceptions, descriptions, and interventions, Pediatr. Nurs. **10**(1):20-23, 1984.

Hester, N., and Barcus, C.: Assessment and management of pain in children. In Pediatrics: nursing update. **1**(14):3, Princeton, NJ, 1986, Continuing Professional Education Center, Inc.
Hurley, A., and Whelan, E.G.: Cognitive development and children's perception of pain, Pediatr. Nurs. **14**(1):21-24, 1988.
Jerrett, M.D.: Children and their pain experience, Child. Health Care **14**(2):83-89, 1985.
Korberly, B.H.: Pharmacologic treatment of children's pain, Pediatr. Nurs. **11**(4):292-294, 1985.
Lutz, W.J.: Helping hospitalized children and their parents cope with painful procedures, J. Pediatr. Nurs. **1**(1):24-32, 1986.
Lynn, M.R.: Pain in the pediatric patient: a review of research, J. Pediatr Nurs. **1**(3):198-201, 1986.
McGrath, P.: Pain in children and adolescents, New York, 1988, Elsevier Science.
McGuire, L., and Dizard, S.: Managing pain in the young patient, Nursing 82 **12**(8):52-57, 1982.
Owens, M.E.: Assessment of infant pain in clinical settings, J. Pain Sympt. Manag. **1**(1):29-31, 1986.
Ross, D.M.: Thought-stopping: a coping strategy for impending feared events, Issues Compr. Pediatr. Nurs. **7**(2-3):83-89, 1984.
Ross, D.M., and Ross, S.A.: Childhood pain: current issues, research, and management, Baltimore, 1988, Urban & Schwarzenberg.
Ross, D.M., and Ross, S.A.: Stress reduction procedures for the school-age hospitalized leukemic child, Pediatr. Nurs. **10**(6):393-395, 1984.
Scott, J.G., and Rigney-Radford, K.: Factors affecting the management of pain, MCN **9**(4):253-255, 1984.
Sheredy, C.: Factors to consider when assessing responses to pain, MCN **9**(4):250-252, 1984.
Smith, D.: Using humor to help children with pain, Child. Health Care **14**(3):187-188, 1986.
Wright, Z.: From IV to PO: titrating your patient's pain medication, Nursing 81 **11:**39-43, 1981.
Young, M.R., and Fu, V.R.: Influence of play and temperament on the young child's response to pain, Child. Health Care **16**(3):209-215, 1988.
Zollo, M.: Management of pain in critically ill children, MCN **9**(4):258-261, 1984.

Special Hospital Situations

Alcock, D., and others: Environment and waiting behaviors in emergency waiting areas, Child. Health Care **13**(4):174-180, 1985.
Baker, C.F.: Sensory overload and noise in the ICU: sources of environmental stress, Crit. Care Q. **6**(4):66-80, 1984.
Bellack, J.P., and Fore, C.V.: The young children in the critical care unit, Crit. Care Update **8**(5):26-38, 1981.
Bozett, F.W., and Gibbons, R.: The nursing management of families in the critical care setting, Crit. Care Update **10**(2):22-27, 1983.
Broome, M.E.: Working with the family of a critically ill child, Heart Lung **14**(4):368-372, 1985.
Byers, M.L.: Same day surgery: a preschooler's experience, Matern. Child Nurs. J. **16**(3):277-282, 1987.
Canright, P., and Campbell, M.J.: Nursing care of the child and his family in the emergency department, Pediatr. Nurs. **3**(4):43-45, 1977.
Carty, R.: Observed behaviors of preschoolers to intensive care, Pediatr. Nurs. **6**(4):21-25, 1980.
deChesnay, M.: Promoting healthy family functioning in acute care units, J. Pediatr. Nurs. **1**(2):96-101, 1986.
Epsersen, S., and Hardy, C.D.: Pediatric care plan for adult ICU nurses, Crit. Care Nurse **5**(2):14-18, 1985.
Etzler, C.A.: Parents' reaction to pediatric critical care settings: a review of the literature, Issues Compr. Pediatr. Nurs. **7:**319-331, 1984.
Ferguson, C.K.: Childhood coping: adaptive behavior during intensive care hospitalization, Crit. Care Q. **6**(4):81-93, 1984.
Hedenkamp, E.A.: Humanizing the intensive care unit for children, Crit. Care Q. **3**(1):63-73, 1980.
Hedenkamp, E.A.: Preparing parents for a visit to the intensive care unit. In Preparing children and families for health care encounters, Washington, DC, 1980, Association for the Care of Children's Health.
King, S.L., and Gregor, F.M.: Stress and coping in families of the critically ill, Crit. Care Nurse **5**(4):48-51, 1985.
Lewandowski, L.: Psychosocial aspects of pediatric critical care. In Hazinski, M.F., editor: Nursing care of the critically ill child, St. Louis, 1984, The C.V. Mosby Co.
McGuire, M., Shepherd, R., and Greco, A.: Hospitalized children in confinement, Pediatr. Nurs. **4**(6):31-35, 1978.
Miles, M.S., and Carter, M.C.: Assssing parental stress in intensive care units, MCN **8**(5):354-359, 1983.
Miles, M.S., and Carter, M.C.: Coping strategies used by parents during their child's hospitalization in an intensive care unit, Child. Health Care **14**(1):14-21, 1985.
Miles, M.S., and Carter, M.C.: Sources of parental stress in pediatric intensive care units, Child. Health Care **11**(2):65-69, 1982.
Miles, M.S., and others: Maternal and paternal stress reactions when a child is hospitalized in a pediatric care unit, Issues Compr. Pediatr. Nurs. **7:**333-342, 1984.
Munn, V.A., and Tichy, A.M.: Nurses' perceptions of stressors in pediatric intensive care, J. Pediatr. Nurs. **2**(6):405-411, 1987.
Orsuto, Sr. J., and Corbo, B.H.: Approaches of health caregivers to young children in a pediatric intensive care unit, Matern. Child Nurs. J. **16**(2):157-175, 1987.
Proctor, D.L.: Relationship between visitation policy in a pediatric intensive care unit and parental anxiety, Child. Health Care **16**(1):13-17, 1987.
Rennick, J.: Reestablishing the parental role in a pediatric intensive care unit, J. Pediatr. Nurs. **1**(1):40-44, 1986.
Shonkwiler, M.A.: Sibling visits in the pediatric intensive care unit, Crit. Care Q. **8**(1):67-72, 1985.
Tse, A.M., Perez-Woods, R.C., and Opie, N.D.: Children's admissions to the intensive care unit: parents' attitudes and expectations of outcome, Child. Health Care **16**(2):68-75, 1987.
Wyckoff, P.M., and Erickson, M.T.: Mediating factors of stress on mothers of seriously ill, hospitalized children, Child. Health Care **16**(1):4-12, 1987.

SELECTED BOOKS FOR CHILDREN

Chase, F., and Coleman, L.: A visit to the hospital, New York, 1974, Grosset & Dunlap.
Clark B.: Pop-up going to the hospital, New York, 1970, Random House, Inc.
Collier, J.: Danny goes to the hospital, New York, 1970, W.W. Norton & Co., Inc.
Howe, J.: The hospital book, New York, 1981, Crown Publishers Inc.
Rey, M., and Rey, H.: Curious George goes to the hospital, New York, 1966, Houghton Mifflin Co.
Stein, S.: A hospital story, New York, 1974, Walker & Co.
Weber, A.: Elizabeth gets well, New York, 1970, Thomas Y. Crowell Co.

OTHER RESOURCES

Association for Care of Children's Health, 3615 Wisconsin Avenue, N.W., Washington, DC 20016.

Talks About the Hospital, a series written by Fred Rogers, is available from Family Communications, Inc., 4802 Fifth Avenue, Pittsburgh, PA 15213.

Bibliographies for children about health and illness are available from Pediatric Projects, Inc., P.O. Box 1880, Santa Monica, CA 90406.

An annotated list of books on various aspects of illness and hospitalization can be found in Fassler, J.: Helping children cope: mastering stress through books and stories, New York, 1978, The Free Press.

CHAPTER 21

Pediatric Variations of Nursing Interventions

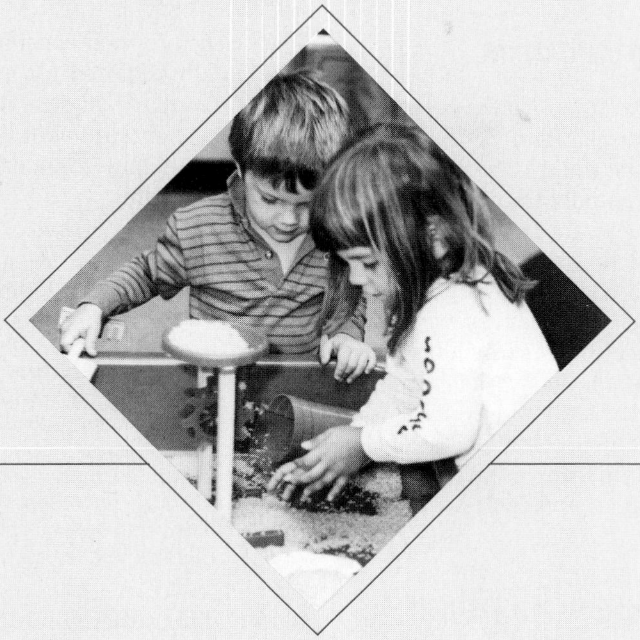

LEARNING OBJECTIVES

On completion of this chapter the reader will be able to:

- Identify those instances in which informed consent is required and in which minors may be considered emancipated
- Formulate general guidelines for preparing children for procedures, including surgery
- Implement uses of play in therapeutic procedures
- List general strategies for enhancing compliance in children and families
- Outline general hygiene and care procedures for hospitalized children
- Implement feeding techniques that encourage food and fluid intake
- Describe methods of reducing temperature in a febrile or hyperthermic child
- Describe the three systems that can be used for infection control
- Describe safe methods of administering oral, parenteral, rectal, optic, otic, and nasal medications to children
- Identify nursing responsibilities in maintaining fluid balance
- Demonstrate correct procedures for postural drainage and tracheostomy care
- Describe the procedures involved in providing nutrition via gavage, gastrostomy, and hyperalimentation
- Describe the procedures involved in administering an enema and ostomy care to children

Children are not simply small adults. They differ from their older counterparts in the areas of biologic, cognitive, and emotional function and response. Consequently many of the standard techniques employed in nursing practice must be altered to meet the special needs of children at various developmental stages. This chapter presents an overview of psychologic preparation of children for procedures, strategies to enhance compliance, application of principles of growth and development in planning, implementing, and evaluating nursing procedures, and selected aspects of skills that require modification in caring for infants and children.

◆ *Preparation for Procedures*

Children, regardless of their age, require preparation for procedures. With appropriate preparation the fear and discomfort are minimized and the child is helped to feel success and mastery from a potentially traumatic experience. However, nurses must be aware that a child's responses are strongly influenced by developmental characteristics, such as physical and cognitive abilities; environmental factors, including past experiences with hospitalization, procedures, and health personnel; and his perception of the present situation. The child's general temperament and behavior patterns should be assessed, as well as his condition and the degree of regression he has experienced as a result of his illness. All of these areas are considered in planning an approach best suited to the child as an individual.

INFORMED CONSENT FOR PROCEDURES

Informed consent refers to the legal and ethical requirement that the patient clearly, fully, and completely understand the medical treatment to be performed and all the risks, consequences, or results that may or may not occur from the medical treatment. The patient must also be informed of alternative treatments that could be offered, including their benefits and risks. For an informed consent to be valid, three conditions must be met (Hogue, 1986):

1. The person must be capable of giving consent; he must be over the age of majority and must be considered competent—that is, possess the mental capacity to make choices and understand their consequences.
2. The person must receive the information needed to make an intelligent decision.
3. The person must act voluntarily when exercising freedom of choice without force, fraud, deceit, duress, or other forms of constraint or coercion.

Because of the numerous variations of the laws within different regions of the United States, the following discussion of informed consent is presented in general terms and is not to be interpreted as legal advice. Although informing patients of the risks, benefits, and alternatives of a procedure is the physician's responsibility, nurses frequently are responsible for securing the person's signature on the consent form (Cushing, 1984). In caring for children special dilemmas may arise regarding who may sign the consent for treatment when parental consent is not available. The age of majority is especially important when caring for adolescents, and competence is a key issue in decisions involving minors who are retarded. Consequently, nurses need to be familiar with the issues involved in this highly significant and complex subject and must keep current on legal aspects of practice within their community.

Requirements for Obtaining Informed Consent

Written informed consent of the parent or legal guardian is usually required for medical or surgical treatment, including many diagnostic procedures. One blanket consent is not sufficient. Separate informed permissions must be obtained for each surgical or diagnostic procedure, including:

1. Major surgery
2. Minor surgery; for example, cutdown, biopsy, dental extraction, suturing a laceration (especially one that may have a cosmetic effect), removal of a cyst, and closed reduction of a fracture
3. Diagnostic tests with an element of risk; for example, bronchoscopy, needle biopsy, angiography, electroencephalogram, lumbar puncture, cardiac catheterization, ventriculography, and bone marrow aspiration
4. Medical treatments with an element of risk; for example, blood transfusion, thoracentesis or paracentesis, radiation therapy, and shock therapies

In addition, there are certain situations, such as the following, that are not directly related to medical treatment but that require parental consent:

1. Taking photographs for medical, educational, or other public use
2. Removal of the child from the hospital against the advice of the physician
3. Postmortem examinations, except in unexplained deaths, such as sudden infant death, violent death, or suspected suicide
4. Examination of medical records by unauthorized persons, such as attorneys or insurance representatives (family members have legal right to medical records)

The need for informed consent is also an issue in research involving children. While parents of minor children must give written informed consent, the researcher must also obtain *assent* from children with a mental age of 7 years or older. Informed assent, which refers to the child's express permission to participate in the research after the purposes and procedures have been explained, is not a legal requirement but an ethical one to protect the rights of children.

Eligibility for Giving Informed Consent

In most situations the parent or legal guardian gives informed consent. However, problems may arise when parents are not available to give informed consent, the child is a borderline or emancipated minor, or the parents neglect or refuse care for their minor children.

Informed consent of parents or legal guardian. Parents have been considered to have full responsibility for the care and rearing of their minor children, including legal control over them. Therefore as long as a child remains classified as a minor, the parent or the person designated as legal guardian for the child is required to give informed consent before medical treatment is implemented or any procedure is performed on the child. If the parents are legally divorced or separated, the custodial parent's consent is usually required.

Informed consent of persons other than parents or legal guardian. In the absence of the parents or legal guardian, a person in charge of the child is usually allowed to give informed consent for treatment. Depending on state law, this person, *in loco parentis*, may be a relative or other person who is caring for the child while the parents are away.

Temporary caregivers, such as school officials, camp counselors, neighbors, baby-sitters, foster parents, and court-appointed welfare workers, need written permission from parents for treatment in the event of an emergency. Special forms are available in many hospitals to authorize emergency care to minors. At the least these individuals should know the location of the parents and the child's home address to contact the persons able to give consent.

Oral informed consent. When the parent is not immediately available to sign a consent form, oral informed consent may be obtained. This may be a telephone consent or an oral consent from a parent who is for some reason unable to sign, such as because of an injury following an accident. When oral informed consent is being secured, it is wise to have a witness, such as another nurse, on a telephone extension. Both nurses can record that informed consent was given and the name, address, and relationship of the person giving consent, together with their signatures indicating that they witnessed the consent. As in any other situation, the nurse must be aware of state laws governing oral informed consent.

Informed consent of mature and emancipated minors. One of the areas in which modifications have been made in the usual view of parental obligation is in regard to borderline minors, that is, youngsters who are legally minors but who are considered to possess the maturity to give consent for their own medical care. Most states have enacted legislation that permits young people to give consent for their medical and surgical treatment.

An *emancipated minor* is one who is legally underage but is recognized as having the legal capacity of an adult under circumstances prescribed by state law. Minors may become emancipated by pregnancy, marriage, high school graduation, living independently, or military service.

The majority of states provide a specific statutory age (usually 15 or 16 years) at which a minor may consent to medical or surgical treatment without parental consent. In this case the child is known as a *mature minor* even though he is not considered emancipated (Leiken, 1983). Examples of medical conditions that can be treated without parental consent include sexually transmitted disease, pregnancy, drug or alcohol abuse, or life-threatening illness or injury. Consent regarding abortion is more complex. Although state laws vary, the U.S. Supreme Court has held that parents have no veto over a daughter's decision for an abortion.

State laws differ in their interpretation of when a child attains the age of majority. Even within the same state a child may be considered an adult in certain situations, for instance, in being responsible for necessities of life (food, clothing, and shelter) but may not be considered an adult in other situations. Many states now consider a child, male or female, an adult upon the eighteenth birthday. However, this may vary; some states may even differentiate between the sexes on attainment of maturity. Because the age of majority and definitions of emancipation vary within jurisdictions, nurses need to be aware of the way in which the law functions in their state regarding medical care to children.

Treatment without parental consent. Exceptions to requiring parental consent before treating minor children occur in situations in which children need prompt medical or surgical treatment and a parent is not readily available to give consent or refuses to give consent. Refusal to give consent can occur when the treatment, such as blood transfusions, conflicts with the parents' religious beliefs. All states recognize such exceptions and have statutory procedures to permit treatment if the life or health of such a minor is in jeopardy or if delayed treatment would create a risk to the health of the minor. The state is also able to intervene in situations that jeopardize the health and welfare of children, as in cases in which parents neglect or impose excessive or improper punishment on a child. In most communities there are procedures by which custody of the child can be transferred to a governmental or a private agency when parental neglect or abuse can be proved.

PHYSICAL PREPARATION FOR PROCEDURES

For most procedures no special physical preparation is needed. However, some procedures require physical preparation before the procedure, such as cleansing and shaving of the skin before surgery (see p. 630). One area of special concern is the administration of appropriate sedation and/or analgesia prior to stressful procedures. The drug is given before the procedure to allow time for the medication to reach its peak effect. Whenever possible, the intravenous (through an existing infusion), oral, or rectal route is used rather than the intramuscular route because children dislike injections. Some institutions are using short-acting anesthetics, such as ketamine, or potent analgesics, such as fentanyl, to eliminate the pain and trauma associated with treatments, such as bone marrow tests, lumbar punctures, burn debridement, and suturing (Forlini, Morin, and Treacy, 1987; Billmire, Neale, and Gregory, 1985).

PSYCHOLOGIC PREPARATION FOR PROCEDURES

The principles governing preparation for hospital procedures, such as diagnostic tests, medical treatments, surgery, and other therapeutic interventions, are similar and include the following:

1. Determine the details of the exact procedure to be performed
2. Review the parents' and child's present level of understanding
3. Plan the actual teaching based on the child's developmental age and existing level of knowledge
4. Incorporate parents in the teaching if they desire and especially if they plan to participate in the care
5. While preparing the child, allow for ample discussion to prevent information overload and ensure feedback

The exact timing of the preparation for a procedure varies with the child's age and the type of procedure. There are no exact guidelines to govern timing, but in general, the younger the child, the closer the explanation should be to the actual procedure to prevent undue fantasizing and worrying. With complex procedures more time may be needed for assimilation of information, especially with older children. For example, the explanation for an injection can immediately precede the procedure for all ages, but preparation for surgery may begin the day before for young children and a few days before for older children, although older children's preferences should be elicited.

In addition, certain guidelines apply to the actual preparation process and are discussed here. Specific suggestions for each age-group, based on developmental characteristics, are included in Table 21-1.

Establish Trust and Provide Support

The nurse who has spent time with and who has established a positive relationship with a child will usually find it easy to gain the child's cooperation. If the relationship is based on trust, the child will associate the nurse with caregiving activities that give him comfort and pleasure most of the time and not as someone who brings discomfort and stress. If the nurse does not know the child, it is best if she is introduced by another staff person whom the child trusts. The first visit with the child should not include any painful procedure and ideally should focus on the child first, then on the explanation of the procedure. When talking with the child, the nurse uses the same guidelines for communicating with children that are discussed in Chapter 6.

Parental support. Children need support during procedures, and for young children the greatest source of comfort is the parents. However, controversy exists regarding the role parents should assume during the procedure, especially if discomfort is involved. Health professionals have basically adopted two opposing philosophies in relation to parental presence during procedures. One view suggests that parents should not be present during stressful procedures as the child may blame the parent for allowing the discomfort to be inflicted on him. Since children normally associate parents with a comforting, "make it better" role, these professionals feel that parents should be a source of comfort and security to the child, which is best served by reuniting the child and parents after the procedure. However, others believe that not allowing the parents to be present inflicts the additional stress of separation on the child and deprives him of his parent's support. There is no consensus on whether parents who are present with the child should participate in the procedure, such as assisting in restraint.

While relatively little research has focused on this important issue, most of the available research provides evidence that parental presence is supportive (see also p. 630) and that most parents choose to participate, do not disrupt the procedure, and even when they find the experience difficult and stressful, are able to comfort their children (Savedra, 1981). Consequently, the parents' preferences for assisting, observing, or waiting outside the room should be assessed. Parents who wish to stay need preparation for what will occur and how they can help. Simple instructions, such as clarifying where parents can stay in the room and positioning them where they have eye contact with the child, provide reassurance and lessen anxiety. Parents who do not wish to be present or participate are supported in their decision and encouraged to remain close by so that they can be available to console the child immediately following the procedure.

Provide an Explanation

Children need an explanation for anything that involves them directly. Before performing a procedure, the nurse explains to the child what is to be done and what is expected of him. The explanation should be short, simple, and appropriate to the child's level of comprehension. Long explanations are not necessary and may only increase anxiety in a child. This is especially true regarding painful procedures. When explaining the procedure to parents with the child present, the nurse uses language appropriate to the child because unfamiliar words can be misunderstood. If the parents need additional preparation, this is done in an area away from the child. Teaching sessions are planned at times most conducive to the child's learning, for example, after a rest period, and for the usual span of attention.

Special equipment is not necessary for preparing a child, but for young children who cannot yet think in concepts, using objects to supplement verbal explanation is important. Allowing children to handle actual items that will be used in their care or comparing the strange equipment with familiar objects, such as likening a stethoscope to audio earphones, helps them to develop familiarity with these items and to reduce the threat often associated with their use. Miniature versions of hospital items such as gurneys and x-ray and intravenous equipment can be used to explain what the children can ex-

TABLE 21-1

Guidelines for Preparing Children for Procedures

Developmental Characteristics	Responsibilities
Infancy: Developing Trust	
Attachment to parent	*Involve parent in procedure if desired Keep parent in infant's line of vision If parent is unable to be with infant, place familiar object with infant, such as stuffed toy
Stranger anxiety	*Have usual caregivers perform or assist with procedure Make advances slowly and in nonthreatening manner *Limit number of strangers entering room during procedure
Sensorimotor phase of learning	During procedure use sensory soothing measures (e.g., stroking skin, talking softly, giving pacifier) *Use analgesics (e.g., local anesthetic, intravenous narcotic) to control discomfort Cuddle and hug child after stressful procedure; encourage parent to comfort child
Increased muscle control	Expect older infants to resist Restrain adequately Keep harmful objects out of reach
Memory for past experiences	Realize that older infants may associate objects or persons with prior painful experiences Keep in mind that older infants will cry and resist at sight of objects or persons that inflict pain *Keep frightening objects out of view *Perform painful procedures in a separate room, not in crib (or bed)
Imitation of gestures	Model desired behavior (e.g., opening mouth)
Toddler: Developing Autonomy	Use same approaches as above in addition to following:
Egocentric	Explain procedure in relation to what child will see, hear, taste, smell, and feel Emphasize those aspects of procedure that require cooperation, such as lying still Tell child it's okay to cry, yell, or use other means to verbally express discomfort
Negative behavior	Expect treatments to be resisted; child may try to run away Use firm, direct approach Ignore temper tantrums Use distraction techniques Restrain adequately
Limited language skills	Communicate using behaviors Use few and simple terms that are familiar to child Give one direction at a time, such as "Lie down" and then "Hold my hand" Use small replicas of equipment; allow child to handle equipment Use play; demonstrate on doll but avoid child's favorite doll as child may think doll is really "feeling" procedure Prepare parents separately to avoid child's misinterpreting words
Limited concept of time	Prepare child shortly or immediately before procedure Keep teaching sessions short (about 5 to 10 minutes) Have preparations completed before involving child in procedure Have extra equipment nearby (e.g., alcohol swabs, new needle, or Band-Aids) to avoid delays Tell child when procedure is completed
Striving for independence	Allow choices whenever possible but realize that child may still be resistant and negative Allow child to participate in care and to help whenever possible (e.g., drink medicine from a cup, hold a dressing)
Preschooler: Developing Initiative	
Preoperational thought; egocentric	Explain procedure in simple terms and in relation to how it affects child (as with toddler, stress sensory aspects) Demonstrate use of equipment Allow child to play with miniature or actual equipment Encourage "playing out" experience on a doll both before and after procedure to clarify misconceptions Use neutral words to describe the procedure (see box, p. 627)
Increased language skills	Use verbal explanation but avoid overestimating child's comprehension of words Encourage child to verbalize ideas and feelings
Concept of time and frustration tolerance still limited	Implement same approaches as for toddler but may plan longer teaching session (10 to 15 minutes); may divide information into more than one session

*Applies to any age.

Continued.

TABLE 21-1

Guidelines for Preparing Children for Procedures—cont'd

Developmental Characteristics	Responsibilities
Illness and hospitalization often viewed as punishment	Clarify why all procedures are performed, such as "This medicine will make you feel better" Ask child his thoughts regarding why a procedure is performed State directly that procedures are never a form of punishment
Fears of bodily harm, intrusion, and castration	Point out on drawing, doll, or child where procedure is performed Emphasize that no other body part will be involved Use nonintrusive procedures whenever possible (e.g., axillary temperatures, oral medication) Apply a Band-Aid over puncture site Realize that procedures involving genitals provoke anxiety Allow child to wear underpants with gown Explain unfamiliar situations, especially noises or lights
Striving for initiative	Involve child in care whenever possible (e.g., hold equipment, remove dressing) Give choices whenever possible but avoid excessive delays Praise child for helping and cooperating; never shame child for lack of cooperation
School-Age: Developing Industry	
Increased language skills; interest in acquiring knowledge	Explain procedures using correct scientific/medical terminology Explain reason for procedure using simple diagrams of anatomy and physiology Explain functioning and mechanism of equipment in concrete terms Allow child to manipulate equipment; use doll or another person as model to practice using equipment whenever possible (doll play may be considered "childish" by older school-age child) Allow time before and after procedure for questions and discussion
Improved concept of time	Plan for longer teaching sessions (about 20 minutes) Prepare in advance of procedure
Increased self-control	Gain child's cooperation Tell child what is expected Suggest ways of maintaining control (e.g., deep breathing, relaxation, counting)
Striving for industry	Allow responsibility for simple tasks, such as collecting specimens Include in decision making, such as time of day to perform procedure, preferred site Encourage active participation, such as removing dressings, handling equipment, opening packages
Developing relationships with peers	May prepare two or more children for same procedure or encourage one to help prepare another peer Provide privacy from peers during procedure to maintain self-esteem
Adolescents: developing identity	
Increasingly capable of abstract thought and reasoning	Supplement explanations with reasons why procedure is necessary or beneficial Explain long-term consequences of procedures Realize that adolescent may fear death, disability, or other potential risks Encourage questioning regarding fears, options, and alternatives
Conscious of appearance	Provide privacy Discuss how procedure may affect appearance, such as scar, and what can be done to minimize it Emphasize any physical benefits of procedure
Concerned more with present than future	Realize that immediate effects of procedure are more significant than future benefits
Striving for independence	Involve in decison making and planning, for example, choice of time, place, individuals present during procedure (such as parents), clothing to wear Impose as few restrictions as possible Suggest methods of maintaining control Accept regression to more childish methods of coping Realize that adolescent may have difficulty in accepting new authority figures and may resist complying with procedures
Developing peer relationships and group identity	Same as for school-age child but assumes even greater significance

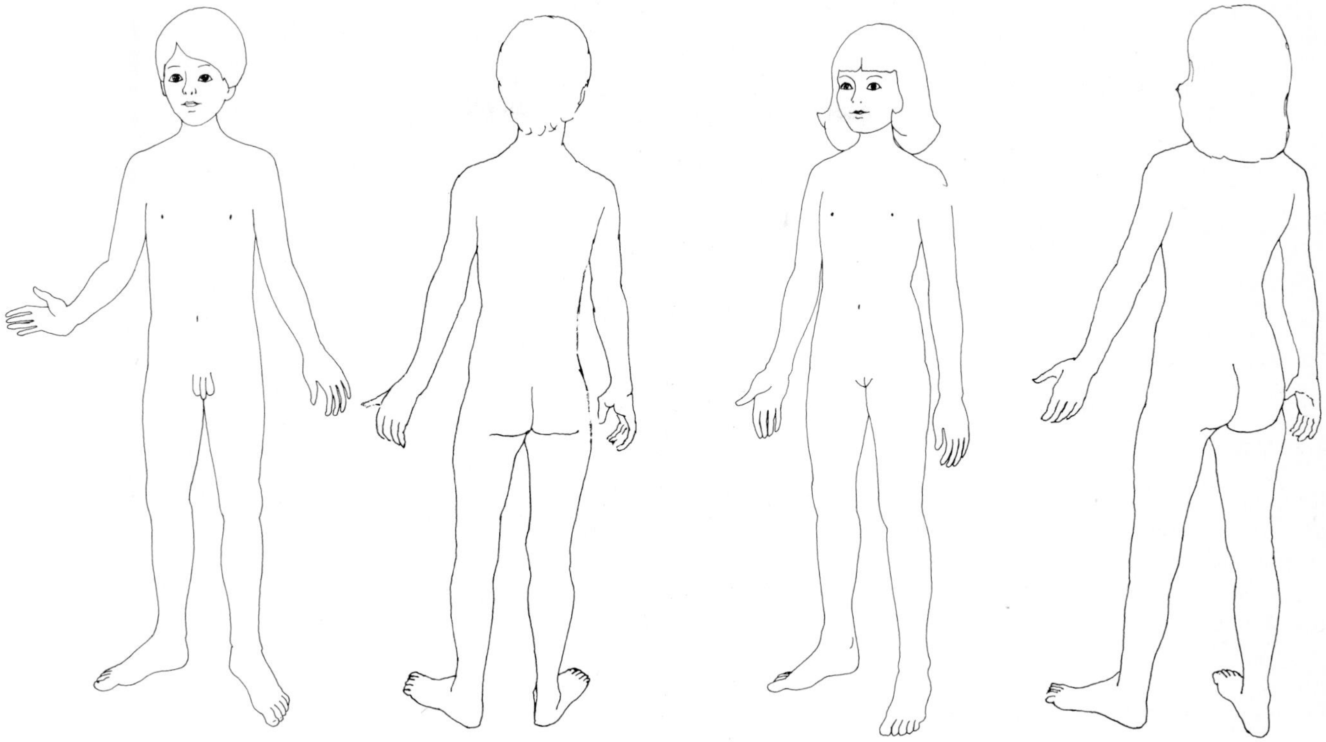

FIG. 21-1 Examples of line drawings to be used in preparing child for procedures.

pect and permit them to safely experience the situations that are unfamiliar and potentially frightening. Written and illustrated materials are also valuable aids to preparation.*

Although the precise words used to describe a procedure will vary for children in each age-group and for each specific event, the following general guidelines apply to any situation:

1. Use concrete, not abstract, terms and visual aids to describe the procedure. For example, use a simple line drawing of a boy or girl (Fig. 21-1) and mark the body part that will be involved in the procedure.
2. Emphasize that no other body part will be involved.
3. Use words appropriate to the child's level of understanding (a rule of thumb for number of words is the age in years plus 1).
4. Avoid words/phrases with dual meanings (see box) unless the child understands such words.
5. Clarify all unfamiliar words, such as "anesthesia is a *special* sleep."
6. Allow children to practice those procedures that will require their cooperation, such as turning, coughing, deep breathing, using a blow bottle or mask, or breathing on an intermittent positive pressure (IPPB) machine.
7. Emphasize the sensory aspects of the procedure—what the child will feel, see, smell, and touch and what he can do during the procedure, such as lie still, count out loud, squeeze a hand, or hug a doll.
8. If the body part is associated with a specific function, stress the change or noninvolvement of that ability, for

*Sources of preparatory materials are the You're gonna do what? series of diagnosis and treatment procedures, available from Arkansas Children's Hospital Companies, 1916 Maryland Ave., Little Rock, AR 72202; Talks about the hospital series by Fred Rogers, available from Family Communications, Inc., 4802 Fifth Ave., Pittsburgh, PA 15213; and Child care series—patient education for children, available from the Centering Corp., P.O. Box 3367, Omaha, NE 68103-0367.

Guidelines for Selecting Nonthreatening Words or Phrases

Words to Avoid	Suggested Substitutions
Shot, bee sting	Medicine under the skin
Organ	Special place in body
Test	See how ______ is working
Incision	Special opening
Fissure	Opening
Stretcher, gurney	Rolling bed
Stool	Child's usual term
Dye	Special medicine
Pain	Hurt, discomfort, "owie," "boo-boo"
Deaden	Numb, make sleepy
Cut, fix	Make better
Take (e.g., temperature)	See how warm you are
Put to sleep, anesthesia	Special sleep
Catheter	Tube
Monitor	TV screen
Specimen	Sample

example, following tonsillectomy, the child can still speak.

9. Introduce anxiety-laden information last, such as the preoperative injection.
10. Be honest with the child about the unpleasant aspects of a procedure but avoid creating undue concern. When discussing that a procedure may be uncomfortable, state that it feels different to different people and the child can tell you how it felt.
11. Emphasize the end of the procedure and any pleasurable events afterward, such as going home or seeing the parent. Stress the positive benefits of the procedure, for example, "After your tonsils are made better, you won't have as many sore throats."

PERFORMANCE OF PROCEDURE

Supportive care continues during the procedure and can be a major factor in a child's ability to cooperate and achieve mastery. Ideally the same nurse who explains the procedure should perform it or assist. Before the procedure is begun, all equipment is assembled and the room is readied to prevent unnecessary delays and interruptions that only serve to increase the child's anxiety. If at all possible, procedures should be performed in a special treatment room rather than the child's bedroom. Procedures should never be performed in "safe" areas, such as the playroom. If the procedure is lengthy, conversation that could be misinterpreted by the child is avoided. As the procedure is nearing completion, the nurse should inform the child that it is almost over.

Expect Success

Nurses who approach children with confidence and who convey the impression that they expect to be successful are less likely to encounter difficulty. It is best to approach children as though they are expected to cooperate. Children sense anxiety in another and will respond to a perceived threat by striking out or with active resistance. Although it is not possible to eliminate such behavior in every child, a firm approach with a positive attitude on the part of the nurse tends to convey a feeling of security to most children.

Involve the Child

As in any other aspect of care, involving children helps to gain their cooperation. Permitting them to make choices gives them some measure of control. However, a choice is given only in situations in which one is available. To ask a child, "Do you want to take your medicine now?" or "I'm going to give you an injection now, okay?" leads him to believe that there is an option and provides him with the opportunity to legitimately refuse or delay the medication. This places the nurse in an awkward, if not impossible, position. It is much better to state firmly, "It's time to drink your medicine now." Children usually like to make choices, but the choice must be one that they do indeed have, for example, "It's time for your medicine. Do you want to drink it plain or with a little water?"

Many children respond to tactics that appeal to their maturity or courage. This also gives them a sense of participation and achievement. For example, preschool children will be proud that they can hold the dressing during the procedure or remove the tape. The same is true for the school-age child who cooperates with a minimum of resistance.

Provide Distraction

When children are occupied with some activity that interests them, they are less likely to focus on the procedure. For example, when an injection is given, it is helpful to give the child something to do or something on which to focus his attention. For example, asking the child to point the toes inward and wiggle them not only helps relax the gluteal muscles but provides a diversion. Other strategies for diverting attention are to have the child tightly squeeze the hands of a parent or an assistant, count aloud, sing a familiar song such as a nursery rhyme, or verbally express his discomfort. Other interventions that may lessen the discomfort are relaxation, imagery, and cutaneous stimulation (see box, p. 598).

When speaking to a child during an anxiety-provoking procedure, the nurse should speak quietly and directly into the child's ear. Speaking loudly, or (worse) shouting, has very little impact and can add to the child's stress. The calm voice usually causes the child to quiet down in an attempt to hear the person's message.

Allow Expression of Feelings

The child should be allowed to express feelings of anger, anxiety, fear, frustration, or any other emotion. It is natural for children to strike out in frustration or to try to avoid stress-provoking situations. The child needs to know that it is all right to cry. Whatever the response, it is important that the nurse accept the behavior for what it is. Telling a child with limited verbal skills, such as a toddler, to stop kicking, biting, or otherwise expressing his frustration conveys to him that he is not being understood. Behavior is his primary means of communication and coping and should be permitted unless it inflicts harm on the child or those caring for him.

POSTPROCEDURAL SUPPORT

After the procedure the child continues to need reassurance that he performed well and is accepted and loved. If the parents did not participate, the child is united with them as soon as possible so that they can comfort him.

Encourage Expression of Feelings

Some planned activity after the procedure is helpful in encouraging expression of feelings in a constructive way.

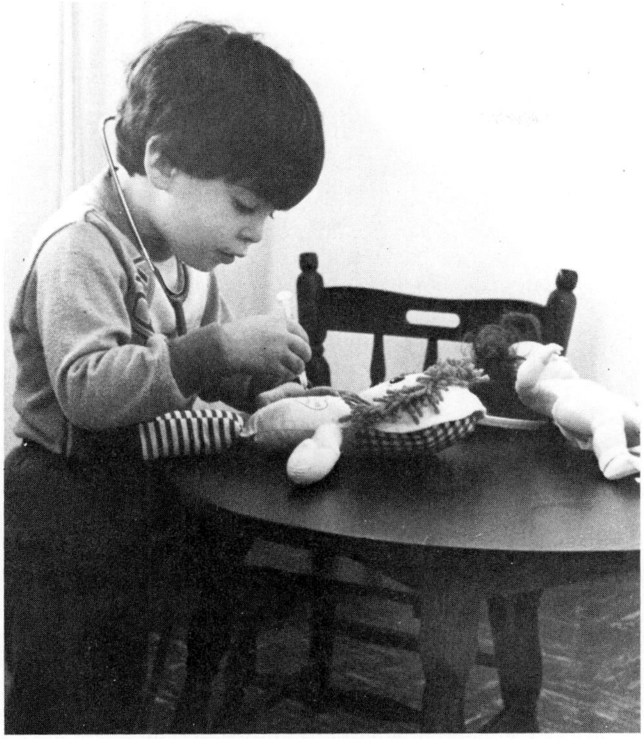

FIG. 21-2 Needle play provides a child with the opportunity to play out fears and concerns.

For verbal children, reviewing the details of the procedure can help clarify misconceptions (see Therapeutic dialogue, p. 615) and provide feedback for improving the nurse's preparatory strategies. Play is an excellent activity for all children. Infants and young children are given the opportunity for gross motor movement. Older children can vent their anger and frustration in acceptable pounding or throwing activities. Play-Doh is a remarkably versatile medium for pounding and shaping. Dramatic play provides an outlet for anger and places the child in a position of control, in contrast to his position of helplessness in the real situation. One of the most effective interventions is therapeutic play, which includes activities such as permitting the child to give a "shot" to a doll or stuffed toy to reduce the stress of injections (Fig. 21-2).

Praise Child

The child needs to hear from others that they know that he did the best he could in the situation—no matter how he behaved. It is important for the child to know that his worth is not being judged on the basis of his behavior in a stressful situation. Reward systems, such as earning stars or tokens or saving the empty medicine cup as evidence of achievement, are often helpful. Children who require distasteful medications or injections over a period of time can look with pride on a series of stars or stickers on a calendar, especially if an accumulated number represents a special privilege or reward.

Returning to the child a short while after the procedure helps the nurse to strengthen a supportive relationship. Relating with the child in a relaxed and nonstressful period allows him to see the nurse not only as someone associated with stressful situations but as someone with whom to share pleasurable experiences as well.

PREPARATION FOR SURGERY

Some of the most traumatic procedures for children involve surgery. Both the psychologic and physical aspects of care are significant in the child's adjustment and recovery. Although procedures related to surgery differ according to the type of surgery, the following is an overview of general nursing interventions.

Psychologic Preparation

In general, psychologic preparation is similar to that discussed for any procedure and may employ many of the same techniques used in preparing a child for hospitalization, such as films, books, play, and tours. However, there are some important differences. Even though children are asleep for the actual surgical intervention, they are subjected to numerous preoperative and postoperative procedures, which require a series of preparatory sessions to prevent overstressing the child with too much information. The following six stress points before and after surgery have been identified as being significant in terms of causing anxiety (Visintainer and Wolfer, 1975): (1) admission, (2) the blood test, (3) afternoon of the day before surgery, (4) injection of preoperative medication, (5) before and during transport to the operating room, and (6) return from the recovery room.

Psychologic intervention consisting of systematic preparation, rehearsal of the forthcoming events, and supportive care at each of these points has been shown to be more effective than a single-session preparation (which is a common method of preoperative preparation) or consistent supportive care without systematic preparation and rehearsal. Play is always an effective strategy in preparing children, and increased familiarity with medical procedures decreases anxiety.

Another stress often imposed on the child undergoing surgery is that more than one nurse is often responsible for different aspects of care. Although the same supportive nurse should remain with the child through as many of the procedures as possible, the child may have other nurses, especially if he returns to a special care unit postoperatively. However, joint planning of care between the various nursing staffs, such as in pediatrics and the recovery room, can overcome some of the disadvantages of unfamiliar nurses caring for the child. Many hospitals have surgical tours for children and parents to familiarize them with the strange environment and to introduce them to other individuals who will be involved in their care.

Special fears are often associated with surgery that are not present with other procedures. One special fear is of anesthesia. Children under 5 years of age primarily worry about what will happen when they wake up, such as where they will be and who will be with them. Showing youngsters the recovery room whenever possible, telling them where their parents will visit them after surgery, and encouraging the parents to be with the children as soon as possible after surgery decrease these fears. School-age children fear the anesthesia itself. Seeing the mask and learning how the "gas" or "medicine" works help minimize their concerns. Children about age 9 years and older fear the anesthesia, the operation itself, and possible death. They may ask, "Will I wake up?" or "What happens if I don't wake up?" Adolescents share these concerns, with a special anxiety for change in body image. They fear the loss of control while under anesthesia, both in terms of their behavior and for their body integrity. Reassuring them that only what is supposed to be done will be performed is essential.

Because anesthesia is a type of sleep, children often supply their own definitions to this concept. Children worry about whether they will awaken during the procedure and how the doctor knows when to awaken them. Stressing that anesthesia is a "special sleep," caused by the mask and gas or medicine that is controlled by a special person, called the anesthesiologist, is important in minimizing children's fear-provoking fantasies.

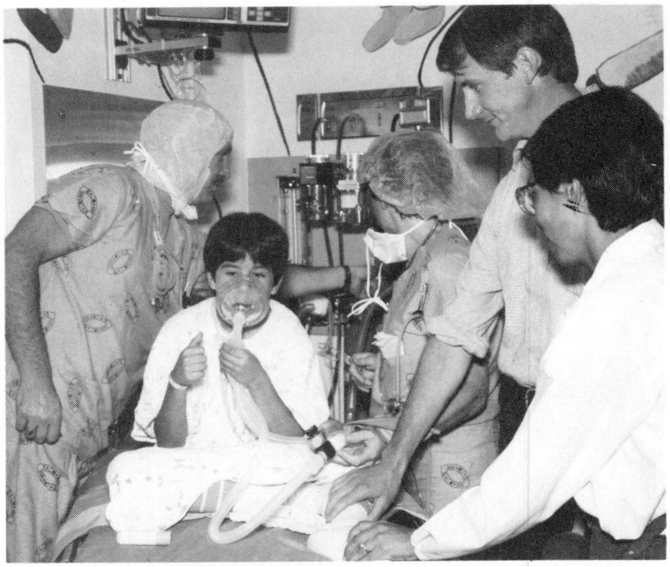

FIG. 21-3 Parental presence during induction of anesthesia can minimize the child's and parents' anxiety during the preoperative period.

Preoperative Care

Besides psychologic preparation, children usually require various types of physical care before surgery, such as those procedures listed in the nursing care plan. Infants require special attention to fluid needs. They should not be without oral fluids for an extended period and should receive carbohydrates in an oral mixture until 3 hours preoperatively to avoid glycogen depletion and dehydration.

Although most of the preoperative care procedures are routine, nurses should keep in mind that they can be anxiety provoking for children and parents. For example, for young children, having to wear a loose-fitting hospital gown without the security of underpants or pajama bottoms can be traumatic. The most upsetting event for children is generally the preoperative injection. Unfortunately, little research has been done on the value of this practice, but there is evidence to suggest that the injection does little to relieve anxiety in adult patients (Catchpole, 1984). Also, the commonly used combination of meperidine (Demerol), promethazine (Phenergan), and chlorpromazine (Thorazine) (known as "DPT") actually has antianalgesic properties (Ros, 1987). Sedation and/or analgesia can be produced with oral or rectal drug administration or with intravenous administration through an existing parenteral line.

Like the preoperative injection, the practice of separating the child and parent before the child enters the surgical unit has been accepted as standard policy. However, there is no theoretical basis for the practice, since the effects of separation on children are well known. In addition, parents are able to support their child and the child has less anxiety when parents remain until induction of anesthesia is under way, thus minimizing or eliminating the need for preoperative sedation (Fig. 21-3) (Hannallah and Rosales, 1983).

Postoperative Care

After surgical procedures, various psychologic and physical interventions are important to facilitate the child's optimum recovery. Ideally, the child should be reunited with the parents as soon as possible after awakening from anesthesia. Whenever possible, the parents should be allowed in the post-anesthesia recovery unit to be with the child.

Several observations are required to prevent or minimize possible untoward effects from anesthesia and the surgical procedure (see Nursing care plan). Although most of these interventions are prescribed by physicians, it is the nurse's responsibility to exercise judgment in their implementation. For example, vital signs are taken as frequently as necessary until they are stable. Each vital sign is evaluated in terms of side effects from anesthesia and possible shock.

Providing comfort is a major nursing responsibility after surgery. Pain is assessed and analgesics are administered to provide comfort and to facilitate the child's cooperation with postoperative procedures, such as ambulating, coughing, and deep breathing. Routinely scheduled analgesics, rather than p.r.n. orders, afford more satisfactory pain control (see pp. 597 to 599). Mouth care is an-

Text continued on p. 636.

NURSING CARE PLAN

The Child Undergoing Surgery

Preoperative Care

Nursing Goals	Nursing Interventions	Expected Patient/Family Outcomes
HP-HMP* **Potential for injury** **Etiology: surgical procedure**		
Ensure legal authorization	Check chart for signed informed consent form Obtain informed consent Contact physician to determine if parents have been informed of procedure (informed consent is physician's responsibility) Obtain and/or witness signature if not obtained earlier	†Appropriate permissions are obtained
Provide hygienic preparation	Bathe child, groom hair Provide mouth care Check for loose teeth Inform anesthesiologist if detected Cleanse operative site according to prescribed method, if ordered	Child is cleansed and prepared appropriately (specify)
Provide physical preparation	Attire child appropriately (e.g., special operating room gown) Allow child to wear underwear or pajama bottoms, if possible Label personal articles and clothing Remove any makeup and/or nail polish (to observe for cyanosis) Remove jewelry and/or prosthetic devices (e.g., mouth retainers)	Child is prepared appropriately (specify)
Prevent complications	Maintain child NPO (nothing by mouth) usually 12 hours before surgery (prevents aspiration from vomiting during anesthesia [gag reflex is depressed]; last feeding indicated by physician) Infants NPO 2-4 hours Be sure child is well hydrated before NPO begins, especially infants Take and record vital signs Report any deviations from admission readings, especially elevated temperature, which may indicate infection	Child is NPO for designated time preoperatively
	Have child void before preoperative medication is administered to prevent bladder distention or incontinence during anesthesia Record time of last voiding if unable to void	Child voids
	Be certain allergies are clearly indicated on chart Check laboratory values for any sign of systemic abnormality, such as infection (increased white blood cells), anemia (decreased hemoglobin and/or hematocrit), or bleeding tendencies (reduced platelets or prolonged bleeding or clotting time	Pertinent information about child is visible
	Be certain physical preparation is completed	†Child is physically prepared
Ensure safety	Ascertain that identification band is securely fastened Check identification band with surgical personnel Fasten side rails of bed or crib Use restraints during transport by use of stretcher (or other conveyance) Do not leave child unattended Explain what is happening, unless child is asleep	Child is safe from immediate harm

*For an explanation of abbreviations, see p. 20.
†Nursing outcome.

Continued.

NURSING CARE PLAN

The Child Undergoing Surgery—cont'd

Preoperative Care—cont'd

Nursing Goals	Nursing Interventions	Expected Patient/Family Outcomes
SP-SCP Anxiety/fear **Etiology: separation from support system, unfamiliar environment, knowledge deficit**		
Increase child's sense of security	Institute preoperative teaching Orient child to strange surroundings Explain where parents will be while child is in operating room	Child demonstrates minimum insecurity or anxiety
Prepare child and parents for expected surgical procedure and postoperative care	Prepare for postoperative procedures, as indicated, such as nasogastric tube, intravenous fluids, nothing by mouth, dressing changes, and wound drains if necessary Explain reason for surgery; if bowel diversion is to be performed, explain basic principle of ostomy and brief outline of bowel care Explain all preoperative procedures, such as blood work, nasogastric tube, bowel preparation, and any other laboratory test In emergency situation, explain most essential components of surgery, such as where child will be before and after surgery, anesthesia, and dressing on abdomen	Child and family demonstrate an understanding of forthcoming events (specify methods of learning and evaluation)
	Accept behavioral reactions of parents and child	†Family's behavioral reactions are accepted and supported
Achieve optimum relaxation and sedation before child arrives in operating room	Place child in quiet room with minimal distraction Do not leave child unattended Explain what is happening, unless child is asleep Encourage parents to stay with child as long as permitted Permit parent to hold child until he falls asleep, if desired Encourage parents to accompany child as far as possible, preferably through induction of anesthesia Allow for significant objects to accompany child (e.g., a favorite toy)	Child falls asleep or lies quietly Child is not left alone
RRP Altered family processes **Etiology: child who is undergoing a surgical procedure**		
Keep family informed	Explain preparation procedures Direct family to appropriate waiting area Be available to family	Family complies with directives (specify)
HP-HMP Potential for injury **Etiology: surgical procedure, anesthesia**		
Prepare room and bedside area to receive child on return from surgery	Collect needed equipment for assessment and recording (e.g., record sheets, IV pole, restraints, thermometer, BP apparatus, etc.) Turn down covers or prepare surgical bed as appropriate	Room is prepared to receive child
Admit to room	Place child in bed (unless transported in own bed or crib) Hang IV and connect any needed equipment (e.g., suction apparatus, traction) Place in position of comfort in accordance with surgeon's orders	Child is transferred to bed with minimum stress

†Nursing outcome.

NURSING CARE PLAN

The Child Undergoing Surgery—cont'd

Postoperative Care—cont'd

Nursing Goals	Nursing Interventions	Expected Patient/Family Outcomes
Acquire baseline information	Take vital signs, including BP; keep BP cuff in place, deflated in order to lessen amount of disturbance to child Take and record more frequently if any value fluctuates Inspect operative area Check dressing if present Outline any bleeding area on dressing or cast with pen Reinforce, but do not remove, loose dressing Observe areas below surgical site for blood that may have drained toward bed Assess for bleeding and other symptoms in areas not covered with a dressing, such as throat following tonsillectomy Assess skin color and characteristic Assess level of consciousness, activity Notify physician of any irregularities	†Child's baseline status is determined Vital signs are within expected limits for age (see inside front cover); skin is pink and dry Operative area is clean and intact Child responds appropriately (for age) when stimulated; is not unduly agitated
Monitor physiologic status	Monitor vital signs as ordered Check dressings for bleeding or other abnormalities Check bowel sounds Report any deviations from normal	†Alterations in physical status are determined early and interventions initiated
Detect early signs of complications	Observe for signs of shock, abdominal distention	Complications are detected and reported
Prevent other complications	Ambulate as prescribed Maintain child NPO until fully awake Assess for bladder distention Encourage to void when awake Offer bedpan Boys may be allowed to stand at bedside Notify physician if unable to void	Child does not exhibit signs of complications
Observe for signs of dehydration	Record all output (urinary, stool, vomiting, nasogastric) and input (intravenous, oral if allowed, and nasogastric irrigant); notify physician of marked discrepancies	Child remains well hydrated
HP-HMP	**Potential for infection** **Etiology: presence of infective organisms**	
Prevent wound infection	Use proper hand washing techniques, especially if wound drainage is present Change dressings if indicated, whenever soiled; carefully dispose of soiled dressings Pin diapers below abdominal dressing to prevent contamination Report any unusual appearance or drainage Carry out special wound care as prescribed: irrigation, drain care, etc.	No signs of wound infection are evident
Detect presence of infection	Take vital signs every 2-4 hours Collect or request needed specimens Inspect wound for signs of infection—redness, swelling, heat, pain, purulent drainage	†Evidence of infection is detected early and appropriate interventions implemented

†Nursing outcome.

Continued.

NURSING CARE PLAN

The Child Undergoing Surgery—cont'd

Postoperative Care—cont'd

Nursing Goals	Nursing Interventions	Expected Patient/Family Outcomes
Prevent respiratory complications	Assess need for pain medication before respiratory hygiene Assist to turn, cough, deep breathe Splint operative site with hand or pillow if possible before coughing Stimulate infant to cry Assist with use of spirometer or blow bottle Perform percussion and vibration, if indicated Suction secretions if needed	Lungs remain clear
N-MP Potential fluid volume deficit **Risk factors: NPO prior to and/or after surgery, loss of appetite, vomiting**		
Promote adequate hydration	Monitor intravenous infusion (if any) Offer fluids as soon as ordered or child tolerates Start with small sips of water and advance as tolerated Avoid brown- or red-colored fluids (to distinguish old and fresh blood from oral fluids) in oral or abdominal surgery Encourage to drink Tempt with favorite fluids	Child exhibits no evidence of dehydration Child takes and retains fluid when allowed (specify)
CPP Pain **Etiology: surgical incision**		
Provide comfort measures	Assess need for pain medication (see p. 587) Implement appropriate nonpharmacologic pain reduction techniques (see p. 598) Monitor effectiveness of interventions Avoid palpating the abdomen unless necessary Insert rectal tube, if indicated Encourage to void, if appropriate Administer mouth care Lubricate nostril to decrease irritation from nasogastric tube, if present Allow the child position of comfort if not contraindicated Perform procedures (e.g., dressing change, deep breathing) after administering analgesics	Child rests quietly and exhibits minimum evidence of pain (specify)
SP-SCP Anxiety/fear **Etiology: separation from support system unfamiliar environment, discomfort**		
Relieve anxiety in child and parents	Maintain calm, reassuring manner Explain procedures and other activities before initiating Answer questions and explain purposes of activities Keep informed of progress	Child rests quietly and calmly Discusses procedures and activities without evidence of anxiety
Provide reassurance	Remain with child as much as possible Explain activities and procedures Give encouragement and positive feedback for cooperation in care See also The child in the hospital, p. 603 Encourage parental visiting as soon as child is awake If emergency procedure, review child's memory of previous events	

†Nursing outcome.

NURSING CARE PLAN

The Child Undergoing Surgery—cont'd

Postoperative Care—cont'd

Nursing Goals	Nursing Interventions	Expected Patient/Family Outcomes
RRP Altered family processes **Etiology: situational crisis (emergency hospitalization of child), knowledge deficit**		
Support and reassure child and family	Explain all procedures Prepare child and family for surgery Keep family informed of child's progress Encourage expression of feelings Review child's memory of events, if an emergency procedure Refer to public health nurse if indicated Refer to appropriate agency or persons for specific help (e.g., social service, clergy) See also Family of the hospitalized child p. 610.	Family discusses child's condition and therapies comfortably Family demonstrates an awareness of child's progress (specify method of evaluation) Family members avail themselves of appropriate assistance
Instruct family regarding home care		
Wound care	If dressing changes are required at home, teach parents sterile or aseptic procedures; provide written list of necessary equipment and instructions	Family demonstrates an understanding of instructions (specify methods of learning and evaluation)
Administration of medications	Instruct parents regarding administration of medications (if ordered)	
Special procedures	Instruct parents in care and management of special procedures such as ostomy care, irrigations	

Nursing interventions related to medical management

Preoperative

Assist with diagnosis
- Obtain history, if appropriate
- Order or collect necessary specimens
  - Collect urine specimens
  - Order blood work

Anticipate possible surgery (if in doubt)
- Administer analgesics cautiously (if ordered) to prevent masking of symptoms
- Initiate nothing by mouth
- Collect and order needed specimens
- Relieve discomfort
  - Administer analgesics as prescribed
  - Record effectiveness of analgesics

Assist in preparing bowel for surgery (if indicated)
- Administer colonic enemas as ordered, using only saline solution
- Administer antibiotics as ordered, observing for known side efects
- Order and/or assist with special tests such as radiographs

Prevent complications
- Consult with physician for appropriate change in schedule or route of administration of any medication child ordinarily receives

Achieve relaxation
- Administer preoperative sedation (preferably oral), as ordered

Provide information needed
- Make certain the following procedures have been performed and evidence is in chart
  - Urinalysis
  - Blood work such as blood count, bleeding and clotting times, and type and cross-match, if ordered
  - Radiographs
  - Electrocardiogram
  - Note by anesthesiologist

Postoperative

Determine specifics of care
- Review surgeon's orders after completing initial assessment
- Perform stat (immediate) activities

Prevent abdominal distention
- Maintain abdominal decompression as ordered
  - Assess and ensure patency of nasogastric tube; irrigate with normal saline solution as indicated
  - Maintain intermittent suction at appropriate negative pressure

Relieve discomfort
- Administer analgesics prescribed
- Administer antiemetics as ordered
- Monitor effectiveness of analgesics

Provide for hydration
- Monitor intravenous infusion at prescribed rate
  - Attach pediatric intravenous apparatus if not done in operating room
  - Begin oral intake as ordered

Provide for nutrition
- Feed diet as ordered
- Advance as appropriate

Facilitate wound healing
- When child begins oral feedings, provide nutritious diet as ordered
- Careful wound care
  - Keep wound clean and dry
  - Cleanse with prescribed preparation (if ordered)
  - Apply antibacterial solutions and/or ointments as ordered

Prevent infection or eradicate organisms
- Administer antibiotics as prescribed

other important aspect of care, since most children are allowed nothing orally until bowel sounds return (see p. 670).

Since respiratory infections are a potential complication, every effort is taken to aerate the lungs and remove secretions. The lungs are auscultated regularly to identify abnormal sounds or any areas of diminished or absent breath sounds. Early signs of respiratory involvement are abnormal rate, shallow depth, and cough. These findings are reported immediately. To prevent hypostatic pneumonia, respiratory excursion can be encouraged with incentive spirometers or other motivating activities (see p. 637). If these measures are presented as games, the child is more likely to comply. The child's position is changed every 2 hours, and coughing is encouraged (see Nursing tip).

Nursing Tip: Coughing

Because coughing is usually painful after surgery, have the child splint the operative site (depending on its location) by hugging a small pillow or a favorite stuffed animal.

During the recovery period the nurse should spend time with the child to assess his perception of surgery. Play, drawing, and story telling are excellent methods of discovering the child's thoughts. With such information the nurse can support or correct his perceptions and assist the child in achieving mastery for having endured a stressful procedure (see Therapeutic dialogue, p. 615).

USE OF PLAY IN PROCEDURES

The use of play is an integral part of relationships with children, and, as such, its value in specific situations is discussed throughout this book, such as in Chapter 20 in relation to hospitalization. Many institutions have very elaborate and well-organized play areas and programs under the direction of child-life specialists, while other institutions have limited facilities and rely on families to provide the bulk of play materials. However, no matter what the institution provides for children, nurses can still include play activities as part of nursing care. Play can be used to teach, for expression of feelings, or as a method to achieve a therapeutic goal. Consequently, it should be included in preparing children for and encouraging their cooperation during procedures. Play sessions after procedures can be structured, such as directed toward needle play, or general, with a wide variety of equipment available for children to play with. Even "routine" procedures such as temperature taking and oral administration of medication may be of concern to children. The box on p. 637 presents suggestions for incorporating play into nursing procedures and activities for the hospitalized child that facilitate learning and adjustment to a new situation.

◆ *Compliance*

Compliance refers to the extent to which the patient's behavior in terms of taking medication, following diets, or executing other life-style changes coincides with the prescribed regimen. Estimates of noncompliance in children with chronic diseases may be as high as 88% (Rapoff and Christophersen, 1982). Since nurses are frequently responsible for teaching families about treatment protocols, they must have knowledge of factors that influence compliance, methods to measure compliance, and strategies to enhance adherence to prescribed treatment.

ASSESSMENT OF COMPLIANCE

In developing strategies to provide compliance, the nurse must first assess factors that influence compliance in the patient. Since many children are too young to assume partial or total responsibility for their care, parents are usually the primary caregivers in terms of home management. Consequently, the nurse needs to assess their ability to carry out instructions. The first approach to assessment is knowledge of those factors that influence compliance and the second is to apply methods to more objectively assess compliance.

Several factors influence compliance (see box), although there are no sets of characteristics to predict who will or will not comply. Basically, any aspect of the health care environment that increases the family's satisfaction with the care they are receiving positively influences adherence to the treatment regimen. However, the more complex, expensive, inconvenient, and disruptive the treatment protocol, the less likely the family is to comply. Long-term conditions that involve multiple treatments

Factors That Positively Influence Compliance

Individual/family factors
High self-esteem
Positive body image
High degree of autonomy (increased locus of control)
Supportive and well-adjusted family
Effective family communication
Family expectation for successful completion of therapy
Care setting factors
Perceived satisfaction with care
Positive interactions with practitioners
Continuity of care
Individualized care
Minimum waiting time for appointments
Convenient care setting
Treatment factors
Simple
Minimum disruption in usual life-style
Short duration
Inexpensive
Visible benefits
Tolerable side effects

Play Activities for Specific Procedures

Fluid Intake
Make freezer pops using child's favorite juice
Cut Jell-O into fun shapes
Make game of taking sip when turning page of book or in games like "Simon Says"
Use small medicine cups; decorate the cups
Color water with food coloring or Kool Aid
Have tea party; pour at small table
Let child fill a syringe and squirt it into his mouth or use it to fill small decorated cups
Cut straws in half and place in small container (much easier for child to suck liquid)
Decorate straw—cut out small design with two holes and pass straw through; place small sticker on straw
Use a "crazy" straw
Make a "progress poster"; give rewards for drinking a predetermined quantity

Deep Breathing
Blow bubbles with bubble blower
Blow bubbles with straw (no soap)
Blow on pinwheel, feathers, whistle, harmonica, balloons, toy horns
Practice band instruments
Draw face on rubber glove to expand when blown up
Have blowing contest using balloons, boats, cotton balls, feathers, marbles, Ping-Pong balls, pieces of paper; blow such objects on a table top over a goal line, over water, through an obstacle course, up in the air, against an opponent, or up and down a string
Suck paper or cloth from one container to another using a straw
Use blow bottles with colored water to transfer water from one side to the other
Dramatize stories, as "I'll huff and puff and blow your house down" from the Three Little Pigs
Do straw blowing painting
Take a deep breath and "blow out the candles" on a birthday cake

Range of Motion and Use of Extremities
Throw bean bags at fixed or movable target, wadded paper into wastebasket
Touch or kick mylar balloons held or hung in different positions (if child is in traction, hang balloon from trapeze)
Play "tickle toes"; wiggle them on request
Play Twister game or "Simon Says"
Play pretend and guess games, such as imitate a bird, butterfly, horse
Have tricycle or wheelchair races in safe area
Play kick or throw ball with soft foam ball in safe area
Position bed so that child must turn to view television or doorway
Climb wall like "spider"
Pretend to teach "aerobic" dancing or exercises; encourage parents to participate
Encourage swimming, if feasible
Play video games or pinball (fine motor movement)
Play "hide and seek" game—hide toy somewhere in bed (or room, if ambulatory) and have child find using specified hand or foot
Provide clay to mold with fingers
Paint or draw on large sheets of paper placed on floor or wall
Encourage combing own hair; play "beauty shop" with "customer" in different positions

Soaks
Play with small toys or objects (cups, syringes, soap dishes) in water
Wash dolls or toys
Bubbles may be added to bath water if permissible; move bubbles to create shapes or "monsters"
Pick up marbles, pennies* from bottom of bath container
Make designs with coins on bottom of container
Pretend to make a boat or submarine by keeping it immersed
Have "Instant Products"† (a capsule filled with a design that when immersed in warm water dissolves and foam rubber animals or other surprises appear) for child over age 3 years
Read to child during soaks, sing with child, or play game, such as cards, checkers, or other board game (if both hands are immersed, move the board pieces for the child)
Sitz bath—give child something to listen to (music, stories) or look at (Viewmaster, book, etc.)

Injections
Let child handle syringe, vial, alcohol swab and give an injection to doll or stuffed animal
Use syringes to decorate cookies with frosting, squirt paint, or target shoot into a container
Draw a "magic circle" on area before injection; draw smiling face in circle after injection
Allow child to have a "collection" of syringes (without needles); make "wild" creative objects with syringes
If multiple injections or venipunctures, make a "progress poster;" give rewards for predetermined number of injections

Ambulation
Give child something to push
- Toddler—push-pull toy
- School age—wagon or decorated IV
- Teenage—a baby in a stroller or wheelchair

Have a parade—make hats, drums, etc.

Extending Environment (patients in traction, etc.)
Make bed into a pirate ship or airplane with decorations
Put up mirrors so patient can see around room
Move patient's bed frequently, especially to playroom, hallway, or outside

*Small objects such as marbles or coins are unsafe for young children.
†Instant Products, Inc., P.O. Box 33068, Louisville, KY 40232.

and considerable rearrangement of life-style most severely affect compliance.

While it is helpful to know those factors that influence compliance, assessment must include more direct measurement techniques. A number of methods exist, although no one method is totally reliable. The most successful approach combines at least two of the following methods:

self-reporting The family is asked about their ability to carry out the prescribed treatments, although most people overestimate their compliance.
direct observation The nurse directly observes the patient

or family perform the treatment. This method is difficult to employ outside the health care setting, and the family's awareness of being observed frequently affects their performance.

monitoring appointments The family's attendance at scheduled appointments is recorded, although this method only indirectly indicates compliance with the prescribed care.

monitoring therapeutic response The child's response in terms of benefit from treatment is monitored, preferably recorded on a graph or chart. Unfortunately, few treatments yield directly measurable results.

pill counts The nurse counts the number of pills remaining in the original container and compares the amount missing to the number of days the medication should have been taken. Although this is a simple method, families may forget to bring the container or deliberately alter the number of pills to avoid detection. This method is also poorly suited to liquid medication, which is so commonly prescribed in pediatrics.

chemical assay For certain drugs, such as digoxin and phenytoin, measurement of plasma drug levels provides information on the amount of drug recently ingested. However, this method is expensive, indicates only short-term compliance, requires precise timing of the assay for accurate results, and is limited to certain kinds of treatments.

STRATEGIES TO ENHANCE COMPLIANCE

Strategies to improve compliance are concerned with those interventions that encourage families to follow the prescribed treatment regimen. Ideally such strategies should be implemented before or concurrent with the initiation of therapy to avoid compliance problems. A number of strategies have been identified as effective, but, like measurement methods, no one approach is always successful and the best results occur when at least two strategies are employed. The following is an overview of compliance strategies.

Organizational Strategies

Organizational strategies refer to those interventions that are concerned with the care setting and the therapeutic plan. They include manipulating the factors listed in the box on p. 636 that are known to positively affect compliance (Young, 1986). Depending on the individual situation, this may involve increasing the frequency of appointments, designating a primary practitioner, reducing the cost of medication by purchasing generic brands, reducing the treatment's disruption of the family's life-style, and using "cues" to minimize forgetting. Numerous devices are available commercially or can be improvised for cueing, such as pill dispensers; watches with alarms; charts to record completed therapy; reminders, such as messages on the refrigerator or morning coffee pot; and treatment schedules that incorporate the treatment plan into the daily routine, such as physical therapy after the evening bath.

Nursing Guidelines for Effective Teaching

- Establish rapport; reduce anxiety and fear
- Assess what family knows and expects to learn, especially if they have concerns and address their concerns before beginning teaching
- Assess family's learning style; ask if they like to have everything explained in detail or if they prefer knowing only the major facts
- Use a variety of teaching materials (lecture, demonstration, video or slide presentation, written material)
- Speak the family's language, avoid jargon, and clarify all terms
- Be specific when giving information
- Divide the information into small steps
- Keep information short, simple, and concrete
- Introduce most important information first
- Use "verbal" headings to organize information, such as "There are two things you need to learn: how to give the medicine and what side effects to look for. First, how to give . . . . Second, what side effects . . ."
- Stress how important the instructions are and the expected benefits; explain the detrimental effects of inadequate treatment but avoid fear tactics
- Evaluate the teaching by eliciting feedback to ensure that the family understands the information
- Repeat information as needed
- Reward the family for learning through verbal praise

Educational Strategies

Educational strategies are concerned with instructing the family about the treatment plan. Although education is an important component in enhancing compliance and patients who are more knowledgeable about their condition are more likely to comply, education alone does not ensure compliant behavior. Also, for education to be effective it must incorporate teaching principles known to enhance understanding and retention of material (see box). Written materials are essential, especially in any regimen requiring multiple or complex treatments, and need to be understandable to the average individual, who reads at about the fourth grade level.

Behavioral Strategies

Behavioral strategies encompass those interventions designed to directly modify behavior. Several strategies exist that are effective in encouraging the desired behavior and are very useful with children. Ideally, positive reinforcement should be employed to strengthen the behavior; this may consist of earning stars or tokens, which gains the child a special privilege or gift. A more formal method is the use of contracting (see p. 66). However, at times disciplinary techniques, such as time out for young children (see p. 66) or withholding privileges for older children, may be needed to reduce noncompliance (Rapoff, 1986).

◆ *General Hygiene and Care*

Hygienic care is continued throughout the child's hospital stay and is essentially no different from that provided to persons of any age. The primary differences are those related to the size of the patient. Grooming aids and attractive attire are important adjuncts to hygienic care. Children are delighted with anything that makes them feel more attractive.

Certain caregiving activities present special challenges, especially feeding the sick child. In addition children often have high fevers that require attention. Any of these activities present excellent opportunities for family health teaching.

BATHING

Unless contraindicated, most infants and children can be bathed in a tub at the bedside, on the bed, or in a standard bathtub located on the unit, which is often conveniently adapted for pediatric use. For infants and young children confined to bed the towel method can be used. Two towels are immersed in a dilute soap solution and wrung damp. With the child lying supine on a dry towel, one damp towel is placed on top of the child and used to gently clean the body. This towel is discarded, then the child is dried and turned prone. The procedure is repeated using the second damp towel.

Infants and small children are *never* left unattended in a bathtub, and infants who are unable to sit alone are securely held with one hand during the bath. The infant's head is supported securely with one hand or the farther arm is firmly grasped in the nurse's hand while the head rests comfortably on the wrist. This provides secure control of the infant while the other hand is free to wash the infant's body (Fig. 21-4). Infants or children who are able to sit without assistance need only close supervision and a pad placed in the bottom of the tub to prevent slipping and loss of balance, which could result in a bumped head or submersion of the face.

Older children may enjoy a shower if it is available. School-age children may be reluctant to bathe, and many are not accustomed to a daily bath. However, most children who feel well require little encouragement to participate in their daily care. Nurses will need to use judgment regarding the amount of supervision the child requires. Some can be trusted to assume this responsibility unaided, whereas others will need someone in constant attendance. Children with mental or physical limitations and suicidal or psychotic children (who may commit bodily harm) require close supervision.

Areas that require special attention during bed baths and for children performing their own care are the ears, between skin folds, the neck, the back, and the genital area. The genital area should be carefully cleansed and dried with particular care to skin folds, and in uncircumcised boys the foreskin should be gently retracted and the exposed surfaces cleansed and then the foreskin replaced. Older children have the tendency to avoid these areas; therefore they may need a gentle reminder.

Children who are ill or debilitated will need more extensive assistance with bathing and other aspects of hygienic care, but they should be encouraged to perform as much as they can without overtaxing their energies. Increasing involvement can be expected with improved strength and endurance. Children who are limited in the

A

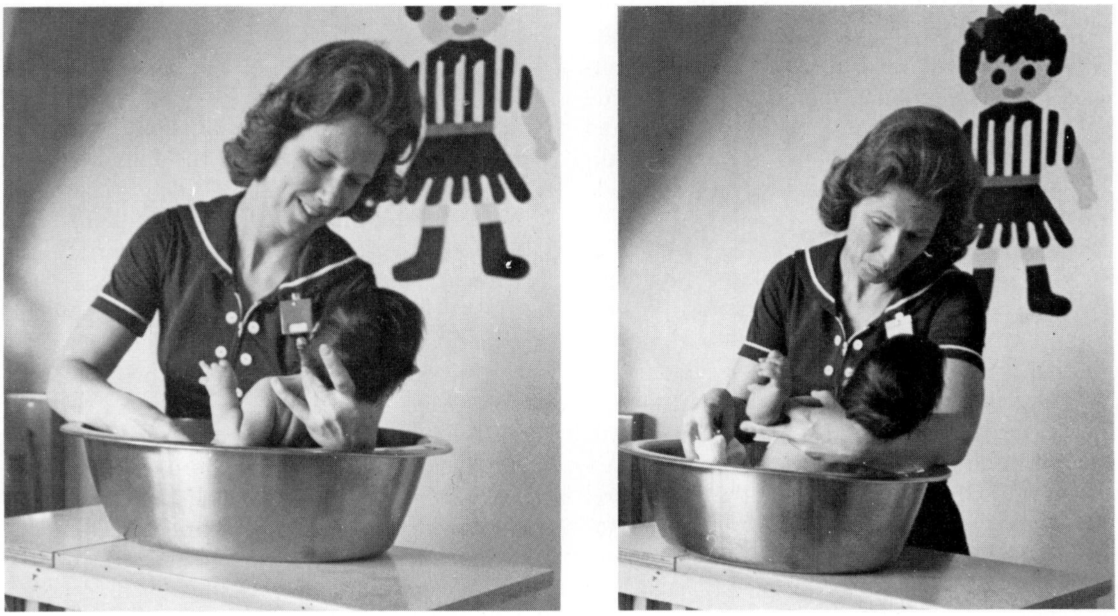

B

FIG. 21-4 Proper method for holding infant for tub bath. **A,** Supporting neck, **B,** Neck supported on wrist.

capacity for self-help and who have no other contraindications benefit a great deal from tub baths. They can be transported to the tub and, with the aid of lifting devices and/or an appropriate number of persons to assist, gain the advantages of a tub bath.

ORAL HYGIENE

Mouth care is an integral part of daily hygiene and should be continued in the hospital. Infants and debilitated children will require the nurse to perform mouth care. Although small children can manage a toothbrush and should be encouraged to use it, most will need assistance to perform a satisfactory job. Older children, although capable of brushing without assistance, sometimes need to be reminded that this is a part of their hygienic care. Most hospitals have equipment available for those children who do not have a toothbrush or toothpaste of their own. (See p. 355 for specific oral hygiene techniques and p. 843 for mouth care of children with mucosal ulcers.)

HAIR CARE

Brushing and combing hair are a part of the daily care for all persons in the hospital, including infants and children. If the child does not have a brush or comb, many hospitals provide one as part of the usual admission kit. If not, the parents should be asked to bring hair care equipment for the child's use. Both boys and girls should be helped to comb or brush their hair, or it should be done for them, at least once daily. There is no special hairstyle that is prescribed for hospitalized children. The hair should be styled for comfort and in a manner pleasing to the child and parents. A satisfactory style for girls with longer hair is the French braid, which is created by starting with three equal portions of hair from the top of one side of the scalp; as the hair is braided, segments of hair are added at successive intervals until all the hair has been incorporated into one neat, head-hugging braid on each side of the head. The ends are firmly anchored with a coated elastic band or barrette. The hair should not be cut without parental permission, although shaving hair to provide access to a scalp vein for intravenous needle insertion is frequently carried out without permission.

If children are hospitalized for more than a few days, the hair may need shampooing. With infants, the hair may be washed during the daily bath or less frequently. For most children washing the hair and scalp once or twice weekly is sufficient, unless there is an indication to wash it more frequently, such as following a high fever and profuse sweating. Some hospitals have shampoo basins, but almost any child can be conveniently transported by a gurney to an accessible sink or washbasin for shampooing. Those who are unable to be transported can receive a shampoo in their beds with adequate protection and/or specially adapted equipment or positioning. A convenient method involves positioning the child near the edge of the bed, placing towels under the shoulders, and draping a large plastic garbage bag at the edge of the bed with one open side under the shoulders and the other side opened away from the head so that the hair is inside the opening. Water can be transported in a basin (see also Nursing tip).

Nursing Tip: Shampooing Hair in Bed

For a convenient source of water, fill an empty enema bag with warm water and hang the bag from an intravenous pole; use the clamp on the bag's tubing to adjust the flow of water (Bourgault, 1985).

Teenagers, with their normally increased oily sebaceous secretions, are particularly in need of frequent hair care and usually require more frequent shampoos. Commercial "dry shampoo" products also may prove useful on a short-term basis.

Black children require special hair care, and this need is frequently neglected or inadequately managed. For the black child with kinky hair, most standard combs are inadequate and may cause hair breakage and discomfort to the child. If a special comb with widely spaced teeth is not available on the unit, the parent can be reminded to bring a comb, if possible, for the child's use. This type of hair also requires a special hair dressing or pomade, which usually has a coconut oil base. The preparation is rubbed on the hands and then transferred to the hair to make it more pliable and manageable. The child's parents should be consulted regarding the preparation they wish to be used on their child's hair, and they should be asked if they can provide some for use during the child's hospitalization. Petroleum jelly should *not* be used.

FEEDING THE SICK CHILD

Loss of appetite is a symptom common to most childhood illnesses and is frequently the initial evidence of illness, preceding fever and other overt signs of infection. In most cases children can be permitted to determine their own need for food. Since an acute illness is usually short, the nutritional state is seldom compromised. In fact, urging foods on the sick child may precipitate nausea and vomiting and in some cases even cause an aversion to the feeding situation that can extend into the convalescent period and beyond.

Refusing to eat may also be one way children can exert power and control in an otherwise helpless situation. For young children, loss of appetite may be related to the depression of separation from their parents and their natural tendency toward negativism. Parents' concern with eating can intensify the problem. Forcing a child to eat only meets with rebellion and reinforces the behavior as a control mechanism. Parents are encouraged to relax any pressure during the period of acute illness. Although it is best to encourage high-quality nutritious foods, the child may desire foods and liquids that contain mostly calories. Some well-tolerated foods include gelatin, clear soups, carbonated drinks, popsicles, dry toast, crackers, and hard candy. Even though these substances are not nutritious, they can provide necessary fluid and calories.

Dehydration is always a hazard when children are febrile or anorexic, especially when this is accompanied by vomiting or diarrhea. An adequate fluid intake should be encouraged by offering small amounts of favored fluids at frequent intervals and by salty foods if allowed. High-calorie liquids, such as colas, fruit juices, water flavored and sweetened with corn syrup, or similar drinks help prevent catabolism and dehydration. Fluids should not be forced, and the child should not be wakened from rest to take fluids. Forcing fluids may create the same difficulties as urging unwanted food. Gentle persuasion with preferred beverages will usually meet with success. Using play techniques can also be very effective (see box on p. 637).

In general, hot dogs, hamburgers, peanut butter and jelly sandwiches, spaghetti, and pizza are favorite foods of most children. Although alone they may not typify well-balanced diets, they can be adjusted to include sufficient amounts from the basic four food groups. It is better to work with preferred food choices than with selections that children rarely eat. A number of creative approaches to food preparation can increase the child's interest in eating (see box).

Once the child is feeling better, the appetite usually begins to improve. It is best to take advantage of any hungry period by serving high-quality foods and snacks. If the child still refuses to eat, nutritious fluids, such as milk shakes, should be encouraged. Parents can be very helpful by bringing in favorite food items from home, especially if the family's cultural eating habits differ from the hospital's food services.

Regardless of the type of diet, charting of the amount consumed is an important nursing responsibility. Descriptions need to be detailed and accurate, such as "4 ounces of orange juice, one pancake, no bacon, and 8 ounces of milk." Comments such as "ate well" or "ate poorly" are inadequate. If parents are involved in the child's care, they are encouraged to keep a list of everything eaten. Using a premeasured cup for fluids ensures a more accurate estimate of intake. A comparison of the intake at each meal can isolate food deficiencies, such as insufficient intake of meat or vegetables. Behaviors associated with mealtime also identify possible factors influencing appetite. For example, the observation that "Child eats well when with other children but plays with food if

Guidelines for Feeding the Sick Child

- Take a dietary history (see p. 122) and use information to make eating time as much like home as possible.
- Encourage parents or other family members to feed child or to be present at mealtimes.
- Have children eat at tables in groups; bring nonambulatory children to eating area in wheelchairs, beds, strollers, gurneys, or wagons.
- Use familiar eating utensils, such as a favorite plate, cup, or bottle for small children.
- Make mealtimes pleasant; avoid any procedures immediately before or after eating; make sure child is rested and pain free.
- Have a nurse present at mealtimes to offer assistance, prevent disruptions, and praise children for their eating.
- Serve small, frequent meals rather than three large meals or serve three meals and nutritious between-meal snacks.
- Bring in foods from home, especially if food preparation is markedly different from hospital; consider cultural differences.
- Provide finger foods for young children.
- Involve children in food selection and preparation whenever possible.
- Serve small portions, and serve each course separately, such as soup first, followed by meat, potatoes, and vegetables, and ending with dessert; with young children camouflage size of food by cutting meat thicker so less appears on plate or by folding a cheese slice in half; offer second helpings; ensure a variety of foods, textures, and colors.
- Provide food selections that are favorites of most children, such as peanut butter/jelly sandwiches, hot dogs, hamburgers, macaroni and cheese, pizza, spaghetti, tacos, fried chicken, and corn on the cob.
- Avoid foods that are highly seasoned, have strong odors, are served hot, or are all mixed together, unless typical of cultural practices.
- Provide fluid selections that are favorites of most children, such as fruit punch, cola, ginger ale, sweetened tea, ice pops, sherbet, ice cream, milk and milk shakes, eggnog, pudding, gelatin, clear broth, or creamed soups. (See also Play activities, p. 637.)
- Offer nutritious snacks, such as frozen yogurt or pudding, ice cream, oatmeal or peanut butter cookies, hot cocoa, cheese slices or "kisses," pieces of raw vegetable or fruit, and dried fruit or cereal.
- Make food attractive and different, for example:
  - Serve a "picnic lunch" in a paper bag.
  - Pack food in a Chinese-food container; decorate container.
  - Put a "face" or a "flower" on a hamburger or sandwich with pieces of vegetable.
  - Use a cookie-cutter to shape a sandwich.
  - Serve pudding, yogurt, or juice frozen as a popsicle.
  - Make slurpies or snowcones by pouring flavored syrup on crushed ice.
  - Add vegetable coloring to water or milk.
  - Serve fluids through brightly colored or unusually shaped straws.
  - Make "bowtie" sandwiches by cutting them in triangles and placing two points together.
  - Slice sandwiches into "fingers."
  - Grate mounds of cheese.
  - Cut apples horizontally to make circles.
  - Put a banana on a hotdog bun and spread with peanut butter.
  - Break uncooked spaghetti into toothpick lengths and skewer cheese, cold meat, vegetables or fruit chunks.
  - Praise children for what they do eat.
  - Do *not* punish children for not eating by removing their dessert or putting them to bed.

left alone in room" helps the nurse plan mealtime activities that stimulate the appetite.

CONTROLLING ELEVATED TEMPERATURE

Elevated temperature is a frequent occurrence in children, especially due to fever and, less commonly, from hyperthermia. To facilitate an understanding of the treatment of elevated temperature, the following terms are defined (McCarthy, 1985):

set point The temperature around which body temperature is regulated by a thermostat-like mechanism in the hypothalamus
fever An elevation in set point such that body temperature is regulated at a higher level
hyperthermia A situation in which body temperature exceeds the set point, which usually results from the body creating more heat than it can eliminate, such as in heat stroke, aspirin toxicity, or hyperthyroidism

Although definitions of temperature elevation to describe fever vary, the following are generally accepted:

fever Rectal temperature above 38° C (100.4° F); oral temperature above 37.8° C (100° F); axillary temperature above 37.2° C (99° F)
high fever Temperature above 40.4° C (105° F)
harmful fever Temperature at or above 41.7° C (107° F)

Fever, one of the most common symptoms of illness in children, is also one of the most frequently misunderstood manifestations of disease and a great source of unnecessary concern to parents. Most fevers in children are of viral origin, relatively brief in duration, and have limited consequences. In addition, fever probably plays a beneficial role in enhancing the development of both specific and nonspecific immunity and in aiding recovery and survival from infection. Contrary to popular belief, high fevers do not always indicate the severity of infection.

Measures to Reduce Elevated Temperature

Treatment of elevated temperature depends on whether it is due to a fever or to hyperthermia. Because the set point is normal in hyperthermia, but increased in fever, different approaches must be used to successfully lower body temperature.

Fever. The principal reason for treating fever is the relief of discomfort; there is no specific degree of fever that requires treatment. Relief measures include pharmacologic and/or environmental intervention. The most effective intervention is the use of antipyretics to lower the set point.

Antipyretic drugs include acetaminophen, aspirin, and nonprescription ibuprofen (Nuprin, Advil). Acetaminophen is the preferred drug; aspirin should not be given to children because of the association between aspirin use in children with influenza virus or chickenpox and Reye syndrome. Ibuprofen is not recommended for children under 12 years of age. The recommended dosage of acetaminophen is given in Table 21-2. It should be given every 4 hours, but no more than five times in 24 hours. Since body temperature normally decreases at night, three to four doses in 24 hours are usually sufficient to control most fevers. The temperature is usually retaken 30 minutes after the antipyretic is given to assess its effect but should not be repeatedly measured; the child's level of discomfort is the best indication for continued treatment.

TABLE 21-2

*Dosage Recommendations for Acetaminophen (Tylenol)**

Age	Weight (pounds)	Dose (mg)	Form†
Under 3 months	6-11	40	½ dropper
4-11 months	12-17	80	1 dropper or ½ tsp elixir
12-23 months	18-23	120	1½ dropper or ¾ tsp elixir or 1½ chewable tablet
2-3 years	24-35	160	2 droppersful or 1 tsp elixir or 2 chewable tablets
4-5 years	36-47	240	1½ tsp elixir or 3 chewable tablets
6-8 years	48-59	320	2 tsp elixir or 4 chewable tablets or 2 swallowable tablets
9-10 years	60-71	400	2½ tsp elixir or 5 chewable tablets or 2½ swallowable tablets
11 years	72-95	480	3 tsp elixir or 6 chewable tablets or 3 swallowable tablets
12-14 years	96+	640	4 swallowable tablets

*Doses should be administered four or five times daily, but not to exceed five doses in 24 hours.
†1 dropper = 80 mg/0.8 ml; elixir = 160 mg/5 ml; chewable tablet = 80 mg each; junior strength swallowable tablets = 160 mg each.

Environmental measures to reduce fever are used if tolerated by the child and if they do not induce shivering. Shivering is the body's way of maintaining the set point by producing heat. Environmental measures such as minimum clothing, exposing the skin to the air, reducing room temperature, increasing air circulation, and cool moist compresses to the skin, such as the forehead, are most effective if employed approximately 1 hour *after* an antipyretic is given so that the set point is lowered. Cooling procedures such as sponging or tepid baths have been shown to be ineffective in treating febrile children either when used alone or in combination with antipyretics, and they inflict considerable discomfort on the child (Newman, 1985).

Hyperthermia. Unlike in fever, antipyretics are of no value in hyperthermia, because the set point is already normal. Consequently, cooling measures are used. Cool applications to the skin help to reduce the core temperature. Cooled blood from the skin surface is conducted to inner organs and tissues, and warm blood is circulated to the surface, where it is cooled and recirculated. The surface blood vessels dilate as the body attempts to dissipate heat to the environment and facilitate this cooling process.

Commercial cooling devices, such as cooling blankets or mattresses, are available to reduce body temperature. They are placed on the bed and covered with a sheet or lightweight blanket. Frequent temperature monitoring is essential to prevent excessive cooling of the body.

Cool applications can also be given in a tub or in the bed or crib. For tepid tub baths, it is usually best to start with warm water and gradually add cool water until the desired water temperature of 37° C (98.6° F) is reached to accustom the child to the lower water temperature. The child is placed directly into the tub of tepid water for 20 to 30 minutes while water is gently squeezed from a washcloth over his back and chest or gently sprayed over his body from a sprayer. The bath is even more effective if the child can tolerate lying down in the water with his head supported on the nurse's arm or a padded support. This is more easily accomplished with a small infant or an older child. Small children dislike lying down and often resist any efforts to force them into the horizontal position. For conscious children a floating toy or other distraction can be employed during the bath. The child is never left alone in the tub.

The cooling bath can also be given in the bed or crib. The child is completely undressed and placed on an absorbent blanket or towel spread over the bed. He is covered with a large towel or lightweight, absorbent cotton blanket. A cool washcloth or ice pack is placed on the child's forehead and changed as it warms. One area of the body is exposed at a time and sponged with a washcloth soaked in tepid water. Special care is taken where two body surfaces touch. The sponge bath is continued for approximately 30 minutes.

An alternate approach is the towel method. The child is undressed and placed on an absorbent towel or blanket, and a cool cloth or ice bag is applied to the forehead. Each extremity is wrapped in a towel moistened in tepid water, one is placed under the back, and another covers the neck and torso. Special care is taken to make certain that opposing body surfaces, such as the groin and lateral torso between the arms and chest, are covered. The towels are changed as they warm. This is continued for approximately 30 minutes.

After the tub or sponge bath, the child is dried and dressed in lightweight pajamas, nightgown, or diaper and placed in a dry bed. The temperature is retaken 30 minutes after the tub bath or sponge bath. The child is dried by gently rubbing the skin surface with a towel to stimulate circulation. The bath or sponge should not be continued or restarted until the skin surface is warm or if the child feels chilled. Chilling causes vasoconstriction, which defeats the purpose of the cool applications. In this condition little blood is carried to the skin surface; the blood remains primarily in the viscera to become heated.

FAMILY TEACHING AND HOME CARE

Nurses have a unique opportunity for teaching the family about health care practices while the child is hospitalized. Although most children have learned self-care and hygiene in the home or at school, many have not. For some young children this is their first introduction to the use of a toothbrush. A great deal of health teaching can be accomplished even when the child is hospitalized for only a short time. The daily bath, handwashing before meals and after bowel and bladder evacuation, and conscientious dental hygiene are taught by example during routine care. Clean hair, nails, and clothing, as well as good grooming, are emphasized as essential to a pleasing appearance. Positive reinforcement of good hygiene practices helps to create a positive body image, promote the development of self-esteem, and prevent health problems (for example, teaching girls to wipe the genital area from front to back after toileting).

While sick children's appetites may be poor and not characteristic of their home eating habits, the hospital stay provides numerous opportunities for nurses to assess the family's knowledge of good nutrition and to implement teaching as needed to improve nutritional intake. Creative games can be employed that not only teach but provide diversion as well (Dininny, 1977; Mandelbaum, 1983).

Parental education about fever is essential, since many parents are unaware of what constitutes a fever, have unrealistic fears about the dangers of fever, and are apt to overmedicate the febrile child. Parents should know how to take the child's temperature and read the thermometer accurately.* Some of the newer temperature measuring devices, such as plastic strip or digital thermometers, may be better suited for home use (see p. 136). If the use of acetaminophen is indicated, the parents may need instruction in administering the drug.* It is important to emphasize accuracy in both the amount of drug given and the time intervals at which the drug is administered. Since many forms of acetaminophen are available, the nurse must be certain of the type being used in the home when discussing dosage. For example, the specially coated swallowable tablets for older children contain *twice* the amount of drug of the chewable tablets.

◆ *Safety*

Safety is an essential component of any patient's care, but children have special characteristics that require an even greater concern for safety. Since small children are sepa-

*Home care instructions on measuring your child's temperature and giving medications to children are available in Wong, D., and Whaley, L.: Clinical handbook of pediatric nursing, ed. 2, St. Louis, 1986, The C.V. Mosby Co.

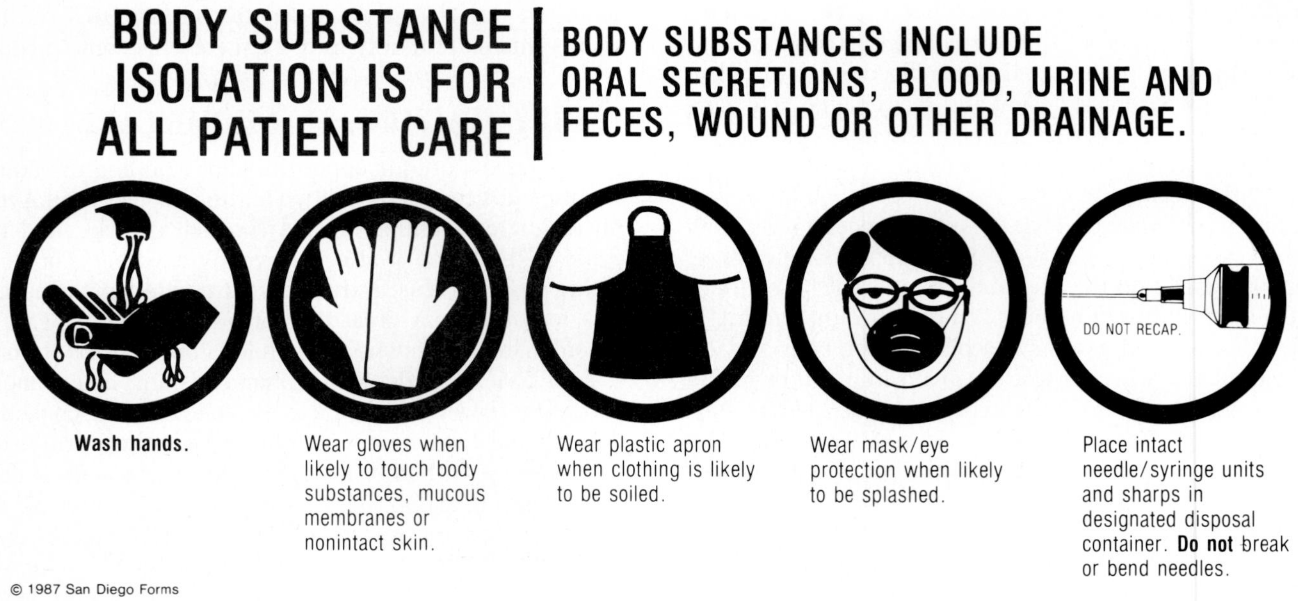
BODY SUBSTANCE ISOLATION IS FOR ALL PATIENT CARE
BODY SUBSTANCES INCLUDE ORAL SECRETIONS, BLOOD, URINE AND FECES, WOUND OR OTHER DRAINAGE.
DO NOT RECAP.
Wash hands.
Wear gloves when likely to touch body substances, mucous membranes or nonintact skin.
Wear plastic apron when clothing is likely to be soiled.
Wear mask/eye protection when likely to be splashed.
Place intact needle/syringe units and sharps in designated disposal container. Do not break or bend needles.
© 1987 San Diego Forms

FIG. 21-5 A, A decal can be displayed in a prominent location, such as on a towel dispenser, to remind personnel to use precautions with all body substances.

rated from their usual environment and do not possess the capacity for abstract thinking and reasoning, it is the responsibility of everyone who comes in contact with them to maintain protective measures throughout their hospital stay. Nurses need a good understanding of the age level at which each child is operating to plan for safety accordingly.

INFECTION CONTROL

The need for medical asepsis and appropriate barrier precautions to reduce the risk of nosocomial (hospital-acquired) infections are paramount in caring for children. Children are infected frequently with organisms, such as varicella (chickenpox), that can be dangerous to others, especially immunocompromised patients. In addition, children may not have developed good hygiene habits, such as handwashing after toileting. Young children are especially at risk for infection because of their high oral activity. Children in diapers present infection risks if caregivers do not practice meticulous cleaning techniques. Because of the importance of reducing the risk of nosocomial infection in children, a brief overview of the traditional and current trends in isolation practices is presented.

Although institutions can design their own system, most hospitals have adopted one of the following two basic systems for isolation precautions recommended by the Centers for Disease Control (1983):

category-specific isolation precautions Isolation categories group diseases for which similar isolation precautions are indicated. Instructions for each category include taking all the precautions necessary to prevent transmission of the most infectious disease in each category. Seven categories are used: strict isolation, contact isolation, respiratory isolation, tuberculosis isolation, enteric precautions, drainage/secretion precautions, and blood/body fluid precautions.

disease-specific isolation precautions Each disease is listed with only the precautions needed to prevent transmission of that disease. Consequently, there is more variability in instructions with this system.

Both of these systems are *diagnosis-driven;* that is, the patient's diagnosis determines the type of precautions needed to interrupt the transmission of the infectious agent. However, these systems are not designed to provide protection when the infected person is undiagnosed. A problem with any diagnosis-driven approach to isolation precautions is that all communicable diseases are infectious before the diagnosis is made (Lynch and others, 1987).

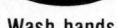

Recent concern for possible transmission of infection, such as hepatitis B and human immunodeficiency virus (the virus that causes the disease AIDS), from undiagnosed patients to other patients and health care workers has prompted the Centers for Disease Control (1987) and other organizations to issue guidelines for treating all patients as potentially infectious. This system is known as *universal precautions.* One type of universal precautions is the *body substance isolation (BSI) system,* which

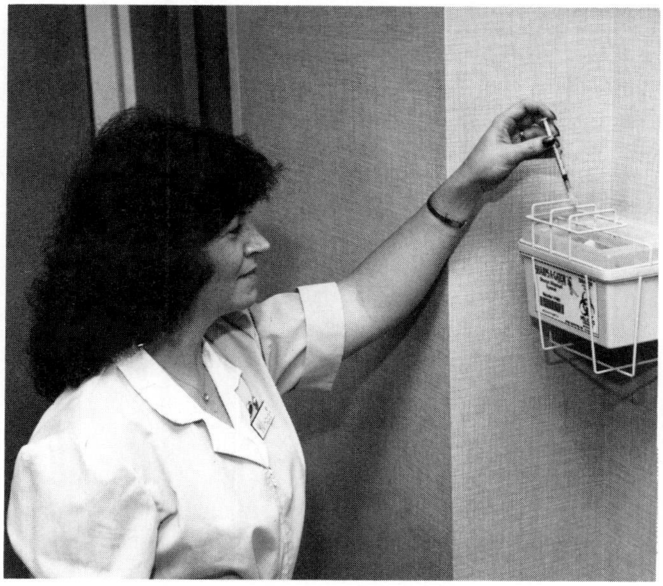

B, To prevent needlestick injuries, used needles (and other sharps) are not capped or broken and are disposed of in a rigid, puncture-resistant container located near the site of use. Note the placement of the container and the use of a protective cage to discourage children's access to the contents.

Universal Precautions for Infection Control

Gloves—worn when contact with mucous membranes, non-intact skin, or moist body substances is likely to occur; changed between patient contacts

Handwashing—performed for 10 seconds with soap, running water, and friction anytime the hands are visibly soiled and between most patient contacts even if gloves are worn; not necessary between sequential low-risk patient contacts involving intact skin, such as taking vital signs or administering medication

Gowns or plastic aprons—worn when it is likely that body substances will soil the clothing; changed between patient contacts

Masks and/or eye protection—worn when it is likely that the eyes and/or nose and mouth will be splashed with body substances or when personnel are working directly over large open skin lesions; eyeglasses generally provide adequate eye protection; masks may be needed for airborne infections

Needle/syringe units and sharps—needles are not capped or broken; all sharps are disposed of in a rigid, puncture-resistant container located preferably near the site of use, such as patient's room and treatment rooms

Trash and linen—are bagged securely in leak-proof containers and disposed of or cleaned according to institutional policy

Private rooms—desirable for children who soil the environment with body substances; required for children with airborne, communicable diseases unless they can share a room with a roommate/or roommates known to be immune to the disease

focuses on the interaction of the care provider with the body substances, non-intact skin, and mucous membranes of all patients. Body substances include oral secretions, blood, feces, urine, vomitus, and wound or other drainage. Specific guidelines for using BSI are summarized in the box. Special reminders are available to encourage compliance with the BSI system (Fig. 21-5, *A*). Additional precautions, such as a private room and possibly the use of masks, are indicated for those diseases, such as varicella, that are transmitted solely or in part by the airborne route.

Nurses caring for young children are frequently in contact with body substances, especially urine, feces, and vomitus. In using BSI nurses need to exercise judgment for those situations when gloves, gowns, or masks are necessary. For example, gloves and possibly gowns should be worn for changing diapers when there are loose or explosive stools. Otherwise, the plastic lining of disposable diapers provides a sufficient barrier between the hands and body substances. During feedings, gowns should be worn if the child is likely to vomit or spit up, which often occurs during burping. If aprons with minimum shoulder protection are worn, the child should be sitting on the nurse's lap, not upright against the shoulder, when the child is bubbled.

Another essential practice of BSI is that all needles (uncapped and unbroken) should be disposed of in a rigid, puncture-resistant container located near the site of use. Consequently, these containers are installed in patients' rooms. Since children are naturally curious, extra attention is needed in selecting a suitable type of container and a location that discourage access to the disposed needles (Fig. 21-5, *B*).

ENVIRONMENTAL FACTORS

All the environmental safety measures in operation for the protection of adults apply to children as well, such as good illumination; floors clear of fluid or objects that might contribute to falls; nonskid surfaces in showers and tubs; electrical equipment that is maintained in good working order, is operated only by personnel familiar with its use, and is not in contact with moisture or near tubs, where it could prove to be a shock hazard; beds of ambulatory patients locked in place and at a height that allows easy access to the floor; proper care and disposal of small breakable items such as thermometers and bottles; and a well-organized fire plan known to all staff members.

All windows should be securely screened and elevators and stairways made safe. Ideally electrical outlets should be provided with covers to prevent burns in small children whose exploratory activities may extend to inserting objects into the small openings. Bath water is carefully checked before placing the child in it, and children must never be left alone in a bathtub. Infants are helpless in water, and small children (and some older ones) may turn on the hot water faucet and be severely burned.

Furniture is safest when scaled to the child's proportions, sturdy, and well balanced to prevent its being easily tipped over. Infants and small children must be securely strapped into infant seats, feeding chairs, and strollers. Infants and small, agitated, or mentally retarded children should not be left unattended on treatment tables, on scales, or in treatment areas. Even tiny premature infants are capable of surprising mobility; therefore portholes in Isolettes must be securely fastened when not in use.

Crib sides should be kept up and fastened securely unless an adult is at the bedside. It is safer to leave crib sides up, even when the crib is unoccupied, to remove the temptation to climb in. Anyone attending an infant or small child in a crib with the sides down should never turn away without maintaining hand contact with the child; that is, one hand should be kept on the child's back or abdomen to prevent the child from rolling, crawling, or jumping from the open crib (Fig. 21-6). A child who is apt to or has demonstrated the inclination to climb over the sides of the crib is safest when placed in a specially constructed crib with a cover or one that has a safety net placed over the top. If the net is used, it must be tied to the frame in such a manner that there is ready access to the child in case of emergency. Nets are never tied to the movable crib sides, and the knots should be tied in a manner that permits quick release. Cribs should not be placed within reach of heating units, appliances, dangling cords, or other objects that can be grabbed by curious hands, and toys should not be tied to or across crib rails once children are old enough to reach them.

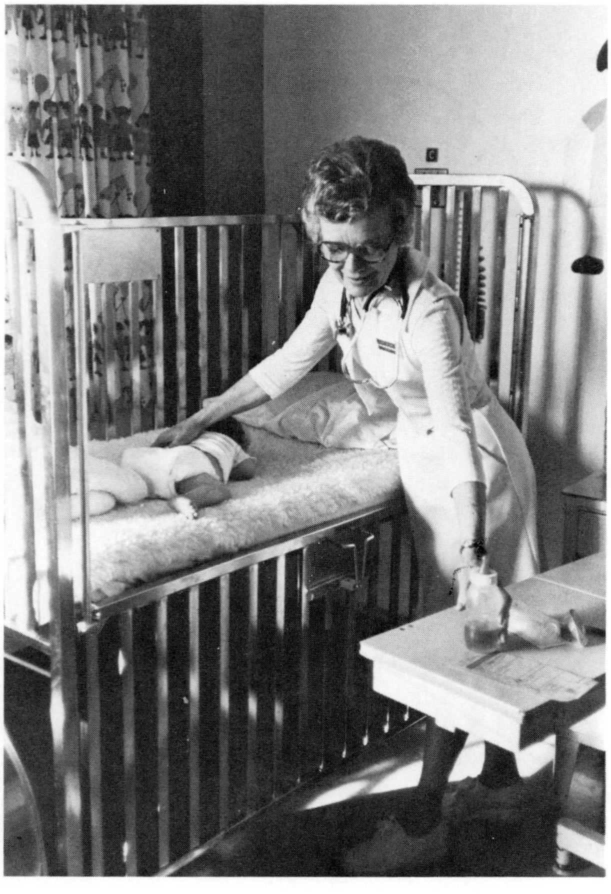

FIG. 21-6 Nurse maintains hand contact when back is turned.

Name bands, a part of hospital safety practices, are particularly important for children in the pediatric age-group. Infants and unconscious patients are unable to tell or respond to their names. Toddlers may answer to any name or to a nickname only. It is not uncommon for older children to exchange places, give an erroneous name, or choose not to respond to their own names as a form of a joke, unaware of the hazards of such practices.

Toys

Toys play a vital role in the everyday life of children, and they are no less important in the hospital setting. However, it is up to nurses to assess the safety of toys brought to the hospital by well-meaning parents and friends. Toys should be appropriate to the child's age, condition, and treatment. For example, if the child is in an oxygen tent, electrical or friction toys cannot be placed in the tent. Toys should be inspected to make certain that they are nonallergenic, washable, and unbreakable and that they have no small, removable parts that can be aspirated or swallowed or that can in other ways inflict injury to a child.

LIMIT-SETTING

Setting limits is essential to a child's safety. Children must understand where they are permitted to go and what they are permitted to do in the hospital. These limitations should be made clear to them, consistently enforced, and repeated as frequently as necessary to make certain that they are understood. The nurse is responsible for where children are at all times. Children can easily wander off unnoticed. Normally active older children often become restless when their activity is restricted and may resort to pillow fights, water fights, and other rough play that might endanger the safety of the involved children or bystanders (other children, staff, visitors). Children in the hospital require surveillance, and appropriate tension-reducing activities can be planned and supervised by nurses and/or by the play therapist. A useful discipline technique is time out (see p. 66).

TRANSPORTING INFANTS AND CHILDREN

In the course of a hospital stay, infants and children usually need to be transported within the unit and to areas outside the pediatric unit. It is ordinarily safe to carry infants and small children for short distances within the unit, but for more extended trips the child should be securely transported in a suitable conveyance.

Small infants can be held or carried in the horizontal position with the back supported and the thigh grasped

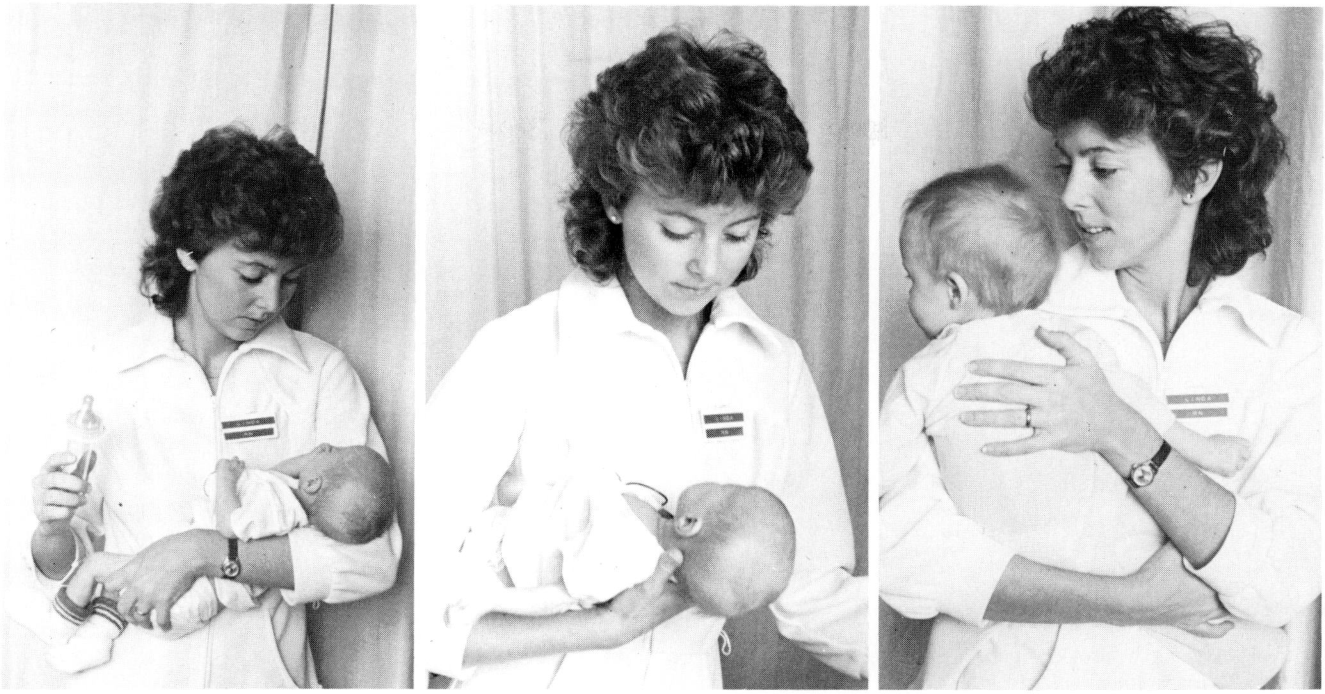

A B C

FIG. 21-7 Transporting infants. **A,** Infant's thigh firmly grasped in nurse's hand; **B,** Football hold; **C,** Back supported.

firmly by the carrying arm (Fig. 21-7, *A*). In the football hold the infant is carried on the nurse's arm with the head supported by the hand and the body held securely between the nurse's body and elbow (Fig. 21-7, *B*). Both of these holds leave the nurse's other arm free for activity. The infant can be held in the upright position with the buttocks on the nurse's forearm and the front of the body resting against the nurse's chest. The infant's head and shoulders are supported by the nurse's other arm to allow for any sudden movement by the infant (Fig. 21-7, *C*). Older infants are able to hold their heads erect but can still make sudden movements.

Infants can be transported to other areas, such as the radiography department, in their bassinets or cribs. Baby carriages are sometimes used for infants who are not likely to stand up. Strollers and wheeled feeding chairs or tables are also convenient transporters in some situations, such as trips to the playroom or nurse's station.

The method of transporting children is determined by their age, condition, and destination. Most older children are safe in wheelchairs or in gurneys. A younger child can be transported in a crib, on a gurney, in a wagon with raised sides, or in a wheelchair with a safety belt. Gurneys should be equipped with high sides and a safety belt, both of which are kept in place during transport.

RESTRAINTS

Frequently some method of restraint is needed for a child's safety or comfort, to facilitate examination, or to carry out diagnostic and therapeutic procedures. Restraint can be accomplished with the hand or with physical devices. Restraining the child with the hand provides an element of human contact that is lacking in restraint by mechanical means. For example, a large infant or small child can be effectively restrained by having him sit astride the lap of an assistant. The assistant hugs him close against the body to provide both comfort and restraint while the nurse safely carries out the necessary procedures (Fig. 21-8).

Mechanical restraints are never used as a punishment or as a substitute for observation. When a child must be restrained, he and his parents need a simple explanation, and if the restraint is applied for an extended time, the explanation must be repeated often to gain his cooperation and to help him understand that it is not a punishment. Restraining devices are not without risk and must be checked frequently to make certain that they are accomplishing the purpose for which they are intended, that they are applied correctly, and that they do not impair circulation.

Parents need to know the purpose of restraints, how to remove and reapply them, and the signs of complications from their use. Parents are sometimes upset when their child must be restrained and need to understand how they can help to ensure the maximum benefit and minimize the stress related to the use of restraints. Children, too, should be prepared for both the procedure or the circumstance for which the restraint is required.

Removing restraints whenever possible (at least every

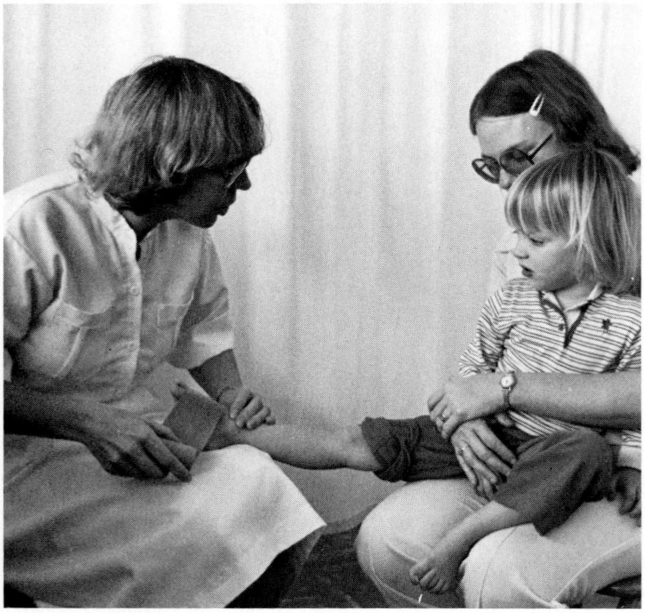

FIG. 21-8 An assistant provides comfort and security to infant while nurse carries out procedure.

2 hours) is an essential part of nursing care of children who are restrained for treatments or other purposes. Alternate methods may be devised to replace the need for passive restraints. Holding the child for periods is a pleasant alternative, as is restraining him in a high chair where he can observe the activities around him. If feasible, distraction techniques such as play and reading to the child should be employed to gain the child's cooperation without resorting to restraints. Parental participation is always encouraged in these efforts.

Jacket Restraint

A jacket restraint is sometimes used as an alternative to the crib net to prevent the child from climbing out of the crib or to keep the child safe in various kinds of chairs. The jacket is put on the child with the ties in back so that the child is unable to manipulate them, and the long tapes, secured to the understructure of the crib, keep the child inside the crib. The jacket restraint is also useful as a means to maintain the child in a desired horizontal position. A Posey belt scaled to fit the child is an alternative device.

FIG. 21-9 Application of mummy restraint. **A,** Infant placed on folded corner of blanket; **B,** One corner of blanket brought across body and secured beneath body.

A

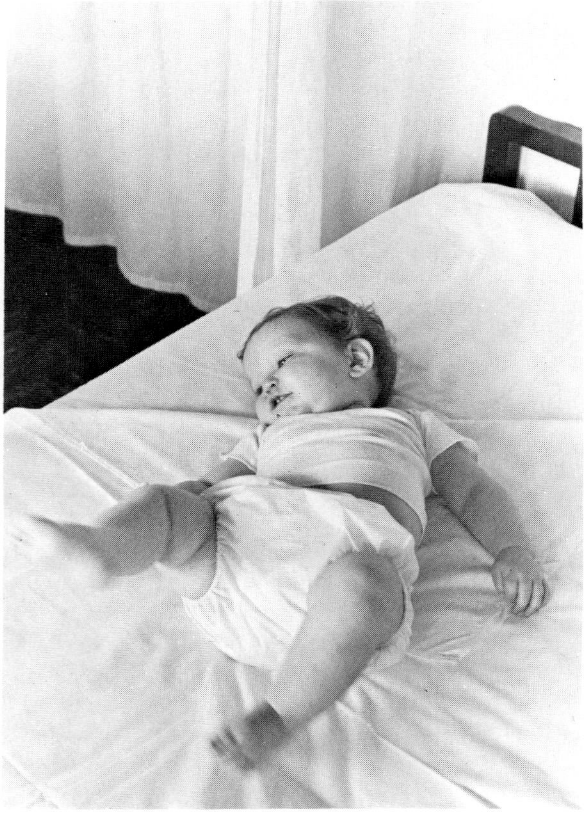

B

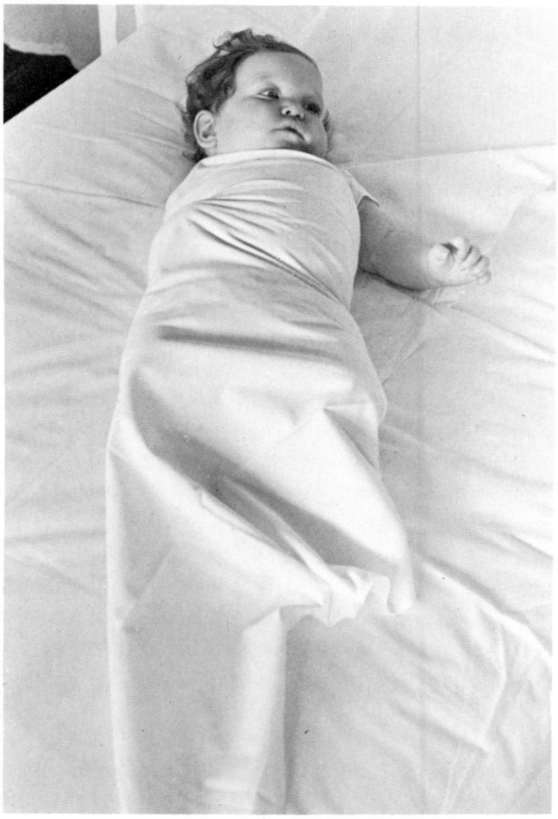

Mummy Restraint

When an infant or small child requires short-term restraint for examination or treatment that involves the head and neck—such as venipuncture, throat examination, and gavage feeding—the mummy device effectively controls the child's movements. A blanket or sheet is opened on the bed or crib with one corner folded to the center. The infant is placed on the blanket with shoulders at the fold and feet toward the opposite corner (Fig. 21-9, *A*). With the infant's right arm straight down against the body, the right side of the blanket is pulled firmly across the infant's right shoulder and chest and secured beneath the left side of the body (Fig. 21-9, *B*). The left arm is placed straight against his side, and the left side of the blanket is brought across the shoulder and chest and locked beneath the child's body on the right side. The lower corner is folded and brought over the body and tucked or fastened securely with safety pins (Fig. 21-9, *C*). Safety pins can be used to fasten the blanket in place at any step in the process.

To modify the mummy restraint for chest examination, the folded edge of the blanket is brought over each arm and under the back, after which the loose edge is folded over and secured at a point below the chest to allow visualization and access to the chest (Fig. 21-9, *D*).

Arm and Leg Restraints

Occasionally one or more extremities must be restrained or limited in motion. A number of commercial restraining devices are available, or a restraint can be fashioned from gauze tape, muslin strips, or a length of narrow stockinette. When this type of restraint is used, it must be appropriate to the size of the child, it must be padded to prevent undue pressure, constriction, or tissue injury, and the extremity must be observed frequently for signs of irritation and/or impairment of circulation. The ends of the restraints are never tied to the crib rails, since lowering of the rail will disturb the extremity, frequently with a jerk that may hurt or injure the child.

The *clove hitch* restraint is fashioned from a length of gauze or muslin tape. When properly applied, the restraint should provide a snug fit with minimum danger of pulling too tightly. Fig. 21-10 illustrates the method of tying and applying a clove hitch restraint.

C, Second corner brought across body and secured, and the lower corner folded and tucked or pinned in place; **D,** Modified mummy restraint with chest uncovered.

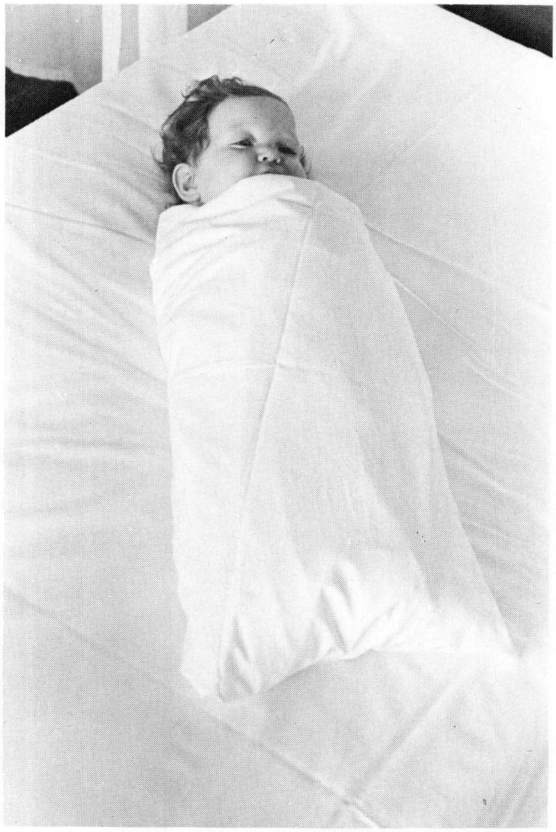

C

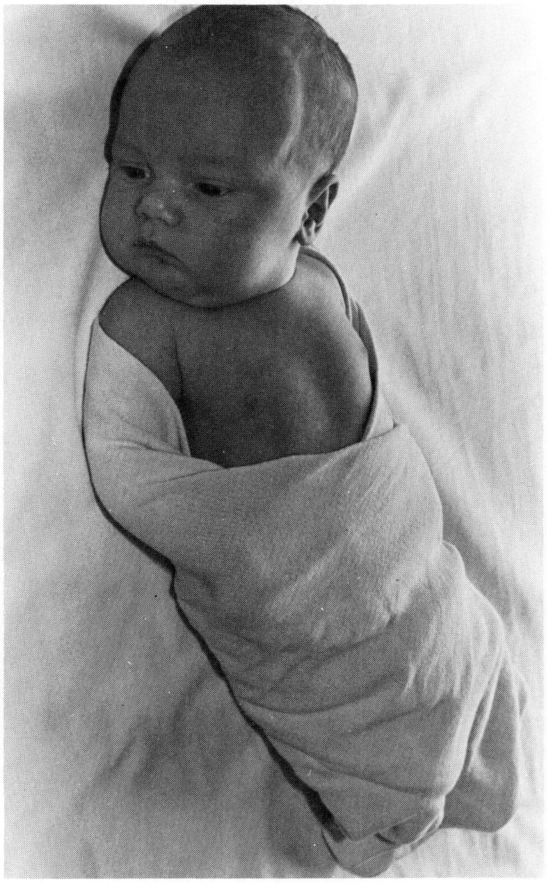

D

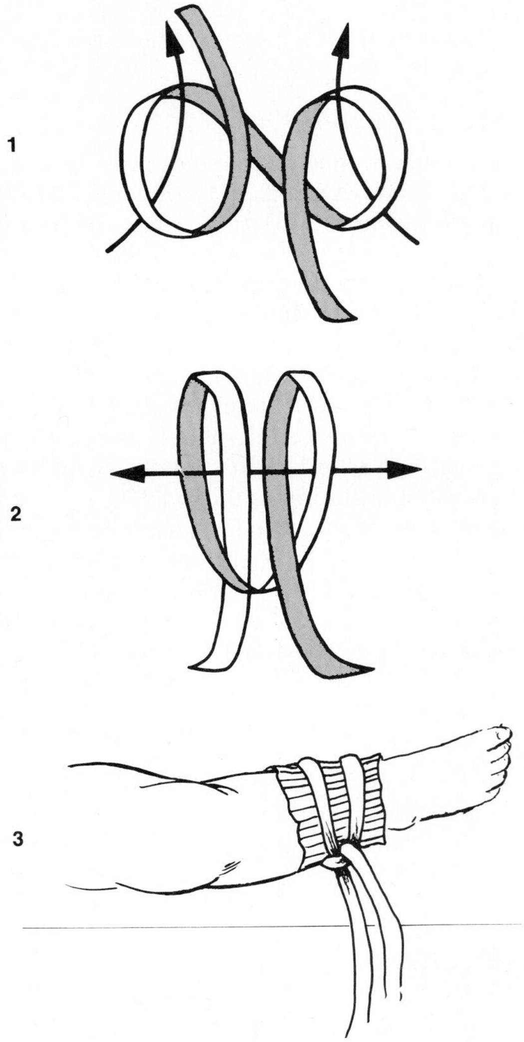

FIG. 21-10 Clove hitch restraint.

Elbow Restraint

Sometimes it is important to prevent the child from reaching his head or face; for example, after lip surgery, when a scalp vein infusion is in place, or to prevent scratching in skin disorders. For this purpose, elbow restraints fashioned from a variety of materials function very well. The most common form of elbow restraint consists of a piece of muslin long enough to reach comfortably from just below the axilla to the wrist with a number of vertical pockets into which tongue depressors are inserted. The restraint is wrapped around the arm and secured with tapes or pins. It may be necessary to pin the top of the restraint to the undershirt sleeve to prevent the restraint from slipping. Similar restraints can be made from commonly available products (see Nursing tip on elbow restraints).

Nursing Tip: Improvised Elbow Restraints

Pad the ends of large-diameter towel rollers or appropriately sized plastic containers from which the tops and bottoms have been removed. Apply adhesive tabs to the top end and pin the tabs to the child's sleeves to prevent the restraint from slipping from the extremity.

Fashion adjustable restraints from tongue blades placed vertically against strips of adhesive and then covered with adhesive; secure with adhesive tabs as described above.

POSITIONING FOR PROCEDURES

Infants and small children are unable to cooperate for many procedures; therefore the nurse is responsible for minimizing their movement and discomfort with proper positioning. Older children usually need only minimum, if any, restraint. Careful explanation and preparation beforehand and support and simple guidance during the procedure are usually sufficient.

Jugular Venipuncture

The large, superficial external jugular vein may be used to obtain blood specimens from infants and young children. For easy access to the vein, the child is first placed in a mummy restraint in which the top edge of the restraint is low enough to permit access to the vein. The child is placed so that the head and shoulders extend over

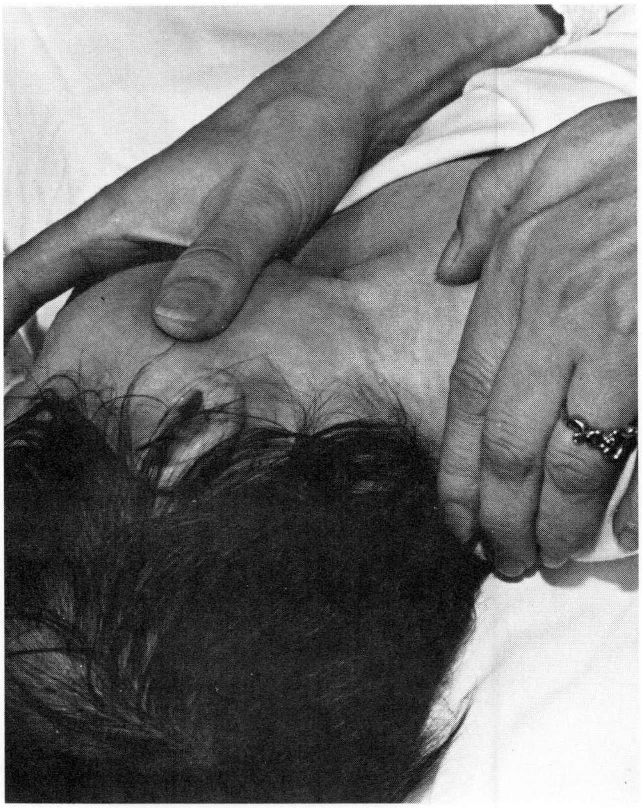

FIG. 21-11 Restraining child for jugular vein puncture.

the edge of a table or a small pillow with the neck extended and the head turned sharply to the side (Fig. 21-11). One alternate method for restraining arms and legs is with the nurse holding the child's arms and legs at the same time that the child's head is restrained and positioned. It is important for the nurse holding the infant to maintain control of the infant's head without interfering with the operator's approach to the vein. The infant's crying during the procedure increases intravenous pressure, which facilitates visualization of the vein. Following venipuncture, digital pressure is applied to the site with a dry gauze square for 3 to 5 minutes or until bleeding stops. Care must be taken not to apply excessive pressure that might compromise circulation or breathing during or following the procedure.

Femoral Venipuncture

Other commonly used sites for venipuncture are the large femoral veins. The nurse restrains the infant by placing him supine with his legs in a frog position to provide extensive exposure of the groin area. Both the arms and the legs of the infant can be effectively controlled by the nurse's forearms and hands (Fig. 21-12). Only the side used for the venipuncture should be uncovered, so that the operator is protected should the child urinate during the procedure. Pressure should be applied to the site after the withdrawal of blood to prevent oozing from the site.

Extremity Venipuncture

The most common sites of venipuncture are the veins of the extremities, especially the arm and hand. A convenient position for restraint is having one person on either side of the bed. The child's outstretched arm is partially stabilized by the technician drawing the blood. The other person leans across the child's upper body, preventing its movement, and uses an arm to immobilize the venipuncture site. This type of restraint also comforts the child because of the close body contact and allows each person to maintain eye contact with him (Fig. 21-13).

Lumbar Puncture

The technique for lumbar puncture in infants and children is similar to that in the adult, although modifications are suggested in premature infants who have less distress in a side-lying position with modified neck extension rather than flexion or in a sitting position. Pediatric lumbar puncture sets contain smaller spinal needles, but sometimes the operator will specify a particular size or type of needle that the nurse should make certain is placed on the tray.

Children are usually controlled best in the side-lying position, with the head flexed and the knees drawn up toward the chest. Even cooperative children need to be restrained to prevent possible trauma from unexpected, involuntary movement. They can be reassured that, al-

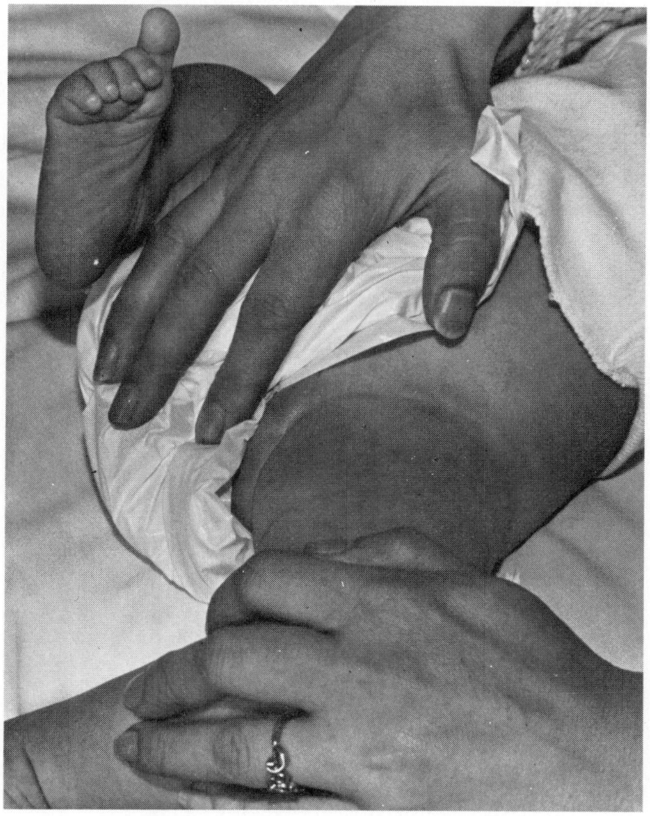

FIG. 21-12 Restraining infant for femoral vein puncture.

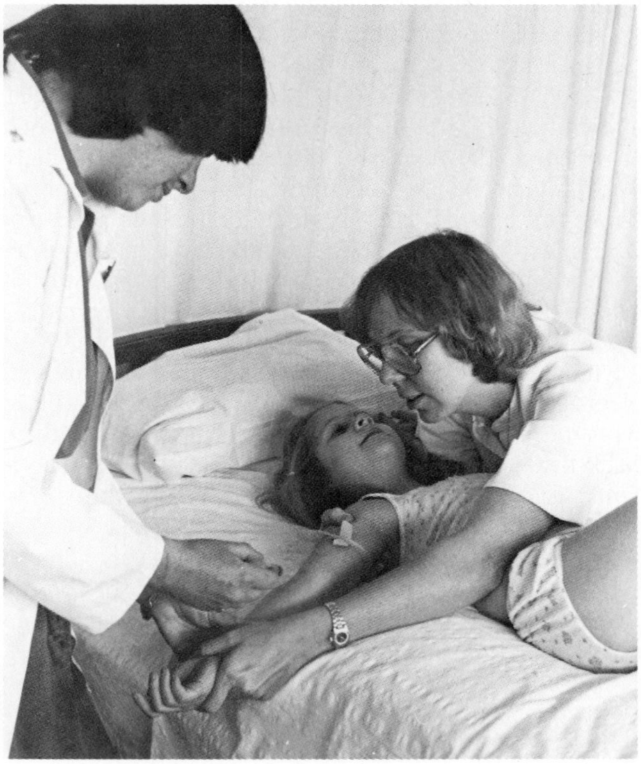

FIG. 21-13 Restraining child for extremity vein puncture.

A

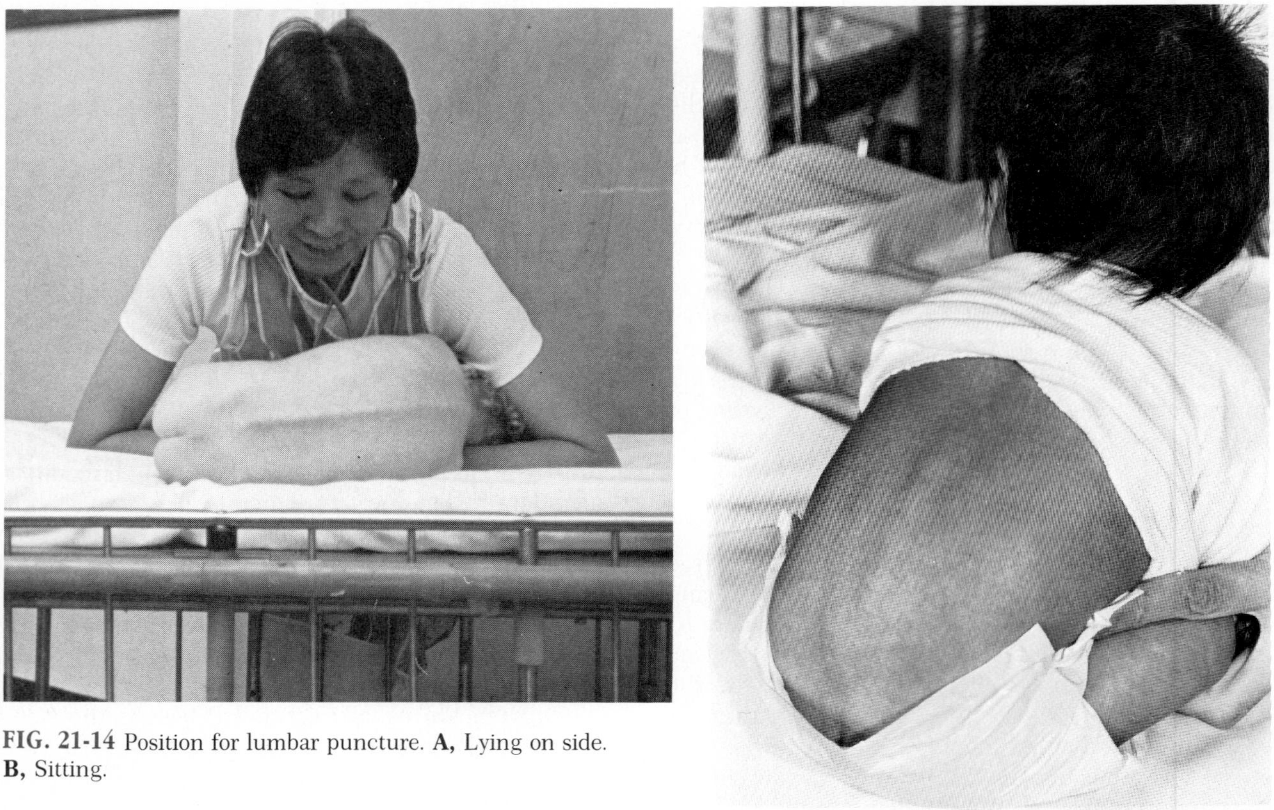

B

FIG. 21-14 Position for lumbar puncture. **A,** Lying on side. **B,** Sitting.

though they are trusted, the restraint will serve as a reminder to maintain the desired position. It also provides a measure of support and reassurance to them.

The child is placed on the side with the back close to the edge of the examining table on the side from which the operator is working. The nurse maintains the child's spine in a flexed position by holding the child with one arm behind the neck and the other behind the thighs. The position can be effectively stabilized if the nurse's hands are clasped in front of the child's abdomen (Fig. 21-14, *A*). The flexed position enlarges the spaces between the lumbar vertebral spines, which facilitates access to the spinal fluid space. It is helpful to wrap the legs before positioning to decrease leg movement.

An alternate position used with small infants and some older children is the sitting position. The child is placed with the buttocks at the edge of the table and with the neck flexed so that the chin rests on the chest. The infant's arms and legs are immobilized by the nurse's hands (Fig. 21-14, *B*). Since this position may interfere with chest expansion and diaphragm excursion, the child is observed for difficulty in breathing. In addition, the soft, pliable trachea of the infant is subject to collapse.

Another position that employs close and comforting contact for the child involves holding the child upright against the nurse's (or parent's) chest with the child's legs wrapped around the adult's waist. The adult's arms are used to hug and restrain the child. For ease of the examiner, the adult should be standing. A small pillow is placed between the child's abdomen and the adult to help arch the child's back. If the pillow proves unsuccessful, a third person can place an arm in this space to achieve the desired position (Brown, 1984).

Specimens and spinal fluid pressure are obtained, measured, and sent for analysis in the same manner as for the adult patient. It is advisable for the child to lie quietly for an hour following the procedure to decrease the likelihood of headache, and he is offered fluids to drink. Vital signs are taken as ordered, and the child is observed for any changes in level of consciousness, motor activity, or other neurologic signs.

Bone Marrow Aspiration/Biopsy

Position for a bone marrow aspiration or biopsy depends on the location of the chosen site. In children the posterior or anterior iliac crest is most frequently used, although in infants the tibia may be selected because of easy access to the site and restraint of the child.

If the posterior iliac crest is used, the child is positioned prone. Sometimes a small pillow or folded blanket is placed under the hips to facilitate the bone marrow specimen. Since few children can be trusted to remain still, restraint is needed and is best applied with two people—one person to immobilize the upper body and a second person to immobilize the lower extremities. If the other sites are used, the child is placed supine and restraint is applied in a similar manner with modifications made for access to the tibia or anterior iliac crest.

Other

For subdural puncture through a fontanel or burr hole, the infant is wrapped in a mummy restraint and placed in the supine position with the head accessible to the examiner. To control the head the nurse uses a firm hold on each side of it. Procedures for immobilizing the head for examining the ears, nose, or throat are discussed in Chapter 7.

◆ *Collection of Specimens*

Many of the specimens needed for diagnostic examination of children are collected in much the same way as they are for adults, and older children are able to cooperate if given proper instruction regarding what is expected from them. Infants and small children, however, are unable to follow directions or control body functions sufficiently to help in collecting some specimens.

URINE SPECIMENS

When children are admitted to the hospital or seen in a clinic or office, a urine specimen may be required as a routine diagnostic procedure. Older children and adolescents will readily use the bedpan or urinal or can be trusted to follow directions for collection in the bathroom. However, they may have special needs. School-age children are cooperative but curious. They are concerned about the reasons behind things and are likely to ask questions regarding the disposition of their specimen and what one expects to discover from it. Self-conscious adolescents may be reluctant to carry a specimen bottle through a hallway or waiting room and appreciate a paper bag or other means for disguising the container. The presence of menses is sometimes an embarrassment to teenage girls; therefore it is a good idea to ask them if it might be that particular time of the month and to make adjustments as necessary. The specimen can be delayed or a notation made on the laboratory slip to explain the presence of red blood cells.

Preschoolers and toddlers are less cooperative primarily because they are usually unable to void on request. It is often best to offer them water or other liquids that they enjoy and wait about 30 minutes until they are ready to void voluntarily or to set a timer to alert the child that he needs to void shortly. The child will better understand what is expected if the nurse uses his terms for the function, such as "pee-pee" or "tinkle." Some children will have difficulty voiding in an unfamiliar receptacle. Potty-chairs or a bedpan placed on the toilet will ordinarily prove satisfactory. Toddlers who have recently acquired bladder control may be especially reluctant, since they undoubtedly have been admonished for "going" in places other than those approved by parents. A useful approach is to enlist the help of parents; they are likely to be successful, and this helps them to feel a part of the child's care.

For infants and toddlers who are not toilet trained, special urine collection devices are used. These devices are clear plastic single-use bags with self-adhering material around the opening at the point of attachment. To prepare the infant, the genitalia, perineum, and surrounding skin are washed and dried thoroughly, since the adhesive will not stick to a moist, powdered, or oily skin surface. The collection bag is easiest to apply if attached first to the perineum, progressing to the symphysis (Fig. 21-15). With little girls the perineum is stretched taut during application to that area to assure a leak-proof fit. With small boys the penis and scrotum are placed inside the bag. The adhesive portion of the bag must be firmly applied to the skin all around the genital area to avoid possible leakage. The diaper is carefully replaced (see Nursing tip). The bag is checked frequently and removed as soon as the specimen is available, since the moist bag may become loosened on an active child. If only a small volume of urine is needed, such as checking specific gravity with a refractometer, the procedure in the Nursing tip box can be used.

Nursing Tip: Urine Collection

When using a urine collection bag, cut a small slit in the diaper and pull the bag through to allow room for urine to collect and to facilitate checking on the contents.

To obtain small amounts of urine, use a syringe without needle to aspirate urine directly from the diaper; if diapers with absorbent gelling material that trap urine are used, place a small gauze dressing or some cotton balls inside the diaper to collect urine and aspirate the urine with a syringe.

At times parents may be requested to bring a urine sample to a health care facility for examination, especially when infants are unable to void during an outpatient visit. In this instance parents need instruction on applying the collection device and storage of the specimen.* Ideally the specimen should be brought to the designated place as soon as possible; if there is a delay, the sample should be refrigerated and the lapsed time reported to the examiner.

Clean-Catch Specimens

Although older children can be instructed in the proper technique, the nurse performs the cleansing procedure on infants and young children. The perineum is cleansed with a soap- or an antiseptic-soaked sterile pad, wiping from front to back only once with each pad. This is re-

*Home care instructions on obtaining a urine sample are available in Wong, D., and Whaley, L.: Clinical handbook of pediatric nursing, ed. 2, St. Louis, 1986, The C.V. Mosby Co.

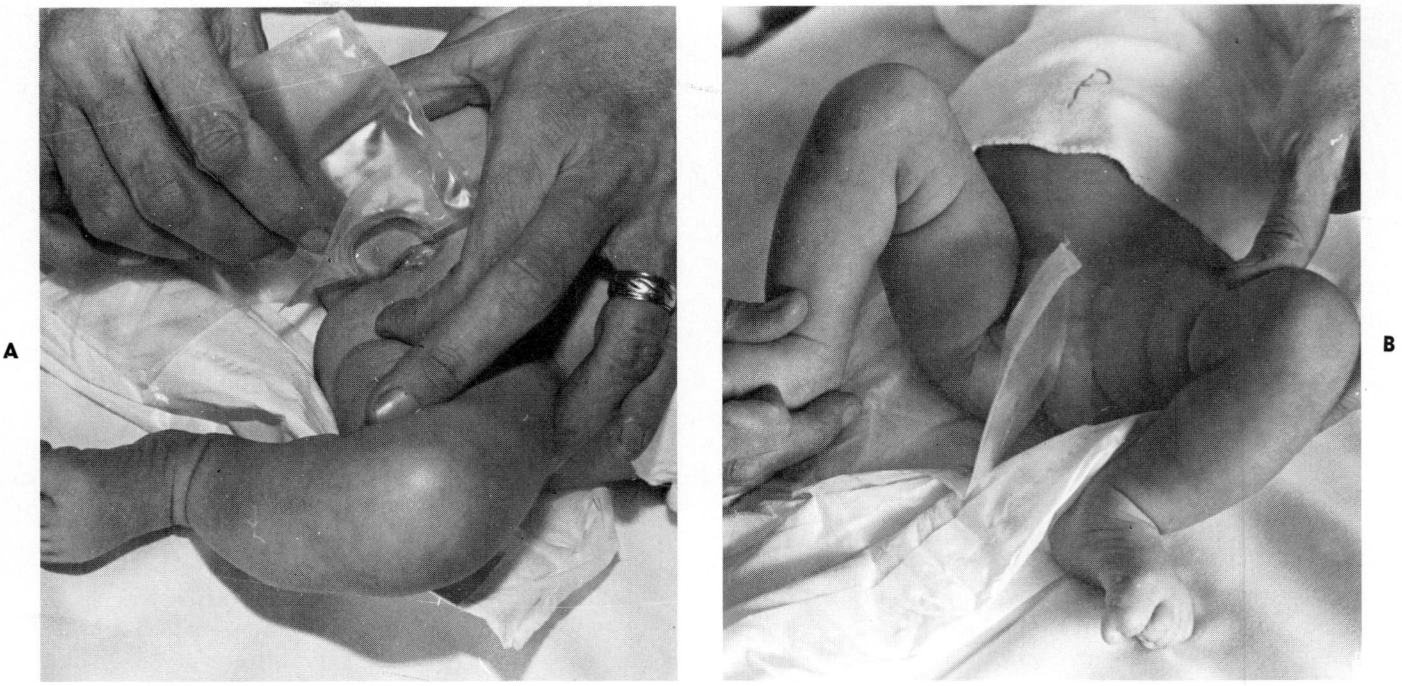

FIG. 21-15 Application of urine collection bag. **A,** On female infants adhesive portion is applied to exposed and dried perineum first. **B,** Bag adheres firmly around perineal area to prevent urine leakage.

peated at least two times. The area is then wiped with sterile water to prevent accidental contamination of the urine with a solution that may destroy the pathogens, although minute amounts of antiseptic such as iodine do not alter bacterial counts.

To collect the urine, the nurse holds the infant over a sterile container or applies a sterile plastic collecting bag. The infant can be encouraged to void by applying pressure over the suprapubic area or by stroking the paraspinal muscles to elicit a Perez reflex. This reflex, which usually disappears by 4 to 6 months of age, results in crying, extension of the back, flexion of the arms and legs, and urination.

When voiding has occurred, the bag is removed immediately. Urine that has been allowed to remain at room temperature is unacceptable as a sample for culture because the number of bacteria doubles every 20 to 30 minutes. If the urine is not tested within 30 minutes, the specimen is refrigerated. If the child has not voided within 45 minutes, the bag must be removed and the cleansing procedure repeated.

Twenty-Four-Hour Collection

Collection of urine voided over a 24-hour period creates some special problems in infants and children. Collection bags and sometimes restraining methods are required to collect specimens from infants and small children. Older children require special instruction about notifying someone when they need to void or have a bowel movement so that urine can be collected separately and not discarded. Some older school-age children and adolescents can be trusted to take responsibility for collection of their own 24-hour specimens. They can keep output records and transfer each voiding to the 24-hour collection container if this is permitted.

As in any 24-hour urine collection, the collection period always starts and ends with an empty bladder. At the time the collection begins, the child is instructed to void and the specimen is discarded. All urine voided in the subsequent 24 hours is saved in a refrigerated container. Twenty-four hours from the time the precollection specimen was discarded, the child is again instructed to void, the specimen is added to the container, and the entire collection is taken to the laboratory for examination.

Infants and small children who are bagged for 24-hour urine collection will require a special collection bag; frequent removal and replacement of adhesive collection devices can produce skin irritation. A thin coating of sealant, such as Skin-Prep, applied to the skin helps to protect it and aids adhesion. Plastic collection bags with collection tubes attached are ideal when the container must be left in place for a time. These can be connected to a collecting device or emptied periodically by aspiration with a syringe. When such devices are not available, a regular bag with a feeding tube inserted through a puncture hole at the top of the bag serves as a satisfactory substitute. However, care must be taken to empty the bag as soon as the infant urinates to prevent leakage and loss of contents.

Special Techniques

Catheterization or *suprapubic aspiration* is employed when a specimen is urgently needed or when the child is unable to void or otherwise provide an adequate specimen. Catheterization is most often used when urethral obstruction or anuria caused by renal failure is believed to be the cause of the child's failure to void. Suprapubic aspiration is useful in clarifying the diagnosis of suspected urinary tract infection in acutely ill infants.

Catheterizing a child requires aseptic technique, good light, and gentle, thorough cleansing of the vulva or glans penis. Most children, including female infants, accommodate a size 8 or 10 French catheter, but in male infants or when the larger catheters cannot be passed, a smaller, soft plastic feeding tube may be needed. Most children are frightened of this procedure, and few small children are entirely cooperative; therefore even when the procedure is adequately explained, an assistant is needed to help restrain and reassure the child. Special care must be exercised when catheterizing young males to avoid trauma to the ductal and glandular openings into the urethra, which might result in sterility.

Suprapubic aspiration, which is performed by a practitioner skilled in the procedure, involves aspirating bladder contents by inserting a 20- or 21-gauge needle in the midline approximately 1 cm above the symphysis and directed vertically downward. The skin is prepared as for any needle insertion, but the bladder should contain an adequate volume of urine. This can be assumed if the infant has not voided for at least 1 hour or the bladder can be palpated above the symphysis. This technique is especially useful for obtaining clean specimens from young infants. The bladder is an abdominal organ at this time and is easily accessible.

STOOL SPECIMENS

Stool specimens are frequently collected in children to identify parasites and other organisms that cause diarrhea, to assess gastrointestinal function, and to check for occult (hidden) blood. Ideally stool should be collected without contamination with urine, but in children wearing diapers this is difficult unless a urine bag is applied. Children who are toilet trained should urinate first, flush the toilet, then defecate in the toilet or in a bedpan (preferably one that is placed on the toilet to avoid embarrassment) (see also Nursing tip, p. 397). An ample amount of stool is collected using a tongue blade and placed in the appropriate container that is covered and labeled. If several specimens are needed, the containers are marked with the date and time and kept in a specimen refrigerator. Special care is exercised in handling the specimen because of the risk of contamination.

BLOOD SPECIMENS

Most blood specimens are obtained by the laboratory staff, physicians, or specially trained nurses, such as those in intensive care units, where specimens are frequently needed. However, all nurses are often responsible for making certain that specimens, such as serial examinations and fasting specimens, are collected on time and that the proper equipment is available, such as correct collection tubes and ice for blood gas samples.

Venous blood samples can be obtained by venipuncture or by aspiration from an intravenous infusion site. When using an intravenous infusion site for specimen collection, it is important to consider the type of fluid being infused. For example, a specimen collected for glucose determination would be inaccurate if removed from a catheter through which glucose-containing solution is being administered (see Nursing tip on blood specimens).

Nursing Tip: Blood Specimens

To obtain a blood specimen from a central venous line or heparin lock when the infusion solution may interfere with tests results, first aspirate a quantity of blood equal to the volume of fluid in the catheter and discard; then aspirate the blood sample.

For a blood culture, use the first sample of blood, since organisms are most likely to collect within the catheter itself (Schreiner, 1987).

Capillary blood samples are taken from children by finger or earlobe stick methods, just as in the adult patient. The best method for taking peripheral blood samples from infants is by a heelstick. Before the blood sample is taken, the heel is warmed with warm, moist compresses for 5 to 10 minutes in order to dilate the vessels in the area. The area is cleansed with alcohol, and with the infant's foot firmly restrained with the free hand, the heel is punctured with a Bard-Parker No. 11 or Redi-Lance blade.

The most serious complication of infant heel puncture is necrotizing osteochondritis from lancet penetration of the underlying calcaneus bone. To avoid this, the puncture should be no deeper than 2.4 mm and should be made at the outer aspect of the heel. The boundaries of the calcaneus can be marked by an imaginary line extending posteriorly from a point between the fourth and fifth toes and running parallel to the lateral aspect of the heel and another line extending posteriorly from the middle of the great toe and running parallel to the medial aspect of the heel (Fig. 21-16).

The needed specimens are collected quickly, and then pressure is applied to the puncture site with a dry gauze square until bleeding stops. The site is then covered with a Band-Aid. Applying warm compresses to ecchymotic areas increases circulation, helps remove extravasated blood, and decreases pain.

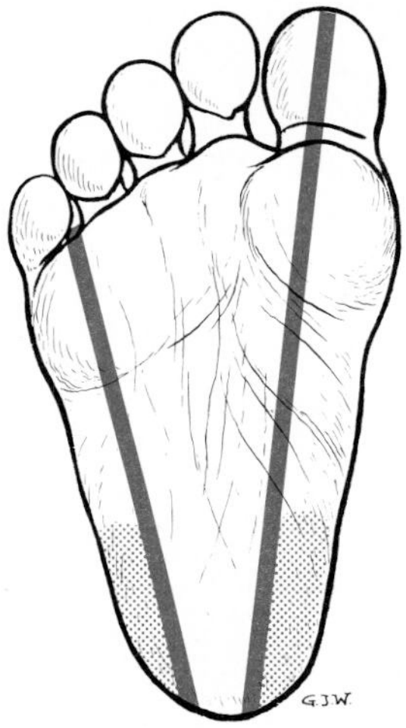

FIG. 21-16 Puncture site (red stippled area) on sole of infant's foot.

Arterial blood samples are sometimes needed for blood gas measurement, although noninvasive techniques, such as transcutaneous oxygen monitoring and pulse oximetry (see p. 224), are being used more frequently. Arterial samples may be obtained by arteriopuncture using the radial, brachial, or femoral arteries; by deep heel puncture; or from indwelling arterial catheters. Since unclotted blood is required, only heparinized collection tubes are used. In addition no air bubbles should enter the tube, since they can alter blood gas concentration. Crying, fear, and agitation also affect blood gas values; therefore, every effort is used to comfort the child. The blood samples are packed in ice to reduce blood cell metabolism and are taken to the laboratory for immediate analysis.

No matter how or by whom the specimen is collected, children, even some older ones, fear the loss of their blood. This is particularly true for children whose condition requires frequent blood specimens. Ignorant about the process of hemopoiesis, they mistakenly believe that blood removed from their bodies is a threat to their lives. Explaining to them that their blood is continually being produced by their bodies provides them with a measure of reassurance regarding this aspect of the stress-provoking procedure. When the blood is drawn, a simple comment such as, "Just look how red it is. You're really making a lot of nice red blood," confirms this information and affords them an opportunity to express their concern. A Band-Aid gives them added assurance that the vital fluids will not leak out through the puncture site.

Children also dislike the discomfort associated with venous, arterial, or capillary punctures. In fact, children have identified these procedures as the ones most frequently causing pain during hospitalization and arterial punctures as being one of the most painful of all procedures experienced (Wong and Baker, 1988). Consequently, nurses need to institute pain reduction techniques to lessen the discomfort of these procedures (see box, p. 664 and Nursing tip on venipuncture).

> *Nursing Tip: Venipuncture*
>
> Keep arm extended, not flexed, while applying pressure for a few minutes after venipuncture in the antecubital fossa to reduce bruising (Dyson and Bogod, 1987).

RESPIRATORY SECRETION SPECIMENS

Collection of sputum or nasal discharge is sometimes required for diagnosis of respiratory infections, especially tuberculosis and respiratory syncytial viruses. Older children and adolescents are able to cough as directed and supply sputum specimens when given proper directions. It must be made clear to them that a coughed specimen, not what is cleared from the throat, is needed. It is helpful to demonstrate a deep cough so that communication is clear. Infants and small children are unable to follow directions to cough and will swallow any sputum produced when they do; therefore gastric washings (lavage) may be used to collect a specimen. Sometimes it is possible to get a satisfactory specimen by using a suction device such as a mucous trap if the catheter is inserted into the trachea and the cough reflex elicited. A catheter that is inserted into the back of the throat is not sufficient. For children with a tracheostomy, a specimen is easily aspirated from the trachea or major bronchi by attaching a collecting device to the suction apparatus.

A nasal washing is needed to collect nasal discharge. The child is placed supine and from 1 to 3 cc of sterile normal saline is instilled with a sterile syringe (without needle) into one nostril. The contents are aspirated using a small, sterile bulb syringe and are placed in a sterile container. To prevent any additional discomfort to the child, all the equipment should be ready before beginning the procedure.

◆ *Administration of Medication*

The administration of medications to children presents a number of problems that are not encountered when giving medication to adult patients. Children vary widely in age, weight, body surface area, and the ability to absorb, metabolize, and excrete medications. Nurses must be particularly alert when computing and administering drugs to infants and children.

DETERMINATION OF DRUG DOSAGE

It is the physician's responsibility to prescribe drugs in the correct dosage to achieve the desired effect without endangering the health of the child. However, nurses must have an understanding of the safe dosage of medications they administer to children, as well as the expected action, possible side effects, and signs of toxicity. Unlike with adult medications, there are few standardized dosage ranges for children in the pediatric age-groups, and, with a few exceptions, drugs are prepared and packaged in average adult-dosage strengths.

Various formulas involving age, weight, and body surface area (BSA) as the basis for calculations have been devised to determine children's drug dosage from a standard adult dose. Since the administration of medication is a nursing responsibility, nurses need not only a knowledge of drug action and patient responses but some resources for estimating safe dosages for children. The method most often used to determine children's dosage is based on surface area.

Body Surface Area

The most reliable method for determining children's dosage is to calculate the proportional amount of body surface area to body weight. The ratio of body surface area to weight varies inversely to length; therefore the infant who is shorter and weighs less than an older child or adult has relatively more surface area than would be expected from his weight.

The usual determination of surface area requires the use of the West nomogram (Fig. 21-17). Body surface

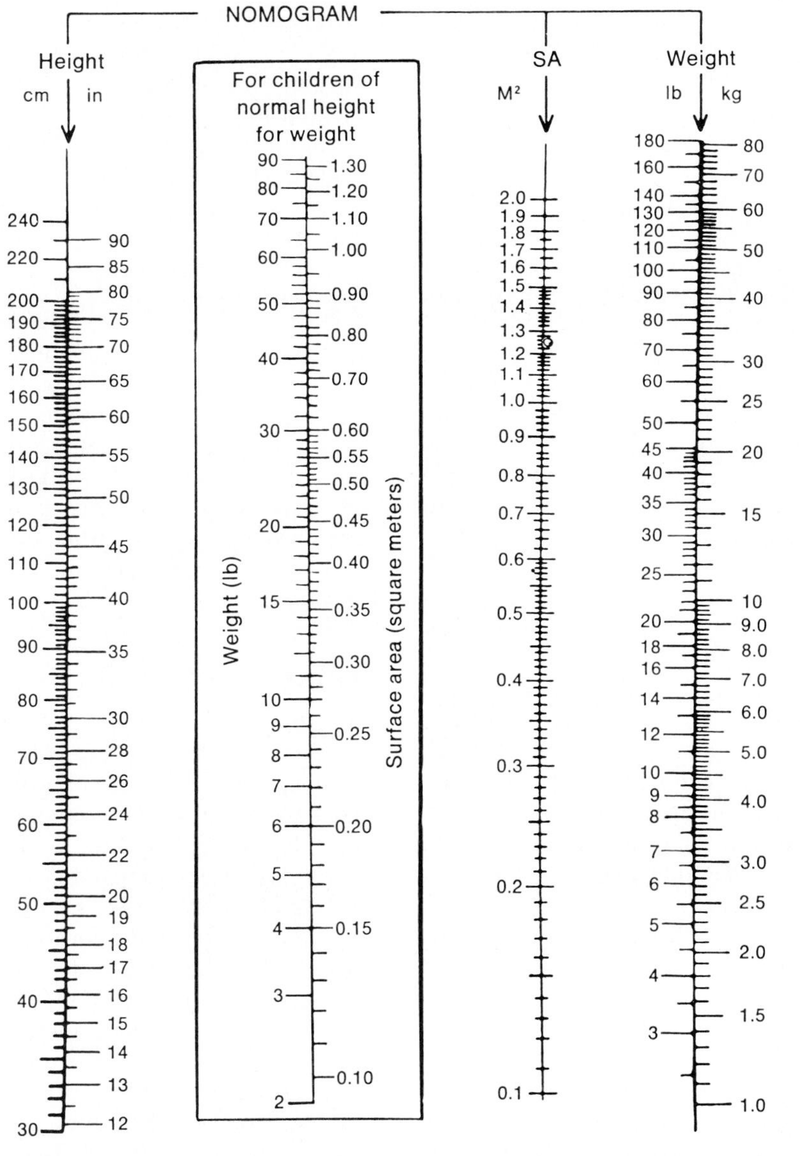

FIG. 21-17 West nomogram (for estimation of surface areas). The surface area is indicated where a straight line connecting the height and weight intersects the surface area *(SA)* column, or if the patient is roughly of normal proportion, from the weight alone *(enclosed area)*. (Nomogram modified from data of E. Boyd by C.D. West; from Behrman, R.E., and Vaughan, V.C., editors: Nelson textbook of pediatrics, ed. 13, Philadelphia, 1987, W.B. Saunders Co.)

area is estimated from height and weight of the child, and then this information is applied to a formula for dosage, such as either of the following formulas, which require different types of information:

$$\frac{\text{Body surface area of child}}{\text{Body surface area of adult}} \times \text{Adult dose} = \begin{array}{c}\text{Estimated}\\\text{child's dose}\end{array}$$

$$\text{Surface area of child (m}^2\text{)} \times \text{Dose/m}^2 = \begin{array}{c}\text{Estimated}\\\text{child's dose}\end{array}$$

PREPARATION FOR SAFE ADMINISTRATION

Unit dose packaging, which is gaining wide usage in hospital pharmacies, frequently does not extend to pediatric medications. Therefore, the ability to calculate fractional doses from larger dosages is absolutely essential. In addition, measuring doses, identifying patients, and gaining cooperation create problems not usually encountered in giving medications to adults.

Checking Dosage

Administering the correct dosage of a drug is a shared responsibility between the physician who orders the drug and the nurse who carries out that order. Children react with unexpected severity to some drugs, and ill children are especially sensitive to drugs. Therefore checking the dose if there is any doubt about its accuracy is a valuable habit to acquire. When a dose is ordered that is outside the usual range or if there is some question regarding the preparation or the route of administration, the nurse should always check with the physician before proceeding with the administration, since the nurse is legally liable for any drug administered.

Administering some medications requires added safeguards. Even when it has been determined that the dosage is correct for a particular child, there are many drugs that are potentially hazardous or lethal. Most hospital units or other facilities where medications are given to children have regulations requiring that specified drugs be double-checked by another nurse before they are given to the child. Among those drugs that require such safeguards are digoxin, heparin, and insulin. Others that are frequently included are epinephrine, narcotics, and sedatives. Even if this precaution is not mandatory, nurses would be wise to take such precautions for their own sense of security.

Identification

Before the administration of any medication, the child must be correctly identified, since children are not totally reliable in giving correct names on request. An infant is unable to give his name, a toddler or preschooler may admit to any name, and a school-age child may deny his identity in an attempt to avoid the medication. Children sometimes exchange beds for a while. Parents may be present to identify their child, but the only safe method for identifying children is to check their hospital identification bands with the medication card.

Parents

Parents can be useful sources of information regarding the child and his capabilities. Nearly all parents have given some kind of medication to their child and can describe the approaches that they have found to be successful. They can also provide information regarding the child's reaction to similar experiences if the child has been hospitalized before or if he has been given medication in a physician's office or clinic. In some cases it is less traumatic for the child if a parent gives the medication, provided the nurse prepares the medication and supervises its administration and the practice is consistent with hospital or ward policy. Children being given daily medications at home are accustomed to the parent functioning in this capacity and are less apt to fuss than they would if the medication were administered by a stranger. Individual decisions need to be made regarding parental presence and participation, such as in helping with restraint during injections (see p. 624).

Child

Every child requires psychologic preparation for parenteral administration of medication and supportive care during the procedure (see p. 628). Even if children have received several injections, they rarely become accustomed to the discomfort and have as much right to understanding and patience from those involved in giving the injection as any other child. Safe administration of any drug requires meticulous attention to the safeguards discussed here.

ORAL ADMINISTRATION

The oral route is preferred for administering medications to children whenever possible. Because of the ease of administration of oral medications, most are dissolved or suspended in liquid preparations. Although some children are able to swallow or chew solid medications at an early age, solid preparations are not recommended for young children. There is danger of aspiration in any oral preparation, but solid forms (pills, tablets, capsules) are especially hazardous if their administration causes marked resistance or crying.

Most pediatric medications come in palatable and colorful preparations for added ease of administration. Some have a slightly unpleasant aftertaste, but the majority of children will swallow these liquids with little if any resistance. The nurse should taste a minute amount of an oral preparation to ascertain if it is palatable or bitter. In this way legitimate complaints of dislike from the child can be accepted and the taste camouflaged whenever possible. Most pediatric units have preparations available for this purpose (see Nursing tip for oral medication).

Nursing Tip: Oral Medication

To encourage the child's acceptance of oral medications:

- Give the child an ice pop or small ice cube to suck to numb the tongue before giving the drug
- Mix the drug with a small amount (about 1 tsp) of sweet-tasting substances, such as honey (except in infants because of the risk of botulism), flavored syrups, jam, fruit purees, or ice cream; avoid essential food items, since the child may later refuse to eat them
- Give a "chaser" of water, juice, a soft drink, or a Popsicle or frozen juice bar after the drug
- If nausea is a problem, give a carbonated beverage poured over finely crushed ice before or immediately after the medication

Preparation

Selecting a vehicle to measure and administer a medication requires careful consideration. The devices available to measure medicines are not always sufficiently accurate for measuring the small amounts needed in pediatric nursing practice (Fig. 21-18). Standard medicine glasses have been replaced by disposable plastic or paper cups. Although the molded plastic cups offer reasonable accuracy in measuring moderate or large doses of liquids, the paper cups are likely to have irregularly shaped or crumpled bottoms. Calibrations on the cups (especially the teaspoon mark) and the personal equation or interpretation of a given measure are highly variable. Measures less than a teaspoon are impossible to determine accurately with a cup.

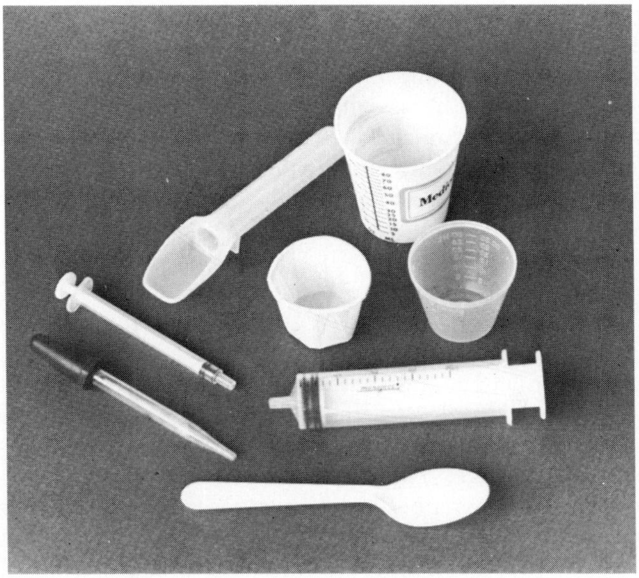

FIG. 21-18 Devices for administration of medications to children. Unacceptable devices for measurement are paper cups, household spoon, and uncalibrated dropper. Acceptable devices for measurement are plastic medicine cup, syringes, and hollow-handled medicine spoon.

Many liquid preparations are prescribed in measurements of teaspoons. However, the teaspoon (and other household measures) is an inaccurate measuring device and is subject to error from a number of variables. For example, household teaspoons vary greatly in capacity, and different persons using the same spoon will pour different amounts. Therefore a drug ordered in teaspoons should be measured in milliliters—the established standard is 5 ml per teaspoon. A convenient hollow-handled medicine spoon is available to accurately measure and administer the drug* (see Fig. 21-18).

Another unreliable device for measuring liquids is the dropper, which varies to a greater extent than the teaspoon or measuring cup. Droppers are available in numerous sizes but, even with the standard USP dropper, the volume of a drop will vary according to the viscosity of the liquid measured. Viscid fluids produce much larger drops than thin liquids. Many medications are supplied with caps or droppers designed for measuring each specific preparation. These are accurate when used to measure that specific medication but are not reliable for measuring other liquids. Emptying dropper contents into a medicine cup invites additional error. Since some of the liquid clings to the sides of the cup, a significant amount of the drug can be lost.

The most accurate means for measuring small amounts of medication is the plastic disposable (never glass) syringe, especially the tuberculin syringe for volumes less than 1 ml. Not only does the syringe provide a reliable measure, it also serves as a convenient means for transporting and administering the medication. The medication can be placed directly into the child's mouth from the syringe. For added safety, a short length of flexible tubing can be placed on the tip of the syringe to prevent injury to the mouth, although the tubing must be completely emptied of medication.

Small children and some older children as well have difficulty in swallowing tablets. Since a number of drugs are not available in pediatric preparations, the tablet will need to be crushed before it can be given to these children (see Nursing tip on crushing tablets). Another alternative is to have the pharmacist prepare the drug in a flavored, chewable troche or lozenge (Wong, 1987).

Not all drugs can be crushed (for example, medication with an enteric or protective coating or formulated for

*Manufactured by Apex Medical Corp., P.O. Box 20171, Bloomington, MN 55420.

Nursing Tip: Crushing Tablets

To minimize loss of the drug, crush the tablet between two spoons or place the tablet in either a medicine cup or between two small paper soufflé cups and use a pestle for crushing; collect the bits of pulverized medication that tend to cling to the sides of the cup or spoon and mix the crushed tablet with a palatable substance.

slow release). For some children it may be possible to encourage swallowing the tablet or capsule by using a special glass designed with a shelf that holds the drug.* The child drinks normally, and the tablet is carried to the back of the throat. For children who must take solid oral medication for an extended period, training sessions using progressively larger candy to teach the child to swallow can be beneficial (Funk, Mullins, and Olson, 1984).

Since pediatric doses often require dividing adult preparations of medication, the nurse may be faced with the dilemma of accurate dosage. With tablets, only those that are scored can be halved or quartered accurately. If the medication is soluble, the tablet or contents of a capsule can be mixed in a small premeasured amount of liquid and the appropriate portion given. If half a dose is required, the tablet is dissolved in 5 ml of water or flavored liquid and 2.5 ml is given.

Administration

While administering liquids to infants is relatively easy, the nurse must be careful to prevent aspiration. With the infant held in a semireclining position, the medication is placed in the mouth from a spoon, plastic cup, plastic dropper, or plastic syringe (without needle). The dropper or syringe is best placed along the side of the infant's tongue and the contents administered slowly to avoid causing the infant to choke. Medicine cups can be used effectively for older infants who are able to drink from a cup. Because of the natural outward tongue thrust in infancy, medications may need to be retrieved from lips or chin and refed. Allowing the infant to suck the medication that has been placed in any empty nipple† or inserting the syringe or dropper into the side of the mouth, parallel to the nipple, while the infant nurses are other convenient methods for giving liquid medications to infants. Medication is not added to the infant's formula feeding.

The small child who refuses to cooperate or resists consistently despite explanation and encouragement may require mild physical coercion. If so, it is carried out quickly and carefully. Every effort is made to determine why the child resists, and the reasons for this alternative are explained to the child in such a way that he will know that it is being carried out for his well-being and is not a form of punishment. There is always a risk in using even mild forceful techniques. A crying child can aspirate a medication, particularly when he is lying on the back. If the nurse holds the child in the lap with the child's right arm behind the nurse, the left hand firmly grasped by the nurse's left hand, and the head securely restrained between the nurse's arm and body, the medication can be slowly poured into the mouth (Fig. 21-19).

*Manufactured by Apex Medical Corp., P.O. Box 20171, Bloomington, MN 55420.

†A commercial nipple (NUK Medi-Nurser) is designed with a reservoir to hold the liquid and is available from Reliance Products Corp., 108 Mason St., P.O. Box 1220, Woonsocket, RI 02895.

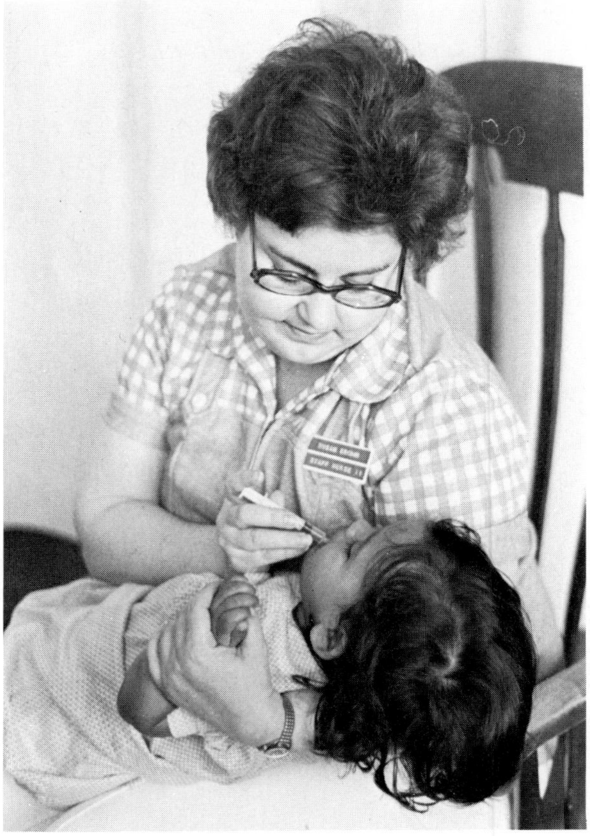

FIG. 21-19 Nurse partially restrains child for easy and comfortable administration of oral medication.

INTRAMUSCULAR ADMINISTRATION

Injections constitute some of the most traumatic health-related experiences for children. No one likes an injection, especially young children, who may associate the procedure with other meanings, such as fear of body mutilation and punishment. At times it can be no less stressful to the nurse who must inflict the distress. Consequently, injections are given only when the drug cannot be given by any other route.

Selecting Syringe and Needle

The volume of medication prescribed for small children and the small amount of tissue for injection require that a syringe be selected that can measure very small amounts of solution. For volumes less than 1 ml the tuberculin syringe, calibrated in one-hundredth increments, is appropriate. Very minute doses may require the use of a 0.5 ml, low-dose syringe. These syringes with specially constructed needles minimize the possibility of inadvertently administering incorrect amounts of a drug because of dead space, which allows fluid to remain in the syringe and needle after the plunger is pushed completely forward. A minimum of 0.2 ml of solution remains in a standard needle hub, therefore when very small amounts of two drugs are combined in the syringe, such as mixtures of insulin, the ratio of the two drugs can be altered significantly.

Dead space is also a significant factor to consider when injecting medication, since flushing the syringe with an air bubble or parenteral fluid adds an additional amount of medication to the prescribed dose. This can be hazardous when very small amounts of a drug are given. For example, a tuberculin syringe filled to the 0.05 ml mark can deliver *more than twice* the calculated dose of medication when it is flushed with parenteral fluid from an intravenous line. Consequently, flushing is not advisable, especially when less than 1 ml of medication is given. Syringes are calibrated to deliver a prescribed drug dose, and the amount of medication left in the hub and needle is not part of the syringe barrel calibrations. However, the air-bubble technique (drawing up about 0.2 ml of air into the syringe after withdrawing the medication) may be beneficial with certain drugs, such as iron dextran and diphtheria and tetanus toxoid, to avoid tracking the drug through the tissue. Another technique to minimize tracking is using the Z track method.

The needle length must be sufficient to penetrate the subcutaneous tissue and deposit the medication well in the body of the muscle (see Nursing tip on needle length). The most satisfactory needles for intramuscular injections in children are the 25- to 21-gauge needles with a length of ½ to 1 inch. Regular intramuscular needles are too large, in both length and gauge, for pediatric use except for very large, obese children.

Nursing Tip: Needle Length

To estimate needle length for intramuscular injection, first grasp lateralis or deltoid muscle and choose needle length that is approximately half the distance between thumb and index finger.

With ventrogluteal or dorsogluteal site, only subcutaneous tissue is grasped, so choose needle length that is slightly more than half the distance.

Choose a final needle length that allows for small portion of needle to be exposed at skin surface as precaution if needle should break off from hub (Lenz, 1983).

Determining Site

Factors that are considered when selecting a site for an intramuscular injection on an infant or child include:

1. The amount and character of the medication to be injected
2. The amount and general condition of the muscle mass
3. The frequency or number of injections to be given during the course of treatment
4. The type of medication being given
5. Factors that may impede access to or cause contamination of the site
6. The ability of the child to assume the required position safely

Ordinarily, older children and adolescents pose few problems in selecting a suitable site for intramuscular injections, but infants with their small and underdeveloped muscles have fewer available sites. It is sometimes difficult to assess the amount of fluid that can be safely injected into a single site. Usually 1 ml is the maximum volume that should be administered in a single site to small children and older infants. The muscles of small infants may not tolerate more than 0.5 ml. As the child approaches adult size, volumes approaching those given to adults may be used. However, the larger the amount of solution, the larger must be the muscle into which it is injected.

Injections must be placed in muscles large enough to accommodate the medication, yet major nerves and blood vessels must be avoided. There is no universal agreement regarding the best intramuscular injection site for children. The preferred site for infants is the vastus lateralis. The general recommendation for using the gluteal sites is after a child has been walking (length of suggested time varies), since the muscle develops with locomotion. Unfortunately, this recommendation is often applied to the ventrogluteal muscle site as well as the dorsogluteal site. However, there are significant differences between these two sites that warrant recognition. The ventrogluteal site is relatively free of major nerves and blood vessels, is a relatively large muscle with less subcutaneous tissue than the dorsal site, has well-defined landmarks for safe site location, and is easily accessible in several positions (Intramuscular injections, 1985). These advantages make it a preferred site over the dorsogluteal muscle and challenge the recommendation that the ventrogluteal site not be used until children have been walking. In older children and adolescents the preferred sites are much the same as in the adult. Table 21-3 summarizes the four major injection sites and illustrates the location of the preferred intramuscular injection sites for children.

Administration

Although injections that are executed with care seldom produce trauma to the child, there have been reports of serious disability related to intramuscular injections in children. Repeated use of a single site has been associated with fibrosis of the muscle with subsequent muscle contracture, and injections in the neighborhood of large nerves, such as the sciatic nerve, have been responsible for permanent disability, especially when potentially neurotoxic drugs are administered. There are several reports of tissue damage from penicillin; one of the difficulties in administering the opaque preparations, such as Bicillin, is that aspirated blood cannot be detected at the bottom of the syringe, thus increasing the risk of injecting into a blood vessel. When such drugs are injected, great care must be used in locating the correct site. When aspirating, the nurse should look for blood at the *top* of the syringe near the plunger since blood may be drawn up through the column of penicillin (Stoller and Losey, 1985).

TABLE 21-3

Intramuscular Injection Sites in Children

Site — **Discussion**

Vastus lateralis

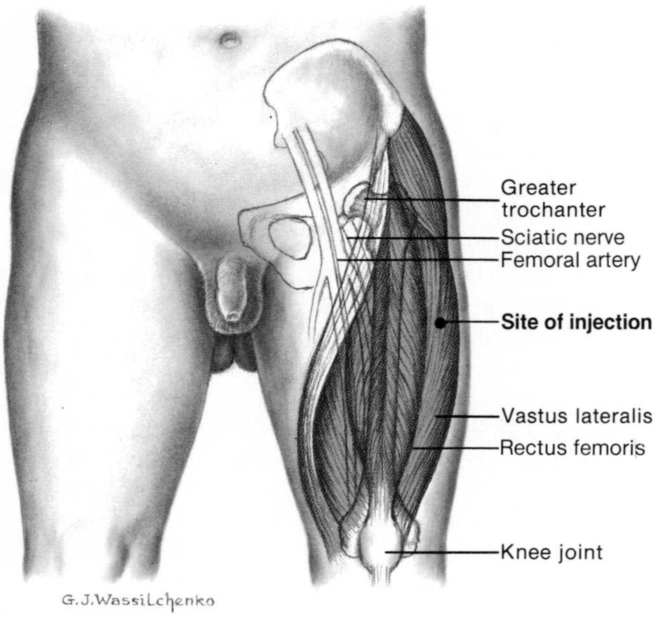

Location
Palpate to find greater trochanter and knee joints; divide vertical distance between these two landmarks into quadrants; inject into middle of upper quadrant.

Needle Insertion
Insert needle at 45-degree angle toward knee in infants and in young children or needle perpendicular to thigh or slightly angled toward anterior thigh.

Advantages
Large, well-developed muscle that can tolerate larger quantities of fluid
No important nerves or blood vessels in this location
Easily accessible if child is supine, side-lying, or sitting
A tourniquet can be applied above injection site to delay drug hypersensitivity reaction if necessary

Disadvantages
Thrombosis of femoral artery from injection in midthigh area
Sciatic nerve damage from long needle injected posteriorly and medially into small extremity

Ventrogluteal

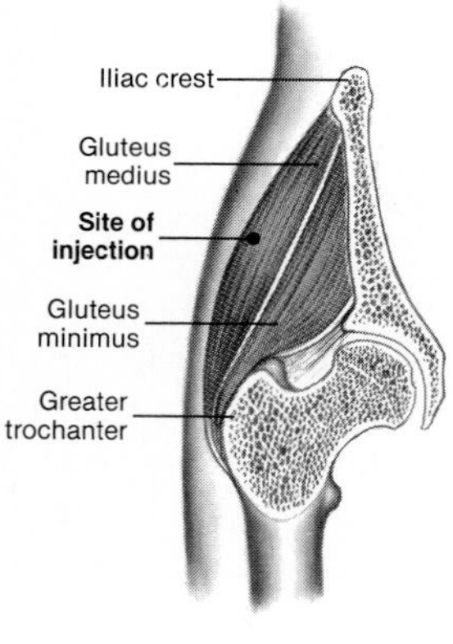

Ventrogluteal site of injection

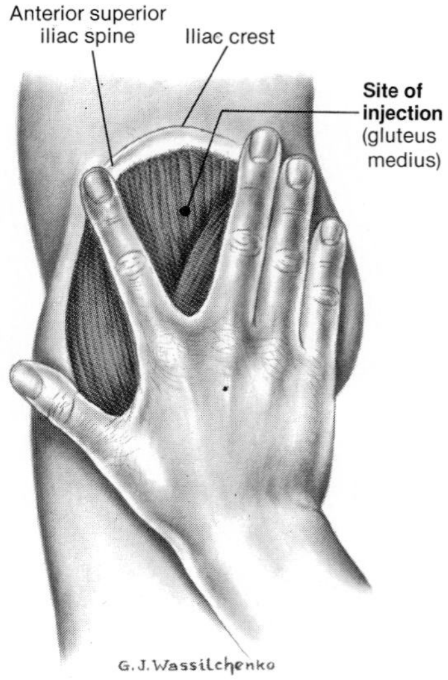

Location
Palpate to locate greater trochanter, anterior superior iliac tubercle (found by flexing thigh at hip and measuring up to 1 to 2 cm above crease formed in groin), and posterior iliac crest; place palm of hand over greater trochanter, index finger over anterior superior ilac tubercle, and middle finger along crest of ilium posteriorly as far as possible; inject into center of V formed by fingers.

Needle Insertion
Insert needle perpendicular to site but angled slightly toward iliac crest.

Advantages
Free of important nerves and vascular structures
Easily identified by prominent bony landmarks
Thinner layer of subcutaneous tissue than in dorsogluteal site, thus less chance of depositing drug subcutaneously rather than intramuscularly
Easily accessible if child is supine, prone, or side-lying
Less painful than vastus lateralis

Disadvantages
Health professionals' unfamiliarity with site
Not suitable for use of a tourniquet

TABLE 21-3

Intramuscular Injection Sites in Children—cont'd

Site	Discussion
Dorsogluteal 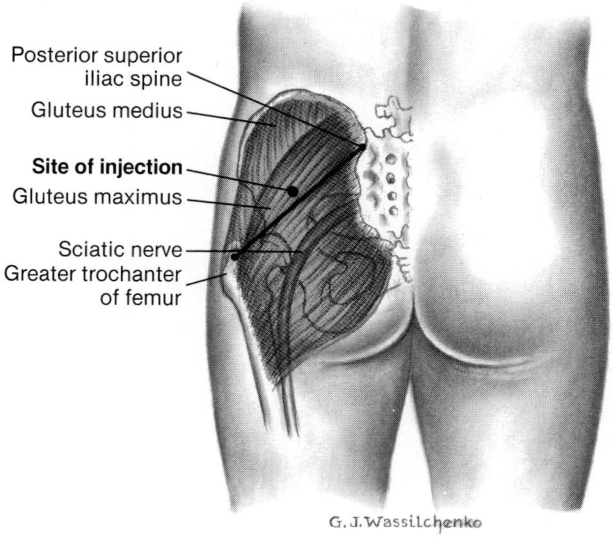	**Location** Locate greater trochanter and posterior superior iliac spine; draw imaginary line between these two points and inject lateral and superior to line into gluteus muscle. **Needle Insertion** Insert needle perpendicular to surface on which child is lying when prone. **Advantages** In older child large muscle mass; well-developed muscle can tolerate greater volume of fluid Child does not see needle and syringe Easily accessible if child is prone or side-lying **Disadvantages** Contraindicated in children who have not been walking for at least 1 year Danger of injury to sciatic nerve Thick, subcutaneous fat, predisposing to deposition of drug subcutaneously rather than intramuscularly Not suitable for use of a tourniquet Inaccessible if child is supine Exposure of site may cause embarrassment in older child
Deltoid 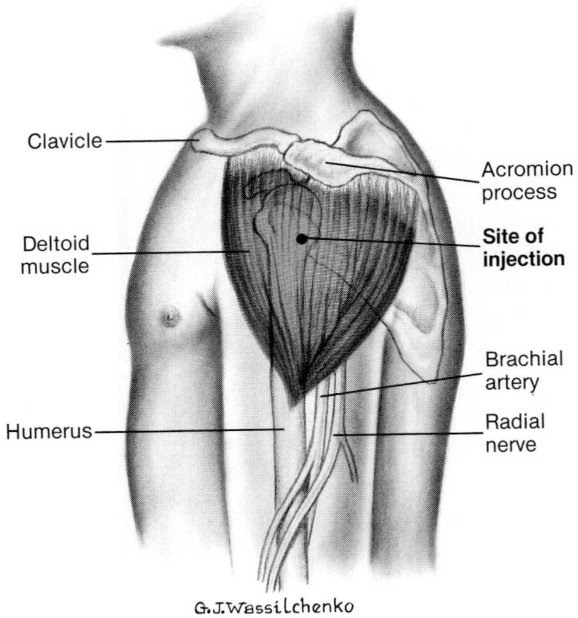	**Location** Locate acromion process; inject only into upper third of muscle that begins about 2 finger-breadths below acromion. **Needle Insertion** Insert needle perpendicular to site but angled slightly toward shoulder. **Advantages** Faster absorption rates than gluteal sites Tourniquet can be applied above injection site Easily accessible with minimum removal of clothing **Disadvantages** Small muscle mass; only limited amounts of drug can be injected Small margins of safety with possible damage to radial nerve Pain with repeated injections

A reported potential hazard with medication in glass ampules is the presence of glass particles in the ampule after the container is broken. When the medication is withdrawn into the syringe, the glass particles are also withdrawn and are subsequently injected into the patient. As a precaution, medication from glass ampules should only be drawn up through a needle with a filter or injected intravenously through a site in the tubing that is distal to an intravenous filter. Another precaution that does not relate to patient safety but to nursing safety is proper disposal of the uncapped, unbroken needle/syringe unit to prevent contamination with organisms such as hepatitis or acquired immune deficiency syndrome (see box on p. 645 and Fig. 21-5).

Most children are unpredictable and few are totally cooperative when receiving an injection. Even children who appear to be relaxed and constrained can lose control under the stress of the procedure. It is advisable to have someone available to help restrain the child if needed. Since children often jerk or pull away unexpectedly, it is a good idea to carry an extra needle to exchange for a contaminated one so that there is a minimum of delay. The child, even a small one, is told that he is getting an injection (preferably using a phrase such as "putting medicine under the skin"), and then the procedure is carried out as quickly and skillfully as possible to avoid prolonging the stressful experience. Delay caused by lengthy explanations, attempts to hide the syringe from sight, or efforts to soothe the child will only serve to increase his anxiety. It must be kept in mind that intrusive procedures such as injections are especially anxiety provoking in preschool children and that small children usually associate any assault to the "behind" area with punishment. Since injections are painful, the nurse should employ excellent injection technique and effective pain-reduction measures to reduce discomfort (see Nursing guidelines).

Small infants offer little resistance to injections. Although they squirm and may be difficult to hold in position, they can usually be restrained without assistance. The body of a larger infant can be securely restrained between the nurse's elbow and body (Fig. 21-20). To inject into the body of the muscle, the muscle mass is firmly grasped between the thumb and fingers to isolate and stabilize the site. However, in obese children it is prefer-

Nursing Guidelines to Reduce Discomfort from Injections

- Prepare child for procedure; allow choice of site if possible
- Allow parent to stay with child if parent and child wish
- Select site where skin is free of irritation and hypersensitive or fibrotic areas
- Use new sharp needle with smallest diameter that permits free flow of medication or blood
- Allow skin preparation, especially alcohol, to dry completely before penetrating skin
- Have medication near room temperature
- Decrease perception of pain during needle insertion (see also Nonpharmacologic interventions on p. 598)
  - Distract child with conversation
  - Give child something on which to concentrate, such as squeezing a hand or bed rail, pinching own nose, humming, or yelling "ouch"
  - Place a cold compress or wrapped ice cube on site about a minute or spray site with an aerosal coolant (Frigiderm) prior to injection (Eland, 1981); for venipuncture, apply cold to contralateral site
  - Apply a topical anesthetic patch to venipuncture site one hour before performing procedure (Clarke and Radford, 1986)
- Insert needle with quick, darting action into muscle
- Inject into relaxed muscle
  - Dorsogluteal—lay child on abdomen with legs and toes rotated inward
  - Ventrogluteal—lay child on side with upper leg flexed and placed in front of lower leg
- Avoid tracking any medication through superficial tissues
  - Replace needle after withdrawing medication or wipe medication from needle tip with sterile gauze
  - Use Z-track method of injection
  - Avoid any depression of plunger during insertion of needle
  - Use an air bubble to clear needle if not contraindicated
- Inject medication slowly into muscle (over a period of 20 seconds)
- Remove needle quickly; hold dry, sterile gauze sponge firmly against the skin near needle when removing it to avoid needle's pulling on tissue
- Hold and cuddle young child and encourage parents to comfort child; praise older child

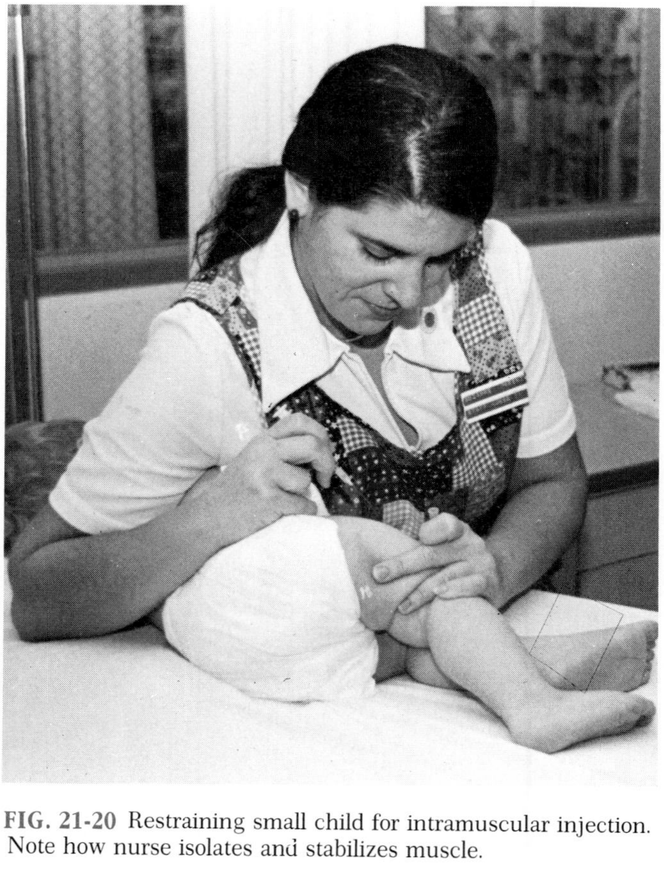

FIG. 21-20 Restraining small child for intramuscular injection. Note how nurse isolates and stabilizes muscle.

able to first spread the skin with the thumb and index finger to displace subcutaneous tissue and then grasp the muscle deeply on each side.

If medication is given around the clock, the nurse should wake the child before giving the injection. Although it may seem easier to surprise the sleeping child and give the injection as quickly as possible, this practice can cause the child to fear going back to sleep. When awakened first, the child knows that nothing will be done to him unless he is forewarned.

INTRAVENOUS ADMINISTRATION

The intravenous route for administering medications has gained widespread use in pediatric therapy. For some important drugs it is the only effective route of administration. This method is used for giving drugs to children who have poor absorption as a result of diarrhea, dehydration, or peripheral vascular collapse; children who need a high serum concentration of a drug; and those with resistant infections that require parenteral medication over an extended time.

Insertion sites and observation of the intravenous infusion are discussed on p. 671. However, there are a number of factors that need to be considered in relation to intravenous medication. When a drug is administered intravenously, the effect is almost instantaneous and further control is limited. Most drugs for intravenous administration require a specified minimum dilution and/or rate of flow, and many are highly irritating or toxic to tissues outside the vascular system. In addition to the precautions and nursing observations related to intravenous therapy, factors to consider when preparing and administering intravenous drugs to infants and children include:

1. Amount of drug to be administered
2. Minimum dilution of drug
3. Type of solution in which drug can be diluted
4. Length of time over which drug can be safely administered
5. Rate of infusion that child and his vessels can tolerate safely
6. Time that this or another drug is to be administered
7. Compatibility of all drugs that child is receiving intravenously

Before any intravenous infusion the site of insertion is checked for patency. Medications are never administered by way of blood products.

When a drug is to be administered within a specific period of time, the infusion rate should take into account the volume of fluid in the tubing from the point that the drug is injected that must infuse before the drug reaches the bloodstream. For example, if a drug is added to 10 ml in the gravity drainage apparatus (such as the Volutrol, Burette, Soluset, or Metriset) and the tubing contains 10 ml of fluid, the infusion rate on the microdropper must be set at 20 drops/minute (to infuse the 10 ml in the tubing and the 10 ml in the Volutrol) for all of the medication to enter the bloodstream in 1 hour. A formula for estimating the length of time *before* the medication reaches the patient is (Axton and Fugate, 1987):

$$\frac{\text{Tubing volume} \times 60 \text{ minutes}}{\text{Hourly IV rate}} = \text{Minutes drug will take to enter patient's vein}$$

Other methods of intravenous infusion are the *bolus technique*, in which medication is injected into the tubing at the site of the Y connection in the direction of the vein; and the *retrograde technique*, in which the medication is also injected into the intravenous tubing but *away* from the vein while the tubing is pinched between the Y connection and the venipuncture site. After the drug is injected, the tubing is no longer pinched and the intravenous infusion is allowed to flow. This allows for slower administration of the drug and greater dilution in the fluid than the bolus method. These techniques are advantageous in administering medication when fluid intake is limited, such as in neonates with congestive heart failure, and the drug must infuse in a short period.

To further conserve fluid and infuse the drug slowly but in less than 1 hour, the *two-syringe method* can be used. The intravenous line must have two Y connection sites (one above and one below the filter set). The syringe containing the diluted medication is attached to the Y connection above the filter, and an empty syringe is attached to the Y connection below the filter. The tubing is clamped above the first syringe and below the second (empty) syringe. As the medication is rapidly injected into the tubing, the equivalent amount of intravenous solution is displaced into the empty syringe. The syringes are removed, and the tubing is unclamped (Axton and Fugate, 1987).

Only one antibiotic should be administered at a time. If the intravenous solution contains other medications such as some electrolytes or vitamins, an antibiotic is not added because the other drugs may inactivate it. To prevent mixing, another bottle of intravenous solution can be hung and attached via a stopcock to the main infusion line. This "piggyback" setup allows antibiotics to be infused without mixing with the other solution. When the piggyback setup cannot be used, the drug can be injected directly into the tubing using the "two-syringe" approach described above. The only difference is that two syringes are used at the distal connector: one syringe contains normal saline, and the other syringe is filled with the diluted medication. First, a small amount of saline is injected into the tubing, followed by the drug, and finally by another amount of saline. With this method the saline "blocks" the drug from the infusion solution (Axton and Fugate, 1987).

Venous access devices. For infusion of intravenous drugs or collection of blood specimens when a continuous infusion is not needed, several venous access devices (VAD) are available. For short-term venous access a *heparin-lock* is ideal. The device consists of a short, flexible catheter or scalp vein needle inserted into a peripheral vein. The visible end of the catheter is occluded with a

A
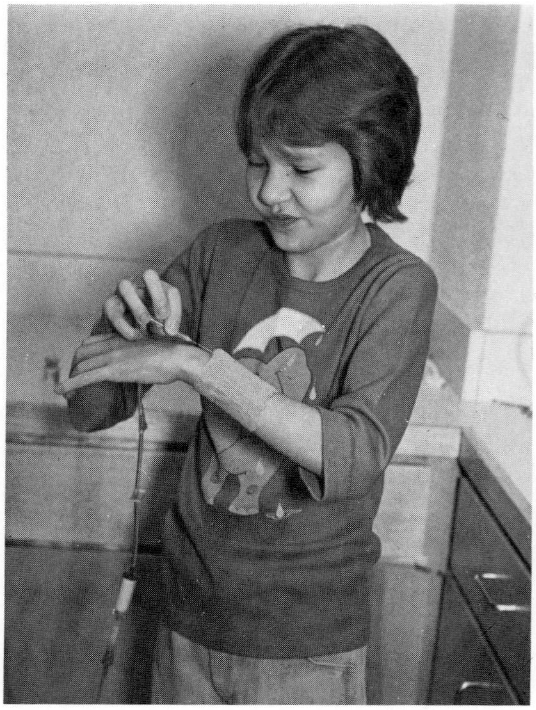
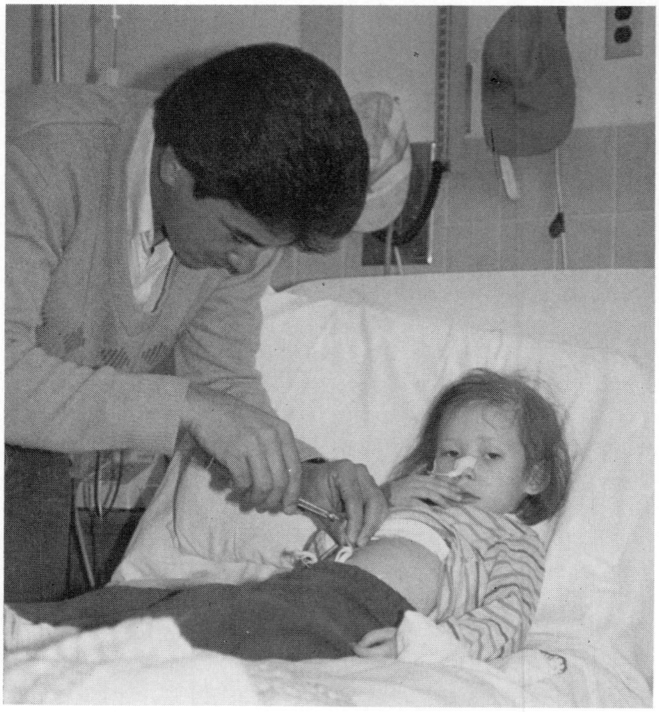
B

rubber diaphragm, and the line is kept patent with heparin or saline flushes (Fig. 21-21, *A*).

Central venous catheters and implantable infusion ports are available for long-term venous access (Fig. 21-21, *B* and *C*). These devices are described and compared in Table 21-4. With the heparin lock or any of the central venous catheters, instilling medication through the injection cap is easily accomplished. With the implanted device the port must be palpated for placement and stabilized, the overlying skin cleansed, and only special Huber needles used to pierce the port's diaphragm. To avoid repeated skin punctures, a special infusion set with a 90-degree prebent Huber needle and extension tubing with Luer connection can be used. With this attached, the injection procedure is the same as for the heparin device or venous catheters. To prevent infection, meticulous aseptic technique must be used anytime the devices are entered, including instillation of heparin or saline to prevent clotting. Because these methods of venous access are preferred for long-term administration of medication, families are usually required to learn the skills necessary for their care at home.*

*Home care instructions on caring for heparin lock and caring for a Hickman/Broviac catheter are available in Wong, D., and Whaley, L.: Clinical handbook of pediatric nursing, ed. 2, St. Louis, 1986, The C.V. Mosby Co.

RECTAL ADMINISTRATION

The rectal route for administration is less reliable but sometimes used when the oral route is difficult or contraindicated. Some of the drugs available in suppository form are aspirin, sedatives, analgesics (morphine), and antiemetics. The difficulty in using the rectal route is that, unless the rectal ampulla is empty at the time of insertion, the absorption of the drug may be delayed, diminished, or prevented by the presence of feces. Sometimes the drug is later evacuated, securely surrounded by stool. However, the rectal route is used most frequently in children who are unable to take anything by mouth and are unlikely to have large amounts of stool. It is also used when oral preparations are unsuitable to control vomiting.

To insert a suppository, the wrapper is removed and a gloved finger is used to quickly but gently place the suppository into the rectum, beyond both of the rectal sphincters. The buttocks are then held or taped together firmly to relieve pressure on the anal sphincter until the urge to expel the suppository has passed—5 to 10 minutes. Sometimes the amount of drug ordered is less than the dosage available. The irregular shape of most suppositories makes the process of dividing them into a desired dose difficult if not dangerous. If the suppository must be halved, it should be cut lengthwise. However, there is no guarantee that the drug is evenly dispersed throughout the petrolatum base.

C

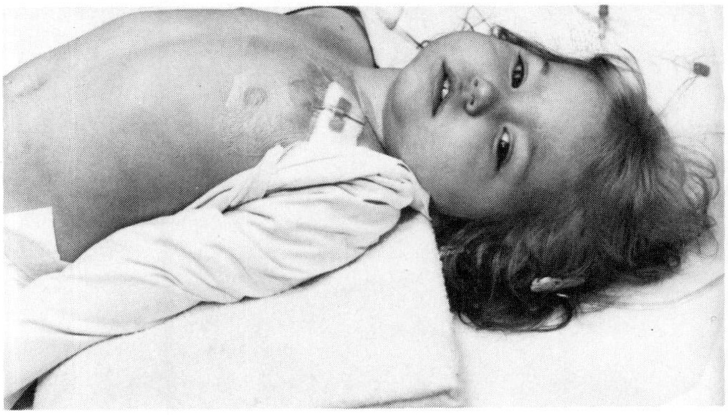

FIG. 21-21 Venous access devices. **A,** Child injecting medication by way of heparin lock; **B,** A parent flushing a central venous (Broviac) catheter; **C,** Child receiving medication by way of an implantable port. Note the bent Huber needle inserted into the port and secured with a transparent dressing.

TABLE 21-4

Comparison of Long-Term Venous Access Devices

Device	Description	Advantages	Disadvantages
Hickman/Broviac catheter	Silicone, radiopaque, flexible catheter with open ends One or two Dacron cuffs on catheter(s) enhances tissue ingrowth	Reduced risk of bacterial migration after tissue adheres to Dacron cuff Easy to use for self-administered infusions	Requires daily heparin flushes Must be clamped or have clamp nearby at all times Must keep exit site dry Heavy activity restricted until tissue adheres to cuff Risk of infection still present Protrudes outside body; susceptible to damage from sharp instruments and may be pulled out; may affect body image More difficult to repair Patient/family must learn catheter care
Groshong catheter	Clear, flexible, silicone, radiopaque catheter with closed tip and two-way valve at proximal end Dacron cuff on catheter enhances tissue ingrowth	Reduced time and cost for maintenance care; no heparin flushes needed Reduced catheter damage—no clamping needed because of two-way valve Increased patient safety due to minimum potential for blood backflow or air embolism Reduced risk of bacterial migration after tissue adheres to Dacron cuff Easily repaired Easy to use for self-administered IV infusions	Requires weekly irrigation with normal saline Must keep exit site dry Heavy activity restricted until tissue adheres to cuff Risk of infection still present Protrudes outside body; susceptible to damage from sharp instruments and may be pulled out; can affect body image Patient/family must learn catheter care
Implanted ports (Port-a-Cath, Infus-A-Port, MediPort)	Totally implantable metal or plastic device that consists of self-sealing injection port with preconnected or attachable silicon catheter that is placed in large blood vessel Port-a-Cath has greater surface and thicker septum that increase ease of cannulation and provide more secure placement of needle in port	Reduced risk of infection Placed completely under the skin; therefore, can not be pulled out or damaged No maintenance care and reduced cost for family Heparinized monthly and after each infusion to maintain patency No limitations on regular physical activity, including swimming No dressing needed No or only slight change in body appearance (slight bulge on chest)	Must pierce skin for access; pain with insertion of needle; can use local anesthetic before accessing port Special needle (Huber) with angled tip must be used to inject into port Skin preparation needed before injection Hard to manipulate for self-administered infusions Catheter may dislodge from port, especially if child "plays" with port site (Twiddler syndrome) Vigorous contact sports (football, soccer, hockey) generally not allowed

If medication is administered via a retention enema, the same procedure is used. Drugs given by enema are diluted in the smallest amount of solution possible to minimize the likelihood of being evacuated.

OPTIC, OTIC, AND NASAL ADMINISTRATION

There are few differences in administering eye, ear, and nose medication to children than to adults. The major difficulty is in gaining children's cooperation or employing restraining techniques. The infant or young child's head is immobilized in the same manner as described in Fig. 7-22. Older children need only explanation and direction. Although the administration of optic, otic, and nasal medication is not painful, these drugs can cause unpleasant sensations that can be eliminated with various techniques (see Nursing tips for eye, ear, and nose drops).

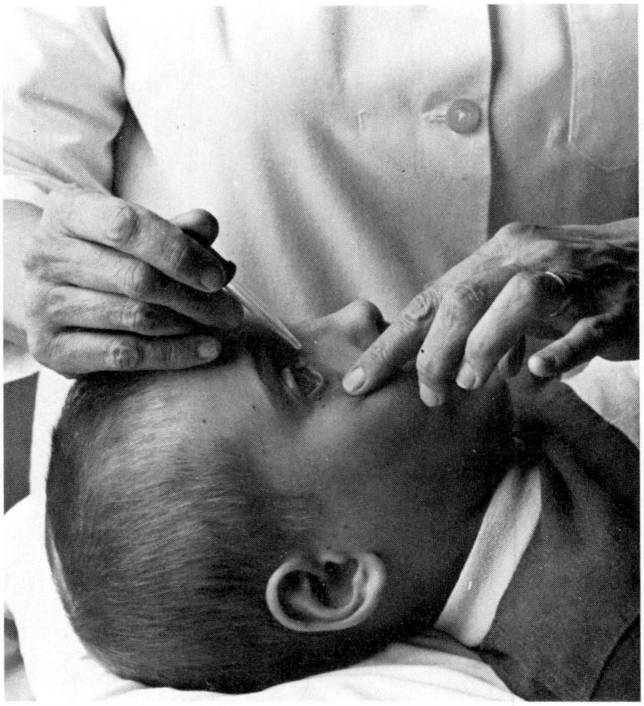

FIG. 21-22 Administering eye drops.

Nursing Tips: Eye/Ear/Nose Drops

To reduce unpleasant sensations:

Eye: Apply finger pressure to the lacrimal punctum at the inner aspect of the lid for 1 minute to prevent drainage of medication to the nasopharynx and the unpleasant "tasting" of the drug

Ear: Allow medications stored in the refrigerator to warm to room temperature before instillation

Nose: Position the child with the head hyperextended to prevent strangling sensations caused by medication trickling into the throat rather than up into the nasal passages

To instill eye medication, the child is placed supine or sitting with the head extended and the child is asked to look up. One hand is used to pull the lower lid downward; the hand that holds the dropper rests on the head so that it may move synchronously with the child's head, thus reducing the possibility of trauma to a struggling child or of dropping medication on the face (Fig. 21-22). As the lower lid is pulled down, a small conjunctival sac is formed; the solution or ointment is applied to this area, never directly on the eyeball. Another effective technique is to pull the lower lid down and out to form a cup, into which the medication is dropped. The lids are gently closed to prevent expression of the medication, and the child is asked to look in all directions to enhance even distribution of the preparation. Excess medication is wiped from the inner canthus outward to prevent contamination to the contralateral eye.

Instilling eye drops in infants can be most difficult, since they often clench the lids tightly closed. One approach is to place the drops in the nasal corner where the lids meet. The medication pools in this area, and when the child opens the lids, the medication flows onto the conjunctiva. For young children, playing a game can be helpful, such as instructing the child to keep the eyes closed until the count of 3, then to open them, at which time the drops are quickly instilled. Ointment can be applied when the child is sleeping by gently pulling down the lower lid and placing the ointment in the lower conjunctival sac.

Ear drops are instilled with the child restrained in the supine position and the head turned to the appropriate side. For children younger than 3 years of age, the external auditory canal is straightened by gently pulling the pinna downward and straight back. The pinna is pulled upward and back in children older than 3 years of age (see Fig. 7-19). After instillation, the child should remain lying on the unaffected side for a few minutes. Gentle massage of the area immediately anterior to the ear facilitates the entry of drops into the ear canal. The use of cotton pledgets prevents medication from flowing out of the external canal. However, the pledgets should be loose enough to allow any discharge to exit from the ear. Premoistening the cotton with a few drops of medication prevents the wicking action from absorbing the medication instilled in the ear.

Nose drops are instilled in the same manner as in the adult patient. Depending on his size, the infant can be positioned in the football hold (p. 647), in the nurse's arm with the head extended and stabilized between the nurse's body and elbow and the arms and hands immobilized with the nurse's hands, or with the head extended over the edge of the bed or a pillow (Fig. 21-23). Following instillation of the drops, the child should remain in position for 1 minute to allow the drops to come in contact with the nasal surfaces.

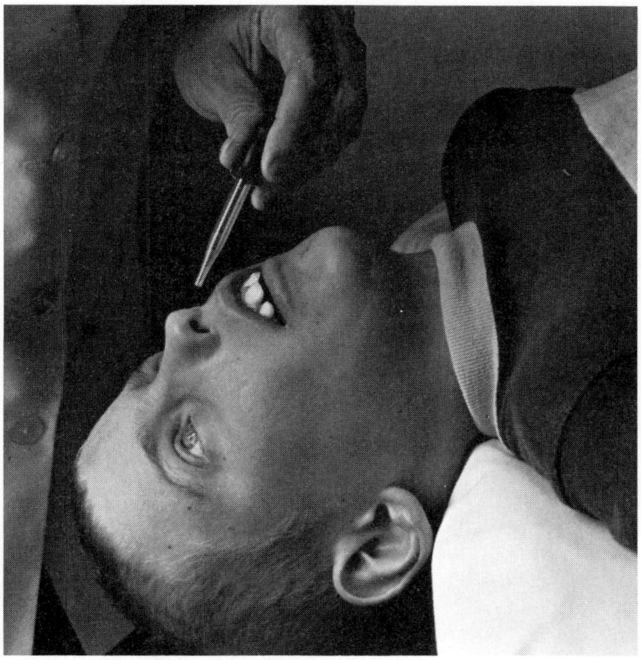

FIG. 21-23 Proper position for instilling nose drops.

FAMILY TEACHING AND HOME CARE

It is usually the nurse who assumes the responsibility for preparing families to administer medications at home. The family should have an understanding of why the child is receiving the medication and the effects that might be expected, as well as the amount, frequency, and length of time the drug is to be administered. Instruction should be carried out in an unhurried, relaxed manner, preferably in an area away from busy ward or office routine, following the same guidelines for teaching as outlined on p. 638.

The caregiver is carefully instructed regarding the correct dosage, and it is the nurse's responsibility to prepare parents for the specifics of the task. Some persons have difficulty understanding or interpreting terminology from the pharmacy, and just because they nod or otherwise indicate an understanding, it cannot be assumed that the message is clear. It is important to ascertain their interpretation of a teaspoon, for example, and to be certain they have acceptable devices for measuring the drug. If the drug is packaged with a dropper, syringe, or plastic cup, the nurse should show the point on the device that indicates the prescribed dose and demonstrate how the dose is drawn up into a dropper or syringe and measured and the bubbles eliminated. If the nurse has any doubts about the parent's ability to administer the correct dose, the parent should give a return demonstration. This is especially important when the drug has potentially serious consequences from incorrect dosage, such as insulin or digoxin, or when more complex administration is required, such as parenteral injections. When teaching a parent to give an injection, adequate time for instruction and practice must be allotted.

Home modifications are often necessary, because the availability of equipment or assistance can differ from the hospital setting. For example, restraint is often necessary when giving medications to children, and the parent may need guidance in devising methods that allow for one person to restrain the child and safely give the drug. One successful method is described in the Nursing tip on one-person restraint.

Nursing Tip: One-Person Restraint

To administer oral, nasal, or optic medication when you are the only person available to restrain the child, use the following procedure:

- Place child supine on flat surface (bed, couch, floor)
- Sit facing child so that his head is between operator's thighs and his arms are under operator's legs
- Place lower legs over child's legs to restrain lower body, if necessary
- To administer oral medication, place small pillow under child's head to reduce risk of aspiration
- To administer nasal medication, place small pillow under child's shoulders to aid flow of liquid through nasal passages

The time that the drug is to be administered is clarified with the parent. For instance, when a drug is prescribed in association with meals, the number of meals that the family is accustomed to eating influences the amount of drug the child receives; do they have meals twice a day or five times a day? When a drug is to be given several times during the day, together the nurse and parents can work out a schedule that accommodates the family routine. This is particularly significant if the drug must be given at equal intervals throughout a 24-hour period. For example, telling parents that the child needs 1 teaspoon of medicine four times a day is subject to misinterpretation, since parents may routinely schedule the doses at incorrect times. Instead, a preplanned schedule based on 6-hour intervals should be set up with the number of days required for therapeutic dosage listed. Written instruction should accompany all drug prescriptions (see Nursing tip on color-coded medication instructions).*

*Home care instructions on giving medications to children are available in Wong, D., and Whaley, L.: Clinical handbook of pediatric nursing, ed. 2, St. Louis, 1986, The C.V. Mosby Co.

Nursing Tip: Color-Coded Medication Instructions

If parents have difficulty reading or understanding English, use colors to convey instructions. For example, mark each drug with a color and place the appropriate color on a calendar chart or on a drawing of a clock to identify when the drug needs to be given.

◆ *Procedures Related to Maintaining Fluid Balance*

Nursing observation and intervention are essential to the detection and therapeutic management of changes in the fluid and electrolyte balance. Nurses need to be comfortable with equipment used to deliver fluids to infants and children and have the knowledge and techniques for assessment.

MEASUREMENT OF INTAKE AND OUTPUT

One of the most important roles of the nurse in maintaining fluid balance is accurate measurement of fluid balance. Although the physician usually indicates when intake and output (I & O) are to be recorded, it is a nursing responsibility to keep an accurate intake and output record on patients in the following situations:

After major surgery
Intravenous, diuretic, or corticosteroid therapy
Severe thermal burns or injuries
Renal disease or damage
Congestive heart failure
Dehydration (vomiting and diarrhea)
Diabetes mellitus
Oliguria

Infants or small children who are unable to use a bedpan or those who have bowel movements with every voiding will require the application of a collecting device (p. 654). If collecting bags are not used, wet diapers or pads are carefully weighed to ascertain the amount of fluid lost. This includes liquid stool, vomitus, and other losses. The volume of fluid in milliliters is equivalent to the weight of the fluid measured in grams. The specific gravity as a measure of osmolality is determined with a urinometer or a refractometer and assists in assessing the degree of hydration.

The weighed diaper method of fluid measurement has disadvantages, including (1) inability to differentiate one type of loss from another because of admixture; (2) loss of urine or liquid stool from leakage or evaporation (especially if the infant is under a radiant warmer); (3) additional fluid in diaper (superabsorbent disposable type) from absorption of atmospheric moisture (from high humidity incubators) (Hermansen and Buches, 1987 and 1988). To avoid the problem of evaporative losses and leakage of excreta, diapers should be weighed as soon as possible after becoming soiled.

It is important to measure and record all intake, oral and parenteral, and output from all sources, including urine, stool, emesis, drainage tubes, fistulas, and wounds from which appreciable amounts of fluid are lost.

Special Needs When the Child Is NPO

Infants or children who are unable or not permitted to take fluids by mouth (NPO) have special needs. To ensure that they do not receive fluids, a sign can be placed in some obvious place, such as over their beds or on their shirts, to alert others to their status. To prevent temptation to drink, fluids should not be left at the bedside.

Oral hygiene, a part of routine hygienic care, is especially important when fluids are restricted or withheld (see p. 640). For the young child who cannot brush the teeth or rinse the mouth without swallowing fluid, the nurse can institute oral hygiene by wiping the teeth, gums, and tongue with a cloth moistened with saline (see Nursing tip). The lips are kept moist with petrolatum (Vaseline) or another commercial lip aid. To meet the need to suck, the infant is provided with a pacifier.

> *Nursing Tip: Mouth Care*
>
> To keep the mouth feeling moist when the child is NPO, give ice chips (if this is permitted by the physician) or spray the mouth with a fine mist of cool water (a perfume atomizer works well).

PARENTERAL FLUID THERAPY

Since most hospitalized infants and children with serious disturbance of fluid and electrolyte balance are almost always maintained on intravenous fluids, monitoring intravenous fluid replacement is a major nursing responsibility. Most of the general principles of intravenous therapy apply to infants and children, but with a number of important variations.

Site

The site selected for intravenous infusion depends on accessibility and convenience. In older children any accessible vein may be used. In small infants a scalp vein or a superficial vein of the wrist, hand, foot, or arm is usually most convenient and most easily stabilized (Fig. 21-24). Since superficial veins of the scalp have no valves, they can be infused in either direction and are used frequently for intravenous therapy in infants.

Equipment

There are several modifications in equipment used for intravenous infusion for children. A gravity drainage apparatus used for children is much the same as that for adults except that it is designed to deliver a reduced drop size (60 drops/ml) and contains a calibrated volume control chamber that limits the maximum amount of fluid that can be infused. A microdropper greatly facilitates calculation of flow rate, because a prescribed *number of milliliters per hour equals the number of drops per minute.* For example, if the solution is to infuse at a rate of 30 ml/hour, the infusion is regulated to deliver 30 drops per minute. A variety of types are available, but all have a

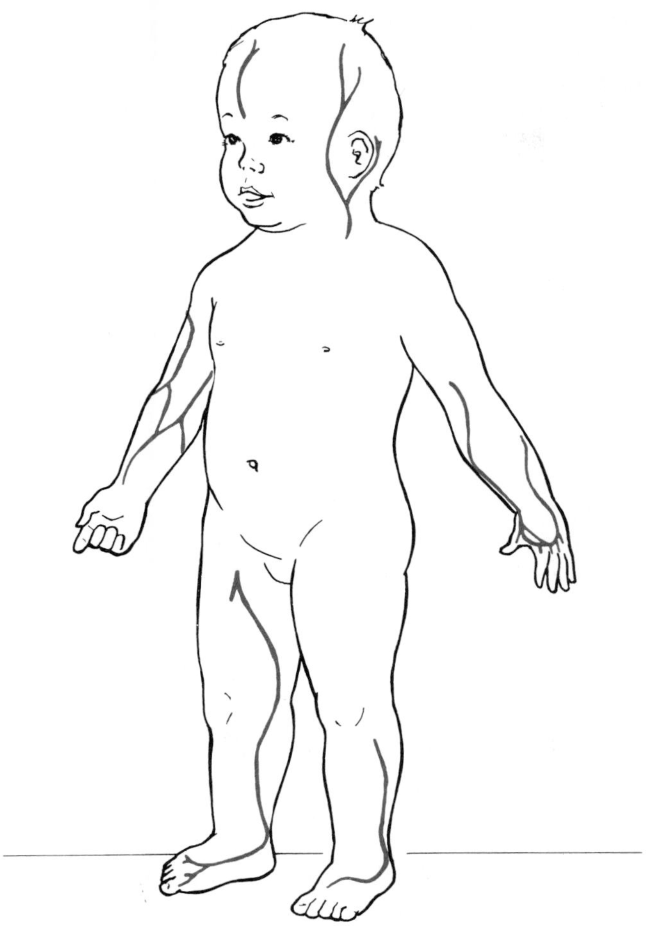

FIG. 21-24 Superficial veins used most often for intravenous infusion. (From Kempe, C.H., Silver, H.K., and O'Brien, D.: Current pediatric diagnosis and treatment, ed. 9, Los Altos, CA, 1986, Lange Medical Publications.)

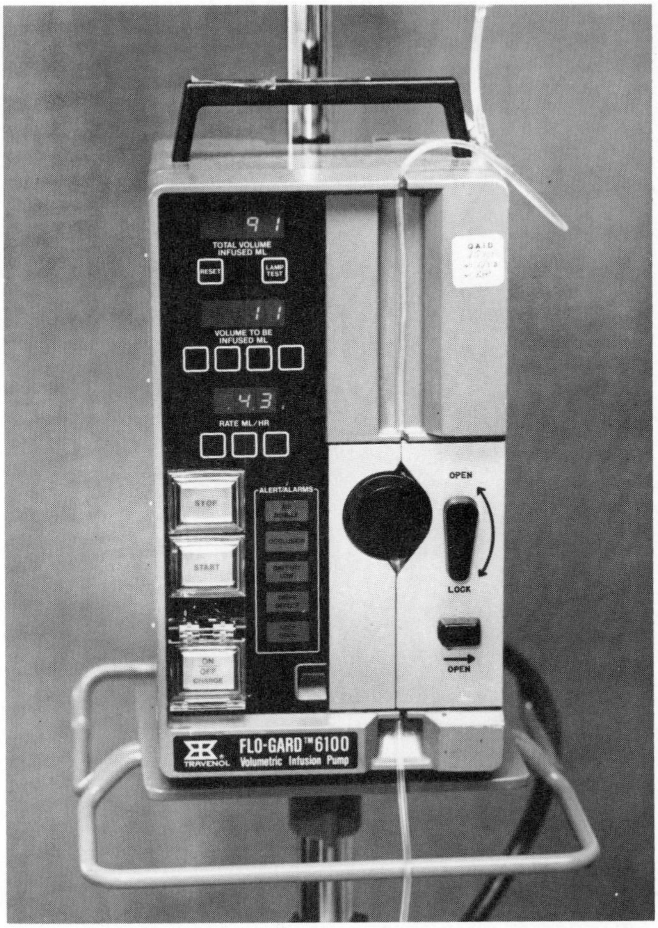

FIG. 21-25 Mechanical infusion pump for administration of intravenous fluids (Travenol).

limited capacity, refillable from the bottle above, to minimize the possibility of overloading the circulation. When such a device is used, it is important that the tubing between the bottle and the chamber is firmly clamped to prevent additional fluid from dripping into the chamber. When sets with collapsible chambers and rigid cylinders with an automatic shut-off valve are employed, the infusion stops automatically when the chamber is empty. It is an important nursing responsibility to calculate the amount to be infused in a given length of time, set the infusion rate, and monitor the apparatus frequently to make certain that the desired rate is maintained and that the infusion does not stop.

To facilitate a more precise flow rate, mechanical infusion pumps are used extensively for pediatric intravenous fluid administration (Fig. 21-25). Most of these devices pump a given amount of fluid by peristaltic action on the tubing, governed by a flow rate setting and regulated by a drop sensor that activates an alarm when no drops are formed. For administering a very small amount of fluid over a specific period of time, precision-controlled syringe pumps may be preferable. These devices, although convenient and efficient, are not without attendant risks. Over-reliance on the accuracy of the machine can cause either too much or too little fluid to be infused. Excess pressure can build up if the machine is set at a rate faster than the vein is able to accommodate (or continues to pump when the needle is out of the lumen). This is especially true in very small infants and when circumstances necessitate the use of a capillary. No matter what device is used, a thorough understanding of the apparatus and careful periodic assessment of the infusion are essential for safe fluid administration.

For most intravenous infusions in children, a scalp-vein size 21 or 23 needle is used with flexible winged tabs that are easily secured to the skin (Fig. 21-26). In situations in which fluids are urgently needed and there is difficulty in entering a vein, a polyethylene tube inserted by the surgical cutdown procedure may be necessary. The vein of choice for this alternative is the internal saphenous vein located just anterior to the medial malleolus of the tibia. For long-term intravenous therapy a number of other techniques may be used (see p. 667).

Selection of a scalp vein as the venipuncture site re-

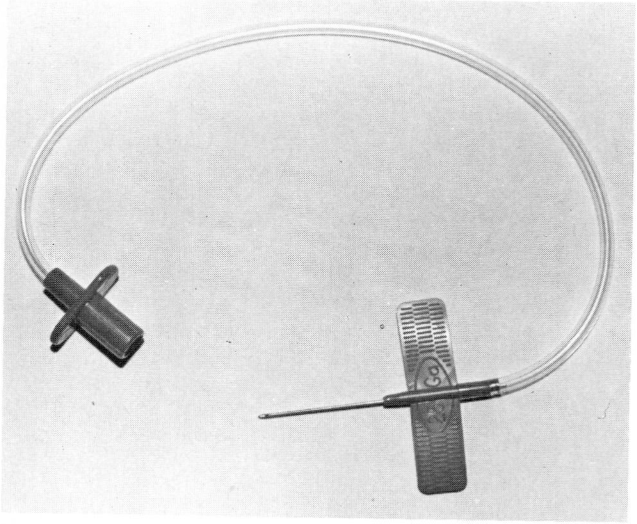

FIG. 21-26 Scalp vein needle.

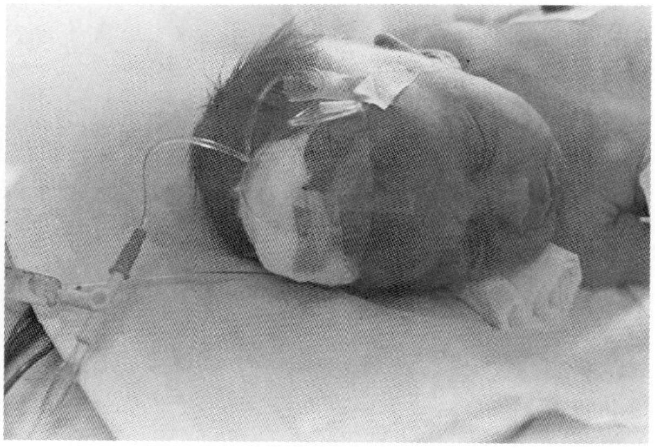

FIG. 21-27 Scalp vein infusion.

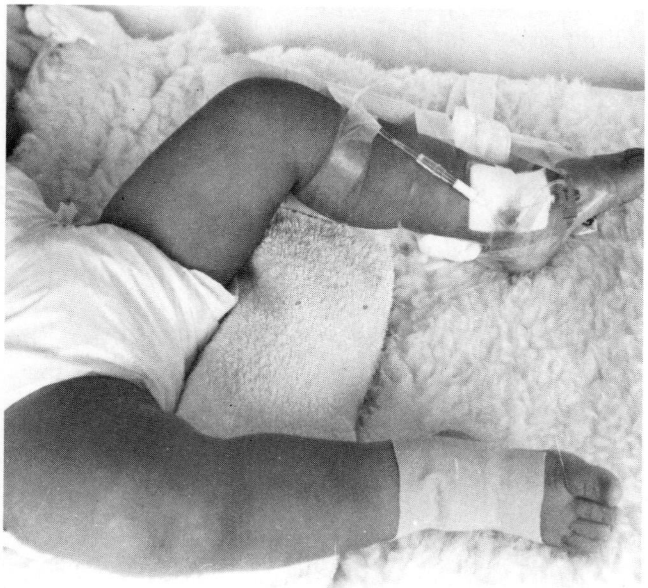

FIG. 21-28 Extremity immobilized with a board and firmly secured to bedding with pins. Note sheepskin, which protects bony prominences.

quires shaving the area around the site to better visualize the vein and provide a smooth surface on which to tape the tubing (Fig. 21-27). A rubber band slipped onto the head from brow to occiput will usually suffice as a tourniquet. Shaving off a portion of the infant's hair is very upsetting to parents; therefore, they should be told what to expect and reassured that the hair will grow in again rapidly.

Special Precautions

To maintain the integrity of the intravenous site, the child will require adequate restraint. The needle is secured firmly at the puncture site with nonallergenic tape or a transparent dressing and is protected from becoming dislodged by immobilization of the extremity. To prevent trauma to the skin from removal of tape, the nurse can place some gauze between the skin and adhesive. A plastic cup applied directly over the needle site will further protect the infusion. The head can be immobilized with covered sandbags. A sandbag or a small board, well padded with plastic foam and a cloth or stockinette cover, provides a suitable means for immobilization (Fig. 21-28). Some form of resilient padding is required to prevent areas of pressure necrosis over bony prominences, such as the ankle; however, the covering should be changed regularly to prevent infection, especially in immunocompromised children (McCarty and others, 1986).

Older children who are alert and cooperative can usually be trusted to protect the intravenous site. Infants, small children, and uncooperative children require restraint. A board used to stabilize a joint is secured to the bed, and the remaining extremities that might be used to dislodge the needle are restrained as described previously (p. 649). This includes feet as well as hands, since most infants will attempt to brush away the offending attachment by rubbing it against another extremity or body part. Range of motion exercises are employed on infants and children who are too ill or unable to move their extremities, but others should be encouraged to move their arms and legs in response to a natural stimulus. Most infants or small children will instinctively move their extremities when released. If not, a toy or other stimulus can be provided for an incentive.

The same precautions regarding maintenance of asepsis, prevention of infection, and observation for infiltration are carried out with patients of any age. However, infiltration is more difficult to detect in infants and small children than it is in adults. The increased amount of subcutaneous fat and the amount of tape used to secure the needle often obscure the signs of early infiltration. When the usual assessment techniques fail to detect the problem, it may be necessary to remove carefully some of the tape and other material that obscure a clear view of the venipuncture site. Dependent areas, such as the palm and undersides of the extremity, or the occiput and behind the ears with a scalp vein infusion, are examined for signs of infiltration.

FAMILY TEACHING AND HOME CARE

Since maintaining fluid balance is so critical, especially in young children, families may need to continue some procedures, such as measuring intake, output, and daily weight, at home. While these are simple skills, families require time to learn and practice them before discharge. With the widespread use of superabsorbent disposable diapers, parents are advised that the diaper may be wet but still feel dry. Placing some cotton balls or tissues in the diaper facilitates checking for wetness.

Intravenous therapy for fluid replacement is rarely carried out in the home, although parenteral administration of drugs or hyperalimentation is much more common. Home care of the child with home hyperalimentation is discussed on p. 683.

◆ *Procedures for Maintaining Respiratory Function*

Procedures to improve ventilation are employed with increasing frequency in the prevention and management of pulmonary dysfunction. Most of these procedures involve the nurse in the hospital or the home situation.

INHALATION THERAPY

The term *inhalation therapy* is an all-inclusive term that encompasses a variety of therapies that involve changing the composition, volume, or pressure of inspired gases. This includes primarily increasing the oxygen concentration of inspired gas (oxygen therapy), increasing the water vapor content of inspired gas (humidification), addition of airborne particles with beneficial properties (aerosol therapy), and various means for controlling or assisting respiration (artificial ventilation, intermittent positive pressure breathing).

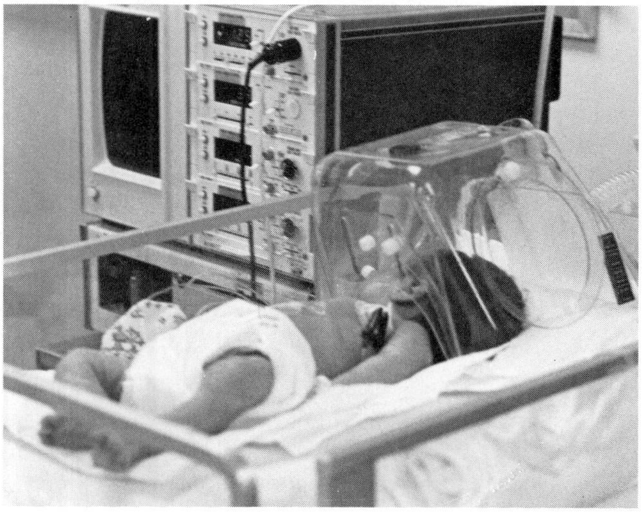

FIG. 21-29 Oxygen administered to an infant by a plastic hood.

Oxygen Therapy

Oxygen therapy is primarily carried out in the hospital, although increasing numbers of children are receiving oxygen in the home. Oxygen delivered to the infant via the Isolette is satisfactory when lower levels are adequate to prevent cyanosis, but the highest concentration (almost 100%) is supplied by way of a plastic hood (Fig. 21-29). The gas should not be allowed to blow directly into the infant's face, and the hood should not rub against the infant's neck, chin, or shoulder. Older cooperative children can use a nasal cannula or prongs, which can supply a concentration of about 50%, but a nasal catheter or a mask is not well tolerated by children.

For most children beyond early infancy, the oxygen tent, or canopy, is the most satisfactory means for administration of oxygen (Fig. 21-30). A tent does not require any device to come into direct contact with the face, but the concentration of oxygen within the tent is difficult to control and to maintain above about 40%. The comfort to the child makes it the method of choice except in cases of marked respiratory distress. A major difficulty with the use of the tent is keeping the tent closed so that oxygen concentration is maintained.

To reduce oxygen loss, nursing care is planned carefully so that the tent is opened as little as possible. Since oxygen is heavier than air, loss will be greater at the bottom of the tent; therefore the tent should be tucked in

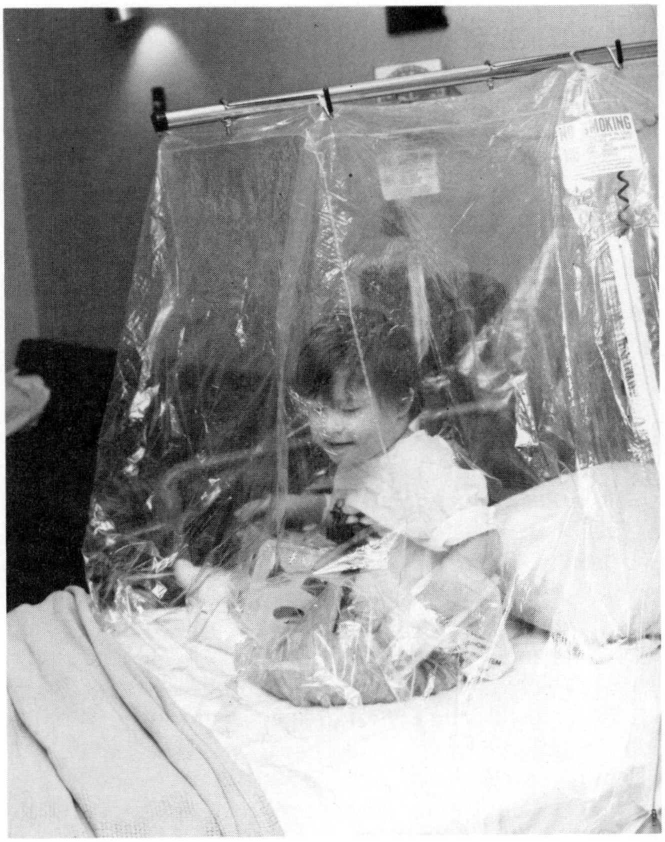

FIG. 21-30 The tent provides a comfortable method for oxygen administration to a child.

snugly without open edges. The bottom of the tent should be examined more often when the child is restless and fussy and liable to pull the covers loose. Some tents are even open at the top. Because of the rapid diffusing qualities of carbon dioxide, the levels of the gas do not build up within these enclosures.

After the tent has been opened for an extended period of time, it is flushed with oxygen by increasing the flow meter for a few minutes to quickly raise the oxygen and mist concentration. The flow meter is then reset to the prescribed number of liters.

The enclosed tent becomes very warm; therefore, some type of cooling mechanism is provided. The temperature inside the tent must be checked periodically to be certain that it is maintained at the desired level. It is important to make certain that the child is kept warm and dry. Mist is usually prescribed in conjunction with oxygen therapy, and the moisture condenses on the tent walls. The child's bedding and clothing are examined periodically and changed as needed to prevent chilling.

The reactions of children to the oxygen tent are variable. Some, especially older children, feel comfortable in the tent and like the cozy, close privacy it affords. Others, more often younger children, may be frightened by the forced enclosure. The plastic walls distort their view of the world and constitute a barrier between them and their source of comfort, their parent. Their distress can be minimized if they are able to see someone nearby and are reassured that they will not be left alone. A favorite toy or object can accompany the child inside the tent. However, all toys should be inspected for safety and suitability. The high oxygen environment makes any source of sparks (such as mechanical or electrical toys) a potential fire hazard. Other familiar items can be placed at the foot of the bed or otherwise in view.

No matter what method is used to administer the oxygen, the child's color and respiratory status are monitored frequently and evaluated in terms of efficacy of treatment. The oxygen content within the device is analyzed periodically (always at a point near the child's head) to determine the rate of flow needed to maintain the desired concentration. The equipment is changed and/or cleaned at regular intervals (at least once weekly) to prevent bacterial growth when the child requires oxygen over an extended period.

In most instances the child can be removed from the oxygen tent for activities such as feeding and bathing, whereas in other cases the child is placed in the tent only during periods of rest. Still other children may require oxygen continuously and can be removed from the tent or Isolette only if an oxygen source is held close to the child's face. Any change in color, increased respiratory effort, or restlessness is an indication to return the child to the oxygen tent.

Oxygen toxicity. Oxygen is essential to life and a valuable therapeutic aid. However, prolonged exposure to high oxygen tensions can be damaging to some body tissues and functions. The organs most vulnerable to the adverse effects of excessive oxygenation are the retina of the premature infant and the lungs of persons at any age.

Oxygen-induced carbon dioxide narcosis is a physiologic hazard of oxygen therapy that may occur in persons with chronic pulmonary disease. It is seldom encountered in children, except those with cystic fibrosis. These children have chronic alveolar hypoventilation with a concomitant chronic carbon dioxide retention and hypoxemia. In these patients the respiratory center has adapted to the continuously higher P_{CO_2} levels, and, therefore, hypoxia becomes the more powerful stimulus to respiration. When the P_{O_2} is elevated during oxygen administration, the hypoxic drive is removed, causing increasing hypoventilation and increased P_{CO_2} levels, and the child rapidly becomes unconscious.

Aerosol Therapy

The inhalation and subsequent deposition of airborne water particles within the airway is the function of aerosol therapy. Saline may be used to help moisten the airway and help liquefy secretions, or the particles may contain mucolytic, bronchodilating, decongestant, or antimicrobial agents.

For continuous aerosol therapy a misting device is attached to or incorporated into the mist tent. Distilled water is used most commonly, although propylene glycol in aqueous solution is often employed, especially in jet-type nebulizers. For intermittent administration of small quantities of an agent with specific pharmacologic action, a small nebulizer can be used powered by a small electric motor or in association with a positive pressure breathing apparatus.

Aerosol therapy is widely used in treatment of both upper and lower respiratory tract disease and of conditions in which there is weakness of the muscles of respiration. In some instances aerosol therapy is employed prophylactically (for example, cystic fibrosis) to prevent complicating pulmonary problems. There is a decided relationship between aerosol therapy and bronchial drainage. Drainage is much more effective immediately after aerosol therapy.

Aerosol therapy is usually performed under the guidance of a respiratory therapist, although nurses may assume this responsibility in the home or in association with the therapist. Nurses need to know how the apparatus works and to recognize when it is functioning improperly. Because of the danger of bacterial growth, the equipment is thoroughly cleaned daily.

BRONCHIAL (POSTURAL) DRAINAGE

Bronchial drainage is indicated whenever excessive fluid or mucus in the bronchi is not being removed by normal ciliary activity and cough. The techniques of segmental drainage, percussion, and vibration assist the normal cleansing mechanisms of the lung. Positioning the child to take maximum advantage of gravity further facilitates removal of secretions.

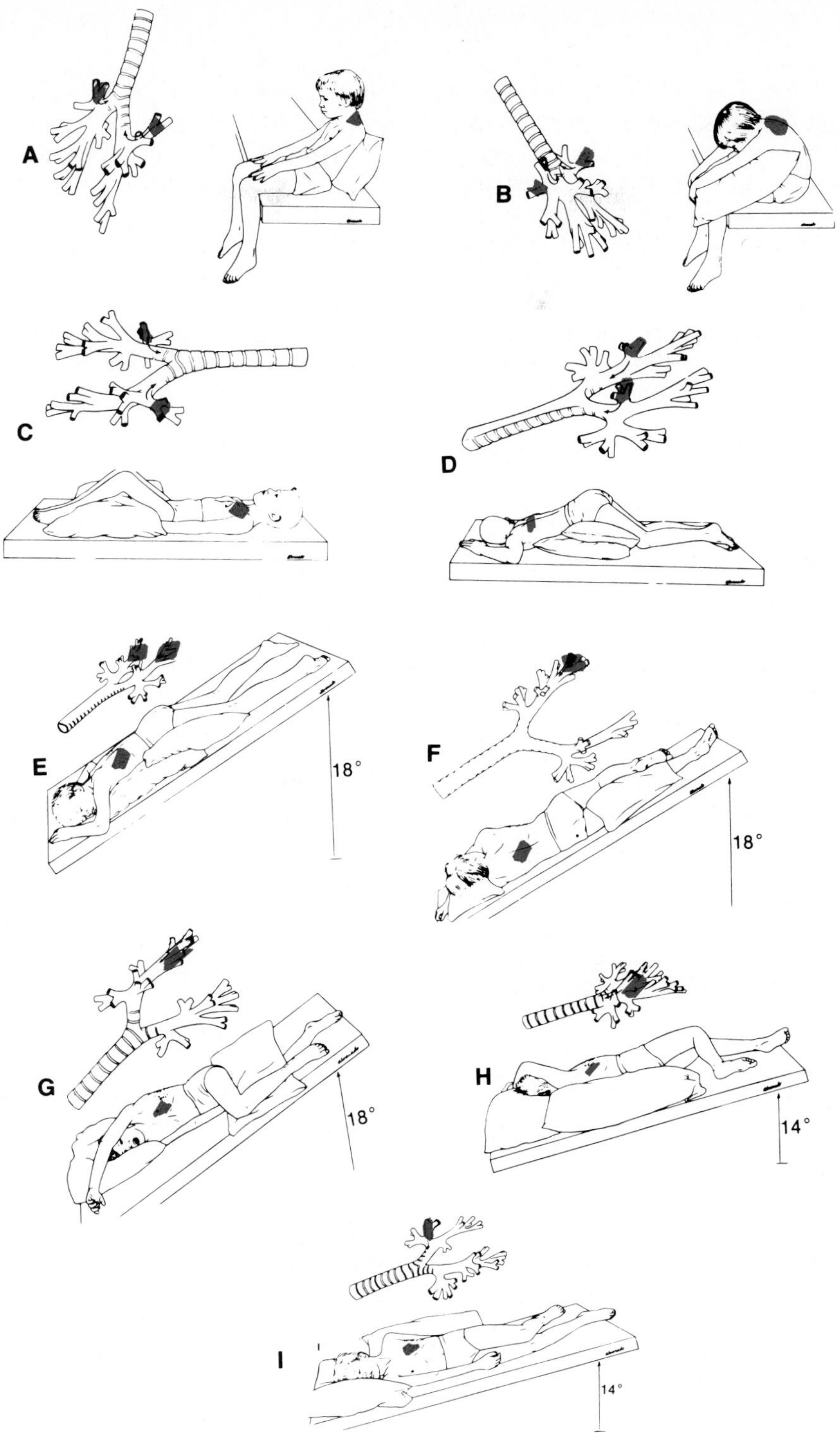

FIG. 21-31 Bronchial drainage positions for all major segments of lung. For each position, model of tracheobronchial tree is projected beside child in order to show segmental bronchus *(colored areas)* being drained and pathway *(arrow)* of secretions out of bronchus. Drainage platform is horizontal unless otherwise noted. **A,** Apical segment of right upper lobe and apical subsegment of apical-posterior segment of left upper lobe. **B,** Posterior segment of right upper lobe and posterior subsegment of apical-posterior segment of left upper lobe. **C,** Anterior segments of both upper lobes; child should be rotated slightly away from side being drained. **D,** Superior segments of both lower lobes. **E,** Posterior basal segments of both lower lobes. **F,** Lateral basal segments of right lower lobe; left lateral basal segment would be drained by mirror image of this position (right side down). **G,** Anterior basal segment of left lower lobe; right anterior basal segment would be drained by mirror image of this position (left side down). **H,** Medial and lateral segments of right middle lobe. **I,** Lingular segments (superior and inferior) of left upper lobe (homologue of right middle lobe). (From Kendig, E.L., Jr., editor: Disorders of the respiratory tract of children, ed. 4, Philadelphia, 1983, W.B. Saunders Co.)

Postural drainage is carried out three to four times daily or as often as every 2 hours and is more effective when it follows other respiratory therapy, such as bronchodilator and/or nebulization medication. Bronchial drainage is generally performed before meals (or 1 to 1½ hours after meals) to minimize the chance of vomiting and at bedtime. The length and duration of treatment depend on the child's condition and tolerance level—usually 20 to 30 minutes. Different positions are used to facilitate drainage from all major lung segments (Fig. 21-31), but all positions are not employed at each session. Children will usually cooperate for four to six positions, but more than six tend to exceed their limits of tolerance. In older children longer periods can be reasonably expected.

In the hospital an older child can be positioned over the elevated knee rest. Small children and infants can be positioned with pillows or on the therapist's lap and legs (Fig. 21-32). Special modifications of the techniques are required in children whose conditions contraindicate the standard positioning, such as head injuries, some types of

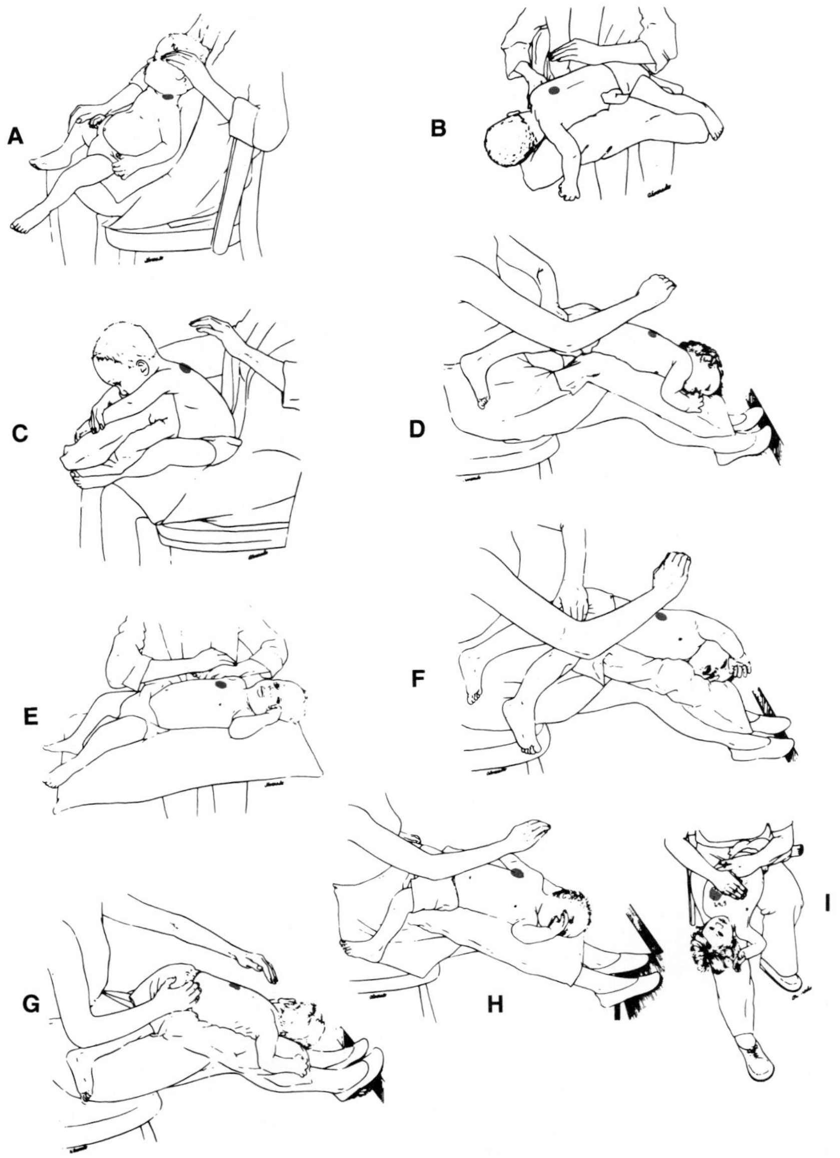

FIG. 21-32 Bronchial drainage positions for major segments of all lobes in infant. Procedure is most easily carried out in therapist's lap. Therapist's hand on chest indicates area to be cupped or vibrated. **A,** Apical segment of left upper lobe. **B,** Posterior segment of left upper lobe. **C,** Anterior segment of left upper lobe. **D,** Superior segment of right lower lobe. **E,** Posterior basal segment of right lower lobe. **F,** Lateral basal segment of right lower lobe. **G,** Anterior basal segment of right lower lobe. **H,** Medial and lateral segments of right middle lobe. **I,** Lingular segments (superior and inferior) of left upper lobe. (Modified from Infant segmental bronchial drainage. Reprinted with permission of Cystic Fibrosis Foundation, Rockville, MD.)

surgical incisions or burns, and casts or traction. At home small children can be positioned on a padded ironing board. Children who require postural drainage over a period of months or years may benefit from specially constructed tables padded and adjusted to their individual needs. The position used and the frequency and duration of treatment are individualized.

Since viscid secretions may not drain by gravity alone, various maneuvers, including deep breathing, reinforced cough, "cupping," or "clapping," and vibration, are performed in association with drainage to assist in their removal.

Percussion

Percussion—clapping or cupping—is performed intermittently during postural drainage. The operator's hands are held in the cupped position (Fig. 21-33) and vigorously and repeatedly strike the chest wall under which the specific lung segment to be drained is situated. The analogy used to illustrate this concept is that of a freshly opened catsup bottle. Even inverted, the catsup will not flow until it is loosened and ejected by repeated blows to the bottom of the bottle.

Performed properly, percussion is painless. The operator's hand should not strike the bare skin. A light cotton undershirt or gown is an appropriate covering to protect the skin from possible irritation. The hand does not slap but conforms to the contour of the chest wall, the entire circumference of the cupped hand touching the chest wall at the same instant. When correctly applied the clapping emits a loud, hollow sound. Care is exerted to clap over the *rib cage only*. For an infant whose chest is too small for conventional hand percussion, a small face mask is substituted for the operator's hand (see Fig. 9-14).

Vibration

Vibration, a more difficult procedure, is performed only during the exhalation phase of breathing. The child is instructed to take a deep breath and exhale slowly through pursed lips. The operator places one hand on top of the other over the target lung segment and, as the child exhales, transmits a rapid vibratory impulse through the chest wall by a tensing contraction of the forearm flexor and extensor muscles. After full expiration, pressure is released. In infants whose respirations are rapid, the padded handle of an electric toothbrush serves as an excellent mechanical vibrator.

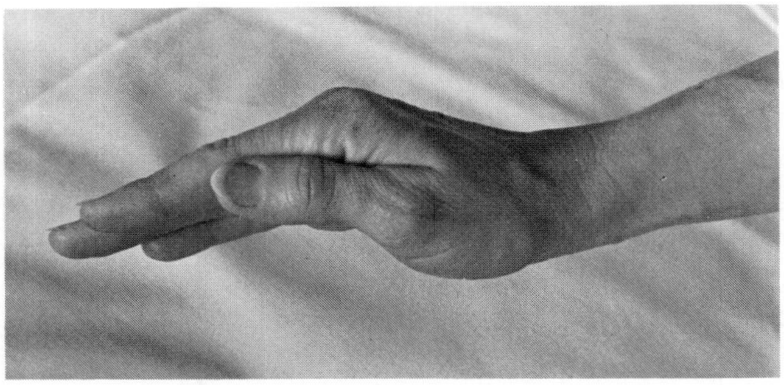

FIG. 21-33 Cupped hand position for percussion.

ARTIFICIAL VENTILATION

The regulation and maintenance of mechanical ventilators are the responsibility of respiratory therapists. However, nurses should understand the function of the ventilator in use and be able to detect signs of malfunction and deviations from the desired settings. The nurse also promotes the effectiveness of ventilation by suctioning, positioning, and providing support and reassurance to the child receiving mechanical respiration. See p. 244 for assisted and controlled respiration in the neonate.

Artificial Airways

An artificial airway is usually used in association with artificial ventilation and in children with upper airway obstruction. Endotracheal intubation can be accomplished by the nasal (nasotracheal), oral (orotracheal), or direct tracheal (tracheostomy) routes. Although it is more difficult to place technically, nasotracheal intubation is preferred to orotracheal intubation because it facilitates oral hygiene and provides more stable fixation, which reduces the complication of tracheal erosion and the danger of accidental extubation. Endotracheal tubes may be cuffed, to provide an airtight seal, or uncuffed. However, pressure cuffs are rarely used in children. Air or gas delivered directly to the trachea must be humidified as in tracheostomy.

Tracheostomy

Tracheostomy can be a lifesaving procedure. It is an emergency or an elective procedure and may be combined with mechanical ventilation.

Plastic and silastic have largely replaced silver as the preferred material for tracheostomy tubes, especially for pediatric use (Fig. 21-34). These materials can be constructed with a more acute angle and, since they soften at room temperature, are better able to conform to the contours of the airway. The flexibility of the material resists kinking, and the smooth surface reduces crust formation; therefore, most tubes are constructed without an inner cannula. The tube is held in place by an appropriate length of sturdy cloth twill tape around the child's neck. Umbilical cord tape is ideal. A better fit can be achieved if the child's head is flexed, rather than extended, while the tape is fixed. If the cord is too loose, the tube may be coughed out. The ties should fit snugly enough that one finger can be inserted with difficulty between the tape and the child's neck (Fig. 21-35). New tapes are attached before the old ones are removed to re-

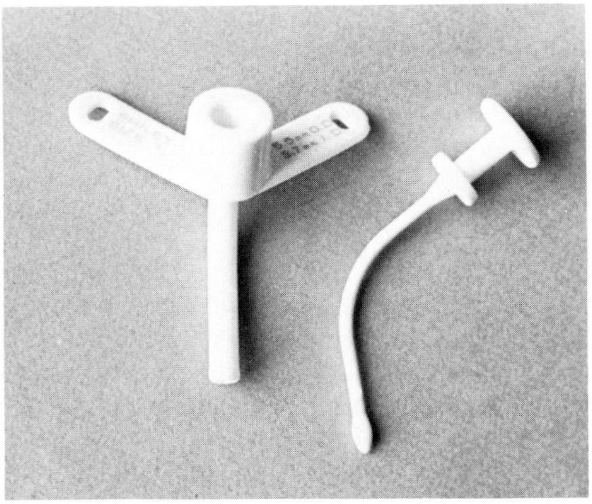

FIG. 21-34 Silastic pediatric tracheostomy tube and obturator for insertion of tube.

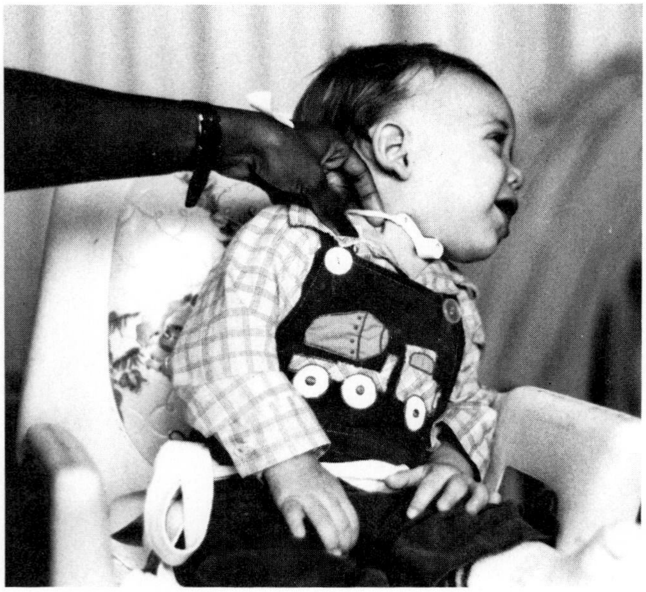

FIG. 21-35 Tracheostomy ties are snug but allow one finger to be inserted.

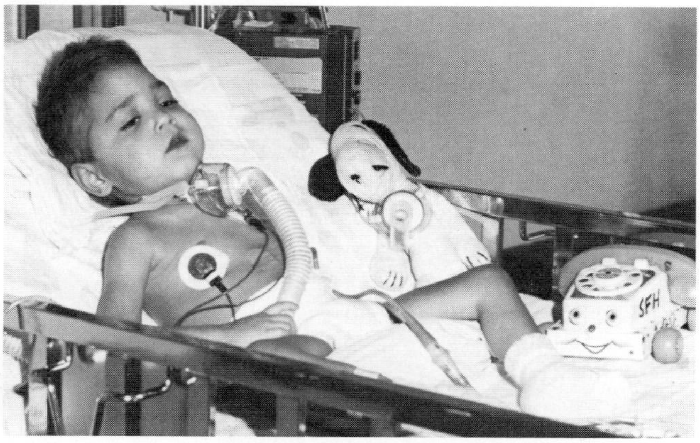

FIG. 21-36 Child with a tracheostomy and a mist collar.

duce the possibility of the tracheostomy tube becoming dislodged. The tapes should be tied at the side of the neck and the position of the knot changed at each tape change. For safety purposes, two operators should change the track tapes, especially if the child is uncooperative. The obturator is kept in a sterile package taped to the head of the bed in case of accidental decannulation.

Since the normal warming, wetting, and filtering functions of the upper airway are inoperative, air entering the tracheostomy opening is humidified by placing the child in a mist tent, by attaching a special tracheostomy mask or "collar" to deliver humidified gas directly to the tracheostomy opening (Fig. 21-36), or by direct attachment to a mechanical ventilator. The humid gas helps to loosen mucus and reduce the chances of crust formation and a mucous plug. Moisture from the humidified gas tends to accumulate on the inner surface of the flexible plastic tubing and must be eliminated periodically to prevent occlusion of the tube and/or accidental aspiration. The tubing is disconnected at the collar or tracheostomy tube and drained into a container. It is not allowed to flow back into the humidifying receptacle.

Suctioning. The airway must remain patent and requires frequent suctioning during the first few hours after tracheostomy to remove mucous plugs and excess secretions. Tracheal suction catheters are available in a variety of sizes. The catheter selected should have a diameter one half the diameter of the tracheostomy tube. If the catheter is too large, it can obliterate the airway. The catheter is constructed with a side port so that the catheter is introduced without suction and removed while simultaneous intermittent suction is applied by obliterating the port with the thumb (Fig. 21-37). The catheter is inserted to 0.5 cm beyond the end of the tracheostomy tube (see Nursing tip). A small amount of sterile isotonic saline (a few drops to 0.5 to 2 ml, depending on the size of the child) injected into the tube helps to loosen the secretions and crusts for easier aspiration.

Nursing Tip: Catheter Insertion

To measure the length for catheter insertion, place the catheter near a sample tracheostomy tube (same size as child's tube) with the end of the catheter 0.5 cm beyond the end of the tube; grasp catheter with sterile-gloved hand to mark the length and insert catheter until hand reaches stoma.

Suctioning should require no more than 3 to 4 seconds (American Heart Association, 1988). Counting 1-one thousand, 2-one thousand, 3-one thousand, while suctioning, is a simple means for monitoring the time. Without a safeguard the airway may be obstructed for too long a period of time. Hyperventilation of the child with 100% oxygen before and after suctioning should also be performed to prevent hypoxia.

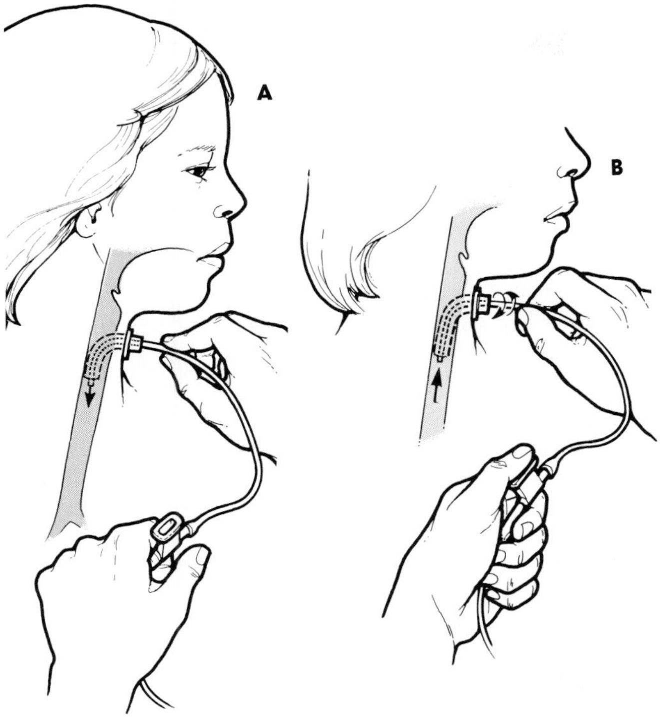

FIG. 21-37 Tracheostomy suctioning. **A,** Insertion, port open. **B,** Withdrawal, port occluded. Note that the catheter is inserted just slightly (0.5 cm) beyond the end of the tracheostomy tube.

Suctioning is carried out at frequent intervals to prevent buildup of crusts and as often as needed for signs of mucus in the airway, such as bubbling, noisy breathing, or coughing. The cough, although noisy, is ineffectual, because the glottis, which normally closes and releases suddenly to effect a cough, is bypassed by the tracheostomy. The child is allowed to rest for 30 to 60 seconds after each aspiration to allow oxygen tension to return to normal, then the process is repeated until the trachea is clear. Suctioning should be limited to about 3 aspirations in one period.

Aseptic technique is essential during care of the tracheostomy. Secondary infection is a major concern, since the air entering the lower airway bypasses the natural defenses of the upper airway. Two gloves are worn during the aspiration procedure, although a sterile glove is needed only on the hand touching the catheter. A new tube, gloves, and sterile saline solution are used each time.

Routine care. A duplicate tracheostomy tube (with obturator) and equipment needed for its insertion are kept at the bedside in the event that the tube becomes dislodged and needs to be replaced. For a "fresh" tracheostomy a tube one size smaller is also placed at the bedside in the event the duplicate cannot be replaced. If the tube accidentally becomes dislodged, the attending nurse should maintain the patency of the incision by spreading the edges with a sterile clamp until the tube can be replaced. The child's head is *gently* extended with a towel roll or small pillow under the shoulders to help keep the stoma open. In an emergency when the child is in distress and unable to move air, a large size (number 10 to 14) French catheter can be inserted about 4 inches and cut off a few inches above the stoma to provide an airway until a tracheostomy tube can be replaced. Children with tracheostomies that must remain in place for months or years require a weekly tube change.

A child with a tracheostomy requires continuous nursing attendance. Vital signs are monitored regularly, and the patency of the tube is maintained. The child is observed closely for any signs of distress or complications. Nursing observation is vital to the child who is unable to verbally signal for help. Signs of impending difficulty include restlessness, dyspnea, pallor or cyanosis, changes in pulse or blood pressure, overt bleeding from the trachea or around the incision site, retractions, and noisy respirations.

FAMILY TEACHING AND HOME CARE

Some of the treatments families need to continue at home are often related to respiratory procedures. Some of the treatments, such as postural drainage, require less preparation than others, such as tracheostomy care. Regardless of the home therapy, the family needs ample time to learn the skills and demonstrate them before discharge. The more comfortable they are with all the aspects of care, the more confident and less anxious they will be when faced with total care of the child at home. For example, the family may require weeks of preparation before they feel comfortable with suctioning, cleaning, and changing a tracheostomy tube and performing cardiopulmonary resuscitation in case of an emergency. Instructions should be detailed and explicit.* To facilitate the family's adjustment, supplies identical to the ones to which they are accustomed should be available in the home. In the event of substitution, parents need to be reassured that the unfamiliar equipment is safe to use on their child.

A nurse from the public health department or other home care service should be available to the family and should periodically assess the family's ability to carry out the activities needed in care of the child. The parents may find it helpful to talk to other parents of children with similar needs. They also need to know whom to call and where they can get help and support in times of uncertainty or in an emergency.

When a child has a tracheostomy, parents are encouraged to provide as normal a life as possible for their child and other family members. The child who is physically able (e.g., a child with a tracheostomy without respiratory disability such as recurrent laryngeal polyps) can usually be allowed to engage in most activities that are appropriate for his age. He may even play outdoors with a scarf or other protection to cover loosely the tracheostomy

*See home care instructions in Wong, D.L, and Whaley, L.F.: Clinical handbook of pediatric nursing, ed. 2, St. Louis, 1986, The C.V. Mosby Co.

stoma. Both child and parents must be cautioned regarding play near any collection of water, such as a swimming pool or stream, and informed about safety precautions in the bathtub. The child should not be exposed to noxious fumes (e.g., paint, varnish, hair spray) and baby powder. Young children who may spill food near the stoma should wear a fabric bib (without plastic lining) or other device to prevent dribbled food or crumbs from being aspirated.

◆ *Procedures Related to Alternative Feeding Techniques*

Children who are unable to take nourishment by mouth because of conditions such as anomalies of the throat, esophagus, or bowel, impaired swallowing capacity, severe debilitation, respiratory distress, or unconsciousness are frequently fed by way of a tube inserted orally or nasally to the stomach (gastric gavage) or duodenum/jejunum (enteral gavage) or by a tube inserted directly into the stomach (gastrostomy) or jejunum (jejunostomy). At times the entire alimentary tract must be bypassed, using intravenous feedings. Such feedings may be intermittent or by continuous drip. Because enteral feedings are used less often than gastric or intravenous feedings, the following discussion is limited to gastric gavage, gastrostomy, and hyperalimentation.

GAVAGE FEEDING

Infants and children can be fed simply and safely by a tube passed into the stomach through either the nares or the mouth. The tube can be left in place or inserted and removed with each feeding. In older children it is usually less traumatic to tape the tube securely in place between feedings. When this alternative is used, the tube should be removed and replaced with a new tube according to hospital policy, specific orders, and the type of tube used. Meticulous handwashing should be practiced during the procedure to prevent bacterial contamination of the feeding, especially during continuous drip feedings.

Preparation

The equipment needed for gavage feeding includes:

- A suitable tube selected according to the size of the child and the viscosity of the solution being fed.
- A receptacle for the fluid; for small amounts a 10 to 30 ml syringe barrel or Asepto syringe is satisfactory; for larger amounts a 50 ml syringe with a catheter tip is more convenient.
- A syringe to aspirate stomach contents and/or to inject air after the tube has been placed.
- Water or water-soluble lubricant to lubricate the tube; sterile water is used for infants.
- Paper or nonallergenic tape to mark the tube and to attach the tube to the infant's or child's cheek.
- A stethoscope to determine the correct placement in the stomach.
- The solution for feeding.

A number of types of feeding tubes are available, including those made of silicone rubber, polyurethane, polyethylene, or polyvinylchloride. The last two types lose their flexibility and need to be replaced frequently, usually every 3 to 4 days. The polyurethane and silicone rubber tubes remain flexible so that they can remain in place longer and afford more patient comfort. They are smaller in diameter than the less flexible tubes and are often referred to as *small bore tubes,* although the diameter inside the polyurethane tube is wider than the silicone tube with equivalent outside diameters. While the increased softness and flexibility are advantages, they can also cause difficulties, such as difficult insertion (may require a stylet—a metal guide wire), collapse of tube during aspiration of gastric contents to test for correct placement, dislodgment during forceful coughing, and unsuitability for thick feedings (Moore and Greene, 1985).

Procedure

Infants will be easier to control if they are first wrapped in a mummy restraint (p. 648). Even tiny infants with

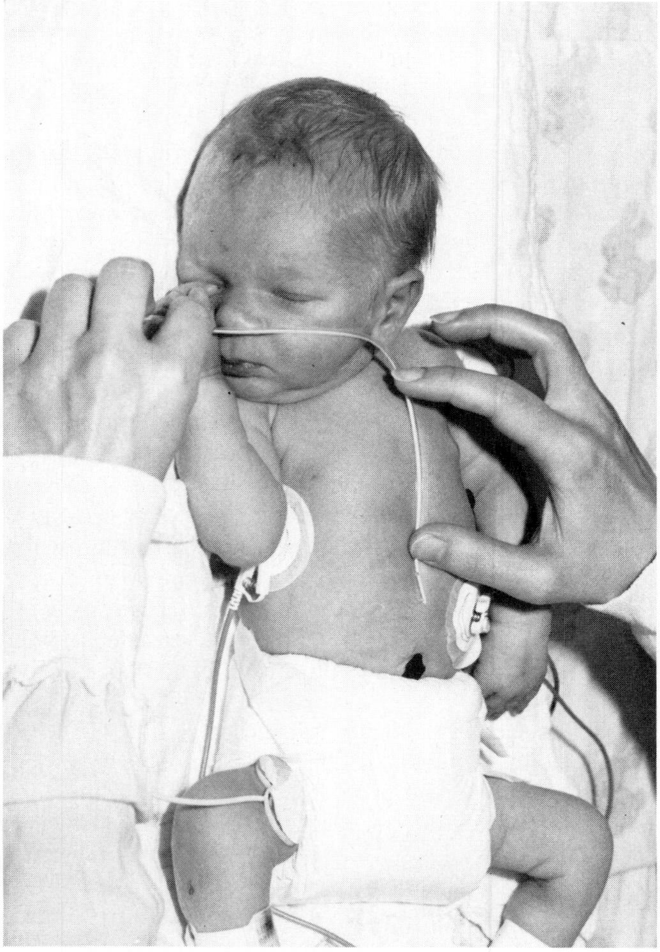

FIG. 21-38 Measuring tube for nasogastric feeding from tip of nose to earlobe and to the midpoint between the end of the xiphoid process and umbilicus.

random movements can grasp and remove the tube.

Premature infants do not ordinarily require restraint. However, if they do, a small towel folded across the chest and secured beneath the shoulders is usually sufficient. Care must be taken so that breathing is not compromised.

Whenever possible the infant should be held during the procedure to associate the comfort of physical contact with the feeding. When this is not possible, gavage feeding is carried out with the infant or child lying on the back or toward the right side with the head and chest elevated slightly. A folded blanket under the head and shoulders is satisfactory for infants, and a pillow is useful for small children. The head of the bed is raised for larger children.

The feeding tube can be passed through either the nose or the mouth. Since most young infants are obligatory nose breathers, insertion through the mouth causes less distress and helps to stimulate sucking. A tube passed through one of the nares in older infants and children is satisfactory once the tube is in place. An indwelling tube is almost always placed through the nose; the tube is alternated between nares with each insertion to minimize irritation, chance of infection, and possible breakdown of mucous membranes from pressure that occurs over a period of time. Between feedings infants should be given a pacifier; non-nutritive sucking has been shown to have several advantages, such as increased weight gain and decreased crying (Anderson, 1986).

The procedure for gavage feeding is carried out as follows:

1. Measure the tube for approximate length of insertion and mark the point with a small piece of tape. Two standard methods of measuring length are (a) measuring from the nose to the earlobe and then to the end of the xiphoid process, or (b) measuring from the nose to the earlobe and then to a point midway between the xiphoid process and umbilicus (Fig. 21-38). However, research on using these methods in premature infants has found both placements to be too high (in the esophagus), although the latter method provided better placement (Weibley and others, 1987).
2. Insert the tube (which has been lubricated with sterile water or water-soluble lubricant) through either the mouth or one of the nares to the predetermined mark. Since the esophagus is situated behind the trachea, the tube is more easily inserted when the child's head is hyperflexed. This reduces the chance of the tube entering the trachea. When using the nose, the tube is slipped along the base of the nose and directed straight back toward the occiput; when entering through the mouth, the tube is directed toward the back of the throat (Fig. 21-39, *A*). The tube is passed quickly and, if the child is able to swallow on command, synchronized with swallowing.
3. Check the position of the tube by using *both* of the following:
   a. Attach the syringe to the feeding tube and apply negative pressure. Aspiration of stomach contents indicates proper placement. However, absence of fluid is not necessarily evidence of improper placement. The

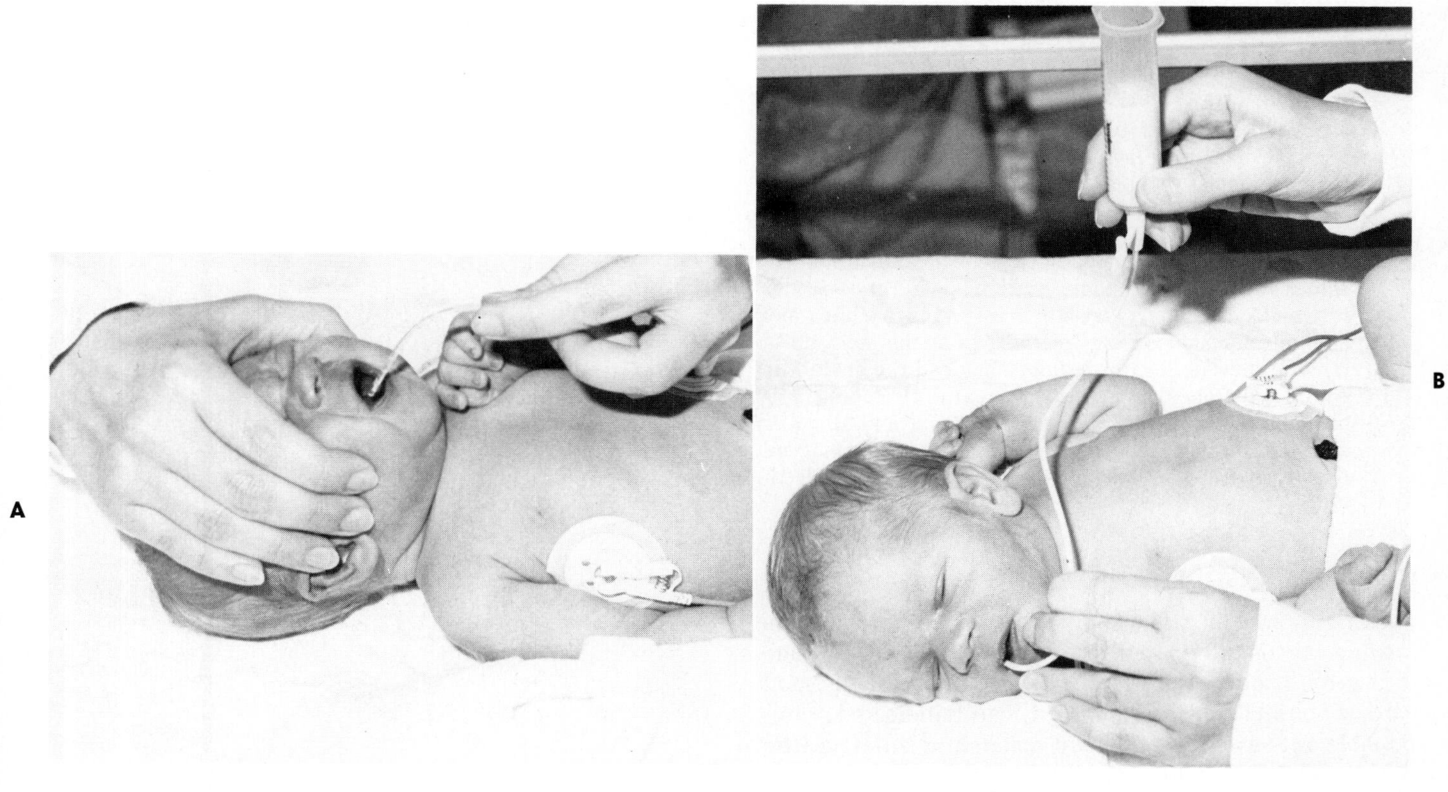

FIG. 21-39 Gavage feeding. **A,** Inserting tube. **B,** Allowing formula to flow into tube by gravity.

stomach may be empty, or the tube may not be in contact with stomach contents. Note the amount and character of any fluid aspirated and return the fluid to the stomach.
   b. With the syringe, inject a small amount of air (0.5 to 1 ml in premature or very small infants to 5 ml in larger children) into the tube while simultaneously listening with a stethoscope over the stomach area. Sounds of gurgling or growling will be heard if the tube is properly situated in the stomach, although it is possible to hear the air entering the stomach even when the tube is positioned above the gastroesophageal sphincter. Withdraw the amount of air injected.
4. Stabilize the tube by holding or taping it to the cheek, not to the forehead because of possible damage to the nostril. To maintain correct placement, measure and record the amount of tubing extending from the nose or mouth to the distal port when the tube is first positioned. Recheck this measurement before each feeding.
5. Feed the formula, which has been warmed to room temperature. Formula is poured into the barrel of the syringe attached to the feeding tube (Fig. 21-39, *B*). To start the flow, a gentle push with the plunger may be required, but the plunger should then be removed and the fluid allowed to flow into the stomach by gravity. The rate of flow should not exceed 5 ml every 5 to 10 minutes in premature and very small infants and 10 ml per minute in older infants and children to prevent nausea and regurgitation. The rate is determined by the diameter of the tubing and the height of the reservoir containing the feeding and is regulated by adjusting the height of the syringe. A usual feeding may take from 15 to 30 minutes to complete.
6. Flush the tube with sterile water (1 or 2 ml for small tubes to 5 ml or more for large ones) to clear it of formula. Indwelling catheters are capped or clamped to prevent loss of feeding and entry of air into the stomach.
7. If the tube is to be removed, first pinch it firmly to prevent escape of fluid as the tube is withdrawn. Withdraw the tube quickly.
8. Position the child on the right side or abdomen for at least 1 hour in the same manner as following any infant feeding to minimize the possibility of regurgitation and aspiration. If the child's condition permits, he can be bubbled after the feeding.
9. Record the feeding, including the type and amount of residual, the type and amount of formula, and the manner in which it was tolerated. For most infant feedings any amount of residual fluid aspirated from the stomach is refed to prevent electrolyte imbalance and the amount is subtracted from the prescribed amount of feeding. For example, if the infant is to receive 30 ml and 10 ml is aspirated from the stomach before the feeding, the 10 ml of aspirated stomach contents is refed plus 20 ml of feeding.

GASTROSTOMY FEEDING

Feeding by way of gastrostomy tube is a variation of tube feeding that is often used for children in whom passage of a tube through the mouth, pharynx, esophagus, and cardiac sphincter of the stomach is contraindicated or impossible or to avoid the constant irritation of a nasogastric tube in children who require tube feeding over an extended period. Placement of a gastrostomy tube may be performed under general anesthesia or percutaneously using an endoscope under local anesthesia (Starkey, Jefferson, and Kirby, 1988). The tube is inserted through the abdominal wall into the stomach about midway along the greater curvature and secured by a purse-string suture. The stomach is anchored to the peritoneum at the operative site. The tube used can be a Foley, wing-tip, or mushroom catheter.

Immediately after surgery the catheter is left open and attached to gravity drainage for 24 hours or more. Postoperative care of the wound site is directed toward prevention of infection and irritation. The area is cleansed and covered with a sterile dressing daily or as often as needed to keep the area dry. After healing takes place, meticulous care is needed to keep the area surrounding the tube clean and dry to prevent excoriation and infection. Daily applications of antibiotic ointment or other preparations may be prescribed to aid in healing and prevention of irritation. Care is exercised to prevent excessive pull on the catheter that might cause widening of the opening and subsequent leakage of highly irritating gastric juices. Sliding the tube through a sterile disposable nipple whose tip is cut off and whose base is then taped to the abdomen keeps the tube from rotating and causing erosion and enlargement of the skin opening (Perez and others, 1984).

For children on long-term gastrostomy feeding, the recently developed feeding button offers several advantages (Fig. 21-40). The button, a small, flexible silicone device that protrudes slightly from the abdomen, is cosmetically pleasing in appearance, affords increased comfort and mobility to the child, is easy to care for, and is fully immersible in water. The one-way valve at the proximal end minimizes reflux and eliminates the need for clamping. However, the button requires a well-established gastrostomy site and is more expensive than the conventional tube. In addition, the valve may become clogged and, when functioning, prevents air from escaping. Therefore, the child requires frequent bubbling. During feeding the

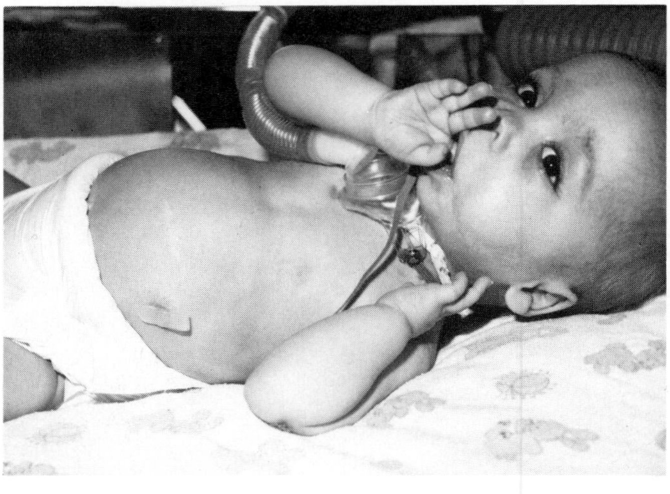

FIG. 21-40 Gastrostomy feeding button. Note child sucking on finger for oral gratification.

child must remain fairly still, since the tubing easily disconnects from the button if the child moves (Huth and O'Brien, 1987).

Positioning and feeding of water, formula, or pureed foods are carried out in the same manner and rate as gavage feeding. However, residual may not be aspirated and is measured as the amount of feeding left in the tube and syringe. After feedings the infant or child is positioned on the right side or in Fowler position, and the tube may be left open and suspended or clamped between feedings, depending on the child's condition. A clamped tube allows more mobility but is only appropriate if the child can tolerate intermittent feedings without vomiting or prolonged backup of feeding into the tube. Sometimes a Y tube is used to allow for simultaneous decompression during feeding. If a Foley catheter is used as the gastrostomy tube, very slight tension is applied and the tube securely taped to maintain the balloon at the gastrostomy opening and prevent its progression toward the pyloric sphincter, where it may occlude the stomach outlet. As a precaution the length of the tube should be measured postoperatively and then remeasured each shift to be sure it has not slipped. When the gastrostomy tube is no longer needed, it is removed; the skin opening ordinarily closes spontaneously by contracture.

TOTAL PARENTERAL NUTRITION

Total parenteral nutrition (TPN), also known as intravenous alimentation or hyperalimentation, provides for the total nutritional needs of infants or children whose lives are threatened because feeding by way of the gastrointestinal tract is impossible, inadequate, or hazardous.

Hyperalimentation therapy involves intravenous infusion of highly concentrated solutions of protein, glucose, and other nutrients. The hyperalimentation solution is infused through conventional tubing with a special filter attached to remove particulate matter or microorganisms that may have contaminated the solution. The highly concentrated solutions require infusion into a vessel with sufficient volume and turbulence to allow for rapid dilution. The wide-diameter vessels selected are the superior vena cava and innominate or intrathoracic subclavian veins approached by way of the external or internal jugular veins. For long-term alimentation, venous access devices are usually used (see p. 667).

The highly irritating nature of concentrated glucose precludes the use of the small peripheral veins in most instances. However, dilute glucose-protein hydrolysates that are appropriate for infusing into peripheral veins are being used with increasing frequency. When peripheral veins are used, intralipids become the major calorie source. Since this fat solution cannot be mixed with the glucose solutions, it requires administration through a separate bottle and tubing that enters the circuit near the venous entry site through a Y-type of injection adaptor.

The major nursing responsibilities are the same as for any intravenous therapy: control of sepsis, monitoring of infusion rate, and continuous observations. The TPN solution must be prepared under rigid aseptic conditions best accomplished by specially trained technicians. The solution and tubing are changed and the infusion site redressed by specially trained nurses, using meticulous aseptic precautions. In some institutions this may be a nursing responsibility. If so, the procedure is carried out according to hospital protocol.

The infusion is maintained at a slow, uniform rate by means of a constant infusion pump to ensure the proper concentrations of glucose and amino acids. Accurate calculation of the rate is required to deliver a measured amount in a given length of time. Since alterations in flow rate are relatively common, the drip should be checked frequently to ensure an even, continuous infusion. If for some reason the infusion rate slows, the rate should not be increased to compensate for the uninfused amount.

General assessments such as vital signs, intake and output measurements, and checking results of laboratory tests facilitate early detection of infection or fluid and electrolyte imbalance. Additional amounts of potassium and sodium chloride are often required in hyperalimentation; therefore, observation for signs of potassium or sodium deficit or excess is part of nursing care. This is rarely a problem except in children with reduced renal function or metabolic defects. Hyperglycemia may occur during the first day or two, as the child adapts to the high-glucose load of the hyperalimentation solution. The addition of insulin may be required to assist the body's adjustment to the hyperglycemia. Nursing responsibilities include blood glucose testing to monitor the effectiveness of the insulin therapy. To prevent hypoglycemia at the time the hyperalimentation is disconnected, the rate of the infusion and the amount of insulin are decreased gradually.

In addition to children's physical needs, their developmental needs must also be considered during the often long-term use of TPN. Regular assessment of development should be performed to assess the child's progress, and appropriate interventions should be instituted to encourage expected milestones. Delays in the areas of gross motor and language skills are found most often (Allen and Harper, 1983); therefore, special attention should be directed to these areas.

FAMILY TEACHING AND HOME CARE

When alternative feedings are needed for an extended period, the family may need to learn how to feed the child with a nasogastric, gastrostomy, or TPN feeding regimen. The same principles discussed earlier in this chapter for compliance, especially in terms of education (see p. 638), and in Chapter 20 for discharge planning and home care are applied.* Because of the numerous skills

*Home care instructions for gavage and gastrostomy feeding are available in Wong, D., and Whaley, L.: Clinical handbook of pediatric nursing, ed. 2, St. Louis, 1986, The C.V. Mosby Co.

the family must learn for home total parenteral nutrition, ample time must be planned for the family to learn and perform the procedures under supervision before assuming full responsibility for the child's care.

◆ *Procedures Related to Elimination*

Children seldom have problems with elimination, but in cases of severe constipation or when an empty rectum is needed before surgery or diagnostic procedures, an enema may be administered to stimulate rectal emptying. A number of conditions in the newborn and childhood period also require formation of an ostomy for purposes of elimination.

ENEMA

The procedure for giving an enema to an infant or child does not differ essentially from that for an adult with the exception of the type and amount of fluid administered and the distance for inserting the tube into the rectum (see box). An isotonic solution is used in children; if prepared saline is not available, it can be made by adding 1 teaspoon of table salt to 500 ml (1 pint) of tap water. Plain water is not used in children because, being hypotonic, it can cause rapid fluid shift and fluid overload.

The Fleet enema is not advised for children because of the potential side effects of sodium biphosphate and sodium phosphate, which include diarrhea, hyperphosphatemia, hypernatremia, and hypocalcemia.

Since infants and small children are unable to retain the solution after it is administered, the buttocks must be held together for a short time to retain the fluid. The enema is administered and expelled while the child is lying with the buttocks over the bedpan and the head and back supported with pillows. Older children are ordinarily able to hold the solution if they understand what to do and if they are not expected to hold it for too long a period. It is well to have the bedpan handy or, for the ambulatory child, to make certain that the bathroom is readily available before beginning the procedure. An enema is an intrusive procedure and thus threatening to the preschool child; therefore a careful explanation is especially important to ease possible distress.

Guidelines for Administration of Enemas to Children

Age	Amount (ml)	Insertion distance (cm/inches)
Infant	120-240	2.5 (1 inch)
2-4 years	240-360	5.0 (2 inches)
4-10 years	360-480	7.5 (3 inches)
11 years	480-720	10.0 (4 inches)

OSTOMIES

Children may require ostomies for various health problems. The most frequent causes are necrotizing enterocolitis and imperforate anus in the infant, less often Hirschsprung disease. In the older child the most frequent causes are inflammatory bowel disease, especially Crohn disease, and ureterostomies for distal ureter or bladder defects.

Care and management of ostomies in the older child differ little from the care of ostomies in the adult patient. The major emphasis in pediatric care is the preparation of the child for the procedure and teaching care of the ostomy to the child and family. The basic principles of preparation are the same as for any procedure (p. 624). Simple, straightforward language is most effective, together with the use of illustrations and a replica model; for example, drawing a picture of a child with a stoma on the abdomen and explaining it as "another opening where bowel movements [or any other term the child uses] will come out." At another time the nurse can draw a pouch over the opening to demonstrate how the contents are collected. Using a doll to demonstrate the process is an excellent teaching strategy (Fig. 21-41) and special books are available.*

Except in infants, an appliance is usually fitted immediately after surgery. Once an appliance is in place, drainage is directly measured from the collecting pouch. In order to accurately measure colostomy drainage when a collecting appliance is not used, the nurse weighs the dry dressing and reweighs it when wet. The difference in weight is calculated as fluid because 1 g equals 1 ml. If formed stool is passed, it is not weighed and calculated as part of fluid loss.

Ostomies performed on infants create special prob-

**Chris Has an Ostomy,* available from United Ostomy Association, Inc., 2001 W. Beverly Blvd., Los Angeles, CA 90057.

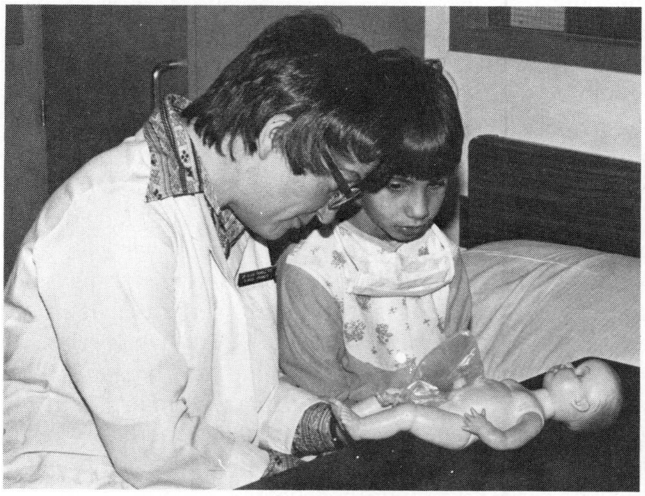

FIG. 21-41 Preparing child for colostomy. Note use of urine-collecting bag as part of colostomy equipment.

lems. The fragile nature of the skin increases the risk of breakdown, and the small surface area of the abdomen is ill suited to the standard appliances. Regardless of the type of ostomy (ileostomy or colostomy), initially most infants are left with a gauze dressing over the stoma. The dressing may or may not be saturated with petroleum jelly or other protective material. The skin is cleansed well after each bowel movement; a nonporous substance, (e.g., zinc oxide ointment [Desitin], karaya products, or a mixture of the zinc oxide ointment and karaya powder) is applied.

A variety of inexpensive techniques have been devised to absorb drainage around the stoma. Squares of paper towel, disposable diaper, or gauze with openings cut to fit the stoma are gently pressed against the layer of protective substance on the area around the stoma. They can be kept in place with a variety of methods that avoid repeated use of tape on the skin (see Nursing tips on colostomy dressing). As a rule, if a sigmoid colostomy is to be performed on an infant, a colostomy appliance is usually not used because the stools are formed and less likely to irritate the skin. Usually only diapers and a nonporous ointment such as zinc oxide around the stoma are used.

Nursing Tips: Colostomy Dressing

To secure a dressing over the colostomy site:

Use a self-adhering wrap (Coban) or an expansible wrap (Kerlix or Ace) around the abdomen and secure the end of the wrap with tape or a safety pin

Use a diaper (may be applied alone or with a dressing over the site)

Use Montgomery straps: on either side of the dressing, apply one or more strips of nonirritating tape to the skin and attach cloth ties to the end of the tapes; lace the ties across the dressing

When the stoma has healed and the infant has grown to a size that permits its use, an appropriate-sized infant pouch with skin barrier water is introduced. Before the pouch is applied, the skin is prepared with a skin sealant that is allowed to dry. Then stoma paste is applied around the base of the stoma. The sealant and paste work together to prevent peristomal breakdown.

FAMILY TEACHING AND HOME CARE

Since these children are almost always discharged with a functioning colostomy, preparation of the family should begin as early as possible in the hospital. The family is instructed in the application of the device (if used), care of the skin, and instructions regarding appropriate action in case skin problems develop. Early evidence of skin breakdown or stomal complications, such as ribbonlike stools, excessive diarrhea, bleeding, prolapse, or failure to pass flatus or stool, should be brought to the attention of the physician, the nurse, or the stoma specialist. The same principles discussed earlier in this chapter for compliance, especially in terms of education (see p. 638), and in Chapter 20 for discharge planning and home care are applied.*

SUMMARY

All children experience some type of medical procedure, although this varies from routine injections for immunizations to distressful tests, such as a bone marrow aspiration or biopsy. Regardless of the type of procedure, children benefit from preparation before and sensitive care during and after the event. Preparation for procedures must be individualized and based on knowledge of children's developmental characteristics at each age.

While the skills needed to perform many procedures in children differ little from those needed to execute procedures with adults, several additional precautions are often necessary with pediatric patients. Safety is always a concern, since even older children may not cooperate fully, and some type of restraint may be necessary. Special equipment, such as intravenous devices, and guidelines, such as measuring nasogastric tubes or insertion of enema tubes, are required to accommodate the anatomic and physiologic differences of children's bodies. Nurses must be aware of these unique variations to perform procedures competently and safely.

*Home care instructions on caring for the child with a colostomy are available in Wong, D., and Whaley, L.: Clinical handbook of pediatric nursing, ed. 2, St. Louis, 1986, The C.V. Mosby Co.

KEY CONCEPTS

- Informed consent is valid when the person is capable of giving consent (is over the age of majority and is competent), is supplied with information needed to make an intelligent decision, and acts voluntarily when exercising freedom of choice.
- Informed consent is needed for major surgery, minor surgery, and diagnostic tests and medical treatments with an element of risk.
- The major principles in psychologic preparation of the child for procedures are to establish trust, provide support, and give an explanation in easy-to-understand terms.
- In the performance of a procedure the nurse should expect success, involve the child when possible in the procedure, provide distraction, and allow for expression of feelings.
- In giving postprocedural support, the nurse should encourage the child to express his feelings and praise him for completion of the procedure.
- Six stressful times before and after surgery that produce anxiety in children are the day of admission, blood tests, the afternoon of the day before surgery, injection of preoperative medication, transportation to the operating room, and return from the recovery room.

- Assessment of compliance entails measuring factors that affect compliance through self-reporting, direct observation, monitoring appointments and therapeutic response, taking pill counts, and performing chemical assay.
- Compliance strategies may be classified as organizational, educational, and behavioral.
- Knowledge of the sick child's eating habits and favorite foods can help in maintaining adequate nutrition.
- Control of fever may be accomplished by pharmacologic means (administration of antipyretics) and environmental means (minimum clothing, increased air circulation, or cool compresses).
- Infection control may be based on one of three basic systems: category-specific isolation precautions, disease-specific isolation precautions, or universal precautions. Only the system of universal precautions provides protection when the infected person is undiagnosed.
- Ensuring safety in the hospital setting is a major concern and can be achieved through environmental measures, limit-setting, and safe transportation.
- Common types of physical restraints for children are jacket, mummy, arm and leg, and elbow.
- Factors that affect drug dosage determination are growth and maturation, difficulty in evaluating drug response, and body surface area.
- The preferred sites for intramuscular injection in children are the vastus lateralis and ventrogluteal areas.
- Intermittent venous access is accomplished by heparin lock, indwelling central venous catheters, or implantable ports.
- Nursing assessment of fluid and electrolyte disturbances entails observation of general appearance, vital signs, and intake and output measurement.
- Oxygen can be administered by Isolette mask, nasal cannula, or oxygen tent.
- Techniques for improving ventilatory capacity include postural drainage, percussion, and vibration.
- Tracheostomy suctioning requires use of sterile normal saline to loosen secretions, correct insertion of catheter, application of suction for 3 to 4 seconds when withdrawing the catheter, and supplemental oxygen before and after suctioning.
- Alternative forms of feeding include gavage feeding, gastrostomy feeding, and total parenteral nutrition.
- Intravenous alimentation provides total nutritional needs when feeding via the gastrointestinal tract is impossible, inadequate, or hazardous.
- In the care of children with ostomies, nurses play an important role in family support and instruction in care of the stoma site.

STUDY QUESTIONS AND ACTIVITIES

1. Outline plans to prepare a preschooler and a school-age child for a venipuncture to draw a blood specimen. Compare the approaches used with these two children of different ages.
2. Select one of the procedures listed in the box on p. 637 and use the play activities with a child who has undergone the procedure, such as some type of injection, or is currently receiving similar therapy, such as deep breathing after surgery.
3. Interview three parents and three children regarding their preferences for parental presence during procedures. Compare their responses to the agency's policy regarding this issue.
4. Compare the equipment (such as intravenous, nasogastric, respiratory) used with adult patients with that used with pediatric patients.
5. Outline the procedure for administering an intramuscular injection and include appropriate pain-reduction techniques (see box on p. 664) that can be used to minimize the discomfort.
6. Describe the two procedures used to check for correct placement of a nasogastric tube and the reasons why each may yield questionable results.

REFERENCES

Allen, S.S., and Harper, K.L.: Developmental delays in infants on long-term TPN, Nutr. Support Serv. **3:**42-43, 1983.

American Heart Association and American Academy of Pediatrics: Instructor's manual for pediatric advanced life support, Dallas, 1988, American Heart Association.

Anderson, G.C.: Pacifiers: the positive side, MCN **11**(2):122-124, 1986.

Axton, S.E., and Fugate, T.: A protocol for pediatric IV meds, Am. J. Nurs. **87**(7):943-945, 1987.

Billmire, D., Neale, H., and Gregory, R.: Use of IV fentanyl in the outpatient treatment of pediatric facial trauma, J. Trauma **25**(11):1079-1080, 1985.

Bourgault, A.: A hair piece, Nursing 85 **15**(9):80, 1985.

Brown, S.R.: An anxiety reduction technique during lumbar punctures in infants and toddlers, J. Assoc. Pediatr. Oncol. Nurses **1**(3):24-25, 1984.

Catchpole, M.: Does preop medication promote stress? Am. J. Nurs. **84**(10):1202, 1984.

Centers for Disease Control: Guidelines for the prevention and control of nosocomial infections, Atlanta, GA, 1983, Centers for Disease Control.

Centers for Disease Control: Recommendations for prevention of HIV transmission in health-care settings, Morbid. Mortal. Weekly Rep. **36**(25):3-18, 1987.

Clarke, S., and Radford, M.: Topical anaesthesia for venipuncture, Arch. Dis. Child. **61**(11):1132-1134, 1986.

Cushing, M.: Informed consent: an MD responsibility? Am. J. Nurs. **84**(4):437-440, 1984.

Dininny, J.B.: Food rummy, the game of nutrition, MCN **2**(2):90-91, 1977.

Dyson, A. and Bogod, D.: Minimizing bruising in the antecubital fossa after venepuncture, Br. Med. J. **294**(6588):1659, 1987.

Eland, J.: Minimizing pain associated with prekindergarten intramuscular injections, Issues Compr. Pediatr. Nurs. **5:**361-372, 1981.

Forlini, J., Morin, D.M., and Treacy, S.: Painless peds procedures, Am. J. Nurs. **87**(3):321-323, 1987.

Funk, M.J., Mullins, L.L., and Olson, R.A.: Teaching children to swallow pills: a case study, Child. Health Care **13**(1):20-23, 1984.

Hannallah, R., and Rosales, J.: Experience with parents' presence during anaesthesia induction in children, Can. Anaesth. Soc. J. **30**(3):287-290, 1983.

Hermansen, M.C., and Buches, M.: Super diapers and premature infants, Pediatrics **79**(6):1056-1057, 1987.
Hermansen, M.C., and Buches, M.: Urine output determination from superabsorbent and regular diapers under radiant heat, Pediatrics **81**(3):428-431, 1988.
Hogue, E.: What you should know about informed consent, Nursing 86 **16**(6):46-48, 1986.
Huth, M.M., and O'Brien, M.E.: The gastrostomy feeding button, Pediatr. Nurs. **13**(4):241-245, 1987.
Intramuscular injections: a guide to sites and techniques, Philadelphia, 1985, Wyeth Laboratories.
Leikin, S.L.: Minors' assent or dissent to medical treatment, J. Pediatr. **102**(2):169-176, 1983.
Lenz, C.L.: Make your needle selection right to the point, Nursing 83 **13**(2):50-51, 1983.
Lynch, P., and others: Rethinking the role of isolation practices in the prevention of nosocomial infections, Ann. Intern. Med. **107:**243-246, 1987.
Mandelbaum, J.: The food square: helping people of different cultures understand balanced diets, Pediatr. Nurs. **9**(1): 20-21, 1983.
McCarthy, D.O.: The adaptive value of fever during infection, Diet. Curr. **12**(3):13-18, 1985.
McCarty, J.M., and others: Outbreak of primary cutaneous aspergillosis related to intravenous arm boards, J. Pediatr. **5**(108):721-724, 1986.
Moore, M.C., and Greene, H.L.: Tube feeding of infants and children, Pediatr. Clin. North Am. **32**(2):401-417, 1985.
Newman, J.: Evaluation of sponging to reduce body temperature in febrile children, Can. Med. Assoc. J. **132:**641-642, 1985.
Perez, R.C., and others: Care of the child with a gastrostomy tube: common and practical concerns, Issues Compr. Pediatr. Nurs. **7**(2-3):107-119, 1984.
Rapoff, M.A.: Helping parents to help their children comply with treatment regimens for chronic diseases, Issues Compr. Pediatr. Nurs. **9**(3):147-156, 1986.
Rapoff, M.A., and Christophersen, E.R.: Improving compliance in pediatric practice, Pediatr. Clin. North Am. **29**(2):339-357, 1982.
Ros, S.: Outpatient pediatric analgesia—a tale of two regimens, Pediatr. Emerg. Care **3**(4):228-230, 1987.
Savedra, M.: Parental responses to a painful procedure performed on their child. In Azarnoff, P., and Hardgrove, C., editors: The family in child health care, New York, 1981, John Wiley & Sons.
Schreiner, V.: Don't discard this specimen, Nursing 87 **17**(10):5, 1987.
Starkey, J.F., Jefferson, P.A., and Kirby, D.F.: Taking care of percutaneous endoscopic gastrostomy, Am. J. Nurs. **88**(1):42-45, 1988.
Stoller, K.P., and Losey, R.: Inadvertent intra-arterial injection of penicillin: an unseen danger, Pediatrics **75**(4):785-786, 1985.
Visintainer, M.A., and Wolfer, J.A.: Psychological preparation for surgical pediatric patients: the effect of children's and parents' stress responses and adjustment, Pediatrics **56**(2):187-202, 1975.
Weibley, T.T., and others: Gavage tube insertion in the premature infant, MCN **12:**24-27, 1987.
Wong, D.L.: Lozenges can be "lifesavers," Am. J. Nurs. **87**(9):1129-1130, 1987.
Wong, D.L. and Baker, C.M.: Pain in children: comparison of assessment scales, Pediatr. Nurs. **14**(1):9-17, 1988.
Young, M.S.: Strategies for improving compliance, Top. Clin. Nurs. **7**(4):31-38, 1986.

BIBLIOGRAPHY

Informed Consent

Dunn, L.J.: Legal aspects of communication with and about the pediatric patient, Issues Compr. Pediatr. Nurs. **4:**13-18, 1980.
Erickson, S., and others: Gray areas: informed consent in pediatric and comatose adult patients, Heart Lung **16**(3):323-325, 1987.
Frost, N.: Parental control over children, J. Pediatr. **103**(4):571-572, 1983.
Holder, A.R.: Parents, courts, and refusal of treatment, J. Pediatr. **103**(4):515-520, 1983.
Laken, D.D.: Protecting patients against themselves: what to do when patients refuse treatment, Nursing 83 **13:**90-94, 1983.
Northrop, C.E., and Kelly, M.E.: Legal issues in nursing, St. Louis, 1987, The C.V. Mosby Co.
Rhodes, A.M.: Consent for medical treatment, MCN **12**(2):133, 1987.
Rhodes, A.M.: Obtaining consent to treat minors, MCN **12**(3):209, 1987.
Rhodes, A.M.: When parents refuse to consent, MCN **12**(4):289, 1987.
Siantz, M.L.D.: Defining informed consent, MCN **13**(2):94, 1988.
Silva, M.C.: Assessing competency for informed consent with mentally retarded minors, Pediatr. Nurs. **10**(4):261-265, 306, 1984.
Silva, M., and Zeccolo, R.: Informed consent: the right to know and the right to choose, Nurs. Manage. **17**(8):18-19, 1986.

Preparing for Hospital Procedures and Surgery/Use of Play

Bates, T.A., and Broome, M.: Preparation of children for hospitalization and surgery: a review of the literature, J. Pediatr. Nurs. **1**(4):230-239, 1986.
Beckemeyer, P., and Bahr, J.E.: Helping toddlers and preschoolers cope while suturing their minor lacerations, MCN **5**(5):326-330, 1980.
Broome, M.E.: The relationship between children's fears and behavior during a painful event, Child. Health Care **14**(3):142-145, 1986.
Crawford, C., Finke, L., and Henning, M.A.: Nursing management of the postoperative pediatric patient, Issues Compr. Pediatr. Nurs. **6:**157-165, 1983.
Demarest, D.S., Hooke, J.F., and Erickson, M.T.: Preoperative intervention for the reduction of anxiety in pediatric surgery patients, Child. Health Care **12**(4):179-183, 1984.
Droske, S.C., and Francis, S.A.: Pediatric diagnostic procedures: with guidelines for preparing children for clinical tests, New York, 1981, John Wiley & Sons, Inc.
Ellerton, M.L., Caty, S., and Ritchie, J.A.: Helping young children master intrusive procedures through play, Child. Health Care **13**(4):167-173, 1985.
Fernald, C.D., and Corry, J.J.: Empathic versus directive preparation of children for needles, Child. Health Care **10**(2):44-47, 1981.
Gatch, G.: Caring for children needing anesthesia, AORN J. **35**(2):218-226, 1982.
Gelfant, B.B.: Minimizing the stress of surgery through patient and family orientation and education, Point View **23**(1):9, 1986.
Hunsberger, M., Love, B., and Byrne, C.: A review of current approaches used to help children and parents cope with health care procedures, MCN **13**(3):145-165, 1984.
Ireland, D.W.: Put some roar in your pediatric program, J. Post Anesth. Nurs. **I**(4):255-257, 1986.
Johnson, J.E.: Coping with elective surgery. In Werley, H.H., and Fitzpatrick, J.J., editors: Annual review of nursing research, vol. 2, New York, 1984, Springer Publishing Co.
Kline, J.: Recovery room care for the child in pain, MCN **9**(4):261-264, 1984.
Mitiguy, J.S.: A surgical liaison program: making the wait more bearable, MCN **11:**388-392, 1986.
Petrillo, M., and Sanger, S.: Emotional care of hospitalized children, ed. 2, Philadelphia, 1980, J.B. Lippincott Co.
Play and preparation: an annotated bibliography, Washington, DC, 1984, Association for the Care of Children's Health.

Pontious, S.L.: Practical Piaget: helping children understand, Am. J. Nurs. **82**(2):114-117, 1982.
Pridham, K.F., Adelson, F., and Hansen, M.F.: Helping children deal with procedures in a clinic setting: a developmental approach, J. Pediatr. Nurs. **2**(1):13-22, 1987.
Ritchie, J.A.: Preparation of toddlers and preschool children for hospital procedures, Can. Nurse **75**(11):30-32, 1979.
Robinson, S.J.: A nurse's role in preparing children for surgery, AORN J. **30**(4):619-621, 1979.
Rushton, C.H.: The surgical neonate: principles of nursing management, Pediatr. Nurs. **14**(2):141-151, 1988.
Schulz, J.B., and others: The effects of a preoperational puppet show on anxiety levels of hospitalized children, Child. Health Care **9**(4):118-121, 1981.
Stevens, M.S.: Which adolescents breeze through surgery?, Am. J. Nurs. **87**(12):1564-1565, 1987.
Streiff, L.D.: Can clients understand our instructions, Image J. Nurs. Sch. **18**(2):48-52, 1986.
Waidley, E.K.: Show and tell: preparing children for invasive procedures, Am. J. Nurs. **85**(7):811-812, 1985.

Compliance

Baer, C.L.: Compliance: the challenge for the future, Top. Clin. Nurs. **7**(4):77-85, 1986.
Burckhardt, C.S.: Ethical issues in compliance, Top. Clin. Nurs. **7**(4):9-16, 1986.
Clark, S.R.: Compliance and health behaviors, Top. Clin. Nurs. **7**(4):39-46, 1986.
Connaway, N.: My patient won't follow the medical plan treatment. what should I do to protect myself—legally? . . . home health care, Home Healthc. Nurse **3**(4):6-8, 1985.
DiFlorio, I.A., and Duncan, P.A.: Design for successful patient teaching, MCN **11**:246-249, 1986.
Kaufman, D.H.: An interview guide for helping children make health-care decisions, Pediatr. Nurs. **11**(5):365-367, 1985.
Klopovich, P.M., and others: Adherence to chemotherapy regimens among children with cancer, Top. Clin. Nurs. **7**(1):19-25, 1985.
Littlefield, L.C.: Therapeutic drug monitoring in ambulatory pediatrics, J. Pediatr. Health Care **1**(2):113-116, 1987.
Lucas, C.M.: Compliance and illness responses, Top. Clin. Nurs. **7**(4):47-56, 1986.
McCord, M.A.: Compliance: self care or compromise? Top. Clin. Nurs. **7**(4):1-8, 1986.
McHatton, M.: A theory for timely teaching, Am. J. Nurs. **85**(7):798-800, 1985.
McLean, J.C., and others: Improving patient compliance in pediatric outpatient surgery . . . nurse practitioner telephones the parents one to two days before the appointment, AORN J. **40**(5):676-680, 1984.
Miller, A.: When is the time ripe for teaching? Am. J. Nurs. **85**(7):801-804, 1985.
Oberst, B.B.: Patient and parent education: why? what? how? Pediatr. Basics **46:**11-15, 1987.
Padrick, K.P.: Compliance: myths and motivators, Top. Clin. Nurs. **7**(4):17-22, 1986.
Sallis, J.F.: Improving adherence to pediatric therapeutic regimens, Pediatr. Nurs. **11**(2):118-120, 1985.
Sloan, M.R., and Schommer, B.T.: Want to get your patient involved in his care? use a contract, Nursing 82 **12**(12): 48-49, 1982.
Westfall, U.E.: Methods for assessing compliance, Top. Clin. Nurs. **7**(4):23-30, 1986.
Yoos, L.: Factors influencing maternal compliance to antibiotic regimens, Pediatr. Nurs. **10**(2):141-147, 1984.

General Care and Hygiene/Safety/Collection of Specimens

Brown, B.S., and Younger, J.B.: Facts about fever, Child. Nurse **2**(3):1-3, 1984.
Burson, J.Z., and Brannigan, C.N.: The use of play in the nutritional support of hospitalized children, Issues Compr. Pediatr. Nurs. **7**(4-5):283-289, 1984.
How to take your child's temperature, Patient Care **14:** 141-148, Sept. 1980.
Jackson, M.M., and McPherson, D.C.: Infection control: keeping current, Nurse Educ. **11**(4):38-40, 1986.
Jackson, M.M., and others: Why not treat all body substances as infectious? Am. J. Nurs. **87**(9):1137-1139, 1987.
Kilmon, C.A.: Home management of children's fevers, J. Pediatr. Nurs. **II**(6):400-404, 1987.
Kilmon, C.A.: Parents' knowledge and practices related to fever management, J. Pediatr. Health Care **1**(4):173-179, 1987.
Long, S., and Henretig, F.: Fever in children, Pediatr. Consult **6**(1):1-8, 1987.
Millam, D.A.: Venous blood samples: sharpen your drawing skills, Nursing 87 **17**(12):56-61, 1987.
Misik, I.: About using restraints—with restraint, Nursing 81 **11**(8):50-55, 1981.
Perry, A.G., and Potter, P.A.: Clinical nursing skills and techniques: basic, intermediate, and advanced, St. Louis, 1986, The C.V. Mosby Co.
Strohbach, M.E., and Kratina, S.H.: Diaper versus bag specimens: a comparison of urine specific gravity values, MCN **7:**198-201, 1982.
Utley, R.M.: A collector's item, Nursing 85 **15**(1):94, 1985.
Younger, J.B., and Brown, B.S.: Fever management: rational or ritual? Pediatr. Nurs. **11**(1):26-28, 1985.

Administration of Medications

Bergman, T.: Verbal responses of adolescents to right atrial catheters, J. Assoc. Pediatr. Oncol. Nurses **3:**31-36, 1985.
Birdsall, C., and Uretsky, S.: How do I administer medication by NG? Am. J. Nurs. **84**(10):1259-1260, 1984.
Chaplin, G., Shull, H., and Welk, P.C., III: How safe is the air-bubble technique for I.M. injections? Nursing 85 **15** (9):59, 1985.
Evans, M.L., and Hansen, B.D.: Administering injections to different-aged children, MCN **6**(3):194-199, 1981.
Favazza, P., Brennan, M., and Carney, K.: The pediatric approach to home IV therapy: a case study, Rx Home Care **9**(6):51-57, 1987.
Frank, T., and Fischer, R.G.: What are some of the most common reasons for medication errors? Pediatr. Nurs. **10**(4): 294, 1984.
Goodman, M.S., and Wickham, R.: Venous access devices: an overview, Oncol. Nurs. Forum **11**(5):16-23, 1984.
Harris, L.C., Rushton, C.H., and Hale, S.J.: Implantable infusion devices in the pediatric patient: a viable alternative, J. Pediatr. Nurs **2**(3):174-183, 1987.
Jerrett, M.D.: Taking the ouch out of injections, Can. Nurse **79**(1):24-27, 1983.
McConnell, E.A.: The subtle art of really good injections, RN **45**(2):24-34, 1982.
McGovern, K.: Take the first step toward reducing medication errors, Nursing 87 **17**(12):49, 1987.
Nortridge, J.A.: Calculating I.V. medications with confidence, Nursing 87 **87**(9):55-57, 1987.
Penatzer, M., and others: Common pediatric IV meds at a glance, Pediatr. Nurs. **14**(1):56-58, 1988.
Perez, S.: Reducing injection pain, Am. J. Nurs. **84**(5):645, 1984.
Rettig, F.M., and Southby, J.R.: Using different body positions to reduce discomfort from dorsogluteal injection, Nurs. Res. **31**(4):219-221, 1982.
Rimar, J.M.: Guidelines for the intravenous administration of medications used in pediatrics, MCN **12:**322-340, 1987.
Shepherd, M.J., and Swearington, P.L.: Z-track injections, Am. J. Nurs. **84**(6):746-747, 1984.
Vogel, T.C., and McSkimming, S.A.: Teaching parents to give indwelling C.V. catheter care, Nursing 83 **13**(1):55-56, 1983.
Walson, P.D.: Giving medicine to children, Pediatr. Consult **2**(4):1-7, 1984.
Wezel-Bolen, G.: Technological advances in the care of children with chronic illness, Pediatrics: Nursing Update Series **1**(11), Princeton, NJ, 1986, Continuing Professional Education Center, Inc.
Wildblood, R.A., and Strezo, P.L.: The how-to's of home IV therapy, Pediatr. Nurs. **13**(1):42-46, 1987.
Wilkes, G., Vannicola, P., and Starck, P.: Long-term venous access, Am. J. Nurs. **85**(7):793-796, 1985.

Wong, D.L.: Significance of dead space in syringes, Am. J. Nurs. **82**(8):1237, 1982.

Wordell, D.C.: Should you crush that tablet?, Nursing 88 **18**(1):48-49, 1988.

Zeanah, P.D., and Bross, R.A.: Emergency drug guidelines: a pediatric reference, Pediatr. Nurs. **11**(3):194-202, 1985.

Procedures Related to Maintaining Fluid Balance/IV Therapy

Cyganski, J.M., Donahue, J.M., and Heaton, J.S.: The case for the heparin flush, Am. J. Nurs. **87**(6):796-797, 1987.

Dunn, D.L., and Lenihan, S.F.: The case for the saline flush, Am. J. Nurs. **87**(6):798-799, 1987.

Fay, M.J.: The special challenges of pediatric IVs, Dimens. Crit. Care Nurs. **2:**23-29, 1983.

Feldstein, A.: Detect phlebitis and infiltration before they harm your patient, Nursing 86 **16**(1):44-47, 1986.

Folk-Lighty, M.: Solving the puzzles of patients' fluid imbalances, Nursing 84 **14**(2):34-41, 1984.

Hook, M.L., and others: Arterial line patency maintained with non-heparinized flush solution, Heart Lung **16:**693-699, 1987.

Koszuta, L.E.: Choosing the right infusion control device for your patient, Nursing 84 **14**(3):55-57, 1984.

Nelson, R., and Miller, H.: Keeping air out of I.V. lines, Nursing 86 **16**(3):57-59, 1986.

Webb, A.A.: Methods of intravenous therapy in preterm infants, Issues Compr. Pediatr. Nurs. **10:**215-221, 1987.

Wittig, P., and Semmler-Bertanzi, D.J.: Pumps and controllers—a nurse's assessment guide, Am. J. Nurs. **83:**1022-1025, 1983.

Procedures Related to Respiratory Function

Aradine, C.: Young children with long-term tracheostomies: health and development, West. J. Nurs. Res. **5:**115-124, 1983.

Czarniecki, L.: Caring for a young child with a tracheostomy, Caring **4**(5):30-32, 1985.

Fuchs, P.L.: Streamlining your suctioning techniques, Part I. Nasotracheal suctioning, Nursing 84 **14**(5):55-61, 1984.

Harris, R., and Hyman, R.: Clean vs. sterile tracheostomy care and level of pulmonary infection, Nurs. Res. **33:**80-85, 1984.

Hartsell, M.B.: Chest physiotherapy and mechanical vibration, J. Pediatr. Nurs. **2**(2):135-137, 1987.

Hazinski, M.F.: Pediatric home tracheostomy care: a parent's guide, Pediatr. Nurs. **12:**41-48, 69, 1986.

Kennelly, C.: Tracheostomy care: parents as learners, MCN **12**(4):264-267, 1987.

Kleiber, C., Krutzfield, N., and Rose, E.F.: Acute histologic changes in the tracheobronchial tree associated with different suction catheter insertion techniques, Heart Lung **17**(1):10-14, 1988.

Nieves, J.: Avoiding spontaneous extubation of nasotracheal or oral tracheal tubes, Pediatr. Nurs. **12:**215-218, 1986.

Paulson, P.R.: Nursing considerations for discharging children home on low-flow oxygen, Issues Compr. Pediatr. Nurs. **10:**209-214, 1987.

Riegel, B., and Forshee, T.: A review and critique of the literature on preoxygenation for endotracheal suctioning, Heart Lung **14:**507-518, 1985.

Spearing, C., and Cornell, D.J.: Inspiring your patient to breathe deeply, Nursing 87 **17**(9):50-51, 1987.

Wills, J.: Concerns and needs of mothers providing home care for children with tracheostomies, MCN **12:**89-107, 1983.

Procedures Related to Alternative Feeding Techniques/Elimination

Ament, M.E.: Home parenteral nutrition in infants and children. In Rombeau, J.L., and Caldwell, M.D., editors: Parenteral nutrition, Philadelphia, 1986, W.B. Saunders Co.

Bayer, L.M., Scholl, D.E., and Ford, E.G.: Tube feeding at home, Am. J. Nurs. **83**(9):1321-1325, 1983.

Berry, R.K., and Jorgensen, S.: Growing with home parenteral nutrition: adjusting to family life and child development (part 1), Pediatr. Nurs. **14**(1):43-45, 1988.

Berry, R.K., and Jorgensen, S.: Growing with home parenteral nutrition: maintaining a safe environment (part 2), Pediatr. Nurs. **14**(2):155-157, 1988.

Guiness, R.: How to use the new small-bore feeding tubes, Nursing 86 **16**(4):51-56, 1986.

Hummel, P.: More on gavage tubes (letter), MCN **13**(1):14, 1988.

Metheny, N.M.: 20 ways to prevent tube-feeding complications, Nursing 85 **15**(1):47-50, 1985.

Paarlberg, J., and Balint, J.P.: Gastrostomy tubes: practical guidelines for home care, Pediatr. Nurs. **11**(2):99-102, 1985.

Perry, S., Johnson, S., and Trump, D.: Gastrostomy and the neonate, Am. J. Nurs. **83**(7):1030-1033, 1983.

Smith, D.B.: The ostomy: how is it managed? Am. J. Nurs. **85**(11):1246-1249, 1985.

Wilson, V.: How to make a feeding tube go down easily, RN **49**(11):40-43, 1986.

Wink, D.M.: The physical and emotional care of infants with gastrostomy tubes, Issues Compr. Pediatr. Nurs. **6:**195-203, 1983.

Zlotkin, S.H., Stallings, V.A., and Pencharz, P.B.: Total parenteral nutrition in children, Pediatr. Clin. North Am. **32:**381-400, 1985.

UNIT

X

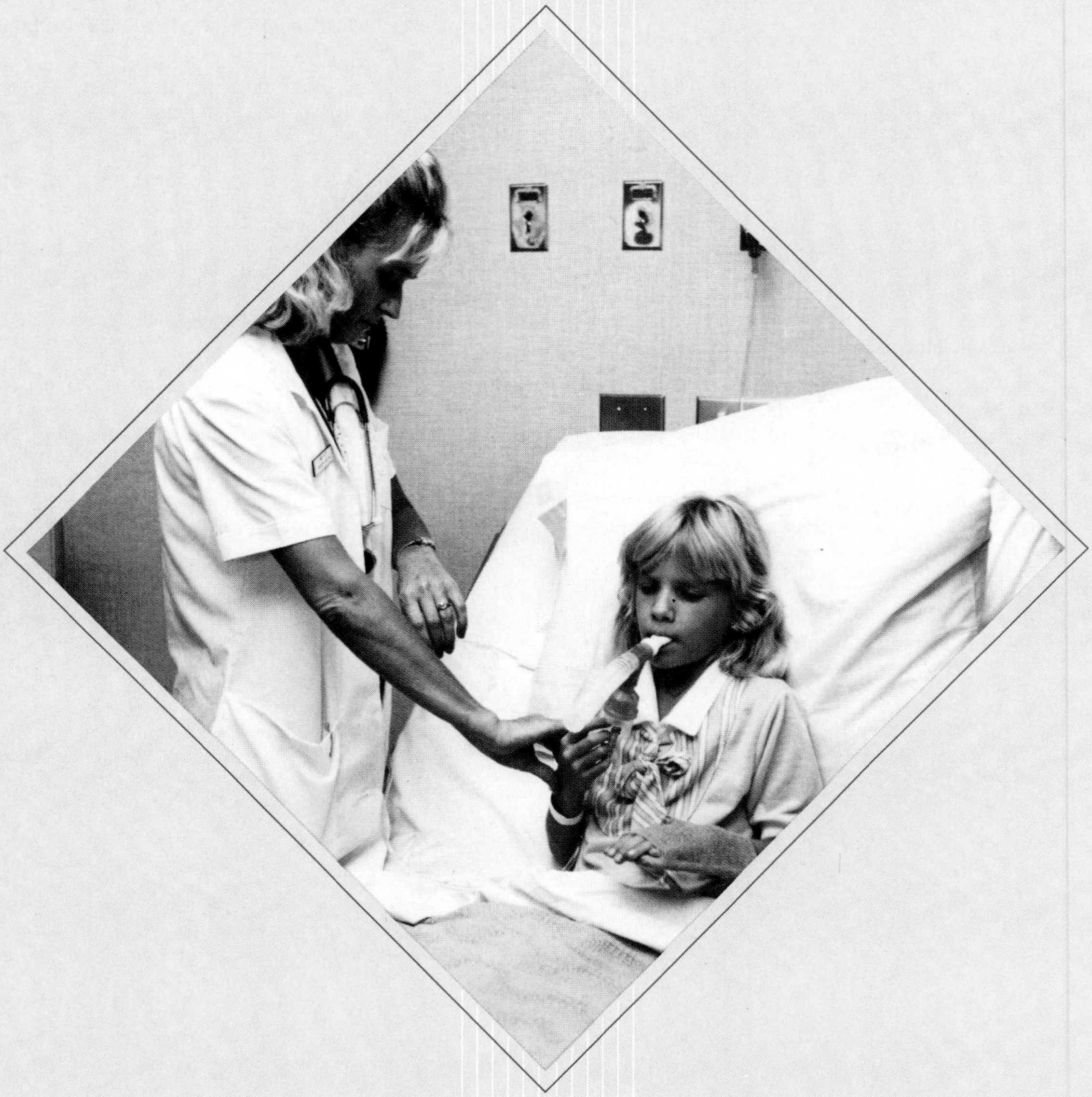

The Child with Problems Related to the Transfer of Oxygen and Nutrients

The survival of an individual depends on a continuous supply of energy for maintaining the function of all the cells in the body. This energy is obtained through oxygen and nutrients, which are incorporated by the body and converted to energy by the process of oxygenation-reduction. Any circumstance or condition that requires an increase in energy requires a concomitant increase in the materials that the body converts into energy. The need for oxygen is most acute, and without this vital substance the body is unable to survive more than a few minutes without permanent damage to vital structures or death. Therefore, oxygen must be supplied constantly. Nutrients and water, on the other hand, can be stored within the body for use at times of increased need or diminished supply.

Alterations in the ability to supply oxygen or nutrients are some of the most common health problems of childhood. Interference with respiratory and gastrointestinal function is encountered at all ages, but very young children are especially vulnerable to dysfunctions in these systems. Chapter 22, *The Child with Respiratory Dysfunction*, describes the more common conditions that impair the exchange of oxygen and carbon dioxide. Chapter 23, *The Child with Gastrointestinal Dysfunction*, is concerned with factors that interfere with digestion or absorption of body nutrients. There are other situations in which there are disturbances in the availability of oxygen and nutrients for energy (for example, diabetes mellitus and disorders of fluid and electrolyte balance), but these are more appropriately discussed elsewhere.

CHAPTER 22

The Child with Respiratory Dysfunction

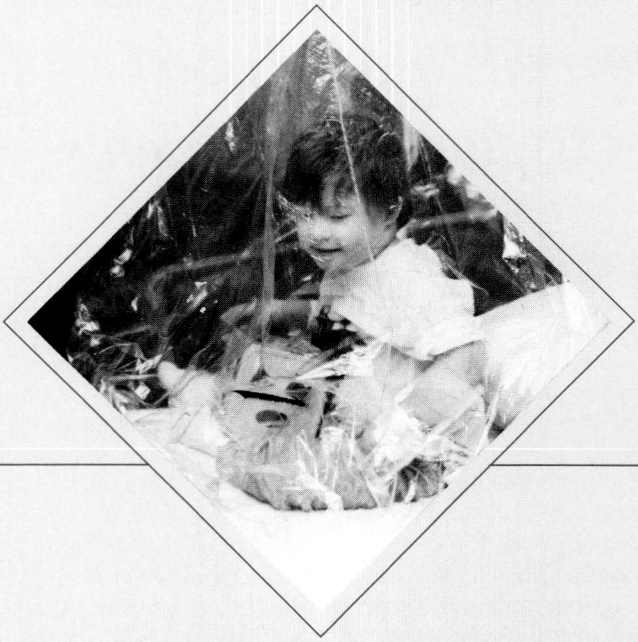

LEARNING OBJECTIVES

On completion of this chapter the reader will be able to:

- Identify the significant differences between the respiratory tract of the infant or young child and that of the adult
- Contrast the effects of various respiratory infections observed in infants and children
- Describe the postoperative nursing care of the child with a tonsillectomy
- Outline a nursing care plan for a child with croup
- Outline a nursing care plan for a child with acute otitis media
- Demonstrate an understanding of the ways in which inhalation of noninfectious irritants produces pulmonary dysfunction
- Describe the ways in which the various therapeutic measures relieve the symptoms of asthma
- Outline a plan for teaching home care for the child with bronchial asthma
- Describe the physiologic effects of cystic fibrosis on the gastrointestinal and pulmonary systems
- Outline a plan of care for the child with cystic fibrosis
- List the major signs of respiratory distress in infants and children

Some of the most common problems in the pediatric age-group are related to disturbed respiratory function, and respiratory failure is the chief cause of morbidity in the newborn period. Respiratory illness can be caused by disease, trauma, or physical anomalies, or it can be seen as a manifestation of a disturbance in another organ or system, such as neurologic disorders involving the respiratory center or innervation to the respiratory musculature. Most communicable diseases have respiratory symptoms. The type and pattern of respiratory disturbances also vary tremendously according to the age of the child. There are differences in susceptibility to infections and in responses to various organisms and conditions at various ages. Moreover, manifestations of illness vary according to the age of the child and may involve different organ systems. This chapter is concerned primarily with infectious, allergic, and mechanical disturbances.

◆ *Respiratory Infection*

Acute infection of the respiratory tract is the most common cause of illness in infancy and childhood. Young children ordinarily have four or five such infections each year that manifest a wide range of severity from trivial to severe or even fatal illness.

ACUTE RESPIRATORY INFECTIONS IN CHILDREN: GENERAL ASPECTS

Acute infections of the respiratory tract are described according to the general areas of involvement in the more common infections: the *upper respiratory tract* or upper airway, which consists primarily of the nose and pharynx; the *croup syndromes,* involving the structurally stable, nonreactive portion of the airway, the epiglottis and larynx; the *lower respiratory tract,* composed of the rigid trachea and the bronchi and bronchioles, whose smooth muscle content has the ability to constrict; and the *primary respiratory unit,* the lungs.

Etiology and Characteristics

The respiratory tract is subject to a wide variety of infective organisms, but the largest number of infections is caused by viruses, especially the respiratory syncytial viruses (RSV), in the upper respiratory passages. Other organisms that may be involved in primary or secondary invasion are group A β-hemolytic *Streptococcus, Staphylococcus aureus, Haemophilus influenzae,* and pneumococci. Of special significance is the β-hemolytic *Streptococcus* because of the relationship between respiratory infection with this organism and the incidence of subsequent nephritis or rheumatic fever.

Infections are seldom localized to a single anatomic structure or area but tend to spread to a variable extent as a result of the continuous nature of the mucous membrane lining the respiratory tract. Consequently infections of the respiratory tract generally involve several areas rather than a single structure, although the effect on one may predominate in any given illness.

The type of illness and the physical response are also related to a variety of factors, including:

1. *The nature of the infectious agent.* The respiratory tract is subject to a wide variety of infectious agents
2. *The size and frequency of the dose.* The larger the dose and the more frequent the exposure, the greater the likelihood of a significant infection
3. *The age of the child.* Children of nursery and grade-school age are more often exposed to infectious agents; infants have less resistance to infections
4. *The size of the child.* Airways are smaller in young children and are subject to considerable narrowing from edema
5. *The ability to resist invading organisms.* School-age children have greater resistance to infection than infants and young children
6. *The presence of general conditions.* Malnutrition, anemia, fatigue, chilling of the body, and immune deficiencies decrease normal resistance to infection
7. *The presence of disorders that affect the respiratory tract.* Allergies, cardiac abnormalities, and cystic fibrosis weaken respiratory defense mechanisms

Diagnostic Evaluation

Most respiratory infections are diagnosed on the basis of clinical manifestations and physical examination. An infant or child may display any or all of the signs and symptoms listed in the accompanying box. Radiograms are frequently employed to evaluate lower tract involvement, and laboratory cultures identify specific organisms.

General Clinical Manifestations of Acute Respiratory Tract Infection in Children

Altered breathing Respirations may be altered to a greater or lesser degree depending on the location and extent of the infective process

Cough Coughing is a common manifestation. A cough may be described as dry, moist, hacking, barking, brassy, croupy, productive, or nonproductive

Nasal blockage The small nasal passages of the infant are easily blocked by mucosal swelling and exudation. Infants have difficulty breathing through their mouths; therefore, this occlusion can interfere with respiration and feeding

Fever Most children manifest an elevated temperature with respiratory infections. In children 6 months to 3 years, the temperature may reach 39.5° to 40.5° C (103° to 105° F), even with mild infections

Febrile seizures In some small children, a sudden temperature rise to 40° C (104° F) or higher will precipitate febrile convulsions (p. 927)

Anorexia Loss of appetite is a symptom common to most childhood illnesses, and it almost invariably accompanies acute infections in small children

Vomiting Small children vomit readily with illness, and vomiting occurs so frequently at the onset of infection that its appearance for no obvious reason is a clue to the advent of infection

Meningism Signs associated with meningitis but without actual inflammation of the meninges include headache, stiffness in the back and neck, and positive Kernig and Brudzinski signs

Diarrhea Mild, transient diarrhea often accompanies respiratory infections in small children, particularly viral infections

Abdominal pain Abdominal pain, sometimes indistinguishable from the pain of appendicitis, is a common complaint in small children with acute respiratory infections

Therapeutic Management

Most children with respiratory infections are treated at home, especially those with upper respiratory infection (URI). Hospitalization is usually recommended for the child with suspected epiglottitis, serious complications, or severe cases of pneumonia. Treatment for URIs is important, however, to prevent or minimize complications. The usual recommendations are (1) have the child rest in bed until he is free of fever for at least 1 day, (2) encourage intake of liquids, and (3) manage temperature.

Effective antimicrobial therapy is available for the eradication of most microorganisms (except viruses) responsible for URIs in children. The penicillins are the drugs of choice for bacterial pneumonia and are available in both oral and parenteral forms. At present there are few specific therapies for viral infections or their symptoms. Other management consists of systematic relief of symptoms and prevention of other complications.

Nursing Considerations

Infants and young children react more severely to acute URI than older children, and they appear to be much more ill than their local manifestations would indicate. This is especially true regarding children between 6 months and 3 years of age. Young children display a number of generalized signs and symptoms as well as local manifestations that differ from those seen in older children and adults (see box, p. 693).

ASSESSMENT

The general assessment of the respiratory system follows the guidelines described in Chapter 7 (see Nose, p. 152; Mouth and throat, p. 153; and Lungs, p. 156), and normal vital signs can be found on the inside front cover.

Respirations. The pattern of respirations is observed for rate, depth, ease, and rhythm of breathing:

Rate—rapid (tachypnea), normal, or slow for the particular child
Depth—normal depth, too shallow (hypopnea), too deep (hyperpnea); usually estimated from the amplitude of thoracic and abdominal excursion
Ease—effortless, labored (dyspnea), orthopnea, associated with intercostal and/or substernal retractions (inspiratory "sinking in" of soft tissues in relation to the cartilaginous and bony thorax), pulsus paradoxus (blood pressure falls with inspiration and rises with expiration), flaring nares, head bobbing (head of sleeping child with suboccipital area supported on mother's forearm bobs forward in synchrony with each inspiration), grunting, or wheezing
Labored breathing—continuous, intermittent, becoming steadily worsening, sudden onset, at rest or on exertion, associated with wheezing, grunting, associated with pain
Rhythm—variation in rate and depth of respirations

Other observations. In addition to respirations, particular attention is addressed to the following:

Evidence of infection—check for elevated temperature, enlarged cervical lymph nodes, inflamed mucous membranes, and purulent discharges from the nose, ears, or lungs (sputum)
Cough—observe the characteristics of the cough (if present); for example, under what circumstances the cough is heard (e.g., night only, on arising), the nature of the cough (paroxysmal, with or without wheeze, "croupy" or "brassy"), frequency of cough, associated with swallowing or other activity
Wheeze—expiratory or inspiratory, high-pitched or musical, prolonged, slowly progressive or sudden, associated with labored breathing
Cyanosis—note distribution (peripheral, perioral, facial, trunk as well as face), degree, duration, associated with activity
Chest pain—may be a complaint of older children. Note location and circumstances: localized or generalized, referred to base of neck or abdomen, dull or sharp, deep or superficial, associated with rapid, shallow respirations or grunting
Sputum—supervised older children may provide sputum sample. Note volume, color, viscosity, and odor
Bad breath—may be associated with some lung infections

NURSING DIAGNOSES

After a thorough patient assessment a number of nursing diagnoses may be identified. The most likely diagnoses are outlined and discussed in the Nursing Care Plan on p. 696. Others may be apparent in individual cases.

PLANNING

The nursing goals for care of the child with an acute respiratory infection are:

1. Facilitate respiratory efforts
2. Promote rest
3. Promote comfort
4. Prevent spread of primary infection to others
5. Reduce temperature (if significantly elevated)
6. Prevent dehydration and provide nourishment
7. Prevent complications
8. Educate and support family

IMPLEMENTATION

Since the majority of children with URIs are treated at home, most of the nursing care is directed toward education and guidance of parents in caring for their child and serving as resources for problem solving. If the practitioner has given the parents written instructions, these can be explained and reinforced as appropriate. If written instructions have not been furnished, the nurse should provide the parents with written guidelines and, in some cases, outlines of procedures to be employed.

Ease respiratory efforts. Most acute respiratory infections are mild and cause few distressing symptoms. Although the child may be uncomfortable and suffer from a "stuffy" nose and some mucosal swelling, respiratory distress is uncommon. The interventions described in the remainder of the discussion are usually sufficient to relieve most minor discomfort. However, the child with croup or epiglottitis may develop sufficient swelling to obstruct the airway. These children are hospitalized for observation and therapy (see discussion on p. 704 and Nursing Care Plan on p. 708). Positioning for optimum respiration and observation for signs of respiratory distress (p. 730) are primary nursing functions.

Promote rest. Any child who has an acute febrile illness should be placed on bed rest. This is usually not difficult while the temperature is elevated but may be difficult, particularly in young children, when the child feels fairly well. When parents take the advice seriously and consistently keep the child in bed, most children learn to cooperate during illness. A number of entertainment devices can be employed to keep the child quiet, based on the child's individual interests.

Promote comfort. Older children are usually able to manage nasal secretions with little difficulty. For very young infants, who normally breathe through their noses, an infant nasal aspirator or a rubber ear syringe is helpful in removing nasal secretions before feeding. This, in conjunction with instillation of saline nose drops, often clears nasal passages and facilitates feeding.

For older infants and children who can better tolerate decongestants, phenylephrine nose drops may be administered 15 to 20 minutes before feeding and at bedtime. Two drops are instilled, and since this shrinks only the anterior mucous membranes, two more drops are instilled 5 to 10 minutes later. The parents are instructed concerning the correct administration of nose drops and throat irrigations, if ordered. Older cooperative children often prefer nasal sprays. They are taught to compress the plastic container at the moment of inspiration to gain relief. Spray bottles and bottles of nose drops should be used for one child only and only for one illness, since they easily become contaminated with bacteria.

Hot or cold applications sometimes provide relief to older children with painful cervical adenitis. An ice bag or heating pad applied to the neck may decrease the discomfort, but safety precautions must be observed in order to prevent burns. The ice bag or heating device must be covered, and the heating pad should not be set at the high ranges.

Warm or cool mist has been a common therapeutic measure for symptomatic relief of respiratory discomfort. The moisture soothes inflamed membranes and seems especially beneficial when there is hoarseness or any laryngeal involvement. Mist tents and hoods are frequently employed in the hospital for liquefying secretions and relieving discomfort. However, moisturizing air by use of steam vaporizers in the home is not advised and should be discouraged because of the hazards related to their use and the little evidence to support their efficacy (Colombo, Hopkins, and Waring, 1981). Alternate suggestions are available, such as humidification systems and cool-mist vaporizers. Shallow pans with wide surface areas for evaporation increase humidity but should be placed where they do not pose a safety hazard (see also Nursing tip box on humidification).

A time-honored method of producing steam is the shower. Running the shower of hot water into the empty bathtub or open shower stall with the bathroom door closed produces a quick source of steam. Ten to fifteen minutes in this environment offers the same advantages as the croup tent without the fear and restraint often associated with the confines of a tent. A small child can be held on the lap of a parent or other adult. Older children can sit in the bathroom under the supervision of an adult.

> ### *Nursing Tip: Humidification*
>
> A large, wet beach towel hung with one end in shallow water in the bathtub will increase humidity if the bathroom door remains open.

Prevent spread of infection. Careful handwashing should be carried out when caring for a child with a respiratory infection. The child and family are taught the correct disposal of respiratory secretions and proper behavior related to airborne droplets (coughing and sneezing). They should be taught to use a tissue or their hand to cover their nose and mouth when they cough or sneeze and to dispose of the tissues properly.

Every endeavor should be made to remove the child from contact with other children. Ideally the ill child should be isolated in a separate bedroom at the first sign of illness. This is seldom a problem with an only child but is often difficult when living arrangements are crowded and there are several children in the family. If the child has no bedroom of his own, sometimes another child can sleep on a couch or cot or at the home of a relative or friend. Well children can be taught to stay away from the ill child if the living conditions allow for segregation and if the rule is rigidly enforced.

Reduce temperature. If the child has a significantly elevated temperature, controlling the temperature becomes a major nursing task. The parent should know how to take the child's temperature and read the thermometer accurately. Most parents are able to do this, but nurses cannot make this assumption. Those parents who cannot will require instruction in use of the thermometer. The reader is referred to Chapter 21 for an extensive discussion of temperature, its assessment, and its management. Intake of cool liquids is encouraged to help reduce the temperature and to minimize the chances of dehydration.

Promote hydration and provide nutrition. Dehydration is always a hazard when children are febrile or anorexic, especially when vomiting or diarrhea also occur. An adequate fluid intake should be encouraged by offering small amounts of favored fluids at frequent intervals. High-calorie liquids such as colas, fruit juices, water flavored and sweetened with corn syrup, or similar drinks help prevent catabolism and dehydration. Fluids should not be forced, and the child should not be wakened from his rest to take fluids.

Anorexia is characteristic of acute infections in children, and in most cases the child can be permitted to

NURSING CARE PLAN

The Child with Acute Respiratory Infection

Nursing Goals	Nursing Interventions	Expected Patient/Family Outcomes
NDX HP-HMP* Potential for infection	**Risk factors: presence of infective organisms (others); weakened condition (patient)**	
Prevent spread of infection	Isolate child from other family members as much as possible Provide separate bedroom if possible Avoid close contact between well persons and ill child Discourage parents and others from lying down with ill child Keep others from using child's eating and drinking utensils Use separate washcloth and towel for ill child Teach child proper behavior when coughing or sneezing and proper disposal of tissues Teach all family members good handwashing technique and encourage frequent use	Others remain free from infection
Prevent secondary infection	Observe good handwashing Prevent contact with infected persons	Child does not acquire a secondary infection
NDX HP-HMP Potential for suffocation (airway obstruction)	**Risk factors: inflammatory process (croup, epiglottitis)**	
Monitor respiratory status	Observe respiratory rate and pattern Auscultate to determine type and location Breath sounds Presence of rales, rhonchi, wheezing Areas of consolidation Effectiveness of chest therapy Assess skin color, presence or absence of retractions, nasal flaring	†Deviations from normal (for the individual child) are detected early (see inside front cover for normal variations) Color remains pink; no visible retractions
Detect complications early	Carry out periodic assessment of respiratory status Change position every 2 hours Observe for signs of Chest pain Abdominal pain Dyspnea Observe color of skin and mucous membranes for pallor and cyanosis Observe for presence of hoarseness, stridor, and cough Monitor heart rate and regularity Observe behavior Restlessness Irritability Apprehension Report and record significant observations	Respirations are unlabored Child exhibits no evidence of discomfort Color remains pink †Any deviations from normal (for the individual child) are detected (specify parameters)
Prevent respiratory arrest	Avoid throat examination (epiglottis) Have emergency equipment available	Child breathes without significant difficulty
NDX N-MP Potential fluid volume deficit	**Risk factors: difficulty swallowing due to inflammatory process, increased metabolic rate, insensible fluid losses**	
Prevent dehydration	Observe for signs of dehydration Monitor intake, output, urine specific gravity, and daily weight Encourage fluids when tolerated	Child remains well hydrated and exhibits no evidence of dehydration Child drinks adequate amounts of fluid (specify)
NDX N-MP Hyperthermia related to the inflammatory process		
Reduce body temperature	Implement measures to decrease temperature Provide cool environment Monitor temperature to detect status of temperature	Body temperature remains within the acceptable limits—between 37.8° and 38.0° C (100° and 100.4° F)

NURSING CARE PLAN

The Child with Acute Respiratory Infection—cont'd

Nursing Goals	Nursing Interventions	Expected Patient/Family Outcomes
	Place in lightweight clothing and bed linen Encourage cool liquids	
A-EP Ineffective airway clearance **Etiology: increased secretions, inflammation**		
Prevent aspiration of secretions	Administer nothing by mouth during acute stage of dyspnea Position to promote drainage of secretions from airway Prevent aspiration of secretions	Airways remain clear
Maintain patent airway	Suction secretions as needed Perform percussion, vibrations, and drainage if prescribed	Airway remains clear
A-EP Ineffective breathing pattern **Etiology: inflammatory process, tracheobronchial obstruction**		
Ease respiratory efforts	Promote rest Maintain patent airway Allow position of comfort Provide high-humidity atmosphere Position for comfort and maximum lung expansion Remove secretions, e.g., encourage cough and expectoration; suction nasal pharynx Reduce anxiety Organize activities to allow for minimal expenditure of energy	Child rests and sleeps quietly Respirations unlabored Respirations remain within normal limits (see inside front cover for normal variations) Child rests and sleeps quietly
Reduce anxiety and apprehension	Provide constant attendance during acute phase of illness Encourage presence of parents Provide comfort and cuddling when possible Remove restraining devices when and as often as possible Provide quiet diversion appropriate to child's age and condition	Child exhibits no signs of distress Parents remain with child and provide comfort Child engages in quiet activities appropriate for age, interest, and condition
CPP Pain **Etiology: inflammatory process**		
Relieve pain	Assess for need of pain medication Implement nonpharmacologic pain reduction techniques (see p. 597)	Child verbalizes pain reduction in discomfort Child's behaviors indicate reduced pain (see p. 590)
SP-SCP Anxiety/fear **Etiology: hospitalization, difficulty breathing**		
Reduce child's apprehension	Remain in constant attendance Hold and cuddle child whenever possible—preferably by parent or other familiar person Provide security devices (e.g., familiar toy, blanket) Encourage parental attendance and, when possible, involvement in child's care	Child responds positively to comforting measures
Keep child calm	Do nothing to make child more anxious Maintain relaxed manner Establish rapport with child and parents Instill confidence in both parents and child Try to avoid intrusive procedures	Child exhibits no signs of apprehension Parents relate readily with personnel and calmly with child
Facilitate nonverbal communication	Observe child's behavior closely to detect nonverbal messages Teach signing, use pictures or other means to communicate needs and concerns	Child communicates needs and concerns

Continued.

NURSING CARE PLAN

The Child with Acute Respiratory Infection—cont'd

Nursing Goals	Nursing Interventions	Expected Patient/Family Outcomes
ND RRP Altered family processes related to situational crisis (hospitalization of child)		
Reduce parental anxiety	Recognize parental concern and need for information and support Explain therapy and child's behavior Provide support as needed Encourage to become involved in child's care	Parents ask appropriate questions, discuss child's condition and care calmly, and become involved positively in child's care
Educate family	Explain procedures and therapies to family (specify) Encourage questions	Family members ask questions and demonstrate an understanding of teaching (specify)
Prepare parents for child's discharge	Teach parents needed skills for home care, e.g., administration of medications Refer to appropriate health agency as indicated	Family members demonstrate evidence of understanding instructions for care

Nursing interventions related to medical management

Ease respiratory efforts
- Place in mist tent or Croupette with cool vapor
- Provide oxygen as prescribed and/or needed
- Give nothing by mouth to prevent aspiration of fluids (severe tachypnea)

Be prepared to assist with tracheostomy (croup)
- Have tracheostomy equipment at bedside
- Obtain parental permission for procedure

Control fever
- Administer antipyretics as indicated (acetaminophen)

Promote rest
- Administer sedatives as indicated if ordered for restlessness and pain

Eradicate causative organisms
- Administer antimicrobial medications if prescribed
- Support body's natural defenses

Ease discomfort
- Administer analgesic medication

Prevent dehydration
- Administer fluids as prescribed
- Monitor intravenous infusion during acute phase

Provide nutrition
- Administer intravenous glucose during acute phase (if prescribed)

Determine causative organisms
- Collect specimens as needed
- Assist with diagnostic procedures
  - Radiographs
  - Thoracentesis
  - Venipuncture

*For an explanation of abbreviations, see p. 20.
†Nursing outcome.

determine his own need for food. Many children show no decrease in appetite, and others respond well to certain foods such as gelatin, soup, and puddings (see also Feeding the sick child, p. 640). Since the illness is relatively short, the nutritional state is seldom compromised. Sometimes reducing the milk intake of formula-fed infants is helpful during the initial phase of an acute respiratory infection.

Support and educate family. The child with a URI is irritable and difficult to comfort. Therefore the family needs support, encouragement, and practical suggestions for the child's care. Since most care involves administration of medication, a primary goal of education is related to this aspect of management. In addition to antipyretics and nose drops, the child may require antibiotic therapy if the infection is caused by group A β-hemolytic *Streptococcus*. The nurse is often the one who collects the throat-culture specimens, administers medication, and instructs the parents regarding continuing the medication. Parents of children who are sent home with oral antibiotics need to understand the importance of regular administration and of continuing the drug for the prescribed length of time, regardless of whether the child appears ill (see p. 669 for teaching parents to administer medications). Caution parents against giving a child any medication that is not approved by the health practitioner. Adverse effects have been noted in children who received some preparations intended for adults, for example, long-acting nose drops and cough squares or lozenges (mistaken for candy).

EVALUATION

The effectiveness of nursing intervention is determined by continued reassessment according to the following observational guidelines and expected outcomes:

1. Observe child's behavior and respiratory movement
2. Observe signs and symptoms for progress toward pre-illness status
3. Observe child's behavior and activity

4. Observe other family members and contacts for evidence of infection
5. Take temperature
6. Observe eating behavior and observe for signs of adequate hydration
7. Assess child for evidence of complications, such as dehydration, weight loss, spread of infection to other areas of the body
8. Observe family's behavior and interview members regarding their feelings and concerns

Expected outcomes:
See Nursing Care Plan on pp. 696 to 698.

ACUTE UPPER RESPIRATORY INFECTIONS

Upper respiratory infections (URIs) include infectious processes involving any or all of the structures in the upper respiratory tract. Most are caused by viruses and are self-limited. Acute nasopharyngitis and pharyngitis (including tonsillitis) are extremely common in pediatric age-groups. These disorders can be merely a part of a generalized upper respiratory infection, or they can be the dominant feature of an infection. Secondary infection or extension of URIs can cause serious or long-lasting effects, especially in infants and very young children. A primary site for extension is the middle ear. The major manifestations of these disorders are compared in the accompanying box.

Nasopharyngitis

Nasopharyngitis, a viral (principally rhinovirus) infection of the nose and throat, is the most common URI. The equivalent of the "common cold" in adults and also termed *acute rhinitis* or *coryza*, the disease occurs throughout the year. Complications of nasopharyngitis in infants are more often otitis media and lower respiratory tract infection; the older child may develop sinusitis as a complication.

Pharyngitis

The throat (including the tonsils) is the principal anatomic site of pharyngitis (sore throat). Although uncommon in children under 1 year of age, the disease is prevalent throughout childhood, with a peak incidence between 4 and 7 years of age. The etiologic agents are either viruses or the group A β-hemolytic *Streptococcus*. Complications can include otitis media, acute cervical adenitis, retropharyngeal abscess, and lower respiratory tract infection. Streptococcal infection sometimes triggers a response in the heart (rheumatic fever) or kidneys (acute glomerulonephritis).

Tonsillitis

The *tonsils* are masses of lymphoid tissue encircling the pharyngeal cavity (Fig. 22-1). The *palatine* or *faucial* tonsils are located on each side of the oropharynx and are usually visible during oral examination (see p. 154). The

Clinical Manifestations of Nasopharyngitis and Pharyngitis

Nasopharyngitis	Pharyngitis
Younger child	*Younger child*
Fever	Fever
Irritability, restlessness	General malaise
Sneezing	Anorexia
Vomiting and/or diarrhea, sometimes	Moderate sore throat
	Headache
Older child	*Older child*
Dryness and irritation of nose and throat	Fever (may reach 40° C)
	Headache
Sneezing, chilly sensation	Anorexia
	Dysphagia
Muscular aches	Abdominal pain
Cough, sometimes	Vomiting
Physical signs	
Edema and vasodilation of mucosa	*Younger child*
	Mild to moderate hyperemia
	Older child
	Mild to fiery red, edematous pharynx
	Hyperemia of tonsils and pharynx; may extend to soft palate and uvula
	Often abundant follicular exudate that spreads and coalesces to form pseudomembrane on tonsils
	Cervical glands enlarged and tender

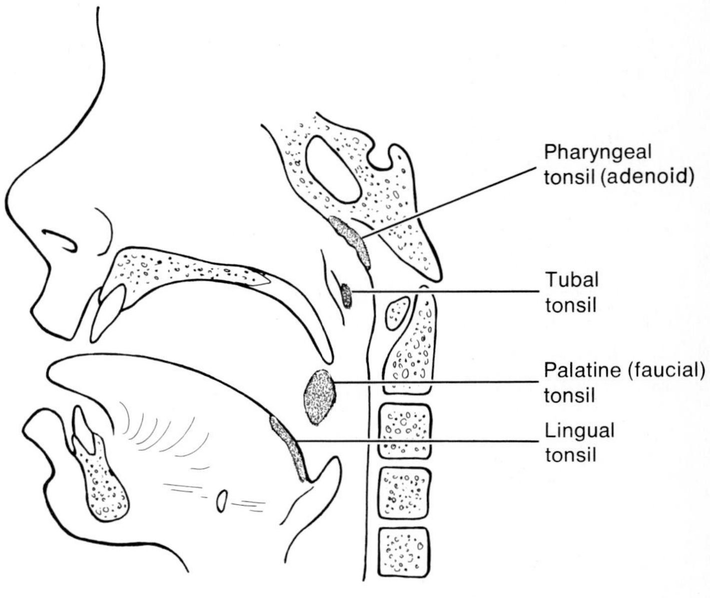

FIG. 22-1 Location of the various tonsillar masses.

pharyngeal tonsils, also known as the *adenoids,* are located in the posterior wall of the nasopharynx, opposite the posterior nares. Their proximity to the nares and eustachian tubes contributes to obstruction of passages during inflammation. The *lingual* tonsils are located at the base of the tongue. The *tubal* tonsils are found near the posterior nasopharyngeal opening of the eustachian tubes.

The filtering function of the tonsils is believed to protect the respiratory and alimentary tracts from invasion by pathogenic organisms. They also may have a role in antibody formation. Although the size of tonsils varies, children generally have much larger tonsils than adolescents or adults. This difference is thought to be a protective mechanism at a time when young children are especially susceptible to URI.

Therapeutic Management

Treatment of a child with viral pharyngitis is symptomatic, because the illness is short and self-limiting. If streptococcal sore throat infection is present, penicillin VK is prescribed in a dosage sufficient to control the acute local manifestations and to maintain an adequate level for at least 10 days to eliminate any organisms that might remain to initiate symptoms of rheumatic fever. Some authorities believe a combination of penicillin and rifampin is more effective in eradicating the organisms.

Surgical treatment of chronic tonsillitis is a controversial subject. *Tonsillectomy* has been the most frequently performed pediatric surgical procedure, but many authorities believe removal of the palatine tonsils is unnecessary. Others continue to recommend the procedure for selected patients. Generally, tonsils should not be removed before 3 or 4 years of age because of the problem of excessive blood loss in small children and the possibility of regrowth or hypertrophy of lymphoid tissue. The tubal and lingual tonsils, which are rarely removed, often enlarge to compensate for the lost lymphoid tissue, resulting in continued pharyngeal and eustachian tube obstruction. Tonsillectomy is indicated for massive hypertrophy that results in difficulty eating or in extreme breathing discomfort.

Adenoidectomy is recommended for children with recurrent otitis media to prevent hearing loss and for those children in whom hypertrophied adenoids obstruct nasal breathing. Removal may be warranted in the child under 3 years of age and should be performed without a tonsillectomy. Follow-up after adenoidectomy should include assessment of hearing, smell, and taste for expected improvement.

Nursing Considerations

Nursing care of the child with tonsillitis and/or pharyngitis mainly involves providing comfort. A soft to liquid diet is generally preferred. A cool-mist vaporizer helps keep the mucous membranes moist during periods of mouth breathing. Warm, salt-water gargles, throat lozenges, and analgesic/antipyretic drugs such as acetaminophen (Tylenol) are useful to promote comfort. If antibiotics are prescribed, parents need counseling regarding their correct administration (see p. 669) and the necessity of completing the treatment period.

If surgery is indicated, the child requires the same psychologic preparation and physical care needed for any other operation (see Chapter 21). The following discussion focuses on the nursing care specific for tonsillectomy and adenoidectomy (T & A).

ASSESSMENT

A complete history is taken preoperatively with special notation of any bleeding tendencies, since the operative site is highly vascular. Baseline vital signs are important for postoperative monitoring and observation. Signs of any URI are noted and reported, and bleeding and clotting times are included in the usual laboratory work requests. During physical assessment the presence of any loose teeth is noted. (See also Preparation for surgery, p. 629.)

Postoperative assessment includes monitoring vital signs, observing for hemorrhage, and assessing general response to surgery.

NURSING DIAGNOSES

Based on a careful assessment a number of nursing diagnoses become apparent. Some are common to all children; others are not. The usual diagnoses associated with care of the child with a T & A are listed in the accompanying box.

PLANNING

Nursing objectives for postoperative care of the child with a T & A are:

1. Facilitate drainage of secretions
2. Promote comfort and relieve pain
3. Observe for evidence of bleeding
4. Prevent complications
5. Provide fluids and nutrition
6. Instruct family for home care
7. Support child and family

Nursing Diagnoses: Child with a Tonsillectomy

Impaired swallowing related to inflammation and discomfort
Pain related to surgery
Altered oral mucous membranes related to operative site
Potential fluid volume deficit related to NPO preoperatively, reluctance to swallow because of pain
Potential for hemorrhage related to raw, denuded surfaces of tonsil sockets
Altered family processes related to hospitalization of child

IMPLEMENTATION

Before the child is fully awake he is placed on his abdomen or side to facilitate drainage of secretions. If suctioning is needed, it is performed carefully to avoid any trauma to the oropharynx. When alert the child may prefer sitting up, although he should remain in bed for the remainder of the day. He is discouraged from coughing frequently or clearing the throat, which may aggravate the operative site.

Some secretions are common, particularly dried blood from surgery. All secretions and vomitus are inspected for evidence of fresh bleeding (some blood-tinged mucus is expected). Also dark-brown (old) blood is usually present in the emesis and in the nose and between the teeth. If parents do not expect this, they may be frightened at a time when they need to be calm and reassuring.

The throat is very sore after surgery. An ice collar may provide relief, but many children find it bothersome and prefer not to have it. Analgesics are usually ordered but may need to be given rectally or parenterally to avoid the oral route. If the child is very irritable, mild sedation is helpful to lessen crying, which irritates the operative site, increasing the chance of bleeding.

Food and fluid are restricted until the child is fully alert and there are no signs of hemorrhage. Cool water or fruit juice is given first, although fluids with a red or brown color are avoided in order to distinguish fresh or old blood in emesis from the ingested liquid. The use of straws has been advised against because sucking may precipitate bleeding; however, this is not universally accepted. Citrus juice is usually poorly tolerated because of the discomfort it causes to denuded areas. Milk, ice cream, and pudding are not offered until after clear fluids are retained because milk products coat the mouth and throat, causing the child to clear the throat more often, which may initiate bleeding. Soft foods, particularly gelatin, cooked fruits, sherbet, soup, and mashed potatoes, are started on the first or second postoperative day or as the child tolerates them. Eating promotes healing because it increases the blood supply to the tissues.

Postoperative hemorrhage is not usual but can occur. The most obvious early sign is the child's continuous swallowing of the trickling blood. The nurse directly observes the throat for bleeding, using a good source of light and if necessary, carefully inserting a tongue depressor. If the child is asleep, frequency of swallowing is noted. Other signs of hemorrhage are increased pulse (above 120 beats/min), pallor, frequent clearing of the throat, and vomiting of bright-red blood. Restlessness, an indication of hemorrhage, may be difficult to differentiate from general discomfort after surgery. Decreasing blood pressure, a later sign, signals impending shock.

If continuous bleeding is suspected, the physician is notified immediately since surgery may be required to ligate the bleeding vessel. Airway obstruction may occur as a result of edema or accumulated secretions and is indicated by progressive cyanosis. Suction equipment should always be set up at the bedside after tonsillectomy.

Discharge instructions include (1) avoiding foods that are irritating or highly seasoned, (2) avoiding the use of gargles or vigorous toothbrushing, (3) discouraging the child from coughing or clearing the throat, and (4) using mild analgesics or an ice collar for pain. Hemorrhage may occur 5 to 10 days after surgery, as a result of tissue sloughing from the healing process. Any sign of bleeding warrants immediate medical attention. Objectionable mouth odor and slight ear pain with a low-grade fever are common occurrences lasting a few days postoperatively. However, persistent severe earache, fever, or cough necessitates medical evaluation. The child's voice may be altered for some time after surgery. Most children are ready to resume normal activity within 1 to 2 weeks.

Family care. A tonsillectomy and/or adenoidectomy often represents the first hospitalization experience for the child. Since the surgery is usually an elective procedure, there is ample opportunity to prepare both the child and parents for this event. Both need reassurance regarding what to expect at the time of admission, before and after surgery, and at discharge. Parents are encouraged to visit often or room-in if possible and participate in the child's care if they wish. The child is honestly apprised of postoperative discomfort and reassured that he will be able to talk. Sometimes children believe that the operation will immediately "make the throat all better" and are dismayed to find that it still hurts after the surgery. Ideally, the child should have an opportunity to discuss his experiences to gain a feeling of mastery and to overcome any fears or misconceptions.

EVALUATION

The effectiveness of nursing care is determined by continued reassessment according to the following observational guidelines and expected outcomes:

1. Monitor the child's vital signs and behavior
2. Observe for evidence of bleeding
3. Observe and interviewing family regarding their understanding of the child's condition
4. Have family demonstrate an understanding of home care
5. Encourage family to discuss concerns that provide some insight into their ability to comply with instructions

Expected outcomes:

1. Vital signs remain within acceptable limits for age (see inside front cover); child rests quietly
2. Child exhibits no evidence of restlessness, frequent swallowing or clearing the throat, or nausea and vomiting
3. Family demonstrates an understanding of the child's condition (specify)
4. Family demonstrates an understanding of and ability to carry out needed home care (specify knowledge and method of demonstration)
5. Family members are able to express their feelings and concerns

INFLUENZA

Influenza, or "flu," is caused by three antigenically distinct orthomyxoviruses: types A and B, which cause epidemic disease, and type C, which is unimportant epide-

Clinical Manifestations of Influenza

May be subclinical, mild, moderate, or severe
Overt illness:
- Dry throat and nasal mucosa
- Dry cough
- Tendency toward hoarseness
- Sudden onset of fever
- Flushed face
- Photophobia
- Myalgia
- Hyperesthesia
- Prostration (sometimes)
- Subglottal croup common (especially in infants)

miologically. The disease is spread from one individual to another by direct contact or by articles recently contaminated by nasopharyngeal secretions. No specific age-group is at risk, but attack rates are highest in young children who have not had previous contact with a strain. During epidemics, infection among school-age children is believed to be a major source of transmission in a community. Influenza is more common during the winter.

Therapeutic Management

The diagnosis of influenza is made on the basis of clinical manifestations (see box). Uncomplicated disease requires only symptomatic treatment, and symptoms last for 4 to 5 days. Amantadine hydrochloride (Symmetrel) has been effective in reducing symptoms associated with type A disease if administered within 24 to 48 hours after onset. It is ineffective against type B or C influenza or other viral disease, and it should not be given to children under 1 year of age. Ribavirin (Virazole), an antiviral agent, has been used successfully in the treatment of patients with acute influenza when administered as an aerosol.

Complications of influenza including severe viral pneumonia, encephalitis, and secondary bacterial infections, such as otitis media, sinusitis, or pneumonia, may develop. Reye syndrome can be a serious complication of type A or B; therefore, children with influenza should not receive aspirin.

Prevention. Immunization against influenza is available and recommended for children with chronic or acute conditions that make them susceptible to serious complications of the disease. (See also Chapter 10.)

Nursing Considerations

The nursing care of the child with influenza includes the measures described on p. 694.

OTITIS MEDIA

Otitis media (OM), middle ear infection, is one of the most prevalent diseases of early childhood. The incidence is highest in children age 6 months to 2 years, then it gradually decreases with age, except for a small increase at age 5 and 6 years, the time of entry into school. OM is uncommon in children over 7 years of age. The incidence of OM is highest in the winter months, and children living in households with many members (especially smokers) are more likely to have OM than those living with fewer persons.

The disorder has been classified in a number of ways, but the current accepted terminology is:

Otitis media—an inflammation of the middle ear without reference to etiology or pathogenesis
Acute otitis media (AOM)—a rapid and short onset of signs and symptoms lasting approximately 3 weeks
Otitis media with effusion (OME)—an inflammation of the middle ear in which a collection of fluid is present in the middle ear space
Subacute otitis media—middle ear effusion lasting from 3 weeks to 3 months
Chronic otitis media with effusion—middle ear effusion that persists beyond 3 months

Etiology/Pathophysiology

AOM is most frequently caused by *Streptococcus pneumoniae, Haemophilus influenzae,* and *Staphylococcus aureus*. The etiology of the noninfectious type is unknown, although it is frequently associated with blocked eustachian tubes caused by the edema of allergic rhinitis or hypertrophic adenoids. A relationship has also been noted between OM and infant feeding methods. Breast-fed infants have a lower incidence of OM compared to formula-fed infants.

OM is primarily the result of dysfunctioning eustachian tubes. The eustachian tube, which connects the middle ear to the nasopharynx, is normally closed and flat, preventing organisms from the pharyngeal cavity from entering the middle ear. It opens to allow drainage of secretions produced by the middle ear mucosa and to equalize air pressure between the middle ear and outside environment. Impaired drainage causes retention of secretions in the middle ear. Air, unable to escape through the obstructed tubes, is absorbed into the circulation, causing negative pressure within the middle ear. If the tube opens, this difference in pressure causes bacteria to be swept into the middle ear chamber, where the organisms quickly proliferate and invade the mucosa.

Diagnostic Evaluation

In AOM otoscopy reveals an intact membrane that appears bright red and bulging, with no visible bony landmarks or light reflex. In OM otoscopic findings may include a slightly injected, dull-gray membrane, obscured landmarks, and a visible fluid level or meniscus behind the eardrum, if air is present above the fluid. Diagnosis usually based on clinical manifestations (see box), but if purulent discharge is present, it should be cultured to assist in therapy.

Clinical Manifestations of Otitis Media

Acute
- Follows an upper respiratory infection
- Otalgia (earache)
- Purulent otorrhea may be present
- Fever
- Purulent discharge may or may not be present

Infant or very young child
- Crying
- Fussy, restless, irritable
- Tendency to rub, hold, or pull affected ear
- Rolls head side to side
- Difficulty comforting child
- Loss of appetite

Older child
- Crying and/or verbalizes feelings of discomfort
- Irritability
- Lethargy
- Loss of appetite

Chronic
- Hearing loss
- Difficulty communicating
- Feeling of fullness, tinnitus, vertigo may be present

Tympanometry may be used to measure the change in air pressure in the external auditory canal from movement of the eardrum. Pneumatic otoscopy also provides an assessment of typanic membrane mobility. Acoustic reflectometry measures the level of sound transmission.

Therapeutic Management

Treatment of AOM is administration of antibiotics, especially ampicillin or amoxicillin. Myringotomy (surgical incision of the eardrum) may be required to relieve the symptoms in some children, especially those with acute suppuration who are in severe pain. Children with AOM should be seen after antibiotic therapy is complete to evaluate the effectiveness of the treatment and to identify potential complications, such as effusion or hearing impairment. Analgesic/antipyretic drugs are used to alleviate discomfort and reduce an elevated temperature.

The major goal in the management of OME is to establish and maintain an aerated middle ear that is free of fluid and that has a normal mucosa and to achieve normal hearing. The medical management is uncertain and controversial. The widespread use of decongestants and antihistamines to shrink the mucous membranes and increase eustachian tube function is of unproven benefit. Many children require surgical intervention. Some children benefit from adenoidectomy alone or in combination with tonsillectomy. More often the surgical treatment involves tympanoplasty or insertion of ventilating tubes. Tympanostomy tubes (pressure-equalizer [PE] tubes, grommets, or dottles), applied under general anesthesia, facilitate continued drainage of fluid and allow ventilation of the middle ear.

Nursing Diagnoses: Child with Acute Otitis Media

Pain related to pressure caused by inflammatory process
Potential impaired skin integrity related to drainage
Altered family processes related to ill child

Nursing Considerations

Since OM is such a common aftermath of URIs, nurses are continually alert to this possibility when caring for a child with such infections.

ASSESSMENT

Examination of the external auditory canal is an integral part of the physical assessment (see p. 147). Nurses should be alert to the possibility of middle ear involvement in any child who has or is recovering from a URI or who displays evidence of hearing difficulty (see p. 151).

NURSING DIAGNOSES

Based on a careful assessment, several nursing diagnoses become evident (see box). Others may apply in specific situations and in the case of chronic OM or OME.

PLANNING

Nursing objectives for the care of children with acute OM include:

1. Relieve pain
2. Facilitate drainage when possible
3. Prevent complications or recurrence
4. Educate family in care of the child
5. Provide emotional support to child and family

IMPLEMENTATION

Analgesics are often very helpful in reducing the severe earache. Although acetaminophen is usually recommended for children, aspirin may be more effective in alleviating the pain. High fever, particularly in infants, should be reduced with antipyretic drugs to avoid febrile convulsions. The application of heat with a heating pad or hot water bottle wrapped in a towel may reduce the discomfort. Local heat should be placed over the ear with the child lying on the affected side. This position also facilitates drainage of the exudate if the eardrum has ruptured or if myringotomy was performed. An ice bag placed over the affected ear may also be beneficial since it reduces edema and pressure. If the child is cooperative, either procedure can be tried to determine which offers maximum relief.

If the ear is draining, the external canal may be cleaned with sterile cotton swabs or pledgets soaked in hydrogen peroxide. If ear wicks or lightly rolled sterile gauze packs are placed in the ear after surgical treatment, they should be loose enough to allow accumulated drainage to flow out of the ear; otherwise the infection may be transferred to the mastoid process. Parents should be told to keep these wicks dry during shampoos or baths. Occasionally drainage is so profuse that the auricle and the skin surrounding the ear become excoriated from the exudate. This is prevented by frequent cleansing and application of petrolatum or zinc oxide to the area.

A concern presented with the use of myringotomy tubes is the possibility of water entering the middle ear. Small amounts of water pose little hazard. However, a factor affecting the danger of water entering the ear is potential for introducing bacteria. Water from baths, showers, swimming pools, and fresh-water lakes is contaminated. In these situations, most earplugs, while not watertight, prevent total flooding of the external canal and provide sufficient protection (Strome, 1983). Parents should be aware of the appearance of a grommet (usually tiny, white, plastic spool-shaped tube) so that they can observe if it falls out. They are reassured that this is normal and requires no immediate intervention, although they should notify the physician.

Prevention of recurrence requires adequate parent education regarding antibiotic therapy. Antibiotics are frequently regarded as "miracle" drugs or as the "one-dose" cure for everything. Since the symptoms of pain and fever usually subside within 24 to 48 hours, the rapid outward signs of recovery support such thinking. Nurses must emphasize that, although the child appears well, the infection is not completely eradicated until all the prescribed medication is taken. Although one does not want to alarm parents, it is important to stress the potential complications of OM that can be prevented with adequate treatment and follow-up care. Such complications include (1) conductive hearing loss, (2) a perforated and scarred eardrum, (3) mastoiditis, an inflammation of the mastoid air cell system, (4) cholesteatoma, a cystlike lesion that can invade and destroy surrounding auditory structures, and (5) intracranial infections, such as meningitis.

The chances of OM occurring may be reduced by sitting or holding the child upright for feedings, encouraging gentle nose blowing, especially during a cold, and promoting aeration of the middle ear through the modified Valsalva maneuver, which consists of pinching the nose, closing the lips, and forcing air up the eustachian tube. Young children can blow balloons or chew sugarless gum to accomplish the same goal. Eliminating tobacco smoke and known allergens is also recommended.

EVALUATION

The efficacy of nursing intervention is determined by these observational guidelines and expected outcomes:

1. Observe behaviors that indicate pain relief; seek verbal confirmation
2. Observe skin in and around external auditory canal
3. Interview family regarding practices that prevent recurrence of infection
4. Observe and interview family regarding their understanding of OM and therapies
5. Interview family regarding their feelings and concerns

Expected outcomes:

1. The child exhibits no evidence of discomfort
2. The child exhibits no evidence of excoriated skin
3. The child develops no complications or recurrence
4. The family demonstrates the ability to care for the child's condition
5. The family express their feelings and concerns

◆ *Croup Syndromes*

Croup is a general term applied to a symptom complex involving the epiglottis, glottis, and larynx and characterized by hoarseness, a resonant cough described as rasping, "barking," or "brassy" (croupy), inspiratory stridor, and varying degrees of respiratory distress resulting from swelling of the airway. Rales, wheezing, or rhonchi are evident on auscultation. Acute infections involve all areas to some extent and are seldom restricted to one but are usually described according to the primary anatomic area affected. Table 22-1 compares and contrasts the major types of infection in these nonreactive airways.

The laryngeal involvement often dominates the clinical picture because of the severe effects on the voice and breathing. Also, acute subglottic infections are of greater importance in infants and small children than they are in older children, in part because of the increased incidence in children in this age-group and partly because of the smaller diameter of the airway, which renders it subject to significantly greater narrowing with the same degree of inflammation.

Laryngotracheobronchitis

Laryngitis, laryngotracheitis, and *laryngotracheobronchitis* are all considered together because of their similarity in manifestations and therapy. The principal etiologic agents in croup are viruses, except in those cases associated with diphtheria, pertussis, and acute epiglottitis. In most children the disease is relatively mild, with cough, stridor, and mild retractions and gradual improvement to recovery in 3 to 7 days. However, complications of viral croup occur in a number of children, the most common of which are extensions of the infection to other areas of the respiratory tract, e.g., OM, bronchiolitis, and pneumonia. The most serious complication, and the one responsible for most deaths from croup, is laryngeal obstruction.

Epiglottitis

Acute epiglottitis, or acute supraglottitis, is a serious obstructive inflammatory process. The obstruction is supra-

TABLE 22-1

Comparison of Croup Syndromes

Description/Etiology	Manifestations/Characteristics	Therapeutic Management
ACUTE EPIGLOTTITIS (SUPRAGLOTTITIS)		
Severe, rapidly progressive infection of the epiglottis and surrounding area Usually in good health before onset May be preceded by URI Chiefly ages 3-7 years Organism: generally *Haemophilus influenzae,* type B	Abrupt onset; rapidly progressive High fever; appears ill Sore throat Difficulty or inability to swallow Drooling of saliva; retching Difficulty in breathing progressing to severe respiratory distress in minutes or hours Child will sit upright, leaning forward, with chin thrust out and mouth open—tripod position Thick, muffled voice Croaking, "froglike" sound on inspiration Anxious and frightened expression Suprasternal and substernal retractions may be visible Seldom struggle to breathe (breathing slowly and quietly provides better air exchange) Sallow color of mild hypoxia to frank cyanosis Throat red, inflamed Distinctive large, cherry-red, edematous epiglottis	Minimal disturbance Avoid visualization of epiglottis without skilled personnel Establishment of an airway is urgent—endotracheal tube or tracheostomy often necessary Humidification with oxygen Vigorous antibiotic therapy intravenously Nasopharyngeal culture Blood culture Rest
ACUTE LARYNGITIS, LARYNGOTRACHEITIS, LARYNGOTRACHEOBRONCHITIS		
Most common form of croup May be localized or one manifestation of a variety of conditions Preceded by URI Most common at ages 3 months to 3 years; mean age—21 months Organisms: viral agents, especially parainfluenza viruses	Wide range of manifestations from few symptoms to severe obstructive laryngitis Infection rapidly descends, with first laryngeal symptoms—hoarseness, brassy cough, stridor, respiratory distress Fever and prostration increase Respiratory distress, especially inspiratory dyspnea with substernal and suprasternal retractions Bronchi involvement becomes evident with increased dyspnea Expiratory difficulty with labored and prolonged expirations Scattered rales of various types; rhonchi Diminished breath sounds bilaterally Pallor or cyanosis Irritability and restlessness	If mild, treated at home If severe, hospitalized High-humidity therapy with high oxygen concentration Tracheostomy set at bedside Rest; disturb as little as possible; reduce need to talk or cry Adequate fluid intake: intravenous fluids to save strength and decrease possibility of vomiting; less severely affected—oral fluids
ACUTE SPASMODIC LARYNGITIS (SPASMODIC CROUP)		
Distinct clinical entity characterized by sudden paroxysmal attacks of laryngeal obstruction that occur chiefly at night Usually preceded by mild to moderate nasopharyngitis or slight laryngitis Usually affects small children ages 1 to 3 years Organism: viral agents In some cases, allergy and psychogenic factors have been implicated Certain children appear to be predisposed	Appears primarily at night Child suddenly wakens with characteristic barking, metallic cough, hoarseness, noisy inspirations, and restlessness; child appears anxious, frightened, and prostrated Accessory muscles of respiration used and inspiratory retractions sometimes evident Dyspnea aggravated by excitement May be some cyanosis Attack wears off in a few hours and child appears well the following day except for some hoarseness and cough May be repeated 1 or 2 nights in succession No fever Usually self-limited	High-humidity atmosphere Induction of expectoration with single dose of ipecac (1 drop per month of age up to 2 years; 2-5 ml for older children) Mild sedation with phenobarbital

glottic as opposed to subglottic obstruction of laryngitis. It is one of the most dramatic diseases of childhood and must be recognized early and treated vigorously to avoid a fatal outcome. The causative organism is almost always *Haemophilus influenzae*, and the onset is very rapid in a previously healthy child.

Therapeutic Management

The major objective in medical management of infectious croup is maintaining an airway and providing for adequate respiratory exchange. Afebrile children with mild laryngitis and a croupy cough are usually managed at home with treatment of symptoms. Bed rest and humidified air during sleep may be helpful.

Children with spasmodic croup are managed at home. Mist inhalation as described for upper respiratory infection is recommended, especially the quick vaporization that is afforded by steam from hot running water in a closed bathroom (a shower is recommended if available). This quick and easy treatment usually provides almost immediate relief of acute laryngeal spasm and respiratory distress. Sometimes the spasm is relieved by sudden exposure to cold air (as when the child is taken out into the night air for medical care). Parents are usually advised to have the child sleep with cool humidified air until the cough has subsided so that subsequent episodes might be prevented.

Although many children with croup and temperatures significantly elevated above 39° C (102.2° F) can be managed at home, hospitalization is often advised. Those for whom hospitalization is indicated are children with:

- Presence or suspicion of epiglottitis, progressive stridor, and respiratory distress (especially during the daytime)
- Presence of hypoxia, restlessness, cyanosis, pallor, and/or depressed sensorium
- A high temperature and toxic appearance

Facilities and equipment for tracheostomy and reliable observation are readily available in the hospital setting. If the hospital does not provide close, skilled observation, the child may be safer at home where the parents can maintain vigilance.

In cases of suspected epiglottitis, attempts to visualize the epiglottis directly with a tongue depressor may precipitate sudden laryngospasm, complete obstruction, and death. Therefore, the nurse does not attempt examination of the throat. Examination is made by a trained practitioner with intubation or tracheostomy equipment at hand.

Children with croup, whether treated at home or in the hospital, require close observation for signs of respiratory obstruction. They are placed in high humidity, preferably in a mist tent or Croupette with cool-mist vapor. Since a rapidly rising heart rate is an early signal of hypoxia and impending airway obstruction, regular monitoring of cardiac rate is instituted, preferably with a cardiac monitor. Oxygen therapy is also indicated to alleviate hypoxia and reduce apprehension.

Fluid by the intravenous route is indicated to lessen physical exertion and to reduce the likelihood of vomiting with the attendant risk of aspiration. Infants with rapid respirations may aspirate feedings.

Medications. Children with suspected bacterial epiglottitis are given ampicillin intravenously. The use of corticosteroids for reducing edema has not been determined to be of benefit. Expectorants, bronchodilators, and antihistamines are rarely helpful in treating the patient with croup, and sedatives are contraindicated because of their depressant effect on the respiratory center. Dramatic relief of laryngeal stridor has been achieved in treatment of croup with the use of racemic epinephrine (Vaponefrin) in nebulized mist or with intermittent positive-pressure breathing.

Nursing Considerations

Although some children with URIs are ill enough to be hospitalized, most are managed at home. Consequently, most of the nursing interventions are directed toward helping families with the care of their child. Some interventions used in acute care are included in the Nursing Care Plan on p. 696.

ASSESSMENT

Assessment is the same as that described for children with acute respiratory infection (p. 694), with particular attention to signs of respiratory embarrassment. As distress increases, the child becomes increasingly restless and anxious. He dozes, wakens startled, and makes visible efforts to draw in air. Tracheostomy or endotracheal intubation is usually performed at this stage of distress. If it is not, the inspiratory stridor and retractions progress until he becomes markedly pale or ashen, his skin is cold and clammy, and all his attention and effort are focused on fighting for air. He becomes increasingly agitated, thrashes about, and tries to climb the sides of the Croupette in his efforts to breathe. His status is critical. An artificial airway is mandatory for survival. The child may or may not be cyanotic; he is often pale to ashen and appears very ill. Cyanosis is often a late sign.

NURSING DIAGNOSES

At the conclusion of a nursing assessment several nursing diagnoses become evident. Not all of those listed in the box are applicable to all children with croup.

PLANNING

The objectives for the care of a child with croup are:

1. Ease respiratory efforts
2. Reduce temperature, if present
3. Prevent dehydration
4. Conserve energy
5. Reduce apprehension of child and family

Nursing Diagnoses: Child with Croup

Ineffective breathing pattern related to obstructed airway
Ineffective airway clearance related to edema and obstruction
Potential for suffocation related to airway obstruction
Anxiety/fear related to difficulty breathing, unfamiliar environment, procedures
Altered family processes related to situational crisis

6. Educate family regarding situation and prepare for home care of the child

IMPLEMENTATION

The most important nursing function in the care of children with croup is vigilant observation for signs of respiratory embarrassment and facilitation of respiratory efforts. The child is placed in a cool high-humidity environment with oxygen, usually administered by way of a mist tent or Croupette, and with skilled nursing personnel in attendance to observe for any indications of respiratory distress.

Vital signs are monitored frequently, and the child's appearance and behavior are observed to detect early signs of impending airway obstruction, such as increased pulse and respiratory rate, substernal, suprasternal, and intercostal retractions, flaring nares, and increased restlessness. Equipment for performing a tracheostomy or endotracheal intubation should be at hand in case an artificial airway must be supplied immediately, and equipment is left there until respiratory difficulty has subsided completely. *Any child with laryngeal stridor requires constant surveillance* (see also Nursing tip box on stridor).

Nursing Tip: Stridor

Laryngeal stridor is recognized as a shrill, harsh respiratory sound, often described as a "crowing" sound, that is particularly marked during inspiration.

Fortunately only a small percentage of children with croup require intubation or tracheostomy. Immediately after the procedure the child becomes more relaxed as a result of the relief from laryngeal obstruction, his breathing becomes regular, and he usually falls asleep from exhaustion. Later he may become frightened to discover that he is unable to speak or to cry. One of the greatest fears is that he will be unable to call someone to his side. He will need continued emotional support as well as the physical vigilance required in tracheostomy care. The tracheostomy is usually left in place only as long as needed to relieve respiratory distress.

To conserve energy, the child is given every opportunity to rest. Fluids are administered intravenously during the acute phase of illness, and other measures are implemented to promote rest and to reduce anxiety. An infant or small child finds that being enclosed within the mist tent, coughing, laryngeal spasms, and restraint for intravenous therapy are additional sources of distress. He needs the security of the parents' or the nurse's presence. When his condition allows, a small child can be removed for short periods for comfort and reassurance, especially to reduce apprehension during coughing spells.

The rapid progression of croup and epiglottitis, the alarming sound of the cough or stridor, and the child's apprehensive behavior and ill appearance combine to create a very frightening experience for the parents. They need reassurance regarding the child's progress and an explanation of treatments. They may feel guilty for not having suspected the seriousness of the condition sooner, especially if an artificial airway is needed. The nurse can provide them with an opportunity to express their feelings, thus minimizing any blame or guilt. Fortunately, as the crisis subsides and as the child responds to therapy, his breathing becomes easier and recovery is generally prompt.

EVALUATION

The extent to which nursing goals are achieved is determined by employing the following observational guidelines and expected outcomes:

1. Observe behaviors that indicate effortless breathing and relief of obstruction
2. Monitor vital signs
3. Assess skin and mucous membranes for signs of dehydration
4. Observe behaviors that indicate unnecessary expenditure of energy
5. Observe behaviors that suggest reduced anxiety in child and family
6. Interview family regarding their understanding of the child's condition and home care instructions

Expected outcomes:

1. The child breathes without apparent difficulty
2. The child's vital signs remain within normal limits
3. The child exhibits no evidence of dehydration
4. The child rests and plays quietly
5. The child and family exhibit no evidence of distress
6. Family demonstrates an understanding of the child's condition and therapies

◆ *Acute Infections of the Lower Respiratory Tract*

The lower portion of the respiratory tract includes the airways (trachea, bronchi, and bronchioles) and the lungs. Infections of these structures are frequently an extension of a URI. Therefore, careful assessment for evidence of these complications is an intergral part of nursing care of children with URIs.

ACUTE INFECTIONS OF THE LOWER AIRWAYS

Infectious disorders of the lower airways are diverse in nature and cause and primarily involve the bronchioles. Bronchial inflammation is usually seen as tracheobronchitis or laryngotracheobronchitis (LTB), but bacterial tracheitis is now recognized as a cause of subglottic obstructive airway disease in children. Table 22-2 compares major characteristics of tracheal, bronchial, and bronchiolar infections.

Bacterial Tracheitis

Bacterial tracheitis, an infection of the mucosa of the upper trachea, is a distinct entity with features of both

TABLE 22-2

Comparison of Lower Airway Infections

Description/Etiology	Manifestations/Characteristics	Therapeutic Management
TRACHEITIS		
Infection of trachea May be a complication of laryngotracheobronchitis Affects children 1 month to 6 years Organisms: bacterial—majority *Staphylococcus aureus, Haemophilus influenzae*	Follows previous URI Begins with signs and symptoms similar to croup Croupy cough, stridor, unaffected by position Copious purulent secretions—may be severe enough to cause respiratory arrest High fever, toxicity No response to laryngotracheobronchitis	Humidified oxygen Tracheal suctioning Antibiotics Often requires artificial airway (endotracheal tube)
ASTHMATIC BRONCHITIS		
Exaggerated response of bronchi to infection Spasm and exudation similar to asthma in older children Occurs in late infancy and early childhood Organisms: most commonly viruses but may be any of a variety of URI pathogens	Sudden onset at night Previous URI Wheezing Productive cough Moderate signs of emphysema	Bronchodilators, such as epinephrine, ephedrine Sedatives, such as phenobarbital Expectorants High-humidity atmosphere
BRONCHITIS		
Seldom occurs as an isolated entity in childhood Usually occurs in association with URI Affects children in first 4 years of life Highest incidence in September and October Organisms: usually viral (same as croup); other agents (e.g., bacteria, fungi, allergic disorders, airborne irritants) can trigger symptoms	Abrupt onset Persistent dry, hacking cough (worse at night) becoming productive in 2-3 days Tachypnea Low-grade fever May have chest pain aggravated by coughing	No specific therapy Symptomatic and supportive therapy
BRONCHIOLITIS		
One of more common infectious diseases of lower respiratory tract Maximum obstruction at bronchiolar level consists of hypersecretion, edema, and inflammatory reaction confined to smaller bronchioles Usually affects children 2-12 months; rare after age 2 years Peak incidence approximately age 6 months Organisms: viral; predominantly respiratory syncytial virus; also, adenoviruses, parainfluenza viruses, and *Mycoplasma pneumoniae*	Begins as simple URI with serous nasal discharge May be accompanied by moderate temperature elevation Gradually develops increasing respiratory distress, paroxysmal cough, dyspnea, and irritability Tachypnea with flaring nares and intercostal and subcostal retractions Emphysema with barrel chest and palpable liver and spleen from depressed diaphragm Shallow respiratory excursion Fine rales and prolonged expiratory phase; diminished breath sounds, hyperresonance, and scattered consolidation May be wheezing	Rest High-humidity atmosphere Oxygen in moderate to severe cases Adequate hydration

croup and epiglottitis. It is believed to be a complication of LTB and may be a serious cause of airway obstruction. Many of the manifestations of bacterial tracheitis are similar to those of LTB but are unresponsive to LTB therapy. Although *Staphylococcus aureus* is the most frequent organism responsible, group A β-hemolytic streptococci and *Haemophilus influenzae* have also been implicated.

Tracheitis requires vigorous management, including antibiotic therapy, antipyretics, and frequent tracheal suctioning to remove copious secretions, and endotracheal intubation is often required to ensure an adequate airway. Humidified oxygen is provided by appropriate means.

Asthmatic Bronchitis

In asthmatic bronchitis the predominant pathologic manifestation is bronchospasm with increased production of mucus. It is often confused with bronchiolitis and represents a peculiar response to a variety of URIs. The affected children are seldom ill, but wheezing, productive cough, and signs of moderate emphysema are apparent. There is usually a history of attacks associated with URIs.

Asthmatic bronchitis is effectively treated with bronchodilators and expectorants. A high-humidity environment is provided and expectorants help liquefy and remove bronchial secretions. Since the majority of attacks are triggered by viral infections, antimicrobials are rarely indicated.

Bronchitis

Bronchitis, an isolated condition that is unusual in childhood, may be associated with either upper or lower respiratory tract conditions. A variety of etiologic agents may initiate the dry, hacking, and nonproductive cough. Noxious chemicals in urban air pollution are becoming an important cause. Bronchitis is a mild, self-limiting disease that requires only symptomatic treatment directed primarily toward cough control.

Bronchiolitis

Bronchiolitis is represented by severe infectious and mechanical changes in the bronchioles. Bronchiole mucosa is swollen, lumina are filled with mucus and exudate, the walls of the bronchi and bronchioles are infiltrated with inflammatory cells, and peribronchiolar interstitial pneumonitis is usually present. The variable degrees of obstruction produced in small air passages by these changes lead to hyperinflation, obstructive emphysema resulting from partial obstruction, and patchy areas of atelectasis. Hospitalization is usually recommended, and the child is placed in a mist tent or Croupette to help loosen tenacious secretions and minimize fluid loss from the lungs. Mist therapy is usually combined with oxygen in concentrations sufficient to alleviate dyspnea and hypoxia. Fluids by mouth may be contraindicated because of tachypnea, weakness, and fatigue; therefore, intravenous fluids are preferred until the crisis of the disease has passed.

Most authorities use the conservative approach regarding medications. Antibiotics are not routinely employed, bronchodilators are ineffectual since bronchospasm is not part of the pathologic picture, corticosteroids have not been proved to be of universal value, cough suppressants and expectorants have not been found useful, and sedatives are contraindicated. The disease lasts about 7 to 10 days, and the prognosis is generally good.

PNEUMONIAS

Pneumonia, inflammation of the pulmonary parenchyma, is common throughout childhood but occurs more frequently in infancy and early childhood. Clinically, pneumonia may occur either as a primary disease or as a complication of some other illness. Morphologically, pneumonias are recognized as: (1) *lobar pneumonia,* involving all or a large segment of one or more pulmonary lobes; (2) *bronchopneumonia* or *lobular pneumonia,* involving the terminal bronchioles and nearby lobules; and (3) *interstitial pneumonia,* involving the alveolar walls (interstitium) and the peribronchial and interlobular tissues.

The pneumonias are more often classified according to the etiologic agent. In general, pneumonia is caused by four processes: viral, atypical (mycoplasma), bacterial, and aspiration of foreign substances (see p. 714). Less often pneumonia may be caused by histomycosis, coccidioidomycosis, and other fungi. The causative agent is identified largely from the clinical history, the child's age, his general health history, the physical examination, radiograms, and laboratory examination.

Viral Pneumonia

Viral pneumonias occur more frequently than bacterial pneumonias and are seen in children of all age-groups. They are often associated with viral URIs, and the respiratory syncytial virus (RSV) accounts for the largest percentage. Others are the influenza virus, parainfluenza virus, psittacosis, rhinovirus, and adenovirus. There are few clinical symptoms to distinguish between the responsible organisms, and differentiations between viruses can be made only by laboratory examination. See box for clinical manifestations.

The prognosis is generally good, although viral infections of the respiratory tract render the affected child more susceptible to secondary bacterial invasion, especially when there is denuded bronchial mucosa. Treatment is usually symptomatic, although some recommend antimicrobial therapy in hope of reducing or preventing secondary bacterial infection. It is usually reserved for cases in which the presence of such infection is demonstrated by appropriate cultures.

Clinical Manifestations of Viral and Atypical Pneumonias

Viral Pneumonia	Atypical Pneumonia
May be acute or insidious Symptoms variable *Mild:* low-grade fever, slight cough, malaise *Severe:* high fever, severe cough, prostration Cough usually unproductive early in disease A few rhonchi or fine crepitant rales heard on auscultation	May be sudden or insidious General systemic symptoms: Fever Chills (older children) Headache Malaise Anorexia Myalgia Followed by: Rhinitis Sore throat Dry, hacking cough Nonproductive early, then seromucoid sputum, to mucopurulent or blood streaked Fine crepitant rales over various lung areas

Primary Atypical Pneumonia

Approximately 10% to 20% of hospital admissions of children with pneumonia are caused by *Mycoplasma pneumoniae*. It occurs principally in the fall and winter months and is more prevalent where there are crowded living conditions. See box for outline of clinical manifestations.

Most affected persons recover from acute illness in 7 to 10 days with symptomatic treatment followed by a week of convalescence. Hospitalization is rarely necessary.

Bacterial Pneumonia

In children beyond the neonatal period, bacterial pneumonias display distinct clinical patterns that facilitate their differentiation from other forms of pneumonia, and individual microorganisms produce a distinct clinical picture. Onset is abrupt and is generally preceded by a viral infection that disturbs the natural defense mechanisms of the upper respiratory tract and allows the pathogenic bacteria normally harbored in the upper passages to increase in number.

Children with bacterial pneumonia appear ill and exhibit both general and localized physical findings. Symptoms and signs include fever, malaise, rapid and shallow respirations, cough, and chest pain that is often exaggerated by deep breathing. The pain may be referred to the abdomen and confused with appendicitis. Chills frequently occur, and meningeal symptoms (meningism) are also common. Pleural reactions and effusions often accompany the disease, and the consolidation process usually proceeds rapidly.

The majority of older children with pneumococcal pneumonia can be treated at home, especially if the condition is recognized and treatment initiated early. Antibiotic therapy, bed rest, liberal oral intake of fluid, and administration of acetaminophen for fever constitute the principal therapeutic measures. Hospitalization is indicated when pleural effusion or empyema accompanies the disease and is mandatory for children with staphylococcal pneumonia. Pneumonia in the infant or young child is best treated in the hospital since the course of illness is more variable and complications are more common in very young patients. Also, fluids are usually given intravenously, and oxygen administration greatly reduces the restlessness associated with respiratory distress.

At the present time the classic features and clinical course of pneumonia are rarely seen because of early and vigorous antibiotic and supportive therapy. However, a large number of children, especially infants, with staphylococcal pneumonia develop empyema, pyopneumothorax, or tension pneumothorax. Pleural effusion is not uncommon in children with lobar (pneumococcal) pneumonia. A diagnostic thoracentesis is performed if fluid is suspected in the pleural cavity. Nonpurulent effusions, such as occur in pneumococcal pneumonia, do not require surgical drainage. Continuous closed-chest drainage is instituted when purulent fluid is aspirated, a frequent finding in staphylococcal infections.

The prognosis for pneumococcal infections is generally good, with rapid recovery when they are recognized and treated early. Streptococcal infections vary in duration but usually resolve spontaneously. The course of staphylococcal pneumonia is generally prolonged. The prognosis varies with the length of illness before treatment is begun, although early recognition and treatment are usually effective. Complications of bacterial pneumonia include pleural effusion, empyema, and tension pneumothorax. The major bacterial pneumonias are compared in Table 22-3.

A vaccine for pneumococcal pneumonia is available (see p. 295). It is not recommended for mass immunization but rather for children over age 2 years who are debilitated and children with diseases that predispose to pneumonia, such as cystic fibrosis.

Nursing Considerations

Nursing care of the child with an infection of the air passages is primarily supportive and symptomatic to meet each child's needs. The child is assigned a bed away from others, frequently in a small, segregated ward used only for children who have respiratory infections. Ideally, the same nurses should be assigned to these children and have responsibility for the care of no other children. It has been shown that many respiratory viruses, especially RSV, are readily transmitted to personnel, families, and other children; therefore appropriate precautions are important (see p. 644).

Rest and conservation of energy are encouraged by relief of physical and psychologic stresses. The child is dis-

TABLE 22-3

Three Major Bacterial Pneumonias

Description/Etiology	Clinical Manifestations
PNEUMOCOCCAL PNEUMONIA **Organism:** pneumococci: most common agent in lobar pneumonia **Involvement:** Usually lobar but may be lobular; areas of consolidation (usually patchy) in one or more lobes Occurs most often in late winter and early spring Highest attack rate during the first 4 years and declines with increasing age; uncommon in infants less than 1 year of age	**Infants** Fretfulness and diminished appetite followed by abrupt onset of fever May be accompanied by convulsions Restlessness, apprehension, respiratory distress, appears acutely ill, flushed cheeks, circumoral cyanosis Decreased breath sounds and crackling rales; exaggerated breath sounds on opposite side; pleural friction rub may be heard **Older children** Usually follows a URI Shaking chill followed by high fever, chest pain, tachypnea Drowsiness with intermittent periods of restlessness, anxiety Occasionally, delirium Circumoral cyanosis Hacking, unproductive cough (initially) Splinting of side caused by pleurisy pain Chest—dullness; diminished breath sounds, tactile and vocal fremitus; consolidation on second or third day evidenced by dullness, increased fremitus, tubular breath sounds, and disappearance of rales With resolution—moist rales; productive cough with large amounts of blood-tinged mucus Resolution begins about 24 hours after initiation of therapy
STAPHYLOCOCCAL PNEUMONIA **Organism:** *S. epidermidis; S. aureus* most common agent in bronchopneumonia **Involvement:** Localized abscesses in older children; more diffuse in infants Formation of peribronchial abscesses, pneumatoceles Greatest incidence in first 2 years of life, usually less than 1 month of age Occurs most often in winter months Usually contracted as primary infection Cross-contamination common in hospitals	Abrupt onset of fever, listlessness and lethargy when undisturbed, irritability on arousal, anorexia, nasal discharge, cough, grunting respirations, progressively severe dyspnea that may include subcostal and sternal retractions and cyanosis Shocklike state may be present Symptoms of complications: for example, pneumothorax, empyema, septicemia Some infants have gastrointestinal disturbances: for example, vomiting, diarrhea, and sometimes abdominal distention Rapid progression of symptoms characteristic Chest—early, diminished breath sounds, rales, and rhonchi with effusion or pneumothorax; dullness on percussion; respiratory lag on affected side; exaggerated excursion on opposite side
STREPTOCOCCAL PNEUMONIA **Organisms:** group A β-hemolytic streptococci, group B streptococcus **Involvement:** Interstitial bronchopneumonia Spreads via lymphatics Although usually lobular, areas of consolidation may coalesce to become lobar Less common than other bacterial pneumonias No seasonal variation Usually occurs as complication of influenza or measles	May appear without evidence of illness Symptoms similar to those of pneumococcal pneumonia Onset sudden High temperature Chills Signs of respiratory distress At times, extreme prostration Occasionally, only mild symptoms Tachypnea, usually mild Rales generally unilateral and exaggerated by deep inspiration

turbed as little as possible. Since rapid improvement is the rule in most types of pneumonia, feedings may be omitted, especially when the respiration is rapid, in order to prevent possible aspiration. To prevent dehydration, fluids are frequently administered intravenously during the acute phase. Oral fluids, if allowed, are given cautiously to avoid aspiration and to decrease the possibility of aggravating a fatiguing cough.

The child is placed in a mist tent with oxygen. Cool mist moistens the airways, helps mobilize secretions, reduces bronchial edema, and provides a cool atmosphere that aids in temperature reduction. The child often requires frequent clothing and linen changes to prevent chilling in the damp atmosphere. He is usually more comfortable in a semierect position but should be allowed to determine his position of comfort. Lying on the affected side (if pneumonia is unilateral) splints the chest on that side and reduces the pleural rubbing that often causes discomfort.

Fever is usually controlled by the cool environment

and administration of antipyretic drugs as prescribed. Temperature is monitored regularly to detect a rapid rise that might trigger a febrile seizure.

Vital signs and chest sounds are monitored to assess the progress of the disease and to detect early signs of complications. Children with ineffectual cough or those with difficulty in handling secretions, especially infants, will require suctioning to maintain a patent airway. A simple bulb syringe is usually sufficient for clearing the nares and nasopharynx of infants, but a suction machine should be readily available if needed. Older children can usually handle secretions without assistance. Percussion, vibration, and suctioning or drainage are generally prescribed every 4 hours or more often depending on the child's condition.

The child in the hospital is apprehensive, and many of the treatments and tests are frightening and stress producing. Reducing anxiety and apprehension not only reduces psychologic distress in the child, but when the child is more relaxed, the respiratory efforts are lessened. Easing respiratory efforts makes the child less apprehensive, and encouraging the presence of the caregiver provides the child with his customary source of comfort and support.

◆ *Other Infections of the Respiratory Tract*

Although less common than the previously described illnesses, several infectious disorders are capable of causing significant morbidity, especially in the infant and very young child. Pertussis (whooping cough) is an acute respiratory infection caused by *Bordetella pertussis* that occurs chiefly in children younger than 4 years of age who have not been immunized. It is highly contagious and is particularly threatening in young infants, in whom there are higher morbidity and mortality rates. (See Table 14-1 for signs, symptoms, and management of pertussis and p. 293 for immunization.) Tuberculosis, an ancient disease, is discussed in the following segment.

PULMONARY TUBERCULOSIS

Tuberculosis (TB, Tbc), although controlled in most developed countries, still remains a health hazard and a leading cause of death throughout many parts of the world. The increasing incidence of tuberculosis in the United States is attributed, in part, to the influx of foreign-born persons and recognition of the disease in the native-born population.

Tuberculosis is caused by *Mycobacterium tuberculosis*. Children are susceptible to both the human *(M. tuberculosis)* and the bovine *(M. bovis)* organisms, and in parts of the world where tuberculosis in cattle is not controlled or pasteurization of milk is not practiced, the bovine type is a common source of infection in children. Although the causative agent is the tubercle bacillus, other factors influence the degree to which the organism is able to produce an altered state in the host, including heredity (resistance to the infection may be genetically transmitted), sex (higher in adolescent girls), age (lower resistance in infants; higher incidence during adolescence), stress (emotional or physical), nutritional state, and intercurrent infection.

The source of infection in children is, in most situations, an infected adult or a teenager, usually a member of the household. It can also be a baby-sitter, domestic worker, or a frequent visitor to the household. The lung is the most frequent portal of entry in human beings; the organism enters less often by ingestion. In the lungs a proliferation of epithelial cells surround and encapsulate the multiplying bacilli in an attempt to wall off the invading organisms, thus forming the typical tubercle. Extension of the primary lesion at the original site causes progressive tissue destruction as it spreads within the lung, discharges material from foci to other areas of the lungs (e.g., bronchi or pleura), or produces pneumonia. Erosion of blood vessels by the primary lesion can cause widespread dissemination of the tubercle bacillus to near and distant sites (miliary tuberculosis). Areas that are frequently affected include lymph nodes, meninges, and bone.

Diagnostic Evaluation

Manifestations of pulmonary tuberculosis in children are extremely variable (see box), and most children have no symptoms when first infected. A history of possible contact may be helpful and radiographic examinations are performed. The diagnosis is confirmed by isolation of the tubercle bacilli by culture from sputum, gastric washings, and/or pleural fluid.

Clinical Manifestations of Pulmonary Tuberculosis

Extremely variable

May be asymptomatic or produce a broad range of symptoms
- Fever
- Malaise
- Anorexia
- Weight loss
- Cough may or may not be present (progresses slowly over weeks to months)
- Aching pain and tightness in the chest
- Hemoptysis (rare)

With progression
- Respiratory rate increases
- Poor expansion of lung on the affected side
- Diminished breath sounds and rales
- Dullness to percussion
- Fever persists
- Generalized symptoms manifest
- Develops pallor, anemia, weakness, and weight loss

Tuberculin test. Tuberculin testing is confined to high-risk population. It is not a routine procedure.

Two types of tuberculin preparations are used for skin tests: *old tuberculin* and *purified protein derivative (PPD)* of tuberculin. The PPD is used most widely, and the standard dose is 5 tuberculin units in 0.1 ml of solution, injected intracutaneously. The techniques for injection are (1) the *Mantoux test,* in which the PPD is injected directly into the dermis, and (2) the *multiple-puncture tests* (tine, Heaf, SclavoTest, Sterneedle, or Mono-Vac).

A positive reaction indicates that the individual has been infected and has developed a sensitivity to the protein of the tubercle bacillus. However, it does not confirm the presence of actual disease. Once persons have reacted positively, they will continue to react positively. A previously negative result that becomes positive indicates that the person has been infected since the last test. Test results are read according to instructions provided by the manufacturer.

Therapeutic Management

Medical management of tuberculous lesions in children consists of adequate nutrition, chemotherapy, general supportive measures, avoidance of unnecessary exposure to other infections that further compromise the body's defenses, prevention of reinfection, and sometimes surgical procedures. The child is placed on bed rest to conserve energy, avoid fatigue, and decrease metabolic demands. Bed rest is continued until the child is free of fever, exhibits evidence of returning strength, has no manifestations that limit ambulation, and desires to be up and about. Since metabolic deficits, particularly negative calcium and nitrogen levels, occur easily in infected children, special attention is given to planning an adequate intake of the necessary nutritional elements.

Chemotherapy. Chemotherapy is the single most important therapeutic modality available for management of tuberculosis. A variety of chemical agents can be employed, and a regimen involving two or more drugs simultaneously has been found to be effective and is usually the mode of choice. The most commonly used combinations of drugs are isoniazid (INH) and rifampin (RMP). Isoniazid with ethambutol (EMB) or another combination of drugs is used if the child is intolerant of the other drug(s). The optimum duration of therapy is unknown, but the usual course of treatment is no less than 12 months for an initial treatment or 18 to 24 months for more serious forms of the disease.

Limited immunity can be produced by administration of the only successful vaccine to date, bacillus Calmette-Guérin (BCG), vaccine containing bovine bacilli with reduced virulence. The freshly prepared vaccine, injected intradermally, produces a definite although incomplete protection against tuberculosis. The distribution of the vaccine is controlled by local or state health departments, but the vaccine is not used extensively, even in areas with a high prevalence of disease. Greater protection is afforded by daily prophylactic administration of isoniazid. The drug is given to children with a high probability of exposure to tuberculosis.

Nursing Considerations

Most children with pulmonary tuberculosis almost always have noninfectious disease; therefore they seldom need to be isolated. There are few bacilli in the sputum, the amount of sputum produced is quite small, and sputum is swallowed rather than expectorated. Hospitalization is seldom necessary except for needed diagnostic tests; most children are managed satisfactorily at home. Therefore the major nursing care of children with tuberculosis involves nurses in ambulatory settings—outpatient departments, schools, and especially public health agencies.

Children without symptoms are able to lead an essentially unrestricted life. They can, and should, attend school (or nursery school), but older children are restricted from vigorous activities such as competitive games and contact sports during the active stage of primary tuberculosis. They should be protected from stresses, including parental anxieties, the tendency toward overprotection, and pressures regarding nutritional intake. The regular immunization schedule should be continued. Care should be exerted to maintain an optimum health status with proper diet, adequate rest, and avoidance of infection.

Nurses assume several important roles in management of the disease, including assisting with radiographic examinations, performing skin tests, and obtaining specimens for laboratory examination. Sputum specimens are difficult or impossible to obtain in an infant or young child, since they swallow any mucus coughed from the lower respiratory tract. Therefore the best means for obtaining material for smears or culture is by gastric washing, that is, aspiration of lavaged contents from the fasting stomach. The procedure is carried out and the specimen obtained early in the morning before the customary breakfast time.

Ambulatory care. Nursing supervision of the child at home involves teaching parents and child about the disease and its ramifications. Since children usually acquire the disease from an adult in the home, parents often feel guilty. Misconceptions regarding the disease need to be clarified. Reducing parental anxieties helps them to deal with the illness more constructively and to collaborate more effectively in planning for the child's continued care. The success of therapy depends on the acceptance and cooperation of the family. The nurse can help the family to understand the rationale of diagnostic procedures and therapy and the importance of maintaining the therapeutic plan over the extended period needed for recovery.

The only certain means to prevent tuberculosis is to avoid contact with the tubercle bacillus. Maintaining an optimum state of health with adequate nutrition and avoidance of fatigue and debilitating infections promotes natural resistance but does not prevent infection. Pasteurization of milk and routine testing and elimination of diseased cattle have helped reduce the incidence of bovine tuberculosis. Infants and children should be given only pasteurized milk from tuberculosis-free cattle.

In general, primary pulmonary tuberculosis in young children is noninfectious for older children or adults. The contagiousness of chronic pulmonary tuberculosis in older children and adolescents is comparable to similar disease in adults. Of concern to hospital personnel is that infected family members may spread the disease when visiting a child in the hospital. Therefore the child and all visitors may be restricted to the child's room until the family can be screened for evidence of the disease.

◆ *Pulmonary Dysfunction Caused by Noninfectious Irritants*

Inflammation of lung tissue can occur occasionally as the result of irritation from foreign material. Aspiration of food, oral secretions, smoke, or other substances by otherwise healthy infants or children can set up an inflammatory response or chemical pneumonia. Young children are especially prone to aspiration of foreign substances, and weak and debilitated children are subject to aspiration of food or secretions. The major problems associated with aspiration in children are asphyxia or respiratory tract inflammation as the result of inhaling foreign material. Medical and nursing care of a subsequent pneumonitis and/or bronchitis is similar to that for lower respiratory tract inflammation resulting from infectious agents.

FOREIGN BODY ASPIRATION

Small children characteristically explore matter with their mouths and are therefore particularly prone to aspirate a foreign body (FB) into the air passages. Aspiration of an FB can occur at any age but is most commonly seen in children ages 1 to 3 years. The signs and changes produced depend on the degree of obstruction and the nature of the foreign body. For example, dry vegetable matter, such as a seed, nut, or piece of carrot or popcorn, that does not dissolve and that may swell when wet creates a particularly difficult problem. The high fat content of potato chips and peanuts may cause the added risk of lipoid pneumonia. "Fun foods" of any kind are among the worst offenders. Offending foods in the order of frequency of aspiration are: hot dog, round candy, peanut or other nut, grape, cooky or biscuit, other meat, carrot, apple, and peanut butter.

Round foods are the most frequent offenders. The first four items together contribute more than 40% of all specified food items. A sharp or irritating object produces irritation and edema. A round, pliable object that does not readily break apart is more likely to occlude an airway than an object with a different shape. Balloons are especially hazardous. A small object may cause little if any pathologic changes, whereas an object of sufficient size to obstruct a passage can produce various changes, including atelectasis, emphysema, inflammation, and abscess.

Diagnostic Evaluation

The diagnosis of FB aspiration is usually suspected on the basis of history and physical signs. Initially a foreign body in the air passages produces choking, gagging, wheezing, or coughing. After the initial period there is often an interval of hours, days, or even weeks without symptoms. Secondary symptoms are related to the anatomic area in which the object is lodged and are usually caused by a persistent respiratory infection focused distal to the obstruction. An FB is always a possibility in acute or chronic pulmonary lesions.

The most common symptoms of laryngotracheal obstruction are dyspnea, cough, and inspiratory stridor. When the object is lodged in the larynx there is inability to speak. An object in the bronchi produces cough, decreased airway entry, wheezing, and dyspnea. A nonobstructive, nonirritating object may cause few symptoms; an obstructive object quickly produces pathologic changes; a slight obstruction may be evidenced only by a wheeze.

Radiographic examination reveals opaque foreign bodies but may be of limited use in localizing vegetable matter. Bronchoscopy is usually required for definitive diagnosis of an object in the larynx and trachea. Fluoroscopic examination is a valuable aid in detecting and localizing an object in the bronchi.

Therapeutic Management

A foreign body is rarely coughed up spontaneously; therefore, it must be removed instrumentally by direct laryngoscopy or bronchoscopy. This should be carried out as soon as possible since the progressive local inflammatory process triggered by the foreign material hampers removal, a chemical pneumonia soon develops, and vegetable matter begins to macerate within a few days, causing it to be even more difficult to remove. Some advocate removal with a Foley catheter inserted to a point beyond the object, inflated, and used to draw the object into the bronchoscope, or the object may be withdrawn simultaneously with the scope. After the object is removed, the child is placed in a high-humidity atmosphere and any secondary infection is treated with appropriate antibiotics.

Nursing Considerations

All persons working with children should be prepared to deal effectively with aspiration of a foreign body. Choking on food or other material should not be fatal. Two very simple procedures, back blows and the Heimlich maneuver, which can be used by both health professionals and lay persons, can save lives. It is the obligation of nurses to learn the techniques and teach them to parents and other groups. (See p. 733 for the procedure.)

To aid a child who is choking, nurses need to recognize when he is indeed in distress. Not every child who gags or coughs while eating is truly choking. The child in distress (1) *cannot speak,* (2) *becomes cyanotic,* and (3) *collapses.* These three signs indicate that the child is truly choking and requires immediate and quick action to save his life. He can die within 4 minutes.

Prevention. Small children should not be allowed access to enticing small objects that they might place in their mouths. Nurses, as child advocates, are in a position to teach prevention in a variety of settings. They can educate parents singly or in groups about hazards of aspiration in relation to the developmental level of their children and encourage them to teach their children safety. Parents teach by example; therefore they should be cautioned about behaviors that their children might imitate, for example, holding foreign objects, such as pins, nails, and toothpicks, in their lips or mouths. See Chapters 10 and 12 for further discussion of aspiration.

SMOKE INHALATION INJURY

A number of noxious substances that may be inhaled are toxic to humans. They are primarily products of incomplete combustion and are believed to cause more deaths from fires than do flame injuries. The severity of the injury depends on the nature of the substances generated by the material being burned and whether the victim is confined in a closed space. Inhaled substances produce injuries (1) locally by irritation, inflammation, and damage to pulmonary tissues or (2) systemically.

Local Injury

A wide variety of gases may be generated during the combustion of materials such as clothing, furniture, and floor coverings. The synthetic materials are especially toxic. Irritant gases such as nitrous oxide or carbon dioxide combine with water in the lungs to form corrosive acids; aldehydes cause denaturation of proteins, cellular damage, and edema of pulmonary tissues.

Possible inhalation injury is suspected when there is a history of flames in a closed space whether burns are present or not. Sooty material around the nose or in the sputum, singed nasal hairs, or mucosal burns of the nose, lips, mouth, or throat are all signs that the affected person demands observation for possible pulmonary injury from inhalants. A hoarse voice and cough, inspiratory and expiratory stridor, and signs of respiratory distress are further evidence of airway involvement.

Systemic Injury

Gases that are nontoxic to the airways (e.g., carbon monoxide and hydrogen cyanide) can cause injury and death by interfering with or inhibiting cellular respiration. Carbon monoxide is an extremely dangerous gas and is responsible for more than half of all fatal inhalation poisonings in the United States. It is a colorless, odorless gas with an affinity for hemoglobin 230 times greater than that of oxygen. When it enters the bloodstream, carbon monoxide combines readily with hemoglobin to form carboxyhemoglobin, but is released less readily. Therefore, tissue hypoxia reaches dangerous levels before oxygen is available to meet tissue needs.

Accidental poisoning is most often the result of exposure to fumes of heaters or smoke from structural fires, although poorly ventilated recreational vehicles with improperly operated or maintained gas lamps or stoves and cooking in underventilated areas with charcoal grills or hibachis are also frequent causes. Carbon monoxide is produced by incomplete combustion of carbon or carbonaceous material such as wood or charcoal.

The signs and symptoms of carbon monoxide poisoning are secondary to tissue hypoxia and vary with the level of carboxyhemoglobin. Mild manifestations may produce headache, visual disturbances, irritability, and nausea, whereas more severe intoxication causes confusion, hallucinations, ataxia, and coma. The bright, cherry-red lips and skin often described are less often observed; pallor and cyanosis are seen more frequently.

Therapeutic Management

When inhalation injury is suspected, the patient is given humidified 100% oxygen by mask until carboxyhemoglobin levels fall to the nontoxic range, and artificial ventilation may be implemented in selected cases. Where a hyperbaric oxygen chamber is available, the breakdown of the carbon monoxide–hemoglobin bond is greatly accelerated.

Respiratory distress may occur early in the course of smoke inhalation as a result of hypoxia, or patients who are breathing well on admission may later develop sudden respiratory distress. Therefore, intubation and/or tracheostomy equipment should be available at the bedside. There is a good deal of controversy regarding tracheostomy, but many prefer this procedure when the obstruction is proximal to the larynx and reserve nasotracheal intubation for lower tract involvement.

Use of corticosteroids, although controversial, may be of value in reducing edema, and bronchodilators (usually isoproterenol) are often given intravenously or by nebulizer. A broad-spectrum antibiotic is sometimes administered prophylactically, but this too is controversial.

Nursing Considerations

Nursing care of the child with inhalation injury is the same as that for any child with respiratory distress. Vital signs and other respiratory assessments are performed frequently, and the pulmonary status is carefully observed and maintained. Pulmonary physical therapy is usually part of the therapeutic program, and mechanical ventilation or periodic intermittent positive-pressure breathing with bronchodilators is employed.

In addition to the observation and management of the physical aspects of inhalation injury, the nurse also deals with the psychologic needs of a frightened child and distraught parents. As with any accidental injury, the parents feel overwhelming guilt, even when the injury occurred through no fault of their own. More often, however, the injury could have been prevented, which compounds their guilt feelings. They need a great deal of support, reassurance, and information regarding the child's condition, treatment, and progress.

PASSIVE SMOKING

There is increasing evidence that children in families with cigarette smokers "passively" inhale sufficient smoke to adversely affect their health. Children living in these families (especially in families where the mother smokes) show lower performance on pulmonary function tests, have an increased number of respiratory infections, and develop symptoms of rhinitis and asthma at an earlier age than children in nonsmoking households (Ogston, 1985; Pedreira and others, 1985).

Nursing Considerations

Passive smoking during childhood may well be the most important precursor of chronic lung disease in the adult. Nurses and other health professionals need to be aware of the problem and include this information in all health assessments of children, especially those with respiratory illnesses. The American Academy of Pediatrics has renewed its statement on hazards of passive smoking (Committee on Environmental Hazards, 1986). Armed with this knowledge, nurses should play a stronger role in ridding children's environments of tobacco smoke by informing parents, setting an example for children and families, and advocating "no smoking" ordinances in public places.

◆ *Long-Term Respiratory Dysfunction*

Some respiratory disorders, although they may have acute episodes, are primarily long-term conditions. Children and families must adjust to the effects of these disorders including the way in which they can alter the lifestyle of the families. The most common of these long-term respiratory disorders are bronchial asthma and cystic fibrosis.

BRONCHIAL ASTHMA

Bronchial asthma is a reversible obstructive process characterized by an increased responsiveness of the airway, especially the lower airways. It is manifested by labored breathing, bilateral wheezing, prolonged expiration, and an irritative tight cough caused by a reduction in the diameter of the airway. The symptoms can vary from a mild cough to severe respiratory distress with hypoxemia, retention of carbon dioxide, and respiratory acidosis that may result in prostration and even fatal asphyxia.

Asthma is a common disorder and the leading cause of chronic illness in childhood. It is believed by many to be the single most important cause of morbidity in childhood.

Etiology

The usual cause of the asthmatic manifestations is an allergic hypersensitivity to foreign substances, usually those carried in the air, such as plant pollens. However, in some instances no allergic process can be detected. Most asthma in children is caused by an allergic reaction in the bronchi, but there may be nonallergic precipitating factors such as bronchial compression from external pressure, a foreign body in the airway, a diffuse endobronchial inflammation, or postexercise bronchial constriction.

There is a heritable tendency in asthma. The familial association among asthma, allergic rhinitis, and atopic dermatitis suggests a common genetic basis for these disorders. There is frequently a family history of allergy although the specific form may vary. Usually the child has other manifestations of allergy such as nasal allergy, eczema, or urticaria.

Pathophysiology

There is general agreement that heightened airway reactivity is characteristic of children with asthma. The reasons for this are less clear, and most theories do not explain all types and causes of asthma. However, the mechanisms responsible for the obstructive symptoms of asthma are (Fig. 22-2):

1. Edema of the mucous membranes

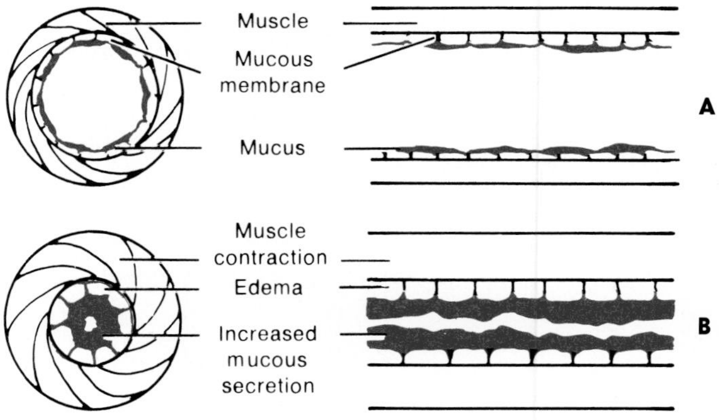

FIG. 22-2 Mechanisms of obstruction in asthma. **A,** Normal bronchus. **B,** Asthmatic bronchus.

2. Accumulation of tenacious secretions from mucous glands
3. Spasm of the smooth muscle of the bronchi and bronchioles, which decreases the caliber of the bronchioles

The role that each of these mechanisms plays varies from patient to patient and during the course of the disease in a given patient. In some patients, smooth muscle contraction is the major factor early in the episode, followed by mucosal edema and increased mucous secretion. In others the sequence of the responses is reversed.

Many of the stimuli that provoke asthmatic episodes may do so by being directly toxic or irritative, such as smoke, fumes, odors, or infection; by eliciting the immune response; or by a combination of mechanisms. Other factors that contribute to the responses are rapid changes in environmental temperature (especially cold), physical stress (fatigue, exertion), psychologic stress (tension, fear, anxiety), or infections in the respiratory tract or nearby structures (such as the ears or sinuses).

Bronchial constriction is a normal reaction to foreign stimuli, but in the asthmatic child it is abnormally severe, producing impaired respiratory function. The smooth muscle, arranged in spiral bundles around the airway, causes narrowing and shortening of the airway, which significantly increase airway resistance to airflow. Since the bronchi normally dilate and elongate during inspiration and contract and shorten on expiration, the respiratory difficulty is more pronounced during the expiratory phase of respiration.

Increased resistance in the airway causes forced expiration through the narrowed lumen. The volume of air trapped in the lungs increases as airways are functionally closed at a point between the alveoli and the lobar bronchi by the combined mechanisms just described. This trapping of gas forces the individual to breathe at higher and higher lung volumes. Consequently the person with asthma fights to inspire sufficient air. This expenditure of effort for breathing causes fatigue, decreased respiratory effectiveness, and increased oxygen consumption. Also, the inspiration occurring at higher lung volumes hyperinflates the alveoli and reduces the effectiveness of the cough. As the severity of obstruction increases, there is a reduced alveolar ventilation with carbon dioxide retention, hypoxemia, respiratory acidosis, and, eventually, respiratory failure.

Diagnostic Evaluation

Children with bronchial asthma may show signs and experience symptoms that range from acute episodes of shortness of breath, wheezing, and cough followed by a quiet period to a relatively continuous pattern of chronic symptoms that fluctuate in severity (see box). An attack may develop gradually or appear abruptly and may be preceded by a URI. The age of the child is often a significant factor, since the first attack in most cases occurs between ages 3 and 8 years. In infancy an attack usually follows a respiratory infection. Some children may experience a prodromal itching at the front of the neck or over the upper part of the back just before an attack.

The diagnosis is determined primarily on the basis of clinical manifestations, history, physical examination, and, to a lesser extent, laboratory tests. Radiographic examinations are used primarily to rule out other diseases and to evaluate coexisting disease.

Clinical Manifestations of Bronchial Asthma

- Cough:
  - Hacking, paroxysmal, irritative, and nonproductive
  - Becomes rattling and productive of frothy, clear, gelatinous sputum
- Shortness of breath
- Prolonged expiratory phase
- Audible wheeze
- Often appears pale
- May have a malar flush and red ears
- Lips deep, dark-red color
- May progress to cyanosis of nail beds, circumoral
- Restlessness
- Apprehension
- Anxious facial expression
- Sweating may be prominent as the attack progresses
- Older children may sit upright with shoulders in a hunched-over position, hands on the bed or chair, and arms braced
- Speaks with short, panting, broken phrases
- Chest:
  - Hyperresonance on percussion
  - Coarse, loud breath sounds
  - Sonorous rales throughout the lung fields
  - Prolonged expiration
  - Coarse rhonchi
  - Generalized inspiratory and expiratory wheezing; increasingly high pitched
- With repeated episodes:
  - Barrel chest
  - Elevated shoulders
  - Use of accessory muscles of respiration
  - Facial appearance—flattened malar bones, circles beneath the eyes, narrow nose, prominent upper teeth

Therapeutic Management

The overall goal of asthma management is to prevent disability and to minimize physical and psychologic morbidity—to assist the child to live as normal and happy a life as possible. This includes facilitating the child's social adjustments in the family, school, and community and normal participation in recreational activities and sports (Bierman and Pearlman, 1983). To accomplish these goals efforts are directed toward recognizing acute episodes early and implementing appropriate therapy, identifying and eliminating irritant and allergic factors from the child's environment, educating parents to the long-term nature of the disease and how to manage exacerbations, and helping the child to deal constructively with the disease. Compliance to the prescribed regimen is essential to successful management.

Allergen control. It is essential to determine the specific allergenic factors and the nonspecific factors that precipitate symptoms. Once the specific allergens are identified and confirmed, steps are taken to eliminate or avoid the offending allergens. Often, simply removing environmental factors will provide protection from attacks, for example, removal of a dog or cat from the home of a child sensitive to dogs or cats. Allergenic foods are eliminated from the diet. Nonspecific factors that may trigger an attack, such as extremes of temperature, are sometimes controlled by humidifiers or air conditioners, and the child can be helped to develop a tolerance to temperature fluctuations by gradual or systematic exposure to temperature differences.

Drug therapy. Most children do not require medication continuously. The goal is to control the acute attack; therefore early recognition and treatment at the onset are most important. Rapid relief of the bronchospasm reduces the need for drastic measures and increases the likelihood that relief will be complete. Parents and older asthmatic children are taught to implement therapy at the onset of symptoms or when exposed to symptom-provoking situations.

The rapid-acting bronchodilators, β-adrenergic agonists and methylxanthines, are the major therapeutic agents for the relief of bronchospasm. Each appears to work differently, and they may be synergistic in their actions on the airways. The *β-adrenergic agonists,* especially epinephrine, provide relief from an acute attack and can be used to prevent exercise-induced asthma. They are available in syrups, tablets, injectable solutions, metered-dose inhalers, and solutions for inhalation therapy. The most effective method of administration is by metered-dose inhaler (metaproterenol, fenoterol, and albuterol) (Fig. 22-3). Since inhalers are difficult to use in very young children, those ages 3 to 6 years are best managed with a spacer or other device that does not require coordinating delivery of the agents used in the treatment of asthma.

The *methylxanthines,* principally theophylline, are probably the most effective and versatile asthma drugs. They are prepared for intravenous, intramuscular, oral, or rectal administration.

A *corticosteroid* preparation may provide significant relief of an attack when symptoms are not controlled by other therapies. The drugs can be given intravenously, orally, or topically by aerosol. The corticosteroids are not actually drugs but act by their hormonal effect; therefore results are delayed for up to 6 hours. The antiinflammatory effect diminishes the inflammatory component of asthma and thereby reduces the airway obstruction. Corticosteroids are lifesaving in status asthmaticus.

Cromolyn sodium is neither a bronchodilator nor an antiinflammatory agent but acts superficially to inhibit the release of chemical mediators, especially histamine, in the human lung. The action is essentially prophylactic and is of no value when administered after the allergic reaction. Its chief value is to prevent an attack, and it is especially useful in preventing exercise-induced bronchospasm.

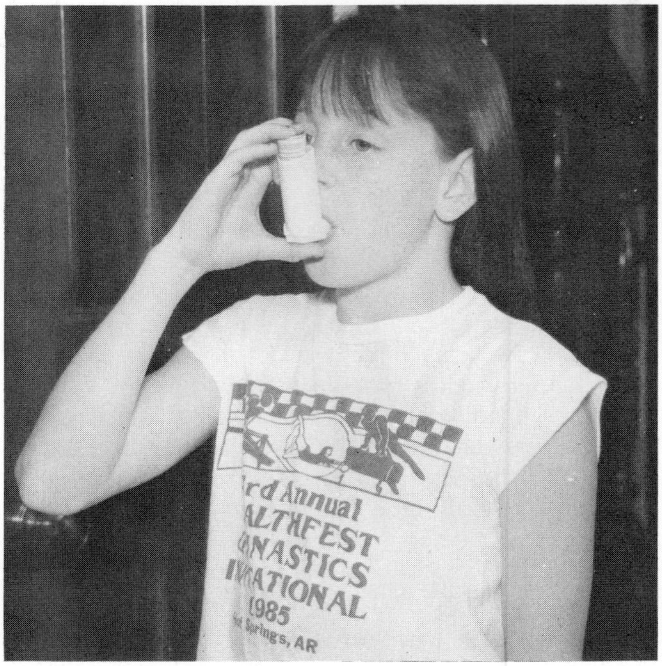

FIG. 22-3 Child using metered-dose inhaler.

Antihistamines are sometimes useful by decreasing postnasal drip–induced cough that may lead to bronchospasm, but they are not a routine part of medical management. In the case of infection the appropriate antibiotic is administered. Expectorants, long used in asthma therapy, have not been shown to be effective.

Exercise. Vigorous physical activity is frequently followed by an asthma attack; therefore children with asthma are often excluded from exercise by parents, teachers, and physicians as well as the children themselves because they are reluctant to provoke an attack. This can seriously hamper peer interaction. It has been found that moderate exercise or even strenuous exercise is advantageous for children with asthma.

The Committee on Children with Disabilities and the Committee on Sports Medicine of the American Academy of Pediatrics (1984) agree that physical activities are useful to asthmatic children and that the majority can participate in activities at school and in sports with minimum difficulty, provided the asthma is under control. Participation is encouraged but should be evaluated on an individual basis in terms of tolerance for duration and intensity of effort. Appropriate prophylactic treatment with β-adrenergic agents administered by aerosol or orally before exercise will usually permit full participation in strenuous exertion. Restrictions are invoked only when the condition of the child makes it necessary.

Asthma camps have become popular in recent years as a means of encouraging physical activity in a more homogeneous, controlled, and less competitive environment. Not all persons subscribe to this practice. There are those who support the positive benefits, which are primarily that the denominator of asthma is removed as a factor. Everyone at the camp has asthma; therefore no child is different from the others. On the other hand, many believe that such segregation from family and peers serves only to reinforce the sick role.

Physical therapy. Physical therapy is one of the standard adjuncts to treatment of chronic, or frequent, asthma. This includes breathing exercises, physical training, and inhalation therapy. These therapies help to produce physical and mental relaxation, improve posture, strengthen respiratory musculature, and develop more efficient patterns of breathing. For the motivated child, breathing exercises and controlled breathing are of value in preventing overinflation and in improving the strength of respiratory muscles and the efficiency of the cough. Stretch exercises sometimes help to increase the flexibility of the ribs. Sit-ups and leg exercises strengthen abdominal muscles and aid expiration.

Hyposensitization. The role of hyposensitization in childhood asthma has not been clarified. When the allergen can be defined and is one that cannot be avoided or controlled satisfactorily by drugs, specific hyposensitization is seriously considered. Immune therapy is not recommended for allergens that can be eliminated effectively, for example, food sensitivities, drugs, and animal dander. Inhalant allergens such as house dust, pollens, and molds are most often the allergens considered for immune therapy.

Prognosis. The outlook for children with asthma varies widely. An impressive number of children lose their symptoms at puberty, but there is no factor that can predict which children will "outgrow" their asthma. Some develop other forms of allergy in adulthood. It has been postulated that, just as the skin manifestations of infancy (eczema) shift to the bronchi in childhood, there may be another shift in the susceptible tissues (shock organ) at adulthood—most frequently to the nose.

The prognosis for control of symptoms or disappearance of symptoms will differ from children who have rare and infrequent attacks to those who are constantly wheezing or some who are subject to status asthmaticus. In general the more severe and numerous the symptoms, the longer they have been present, and when there is a family history of allergy, the poorer is the prognosis for improvement. Many who outgrow them are subject to exercise-induced asthma as adults, and the associated disorders such as growth impairment, chest deformity, and airway obstruction are maintained throughout life.

Status asthmaticus. Children who continue to display respiratory distress despite vigorous therapeutic measures, especially sympathomimetics, are considered to be in status asthmaticus. The condition may develop gradually or rapidly, often coincident with complicating conditions such as pneumonia that can influence the duration and treatment of the attack. These children are acutely ill and require hospitalization, preferably where intensive care is available. They need continuous nursing attendance with frequent monitoring and observation.

Therapy of status asthmaticus is directed toward correction of dehydration and acidosis, improvement of ventilation, and treatment of any concurrent infection. The drug most frequently prescribed in emergency rooms is aqueous epinephrine 1:1000 followed by epinephrine 1:200 (Sus-Phrine). Failure to respond to these drugs establishes the diagnosis of status asthmaticus.

The child is given intravenous fluids and nothing by mouth except liquids if his condition permits. The intravenous infusion provides a means for hydration, liquefying secretions, and administering medications. The correction of dehydration, acidosis, hypoxia, and electrolyte derangements is guided by frequent determination of arterial pH, Po_2, Pco_2, and serum electrolytes. Acidosis is corrected by administration of sodium bicarbonate in sufficient amounts to maintain pH at acceptable levels.

Aminophylline and corticosteroids are administered intravenously, and isoproterenol may also be given to children less than 14 years of age. Sedatives, tranquilizers, morphine, and antihistamines are contraindicated (Sly, 1986), although a mild sedative or tranquilizing agent may be given with caution to children whose agitation is not caused by anoxia.

Humidified oxygen is administered by tent, face mask, or cannula to maintain satisfactory oxygenation. Since oxygen is a stimulus for respiration, high levels may significantly depress respirations.

Administration of antibiotics is frequently advisable in therapy, since infection may be masked or may not always be evident and is always a threatening complication. As the attack subsides, fluids and medication are given orally and breathing exercises help remove secretions. Administration of steroids is discontinued as rapidly as possible.

Psychologic Aspects

Emotional factors are known to be associated with childhood asthma; however, it is not known whether emotional disturbance is present before the onset of asthma and is a probable causative factor in its development or whether it occurs as a result of the asthma. Although no decisive evidence is available regarding the relative importance of all etiologic factors, the consensus accepts a multicausal etiology for childhood asthma in which hereditary, allergic, infectious, and psychologic factors assume importance independently or, more often, in combination.

Behavioral problems are apt to occur in asthmatic children whose attacks commenced before age 2 years and those with continuing asthma and symptoms that are more severe and prolonged. It is unclear whether the emotional disturbances are peculiar to children with asthma or are similar to those that may occur in children with other chronic diseases. Children with any chronic condition are at higher risk to develop adjustment problems than are healthy children.

Both short- and long-term adaptation of the asthmatic child to his disease depends to a great extent on the family's acceptance of his disorder. The task of living day to day with an affected child involves the family continually. There are periodic crises and the ever-present threat of a crisis, requiring parental vigilance, sleepless nights, frequent emergency trips to the hospital, and often overwhelming medical expenses. Throughout these stresses the parents are expected and encouraged to promote as normal a life as possible for the child with asthma without neglecting the needs of the siblings.

Where family relationships are determined to produce an adverse effect on the child with asthma, psychiatric help is recommended, and where disturbances are marked, foster placement or respite care in a residential facility for asthmatic children is advised. When a child repeatedly improves during separation from family members, it is strongly suspected that emotional and family interactional factors are contributing to the course of the disease.

Nursing Considerations

Nursing care of children with bronchial asthma involves both acute and long-term care and includes therapies and observations described in previous discussions of respiratory disturbances. Nurses who are involved with children with asthma in the home, clinic, or physician's office play an important role in helping the children and their families learn to live with the condition. The disease can be tolerated if it does not interfere with family life, physical activity, or school attendance or if it does not require hospitalization.

ASSESSMENT

Physical assessment of asthma involves the same observations and techniques described in the general discussion of assessment of respiratory infection (p. 694) and physical assessment of the chest (p. 154). In addition, some physical characteristics of chronic respiratory involvement are noted and evaluated. These include chest configuration and finger clubbing. The chests of children with chronic obstructive respiratory disease often assume a "barrel" shape from chronic hyperinflation. Clubbing, the proliferation of tissue about the terminal phalanges, reflects the severity of the hypoxia. Increased clubbing correlates with worsening of the condition.

Psychologic assessment consists of assessing the degree to which the disorder interferes with everyday activities, the child and the family cope with the condition, the disorder alters the child's self-concept, and the child and family comply with the therapeutic management.

NURSING DIAGNOSES

After a thorough assessment numerous nursing diagnoses are identified. The more common diagnoses for the child with asthma are included in the Nursing Care Plan on pp. 722 to 724.

PLANNING

The plan of care for the child with asthma and family includes:

1. Relieve bronchospasm
2. Eliminate or avoid proved or suspected irritants and allergens
3. Maintain optimum health
4. Prevent and relieve respiratory symptoms
5. Promote normal activities
6. Prevent complications
7. Support and educate child and family regarding the disease and its management
8. Support child and family

IMPLEMENTATION

Nurses are involved in both acute and long-term management of children with bronchial asthma. Acute care usually takes place in the hospital setting.

Acute Asthma

Children who are admitted to the hospital with acute asthma are ill, anxious, and uncomfortable. In most instances the child is admitted on an emergency basis with status asthmaticus and is in acute distress. An intravenous infusion is begun immediately, and medication, usually corticosteroids and aminophylline, is administered to relieve bronchospasm. The child is monitored closely and continuously during aminophylline administration for relief of respiratory distress and signs of side effects or toxicity. The pulse, respiration, and blood pressure are taken and recorded every 5 minutes during rapid infusion and every 15 minutes for at least an hour after the drug has been absorbed.

It is especially important that the child receive sufficient fluid either orally or intravenously to replace losses through diaphoresis and hyperventilation (see Nursing tip box on liquids). Cold liquids can trigger reflex bronchospasm and should be avoided. Nourishment is provided in small, frequent feedings to avoid abdominal distention that might interfere with diaphragm excursion.

The child usually prefers the high-Fowler position, and he is placed in a mist tent for relief of dyspnea and cyanosis (an older child may prefer a nasal cannula). Asso-

> ***Nursing Tip: Liquids***
>
> Liquids are best tolerated if they are warm or room temperature. Cold liquids can trigger reflex bronchospasm and should be avoided (Seaman-Bates, 1980).

ciated treatments such as intermittent positive-pressure breathing and tests, such as blood gases or pulmonary function tests, are often performed by specialized personnel, or they may be the nurse's responsibility.

The child with status asthmaticus is apprehensive and anxious. The calm, efficient presence of a nurse helps to reassure him that he is safe and will be cared for during this stressful period. It is important to assure the child that he will not be left alone and that his parents are allowed to be near and available when he needs them.

Family support. Parents need reassurance too. They want to be informed of their child's condition and the therapies being employed. Often they feel that they may have in some way contributed to the child's condition or could have prevented the attack. Reassurance regarding their efforts expended on the child's behalf and their parenting capabilities can help alleviate their stress. All efforts to reduce the parental apprehension will, in turn, help reduce the child's distress. Anxiety is easily communicated to the child from parents and members of the staff.

Long-Term Support

Nurses are involved in the initial assessment and workup to determine the cause and extent of the asthma. They assist with diagnostic tests, pulmonary function tests, and general health assessment. Parents need to know the nature of the disease and, when the allergens are determined, how they can avoid and/or relieve asthmatic attacks.

The parents and the older child need to learn how to use the medications prescribed to relieve bronchospasm. They are taught to recognize early signs and symptoms of an impending attack so that it can be controlled before symptoms become distressful. Many children are given theophylline or other medication, and parents should understand the importance of taking the drugs as prescribed. Older children who use a nebulizer or aerosol device to deliver adrenergic drugs need to be taught how to use the device. The child and parents also need to be cautioned about the adverse effects of the drugs and the dangers of overuse. They should know that it is important to use them when needed but not indiscriminately or as a substitute for avoiding the symptom-provoking allergen.

The family can acquire a peak flow meter that measures the maximum peak expiratory flow rate to predict an attack. This provides information for adjusting medication dosage.

The parents are cautioned to avoid exposing the child to excessive cold, wind, or other extremes of weather and to smoke, sprays, or other irritants. Although foods are an unusual cause of asthma, foods known to provoke symptoms should be eliminated from the diet. The foods most frequently allergenic are eggs, milk, grains, peanuts, and chocolate. Parents should be advised to read labels on prepared foods and snacks to determine the presence of allergens. For example, a tremendous number of foods contain sodium caseinate or dried milk products. Since approximately 2% to 6% of asthmatic children are sensitive to aspirin, nurses caution the parents to use other analgesic/antipyretic drugs for discomfort or fever.

Nursing Tip: Breathing Cold Air

To reduce the probability of an attack triggered by cold air, teach the child to breathe through the nose (not the mouth). Also, a reservoir of warm air can be created by having the child wear a mask or swaddling the nose and mouth in a scarf when in cold air.

The child should be protected from a respiratory infection that can trigger an attack or aggravate the asthmatic state, especially in young children. Their airways are mechanically smaller and more reactive; therefore, edema from infection causes wheezing and other signs of respiratory obstruction. Also, the equipment used for the child, such as nebulizers, must be kept absolutely clean to decrease the chances of contamination with bacteria and fungi.

Breathing exercises and controlled breathing are taught and encouraged for the motivated youngster, and the nurse can help him select activities suitable to his capacity.* (See Nursing tip box on breathing exercises.) Anything that promotes proper diaphragmatic breathing, side expansion, and generally improved mobility of the chest wall is encouraged. If the child requires segmental drainage and percussion, someone in the family must assume responsibility of carrying out the procedure. It is the responsibility of the physical therapist or the nurse to teach the parent the proper technique.

Nursing Tip: Breathing Exercises

Play techniques that can be employed for younger children to extend their expiratory time and increase expiratory pressure include blowing cotton balls or a Ping-Pong ball on a table, blowing a pinwheel, or preventing a tissue from falling by blowing it against the wall.

Children with emotional overtones associated with their asthma create additional problems. In these children an attack can be triggered by emotional experiences. Even some respiratory behaviors (such as crying, laughing, coughing, and hyperventilation) that accompany strong emotions may trigger a mechanical or reflex narrowing of the airway.

The interactions of members of the family need careful assessment to identify maladaptive behaviors and precip-

*A comic book explaining breathing exercises for asthmatic children, *Captain Wonderlung,* is available from the American Academy of Pediatrics, P.O. Box 927, Elk Grove Village, IL 60009.

NURSING CARE PLAN

The Child with Bronchial Asthma

Nursing Goals	Nursing Interventions	Expected Patient/Family Outcomes
HP-HMP* **Potential for suffocation** **Risk factor: interaction between individual and environmental allergen**		
Determine causative factor(s)	Take careful history to identify possible precipitating factor(s) Assess environment for presence of possible allergenic factors Explore parent-child relationships	†Causes and possible causes of allergic reaction are determined.
Maintain optimum health	Encourage sound health practices Balanced, nutritious diet Adequate rest Hygiene Appropriate exercise	Child and parents conform to sound health practices
Control allergens	Assist parents in eliminating or avoiding allergens that trigger attack Meal planning to eliminate allergenic foods Removal of pets Modification of environment ("allergy proof" the home) Assist parents in obtaining and/or installing device to control environment (humidifier, air conditioner, electronic air filter)	Family makes every effort to remove or avoid possible allergens or precipitating events
HP-HMP **Potential for infection** **Risk factors: weakened respiratory defenses, presence of large volumes of sputum**		
Prevent infection	Avoid exposure to infection Employ meticulous care of equipment to avoid bacterial and/or fungal growth Employ good handwashing	Child exhibits no evidence of infection
A-EP **Activity intolerance** **Etiology: imbalance between oxygen supply and demand**		
Promote rest	Encourage activities appropriate to the child's capabilities (specify) Provide ample opportunities for rest and quiet activities	Child engages in appropriate activities (specify) Child appears rested
Prevent attack	Discuss appropriate exercises and activities and encourage participation Teach importance of preexercise protocol Avoid activities that precipitate attack (specify)	Child does not have an attack during or after exercise
A-EP **Ineffective breathing pattern (acute attack)** **Etiology: bronchospasm, mucous secretions, edema**		
Detect status of respiratory distress	Assess skin color for cyanosis Assess character of respirations	†Signs of respiratory distress are recognized and correctly evaluated early
Improve ventilatory capacity	Instruct and/or supervise Breathing exercises Controlled breathing Assist child and family in selecting physical exercises appropriate to the child's capabilities Encourage regular exercise	Respirations are unlabored
Prevent bronchospasm	Avoid extremes of environmental temperature Avoid cold liquid drinks	Child avoids precipitating bronchospasm
Increase oxygen supply to lungs	Position for maximum ventilatory efficiency such as high-Fowler position or sitting, leaning forward Avoid constricting clothing, linens, restraints	Respiratory rate slows and becomes steady (see inside front cover for normal variations) Child can converse easily
Reduce anxiety during attack	Remain with child and assure him that he will not be left alone	Facial expression does not appear tense or anxious

*For an explanation of abbreviations, see p. 20.
†Nursing outcome.

NURSING CARE PLAN

The Child with Bronchial Asthma—cont'd

Nursing Goals	Nursing Interventions	Expected Patient/Family Outcomes
Reduce anxiety during diagnostic procedures	Explain unfamiliar procedures and equipment to the child Remain with child during procedures Employ calm, reassuring manner	Child remains calm and cooperative
Promote expectoration of mucous secretions	Ensure adequate fluid intake Provide humidified atmosphere Assist child to cough effectively Remove accumulated mucus; suction, if needed	Older child expectorates secretions appropriately and without undue stress and fatigue
Increase ventilatory capacity	Position for optimum lung expansion High-Fowler position Provide overbed table with pillows on which to lean if more comfortable for child	Respirations are less labored

A-EP **Ineffective breathing pattern (long-term)**
Etiology: bronchospasm, mucous secretions, edema

Nursing Goals	Nursing Interventions	Expected Patient/Family Outcomes
Promote respiration	Teach correct use of inhalator Supervise breathing exercises Avoid contacts or activities that precipitate asthmatic attack (specify)	Child breathes without stress

RRP **Altered family processes**
Etiology: situational crisis (emergency hospitalization of child; chronic illness of child)

Nursing Goals	Nursing Interventions	Expected Patient/Family Outcomes
Increase family's understanding of disease and its ramifications	Explain disease, procedures, therapies Encourage family to ask questions and discuss their concerns	Family demonstrates an understanding of the disease (specify knowledge and physical condition)
Reduce parental anxiety (acute attack)	Keep parents informed of child's condition Encourage expression of feelings Allow parents to be with the child as much as possible Point out any evidence of improvement	Parents verbalize feelings and concerns
Provide support and reassurance to parents	Provide comfortable room for parents when they are not with child Be available to parents Answer questions and reinforce medical information See also The family of the hospitalized child (p. 610)	Parents avail themselves of services offered
Promote positive adaptation to the disorder	Foster positive family relationships Be alert to signs of parental rejection or overprotection Intervene appropriately if there is evidence of maladaptation Use every opportunity to increase the parents' and child's understanding of the disease and its therapies Be alert to signs that the child may be using his symptoms to manipulate his interpersonal relationships See also The child with a chronic illness or disability, p. 531	Child demonstrates an understanding of his strengths and limitations and engages in age-appropriate activities Child is able to handle his limitations, discusses his concerns and fears
Prepare for discharge	Teach skills needed for home care Collaborate with school nurse to assure continuity of care plan	Family demonstrates an understanding of needed skills Family members avail themselves of community services (specify)
Educate family and child to prevent acute attack	Avoid contact with offending allergens Avoid extremes of environmental temperature Avoid undue excitement and/or physical exertion Implement therapeutic measures at earliest symptoms Teach child and family to recognize early signs and symptoms so that an impending attack can be controlled before it becomes distressful Teach child to understand how equipment works Teach child correct use of inhalators	Family "allergy proofs" the child's controllable environment Family is able to detect signs of an impending attack early and implement appropriate actions
Educate family regarding outside support	Refer to other agencies and persons for additional interpersonal support Refer to agencies for financial support	Family avails itself of support

Continued.

NURSING CARE PLAN

The Child with Bronchial Asthma—cont'd

Nursing Goals	Nursing Interventions	Expected Patient/Family Outcomes
Support, assist, and reassure family	Be available to family Allow for expression of feelings Support and emphasize strengths and abilities of parents Discuss age-appropriate behaviors and activities for the child Help parents establish and/or maintain a nonstressful environment for the child	Family and child display an attitude of understanding complicity

Nursing Interventions Related to Medical Management

Acute care

- Relieve symptoms immediately
  - Assist with starting intravenous infusion
  - Initiate oxygen therapy with appropriate equipment
    - Tent
    - Cannula
    - Mask
  - Administer bronchodilators and corticosteroids as prescribed
- Relieve bronchospasm
  - Administer prescribed bronchodilator (usually aminophylline)
  - Carefully regulate flow rate of aminophyline infusion; monitor pulse, respiration, and blood pressure before, during, and after administration
- Reduce mucosal inflammation and edema
  - Administer corticosteroids
  - Provide cool, moist environment
  - Administer antibiotics as prescribed
- Correct acidosis
  - Administer sodium bicarbonate or tromethamine as ordered
  - Administer oxygen to reduce anaerobic metabolism (and subsequent increase in acid metabolites)
- Detect drug toxicity
  - Interview parents to determine medications given before admission to avoid possible overdose
  - Monitor condition frequently during and after administration of drugs, including oxygen
  - Monitor serum blood levels
- Liquefy secretions
  - Administer expectorants
- Promote adequate hydration
  - Maintain intravenous infusion
- Detect status of respiratory distress
  - Collect or assist in collection of blood gases
- Increase ventilatory capacity
  - Administer or arrange for positive-pressure breathing if ordered
  - Perform percussion and vibration
  - Perform postural drainage when condition allows
  - Facilitate removal of secretions with percussion and administration of expectorant drugs
  - Administer bronchodilators, antiinflammatory agents, mucolytic agents, and oxygen
- Determine effectiveness of therapy
  - Take vital signs frequently (every 1-2 hours)
  - Observe
    - Type and rate of respirations
    - Color
    - Apprehensiveness
- Prevent infection
  - Administer prophylactic antibiotics if ordered

Long-term care

- Determine causative agent
  - Assist with sensitivity testing
  - Supervise elimination diet
- Determine extent of respiratory involvement
  - Assist with diagnostic procedures
    - Pulmonary function tests
    - Radiographs
    - Blood work
- Prevent asthmatic attack
  - Use prophylactic medication(s) according to instructions

itating factors. Sometimes it is necessary to remove the child from the family for short-term respite care and provide the family with crisis therapy. In severe cases long-term respite care is the only satisfactory solution. The children live in one of the residential treatment centers throughout the country in which the needs of the child are met by professionals. Several organizations provide education and services for health professionals and families of asthmatic children.*

*__Asthma and Allergy Foundation of America (AAFA),__ 1717 Massachusetts Avenue NW, Suite 305, Washington, DC 20036. **American Lung Association,** 1740 Broadway, New York, NY 10019. **Canadian Lung Association,** 75 Albert St., Suite 908, Ottawa, Ontario K1P 5E7. **The Lung Association,** 573 King St. East, Suite 201, Toronto, Ontario M5A 1M5.

Self-care is a hallmark of effective asthma management, and self-management programs are important in helping the child and family cope with the disease. The principles that are conveyed are:

1. Asthma is a very common disease and to have asthma is annoying but not disgraceful
2. Persons with asthma are able to live full and active lives
3. It is much easier to prevent than to treat an asthmatic attack
4. Individuals do not become addicted to asthma medication, but they do prefer to breathe more freely whenever possible

Self-contained programs and brochures for patient education are available through the national organizations.

Asthma education and awareness are important aspects of asthma management. Although the principles of self-management are very general and the programs are designed for general use, each child and his family have their own special needs that require individualized care and attention.

EVALUATION

The effectiveness of nursing interventions is determined by continual reassessment and evaluation of care based on the following observational guidelines and expected outcomes:

1. Observe child for evidence of respiratory symptoms
2. Interview family regarding removal or avoidance of known allergens
3. Assess child's general health
4. Interview child and family regarding the frequency and duration of symptoms
5. Interview child regarding daily activities
6. Observe child and interview family concerning any infections or other complications
7. Determine the degree to which the family and child understand the child's condition and the extent to which the therapies are carried out
8. Encourage child and family to discuss their feelings and concerns regarding the disease and its impact on their lives

Expected outcomes:
See Nursing Care Plan on pp. 722 to 724.

CYSTIC FIBROSIS

Cystic fibrosis (CF), the most common serious pulmonary and gastric disease of children, is a multisystem disorder primarily affecting the exocrine (mucus-producing) glands and accounts for a large percentage of lung disease in children. It appears in varying degrees of severity, which presents some problems with early recognition.

Etiology

Cystic fibrosis is inherited as an autosomal-recessive trait, and as such, the affected child inherits the defective genes from both parents with an overall incidence of 1 in 4 (see inheritance patterns, Appendix B). The incidence of the disease is estimated to be 1 in 1600 births in predominantly white populations and has an equal sex distribution.

Pathophysiology

The basic biochemical defect in CF is unknown, although the prominent feature is an impermeability of epithelial cells to chloride. It is assumed that the defect is caused by alteration in a protein, probably an enzyme. The defect gives rise to several apparently unrelated clinical features—increased viscosity of mucous gland secretions, a striking elevation of sweat electrolytes, an increase in several organic and enzymatic constituents of saliva, and possible abnormalities in autonomic nervous system function.

The primary factor, and the one that is responsible for the multiple clinical manifestations of the disease, is mechanical obstruction caused by the increased viscosity of mucous gland secretions (Fig. 22-4). Instead of forming a thin, freely flowing secretion, the mucous glands produce a thick, inspissated mucoprotein that accumulates and dilates them. Small passages in organs such as the pancreas and bronchioles become obstructed as secretions precipitate or coagulate to form concretions in glands and ducts. The earliest manifestation of cystic fibrosis is *meconium ileus* in the newborn, in which the small intestine is blocked with thick, puttylike, tenacious, mucilaginous meconium.

In the pancreas the thick secretions block the ducts. This blockage (1) leads to cystic dilations of the acini (small lobes of the gland), which then undergo degeneration and progressive diffuse fibrosis, and (2) prevents essential pancreatic enzymes from reaching the duodenum, which causes marked impairment in the digestion and absorption of nutrients. The disturbed function is reflected in bulky stools that are frothy from undigested fat and foul-smelling from putrified protein. The islands of Langerhans may decrease in number as pancreatic fibrosis progresses, and in the liver localized biliary obstruction and fibrosis are common and become more extensive with time.

The most common gastrointestinal complication associated with CF is *prolapse of the rectum,* which occurs most often in infancy and childhood. Affected children of all ages are subject to intestinal obstruction from inspissated or impacted feces.

Pulmonary complications are present in almost all children with CF and constitute the most serious threat to life. However, the time of appearance is variable. The majority of children show evidence before 1 year of age; others may not develop symptoms for weeks, months, or years. Bronchial and bronchiolar obstruction by the abnormally thick, tenacious mucus causes patchy atelectasis with hyperinflation. The child is unable to expectorate the mucus because of its increased viscosity. This retained mucus serves as an excellent medium for any bacterial growth. Reduced oxygen–carbon dioxide exchange causes variable degrees of hypoxia, hypercapnia, and acidosis.

Diagnostic Evaluation

An initial evaluation is conducted with general appraisal in the areas of general activity, physical findings, nutritional status, and findings on chest radiograms (see box). The diagnosis of CF is established on the basis of (1) a history of the disease in the family, (2) absence of pancreatic enzymes, (3) increase in electrolyte concentration of sweat, and (4) chronic pulmonary involvement.

The consistent finding of abnormally high sodium and

chloride concentrations in the sweat is a unique characteristic of CF. Mothers frequently observe that their infants taste "salty" when they kiss them. For diagnostic purposes the quantitative test is performed on sweat usually obtained by electrophoresis of pilocarpine. Normally the sweat chloride content is less than 40 mEq/liter; a chloride concentration greater than 60 mEq/liter is diagnostic of CF.

Therapeutic Management

Wherever possible the goals of care are aimed at promoting a normal life for the affected child. This includes maintaining good nutrition, preventing and controlling pulmonary infections, and promoting a satisfactory psychologic adjustment to the disease and all of its ramifications.

No diet restrictions are imposed on the child, but he is encouraged to eat foods high in protein and carbohydrate.

Water-miscible preparations of vitamins A, D, and E are provided daily in twice the usual recommended dosage. Vitamin K is indicated if hypoprothrombinemia is present as a result of accompanying liver involvement. Supplementary iron is also prescribed, and diet supplements are frequently given to provide additional protein, vitamins, and calories.

Clinical Manifestations of Cystic Fibrosis

Meconium ileus:
- Abdominal distention
- Vomiting
- Failure to pass stools
- Rapid development of dehydration

Gastrointestinal:
- Large, bulky, loose, frothy, extremely foul-smelling stools
- Voracious appetite (early in disease)
- Loss of appetite (later disease)
- Weight loss
- Marked tissue wasting
- Failure to grow
- Distended abdomen
- Thin extremities
- Sallow skin
- Evidence of deficiency of fat-soluble vitamins A, D, E, K
- Anemia

Pulmonary:
- Initial manifestations:
  - Wheezy respirations
  - Dry, nonproductive cough
- Eventually:
  - Increased dyspnea
  - Paroxysmal cough
  - Evidence of obstructive emphysema and patchy areas of atelectasis
- Progressive involvement:
  - Overinflated, barrel-shaped chest
  - Cyanosis
  - Clubbing of fingers and toes
  - Repeated episodes of bronchitis and bronchopneumonia

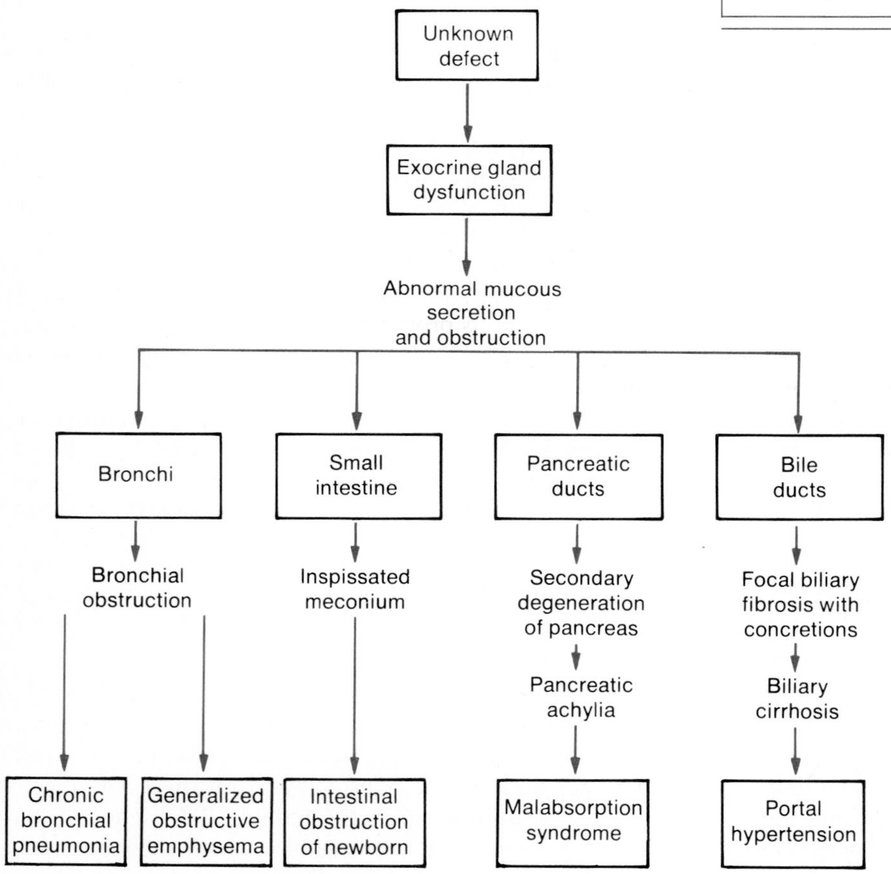

FIG. 22-4 Various effects of exocrine gland dysfunction in CF.

Pancreatic enzyme replacement is given in conjunction with meals and snacks and is regulated in order to obtain normal bowel movements, nutrition, and growth. A variety of preparations are available but the preferred preparation consists of enteric-coated microspheres contained in a capsule. The enteric coating delays release of the enzyme and its destruction in the acid environment of the stomach. The capsules may be swallowed intact or broken apart and the contents sprinkled on soft foods, which do not require chewing, such as applesauce or pudding. Sometimes antacids (such as Maalox) or cimetidine is administered with the enzymes to lower the gastric acidity.

Since salt depletion through sweating is a hazard, children are allowed to use salt generously. Most children are able to adjust this to their needs, and older children often exhibit a preference for salty foods. Additional salt should be taken during hot weather or febrile periods.

Pulmonary therapy. Pulmonary therapy to improve pulmonary function and loosen and eliminate bronchial secretions is probably the most important aspect of treatment. Postural drainage through positioning, clapping, and vibration (see p. 674) assists in removal of mucus and exudate. The procedure should be carried out several times a day as often as the child is able to tolerate it without undue fatigue. Chest physiotherapy should not be performed before or immediately after meals; therefore activities should be planned so that they do not coincide with meals.

Breathing exercises are recommended for the majority of children with CF, even for those with minimal pulmonary involvement. The exercises are usually performed twice daily, and they are preceded by postural drainage. Exercises to improve posture and mobilize the thorax are included, such as swinging the arms and bending and twisting the trunk. The ultimate aim of these exercises and physical activities is to establish a good habitual breathing pattern.

Aerosol therapy has proved beneficial for children who cough and produce sputum. The therapy attempts to liquefy tenacious secretions in the lower airways. It also provides a means for delivering medication to the lower respiratory tract and enhances its effectiveness when employed just before chest physiotherapy.

Oxygen therapy is usually recommended for children with acute episodes, and since many of these children have chronic carbon dioxide retention, the unsupervised use of oxygen can be harmful. Expectorants and mucolytic agents may be used to relieve bronchial obstruction, and intensive antibiotic therapy is used to control pulmonary infection.

Exercise. Numerous investigations have reported that exercise training is often effective in improving the ability of a patient to clear accumulated lung secretions and in increasing the capacity to endure exercise before experiencing dyspnea. Therefore, an exercise program is often included as an intergal part of the therapeutic regimen (Edlund and others, 1986). Children are encouraged to increase physical activity and participate in sports. Activities that are encouraged are swimming and walking/jogging. The exercise and increased feeling of well-being have the added benefit of improving self-image, self-confidence, and quality of life for the youngster with CF.

Complications. During acute exacerbations of pulmonary disease, intensive antibiotics are employed to control pulmonary infection. Many physicians prefer to use antibiotics only when there is evidence of infection, whereas others prescribe their use as a prophylactic measure. When used therapeutically, it is important that the drugs be given over a long enough period of time and in sufficient dosage to be effective.

Other complications are treated symptomatically. Meconium ileus usually responds to administration of diatrizoate methylglucamine (Gastrografin) or acetylcysteine (Mucomyst) enemas. Rectal prolapse is reduced by gently pressing against the everted rectum with a gloved, lubricated finger while the child is in the knee-chest position. The buttocks are then strapped together with tape for 20 to 30 minutes.

Prognosis

It is the pulmonary involvement that determines the ultimate outcome of the disease. Pancreatic enzyme deficiency is less of a problem if adequate nutrition is assured. Hemorrhage from liver cirrhosis and massive salt depletion in hot weather are occasional hazards. With early diagnosis and improved therapeutic measures, the life expectancy has improved. Many more children are reaching adulthood; however, the variation in severity of the disease is an important factor in determining the ultimate outcome.

Nursing Considerations

The nurse's contact with an affected child usually begins when the child is brought to the hospital or clinic for confirmation of the diagnosis. Perhaps the reason for hospitalization is failure to thrive or recurrent respiratory infections. Later, during recurrent admissions to the hospital or during ongoing follow-up in the clinic or at home, the nurse and the child develop a sustained relationship.

ASSESSMENT

Assessment of the child with CF involves both pulmonary and gastrointestinal observations. Pulmonary assessment is the same as that described for bronchial asthma (p. 720), with special attention to lung sounds, observation of cough, and evidence or degree of finger clubbing. Gastrointestinal observations are primarily observation of the frequency and nature of the stools and abdominal distention. The observer is also alert to evidence of failure to thrive, e.g., weight loss, wasting, pallor, and poor appetite. The family members are interviewed to determine the child's eating and elimination habits, observation of

Nursing Diagnosis: Child with Cystic Fibrosis

Ineffective airway clearance related to secretion of thick, tenacious mucus
Impaired gas exchange related to airway obstruction
Ineffective breathing pattern related to tracheobronchial obstruction
Altered nutrition: less than body requirements related to inability to digest nutrients, loss of appetite (advanced disease)
Altered growth and development related to inadequate digestion of nutrients
Potential for infection related to impaired body defenses, presence of mucus as medium for growth or organisms
Activity intolerance related to imbalance between oxygen supply and demand
Altered family processes related to situational crises
Impaired social interaction related to frequent hospitalizations, confinement to home, fatigue
Anticipatory grieving related to perceived potential loss of child

salty perspiration, and history of frequent respiratory infections and/or bowel obstruction in infancy.

NURSING DIAGNOSES

After a careful assessment numerous nursing diagnoses will become evident. The degree of both pulmonary and gastrointestinal involvement varies among affected children; therefore, nursing diagnoses will also vary according to the individual case. See box for most common nursing diagnoses.

PLANNING

The plan of care for the child with CF involves both child and family. Major goals include, but are not limited to, the following:

1. Improve pulmonary aeration
2. Facilitate lung clearance
3. Encourage compliance
4. Prevent and/or manage complications
5. Facilitate growth and maintain optimum health
6. Educate child and family regarding disease and its management
7. Provide long-term support and follow-up

IMPLEMENTATION

On the initial contact, frequently in the hospital setting, nurses are involved in performing or assisting with diagnostic tests and obtaining sweat for laboratory analysis of chloride content and, occasionally, collecting stool specimens for analysis of trypsin and fat. The child, usually an infant, needs comfort during these procedures; young children need distraction while they are confined during collection of sweat for testing.

Hospital care. When the child is hospitalized for confirmation of the diagnosis or for pulmonary complications, aerosol therapy is instituted or continued. The child may or may not be placed in an oxygen tent, but nebulization is almost always central to hospital management. Respiratory therapy is usually initiated and supervised by a trained respiratory therapist or physiotherapist. In institutions with large support staffs, the therapists may provide all treatments. If not, it becomes the responsibility of the nurse to perform the prescribed nebulization, postural drainage, percussion, and vibration and to teach supervised breathing exercises. (See Chapter 21 for care of the child in an oxygen tent.)

The hazard of oxygen narcosis is a concern in children with long-standing disease who receive oxygen. Intensive aerosol therapy may cause large volumes of sputum to be thinned suddenly in the early hours of treatment; therefore, the child requires close observation to assist him with expectoration and to prevent deeper aspiration. Expectorant drugs are administered orally, which further facilitates the expectoration of mucus.

A diet is implemented for the child with newly diagnosed disease or continued for the child who is hospitalized for pulmonary disease. Enzymes are supplied for each meal or snack, and adequate salt is provided, especially for febrile children. Unless the child is ill, his appetite is usually satisfactory. An ample supply of food should be made available to satisfy the voracious appetite characteristic of many of these children. However, some younger children may object to the extra fluids that are encouraged to promote thinning of mucous secretions.

Special efforts are made to protect the child from further infection, even though a respiratory infection is probably the reason for hospitalization. These children are particularly vulnerable to cross-contamination. Therefore appropriate infection control measures are employed, such as assigning the child to a room with noninfectious children.

The child will need support for the many treatments and tests that are a necessary part of the hospital therapy. Intravenous fluids and blood tests are almost always a part of the treatment, and the child soon associates hospitalization with these stress-provoking procedures. Most children are provided with central venous catheters for administration of medications, which reduces the stress related to many invasive therapies.

Home care. After the diagnosis is confirmed and a treatment program determined, parents will need help in finding inhalation equipment for home use that best meets their needs. They will need to learn about and practice the use of the equipment and will need to be informed of some of the problems they may encounter.

Parents need to learn about a healthful diet and any dietary modifications that may be prescribed and the administration of pancreatic enzymes. They need to be taught to perform percussion, vibration, and drainage. The nurse will be responsible for teaching the technique to those children and families who are selected to administer antibiotics by the intravenous route at home. The nurse can assist the family to contact resources that provide help to families with affected children. The various **Crippled children's services,** many local clinics, private agencies, service clubs, and other community groups often offer equipment and medications either free or at reduced rates. The **Cystic Fibrosis Foundation*** and the **Canadian Cystic Fibrosis Foundation†** have chapters throughout the United States and Canada to provide education and services to families and professionals.

Family support. One of the most important aspects of providing care for the family of a child with CF is coping with the emotional needs of the child and family. The shock associated with the diagnosis is overwhelming to parents and fraught with a multiplicity of problems, frustrations, and feelings.

They must face the impact of the chronic, life-threatening nature of the disease and the prospect of intensive treatment, for which they must assume a major part of the responsibility and for which they are ill prepared. They often fear that they will be unable to provide the care the child needs. One of the most difficult aspects of the diagnosis is the implications inherent in its cause; that is, the recognition that each parent contributed the gene responsible for the defect in their child. This often evokes feelings of guilt and self-recrimination in the parents. These feelings may be particularly marked if the child with newly diagnosed disease is the second affected child in the family and if the parents had been counseled regarding the 1 in 4 risk of such an event occurring.

The family needs patient and careful explanations of the disease, how it might affect them as a family, and what they can do to provide the best possible care for their child. The progressive nature of the disease makes each illness requiring hospitalization a potentially life-threatening event. Skilled nursing care and sympathetic attention to the emotional needs of the child and family help them cope with the stresses associated with repeated respiratory infections and hospitalization.

For the family the illness means modification of numerous family activities. Postural drainage must be continued wherever the child may be. Also, members of the family hesitate to take the child too far from familiar and trusted medical care. The illness even determines the family's place of residence and employment, since the child's condition dictates that he should remain near medical care facilities that offer the specialized care he needs.

The long-range problems are those encountered in the care of a child with a chronic illness (see Chapter 18). Both the child and the family must make many adjustments, the success of which depends on their ability to cope and on the quality and quantity of support they receive from sources outside the family.

A constant source of anxiety for both parents and child is the ever-present fear of death. The expected life span, although significantly increased during the past years, offers only limited encouragement regarding prognosis. The future is always uncertain. These families need all the support and skill the nurse can offer to cope with the guarded prognosis (see Chapter 18).

EVALUATION

Evaluation of the efficacy of nursing management can be determined by application of observational guidelines, which might include the following:

1. Monitor vital signs, especially respiratory parameters
2. Monitor chest physical therapy and other procedures to assess the expected outcomes, e.g., expectoration of secretions, increased lung expansion
3. Monitor meals to assure that enzymes are taken
4. Monitor child for evidence of respiratory infection, gastrointestinal dysfunction, and other complications
5. Observe nutrition intake. For the child at home, interview the family regarding child's intake or have child maintain a log of nutritional intake. Obtain regular measurements of growth, and interview the child and family regarding school attendance, interaction with peers, and participation in sports and other activities
6. Explore family's understanding of the disease and its therapies and their ability to carry out the treatment plan
7. Maintain contact with family (if feasible) at follow-up evaluations, home care. Observe for readmissions. Interview child and family regarding involvement with agencies and services for children with CF

Expected outcomes:

1. Child breathes easily and without dyspnea
2. Child manages secretions with minimum distress
3. Child takes pancreatic enzymes as prescribed
4. Child displays no evidence of an infective process
5. Child is well nourished, exhibits a satisfactory weight gain, and engages in appropriate activities
6. Child and family demonstrate an understanding of the disease and comply with the therapeutic regimen (specify knowledge and method of demonstration)
7. Family maintains contact with health care providers

◆ *Respiratory Emergency*

Nurses must be prepared to deal effectively with respiratory emergencies. Although the interventions are similar to those used for adults, there are some variations for infants and children.

RESPIRATORY FAILURE

In general, the term *respiratory insufficiency* is applied to two conditions: (1) children with increased work of breathing but with gas exchange function near normal (ventilatory insufficiency) and (2) children who are unable to maintain normal blood gas tensions and develop hypoxemia and acidosis as a result of carbon dioxide retention.

Respiratory failure is defined as the inability of the

*6931 Arlington Rd., Bethesda, MD 20814-3205.
†586 Eglinton Ave. East, Suite 204, Toronto, Ontario M4P 1P2.

respiratory apparatus to maintain adequate oxygenation of the blood, with or without carbon dioxide retention.

Respiratory arrest is the cessation of respiration.

Effective pulmonary gas exchange requires clear airways, normal lungs and chest wall, and adequate pulmonary circulation. Anything that affects these functions or their relationships can compromise respiration.

Diagnostic Evaluation

Respiratory failure that occurs as a result of acute obstruction of a major airway or cardiac arrest is sudden and readily apparent. Gradual or progressive deterioration of respiratory function is less easily recognized. Therefore, nursing observation and judgment are vital to the recognition and early management of respiratory failure. Nurses must be able to assess a situation and initiate appropriate action within moments. Signs of respiratory failure are listed in the accompanying box.

Management

The interventions used in the management of respiratory failure are frequently dramatic, requiring special skills, and are often emergency procedures. Some of the techniques employed to assist ventilation include artificial ventilation, artificial airway, and cardiopulmonary resuscitation.

Clinical Manifestations of Respiratory Failure

Cardinal Signs
- Restlessness
- Tachypnea
- Tachycardia
- Diaphoresis

Early but Less Obvious Signs
- Mood changes, such as euphoria or depression
- Headache
- Altered depth and pattern of respirations
- Hypertension
- Exertional dyspnea
- Anorexia
- Increased cardiac output and renal output
- Central nervous system symptoms (decreased efficiency, impaired judgment, anxiety, confusion, restlessness, and irritability)
- Flaring nares
- Chest wall retractions
- Expiratory grunt
- Wheezing and/or prolonged expiration

Signs of More Severe Hypoxia
- Hypotension or hypertension
- Dimness of vision
- Somnolence
- Stupor
- Coma
- Dyspnea
- Depressed respirations
- Bradycardia
- Cyanosis, peripheral or central

Artificial ventilation. There are a variety of methods for controlling or assisting ventilation. Temporary assistance can be provided by a hand-operated self-inflating ventilation bag with mask and a nonreturnable valve to prevent rebreathing (AMBU bag). With the mask placed on the child's nose and mouth (an open airway is established by correct positioning with the chin forward and the neck extended to the "sniffing" position), the bag is rhythmically compressed, forcing the gas from the bag into the patient's lungs.

For more prolonged assistance, mechanical ventilation is employed to replace the bellows function of the diaphragm and thoracic wall muscles. The lungs are inflated by the application of either positive or negative pressure. The positive-pressure machine inflates the lung by increasing airway pressure above atmospheric pressure, and a negative-pressure ventilator creates a subatmosperic pressure around the chest wall, whereas airway pressure remains atmospheric. Application of positive pressure by mechanical means usually improves the distribution of gas within the lung and often reinflates partially collapsed lung segments. The overall effect is the improvement of gas exchange.

Cardiopulmonary Resuscitation

Complete apnea signals the need for rapid and vigorous action to prevent cardiac arrest. In such situations nurses must be prepared to initiate action immediately. In the hospital emergency equipment should be readily available in areas in which respiratory arrest might take place, and the status of this resuscitation equipment should be checked at least daily. Regardless of the cause of the arrest, some very basic procedures are carried out, modified somewhat according to the size of the child. The following actions are based on the *Standards for Cardiopulmonary Resuscitation (CPR) and Emergency Cardiac Care (ECC)* published by the American Medical Association (1986).

Outside the hospital situation, the first action in an emergency is to assess quickly the extent of any injury and determine whether the child is unconscious. A child who is struggling to breathe but conscious should be transported immediately to an advanced life support facility; the child should be allowed to maintain whatever position affords the most comfort. An unconscious child is managed with care to prevent additional trauma if the child has sustained a head or spinal cord injury. The circumstances in which the child is found offer some clues to a possible injury. For example, a child who has been thrown from a bicycle or fallen from a tree is more likely to sustain trauma than a child who is discovered in bed. The child should be turned as a unit with firm support to the head and neck to prevent rolling, twisting, or tilting backward or forward.

Resuscitation. For effective CPR the victim is placed on the back on a firm, flat surface, and appropriate precautions are employed (see Emergency Treatment: Child with Cardiopulmonary Arrest for outline of procedure).

EMERGENCY TREATMENT

Child with Cardiopulmonary Arrest

Assessment

1. Determine responsiveness or respiratory difficulty.
2. Call for help.
3. If alone with child: perform CPR for 1 minute before calling for help.
4. If second rescuer present: one rescuer continue CPR; second rescuer call emergency medical systems, giving the following information:
   Location of emergency
   Telephone number from which call is being made
   Circumstances of emergency
   Condition of victim
   Nature of aid being given
   Any other information requested (caller should hang up last)

Resuscitation

1. Position victim on back on firm, flat surface, taking precautions if evidence of head and/or neck injury.
2. Check mouth and remove foreign material, e.g., vomitus or foreign body.
3. Open airway.
   No neck injury: tilt head gently back to "sniffing" or neutral position. Lift chin from airway.
   Suspected neck injury: lift jaw by placing two or three fingers at its angle and lifting upward.
4. Check for evidence of breathing.
   a. Look at chest for movement.
   b. Listen for exhaled air.
   c. Feel for exhaled airflow.
5. Breathe for victim.
   a. Take a breath.
   b. Open mouth wide and place over mouth and nose of child. For larger child place mouth over child's mouth and occlude nostrils with rescuer's cheek or pinch nares tightly with fingers.
   c. Force breaths into victim's mouth, using just enough air pressure to cause child's chest to rise.
   d. Give two slow breaths (1 to 1.5 seconds per breath), pausing to inhale between breaths.
6. Check pulse of a large central artery.
   Children—carotid artery
   Infants—brachial artery
7. Continue as follows:
   If pulse present: initiate rescue breathing and continue until spontaneous breathing resumes.
   Infant—every 3 seconds, or 20 times per minute.
   Child—every 4 seconds, or 15 times per minute.
   If pulse not present: initiate chest compressions and coordinate with breathing.

Note: If second rescuer present, breathing and compressions are shared.

Chest Compressions

Infants:

1. Place index finger of hand farthest from infant's head just under imaginary line drawn between nipples.
2. Move index finger to a position one fingerbreadth below this intersection (compression area).
3. Using two or three fingers, compress sternum to depth of ½ to 1 inch (1.3 to 2.5 cm).
4. Release pressure without moving fingers from position.
5. Repeat at rate of at least 100 times per minute.

Children:

1. Using hand farthest from child's head, locate notch on child's chest where rib cage meets sternum.
2. With middle finger on notch, place index finger next to middle finger.
3. Place heel of other hand next to index finger with long axis of heel of hand parallel to sternum.
4. Compress chest with one hand to depth of 1 to 1½ inches (2.5 to 3.8 cm).
5. Compress at rate of 80 to 100 times per minute.

Coordinate Compression and Breathing

1. Pause at end of every fifth compression to allow for a ventilation.
2. Maintain 5:1 ratio for one or two rescuers.
3. Reassess after 10 cycles of compression and ventilation and every few minutes thereafter.

Note: Adult standards are applied to children over 8 years of age.

EMERGENCY TREATMENT

With loss of consciousness the tongue, which is attached to the lower jaw, relaxes and falls back, obstructing the airway. To open the airway, the head is positioned with either head tilt/chin lift (Fig. 22-5, *A*) or jaw thrust (Fig. 22-5, *B*). After a patent airway is restored by removal of foreign material and secretions (if indicated), and if the child is not breathing, continuation of the airway is maintained and rescue breathing is initiated. To ventilate the lungs in the infant and small child, the mouth of the operator is placed in such a way that both the mouth and the nostrils are included (Fig. 22-5, *C*). Older children are ventilated through the mouth while the nostrils are firmly pinched for airtight contact (Fig. 22-5, *D*).

The volume of air in an infant's lungs is small, and the air passages are considerably smaller, with resistance to flow potentially higher than in adults. However, since the differences are relative and vary according to the size of the child, the correct volume of air and force of the rescue breaths cannot be stated with certainty. If air enters freely and the chest rises, the airway is assumed to be clear. Breaths should be given slowly; the necessary volume can be provided without causing abdominal distention. Gastric distention, which interferes with diaphragmatic excursion, frequently occurs when breaths are delivered too rapidly.

After an initial two breaths, a peripheral pulse is palpated to ascertain the presence of a heartbeat. The carotid is the most central and accessible artery (Fig. 22-5, *E*). The very short and often fat neck of the infant renders the carotid pulse (ordinarily used in the adult) difficult to palpate. Therefore it is preferable to use the brachial pulse, located on the inner side of the upper arm midway between the elbow and shoulder (Fig. 22-5, *F*).

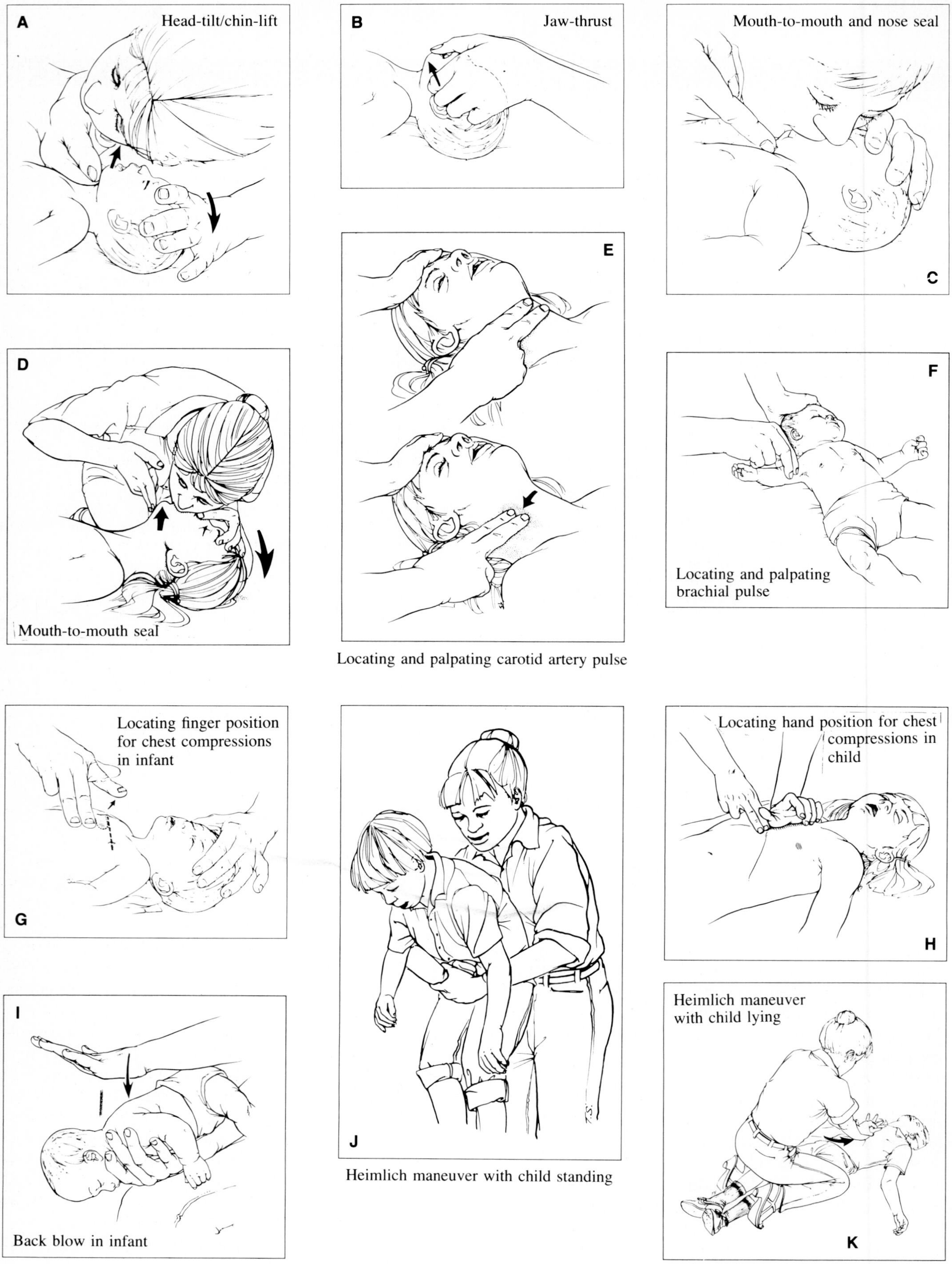

FIG. 22-5 Procedures for CPR *(A-H)* and airway obstruction *(I-K)*. (From Standards for Cardiopulmonary Resuscitation [CPR] and Emergency Cardiac Care [ECC]: Part IV. Pediatric basic life support, JAMA **225**(21):2954-2960, 1986.)

EMERGENCY TREATMENT

Airway Obstruction

Infant

1. Check inside of infant's mouth for foreign object.
2. If foreign body is observed, insert middle finger inside child's mouth on side farthest from rescuer, taking great care not to push object farther into throat. *No blind finger sweeps should be used.*
3. Place infant face down on rescuer's forearm in a 60-degree head-down position with head and neck stabilized.
4. Rest supporting arm on thigh.
5. Deliver four back blows forcefully with heel of free hand between infant's shoulder blades.
6. Place free hand on infant's back so infant is sandwiched between both hands; one supporting neck, jaw, and chest, the other supporting back.
7. If obstruction is not relieved, turn infant and place supine head down, with head and neck supported, and apply four chest thrusts to same location as chest compressions using two fingers but at a slower rate.

Alternative position: Place infant face down on rescuer's lap, head lower than trunk, and head firmly supported. Apply back blows, turn infant, and apply chest thrusts as above.

8. If breathing has not resumed:
   Grasp both tongue and lower jaw between thumb and finger and lift (tongue-jaw lift technique).
   If foreign body is visible, extract manually by finger sweep.
   No blind sweeps.
9. If there is no spontaneous breathing:
   Attempt ventilation with two breaths by mouth-to-mouth or mouth-to-mouth and nose technique.
10. Repeat steps 3 to 9.

Note: The Heimlich maneuver is not recommended for infants under 1 year of age.

Child

Heimlich maneuver with victim standing or sitting (older, larger child)

1. Stand behind victim.
2. Wrap arms around victim's waist with one hand made into fist.
3. Place fist on victim's abdomen in midline slightly above navel and well below tip of sternum with thumb side of fist resting against victim's abdomen.
4. Grasp fist with other hand and press into victim's abdomen with a series of 6 to 10 quick upward thrusts.
5. Each thrust should be a separate and distinct movement.
6. If obstruction is not relieved, open victim's mouth using tongue-jaw lift to draw tongue away from back of throat.
7. If foreign body is visualized, attempt to remove manually by a finger sweep. Avoid sweeps, which may cause further obstruction.
8. Repeat above sequences while rapidly seeking aid.

Heimlich maneuver with victim lying (conscious or unconscious)

1. Position child face up, on back.
2. Kneel *next to* child.
3. Place heel of *one hand* on child's abdomen in midline slightly above navel and well below rib cage.
4. Place other hand on top of first hand and press into victim's abdomen with a quick upward thrust.
5. Repeat thrusts if needed (6 to 10 in rapid succession).

Note: The astride position is not recommended for a small child but may be used for a large one.

From Committee on Accidents and Poison Prevention: First aid for the choking child, Pediatrics **81:**740-742, 1988.

Absence of carotid or temporal pulse is considered sufficient indication to begin external cardiac massage.

Chest compression. External chest compression consists of serial, rhythmic compressions of the chest to maintain circulation to vital organs until the child achieves spontaneous vital signs or advanced life support can be provided. Chest compressions are always accompanied by simultaneous ventilation of the lungs. For optimum compressions it is essential that the child's spine is supported during compression of the sternum, and sternal pressure must be forceful but not traumatic. In an infant the hard surface can be the palm of the hand not performing compressions, with head tilt provided by the weight of the head and a slight uplift of the shoulders.

The placement of the fingers for compression in infants is now determined to be lower than previously thought, that is, at a point on the lower rather than the middle sternum. The site is one fingerbreadth below the intersection of the sternum and an imaginary line drawn between the nipples (Fig. 22-5, *G*) (see Emergency treatment). Compressions on the child 1 to 8 years of age are applied to the lower sternum two fingerbreadths above the sternal notch (Fig. 22-5, *H*) (see also Emergency treatment). Sternal compression to infants is applied with two or three fingers on the sternum exerting a sharp downward thrust; on children pressure is applied with the heel of one hand. The depth of compression is also adapted to the size of the child (see Emergency treatment). The location, rate, and depth for children over 8 years are the same as for adults (*Standards for CPR and ECC,* 1986). There previously was concern regarding the possibility of rib fractures during CPR; this has been found to be a rare occurrence (Feldman and Brewer, 1984).

Ventilation and compression are continued by the mouth-to-mouth method or by artificial ventilator at a ratio of one breath for five compressions until there are signs of recovery, as evidenced by palpable peripheral pulses, return of pupils to normal size, and the disappearance of mottling and cyanosis.

AIRWAY OBSTRUCTION

Attempts at clearing the airway should be considered for (1) children in whom aspiration is witnessed or strongly suspected and (2) unconscious, nonbreathing children whose airways remain obstructed despite the usual maneuvers to open them (*Standards of CPR and ECC*, 1986). When a child is obviously choking, the initial step is to open his mouth and attempt to visualize and remove the object. *No blind finger sweeps should be used.* If this fails, the next step is to apply mechanical force in an attempt to dislodge the object.

There is strong controversy concerning the optimum method for relieving foreign-body obstruction in children. The methods currently offered are a combination of *back blows* and *chest thrusts* and the *Heimlich maneuver*. Because of the risk of injury to abdominal organs, abdominal thrusts are not recommended for infants.

Infants

A choking infant is placed face down over the rescuer's arm, with his head lower than his trunk and his head supported (Fig. 22-5, *I*). Additional support can be achieved if the rescuer supports his arm firmly against his thigh (Committee on Accidents and Poison Prevention, 1986). Four quick, sharp back blows are delivered between the infant's shoulder blades with the heel of the rescuer's hand. Less force is required than would be applied to an adult. After delivery of the back blows, the rescuer's free hand is placed flat on the infant's back so that the infant is "sandwiched" between the two hands, making certain the neck and chin are well supported. While the rescuer maintains support with the infant's head lower than the trunk, the infant is turned and placed supine on the rescuer's thigh, where four chest thrusts are applied in rapid succession in the same manner as external chest compressions described for CPR (see Emergency treatment, p. 731).

Children

The Heimlich maneuver, a series of subdiaphragmatic abdominal thrusts, is recommended for children. The maneuver creates an artificial cough that forces air, and with it the foreign body, out of the airway. The procedure is carried out with the child in a standing, sitting, or lying position (Fig. 22-5, *J* and *K*). Upward thrusts are delivered to the upper abdomen with the fisted hand at a point just below the rib cage (see Emergency treatment). To prevent damage to the internal organs, the rescuer's hands should not touch the xiphoid process of the sternum or the lower margins of the ribs. Six to 10 thrusts are repeated in rapid succession until the foreign body is expelled.

It is neither necessary nor desirable to squeeze or compress the arms during the procedure. It is not a punch or a bear hug. The child may vomit after relief of the obstruction and should be positioned to prevent aspiration. After breathing is restored, the child should receive medical attention so he can be assessed for complications.

The success of the technique is primarily a result of the fact that obstruction takes place at the end of a maximum respiration. The victim is most likely to choke on food during inspiration; therefore the tidal volume plus expiratory reserve volume is present in the lungs. When pressure is exerted on the diaphragm by the maneuver, the food bolus is ejected with considerable force by this trapped air.

SUMMARY

Respiratory dysfunction in childhood can be acute or chronic. Upper respiratory infections are the most common disorders that affect children, are subject to invasion by a variety of infective organisms, and can be focused on any structure within the respiratory tract. Most disorders are amenable to home care and management. Tonsillitis and otitis media are the infections most frequently requiring surgical intervention, and asthma is responsible for more school absences than any other chronic illness.

Respiratory emergencies, choking and respiratory arrest, are situations that require immediate action. Nurses should be prepared to respond to these emergencies and encourage parents to learn the lifesaving techniques.

KEY CONCEPTS

- Acute infection of the respiratory tract is the most common cause of illness in infancy and childhood.
- The incidence and severity of respiratory tract infections are influenced by the infectious agents involved, the child's age, and the child's natural defenses.
- Common respiratory tract infections of childhood include acute nasopharyngitis, acute pharyngitis (including tonsillitis), influenza, and otitis media.
- Croup syndromes involve acute inflammation and variable degrees of obstruction of the epiglottis, larynx, and/or trachea.
- The primary goals in the care of children with croup are observation for signs of respiratory embarrassment and relief of laryngeal obstruction.
- Common infections of the lower airways are bacterial tracheitis, asthmatic bronchitis, bronchitis, and bronchiolitis.
- Pneumonias are classified according to site (lobar, bronchial, or interstitial) or by etiologic agent (viruses, bacteria, mycoplasms, or associated with aspiration of foreign material).
- In tuberculosis, susceptibility to the bacillus can be influenced by heredity, age, stress, poor nutrition, and intercurrent infection.
- Passive inhalation of cigarette smoke is one of the primary environmental pollutants contributing to respiratory disease in children.
- Bronchial asthma is the leading cause of chronic illness in children.
- General therapeutic management of asthma includes allergen control, drug therapy, controlled exercise, physical therapy, and hyposensitization.
- Support for the family of the child with asthma includes education about the disease and its therapy and facilitation of self-management.
- Cystic fibrosis is the most common inherited disease in children.
- The diagnosis of cystic fibrosis is based on family history, increased sweat electrolyte content, absent pancreatic enzymes, and chronic pulmonary involvement.
- Choking and respiratory failure are respiratory emergencies that necessitate immediate intervention.

STUDY QUESTIONS AND ACTIVITIES

1. Outline a plan of care for a child with an acute respiratory infection.
2. Outline a teaching plan for the parents of a child being discharged after a tonsillectomy and adenoidectomy.
3. Visit a pharmacy, supermarket, or discount department store and make a list of the categories (e.g., antitussives, antihistamines, decongestants) of over-the-counter drugs on display; then count the the number of different brands within each category. How many are not recommended for children?
4. Investigate the community resources for children with chronic lung disease.
5. Assess the home of a friend, relative, or self for possible allergens. Make recommendations for making the environment as allergy-proof as possible for a child with asthma.

REFERENCES

American Academy of Pediatrics Committee on Accident and Poison Prevention: Revised first aid for the choking child, Pediatrics **78:**177-178, 1986.

Bierman, C.W., and Pearlman, D.S.: Asthma. In Kendig, E.L., and Chernick, V., editors: Disorders of the respiratory tract in children, ed. 2, Philadelphia, 1983, W.B. Saunders Co.

Colombo, J.L., Hopkins, R.L., and Waring, W.W.: Steam vaporizer injuries, Pediatrics **67:**661-663, 1981.

Committee on Accidents and Poison Prevention, American Academy of Pediatrics: Revised first aid for the choking child, Pediatrics **78:**177-178, 1986.

Committee on Children with Disabilities and Committee on Sports Medicine: The asthmatic child's participation in sports and physical education, Pediatrics **74:**155-156, 1984.

Committee of Environmental Hazards: Involuntary smoking—a hazard to children, Pediatrics **77:**755-757, 1986.

Edlund, L.D., and others: Effects of swimming program on children with cystic fibrosis, Am. J. Dis. Child. **140:**880-883, 1986.

Feldman, K.W., and Brewer, D.K.: Child abuse, cardiopulmonary resuscitation and rib fractures, Pediatrics **73:**339-342, 1984.

Ogston, S.A.: The Tayside infant morbidity and mortality study: effect on health of using gas for cooking, Br. Med. J. **290:**957-960, 1985.

Pedreira, F.A., and others: Involuntary smoking and incidence of respiratory illness during the first year of life, Pediatrics **75:**594-597, 1985.

Sly, R.M.: Asthma. In Gellis, S.S., and Kagon, B.M., editors: Current pediatric therapy 12, Philadelphia, 1986, W.B. Saunders Co.

Standards for Cardiopulmonary Resuscitation (CPR) and Emergency Cardiac Care (ECC): Part IV. Pediatric basic life support, JAMA **255**(21):2954-2960, 1986.

Strome, M.: Must children with tympanostomy tubes avoid swimming? Pediatr. Alert **8**(7):28, 1983.

BIBLIOGRAPHY

General

Anton, B.: Pediataric respiratory therapy beyond the neonatal ICU, Resp. Therapy **14**(4):19-26, 1984.

Belitz, J.: Minimizing the psychological complications of patients who require mechanical ventilation, Crit. Care Nurse **3**(3):42-46, 1983.

Curley, M.A.Q., and Vaughan, S.M.: Assessment and resuscitation of the pediatric patient, Crit. Care Nurse **7**(3):26-42, 1987.

Diamond, L.: Triaging pediatric emergencies, Crit. Care Update **7**(2):28-32, 1980.

Eigen, H.: The clinical evaluation of chronic cough, Pediatr. Clin. North Am. **29:**67-78, 1982:

Finer, N.N., and others: Limitations of self-inflating resuscitators, Pediatrics **77:**417-420, 1986.

Gammon, S.S.: Respiratory acidosis, Nursing 82 **12**(8):65, 1982.

Hess, D.: Bedside monitoring of the patient on a ventilator, Crit. Care Q. **6**(2):23-31, 1983.

Janowsky, M.J.: Accidental disconnections from breathing systems, Am. J. Nurs. **84:**241-244, 1984.

Landis, K., and Smith, S.: The mechanically ventilated patient: a comprehensive nursing care plan, Crit. Care Q. **6**(2):43-52, 1983.

McCarthy, M.F.: Home discharge program for ventilator-assisted children, Pediatr. Nurs. **12:**331-380, 1986.

Nielsen, L.: Assessing patients' respiratory problems, Am. J. Nurs. **80:**2192-2196, 1980.

Nielsen, L.: Interpreting arterial blood gases, Am. J. Nurs. **80:**2197-2201, 1980.

Nielsen, L.: Pulmonary oxygen toxicity and other hazards of oxygen therapy, Am. J. Nurs. **80:**2213-2215, 1980.

Raulin, A.M., and Shannon, K.A.: PNPs: case managers for technology-dependent children, Pediatr. Nurs. **12:**338-340, 1986.

Rokosky, J.S.: Assessment of the individual with altered respiratory function, Nurs. Clin. North Am. **16:**195-209, 1981.

Signor, G., and Del Bueno, D.J.: A sinfully easy way to interpret ABGs, RN **45**(9):45-49, 1982.

Weaver, T.E.: New life for lungs through incentive spirometers, Nursing 81 **11**(2):54-58, 1981.

Respiratory Infections

Antibiotic therapy at home, Am. J. Nurs. **84:**348-350, 1984.

Castiglia, P.T., and Aquilina, S.: Streptococcal pharyngitis: a persistent challenge, Pediatr. Nurs. **8:**377-381, 1982.

Casto, D.T.: Amantadine hydrochloride: an agent for the prevention and treatment of influenza A infection, J. Pediatr. Health Care **1:**51-53, 1987.

Coleman, D.A.: TB: the disease that's not dead yet, RN **47**(9):49-59, 1984.

Dupont, J.: EENT emergencies, Nursing 79 **9**(11):65-70, 1979.

Fathers, B.: Mycoplasma pneumonia, Nurs. Times **77:**1661-1664, 1981.

Fried, W.: Acute epiglottitis, Issues Compreh. Pediatr. Nurs. **4:**29-36, 1980.

Gladwin, B.: Adenotonsillectomy: bearing up with Paddington, Nurs. Mirror **150**(6):42-44, 1980.

Langslet, J., and Habel, M.L.: The aminoglycoside antibiotics, Am. J. Nurs. **81:**1144-1146, 1981.

Mansell, K.A.: New immunization against *H. influenzae* type b, Pediatr. Nurs. **11:**433-435, 1985.

Maurer, J.A.: The care and feeding of a T & A, Point of View **18**(4):10, 1981.

Pantell, R.H., and others: Fever in the first six months of life, Clin. Pediatr. **19:**77-82, 1980.

Ryan, A.M.: Pneumonia: aggressive treatment is the key, RN **45**(8):44-50, 1982.

Safety precautions in home chemotherapy, Am. J. Nurs. **84:**346-347, 1984.

Thomas, D.O.: Are you sure it's only croup? RN **47**(12):40-43, 1984.

Yoos, L.: Factors influencing maternal compliance to antibiotic regimens, Pediatr. Nurs. **10:**141-147, 1984.

Otitis Media

Adams, J.L., Evans, G.A., and Roberts, J.E.: Diagnosing and treating otitis media with effusion, Am. J. Maternal Child Nurs. **9:**22-28, 1984.

Castiglia, P.T., Aquilina, S.S., and Kemsley, M.: Focus: nonsuppurative otitis media, Pediatr. Nurs. **9:**427-430, 1983.

Dyson, A.T., Holmes, A.E., and Duffitt, D.V.: Speech characteristics of children after otitis media, J. Pediatr. Health Care **1:**261-265, 1987.

Sataloff, R.T., and Colton, C.M.: Otitis media: a common childhood infection, Am. J. Nurs. **81**(8):1480-1483, 1981.

Study identifies children at risk for otitis media, AORN J. **31**(6):1014-1015, 1980.

Noninfectious Irritants

Barker-Stotis, K.: CO poisoning, Nursing 87 **17**(12):33, 1987.

Blazer, S., Naveh, Y., and Friedman, A.: Foreign body in the airway, Am. J. Dis. Child. **134:**68-71, 1980.

Brandeburg, J.: Inhalation injury: carbon monoxide poisoning, Am. J. Nurs. **80:**98-100, 1980.

Breslin, E.H., and Lery, M.J.: Prevention and treatment of aspiration pneumonitis secondary to massive gastric aspiration, Crit. Care Q. **6**(2):73-82, 1983.

Burton, J.: Carbon monoxide poisoning, Crit. Care Update **10**(2):19-21, 1983.

Desai, M.H.: Inhalation injuries in burn victims, Crit. Care Q. **7**(3):1-7, 1984.

Friedman, G.D., Petitti, D.B., and Bawol, R.D.: Prevalence and correlates of passive smoking, Am. J. Public Health **73:**401-405, 1983.

Gaston, S.F., and Schuman, L.L: Inhalation injury: smoke inhalation, Am. J. Nurs. **80:**94-97, 1980.

Gozal, D., and others: Accidental carbon monoxide poisoning: emphasis on hyperbaric oxygen treatment, Clin. Pediatr. **24:**132-135, 1985.

Lybarger, P.M.: Inhalation injury in children: nursing care, Issues Compreh. Pediatr. Nurs. **10:**33-50, 1987.

Mohler, S.E.: Passive smoking: a danger to children's health, J. Pediatr. Health Care **1**:298-304, 1987.

Wagner, T.J., and Hindi-Alexander, M.: Hazards of baby powder? Pediatr. Nurs. **10:**124-125, 1984.

Bronchial Asthma

Bowers, K., and Koviach, J.: Self-care management of asthma, Child. Nurse **5**(1):1-4, 1987.
Burton, J.: Extrinsic allergic alveolitis, Crit. Care Update **10**(1):33-37, 1983.
Conboy, K.: Nursing care plan for the child with status asthmaticus, Crit. Care Nurse **5**(2):8-9, 12, 1985.
Duffy, D.M., and Halloran, M.C.: Effect of an educational program on parents of children with asthma, Child. Health Care **16:**76-80, 1987.
Foster, S.D.: Theophylline, Am. J. Maternal Child Nurs. **5:**136, 1981.
Gever, L.N.: Theophylline: know how to handle this potent bronchodilator, Nursing 80 **10**(11):50-53, 1980.
Hudgel, D.W., and Madsen, L.A.: Acute and chronic asthma: a guide to intervention, Am. J. Nurs. **80:**1791-1795, 1980.
Jennings, C.: Controlling the home environment of the allergic child, MCN **7:**376-381, 1982.
Kirilloff, L.H., and Tibbals, S.C.: Drugs for asthma. A complete guide, Am. J. Nurs. **83:**55-61, 1983.
Kubly, L.S., and McClellan, M.S.: Effects of self-care instruction on asthmatic children, Issues Compreh. Pediatr. Nurs. **7:**121-130, 1984.
McCaully, H.E.: Breathing exercises as play for asthmatic children, Am. J. Maternal Child Nurs. **5:**340-344, 1980.
Nemec, M.A.: Inhalation medications for chronic asthma, J. Pediatr. Health Care **1:**223-227, 1987.
Nursing Grand Rounds: Fighting the frustrations of status asthmaticus, Nursing 82 **12**(3):58-63, 1982.
Odom, J.D., and Taylor, R.W.: Environmental variables and acute asthmatic attacks in children, J. Pediatr. Nurs. **1:**335-341, 1986.
Rachelefsky, G.S.: Asthma self-management programs for children, Child Care Newsletter **3**(2):5-8, 1984.
Rew, L.: The relationship between self-care behaviors and selected psychosocial variables in children with asthma, J. Pediatr. Nurs. **2:**333-341, 1987.
Rimar, J.M.: Albuterol: a selective beta$_2$ bronchodilator, MCN **11:**169, 1986.
Saucier, C.P.: Self-concept and self-care management in school-age children with diabetes, Pediatr. Nurs. **10:**135-138, 1984.
Sedlacek, K.K.: Asthma in children: facilitating self-care, Pediatr. Nurs. Update **1**(1):1-8, 1985.
Shultz, C.M.: Sulfite sensitivity, Am. J. Nurs. **86:**914, 1986.
Webber-Jones, J.E., and Bryant, M.K.: Over-the-counter bronchodilators, Nursing 80 **10**(1):34-39, 1980.
Weeks, H.F.: The xanthines, Am. J. Nurs. **5:**206, 1980.
Wolf, S.I.: Exercise and the asthmatic child and PL 94-142, Pediatr. Nurs. **6**(6):21-23, 1980.

Cystic Fibrosis

Brissette, S., and others: Nursing care plan for adolescents and young adults with advanced cystic fibrosis, Issues Compreh. Pediatr. Nurs. **10:**87-97, 1987.
Canam, C.: Talking about cystic fibrosis within the family—what parents need to know, Issues Compreh. Pediatr. Nurs. **9:**167-178, 1986.
Glendon, M.: Teaching Harry what we'd thought he knew, Nursing 85 **15**(7):44-46, 1985.
Harder, L., and Bowditch, B.: Siblings of children with cystic fibrosis: perceptions of the impact of the disease, Child. Health Care **10:**116-120, 1982.
Johnson, M.P.: Self-instruction for the family of a child with cystic fibrosis, MCN **5:**345-348, 1980.
Kruger, S., Shawyer, M., and Jones, L.: Reactions of families to the child with cystic fibrosis, Image **12:**67-72, 1980.
Myer, P.A.: Parental adaptation to cystic fibrosis, J. Pediatr. Health Care **2**:20-28, 1988.
Patton, A.C., Ventura, J.N., and Savedra, M.: Stress and coping responses of adolescents with cystic fibrosis, Child. Health Care **14:**153-156, 1986.
Pumariega, A.J.: The adolescent with cystic fibrosis: developmental issues, Child. Health Care **11:**78-81, 1982.
Rose, J., and Jay, S.: A comprehensive exercise program for persons with cystic fibrosis, J. Pediatr. Nurs. **1:**323-334, 1986.
Spotting and sustaining patients with CF, Patient Care **16:**16-53, 1982.
Stewart, A.: Care in the hospital: cystic fibrosis. Part 3, Nurs. Times **80**(22):44-45, 1984.
Walker, L.S., Ford, M.B., and Donald, W.D.: Cystic fibrosis and family stress: effects of age and severity of illness, Pediatrics **79:**239-246, 1986.

Respiratory Emergencies

Brill, J.E.: Cardiopulmonary resuscitation, Pediatr. Ann. **15:**24-29, 1986.
Carlile, T.: Self-administered Heimlich maneuver (letter), JAMA **249:**3175, 1983.
Carter, J.H.: CPR: breathing life back into a child, Nursing 86 **16**(10):50-57, 1986.
Dixon, M., and Holmes, R.B.: The care of a ventilator-dependent child on a general pediatric unit, J. Pediatr. Nurs. **2:**184-192, 1987.
Hazinski, M.F.: New guidelines for pediatric and neonatal cardiopulmonary resuscitation and advanced life support. Part I: Basic CPR for adults and children, Pediatr. Nurs. **12:**373-376, 1986.
Hazinski, M.F.: New guidelines for pediatric and neonatal cardiopulmonary resuscitation and advanced life support. Part II: Pediatric advanced life support, Pediatr. Nurs. **12:**445-448, 1986.
Hazinski, M.F.: New guidelines for pediatric and neonatal cardiopulmonary resuscitation and advanced life support. Part III: Neonatal advanced life support, Pediatr. Nurs. **12:**57-60, 1987.
New CPR guidelines: bicarb now a last resort, Am. J. Nurs. **86:**889, 1986.
Phillips, G.W.L., and Zideman, D.A.: Relation of infant heart to sternum: its significance in cardiopulmonary resuscitation, Lancet **1:**1024-1025, 1986.
Rehm, R.S.: Teaching cardiopulmonary resuscitation to parents, J. Maternal Child Nurs. **8:**411-414, 1983.
Scientific Board, California Medical Association: Transmission of disease via mouth-to-mouth resuscitation, West. J. Med. **143:**468, 1985.
Steele, N.F., and Harrison, B.: Technology-assisted children: assessing discharge preparation, J. Pediatr. Nurs. **1**(3):150-158, 1986.

CHAPTER 23

The Child with Gastrointestinal Dysfunction

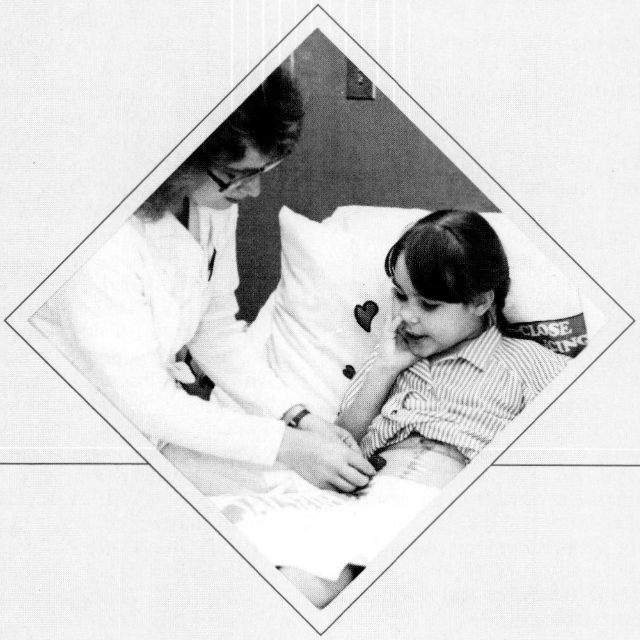

LEARNING OBJECTIVES

On completion of this chapter the reader will be able to:

- Describe the characteristics of infants that affect their ability to adapt to fluid loss or gain
- Outline a plan of care for the infant with acute diarrhea
- Outline a plan for teaching the parents pre- and postoperative care of a child with a cleft lip and/or palate
- Compare the pre- and postoperative care of an infant with a structural defect of the gastrointestinal tract
- Plan the diet for a child with a malabsorption syndrome
- Outline a plan of care for a child with an obstructive disorder
- Compare and contrast the inflammatory diseases of the gastrointestinal tract
- Discuss the cause, prevention, and nursing care of the child with hepatitis

Disorders of the gastrointestinal (GI) tract are very common and constitute one of the largest categories of illnesses that occur in infancy and childhood. These GI disturbances can be acute or chronic conditions that often interfere with usual daily activities and may even require an altered life-style. This chapter is concerned with those conditions that in some way interfere with normal digestion and absorption of nutrients.

◆ *Gastrointestinal Dysfunction*

The gastrointestinal (GI) system serves to process and absorb nutrients necessary to maintain metabolic processes and to support growth and development. All actions of the gastrointestinal tract are subject to a variety of outside influences. At all ages children are sensitive to tensions and anxieties, and many diseases and disorders are reflected in altered GI function.

Some GI disorders, e.g., vomiting and/or diarrhea, occur as primary and isolated disturbances but are also among the manifestations often associated with a variety of childhood illnesses. Structural and obstructive defects interfere with the ingestion and transport of ingested foodstuffs, and inflammatory, malabsorptive, and maldigestive disturbances impair the functional integrity of the gastrointestinal tract. Furthermore, in most of the disorders the primary defect can produce additional complications. For example, loss of gastrointestinal contents causes significant alterations in fluid and electrolytes, and obstructive or inflammatory conditions affect digestion and absorption because bowel motility, mucosal functioning, enzymatic activity, and bacterial flora are altered.

Numerous general observations provide possible clues to specific gastrointestinal problems (see box). In some cases only one manifestation may be observed; others may involve a number of signs and symptoms as part of the disease complex. In any disorder that involves GI losses, particularly large amounts of fluid, dehydration poses a serious threat to life and often dominates the clinical picture. Because many of the abdominal disorders require surgical intervention, the major focus of nursing care is related to pre- and postoperative management.

Clinical Manifestations of Gastrointestinal Dysfunction in Children

Failure to thrive, as evidenced by deceleration from established growth pattern or consistently below the fifth percentile for height and weight on standard growth charts.

Spitting up and/or regurgitation, characteristic of infants, are discussed on p. 324.

Vomiting, the forceful ejection of stomach contents, involves a complex reflex that is associated with widespread autonomic discharge that causes salivation, pallor, sweating, and tachycardia. Vomiting is ordinarily accompanied by nausea.

Projectile vomiting, vomiting in which the vomitus is forcefully ejected as far as 2 to 4 feet (0.6 to 1.2 m) from the child and is not associated with nausea.

Hematemesis, the vomiting of blood that may result from swallowing blood from the oropharynx or from bleeding in the upper GI tract.

Nausea, an unpleasant sensation vaguely referred to the epigastrium, with an inclination to vomit.

Stools, the number, type, consistency, presence or absence of blood, and associated signs and symptoms provide clues to the etiology of gastrointestinal dysfunction.

Constipation, the regular passage of firm or hard stools or of small, hard masses with associated symptoms such as difficulty expelling the stools, blood-streaked bowel movements, and abdominal discomfort. Suggested lower limit of frequency is six movements per week in children less than 3 years and 4 per week in older children. The apparent difficulty in passing stools is not a reliable sign, especially in infancy.

Diarrhea, an increase in the number of stools or a decrease in their consistency as a result of alterations of water and electrolyte transport by the alimentary tract. Diarrhea may be acute or chronic.

Abdominal pain, specific or nonspecific, is associated with a number of GI disorders.

Abdominal enlargement or distention, is a common observation in a child with GI dysfunction.

Dysphagia, difficulty in swallowing, can be the result of structural abnormalities or neurologic or neuromuscular impairment.

Bowel sounds, or their absence, can provide information about some GI disorders.

Jaundice, the yellow discoloration of the skin associated with liver dysfunction.

Disability in sucking and swallowing are manifestations often observed in infants.

DEHYDRATION

Dehydration is a common disturbance in infants and children and occurs whenever the total output of fluid exceeds the total intake, regardless of the underlying cause. It occurs most often as a result of abnormal GI losses.

Water Balance in Infants

Because of several characteristics, infants and young children have a greater need for water and are more vulnerable to alterations in fluid and electrolyte balance. Compared to older children and adults, they have a greater fluid intake and output relative to size, water and electrolyte disturbances occur more frequently and more rapidly, and they adjust less promptly to these alterations.

The fluid compartments in the infant vary significantly from those in the adult primarily because of an expanded extracellular compartment. The extracellular fluid compartment comprises over half of the total body water at birth and, accompanying this, a greater relative content of extracellular sodium and chloride. The infant loses a large amount of fluid at birth and still maintains a larger amount of extracellular fluid than the adult until about 2 years of age. This contributes to greater and more rapid water loss and poorer compensatory adjustment during this age period.

Surface area. The infant's relatively greater surface area allows larger quantities of fluid to be lost in insensible perspiration through the skin. It is estimated that the body surface area of the premature infant is five times as great, and that of the newborn is two to three times as great, as that of the older child or adult. The proportionately longer gastrointestinal tract in infancy is also a source of relatively greater fluid loss, especially from diarrhea. Also, the daily volume of secretions into the gastrointestinal tract is much higher in infants than in children.

Metabolic rate. The rate of metabolism in infancy is significantly higher because of the larger surface area in relation to the mass of active tissue. Consequently there is a greater production of metabolic wastes that must be excreted by the kidneys. Any condition that increases metabolism causes greater heat production, with its concomitant insensible fluid loss and an increased need for water for excretion.

Kidney function. The kidneys of the infant are functionally immature at birth and are, therefore, inefficient in excreting waste products of metabolism. Of particular importance for fluid balance is the inability of the infant's kidneys to concentrate or dilute urine, to conserve or excrete sodium, and to acidify urine. Therefore, the infant is less able to handle large quantities of solute-free water than the older child.

Fluid requirements. As a result of these characteristics, infants ingest and excrete a greater amount of fluid per kilogram of body weight than older children. Since electrolytes are excreted with water and the infant has limited ability for conservation, maintenance requirements include both water and electrolytes. The daily exchange of extracellular fluid in the infant is greatly increased over that of older children, which leaves them little fluid volume reserve in dehydrated states.

Types of Dehydration

Sodium is the primary osmotic force that controls fluid movement between the major fluid compartments; however, other osmotic forces (e.g., protein, glucose) may play a dominant role. Consequently, dehydration is conveniently classified according to the compositional changes in the plasma, or tonicity: (1) isotonic, (2) hypotonic, and (3) hypertonic.

Isotonic. Isotonic (isonatremic) dehydration occurs in conditions in which the electrolyte and water deficits are present in approximately balanced proportion, i.e. salt and water lost in equal amounts. Shock is the greatest threat to life in isotonic dehydration, and the child displays the symptoms characteristic of hypovolemic shock. Plasma sodium remains within normal limits, between 130 and 150 mEq/liter.

Hypotonic. Hypotonic (hyponatremic) dehydration occurs when the electrolyte deficit exceeds the water deficit, leaving the serum hypotonic. Since intracellular fluid is more concentrated than extracellular fluid in hypotonic dehydration, water moves from the extracellular to the intracellular fluid to establish osmotic equilibrium. Therefore, this further increases the extracellular fluid volume loss, and shock is a frequent finding. Since there is a greater proportional loss of extracellular fluid in hypotonic dehydration, the physical signs tend to be more severe with smaller fluid losses than isotonic or hypertonic dehydration. Plasma sodium concentration is less than 130 mEq/liter.

Hypertonic. Hypertonic (hypernatremic) dehydration results from water loss in excess of electrolyte loss and is usually caused by either a proportionately larger loss of water and/or a larger intake of electrolytes. This sometimes occurs in infants with diarrhea who are given fluids by mouth that contain large amounts of solute or in children receiving high-protein nasogastric tube feedings that place an excessive solute load on the kidneys. In hypertonic dehydration fluid shifts from the lesser concentration of the intracellular to the extracellular fluid. Plasma sodium concentration is greater than 150 mEq/liter. Since the extra-cellular fluid volume is proportionately larger, hypertonic dehydration has a larger degree of water loss for the same intensity of physical signs. Shock is less apparent in hypertonic dehydration. However, neurologic disturbances, such as seizures, are more likely to occur. Cerebral changes are serious and may result in permanent damage.

Clinical Manifestations of Dehydration

	Isotonic (loss of water and salt)	Hypotonic (loss of salt in excess of water)	Hypertonic (loss of water in excess of salt)
Skin			
Color	Gray	Gray	Gray
Temperature	Cold	Cold	Cold or hot
Turgor	Poor	Very poor	Fair
Feel	Dry	Clammy	Thickened, doughy
Mucous membranes	Dry	Slightly moist	Parched
Tearing and salivation	Absent	Absent	Absent
Eyeball	Sunken and soft	Sunken and soft	Sunken
Fontanel	Sunken	Sunken	Sunken
Body temperature	Subnormal or elevated	Abnormal	Subnormal or elevated
Pulse	Rapid	Very rapid	Moderately rapid
Respirations	Rapid	Rapid	Rapid
Behavior	Irritable to lethargic	Lethargic to comatose; convulsions	Marked lethargy with extreme hyperirritability on stimulation

Diagnostic Evaluation

Diagnosis of dehydration is made on the basis of clinical manifestations (see box). In infants, isotonic dehydration is usually described as 5% (mild), 10% (moderate), and 15% (severe). Older children and adolescents, with proportionately less total body water, display smaller proportional losses; therefore, the estimates of 3%, 6%, and 9% more nearly describe mild, moderate, and severe dehydration, respectively, in these age-groups (Table 23-1).

Shock is a common feature of severe depletion of extracellular fluid volume with tachycardia and low blood pressure (see p. 811). A fissured tongue and soft eyeballs are additional signs of severe deydration, and in infants, the anterior fontanel is depressed.

Therapeutic Management

See Therapeutic management of diarrhea, p. 743.

Nursing Considerations

Nursing observation and intervention are essential to the detection and therapeutic managment of dehydration. There are a wide variety of circumstances in which fluid loss may be precipitated, especially in infants, and changes can take place in a very short time. Therefore, an important nursing responsibility is perceptive observation for any signs of dehydration, particularly in those situations and conditions in which depletion is likely to occur, such as vomiting, sweating, diarrhea, elevated temperature, and major surgery.

The nursing assessment of suspected or potential fluid loss begins with the observation of general appearance, then proceeds with specific observations.

Intake and output. Accurate measurements of fluid intake and output are vital to the assessment of dehydration. This includes oral and parenteral intake and losses from urine, stools, vomiting, fistulas, nasogastric suction, sweat, and wound drainage.

Urine—assess frequency, volume, and consistency of urine
Stools—assess frequency, volume, and consistency of stools
Vomitus—assess for volume, frequency, and type of vomiting
Sweating—can be only estimated from frequency of clothing and linen changes

Other observations. In addition to fluid intake and output the following observations assist in assessment of dehydration:

Vital signs—temperature (normal, elevated, or lowered depending on degree of dehydration), pulse, and blood pressure
Skin—assess for color, temperature, feel, turgor, and presence or absence of edema
Mucous membranes—assess for moisture, color, and presence of and consistency of secretions; condition of tongue
Fontanel (infants)—sunken, soft, normal
Sensory alterations—presence of thirst

For nursing interventions, see discussion under specific disorders.

◆ *Disorders of Motility*

Acute attacks of vomiting and diarrhea are so common in the pediatric age-group that they can almost be regarded as part of the normal way of life. However, the nature of the anatomic and physiologic structure of the infant and small child renders them particularly vulnerable to fluid and electrolyte imbalances when pathologic changes affect the fluid compartments. Most illnesses create some disturbance in body fluids and/or electrolytes, and, in vomiting and diarrhea, these disturbances are more threatening than the primary pathology.

ACUTE DIARRHEA

Diarrhea is a symptom that can result from disorders involving digestive, absorptive, and secretory functions. There are wide variations in colonic function among different individuals; therefore, a precise definition and identification of what constitutes diarrhea pose a problem in terms of number or consistency of stools. For example, one infant may have one firm stool every second or third day, whereas another normally passes from five to eight small, soft stools daily. More important are (1) a noticeable or sudden increase in number of stools, (2) a reduc-

TABLE 23-1

Intensity of Clinical Signs Associated with Varying Degrees of Isotonic Dehydration in Infants

	Degree of Dehydration		
	Mild	**Moderate**	**Severe**
Body weight	Up to 5%	5%-9%	10%-15%
Skin color	Pale	Gray	Mottled
Skin turgor	Decreased	Poor	Very poor
Mucous membranes	Dry	Very dry	Parched
Urine output	Decreased	Oliguria	Marked oliguria and azotemia
Blood pressure	Normal	Normal or lowered	Lowered
Pulse	Normal or increased	Increased	Rapid and thready

tion in their consistency with an increase in fluid content, and (3) a tendency for the stools to be greenish in color.

Diarrhea may be acute or chronic, inflammatory or noninflammatory, and the physiologic consequences vary considerably in relation to its severity, duration, associated symptoms, the age of the child, and the child's nutritional status before the onset of diarrhea.

Etiology

Diarrhea can be attributed to a large number of specific causes, mechanisms, and predisposing factors. Factors that predispose a child to diarrhea and its physiologic consequences include: (1) the younger the child, the more susceptible he is to diarrhea and the more severe the diarrhea is likely to be; (2) children who are malnourished or debilitated from disease are more susceptible to diarrhea; (3) warm climates (and warm weather) where sanitation and refrigeration are a problem promote growth of bacteria; and (4) crowded and substandard environment with poor facilities for preparation and refrigeration of food contribute to contamination.

Specific causes. A variety of factors can produce diarrhea in the infant or child either as the presenting symptom or as an associated symptom. Often a specific etiologic diagnosis is lacking. *Acute* diarrhea, a sudden change in frequency and consistency of stools, is more often caused by an inflammatory process of infectious origin but may also be the result of a toxic reaction to ingestion of poisons, dietary indiscretions, or infection outside the alimentary tract, for example, communicable diseases, infections of the respiratory or urinary tracts, and emotional tension. Most are self-limited and will ultimately subside without specific treatment if consequent dehydration does not create a serious complication.

Chronic diarrhea, the passage of loose stools with increased frequency that lasts for more than 2 weeks, is more apt to be associated with disorders of malabsorption, anatomic defects, abnormal bowel motility, hypersensitivity (allergic) reaction, or an inflammatory response.

Diarrheal disturbances can involve the stomach and intestine *(gastroenteritis)*, the small intestine *(enteritis)*, the colon *(colitis)*, or the colon and intestine *(enterocolitis)*. *Dysentery* is a term that describes intestinal inflammation, especially of the colon, that is accompanied by cramping abdominal pain, tenesmus, and watery stools, containing blood and mucus. Enteropathologic organisms are frequent causes of diarrhea in infancy and childhood and are further discussed in relation to gastroenteritis (p. 747).

Common causes of diarrhea are dietary indiscretions (e.g., green apples or fruits in large amounts), food sensitivities, and high osmolar formulas in infancy. Also sorbitol, the sweetener used in some "sugar free" gum and other products, is poorly absorbed in the gastrointestinal tract and may produce osmotic diarrhea if ingested in large amounts.

Pathophysiology

Invasion of the gastrointestinal tract by pathogens produces diarrhea by (1) production of enterotoxins that stimulate secretion of water and electrolytes, (2) direct invasion and destruction of intestinal epithelial cells, and (3) local inflammation and systemic invasion by the organisms. However, the most serious and immediate physiologic disturbances associated with severe diarrheal disease are (1) dehydration, (2) acid-base derangements with acidosis, and (3) shock that occurs when dehydration progresses to the point that circulatory status is seriously disturbed.

Diagnostic Evaluation

The history provides valuable information regarding exposure to infectious agents, personal contact, travel, or probable contact with contaminated foods. Allergic and dietary history may indicate food allergies.

The age of the child provides clues to the cause of diarrheal disturbances. For example, milk allergy or intolerance of other formula constituents is suspected in early infancy. In later infancy new foods added to the diet are frequent offenders. Parenteral infections are very common causes of diarrhea in infancy. Most acute, inflammatory diarrheas are infectious, and the type of stools and symptoms associated with diarrhea provide clues to the organism (see p. 748).

The clinical manifestations of diarrhea are outlined in the accompanying box. Manifestations of severe diarrhea are primarily those of dehydration (see dehydration). Although vomiting may occur in all infectious diarrheas, it is not a major feature.

Although the child may not gain weight or may even show a slight loss in mild diarrhea, signs of dehydration are usually absent. If the diarrhea persists, if the child

Clinical Manifestations of Diarrhea

- Mild diarrhea—few loose stools each day without other evidence of illness
- Moderate diarrhea—several loose or watery stools daily
  - Elevated temperature, often
  - Vomiting
  - Fretfulness and irritability
  - Signs of dehydration usually absent, although may not gain weight or may even show weight loss
- Severe diarrhea—numerous to continuous stools
  - Signs of moderate to severe dehydration evident (see Table 23-1)
  - Drawn, flaccid expressions
  - Eyes lack luster
  - Cry lacks vigor, is often whining and higher pitched than usual
  - Irritable
  - Seeks comfort and attention of parent
  - Displays purposeless movements and inappropriate responses to people and familiar things
  - May become lethargic, moribund, or comatose

loses weight, if there is blood in the stools, or if the child develops associated signs such as deep breathing, listlessness, or reduced urinary output that may signal complications, the child should be seen by the physician.

Laboratory examination. Stools are examined for pH, blood, and evidence of bacterial invasion. The stool specimen obtained from evacuated stool should include mucus or tissue shreds, if present. The specimen is examined with indicator paper for pH, and a Clinitest tablet will detect the acid stool containing sugar that is characteristic of disaccharide intolerance. Bulky stools containing fat suggest malabsorption diarrhea.

The specimen is also examined for the presence of red blood cells. Serum electrolyte values are obtained in the young infant who is hospitalized with diarrhea because of the likelihood of complicating dehydration and associated electrolyte imbalances, particularly in relation to sodium and potassium alterations. Dehydrated infants will have an elevated hematocrit as a result of volume loss, and an elevated blood urea nitrogen will be found in the presence of reduced renal circulation.

Therapeutic Management

Medical management is directed at correcting the fluid imbalance and treating the underlying cause. The therapeutic plan must consider the degree of dehydration, the type of dehydration, and associated electrolyte (especially serum potassium) and acid-base imbalances. Initial and regular ongoing evaluations are carried out to assess the patient's progress toward equilibrium and the effectiveness of therapy.

Mild or moderate diarrhea. Mild or moderate diarrhea is usually managed by simple measures and seldom requires hospitalization. When the moderate diarrhea becomes worse or does not respond to simple measures, hospitalization is indicated.

When the child is alert, awake, and not in shock dehydration can be corrected with oral fluid administration. Most dehydration is mild and can be managed at home by this method. Several oral rehydration solutions (ORS) are available for rapid rehydration. Amounts and rates are calculated according to body weight and degree of dehydration, and are increased if rehydration is incomplete or if excess losses continue. When oral rehydration is complete, maintenance therapy is begun, although full diet is usually withheld until the child is well hydrated and the basic problem is under control.

Parenteral fluid therapy is instigated whenever the child is unable to ingest sufficient amounts of fluid and electrolytes to (1) meet ongoing daily physiologic losses, (2) replace previous deficits, and (3) replace ongoing abnormal losses. Patients who usually require intravenous fluids are those with severe dehydration, those with uncontrollable vomiting, those who are unable to drink for any reason (such as extreme fatigue or coma), and those with severe gastric distention.

Severe diarrhea. Severe diarrhea is largely a problem of infants and very young children, and, regardless of the cause, successful management relies primarily on appropriate treatment of physiologic disturbances and is only secondarily concerned with specific treatment of the causative agent. Severe diarrhea warrants hospitalization, comprehensive evaluation, and parenteral fluid therapy. Fluid therapy is directed toward replacement of (1) the fluid deficit as determined by weight loss and clinical signs, (2) ongoing normal losses from urine, lungs, and sweat, and (3) continued abnormal gastrointestinal losses.

Intravenous administration of fluid is begun immediately, and the solution selected based on what is known regarding the probable type and cause of the dehydration—usually a saline solution. Sodium bicarbonate may be added, since acidosis is usually associated with severe dehydration, but potassium is not administered until kidney function is restored. Although the initial phase of fluid replacement is rapid in both isotonic and hypotonic dehydration, it is contraindicated in hypertonic dehydration because of the risk of water intoxication, especially in the brain cells.

Once the severe effects of dehydration are under control, specific diagnostic and therapeutic measures are instigated to detect and treat the cause of the diarrhea. This includes mild sedation, antimicrobial therapy where indicated, and treatment of secondary effects of the illness or its therapy. For example, secondary bacterial growth may be countered with a short course of nonabsorbable antibiotics and/or the oral administration of lactobacilli to recolonize the normal flora of the gastrointestinal tract.

Nursing Considerations

Nursing observation and care are essential to the management of diarrheal disease. Most of the management is directed toward evaluation and management of dehydration (see p. 741), and may include specific nursing considerations related to any etiology.

ASSESSMENT

The nursing assessment of diarrhea begins with observation of the infant's or child's general appearance and behavior. The physical assessment includes all the parameters described for assessment of dehydration (p. 740). A history provides valuable information regarding probable etiologic agents, such as introduction of a new food, exposure to infectious agents, travel to an area of high susceptibility, contact with foods that might be contaminated, and contact with pets that are known to be sources of enteric infections. Allergic and dietary history may indicate food allergies.

NURSING DIAGNOSES

Several nursing diagnoses become apparent based on a thorough physical assessment. The major diagnoses appropriate for the infant or child are described in the Nursing Care Plan on p. 745. Other diagnoses will be evident depending on the age, condition, and etiology of the diarrhea.

PLANNING

The goals of nursing care for the dehydrated infant or child are:

1. Provide fluid to replace losses, prevent further fluid losses, and meet ongoing fluid requirements
2. Provide nutrition appropriate to age and condition of the child
3. Prevent spread of diarrhea (if infectious etiology)
4. Prevent complications
5. Support and educate child and family

IMPLEMENTATION

Mild or moderate diarrhea is usually managed at home under the supervision of the nurse. The parents are allowed to give fluids to the child. Fluids are usually tolerated best at room temperature, and the parent is cautioned against giving other than those prescribed by the physician. The ORS is usually well accepted by infants, but older children find them unpalatable. Some type of flavoring may improve the taste.

When the diet is advanced to include clear liquids, diluted fruit juice, liquid or solid Jell-O, sweetened tea, Popsicles, and decarbonated cola or ginger ale are well tolerated. Broth or other high-sodium liquids are used with caution to avoid the possibility of hypernatremia. Diet consistent with the age and condition of the child is allowed when liquids are well tolerated, as evidenced by no vomiting and an increased consistency and decrease in number of stools. Appropriate soft foods include gelatin desserts, soups (not creamed), bananas, applesauce, strained carrots, crackers (including pretzels), rice, and toast with jelly. Because mucosal damage interferes with digestion and absorption of lactose for a time, milk and lactose-containing formulas are usually withheld for infants with severe diarrhea until return of normal function. Soybean formulas (such as Isomil and ProSobee) or hydrolyzed protein formulas with nonlactose sugar (such as Nutramigen or Pregestimil) are substituted until the gastrointestinal tract is again able to tolerate milk and milk products.

> ### *Nursing Tip: Decarbonating Beverages*
>
> To decarbonate beverages, pour the beverage into a cup and place in a microwave oven for 15 seconds. Allow the beverage to cool before serving it.

Severe diarrhea. The infant or child admitted to the hospital with diarrhea is usually isolated from children who do not have diarrhea, and appropriate precautions are implemented to prevent possible spread to other patients and personnel. Each hospital has a policy regarding necessary precautions.

The child is weighed on admission and frequently during the initial rehydration period. Accurate intake and output measurement is imperative, and (if needed) a urine collection bag is placed to determine the volume of output, to measure specific gravity, and as an indication that renal blood flow is sufficient to permit administration of potassium. Unless urine is separated from stool, this essential information cannot be obtained.

Children who are sufficiently ill to require hospitalization are almost always placed on parenteral fluid therapy with nothing by mouth for 12 to 48 hours, although this varies with institutions and practitioners. Monitoring the intravenous infusion is a primary nursing function, with careful attention to ascertain that the correct fluid and electrolyte concentration is infused, the flow rate is adjusted to deliver the desired volume in a given period of time, and the intravenous site is maintained. Restraint of some type is needed with infants and small children, whose purposeful or random movements might disturb the needle placement.

The nurse is responsible for examination of stools and the collection of specimens for laboratory examination. Care is exerted in obtaining and transporting stools to prevent possible spread of infection. Stool specimens are transported to the laboratory in appropriate containers and media according to hospital policy. A clean tongue depressor can be used to obtain specimens for laboratory examination when a larger volume is needed or as an applicator for transfer to a culture medium. Tests for pH, blood, and sugar can be done without removing the stool from the diaper.

Since diarrheal stools are highly irritating to the skin, extra care is needed to protect the skin of the diaper region from becoming excoriated. The diaper area should be bathed frequently. A gentle cleansing with mild soap and warm water followed by thorough rinsing and drying after each stool is ideal.

Exposing the reddened areas to heat and light is also an effective method to facilitate healing although difficult to accomplish in the home. In the hospital an excellent

> ### *Nursing Tip: Drying the Buttocks*
>
> Using a hair dryer on a low or cool setting is helpful for drying the skin of the diaper area.

> ### *Nursing Tip: Commercial Wipes*
>
> Many commercial baby wipes contain alcohol, which can sting. Therefore nurses and families should be cautioned against their use on excoriated or denuded areas of skin.

NURSING CARE PLAN

The Child with Gastroenteritis (Acute Diarrhea)

Nursing Goals	Nursing Interventions	Expected Patient/Family Outcomes
HP-HMP* Potential for infection **Risk factors: presence of infectious organisms**		
Prevent spread of infection	Isolate affected child from contact with others Implement protective techniques as dictated by hospital policy, including Disposal of excreta and laundry Appropriate handling of specimens Maintain careful handwashing Apply diaper snugly to reduce likelihood of fecal spread Instruct others (parents, members of staff) in protective procedures Teach affected children protective methods to prevent spread of infection, for example, remaining in restricted area, hand washing, handling genital area, care after using bedpan or toilet Endeavor to keep infants and small children from placing hand and objects in contaminated areas Assess home situation and implement protective measures as feasible in individual circumstances	Infection does not spread to others
HP-HMP Potential for trauma **Risk factors: therapies**		
Prevent complications from restraining devices	Remove restraints from extremities as often as possible Change position at least every 2 hours Frequently observe circulation, position, and pressure points	Extremities remain free of construction and pressure
Observe for signs of complications	Assess frequently Vital signs—temperature, pulse, respiration, and blood pressure Skin characteristics Sensory response Neurologic signs Behavior	Vital signs remain within normal limits for age (see inside front cover for normal variations)
N-MP Fluid volume deficit (2) **Etiology: excessive losses**		
Promote hydration	Offer appropriate fluids as tolerated	Child exhibits signs of adequate hydration (specify)
Assess progress of hydration	Maintain accurate record of intake Weigh child daily or as ordered Assess all parameters, for example, vital signs, skin characteristics Apply urine collection device when indicated Measure urine volume and specific gravity	
Prevent interference with therapeutic regimen	Apply appropriate restraining methods where indicated	†Therapy(ies) are maintained
N-MP Altered nutrition: less than body requirements **Risk factors: nothing by mouth, diarrheal losses**		
Reestablish diet appropriate for age	Gradually reintroduce foods as indicated (specify) Observe response to feedings Describe feeding behavior	Child takes prescribed nourishment †Observations are recorded accurately

*For an explanation of abbreviations, see p. 20.
†Nursing outcome.

Continued.

NURSING CARE PLAN

The Child with Gastroenteritis (Acute Diarrhea)—cont'd

Nursing Goals	Nursing Interventions	Expected Patient/Family Outcomes
NDx N-MP Altered oral mucous membranes **Risk factors: dehydration, nothing by mouth**		
Relieve dryness	Administer special mouth care while fluids by mouth are restricted	Mucous membranes remain moist and clean
NDx N-MP Potential impaired skin integrity **Risk factors: frequent loose stools**		
Prevent skin breakdown	Change diaper and wash and dry area thoroughly after each soiling Cleanse buttocks and genital area well Apply protective lotion or ointment Expose reddened area to heat and air where feasible (risk of contamination great in explosive diarrhea)	Skin exhibits no evidence of discoloration or irritation
NDx EP Diarrhea **Etiology: inflammation, irritation**		
Assess status of diarrhea	Record urine output Record fecal output—number, volume, characteristics Observe and record presence of associated signs—tenesmus, cramping, vomiting	†Extent of intestinal losses is determined
NDx SP-SCP Anxiety/fear **Etiology: separation from parents, strange environment, distressing procedures**		
Provide comfort measures	Provide pacifier for infants who are receiving nothing by mouth Bubble child periodically to help expel swallowed air Hold infant or child when this does not interfere with therapy Touch, talk, and otherwise comfort child who cannot be held Provide sensory stimulation and diversion appropriate to child's level of development Encourage family members to visit and allow them to comfort and care for child to the extent possible	Child engages in nonnutritive sucking Child exhibits no signs of distress
NDx RRP Altered family processes **Etiology: situational crisis (child's illness and/or hospitalization), knowledge deficit**		
Support family	Reassure family, especially mother Explain therapeutic measures that may be distressing to family Nothing by mouth Parenteral fluids Restraints necessary Shaving of infant's head for intravenous therapy Isolation from other children Need for precautions that family must observe Help family provide comfort and support for child See also The family of the hospitalized child, p. 610.	Family displays an understanding of the child's condition and therapies and becomes actively involved in physical and emotional care
Educate family	Instruct in diet planning (see general plan for dietary management, which follows) Help caregiver plan diet to meet needs of affected child in relation to family diet plan Instruct in preparation and storage of food, based on assessment of individual family needs and facilities Instruct in care and disposal of waste materials Teach and emphasize importance of good hygiene and sanitation	Family demonstrates and understands child's care and management (specify)

†Nursing outcome.

NURSING CARE PLAN

The Child with Gastroenteritis (Acute Diarrhea)—cont'd

Nursing Goals	Nursing Interventions	Expected Patient/Family Outcomes
Arrange for follow-up care	Emphasize importance of posthospitalization health assessment Refer to community health agency for care and instruction when indicated	Family complies with instructions

Nursing interventions related to medical management

Rehydrate child
- Administer fluids as ordered
  - Intravenous
    - Administer correct fluid
    - Maintain desired drip rate
    - Add appropriate electrolytes as prescribed
    - Maintain integrity of infusion site
  - Oral
    - Feed electrolyte-containing solutions as prescribed

Eradicate infectious agent
- Administer antimicrobial medications as prescribed
- Administer other medications as prescribed

Assess progress of diarrhea
- Collect specimens as needed
- Make appropriate diagnostic tests and record
  - Stools—pH, blood, sugar, frequency
  - Urine—pH, specific gravity, frequency

Detect source of infection
- Examine other members of household and refer for treatment where indicated
  - Collect stool specimens from household members where indicated

way to provide dry heat to the area is by means of a goose-necked lamp, but the lamp must be placed at a distance sufficient that the child is unable to reach any part of it. The heat source should be no closer than 18 inches. The child will require close observation during treatment, and the length of each application should not exceed 20 minutes.

Support for the child and family involves the same care and consideration as for all children. The child who is restrained to maintain an intravenous infusion must have the restraints removed periodically (under supervision). An intravenous insertion site that is well-situated allows for the child to be held and comforted with only moderate adjustment. The tenuously situated intravenous presents more complex problems (see p. 670). Alternative means for providing comfort include sensory contact, visual and auditory stimulation with environmental decoration, situating the bed for maximum view of the environment and encouraging family and others to be physically involved with the child. Parents are kept informed of the child's progress and instructed in special care behaviors such as handwashing.

EVALUATION

The effectiveness of nursing interventions is determined by continued reassessment according to the following observational guidelines and expected outcomes:

1. Monitor fluid losses with careful intake and output measurements and daily weights
2. Monitor food intake
3. Observe for evidence of complications from underlying disease (specify) and/or therapy
4. Observe and interview family to determine extent and effectiveness of care

Expected outcomes:
See Nursing Care Plan, pp. 745 to 747.

ACUTE INFECTIOUS GASTROENTERITIS

When diarrhea is presumed or established to be caused by a microorganism, the terms *infectious gastroenteritis* or *bacterial gastroenteritis* are applied. In the pediatric age-group infectious gastroenteritis is second only to upper respiratory tract infections as a cause of illness. Although they are ordinarily benign and self-limited, they are a major pediatric problem and account for a significant number of hospital admissions.

Etiology/Epidemiology

Most organisms that cause diarrhea are spread by the fecal-oral route. Some are transmitted by direct person-to-person contact, especially where sizable groups are in direct contact such as in daycare centers. Viral disease is more frequent in winter months; bacterial disorders are more prevalent during summer and fall. Although acute gastroenteritis affects all age groups, there is a greater frequency of diarrheal disease in younger children; *E. coli* is the prominent pathogen in the newborn; rotaviruses are the most common cause of winter diarrhea in children younger than 2 years; and, *Shigella* is a common

TABLE 23-2

Enteropathologic Causes of Infectious Gastroenteritis

Organism	Characteristics/Manifestations	Comments
Viral Agents		
Rotavirus Incubation period: 2-3 days	Abrupt onset Fever (38° C or above) lasting approximately 48 hours Associated upper respiratory tract infection Diarrhea may persist for more than a week	Incidence higher in cool weather (80% in winter) Affects all age groups; 6- to 24-month-old infants more vulnerable Usually mild and self-limited
Norwalk-like organisms Incubation period: 1-2 days	Fever Loss of appetite Nausea/vomiting Abdominal pain Diarrhea Malaise	Source of infection: drinking water, recreation water, food (including shellfish) Affects all ages Benign; seldom lasts more than 3 days Self-limited
Bacterial Agents		
Pathogenic		
Escherichia coli Incubation period: highly variable	Onset gradual or abrupt Variable clinical manifestations Moist—green, watery diarrhea with mucus; becomes explosive Vomiting may be present from onset Abdominal distention Diarrhea Fever; appears toxic	Incidence higher in summer Usually interpersonal transmission but may transmit via inanimate objects A cause of nursery epidemics With symptomatic treatment only, may continue for weeks Full breast-feeding has a protective effect Symptoms generally subside in 3-7 days Relapse rate approximately 20%
Salmonella groups (nontyphoidae)—gram-negative, nonencapsulated, nonsporulating Incubation period: 6-72 hours for intraluminal 7-21 days for extraluminal	Rapid onset Variable symptoms—mild to severe Nausea, vomiting, and colicky abdominal pain followed by diarrhea, occasionally with blood and mucus Chills not uncommon Hyperactive peristalsis and mild abdominal tenderness Symptoms usually subside within 5 days May have fever, headache, and cerebral manifestations, e.g., drowsiness, confusion, meningismus, or seizures Infants may be afebrile and nontoxic May result in life-threatening septicemia and meningitis	Two thirds of patients are younger than 20 years of age Highest incidence in children younger than 9 years of age, especially infants More prevalent July through October, lowest from January through April Transmission primarily via contaminated food and drink Most common sources are poultry and eggs In children—pets, e.g., dogs, cats, hamsters, and especially pet turtles Communicable as long as organisms are excreted
S. typhi	Variable in infants Older children—irregular fever, headache, malaise, lethargy Diarrhea occurs in 50% at early stage Cough is common In a few days, fever rises and is consistent; fatigue, cough, abdominal pain, anorexia, and weight loss develop; diarrhea begins	Rapid invasion of bloodstream from minor sites of inflammation Decreased incidence in last decade Acute symptoms may persist for a week or more
Shigella groups—gram-negative, nonmotile, anaerobic bacilli Incubation period: 1-7 days	Onset variable but usually abrupt Fever and cramping abdominal pain initially Fever—may reach 40.5° C Convulsions in about 10%—usually associated with fever Patient appears sick Headache, nuchal rigidity, delirium	Approximately 60% of cases in children younger than age 9 years with more than one third between ages 1 and 4 years Peak incidence late summer Transmitted directly or indirectly from infected persons Communicable for 1-4 weeks
Vibrio cholerae (cholera) groups Incubation period: usually 1-3 days; range from few hours to 5 days	Sudden onset of profuse, watery diarrhea without cramping, tenesmus, or anal irritation, although children may complain of cramping Stools are intermittent at first, then almost continuous Stools are whitish, almost clear, with flecks of mucus—"rice water stools"	Rare in infants younger than 1 year old Mortality high in both treated and untreated infants and small children Transmitted via contaminated food and water Attack confers immunity

TABLE 23-2

Enteropathologic Causes of Infectious Gastroenteritis—cont'd

Organism	Characteristics/Manifestations	Comments
Food Poisoning		
Staphylococcus Incubation period: 4-6 hours	Nausea, vomiting Severe abdominal cramps Profuse diarrhea Shock may occur in severe cases May be a mild fever	Transferred via contaminated food—inadequately cooked or refrigerated, e.g., custards, mayonnaise, cream-filled or -topped desserts Self-limited; improvement apparent within 24 hours Excellent prognosis
Clostridium perfringens Incubation period: 8-24 hours	Moderate to severe crampy, midepigastric pain	Self-limited illness Transmission by commercial food products—most often meat and poultry
Botulism		
Clostridium botulinum Incubation period: 12 hr–3 days	Nausea, vomiting Diarrhea CNS symptoms with curarelike effect (see p. 000) Dry mouth, dysphagia	Transmitted by contaminated food products Variable severity—mild symptoms to rapidly fatal within a few hours Antitoxin administration

pathogen in toddlers 13 to 24 months old. The chance of *C. jejuni* being the cause of illness is greater in older children, and the Norwalk-like viruses are a frequent cause of epidemics in school-age children (Guerran, Lohr, and Williams, 1986). Daycare centers are a prime source of infection in younger children, especially centers that care for children in diapers. Sexually active adolescents are subject to enteric pathogens that are transmitted by sexual contact, and traveler's diarrhea is a common problem for some persons traveling to other countries.

Organisms that are considered "normal flora" in most situations are enteropathic under certain conditions and in susceptible children, particularly newborn and young infants. For example, some strains of *E. coli* produce diarrhea by invasion of the intestinal mucosa, and others by elaboration of enterotoxins. *S. aureus* can cause diarrhea by (1) food poisoning from contamination (especially milk or egg products) with exotoxin production, (2) enteritis as a result of prolonged broad-spectrum antibiotic therapy that destroys and eliminates enteric organisms that normally control staphylococcal invasion, (3) enteritis as a complication of staphylococcal infection elsewhere (skin or lungs), and (4) primary staphylococcal infection in newborn infants who have not yet established competing enteric flora.

The enteropathic organisms are briefly outlined in Table 23-2. Other agents such as *Pseudomonas, Klebsiella,* and *Proteus* may cause diarrhea but do not ordinarily have a tendency to do so. Amebic dysentery seldom occurs in infants.

Diagnostic Evaluation

Infectious diarrheas have some features in common, such as vomiting, and frequently there is abdominal discomfort. Bacterial infections and some viral infections are accompanied by fever. The manifestations and severity are variable among the various forms (see Table 23-1). Laboratory confirmation of the specific organism confirms the diagnosis and serves as a guideline for appropriate medical therapy.

Therapeutic Management

The primary concern in infectious gastroenteritis, as in all conditions in which fluid is lost in large amounts, is dehydration and the attendant deterioration. Fluid replacement and monitoring of electrolyte status with replacement are the same as for any diarrheal disorder. When the organism is identified appropriate antibiotics are prescribed for those diarrheas for which specific therapy has been found to be effective.

Nursing Considerations

Basic nursing care for the infant or child with infectious gastroenteritis is the same as for any diarrheal disease. However, appropriate isolation precautions are carried out to prevent the spread of the infection to others.

It may be necessary to obtain stool specimens from the child and other family members who are affected or suspected to be carriers of infectious organisms. The parents are provided with specimen containers and instructed in collection and disposition of stool samples.

There are some medications that appear to be safe for adults in preventing traveler's diarrhea; however, parents should be cautioned against giving any of the drugs to children. Until vaccines or other prophylactic measures are proved safe for children, the best prevention is to allow children to drink only bottled water and carbonated beverages (from the container through a straw supply brought from home). Tap water, ice, unpasteurized dairy products, raw vegetables, and unpeeled fruits should be avoided. Meats and seafoods may be risky as well.

CONSTIPATION

Constipation can be a symptom of a number of abdominal disorders, primarily those that cause an obstruction in the lower intestinal tract, such as Hirschsprung disease or imperforate anus. Physical and mental disorders are often associated with defecation problems, for example, neurologic or anatomic disorders, mental retardation, hypothyroidism, and hypercalcemia. The apparent difficulty in passing stools is not a reliable sign, especially in infancy. The development and course of constipation can be influenced by a number of familial, cultural, and social factors. Psychologic factors, as well as toilet-training techniques, diet, overuse of laxatives, and enemas play an important role in bowel habits.

Newborn

Normally the newborn infant passes a first meconium stool within 24 to 36 hours of birth. Any infant who does not do so should be assessed for evidence of intestinal atresia or stenosis, congenital aganglionic megacolon (50% of cases), hypothyroidism, meconium plugs, or meconium ileus. *Meconium plugs* are caused by meconium that has reduced water content and are usually evacuated following digital examination but may require irrigations of normal saline or the iodinated contrast medium diatrizoate meglumine *(Gastrografin)*.

Meconium ileus, the initial manifestation of cystic fibrosis, is the presence of thick, mucilagenous meconium that clings to the abdominal wall making it difficult, if not impossible, to pass. Treatment is the same as for a meconium plug. Rarely, surgical intervention may be necessary.

Infancy

Medical causes such as Hirschsprung disease, hypothyroidism, and strictures must be ruled out in chronic cases of constipation. However, the most frequent cause in infancy is dietary mismanagement. It is almost unknown in breast-fed infants who typically have fewer stools than bottle-fed infants. Constipation may accompany a change from human milk or modified cow's milk to whole cow's milk.

Simple measures ordinarily correct the problem, such as increasing the amount of fluid in the formula in the very young infant, adding or increasing the amount of cereal, vegetables, and fruit in the diet of the older infant. Very dilute fruit can be given to younger infants.

Childhood

Children between 1 and 3 years of age are most likely to have constipation, usually due to enviromental changes. It may be the result of some medications (e.g., iron preparations, diuretics, antacids, or anticonvulsant agents). If there are associated manifestations, such as vomiting, abdominal distention or pain, and evidence of growth failure, the condition merits further investigation.

The management of simple constipation consists of a plan to keep the bowel relatively empty of stool, and dietary management to prevent further constipation. There is not total agreement on the most effective means to clean the bowel, although most agree that the use of laxatives is not usually recommended because of their tendency to create dependency. Enemas are sometimes used to empty the bowel and repeated if voluntary evacuation does not occur within 48 hours.

In addition, increasing intake of fluids and implementing a high-fiber diet (including supplemental bran, if needed) are advised. Any foods known to be constipating are eliminated. Sometimes a stool softener such as dioctyl sodium sulfosuccinate (Colace) is of benefit.

Nursing Considerations

Constipation, unfortunately, tends to be self-perpetuating. If the child has difficulty or discomfort when attempting to evacuate his bowels he has a tendency to retain the bowel contents, and thus begins a vicious cycle. Nursing assessment begins with an accurate history of bowel habits, diet, events that may be associated with the onset of constipation, drugs or other substances that the child may be taking, and the consistency, color, frequency, and other characteristics of the stool. If there is no evidence of a pathologic condition that requires further investigation, the major task of the nurse is to educate the parents regarding normal stool patterns and to relieve the cause of the constipation.

Dietary modifications are usually essential in preventing constipation. During infancy simply increasing the carbohydrate (sugar or corn syrup) in an infant formula will often relieve the problem. During childhood the diet should contain increased amounts of fiber and fluid. Par-

TABLE 23-3

High-Fiber Foods

Food Group	Selections
Bread, grains	Whole-grain bread or rolls Whole-grain cereals Bran Pancakes, waffles and muffins with fruit or bran Unrefined (brown) rice
Vegetables	Raw vegetables, especially broccoli, cabbage, carrots, cauliflower, celery, lettuce, and spinach Cooked vegetables, such as those listed above and asparagus, beans, brussels sprouts, corn, potatoes, rhubarb, squash, string beans, turnips
Fruits	Raw fruits, especially those with skins or seeds, other than ripe banana or avocado Raisins, prunes, or other dried fruits
Miscellaneous	Nuts, seeds, legumes, popcorn

ents will benefit from guidance in dietary planning especially regarding foods that facilitate bowel movements (see Table 23-3). They will need reassurance concerning the benign nature of the condition. It is important to discuss with them their attitudes and expectations regarding toilet habits and to discourage the use of stool softeners, laxatives, and enemas. If such measures have been prescribed by a physician they should understand that these are merely temporary measures and not to be continued beyond the current need.

HIRSCHSPRUNG DISEASE

Hirschsprung disease (congenital aganglionic megacolon) is a mechanical obstruction caused by inadequate motility in part of the intestine. It accounts for about one fourth of all cases of neonatal obstruction, although it may not be diagnosed until later in infancy or childhood. It is four times more common in males than females, follows a familial pattern in a small number of cases, and is considerably more common in children with Down syndrome. Depending on its presentation, it may be an acute, life-threatening condition or a chronic disorder.

Pathophysiology

The term *congenital aganglionic megacolon* describes the pathology. The primary defect is absence of parasympathetic ganglion cells in one segment of colon. The functional defect as a result of lack of innervation is absence of propulsive movements (peristalsis), causing accumulation of intestinal contents and distention of the bowel proximal to the defect, hence the term "megacolon," or large colon. In addition there is failure of the internal rectal sphincter to relax, which prevents evacuation of solids, liquids, and gas and, thus, contributes to the manifestations of obstruction (Fig. 23-1).

Diagnostic Evaluation

Clinical manifestations vary according to the age when symptoms are first recognized and the presence of complications, such as enterocolitis (see box). In the neonate diagnosis is usually made based on clinical signs of intestinal obstruction and failure to pass meconium. Radiographs, barium enema, and anorectal manometric examinations assist in the differential diagnosis, which is then confirmed by histologic examination of a full-thickness rectal biopsy demonstrating absence of ganglia.

Therapeutic Management

Treatment is primarily surgical to remove the aganglionic portion of the bowel in order to permit normal bowel motility and establish continence by improved functioning of the internal anal sphincter. In most cases this is accomplished in three stages. First, a temporary colostomy of the sigmoid or transverse colon is performed to allow the normal bowel a period of time to rest and resume its normal caliber and tonicity.

Second, complete correction is accomplished with a pull-through anastomosis of the bowel, which consists of "pulling" the end of functioning ganglionated bowel down to a point near the rectum from which it can propel stool through the anus. In many cases a sphincterotomy of the internal sphincter is performed to improve anal control. Third, closure of the colostomy is usually performed within a few months to a year.

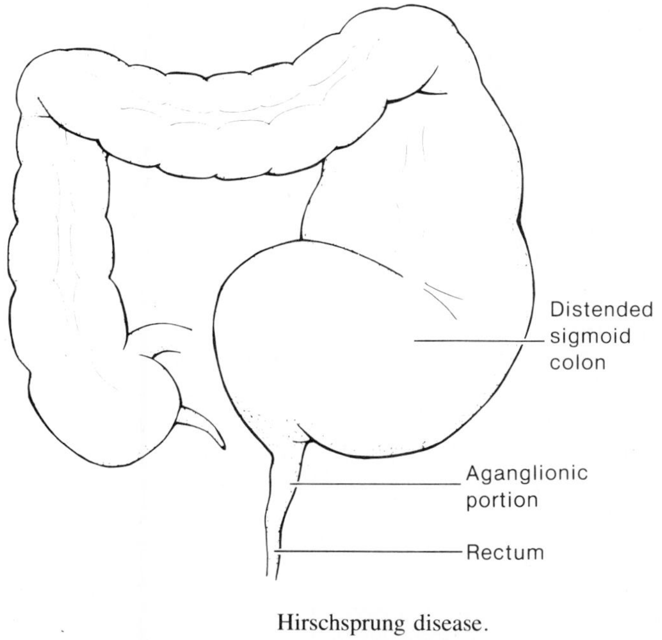

FIG. 23-1 Hirschsprung disease.

Clinical Manifestations of Hirschsprung Disease

Newborn period
- Failure to pass meconium within 24 to 48 hours after birth
- Reluctance to ingest fluids
- Bile-stained vomitus
- Abdominal distention

Infancy
- Failure to thrive
- Constipation
- Abdominal distention
- Episodes of diarrhea and vomiting
- Ominous signs (often signify the presence of enterocolitis)
  - Explosive, watery diarrhea
  - Fever
  - Severe prostration

Childhood (symptoms more chronic)
- Constipation
- Ribbonlike, foul-smelling stools
- Abdominal distention
- Visible peristalsis
- Fecal masses easily palpable
- Child usually poorly nourished and anemic

Nursing Considerations

Many of the nursing concerns depend on the child's age and the type of treatment. If the disorder is diagnosed during the neonatal period, the main objectives are: (1) to help the parents adjust to a congenital defect in their child, (2) to foster infant-parent bonding, (3) to prepare them for the medical/surgical intervention, and (4) to assist them in colostomy care after discharge.

Preoperative care. Much of the child's preoperative care depends on his age and clinical condition. If the child is malnourished, he may not be able to withstand surgery until his physical status improves. Often this involves symptomatic treatment with enemas, a low-fiber, high-calorie and high-protein diet, and, in severe situations, the use of parenteral alimentation.

Physical preoperative preparation entails the same measures that are common to any surgery (p. 630). In the newborn, whose bowel is sterile, no additional preparation is necessary. However, in other children emptying the bowel with repeated saline enemas and decreasing bacterial flora with systemic antibiotics and colonic irrigations using antibiotic solution are usually ordered. A nasogastric tube is sometimes inserted to prevent abdominal distention, and antibiotic solution may be instilled through the tube to further prepare the gastrointestinal tract. The nurse records all intake and output of irrigant and drainage, noting particularly any marked discrepancy in retention or loss of fluid.

Since progressive distention of the abdomen is a serious sign, the nurse measures abdominal circumference with a paper tape measure at the level of the umbilicus. The point of measurement is marked with a pen to assure reliability of subsequent measurements. As a rule of thumb, abdominal measurement can be performed at the same time that vital signs are taken, and recorded in serial order so that a change will be readily apparent.

> ### *Nursing Tip: Abdominal Circumference Measurements*
>
> In order to reduce any stress to the acutely ill child when frequent measurements of abdominal circumference are needed, the tape measure can be left in place beneath the child, rather than removed each time.

The age of the child dictates the type and extent of psychologic preparation necessary for child and parents. Since a colostomy is usually performed, the child who is of at least preschool age is told about the procedure in concrete terms, with the use of visual aids (see p. 684 for preparing a child for a colostomy). It is important to space explanations in order to prevent the anxiety and confusion that could result from too much information.

It is important to stress to parents and older children that the colostomy for Hirschsprung disease is temporary, unless so much bowel is involved that a permanent ileostomy must be performed. In most instances the physician is fairly certain of the extent of bowel resection prior to surgery, although the nurse should be aware of those instances when there is doubt concerning repair. The nurse should also keep in mind that, although a temporary colostomy is favorable in terms of future health and adjustment, it also requires additional surgery, which may be very stressful to parents and children.

Postoperative care. Postoperative care is the same as for any child or infant with abdominal surgery (p. 630). When a colostomy is part of the corrective procedure, stomal care becomes a major nursing problem (p. 684). To prevent contamination of the abdominal wound with urine in the infant, the diaper should be pinned below the dressing. Sometimes a Foley catheter is used in the immediate postoperative period to divert the flow of urine away from the abdomen.

Discharge care. Postoperatively parents need instruction concerning colostomy care. Even a preschooler can be included in the care by handing articles to the parent, rolling up the colostomy bag after emptying, or applying cream to the surrounding skin. Although diagnosis of Hirschsprung disease is less frequent in school-age children or adolescents, if discovered in older children, they should be involved in colostomy care to the point of total responsibility.

Referral to a public health nurse establishes continuity of care, especially in relation to colostomy care and dietary management. The community nurse can also assist parents and children in anticipating subsequent surgery. Sometimes families require financial assistance and additional psychologic support. Therefore, a referral to a social worker or other service agency may be necessary.

VOMITING

Vomiting, a very common symptom in childhood, is usually of little concern. Often it is of a minor and temporary nature, but when vomiting is persistent and prolonged, the consequences to the infant or child can be rapid and serious. Vomiting in childhood can be caused by numerous intrinsic and extrinsic factors but is usually the result of readily detectable infections or psychologic causes.

Therapeutic Management

Medical management is directed toward detection and treatment of the cause of the vomiting and prevention of complications from the loss of fluid. Fluids are administered in the same manner and in a similar electrolyte composition to those administered in diarrhea (p. 743). Although most children respond well to these measures, centrally acting antiemetic drugs such as promethazine (Phenergan), diphenidol (Vontrol), or trimethobenzamide hydrochloride (Tigan) may be recommended. For children who are prone to motion sickness, it is often helpful to administer an appropriate dose of dimenhydrinate (Dramamine) before a journey.

Nursing Considerations

The major emphasis of nursing care of the vomiting infant or child is on observation and reporting of vomiting behavior and associated symptoms, and the implementation of measures to reduce the vomiting. Accurate assessment of the type of vomiting, the appearance of the vomitus, and the child's behavior associated with the vomiting greatly aids in establishing a diagnosis of disorders that have vomiting as a clinical feature.

Nursing interventions are determined by the cause of the vomiting. When the vomiting is identified as a manifestation of improper feeding methods, establishing proper techniques through teaching and example will ordinarily correct the situation. If the vomiting is assessed as a probable sign of a gastrointestinal obstruction, food is usually withheld or special feeding techniques are implemented. In situations in which vomiting is related to concurrent infection, dietary indiscretion, or emotional factors, efforts are directed toward maintaining hydration or preventing dehydration.

The thirst mechanism is the most sensitive guide to fluid needs, and ad libitum administration of a glucose-electrolyte solution to an alert child will restore water and electrolytes satisfactorily. It is important to include carbohydrate to spare body protein and to avoid ketosis resulting from exhaustion of glycogen stores. Once vomiting has abated, more liberal amounts of fluids can be offered, followed by simple foods such as gelatin, crackers, clear broth, and buttered toast in small portions, when the child desires, followed by gradual resumption of the regular diet.

GASTROESOPHAGEAL REFLUX

Gastroesophageal reflux (GER) (chalasia, cardiochalasia) is relaxation or incompetence of the lower esophageal sphincter, which results in frequent return of stomach contents into the esophagus. In newborns this is considered a normal phenomenon because of immature neuromuscular control of the gastroesophageal sphincter. However, in a small percentage of infants reflux continues, producing symptoms that warrant investigation. The exact cause is not known, although it is thought to result from delayed maturation of lower esophageal neuromuscular function or impaired local hormonal control mechanisms.

Clinical Manifestations of Gastroesophageal Reflux

Vomiting—can be quite forceful
Weight loss
Respiratory problems
Bleeding

Reflux of stomach contents to the pharynx predisposes to aspiration and the development of respiratory symptoms, particularly pneumonia. Repeated irritation of the esophageal lining with gastric acid can lead to esophagitis and subsequent bleeding. Blood loss produces anemia and is seen as hematemesis or melena (blood in stools). Heartburn is also a frequent symptom in older children who are able to describe it, but it may go unrecognized in infants.

Diagnostic Evaluation

In addition to a history, several tests are available to establish the presence of reflux: fluoroscopc observation of reflux following a barium swallow, manometry (which measures esophageal sphincter pressure), direct measurement of the pH of the distal esophagus, and scintigraphy (detects radioactive substances in the esophagus after a feeding of the compound).

Therapeutic Management

Therapeutic management of GER depends on its severity. No therapy is needed for the infant who is thriving. For the symptomatic child modification of feeding with small, frequent feedings of thickened formula and positioning may help minimize the symptoms until the child grows and a normal physiologic barrier to reflux develops.

Traditionally, the upright position (usually in an infant seat) has been recommended, but it has been demonstrated that, in infants less than 6 months of age, positioning the child prone with the head elevated at about a 30-degree angle for 24 hours a day, is more effective. The position can be maintained by use of an upper body harness (Fig. 23-2). The therapy is usually effective in approximately two weeks although it may require more lengthy treatment.

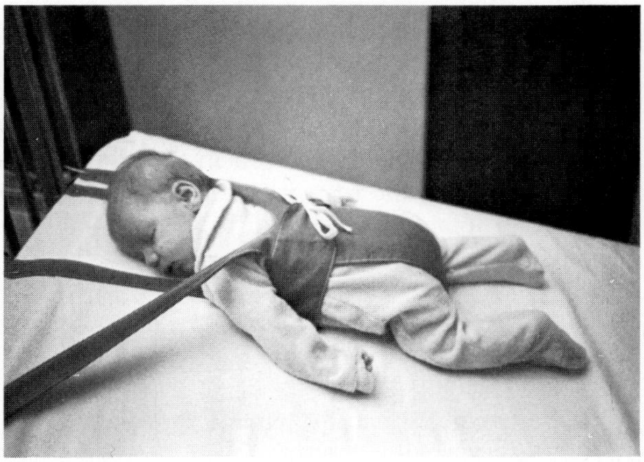

FIG. 23-2 Five-week-old infant positioned in harness. (From Orenstein, S.R., and Whitington, P.F.: Positioning for prevention of infant gastroesophageal reflux, J. Pediatr. **103:** 534-537, 1983.)

Drugs that promote gastric emptying and/or relax the pyloric sphincter are sometimes useful. Surgical intervention is selected for those children with severe complications, such as respiratory distress (choking, aspiration, recurrent apnea), esophagitis, or esophageal stricture. A commonly used surgical procedure is one that creates a valve mechanism at the distal esophagus.

Nursing Considerations

Nursing care is directed toward (1) identifying children with symptoms that suggest GER, (2) helping parents with positioning and feeding at home, (3) providing reassurance to parents regarding the usually benign nature of the condition, and (4) if appropriate, providing care for the child undergoing surgical repair.

To help parents cope with the inconvenience of dealing with a child who vomits frequently, simple measures such as using bibs and protective cloths during and after feeding are beneficial. The greatest challenge lies in maintaining the desired position for the child and adhering to a frequent feeding schedule. The 30-degree angle can be provided by elevating the head of the infant's crib with extra bedding, a wood or metal frame, or a wedge constructed from a cardboard box. An alternative is a specially constructed frame that can be moved about to allow the child a change of environment with minimum disturbance. The child is suspended from the head of the crib or frame in a prepared or improvised harness.

When the infant is older and more mobile, maintaining correct positioning becomes increasingly difficult. An alternative frame has been described that consists of a cradle bed, bassinet, or board with a firm wooden base and a wooden spindle or large dowel that protrudes through the center of the mattress. The infant is positioned prone with his legs straddling the well-padded spindle and secured to the mattress with a harness or folded diaper across his back and pinned to the mattress (Kurfiss-Daniels, 1982). To prevent undue pressure on areas such as the infant's knees and elbows the mattress is covered with a sheepskin or egg-crate pad.

Early in the treatment program both parents and other available family members should be encouraged to participate in the feeding regimen, especially with alternate night shifts. Nurses need to be sensitive to the demands placed on the family and recognize those situations when hospitalization may be required to ensure continued treatment.

◆ *Inflammatory Disorders*

Inflammatory conditions involving large or small segments of the gastrointestinal tract are not uncommon in childhood. They may be acute or chronic and some are more likely to affect one age-group more than another; for example, necrotizing enterocolitis is seen in the newborn, ulcerative colitis occurs most frequently in the prepubescent and adolescent child, whereas acute appendicitis presents at any age.

ACUTE APPENDICITIS

Appendicitis, inflammation of the vermiform appendix or blind sac at the end of the cecum, is the most common condition requiring abdominal surgery during childhood. Although rare in children younger than 2 years of age, it is associated with increased complications and mortality in this age-group. Primarily an acute condition, appendicitis rapidly progresses to perforation and peritonitis if it remains undiagnosed. It is a significant pediatric problem, because early diagnosis is frequently delayed as a result of the child's inability to verbalize his symptoms and the failure of professionals to interpret behavioral clues correctly.

Etiology

The exact cause of appendicitis is poorly understood but it is almost always a result of obstruction of the lumen, usually by a fecalith (a hard fecal concretion). Sometimes a fold of peritoneum causes the appendix to adhere to the cecum resulting in an obstructive kink. Other causes include lymphoid hyperplasia, fibrous stenosis from an earlier inflammation, and tumors. Although worms are frequently found in the appendix, their role in the pathology is unclear. There is mounting evidence that dietary habits play a role; children with diets high in fiber foods have a lower incidence of appendicitis than those whose fiber intake is low (Barker, Morris, and Nelson, 1986).

Pathophysiology

With acute obstruction the outflow of mucous secretions is blocked, pressure builds within the lumen, resulting in compression of blood vessels. The resulting ischemia is followed by ulceration of the epithelial lining and bacterial invasion. Subsequent necrosis causes perforation or rupture with fecal and bacterial contamination of the peritoneal cavity. The resulting inflammation spreads rapidly throughout the abdomen (*peritonitis*)—especially in young children who are unable to localize infection. Progressive peritoneal inflammation results in functional intestinal obstruction of the small bowel, since intense gastrointestinal reflexes severely inhibit bowel motility.

Diagnostic Evaluation

Diagnosis is based primarily on history and examination (see box). The white blood cell count is usually elevated but is seldom higher than 15,000 to 20,000/mm^3, and radiographic studies of the abdomen may reveal possible contributing causes of appendicitis, such as fecaliths or a foreign body.

Pain, the cardinal feature, is initially generalized (usually periumbilical); however it usually descends to the

Clinical Manifestations of Appendicitis

Colicky abdominal pain
Rebound tenderness
Fever
Rigid abdomen
Decreased or absent bowel sounds
Vomiting (commonly follows onset of pain)
Constipation or diarrhea may be present
Anorexia
Tachycardia, rapid shallow breathing
Pallor
Restlessness
Irritability

lower right quadrant. The most intense site of pain may be at McBurney point, located at a point midway between the anterior superior iliac crest and the umbilicus. Rebound tenderness is not a reliable sign and is extremely painful to the child. Referred pain, elicited by light percussion around the perimeter of the abdomen, indicates the presence of peritoneal irritation. Jarring on the heels or riding over bumps in an automobile or gurney aggravates the pain. In addition to pain, probably the most significant clinical manifestations are a change in behavior and anorexia.

Diagnosis is not always straightforward. Numerous infectious processes have features in common. For example, fever, vomiting, abdominal pain and elevated blood count are associated with inflammatory bowel disease, pelvic inflammatory disease, gastroenteritis, urinary tract infection, right lower lobe pneumonia, constipation, mesenteric adenitis, Meckel diverticulum, and intussusception. Also, diagnosis may be delayed in infants and small children because they do not localize infections well and can become sick more rapidly than older children. Consequently the risk of perforation is greater.

Therapeutic Management

The definitive treatment of appendicitis before perforation is surgical removal of the appendix (appendectomy). However, fluid and electrolyte imbalances need to be corrected before surgery since the child is likely to be dehydrated as a result of the marked anorexia characteristic of appendicitis. Recovery is rapid and, if there are no complications, the child is discharged within a day or two, often as early as the first day postsurgery.

Ruptured appendix. Management of the child diagnosed with peritonitis caused by a ruptured appendix often begins preoperatively with intravenous administration of fluid and electrolytes, systemic antibiotics, and nasogastric suction. Postoperative management includes fluid and electrolyte balance maintenance, continued administration of antibiotics, and nasogastric suction for abdominal decompression until intestinal activity returns.

The child with peritonitis is given antibiotics until he is no longer febrile. In the presence of infection (abscess formation, necrotic or severely damaged tissue, or purulent collections within the peritoneum) the wound is left open for a few days; some surgeons provide for external drainage from a separate incision. Wound irrigations may be prescribed. The child is maintained in semi-Fowler position to reduce spread of the infection to other parts of the peritoneum, one of the most common of which is the subdiaphragmatic area.

Nursing Considerations

Because successful treatment of appendicitis is based on prompt recognition of the disorder, a primary nursing objective is assisting in establishing a diagnosis. Since the treatment is universally surgical, pre- and postoperative care are major nursing functions.

ASSESSMENT

Since abdominal pain is the most common childhood complaint, the nurse needs to make some preliminary evaluation of the severity of pain (see p. 587 for assessment of pain). One of the most reliable estimates is the degree of change in behavior. For example, a child who stays home from school and voluntarily lies down or refuses to play is much more likely to have considerable discomfort than the child who is absent from school but plays contentedly at home. The younger, nonverbal child will assume a rigid, motionless, side-lying posture with the knees flexed on the abdomen, and there is decreased range of motion of the right hip. The older child may exhibit all of these behaviors, while complaining of abdominal pain. He can always indicate a point at which the pain is worse than at any other.

NURSING DIAGNOSES

Following a thorough assessment a number of nursing diagnoses become evident. The more likely diagnoses are listed in the accompanying box. Others will be apparent in specific circumstances.

Nursing Diagnoses: The Child with Appendicitis

Pain related to inflamed appendix
Potential fluid volume deficit related to decreased intake secondary to loss of appetite, vomiting
Potential for infection related to possibility of rupture
Altered family processes related to illness and hospitalization of a child

PLANNING

The goals of nursing care for the child with a simple appendectomy include:

1. Prepare the child and family for surgical removal of appendix
2. Provide competent postoperative care as described for the child with abdominal surgery

Goals for the child with peritonitis include the above plus:

3. Prevent dehydration
4. Prevent spread of infection
5. Provide support to child and family

IMPLEMENTATION

Physical preparation of the child with appendicitis is the same as that for any child undergoing surgery (see p. 630). In any instance when severe abdominal pain is expected, the nurse must be aware of the danger of administering laxatives, enemas, or applying heat to the area. Such measures stimulate bowel motility and increase the risk of perforation.

Postoperative care. Postoperative care for the nonperforated appendix is the same as for most abdominal operations. Care of the child with a ruptured appendix and peritonitis involves more complex care. The course of recovery is considerably longer, usually 7 to 10 days of hospitalization.

The child is maintained on intravenous fluids, allowed nothing by mouth, and remains on low intermittent gastric decompression until there is evidence of intestinal activity. Listening for bowel sounds and observing for other signs of bowel activity (such as passage of stool) are part of the routine assessment. Management of intravenous therapy is the same as for any child receiving fluids and parenteral antibiotics.

Positioning the child in semi-Fowler position or lying on the right side after surgery for a ruptured appendix facilitates drainage from the peritoneal cavity as well as prevents the formation of a subdiaphragmatic abscess. Frequent dressing changes are usually needed, these include meticulous skin care to prevent excoriation of the area surrounding the surgical site. Often wound care includes irrigations with antibacterial solution.

Psychologic care of the child and parents is similar to that used in other emergency situations. Parents and older children need an opportunity to express their feelings postoperatively. It is especially important for the nurse to encourage the child to relate all the events he remembers concerning admission and treatment in order to clarify misconceptions.

EVALUATION

The efficacy with which nursing interventions meet the goals of care is determined by reassessment based on the following observational guidelines and expected outcomes:

1. Observe the child preoperatively for reaction to situation and compliance with care
2. Monitor child's physical and emotional reaction to hospitalization and surgery
3. Observe child's physical indications of good hydration
4. Observe child for evidence of infection
5. Interview and observe child and family for evidence of understanding the illness

Expected outcomes:

1. Child complies with directives and exhibits evidence of understanding the rationale for care appropriate to his age and developmental level (specify)
2. The child is relaxed and exhibits no evidence of distress (specify expected behaviors based on the characteristics of the child)
3. The child exhibits no evidence of dehydration
4. The child exhibits no evidence of infection at other body sites
5. Child and family readily express feelings and concerns and appear relaxed within the limitations imposed by the hospitalization (specify behaviors identified for specific case)

MECKEL DIVERTICULUM

Meckel diverticulum is a vestigial remnant of a fetal structure that connects the yolk sac with the intestinal cavity during fetal life. The diverticulum is located at the distal ileum and varies in size from a small appendiceal process to a pouch several inches long and almost as wide. At times it may be connected to the umbilicus by a cord.

Meckel diverticulum is the most common congenital malformation of the gastrointestinal tract and is present in 1% to 2% of the population. It is twice as common in males as in females, and complications are several times more frequent in males. Most symptomatic cases are seen in the first 2 years of life, but it frequently exists without causing symptoms.

Pathophysiology

Meckel diverticulum is a sac subject to inflammation (diverticulitis) in the same manner as appendicitis. In over half the cases the diverticulum contains gastric mucosa, which produces hydrochloric acid and pepsin. The acid continually irritates the bowel and erodes the surface resulting in bleeding and, in some instances, may lead to perforation. Mechanical obstruction can occur as a result of volvulus, or twisting of the bowel around the fibrotic Meckel cord.

Diagnostic Evaluation

Diagnosis is ordinarily based on the history. Over half of the individuals with Meckel diverticulum are symptomatic, and the signs and symptoms reflect the pathologic process as, for example, intestinal obstruction. Acute diverticulitis presents the same clinical picture as acute appendicitis, although the pain may be vague and recurrent (see box). Rectosigmoidoscopy and barium enema are usually performed to eliminate other possible diagnoses, such as anal fissure, polyps, and intussusception. Radio-

Clinical Manifestations of Meckel Diverticulum

- Abdominal pain
  - Similar to appendicitis
  - May be vague and recurrent
- Rectal bleeding—often presenting sign
  - Painless
  - Bright or dark red
  - In infants, bleeding may be accompanied by pain
- Sometimes:
  - Severe anemia
  - Shock

logic studies are not helpful in confirming the diagnosis, because the diverticulum may be too small to be visualized or may fail to fill with barium. Blood studies are usually part of the general laboratory workup to rule out any bleeding disorders and to evaluate the severity of the anemia.

Therapeutic Management

Treatment is surgical removal of the diverticulum. In instances in which severe hemorrhage increases the surgical risk, medical intervention to correct hypovolemic shock, such as blood replacement, intravenous fluids, and oxygen, may be necessary. In diverticulitis antibiotics may be used preoperatively to control infection. If intestinal obstruction has occurred, appropriate preoperative measures are used to reverse electrolyte imbalances and prevent abdominal distention.

Nursing Considerations

Nursing objectives are similar to those for the child with appendicitis. Since the onset is usually rapid, psychologic support parallels that for other conditions, such as appendicitis. It is important to remember that the the massive rectal bleeding is most often traumatic to both the child and the parent and may significantly affect their emotional reaction to hospitalization and surgery.

Specific preoperative considerations when rectal bleeding is present include (1) frequent monitoring of vital signs and blood pressure for shock, (2) keeping the child on bed rest, and (3) recording the approximate amount of blood lost in stools. In the absence of frank rectal hemorrhage, the nurse tests the stools for occult blood.

INFLAMMATORY BOWEL DISEASE

Inflammatory bowel disease (IBD) is a general term used to designate two chronic intestinal disorders—*ulcerative colitis* and *Crohn disease*. Although these two diseases are classified as IBD because of their similar epidemiologic, immunologic, and clinical features, they are two distinct conditions with very significant differences (see Table 23-4). The most important reason for differentiating between the two is prognosis. Crohn disease is considered to be the more serious and disabling disorder, and medical/surgical treatment is much less effective than in ulcerative colitis.

TABLE 23-4

Clinical Manifestations of Inflammatory Bowel Diseases

Characteristics	Ulcerative Colitis	Crohn Disease
Rectal bleeding	Common	Uncommon
Diarrhea	Often severe	Moderate to absent
Pain	Less frequent	Common
Anorexia	Mild or moderate	Can be severe
Weight loss	Moderate	Severe
Growth retardation	Usually mild	Often marked
Anal and perianal lesions	Rare	Common
Fistulas and strictures	Rare	Common

Etiology

The cause of IBD is unknown, although infectious, nutritional, immunologic, and psychogenic etiologies have been proposed. The current thinking is that IBD is the result of a genetically conditioned susceptibility to one or more environmental influences. Psychologic factors such as stress or personality characteristics do not play a role in the pathogenesis of the disease but may accentuate symptoms and the severity of a relapse (Silverman and Roy, 1983).

Several genetic and environmental factors influence the incidence of IBD: (1) there is a familial tendency in about 5% to 15% of the cases, (2) individuals from higher socioeconomic levels and more whites than nonwhites are affected, (3) the incidence is several times greater in Jews living in Europe and North America than in the general population, and (4) there is a higher occurrence of the disease in children living in urban settings than rural areas.

Pathophysiology: Ulcerative Colitis

The mucous membranes of the bowel become hyperemic and edematous with the formation of patchy granulations over the intestinal surface that bleed easily and eventually develop irregular areas of superficial ulcerations. In long-standing disease, the bowel becomes narrowed, smooth, and inflexible with thin or absent mucosa heavily infiltrated by scar tissue.

Pathophysiology: Crohn Disease

Crohn disease (also known as regional enteritis) may involve any part of the gastrointestinal tract but most commonly affects the terminal ileum. The disease characteristically involves all layers of the bowel wall (transmural). Acute edema and inflammation eventually progress to deep, transverse, or longitudinal ulcerations often associated with fissure formation. The thickened bowel wall may lead to obstruction. The asymmetric and patchy distribution of the lesions helps to differentiate Crohn disease from the contiguous and symmetric lesions of ulcerative colitis. Local lymph nodes are enlarged.

Diagnostic Evaluation

Diagnosis is suspected on the basis of history and physical examination and is usually confirmed by rectosigmoidoscopy. Barium enema and small bowel series are often helpful and mucosal biopsy is useful in demonstrating characteristic bowel changes. Stool examination is carried out to rule out infections and malabsorptive defects, and blood studies determine the state of anemia, electrolytes, and immunoglobulin levels.

Therapeutic Management

The goals of therapy are: (1) control the inflammatory process in order to reduce or eliminate the symptoms, (2) maintain long-term remission, and (3) allow as normal a lifestyle as possible (Biller, 1986). Treatment must be individualized and managed according to the severity of the disease, its location, and the response to therapy.

Medical treatment. The drug sulfasalazine has proven useful in decreasing the frequency of recurrences in patients with mild cases of IBD. Because it interferes with the absorption and utilization of folic acid, daily supplements of folic acid are prescribed.

Corticosteroids are the most important and effective drugs for treating moderate and severe IBD. High doses are administered for acute episodes, then tapered according to the clinical response. Although high doses of corticosteroids interfere with growth, significant growth can be achieved with judicious management and maintenance of optimum nutrition. Sometimes steroid enemas are helpful in reducing the need for systemic administration for children with rectosigmoid involvement.

Other drugs include metronidazole for treatment of perianal Crohn disease, antispasmodic agents, which sometimes help relieve the discomfort of diarrhea and cramping, and immunosuppressive agents, which are efficacious in patients on high-dose corticosteroids.

Dietary treatment. Dietary management is often vigorous because of the child's poorly nourished state. The goals are to replace nutrient losses associated with the inflammatory processes, to correct body deficits, and to provide sufficient nutrients to promote energy and nitrogen balance for normal metabolic function (Motil and Grand, 1985). These goals can be accomplished by enteral and/or parenteral routes. The therapeutic diet consists of high protein, high calorie, normal to low fat, and low fiber. Vitamin and mineral supplements are usually provided to correct anemia and other deficiencies.

During the acute stage supplemental nutrition by way of intermittent or continuous drip gastric feedings, intravenous fluids to correct dehydration and associated electrolyte imbalances, and/or parenteral alimentation may be required.

Surgical treatment. In some instances elective surgery is required. A temporary colostomy may be performed to allow the bowel a period of rest, or to arrest the disease process by removing the entire section of ulcerated bowel, in which case a total colectomy and ileostomy are usually required. Advances in surgical techniques over the incontinent abdominal stoma now provide options for some children. Surgical alternatives include a *continent (Koch) ileostomy* in which an intra-abdominal pouch or reservoir is created to allow continence, or an *ileo-anal anastomosis,* which preserves the normal pathway for defecation and eliminates the abdominal stoma.

Removal of the diseased bowel is a permanent remedy for ulcerative colitis and prevents possible development of carcinoma. However, in Crohn disease surgical removal of the affected bowel is not curative since the disease tends to recur and the risk of cancer of the bowel is not affected, which requires appropriate screening for early detection.

Nursing Considerations

Many of the nursing considerations relate directly to the therapeutic management in treating colitis. However, the scope of nursing responsibilities extends beyond the immediate period of hospitalization and involves (1) continued guidance of families in terms of dietary management, (2) coping with those factors that increase stress and emotional lability, (3) adjusting to a disease of remission and exacerbations or one of chronic ill health, and (4) when indicated, preparing the child and parents for the possibility of diversionary bowel surgery.

Since diet therapy is a very important component of therapy, encouraging the anorexic child to consume sufficient quantities of this diet is of primary importance and is frequently a nursing challenge. An approach that is more likely to meet with success involves including the child in meal planning; encouraging small, frequent meals or snacks rather than three large meals a day; serving meals around medication schedules when diarrhea, mouth pain, and intestinal spasm are controlled; and preparing high-protein, high-calorie foods, such as eggnog, milk shakes, cream soups, puddings, or custard (if lactose is tolerated) (see also Feeding the sick child, p. 640). Foods that are known to aggravate the condition are avoided as are high-fiber foods (see Table 23-4). Occasionally the occurrence of aphthous stomatitis further complicates adherence to dietary management. Good mouth care before eating and the selection of bland foods help relieve the discomfort of mouth sores.

The importance of continued drug therapy despite remission of symptoms must be stressed to the parents and child. Failure to adhere to the pharmacologic regimen can result in exacerbation of the disease process (see Chapter 21 for a discussion of compliance).

Family support. Attending to the emotional components of a chronic disease requires a thorough assessment of those stress factors that are disease related. Frequently the nurse can be instrumental in helping these children adjust to the problems of growth retardation, delayed sexual maturation, dietary restrictions, feelings of being "different" or "sickly," inability to compete with peers, and necessary absence from school during exacerbations of the illness (see Chapter 18).

In the event that a permanent colectomy/ileostomy is required, the nurse can assist the child and family in accepting and adjusting to the change by teaching them how to care for the ileostomy, by emphasizing the positive aspects of surgery, particularly accelerated growth and sexual development; permanent recovery and eliminated risk of colonic cancer in ulcerative colitis; and by stressing the normality of life despite bowel diversion. Introducing the child and parents to other ostomy patients, especially those of the child's age, can be the greatest therapeutic measure in fostering eventual acceptance. Whenever possible the newer continent ostomies should be offered as options to the child, although they are not performed in all centers throughout the United States.

Because of the chronic and often life-long nature of the disease, families benefit from many of the services provided by organizations such as the **National Foundation for Ileitis and Colitis, Inc.,*** which has branches in many major communities and provides education regarding the management of inflammatory bowel disease. If diversionary bowel surgery is indicated, the **United Ostomy Association†** is available to assist the ileostomy care and provides important psychologic support through its self-help groups.

PEPTIC ULCER

A peptic ulcer, or peptic ulcer disease (PUD), is an erosion of the mucosal wall of the stomach, pylorus, or duodenum. *Gastric ulcers* affect the lining of the stomach, whereas *duodenal ulcers* involve the pylorus or duodenum. Although peptic ulcers are more common in adults, they are also a significant pediatric problem, occurring at any age but most frequently between the ages of 12 and 18 years. Males are affected more than three times as often as females.

Etiology

The exact cause of peptic ulcer is not known, although both genetic and environmental factors appear to be important in the etiology of peptic ulcers. There is an increased frequency among relatives and a positive relationship to blood group O. However, emotional stress has been implicated as an important contributing factor toward the development, severity, and prognosis of peptic ulcers.

Pathophysiology

The precise mechanism is not understood, but one of two mechanisms probably reflects the basic defect: (1) an increase in the rate of production of gastric juice or (2) interference with the normal protective mechanisms of the mucosal lining. As a result of either of these two conditions, the gastric mucosa is highly vulnerable to the digestive effects of gastric juice. Prolonged contact with the highly acidic contents of the stomach and duodenum causes an erosion of the mucosal wall, especially in those areas least protected, such as the cardiac and lesser curve of the stomach and the area immediately beyond the pylorus.

Secondary or *stress ulcers* are also known to occur as a complication of a number of acute disorders (such as encephalitis, meningitis, or sepsis) and several chronic conditions (for example, burns, rheumatoid arthritis, cirrhosis of the liver, or chronic obstructive lung disease). Also, certain drugs, particularly aspirin and corticosteroids, are ulcerogenic.

Diagnostic Evaluation

Diagnosis is based on the history (pattern of pain)(see box), physical examination (pain in the epigastric area), and diagnostic testing such as radiologic studies, barium

Clinical Manifestations of Peptic Ulcer

Neonates (usually gastric)
Usually perforation
Often massive hemorrhage
Almost the same as seen in stress ulcers

Infants to 2-year-old children (gastric or duodenal, primary or secondary)
Poor eating, vomiting, crying spells after feeding, abdominal distention, tarry stools, melena
Vague discomfort
Irritability
Usually bleed rather than perforate

2- to 6-year-old children (gastric or duodenal)
No really positive physical findings
May have vomiting related to eating, generalized or periumbilical pain, melena, hematemesis
Wake at night crying with pain
Perforation more likely in secondary ulcers

6- to 9-year-old children (usually duodenal and primary)
Pain—burning or gnawing sensation in epigastrium related to fasting state, melena, hematemesis, vomiting
Often with obstruction

Over 9 years (usually duodenal)
Same as above
More typical of adult type

*44 Park Ave. South, New York, NY 10016. In Canada: **Canadian Foundation for Ileitis and Colitis,** 21 St. Clair Ave. E., Suite 301, Toronto, Ontario M4T 1L9.

†2001 W. Beverly Blvd., Los Angeles, CA 90057. In Canada: **United Ostomy Association, Canada,** 5 Hamilton Ave., Hamilton, Ontario L8V 2S3.

swallow, and panendoscopy (visualization of the gastric wall with a fiberoptic instrument). Other tests include blood studies (anemia), stool samples (occult blood), and, occasionally, gastric acid measurements (to isolate hypersecretors).

Therapeutic Management

The objectives of therapy for children with peptic ulcers is to relieve discomfort, promote healing, prevent complications, and prevent recurrence. The management of ulcers is primarily medical and consists of administration of medications that reduce or neutralize gastric acid secretion and, when possible, implement measures to eliminate or reduce stresses.

Antacids are the principal agents used in the initial treatment of peptic ulcers. The antacid of choice, usually a liquid magnesium preparation, is administered every 1 and 3 hours after each meal and at bedtime. The dosage is determined by the size of the child. As healing progresses, the frequency of administration is gradually reduced but not usually discontinued for several weeks.

The histamine (H_2) blocking agent cimetidine (Tagamet) is effective in the management of acute episodes and the newer histamine(H_2) antagonist, ranitidine (Zantac), offers the benefits of increased potency and longer duration of action. Both drugs suppress pepsin and gastric acid secretion and provide for greater compliance because of the reduced frequency of administration. Diazepam (Valium) has been used successfully in children with stress ulcers who have underlying or associated anxiety problems. Psychologic assistance may be required for those children with overlying anxiety problems.

The child is provided with a nutritious diet but advised to avoid foods that are associated with aggravation of symptoms. Sedatives are seldom helpful and are not generally prescribed. Since aspirin is known to have a damaging effect on gastric mucosa, acetaminophen is recommended as a substitute.

A child with an acute ulcer who has developed complications, such as massive hemorrhage, requires emergency care. Gastric lavage with saline and buffering with antacids usually stops bleeding in most instances. Administration of intravenous fluids, blood, or plasma depends on the amount of blood loss. Blood replacement with whole blood or packed cells may be necessary for significant loss.

Surgical management is *very* uncommon, except for the catastrophic ulcerations of the newborn. For intractable ulcers (those that do not respond to medical therapy) vagotomy and pyloroplasty are the preferred procedures. A gastric resection is seldom done unless absolutely necessary and usually only for stress ulcers.

Nursing Considerations

The main nursing objective is to promote healing of the ulcer through compliance with the dietary and medication regimen. The diet is usually quite liberal, with avoidance of those foods that enhance gastric secretion, such as tea, coffee, spices, carbonated beverages, and meat extractives (beef broth), and any food that causes the child discomfort. Substances that irritate the gastric wall are also avoided, such as alcohol, tobacco, and aspirin. However, these present no problem in children, although use of alcohol and tobacco may be an issue in adolescents with ulcers.

Drug compliance is essential and can be a problem with frequent administration of antacids. Therefore strategies to improve compliance are instituted early in the course of therapy (see Chapter 21). For traveling and during school the use of antacid tablets rather than liquid is more convenient.

Although the exact role stress plays in the pathogenesis of ulcers in children is unclear, especially since many ulcers occur secondary to other conditions, the nurse should be aware of those family and environmental conditions that may have precipitated or may aggravate the condition. Children may benefit from psychologic counseling and from learning how to cope more constructively with stresses in their lives, such as school, family, and friends (Sibinga, 1983).

◆ *Hepatic Disorders*

The liver is a vital organ that performs multiple important functions: (1) secretion of bile, (2) enzyme secretion, (3) storage depot, (4) detoxification, (5) synthesis of blood proteins, and (6) heat production. Inflammatory, obstructive, or degenerative disorders that affect the liver will also interfere with all or some of these functions with greater or lesser consequences for the affected child.

ACUTE HEPATITIS

Hepatitis, or inflammation of the liver, is rapidly emerging as one of the major causes of morbidity and a significant cause of mortality in children. The discussion that follows is focused primarily on acute hepatitis, although the chronic disease may involve many of the same mechanisms.

Etiology

Hepatitis of viral etiology is caused by at least four types of virus. These are:

Hepatitis virus A (HAV), formerly referred to as "infectious hepatitis"
Hepatitis virus B (HBV), formerly referred to as "serum hepatitis"
Hepatitis D (HDV)
Non-A, non-B virus (NANBV)

HDV is a newly described, unique viral agent that replicates only in the presence of HBV. NANBV agents have not been identified but are referred to when other viral agents are excluded. They are the most common cause of posttransfusion hepatitis. The remaining discussion is confined to HAV and HBV. Although these viruses produce the same pathologic changes in the liver and very similar clinical manifestations, they are distinct in their epidemiologic and immunologic characteristics.

Hepatitis A. HAV is highly contagious and is transmitted from one person to another primarily by the oral route, usually from ingestion of contaminated food or water. This includes eating shellfish caught in contaminated water and from swimming in such water. HAV can affect individuals at any age but is seen primarily in children under 15 years of age. Additional sources for children are daycare centers (especially those that have children in diapers) and in custodial care facilities. School contacts are considered a relatively low risk. Incubation period is 15 to 40 days (average 25 days).

Hepatitis B. HBV, a more insidious and serious disease, is transmitted by direct (needles) or indirect (cuts, burns, abrasions) parenteral means although it can be spread to mucous surfaces (intimate contact, contaminated secretions splashed into mouth or eyes during irrigations) and certain fomites (contaminated equipment). The virus can also be found in other body fluids and secretions—saliva, tears, sweat, urine, genital secretions, nasopharyngeal secretions, and breast milk, although these secretions are low-risk sources of transmittable HBV. Persons at risk for HBV include close family contacts, especially sex partners, clients and staff of custodial institutions for retarded children, those requiring frequent blood transfusions and hemodialysis, and health workers—especially those in operating rooms, emergency rooms, dialysis units, intensive care units, and laboratories, and personnel of dental offices. With the abuse of parenteral drugs, the incidence of HBV is significant in adolescent drug users and their contacts. Newborn infants are also at risk for neonatal hepatitis, especially if the mother is infected with HBV or was a carrier of HBV during pregnancy. Incubation period is 6 weeks to 6 months.

Pathophysiology

The pathologic changes occur primarily in the parenchymal cells of the liver and result in variable degrees of swelling, infiltration of liver cells by mononuclear cells, subsequent degeneration, necrosis, and autolysis. Structural changes within the hepatocyte are thought to account for altered liver functions.

Hepatitis is usually self-limited and complete regeneration of liver cells without scarring occurs within 2 to 3 months. However, some forms of hepatitis do not result in complete return of liver function. These include *fulminant hepatitis,* which is characterized by a severe, acute course with death frequently occurring within 1 to 2 weeks, and *subacute* or *chronic active hepatitis,* characterized by progressive liver destruction and uncertain regeneration with the possibility of scarring.

TABLE 23-5

Clinical Manifestations of Types A and B Hepatitis

Characteristics	Type A	Type B
Onset	Usually rapid, acute	More insidious
Fever	Common and early	Less frequent
Anorexia	Extreme	Mild to moderate
Nausea and vomiting	Common	Less common
Rash	Rare	Common
Arthralgia	Rare	Common
Pruritus	Rare	Sometimes present
Jaundice	Present	Present

Diagnostic Evaluation

The clinical manifestations for both types of viral hepatitis are similar except for a more rapid, acute onset in type A and a slower, more insidious onset in type B (Table 23-5). Both types may present with the flu-like symptoms. Some may never be recognized as actual cases of hepatitis.

Diagnosis of hepatitis is based on history (especially regarding possible exposure to a hepatitis virus), physical examination, laboratory evidence of the virus, and liver function tests. The diagnosis is confirmed by detection of antibodies or antigens formed in response to the specific virus, such as HBsAg (the hepatitis B surface antigen).

No liver function test is specific for hepatitis. Serum glutamic-oxaloacetic transaminase (SGOT) and serum glutamic-pyruvic transaminase (SGPT) levels are markedly elevated. Serum bilirubin levels peak 5 to 10 days after clinical jaundice appears.

Therapeutic Management

There is no specific treatment for either type of viral hepatitis. Management is primarily treatment of symptoms. For example, antiemetics may be helpful to reduce the nausea or vomiting. The value of bed rest in promoting overall recovery is controversial. Since the child feels ili and tired in the anicteric phase, he usually chooses to stay in bed. However, once improvement of physical complaints begins, the child prefers to resume normal activity gradually. The best approach is probably to allow the child to regulate his own pace. Hospitalization is rarely necessary, although proper isolation practices at home are imperative.

The child is allowed to choose foods he prefers, especially during the initial stage when anorexia is severe. Generally low-fat foods cause less stomach distention and are better tolerated than foods high in fat content. Carbohydrates should be encouraged to ensure an adequate caloric intake to spare proteins for cell growth. Vitamin K is administered if prothrombin time is prolonged.

Prevention. Isolation or quarantine of the infected child is not necessary as long as measures are used to prevent spread of the virus. An attack of either virus confers long-lasting immunity to that virus, however, there is no cross-over protection to the other virus. Prophylactic use of immune serum globulin (ISG) is effective in preventing hepatitis virus A in situations of preexposure (such as anticipated travel to areas where HAV is prevalent) or in situations of postexposure during the early part of the incubation period and, to a lesser extent, before the onset of the disease. It is of inconsistent benefit in preventing type B virus.

Passive immunity to HBV can be achieved with hyperimmune gamma globulin (hepatitis B immune serum globulin, HBIG) but it is very expensive. However, it is used for postexposure prophylaxis in specific situations such as newborn infants born to HBsAg-positive mothers, accidental needlestick or mucosal exposure to HBsAg-positive blood, or sexual contact with an HBsAg-positive person. Hepatitis B vaccines are highly effective in providing protection against HBV. At present the vaccine is recommended for a variety of persons at risk, including health care workers with frequent exposure to blood.

Nursing Considerations

Nursing objectives depend largely on the severity of the hepatitis, the rigidity of medical management, and factors influencing the control and transmission of the disease. Since children with benign viral hepatitis are frequently cared for at home, the responsibility of explaining any medical therapies and control measures is frequently left to the clinic or office nurse. In instances in which further assistance is needed for parents to comply with such instructions, a public health nursing referral may be necessary.

The emphasis is on encouraging a well-balanced diet and a realistic schedule of rest and activity adjusted to the child's condition. Since hepatitis type A is not infectious within a week or so after onset of jaundice, the child may feel well enough to resume school shortly thereafter. The parents are also cautioned about administering any medication to the child without the physician's knowledge, since normal doses of many drugs may become dangerous because of the liver's inability to detoxify and excrete them. Common drugs that are affected by hepatic failure include acetaminophen (Tylenol), ferrous sulfate (oral iron), and propoxyphene hydrochloride (Darvon).

Handwashing is the single most critical measure in reducing risk of hepatitis transmission in any setting. The nurse explains to parents and children the usual ways in which hepatitis virus A (oral-fecal route) and hepatitis virus B (parenteral route) are spread.

Hospitalized children are not usually isolated in a separate room unless they are fecally unreliable or incontinent or if their toys and other items might become contaminated with feces. They are discouraged from sharing their toys. For further discussion of infection control see p. 644.

In those children with HBV who have a known or suspected history of illicit drug use, the nurse has the additional responsibility of helping them realize the associated dangers of drug abuse, stressing the parenteral mode of transmission, and encouraging them to seek counseling from a drug program.

CIRRHOSIS

Cirrhosis, which means "yellow" and refers to the typical orange-colored nodules of a fibrotic liver, is a result, not a primary cause, of liver dysfunction. It represents the end stage of chronic disease in which there is generalized destruction of hepatic cells. Cirrhosis is not a common cause of morbidity in children; therefore, the diagnosis may be easily missed.

The three major complications of chronic liver disease are (1) bleeding from esophageal varices, (2) ascites, and (3) hepatic encephalopathy (hepatic coma). Not infrequently the first evidence of severe liver decompensation is failure to thrive, ascites, or bleeding esophageal varices.

Clinical manifestations depend on the etiology and reflect the consequences of liver malfunction. In cirrhosis from congenital biliary atresia, jaundice is usually the first sign, although all the pathologic effects eventually become evident, especially since most cases are not amenable to surgical correction. In cirrhosis from other causes, the symptoms are usually vague and the onset insidious. Liver function tests are abnormal, and definitive diagnosis is made on the basis of histologic changes observed from liver biopsy.

Therapeutic Management

There is no specific treatment for cirrhosis, except in those cases in which a treatable cause, such as an infection, exists. Therapy is directed primarily toward (1) frequent assessment of liver status with physical examination and liver function tests and (2) management of pathologic changes based on these findings. Complications of cirrhosis, including hemorrhage from esophageal varices, ascites, and hepatic encephalopathy, are managed appropriately.

Nursing Considerations

Nursing objectives in caring for the child with cirrhosis depend on several factors, including the precipitating cause of the cirrhosis, the severity of complications, and the prognosis. Overall the last factor has the greatest impact because the prognosis for life is poor. Since treatment of cirrhosis ideally is treatment of the cause, in many instances a fatal outcome is determined by the inability to surgically correct biliary atresia (see next section), reverse hepatic necrosis, or stop the progressive damage as a result of cystic fibrosis. Therefore, nursing care of this child is the same as that for a potentially terminally ill child (see Chapter 18). Hospitalization is usually required when complications occur.

BILIARY ATRESIA

Biliary atresia is the congenital obstruction or absence of a portion of the bile ducts. Blockage may be either *intrahepatic,* the absence of bile ducts within the liver, or *extrahepatic,* in which there is absence or obstruction of the main bile passages outside the liver. Numerous variations are encountered but the most common abnormality is complete atresia of the extrahepatic structures. The cause is unknown but recent evidence favors a viral infection before or shortly after birth. The predictable course of the disease terminates in complete and irreversible obliteration of the extrahepatic bile ducts.

Diagnostic Evaluation

No single test or combination of tests is diagnostic. The disease is suspected on the basis of clinical signs (see box) but surgical exploration is needed for confirmation.

Therapeutic Management

The major hope in care of these children is that the condition will benefit from surgery. Although surgical correction is possible in only a few cases of extrahepatic atresia, surgery is most successful when performed early; therefore, diagnosis is urgent. Occasionally a duct obstruction can be relieved. More often the Kasai procedure is used in which a substitute duct is formed from a segment of jejunum if there are any hepatic duct remnants. Liver transplantation offers hope for some.

Medical management is primarily supportive. It is the method of choice for intrahepatic atresia and supplemental to surgical therapy in extrahepatic atresia. Medical management consists of a high-calorie formula containing fats that can be digested without bile (Pregestimil, Portagen) and water-miscible vitamins. The bile acid-binding drug cholestyramine (Questran, Cuemid) is sometimes useful in reducing pruritis and improving liver function. Phenobarbital helps reduce irritability. A low-salt diet and diuretics may reduce ascites formation. Phototherapy is not effective in reducing the jaundice of unconjugated bilirubin.

Clinical Manifestations of Biliary Atresia

- Jaundice
  - Earliest manifestation and most striking feature of disorder
  - First observed in sclera
  - May be present at birth
  - Usually not apparent until age 2 to 3 weeks
- Urine dark and stains diaper
- Stools lighter than expected
- Hepatomegaly and abdominal distention common
- Splenomegaly occurs later
- Poor fat metabolism results in
  - Poor weight gain
  - General failure to thrive
- Pruritis
- Irritability
- Difficult to comfort infant

Nursing Considerations

Nursing care of the infant with biliary atresia is primarily supportive. Initially the infant is not uncomfortable and requires care suited to any infant of the same age. As the disease progresses the accumulation of toxic products causes the child to become irritable, restless, and difficult to comfort. Efforts are extended to allow as much sleep and rest as possible. The child is cared for when he awakens and provided with sedatives and comforting measures that he is able to tolerate.

During the diagnostic phase of the illness the nurse assists with tests and procedures as ordered. The child who has undergone exploratory or corrective surgery is given the same care as any infant following abdominal surgery. Infants with the Kasai operation require care of the double stoma and collection, measurement, and replacement of bile via the stomal openings. Parental teaching includes this practice, administration of antibiotics, and observation for signs of cholangitis. Children who are candidates for liver transplantation can avail themselves of help from the **Children's Liver Foundation***, which provides educational materials, programs, and support systems for families of children with liver disease.

◆ *Structural Defects*

There are numerous congenital abnormalities that involve any segment of the gastrointestinal tract. They are attributed to defective development during cell division and organ formation in the embryo. Most are apparent at birth or shortly after and are anomalies in which normal growth ceased at a crucial stage of development, leaving the structure in an embryonic form or only partially completed.

CLEFT LIP AND/OR CLEFT PALATE

Clefts of the lip and cleft palate are facial malformations that occur during embryonic development, are common to all human populations, and can constitute a severe disability to the affected individual. They may appear separately or, more commonly, together. Cleft lip (CL) results from failure of the maxillary and median nasal processes to fuse; cleft palate (CP) is a midline fissure of the palate that results from failure of the two sides to fuse. This discussion is concerned primarily with cleft lip and palate (CL/P). The incidence of CL/P shows a wide variation in races: it occurs in about 1:750 to 1:1000 live births. The defect appears more often in Orientals and certain tribes of Native Americans than in whites and less frequently in American blacks.

*Suite 202, South Orange, NJ 07079 or 139 S. Beverly Drive #312, Beverly Hills, CA 90212.

Etiology

In the majority of cases, CL/P appears to have a mixed genetic and environmental cause. There is an increased incidence in relatives, and identical twins are more apt to share the disorder than fraternal twins. Many recognized syndromes include these defects as a feature.

Pathophysiology

CL/P results from failure of the maxillary and premaxillary processes to come in contact during early embryonic life. Although often appearing together, cleft lip and cleft palate are distinct malformations embryologically, occurring at different times during the developmental process. Merging of the upper lip at the midline is completed between the seventh and eighth weeks of gestation. Fusion of the secondary palate (hard and soft palate) takes place later in development, between the seventh and twelfth weeks of gestation.

Diagnostic Evaluation

The cleft that involves the lip with or without cleft palate is readily apparent at birth and is one of the defects that elicits the most severe emotional reactions in parents. Clefts of the lip may be unilateral or bilateral and may range from a notch in the vermilion border of the lip to complete separation extending to the floor of the nose (Fig. 23-3). Varying degrees of nasal distortion usually accompany cleft lip with or without cleft palate, and the defect frequently involves supernumerary, deformed, or absent teeth.

Clefts of the palate may occur as an isolated defect or in association with cleft lip. Less obvious than cleft lip, the defect may not be detected without a thorough assessment of the mouth. The deformity can be identified by placing the examiner's fingers directly on the palate. Clefts of the hard palate form a continuous opening between the mouth and the nasal cavity. This creates special feeding problems. The infant is unable to develop suction because of the defect and has difficulty in swallowing. The open pathway must be closed in order to provide sufficient pressure for the swallowing sequence.

Therapeutic Management

Treatment of the child with CL/P involves the cooperative efforts of a number of specialists—pediatrician, nurses,

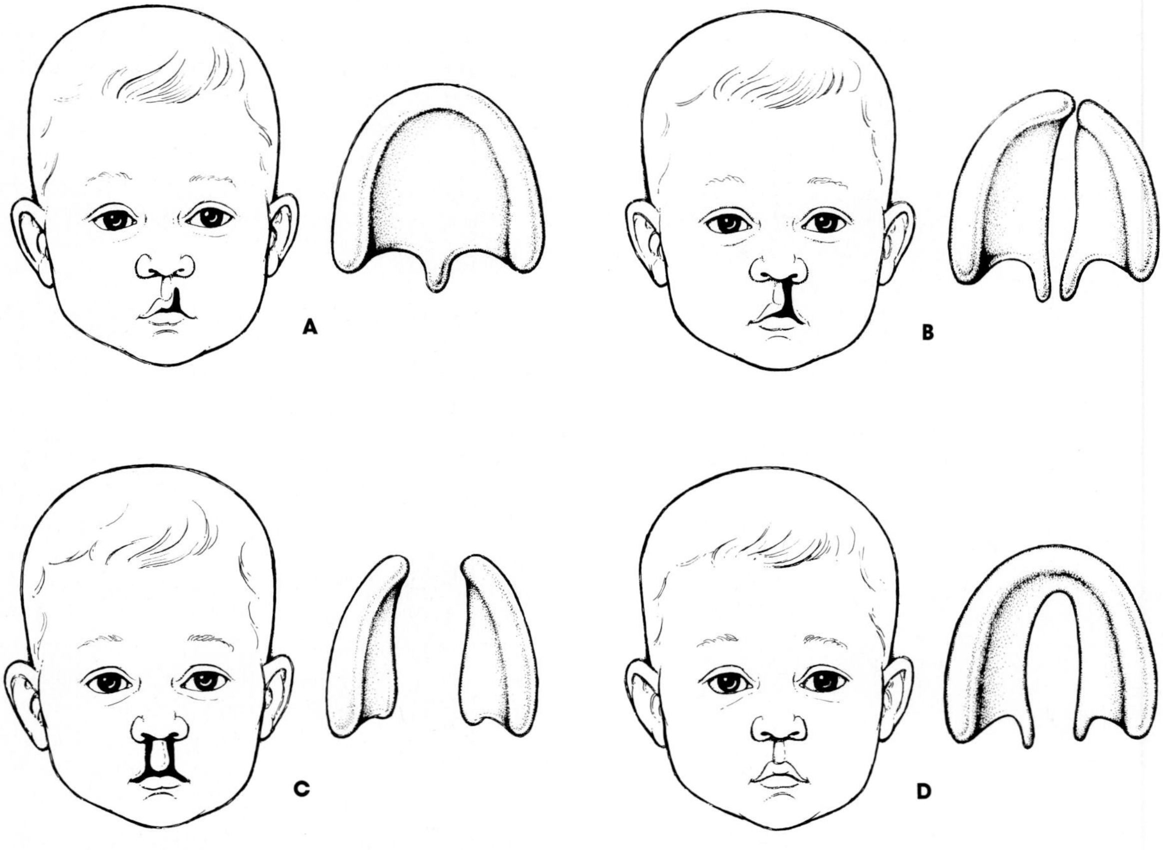

FIG. 23-3 Variations in clefts of the lip and palate at birth. **A,** Notch in vermilion border. **B,** Unilateral cleft lip and palate. **C,** Bilateral cleft lip and palate. **D,** Cleft palate.

plastic surgeon, orthodontist, prosthodontist, otolaryngologist, speech therapist, and, sometimes, a psychiatrist. Medical management is directed toward closure of the cleft(s), prevention of complications, habilitation, and facilitation of normal growth and development of the child.

Surgical correction: cleft lip. Closure of the lip defect precedes that of the palate, although the optimum times for surgery are still being debated. Those who favor immediate repair of the lip argue that it makes the infant more acceptable to the parents before discharge from the hospital, thereby improving establishment of satisfactory parent-child relationships. Others prefer to wait until the infant shows a steady weight gain and a hemoglobin level of at least 10 g/100 ml, usually at 6 to 12 weeks of age. They believe that the delay helps the infant better withstand the surgery.

Immediately after surgery the suture line is protected from tension by a thin, arched metal device (the Logan bow) taped to the cheeks or a butterfly-type adhesive restraint, and the arms are restrained at the elbows to prevent the infant from rubbing the incision with his hands. In the absence of infection or trauma, healing takes place with little scar formation.

Surgical correction: cleft palate. Cleft palate repair is generally postponed until later in order to take advantage of palatal changes that take place with normal growth, sometime between the ages of 6 months and 5 years. Most surgeons prefer to close the cleft between 1 and 2 years of age, before the child develops faulty speech habits.

Long-term problems. Even with good anatomic closure, the majority of children with CL/P have some degree of speech impairment, which requires speech therapy. Physical problems result from inefficient functioning of the muscles of the soft palate and nasopharynx, improper tooth alignment, and varying degrees of hearing loss. Improper drainage of the middle ear, as the result of inefficient function of the eustachian tube, contributes to recurrent otitis media with scarring of the tympanic membrane, which leads to hearing impairment in a large proportion of children with palatal clefts. Upper respiratory infections require immediate and meticulous attention, and extensive orthodontics and prosthodontics are needed to correct problems of malposition of teeth and maxillary arches.

Nursing Considerations

In addition to the general management of the child with a developmental defect, the infant with cleft lip with or without cleft palate offers some special challenges to both nurses and families.

ASSESSMENT

Since the lip defect is readily visible at birth, assessment consists of describing the location and extent of the defect, and the palatine cleft is estimated by visualization during crying. Cleft palate without cleft lip is detected by palpating the palate with the finger during the newborn assessment.

The emotional impact of the birth of a child with a cosmetic as well as a functional disability is especially traumatic to the family. Consequently, the nursing assessment is also concerned with the emotional reaction of the family to the child and the defect (see p. 506).

NURSING DIAGNOSES

Following a thorough physical assessment a number of nursing diagnoses are evident. These are described in the Nursing Care Plan on p. 768.

PLANNING

The goals of care for the infant with a cleft lip and/or palate include preoperative care, short-term postoperative care, and long-term management. The major goals of care include:

Preoperative care:

1. Prepare infant and family for surgery
2. Implement a feeding method

Postoperative care:

3. Prevent injury to operative site
4. Provide nutrition
5. Prevent complications
6. Support child and family

IMPLEMENTATION

The immediate nursing problems in the care of an infant with CL/P deformities are related to feeding the infant and dealing with the severe parental reaction to the defect. A cleft lip is the most disfiguring of the visible defects and one that generates strong negative responses in both nurses and parents. It is especially important for nurses to emphasize the positive aspects of the infant's physical appearance and optimism regarding surgical correction. Sometimes showing parents a photograph of the possible cosmetic improvement as a result of surgery does much to relieve their anxiety. The manner of the nurse in handling the infant should convey to the parents that the infant is indeed a precious human being. (See Chapter 18 for interventions in assisting parents to accept a birth defect.)

Throughout the course of therapy parents need an explanation of the immediate and long-range problems frequently associated with cleft palate. Often they are unaware that more is involved than merely repairing the defect. Whenever possible, they should be referred to a comprehensive cleft palate team.

Feeding. Feeding the infant offers a special challenge to nurses. Clefts of lip or palate reduce the infant's ability to suck, which interferes with compression of the areola and renders breast-feeding and bottle-feeding difficult.

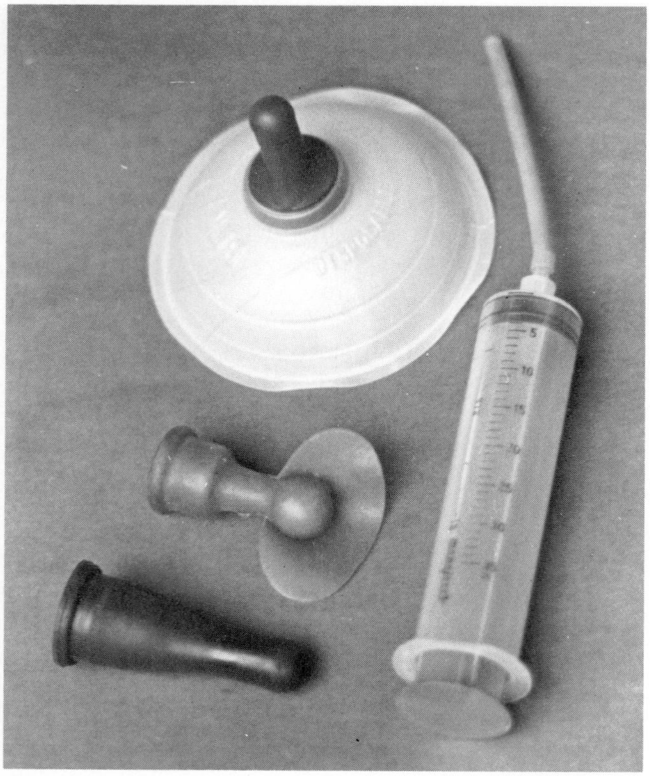

FIG. 23-4 Some devices used to feed an infant with a cleft palate. *Clockwise*: lamb's nipple, flanged nipple, special nurser, and syringe with rubber tubing (Breck feeder).

Liquid taken into the mouth has a tendency to escape via the cleft through the nose. Feeding is usually best accomplished with the infant's head in an upright position, either held in the caregiver's hand or cradled in the arm. Normal nipples are unsuitable for these infants, who are unable to generate the suction required; therefore, special nipples or other feeding devices are needed. A variety of special "cleft palate" nipples have been devised and used with some success. However, large, soft nipples with large holes, Nursettes, or the long, soft lamb's nipples appear to offer the best means for nipple feeding (Fig. 23-4). The newer "gravity flow" nipple* attached to a squeezable plastic bottle allows formula to be deposited directly into the pharynx in much the same manner as a bulb syringe. Success has also been achieved by the modification of a standard nipple. A single small slit or crosscut is made in the end of the nipple with a sharp surgical blade or a pair of scissors with sharp, thin blades. This allows the infant to express the formula readily. The size of the slit is adjusted to the needs of the infant.

Using these various types of nipples for feeding also has the advantage of helping to meet the infant's sucking needs and, when placed in the normal sucking position (not through the cleft), encourage use of the sucking muscles. Muscle development is especially important for later development of speech. The nipple should be positioned in such a way that it is compressed by the infant's tongue and existing palate. If a single-slit nipple is used, the slit should be placed vertically so that the infant will be able to produce and stop a flow of milk by alternately opening and closing the opening. No matter which type of nipple is used, gentle, steady pressure on the base of the bottle reduces the chance of choking or coughing, and the person feeding should resist the temptation to remove the nipple because of the noise the infant makes or for fear that he will choke. Since these infants have a tendency to swallow excessive amounts of air, they require frequent bubbling.

When the infant has trouble with nipple feeding, a rubber-tipped medicine dropper, Asepto syringe, or "Breck feeder" often provides an efficient, safe feeding device. The rubber extension should be sufficiently long to extend well back into the mouth to reduce the likelihood of regurgitation through the nose. The formula is deposited on the back of the tongue and the flow controlled by bulb compression that is adjusted to the infant's capacity to handle it. With some infants, spoon feeding works best, especially if the formula is slightly thickened with cereal. After feeding the infant is given water to rinse the mouth.

The mother should begin to feed the infant as soon as possible, preferably after the initial nursery feeding. In this way she is able to help determine the method best suited to her and the infant and to become adept in the technique before they are discharged from the hospital.

Preoperative care. In preparation for surgical repair, the parent is frequently instructed to accustom the infant to some of the needs of the early postoperative period, particularly if surgery is delayed several months. Since it is mandatory for the infant to be positioned on the back or side postoperatively, it is helpful to train him to lie in these positions a great deal of the time to reduce the irritability and resistance associated with any change in routine. It is also helpful to place the infant or child in arm restraints periodically prior to admission and, after admission, to feed him with a rubber-tipped Asepto syringe or other device in the manner to be used postoperatively. No special formula is required, and the infant is usually allowed to eat up to about 6 hours preoperatively. Preoperative preparation, including medication, is determined by the surgeon and anesthesiologist.

Postoperative care: cleft lip. The major efforts in the postoperative period are directed toward protecting the operative site. Before the infant leaves the operating room the metal appliance is securely taped to the cheeks to relax the operative site and prevent tension on the suture line caused by crying or other facial movement. Arm restraints are needed to prevent the infant from rubbing or otherwise disturbing the suture line and are ready at the bedside for immediate application on his arrival at the unit. It is advisable to pin the cuff of the restraints to the

*Ross Laboratories, Columbus, OH 43216.

infant's clothing or bed to prevent rubbing the face with the upper arms. The older infant who is able to roll over will require a jacket restraint in addition to restricting arm movement to prevent his rolling on the abdomen and rubbing his face on the sheet, especially if the repair involves the lip. It is important to remove the restraints periodically to exercise the arms, to provide relief from restrictions, and to observe the skin for signs of irritation. It is advisable to release the restraints one at a time, especially in a very vigorous, active infant. Removing restraints also offers an opportunity for cuddling and body contact. Sitting him in an infant seat provides a change of position and a different perspective of the environment. Sedation is sometimes needed for a very restless, anxious infant. Rooming-in is always encouraged because preserving parent contact greatly increases the child's comfort.

Feeding is essentially the same as before surgery. It is safe to offer clear liquids when the infant has fully recovered from the anesthesia, and formula feeding is usually resumed when tolerated. Asepto-syringe feeding is preferred in most cases. Care is taken to slip the rubber tip in from the side of the mouth to avoid the operative area and to prevent the infant from sucking on the tubing. This method is continued until the lip is well healed, after which bottle-feeding can be resumed if this has been the infant's mode of feeding. The mouth should be rinsed with water after each feeding. The suture site is carefully cleansed of formula or serosanguineous drainage as needed with a gauze- or cotton-tipped swab dipped in saline. Meticulous care of the suture line is a nursing responsibility since inflammation or sloughing will interfere with optimum healing and the ultimate cosmetic effect of the surgical repair.

Gentle aspiration of mouth and nasopharynx secretions may be necessary to prevent aspiration and respiratory complications. A side-lying or partial side-lying position is helpful for the infant in the immediate postoperative period and for one who has difficulty in handling secretions. As with any infant, the child with cleft palate repair is placed on the right side after feedings to reduce the chance of aspirating regurgitated formula.

Postoperative care: cleft palate. The child with a cleft palate repair is allowed to lie on the abdomen, especially immediately postoperatively. The nurse avoids the use of suction or other objects in the mouth, such as a tongue depressor when the suture lines are being checked or straws when the child is given liquids. Fluids are best taken from a cup. Young children are not given a pacifier and children old enough to understand are cautioned against rubbing their tongue against the roof of the mouth. Spoons should not be allowed in the mouth. The child with a cleft palate repair may be fed with a wide-bowl spoon (such as a soup spoon) that cannot enter the mouth.

As with cleft lip repair, the elbows are immobilized to keep the hands away from the mouth, and the parents are instructed to continue this precaution at home until the palate is healed. They are instructed to remove the restraints (usually one at a time) at frequent intervals to allow the child to exercise the arms. It is important to stress that the child should be closely supervised during this time.

The child is generally discharged on a soft diet, which parents are instructed to continue until the surgeon directs them otherwise. They are cautioned against allowing the child to eat hard items such as toast, hard cookies, and potato chips, which could damage the newly repaired palate. The nurse might suggest that the parents not offer the child any food harder than mashed potatoes.

Occasionally the child will have difficulty in breathing following surgery, especially the child with cleft palate repair who must alter an established pattern of breathing and adjust to breathing through the nose. This is frustrating but seldom requires more than positioning and support. Sometimes the infant or child is placed in a mist tent for a short period after surgery.

Long-term care. Children with CL/P often require a variety of services during the process of habilitation. Families of these children need support and encouragement by health professionals and guidance in activities that facilitate the most normal outcome for their children. With the combined efforts of family and the health team the majority of these children achieve a satisfactory habilitation. Parents need to understand the function of therapy and the purpose and care of any appliance and of establishing good mouth care and proper brushing habits.

Throughout the child's habilitation the ultimate goal should be the development of a healthy personality and self-esteem. Many local areas have Cleft Palate Parents groups who offer help and support to families. Several specialized agencies provide education and services for children with CL/P, their families, and health professionals. These include the **American Cleft Palate Association*** and the **Canadian Cleft Lip and Palate Family Association.**†

EVALUATION

The effectiveness of nursing interventions is determined by continual reassessment and evaluation of care based on the following observational guidelines and expected outcomes:

Preoperative care:

1. Observe and interview family regarding their understandings, feelings, and concerns of the defect and surgery
2. Observe the infant during feeding

Postoperative care:

3. Inspect operative site including the protective tape or device

*1218 Grandview Ave., Pittsburgh, PA 15261.

†180 Dungas St. W., Suite 1508, Toronto, Ontario M5G 1X8, (416) 598-2311.

NURSING CARE PLAN

The Infant with Cleft Lip/Palate

Nursing Goals	Nursing Interventions	Expected Patient/Family Outcomes
NDx HP-HMP* **Potential for trauma or aspiration** **Risk factors: fresh operative site, immature reasoning**		
Prevent trauma to suture line	Position on back or side Maintain lip protective device Use nontraumatic feeding techniques Restrain arms to prevent access to operative site Use jacket restraints on older infant Avoid placing objects in the mouth following cleft palate repair (suction catheter, tongue depressor, straw, pacifier, small spoon)	Operative site remains undamaged
Prevent aspiration of secretions	Position to allow for mucus drainage (partial side-lying position)	Secretions are managed without aspiration
NDx N-MP **Altered nutrition: less than body requirements** **Etiology: difficulty eating**		
Provide adequate nutritional intake	Administer diet appropriate for age Modify feeding techniques to adjust to defect Feed in sitting position Use special appliances Encourage frequent bubbling Assist with breast-feeding if method of choice	Infant consumes an adequate amount of nutrients (specify amounts)
NDx N-MP **Potential impaired skin integrity** **Risk factors: mouth secretions, application of restraining devices**		
Prevent tissue infection and breakdown	Keep suture line dry Cleanse suture line gently after feeding and as necessary	Skin remains clean and free of irritation
NDx RRP **Altered family processes** **Etiology: situational crisis (child with a physical defect) temporary family disorganization, knowledge deficit**		
Facilitate family's acceptance of infant	Allow expression of feelings Convey attitude of acceptance of infant and family Indicate by behavior that child is a valuable human being	Family discusses feelings and concerns regarding the child's defect, its repair, and future prospects
Educate family	Describe surgical results Use photographs of satisfactory results Involve family in determining best feeding methods Teach feeding and suctioning techniques Teach cleansing and restraining procedures, especially when infant will be discharged before suture removal	Family demonstrates ability to carry out postoperative care
Provide for continued support	Refer to public health agency for continuity of care Refer to social service Refer to Crippled Children's Services for financial assistance Refer to local cleft palate parent group and other agencies Ensure follow-up care and management See also The family of the hospitalized child, p 610	Family uses appropriate resources

*For an explanation of abbreviations, see p. 20.

4. Observe infant during feeding; measure intake and output; weigh infant daily
5. Observe operative site for evidence of infection, bleeding, sloughing, or irritation
6. Observe and interview family regarding their understandings and concerns about the child and his long-term needs

Expected outcomes:
See Nursing Care Plan above.

ESOPHAGEAL ATRESIA WITH TRACHEOESOPHAGEAL FISTULA

Congenital atresia of the esophagus and tracheoesophageal fistula (TEF) are rare malformations that represent a failure of the esophagus to develop as a continuous passage. These defects may occur as separate entities or in combination (Fig. 23-5) and, without early diagnosis and treatment, are rapidly fatal.

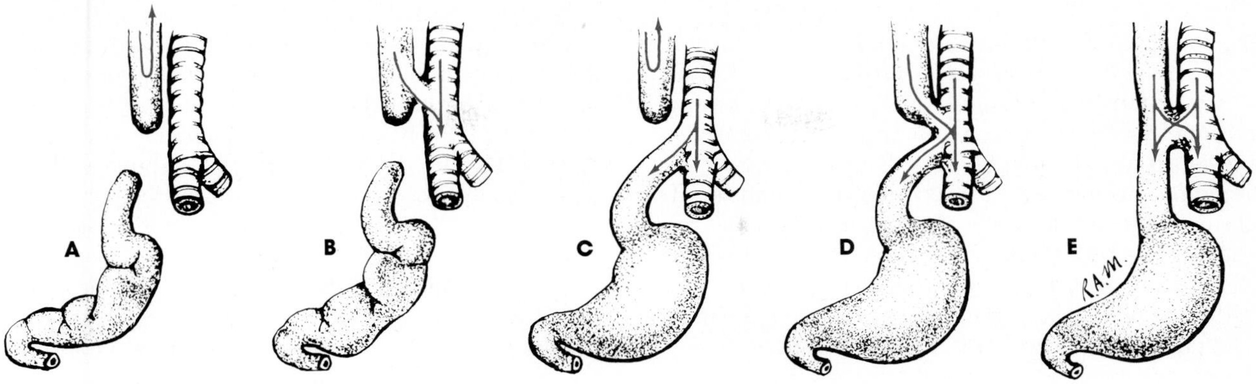

FIG. 23-5 Five most common types of esophageal atresia and tracheoesophageal fistula.

Etiology

The cause of esophageal atresia and TEF is not known. The incidence has been estimated to be from 1:800 to 1:5000 live births. There appear to be no sex differences, but the birth weight of most affected infants is significantly lower than average and there is an unusually high percentage of prematurity.

Pathophysiology

The most commonly encountered form of esophageal atresia and TEF (80% to 95% of cases) is one in which the proximal esophageal segment terminates in a blind pouch and the distal segment is connected to the trachea or primary bronchus by a short fistula at or near the bifurcation (Fig. 23-5, *C*). The second most common variety (5% to 8%) consists of a blind pouch at each end, widely separated and with no communication to the trachea (Fig. 23-5, *A*). Less frequently an otherwise normal trachea and esophagus are connected by a common fistula (Fig. 23-5, *E*). Extremely rare anomalies involve a fistula from the trachea to the upper esophageal segment (Fig. 23-5, *B*) or to both the upper and lower segments (Fig. 23-5, *D*).

Diagnostic Evaluation

The disorder is suspected on the basis of clinical manifestations (see box). To rule out esophageal atresia a catheter, gently passed into the esophagus, meets with resistance if the lumen is blocked but passes unobstructed if the lumen is patent. A moderately stiff catheter is used to avoid coiling in the esophageal pouch. Aspiration of stomach contents or auscultation over the stomach as air is introduced through the catheter confirms a patent esophagus. Radiopaque fluid carefully instilled in the esophagus under fluoroscopy will readily establish the diagnosis. Sometimes fistulas are not patent, which makes their presence more difficult to diagnose.

Clinical Manifestations of Tracheoesophageal Fistula (TEF)

Excessive salivation and drooling
Three Cs of TEF:
- Coughing
- Choking
- Cyanosis

May stop breathing

Therapeutic Management

The treatment of esophageal atresia and TEF consists of prevention of pneumonia and surgical repair of the anomaly. When a TEF is suspected, the infant is immediately deprived of oral intake, started on intravenous fluids, and placed in the position least likely to cause aspiration of either mouth or stomach secretions. A gastrostomy is usually performed to decompress the stomach and prevent further aspiration of gastric contents by way of the fistula. Since aspiration pneumonia is almost inevitable and appears early, broad-spectrum antibiotic therapy is instituted.

Surgical correction consists of a thoracotomy with division and ligation of the TEF and an end-to-end anastomosis of the esophagus. For infants who are premature, have multiple anomalies, or are in very poor condition, a staged operation is preferred that involves palliative measures including gastrostomy, ligation of the TEF, and provision of constant drainage of the esophageal pouch.

There are rare instances in which a primary anastomosis cannot be accomplished because of insufficient length of the two segments of esophagus. In these cases the defect must be bridged with a segment of intestine. This esophageal replacement is usually deferred until the child is 18 to 24 months old. In the meantime the fistula is closed and the child fed directly by gastrostomy, whereas the upper esophageal segment is drained by means of a cervical esophagostomy, an artificial opening made in the neck to allow the escape of saliva.

Nursing Considerations

Nursing responsibility for detection of this serious malformation begins *immediately* after birth. Nurses should suspect any infant who has an excessive amount of mucus or difficulty with secretions and unexplained episodes of cyanosis. Ideally the condition is diagnosed before the initial feeding, but often it is not. If fed, the infant swallows normally but suddenly coughs and struggles and the fluid returns through the nose and mouth. For this reason it is customary for the nurse to give the infant the first feeding of plain water or to be present when a parent feeds the child in order to observe his reactions.

Cyanosis is usually the result of laryngospasm caused by overflow of saliva into the larynx from the proximal esophageal pouch, and it normally clears after removal of the secretions from the oropharynx by suctioning. Any such suspicion is reported to the physician immediately. The infant is placed in an Isolette or under a radiant warmer, and oxygen is administered to help relieve respiratory distress. Positive pressure is contraindicated since it may add to air pressure in the stomach.

The most desirable position for a newborn who is suspected of having a TEF is supine with the head elevated on an inclined plane of at least 30 degrees. This positioning serves to minimize the reflux of gastric secretions up the distal esophagus into the trachea and bronchi, especially when intra-abdominal pressure is elevated during crying.

It is imperative that the source of aspiration be removed at once. Oral fluids are withheld and the infant's fluid needs are met parenterally or via gastrostomy. Until surgery the blind pouch is kept empty by intermittent or continuous suction through an indwelling nasal catheter that extends to the end of the pouch. The catheter needs attention since it has a tendency to become clogged with mucus. It is usually replaced daily by the physician. On diagnosis the gastrostomy tube is inserted and left open so that air entering the stomach through the fistula can escape, thus minimizing the danger that gastric contents will be regurgitated into the trachea. The tube empties by gravity drainage.

Postoperative care. Postoperative care for these infants is essentially the same as the care of any high-risk newborn (see p. 221). The infant is returned to the warm, high-humidity atmosphere of the Isolette, and the gastrostomy tube is returned to gravity drainage until the infant can tolerate feedings, usually the second or third postoperative day. At this time the tube is elevated and secured at a point above the level of the stomach. This allows gastric secretions to pass to the duodenum, whereas swallowed air can escape through the open tube. If tolerated, gastrostomy feedings are continued until the esophageal anastomosis is healed, about the tenth to fourteenth day, after which oral feedings are initiated.

The initial attempt at oral feeding must be carefully observed to make certain that the infant is able to swallow without choking. Until the infant is able to take a sufficient amount by mouth, oral intake may need to be supplemented by gastrostomy feedings. Ordinarily the infant is not discharged until he is taking oral fluids well and the gastrostomy tube has been removed. However, the infant who has undergone palliative surgery will be discharged with the gastrostomy tube in place. The nurse is responsible for making certain that the caregiver is educated and practiced in the care of the gastrostomy (p. 682).

Special problems. Upper respiratory complications are a threat to life in both the preoperative and postoperative period. In addition to pneumonia, there is a constant danger of respiratory embarrassment resulting from atelectasis, pneumothorax, and laryngeal edema. Any persistent respiratory difficulty after removal of secretions is reported to the surgeon immediately.

In the infant awaiting esophageal replacement surgery and the upper esophageal segment is drained through a cervical esophagostomy. This is a source of annoyance as the skin may become irritated by moisture from the continual discharge of saliva. Frequent removal of drainage and application of a thin layer of protective ointment are usually sufficient treatment.

Meeting the oral needs of infants who are unable to suck on a bottle should not be overlooked. A pacifier offered periodically is an acceptable substitute until oral feedings are instituted. The child who has corrective surgery delayed until 18 to 24 months of age may have a different problem. Some children who have not been able to go through the processes of eating in the normal manner have difficulty with this new task and require patient, firm guidance in learning the techniques of taking food into the mouth and swallowing.

As with any congenital anomaly parents need support in adjusting to the child (see Chapter 18). One of the difficulties in TEF is the immediate transfer of the sick newborn to the intensive care unit and sometimes lengthy hospitalization. The attachment process is facilitated by encouraging parents to visit the infant, participate in his care where appropriate, and express their feelings regarding his defect. The nurse in the intensive care unit should assume responsibility for ensuring that the parents are kept fully informed of the infant's progress.

HERNIAS

A hernia is a protrusion of a portion of an organ or organs through an abnormal opening. The danger from herniation arises when the organ protruding through the opening is constricted to the extent that circulation is impaired or when the protruding organs encroach upon and impair the function of other structures. The herniations of concern are those that protrude through the diaphragm, the abdominal wall, or the inguinal canal (see p. 884). The other hernias of significance to the pediatric age groups are outlined in Table 23-6.

Table 23-6

Summary Outline of Diaphragmatic and Abdominal Hernias

Type	Manifestations/Diagnostic Evaluation	Management
Diaphragmatic		
Through foramen of Bochdalek: Protrusion of part of the stomach through an opening in the diaphragm	Symptoms—mild to severe respiratory distress within a few hours after birth; tachypnea, cyanosis, dyspnea, and severe acidosis Breath sounds absent in affected area; bowel sounds may be present Rarely asymptomatic Diagnosis made by radiographic study	Therapeutic: Supportive treatment of respiratory distress and correction of acidosis Prophylactic antibiotic administration Surgical reduction of hernia and repair of defect Nursing: Preoperative Prevent crying Maintain suction, oxygen, and intravenous fluids Place in semi-Fowler position Assist with diagnostic and preoperative procedures Administer medications Postoperative Carry out routine postoperative care and observation Use comfort measures Support parents
Hiatal		
Sliding: Protrusion of an abdominal structure (usually the stomach) through the esophageal hiatus	Symptoms—dysphagia, failure to thrive, vomiting, neck contortions, frequent unexplained respiratory problems, bleeding, incompetent cardiac sphincter Diagnosis made by fluoroscopy	Therapeutic: Surgical repair of defect Nursing: Be alert to significant signs Carry out routine postoperative care
Abdominal		
Umbilical: Soft skin-covered protrusion of intestine and omentum through a weakness in the abdominal wall around the umbilicus	Inspection and palpation of abdomen High incidence in black infants Spontaneous closure by age 1 to 2 years	Therapeutic: No treatment of small defects Operative repair if persists to age 2 to 5 years Strangulation requires immediate attention Nursing: Discourage use of home remedies, e.g., belly bands, coins Reassure parents
Omphalocele: Protrusion of intra-abdominal viscera into the base of the umbilical cord *Gastroschisis:* Protrusion of intra-abdominal contents through a defect in the abdominal wall	Obvious on inspection Observation for other malformations	Therapeutic: Surgical repair of defect Preoperative Large lesions—gradual reduction of abdominal contents Prophylactic antibiotic administration Nursing: Preoperative Keep sac or viscera moist Use overhead warming unit Carry out routine care of intravenous line, nasogastric suction Give nothing by mouth Use comfort measures

◆ *Obstructive Disorders*

Obstruction of the bowel occurs when the passage of intestinal contents is mechanically impeded by a constricted or an occluded lumen or when there is interference with normal muscular contraction. Intestinal obstruction from any cause is characterized by similar signs and symptoms (see box), although the progression may vary greatly. For example, in acute conditions, such as intussusception, the clinical manifestations are apparent within a few hours of the onset of the disorder. In other conditions, such as pyloric stenosis, the signs and symptoms usually develop more gradually and can be missed in the early stages.

Clinical Manifestations of Mechanical Intestinal Obstruction

Colicky abdominal pain—from peristalsis attempting to overcome the obstruction
Abdominal distention—as a result of accumulation of gas and fluid above the level of the obstruction.
Vomiting—often the earliest sign of a high obstruction; a later sign of lower obstruction
Constipation and obstipation—early signs of low obstructions; later signs of higher obstructions
Dehydration—from losses of large quantities of fluid and electrolytes
Rigid and boardlike abdomen—from increased distention
Bowel sounds—gradually diminish and cease
Respiratory distress—occurs as the diaphragm is pushed up into the pleural cavity
Shock—plasma volume diminishes as proteins are lost from the bloodstream into the intestinal lumen

HYPERTROPHIC PYLORIC STENOSIS

Pyloric stenosis (PS), obstruction at the pyloric sphincter by hypertrophy of the circular muscle of the pylorus, is one of the most common surgical disorders of early infancy. This functional anomaly is seen soon after birth with vomiting that becomes progressively more severe and projectile. It is five times more common in male than female infants, affecting approximately five of every 1000 males and only one of every 1000 females. It is seen less frequently in black and Oriental than in white infants. It is more likely to affect a full-term than a premature infant.

The cause of the increased size of the pyloric musculature is unknown. A higher incidence in first-degree relatives and in monozygotic as opposed to dizygotic twins implicates heredity in the etiology, although the nature of the hereditary factors is only speculative.

Pathophysiology

The circular muscle of the pylorus is grossly enlarged as a result of both hypertrophy and hyperplasia. This produces severe narrowing of the pyloric canal between the stomach and duodenum. Consequently the lumen at this point is partially obstructed. Over a period of time inflammation and edema further reduce the size of the opening until the partial obstruction may progress to complete obstruction. The muscle is thickened to as much as twice its usual size—2 to 3 cm long—and is almost cartilaginous in consistency. The distal portion ends abruptly and is externally distinct and easily palpated, but the proximal end merges into the gastric antrum. The stomach is usually dilated (Fig. 23-6, *A*).

Diagnostic Evaluation

The age of onset and pattern of vomiting are variable. Typically the infants with pyloric stenosis are well during the first weeks of life. Initially there is only regurgitation or occasional nonprojectile vomiting that begins about the second to the fourth week after birth, although in a few infants symptoms begin at birth. Others do well for the first few weeks and then suddenly develop projectile vomiting that rapidly leads to dehydration. The projectile vomiting usually develops within a week and may lead to complete obstruction by 4 to 6 weeks.

If diagnosis is inconclusive from the history and physical signs (see box), upper gastrointestinal radiographic studies will reveal delayed gastric emptying and an elongated, threadlike pyloric channel. Many are finding that ultrasound is as accurate and less traumatic for diagnosis

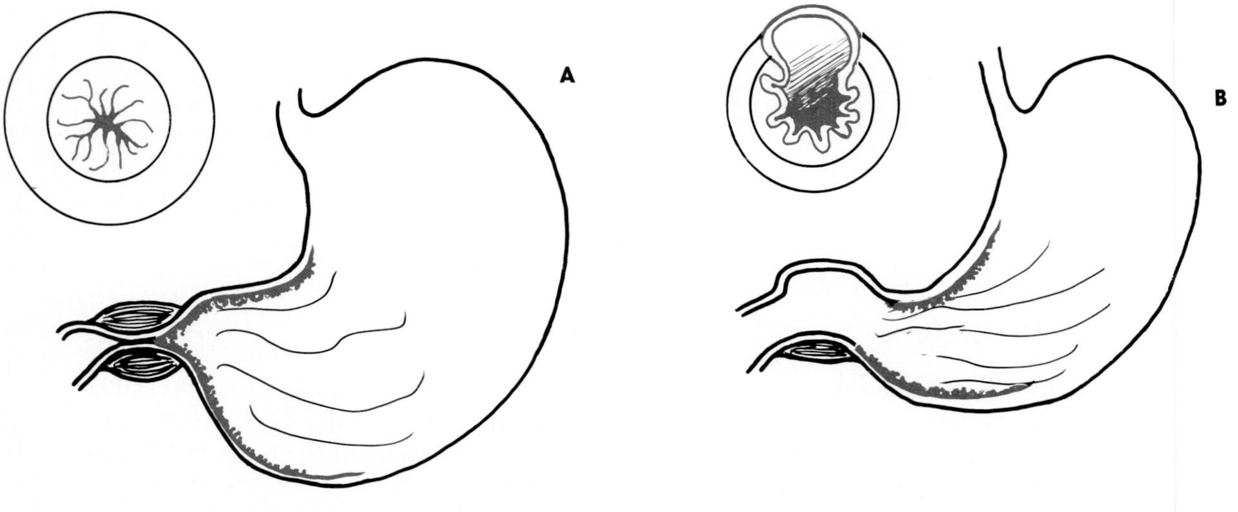

FIG. 23-6 Hypertrophic pyloric stenosis. **A,** Enlarged muscular tumor nearly obliterates pyloric channel. **B,** Longitudinal surgical division of muscle down to submucosa establishes adequate passageway.

Clinical Manifestations of Hypertrophic Pyloric Stenosis

Projectile vomiting
- May be ejected 3 to 4 feet from the child when side-lying, 1 foot or more when back-lying
- Occurs shortly after a feeding (may not occur for several hours)
- May follow each feeding or appear intermittently
- Nonbilious vomitus; may be blood-tinged

Infant hungry, avid nurser, eagerly accepts a second feeding after vomiting episode
No evidence of pain or discomfort except that of chronic hunger
Weight loss
Signs of dehydration
Distended upper abdomen
Readily palpable olive-shaped tumor in the epigastrium just to the right of the umbilicus
Visible gastric peristaltic waves that move from left to right across the epigastrium

of PS. Laboratory findings reflect the metabolic alterations created by severe depletion of both water and electrolytes from extensive and prolonged vomiting. There are decreased serum levels of both sodium and potassium, although these may be masked by the hemoconcentration from extracellular fluid depletion. Of greater diagnostic value are a decrease in serum chloride levels and increases in pH and bicarbonate (carbon dioxide content) characteristic of metabolic alkalosis.

Therapeutic Management

Surgical relief of the pyloric obstruction by pyloromyotomy is simple, safe, and effective and is, with very few exceptions, the standard treatment for this disorder. The surgical procedure is performed through a right upper quadrant muscle-splitting incision and consists of a longitudinal incision through the circular muscle fibers of the pylorus down to, but not including, the submucosa (Fredet-Ramstedt operation, Fig. 23-6, *B*). The procedure has a very high success rate when infants receive careful preoperative preparation to correct fluid and electrolyte imbalances.

Feedings are usually begun 4 to 6 hours postoperatively, beginning with small, frequent feedings of glucose in water or electrolyte solutions. If clear fluids are retained, about 24 hours after surgery formula is started in the same stepwise increments, gradually increasing the amount and the interval between feedings until a full feeding schedule is reinstated, which usually takes about 48 hours. The infant is ready to be discharged from the hospital by about the fourth postoperative day. The prognosis is excellent, and the mortality rate is low.

Nursing Diagnoses: The Infant with Hypertrophic Pyloric Stenosis

Potential fluid volume deficit related to persistent vomiting
Altered nutrition: less than body requirements related to persistent vomiting
Altered family processes related to hospitalization of infant

Nursing Considerations

Nursing care of the infant with hypertrophic PS involves primarily observation for physical signs and behaviors that help establish the diagnosis, careful regulation of fluid therapy, and reestablishment of normal feeding behaviors.

ASSESSMENT

Hypertrophic PS should be considered as a possibility in the very young infant who appears alert but fails to gain weight and has a history of vomiting after meals. Assessment is based on observation of eating behaviors and evidence of other characteristic clinical manifestations.

NURSING DIAGNOSES

Based on a thorough assessment, a number of nursing diagnoses are evident. The most typical are those listed in the accompanying box.

PLANNING

The goals of nursing care for the child with hypertrophic PS are primarily related to pre- and postsurgical care of the infant. These include:

1. Provide nutrition
2. Prevent vomiting
3. Prevent complications
4. Support and educate family

IMPLEMENTATION

Preoperatively the emphasis is placed on restoring hydration and electrolyte balance and beginning replacement of depleted body fat and protein stores. These infants are usually given no oral feedings and placed on intravenous fluids with glucose and electrolyte replacement based on laboratory serum electrolyte values. Careful monitoring of the intravenous infusion and diligent attention to intake, output, and urine-specific gravity measurements are important to the success of fluid replacement. Any vomiting, as well as the number and character of stools, is observed and recorded accurately.

No matter what the infant is fed, special techniques are needed to minimize the likelihood of vomiting. Feedings are given slowly with the infant held in a semi-upright position. Because these infants tend to suck their fingers and hands, they swallow a good deal of air; therefore, bubbling before and frequently during feedings will lessen gastric distention. After a feeding the infant is turned slightly on the right side in high-Fowler position in an infant seat or propped in the crib to facilitate gastric emptying. Minimum handling, especially after a feeding, helps prevent vomiting. If vomiting occurs, the type, amount, character, and its relationship to the feeding are observed and recorded. Refeeding of formula is usually ordered in an amount equivalent to the volume lost.

Observations include assessment of vital signs, particularly those that might indicate fluid or electrolyte imbalances. These infants are especially prone to metabolic alkalosis from loss of hydrogen ions and to potassium, sodium, and chloride depletion. The skin and mucous membranes are assessed for alterations in hydration status, and daily weight provides added clues to water gain or loss.

When stomach decompression and gastric lavage are part of preoperative management, it is the responsibility of the nurse to ensure that the tube is patent and functioning properly and to measure and record the type and amount of drainage. The infant is usually positioned flat or with the head slightly elevated. The infant who is receiving intravenous fluids and/or has a nasogastric tube to continuous drainage must be adequately restrained to prevent the needle and/or tube from becoming dislodged.

General hygienic care, with particular attention to skin and mouth in dehydrated infants, is an important part of care. Protection from infection is also important, since infants with impaired nutritional status are even more susceptible than normal newborn infants. Sensory stimulation is incorporated into nursing care, and parental involvement is encouraged and promoted.

Postoperative care. Postoperative vomiting is not uncommon, and most infants, even with successful surgery, exhibit some vomiting during the first 24 to 48 hours. Intravenous fluids are administered until the infant is taking and retaining adequate amounts by mouth. Therefore, much of the same care that was instituted prior to surgery is continued postoperatively, that is, observation of physical signs, monitoring intravenous fluids, and careful observation and recording of intake and output. In addition the infant is observed for responses to the stress of surgery. The nasogastric tube may be maintained after surgery for a variable length of time.

Feedings are usually instituted relatively soon, beginning with clear liquids containing glucose and electrolytes. They are offered slowly, in small amounts, and at frequent intervals as ordered by the physician. If the infant has been breast-fed, breast milk, expressed by the mother, is given by bottle when the infant is able to tolerate feedings, and breast-feeding is resumed as soon as feasible. Observation and recording of feedings and the infant's responses to feedings and feeding techniques are a vital part of postoperative care. Positioning with the head elevated is usually continued postoperatively. Care of the operative site consists of observation for any drainage or signs of inflammation and care of the incision as directed by the surgeon.

As with any child in the hospital, parents are encouraged to remain with their child and become involved in the child's care. Vomiting of a projectile nature is frightening to parents, and they often believe that they may have done something wrong. Most parents need support and reassurance that the condition is caused by a structural problem and is in no way a reflection on their parenting skills and capacities.

EVALUATION

The effectiveness of nursing interventions is determined by reassessment based on the following observational guidelines and expected outcomes:

1. Observe feeding behavior, especially vomiting episodes
2. Weigh infant daily
3. Observe for evidence of complications
4. Observe and interview family regarding feelings, understanding, and concerns

Expected outcomes:

1. Infant consumes a sufficient amount of formula
2. Infant takes and retains feedings
3. Infant recovers with no evidence of complications
4. Family express their feelings and concerns, demonstrate an understanding of the infant's condition, and are actively involved in the infant's care.

INTUSSUSCEPTION

Intussusception is one of the most frequent causes of intestinal obstruction during infancy. Half of the cases occur in children younger than age 1 year, more commonly between 3 and 12 months of age, and most of the others occur in children during the second year. Intussusception is three times more common in males than females. Although specific intestinal lesions can be found in a small percentage of the children, generally the cause is not known.

Pathophysiology

Intussusception is an invagination or telescoping of one portion of the intestine into another. The most common site is the ileocecal valve, where the ileum invaginates into the cecum and colon (Fig. 23-7) producing an obstruction to the passage of intestinal contents beyond the defect. In addition the two walls of the intestine press against each other, causing inflammation, edema, and eventually decreased blood flow. Because fecal material is unable to move beyond the obstruction the stools contain primarily blood and mucous, the "current-jelly" stools characteristic of the disorder. Continued incarceration results in necrosis with hemorrhage, perforation, and peri-

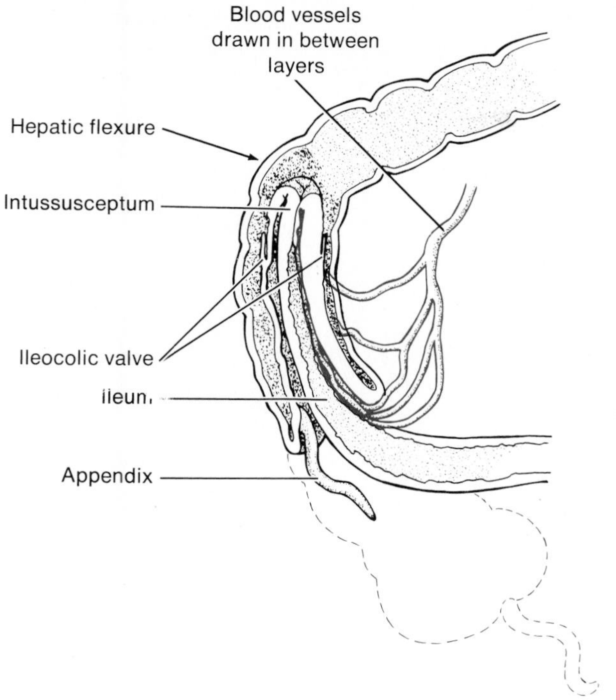

FIG. 23-7 Ileocolic intussusception.

tonitis. If left untreated this condition is incompatible with life.

Diagnostic Evaluation

Frequently the diagnosis can be made on subjective findings alone (see box). The classic presentation of intussusception is a healthy, thriving child, usually between 3 and 12 months of age, who suddenly develops an episode of acute abdominal pain, vomiting, and passing of one normal brown stool. However, definitive diagnosis is based on a barium enema, which clearly demonstrates the obstruction to the flow of barium. A rectal examination reveals mucus, blood, and, occasionally, a low intussusception itself.

Therapeutic Management

In most cases the initial treatment of choice is nonsurgical hydrostatic reduction by barium enema at the time of diagnostic testing. The force exerted by the flowing barium is usually sufficient enough to push the invaginated portion of the bowel into its original position, similar to pushing an inverted "finger" out of a glove. Successful reduction is accomplished in about 75% to 85% of uncomplicated cases. This procedure is not recommended if there are clinical signs of shock or perforation.

Since this procedure is not always successful, the child is prepared for surgery before the barium enema. Surgical intervention consists of reducing the invagination manually and, where indicated, resecting any nonviable intestine.

Clinical Manifestations of Intussusception

- Sudden acute abdominal pain
  - Child screams and draws the knees onto the chest
  - Child appears normal and comfortable during intervals between episodes of pain
- Vomiting
- Apathy
- Passage of red currant jelly-like stools (stool mixed with blood and mucus)
- Tender, distended abdomen
- Palpable sausage-shaped mass in upper right quadrant
- Empty lower right quadrant (Dance sign)
- Eventual fever, prostration, and other signs of peritonitis

Nursing Considerations

The nurse can assist in establishing a diagnosis by carefully listening to the parent's description of the child's physical and behavioral symptoms. Parents are astute in detecting that something is wrong with their child and it is not unusual for parents to express that they felt something was seriously wrong with their child before the physician shared their concerns. The description of the child's severe colicky abdominal pain combined with vomiting is a significant sign of intussusception.

As soon as a possible diagnosis of intussusception is made, the nurse begins to prepare the parents for the immediate need for hospitalization, the usual nonsurgical technique of barium enema, and the possibility of surgery. It is important at this time to explain the basic defect of intussusception, which is easily demonstrated by pushing the end of a finger on a rubber glove back into itself or using the example of a telescoping rod.

Nursing Tip: Family Teaching

The principle of reduction by hydrostatic pressure can be simulated by filling the glove with water, which pushes the "finger" into a fully extended position.

Since this hospitalization may be the child's first separation from his parents, it is especially important to preserve the parent-child relationship by encouraging rooming-in or extended visiting. It may also be the parents' first experience with hospital care for their child, necessitating their preparation for procedures such as intravenous therapy, frequent vital sign and blood pressure monitoring, dressings, and special orders, such as nothing by mouth. Because of the rapidity of the onset, diagnosis, and treatment, parents may be left with the feeling of stunned numbness. They may ask few questions or they may constantly make inquiries, sometimes the same ones several times. If the nurse realizes the circumstances surrounding this condition, the parents' reactions are more likely to be understood and accepted.

Physical care of the child with intussusception differs little from that for any child undergoing abdominal surgery. Even though nonsurgical intervention may be successful, usual preoperative procedures, such as withholding fluids, routine laboratory testing (complete blood count and urinalysis), signed parental consent, and preanesthetic sedation, are carried out. For the child with signs of electrolyte imbalance, hemorrhage, or peritonitis, additional medical preparation such as replacement fluids, whole blood or plasma, and nasogastric suctioning may be performed. Before surgery the nurse monitors all stools. Passage of a normal brown stool usually indicates that the intussusception has reduced itself. This is immediately reported to the physician, who may choose to alter the diagnostic/therapeutic plan of care.

Postprocedural care includes the usual postoperative observations, such as vital signs, blood pressure, intact sutures and dressing, and the return of bowel sounds. In the case of hydrostatic reduction or autoreduction, the nurse observes for passage of barium and the stool patterns, since recurrences of the intussusception are most likely to occur within the first 36 hours after reduction. For this reason the child may be kept in the hospital for 2 to 3 days.

ANORECTAL MALFORMATIONS

Malformations in the anorectal region of the gastrointestinal tract are among the more common congenital malformations caused by abnormal development (approximately 1 in 5000). All are classified as *imperforate anus*. Distinction between these categories is important for planning therapy and determining a prognosis.

Clinically anorectal malformations can be divided into three categories according to the relationship of the rectum to the puborectalis muscle:

low anomalies Rectum has descended normally through the puborectalis muscle, the internal and external sphincters are present and well developed with normal function, and there is no connection to the genitourinary tract (Fig. 23-8, *A* or *B*.)

intermediate anomalies Rectum is at or below the level of the puborectalis muscle, the anal dimple and external sphincter are positioned normally.

high anomalies Rectum ends above the puborectalis muscle and there is absence of internal and external sphincters. This is usually associated with genitourinary fistulae—rectourethral (male) or rectovaginal (female) (Fig. 23-8, *F*).

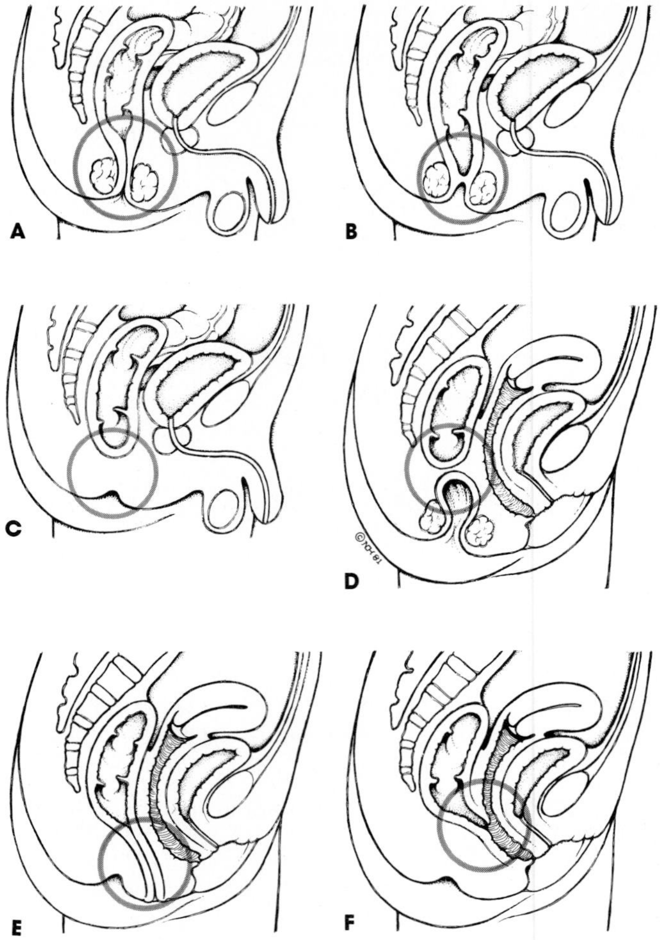

FIG. 23-8 Anorectal stenosis and imperforate anus. **A,** Congenital anal stenosis. **B,** Anal membrane atresia. **C,** Anal agenesis. **D,** Rectal atresia. **E,** Rectoperineal fistula. **F,** Rectovaginal fistula.

Diagnostic Evaluation

Inspection of the perineal area and checking for patency of the anus and rectum are a routine part of the newborn assessment, including observation or inquiries regarding the passage of meconium. Failure to pass meconium is cause for investigation. Digital and endoscopic examinations identify constriction or the blind pouch of rectal atresia. Stenosis may not become apparent until 1 year of age or older when the child has a history of difficult defecation, abdominal distention, and ribbonlike stools.

Fistulas associated with types B and C anomalies are not usually apparent at birth, but as peristalsis gradually forces the meconium through the fistula they can be identified by careful examination. With a rectourinary fistula, meconium appears in the urine.

Definitive diagnosis of the extent and location of the rectal pouch is made by radiographic examination. With the infant inverted and an opaque marker at the anal dimple, air ascending into the rectum and lower bowel will outline the location of the pouch in relation to the anal depression.

Therapeutic Management

Successful treatment for anal stenosis is generally accomplished by manual dilations. The procedure, begun by the physician, is repeated on a regular basis by the nurses in the hospital and continued at home by the parents, after they are carefully instructed in the technique. An imperforate anal membrane is excised and followed by daily anal dilations.

Reconstruction of an anus in the proper position is the goal of surgical treatment of other anorectal malformations. Malformations of the lower rectum often can be corrected in the neonatal period by way of an abdominal-perineal pull-through procedure and/or anoplasty. Infants with higher anomalies require a divided sigmoid colostomy in the newborn period. Final correction of higher defects is usually postponed for a year.

Nursing Considerations

The first nursing responsibility is identification of undetected anorectal malformations. A newborn who does not pass a stool within 24 to 36 hours of birth requires further assessment, and meconium that appears at an inappropriate orifice is reported.

Postoperative nursing care ordinarily presents few problems and is primarily directed toward healing of the anoplasty without infection or other complications. Where the infant has undergone a pull-through procedure with anoplasty, special nursing care involves maintaining the anal area as clean as possible with scrupulous perineal care. There may or may not be a temporary dressing and drain, but, when the infant is passing stool, dressings are of little value. The preferred position is a side-lying prone position with the hips elevated or a supine position with the legs suspended at a 90-degree angle to the trunk to prevent pressure on perineal sutures. Periodic application of a heat lamp facilitates healing.

The infant is administered regular infant formula as soon as peristalsis returns. In the meantime there may be a nasogastric tube for abdominal decompression and intravenous feedings. Care of the infant with a colostomy involves frequent dressing changes, meticulous skin care, and correct application of a collection device (p. 684).

◆ *Malabsorption Syndromes*

The term "malabsorption syndrome" is applied to a long list of disorders associated with some degree of impaired digestion and/or absorption. Most are classified according to the locations of the supposed anatomic and/or biochemical defect. The term *celiac syndrome* is often used to describe a symptom complex that has four characteristics in common: (1) steatorrhea (fat, foul, frothy, bulky stools), (2) general malnutrition, (3) abdominal distention, and (4) secondary vitamin deficiencies.

Digestive defects mainly include those conditions in which the enzymes necessary for digestion are diminished or absent, such as (1) cystic fibrosis, in which pancreatic enzymes are absent, (2) biliary or liver disease, in which bile production is affected, or (3) lactase deficiency, in which there is congenital or secondary lactose intolerance.

Absorptive defects include those conditions in which the intestinal mucosal transport system is impaired. It may be because of a primary defect (such as in celiac disease) or secondary to inflammatory disease of the bowel that results in impaired absorption because bowel motility is accelerated (such as ulcerative colitis). Obstructive disorders (such as Hirschsprung disease) can also cause secondary malabsorption from enterocolitis.

Anatomic defects, such as extensive resection of the bowel or "short bowel syndrome," affect digestion by decreasing the transit time of substances with the digestive juices and affects absorption by severely compromising the absorptive surface.

CELIAC DISEASE

Celiac disease (CD), also known as gluten-induced enteropathy, gluten-sensitive enteropathy (GSE), and celiac sprue, is second only to cystic fibrosis as a cause of malabsorption in children. The incidence is variously reported as one in 300 to one in 4000, and appears to be declining—possibly related to the current practice of delayed introduction of solid food. It is seen more frequently in Europe than in America and is rarely reported in Orientals or blacks. The exact cause of celiac disease and mode of transmission are not known, but there is a tendency for the disease to occur in several members of the same family.

Pathophysiology

The disease is characterized by an intolerance for gluten, one of the proteins found in wheat, barley, rye, and oats. Gluten consists of two fractions, glutenin and gliadin. Although the pathologic process is still obscure, susceptible individuals are unable to digest the gliadin faction, resulting in an accumulation of a toxic substance that is damaging to the mucosal cells. Eventually villi atrophy, reducing the absorptive surface of the small intestine.

Diagnostic Evaluation

Symptoms of celiac disease are first noted about 3 to 6 months following the introduction of gluten-containing grains into the diet, typically at 9 to 12 months of age, although it may not be evident until early childhood (see box). The clinical manifestations are usually insidious and chronic. The first evidence of the disease may be failure to regain weight or appetite after a bout of diarrhea.

A definitive diagnosis is based on a peroral jejunal biopsy, which demonstrates the atrophic changes in the architecture of the mucosal wall. This procedure is performed by passing a polyethylene tube through the mouth along the alimentary tract to the jejunum of the small bowel.

The other essential criterion of diagnosis is dramatic clinical improvement after adherence to a gluten-restricted diet. Within a day or two after instituting the diet, most children with celiac disease demonstrate a favorable

Clinical Manifestations of Celiac Disease

- Impaired fat absorption:
  - Steatorrhea (excessively large, pale, oily, frothy stools)
  - Exceedingly foul-smelling stools
- Impaired absorption of nutrients:
  - Malnutrition
  - Muscle wasting (especially prominent in legs and buttocks)
  - Anemia
  - General wasting
  - Abdominal distention
- Behavioral changes common:
  - Irritability
  - Fretfulness
  - Uncooperativeness
  - Apathy
- Celiac crisis (in very young children)
  - Acute, severe episodes of profuse watery diarrhea and vomiting
  - May be precipitated by
    - Infections (especially gastrointestinal)
    - Prolonged fluid and electrolyte depletion
    - Emotional disturbance

personality change. Weight gain, improved appetite, and disappearance of diarrhea and steatorrhea usually do not occur for several days or weeks.

Therapeutic Management

Treatment of chronic celiac disease is primarily dietary management. Although the diet is called "gluten free" it is in reality low in gluten, since it is impossible to remove every source of this protein. Also, studies demonstrate that most patients are able to tolerate restricted amounts of gluten. Because gluten is found primarily in the grains of wheat and rye, but also in smaller quantities in barley and oats, these four foods are eliminated. Corn and rice become substitute grain foods.

In children with severe malnutrition, specific deficiencies may be treated with supplemental vitamins, iron, and calories and, because absorption of fat-soluble vitamins is impaired, these are supplied in a water-miscible form.

Nursing Considerations

The main nursing consideration is helping the parents and child adhere to the prescribed diet. A considerable amount of time is involved in explaining the disease process, the specific role of gluten in aggravating the pathology, and those foods that must be restricted. Although the chief source of grain is cereal and baked goods, grains are frequently added to processed foods as thickeners or fillers. To add to the difficulty, gluten is added to many foods but obscurely listed on the label as "hydrolyzed vegetable protein." The nurse must advise parents to carefully read all ingredients on labels in order to avoid hidden sources of gluten. Many of the gluten-containing products can be eliminated from the infant's or young child's diet fairly easily, but monitoring the diet of a school-age child or adolescent is a much more difficult situation. Many "favorite" foods, such as hot dogs, pizza, and spaghetti, are chief offenders. Luncheon preparation away from home is particularly difficult, since bread, luncheon meats, and instant soups are not allowed.

In addition to restricting gluten, other dietary alterations may also be necessary in the beginning. For example, in some children who have more severe mucosal damage, the digestion of disaccharides is impaired, especially in relation to lactose. Therefore, these children often need a temporary lactose-free diet, which necessitates eliminating all milk products.

Generally management includes a diet high in calories and proteins, with simple carbohydrates, such as fruits and vegetables, but low in fats. Since the bowel is usually inflamed as a result of the pathologic processes in absorption, coarse, rough foods with high fiber, such as nuts, raisins, raw vegetables, and raw fruits with skin, are avoided until inflammation has subsided.

It is the recommendation that the child continue the diet indefinitely. This is especially difficult for parents and children to understand when there have been no symptoms of the disease for an extended period of time and occasional dietary indiscretions, probably the result of increased tolerance to glutens, have not caused untoward effects. However, evidence demonstrates that the majority of individuals who relax their diet will experience a relapse of their disease and possibly exhibit growth retardation, anemia, or osteomalacia. There is also the risk of developing malignant lymphoma of the small intestine, esophageal cancer, and other gastrointestinal malignancies.

Several resources are available to assist parents in all aspects of coping with celiac disease. The **American Celiac Society*** and the **Celiac Sprue Association/United States of America†** are organizations that provide support and guidance to families and supply educational materials concerning gluten-free diet, food sources, and recipes, and travel information. A booklet, *Pointers for Parents: Coping with Celiac Sprue,* is available‡ that provides information on shopping, cooking, and otherwise living with an affected child.

SHORT GUT (BOWEL) SYNDROME

The short gut syndrome is a condition in which there is a loss of intestine resulting in a diminished ability to digest and absorb a regular diet normally. The major causes in children are: (1) congenital, such as small intestine atresias or gastroschisis, (2) volvulus involving a large segment of bowel, and (3) inflammation, such as that of necrotizing enterocolitis or Crohn disease.

*Dept. N83, 45 Gifford Ave., Jersey City, NJ 07304.

†3213 Rocklyn Dr., Des Moines, IA 50322. In Canada: **The Canadian Celiac Association, Inc.,** 1087 Meyerside Dr., Suite 5, Mississauga, Ontario L5T 1M5, (416) 673-8200.

‡Clinical Dietetics Department, Children's Memorial Hospital, 2300 Children's Plaza, Chicago, IL 60614

Both the amount and location of gut lost are important in determining the severity of the condition. Up to 50% of the intestine can be lost without affecting the health of the child, unless it includes the distal ileum. A loss of greater than 75% of the small bowel results in malabsorption. However, the remaining intestine and stomach can adapt to the loss through compensatory growth provided the child is kept alive with special nutritional support.

Therapeutic Management

The goals of treatment are (1) to preserve as much length of bowel as possible during surgery and (2) to maintain the child's nutritional status until adaptation to the altered bowel takes place. For the severely affected child total parenteral nutrition is the treatment of choice.

Nursing Considerations

Nursing care is directed toward maintaining the child's nutritional state. Every effort is made to preserve the intravenous line in parenteral alimentation and to prevent complications such as infection. When long-term parenteral nutrition is required, preparing the family for home care of the child is a major nursing responsibility. Since hospitalization may be prolonged, the child's developmental and emotional needs must be met as well.

SUMMARY

Some of the most common disorders of childhood are those related to GI function. Diarrhea and vomiting are both isolated problems and symptoms of a variety of diseases and conditions. However, the major hazard associated with GI losses is dehydration, which can assume dangerous proportions with surprising rapidity. The most common causes of GI losses are organisms, food indiscretions, and structural or functional defects of the GI tract.

The GI tract is subject to numerous structural or mechanical abnormalities that interfere with the ingestion and passage of nutrients through the alimentary canal. The type of defect in many cases is related to the age of the child; for example, pyloric stenosis in very early infancy, intussusception in later infancy, and peptic ulcers in later childhood. However, inflammatory conditions, especially appendicitis and inflammatory bowel disease, are as common in childhood as in early adulthood. Careful assessment and evaluation often alert perceptive nurses to the possibility of some of these conditions in their infant or child patients.

KEY CONCEPTS

- Infants are subject to fluid depletion because of their greater surface area relative to body mass, high rate of metabolism, and immature kidney function.
- Dehydration can be classified as isotonic, hypotonic, and hypertonic.
- Vomiting and diarrhea account for significant fluid depletion, especially in infants and small children.
- The amount, frequency, and characteristics of stool and vomitus are important nursing observations.
- Acute diarrhea can be caused by an inflammatory process of infectious origin, a toxic reaction to ingestion of poisonous substances, dietary indiscretions, or can be associated with infections outside the alimentary tract.
- Postoperative care of the child with abdominal surgery involves providing hydration and nutrition, IV fluids, proper positioning, and psychologic support.
- Nursing care of gastrointestinal reflux is aimed at identifying children with suggestive symptoms, helping parents with home care feeding and positioning, and caring for the child undergoing surgical intervention.
- Surgical correction in Hirschsprung disease is a three-stage approach: a temporary colostomy, reanastomosis at 8 months to 1 year of age, and closure of colostomy a few months later.
- Although the cause of appendicitis is poorly understood, it is commonly a result of obstruction of the lumen, usually by a fecalith. Common signs and symptoms are colicky abdominal pain, tenderness, and fever.
- Meckel diverticulum, the most common congenital malformation of the GI tract, is characterized by rectal bleeding.
- Inflammatory bowel disease refers to ulcerative colitis and Crohn disease of which persistent and recurring diarrhea is the most common feature. It is treated by dietary management and medication, although surgery is needed in a number of cases.
- Peptic ulcers are poorly understood, but one of two mechanisms probably reflects the basic defect: an increase in the rate of production of gastric juice, or interference with the normal protective mechanisms of the mucosal lining.
- Viral hepatitis is caused by at least four types of virus—hepatitis A virus, hepatitis B virus, hepatitis D virus, and non-A, non-B virus.
- Hepatitis A virus is spread by the fecal-oral route, whereas hepatitis B virus is transmitted primarily by the parenteral route. The single most effective measure in prevention and control of hepatitis in any setting is handwashing.
- Structural disorders of the gastrointestinal tract include cleft lip, cleft palate, esophageal atresia with tracheoesophageal fistula, anorectal malformations, and biliary atresia.
- Cleft lip and palate, the most common facial malformation, may involve nutritional, dental, and speech problems.
- Hernias related to the gastrointestinal tract can be minor (umbilical hernia) or life-threatening (hiatal, gastroschisis, omphalocele).
- General signs of obstruction include colicky abdominal pain, nausea and vomiting, abdominal distention, and constipation.

- Hypertrophic pyloric stenosis is recognized by characteristic projectile vomiting and a palpable mass in the epigastrium and is relieved by pyloromyotomy.
- Intussusception is one of the most common causes of intestinal obstruction during infancy. Treatment is either nonsurgical hydrostatic reduction by barium enema or surgical reduction.
- Malabsorption syndromes are disorders associated with some degree of impaired digestion and/or absorption. They include digestive defects, absorptive defects, and anatomic defects.
- Celiac disease, the second leading cause of malabsorption in children, is characterized by an intolerance for gluten. It is thought to be either an inborn error of metabolism or an immunologic response.

STUDY QUESTIONS AND ACTIVITIES

1 Design a low fiber diet for an adolescent with inflammatory bowel disease, keeping in mind the normal needs and developmental characteristics of the adolescent.
2 Interview a child recovering from surgery for acute appendicitis to determine his understanding of the reason for the surgery—what he believes to have caused the appendicitis.
3 Outline a nursing care plan for the infant with pyloric stenosis.
4 Select a specified number of common packaged foods and scrutinize the labels for evidence of ingredients that would be contraindicated in a diet for a child with celiac disease.
5 Compare and contrast the nursing needs of an infant with cleft lip and one with cleft palate.

REFERENCES

Barker, D.J.P., Morris, J., and Nelson, M.: Vegetable consumption and acute appendicitis in 59 areas in England and Wales, Br. Med. J. **292:**927-930, 1986.

Biller, J.A.: Ulcerative colitis and Crohn's disease. In Gellis, S.S., and Kagan, B.M.: Current pediatric therapy, ed. 12, Philadelphia, 1986, W.B. Saunders Co.

Guerrant, R.L., Lohr, J.A., and Williams, E.K.: Acute infectious diarrhea. I. Epidemiology, etiology and pathogenesis, Pediatr. Infect. Dis. **5:**353-349, 1986.

Kurfiss-Daniels, D.: Positioning as treatment for infant gastroesophageal reflux, Am. J. Nurs. **82:**1535-1537, 1982.

Motil, K.J., and Grand, R.J.: Nutritional management of inflammatory bowel disease, Pediatr. Clin. North Am. **32:**447-469, 1985.

Sibinga, M.S.: The gastrointestinal tract. In Levine, M.D., and others, editors: Developmental-behavioral pediatrics, Philadelphia, 1983, W.B. Saunders Co.

Silverman, A., and Roy, C.C.: Pediatric clinical gastroenterology, ed. 3, St. Louis, 1983, The C.V. Mosby Co.

BIBLIOGRAPHY

Disorders of Motility

Alterescu, K.B.: The ostomy: what about special procedures? Am. J. Nurs. **85**(12):1363-1367, 1985.

Aquilina, S.S.: Gastroesophageal reflux: problem or nuisance? J. Pediatr. Health Care **1:**233-239, 1987.

Boarini, J.: The ostomy: what can go wrong? Am. J. Nurs. **85**(12):1358-1362, 1985.

Boyd, C.W.: A bed for infants with gastroesophageal reflux, Pediatr. Nurs. **7**(5):53-55, 1981.

Boyd, C.W.: Postural therapy at home for infants with gastroesophageal reflux, Pediatr. Nurs. **8:**395-398, 1982.

Cerrato, P.L.: What to tell your patients about dietary fiber, RN **50**(1):63-64, 1987.

Copeland, L.: Chronic diarrhea in infancy, Am. J. Nurs. **77:**461-463, 1977.

Hamm, P., and Jemison-Smith, P.: Salmonella, Crit. Care Update **9**(1):41-44, 1982.

Ling, L., and McCamman, S.P.: Dietary treatment of diarrhea and constipation in infants and children, Issues Compr. Pediatr. Nurs. **3**(4):17-28, 1978.

Lynn, M.R.: Use of infant seats for gastroesophageal reflux, J. Pediatr. Nurs. **1**(2):127-129, 1986.

Petersen, M.: Esophageal pH monitoring, J. Pediatr. Nurs. **1:**354-357, 1986.

Sasso, S.C.: Metoclopramide and chalasia, MCN **8**(5):361, 1983.

Sugar, E.C.: Hirschsprung's disease, Am. J. Nurs. **81:**2065-2067, 1981.

Trowell, H., and Burkitt, D.: Physiological role of dietary fiber: a ten-year review, Contemp. Nutr. **11**(7):1-2, 1986.

Tucker, J.A., and Sussman-Karten, K.: Treating acute diarrhea and dehydration with an oral rehydration solution, Pediatr. Nurs. **13:**169-174, 1987.

Inflammatory Disorders

Brender, J.D., and others: Fiber intake and childhood appendicitis, Am. J. Public Health **75**(4):399-400, 1985.

Broadwell, D.C., and Woodruff, N.H.: Continent ileostomy and ileoanal reservoir: two surgical alternatives for patients once requiring conventional ileostomies, Point of View **23**(3):12-15, 1986.

Cassell, B.L.: The new trend in ileostomy surgery, RN **47** (1):48-51, 1984.

Deters, G.E.: Managing complications after abdominal surgery, RN **50**(3):27-32, 1987.

Ellett, M.L., and Schibler, K.: Adolescent psychosocial adaptation to inflammatory bowel disease, J. Pediatr. Health Care **2:**57-66, 1988.

Gryboski, J.D.: Crohn's disease in children, Pediatr. Rev. **2**(8):239-244, 1981.

Hagenah, G.C., Harrigan, J.F., and Campbell, M.: Inflammatory bowel disease in children, Nurs. Clin. North Am. **19**(1):27-39, 1984.

Hartter, C.: What's a continent ileostomy? When Karen found out, so did we, Nursing 81 **11**(11):84-89, 1981.

Lessman, M.: Painful chronicle, Am. J. Nurs. **85**(5):551-552, 1985.

Lewicki, L.J., and Leeson, M.J.: The multisystem impact on physiologic processes of inflammatory bowel disease, Nurs. Clin. North Am. **19**(1):71-80, 1984.

Mathewson, M., and Farnham, C.: Milk therapy in ulcer disease: yes or no? Home Healthcare Nurse **2**(4):8, 1984.

Neufeldt, J.: Helping the I.B.D. patient cope with the unpredictable, Nursing 87 **17**(8):47-49, 1987.

Nursing grand rounds: supporting the patient with Crohn's disease, Nursing 83 **13**(11):46-51, 1983.

Rosenberg, J.M., and Kirschenbaum, H.L.: Antacids, Am. J. Nurs. **82:**54-56, 1982.

Samelson, S.L., and Reyes, H.M.: Management of perforated appendicitis in children—revisited, Arch. Surg. **122:**691-696, 1987.

Simmons, M.A.: Using the nursing process in treating inflammatory bowel disease, Nurs. Clin. North Am. **19**(1):11-25, 1984.

Sparacino, L.L.: Psychosocial considerations for the adolescent and young adult with inflammatory bowel disease, Nurs. Clin. North Am. **19**(1):41-49, 1984.

Stotts, N.A., Fitzgerald, K.A., and Williams, K.R.: Care of the patient critically ill with inflammatory bowel disease, Nurs. Clin. North Am. **19**(1):61-70, 1984.

Wilson, C.: The diagnostic work-up for the patient with inflammatory bowel disease, Nurs. Clin. North Am. **19**(1):51-59, 1984.

Hepatic Disorders

Brainerd, E.: Nursing management of chronic infectious diseases in children, Pediatrics Nurs. Update **1**(17):2-7, 1986.

Barkin, R.M., and Lilly, J.R.: Biliary atresia and the Kasai operation: continuing care, J. Pediatr. **96:**1015-1019, 1980.

Fredette, S.L.: When the liver fails, Am. J. Nurs. **84:**64-67, 1984.

Guenter, P.: Hepatic disease: nutritional implications, Nurs. Clin. North Am. **18:**71-80, 1983.

Gurevich, I.: Hepatitis in critical care: area of concern, Crit. Care Update **10**(4):14-17, 1983.

Gurevich, I.: Viral hepatitis, Am. J. Nurs. **83:**572-586, 1983.

Hamm, P., and Jemison-Smith, P.: Viral hepatitis, Crit. Care Update **10**(2):37-44, 1983.

Keith, J.S.: Hepatic failure: etiologies, manifestations, and management, Crit. Care Nurse **5**(1):60-86, 1985.

Kirkman-Liff, B., and Dandoy, S.: Hepatitis B: what price exposure? Am. J. Nurs. **84**(4):988-990, 1984.

Mar, D.D.: New hepatitis B vaccine: a breakthrough in hepatitis prevention, Am. J. Nurs. **82**(2):306-307, 1982.

Oellrich, R.G., and Cusumano, M.M.: Biliary atresia, Neonatal Network **5**(5):25-32, 1987.

Williams, L.: Care of the pediatric liver transplant patient in the ICU, Crit. Care Q. **8**(1):13-25, 1985.

Wimpsett, J.: Trace your patient's liver dysfunction, Nursing 84 **14**(8):56-57, 1984.

Structural Defects

Colburn, N., and Cherry, R.S.: Community-based team approach to the management of children with cleft palate, Child. Health Care **13:**122-128, 1985.

Dixon, A.G.: Jeff's story: a unique approach to the care of an infant with esophageal atresia and a cervical esophagostomy, Neonatal Network, **4**(6):7-12, 1986.

Frentner, S.: Abdominal wall defects: omphalocele and gastroschisis, Neonatal Network **6**(3):29-41, 1987.

Hazle, N.: An infant who survived gastroschisis, MCN **6**(1):35-40, 1981.

Huth, M.M., and O'Brien, M.E.: The gastrostomy feeding button, Pediatr. Nurs. **13:**241-245, 1987.

Martin, L.W.: A new "gravity-flow" nipple for feeding infants with congenital cleft palate, Pediatrics **72:**244, 1983.

Moynihan, P., and Gerraughty, A.: Diaphragmatic hernia: low stress = higher survival, Am. J. Nurs. **85:**662-665, 1985.

Pate, C.M.H.: Care of the family following the birth of a child with a cleft lip and/or palate, Neonatal Network **5**(6):30-37, 1987.

Scheuerle, J., and others: A survey of nursing care for parents and infants with cleft lip and palate, Cleft Palate J. **21:**110-114, 1984.

Styer, G.W., and Freeh, K.: Feeding infants with cleft lip and/or palate, JOGNN **10:**329-331, 1981.

Zissermann, L.: Feeding problems: weaning an infant from a transpyloric tube, Pediatr. Nurs. **12:**33-37, 1986.

Obstructive Disorders

Cargile, N.D.: Buying time when you face a bowel obstruction, RN **48**(8):40-46, 1985.

Literte, J.W.: Nursing care of patients with intestinal obstruction, Am. J. Nurs. **77**(6):1003-1006, 1977.

McConnell, E.A.: Meeting the challenge of intestinal obstruction, Nursing 87 **17**(7):34-41, 1987.

Malabsorption Syndromes

Gantt, L., and Thompson, C.: Short gut syndrome in the infant, Am. J. Nurs. **85**(11):1263-1266, 1985.

Hartwig, M.S.: Sticking to a gluten free diet, Am. J. Nurs. **83:**1308-1310, 1983.

Lamb, C.: Simplifying diagnosis of malabsorption, Patient Care **15**(17):128-178, 1981.

Robinson, L.A.: Nontropical sprue (gluten intolerance and vitamins), Pediatr. Nurs. **7**(5):61, 1981.

UNIT XI

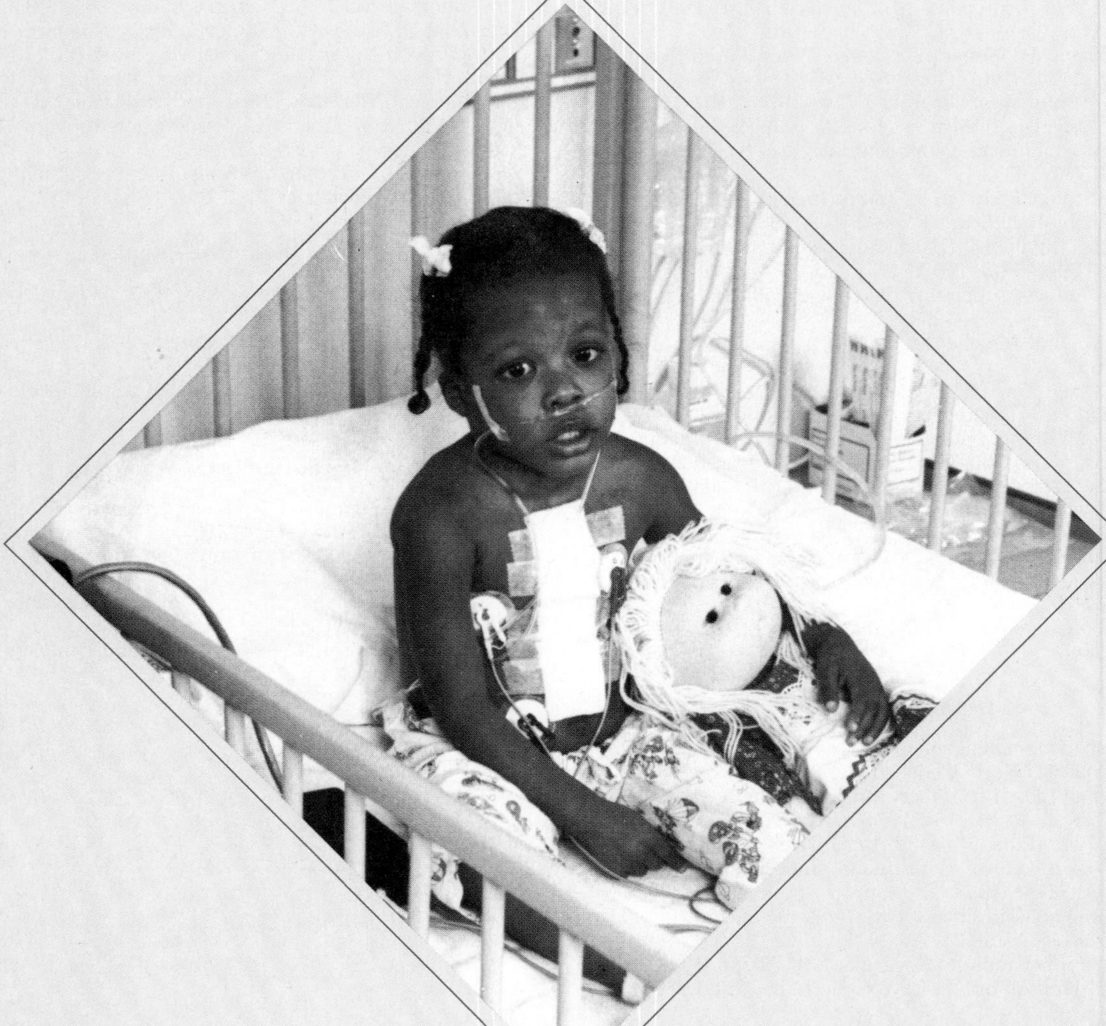

The Child with Problems Related to Production and Circulation of Blood

Some of the most common and serious childhood conditions are related to the heart and the formed elements of the blood. Many of these disorders are inherited and present at birth, whereas others are acquired. Most of them necessitate medical/surgical intervention to prevent complications and permit normal growth. Nursing care at the time of diagnosis, prior to and during corrective or palliative procedures, and after treatment is essential to promote physical and emotional recovery.

Chapter 24, *The Child with Cardiovascular Dysfunction,* discusses the types of congenital and acquired cardiac disorders and the physical consequences of impaired functioning. It focuses on caring for the child with heart disease, preparation of the family for surgery, diagnostic procedures, and postoperative nursing interventions. It also discusses problems of short- and long-term circulatory impairment in children. Chapter 25, *The Child with Hematologic or Immunologic Dysfunction,* deals with several disorders related to the formed elements of the blood. Since most of these conditions are inherited and chronic, nursing interventions stress helping the family adjust to the disorder and cope with and prevent its complications.

CHAPTER 24

The Child with Cardiovascular Dysfunction

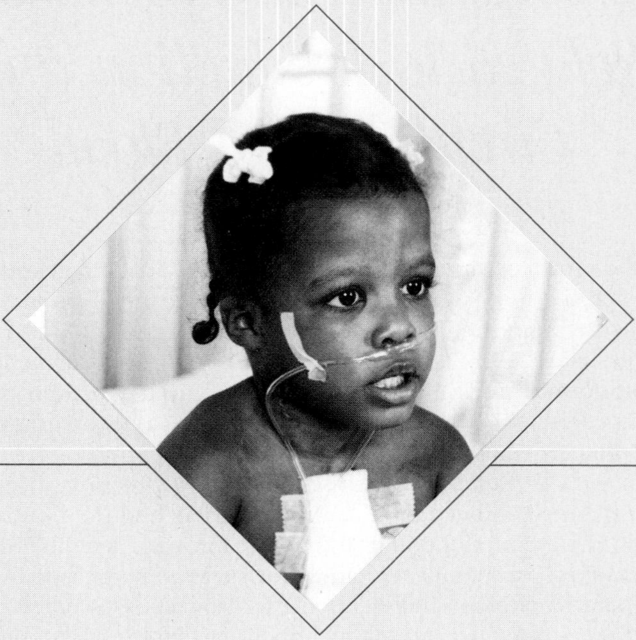

LEARNING OBJECTIVES

On completion of this chapter the reader will be able to:

- Design a plan for assisting a child during a cardiac diagnostic procedure
- Demonstrate an understanding of the hemodynamics, distinctive manifestations, and therapeutic management of congenital heart disease
- Describe the care for an infant or a child with a congenital heart defect
- Outline a plan of care for an infant or child with congestive heart failure
- Discuss the role of the nurse in assisting the child and family to cope with congenital heart disease
- Discuss the assessment and management of hypertension in children and adolescents
- Contrast the causes and mechanisms of shock in children
- Outline a plan of care for the child with Kawasaki disease

*D*isorders involving the heart and blood vessels include those that are present at birth and those that are acquired as the result of some disease process that directly or indirectly affects cardiovascular function. Some conditions are asymptomatic and detected only on examination. Many conditions place minimal limitations on a child's activities, while others are serious enough to impose severe restrictions. A few are incompatible with life.

◆ *Cardiovascular Dysfunction*

The most common form of heart disease in children is congenital heart disease, predominantly structural defects that result from developmental arrest or deviation. The acquired heart lesion most frequently encountered in pediatrics is carditis and subsequent valvular stenosis related to childhood rheumatic fever. Congestive heart failure is a serious consequence of congenital or acquired heart disease, and it is also a complication of other diseases, including chronic lung disease, muscular dystrophy, advanced kidney disease, and a variety of acute disorders and infections that place undue demands on the heart.

Rhythm disturbances are relatively uncommon in children. Occasionally, bradycardia is recognized during the prenatal period and the infant is closely monitored before and after birth for any untoward effects. Paroxysmal atrial tachycardia, a potentially serious disorder, is amenable to therapy when it is recognized early.

Disorders of the peripheral circulation include those that increase blood pressure, those that decrease blood pressure (shock), and those that affect the vessels directly (Kawasaki disease, purpura).

Any disorder that affects the heart provokes anxiety in the family, the nurse, and, subsequently, the child. In many instances this anxiety is not unfounded, but in some cases it is greater than that called for by the seriousness of the condition. To help the child and his family to adjust to a heart condition and to live a life without overprotection and excessive restriction requires guidance and support from many health professionals, particularly nurses.

TABLE 24-1

Procedures for Cardiac Diagnosis

Procedure	Description
Electrocardiography	Measures electrical potential generated from heart muscle
Echocardiography	Short pulses of ultrasound transmitted through the heart bounce off heart structures; reflected on a screen
Ultrasonography	Similar to echocardiography; it is synchronized with ECG to provide a three-dimensional recording of heart structures
Roentgenography	
Fluoroscopy	Provides direct observation of heart size, position, contour, and relationships
Radiography	Provides permanent record of heart size and configuration
Angiocardiography	Opaque media injected into circulatory system outlines blood flow through the heart and vessels performed in conjunction with cardiac catheterization
Cardiac catheterization	Opaque catheter introduced into the heart chambers via large peripheral vessels is observed by fluoroscopy or image intensification; pressure measurements and blood samples provide additional source of information
Digital subtraction angiography (DSA)	Opaque media injected into circulatory system Provides computerized images of vessels and tissues containing dye—"subtracts" all tissues not containing dye

ASSESSMENT OF CARDIAC FUNCTION

Diagnosis of congenital or acquired heart disease is based on a comprehensive history and physical examination and on a variety of specific and related diagnostic procedures. Physical assessment also assumes a prominent position in evaluation of cardiac status. Cardiac catheterization, which generates more anxiety than any other test, is discussed in detail. Specific findings are included in the discussions of the various heart defects presented in this chapter.

Diagnostic Evaluation

A variety of techniques are employed for evaluating cardiac function in infants and children. Objective evaluation is an essential aspect of medical and nursing assessment and is described in the following section. Laboratory tests of significance include complete blood count, hemoglobin, hematocrit, and sometimes blood gas analysis. Special tests are briefly outlined in Table 24-1.

Nursing Considerations

Nursing assessment of children for evidence of cardiac dysfunction begins with a careful history to elicit information regarding possible causes of heart disease: (1) history of heart disease in other family members, such as a parent or sibling; (2) contact with known teratogens, such as rubella, during pregnancy; (3) poor weight gain and/or feeding behavior; (4) frequent respiratory infections; (5) prior murmurs; (6) respiratory difficulties, such as tachypnea, dyspnea, shortness of breath; or (7) recent streptococcal infection in the child. Exercise intolerance and fatigue (such as during feeding in the infant) are characteristic features of heart disease.

The physical assessment of suspected cardiac disease begins with observation of general appearance, then proceeds with more specific observations. The following are supplementary to the general assessment techniques described for physical assessment of the chest on p. 154.

INSPECTION

Nutritional state—failure to thrive or poor weight gain are associated with heart disease

Color—cyanosis is a common feature of congenital heart disease and pallor is associated with anemia, which frequently accompanies heart disease

Chest deformities—an enlarged heart sometimes distorts the chest configuration
Unusual pulsations—visible pulsations are seen in some patients
Respiratory excursion—the ease or difficulty of respiration, e.g., tachypnea, dyspnea, presence of expiratory grunt
Clubbing of fingers—are associated with some types of congenital heart disease
Behavior—squatting is typical of some types of heart disease

PALPATION AND PERCUSSION
Chest—helps discern heart size and other characteristics (such as thrills) associated with heart disease
Abdomen—hepatomegaly and/or splenomegaly may be evident
Peripheral pulses—rate, regularity, and amplitude (strength) may reveal discrepancies

AUSCULTATION
Heart—detect presence of heart murmurs
Heart rate and rhythm—observe for discrepancies between apical and peripheral pulse
Character of heart sounds—reveals deviations in heart sounds and intensity that help localize heart defects
Lungs—may reveal rales, ronchi
Blood pressure—deviations present in some cardiac conditions, e.g., discrepancies between upper and lower extremities

CARDIAC CATHETERIZATION

The most valuable diagnostic procedure is cardiac catheterization, in which a radiopaque catheter is inserted through a peripheral blood vessel into the heart. The catheter is usually introduced by way of the femoral vein—either through a cutdown procedure, in which a small incision is made to expose the vessel, or through a percutaneous technique, in which the catheter is threaded through a large-bore needle that is inserted into the vein. The catheter is guided through the heart with the aid of fluoroscopy. Once the tip of the catheter is within a heart chamber, dye is injected and films are taken of the dilution and circulation of the material. At various times blood samples are taken and oxygen concentrations and blood pressures within the chambers are measured and recorded.

There are two main types of cardiac catheterization: (1) right-sided catheterization, in which the catheter is introduced from a vein into the right atrium, and (2) left-sided catheterization, in which the catheter is threaded by way of a systemic artery retrograde into the aorta and left ventricle or, from a right-sided approach, into the left atrium by means of a septal puncture. In children the most common method is right-sided catheterization, since septal defects permit entry into the left side of the heart from the right side.

Nursing Considerations

Although cardiac catheterization has become a routine diagnostic procedure, it is not without risks, especially in neonates, infants, and seriously ill children. Therefore, nursing judgment prior to and after the procedure is essential. Since cardiac catheterization is performed more frequently than cardiac surgery, consideration of this necessary but potentially frightening procedure is of utmost importance for nurses.

Preprocedural care. Preparing the child and his family for the procedure is the joint responsibility of physician, nurse, and parents. The cardiologist usually explains the procedure to the parents, but nurses can reinforce and clarify the information they have received. Many parents of children who undergo both cardiac catheterization and cardiac surgery say in retrospect that they were more anxious about the catheterization than about the surgery.

Little psychologic preparation can be made for infants and toddlers, who comprise the majority of candidates for cardiac catheterization. The preparation of children of preschool age and above must be individualized to their level of development (especially their cognitive skills), their past experiences, and their understanding and perception of the situation. They should be neither underprepared nor overprepared for the experience. Overpreparing the child, especially a preschooler, can *add* to the level of anxiety rather than decrease it.

Preparation for cardiac catheterization requires the same attention to basic principles of preparation for procedures described in Chapter 21. As a general guideline, it is best to inform the child about what he will see, feel, and hear during the procedure and about what he will be expected to do to cooperate. He needs to know what preparations will begin before he goes to the cardiac catheterization laboratory and something about what he will experience during the time he is there. Familiar and strange aspects of the procedure are explained and, whenever possible, related to past experiences, for example, electrocardiograph leads on the chest, a thermometer to monitor body temperature, and restraints to "help him remember to lie very still." It is helpful to include parents and to enlist their aid as participants, since they are often aware of the child's fears and concerns.

The child who is old enough to understand should be told that he will receive medication that will make him "very, very sleepy" and that he will ride on a special bed (if he has not had experience with a gurney) to a special room (some institutions routinely take a child on a brief tour of the area the day before the test). It is important to describe some of the things he will see, feel, or hear that may be anxiety-provoking, such as what the "cath" room looks like, because the x-ray machinery can have a frightening appearance. Since the test is performed under sterile conditions, all health personnel wear surgical garb. If the child is unfamiliar with this, he may become frightened by their masked appearance unless he has been prepared beforehand.

Although the child will be very heavily sedated he can be told about some of the sensations that he will experience during the procedure such as people working and talking close around him. He should be told that a special medicine will make him feel warm for a few seconds and then the lights will go out and a machine that is taking his picture will make a "funny noise." The last point is important to stress, because younger children may associate the lights going off with "causing" the warm feeling from the radiopaque solution. As a result they may become fearful of the dark and the noise from the machines. It is also advisable to avoid using the word "dye" for the radiopaque solution, since children may interpret the word as "die."

Older children may appreciate a more detailed explanation of how the solution aids in the diagnostic procedure, since this point can be elaborated on during the test to prevent boredom. An adequate explanation is helpful in ensuring the older child's cooperation during the long procedure, which may last from 2 to 5 hours. It is often best to explain what is going on and what to expect as the procedure progresses rather than explaining the entire process in detail ahead of time. Reading a younger child stories during the test or allowing him to hold a favorite toy is helpful in maintaining cooperation.

Physical preparation of the child is the same as the preparation for any surgical procedure. He is allowed nothing by mouth for 4 to 6 hours before the catheterization, and he is given sedation, usually a combination analgesic. Usually, the morning dose of oral digoxin is withheld (for those children who are receiving the drug), although this is clarified beforehand with the physician.

Infants are not premedicated and it is not advisable to withhold fluids for more than 2 to 3 hours prior to the scheduled time of the procedure because any state of dehydration will cause difficulty in entering the veins. It is wise to send along extra diapers and a pacifier and/or a bottle of water if these items are not part of the laboratory's inventory.

Postprocedural care. Essentially, the care following cardiac catheterization is the same as postoperative care. However, since children are not anesthetized during the procedure, they usually return directly to their room.

Cardiac catheterization involves several potential complications, including arrhythmias, cardiac perforation, hemorrhage, arterial obstruction, reactions to contrast media, infection, phlebitis, and hypoxia. The most important nursing responsibility is observation of the following: (1) temperature, respirations, and apical pulse; (2) blood pressure; (3) pulses, especially below the catheterization site, which are checked for equality and symmetry (pulse distal to the site may be weaker for the first few hours after catheterization but should gradually increase in strength); (4) temperature and color of the affected extremity, since coolness, cyanosis, or blanching may indicate vessel obstruction; and (5) dressings, which are checked for evidence of bleeding or hematoma formation in the femoral or antecubital area.

Usually, children are kept in bed for up to 24 hours after the procedure. Infants and small children can be held, especially if restless. They are allowed their usual diet as soon as it is tolerated. It is best to begin with sips of water and advance as their condition indicates.

Generally, there is only slight discomfort at the cutdown or percutaneous site. The area is protected from possible contamination, such as that resulting from soiling if the child wears diapers. If keeping the dressing dry is a problem, it can be covered with a piece of plastic film and the edges sealed to the skin with tape. The nurse must be careful, however, to continue to observe the site for any evidence of bleeding.

It is important at this time to evaluate the child's conception of what occurred during the procedure, in order to clarify any misconceptions and allow him a feeling of triumph and satisfaction in having gone through the experience.

◆ *Congenital Heart Disease*

The incidence of congenital heart disease (CHD) in children is generally believed to be 4 to 8 per 1000 live births and is the major cause of death in the first year (other than prematurity). The sexes are affected differently, depending on the defect, and defects are found in a much higher percentage of stillbirths and spontaneous abortions.

GENERAL CONCEPTS

The etiology of most congenital heart defects is not known. However, several factors are associated with a higher than normal incidence of the disease. These include prenatal factors such as (1) maternal rubella during pregnancy, (2) maternal alcoholism, (3) maternal age over 40 years, and (4) maternal insulin-dependent diabetes. Several genetic factors are also implicated. For example, there is an increased risk of congenital heart disease in the child who (1) has a sibling with a heart defect, (2) has a parent with congenital heart disease, (3) has a chromosomal aberration, such as Down syndrome, or (4) is born with other, noncardiac congenital anomalies.

Circulatory Changes at Birth

During fetal life, blood carrying oxygen and nutritive materials from the placenta enters the fetal system through the umbilicus via the large umbilical vein. Oxygenated blood enters the heart by way of the inferior vena cava. Because of the higher pressure of blood entering the right atrium, it is directed posteriorly in a straight pathway across the right atrium and through the *foramen ovale* to the left atrium. In this way the better-oxygenated blood enters the left atrium and ventricle, to be pumped through the aorta to the head and upper extremities. Blood from the head and upper extremities entering the right atrium from the superior vena cava is directed downward through the tricuspid valve into the right ventricle. From here it is pumped through the pulmonary artery, where the major portion is shunted to the descending aorta via the *ductus arteriosus*. Only a small amount

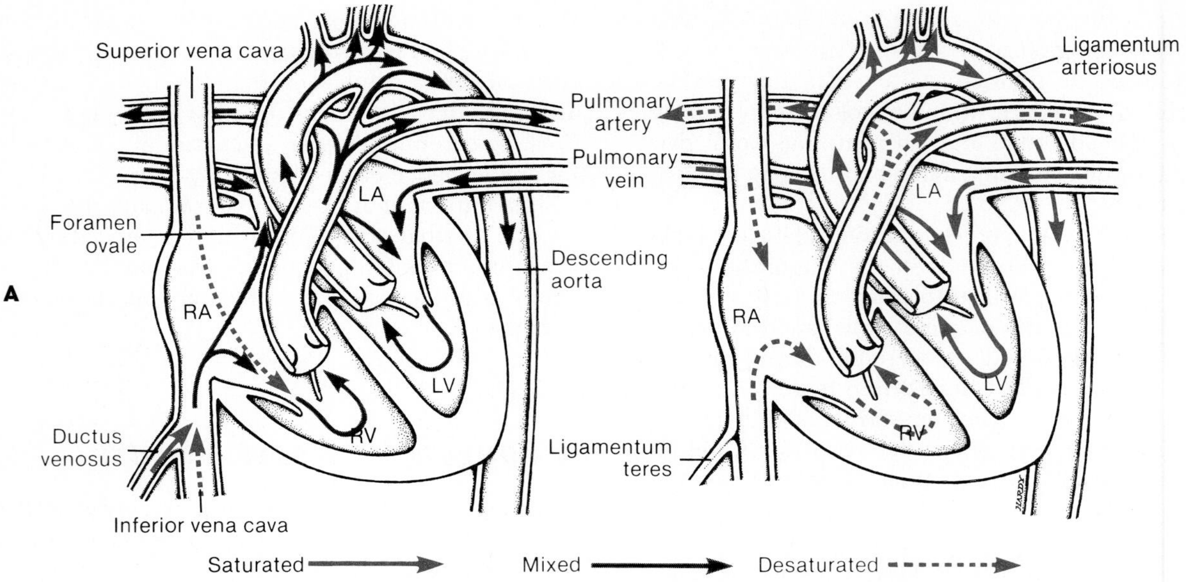

FIG. 24-1 Changes in circulation at birth. **A,** Prenatal circulation. **B,** Postnatal circulation. Arrows indicate direction of blood flow. *RA,* Right atrium. *LA,* Left atrium. *RV,* Right ventricle. *LV,* Left ventricle. *Note:* Although four pulmonary veins enter the left atrium, for simplicity this diagram shows only two.

flows to and from the nonfunctioning fetal lungs (Fig. 24-1, *A*).

Before birth the high pulmonary vascular resistance created by the collapsed fetal lung causes greater pressures in the right side of the heart and the pulmonary arteries. At the same time the free-flowing placental circulation and the ductus arteriosus produce a low vascular resistance in the remainder of the fetal vascular system. With the cessation of placental blood flow from clamping of the umbilical cord and the expansion of the lungs at birth, the hemodynamics of the fetal vascular system undergo pronounced and abrupt changes (Fig. 24-1, *B*).

Types of Defects

Congenital heart defects may be divided into various categories, but two commonly used divisions are based on the altered circulation:

acyanotic in which there is no mixing of desaturated (poorly oxygenated venous) blood in the systemic arterial circulation

cyanotic in which desaturated blood enters the systemic arterial circulation, regardless of whether cyanosis is clinically evident

Clinical manifestations depend on the severity of the defect and the amount of pulmonary blood flow. In acyanotic defects no associated signs and symptoms may be apparent if the defect is small and the heart is able to compensate for the extra workload.

Altered hemodynamics. To appreciate the physiology of heart defects, it is necessary to understand the role of pressure gradients, flow, and resistance within the circulation. Like any fluid, blood flows from an area of high pressure to one of lower pressure and toward the path of least resistance in response to the pumping action of the heart. In general, the higher the pressure gradient, the greater the rate of flow; the higher the resistance, the less is the rate of flow.

Normally the pressure on the right side of the heart is lower than that on the left side, and the resistance in the pulmonary circulation is less than that in the systemic circulation. Vessels entering or exiting these chambers have corresponding pressures. Therefore, if there is an abnormal connection between the heart chambers (such as a septal defect) blood will necessarily flow from an area of higher pressure (left side) to one of lower pressure (right side). Such a flow of blood is termed a *left-to-right shunt.* No desaturated blood flows directly into the left side of the heart; hence the term *acyanotic defect* (Fig. 24-2, *B*). If the opening is small and high on the septum, the amount of blood shunted to the atrium or ventricle may be easily compensated for by a moderately increased cardiac effort.

Cyanotic heart defects may be the result of anomalies that cause a change in pressure so that the blood is shunted from the right to the left side of the heart (*right-to-left shunt*) because of either increased pulmonary vascular resistance or obstruction to blood flow through the pulmonic valve and artery (Fig. 24-2, C). Cyanosis may also result from a defect that allows mixing of blood between the pulmonary and systemic circulations, such as occurs in truncus arteriosus.

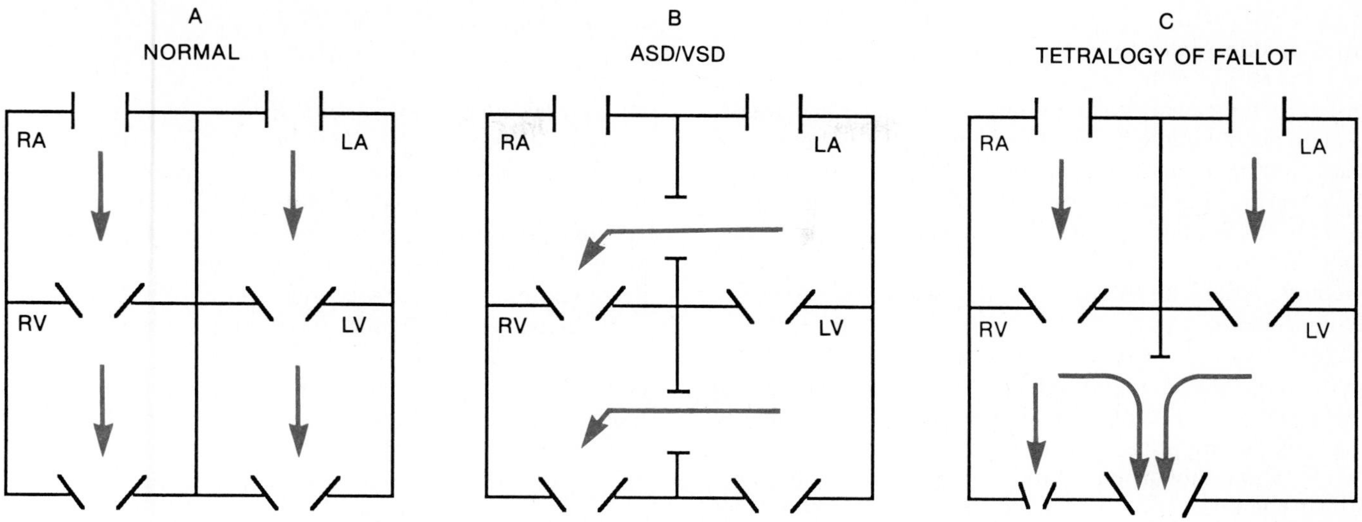

FIG. 24-2 Shunting of blood in congenital heart disease. **A,** Normal. **B,** Acyanotic defect. **C,** Cyanotic defect.

Physical Consequences

The general effects of heart malformation may be summarized as (1) increased workload in terms of systolic or diastolic overloading of the chambers, (2) pulmonary hypertension (increased pulmonary vascular resistance), (3) inadequate systemic cardiac output, and, in cyanotic defects, (4) arterial desaturation from shunting of unoxygenated blood directly into the systemic circulation, which produces hypoxemia and (if severe enough) tissue hypoxia. Although they may vary in severity, the principal physical consequences of these changes are growth retardation, decreased exercise tolerance, dyspnea, tachypnea, tachycardia, cyanosis, and tissue hypoxia (Fig. 24-3).

The body attempts to meet the body's demand for oxygen by improving the cardiac output through increasing the rate of contractions (*tachycardia*). Increased cardiac effort eventually produces an increase in size of the heart muscle (*cardiomegaly*).

Dyspnea occurs as a result of decreased lung compliance and the increased work of breathing or it may be caused by decreased arterial oxygen saturation. It may be associated with *tachypnea* as the lungs try to compensate through an increased respiratory effort. Tachypnea can also be a reflex response to hypoxemia.

Cyanosis results from deoxygenated hemoglobin in the skin blood vessels, especially in the capillaries. Any event that increases metabolism and thus causes a demand for additional oxygen will result in a more severe

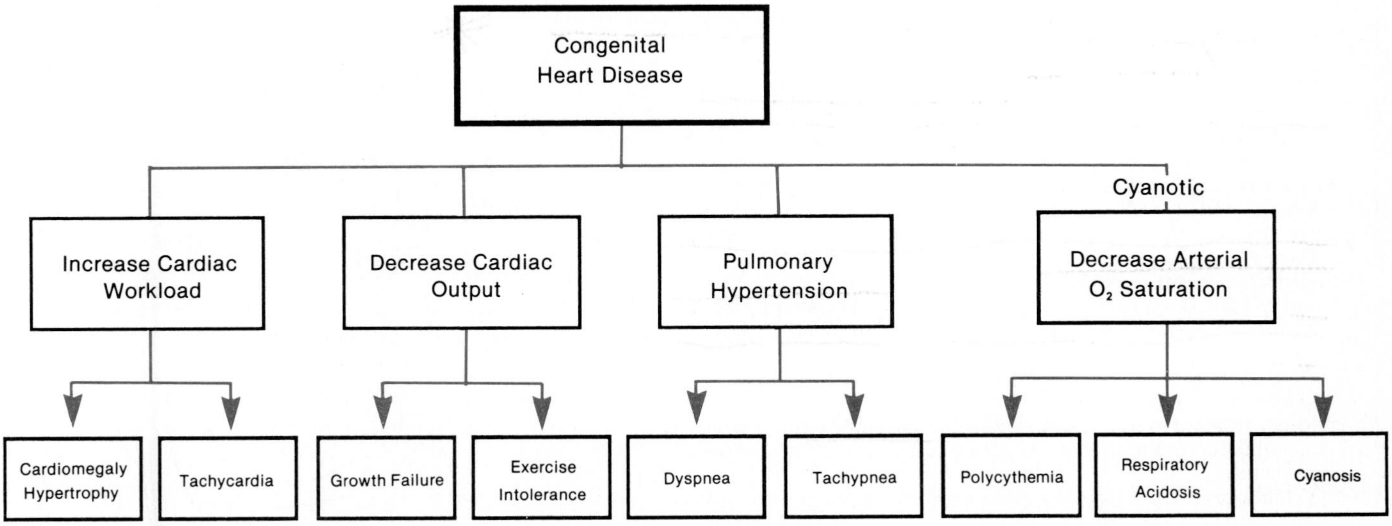

FIG. 24-3 Effects of congenital heart disease.

degree of cyanosis. (See p. 140 for a discussion of evaluation of skin color.)

Growth retardation and *decreased exercise tolerance* are direct consequences of inadequate nutrient intake and oxygen supply for cellular metabolism. Failure to gain weight, even during the neonatal period, is a consistent finding. Decreased exercise tolerance is a direct result of inadequate intake and increased metabolic demands and is usually first noted by the parent during feedings when the infant is too fatigued to consume the entire formula.

Recurrent respiratory infections occur as a result of pulmonary vascular congestion when large amounts of blood pool in the lungs, making it readily susceptible to bacterial or viral invasion and growth.

Murmurs, abnormal sounds produced by vibrations within the heart chambers or vessels, are characteristic of many heart defects. Individual heart defects produce distinctive murmurs that aid in the diagnosis of the anomaly (see box for summary of clinical manifestations).

ACYANOTIC DEFECTS

Most acyanotic defects involve primarily left-to-right shunting through an abnormal opening. Others result from obstructive lesions that reduce the flow of blood to various areas of the body. The more common acyanotic defects, with the distinctive manifestations associated with them and the surgical correction available, are outlined on pp. 790 to 792.

The majority of acyanotic defects are amenable to surgical correction, and the tendency is toward early diagnosis and surgical repair. Patent ductus arteriosus is repaired as soon as the defect is discovered, sometimes in the newborn period in severe conditions. Defects of the septum are corrected surgically sometime before school entry. The child is placed on a regimen of oral digitalis to strengthen heart action and reduce the incidence of congestive heart failure, and some form of iron preparation is prescribed to enhance the iron carrying capacity of hemoglobin. Since children with congenital heart disease are more susceptible to upper respiratory infections than other children are, every effort is exerted to prevent unnecessary exposure to infections.

Palliative surgical procedures may be performed on symptomatic infants until permanent repair can be safely carried out. The usual procedure is banding of the pulmonary artery to decrease the blood flow to the pulmonary circulation.

CYANOTIC DEFECTS

Cyanotic defects are those in which desaturated blood is mixed with saturated blood in the systemic circulation. Diminished circulatory oxygen saturation is usually caused by right-to-left shunting of blood through an abnormal opening and/or vessel configuration. Improvements in surgical techniques have significantly increased the outlook for children with these defects. Some of the most frequently encountered cyanotic disorders are outlined on pp. 793 to 794.

Compensatory Mechanisms Observed in Cyanotic Heart Disease

In addition to the physical consequences of congenital heart defects children with cyanotic lesions often develop other compensatory mechanisms. The body responds to

Text continued on p. 795.

Major Acyanotic Defects

Defect: Patent Ductus Arteriosus (PDA)

Description: Failure of the fetal ductus arteriosus to completely close after birth. Complete anatomic closure may take several weeks.

Altered hemodynamics: Blood from the aorta (a vessel of high pressure) flows into the pulmonary artery (a vessel of lower pressure) to be resaturated with oxygen in the lungs and returned to the left atrium and left ventricle. The effects of this altered circulation are increased workload on the left side of the heart and increased pulmonary vascular congestion.

Distinctive manifestations: Characteristic, machinery-like murmur, which is heard best at the mid to upper left sternal border; widened pulse pressure; cardiomegaly; bounding pulses; tachycardia.

Complications: Congestive heart failure, potential for bacterial (infective) endocarditis.

Medical management: Administration of indomethacin (prostaglandin inhibitor) has proved successful in closing a patent ductus in newborns.

Surgical correction: Surgical division or ligation of the patent vessel.

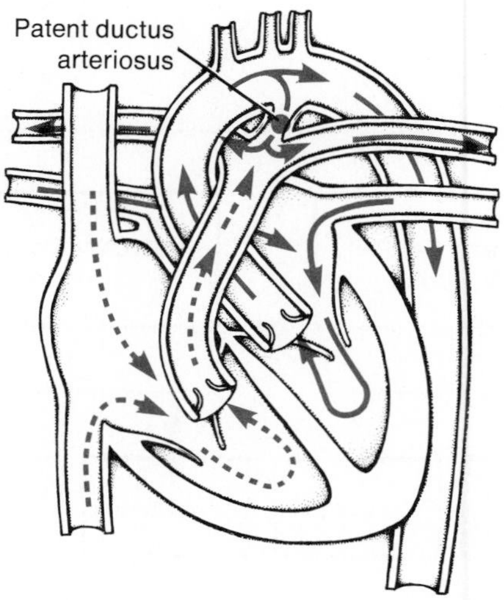

NOTE: Saturated → Mixed → Desaturated - - - →

Major Acyanotic Defects—cont'd

Defect: Coarctation of Aorta

Description: Localized narrowing of the aorta.

Preductal, proximal to the insertion of the ductus arteriosus; *postductal,* distal to the ductus arteriosus.

Altered hemodynamics: Increased pressure proximal to the defect and decreased pressure distal to it.

Distinctive manifestations (postductal): High blood pressure and bounding pulses in areas of the body that receive blood from vessels proximal to the defect. Femoral pulses are weak or absent, the lower extremities may be cooler than the upper ones, and muscle cramps may result during increased exercise from tissue anoxia. Child may experience dizziness, headaches, fainting, and epistaxis caused by hypertension. A murmur may or may not be present.

Complications: Intracranial hemorrhage and stroke, hypertension, ruptured aorta, hypertensive heart disease, congestive heart failure, possibility of a ruptured dissecting aortic aneurysm, and infective endocarditis.

Surgical correction: Resection of the coarcted portion with an end-to-end anastomosis or graft replacement of the constricted section.

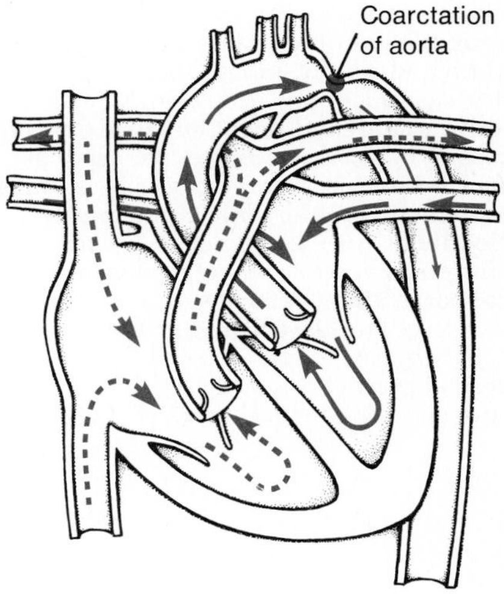

Defect: Atrial Septal Defect (ASD)

Description: Abnormal opening between the two atria.

Altered hemodynamics: Pressure in the left atrium exceeds that in the right atrium, causing blood to flow from left to right. Thus, there is an increased flow of saturated blood into the right side of the heart.

Distinctive manifestations: Characteristic, crescendo-decrescendo type of systolic ejection murmur over the second to third interspace along the left sternal border; dyspnea and fatigue on exertion.

Complications: Congestive heart failure, pulmonary vascular disease, bacterial endocarditis, and atrial arrhythmias (probably from atrial enlargement and effect on conduction system).

Surgical correction: Surgical closure of moderate to large defects similar to closure of ventricular septal defects. Open repair with cardiopulmonary bypass.

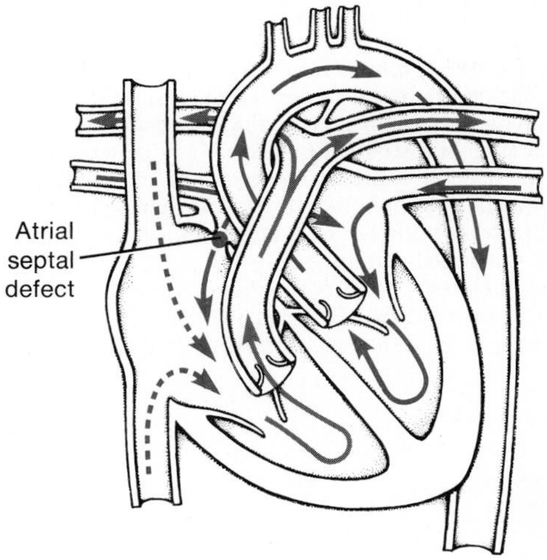

Defect: Ventricular Septal Defect (VSD)

Description: Abnormal opening between the right and left ventricles. May vary in size from a small pinhole to absence of the septum, resulting in a common ventricle. Frequently associated with other defects.

Altered hemodynamics: Pressure within the left ventricle causes blood to flow through the defect to the right ventricle, resulting in increased pulmonary vascular resistance.

Distinctive manifestations: Loud, harsh, pansystolic murmur heard best at the left lower sternal border and radiating throughout the precordium. A systolic thrill is associated with loud murmurs.

Complications: Congestive heart failure, infective endocarditis, aortic insufficiency, pulmonary stenosis, and progressive pulmonary vascular disease.

Surgical correction:

Palliative: Pulmonary banding in symptomatic infants.

Complete repair: Small defects are repaired with a purse-string approach. Large defects usually require a knitted Dacron patch sewn over the opening. Both procedures are performed via cardiopulmonary bypass.

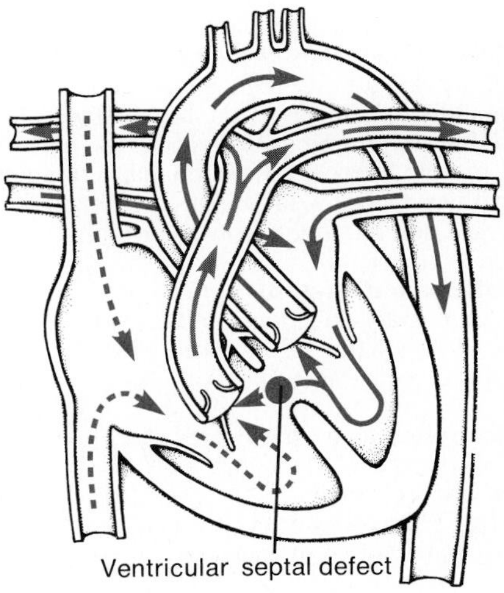

Continued.

Major Acyanotic Defects—cont'd

Defect: Pulmonary Stenosis (PS)

Description: Narrowing at the entrance to the pulmonary artery.

Altered hemodynamics: Resistance to blood flow causes right ventricular hypertrophy and decreased pulmonary blood flow.

Distinctive manifestations: Can range from only the presence of a murmur to cyanosis and congestive heart failure. Systolic ejection murmur is heard best over the second left intercostal space lateral to the sternum. Systolic thrill. Cardiomegaly.

Complications: With severe defects cyanosis, congestive heart failure, decreased systemic output, and increased venous resistance.

Surgical correction: In infants, transventricular (closed) valvotomy (Brock) procedure. In children, pulmonary valvotomy with cardiopulmonary bypass.

Nonsurgical correction: Medical therapy with antibiotics to prevent infective endocarditis (mild stenosis); balloon angioplasty.

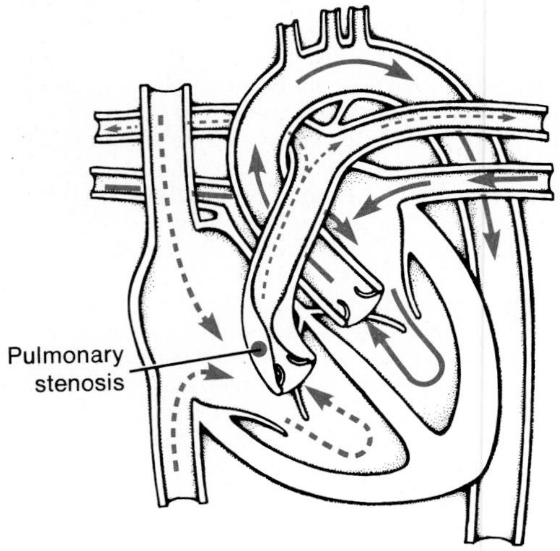

Defect: Aortic Stenosis (AS)

Description: Narrowing or stricture of the aortic valve.

Altered hemodynamics: Stricture causes resistance to blood flow in the left ventricle, decreased cardiac output, left ventricular hypertrophy, and pulmonary vascular congestion.

Distinctive manifestations: Systolic ejection murmur. Infants with severe defects demonstrate evidence of decreased cardiac output, such as faint peripheral pulses, severe physical limitations. Children show exercise intolerance, epigastric or anginal pain, and dizziness after prolonged standing.

Complications: Coronary insufficiency, ventricular failure.

Surgical correction: Opening the valve orifice (commissurotomy); patch graft for extensive narrowing.

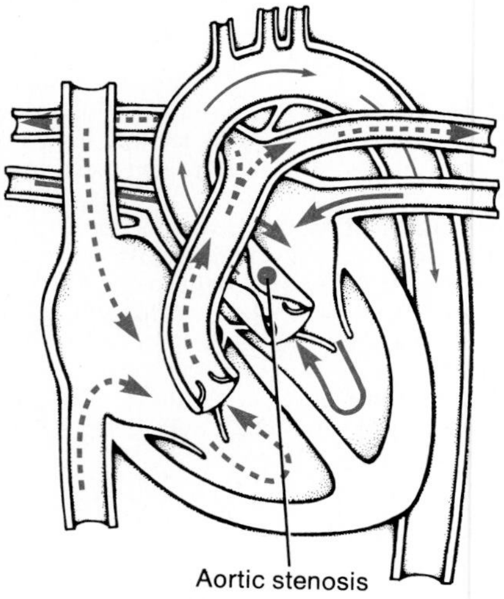

Defect: Endocardial Cushion Defect (ECD)

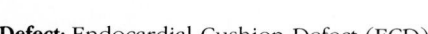

Description: Incomplete fusion of endocardial cushions. Consists of a low atrial septal defect that is continuous with a high ventricular septal defect and clefts of the mitral and tricuspid valves, creating a large central atrioventricular valve that allows blood to flow between all four chambers of the heart. May be complete or partial.

Altered hemodynamics: The openings between chambers allow blood to flow freely from one chamber to another. The directions and pathways of flow are determined by pulmonary and systemic resistance, left and right ventricular pressures, and the compliance of each chamber.

Distinctive manifestations: In the complete form: dyspnea, fatigability, pulmonary infections, and a harsh pansystolic murmur. Cyanosis is generally mild or absent. Gross cardiomegaly is evident. Symptoms occur later and with less severity in the incomplete types.

Complications: Congestive heart failure is common; pulmonary vascular obstruction.

Surgical correction:

Palliative: Pulmonary artery banding for infants with severe symptoms that are caused by increased pulmonary blood flow.

Complete repair: Open repair with cardiopulmonary bypass. Consists of mitral and tricuspid valve repair and patch closure of septal defects.

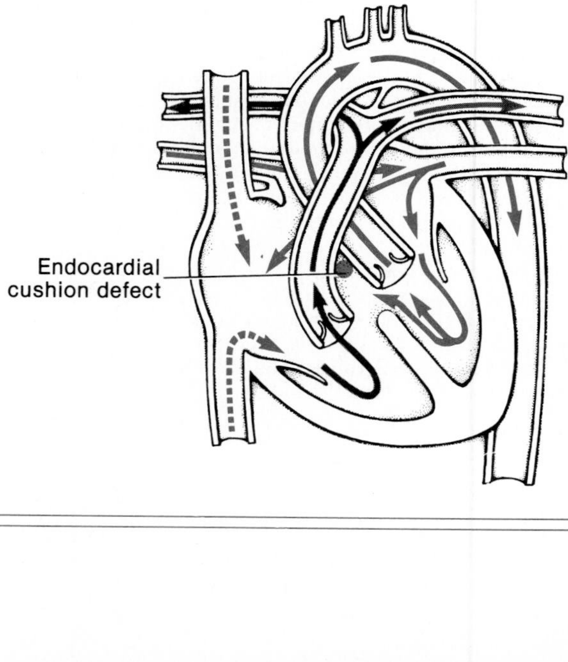

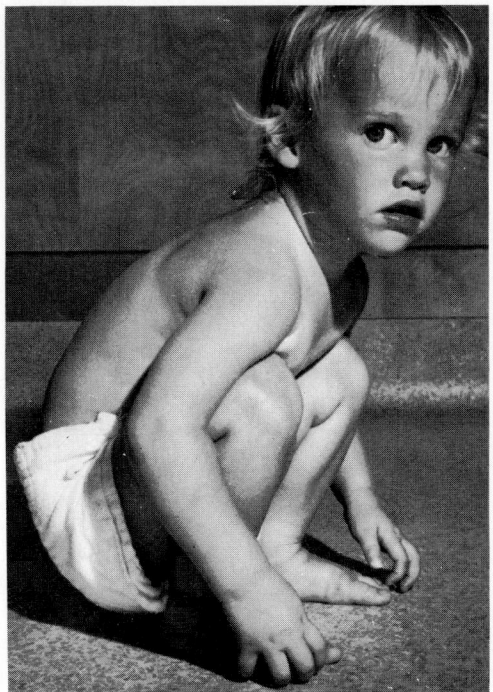

FIG. 24-4 The characteristic squatting position assumed by the child with tetralogy of Fallot. (From Ingalls, A.J., and Salerno, M.C.: Maternal and child health nursing, ed. 6, St. Louis, 1987, The C.V. Mosby Co.)

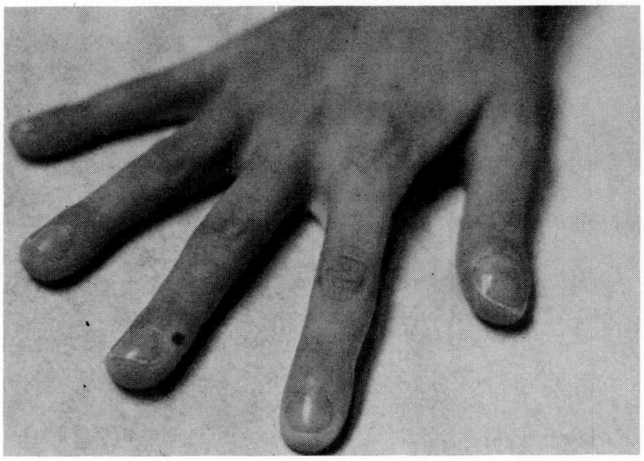

FIG. 24-5 Clubbing of the fingers.

Major Cyanotic Defects

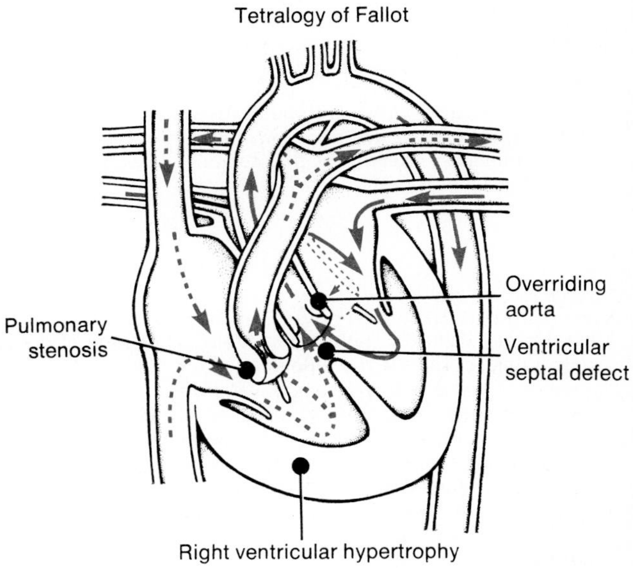

Defect: Tetralogy of Fallot (TOF)

Description: The classic form includes four defects: (1) ventricular septal defect, (2) pulmonic stenosis, (3) overriding aorta, and (4) right ventricular hypertrophy.

Altered hemodynamics: The pulmonic stenosis impedes the flow of blood to the lungs, and thus causes increased pressure in the right ventricle, forcing desaturated blood through the septal defect to the left ventricle. The increased workload on the right ventricle causes hypertrophy. The overriding aorta receives blood directly from both the right and left ventricles.

Distinctive manifestations:

Infants: Acute episodes of cyanosis and hypoxia, often called "blue spells." Anoxic spells occur when the infant's oxygen requirements exceed the blood supply, usually during crying or after feeding. The infant may assume a knee-chest position rather than an extended position.

Children: Physical evidence of cyanosis, markedly delayed physical growth and development, clubbing of the fingers, squatting to relieve the chronic hypoxia. Fainting and/or mental slowness may occur from chronic hypoxia to the brain. Seizures may occur after exertion. A pansystolic murmur is usually heard at the mid to lower left sternal border; usually associated with a thrill. Radiographic studies reveal a "boot-shaped" configuration of heart and great vessels.

Complications: Polycythemia, thrombophlebitis, emboli, cerebrovascular disease, brain abscess. Hyperpnea with severe cyanosis may lead to unconsciousness and death.

Surgical correction:

Palliative: Several procedures available to stimulate a ductus arteriosus, thus increasing oxygen delivery to the systemic circulation. Currently preferred: Blalock-Taussig or a modified Blalock-Taussig procedure, which creates an artificial connection between the pulmonary and systemic circulations by way of a subclavian artery–pulmonary artery anastomosis.

Corrective: Repair of the defects—that is, closure of the ventricular septal defect, pulmonic valvotomy, as well as (when indicated) correction of the overriding aorta.

NOTE: Saturated ⟶ Mixed ⟶ Desaturated - - - - ->

Continued.

Major Cyanotic Defects—cont'd

Defect: Transposition of Great Arteries (TGA), or Vessels (TGV)

Description: Pulmonary artery leaves the left ventricle and the aorta exits from the right ventricle, with no communication between systemic and pulmonary circulations.

Associated defects and hemodynamics: Associated defects such as septal defects or patent ductus arteriosus permit blood to enter the systemic circulation and/or the pulmonary circulation for mixing of saturated and desaturated blood. However, presence of these defects can increase the problems of congestive heart failure, which results from large amounts of blood flowing through the heart to the lungs.

Distinctive manifestations: Depend on the type and size of the associated defects. Children with minimum communication are severely cyanotic and depressed at birth. Those with large septal defects or a patent ductus arteriosus may be less severely cyanotic but may have symptoms of congestive heart failure. Heart sounds vary according to the type of defect present. Cardiomegaly is usually evident a few weeks after birth.

Complications: Congestive heart failure is the main complication; hypoxia is the major cause of death.

Surgical correction:

Palliative: To prevent pulmonary vascular resistance and congestive heart disease until the child is able to tolerate complete cardiac repair: (1) enlargement of an existing atrial septal defect by pulling a balloon through the defect (balloon septotomy) during a cardiac catheterization (Rashkind procedure), (2) creation of a systemic-pulmonary shunt if pulmonic stenosis is present, (3) pulmonary artery banding to decrease blood flow to the lungs, and (4) surgical creation of an atrial septal defect (Blalock-Hanlon operation) (rarely performed).

Complete repair: Several procedures available: (1) creation of an intra-atrial baffle to divert venous blood to the mitral valve and pulmonary venous blood to the tricuspid valve using the patient's atrial septum (Senning procedure) or a prosthetic material (Mustard procedure); (2) switching the great vessels to their correct anatomic position (Jatene operation); (3) baffle closure of the VSD with direction of left ventricular blood through the baffle to the aorta, closure of the pulmonic valve and direction of blood from the right ventricle to the pulmonary artery through a conduit (Rastelli procedure).

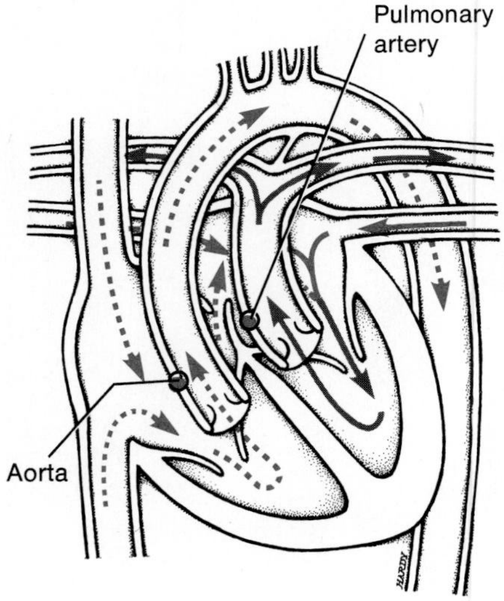

Transposition of the great vessels

Defect: Truncus Arteriosus (TA)

Description: Failure of normal septation and division of the embryonic bulbar trunk into the pulmonary artery and aorta, resulting in a single vessel that overrides both ventricles.

Altered hemodynamics: Blood ejected from the left and right ventricles enters the common artery and flows either to the lungs or to the aortic arch and body. Pressure in both ventricles is high, and blood flow to the lungs is markedly increased.

Distinctive manifestations: Marked cyanosis, left ventricular hypertrophy, dyspnea, marked activity intolerance, and retarded growth.

Complications: Congestive heart failure, hypoxia, infective endocarditis, brain abscess.

Surgical correction:

Palliative: Banding both pulmonary arteries as they arise form the truncus arteriosus, to decrease the amount of blood flow to the lungs.

Corrective: Closing the ventricular septal defect and inserting a prosthetic valved conduit (modified Rastelli operation).

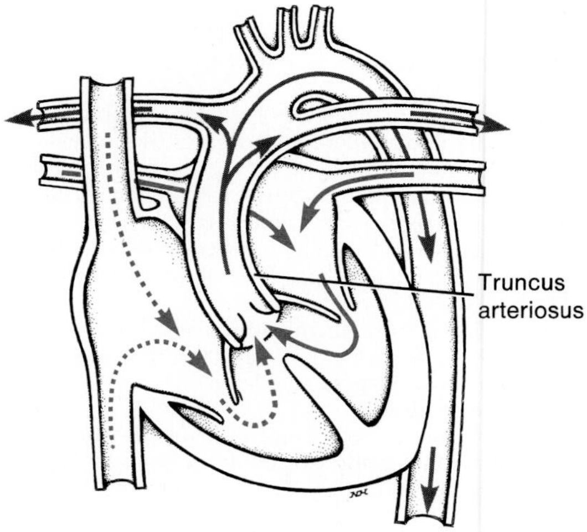

decreased oxygen supply by increased production of erythrocytes, (*polycythemia*), in an attempt to carry more available oxygen to tissues. The additional number of red blood cells increases the viscosity of the blood. As a result circulation becomes sluggish and is often impeded, especially in the capillaries, and blood that is able to carry additional oxygen is not able to reach the peripheral circulation. Because of this increased viscosity the child is at increased risk for complications such as emboli and cerebrovascular accident (stroke). Dehydration presents further hazards to the child because of the increased hemoconcentration.

Decreased oxygen to the brain is often manifested in cerebral changes, such as fainting (*syncope*), mental confusion, seizures, and sometimes mental slowness.

Posturing is a compensatory mechanism automatically learned by the child. Infants assume either a flaccid posture with the extremities extended or a side-lying or prone position with the knees bent toward the chest (knee-chest position). The former position, in contrast to the normal flexed posturing of infants, is a response to tissue hypoxia. Continual muscle contraction demands additional oxygen supply. Flaccidity is usually a sign of progressive heart failure.

The knee-chest position and, later in childhood, the squatting position serve to decrease venous return by occluding the femoral vein through hip flexion, to lessen the workload on the right side of the heart, and to increase arterial oxygen saturation, especially to vital organs in the body (Fig. 24-4).

A characteristic finding in cyanotic cardiac lesions is *clubbing* of the fingers, a thickening and flattening of the distal phalanges (Fig. 24-5). Although the exact cause is unknown, some theories ascribe it to soft tissue fibrosis and hypertrophy from anoxia and formation of increased numbers of capillaries to enhance blood supply to hypoxic tissues.

Clinical Manifestations of CHD

Infants

Cyanosis—generalized, especially mucous membranes, lips and tongue, conjunctiva; highly vascularized areas
Cyanosis during exertion such as crying, feeding, straining, or when immersed in water; peripheral or central
Dyspnea, especially following physical effort such as feeding, crying, straining
Fatigue
Poor growth and development (failure to thrive)
Frequent respiratory tract infections
Feeding difficulties
Hypotonia
Excessive sweating
Syncopal attacks such as paroxysmal hyperpnea, anoxic spells

Older Children

Impaired growth
Delicate, frail body build
Fatigue
Effort dyspnea
Orthopnea
Digital clubbing
Squatting for relief of dyspnea
Headache
Epistaxis
Leg fatigue

NURSING CARE OF THE CHILD WITH CONGENITAL HEART DISEASE

When a child is born with a severe cardiac anomaly, the parents are faced with the immense psychologic and physical tasks of adjusting to the birth and raising a child with physical limitations. Many of the concepts and interventions related to the management of the child with a physical disability or a chronic illness have been discussed in Chapter 18.

ASSESSMENT

Nursing care of the chid with a congenital heart defect begins as soon as the diagnosis is suspected. However, in many instances symptoms that suggest a cardiac anomaly are not present at birth or, if manifest, are so subtle that they are easily overlooked.

Many heart defects are not evident until the child's growth and/or energy expenditure exceeds the heart's ability to supply oxygenated blood. Since the onset is gradual, the child may curtail his activity so that the signs of exercise intolerance are less obvious. However, a careful history yields important clues to this change. For example, toddlers are normally extremely mobile and their energies are directed toward learning gross motor skills. It is very unusual to hear of a toddler who prefers to sit rather than crawl or walk. Such histories should alert the nurse to assess cardiac function. Likewise, a child who needs frequent rests after limited play periods may be exhibiting exercise intolerance.

Other clues, which have already been discussed, are a history of retarded weight gain, poor feeding habits (especially the need to pause during feeding), frequent respiratory infections (particularly when the child is well cared for and isolated from known sources of infection), and any unusual posturing, such as squatting. Since parents may not view any of these findings as abnormal, the nurse must ask about them specifically during a physical assessment. Children with suspected heart murmurs are referred for evaluation.

A vital component of nursing assessment is related to the impact of the disorder on the family, especially the parents. Therefore, the reactions, coping, and concerns of the family are also included in the assessment process (see Chapter 18).

NURSING DIAGNOSES

Many nursing diagnoses are apparent following a thorough assessment of the child and family. Some of these are developed in the Nursing Care Plan on p. 799. Others will be evident based on assessment of individual cases.

PLANNING

The overall plan of care for the infant or child with congenital heart disease will include those listed below. The nursing care not only consists of providing direct care to the infant or child but also includes indirect care through family members.

1. Help parents adjust to the diagnosis
2. Educate family regarding symptoms of the disease and their management
3. Help the child adjust to living with a heart condition
4. Foster growth-promoting family relationships
5. Prepare child and family for surgical repair of a defect
6. Provide competent care to the child undergoing cardiac surgery
7. Prepare child and family for home care

IMPLEMENTATION

Many problems face nurses and families when a child is born with a congenital abnormality, and cardiac defects are especially frightening to families because of the serious connotations that cardiac problems engender in their minds. The specific aspects of general care for a child with congenital heart disease are outlined in the Nursing Care Plan (p. 799) and the care of the infant with congestive heart failure (p. 802).

The present discussion is concerned with the family whose child has a serious heart defect that requires an indefinite period of home care prior to corrective surgery. The overall goal for this child is to live as normal a life as possible within the limitations of his condition. Since the prognosis is often variable, such a goal allows him time to live as a child first and as a patient second. Since many defects are correctable, it also prepares the child to abandon the sick role following surgery and adjust to the privileges and responsibilities of being a well child.

Help Parents and Child Adjust to the Disorder

When parents and older children learn of the heart defect, they are in a period of shock initially, followed by high anxiety. They are especially fearful that the child may die. The diagnosis may be made soon after the child's birth or at a later period in life. Whatever its timing, the family needs a period of grief before assimilating the meaning of the defect. Unfortunately, the demands for medical treatment, which require that the parents be informed of the condition in order to consent to various procedures, may not allow this. However, the nurse can support parents in their loss, assess their level of understanding, supply information as needed, and help other members of the health team to understand the parents' reactions.

Parental adjustment. Once parents are ready to hear about the heart condition, it is essential that they be given a clear explanation, based on their level of understanding. One tool for illustrating heart defects simplistically is to depict the heart as a four-room structure (house) with normal exits and entrances (representing the valves and vessels). A septal defect can then be illustrated as an abnormal entrance to one side of the structure that allows mixing of blood that should remain only in one room. Although this explanation may not suffice for all parents, it does allow for clarification of basic information. Parents also appreciate receiving written information about the specific defect.*

Parents are primarily interested in two kinds of information—the prognosis, and whether surgery will be required—and are upset about indefinite answers to their questions. In addition, all members of the health team may not use the same terms to present identical information. If this is identified as a problem, the nurse should encourage parents to write down the term or ask the informant to clarify it.

Parents also need an explanation regarding the symptoms of the disease. Watching a child become cyanotic and dyspneic is frightening. However, offering parents suggestions of what to do during and after an episode decreases their anxiety by providing them some control. After a cyanotic and/or dyspneic episode, the child needs to rest and attain a position of comfort, which usually consists of lying on his side or on his stomach with knees flexed and the head and chest elevated. An infant is cuddled against an adult's shoulder with his knees and hips flexed. This serves to decrease the volume of deoxygenated blood returning to the heart and to provide comfort. He is kept warm to prevent increased metabolism and vasoconstriction. Most importantly, he should remain calm. The cyanotic spell is treated casually to prevent parental emotions from being transferred to the child.

Medications are often prescribed for the child with CHD to improve heart action and reduce the likelihood of complications. Medications may include digitalis to strengthen cardiac action (see p. 803 for nursing responsibilities), an iron preparation to ensure optimum oxygen-carrying capacity of red blood cells, a diuretic to prevent edema, and potassium chloride to maintain an adequate serum potassium level and prevent cardiac dysrythmia. The family will need instruction in the administration of these medications (see p. 699).

An essential intervention is prevention of cyanosis and dyspnea by tailoring energy expenditure to cardiac output and arterial oxygenation. For older children this involves little difficulty, because activity restrictions are self-imposed. Even in infants there is little need to prevent crying because it usually ceases when hypoxia increases. Deliberate attempts to prevent crying should be avoided because they can establish a maladaptive parental pattern

*Several booklets that are suitable for parents are available from the local or national branch of the **American Heart Association,** 7320 Greenville Ave., Dallas TX 75231, and from the **Canadian Heart Foundation**, 1 Nicholas St., Suite 1200, Ottawa, Ontario K1N 7B7.

of relating to the infant. Strenuous spontaneous activity and competitive sports may be restricted in selected children and adolescents.

An important area of intervention for distressed infants is decreasing energy requirements needed for feeding. The infant may need to be fed small amounts of formula approximately every two hours to ensure an adequate intake. If several nighttime feedings are required, the nurse should discuss with parents the need to share the responsibility and to enlist the help of others whenever possible, including teaching tube-feeding techniques. Parents do not feel confident leaving the child in the care of someone else. They believe that the child will be upset by a change in routine and that the individual will be unable to cope with the child's symptoms.

Since growth retardation is believed to be a result of inadequate caloric intake, the nurse assists parents in finding ways to provide highly nutritious foods. The physician may order protein-calorie supplements. Less energy is required for sucking if the nipple hole is enlarged by cutting a cross in the center to facilitate flow of the formula.

Children with severe cardiac defects are often anorexic and tempting them to eat can be a tremendous challenge. Because of the parents' concern over eating, children learn at an early age to manipulate them through eating behavior, such as making unrealistic demands for foods that are not available. The nurse advises parents of this potential problem, since prevention yields greater success than intervention.

Child adjustment. Children of various ages form different ideas about the heart. Children between 4 and 6 years of age have heard about the heart, know its approximate anatomic location in the chest or back, illustrate it as valentine shaped, and characterize it by its sounds—tick-tock, thump, and so on. Children 7 to 10 years of age have a clearer concept of the heart, realizing that it is not shaped like a valentine and that it has vital functions—for example, "It makes you live." However, their knowledge of its integrated functions in pumping blood through a system of vessels to all parts of the body is still vague. By the age of 10 or 11 years, children have a much more involved concept of the heart, with knowledge of veins, valves, pumping action, and circulation. They are beginning to appreciate its mechanisms and the reason that death occurs when the heart stops.

Information about his condition must be tailored to the child's developmental level. Preschoolers need basic information about what they may experience and what they are allowed to do more than they need information about what is actually occurring physiologically. School-age children benefit from a concrete explanation of the defect. Using the "house" model can be very effective. Preadolescents and adolescents often appreciate a more detailed description of how the defect affects the heart. Children of all ages need an opportunity to express their feelings concerning the diagnosis and its particular meaning to them.

Foster growth-promoting family relationships. The effect of a child with a serious heart defect on the family is complex. No member, regardless of the degree of positive adjustment, is unaffected. The mother frequently feels inadequate in her mothering ability because she is unable to continually satisfy the child. She may view the child's failure to feed well as evidence of *her* failure, not as a direct consequence of the disease. The usual joys of watching a child grow and thrive are limited. Frequently, attainment of gross motor milestones is delayed because of physical inability to practice crawling or sitting unsupported. Mothers often feel constantly exhausted from the pressures of caring for these children and the other members of the family.

The need to maintain discipline and to set limits cannot be overemphasized. Behavior modification techniques, either in the form of concrete rewards, such as a favorite food, or social reinforcement, such as approval, can be effective. However, such techniques are most beneficial if they are employed *before* the child learns to control the family. Therefore, guiding parents toward the need for discipline while the child is in infancy is necessary to prevent problems later on. These children must be taught how to tolerate frustration and delayed gratification, an ability that is difficult to attain because of the early need for immediate satisfaction of all their needs.

Although the child may not be able to participate in physical activity, he is encouraged in acceptable pursuits, such as reading, quiet hobbies, and less demanding physical activities. Allowing the child to watch television as his total means of recreation will not foster his development. If the child enters school prior to corrective surgery, the parents should discuss appropriate activity levels with the teacher, the school nurse, and the principal.

Another problem that frequently develops within family relationships is the child's overdependency, especially on his mother. Mothers, in turn, frequently respond to the dependency with overprotectiveness, which results in a cycle that is mutually satisfying although destructive in terms of developing maturity and responsibility. The nurse should encourage parents to begin early to stimulate the infant toward feasible developmental goals, such as holding his own bottle, learning to amuse himself for short periods rather than always being held, and picking up finger foods. Unless parents are helped to see what the child can do, they often will focus only on his physical limitations.

The child also needs opportunities for social development. Often these children are isolated from known sources of infection and not allowed to play with other children because of overexertion. Such limitations only add to the dangers of increased dependency on the home environment. Parents need to be encouraged to seek appropriate social activity, especially prior to kindergarten. One approach is to introduce the family to other families with similarly affected children who can help them adjust to the daily stresses of coping with a child with a heart defect. Sometimes several parents who have children with heart disease are willing to form a cooperative group to share such responsibilities, form a play group for their children, and provide respite care for one another.* (See Chapter 18 for further approaches to care of chronically ill children and their families.)

Nursing Care of the Child Undergoing Heart Surgery

The child is usually admitted to the hospital for diagnostic tests 1 or 2 days prior to surgery. Few surgical procedures demand as much planning for preoperative and postoperative care; therefore, this interval allows additional time to prepare the child and parents for surgery. Since a great deal of information is conveyed, it is important to schedule teaching to prevent information overload and to be alert to signs of overload (see p. 629 for suggestions on preparing children and parents for surgical procedures).

The preparation is divided into three major categories: environment, equipment, and procedures. Ideally, when the child is admitted he should be assigned to one nurse for each shift—preferably the nurses who will be responsible for his care postoperatively. A visit to the recovery room and/or intensive care unit is desirable for the school-age and older preschool child and should take place when there is least activity in the unit, when the parents can accompany the child, and when the child is well rested. Usually the day before surgery is ample time to allow the child to ask questions but to prevent him from fantasizing unduly about the experience. All positive, nonfrightening aspects of the environment are emphasized, such as the play area, visitors' section, pictures or mobiles in the room, or the television.

Pieces of equipment that are new and unfamiliar are shown to the child and the family, and demonstrated either on him or on a doll. These might include such items as the oxygen mask, the oxygen tent, suction, chest tubes, the endotracheal tube, incentive spirometer, and intravenous tubing. With a preschool child, displaying miniature equipment that is suitable for use with a doll or puppet is often less anxiety-producing than showing the actual objects. If other children in the unit are receiving intravenous infusions or are in oxygen tents, an older child may benefit from seeing them. The more sensations he experiences beforehand, the less likely it is that he will be frightened by them later.

The type and size of dressing the child will have after surgery are discussed and demonstrated on a doll. Usually, one of two types of incisions is made: a median sternotomy (which splits the sternum) or a lateral thoracotomy (which extends from the midaxillary line to the scapula). In either instance the suture line and dressing are extensive. Frequently no sutures are visible because subcuticular, absorbable sutures may be used. If this is done, it should be pointed out to the child and parents, who may fear that the incision might open.

*Many local chapters of the American Heart Association have organized parent groups.

The older child is told about chest tubes, their purpose, and that he will be expected to move while they are in place. He is also told about the presence of a postsurgery endotracheal tube, which will be removed as soon as possible, but he should be assured that, although he will be unable to talk, he will be able to communicate his desires by other means, such as finger or eye signals, that can be determined in advance.

Several postoperative procedures are imperative to prevent postsurgical complications—especially coughing, turning, deep breathing, and postural drainage and percussion. Each of these is practiced several times before surgery. Although they can be presented as a game, the child is told that each procedure will not be as easy after surgery and may cause discomfort.

Deep breathing is demonstrated by having the child watch the nurse's chest rise and fall. The child is told to imitate the nurse's actions, emphasizing that the higher the chest rises, the more air enters the lung. For a young child the nurse can explain that the lungs are like balloons that expand when air is inspired. The use of incentive spirometers is also demonstrated to encourage breathing. If these are not available, the child can blow bubbles through a straw placed in water. Coughing is demonstrated by taking a deep breath and forcibly attempting to bring up secretions. It is emphasized that coughing is not the same as clearing the throat. The nurse also performs percussion and vibration on the child to demonstrate the procedure and clarify that the clapping is not hitting.

The child also practices turning in bed while in a semi-Fowler position and using the bedpan or urinal. He is told that following surgery he will have a special tube (Foley catheter) so that he will not have to urinate for a day or two but after that he will be expected to use the other equipment.

The child is also prepared for preoperative procedures, such as taking nothing by mouth for 12 hours prior to surgery, skin preparation, which includes shaving or the use of a topical depilatory in adolescent males and females, and preoperative sedation. Physical preoperative care differs little from that for any type of surgery. Skin preparation may involve a tub bath with special bactericidal cleanser the day before surgery. The nurse clarifies with the physician exactly what preoperative procedures are to be done, to avoid the hazard of overpreparing or underpreparing the child. (See also the discussion of preparing the child for surgery, p. 629.)

Postoperative care. Immediate postoperative care is usually provided by specially trained nurses in intensive care units (see p. 616). Many of the procedures, such as intra-arterial and central venous pressure monitoring and the observations related to vital functions, require advanced education and technical training. These procedures will not be elaborated here.

The child will be returned to the pediatric unit as soon

NURSING CARE PLAN

The Child with Congenital Heart Disease

Nursing Goals	Nursing Interventions	Expected Patient/Family Outcomes
HP-HMP* Potential for infection **Risk factors: debilitated physical status**		
Prevent infection	Avoid contact with infected persons Provide for adequate rest Provide optimum nutrition	Child remains free of infection
HP-HMP Altered growth and development **Etiology: inadequate oxygen and nutrients to tissues; social isolation**		
Promote physical growth	Provide highly nutritious diet	Child achieves normal growth
Promote development	Encourage activities appropriate to developmental level and capabilities	Child engages in appropriate activities (specify)
Promote interpersonal relationships	Encourage relationships with children his own age Arrange for continued family contacts during hospitalization Promote development of a positive self-image	Child engages in age-appropriate activities within the limits of his capabilities
Prevent overprotection	Encourage family to provide normal life-style for the child including activities, discipline, and expectations	See above
Maintain nutrition Prevent potassium depletion Improve iron-carrying capacity of blood Facilitate feeding	Ensure well-balanced diet Help plan a diet with potassium-rich foods to prevent depletion Encourage iron-rich foods in the diet Administer small, frequent meals Encourage child to eat (see p. 640)	Infant or child consumes an adequate amount of nutrients (specify amounts)
A-EP Activity intolerance **Etiology: imbalance between oxygen supply and demand**		
Reduce energy expenditure	Feed infant slowly Allow for frequent rest periods Encourage quiet games and activities Caution family to consult with child's cardiologist before taking child on an airplane or to a higher altitude	Child rests quietly and breathes easily Child determines and engages in activities commensurate with his capabilities (specify)
SP-SCP Body image disturbance **Etiology: activity intolerance, feeling of differentness**		
Promote a positive self-concept	Allow child to express feelings about heart condition Explore child's feelings regarding his disorder Clarify misconceptions child may have acquired Support positive coping mechanisms and extinguish negative ones	Child openly discusses feelings and concerns about his condition
Help child understand his defect	Assess child's level of understanding Use visual aids to describe heart defect Provide written information Keep technical information simple Convey same information as other health team members Stress that prognosis and plans for surgery may change Base explanation of heart on child's developmental level of understanding	Child demonstrates an understanding of his disease and its implications

*For an explanation of abbreviations, see p. 20.

Continued

NURSING CARE PLAN

The Child with Congenital Heart Disease—cont'd

Nursing Goals	Nursing Interventions	Expected Patient/Family Outcomes
ND CPP Knowledge deficit **Etiology: unfamiliarity with disease and prescribed treatments**		
Increase family's understanding of child's condition	Assess family's understanding of diagnosis Reinforce and clarify physician's description of child's condition and the prognosis Explore their feelings regarding prescribed therapies Reinforce and clarify physician's explanation of suggested diagnostic procedures and palliative or corrective surgeries	Family demonstrates an understanding of the disease (specify)
Help family cope with symptoms of disease	Explore coping strategies with family, such as: During dyspneic/cyanotic spell, place child in knee-chest position, with head and chest elevated or over the shoulder Keep child warm; encourage rest and sleep Decrease child's anxiety by remaining calm Encourage family to include others in child's care to prevent their own exhaustion	Family copes with child's symptoms in a positive way
	Assist family in determining appropriate physical activity and disciplining methods for child	Child engages in appropriate activities for age and condition (specify)
Recognize signs of complicating factors	Be alert for signs of complications Congestive heart failure (CHF) (p. 804) Maintain high index of suspicion regarding digitalis toxicity Increased respiratory effort—tachycardia, retraction, grunting, cough, cyanosis Hypoxemia—cyanosis, restlessness, tachycardia Cerebral thrombosis—compensatory polycythemia (in cyanotic heart disease) is particularly hazardous when child is dehydrated Cardiovascular collapse—pallor, cyanosis, hypotonia	*Evidence of complications is detected early and interventions are implemented without delay
Prepare for diagnostic tests and surgery	Explain or clarify information presented to family by physician and surgeon Prepare child and parents for procedure Assist with family's decision regarding surgery Explore feelings regarding palliative or corrective surgery	Family demonstrates an understanding of tests, surgery, etc. (specify learning and manner of demonstration) Family expresses feelings and concerns
ND RRP Altered family processes **Etiology: situational crisis (child with a defect, hospitalization of child)**		
Help family and child adjust to diagnosis	Allow period of grief Accept initial shock and disbelief Repeat information as often as necessary Encourage family to express their concerns Foster parent-child attachment, especially with newborn Introduce parents to other families who have similarly affected child	Family demonstrates an attitude of acceptance and adjustment (specify)
Reduce family's fears and anxieties	Explore family's concerns and feelings of irritation, guilt, anger, disappointment, inadequacy Help family distinguish between realistic fears and eliminate unfounded fears Discuss with parents their fears regarding child's symptoms, such as pounding heart, cyanotic spells, irritability Deal with child's anxiety about his condition Fear of dreadful developments Fear of death Fear of tests and procedures	Family discusses their fears and concerns

NURSING CARE PLAN

The Child with Congenital Heart Disease—cont'd

Nursing Goals	Nursing Interventions	Expected Patient/Family Outcomes
Foster growth-promoting family relationships	Assess family's support systems Reinforce positive coping mechanisms Encourage family members to discuss their feelings about each other Impress upon parents importance of providing as normal a life as possible for affected child	Family demonstrates positive, growth-promoting behaviors
	Help family feel adequate in their parental roles by emphasizing growth and developmental progress of their child Help family foster child's development by stimulating child to age-appropriate goals consistent with his activity tolerance	Child engages in activities appropriate for his age and capabilities
Prepare family for home care of infant or child	Encourage family to participate in care of child Administration of medications Feeding techniques Interventions for conserving energy and those directed toward relief of frightening symptoms Signs that indicate complications Where and whom to contact for help and guidance Anticipate need for further information and support	Family demonstrates the ability and motivation for home care of the infant
	Refer family to local chapter of the American Red Cross for instruction in cardiopulmonary resuscitation	Family members learn cardiopulmonary resuscitation technique
Support family	Be available to family Refer to family support groups such as those provided through local branch of the American Heart Association See also The family of the hospitalized child, p. 610	Family becomes involved with local support groups
Assist in providing financial support	Investigate state and local agencies that may be able to provide financial assistance, such as state, Special Child Health Services, American Heart Association Collaborate with social service agency to ensure optimum utilization of community services	Parents avail themselves of assistance

Nursing interventions related to medical management

Assist with diagnosis
- Order or draw blood for CBC
- Perform or assist with electrocardiography
- Order and/or assist with x-ray examinations, echocardiography, angiography, fluoroscopy, ultrasonography
- Prepare child and family for and assist with cardiac catheterization

Prevent anemia
- Administer iron preparations as prescribed

Prevent fluid accumulation
- Administer diuretics as prescribed
- Provide low-sodium diet

Prevent hypokalemia
- Provide high-potassium diet
- Administer supplemental potassium as prescribed

Palliate or correct defects
- Perform needed preoperative procedures and tests

as his condition warrants. Physical care is the same as for any child recovering from major surgery. He is encouraged to be as active and as involved in his own care as his age and condition indicate. This seldom creates difficulty, since most children are naturally active, although children with cardiac lesions tend to prefer more quiet activities as a result of their preoperative behavior patterns.

Discharge planning. Ideally, planning for discharge begins on admission, when the nurse assesses the readiness and ability of the parents and child to give up the sick role and adjust to the responsibilities and privileges of a healthy child. If parents have been guided in caring for the child as they would for a normal child, the transition to full recovery is facilitated. Unfortunately, this is not always the case, and requires that the nurse discuss this phase of recovery with the parents.

Emotional adjustment involves a gradual resumption of physical ability as well as responsibility. For an older child who has never had the opportunity to develop athletic competence, a sense of competition, or fine muscle coordination, it may be unrealistic to pursue a goal in this direction, despite the physical ability to do so. In such an instance it is more beneficial to encourage interests that have already been developed. This may be very difficult for fathers who may anticipate that after corrective heart surgery their sons will be able to join them in competitive sports.

Fostering a sense of responsibility is equally difficult. Parents may have a great need to continue a dependent relationship for themselves. Likewise, the child may be unwilling to accept new limits or to give up privileges of the sick role. The nurse investigates the family relationships to identify those roles or needs that may prevent parents or children from establishing a new set of expectations.

The nurse can facilitate adjustment by gradually expecting more from the child in the recovery period and stressing to parents the importance of gradual achievement of new skills and responsibilities. Since the postoperative period is quite short—only 7 to 10 days for an uncomplicated recovery—the nurse should make a referral to a public health nursing agency for follow-up care in the home.

EVALUATION

The effectiveness of nursing interventions is determined by continual reassessment and evaluation of care based on the following observational guidelines and expected outcomes:

1. Interview families and observe their behavior with the infant or child
2. Encourage family to discuss their feelings and concerns; observe their response to education
3. Interview the child and observe his/her behavior and concerns; encourage verbal child to express feelings
4. Interview family and observe family interactions and relationships
5. Interview family regarding their understanding of the condition and the proposed surgery
6. Monitor and observe the infant or child and family preoperatively and postoperatively
7. Observe and interview child and family regarding their understanding of home care needs, their ability to carry out care, and compliance with the plan of care

Expected outcomes:
See Nursing Care Plan, pp. 799 to 801.

◆ *Acquired Heart Disease*

Acquired heart disease, as opposed to congenital heart disease, occurs as a result of a previously existing disease or defect or as a complication of an acute disease. The most common condition classified as acquired heart disease is congestive heart failure—usually as a complication of congenital heart disease. *Cor pulmonale* is the term applied to congestive failure that results from pulmonary hypertension associated with chronic lung disease, principally cystic fibrosis.

CONGESTIVE HEART FAILURE

Congestive heart failure (CHF) is the inability of the heart to pump an adequate amount of blood to the systemic circulation to meet the body's metabolic demands. In children congestive heart failure most frequently occurs secondary to structural abnormalities that result in increased blood volume and pressure. Congestive heart failure is a symptom caused by an underlying cardiac defect, not a disease in itself, since it is usually the result of an excessive workload imposed on a normal myocardium. Most children who experience congestive heart failure are infants.

Pathophysiology

Heart failure is often separated into two categories, right-sided and left-sided failure. In *right-sided failure* the right ventricle is unable to pump blood into the pulmonary artery, resulting in less blood being oxygenated by the lungs and increased pressure in the right atrium and systemic venous circulation. Systemic venous hypertension causes edema in the extremities and viscera. In *left-sided failure* the left ventricle is unable to pump blood into the systemic circulation, resulting in increased pressure in the left atrium and pulmonary veins. The lungs become congested with blood, causing elevated pulmonary pressures and pulmonary edema.

Although each type produces different systemic and pulmonary alterations, clinically it is unusual to observe solely right- or left-sided failure. Since each side of the heart depends on adequate function of the other side, failure of one chamber causes a reciprocal change in the opposite chamber. For example, in left-sided failure an increase in pulmonary vascular congestion will cause back pressure in the right ventricle, resulting in right ventricular hypertrophy, decrease myocardial efficiency, and eventually cause pooling of blood in the systemic venous circulation.

If the abnormalities precipitating heart failure are not corrected, the heart muscle becomes damaged. Despite compensatory mechanisms, the heart is unable to maintain an adequate cardiac output. Decreased blood flow to the kidneys continues to stimulate sodium and water reabsorption, leading to hypervolemia, increased workload on the heart, and congestion in the pulmonary and systemic circulations (Fig. 24-6). Systemic congestion is evidenced by distended neck and peripheral veins, edema (reflected in weight gain), and hepatomegaly. Inappropriate sweating, especially on the head, is a sympathetic response characteristic of infants in congestive failure.

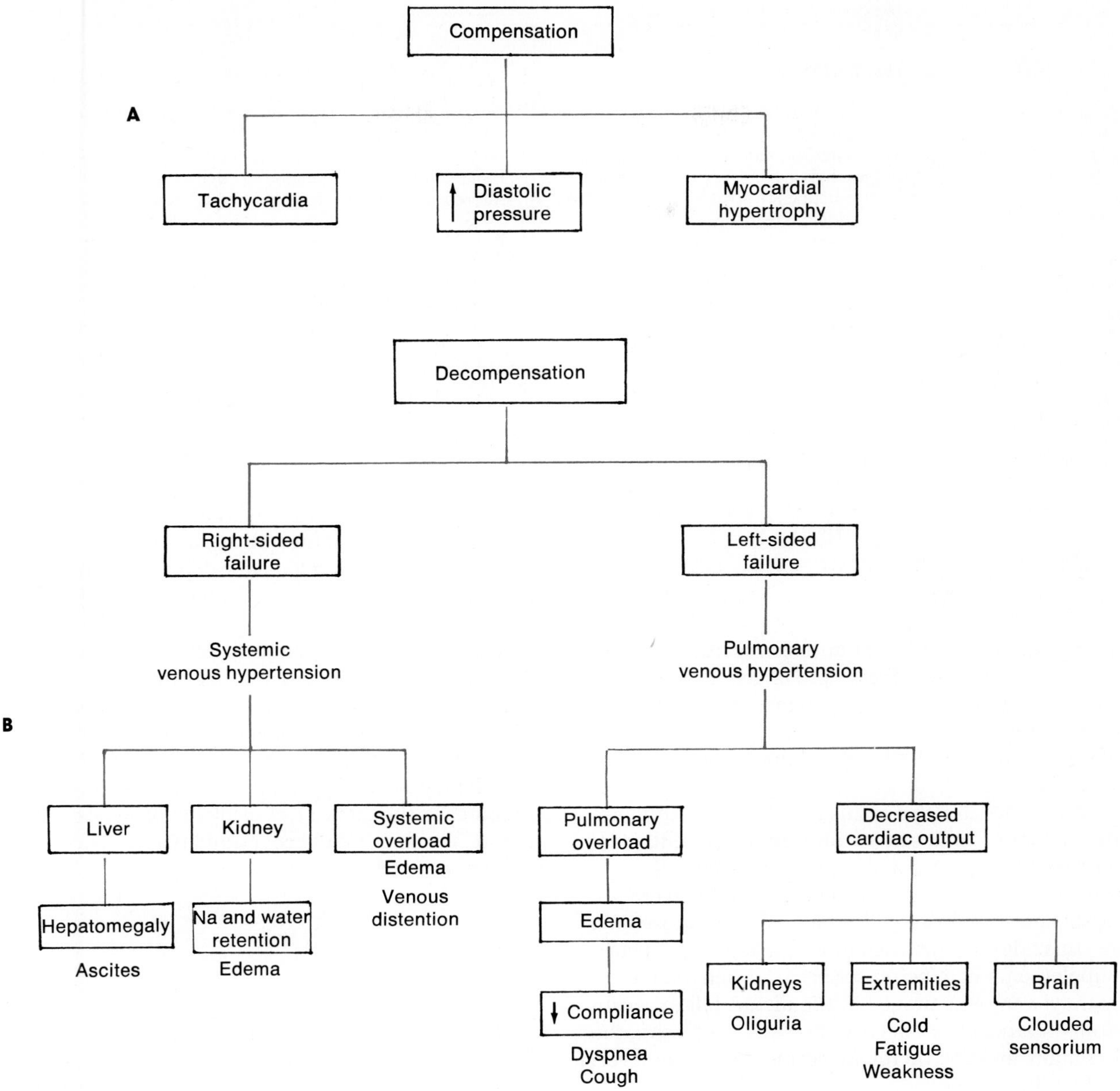

FIG. 24-6 Pathophysiology of heart failure. **A,** Compensated. **B,** Decompensated.

Diagnostic Evaluation

Diagnosis is made on the basis of clinical manifestations (see box).

Therapeutic Management

The goals of treatment are to (1) improve cardiac function, (2) remove accumulated fluid and sodium, (3) decrease cardiac demands, and (4) improve tissue oxygenation.

Improve cardiac function. Myocardial efficiency is improved through administration of digitalis glycosides. The beneficial effects are increased cardiac output, decreased heart size, decreased venous pressure, and relief of edema. In pediatrics digoxin (Lanoxin) is used almost exclusively, because of its more rapid onset and the decreased risk of toxicity as a result of a much shorter half-life. It is available as an elixir (0.05 mg/ml) for oral administration. For infants the dose is often calculated in micrograms (1000 μg = 1 mg).

Treatment consists of a digitalizing dose, given orally, intramuscularly, or intravenously as one large dose or in divided doses over a short time span to produce optimum cardiac effects, and a maintenance dose, usually one fourth to one third the digitalizing dose, given orally twice a day to maintain blood levels. During digitalization the

Clinical Manifestations of CHF

General
Weakness
Fatigue
Poor feeding
Irritability
Pallor
Duskiness
Cyanosis, especially on exertion

Cardiac
Tachycardia (pulse over 140 in sleeping infants, over 100 in sleeping older children)
Cardiomegaly
Gallop rhythm
Pulsus alternans

Pulmonary
Dyspnea
Costal retractions
Tachypnea
Orthopnea
Cardiac wheezing
Cough
Weak cry
Hoarseness
Gasping
Grunting on expiration

Systemic
Hepatomegaly
Weight gain (edema)
Ascites
Pleural effusions
Distended neck and peripheral veins
Sweating, especially on exertion

child is monitored by means of an electrocardiograph, to observe for the desired effects (prolonged P-R interval and reduced ventricular rate) and detect side effects, especially arrhythmias.

Remove accumulated fluid and sodium. Treatment consists of diuretics, fluid restriction, and possible sodium restriction. Diuretics are the mainstay of therapy to eliminate excess water and salt to prevent reaccumulation. The most commonly used agents are furosemide (Lasix), the thiazides (chlorothiazide suspension or hydrochlorothiazide tablets), and spironolactone. Since furosemide and the thiazides are potassium-losing diuretics, potassium supplements may be prescribed and rich sources of the electrolyte are encouraged in the diet. A fall in serum potassium enhances the effects of digitalis, increasing the risk of digitalis toxicity; therefore, serum potassium levels are carefully monitored.

Fluid restriction may be required in the acute states of CHF or if fluid retention is accompanied by loss of sodium. For example, diuretics cause additional sodium loss whereas limited oral fluids preserve the serum sodium levels. Fluids must be carefully calculated to avoid dehydrating the child, especially if significant polycythemia is present.

Sodium-restricted diets are used less often in children than in adults to control congestive heart failure, because of their potential negative effects on appetite. For example, low-sodium milk is unpalatable and poorly tolerated by infants. If salt intake is restricted, the diet usually consists of avoiding additional table salt and highly salted foods.

Decrease cardiac demands. The workload on the heart is reduced when metabolic needs are kept to a minimum. This is accomplished by limiting physical activity (bed rest), preserving body temperature, treating any existing infections, reducing the effort of breathing (semi-Fowler position), and using medication to sedate an irritable child (usually morphine sulfate, 0.1 mg/kg). Since meeting these objectives effectively depends on nursing interventions, they are discussed in more detail in the next section.

Improve tissue oxygenation. All of the preceding measures serve to increase tissue oxygenation, either by improving myocardial function or by lessening tissue oxygen demands. Iron supplements are administered to enhance the oxygen-carrying capacity of red blood cells. Supplemental cool humidified oxygen is usually provided to increase the amount of available oxygen during inspiration. The amount of cool humidity is carefully regulated to prevent overhydration and chilling.

Nursing Diagnoses: The Child with CHF

Decreased cardiac output related to structural defect, myocardial dysfunction
Ineffective breathing pattern related to pulmonary congestion
Fluid volume excess related to edema
Altered growth and development related to cardiac dysfunction
Potential for infection related to pulmonary congestion, reduced body defenses
Altered nutrition: less than body requirements related to fatigue, circulatory impairment
Activity intolerance related to imbalance between oxygen supply and demand
Altered family processes related to hospitalization of child

Nursing Considerations

The infant or child with CHF is usually admitted to the hospital where intensive nursing care is available. The child is positioned for optimum ventilation, is administered oxygen by the most effective means, an intravenous access is established, and cardiac and respiratory function is monitored continuously. Urinary output and serum electrolytes, especially blood gases, are evaluated frequently.

ASSESSMENT

See Assessment of cardiac function, p. 785.

NURSING DIAGNOSES

Following a thorough assessment a number of nursing diagnoses are evident (see box). Others may become apparent in special circumstances and with children in different age groups.

PLANNING

The objectives of nursing care of the infant or child with congestive heart failure include:

1. Assist in measures to improve cardiac function
2. Decrease cardiac demands
3. Reduce respiratory distress
4. Maintain nutritional status
5. Assist in measures to promote fluid loss
6. Support child and family

IMPLEMENTATION

Although the objectives of nursing care are the same, the interventions differ depending on the child's age; interventions for infants are quite different from those for older children.

Improve cardiac function. The responsibility of the nurse in administering digitalis includes calculating and administering the correct dose, observing for signs of toxicity, and instituting parental teaching regarding drug administration in the home.

Digitalis is a potentially dangerous drug because the differences between therapeutic, toxic, and lethal doses are very small. Many toxic responses are extensions of the drug's therapeutic effects. Therefore, when administering digitalis, the nurse must observe carefully for the following signs of toxicity.

The earliest indication of toxicity is vomiting although one episode does not warrant cessation of the drug since it is such a common occurrence in infants. The principal manifestations of cardiac toxicity are abnormalities in heart rate, rhythm, and conduction. An early sign is bradycardia; therefore, the *apical* pulse (counted for one full minute) is always checked before administering digitalis. As a general rule the drug is not given if the pulse is below 90 to 110 beats/minute in infants and young children or below 70 beats/minute in older children. Since the pulse rate varies in children within different age-groups, the physician should specify in the written order at what heart rate the drug is to be withheld. The nurse should also use judgment in evaluating the pulse rate. If it is significantly lower than the previous recording, the dose should be withheld until the physician is notified.

In no other drug is it more important to employ the safe practice of checking for correct drug preparation, dose, patient, time, and route. An accidental overdose can be fatal. As an added safety precaution, the nurse administering the drug always checks the dose with another nurse before giving the drug to the child.

A problem arises when the child vomits or spits out the medication, since regiving it may result in overdose. In general, the physician is notified prior to administering another dose, especially since vomiting may be an early sign of toxicity. To minimize this problem, it is important to administer the drug carefully, by slowly instilling it with a syringe or dropper on the side and back of the mouth. It should not be mixed with foods or fluids, since refusal to consume these substances results in inaccurate dosage of the drug.

Decrease cardiac demands. The infant or child with CHF is placed at complete rest although the manner of attainment varies with the age of the child. The infant requires rest and conservation of energy for the task of feeding; therefore, every effort is made to organize nursing activities to allow for periods of uninterrupted sleep. Whenever possible, the parents are encouraged to stay with their infant to provide the holding, rocking, and cuddling that help children sleep more soundly and to preserve the parent-child relationship.

To minimize disturbing the infant, changing bedclothes and complete bathing are done only when necessary. Feeding is planned to accommodate the infant's sleep and waking patterns. He is fed as soon as he appears hungry, for example, when he is sucking on his fists. He should be fed before he begins to cry for a bottle, since the stress of crying exhausts his limited energy supply. If he is sleeping, he is fed after he awakens.

Usually, the older child is placed on a regimen of complete bed rest to minimize any unnecessary physical activity. This usually means dependence on others for feeding, bathing, and elimination (use of bedpan for older child). Encouraging parents to stay with the child and participate in his care is most beneficial to ensuring bed rest, since the child's physical and emotional needs are anticipated and quickly met. Children need an explanation of what is happening to them, to decrease anxiety about their physical status, for example, an explanation of equipment and procedures. Sometimes the sense of urgency associated with admission of a child in severe congestive heart failure overshadows the need for psychologic preparation. However, the few minutes it takes to reassure a child that electrocardiograph leads do not hurt or to familiarize him with the way the world appears through a plastic tent reduce the physiologic responses to stress.

Temperature is carefully monitored because hyperthermia or hypothermia increases the need for oxygen. Febrile states are reported to the physician, since infection must be promptly treated. Maintaining body temperature is of special importance in children who are receiving cool, humidified oxygen, and in infants, who tend to be diaphoretic and lose heat by way of evaporation.

Reduce respiratory distress. To facilitate respiratory effort, the child is placed in a semi- to high-Fowler position; infants are placed in an infant or cardiac seat. Infants and young children with cyanotic heart disease often breathe better in the knee-chest position, which decreases venous return and reduces the workload of the right side of the heart. An infant can be maintained in this position by placing him on his side (maintaining Fowler position), with the knees bent toward the chest and pillows propped behind the back and buttocks. If he must be transported, either position is maintained. Shirts and diapers are pinned loosely to allow maximum chest expansion. Safety restraints, such as those used with the infant seats, are applied low on the abdomen; they should be secure enough to provide safety but loose enough to allow maximum expansion.

Respiration is carefully monitored, the rate counted for 1 full minute during a resting state, and any unusual breathing patterns or other evidence of respiratory distress are reported to the physician. If morphine sulfate is given, the nurse observes for respiratory depression from the drug.

The child is usually placed in a highly humidified oxygen environment—the infant in an incubator or under an oxygen hood; a child in a Croupette. However, supplemental oxygen may or may not be helpful in relieving the respiratory distress or cyanosis. If a trial period is ordered to determine its effectiveness, the nurse evaluates the child's response by noting respiratory rate, ease of respiration, degree of cyanosis, and interval of sleep. (See p. 673 for care of the child receiving oxygen therapy.)

Since children with congestive heart failure are susceptible to recurrent respiratory infection, they are placed in rooms with patients who have noninfectious conditions. With an older child, it is advantageous to choose a roommate who is also confined to bed and is relatively quiet, in order to promote a restful environment. Visitors and hospital personnel with active respiratory infection are isolated from the child. Good handwashing technique is practiced before and after caring for either an infant or an older child. Antibiotics are given to combat respiratory infection. The nurse ensures that the drug is given at equally divided times over a 24-hour schedule, to maintain high blood levels of the antibiotic.

Maintain nutritional status. Many infants with severe cardiac defects are poorly nourished and physically retarded. Because of the dyspnea on exertion, sucking becomes an exhausting activity and the infant is unable to consume his needed nutrients. To minimize the effort of eating, small frequent feedings are scheduled, allowing for needed rest periods. The nipple should be soft, with a hole that is large enough to permit entry of milk without the danger of aspiration. To reduce the respiratory effort, the infant is fed in an upright position and burped frequently. If these measures are still exhausting to the infant, he may require gavage for all or part of the feedings. For the infant who is unable to tolerate extended periods without supplemental oxygen, the source can be held near his face during feeding or comforting. Gavage or nasogastric feedings may be continued at home, in which case families are instructed in the procedure.

Food selections for older children need to be highly nutritious, easy to ingest, and palatable. They should also provide sufficient fluid to maintain hydration. Blenderized preparations, such as shakes and malted milks, or commercially available food supplements are usually well tolerated by children, especially if prepared with their favorite flavors, such as chocolate or strawberry. The use of a straw, a special cup, or rewards for drinking or eating, such as reading a story or playing a quiet game, can be incentives. To minimize the fatigue of eating, mealtimes should be carefully planned around rest periods and spaced at frequent intervals.

Promote fluid loss. When diuretics are given, the nurse continues to record fluid intake and output and to monitor body weight at the same time each day, to evaluate the effectiveness of the drug. Since profound diuresis may cause dehydration and electrolyte imbalance (loss of sodium, potassium, chloride, and bicarbonate), the nurse observes for signs that indicate either complication. Diuretics are given early in the day to children who are toilet trained, to avoid the need to urinate at night. If potassium-losing diuretics are given, the nurse observes for signs of hypokalemia and encourages foods high in potassium, such as bananas, oranges, whole grains, legumes, and leafy vegetables. A potassium supplement, if given, is mixed with fruit juice (red punch or grape juice works well) to disguise the bitter taste and to prevent intestinal irritation from a concentrated solution.

Fluid restriction is rarely necessary in infants because of their difficulty in feeding. When fluids are restricted, the nurse plans fluid-intake schedules. With toddlers and preschoolers it is psychologically advantageous to give small amounts of liquid in vessels of appropriate size, since young children associate volume with size of the container. Suitable utensils are decorated medicine cups, paper Dixie cups, doll-sized teacups, or measuring cups. It is also important to avoid leaving extra fluids at the bedside, since older children may help themselves to additional servings. The cooperation of older children can be gained by placing them in charge of recording fluid intake.

If salt intake is limited, the nurse discusses food sources of sodium with the parents and discourages their bringing salt-containing treats to the child. At mealtime the nurse checks the child's tray to make sure that salt was not mistakenly given.

Support child and family. CHF is a serious, potentially fatal complication of heart disease and parents and older children are usually acutely aware of the critical nature of the condition. Since stress places additional demands on cardiac function, nurses focus on reducing anxiety through anticipatory preparation, frequent communication with the parents regarding the child's progress, and constant reassurance that everything possible is being done.

The imposed bed rest and placement of the child in an oxygen tent severely limit physical contact between the child and the parents. This separation can be minimized by encouraging parents to participate in care, such as feeding, bathing, positioning, and stimulating the child. As was mentioned earlier, active parent participation also optimally meets the infant's physical and emotional needs, with minimum exertion. However, parents must feel comfortable and well accepted by the staff. For example, positioning the child may be cumbersome because of the interference of the electrocardiogram leads, but, with practice, parents become expert in functioning despite such equipment.

If congestive heart failure is the final stage of a severe heart defect, the nurse cares for the child as for any terminally ill child, using principles discussed in Chapter 18.

EVALUATION

The effectiveness of nursing interventions is determined by continual reassessment and evaluation of care based on the following observational guidelines and expected outcomes:

1. Monitor heart rate and quality, respiratory rate and efforts, and color, and observe behaviors that provide clues to expended effort
2. Observe nutritional intake, feeding behaviors, and weight
3. Monitor intake, output, and weight
4. Interview and observe behaviors of family

Expected outcomes:

1. Vital signs are within normal limits; child breathes easily without compensatory behaviors and displays good skin color
2. Child consumes an adequate amount and exhibits a satisfactory weight gain
3. The child does not exhibit signs of overhydration
4. Family expresses feelings and concerns

Clinical Manifestations of Infective Endocarditis

Onset usually insidious
Unexplained fever
Anorexia
Malaise
Weight loss
Characteristic findings caused by extracardiac emboli formation:
- Splinter hemorrhages (thin black lines) under the nails
- Osler nodes (red, painful intradermal nodes found on pads of phalanges)
- Janeway lesions (painless hemorrhagic areas on palms and soles)
- Petechiae on oral mucous membranes

May be present:
- Congestive heart failure
- Cardiac arrhythmias
- New murmur or change in previously existing one

INFECTIVE (BACTERIAL) ENDOCARDITIS

Infective endocarditis (IE), or bacterial endocarditis (BE), an infection of the valves or inner lining of the heart, is one of the most serious of the cardiac complications and is a significant cause of morbidity in the pediatric age-group. It develops most often as a complication of congenital or rheumatic heart disease but can occur without an underlying heart disorder. The most common causative agents are bacteria (streptococci, especially *Streptococcus viridans,* staphylococci, enterococci, and pneumococci), fungi such as *Candida albicans,* and *Rickettsia.*

Pathophysiology

Organisms usually gain entrance to the bloodstream by: (1) lymphatic spread from a wound site, (2) infected thrombi, which attain direct access into the general circulation, and (3) infected materials inserted into the peripheral circulation during surgical or traumatic procedures. The most common portals of entry are oral, particularly with dental procedures (*S. viridans*); urinary tract infections following catheterization (gram-negative bacilli); and the bloodstream, as a result of long-term infusions.

Following an infection, vegetations (*verrucae*) consisting of deposits of platelets, fibrin, and fibrinoid material form at a weakened spot on the endocardium. Infective endocarditis results when these vegetations become contaminated with microorganisms from the bloodstream. Infected emboli may travel through the bloodstream to other areas of the heart and to other organ systems producing extensive damage.

Diagnostic Evaluation

The diagnosis is suspected on the basis of clinical manifestations (see box). Several laboratory findings may suggest infective endocarditis, for example, electrocardiographic changes (prolonged P-R interval), radiographic evidence of cardiomegaly, anemia, elevated erythrocyte sedimentation rate, leukocytosis, and microscopic hematuria. Definitive diagnosis rests on growth and identification of the causative agent in the blood.

Therapeutic Management

Treatment should be instituted immediately and consists of administration of high doses of appropriate antibiotics intravenously and/or intramuscularly for at least 4 weeks. Blood cultures are taken periodically to evaluate response to antibiotic therapy.

Prevention of infective endocarditis in susceptible children is achieved by administering prophylactic antibiotic therapy both prior to and for a short period after procedures known to increase the risk of entry of organisms, including dental work and any manipulation of the respiratory, genitourinary, or gastrointestinal tract. In female adolescents this includes childbirth.

Nursing Considerations

Ideally, the objective of nursing care is prevention through counseling parents of high-risk children about the need for prophylactic antibiotic therapy prior to procedures such as dental work. Unless parents are aware of the risk inherent in exposing their child to these procedures, they may not be inclined to seek medical treatment beforehand. The family's regular dentist should be advised of existing cardiac problems in the child, as an added precaution and to ensure that preventive treatment is carried out.

Treatment requires hospitalization for the duration of parenteral drug therapy. Nursing goals during this period are (1) preparation of the child for continuous intravenous infusion, possibly for several venipunctures for blood cultures; (2) observation for side effects of antibiotics; and (3) observation for complications, especially from embolism, and the possibility of heart failure. For specific interventions see the nursing care summary for the child with congestive heart failure.

RHEUMATIC FEVER

Rheumatic fever (RF), or acute rheumatic fever (ARF), is an inflammatory disease affecting the heart, joints, central nervous system, and subcutaneous tissue. It derives its name from involvement of joints and the presence of fever in the acute stage. The most significant sequela of RF is *rheumatic heart disease*, especially damage to and scarring of the mitral valve. Although the disease has declined during the past 30 years, recent outbreaks of the disease have been reported in several areas causing some concern for health professionals.

Clinical Manifestations of Rheumatic Fever

General
Low-grade fever, usually spiking in late afternoon
Unexplained epistaxis
Abdominal pain
Arthralgia without arthritic changes
Weakness
Fatigue
Pallor
Loss of appetite
Weight loss

Specific Manifestations
Carditis
- Tachycardia out of proportion to degree of fever
- Cardiomegaly
- New murmurs or change in preexisting murmurs
- Muffled heart sounds
- Precardial friction rub
- Precordial pain
- Changes in ECG (especially prolonged P-R interval)

Migratory polyarthritis
- Swollen, hot, red, painful joint(s)
- After 1 to 2 days affects different joint(s)
- Favors large joints—knees, elbows, hips, shoulders, wrists

Erythema marginatum
- Erythemous macules with clear center and wavy, well-demarcated border
- Transitory
- Nonpruritic
- Primarily affects trunk and proximal extremities

Chorea (St. Vitus dance, Sydenham chorea)
- Sudden aimless, irregular movements of extremities
- Involuntary facial grimaces
- Speech disturbances
- Emotional lability
- Muscle weakness (can be profound)
- Muscle movements exaggerated by anxiety and attempts at fine motor activity; relieved by rest

Subcutaneous nodes
- Nontender swelling
- Located over bony prominences
- May persist for some time, then gradually resolve

Etiology and Pathophysiology

RF occurs primarily in school-age children and environmental, climatic, and familial factors influence the incidence in certain individuals. These factors include a lower socioeconomic standard of living, crowded housing, cold, humid climate, and parental or personal history of rheumatic fever.

In almost all cases of RF a previous infection with group A beta-hemolytic streptococci can be documented by laboratory evidence; therefore prevention or treatment of these infections prevents RF. The mechanism by which the organisms initiate connective tissue damage is believed to be an autoimmune process. Streptococci release several different proteins against which antibodies are formed. These proteins resemble many different tissues in the body.

Diagnostic Evaluation

There is no specific test for RF; therefore a combination of clinical manifestations and laboratory findings is used as a basis for diagnosis. Many general and some specific manifestations are observed (see box). Since RF may affect a number of organs and tissues, a combination of clinical manifestations and laboratory findings as outlined

TABLE 24-2

Jones' Criteria (revised) for Guidance in the Diagnosis of Rheumatic Fever

Major Manifestations	Minor Manifestations
Carditis	Clinical features
Polyarthritis	Fever
Chorea	Arthralgia
Erythema marginatum	History of previous rheumatic fever or rheumatic heart disease
Subcutaneous nodules	Laboratory
	Increased ESR
	C-reactive protein
	Leukocytosis
	Anemia
	Prolonged P-R interval on ECG

Supportive evidence of preceding streptococcal infection:
- Recent scarlet fever
- Positive throat culture for group A β-hemolytic streptococci
- Increased ASO or other streptococcal antibodies

Presence of two major manifestations or one major and two minor manifestations with supportive evidence of recent streptococcal infection indicates a high probability of rheumatic fever.

in Jones' criteria (Table 24-2) is useful in establishing a diagnosis. However, the three major manifestations—arthritis, carditis, and chorea—differ in both frequency and time of appearance in the course of the disease. There are also other conditions that fulfill these criteria.

Children suspected of having RF are tested for streptococcal antibodies. The most reliable and best standardized test is an elevated or rising antistreptolysin-O (ASO) titer, which occurs in 80% of children with RF. Others include anti-DNAse B and anti-DPNase tests, erythrocyte sedimentation rate (ESR), and C-reactive protein. Electrocardiographs and radiographs are obtained to detect any evidence of heart involvement.

Therapeutic Management

The goals of medical management are to (1) eradicate group A β-hemolytic streptococci; (2) prevent permanent cardiac damage; (3) palliate other symptoms; and (4) prevent recurrences of the disease.

Penicillin in sufficient dosage to eradicate the streptococci is the drug of choice for treatment with erythomycin as a substitute in penicillin-sensitive children. Hospitalization is advised and bed rest recommended, the length determined by the severity and duration of the illness.

Manifestations are managed appropriately. Anti-inflammatory drugs, principally salicylates, are used to suppress acute joint inflammation when multiple joints are involved. Acetaminophen may be prescribed when only one joint is involved and diagnosis is uncertain. Corticosteroids are administered to suppress severe myocardial inflammation. Mild sedation is often helpful in alleviating some of the anxiety and restlessness caused by chorea. In some cases the anticonvulsive clonazepam (Clonopin) is prescribed for more distressing symptoms.

Prevention. Prevention of first attacks (primary prevention) is accomplished by identification and adequate treatment of streptococcal upper respiratory tract infection. Because children who have suffered a previous attack of RF are highly susceptible to recurrent attacks following streptococcal upper respiratory infections, they need continuous protection to prevent recurrences (secondary prevention).

Penicillin is the drug of choice for primary prevention. The drug may be given intramuscularly in a single dose or orally for a full 10 days. The oral route is preferred unless there is a question of compliance and the possible risk of rheumatic fever in the population group being served. Other antimicrobial agents are used for penicillin-sensitive children.

Since any streptococcal respiratory infection (even asymptomatic infections) can trigger a recurrent attack of RF in rheumatic subjects, the most effective protection is afforded by long-term *continuous prophylaxis*. Once a month intramuscular injection of long-acting penicillin is the method of choice, especially for children at higher risk of recurrence or those in whom compliance is in doubt. Oral penicillin or sulfadiazine are used for low-risk compliant children (Shulman and others, 1985).

Nursing Considerations

The objectives of nursing care of the child with RF are to (1) facilitate recovery from the illness, (2) encourage compliance with drug regimens, (3) provide emotional support, and (4) prevent primary or secondary disease.

The period of bed rest may be difficult to enforce if the child is feeling well. Therefore, the facts of the situation are discussed frankly with the child and his family. If bed rest or limited activity is continued in the home a public health referral is desirable.

The child with carditis may be hospitalized for an extended period depending on the severity of the disorder and placed on limited activity following discharge. Slow convalescence requires home care and home tutoring, and any athletic activities are usually restricted for some time. The family may need help in coping with the child's enforced inactivity. Therefore, encouraging the child to become involved in quiet activities of interest and to maintain contact with friends are important aspects of nursing care.

Chorea is one of the most frustrating manifestations of the disease. The onset is gradual and may occur weeks to months after the initial illness. The nurse can be helpful by explaining the disturbing, although temporary, nature of the manifestations and protecting the child from stressful situations.

Nurses need to stress to families the importance of compliance with the oral penicillin regimen. If compliance is in doubt this should be reported to the physician so that long-acting penicillin can be administered. If parenteral medication is instituted the child needs preparation for and support during the monthly injections.

◆ *Vascular Dysfunction*

Disorders of the circulatory system in children involve primarily the shock states and hypertension. The vascular degenerative disorders seen in adults are almost nonexistent in children; however, vascular anomalies and cerebrovascular accidents are an uncommon cause of cerebral dysfunction in children.

SYSTEMIC HYPERTENSION

Hypertension is defined as the consistent elevation of blood pressure (BP) beyond values considered to be the upper limits of normal. The Second Task Force on Blood Pressure Control in Children (1987) further defines BP as:

Normal BP—systolic and diastolic pressure below the 90th percentile for age and sex

Normal high BP—Average systolic and/or average diastolic BP between 90th and 95th percentiles for age and sex

High BP—average systolic and/or average diastolic BP at or greater than the 95th percentile for age and sex with measurements obtained on at least three occasions

The two major categories of hypertension are *essential* (no identifiable cause) and *secondary* (subsequent to an identifiable cause) hypertension. Although traditionally considered a primary risk for cerebral vascular accident and a major risk factor for myocardial infarction in adults, in recent years there has been increasing interest in this disorder as it occurs in adolescents and children, particularly in terms of prevention of fatal consequences in adulthood.

Routine blood pressure measurements of children have detected hypertension similar to essential hypertension in adults with surprising frequency in asymptomatic children, especially teenagers. Although the prevalence of the condition in adolescents is difficult to evaluate, evidence is accumulating to indicate that the essential hypertension of adulthood may have its origin in childhood; thus its early detection has significance for prevention and treatment.

Etiology

Most instances of hypertension observed in young children occur secondary to a structural abnormality or an underlying pathologic process, although this is being challenged by screening programs of relatively healthy children. The most common cause of secondary hypertension is renal disease (80%), followed by cardiovascular, endocrine, and some neurologic disorders (Mentser, 1982).

The causes of essential hypertension are undetermined, but there is evidence to indicate that both genetic and environmental factors play a role. The incidence of hypertension has been shown to be higher in children whose parents are hypertensive. American blacks have a higher incidence of hypertension than whites, and in these persons it develops earlier, is frequently more severe, and results in mortality at an earlier age.

Diagnostic Evaluation

Although clinical manifestations associated with hypertension depend largely on the underlying cause, there are some observations that can provide clues to the examiner that an elevated blood pressure may be a factor (see box). In infants and very young children who cannot communicate symptoms, observation of behavior provides clues, although gross behavioral changes may not be apparent until complications are present. A classification of hypertension by age group (Task Force on Blood Pressure in Children, 1987) is provided in Table 24-3. *Significant hypertension* is considered to be a BP persistently between the 95th and 99th percentile for age and sex and *severe blood pressure* is a BP persistently at or above the 99th percentile for age and sex.

Clinical Manifestations of Hypertension

Adolescents and older children:
- Frequent headaches
- Dizziness
- Changes in vision

Infants or young children:
- Irritability
- Head-banging or head-rubbing
- May wake up screaming in the night

Detection of elevated blood pressure calls for a full diagnostic evaluation to determine the etiology. However, when there is a strongly positive family history of hypertension, and in the absence of other signs or symptoms, the youngster with borderline readings is not usually subjected to an intensive barrage of diagnostic tests.

Therapeutic Management

Therapy for secondary hypertension involves diagnosis and treatment of the underlying cause. Children or adolescents who have consistently elevated blood pressure readings with no known etiology or those in whom secondary hypertension is not amenable to surgical correction are placed on hypotensive drug therapy. The type of drug and the dosage are tailored to meet the needs of individual children and are determined by the hypotensive effect produced and the appearance of any side effects. The aim is to achieve a normotensive state throughout the day without any accompanying side effects. The drug regimen is kept simple, preferably with a single an-

TABLE 24-3

Classification of Hypertension by Age-Group

Age-Group	Significant Hypertension (mm Hg)	Severe Hypertension (mm Hg)
Newborn (7 d)	Systolic BP ≥96	Systolic BP ≥106
(8-30 d)	Systolic BP ≥104	Systolic BP ≥110
Infant (<2 yr)	Systolic BP ≥112 Diastolic BP ≥74	Systolic BP ≥118 Diastolic BP ≥82
Children (3-5 yr)	Systolic BP ≥116 Diastolic BP ≥76	Systolic BP ≥124 Diastolic BP ≥84
Children (6-9 yr)	Systolic BP ≥122 Diastolic BP ≥78	Systolic BP ≥130 Diastolic BP ≥86
Children (10-12 yr)	Systolic BP ≥126 Diastolic BP ≥82	Systolic BP ≥134 Diastolic BP ≥90
Adolescents (13-15 yr)	Systolic BP ≥136 Diastolic BP ≥86	Systolic BP ≥144 Diastolic BP ≥92
Adolescents (16-18 yr)	Systolic BP ≥142 Diastolic BP ≥92	Systolic BP ≥150 Diastolic BP ≥98

From Report of the Second Task Force on blood pressure control in children, 1987, Pediatrics **79**(1):1-25, 1987.

tihypertensive agent in combination with a suitable diuretic.

Nursing Considerations

The nurse is a valuable link in the health-care delivery system in relation to hypertension in the pediatric age-group. Blood pressure measurement should always be part of the routine assessment of infants and children. In carrying out the procedure it is most important to make certain that the cuff used is suited to the individual child and that the procedure is repeated if there is a questionable reading, using different instruments if necessary. When an elevated pressure is detected the procedure is carried out in the standing, sitting, and supine positions and comparison readings are made between both upper extremities to ascertain if they are equal.

Blood pressure levels vary widely within a normal range in children of the same age and in the same child on any given day. To obtain an accurate reading, care is taken to quiet the child or relax the adolescent while the measurement is recorded to avoid false readings caused by excitement. The chief cause of falsely elevated blood pressure readings is the use of improperly fitting, narrow cuffs. Sphygmomanometer cuffs must be selected according to the weight and build of the child. (See p. 138 for information on techniques and selection of cuff and inside front cover for expected readings at various ages.)

Home management. Nursing counseling and guidance of the hypertensive teenager pose a number of problems. In the hospital diet and medication regimens can be carefully regulated. Home management necessitates motivating older youngsters and their parents to cooperate in carrying out a treatment plan. The major problem in hypertensive children is compliance in relation to maintaining contact with the physician or clinic for follow-up care, taking antihypertensive drugs as prescribed, and allowing home blood pressure to be taken (see discussion of compliance, p. 636). An important aspect of nursing care is to convince these youngsters that their disorder is probably a lifelong concern and that management must include drug therapy, perhaps some modification in diet and activity, and regular follow-up care.

Home blood pressure measurements greatly facilitate surveillance in youngsters with chronic hypertension. Someone in the hypertensive child's family, such as a parent, sibling, or other responsible person, must be assisted in securing proper equipment and instructed in its use. Also, the drug therapy program, including the need for taking the drug, how the drug works and its duration of action, any side effects that may be expected, and what to do if such effects are experienced, must be explained to the youngster and his family. It is important to impress on the youngster the importance of taking the drug continuously as prescribed and that it is effective only during the time it is taken regularly.

Unfortunately not all children and their families are able to accept the responsibility and the stress of continuous management. In such cases the school nurse may need to assume the responsibility for taking blood pressure measurements regularly or make arrangements for another individual to do so. Both the teenager and the parent will need guidance in the avoidance of high-sodium foods, and preparation and selection of palatable, low-salt foods; exercise prescriptions may be difficult for youngsters to follow unless they are enjoyable.

SHOCK

Shock, or circulatory failure, is a clinical syndrome characterized by prostration and tissue perfusion that is inadequate to meet the metabolic demands of the body, resulting in depressed vital cell function. Although the causes are different, the physiologic consequences are the same: hypotension, tissue hypoxia, and metabolic acidosis.

Stages of Shock

Because of the progressive nature of shock, it can be divided into three stages or phases: *compensated, uncompensated,* and *irreversible* (Perkin and Levine, 1982).

Compensated—vital organ function is maintained by intrinsic compensatory mechanisms; blood flow is usually normal or increased but generally uneven or maldistributed in the microcirculation.

Uncompensated—efficiency of the cardiovascular system gradually diminishes, until perfusion in the microcirculation becomes marginal despite compensatory adjustments.

Irreversible shock or terminal shock—damage to vital organs such as the heart or brain of such magnitude that the entire organism will be disrupted regardless of therapeutic intervention. Death occurs even if cardiovascular measurements return to normal levels with therapy.

Types of Shock

Circulatory failure in children is the result of hypovolemia, altered peripheral vascular resistance, or pump failure.

Hypovolemic shock. The most common type of circulatory failure in children is hypovolemia, or *hypovolemic shock,* which follows a reduction in circulating blood volume. Causes of hypovolemic shock are:

Blood loss (hemorrhagic shock)—caused by trauma, gastrointestinal bleeding, intracranial hemorrhage

Plasma loss—caused by increased capillary permeability associated with sepsis, acidosis, hypoproteinemia, burns, peritonitis

Extracellular fluid loss—caused by vomiting, diarrhea, glycosuric diuresis, sunstroke

Distributive shock. Reduction in peripheral vascular resistance with an associated increase in venous capacity and pooling produces an acute reduction in return blood flow to the heart and a consequent diminished cardiac output. Reduction in peripheral vascular resistance is observed in the following types of shock:

Anaphylaxis *(anaphylactic shock)*—caused by an extreme allergy or hypersensitivity to a foreign substance
Sepsis *(septic shock, bacteremic shock, endotoxic shock)*—caused by overwhelming sepsis and circulating bacterial toxins
Loss of neuronal control *(neurogenic shock)*—caused by interruption of neuronal transmission such as observed in spinal cord injury

Cardiogenic shock. Decreased cardiac output (not common in children) can be caused by the following:

Congenital heart disease—in infancy, usually caused by outflow obstruction or systemic-to-pulmonary shunting
Inflow or outflow obstruction—associated with cardiac tamponade, tension pneumothorax, or pericardial effusion
Primary pump failure—associated with myocarditis, myocardial trauma, biochemical derangements
Dysrhythmias—such as paroxysmal atrial tachycardia, atrioventricular block, and ventricular arrhythmias; may occur secondary to myocarditis or biochemical abnormalities (occasionally)

Pathophysiology

A healthy child's circulatory system is able to transport oxygen and metabolic substrates to body tissues, which require a constant source for these essential needs. The cardiac output and distribution to the various body tissues can change very rapidly in response to intrinsic (myocardial and intravascular) or extrinsic (neuronal) control mechanisms. In shock states these mechanisms are altered or challenged.

Reduced blood flow, as in hypovolemic shock, causes diminished venous return to the heart, low central venous pressure, low cardiac output, and hypotension. Vasomotor centers in the medulla are signaled, causing a compensatory increase in the force and rate of cardiac contraction and constriction of arterioles and veins, thereby increasing peripheral vascular resistance. At the same time the mechanisms are activated in an effort to conserve body fluids. This causes reduced blood flow to the skin, kidneys, muscles, and viscera in order to shunt the available blood to the brain and heart. Consequently the skin feels cold and clammy, there is poor capillary filling, and glomerular filtration and urine output are significantly reduced.

Oxygen depletion in tissue cells as a result of impaired perfusion causes the cells to revert to anaerobic metabolism, thus producing lactic acidosis. The acidosis places an extra burden on the lungs as they attempt to compensate for the metabolic acidosis by increased repiratory rate to remove excess carbon dioxide. Prolonged vasoconstriction results in fatigue and atony of the peripheral arterioles, which leads to vessel dilation. Venules, less sensitive to vasodilator substances, remain constricted for a time, causing massive pooling in the capillary and venular beds, which further depletes blood volume.

Clinical Manifestations of Shock

Early clinical signs
Apprehensiveness
Irritability
Unexplained tachycardia
Normal blood pressure
Narrowing pulse pressure
Thirst
Pallor
Diminished urinary output

Advanced shock
Confusion and somnolence
Tachypnea
Moderate metabolic acidosis
Oliguria
Cool, pale extremities
Decreased skin turgor
Poor capillary filling

Impending cardiopulmonary arrest
Thready, weak pulse
Hypotension
Periodic breathing or apnea
Anuria
Stupor or coma

Diagnostic Evaluation

The etiology of shock can be discerned from the history and the physical examination. The extent of the shock is determined by measurements of vital signs, including central venous pressure and capillary filling (see box). Shock can be regarded as a form of compensation for circulatory failure. Initially, the child's ability to compensate is effective; therefore, early signs are subtle. As the shock state advances, signs are more obvious and indicate early decompensation.

Additional signs may be present depending on the type and etiology of the shock. In early septic shock there are chills, fever, and vasodilation with increased cardiac output that results in warm, flushed skin (hyperdynamic or "hot" shock). A later and ominous development is disseminated intravascular coagulation (p. 837), the major hematologic complication of septic shock. Anaphylactic shock (caused by an extreme allergy or hypersensitivity to a foreign substance) is frequently accompanied by urticaria and angioneurotic edema, which is life-threatening when it involves the respiratory passages.

Laboratory tests that assist in assessment are blood gas measurements, pH, and sometimes liver function tests. Coagulation tests are evaluated when there is evidence of bleeding, such as oozing from a venipuncture site, bleeding from any orifice, or petechiae. Cultures of blood and other sites are indicated when there is a high suspicion of sepsis. Renal function tests are performed when impaired renal function is evident.

Therapeutic Management

Treatment of the child in shock begins with establishment of an airway and administration of oxygen. Once the airway is assured, circulatory stabilization is the major concern. Placement of an intravenous catheter for rapid volume replacement is the most important action for reestablishment of circulation. In the majority of cases rapid restoration of blood volume is all that is needed for resuscitation of the child in shock. Successful resuscitation will be reflected by an increase in blood pressure and a reduction in heart rate; increased cardiac output will result in improved capillary circulation and skin color. Central venous pressure measurements of right atrial pressure help guide fluid therapy, and urinary output measurement is an important indicator of adequacy of circulation. Correction of acidosis, hypoxemia, and any metabolic derangements is mandatory.

Temporary pharmacologic support may be required to enhance myocardial contractility, to reverse metabolic or respiratory acidosis, and/or to maintain arterial pressure. The principal agents used to improve cardiac output and circulation are the sympathetic amines administered by constant infusion pump. Those given most often to pediatric patients are the catecholamines dopamine (Intropin), epinephrine (Adrenalin), and isoproterenol (Isuprel). Vasodilators that are sometimes employed include nitroprusside (Nipride) and hydralazine (Apresoline).

Acidosis is corrected with adequate ventilatory support, including oxygen, and the administration of sodium bicarbonate. Calcium chloride may be administered to improve cardiac function. Appropriate antibiotics are administered to patients with septic shock. In cases of septic shock caused by gram-negative organisms, corticosteroids are of value. Other complicating disorders are treated appropriately.

Nursing Considerations

When shock is a likely complication, the child is observed carefully for any early signs such as irritability, unexplained increase in heart rate, thirst, pallor, or diminished urinary output. Appearance of any of these signs requires further evaluation and initiation of therapy.

The child who is in shock requires intensive observation and care. The initial action is to ensure adequate tissue oxygenation. The nurse should be prepared to administer oxygen by the appropriate route and to assist with any intubation and ventilatory procedures indicated. Other procedures and activities that require immediate attention are establishing an intravenous line, weighing the child, obtaining baseline vital signs, placing an indwelling catheter, obtaining blood gas and other measurements, and administering medications as indicated.

The nurse's responsibilities are to monitor the intravenous infusion, intake and output, vital signs (including central venous pressure), and general systems assessments on a routine basis. Intravenous medications are titrated according to patient responses, and vital signs are taken every 15 minutes during the critical periods and thereafter as needed. Urine output is measured hourly, and blood gases, hematocrit, pH, and electrolytes are monitored frequently to assess the status of the child and the efficacy of therapy. An apnea and cardiac monitor is attached and monitored continuously. In the initial stages of acute shock the care of the child often requires the attendance of more than one nurse in order to manage all the necessary activities that must be carried out simultaneously.

Throughout the intense activity the parents must not be overlooked. Someone should contact them at frequent intervals to inform them about what is being done and if there is any progress. Ideally someone should remain with the parents to serve as liaison between them and the intensive care team. However, this is not always feasible in such a critical situation. As soon as possible they should be allowed to see the child. A clergyman may be called to help provide comfort and support.

TOXIC SHOCK SYNDROME

Toxic shock syndrome (TSS) is a relatively rare disease that occurs predominantly (but not exclusively) in previously healthy young women during their menstrual periods. The organism implicated is the phage group-1 *Staphylococcus aureus*, which is believed to produce an epidermal toxin. The disease has been observed primarily in women who use tampons during a menstrual period. The tampons may carry the organism from the fingers or the vulva into the vagina during insertion, the tampon might traumatize the vaginal wall and provide a focus of infection, or the tampon itself may provide a favorable environment for growth of the organism or elaboration of its toxin.

Diagnostic Evaluation

Diagnosis is established on the basis of the criteria established by the Centers for Disease Control's toxic case definition (see box). A history of tampon use contributes to the diagnosis. Additional laboratory tests include cultures from blood, vagina, cervix, and any discharge. Other laboratory tests are those that facilitate the management of shock.

Therapeutic Management

The management of toxic shock syndrome is the same as management of shock of any etiology, and may involve supportive care in mild cases to hospitalization and intensive care in severe cases. Appropriate parenteral antibiotics are usually administered after cultures are obtained.

Nursing Considerations

Nursing care and observation of the acutely ill patient are the same as those described for shock of any etiology. Since the disease is relatively rare, the major efforts of nursing are directed toward prevention. The association between the disease and the use of tampons provides some direction for education. Avoiding the use of tam-

Case Definition of Toxic Shock Syndrome

1. Fever (temperature at or above 38.9° C, or 102° F)
2. Rash (diffuse macular erythroderma)
3. Desquamation 1 to 2 weeks after onset of illness, particularly of the palms and soles
4. Hypotension (systolic blood pressure at or below 90 mm HG for adults or below the fifth percentile for age for children younger than 16 years of age, or orthostatic syncope)
5. Involvement of three or more of the following organ systems:
   a. Gastrointestinal (vomiting or diarrhea at onset of illness)
   b. Muscular (severe myalgia or creatine phosphokinase level above 2 times the upper limits of normal)
   c. Mucous membrane (vagina, oropharyngeal, or conjunctival hyperemia)
   d. Renal (blood urea nitrogen or creatinine levels above 2 times the upper limits of normal or above 5 white blood cells per high-power field—in the absence of a urinary tract infection)
   e. Hepatic (total bilirubin, SGOT [serum glutamic oxaloacetic transaminase], or SGPT [serum glutamic pyruvic transaminase] above 2 times the upper limits of normal)
   f. Hematologic (platelets below 100,000/mm^3)
   g. Central nervous system (disorientation or alterations in consciousness without focal neurologic signs when fever and hypotension are absent)
6. Negative results on the following tests, if obtained:
   a. Blood, throat, or cerebrospinal fluid cultures
   b. Serologic tests for Rocky Mountain spotted fever, leptospirosis, or measles

From Centers for Disease Control: Morbid. Mortal. Weekly Rep. **29:**442, 1980.

pons offers the most certain preventive measure, although this approach is probably unacceptable to most adolescent girls. Most young women prefer the freedom, comfort, and inconspicuousness that tampons afford and are unlikely to comply with this advice.

Adolescent girls who use tampons can be advised to modify their use. For example, intermittent use of tampons during the menstrual cycle, alternating with sanitary napkins—perhaps using the napkins during the night and tampons during the day. It is probably advisable to encourage young girls not to use superabsorbent tampons and not to leave any tampon in the body for more than 12 hours. Instruction in general hygienic measures, such as hand washing before insertion of the tampon, is an important part of patient teaching.

It is also advisable to teach patients how to recognize the early symptoms of toxic shock syndrome. They should understand that they should remove the tampon and consult their physician if they develop a sudden high fever, vomiting, diarrhea, muscle pain, dizziness, or rash.

HENOCH-SCHÖNLEIN PURPURA

Henoch-Schönlein purpura (HSP, Schönlein-Henoch vasculitis, allergic purpura, anaphylactoid purpura) is a relatively common acquired disorder in children characterized by a nonthrombocytopenic purpura and variable joint and visceral abnormalities. The etiology is unknown but the disease often follows an upper respiratory infection, and allergy or drug sensitivity play a role in some instances. The disease occurs in children aged 6 months to 16 years but more frequently in children between ages 2 to 8 years. It is observed more often in white children, and in boys three times more often than in girls.

Clinical Manifestations of Henoch-Schönlein Purpura

Primary feature: symmetrical purpura
- Involves buttocks and lower extremities
- May extend to include extensor surfaces of upper extremities
- Less commonly, upper trunk and face
- May be associated with maculopapular lesions and variable elements of urticaria and erythema
- Often marked edema of scalp, eyelids, lips, ears, and dorsal surfaces of hands and feet—especially in infants and younger children

Arthritic effects (two thirds of affected children)
- Asymptomatic swelling around a single joint
- Painful tender swelling of several joints, most often the knees and ankles

Gastrointestinal involvement (two thirds of affected children)
- Recurrent colicky midabdominal pain
- Often associated with nausea and vomiting
- Stools contain gross or occult blood and mucus

Renal involvement (up to one half of affected children)
- Hematuria
- Casts
- Proteinuria

Pathophysiology

The disease is characterized by inflammation of small blood vessels and the manifestations observed are influenced by the size and distribution of the affected vessels. A generalized vasculitis of dermal capillaries (and to a lesser extent small arterioles and veins) causing extravasation of red blood cells produce the petechial skin lesions. Inflammation and hemorrhage may also occur in the gastrointestinal tract, synovium, glomeruli, and central nervous system. Renal involvement is potentially the most serious long-term complication. Although the majority of children with renal involvement recover completely, some develop chronic renal disease with eventual renal failure. The arthritic involvement is periarticular and resolves in a few days without permanent damage or deformity.

Diagnostic Evaluation

Diagnosis is usually established on the basis of clinical manifestations (see box). The onset of the disease may be abrupt, with simultaneous appearance of several manifestations, or gradual, with sequential appearance of different manifestations. Laboratory tests are used to assess gastrointestinal and renal involvement and to determine adequacy of hematostatic function.

Therapeutic Management

Management is primarily supportive with close observation for signs of renal or gastrointestinal manifestations. Edema, rash, malaise, and arthralgia are usually managed with appropriate analgesics, such as acetaminophen, and mild sedation if necessary. Corticosteroids may be prescribed for relief of more severe edema, arthralgia, and colicky abdominal pain but are not warranted in all cases.

The majority of children recover without the need for hospitalization and, in most instances, a single acute episode clears spontaneously within a month. Others may have periodic recurrences for as long as 2 to 3 years before permanent remission from symptoms. Rarely death occurs from severe gastrointestinal complications, acute renal failure, or central nervous system involvement.

Nursing Considerations

Nursing care of the child hospitalized with Henoch-Schönlein purpura is primarily supportive with vigilant observation for signs of complications. Vital signs are taken and recorded at regular intervals, specimens obtained for laboratory examination, and medication administered as prescribed. Urine and stools are carefully observed for fresh and occult blood.

If the child suffers from joint pain positioning, careful movement and administration of analgesics help reduce discomfort. Analgesics also relieve the discomfort of fever and malaise. More severe involvement such as gastrointestinal symptoms and nephritis are managed as for any such disorder (see appropriate nursing care).

The child may be concerned about the unsightly appearance of the rash. He and his parents can be reassured that it is only a temporary phenomenon, and the child can be encouraged to wear clothing that helps to hide the rash, such as long sleeves, pants, and robe. Emphasizing good grooming and attractive apparel helps promote a more positive self-image.

MUCOCUTANEOUS LYMPH NODE SYNDROME (KAWASAKI DISEASE)

Mucocutaneous lymph node syndrome (MCLS), or Kawasaki disease (KD), is an acute febrile illness of unknown etiology that occurs primarily in infants and young children. In the United States the peak incidence is 3 years of age, with a slightly higher incidence in males. In Japan, where it was first described, the peak incidence is 9 to 12 months of age. There appears to be no regional, seasonal, or socioeconomic prevalence associated with the disease, and no organism or environmental toxins have been implicated. There is some evidence to indicate that susceptibility is associated with histocompatibility antigens, however.

Clinical Manifestations of Kawasaki Disease

The child must exhibit five of the following six criteria, including fever:

1. Fever for 5 or more days
2. Bilateral congestion of the ocular conjunctiva without exudation
3. Changes of the mucous membranes of the oral cavity, such as erythema, dryness, and fissuring of the lips; oropharyngeal reddening (strawberry tongue)
4. Changes in the extremities, such as peripheral edema, peripheral erythema, and desquamation of palms and soles—particularly periungual peeling
5. Polymorphous rash, primarily of the trunk
6. Cervical lymphadenopathy

Pathophysiology

The principal area of involvement is the cardiovascular system. During the initial stage of the illness there is extensive inflammation of the arterioles, the venules, and the capillaries, which later progresses to include the main coronary arteries, the heart, and the larger veins. When death occurs, it is usually the result of coronary thrombosis or severe scar formation and stenosis of the main coronary artery.

Diagnostic Evaluation

Diagnosis is established on the basis of the clinical findings (see box). No laboratory tests are of significant value in the diagnosis of the disease.

Therapeutic Management

There is no definitive treatment for the disease; therefore, management is primarily supportive and aimed at controlling fever, preventing dehydration, and minimizing possible cardiac complications. Large doses of aspirin are administered in the acute stage to control fever and the symptoms of inflammation, and during the recovery period to prevent platelet aggregation. High doses of salicylates or reduced amounts of salicylates with intravenous gamma globulin may be effective in reducing the risk of coronary disease. Monitoring the cardiac status for possible complications is essential in follow-up care.

Nursing Considerations

The nursing care of children with Kawasaki disease is primarily concerned with assisting in the diagnosis and case finding, supportive treatment as outlined by the physician, and supportive care to the child and family during both the acute and the chronic phases of the illness. Nurses should be aware that children with prolonged fever may be victims of this disorder and should encourage early medical evaluation. Administration of aspirin involves an understanding of the reasons for administration and teaching the family how it can best be administered, the importance of compliance, and the early signs of toxicity. The child requires careful monitoring during the acute phase and conscientious follow-up in the chronic phase. It is during the long-term stage of the disease that the nurse can be especially valuable in monitoring progress and preparing the child for health visits and diagnostic tests that may be ordered to assess cardiac status, such as echocardiography and electrocardiography. The importance of nutrition, hygiene, and normal activities is emphasized.

SUMMARY

Cardiovascular problems in infants and children, although not common in the pediatric age-group, generate considerable concern and anxiety in both health professionals and families. Congenital heart defects are the usual cause of heart disease and may be apparent at birth or not become evident for years. The defects can be cyanotic or acyanotic but either type is capable of producing serious disability in the pediatric patient. Most of the defects are amenable to surgical correction at an increasingly earlier age. However, the prime aim of health professionals is to recognize the presence of a defect and to help the child and family adjust to the disability with minimum disruption of a normal life-style.

The major focus in management of acquired cardiovascular diseases is prevention, since most acquired diseases are conditions that arise as complications of other disorders. Short-term vascular disorders require intense nursing care and observation to prevent serious consequences or death. Teaching and nursing supervision are primary forces in long-term cardiovascular problems that require compliance to a medical regimen.

KEY CONCEPTS

- Congenital heart defects are the most common cause of cardiac disease in children.
- Major categories to investigate in the cardiac history are poor weight gain, poor feeding habits, fatigue during feeding, frequent respiratory infections and difficulties, cyanosis with or without clubbing, and evidence of exercise intolerance.
- Cardiac catheterization provides important information about oxygen saturation of blood within the chambers and great vessels, pressure changes, changes in cardiac output or stroke volume, and anatomic abnormalities.
- Congenital heart disease is usually classified as acyanotic or cyanotic.
- Physical consequences of congenital heart disease are growth retardation, decreased exercise tolerance, dyspnea, tachypnea, tachycardia, cardiomegaly, cyanosis, and clubbing.
- Acyanotic defects in children include ventricular septal defect, atrial septal defect, endocardial cushion defect, patent ductus arteriosus, coarctation of the aorta, pulmonic stenosis, and aortic stenosis.
- Some cyanotic defects affecting children include tetralogy of Fallot, transposition of the great vessels, and truncus arteriosus.
- Goals of nursing care for the infant or child with congenital heart disease are: improve cardiac function, decrease cardiac demands, reduce respiratory distress, maintain nutrition, promote fluid loss, and provide emotional support to child and family.
- Nursing care includes helping parents and child adjust to the disorder and fostering growth-promoting family relationships.
- Preoperative care of the child with a congenital defect involves introducing the child and family to the hospital, preparing them for preoperative and postoperative procedures, and assessing physiologic status to determine baseline data.
- Providing postoperative care includes observing vital signs and arterial venous pressures, maintaining respiratory status, allowing maximum rest, providing comfort, monitoring fluids, planning for progressive stages of activities, giving emotional support, observing for complications of surgery, and planning for discharge and home care.
- Acquired cardiac disorders include congestive heart failure, bacterial endocarditis, and rheumatic fever.
- Serious vascular disorders are systemic hypertension, Kawasaki disease, and Henoch-Schönlein purpura.
- Clinical manifestations of congestive heart failure (CHF) are evidence of impaired myocardial function (tachycardia, cardiomegaly), pulmonary congestion (dyspnea, tachypnea, orthopnea, cyanosis), and systemic congestion (hepatomegaly, edema, distended veins).
- Nursing measures in the care of a child with CHF are to assist in improving cardiac function, decrease cardiac demands, reduce respiratory distress, maintain nutritional status, promote fluid loss, and provide family support.
- Prevention of bacterial endocarditis in certain children with congenital heart disease (CHD) involves administration of prophylactic antibiotics when specific procedures are performed.
- Systemic hypertension is now recognized as an important disorder of childhood.
- Education of the child with hypertension and his family focuses on drug therapy, diet control, and appropriate exercise.
- Stages of shock are: compensated, uncompensated, and irreversible.
- Shock classifications in children are hypovolemic shock, distributive shock, and cardiogenic shock.
- Kawasaki disease is extensive inflammation of small vessels and capillaries that may progress to involve the heart and larger vessels.

STUDY QUESTIONS AND ACTIVITIES

1 Explain fetal circulation and the changes that normally take place at birth to someone who does not have a background in anatomy and physiology.
2 Investigate the services provided for children and their families by the local branch of the American Heart Association.
3 Plan appropriate play activities for a an infant, a preschool child, and a school-age child with a cyanotic heart defect.
4 Interview a cardiovascular nurse specialist to determine the pre- and postoperative care given to the child cardiac surgery patient.
5 Prepare a nursing care plan for a child in hypovolemic shock.
6 Devise a teaching plan for a teenager newly diagnosed with systemic hypertension.

REFERENCES

Centers for Disease Control: Follow-up on toxic shock syndrome, Morbid. Mort. Weekly Rep. **29:**441-445, 1980.
Perkin, R.M., and Levin, D.L.: Shock in the pediatric patient. Part I. J. Pediatr. **101:**163-169, 1982.
Shulman, S.T., and others: Prevention of rheumatic fever (Special Report), Circulation **70:**1118A-1122A, 1985.
Task Force on Blood Pressure Control in Children: Report of the second task force on blood pressure control in children—1987, Pediatrics **79:**1-25, 1987.

BIBLIOGRAPHY

General

Danaher, R.R.: Complete congenital heart block: a case study, Neonatal Network **5**(4):19-23, 1987.
Hazinski, M.F.: Sudden cardiac death in children, Crit. Care Q. **7**(2):59-70, 1984.
Johnson, D.L.: Pediatric arrhythmias: a nursing approach, Dimen. Crit. Care Nurs. **2**(3):147-157, 1983.
Nativio, D.G.: Henoch-Schönlein purpura in childhood, J. Pediatr. Health Care **2:**9-13, 1988.
Vincent, R.N., and Collins, G.F.: Cardiac embryology and fetal cardiovascular physiology, Crit. Care Q. **9**(2):1-5, 1986.
Werner, B.L.: Cardiovascular crises. In Vestal, K.W.: Pediatric critical care nursing, New York, 1981, John Wiley & Sons.

Cardiac Diagnosis

Agamalian, B.: Pediatric cardiac catheterization, J. Pediatr. Nurs. **1**(2):73-79, 1986.
Armstrong, F., and Finesilver, C.: Cardiac catheterization, Crit. Care Update **10**(7):39-46, 1983.
Caire, J.B., and Erickson, S.: Reducing distress in pediatric patients undergoing cardiac catheterization, Child. Health Care **14**(3):146-152, 1986.
Haughey, C.W.: Preparing your patient for echocardiography, Nursing 84 **14**(5):68-71, 1984.
Hinz, E.: Coping strategies of a two year old girl hospitalized for cardiac catheterization, Matern. Child Nurs. J. **9**(1):1-6, 1980.
Malinowski, L.M., and Doyle, J.E.: Cardiac catheterization of the neonate, Am. J. Nurs. **85**(1):60-62, 1985.
Slota, M.: Pediatric cardiac catheterization: complications and interventions, Crit. Care Nurse **2:**22-26, 1982.
Smith, P.A.: Current diagnostic and therapeutic catheterization techniques, Crit. Care Q. **9**(2):24-39, 1986.
Sumner, S.M., and Grau, P.A.: Guidelines for running a 12-lead E.K.G., Nursing 85 **15**(12):30-33, 1985.
Tesler, M., and Hardgrove, C.: Cardiac catheterization: preparing the child, Am J. Nurs. **73**:80-82, 1983.
Vincent, R.N., and Elixson, E.M.: Hemodynamic monitoring, Crit. Care Q. **9**(2):40-48, 1986.
Youssef, M.M.: Self control behaviors of school-age children who are hospitalized for cardiac diagnostic procedures, Matern. Child Nurs. J. **10:**219-284, 1981.

Congenital Heart Disease

Cloutier, J., and Measel, C.P.: Home care for the infant with congenital heart disease, Am. J. Nurs. **82:**100-103, 1982.
Dance, D., and Yates, M.: Nursing assessment and care of children with complications of congenital heart disease, Heart Lung **14**(3):209-214, 1985.
D'Antonio, I.G.: Cardiac infant's feeding difficulties, West. J. Nurs. Res. **1**(1):53-55, 1979.
Furgal, C.L.: Pediatric cardiology: stressors, reactions, and interventions, Issues Compr. Pediatr. Nurs. **5:**21-31, 1981.
Hazinski, M.F.: Critical care of the pediatric cardiovascular patient, Nurs. Clin. North Am. **16**(4):671-697, 1981.
Kashani, I.A., and Higgins, S.S.: Counseling strategies for families of children with congenital heart disease, Pediatr. Nurs. **12**(1):38-40, 1986.
Kotchabhakdi, P., and Beardslee, C.: School-age children's conceptions of the heart and its function: part I. Review of literature, MCN **14**(3):139-152, 1985.
Loeffel, M.: Developmental considerations of infants and children with congenital heart disease, Heart Lung **14**(3):214-217, 1985.
Malinowski, P., and Elixson, E.M.: Transposition of the great arteries, Crit. Care Nurse **5**(3):35-48, 1985.
Malinowski, P., and Yablonski, C.: Congenital heart disease in infants: nursing assessment, Crit. Care Q. **9**(2):6-23, 1986.
Page, G.G.: Tetralogy of Fallot, Heart Lung **15:**390-399, 1986.
Sasso, S.C.: Prostaglandin 1 for infants with congenital heart disease, MCN **8:**29, 1983.
Uzark, K., Messiter, E., and Rosenthal, A.: Promoting dental health care in children with congenital heart disease, Pediatr. Nurs. **12**(2):96-99, 152, 1986.

Cardiac Surgery

Filipek, J.E.: Post-operative care of the pediatric cardiac patient, Crit. Care Q. **3**(1):45-52, 1980.
Fisk, R.: Management of the pediatric cardiovascular patient after surgery, Crit. Care Q. **9**(2):75-82, 1986.
Hazinski, M.F.: Critical care of the pediatric cardiovascular patient, Nurs. Clin. North Am. **16:**671-679, 1981.
Lewandowski, L.A.: Stresses and coping styles of parents of children undergoing open-heart surgery, Crit. Care Q. **3:**75-84, 1980.
Marsden, C.: Ethical issues in a heart transplant program, Heart Lung **14**(5):495-499, 1985.
Mathias, J.M.: Immunosuppression: postoperative management of heart transplant recipients, AORN J. **41**(4):748-753, 1985.
Myrer, M.L.: Respiratory care of the postoperative cardiac surgery patient, Crit. Care Q. **9**(2):64-74, 1986.
Rogers, T.R., and others: Heart surgery in infants: a preliminary assessment of maternal adaptation, Child. Health Care **13**(2):52-58, 1984.
Rotondi, P.: Intensive care unit management of the postoperative cardiac surgery patient, Crit. Care Q. **9**(2):49-63, 1986.
Rushton, C.H.: Preparing children and families for cardiac surgery: nursing interventions, Issues Compr. Pediatr. Nurs. **6:**235-248, 1983.
Schnepf, C.A.: The pediatric heart transplant patient: immunosuppressive drugs and organ rejection, J. Pediatr. Health Care **1:**91-97, 1987.
van Breda, A.: Postoperative care of infants and children who require cardiac surgery, Heart Lung **14**(3):205-208, 1985.

Congestive Heart Failure

Cohen, S.: New concepts in understanding congestive heart failure. I. How the clinical features arise, Am. J. Nurs. **81**(1):119-142, 1981.

Cohen, S.: New concepts in understanding congestive heart failure. II. How the therapeutic approaches work, Am. J. Nurs. **81**(2):357-380, 1981.

McCauley, K.: Probing the ins and outs of congestive heart failure, Nursing 82 **12**(11):60-65, 1982.

Norsen, L.H., and Fox, G.B.: Understanding cardiac output—and the drugs that affect it, Nursing 85 **15**(4):34-41, 1985.

Van Parys, E.: Assessing the failing state of the heart, Nursing 87 **17**(2):42-49, 1987.

Infective Endocarditis

Jenkins, J.: Infective endocarditis: a clinical overview, Crit. Care Update **10**(5):42-47, 1983.

Scrima, D.A.: Infective endocarditis: nursing considerations, Crit. Care Nurse **7**:47-56, 1987.

Updated antibiotic labeling for prevention of bacterial endocarditis, FDA Drug Bull. **10**(2):12-13, 1980.

Rheumatic Fever

Bisno, A.L.: The rise and fall of rheumatic fever, JAMA **254**(4):538-541, 1985.

Diehl, A.M.: Clinical aspects of rheumatic fever: an update, Issues Compr. Pediatr. Nurs. **2**:69-76, April 1980.

Hosier, D.M., and others: Resurgence of acute rheumatic fever, Am. J. Dis. Child. **141**:730-733, 1987.

Kaplan, E.L.: The startling comeback of rheumatic fever, Contemp. Pediatr. **4**(11):20-34, 1987.

Hypertension

Britton, C.V.: Blood pressure measurement and hypertension in children, Pediatr. Nurs. **7**(4):13-17, 1981.

Cranwell, P.D.: Blood pressure teaching and screening programs for school children in grades 5-8, Home Healthc. Nurse **2**(3):42-46, 1984.

Falkner, B.: Hypertension in children, Child Care Newsletter, **6**(1):3-5, 1987.

Grim, C.M., and Grim, C.E.: The nurse's role in hypertension control, Fam. Community Health **4**:29-40, 1981.

Hill, M.N., and Foster, S.B.: Seeking and finding all those patients with high blood pressure, Nursing 82 **12**(2):72-75, 1982.

Hutchins, L.N.: Drug treatment of high blood pressure, Nurs. Clin. North Am. **16**:365-376, 1981.

Loustau, A., and Blair, B.J.: A key to compliance: systematic teaching to help hypertensive patients follow through on treatment, Nursing 81 **11**:84-87, 1981.

Maloney, R.J.: Hypertension update! Crit. Care Update **9**(10):7-18, 1982.

Marcinek, M.A.: Hypertension, Crit. Care Update **9**(3):22-32, 1982.

Marsh B., Dubes, M., and Boosinger, J.K.: Adolescent hypertension and significant variables: weight, height, and skinfold thickness, Pediatr. Nurs. **9**:287-289, 1983.

Moore, L.C., and Pulliam, C.B.: An on-the-spot guide to antihypertensive drugs, Nursing 86 **16**(1):54-57, 1986.

Moser, M.: Hypertension: how therapy works, Am. J. Nurs. **80**:937-941, 1980.

Nauright, L.P., and others: Identifying hypertensive adolescents, Pediatr. Nurs. **5**(2):34-37, 1979.

Shock

Barrows, J.J.: Shock demands drugs, Nursing 82 **12**(2):34-41, 1982.

Cohen, M.R.: Action stat! Drug-induced anaphylaxis, Nursing 85 **15**(2):43, 1985.

Holt, M., McKenny, S., and Pribyl, C.: Shock—detecting it soon enough to save your patient: seven fast refreshers. Part I, Nurs. Life **4**(6):33-40, 1984.

Holt, M., Mc Kenny, S., and Pribyl, C.: Shock—detecting it soon enough to save your patient: nine more fast refreshers. Part II, Nurs. Life **5**(1):33-40, 1985.

Keely, B.R.: Septic shock, Crit. Care Q. **7**(4):59-67, 1985.

Lamb, L.S.: You think you know septic shock, Nursing 82 **12**(1):34-43, 1982.

McConnell, E.A.: Septic shock: recognizing it can be the hardest part of dealing with it, Nurs. Life **3**(5):33-40, 1983.

Purcell, J.A.: Shock drugs. Standardized guidelines, Am. J. Nurs. **82**:965-975, 1982.

Randall, B.J.: Reacting to anaphylaxis, Nursing 85 **16**(3):34-40, 1985.

Rice, V.: Shock management. II. Pharmacologic interventions, Crit. Care Nurse **5**(1):42-46, 48-49, 1985.

Rimar, J.M.: Recognizing shock syndromes in infants and children, MCN **13**:32-37, 1988.

Toxic Shock Syndrome

Brown, B.S.: Tampons, teen-agers, and toxic shock syndrome (editorial), Pediatr. Nurs. **7**(3):7, 1981.

Brown, L.K.: Toxic shock syndrome, MCN **6**:57-60, 1981.

Cestaro-Seifer, D.J.: Developing an instructional unit on toxic shock syndrome for adolescent girls, Issues Compr. Pediatr. Nurs. **6**:107-126, 1983.

Stein, A.P., and Baughman, D.C.: Nursing implications of toxic shock syndrome, Crit. Care Update **8**(6):17-19, 1981.

Toxic shock syndrome: an update, Crit. Care Update **8**(2):33-35, 1981.

Toxic shock syndrome: an update on symptoms and treatment, Nursing 85 **15**(9):74, 1985.

Whettam, J.: Update on toxic shock: how to spot it and treat it, RN **47**(2):55-56, 1984.

Wroblewski, S.S.: Toxic shock syndrome, Am. J. Nurs. **81**:82-85, 1981.

Kawasaki Disease

Anderson, D.J., and Thibault, J.: Nursing management of the pediatric patient with Kawasaki's disease, Issues Compr. Pediatr. Nurs. **5**(1):1-10, 1981.

Hall, C.B.: Exploring clues to Kawasaki disease, Patient Care, Aug. 15, 1980, pp. 64-81.

L'Orange, C.: Kawasaki disease: a new threat to children, Am. J. Nurs. **83**:558-562, 1983.

Lynch, M.H., and Gray, J.L.: Kawasaki disease, Pediatr. Nurs. **8**:96-101, 1982.

Sealy, S.: Kawaski disease: a worldwide problem, MCN **5**:331-334, 1980.

Yanagihara, R., and Todd, J.K.: Acute febrile mucocutaneous lymph node syndrome, Am. J. Dis. Child. **134**:603-614, 1980.

CHAPTER 25

The Child with Hematologic or Immunologic Dysfunction

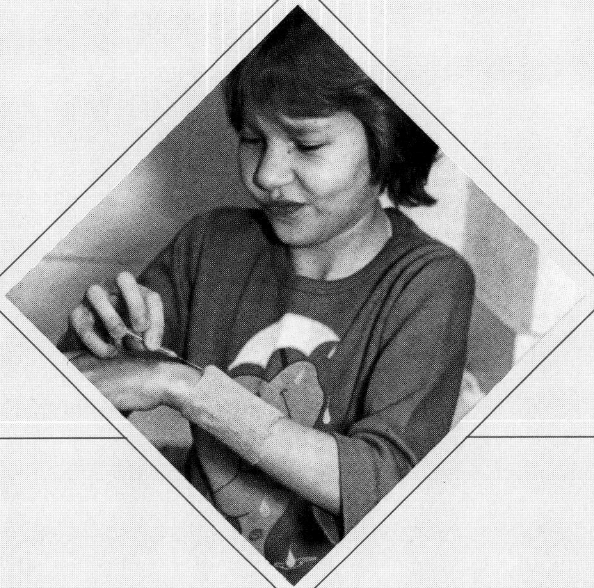

LEARNING OBJECTIVES

On completion of this chapter the reader will be able to:

- Distinguish between the various categories of anemia
- Describe the prevention of and care of the child with iron-deficiency anemia
- Compare the pathophysiology and care of children with sickle cell anemia and thalassemia major
- Describe the mechanisms of inheritance and nursing care of the child with hemophilia
- Relate the pathophysiology and clinical manifestations of leukemia
- Demonstrate an understanding of the rationale of therapies for neoplastic disease
- Outline a plan of care for the child with neoplastic disease and his family
- Contrast the pathophysiology and management of the immune-deficiency disorders

*D*isorders involving the blood and/or blood-forming organs in childhood encompass a wide range of diseases and pathologic states. Since the blood is a multipurpose fluid concerned with the functions of so many tissues and organs, either primary or secondary changes in the blood are reflected in the essential functions of these structures. Hematologic or immunologic disorders in childhood include the anemias, defects in hemostasis, neoplastic disorders, and the immunologic-deficiency disorders.

◆ *Red Blood Cell Disorders*

The most common disorders affecting the blood are those that in some way alter the function or production of red blood cells. In broad terms all of the disorders produce anemia, but the causes of reduction in erythrocyte volume or hemoglobin production vary tremendously.

ANEMIA

Anemia is defined as a condition in which the number of red blood cells and/or the hemoglobin concentration is reduced below normal. As a result of this decrease the oxygen-carrying capacity of the blood is diminished, causing a reduction in the oxygen available to the tissues. Anemia is the most common hematologic disorder of infancy and childhood and is not a disease itself but an indication or manifestation of an underlying pathologic process.

Classification

Anemias are classified in relation to (1) etiology or physiology, manifest by erythrocyte and/or hemoglobin depletion, and (2) morphology, the characteristic changes in red cell size, shape, and/or color. While the morphologic classification is more useful in terms of laboratory evaluation of anemia, the etiologic approach provides direction for planning nursing care. For example, anemia with reduced hemoglobin concentration may be caused by a dietary depletion of iron, and the principal intervention is replenishing iron stores.

Etiology. Etiologic factors responsible for anemia are:

Excessive blood loss—from acute or chronic hemorrhage (internal or external). Until stores are replaced there is usually a normocytic (normal size), normochromic (normal color) anemia, provided there are sufficient iron stores for hemoglobin synthesis

Destruction (hemolysis) of erythrocytes—as a result of an intracorpuscular defect within the RBC (such as sickle cell anemia) or an extracorpuscular factor (such as infectious agents, chemicals, or immune mechanisms) that causes destruction to outpace production

Decreased or impaired production of erythrocytes or their components—as a result of bone marrow failure (caused by factors such as neoplastic diseases, irradiation, chemicals, or disease) or deficiency of essential nutrients (such as iron)

Morphology. Morphologic classification provides an orderly method for establishing an etiology. The major characteristics of the RBC are described according to:

Size—cell size; for example, *normocytes* (normal), *microcytes* (smaller than normal), or *macrocytes* (larger than normal)

Shape—irregularly shaped red blood cells; for example, *poikilocytes* (irregularly shaped cells), *spherocytes* (globular cells), and *drepanocytes* (sickle cells)

Staining characteristics or color—reflects the hemoglobin concentration; for example, *normochromic* (sufficient or normal amount) or *hypochromic* (reduced amount)

Consequences of Anemia

The basic physiologic defect caused by anemia is a decrease in the oxygen-carrying capacity of blood and a reduction in the amount of oxygen available to the tissues. This reduced oxygen-carrying capacity is associated with a compensatory increase in heart rate and cardiac output.

The effects of anemia on the circulatory system can be profound. Because the viscosity of blood depends almost entirely on the concentration of red blood cells, the resulting hemodilution of severe anemia decreases peripheral resistance, causing greater quantities of blood to return to the heart. As a result, the cardiac workload is markedly increased (especially during exercise, infection, or emotional stress), and cardiac failure may ensue.

Children seem to have a remarkable ability to function quite well despite low levels of hemoglobin. Cyanosis (the result of the quantity of deoxygenated hemoglobin in arterial blood) is typically not evident. Growth retardation, resulting from decreased cellular metabolism and coexisting anorexia, is a common finding in chronic severe anemia and is frequently accompanied by delayed sexual maturation in the older child.

Diagnostic Evaluation

The diagnosis of anemia depends largely on its cause. In general, anemia may be suspected from findings of the history and physical examination. Most of the clinical manifestations of anemia are attributed directly to tissue hypoxia (see box). Frequently infants with iron deficiency anemia are overweight because of excessive milk ingestion (so-called milk babies). These children become anemic when milk, a poor source of iron, is given almost

Clinical Manifestations of Anemia

General Manifestations
- Muscle weakness
- Easy fatigability
  - Frequent resting
  - Shortness of breath
  - Poor sucking (infants)
- Pale skin
  - Waxy pallor seen in severe anemia
- Pica—eating clay, ice, paste

Central Nervous System Manifestations
- Headache
- Dizziness
- Light-headedness
- Irritability
- Slowed thought processes
- Decreased attention span
- Apathy
- Depression

Shock (blood loss anemia)
- Poor peripheral perfusion
- Skin moist and cool
- Low blood pressure and central venous pressure
- Increased heart rate

TABLE 25-1

Tests Used in Assessment of Anemia

Test	Description	Comments
Red blood cell (RBC) count	Number of RBCs/mm^3 of blood	Indirectly estimates Hb content of blood Reflects function of bone marrow
Hemoglobin (Hb) determination	Amount of Hb/dl of whole blood	Total blood Hb primarily depends on number of circulating RBCs, but also on amount of Hb in each cell
Hematocrit (Hct)	Percentage or volume of packed RBCs to whole blood	Indirectly measures Hb content Is approximately three times Hb content
Red blood cell indices Mean corpuscular volume (MCV)	Average or mean volume (size) of a single RBC	All indices depend on average cell measurements MCV depends on accurate RBC MCV values expressed as cubic microns (μm^3) or femtoliters (fl)
Mean corpuscular hemoglobin (MCH)	Average or mean quantity (weight) of Hb of a single RBC	MCH depends on accurate RBC MCH values expressed as picograms (pg) or micromicrograms (μμg)
Mean corpuscular hemoglobin concentration (MCHC)	Average concentration of Hb in a single RBC	MCHC does not depend on accurate RBC; therefore is often more reliable than MCV or MCH MCHC values expressed as % Hb/cell or Hb/dl RBC
Reticulocyte count	% Reticulocytes relative to RBCs	Indirectly estimates hypochromic anemia Index of production of mature RBCs by red bone marrow Decreased count indicates depressed bone marrow function Increased count indicates erythrogenesis in response to some stimulus When reticulocyte count is extremely high, other forms of immature RBCs (normoblasts, even erythroblasts) may be present
White blood cell (WBC) count	Number of WBC/mm^3 of blood	Total number of WBCs less important than differential count
Differential WBC count	Inspection and quantification of white blood cell types present in peripheral blood	Values are expressed as percentages. To obtain absolute number of any type of WBCs, multiply its respective percentage by total number of WBCs
Neutrophils (polys)		Primary defense in bacterial infection. Capable of phagocytizing and killing bacteria
Bands		Immature neutrophil Increased numbers in bacterial infection Also capable of phagocytosis and killing
Eosinophils		Named for their staining characteristics with eosin dye Increased in allergic disorders, parasitic diseases, certain neoplasms, and other diseases
Basophils		Named for their characteristic basophilic stippling Contain histamine, but their function is unknown
Lymphocytes		Involved in development of antibody and delayed hypersensitivity reactions
Monocytes		Large phagocytic cells that are involved in early stage of inflammatory reaction
Platelet count		Cellular fragments that are necessary for clotting to occur
Stained peripheral blood smear	Visual estimation of amount of Hb in RBCs and overall size, shape, and structure of RBCs	Various staining properties of RBC structures may be evidence of immature forms of erythrocyte Shows variation in size and shape of RBCs—microcytic, macrocytic, poikilocytic (variable sizes)

to the exclusion of solid foods. Although chubby, these infants are pale, usually demonstrate poor muscle development, and are prone to infection. The skin color is sometimes described as porcelain-like.

Unless the anemia is severe the first clue to the disorder may be alterations in laboratory findings. Several tests are used to evaluate the morphologic and quantitative changes that are observed in anemia (see Table 25-1 for tests and Appendix E for normal values).

Other tests specific to a particular type of anemia are employed to determine the underlying cause of anemia. These are discussed in relation to the particular disorder.

Therapeutic Management

The objective of medical management is to reverse the anemia by treating the underlying cause and to make up for any deficiency of blood, blood component, or substance the blood needs for normal functioning. For example, blood or blood cells are replaced after hemorrhage; in nutritional anemias the specific deficiency is replaced.

Iron deficiency anemia is usually treated with oral iron supplements. Ferrous iron, more readily absorbed than ferric iron, results in higher hemoglobin levels. Dietary addition of iron-rich foods is usually inadequate as a sole treatment for iron deficiency anemia, because the iron is poorly absorbed and provides insufficient supplemental quantities of iron. Therefore, oral iron supplements are prescribed for approximately 3 months to replace body stores. Ascorbic acid appears to facilitate absorption of iron and may be prescribed in addition to the iron preparation.

If the hemoglobin is very low or if levels fail to rise after 1 month of oral therapy, intramuscular injections of iron dextran (Imferon) are administered. Transfusions are indicated for the most severe anemia and in cases of serious infection, cardiac dysfunction, or surgical emergency where anesthesia is required. Packed red cells, not whole blood, should be used to minimize the chance of circulatory overload. Supplemental oxygen is administered when tissue hypoxia is severe.

In cases of severe anemia supportive medical care may include oxygen therapy, bed rest, and replacement of intravascular volume with intravenous fluids. See Table 25-2 for medical management of selected anemias.

TABLE 25-2

Management of Some Anemias

Type of Anemia	Diagnosis	Management
Blood loss anemia	Until 20% or more of blood volume lost with normal vital signs	No therapy needed
	Altered vital signs with losses of 30% to 40% blood volume and signs of shock	Blood replacement Plasma or plasma protein product until blood available
Iron deficiency	Reduced hemoglobin concentration; see discussion	Oral iron (preferred) Parenteral iron by deep IM injection
Anemia of renal disease	Usually not until symptomatic and Hb less than 7 to 8 mg/dl	Transfusion of packed red blood cells
Hemolytic anemias Spherocytosis Elliptocytosis	Shortened survival of red blood cells	Splenectomy
Sickle cell	See discussion	
Thalassemia	See discussion	

Nursing Considerations

Since anemia is not a disorder but a symptom of some underlying problem, nursing care is directed toward determining the cause, fostering appropriate supportive and therapeutic treatments, and decreasing tissue oxygen requirements.

ASSESSMENT

The assessment of anemia includes the basic techniques that are applicable to any condition. The age of the infant or child provides some clues regarding the possible etiology of the anemia. For example, iron deficiency anemia occurs more frequently in infants between 6 and 24 months of age and during the growth spurt of adolescence. The prevalence of iron deficiency in these age-groups is a consequence of the rapid growth rate of each, poor dietary practices, and menstruation. Iron stores present at birth are usually adequate for the first 4 to 5 months but may be depleted earlier in a prematurely born infant. Delayed addition of solid foods in infants and the eating habits of teenagers aggravate the iron depletion in these age-groups.

Racial or ethnic background is significant. For example, the anemias related to abnormal hemoglobins are found in blacks, southeast Asians, and persons of Mediterranean ancestry. Certain ethnic populations (e.g., blacks and Chinese) are genetically deficient in lactase after the period of infancy and are unable to tolerate lactose in the diet, with consequent intestinal irritation and chronic blood loss.

Special emphasis is placed on a careful history to elicit any information that might help identify the cause of the anemia. For example, a statement such as, "The baby drinks lots of milk," is a frequent finding in infants with iron deficiency anemia. An episode of diarrhea may have precipitated a temporary lactose intolerance in infants.

Stool examination for occult blood (guaiac test) often helps identify chronic intestinal bleeding that results from a primary or secondary lactase deficiency. It is also important to understand the significance of various blood tests. Blood loss from overt hemorrhage may be manifest as shock (p. 811).

NURSING DIAGNOSES

A variety of nursing diagnoses may be evident following assessment of anemia. Some of the general aspects of nursing management are included in the Nursing Care Plan on pp. 826 to 827. Others become apparent in specific situations.

PLANNING

The goals of nursing care for the infant or child with anemia include the following:

1. Assist with replacement of deficient blood elements
2. Prevent complications
3. Provide support and education to child and family

IMPLEMENTATION

The nursing care of an infant or child with anemia may involve a number of modalities, primarily administration of blood or blood products (usually packed red blood cells), administration of iron preparations, and diet counseling.

Blood transfusion. Any blood transfusion carries attendant risks. Blood is administered by infusion pump; therefore the usual precautions and management apply. When the blood is started with a standard transfusion set, the filter chamber is filled to allow the total filter to be used. The drip chamber is partially filled with blood to permit counting of the drops. In adjusting the flow rate, it is important to remember that blood administration sets do not use microdrops (60 drops/ml) but regular drops (usually 10 or 15 drops/ml). Therefore, this must be considered when calculating the flow rate. A unit of blood (or the specified amount) should be infused within 4 hours. If the infusion will exceed this time, the blood should be divided into appropriate size quantities by the blood bank and the unused portion refrigerated under controlled conditions.

It is critical for the nurse assisting in this procedure always to be alert for signs that might indicate a reaction. Table 25-3 summarizes the major hazards of transfusions, the signs and symptoms commonly associated with each, and nursing responsibilities. General guidelines that apply to all transfusions include:

1. Take vital signs, including blood pressure, *before* administering blood to establish baseline data for intratransfusion and posttransfusion comparison, then every 15 minutes for 1 hour while blood is infusing
2. Check the identification of the recipient with the donor's blood group and type, regardless of the blood product used
3. Administer the first 50 ml of blood or 1/5 volume (whichever is smaller) *slowly* and stay with the child
4. Administer with normal saline on a piggyback setup
5. Administer blood through an appropriate filter to eliminate particles in the blood and prevent the precipitation of formed elements—gently shake container frequently
6. Use blood within 30 minutes of its arrival from the blood bank; if it is not used, return to blood bank—do not store in regular unit refrigerator
7. If a reaction of any type is suspected, take vital signs, stop the transfusion, maintain a patent intravenous line with normal saline and new tubing, notify the physician, and do not restart the blood until the child's condition has been medically evaluated

While hemolytic reactions are rare, ABO incompatibility remains the most common cause of death from blood transfusion, and human error is usually responsible (administration of wrong type to patient or mislabeling of blood product) (Kasprisin, 1986). Hemolysis can also cause the release of large quantities of phospholipids, which are capable of stimulating disseminated intravascular coagulation (DIC) (p. 837). Acute kidney shutdown and eventual *renal failure* are the result of renal vasoconstriction from antigen-antibody complexes derived from the red cell surface.

Iron administration. There are several considerations in the administration of iron preparations and in the instruction of parents for administration.

An essential nursing responsibility is instructing parents in the administration of iron. It should be given as prescribed in three divided doses between meals, when the presence of free hydrochloric acid is greatest, because more iron is absorbed in the acid environment of the upper gastrointestinal tract. A citrus fruit or juice taken with the medication aids in absorption.

An adequate dosage of oral iron turns the stools a tarry green color. The nurse advises parents of this normally expected change and inquires about its occurrence on follow-up visits. Absence of the greenish black stool may be a clue to poor administration of iron, either in schedule or in dosage. Vomiting and/or diarrhea are not uncommon complications of iron therapy. If the parents report these symptoms, the iron can be given with meals and the dosage reduced, and then gradually increased until tolerated.

Liquid preparations of iron may temporarily stain the teeth. If possible the medication should be taken through a straw or given through a syringe or medicine dropper placed toward the back of the mouth. Brushing the teeth after administration of the drug lessens the discoloration.

When iron dextran is ordered, it must be injected deeply into a large muscle mass using the Z-tract method, and the injection site should *not* be massaged after injection to minimize skin staining and irritation. Since no more than 1 ml should be given in one site, multiple injections are sometimes required.

Diet. A primary nursing objective is to prevent nutritional anemia through parent education. The nurse discusses with parents the importance of using iron-fortified formula and the introduction of solid foods at the appropriate age. The best solid food source of iron is commer-

TABLE 25-3

Nursing Care of the Child Receiving Blood Transfusions

Complication	Signs/Symptoms	Precautions/Nursing Responsibilities
Immediate Reactions		
Hemolytic Reactions—most severe type, but rare Incompatible blood Intradonor incompatibility in multiple transfusions	Chills Shaking Fever Pain at needle site and along venous tract Nausea/vomiting Sensation of tightness in chest Red or black urine Headache Flank pain Progressive signs of shock and/or renal failure	Positively identify donor and recipient blood types and groups before transfusion is begun; verify with one other nurse or physician Transfuse blood slowly for first 15 to 20 minutes and/or initial 1/5 volume of blood; remain with patient In event of signs or symptoms, stop transfusion immediately, maintain patent intravenous line, and notify physician Save donor blood to re-crossmatch with patient's blood Monitor for evidence of shock Insert urinary catheter and monitor hourly outputs Send sample of patient's blood and urine to laboratory for presence of hemoglobin (indicates intravascular hemolysis) Observe for signs of hemorrhage resulting from disseminated intravascular coagulation (DIC) Support medical therapies to reverse shock
Febrile Reactions Leukocyte or platelet antibodies Plasma protein antibodies	Fever Chills	May give acetaminophen for prophylaxis Leukocyte-poor red blood cells are less likely to cause reaction Stop transfusion immediately; report to physician for evaluation
Allergic Reactions—recipient reacts to allergens in donor's blood	Urticaria Flushing Asthmatic wheezing Laryngeal edema	Give antihistamines for prophylaxis to children with tendency toward allergic reactions Stop transfusions immediately Epinephrine for wheezing or anaphylactic reaction
Circulatory Overload Too rapid transfusion (even a small quantity) Excessive quantity of blood transfused (even slowly)	Precordial pain Dyspnea Rales Cyanosis Dry cough Distended neck veins	Transfuse blood slowly Prevent overload by using packed red blood cells or administering divided amounts of blood Use infusion pump to regulate and maintain flow rate If signs of overload, stop transfusion immediately Place child upright with feet in dependent position to increase venous resistance
Air Emboli—may occur when blood is transfused under pressure	Sudden difficulty in breathing Sharp pain in chest Apprehension	When infusing blood under pressure, normalize pressure before container is empty If air is observed in tubing, clamp tubing immediately below air bubble, clear tubing of air by aspirating air with syringe or disconnecting tubing and allowing blood to flow until air has escaped
Hypothermia	Chills Low temperature Irregular heart rate Possible cardiac arrest	Allow blood to warm at room temperature (less than 1 hour) Use an electric warming coil to rapidly warm blood Take temperature if patient complains of chills; if subnormal stop transfusion
Electrolyte Disturbances Hyperkalemia (in massive transfusions or patients with renal problems)	Nausea, diarrhea Muscular weakness Flaccid paralysis Paresthesia of extremities Bradycardia Apprehension Cardiac arrest	Use washed red blood cells or fresh blood if patient at risk
"Citrate" Intoxication (hypocalcemia)	Tingling in fingers Tetany Muscular cramps Carpopedal spasm Hyperactive reflexes Convulsions Laryngeal spasm Respiratory arrest	Infuse blood slowly (citrate reaction less likely to occur) If signs of tetany occur, clamp tubing immediately, maintain patent intravenous line, and notify physician

TABLE 25-3

Nursing Care of the Child Receiving Blood Transfusions—cont'd

Complication	Signs/Symptoms	Precautions/Nursing Responsibilities
Delayed Reactions		
Transmission of Infection Hepatitis AIDS Malaria Syphilis Bacteria or viruses Other	Signs of infection, e.g., jaundice Toxic reaction: high fever, severe headache or substernal pain, hypotension, intense flushing, vomiting/diarrhea	Blood is tested for HB_sAg (hepatitis B), syphilis, and HIV (AIDS); positive units are destroyed. Individuals at risk for carrying certain viruses are deferred from donation Report any sign of infection, and, if occurring during transfusion, stop transfusion immediately, send sample for culture and sensitivity tests, and notify physician
Alloimmunization (antibody formation)	Increased risk of hemolytic, febrile, and allergic reactions	Occurs in patients receiving multiple transfusions Use limited number of donors Observe carefully for signs of reactions
Delayed hemolytic reaction	Destruction of red blood cells and fever 5 to 10 days after transfusion	Observe for posttransfusion anemia and decreasing benefit from successive transfusions

cial infant cereals. It may be difficult at first to teach the infant to accept foods other than milk. The same principles are applied as those for introducing new foods (p. 290), especially feeding the solid food before the milk. Predominantly milk-fed infants rebel against solid foods, and parents are cautioned about this and the need to be firm in not relinquishing control to the child. It may require intense problem solving on the part of both parents and nurse to overcome the child's resistance.

A difficulty encountered in discouraging the parents from feeding milk to the exclusion of other foods is dispelling the popular myth that milk is a "perfect food." Many parents believe that milk is best for the infant and equate the resultant weight gain with a "healthy child." They are not concerned about providing other foods as long as the child continues to take milk. The nurse can also stress that overweight is not synonymous with good health.

Diet education of teenagers is especially difficult, especially when teenage girls are particularly prone to following weight-reduction diets at this time. Emphasizing the effect of anemia on appearance (pallor) and energy level (difficulty maintaining popular activities) may be useful, but adolescents are notoriously adverse to adult counsel.

Prevent complications. The infant or child who is so severely anemic that he requires hospitalization may require oxygen to prevent or reduce tissue hypoxia (see p. 673 for oxygen administration). Since these children are highly susceptible to infection every effort is expended to prevent exposure to infectious agents.

Family support. See Nursing Care Plan on p. 610 for other supportive and educative strategies.

EVALUATION

The effectiveness of nursing interventions is determined by continual reassessment and evaluation of care based on the following observational guidelines and expected outcomes:

1. Monitor therapeutic interventions and interview family regarding adherence to medication and diet
2. Assess child for evidence of infection and/or complications of therapies
3. Interview child and family regarding their feelings and concerns

Expected outcomes:
See Nursing Care Plan on pp. 826 to 827.

SICKLE CELL ANEMIA

Sickle cell anemia is one of a group of diseases collectively termed *hemoglobinopathies,* in which normal adult hemoglobin (hemoglobin A or Hb A) is partly or completely replaced by an abnormal hemoglobin. Sickle cell disease includes all those hereditary disorders, the clinical, hematologic, and pathologic features of which are related to the presence of sickle hemoglobin (Hb S).

The gene that determines the production of Hb S is situated on an autosome and, when present, is always detectable and therefore dominant. Heterozygous persons who have hemoglobin containing both normal Hb A and abnormal Hb S are said to have *sickle cell trait.* Persons who are homozygous have predominantly Hb S and suffer from *sickle cell anemia.* Although the Hb S gene is inherited as autosomal dominant, the inheritance pattern is essentially that of an autosomal recessive disorder (see p. 1083). Therefore, when both parents have sickle cell trait, there is a 25% chance of their producing an offspring with sickle cell anemia.

Sickle cell anemia is observed primarily in blacks, although infrequently it affects Caucasians, especially those of Mediterranean descent. The incidence of the disease varies in different geographic locations. Among American blacks, the incidence of sickle cell trait is about

NURSING CARE PLAN

The Child with Anemia

Nursing Goals	Nursing Interventions	Expected Patient/Family Outcomes
HP-HMP* **Potential for infection** **Risk factors: lowered body defenses**		
Prevent and observe for infection	Place child in room with noninfectious children; restrict visitors with active illnesses Advise visitors (and hospital personnel) to practice good handwashing Report any temperature elevation to physician Observe for leukocytosis Maintain adequate nutrition	Child exhibits no signs of infection
N-MP **Altered nutrition: less than body requirements** **Etiology: reported inadequate iron intake less than RDA**		
Promote adequate intake of iron-rich foods	Take careful diet history to identify deficiencies Provide diet counseling to caregiver; emphasize: Food sources of iron, e.g., meat, liver, fish, green leafy vegetables, legumes, nuts, whole grains Milk is undesirable as entire or predominant food in infant's diet Assist in meal selection	Diet modifications are implemented
A-EP **Activity intolerance** **Etiology: generalized weakness, diminished oxygen delivery to tissues**		
Minimize physical exertion	Assess child's level of physical tolerance Anticipate and assist child in those activities of daily living that may be beyond his tolerance Provide diversional play activities that promote rest and quiet but prevent boredom and withdrawal Choose appropriate roommate of similar age and interests who requires restricted activity Plan nursing activities to provide sufficient rest Assist with activities requiring exertion	Child plays and rests quietly and engages in activities appropriate to his capabilities
Increase oxygen to tissues	Position for optimum air exchange Administer supplemental oxygen if needed	Patient breathes easily; respiratory rate and depth normal (see inside front cover)
Minimize emotional stress	Anticipate child's irritability, short attention span, and fretfulness by offering to assist him in activities rather than waiting for him to ask Assess parents' awareness of child's need for dependency to conserve strength Explain to older children and parents reason for behavioral changes caused by anemia Encourage parents to remain with child	Child remains calm and quiet
RRP **Altered family processes** **Etiology: situational crisis (child in the hospital)**		
Support family	Keep family informed regarding child's progress Explain procedures and precautions related to child's care Encourage expression of feelings and concerns See also The child in the hospital, p. 603	Family demonstrates understanding of information given (specify information and manner of demonstration) Family members verbalize fears and concerns

*For an explanation of abbreviations, see p. 20.

NURSING CARE PLAN

The Child with Anemia—cont'd

Nursing interventions related to medical management

Assist in establishing diagnosis
- Take careful history regarding common causes of anemia in childhood
- Be aware of significance of various blood tests

Improve tissue oxygenation
- Administer oxygen as indicated
- Monitor for benefit of oxygen but avoid prolonged use

Determine cause of anemia
- Assist with diagnostic tests

Iron deficiency anemia

Replace iron
- Administer iron as prescribed
- Instruct family regarding correct administration of oral iron preparation
  - Give in divided doses (specify)
  - Give between meals
  - Administer with fruit juice or multivitamin preparation
  - Do not give with milk, antacids, or tea
- Instruct family to administer liquid preparation with dropper, syringe, or straw to prevent contact with teeth

8%. In West Africa the incidence is reported to be as high as 40% among native blacks. The high incidence of sickle cell trait in these individuals is believed by some to be the result of selective protection afforded trait carriers against one type of malaria.

Of sickle cell diseases, sickle cell anemia is the most common form in black Americans in the United States, followed by sickle cell–hemoglobin C disease. Another beta chain variant, hemoglobin E, is found primarily in people of southeast Asian origin. Persons who carry the trait for hemoglobin E are completely asymptomatic, but those who are homozygous exhibit a disease clinically similar to hemoglobin C disease.

Pathophysiology

The pathologic changes from sickle cell anemia are primarily the result of (1) increased blood viscosity, and (2) increased red blood cell destruction (Fig. 25-1). The entanglement and enmeshing of rigid sickle-shaped cells with one another increases the internal friction of the suspension, thus increasing blood viscosity. The thickened blood slows the circulation, causing capillary stasis, obstruction by elongated and pointed erythrocytes, and thrombosis. The effect of sickling and infarction on organ structures occurs in the following sequence (see also consequences in the box listing clinical manifestations):

1. Stasis with enlargement and engorgement
2. Infarction with ischemia and destruction
3. Replacement with fibrous tissue (scarring)

The most acute symptoms of the disease occur during periods of exacerbation called *sickle cell crises,* which are usually precipitated by infection but can also be triggered by cold, high altitude, or emotional stress. The crisis may be a *vaso-occlusive crisis* (the most frequent variety), characterized by distal ischemia and infarction; *sequestration crisis*, a pooling of blood in liver and spleen with

Clinical Manifestations of Sickle Cell Anemia

General
- Growth retardation
- Chronic anemia (Hb 6.5 to 8 g/dl)
- Delayed sexual maturation
- Marked susceptibility to sepsis

Vaso-occlusive Crisis
- Pain in area(s) of involvement
- Manifestations related to ischemia of involved areas:
  - Extremities: painful swelling of hands and feet (sickle cell dactylitis, or "hand-foot syndrome"), painful joints
  - Abdomen: severe pain resembling acute surgical condition
  - Cerebrum: stroke, visual disturbances
  - Chest: symptoms resemble pneumonia, protracted episodes of pulmonary disease
  - Liver: obstructive jaundice, hepatic coma
  - Kidney: hematuria

Sequestration Crisis
- Pooling of large amounts of blood:
  - Hepatomegaly
  - Splenomegaly
  - Circulatory collapse

Effects of Chronic Vaso-occlusive Phenomena
- Heart: cardiomegaly, systolic murmurs
- Lungs: altered pulmonary function, susceptibility to infections, pulmonary insufficiency
- Kidneys: inability to concentrate urine, progressive renal failure, enuresis
- Genital: priapism (painful constant penile erection)
- Liver: hepatomegaly, cirrhosis, intrahepatic cholestasis
- Spleen: splenomegaly, susceptibility to infection, functional reduction in splenic activity progressing to autosplenectomy
- Eyes: intraocular abnormalities with visual disturbances, sometimes progressive retinal detachment and blindness
- Extremities: skeletal deformities, especially lordosis and kyphosis, chronic leg ulcers, susceptibility to salmonella osteomyelitis
- CNS: hemiparesis, seizures

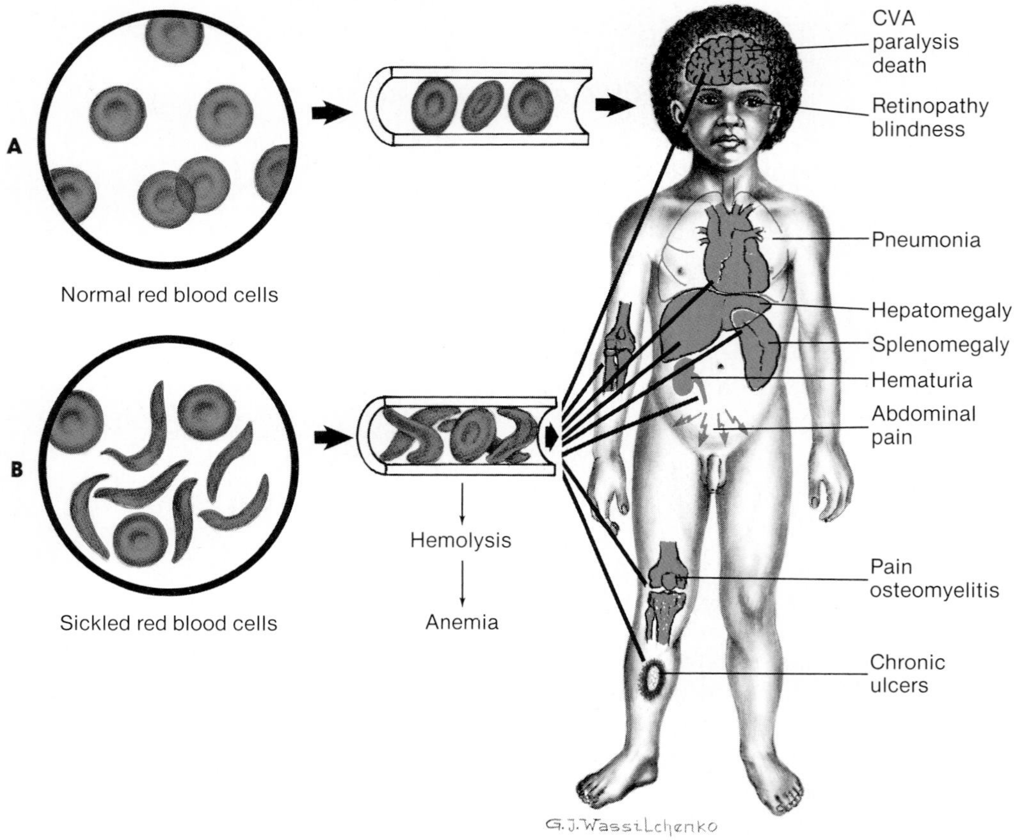

FIG. 25-1 Differences between **A,** normal, and **B,** sickled blood cells on circulation with selected consequences in child with sickling.

decreased blood volume and shock; *aplastic crisis,* diminished red blood cell production resulting in profound anemia; and *hyperhemolytic crisis,* an unusual form that occurs in persons with coincidental G-6-PD deficiency, in which red blood cells are rapidly destroyed.

Diagnostic Evaluation

Although sickle cell anemia has been reported during the neonatal period and early part of infancy, it most commonly is recognized after 4 months of age, when fetal hemoglobin (Hb F) levels are diminished. It is particularly apparent during the toddler and preschool period and is frequently first diagnosed during a crisis that follows acute upper respiratory or gastrointestinal infection. Although growth and maturation are delayed, if the child reaches adulthood, sexual development and adult height are usually achieved (see clinical manifestations in the accompanying box).

Routine hematologic tests are carried out to evaluate the anemia. Several specific tests are used to detect the presence of the abnormal hemoglobin in the heterozygote and/or the homozygote. For screening purposes the sickle-turbidity test (Sickledex) is commonly used, because it can be performed on blood from a fingerstick and yields accurate results in 3 minutes. However, if the test is positive, hemoglobin electrophoresis is necessary to distinguish between those children with the trait and those with the disease. Hemoglobin electrophoresis ("fingerprinting" of the protein) is an accurate, rapid, and specific test for detecting the homozygous and heterozygous forms of the disease, as well as the percentages of the various hemoglobins. Screening for sickle cell trait has become a controversial subject, especially in the black community, since there is no method of preventing the disease other than selective birth procedures.

Therapeutic Management

There is no cure for sickle cell anemia. The aims of therapy are (1) to prevent the sickling phenomenon, which is responsible for the pathologic sequelae, and (2) to treat sickle cell crisis, which constitutes a medical emergency. Prevention consists of promoting adequate oxygenation and maintaining hemodilution. The successful implementation of these two goals depends more often on nursing interventions than on medical therapies.

Medical management of a crisis is usually directed at supportive and symptomatic treatment. The main objectives are to provide (1) bed rest to minimize energy expenditure and oxygen use, (2) hydration through oral and intravenous therapy, (3) electrolyte replacement, (4) analgesics for the severe abdominal and joint pain, (5) blood replacement to treat anemia, and (6) antibiotics to treat any existing infection. Administration of pneumococcal, *Haemophilus influenzae* type B, and meningococcal vaccines is recommended for these children who are over 2 years of age because of their susceptibility to infection as a result of functional asplenia (see p. 293). Oral penicillin prophylaxis by 4 months of age is also recommended (Gaston and others, 1986).

Short-term oxygen therapy may be helpful in severe anoxia, especially in children in cardiac failure. Although oxygen may prevent more sickling, it usually is not effective in reversing sickling, because the oxygen is unable to reach the enmeshed sickled erythrocytes in clogged vessels. In addition, prolonged administration can depress bone marrow, further aggravating the anemia.

Exchange transfusion, which reduces the number of circulating sickle cells and slows down the vicious cycle of hypoxia, thrombosis, tissue ischemia, and injury, has been successful. The procedure is sometimes advocated as a possible preventive technique. However, multiple transfusions carry the risk of hepatitis, hemosiderosis, and transfusion reactions.

In children with recurrent splenic sequestration, splenectomy may be a life-saving measure. However, since the spleen usually atrophies on its own through progressive fibrotic changes, routine splenectomy is not recommended, especially since any procedure that requires anesthesia has increased risk for these children.

Painful priapism may be treated by aspiration of the corpora cavernosum. This complication is particularly frequent in vaso-occlusive crises.

Nursing Considerations

Nursing management of the child with sickle cell anemia is largely related to teaching and supporting the family and providing comfort and pain relief to the child during a sickle cell crisis. The disease is usually first recognized when the child is a toddler, and the lifelong care begins with the diagnosis. This requires awareness of factors that precipitate reactions and active measures to prevent crises.

ASSESSMENT

Many nurses are involved in screening programs for sickle cell anemia to identify persons with the abnormal hemoglobin in order to implement therapy for homozygotes and provide genetic counseling for heterozygotes. Young children from families of at-risk racial or geographic origins who exhibit any of the signs previously described are advised to seek medical attention immediately.

Assessment of the child in sickle cell crisis involves all areas and systems that can be affected by circulatory obstruction, including vital signs, neurologic signs, vision, and hearing assessment, as well as assessment of the respiratory, gastrointestinal, renal, and musculoskeletal systems. It is also important to assess the location and intensity of pain (see p. 587).

Nursing Diagnoses: The Child with Sickle Cell Anemia

Potential for injury related to sickling of red blood cells
Impaired physical mobility related to tissue ischemia, generalized weakness
Potential for infection related to poor tissue oxygenation
Altered family processes related to child with a disabling condition

Sickle Cell Crisis
Pain related to tissue ischemia (sickle cell crisis)
Altered cardiopulmonary tissue perfusion related to impaired arterial blood flow (sickle cell crisis)

NURSING DIAGNOSES

Nursing diagnoses are derived from observation and assessment of children at risk or who demonstrate evidence of sickle cell disease (see box). Others will be apparent depending on the state of the child's health, the organs involved, and the individual needs of the child and family.

PLANNING

The primary nursing goals are to:

1. Educate family and child (when appropriate) regarding the sickling phenomenon and possible consequences
2. Minimize the effects of sickling
3. Encourage genetic counseling
4. Help the child and parents adjust to a lifelong, potentially fatal hereditary disease

IMPLEMENTATION

Many of the measures that prevent sickling are also appropriate when a crisis occurs. In addition, special cautions are mandatory when the child undergoes surgery of any kind. Nurses may also be faced with the dilemmas of sickle cell screening and their role in genetic counseling. Taking time to establish a sound basis of understanding why certain measures are beneficial to the child encourages parents to practice them.

Family education begins with an explanation of the disease and its consequences. To prevent tissue hypoxia the child should avoid situations that cause increased cellular metabolism. This includes (1) strenuous physical activity (especially contact sports if the spleen is enlarged, since rupture will cause massive internal hemorrhage), (2) emotional stress, (3) environments of low oxygen concentration, such as high altitudes or nonpressurized airplane flights, and (4) known sources of infection. If the child has even a mild infection, the parents must seek medical attention at once.

Nursing Tip: Normal and Sickle Cells in Circulation

One simple yet graphic way to demonstrate the effect of sickling is to roll rounded objects, such as marbles or beads, through a tube to simulate normal circulation and then roll pointed objects, such as screws or jacks, through the tube. The effect of sickling and clumping of the pointed objects is especially noticeable at a bend or slight narrowing of the tube.

The nurse emphasizes the importance of adequate hydration to prevent sickling and to delay the stasis–thrombosis–ischemia cycle in a crisis. It is seldom sufficient to advise parents to "force fluids" or "encourage drinking." They need specific instructions on how many glasses or bottles of fluid are required. Many foods are also a source of fluid, particularly soups, gelatin, and puddings. Parents are advised to be particularly alert during situations where dehydration may be a possibility, such as hot weather, and to recognize early signs of reduced intake, such as decreased urine output.

Forced fluids combined with renal diuresis result in the problem of enuresis. Parents who are unaware of this fact frequently employ the usual measures to discourage bed-wetting, such as limiting fluids at night, and many revert to punishment and shame to force bladder control. It is advisable to treat the enuresis as a complication of the disease, such as joint pain or some other symptom, in order to alleviate parental pressure on the child.

Since infection is often a predisposing factor toward a crisis and since the body's natural ability to resist infection is compromised, the nurse stresses to parents the importance of adequate nutrition, immunizations, frequent medical supervision, and isolation from known sources of infection. The last measure must be tempered with an awareness of the child's need for living a normal life.

The need for a surgical procedure poses an additional risk for the child with sickle cell anemia. The main surgical risk is hypoxia from anesthesia. However, emotional stress, the demands of wound healing, and the possibility of infection potentially increase the sickling phenomenon, both in children with the disease and in those with the trait. The primary nursing objectives are aimed at minimizing each of these threats preoperatively and postoperatively.

Promote supportive therapies during crises. The success of many of the medical therapies relies heavily on nursing implementation. Management of pain is an especially difficult problem and often involves experimentation with various analgesics and schedules before relief is achieved (see assessment and management of pain pp. 587 and 597). Heat to the affected area is often soothing. Applying cold compresses to the area is avoided, because this enhances sickling and vasoconstriction.

Bed rest is usually well tolerated during a crisis, although actual rest depends a great deal on pain alleviation and organized schedules of nursing care. Although the object of bed rest is to minimize oxygen consumption, some activity, particularly passive range of motion exercises of non-painful joints, is beneficial to promote circulation. Usually the best course of action is to let the child dictate his positions of comfort and activity tolerance.

Intake, especially intravenous fluids, and output are recorded. The child's admission weight serves as a baseline for evaluating hydration. Vital signs and blood pressure are also closely monitored for impending shock. If blood transfusions or exchange transfusions are administered, the nurse has the responsibility of observing for signs of transfusion reaction. Since hypervolemia from too rapid transfusion can increase the workload of the heart, the nurse also is alert to signs of cardiac failure.

If oxygen is administered, the nurse notes the child's response in terms of decreased pain and improved physical status. However, prolonged oxygen can aggravate the anemia; therefore signs that indicate lack of therapeutic benefit (such as restlessness, increased pallor, and continued pain) are reported.

Provide screening and genetic counseling. Although screening children for sickle cell anemia is generally accepted, since it allows earlier, more prevention-oriented treatment, there is considerable controversy regarding the proposed benefits and potential hazards of screening for the trait. The advantages of trait identification lie in selective reproduction of offspring not afflicted with hemoglobin S. To be effective, screening must be combined with genetic counseling and long-term follow-up. A primary consideration in genetic counseling is informing parents who both carry the trait of the 1-in-4 risk of having a child with the disease (see Appendix B).

Support the family. Families need the opportunity to discuss their feelings regarding transmitting a potentially fatal, chronic illness to their child. Because of the widely publicized prognosis for children with sickle cell anemia, many parents express their prevalent fear of the child's death. Prognosis varies; the greatest risk is usually in children under 5 years of age; the majority of deaths in these children are caused by overwhelming infection. However, as the child grows older, the crises usually become less severe and less frequent. Since there is no way to predict which child will follow a favorable course, nursing care for the family should be the same as for any family with a child with a life-threatening illness. Particular emphasis is placed on the siblings' reactions, the stress on the marital relationship, and the childrearing attitudes displayed toward the child (see Chapter 18). Several resources are available to the family with a sickling disorder.*

*A Sickle Cell Home Study Kit For Families is available from the **National Association for Sickle Cell Disease, Inc.,** 4221 Wilshire Blvd., Los Angeles, CA 90010. Additional resources are **Howard University, Center for Sickle Cell Disease,** 2121 Georgia Ave., N.W., Washington, DC 20059; National Sickle Cell Disease Program, **National Heart, Lung, and Blood Institute,** Bldg 31, Room 4A-21, Rockville Pike, Bethesda, MD 20205, **Canadian Sickle Cell Society,** 1076 Bathurst St., Suite 305, Toronto, Ontario M5R 3G9.

The nurse advises parents to inform all treating personnel of the child's condition. The use of a Medic Alert bracelet is another way of ensuring awareness of the disease. Some people view such identification as "negative labeling." The nurse can stress the positive benefits of displaying this information, especially in emergencies when the use of anesthesia may be required.

EVALUATION

The effectiveness of nursing interventions is determined by continual reassessment and evaluation of care based on the following observational guidelines and expected outcomes:

1. Interview the family regarding their understanding of the disease, the sickling phenomenon, and its consequences
2. Observe the child for any evidence of sickling; monitor preventive strategies and therapies
3. Interview family regarding genetic counseling
4. Interview and observe the child and family regarding the way in which the disease has affected their lives

Expected outcomes:

1. The family demonstrates an understanding of the disease and its consequences (specify knowledge and method of demonstration)
2. Child exhibits few episodes of sickling; pain is effectively controlled
3. Family takes advantage of genetic counseling services
4. Child and family express their feelings and concerns regarding the disease

β-THALASSEMIA (COOLEY ANEMIA)

The term *thalassemia,* which is derived from the Greek word *thalassa,* meaning sea, is applied to a variety of inherited blood disorders characterized by deficiencies in the rate of production of specific globin chains in hemoglobin. The name appropriately refers to descendants of or those people living near the Mediterranean sea who have the highest incidence of the disease, namely, Italians, Greeks, and Syrians. There is evidence to suggest that the high incidence of the disorders among these groups is a result of selective advantage of the trait to malaria, as is postulated in sicklemia.

β-thalassemia is the most common of the thalassemias and occurs in three forms: a heterozygous form, *thalassemia minor* or *thalassemia trait,* which produces a mild microcytic anemia, *thalassemia intermedia,* which manifests as splenomegaly and severe anemia, and a homozygous form, *thalassemia major* (also known as Cooley anemia), which results in an anemia of variable severity that is not compatible with life without transfusion support.

Pathophysiology

Normal postnatal hemoglobin is composed of equal amounts of α- and β-polypeptide chains. In β-thalassemia there is a partial or complete deficiency in the synthesis of the β-chain of the hemoglobin molecule. Consequently, there is a compensatory increase in the synthesis of α-chains, and γ-chain production remains activated, resulting in defective hemoglobin formation. This unbalanced polypeptide unit is very unstable; when it disintegrates it damages the red blood cells, causing severe anemia.

To compensate for the hemolytic process an overabundance of red blood cells is formed. This excessive and largely ineffective erythropoietic activity causes a hyperexpansion of the bone marrow volume that is reflected in skeletal abnormalities of the involved bone. Especially noticeable are those of the frontal, malar, and maxillary bones. Extramedullary hematopoiesis causes enlargement of the liver, spleen, and kidneys. Excess iron from hemolysis of supplemental erythrocytes in transfusions and from the rapid destruction of defective red blood cells is stored in various organs (hemosiderosis).

Diagnostic Evaluation

The onset of thalassemia major is usually insidious and not recognized until the latter half of infancy. The clinical effects of thalassemia major are primarily attributable to (1) defective synthesis of hemoglobin A, (2) structurally impaired red blood cells, and (3) shortened life span of erythrocytes (see box).

Clinical Manifestations of β-Thalassemia

Anemia
Unexplained fever
Poor feeding
Markedly enlarged spleen

Bone Changes (older children)
Enlarged head
Prominent frontal and parietal bosses
Prominent malar eminences
Flat or depressed bridge of the nose
Enlarged maxilla
Protrusion of the lip and upper central incisors and eventual malocclusion
Mongoloid appearance of eyes

Other Features
Small stature
Delayed sexual maturation
Bronzed, freckled complexion
Protrusion of the abdomen (hepatosplenomegaly)

With Progressive Anemia
Signs of chronic hypoxia
- Headache
- Precordial and bone pain
- Decreased exercise tolerance
- Listlessness
- Anorexia

Other Symptoms
Frequent epistaxis
Hyperuricemia and gout
Hemochromatosis
Hemosiderosis

Hematologic studies reveal the characteristic changes in the red blood cells and immature erythrocytes. Low hemoglobin and hematocrit levels are seen in severe anemia, although they are typically lower than the reduction in red blood cell count because of the proliferation of immature erythrocytes. Hemoglobin electrophoresis confirms the diagnosis, and radiographs of involved bones reveal characteristic findings.

Therapeutic Management

There is no specific treatment and no known cure for children with thalassemia major. The objective of supportive therapy is to maintain sufficient hemoglobin levels to prevent tissue hypoxia. A transfusion program to maintain the hemoglobin level at 10.5 g/dl or greater will enable affected children to feel well and engage in most age-appropriate activities. It also decreases cardiomegaly and hepatomegaly, diminishes or prevents development of the bony abnormalities associated with the disease, and seems to improve growth and development.

A potential complication of frequent blood transfusions is iron overload. Because the body has no effective means of eliminating excess iron, the mineral is deposited in body tissues. At the present time there is no completely successful method of preventing excessive iron storage, although the use of the iron-chelating agent deferoxamine (Desferal or DFO), which increases iron excretion, is the current treatment of choice.

In some children with severe splenomegaly who require repeated transfusions, a splenectomy may be necessary to decrease the disabling effects of abdominal pressure and to increase the life span of supplemental red blood cells. A major postsplenectomy complication is severe and overwhelming infection. Therefore, these children are usually kept on prophylactic antibiotics with close medical supervision for many years and are considered candidates for the pneumococcal, meningococcal, and *Haemophilus influenzae* vaccines.

Nursing Considerations

The objectives of nursing care are to (1) observe for complications of multiple blood transfusions, (2) assist the child in coping with the anxiety-provoking treatments and the effects of the illness, and (3) foster the child's and family's adjustment to a life-threatening illness. Basic to each of these goals is explaining to parents and older children the defect responsible for the disorder and its effect on red blood cells. Since the prevalence of this condition is high among families of Mediterranean descent, the nurse also inquires regarding the family's previous knowledge about thalassemia. All families with a child with thalassemia should be tested for the trait and referred for genetic counseling.

The prognosis of thalassemia major is variable and relies heavily on the severity of the anemia. The chief cause of death is heart failure, and, once signs of this complication become evident, death may occur within a year. Unfortunately it is not possible to predict which severely afflicted child will follow a more favorable course. Since many children with the severe form die before puberty and since few survive beyond the third decade, thalassemia is considered a potentially fatal disease.

As with any chronic, life-threatening illness, the needs of the family must be met for optimum adjustment to the stresses imposed by the disorder. These needs are discussed in Chapter 18. Sources of information for the family are the **Cooley's Anemia Foundation*** and the **AHEPA Cooley's Anemia Foundation.**† Genetic counseling for the parents and fertile offspring is mandatory, and both prenatal diagnosis using amniocentesis at 10 weeks of gestation or fetal blood sampling at 20 weeks (Alter, 1985) and screening for thalassemia trait are available.

APLASTIC ANEMIA

Aplastic anemia refers to a condition in which all formed elements of the blood are simultaneously depressed. The peripheral blood smear demonstrates pancytopenia or the triad of profound anemia, leukopenia, and thombocytopenia. *Hypoplastic anemia* is characterized by a profound depression of erythrocytes but normal or slightly decreased white blood cells and platelets.

Etiology

Aplastic anemia can be primary (congenital) or secondary (acquired). The best known congenital disorder of which aplastic anemia is an outstanding feature is *Fanconi syndrome*. The syndrome appears to be inherited as an autosomal-recessive trait with varying penetrance; therefore, affected siblings may demonstrate several different combinations of defects. Prognosis is variable but is better than for acquired types.

Several factors contribute to the development of acquired hypoplastic anemia, including suppressed erythropoiesis from multiple transfusion therapy, hemolytic syndromes, such as sickle cell anemia, infections, toxic substances, drugs, and autoimmune or allergic states. The following discussion, however, focuses on acquired aplastic anemia, which carries a poorer prognosis and follows a more rapidly fatal course than the primary types.

The most common causes of acquired aplastic anemia are (1) irradiation; (2) drugs, such as the chemotherapeutic agents and several antibiotics, most notable of which is chloramphenicol; (3) industrial and household chemicals, including benzene and its derivatives, which are found in petroleum products, dyes, paint remover, shellac, and lacquers; (4) infections, especially hepatitis or overwhelming infection; (5) infiltration and replacement of myeloid elements, such as in leukemia or the

*105 E. 22nd St., New York, NY 10010.
†136-59 39th Ave., Flushing, NY 11354.

lymphomas; and (6) idiopathic causes, in which no identifiable precipitating cause can be found. Prognosis is worse for children in the idiopathic group.

Diagnostic Evaluation

The onset of clinical manifestations, which include anemia, leukopenia, and decreased platelet count, is usually insidious, not unlike that seen in leukemia. Definitive diagnosis is determined from bone marrow aspiration, which demonstrates the conversion of red bone marrow to yellow, fatty bone marrow.

Therapeutic Management

The objectives of treatment are based on the recognition that the underlying disease process is failure of the bone marrow to carry out its hematopoietic functions. Therefore therapy is directed at restoring function to the marrow and involves two main approaches: (1) immunosuppressive therapy to remove the presumed immunologic functions that prolong aplasia, and/or (2) replacement of the bone marrow through transplantation. Bone marrow transplantation is the treatment of choice for severe aplastic anemia when a suitable donor exists.

Two agents have been found to be effective in restoring function to the bone marrow. Currently, antilymphocyte globulin (ALG) or antithymocyte globulin (ATG) is the preferred agent over androgens, which previously constituted the principal treatment for aplastic anemia. The optimum schedule for ATG administration is still under investigation. It is usually given intravenously over 12 to 16 hours, after a test dose to check for hypersensitivity. Subsequent doses are given depending upon the reduction in circulating lymphocytes.

Androgens are ineffective for patients with severe disease but may be given to stimulate erythropoiesis in patients with milder forms of the disease. Although the exact mechanism of erythropoietic action is unclear, testosterone increases production of erythroid elements, converting the fatty, hypocellular bone marrow to one of erythroid hyperplasia. Several testosterone preparations are available. For patients receiving the drug longer than 4 months it may be combined with corticosteroids (usually prednisone) to retard bone maturation stimulated by androgens.

Cyclosporin may be useful in cases refractory to ATG or high doses of corticosteroids and is given in large doses before transplantation to nontransfused patients.

Because of the relatively poor prognosis in aplastic anemia treated with drug therapy, bone marrow transplantation should be considered *early* in the course of the disease if a compatible donor can be found. Transplantation is more successful when performed before multiple transfusions have sensitized the child to leukocyte and HLA antigens. Children who are eligible for transplantation should be transferred to one of the medical centers that specialize in this procedure.

Nursing Considerations

The care of the child with aplastic anemia is similar to that of the child with leukemia (p. 681)—specifically, preparing the child and family for the diagnostic and therapeutic procedures, preventing complications from the severe pancytopenia, and emotionally supporting them in terms of a potentially fatal outcome. Since each of these nursing considerations is discussed in the section on leukemia, only the exceptions are presented here.

The drug ATG is usually administered by way of a central vein. If not, vigilant care must be directed to the intravenous infusion to prevent extravasation. Meticulous care of the venous access is essential because of the child's susceptibility to infection. See p. 670 for care and management of intravenous infusions.

Testosterone produces several undesirable effects that, when combined with the effects of steroid therapy, such as moon face, result in dramatic body image alterations. The virilizing effects of testosterone include deepening of the voice, hirsutism, growth of pubic hair, enlargement of the penis in males, flushing of the skin, and acne. Potentially testosterone can cause muscular and skeletal maturation, resulting in severely retarded height in a young child. Not only are these changes difficult to accept, they are especially difficult to explain to children not approaching puberty. Parents may feel embarrassed because they are unprepared for the sexual changes.

The nurse can help by deemphasizing the sexual nature of the effects and by matter-of-factly explaining each in the same tone as moon face or truncal obesity. Expressing embarrassment or surprise to the child at observing mature sexual characteristics must be avoided. New members of the staff who may be assigned to care for the child need to be prepared for the experience of seeing a sexually mature "6-year-old male with a slight beard and a deep masculine voice."

Since chemotherapeutic agents may be used, many of the reactions, such as nausea and vomiting, alopecia, and painful mucosal ulceration can be encountered. In addition, extensive ecchymotic areas of the oral mucosa that result from thrombocytopenia require meticulous mouth care to prevent breakdown, bleeding, and infection. Local anesthetics are usually not necessary, but anorexia is still a consequence because of the edematous nature of the lesions. Liquid, bland, and soft diets are usually tolerated best (see Feeding the sick child p. 640).

◆ *Defects in Hemostasis*

The body controls excessive bleeding through three processes: (1) vascular spasm, (2) platelet aggregation, and (3) coagulation and clot formation. Defects in platelets and clotting factors are the most common causes of bleeding during childhood. The following discussion focuses on the major conditions that require nursing intervention. The reader is urged to apply these principles to other medical conditions that involve similar nursing considerations.

HEMOPHILIA

The term *hemophilia* refers to a group of bleeding disorders in which there is a deficiency of one of the factors necessary for coagulation of the blood. Although the symptomatology is similar despite the missing factor, the identification of specific factor deficiencies has allowed definitive treatment with replacement agents.

In about 80% of all cases of hemophilia, the inheritance pattern is demonstrated as X-linked recessive (see Appendix B). The two most common forms of the disorder are classic hemophilia (hemophilia A or factor VIII deficiency) and Christmas disease (hemophilia B or factor IX deficiency). The following discussion is primarily concerned with the classic form, which accounts for about 75% of all cases.

Pathophysiology

The basic defect of hemophilia A is a deficiency of factor VIII—antihemophilic factor (AHF) or antihemophilic globulin (AHG). This factor is necessary for the formation of thromboplastin in phase I of blood coagulation. The less antihemophilic globulin found in the blood, the more severe is the disease. The source of the factor in the body is unknown.

Bleeding into tissue can occur anywhere, but hemorrhage into joint cavities is the most frequent type of internal bleeding, often resulting in bone changes and, consequently, crippling, disabling deformities. It is serious if bleeding occurs in the neck, mouth, or thorax, since the airway can become obstructed. Intracranial hemorrhage can result in fatal consequences, although this occurs less frequently than expected because the brain tissue has a high concentration of thromboplastin. Hemorrhage anywhere along the gastrointestinal tract can lead to obstruction, and hematomas in the spinal cord can cause paralysis. Petechiae are uncommon in persons with hemophilia, because repair of small hemorrhages depends on platelet function, not on blood-clotting mechanisms.

Diagnostic Evaluation

Overt, prolonged hemorrhage is readily apparent; bleeding into tissues is less apparent (see box). The diagnosis is usually made on a history of bleeding episodes, evidence of X-linked inheritance (only one third are new mutations), and laboratory findings. The tests specific for hemophilia are those that depend on specific factors for a reaction to occur, such as the partial thromboplastin time test, thromboplastin generation test, and prothrombin consumption test. Specific determination of factor deficiencies requires assay procedures normally performed in specialized laboratories.

Clinical Manifestations of Hemophilia

Prolonged bleeding anywhere from or in the body
Hemorrhage from any trauma—loss of deciduous teeth, circumcision, cuts, epistaxis, injections
Excessive bruising—even from a slight injury, such as a fall
Subcutaneous and intramuscular hemorrhages
Hemarthrosis (bleeding into the joint cavities), especially the knees, ankles, and elbows
Hematomas—pain, swelling, and limited motion
Spontaneous hematuria

Therapeutic Management

The primary therapy for hemophilia is to prevent spontaneous bleeding by replacement of the missing factor VIII, The products currently available are (1) *factor VIII concentrate,* to be reconstituted with sterile water immediately before use, (2) *cryoprecipitate,* a concentrated form of AHF plus fibrinogen, and (3) *fresh frozen plasma,* which contains all coagulation factors. Current treatment of blood products has virtually eliminated the risk of contracting blood-borne infections, such as hepatitis B (p. 760) and acquired immuno-deficiency syndrome (p. 851), to children newly diagnosed with the disease.

Vigorous therapy is instituted to prevent chronic crippling effects from joint bleeding. If replacement therapy is begun immediately, local measures such as ice applications and splinting are seldom needed.

Other drugs may be included in the therapy plan, depending on the source of the hemorrhage. Corticosteroids are administered to reduce inflammation in the joints; nonsteroidal antiinflammatory agents, such as aspirin, indomethacin (Indocin), and phenylbutazone (Butazolidin), should not be used because they inhibit platelet function. Ibuprofen (Motrin, Advil, or Nuprin) has been demonstrated to be safe despite its antiplatelet aggregation effect (Karayalcin, 1985). Local application of epsilon aminocaproic acid (Amicar) prevents clot destruction; however, its use is limited to mouth or trauma surgery.

A regular program of exercise and physical therapy is an important aspect of management. Physical activity, within reasonable limits, strengthens muscles around joints, which will help retard or confine bleeding in the area.

Treatment without delay results in more rapid recovery and a decreased likelihood of complications; therefore, most children are treated at home. The family is taught the technique of venipuncture and to administer the AHF to children over 3 years of age. The child himself learns the procedure for self-administration at 9 to 12 years of age. Home treatment is highly successful and the rewards, in addition to the immediacy, are less disruption of family life, fewer school or work days missed, and enhancement of the child's self-esteem.

Nursing Considerations

Hemophilia is a lifelong health problem; therefore the major emphasis of care is related to patient management of the disorder and genetic counseling of the patient and family.

ASSESSMENT

The earlier a bleeding episode is recognized, the more effectively it can be treated. Signs that indicate internal bleeding are especially important to recognize. Children are aware of internal bleeding and are very reliable in telling the examiner where an internal bleed is. In addition to the manifestations described (see box), the nurse maintains a high level of suspicion when a child with hemophilia demonstrates unlikely signs, such as headache, slurred speech, loss of consciousness (from cerebral bleeding), and black tarry stools (from gastrointestinal bleeding).

NURSING DIAGNOSES

Nursing diagnoses for the child with hemophilia include but are not limited to the diagnoses listed in the accompanying box.

PLANNING

The objectives for nursing care can be divided into immediate needs and long-term goals:

1. Prevent and control bleeding episodes
2. Prevent crippling effects of bleeding
3. Provide support and education to the child and family
4. Identify persons at risk

IMPLEMENTATION

Since hemophilia is a lifelong health problem, the ultimate adjustment and prognosis for the child rely heavily on the child's family's ability to cope with the disorder, to learn effective methods of control and prevention, and to temper childrearing practices with judicious protection from injury while fostering independence and development.

Prevent bleeding. The goals of prevention of bleeding episodes are directed toward decreasing the risk of injury and prophylactic administration of clotting factors. Prevention of bleeding through control of behavior is no easy task. During infancy and toddlerhood the normal acquisition of motor skills creates innumerable opportunities for falls, bruises, and minor wounds. Restraining the child from mastering motor development can herald more serious long-term problems than allowing the behavior. However, the environment can be made as safe as possible to minimize the incidental injuries, with close supervision maintained during playtime.

For older children the family usually needs assistance in preparing for school. A nurse who knows the family can be instrumental in discussing the situation with the school nurse and in jointly planning an appropriate schedule of activity. Since almost all persons with hemophilia are boys, the physical limitations in regard to active sports are a difficult adjustment, and activity restrictions must be tempered with sensitivity to the child's emotional as well as physical needs. Use of protective equipment is particularly important, and noncontact sports, especially swimming, should be encouraged.

To prevent oral bleeding, some readjustment in terms of dental hygiene may be needed to minimize trauma to the gums. For example, the nurse can recommend the use of a water irrigating device, softening the toothbrush in warm water before brushing, or using a sponge-tipped disposable toothbrush available in many drugstores. A regular toothbrush should be soft bristled and small in size. Adolescents also need to be advised of the dangers of shaving with razor blades and encouraged to use an electric shaver.

Since any trauma can lead to a bleeding episode, all persons caring for these children must be aware of their disorder. These children should wear Medic Alert identification, and older children should be encouraged to recognize situations in which disclosing their condition is important, such as dental extraction or injections. Health personnel need to take special precautions to prevent the use of procedures such as intramuscular injections or venipunctures. A peripheral fingerstick is better for blood samples, and the subcutaneous route is substituted for intramuscular injections whenever possible. Neither aspirin nor any aspirin-containing compound should be used. Acetaminophen (Tylenol) is a suitable aspirin substitute, especially for use during control of pain at home. Another common drug that should not be used is glyceryl guaiacolate (guaifenesin), an expectorant found in several over-the-counter cough preparations.

The nurse, who is skilled in venipuncture techniques, is often the person who teaches families to administer AHF concentrates. The nurse must be familiar with the properties of concentrates and their preparation. For example, in reconstituting dried antihemophilic factor with diluent, the process can be hastened by warming the solution or gently rotating the vial. However, excessive heat or shaking will result in loss of the active factor.

Recognize and control bleeding. The earlier a bleeding episode is recognized, the more effectively it can be

---

Nursing Diagnoses: The Child with Hemophilia

- Potential for trauma to tissues
- Pain related to bleeding into tissues
- Impaired physical mobility related to hemorrhages into joints and other tissues
- Altered family processes related to child with a potentially disabling disease

---

treated. Factor replacement therapy should be instituted according to established medical protocol and supportive measures may be implemented, such as (1) applying pressure to the area for at least 10 to 15 minutes to allow clot formation, (2) immobilizing and elevating the area above the level of the heart to decrease blood flow, and (3) applying cold to promote vasoconstriction. When parents and older children are taught such measures beforehand, they can be prepared to initiate immediate treatment before blood loss is excessive. Plastic bags of ice or Cryogel* cold packs should be kept in the freezer for such emergencies. However, such measures should not take the place of factor replacement.

Prevent crippling effects of bleeding. From repeated hemarthrosis, incompletely absorbed blood in the joints, and limitation of motion, bone and muscle changes occur that result in flexion contractures and joint fixation. During bleeding episodes the joint is elevated and immobilized. Passive range of motion exercises are usually instituted after the acute phase. If an exercise program is instituted in the home, a physical therapist or public health nurse may need to supervise compliance with the regimen. Diet is also an important consideration, since excessive body weight can increase the strain on affected joints, especially the knees, and predispose to hemarthrosis. Consequently, calories need to be supplied in accordance with energy requirements.

Support family and educate for home care. The discovery of factor concentrates has greatly changed the outlook for these children. With scheduled infusions of the missing factor, bleeding can be prevented, and the child can live a much more normal, unrestricted life.

Constructive teaching about the disease and measures to control or prevent bleeding must follow a period of parental adjustment to the diagnosis (see Chapter 18 for suggestions for dealing with the parents of a child with chronic illness). Children are taught to take responsibility for their disease at an early age. They learn their limitations and other preventive measures, then self-administration of the prophylactic antihemophilic factor.

The needs of families who have children with hemophilia are best met through a comprehensive team approach of physicians (pediatrician, hematologist, orthopedist), nurse, social worker, and physical therapist. Parent-group discussions are beneficial in meeting those needs often best met by similarly affected families. For example, with the improved prognosis for these children, parents and adolescents with hemophilia are faced with vocational and financial problems, in addition to concern over future childbearing. Once children reach 21 years of age, many insurance companies no longer wish to carry them. This can be disastrous in terms of the cost of treatment. A person with severe hemophilia may require factor replacement therapy and other medical treatments in excess of $10,000 a year. The **National Hemophilia Foundation*** and the **Canadian Hemophilia Society**† provide numerous services and publications for both health providers and families.

The threat of acquired immune deficiency disease (AIDS) is a constant concern of children receiving blood products. Those children who have contracted the disease through transfusions and factor replacement products are faced with the consequences of this dreaded disease. Consequently they need the support of health professionals, especially in the area of public education, regarding the disease and ways to deal with public reactions to persons who have the disease (see p. 851 for a discussion of AIDS).

Identify persons at risk. Genetic counseling is essential as soon as possible after diagnosis. Unlike many other disorders in which both parents carry the trait, the feeling of responsibility for this condition usually rests with the mother. Without an opportunity to discuss her feelings, the marital relationship can suffer. Technology is now available to identify carriers in approximately 80% of cases and may reduce the anxiety regarding childbearing in females who may be at risk of carrying the defective gene, such as sisters or maternal aunts of an affected male.

EVALUATION

The effectiveness of nursing interventions is determined by continual reassessment and evaluation of care based on the following observational guidelines and expected outcomes:

1. Interview the child and family regarding preventive measures implemented and any bleeding episodes the child suffers
2. Reassess the child for evidence of tissue damage from bleeding
3. Observe and interview the family regarding treatments and schedule of prophylactic administration of antihemophilic factor
4. Interview the family and/or consult the genetic counseling service regarding the carrier status of other members of the family

Expected outcomes:

1. The child exhibits no evidence of bleeding
2. The child exhibits no evidence of tissue damage
3. The child and family discuss their feelings and concerns and demonstrate an understanding of the disease and its therapy (specify knowledge and method of demonstration)
4. The family seeks genetic counseling

THROMBOCYTOPENIC PURPURA

Idiopathic thrombocytopenic purpura (ITP) is an acquired hemorrhagic disorder that is characterized by (1) excessive destruction of platelets (thrombocytopenia),

*Manufactured by 3M Co., Medical Products Division, St. Paul, MN

*Soho Bldg, Rm 406, 110 Green St., New York, NY 10012.
†100 King St. West, Suite 210, Hamilton, Ont. L8P 1A2.

Clinical Manifestations of Idiopathic Thrombocytopenic Purpura

- Easy bruising
  - Petechiae
  - Ecchymoses
  - Most commonly over bony prominences
- Bleeding from mucous membranes
  - Epistaxis
  - Bleeding gums
  - Internal hemorrhage evidenced by:
    - Hematuria
    - Hematemesis
    - Melena
    - Hemarthrosis
    - Menorrhagia
- Hematomas over lower extremities

and (2) purpura (a discoloration caused by petechiae beneath the skin). Although the cause is unknown, it is believed to be an autoimmune response to disease-related antigens. It is the most frequently occurring thrombocytopenia of childhood.

The disease occurs in one of two forms: an acute, self-limiting course or a chronic condition interspersed with remissions. The acute form is most commonly seen after upper respiratory infections or after the childhood diseases measles, rubella, mumps, and chickenpox.

Diagnostic Evaluation

The diagnosis is suspected on the basis of clinical manifestations (see box). In ITP the platelet count is reduced to below 20,000 mm^3; therefore tests that depend on platelet function are abnormal, such as the tourniquet test, bleeding time, and clot retraction. Although there is no definitive test on which to establish a diagnosis of ITP, several tests are usually performed to rule out other disorders in which thrombocytopenia is a manifestation, such as systemic lupus erythematosus, lymphoma, or leukemia.

Therapeutic Management

Management is primarily supportive, since the course of the disease is self-limited in the majority of cases. Activity is restricted at the onset while the platelet count is low and while active bleeding or progression of lesions is occurring. This restriction is most easily accomplished in the hospital. Corticosteroids are employed for children with the highest risk for serious bleeding, for chronic cases with increased bleeding tendencies, as an adjunct to life-threatening hemorrhage, or before splenectomy to decrease the risk of surgical bleeding. Administration of intravenous gammaglobulin has proved successful in increasing the platelet count of children with chronic disease. Splenectomy is reserved for symptomatic children with chronic disease or as an emergency measure in the event of life-threatening hemorrhage. Packed red blood cells may be given to replace blood lost in symptomatic children. Platelets are seldom administered.

Nursing Considerations

Nursing care is largely supportive. Children and parents need careful explanations of the rationale behind the therapies employed and support in their efforts to comply. The nursing considerations of controlling bleeding, preventing bruising, and preventing crippling effects of hemarthrosis are similar to those discussed in the section on hemophilia. The deleterious effects of using aspirin to control joint pain are critical for these children; therefore, salicylate substitutes should always be used.

DISSEMINATED INTRAVASCULAR COAGULATION

Disseminated intravascular coagulation (DIC), also known as *consumption coagulopathy,* is not a primary disease. It is a secondary disorder of coagulation that complicates a number of pathologic processes (such as hypoxia, acidosis, shock, and endothelial damage) and many severe systemic disease states (such as congenital heart disease, necrotizing enterocolitis, gram-negative bacterial sepsis, rickettsial infections, and some severe viral infections). The disease is characterized by inappropriate systemic activation and acceleration of the normal clotting mechanism.

Pathophysiology

Disseminated intravascular coagulation occurs when the first stage of the coagulation process is abnormally stimulated. Although there is no well-defined sequence of events, two distinct phases can be identified. First, when the clotting mechanism is triggered in the circulation, thrombin is generated in greater amounts than can be neutralized by the body. Consequently, there is rapid conversion of fibrinogen to fibrin with aggregation and destruction of platelets. If local and widespread fibrin deposition in blood vessels takes place, obstruction and eventual necrosis of tissues occur. Second, the fibrinolytic mechanism is activated, causing extensive destruction of clotting factors. With a deficiency of clotting factors the child is vulnerable to uncontrollable hemorrhage into vital organs. An additional complication is damage and hemolysis of red blood cells (Fig. 25-2).

Diagnostic Evaluation

DIC is suspected when there is an increased tendency to bleed (see box). Hematologic findings include prolonged prothrombin (PT), partial thromboplastin (PTT), and thrombin times. There is a profoundly depressed platelet

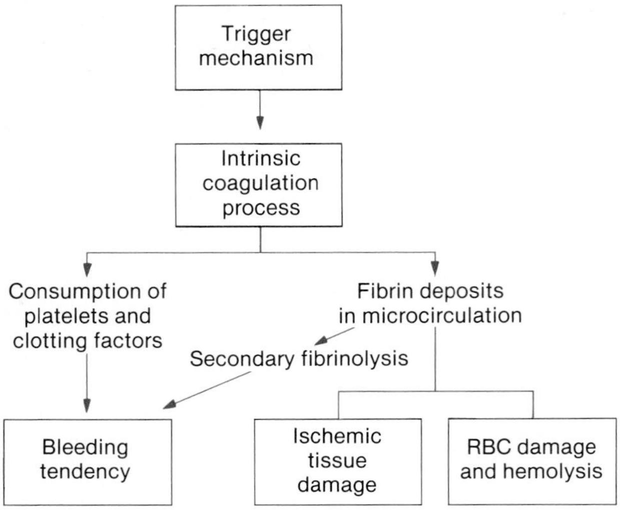

FIG. 25-2 Effects of disseminated intravascular coagulation.

count, fragmented red blood cells, and depleted fibrinogen.

Therapeutic Management

Treatment of DIC is directed toward control of the underlying or initiating cause, which, in most instances, stops the coagulation problem spontaneously. Platelets and fresh frozen plasma may be needed to replace lost plasma components, especially in the child whose underlying disease remains uncontrolled. The extremely ill newborn infant may require exchange transfusion with fresh blood. The administration of heparin to inhibit thrombin formation is most often restricted to severe cases.

Nursing Considerations

The goals of nursing care are to be aware of the possibility of DIC in the severely ill child and to recognize signs that might indicate its presence. The skills needed to monitor intravenous infusion and blood transfusions and to administer heparin are the same as for any child receiving these therapies (see p. 670). See Chapter 18 for care of the child with a life-threatening illness.

EPISTAXIS (NOSEBLEEDING)

Isolated and transient episodes of epistaxis, or nosebleeding, are common in childhood. The nose, especially the septum, is a highly vascular structure, and bleeding usually results from direct trauma, including blows to the nose, foreign bodies, and nose picking, or from mucosal inflammation associated with allergic rhinitis and upper respiratory infections. The bleeding ordinarily stops spontaneously or with minimum pressure and requires no medical evaluation or therapy.

Recurrent epistaxis and severe bleeding may indicate an underlying disease, particularly vascular abnormalities, leukemia, thrombocytopenia, and clotting factor deficiency diseases, such as hemophilia and von Willebrand disease. Nosebleeds are sometimes associated with administration of aspirin, even in normal amounts. Persistent episodes of epistaxis require medical evaluation.

Clinical Manifestations of Disseminated Intravascular Coagulation

Petechiae
Purpura
Bleeding from openings in the skin
- Venipuncture site
- Surgical incision

Bleeding from umbilicus, trachea (newborn)
Evidence of gastrointestinal bleeding
Hypotension
Organ dysfunction from infarction and ischemia

Nursing Considerations

In the event of a nosebleed, the foremost intervention is to remain calm. Otherwise the child becomes more agitated, his blood pressure will increase, and he will not cooperate. To control the bleeding the child is instructed to sit up and lean forward (not to lie down) to avoid aspiration of blood. Most of the nosebleeding originates in the anterior part of the nasal septum and can be controlled by applying pressure to the soft lower portion of the nose with the thumb and forefinger (see Emergency box). During this time the child breathes through his mouth.

In the event that hemorrhage continues, the child should be evaluated by a physician, who may pack the nose with epinephrine-soaked gauze. After a nosebleed, petroleum or water-soluble jelly can be inserted into each nostril to prevent crusting of old blood and to lessen the likelihood of the child's picking at his nose and restarting the hemorrhage. If a child has numerous nosebleeds, factors believed to increase the likelihood of bleeds are eliminated, such as discouraging nose picking or altering the household humidity by placing a cool-mist humidifier in the child's room. Repeated bleeding episodes may be an indication to refer the child for evaluation for the possibility of a bleeding disorder.

◆ *Neoplastic Disorders*

Neoplastic disorders are the leading cause of death from disease in children past infancy, and almost half of all childhood cancer involves the blood or blood-forming organs. Problems related to the various solid tumors of childhood are discussed elsewhere in relation to the tissues or organs involved.

The leukemias are neoplastic diseases of the blood-forming tissues; the lymphomas are a group of neoplastic diseases that arise from the lymphoid and reticuloendothelial system. Lymphomas are more common in males than in females and are usually divided into the Hodgkin and non-Hodgkin lymphomas. This discussion is concerned with the leukemias and the lymphomas.

LEUKEMIAS

Leukemia, cancer of the blood-forming tissues, is the most common form of childhood cancer. It occurs more frequently in males than females after age 1 year, and the peak onset is between 2 and 5 years of age. It is one of the forms of cancer that has demonstrated dramatic improvements in survival rates. Before the use of antileukemic agents in 1948, a child with acute lymphocytic leukemia (ALL) lived only 2 to 3 months. Current 5-year survival rates for children with ALL exceed 50% in major research centers, and a proportion of these children may be cured (Pizzo, 1987).

Classification

Leukemia is the broad term applied to a complex and heterogenous group of malignant diseases of the bone marrow and lymphatic system. Classification of the leukemias is necessary for therapeutic and prognostic purposes and is based on the morphologic (structural), cytochemical, and immunologic characteristics of the cells.

Morphology. Leukemia is classified according to its predominant cell type and level of maturity as follows:

Lympho indicates leukemias involving the lymphoid or lymphatic system
Myelo indicates those leukemias of myeloid (bone marrow) origin
Blastic and acute indicate those leukemias involving immature cells
Cytic and chronic indicate those leukemias involving mature cells

In children two forms of leukemia are generally recognized: (1) *acute lymphoid leukemia (ALL),* and (2) *acute nonlymphoid leukemia (ANLL).* Synonyms for ALL include acute lymphatic, lymphocytic, lymphoblastic, and lymphoblastoid leukemia. The term *stem cell* or *blast cell* usually refers to the lymphoid type of leukemia. Synonyms for ANLL include myelogenous (AML), myelocytic, monocytic, monoblastic, monomyeloblastic, and acute granulocytic leukemia.

Because of the confusion and inconsistency in classifying the leukemias, ALL and ANLL are further subdivided after thorough study of the cell morphology. They are also classified according to whether or not they contain cell elements. These more definitive classifications are significant for purposes of prognosis but will not be discussed here.

Cytochemical. Leukemic cells also demonstrate different reactions when they are exposed to certain chemicals.

Immunology. A number of cell-surface antigens allow for differentiation of ALL into three broad categories: T-lymphocytes (T-cells), B-lymphocytes (B-cells), or "null" cells (those cells that lack T- or B-cell characteristics). This further classification of lymphocytic leukemia appears to have prognostic importance in that persons with leukemias of the "null" category (about 85% of ALL) demonstrate better survival rates.

EMERGENCY TREATMENT

Epistaxis

1. Have child sit up and lean forward (not lying down)
2. Apply continuous pressure to nose with thumb and forefinger for at least 10 minutes
3. Insert cotton or wadded tissue into each nostril and apply ice or cold cloth to bridge of nose if bleeding persists
4. Keep child calm and quiet

Pathophysiology

Leukemia is an unrestricted proliferation of immature white blood cells in the blood-forming tissues of the body. Although not a "tumor" as such, the leukemic cells demonstrate the same neoplastic properties of solid cancers. Therefore, the resulting pathology and clinical manifestations are caused by infiltration and replacement of any tissue of the body with nonfunctional leukemic cells. Highly vascular organs of the reticuloendothelial system are most severely affected.

In order to understand the pathophysiology of the leukemic process, it is important to clarify two common misconceptions. First, although leukemia is an overproduction of white blood cells, most often in the acute form the leukocyte count is low (hence, the term *leukemia*). Second, these immature cells do not deliberately attack and destroy the normal blood cells or vascular tissues. Cellular destruction takes place by infiltration and subsequent competition for metabolic elements (Table 25-4).

In all types of leukemia the proliferating cells depress the production of formed elements of the blood in bone marrow by competing for and depriving the normal cells of the essential nutrients for metabolism. The invasion of the bone marrow with leukemic cells gradually causes a weakening of the bone and a tendency toward physiologic fractures. The most frequent presenting signs and symptoms of leukemia are a result of infiltration of the bone marrow. As leukemic cells invade the periosteum, increasing pressure causes severe pain.

The organs of the reticuloendothelial system—the spleen, liver, and lymph glands—demonstrate marked infiltration, enlargement, and eventually fibrosis. Hepatosplenomegaly is typically more severe than lymphadenopathy. Toxic chemotherapeutic agents seem to account for more liver and spleen damage than the disease process.

The next most important site of involvement is the

TABLE 25-4

Pathology and Related Clinical Manifestations of Leukemia

Organ or Tissue	Consequences	Manifestations
Bone marrow dysfunction	Decreased RBC—anemia	Pallor, fatigue
	Neutropenia—infection	Fever
	Decreased platelets—bleeding tendencies	Hemorrhage (petechiae)
	Invasion of bone marrow—bone weakness; invasion of periosteum	Tendency to fractures Pain
Reticuloendothelial system:		
Liver Spleen Lymph glands	Infiltration, enlargement, eventual fibrosis	Hepatomegaly Splenomegaly Lymphadenopathy
CNS		
Meninges	Increased intracranial pressure, ventricular enlargement	Severe headache Vomiting Irritability, lethargy Papilledema Eventual coma
	Meningeal irritation	Pain Stiff neck and back
Hypermetabolism	Cell deprivation of nutrients by invading cells	Muscle wasting Weight loss Anorexia Fatigue

central nervous system. Initially leukemic cells do not tend to invade this area, probably as a result of the protective blood-brain barrier. However, this normal protective mechanism also prevents the antileukemic drugs, with the exception of steroids, from entering the brain in sufficient therapeutic doses to be effective. The usual effect of leukemic infiltration is increased intracranial pressure, which causes the signs and symptoms normally associated with this condition. Cranial nerves may be involved also, and the signs and symptoms observed reflect the area affected (see p. 170).

Other sites of involvement in long-term disease include the kidneys, testes, prostate, ovaries, gastrointestinal tract, and lungs. With the increased length of survival becoming more common, such sites of leukemic invasion are becoming more important clinically.

The immense metabolic needs of proliferating leukemic cells eventually deprive all body cells of nutrients necessary for survival. Obviously, in addition to the risk of death from infection and hemorrhage, uncontrolled growth of leukemic cells can also terminate in metabolic starvation.

Diagnostic Evaluation

Leukemia is usually suspected by the history, physical manifestations (Table 25-4), and a peripheral blood smear that contains immature forms of leukocytes, frequently combined with low blood counts. Definitive diagnosis is based on bone marrow aspiration or biopsy. Typically the bone marrow is hypercellular, with primarily blast cells. Once the diagnosis is confirmed, a lumbar puncture is performed to determine if there is any central nervous system involvement, although a very small number of children have CNS involvement, and most are asymptomatic.

Therapeutic Management

Treatment of leukemia involves the use of chemotherapeutic agents and irradiation in three phases: (1) *remission induction therapy,* which is determined by absence of clinical evidence of disease and presence of less than 5% blast cells in the bone marrow; (2) *sanctuary therapy*, which prevents leukemic cells from invading or destroying leukemic cells in those areas of the body normally protected from cytotoxic drug levels; and (3) *maintenance therapy,* which serves to maintain the remission phase. Although the combination of drugs and radiation may vary according to institutions and the type of leukemia being treated, the following general principles for each phase are quite consistently employed.

Remission induction. Almost immediately after confirmation of the diagnosis, induction therapy is begun and lasts 4 to 6 weeks. The principal drugs used for induction in ALL are corticosteroids (especially prednisone), intravenous vincristine, and Å-asparaginase, with or without doxorubicin. Drug therapy for AML includes doxorubicin or daunomycin and cytosine arabinoside.

Since many of the drugs also cause suppression of some blood elements, the period immediately following a remission can be critical; the body is defenseless against invading organisms (especially normal bacterial flora) and highly susceptible to spontaneous hemorrhage. Consequently, supportive therapy during this time is essential.

Sanctuary therapy. Sanctuary therapy refers to treatment directed at those anatomic areas that are protected to some degree from systemic chemotherapy—the central nervous system (protected by the blood-brain barrier) and the testes (which lie outside the body). Therapy consists of prophylactic treatment with cranial irradiation and/or intrathecal administration of methotrexate (CNS) and chemotherapy (testes). Therapy is usually begun during the first 6 to 8 weeks after diagnosis and is continued for a specified time period.

Maintenance therapy. Maintenance or continuation therapy is begun after completion of successful induction and sanctuary therapy to preserve the remission and further lessen the number of leukemic cells. It begins when blood values start to approach normal levels. As with induction therapy, combined drug regimens have been more successful in maintaining remissions and preventing drug resistance. Also, during maintenance therapy weekly or monthly complete blood counts are taken to evaluate the marrow's response to the drugs.

Reinduction therapy. For many children a fourth phase of therapy becomes necessary when a relapse occurs, as evidenced by the observed presence of leukemic cells within the bone marrow. Usually reinduction includes the use of prednisone and vincristine with a combination of other drugs not previously used. Sanctuary and maintenance therapy follow as outlined before if a remission is induced.

Bone marrow transplant. Bone marrow transplants have been used successfully for treating children who have ALL and ANLL. Bone marrow transplantation is not recommended for children with ALL during the first remission because of the excellent results possible with chemotherapy. Because of the poorer prognosis in children with ANLL, transplantation may be considered during the first remission (Grier and Weinstein, 1985).

Prognosis

The most important prognostic factors for determining long-term survival for children with ALL (in addition to treatment) are (1) the initial white blood count (WBC), (2) the child's age at the time of diagnosis, (3) the type of cell involved, (4) the sex of the child, and (5) karyotype analysis. Children with normal or low white blood count appear to have a much better prognosis than those with a high count. Children diagnosed between 2 and 9 years of age have consistently demonstrated a better outlook than those diagnosed before 2 or after 10 years of age, and females appear to have a more favorable prognosis than males. The presence of chromosome translocations, found in 40% of ALL cases, is associated with treatment failure. In addition, it appears that the more rapid the induction of a remission in ANLL, the better is the chance for an ultimate long-term continuous remission.

Nursing Considerations

Nursing care of the child with leukemia is directly related to the regimen of therapy. Secondary complications that necessitate supportive physical care are caused by myelosuppression, drug toxicity, and leukemic infiltration. Although this discussion is primarily concerned with the physical problems requiring nursing care, it also focuses on the specific emotional needs during diagnosis, treatment, and relapse. The general psychologic interventions during each phase of therapy are discussed in Chapter 18.

ASSESSMENT

The history and physical examination often yield the first clues to the presence of neoplastic disease. Vague complaints, such as fatigue, pain in a limb, night sweating, lack of appetite, headache, and general malaise, may be the earliest clues and need to be taken seriously. Most children have a great deal of energy and if sick with a cold or other childhood affliction recover quickly and completely. Any evidence of a lingering disorder is often the first sign of leukemia.

NURSING DIAGNOSES

A number of nursing diagnoses become apparent following an assessment of the child with leukemia and his family. Some are considered in the Nursing Care Plan on p. 844. Others will be identified in specific situations.

PLANNING

The goals of nursing care of the child with leukemia and his family include:

1. Prepare the child and family for diagnostic and therapeutic procedures
2. Relieve pain
3. Prevent complications of myelosuppression
4. Manage problems of irradiation and drug toxicity
5. Provide continued emotional support to child and family

IMPLEMENTATION

Nursing care of the child with leukemia is directly related to the regimen of therapy. Nurses working with families of children with cancer have a significant supportive role in helping them understand the various therapies, preventing or managing expected side effects or toxicities, observing for late effects of treatment, and helping the child and family live as normal a life as possible and cope with the emotional aspects of the disease. Education is a constant feature of the nursing role, especially in terms of new treatments, clinical trials, and home care.

Because of the anxiety generated by the diagnosis of leukemia, some families may resort to unproven methods of therapy that are frequently referred to as "cancer quackery." These unorthodox approaches are a threat to every cancer family. Nurses can be instrumental in working against cancer quackery by being aware of factors that increase a family's likelihood of seeking unproven remedies, communicating effectively with families about the diagnosis and forms of therapy, and providing all possible support and reassurance during treatment.

Prepare family for diagnostic and therapeutic procedures. From the time before diagnosis to cessation of therapy, children must undergo several tests, the most traumatic of which are bone marrow aspiration or biopsy and lumbar punctures. Multiple fingersticks and venipunctures for blood analysis and drug infusion are common occurrences for several years after the diagnosis. Therefore, the child needs an explanation of why each procedure is done and what can be expected. In addition effective pharmacologic and non-pharmacologic strategies are used to reduce discomfort associated with these painful procedures (see p. 597).

Relieve pain. The effective use of analgesia is especially important when the malignant process is uncontrolled and causes pain. Bone pain is particularly acute. Dosages of narcotics *titrated to the child's needs* should be administered *around the clock* for optimum pain control. Nonpharmacologic strategies should be implemented as needed but should not be regarded as substitutes for pharmacologic management. The reader is encouraged to review the principles of pain assessment and management presented in Chapter 20 when caring for a child with leukemia.

Prevent complications of myelosuppression. The leukemic process and most of the chemotherapeutic agents cause myelosuppression. The reduced numbers of blood cells result in secondary problems of infection, bleeding tendencies, and anemia. Supportive care involves both medical and nursing management. Because they are so closely linked, they are discussed together rather than separately.

Infection. The most frequent cause of death from leukemia is overwhelming infection. The child is most susceptible to overwhelming infection during three phases of his disease: (1) at the time of diagnosis and relapse when the leukemic process has replaced normal leukocytes, (2) during immunosuppressive therapy, and (3) after prolonged antibiotic therapy that predisposes to the growth of resistant organisms.

Because the usual viral infections of childhood are particularly dangerous, the child is *not* immunized against these diseases (measles, rubella, mumps, and polio) until his immune system is capable of responding appropriately to the vaccine. If given when the immune system is depressed, the attenuated virus can result in an overwhelming infection. Exceptions are the use of Salk (inactivated) vaccine for poliomyelitis and the newly developed investigational varicella (chickenpox) vaccine.

The first defense against infection is prevention. When the child is hospitalized, the nurse employs all measures to control transfer of infection. These typically include the use of a private room, restriction of all visitors and health personnel with active infection, and strict handwashing technique with an antiseptic solution. In some research centers special germ-free environments are available during complete myelosuppression from intensive chemotherapy or for bone marrow transplant.

The child is evaluated for potential sites of infection (e.g., mucosal ulceration, skin abrasion or tear, such as a hangnail) and observed for any elevation in temperature. To identify the source of infection, chest radiographs and blood stool, urine, and nasopharyngeal cultures are taken. Intravenous antibiotics are administered and, if prolonged, venous access device (Broviac/Hickman catheter or implanted infusion port) or a heparin lock is used to maintain an intravenous accesss without undue limitations of activity.

Prevention of infection continues to be a priority after discharge from the hospital. Ordinarily the child is allowed to return to school when the blood count is at a satisfactory level. At all times family members are encouraged to practice good handwashing to prevent introducing pathogens into the home. The child may need to be isolated from school contacts in the event of an outbreak of a childhood disease, especially chickenpox.

Nutrition is another important component of infection prevention. An adequate protein-calorie intake provides the child with better host defenses against infection and increased tolerance to chemotherapy and irradiation. However, providing optimum nutrition during periods of anorexia and vomiting from chemotherapy is a tremendous challenge (see Feeding the sick child, p. 640).

Hemorrhage. Before the use of transfused platelets, hemorrhage was a leading cause of death in leukemia. Now most bleeding episodes can be prevented or controlled with judicious administration of platelet concentrates or platelet-rich plasma.

Since infection increases the tendency toward hemorrhage, and bleeding sites become more easily infected, skin punctures are avoided whenever possible, and when fingersticks, venipunctures, intramuscular injections, and bone marrow aspirations are performed, aseptic technique must be employed as well as continued observation for bleeding. Meticulous mouth care is essential, since gingival bleeding with resultant mucositis is a frequent problem. Since the rectal area is prone to ulceration from various drugs, feces and urine are removed immediately and the perianal area washed. Rectal temperatures are avoided to prevent trauma, and frequent turning, use of a special mattress (egg crate, flotation, or alternating-pressure), and sheepskin under bony prominences prevent development of pressure areas and decubital ulcers.

Platelet transfusions are generally reserved for active bleeding episodes that do not respond to local treatment and that may occur during induction or relapse therapy. Epistaxis and gingival bleeding are the most common. The nurse teaches parents and older children measures to control nosebleeding (see p. 838). Pressure at the site without disturbing clot formation is the general rule.

During bleeding episodes the parents and child need much emotional support. The sight of oozing blood is very upsetting. Often parents will request a platelet transfusion, unaware of the need to trying local measures first. The nurse can be instrumental in allaying anxiety by acknowledging the feelings of the child and family and explaining the reason for delaying a platelet transfusion until absolutely necessary.

Anemia. Initially anemia may be profound, from complete replacement of the bone marrow by leukemic cells. During induction therapy, blood transfusions with packed red cells may be necessary to raise hemoglobin to levels approaching 10 g/dl. The usual precautions in caring for the child with anemia are instituted (see p. 822).

Manage problems of irradiation and drug toxicity. The irradiation and chemotherapy present several nursing challenges. The complexity of the treatment protocols are often overwhelming to families. In addition, each therapy is associated with a number of predictable side effects.

Nurses must be aware of these side effects and use judgment in recognizing which are normal reactions and which indicate toxicity. The reader is referred to more extensive discussions.*

Nausea and vomiting. The nausea and vomiting that occur shortly after administration of several of the drugs and as a result of cranial radiation can be profound. Although a number of antiemetic agents are available, no product is uniformly successful in controlling the vomiting, and some may cause undesirable side effects. Most are available in oral, parenteral, or suppository form.

The most beneficial regimen for antiemetic control has been the administration of the antiemetic *before* the chemotherapy begins. The goal is to prevent the child from ever experiencing nausea or vomiting, thus preventing development of anticipatory symptoms (the conditioned response of developing nausea and vomiting before receiving the drug) (Dolgin and others, 1985).

Anorexia. Loss of appetite is a direct consequence of the chemotherapy, irradiation, and nausea and vomiting. It is a major problem for parents because it is the one area they feel responsible for, particularly when so many other facets of care are outside their control. There are no universally successful techniques for encouraging a sick child to eat. However, the guidelines on p. 640 can be helpful during the anorexic period and can prevent additional problems during the remission.

Some children still do not eat despite these approaches. When loss of appetite and weight persist, the nurse should investigate the family situation to determine if there are any factors (such as conditioned aversion to food, environmental stress related to eating, controlling behavior, or anger) that might be contributing to the problem. Total parenteral nutrition is often implemented for children with significant nutritional problems.

Mucosal ulceration. One of the most distressing side effects of several drugs is gastrointestinal mucosal cell damage, which can produce ulcers anywhere along the alimentary tract. Oral ulcers greatly compound anorexia because eating is extremely uncomfortable, but the following interventions may be helpful: (1) provide a bland, moist, soft diet appropriate for the child's age and preferences, (2) use a soft sponge toothbrush (Toothettes)† or cotton-tipped applicator, (3) provide frequent mouthwashes with normal saline, and (4) apply local anesthetics, such as Chloroseptic spray, viscous lidocaine, or nonprescription preparations, such as Orabase.

Stomatitis may cause such difficulty with eating that the child may require hospitalization for hydration and parenteral nutrition if he refuses fluids. The child will usually choose the foods that are best tolerated, and the nurse should encourage parents to relax any eating pressures. Since the stomatitis is a temporary condition, once the ulcers heal the child can resume good food habits.

*Whaley, L.F., and Wong, D.L.: Nursing care of infants and children, ed. 3, 1987, The C.V. Mosby Company, Chapter 36.
†Manufactured by Halbrand, Inc., Willoughby, OH.

Dental hygiene can become a serious problem for children with orthodontic appliances. Sometimes it may be necessary to remove the braces to allow chemotherapy to continue.

Rectal ulcers are managed by meticulous toilet hygiene, warm sitz baths after each bowel movement, and periodic exposure of the ulcerated area to warm heat to promote healing. Parents should be advised to record bowel movements, since the child may voluntarily avoid defecation to prevent discomfort. Rectal temperatures are contraindicated because the thermometer may further traumatize the area.

Neuropathy. Vincristine and, to a lesser extent, vinblastine can cause various neurotoxic effects. Nursing interventions for management of these effects include (1) administering stool softeners or laxatives for severe constipation caused by decreased bowel innervation, (2) maintaining good body alignment and a footboard to minimize or prevent footdrop, (3) carrying out safety measures during ambulation because of weakness and numbing of the extremities, which may cause difficulty in walking or fine hand movement, and (4) providing a soft or liquid diet for severe jaw pain.

Hemorrhagic cystitis. Sterile hemorrhagic cystitis, a side effect of chemical irritation to the bladder from cyclophosphamide, can be prevented by (1) a liberal fluid intake (at least one and a half times the recommended daily fluid requirement), (2) frequent voiding immediately after feeling the urge, before bed, and after arising, and (3) administering the drug early in the day to allow for sufficient oral intake and voiding. If signs of cystitis occur, such as burning on urination, prompt medical evaluation is needed. If oral home administration is prescribed, the family needs *specific* instructions regarding exactly how much fluid the child must have.

Alopecia. Hair loss is a common side effect of several chemotherapeutic drugs and cranial irradiation, although not all children lose their hair during drug therapy. It is better to warn children and parents of this side effect than to allow them to think that it is only a remote possibility. A soft cotton cap is the most comfortable head wear for children. Polyester increases perspiration and causes itching. Other options include scarves, hats, or a wig. If the child chooses to wear a wig, encouraging a child to select one similar to his own hairstyle and color before the hair falls out is helpful in fostering later adjustment to hair loss. The nurse should also inform the family that hair regrows in 3 to 6 months and may be of a different color and texture. Frequently, the hair is darker, thicker, and curlier than before.

If the child chooses not to wear a wig, attention to some type of head covering, especially in cold climates and in bright sunlight, and scalp hygiene are important. The scalp should be washed like any other body part.

Moon face. Short-term steroid therapy produces no acute toxicities and produces two beneficial reactions—increased appetite and a sense of well-being. However, it does produce alterations in body image, which, although

Text continued on p. 848.

NURSING CARE PLAN

The Child with Leukemia

Nursing Goals	Nursing Interventions	Expected Patient/Family Outcomes
HP-HMP* **Potential for infection** **Risk factors: reduced body defenses (myelosuppression)**		
Minimize risk of infection	Place child in private room or with similarly affected children Advise all visitors and staff to practice handwashing Screen all visitors and staff for signs of infection Use scrupulous aseptic technique for all invasive procedures	Child does not come in contact with infected persons or contaminated articles †Staff and visitors comply with infection precautions
	Evaluate child for any potential sites of infection (needle punctures, mucosal ulceration, minor abrasions, dental problems)	†Signs of infection are recognized and reported. Note: Usual signs of infection may not be present in all immunocompromised children
	Provide nutritionally complete diet for age	Child consumes diet appropriate for age (specify)
	Teach preventive measures at discharge (handwashing and isolation from crowds) Stress importance of isolating child from any known cases of chickenpox or other childhood diseases; work with school nurse and physician to determine optimum time for school reattendance	Family demonstrates knowledge of instructions (specify methods of learning and evaluate)
HP-HMP **Potential for tissue damage, hemorrhage, or neuropathy** **Risk factors: fatigue, antimetabolites**		
Prevent hemorrhagic cystitis	Observe for signs (burning and pain on urination) Give liberal (3000 ml/m^2/day) fluid intake Encourage frequent voiding, including during nighttime	Urine remains clear; voids without discomfort; sufficient output (urinary)
Prevent hemorrhage	Use all measures to prevent infection, especially in ecchymotic areas Use local measures to stop bleeding Restrict strenuous activity that could result in accidental injury Involve child in responsibility for limiting activity when platelet count drops	Child exhibits no evidence of bleeding
Reduce effects of peripheral neuropathy	Encourage ambulation when child is able Alter activity to prevent accidents if weakness occurs, including school attendance Use footboard to prevent footdrop Provide fluids and soft foods to lessen chewing movements	Child ambulates without incident or difficulty
N-MP **Altered nutrition: less than body requirements** **Etiology: loss of appetite**		
Stimulate appetite	Encourage parents to relax; stress legitimate nature of loss of appetite Allow child *any* food he tolerates; plan to improve quality of food selections when appetite increases Stress expected increase in appetite from steroids Take advantage of any hungry period; serve small "snacks" Fortify foods with nutritious supplements, such as powdered milk or commercial supplements Encourage child to be involved in food preparation and selection Make food appealing Apply knowledge of usual food practices typical of children in each age-group, such as food jags or physiologic anorexia in toddlers	Child consumes adequate amounts of appropriate foods

*For an explanation of abbreviations, see p. 20.
†Nursing outcome.

NURSING CARE PLAN

The Child with Leukemia—cont'd

Nursing Goals	Nursing Interventions	Expected Patient/Family Outcomes
	Assess family for additional problems (e.g., use of food by child as a control mechanism if appetite does not improve despite improved physical status) See Feeding the sick child, p. 640	
N-MP Altered oral mucous membranes **Etiology: administration of antimetabolites, disease process**		
Prevent ulceration	Institute meticulous oral hygiene as soon as a drug is used that causes oral ulcers Use soft-sponge toothbrush, cotton-tipped applicator, or gauze-wrapped finger Administer frequent (at least every 4 hours and after meals) mouthwashes (normal saline)	Mucous membranes remain intact
Identify ulceration early	Inspect mouth daily for oral ulcers Report evidence of ulcers to physician	†Any ulceration is detected early and appropriate interventions implemented
Prevent further injury and facilitate healing	Avoid taking oral temperatures Apply local anesthetics to ulcerated areas before meals and as needed Serve bland, moist, soft diet Encourage fluids; use a straw to help bypass painful areas Avoid juices containing ascorbic acid, lemon swabs, and hot or cold foods	Ulcers show evidence of healing
N-MP Potential impaired skin integrity **Risk factors: administration of antimetabolites, radiotherapy, immobility**		
Prevent skin breakdown	Provide meticulous skin care, especially in mouth and perianal regions Change position frequently Encourage adequate calorie-protein intake	Skin remains intact
Reduce undesirable effects of therapy	Suggest and/or implement measures to reduce physical effects of radiotherapy Select loose-fitting clothing over irradiated area to minimize additional irritation Protect area from sunlight and sudden changes in temperature (avoid ice packs, heating pads)	Child and family comply with suggestions (specify)
EP Constipation **Etiology: medications, pain on defecation, rectal ulcers**		
Prevent or reduce effects of rectal ulcers	Wash perianal area after each bowel movement Use warm sitz baths or tub baths as frequently as necessary for comfort Expose ulcerated area to warm heat to hasten healing Observe for constipation resulting from child's voluntary refusal to defecate or from chemotherapy Avoid rectal temperatures and suppositories Record bowel movements; use stool softener to prevent constipation; may need stimulants for evacuation	Rectal mucosa remains clean and intact Ulcerated areas heal without complications Child has regular bowel movements
A-EP Potential activity intolerance **Risk factors: anemia, reduced energy and fatigue**		
Promote rest and reduce fatigue	Allow child to monitor his activity Encourage rest periods throughout day and at least 8 to 10 hours of sleep at night See also Nursing Care Plan for the child with anemia, pp. 826-827	Child engages in activities according to his abilities

†Nursing outcome.

Continued.

NURSING CARE PLAN

The Child with Leukemia—cont'd

Nursing Goals	Nursing Interventions	Expected Patient/Family Outcomes
CPP Pain **Etiology: physiologic effects, neoplasia**		
Relieve pain	Assess need for pain management (see p. 587) Avoid excessive noise or light Place all commodities within easy reach Use gentle, minimal physical manipulation Avoid pressure (bedclothes, sheets) on painful areas Experiment with using heat or cold on painful areas (use cautiously because of easy skin breakdown) Change position frequently; if difficult for child, coordinate with pain relief from analgesics Avoid pressure on bony prominences or painful sites (water bed, bean bag chair, flotation mattress); ensure good body alignment Evaluate effectiveness of pain relief with degree of alertness vs sedation Implement appropriate nonpharmacologic pain reduction techniques (see p. 597)	Child rests quietly, exhibits no evidence of discomfort, verbalizes no complaints of discomfort
SP-SCP Body image disturbance **Etiology: loss of hair, moon face, debilitation**		
Help child and family cope with hair loss	Introduce idea of wig prior to hair loss Administer good scalp hygiene Provide adequate covering during exposure to sunlight, wind, or cold Suggest keeping thin hair clean, short, and fluffy to camouflage partial baldness Stress that hair begins to regrow in 3-6 months and may be a slightly different color or texture Stress that alopecia during a second treatment with same drug may be much less severe	Child verbalizes concern regarding hair loss Child helps determine methods to reduce effects of hair loss and applies these methods
	Encourage good hygiene, grooming, and sex-appropriate items to enhance appearance, such as wig, scarves, hats, makeup, attractive, sex-appropriate clothing	Child appears clean, well-groomed, and attractively dressed
Promote adjustment to altered facial appearance	Encourage rapid reintegration with peers to lessen contrast of changed facial appearance Stress that this reaction is temporary Evaluate weight gain carefully (in weight gain resulting from administration of steroids, extremities remain thin) Encourage visits from friends before discharge to prepare child for reactions and questions Encourage early and consistent interaction with peers	Child resumes former activities and relationships within capabilities
Encourage expression of feelings	Provide opportunities for child to discuss feelings and concerns Provide materials for non-verbal expression, e.g., play, art	Child expresses feelings regarding altered body in words, play, art (specify)
RRP Anticipatory grieving **Etiology: perceived potential loss of child, prospect of loss of limb or other bodily function**		
Help family face possibility of child's death	Provide consistent contact with family Clarify, refocus, and supply information as needed Help family plan care of child, especially at terminal stage (e.g., extent of extraordinary life-saving measures) Provide or help arrange for hospice care if family desires Arrange for spiritual support in accordance with family's beliefs and/or affiliations	Family remains open to counseling and nursing contacts Family and child discuss their fears, concerns, needs, and desires at terminal stage Family investigates hospice care Appropriate religious representative is contacted (specify)

NURSING CARE PLAN

The Child with Leukemia—cont'd

Nursing Goals	Nursing Interventions	Expected Patient/Family Outcomes
NDx RRP Altered family processes **Etiology: situational crisis (child with a life-threatening disease)**		
Support family	Help family plan for future, especially toward helping child live a normal life Encourage family to discuss feelings regarding child's course prior to diagnosis and his prospects for survival	Family discusses feelings and concerns
	Advise family of expected therapy side effects vs toxicities; clarify which demand medical evaluation (mucosal ulceration, hemorrhagic cystitis, peripheral neuropathy, evidence of infection or dehydration) Reassure family that such reactions are not caused by return of cancer cells Interpret prognostic statistics carefully, realizing family's temporary need to interpret them as they see necessary Refer to local chapter of **American Cancer Society,*** **Leukemia Society of America, Inc.,†** or other organizations See also The hospitalized child, p. 603; Family of the hospitalized child, p. 610	Family demonstrates understanding of consequences of therapies
Prepare family for diagnostic/therapeutic procedures	Explain reason for each test (fingersticks, venipunctures, bone marrow aspirations, lumbar punctures, x-ray treatments) Explain basic elements of blood to provide foundational information for tests and therapies Encourage older children and parents to learn meaning of various blood values Explain bone marrow aspiration and lumbar puncture with step-by-step approach	Family demonstrates understanding of procedures (specify learnings and manner of demonstration)
Prepare family for mood changes	Prepare family for expected mood changes from steroids Interpret mood changes based on drugs or reactions to disease/treatment	Family demonstrates understanding of behavior changes
Support child during treatment for myelosuppression	Explain reason for antibiotics and/or transfusions, particularly why platelets are reserved for acute, uncontrolled bleeding episodes	Child demonstrates understanding of procedures and tests (specify method and learnings)
Prepare for discharge	Answer questions regarding posthospital care Teach parents skills and give information necessary for home care	Child and family demonstrate skills needed for home care (specify)
	Arrange for and emphasize importance of maintaining therapy regimen Arrange for acquisition of needed supplies if appropriate	Child and family demonstrate understanding of therapeutic regimen
	Encourage family to allow child to live as normal a life as possible, especially resumption of school Help child prepare for questions from peers regarding hair loss or moon face	Child attends school with reasonable regularity (specify)
	Refer to appropriate agencies and groups to facilitate care and adjustment, such as American Cancer Society, parent groups Maintain contact with family See also The child with a chronic illness, p. 531	Family receives continuing support (specify type and amount)

*777 Third Ave., New York, NY 10017.
†211 East 43rd St., New York, NY 10017.

Continued.

NURSING CARE PLAN

The Child with Leukemia—cont'd

Nursing interventions related to medical management

Assist in establishing diagnosis
Assist with diagnostic procedures and tests
Collect specimens as indicated
Eradicate malignancy
Administer antimetabolites as prescribed
Assist with radiotherapy as ordered
Prevent infection
Administer antibiotics
Prevent hemorrhage
Administer platelets

Relieve pain
Administer analgesics as prescribed
Avoid aspirin or any of its compounds
Administer drugs on preventive schedule
Monitor effectiveness of therapy on pain assessment record (p. 591)
Manage problems of radiotherapy and drug toxicity
Give antiemetic prior to onset of nausea and vomiting
Give drug before bedtime and/or on empty stomach whenever possible

not clinically significant, can be extremely distressing to older children. One of these is moon face in which the child's face becomes rounded and puffy. It is not unusual for other children to make fun of the child with such remarks as "porky-pig" or "fat face." For the child who experiences such name-calling, it is helpful to reassure him that after cessation of the drug the facial changes will return to normal. Unlike hair loss, little can be done to camouflage this obvious change. If the child resumes activity early in the course of treatment, the change may be less noticeable to peers than after a long absence.

Mood changes. Shortly after beginning steroid therapy, children experience a number of mood changes, which range from feelings of well-being and euphoria to depression and irritability. If parents are unaware of these drug-induced changes, they may become unduly concerned. Therefore, the nurse should warn them of the reactions and encourage them to discuss the behavioral changes with each other and the child.

Provide continued emotional support. The preceding discussion of nursing care of the child with leukemia is based on typical problems that confront the family during the treatment phases. It is not unlikely for a child who discontinues therapy after 2 or 3 years and maintains a permanent remission to experience many of these side effects. Therefore, the nurse's role is continually one of support, guidance, clarification, and judgment. Parents need to know how to recognize symptoms that demand medical attention. Although some of the reactions discussed are expected, parents should still report them to their physician. Warning parents of their possible occurrence beforehand, however, allows parents the opportunity to prepare for them. At the same time it reassures them that these reactions are not caused by a return of leukemic cells.

Another aspect of continued emotional support involves prognosis. Although leukemia can no longer be defined as invariably fatal, it must be remembered that survival statistics are only average estimates and apply to those children treated with the latest protocols since diagnosis. For the low-risk child the chances may be better, but for the high-risk child they may be significantly poorer. Of those who do survive after discontinuing therapy, a portion will relapse. Therefore at present only the passage of time is positive confirmation of the child who is ultimately "cured" of the disease. Remission, even in excess of 5 years, cannot be equated with a cure. The nurse who is working with family members must individualize the "numbers" to relate to the people. An understanding of each member's emotional needs, as well as competent care of physical ones, is essential to the positive, growth-promoting support of the family. Comprehensive emotional support for the family of the child with a potentially fatal illness is discussed in Chapter 18.

EVALUATION

The effectiveness of nursing interventions is determined by continual reassessment and evaluation of care based on the following observational guidelines and expected outcomes:

1. Interview child and family regarding their understanding of treatments and diagnostic tests
2. Employ pain assessment techniques
3. Make careful observations of physical status:
   Take vital signs regularly
   Observe for evidence of bleeding, infection, neuropathy, cystitis, mucosal ulceration
   Observe and record intake and output
4. Interview child and family and observe behaviors as a result of complications of therapies
5. Interview child and family and observe behaviors that provide clues to their response to the disease, its therapy, and nursing interventions

Expected outcomes:
See Nursing Care Plan on pp. 844 to 848.

HODGKIN DISEASE

Hodgkin disease is a neoplastic disease that originates in the lymphoid system and primarily involves the lymph nodes. Although Hodgkin disease is extremely rare before 5 years of age, there is a striking increase in children 15 to 19 years, when it occurs with almost the same frequency as leukemia. The malignancy originates in the lymphoid system and primarily involves the lymph nodes. It predictably metastasizes to non-nodal or extralymphatic sites, especially the spleen, liver, bone marrow, and lungs, although no tissue is exempt from involvement (Fig. 25-3).

The disease is usually classified according to four histologic types: (1) lymphocytic predominance, (2) nodular sclerosis, (3) mixed cellularity, and (4) lymphocytic depletion. Accurate staging of the extent of disease is the basis for treatment protocols and expected prognoses. The specific classification for each patient is derived from the history, physical examination, radiographic studies, laboratory tests, and biopsy findings. The staging system proceeds from stages I to IV, or from most to least favorable prognosis, respectively.

Diagnostic Evaluation

The diagnosis is often suspected on the basis of clinical manifestations and detection of enlarged lymph nodes during a physical examination (see box). Because of the multiple organs that can become involved, diagnosis consists of several tests to confirm the presence of Hodgkin disease and to assess the extent of involvement for accurate staging. Tests include complete blood count, uric acid levels, liver function tests, urinalysis, and erythrocyte sedimentation rate. Computerized tomography of the chest, liver, and spleen, and bone scans are performed to detect metastasis.

Although used less frequently, lymphangiography may be performed. This is the visualization of lymphatic circulation of the lower extremities, groin, ileopelvic and abdominal-aortic regions, and the thoracic duct by way of a radiopaque medium injected in the foot.

Lymph node biopsy is essential to diagnosis and staging. A bone marrow aspiration or biopsy is usually performed, also. A laparotomy is recommended for definitive pathologic staging, and the spleen is removed, although this remains a controversial practice because of the risk of overwhelming infections from asplenia.

Clinical Manifestations of Hodgkin Disease

- Painless enlargement of the lymph nodes:
  - Enlarged, firm, nontender, movable nodes in the cervical area are most common
  - "Sentinel" node located near the left clavicle may be first enlarged node
  - Axillary and inguinal lymph nodes less frequently
- Other signs and symptoms of lymphadenopathy:
  - Enlarged mediastinal nodes cause persistent nonproductive cough
  - Enlarged retroperitoneal nodes produce unexplained abdominal pain
- Systemic symptoms (usually indicate advanced involvement):
  - Low-grade and/or intermittent fever
  - Anorexia
  - Nausea
  - Weight loss
  - Night sweats
  - Pruritus

Therapeutic Management

The primary modalities of therapy are radiation and chemotherapy. Each may be used alone or in combination based on the clinical staging. Radiation may involve only the involved field (IF), an extended field (EF) (involved areas plus adjacent nodes), or total nodal irradiation (TNI), depending on the extent of involvement. The most widely used chemotherapeutic regimen is is MOPP (mechlorethamine [Mustargen], vincristine [Oncovin], prednisone, and procarbazine). Other drug combinations may be used in some cases.

Follow-up care of children off therapy is essential to identify relapse. In children with asplenia, prophylactic

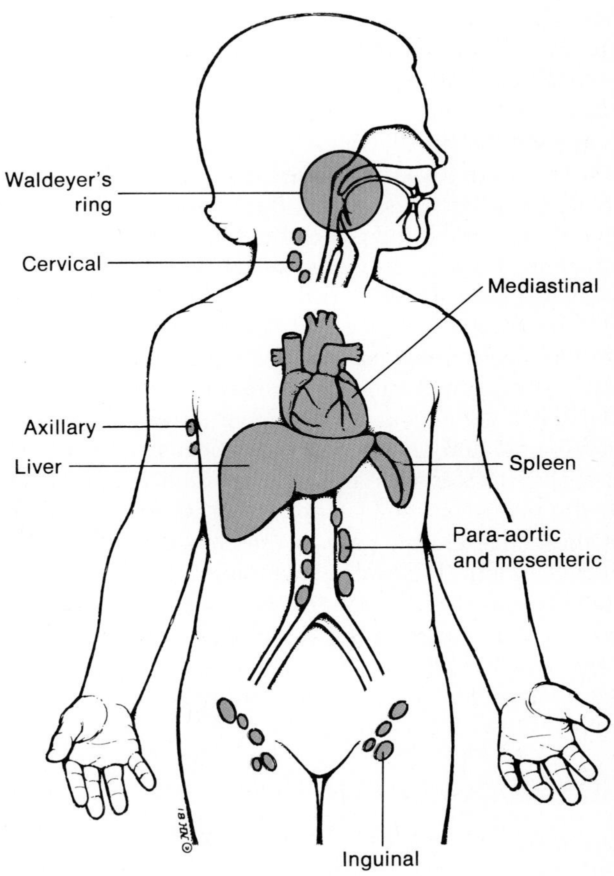

FIG. 25-3 Main ideas of lymphadenopathy and organ involvement in Hodgkin disease.

anitbiotics are administered for an indefinite period, and immunizations against pneumococci, meningococci, and *Haemophilus influenzae* are recommended.

Nursing Considerations

Nursing care involves the same objectives as for patients with other types of cancer—specifically, (1) preparation for diagnostic and operative procedures (see p. 623), (2) explanation of treatment side effects, and (3) child and family support (see Chapter 18). Since this is most often a disease of adolescents and young adults, the nurse must have an appreciation of their psychologic needs and reactions during the diagnostic and treatment phases.

Once the child is hospitalized for suspected Hodgkin disease, a battery of diagnostic tests is ordered. The family needs an explanation of why each test is performed, since many of them, such as a bone marrow aspiration, are not routine. The one test that deserves special explanation is lymphography. If a laparotomy is performed, preparation is similar to that for any other surgery.

The most common side effect of irradiation is malaise, which may last for a year after treatment. This is particularly difficult for active, outgoing school-age children and adolescents, because it prevents them from keeping up with their peers. Sometimes the adolescent will push himself to the point of physical exhaustion rather than admit and succumb to the decreased activity tolerance. The nurse cautions parents to observe for such behavior, such as extreme fatigue at the end of the day, falling asleep at the dinner table, inability to concentrate on homework, or an increased susceptibility to infection. A regular bedtime and scheduled rest periods are important for these children, especially during chemotherapy, when myelosuppression increases the risk of infection and debilitation. Prior to discharge the nurse should discuss a feasible school schedule with the parents and child.

An area of concern for adolescents is the high risk of sterility from irradiation and chemotherapy. Both irradiation to the gonads and drugs, particularly procarbazine and alkylating agents, can lead to infertility. Sexual function is not altered, although the appearance of secondary sexual characteristics and menstruation may be delayed in the pubescent child. Adolescents should be informed of these side effects early in the course of the diagnosis and treatment. Delayed sexual maturation may be an extremely sensitive and painful area for children (see Chapter 17). It is important for the nurse to respect their concern and refrain from casually placating them with expressions such as, "You'll catch up someday."

NON-HODGKIN LYMPHOMA

Non-Hodgkin lymphoma (NHL) in children is strikingly different from Hodgkin disease and adult NHL in several aspects (Gardner and Graham-Pole, 1983):

1. The disease is usually diffuse rather than nodular.
2. The cell type is either undifferentiated or poorly differentiated.
3. Dissemination occurs early, more often, and rapidly.
4. Mediastinal involvement and invasion of meninges are common.

NHL exhibits a variety of morphologic, cytochemical, and immunologic features, not unlike the diversity seen in leukemia. Classification is based on the histologic pattern, either nodular (circumscribed) or diffuse (spread out). Immunologically these cells are also classified as T-cells, B-cells, or null cells (lacking immunologic properties).

The clinical staging system used in Hodgkin disease is of little value in NHL, although it has been modified and other systems have been developed. The prognosis is excellent for children with localized disease, and long-term remissions are possible in many patients, even in those with disseminated disease. Since relapse after 2 years is rare, survival after 24 months is considered a cure.

Diagnostic Evaluation

Because most children with non-Hodgkin lymphoma present with widespread disseminated disease, thorough pathologic staging is unnecessary. Clinical manifestations depend on the anatomic site and extent of involvement. These manifestations include many of those seen in Hodgkin disease, leukemia, and organ symptoms related to pressure from enlargement of adjacent lymph nodes, such as intestinal or airway obstruction, cranial nerve palsies, or spinal paralysis.

Current recommendations for staging include a surgical biopsy, histopathologic confirmation of disease with cytochemical and immunologic evaluation, bone marrow examination, radiographic studies (especially tomograms of lungs and gastrointestinal organs), and lumbar puncture.

Therapeutic Management

The present treatment protocols for NHL include aggressive application of irradiation and chemotherapy. Similar to leukemic therapy, the protocols include induction, consolidation, and maintenance phases, some with intrathecal methotrexate and/or cranial irradiation. Several drug combinations are employed, most of which contain several antineoplastic agents.

Nursing Considerations

Nursing care of the child with NHL is very similar to that required for children with leukemia. Many of the same drugs are employed, although the schedules differ. Because of the intense chemotherapy, nursing care is primarily directed toward managing the side effects of these agents and supportive care to the child and family.

◆ *Immunologic-Deficiency Disorders*

The immune system consists of the *primary lymphoid organs* (thymus, bone marrow, and probably liver) and the *secondary lymphoid organs* (lymph nodes, spleen, and gut-associated lymphoid tissue). The defense functions of the immune system are basically of two types: nonspecific and specific. *Nonspecific immune defenses* are activated on exposure to any foreign substance but react similarly regardless of the type of antigen; they are unable to identify the antigen. *Phagocytosis*, the ingestion and digestion of foreign substances, is the principal process of this system.

Specific (adaptive) defenses are those that have the ability to recognize the antigen and respond selectively. Adaptive immunity consists of (1) *humoral immunity*, which includes antibodies in the form of the immunoglobulins and which is concerned primarily with response to foreign antigens, and (2) *cell-mediated immunity*, which provides protection against most invading organisms. Conditions that cause interference with any or all of these protective mechanisms leave the body vulnerable to disease.

ACQUIRED IMMUNE DEFICIENCY SYNDROME

Acquired immune deficiency syndrome (AIDS) is a disorder that has generated intense medical investigation and even greater public concern and fear. The disease is caused by the human immunodeficiency virus (HIV), and produces a generalized disturbance involving all four major components of the immune mechanism. Reported cases in children constitute only a very small percent of all cases and consist primarily of infants born to mothers with the disease or those who have received transfused blood products. It is common for an affected child to be the index case in a family, and a history reveals a parent who is an individual at risk (see box).

Maternal transmission of HIV can be intrauterine, at delivery, or postnatally. Although the mode of transmission is not entirely clear, the virus can be grown from blood, vaginal secretions, and breast milk. The age at diagnosis is significant. Most infections in children of high-risk mothers are acquired before or during birth (Church, Allen, and Stiehm, 1986). Children of seropositive mothers are diagnosed in the early years, although some not until toddlerhood; in older children the cause is more likely to be transfusion-related. In adolescents the cause is similar to that seen in adults—as a result of high risk behaviors.

The incubation period is shorter in children than it is in adults—about 6 months in children as compared with years in adults. Children with the disease develop recurrent infections and/or chronic infections, usually of the varieties common to all children. A syndrome of morphologic features has also been described for children born to mothers with AIDS, but this is still controversial (see box).

Diagnostic Evaluation

The diagnosis of AIDS in children is suspected on the basis of clinical manifestations (see box) and the presence of risk factors associated with AIDS (see box). Diagnosis of HIV in infancy is complicated by the passage

Congenital AIDS

Dysmorphic Features
- Microcephaly
- Progressive loss of developmental milestones
- Hypertelorism
- Prominent, boxlike forehead
- Mild obliquity of eyes
- Flattened nasal bridge
- Long palpebral fissures with blue sclerae
- Short nose with flattened columella
- Well-formed, triangular philtrum
- Prominent upper vermilion border

From Marion, R.W., and others: Human T-cell lymphotropic virus type III (HTLV-III) embryopathy, Am. J. Dis. Child. **140:**638-640, 1986.

High Risk for AIDS in Children

Maternal factors:
- Intravenous drug use
- Maternal promiscuity
- Diagnosis of AIDS in the mother
- Haitian or central African origin

High-risk groups:
- Intravenous drug abusers
- Recipients of multiple transfusions
- Sexual partners of risk group and members
- Sexually active homosexual males
- Bisexual males

Clinical Manifestations of AIDS in Children

Failure to thrive
*Recurrent bacterial infections
- Pneumonitis
- Otitis media

*Parotitis (often chronic)
Persistent oral candidiasis
Hepatosplenomegaly
Neurologic features
- Seizures
- Truncal ataxia

*Unique to pediatric AIDS.

of maternal IgG across the placenta, which may result in false-positive antibody testing. It takes infants 6 weeks to form antibodies and 9 months for maternal antibodies to disappear. False-negative results have also been seen in seronegative infants whose blood cultures are positive for HIV.

Therapeutic Management

There is no known cure for the disease, but antimicrobial therapy for active infections and supportive measures for other symptoms are implemented. Monthly prophylactic intravenous gammaglobulin has proved of benefit, and prophylactic trimethoprim-sulfa is often given to prevent pneumocystis. The condition is not reversible with present knowledge, and treatment is disappointing.

The use of live-virus vaccines in children with AIDS is controversial. The American Academy of Pediatrics (1987) recommends that children who are symptomatic with HIV infection should not receive live-virus immunizations (measles, mumps, rubella, and poliomyelitis [Sabin]). However, asymptomatic children should receive these vaccines, but the inactive form of polio vaccine (Salk).

Mothers at risk are advised not to breast-feed their infants, and those who deliver an infant that subsequently develops AIDS are advised against having more children.

Nursing Considerations

Nursing considerations are primarily directed at preventing the transmission of the virus, caring for the child with AIDS, and educating the public regarding the *realistic* concerns in terms of communicability of the virus. Recommendations for preventing spread of the virus consist of the use of universal precautions (see box, p. 645).

The nursing care of the child with AIDS is primarily supportive, both physiologically and psychologically. Since the child is immunodeficient, every precaution to prevent infection is implemented. However, the social and psychologic implications of the disease are often overwhelming to the family. Unfortunately, the public is very fearful of contracting the disease from AIDS victims, and criticism and ostracism of the child and family are common. While certain precautions are justified in limiting exposure to sources of infection, they must be tempered with concern for the child's normal developmental needs. Both the family and the community need education about AIDS virus to dispel many of the myths that have been perpetuated by the uninformed (Guidelines, 1988).*

Of major concern for both family and community has been school attendance for children with AIDS. Both the Centers for Disease Control (1985) and the American Academy of Pediatrics (1986) have published guidelines regarding school attendance, which include the following:

1. Unrestricted school attendance for most school-age children and adolescents, with the approval of their personal physician, is recommended, including children with AIDS or AIDS-related complex, or who have antibody to the virus.
2. Students who do not have control of their bodily secretions, who display behaviors such as biting, or who have open sores that cannot be covered may present a greater risk and should be given a more restricted school environment until more is known about the disease.

One of the major concerns of health professionals who work with adolescents is the threat of AIDS to this population. The changing moral standards, increased sexual freedom, and the lack of knowledge about the disease in this age-group render adolescents at high risk for exposure to the disease. As patient advocates, nurses can become involved in educating these people directly by counseling them on matters such as avoiding casual sex and the use of a condom. Nurses also can help promote educational messages in the media (e.g., radio and MTV) and in places that youths frequent (e.g., record stores, concerts, and entertainment events) and by enlisting rock stars and sports figures to help spread the message. Otherwise, adolescents appear to be the group in which the disease is likely to show the most rapid increase in the next few years.

COMBINED IMMUNODEFICIENCY DISEASE

Combined immunodeficiency disease (CID) is a disorder in which there is diminished or absent T- and B-cell function. The exact cause of CID is unknown, but the consequence of the immunodeficiency is an overwhelming susceptibility to infection. The inheritance is either X-linked or autosomal recessive.

Susceptibility to infection occurs early in life, most often by 3 months of age, when prenatal acquired immunity is exhausted. The child suffers from chronic infection, fails to completely recover from an infection, is frequently reinfected, and is infected with unusual agents. Failure to thrive is a consequence of the persistent illnesses.

Diagnosis is usually based on a history of recurrent, severe infections from early infancy and specific laboratory findings, which include lymphopenia, lack of lymphocyte response to antigens, and absence of plasma cells in the bone marrow. Documentation of immunoglobulin deficiency is difficult during infancy because of the normally delayed response of the infant to produce his own immunoglobulins and material transfer of immunoglobulin G.

Therapeutic Management

The only definitive treatment for CID is a bone marrow transplant from a histocompatible donor, usually a sib-

*Information is available from the AIDS hotline: 1-800-FOR-AIDS (Atlanta area: 1-404-329-1295); in Canada, AIDS Information Line, 1-800-972-2437.

ling. Other therapies have been attempted with varying degrees of success, including maintaining the child in a sterile environment. The latter is effective only if instituted prior to the existence of any infectious process in the infant.

Nursing Considerations

Nursing care depends on the type of therapy employed. If bone marrow transplantation is attempted, the care is consistent with that needed for bone marrow transplantation for any condition. Since the prognosis for CID is very poor if a compatible bone marrow donor is not available, nursing care is directed at supporting the family in caring for a child with a life-threatening illness (Chapter 18). Genetic counseling is essential because of the modes of transmission in either form of the disorder.

WISKOTT-ALDRICH SYNDROME

The Wiskott-Aldrich syndrome is an X-linked recessive disorder characterized by a triad of abnormalities: (1) thrombocytopenia, (2) eczema, and (3) immunodeficiency of selective functions of B- and T-lymphocytes. At birth the major effect of the disorder is bleeding as a result of the thrombocytopenia. As the child grows older, recurrent infection and eczema become more severe, and the bleeding becomes less frequent.

Eczema is typical of the allergic type and easily becomes superinfected. Chronic infection with herpes simplex is a frequent problem and may lead to chronic keratitis of the eye with loss of vision. Chronic pulmonary disease, sinusitis, and otitis media result from repeated infections. In those children who survive the bleeding episodes and overwhelming infections, malignancy presents an additional risk to survival.

Specific tests for immunologic function confirm the diagnosis. Medical treatment involves (1) counteracting the bleeding tendencies with platelet transfusions, (2) providing gamma globulin to provide passive immunity, and (3) administering prophylactic antibiotics to prevent and control infection. Bone marrow transplants have been attempted, but even if successful, do not reverse all the defects of this disorder.

Nursing Considerations

Because of the grave prognosis for these children, the main nursing consideration is supporting the family in the care of a fatally ill child (see Chapter 18). Physical care is directed at controlling the problems imposed by the disorder. The measures used to control bleeding are similar to those for hemophilia. Another major goal is prevention or control of infection. Since eczema is a troublesome problem, nursing measures specific to this condition are especially important. The genetic implications of this X-linked recessive disorder differ little from those of any other X-linked disorder.

SUMMARY

Hematologic and immunologic disorders are some of the most serious diseases affecting children. Although some, such as nutritional anemia, are readily amenable to simple therapy, others, such as leukemia and the immune deficiency disorders, are life-threatening. These potentially terminal diseases pose as many psychologic, emotional, social, and financial problems as physical and medical problems. For many of the disorders that were formerly terminal illnesses, therapy has prolonged the life-expectancy for their victims, which offers hope for eventual curative therapy for others.

The hereditary nature of many hematologic and immunologic disorders presents special problems in relation to genetic counseling. Nurses should become aware of counseling services in their community to which these families can be directed. Nurses are prime sources of support and guidance for children with any type of hematologic or immunologic disorder and their families.

KEY CONCEPTS

- The major blood-forming organs of the body are the red bone marrow, lymphatic system, and reticuloendothelial system.
- Anemia is defined as reduction of red cell volume or hemoglobin concentration to levels below normal; disorders are classified either by etiology/physiology or by morphology.
- The role of the nurse in treatment of anemia is to assist in establishing a diagnosis, prepare the child for laboratory tests, administer prescribed medications, decrease tissue oxygen needs, implement safety precautions, and observe for complications.
- The main nursing goal in prevention of nutritional anemia is parent education regarding optimum feeding practices.
- Sickle cell anemia is a hereditary disorder affecting primarily blacks.
- Nursing care of the child with sickle cell disease is aimed at teaching the family how to prevent and recognize sickling, managing pain during crises, and helping the child and parents adjust to a lifelong, potentially fatal disease.
- Nursing care of the child with Cooley anemia involves observing for complications of multiple blood transfusions, assisting the child to cope with the effects of illness, and fostering parent-child adjustment to long-term illness.
- Causes of aplastic anemia include irradiation, drugs, industrial and household chemicals, infections, infiltration and replacement of myeloid elements, and idiopathic conditions.
- The human body controls bleeding through three processes: vascular spasm, platelet aggregation, and coagulation and clot formation.
- Nursing care of the child with hemophilia involves preventing bleeding by decreasing the risk of injury, recognizing and managing bleeding, preventing the crippling effects of joint degeneration, preparing and supporting the child and family for home care.
- Nursing goals in the care of the child with leukemia are to prepare the family for diagnostic and therapeutic procedures, prevent complications of myelosuppression, manage problems of irradiation and drug toxicity, and provide continued emotional support.
- The lymphomas include Hodgkin and non-Hodgkin lymphoma and are disorders involving the lymph glands.
- Immunodeficiency disorders are those that in some way render the affected individual unable to fight infectious organisms.
- Pediatric AIDS is acquired primarily from a parent with AIDS or, until recently, from blood transfusion.

STUDY QUESTIONS AND ACTIVITIES

1 Outline a teaching plan for the family of an infant with iron deficiency anemia.
2 Explain the hereditary nature of sickle cell anemia and the risk of producing an offspring with the abnormal hemoglobin when (a) one parent has the sickle cell trait, and (2) both parents have the sickle cell trait. In each instance, how many offspring will have the trait; how many will have the anemia?
3 Outline a plan for explaining the heredity of hemophilia to female siblings of a boy with hemophilia A.
4 Prepare a list of antineoplastic drugs (antimetabolites) used in the treatment of leukemia and Hodgkin disease and discuss the nursing problems presented by each.
5 Visit the local chapter of the American Cancer Society and find out what programs and services are available to children with leukemia and Hodgkin disease.
6 Interview a grade-school teacher to determine his/her attitude toward having a child with AIDS in his/her classroom. Interview the parent(s) of a school-age child for the same purpose.

REFERENCES

Alter, B.P.: Antenatal diagnosis of thalassemia: a review. In Bank, A., Anderson, W.F., and Zaino, E.C.. editors: Fifth Cooley's anemia symposium, vol. 445, New York, 1985, Ann. N.Y. Acad. Sci.

American Academy of Pediatrics Committee on Infectious Diseases: Health guidelines for the attendance in day care and foster care settings of children affected with human immunodeficiency virus, Pediatrics **79:**466-467, 1987.

American Academy of Pediatrics, Committee on School Health, Committee on Infectious Disease: School attendance of children and adolescents with human T-lymphotropic virus III/lymphadenopathy-associated virus infection, Pediatrics **77:**430-432, 1986.

Centers for Disease Control: Education and foster care of children infected with human T-lymphotropic virus type III/lymphadenopathy-associated virus, MMWR **34:**517-521, 1985.

Church, J.A., Allen, J.R., and Stiehm, E.R.: New scarlet letter(s), pediatric AIDS, Pediatrics **77:**423-427, 1986.

Dolgin, M.J., and others: Anticipatory nausea and vomiting in pediatric cancer patients, Pediatrics **75:**547-552, 1985.

Gardner, R.V., and Graham-Pole, J.: Non-Hodgkin's lymphoma, Pediatr. Ann. **12:**322-335, 1983.

Gaston, M.H., and others: Prophylaxis with oral penicillin in children with sickle cell anemia, N. Engl. J. Med. **314:**1593-1599, 1986.

Guidelines for effective school health education to prevent the spread of AIDS, MMWR Suppl. **37**(S-2)1-13, 1988.

Grier, H.E., and Weinstein, H.J.: Acute nonlymphocytic leukemia, Pediatr. Clin. North Am. **32:**653-668, 1985.

Karayalcin, G.: Current concepts in the management of hemophilia, Pediatr. Ann. **14:**640-659, 1985.

Kasprisin, C.A.: Recipient considerations. In Reynolds, A.W., and Steckler, D., editors: Practical aspects of blood administration, Arlington, VA, 1986, American Association of Blood Banks.

Pizzo, P.A.: Childhood cancer: advances in the past decade, J. Assoc. Pediatr. Oncol. Nurses **4**(1 & 2):34-36, 1987.

BIBLIOGRAPHY

General

Cameron, C.O., and Wallace, N.: Having a bone marrow test: a child's perspective, Child. Health Care **12**(1):41-42, 1983.

Cohen, F.: Clinical genetics in nursing practice, Philadelphia, 1984, J.B. Lippincott Co.

Committee on Transfusion Practices, American Association of Blood Banks: The latest protocols for blood transfusions, Nursing 86 **16**(10):34-41, 1986.

Griffin, J.P.: Be prepared for the bleeding patient, Nursing 86 **16**(6):34-40, 1986.

Hockenberry, M.J., and Coody, D.K.: Pediatric oncology and hematology: perspectives on care, St. Louis, 1986, The C.V. Mosby Co.

Hutchison, M.M., editor: Symposia on bone marrow transplantation, Nurs. Clin. North Am. **18**(3):509-610, 1983.

Landier, W.C., Barrell, M.L., and Styffe, E.J.: How to administer blood components to children, J. Maternal Child Nurs. **12:**178-184, 1987.

McConnell, E.A.: Leukocyte studies: what the counts can tell you, Nursing 86 **16**(3):42-43, 1986.

Silinsky, J.: Understanding white cell morphology, RN **47**(12):82-84, 1984.

Smith, L.G.: Reactions to blood transfusions, Am. J. Nurs. **84:**1096-1101, 1984.

Wiley, F.M., and DeCuir-Whalley, S.: Allogeneic bone marrow transplantation for children with acute leukemia, Oncol. Nurs. Forum **10**(3):49-53, 1983.

Anemia

Dallman, P.R., Siimes, M.A., and Stekel, A.: Iron deficiency in infancy and childhood, Am. J. Clin. Nutr. **33:**86-118, 1980.

Gever, L.N.: New thinking about parenteral iron supplements, Nursing 80 **10**(8):60, 1980.

Hutchison, M.M.: Aplastic anemia. Care of the bone-marrow-failure patient, Nurs. Clin. North Am. **18:**543-551, 1983.

Klopovich, P.M.: An overview of anemia in children, Issues Compr. Pediatr. Nurs. **6**(5-6):277-282, 1983.

Patterson, K.L.: The childhood anemias, Pediatrics: Nursing Update **1**(4):2-7, 1985.

Pipes, P.L.: Nutrition in infancy and childhood, ed. 4, St. Louis, 1989, The C.V. Mosby Co.

Robinson, L.A., Brown, A.L., and Underwood, T.: Iron therapy: helps and hazards, Pediatr. Nurs. **4**(6):9-13, 1978.

Waskerwitz, M.J.: Iron deficiency anemia in children, Issues Compr. Pediatr. Nurs. **6**(5-6):283-294, 1983.

Weeks, H.F.: Iron supplements, MCN **5**(5):354, 1980.

Sickle Cell Anemia

Flanagan, C.: Home management of sickle cell anemia, Pediatr. Nurs. **6**(2):B-D, 1980.

Gibbons, P.T.: Transfusion therapy in sickle cell disease, Nurs. Clin. North Am. **18:**201-205, 1983.

Godwin, M., and Baysinger, M.: Understanding antisickling agents and the sickling process, Nurs. Clin. North Am. **18:**207-214, 1983.

Gradolf, B.: Sickle cell anemia in children, Issues Compr. Pediatr. Nurs. **6**(5-6):295-306, 1983.

Hathaway, G.: The child with sickle cell anemia: implications and management, Nurse Pract. **9**(10):16-22, 1984.

Lamb, C., editor: Managing sickle cell emergencies, Patient Care **19**(1):92-141, 1985.

Reindorf, C.A.: Sickle cell anemias: current concepts, Pediatr. Nurs. **6**(2):E-G, 1980.

Richardson, E.A.W., and Milne, L.S.: Sickle-cell disease and the childbearing family: an update, MCN **8:**417-422, 1983.

Rooks, Y., and Pack, B.: A profile of sickle cell disease, Nurs. Clin. North Am. **18:**131-138, 1983.

Rozzell, M.S., Hijazi, M., and Pack, B.: The painful episode, Nurs. Clin. North Am. **18:**185-199, 1983.

Treiber, F, Mabe P.A., III, and Wilson, G.: Psychological adjustment of sickle cell children and their siblings, Child. Health Care **16:**82-88, 1987.

Walters, I., and others: Complications of sickle cell disease, Nurs. Clin. North Am. **18:**139-184, 1983.

Williams, I., Earles, A.N., and Pack, B.: Psychological considerations in sickle cell disease, Nurs. Clin. North Am. **19:**215-229, 1983.

Thalassemia

Giordano, V.: Psychologic impacts on a thalassemic patient's life. In Bank, A., Anderson, W.F., and Zaino, E.C., editors: Fifth Cooley's anemia symposium, vol. 445, New York, 1985, Ann. N.Y. Acad. Sci.

Ohene-Frempong, K., and Schwartz, E.: Clinical features of thalassemia, Pediatr. Clin. North Am. **27:**403-420, 1980.

Pearson, H.A., and others: Patient age distribution in thalassemia major: changes from 1973 to 1985, Pediatrics **80:**53-57, 1987.

Piomelli, S., and others: Current strategies in the management of Cooley's anemia. In Bank, A., Anderson, W.F., and Zaino, E.C., editors: Fifth Cooley's anemia symposium, vol. 445, New York, 1985, Ann. N.Y. Acad. Sci.

Sherman, M., and others: Thalassemic children's understanding of illness: a study of cognitive and emotional factors. In Bank, A., Anderson, W.F., and Zaino, E.C., editors: Fifth Cooley's anemia symposium, vol. 445, New York, 1985, Ann. N.Y. Acad. Sci.

Wolfe, L., Sallan, D., and Nathan, D.G.: Current therapy and new approaches to the treatment of thalassemia major. In Bank, A., Anderson, W.F., and Zaino, E.C., editors: Fifth Cooley's anemia symposium, vol. 445, New York, 1985, Ann. N.Y. Acad. Sci.

Defects in Hemostasis

Dressler, D.: Understanding and treating hemophilia, Nursing 80 **10**(8):72-73, 1980.

Gaddy-Cohen, D.: Idiopathic thrombocytopenic purpura in children, Issues Compr. Pediatr. Nurs. **6**(5-6):307-316, 1983.

Ingram, N.M.: Stanching nosebleeds: your guide to all the measures available, RN **45**(9):51-53, 115, 1982.

Karpatkin, M.: Screening tests in hemostasis, Pediatr. Clin. North Am. **27**(4):831-841, 1980.

Koch, P.M.: Thrombocytopenia: don't let it make a big problem out of nothing, Nursing 84 **14**(10):55-57, 1984.

Lightsey, A.L., Jr.: Thrombocytopenia in children, Pediatr. Clin. North Am. **27:**293-308, 1980.

McConnell, E.A.: APTT and PT: the tests of time, Nursing 86 **16**(5):47, 1986.

McGillick, K.: DIC: the deadly paradox, RN **45**(8):41-43, 1982.

Sergis-Deavenport, E., Miller, R., and Gomperts, E.: Overview of hemophilia, Issues Compr. Pediatr. Nurs. **6**(5-6):317-328, 1983.

Sergis-Davenport, E., and Varni, J.W.: Behavioral techniques in teaching hemophilia factor replacement to families, Pediatr. Nurs. **8:**416-419, 1982.

Leukemias/Lymphomas

Campbell, J.B., Preston, R., and Smith, K.Y.: The leukemias. Definition, treatment, and nursing care, Nurs. Clin. North Am. **18:**523-541, 1983.

Consalvo, K., and Gallagher, M.: Winning the battle against Hodgkin's disease, RN **49**(12)20-25, 1986.

Craft, M., and others: Nursing care in childhood cancer: coping, Am. J. Nurs. **82:**440-442, 1982.

Daeffler, R.: Oral hygiene measures for patients with cancer, II, Cancer Nurs. **3**(6):427-432, 1980.

Dreyer, K.: The special problems of childhood leukemia, RN **49**(11):37, 1986.

Fergusson, J., and Hobbie, W.: Home visits for the child with cancer, Nurs. Clin. North Am. **20**(1):109-116, 1985.

Fischer, R.G.: Handling antineoplastic drugs, Pediatr. Nurs. **12**(1):59, 1986.

Fochtman, D., and Foley, G.V., editors: Nursing care of the child with cancer, Boston, 1982, Little, Brown & Co.

Gaddy, D.S.: Nursing care in childhood cancer: update, Am. J. Nurs. **82:**416-421, 1982.

Gallagher, M.T., and Wyland, N.L.: Leukemia: when white cells run wild, RN **49**(11)33-37, 1986.

Greene, P.E., and Fergusson, J.H.: Nursing care in childhood cancer: late effects of therapy, Am. J. Nurs. **82**(3):443-446, 1982.

Griffiths, S.S.: Changes in body image caused by antineoplastic drugs, Issues Compr. Pediatr. Nurs. **4**(1):17-27, 1980.

Hagan, S.J.: Bring help and hope to the patient with Hodgkin's disease, Nursing 83 **13**(8):58-63, 1983.

Hockenberry, M.J., and Bologna-Vaughn, S.: Preparation for intrusive procedures using noninvasive techniques in children with cancer: state of the art versus new trends, Cancer Nurs. **8**(2):97-102, 1985.

Houlihan, N.G.: Leukemia: the leukemia process, Cancer Nurs. **4**(2):149-160, 1981.

Houlihan, N.G., and Flaherty, A.M.: Leukemia: a hematology review, Cancer Nurs. **4**(1):61-71, 1981.

Hughes, C.B.: Giving cancer drugs: IV: some guidelines, Am. J. Nurs. **86**(1):34-38, 1986.

Hunt, J.M., Anderson, J.E., and Smith, I.E.: Scalp hypothermia to prevent Adriamycin-induced hair loss, Cancer Nurs. **5**(1):25-31, 1982.

Klopovich, P.M., and Trueworthy, R.C.: Adherence to chemotherapy regimens among children with cancer, Top. Clin. Nurs. **7**(1):19-25, 1985.

Klopovich, P.: Immunosuppression in the child who has cancer, MCN **4:**288-292, 1979.

Koch-Critchfield, M.: When a child needs his parents most, RN **50**(7)17-18, 1987.

Petton, S.: Your role in radiation therapy, RN **48**(2):32-37, 1985.

Potter, S.: Critical infections in the pediatric oncologic patient, Nurs. Clin. North Am. **16**(4):699-706, 1981.

Rahr, V.: Giving intrathecal drugs, Am. J. Nurs. **86**(7):829-831, 1986.

Ruccione, K.: Acute leukemia in children: current perspectives, Issues Compr. Pediatr. Nurs. **6**(5-6):329-362, 1983.

Ruccione, K., and Fergusson, J.: Late effects of childhood cancer and its treatment, Oncol. Nurs. Forum **11**(5):54-64, 1984.

Sutow, W.W., Fernbach, D.J., and Vietti, T.J.: Clinical pediatric oncology, ed. 3, St. Louis, 1984, The C.V. Mosby Co.

Tafuro, P., and Gurevich, I.: Prevention and management of varicella in high-risk individuals, MCN **9**(5):314-317, 1984.

Veninga, K.S.: Improving nutrition in children with cancer, Pediatr. Nurs. **11**(1):18-20, 1985.

Waskerwitz, M.J.: Special nursing care for children receiving chemotherapy, J. Assoc. Pediatr. Oncol. Nurses **1**(1):16-25, 1984.

Waskerwitz, M.J., and Ruccione, K.: An overview of cancer in children in the 1980s, Nurs. Clin. North Am. **20**(1):5-30, 1985.

Wolf, W.J., and Bancroft, B.: Early detection of childhood malignancies, Pediatr. Nurs. **5**(1):43-46, 1980.

Immunodeficiency Disorders

Brainerd, E.: Nursing management of chronic infectious diseases in children, Pediatrics: Nursing Update **1**(17):2-7, 1986.

Dharan, M.: Immunoglobulin abnormalities, Am. J. Nurs. **76**(10):1626-1628, 1976.

Fonger, P.A., and others: Nursing care of the child with severe combined immune deficiency, J. Pediatr. Nurs. **2:**373-380, 1987.

Fidler, R.: Deciphering diagnostic studies: complement assays, Nursing 83 **13**(6):17-19, 1983.

Groenwald, S.L.: Physiology of the immune system, Heart Lung **9**(4):645-650, 1980.

Jemison-Smith, P., and Hamm, P.: Immune responses, Crit. Care Update **10**(8):45-46, 1983.

Lind, M.: The immunologic assessment: a nursing focus, Heart Lung **9**(4):658-661, 1980.

Taylor, D.L.: Immune response: physiology, signs, and symptoms, Nursing 84 **14**(5):52-54, 1984.

AIDS

Bennett, J.: AIDS: what precautions do you take in the hospital? Am. J. Nurs. **86:**952-953, 1986.

Bennett, J.A.: AIDS epidemiology update, Am. J. Nurs. **85**(9):968-972, 1985.

Bennett, J.A.: HTLV-III AIDS link, Am. J. Nurs. **85**(10):1086-1089, 1985.

Black, J.L.: AIDS: preschool and school issues, J. Sch. Health **56**(3):93-95, 1986.

Boland, M., and Gaskill, T.B.: Managing AIDS in children, MCN **9**(6):384-389, 1984.

Brady, M.: AIDS in children, J. Pediatr. Health Care **1:**214-217, 1987.

Centers for Disease Control: Recommendations for assisting in the prevention of perinatal transmission of human T-lymphotropic virus type III/lymphadenopathy-associated virus and acquired immunodeficiency syndrome, MMWR **34**(48):721-732, 1985.

Coleman, D.A.: How to care for an AIDS patient, RN **49**(7):16-21, 1986.

Dhundale, K., and Hubbard, P.M.: Home care for the A.I.D.S. patient: safety first, Nursing 86 **16**(9):34-36, 1986.

Hughes, R.B., and Bailey, F.K.: AIDS from a school health perspective, Pediatr. Nurs. **13:**155-156, 1987.

Kennedy, M.: AIDS. Coping with fear, Nursing 87 **17**(4):45-46, 1987.

Klug, R.: Children with AIDS, Am. J. Nurs. **86:**1126-1132, 1986.

McCutchan, J.A.: What you can do to stop the AIDS panic, RN **49**(10):18-21, 1986.

Miller, D.S.: Intravenous immune globulin for treating primary immunodeficiency disease, MCN **12:**244-248, 1987.

Nelms, B.C.: AIDS and professional responsibility (editorial), J. Pediatr. Health Care **1:**171-172, 1987.

Phillips, A.: Are blood transfusions really safe? Nursing 87 **17**(6):663-664, 1987.

Thompson, S.W., and Gietz, K.R.: Acquired immune deficiency syndrome in infants and children, Pediatr. Nurs. **11**(4):278-280, 1985.

UNIT

XII

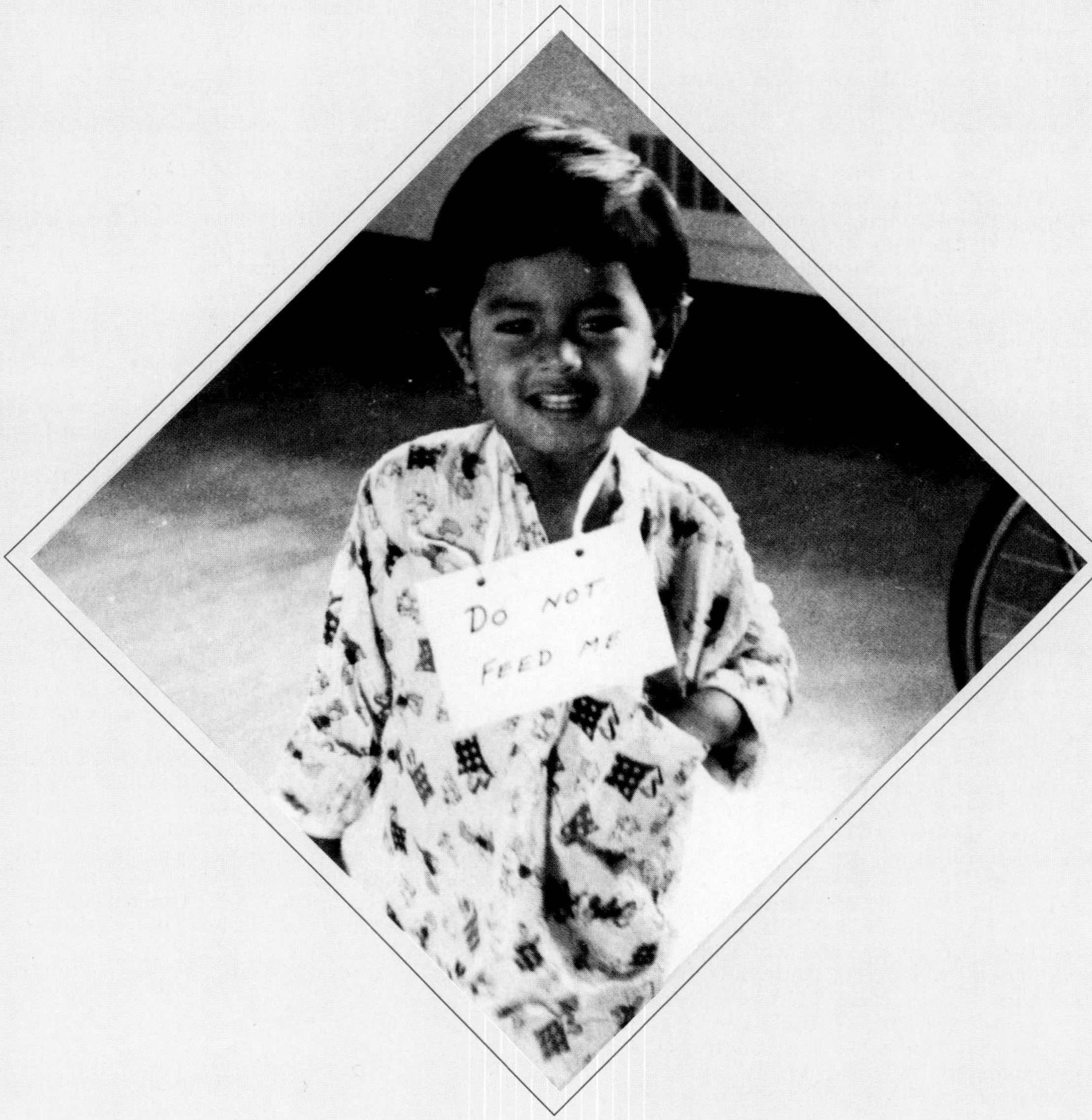

The Child with a Disturbance of Regulatory Mechanisms

Regulation is the function of automatically maintaining an important biologic variable within a narrow range regardless of disturbances that may act on the system, and preventing excessive deviations that are incompatible with life. Regulation enables the organism to maintain the function of cells, tissues, organs, and systems within the parameters described as normal for that system despite changes in the internal or external environment. Communication between the various systems and subsystems is carried by chemical or neural mechanisms. Disturbances in the regulatory processes can create disturbances in one or more of the interrelated component parts of the system with consequences that affect other systems and the organism as a whole.

Genetic and numerous chemical regulatory mechanisms, for example, acid-base equilibrium and oxygen–carbon dioxide disturbances, have been discussed in previous units. The major regulatory mechanisms of the body are the endocrine and neural systems. The portion of the endocrine regulation that involves the pituitary gland is so closely associated with the neurologic system that it is frequently referred to as the neuroendocrine system. It is sometimes difficult to determine whether dysfunctions in this interrelated system are caused by impaired function in the target glands that secrete hormones, the tropic substances that stimulate the target glands to secrete hormones, or the portions of the midbrain that produce releasing factors that stimulate the pituitary gland.

The kidneys are important regulatory organs and are principally concerned with regulation of fluid and acid-base equilibrium. Although the function of the skin is primarily protective, its integrity and metabolism markedly affect the structures encased within this protective shelter.

Renal impairment is discussed in Chapter 26, *The Child with Genitourinary Dysfunction*. Dysfunction of the central nervous system is discussed in Chapter 27, *The Child with Cerebral Dysfunction*. Chapter 28, *The Child with Endocrine Dysfunction,* describes the problems related to impairment of the complex endocrine system and the pancreatic hormones. Chapter 29, *The Child with Integumentary Dysfunction,* is concerned with the multiple disorders of the skin.

CHAPTER 26

The Child with Genitourinary Dysfunction

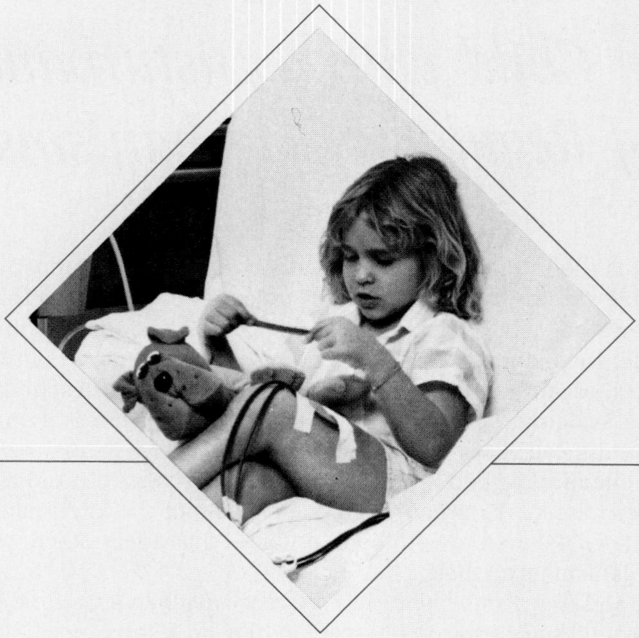

LEARNING OBJECTIVES

On completion of this chapter the reader will be able to:

- Describe the various factors that contribute to urinary tract infections in infants and children
- Demonstrate an understanding of the causes and mechanisms of edema formation in nephrotic syndrome
- Outline a nursing care plan for a child with nephrotic syndrome
- Compare the manifestations and nursing care of the child with minimal-change nephrotic syndrome and a child with acute glomerulonephritis
- Contrast the causes, complications, and management of acute and chronic renal failure
- Discuss the preoperative preparation of the child and parents when the child has a structural defect of the genitourinary tract
- Discuss the role of the nurse in assisting the parents to cope with the problems of a newborn with ambiguous genitalia

The primary responsibility of the kidney is to maintain the composition and volume of the body fluids in equilibrium. To maintain this constant internal environment, the kidney must respond appropriately to alterations in the internal environment caused by variations in dietary intake and extrarenal losses of water and solutes. A secondary function of the kidney is the production of certain humoral substances important in stimulating erythropoiesis in the bone marrow and the regulation of blood pressure.

When pathologic processes interfere with these functions, the consequences are manifest in a variety of systems and processes. Diseases involving the kidneys are relatively common in childhood and are caused by a variety of etiologic factors, including infectious processes and structural abnormalities.

ASSESSMENT OF RENAL FUNCTION

Assessment of kidney and urinary tract integrity and the diagnosis of renal or urinary tract disease are based on several evaluative tools. Physical examination, history, and observation of symptoms are the initial procedures. In suspected urinary tract disorders, further assessment by laboratory, radiologic, and other evaluative methods are carried out. The major evaluative tools used to assess genitourinary function are outlined in Table 26-1.

◆ *Inflammatory Disorders of the Genitourinary Tract*

Kidneys react to tissue injury in the same manner as all other body tissues. Acute inflammation evokes a pattern of exudation, white blood cell accumulation, and tissue damage; chronic long-standing inflammation results in scarring and permanent destruction of tissue elements. This discussion focuses on inflammations of the renal

TABLE 26-1

Diagnostic Tests of Renal Function

Test	Significance
Urine	
Physical Tests	
Specific gravity	Provide information regarding hydration and concentrating and/or reabsorbing ability of nephrons
Osmolality	Same as specific gravity; more sensitive index
Chemical Tests	
pH	Elevated in tubular acidosis, urinary infection
Protein level	Present in altered glomerular permeability
Glucose level	Elevated in impaired tubular reabsorption
Microscopic Tests	
White blood cell count	Elevated in urinary tract inflammatory process
Red blood cell count	Elevated in trauma, stones
Presence of bacteria	Urinary tract infection
Presence of casts	Pronounced renal malfunction, tubular or glomerular disorders, pyelonephritis, glomerulonephritis
Other Tests	
Urine culture and sensitivity	Determines presence of pathogens and the drugs to which they are sensitive
Blood	
Blood urea nitrogen (BUN)	Increased in acute and chronic renal disease
Uric acid	Increased in severe renal disease
Creatinine	Increased in severe, long-standing renal impairment
Radiographic	
Intravenous pyelography (IVP) (intravenous urogram; excretory urogram)	Defines urinary tract Provides information about integrity of kidneys, ureters, and bladder Retroperitoneal masses visualized when they shift position of ureters
Time-sequence IVP	More accurately distinguishes differences between kidneys Differences in times of excretion indicate unilateral disease
Retrograde pyelography	Visualizes pelvic calyces, ureters, and bladder
Renal angiography	Visualizes renal vascular system, especially for renal arterial stenosis
Radioisotope renography and renal scanning	Records appearance and disappearance of radioactivity in each kidney Gives detailed picture of excretory performance Helps define intrarenal masses
Voiding cystourethrography	Visualizes bladder outline and urethra, reveals reflux of urine into ureters, and shows complications of bladder emptying
Scout film (KUB)	Detects and establishes renal outlines, presence of calculi, or opaque foreign bodies in bladder
Miscellaneous	
Cystoscopy	Investigation of bladder and lower tract lesions; visualizes urethral openings, bladder wall, trigone, and urethra
Renal biopsy	Yields histologic and microscopic information about glomeruli and tubules; helps to distinguish between types of nephrotic syndromes Distinguishes other renal disorders
Nephrosonography	Distinguishes between cystic and solid masses and renal and nonrenal masses, localizes kidneys, and delineates nonfunctional kidney
Tomography	Visualizes vertical or horizontal cross section of kidney Especially valuable to distinguish tumors and cysts

system, including bacterial infections and those nonsuppurative disorders, collectively described as *nephritis*.

URINARY TRACT INFECTION

Urinary tract infection (UTI) is the term used to describe a clinical condition that may involve the urethra, bladder (lower urinary tract), and/or the ureters, renal pelvis, calyces, and renal parenchyma (upper urinary tract). Because it is often impossible to localize the infection, the broad designation UTI is applied to the presence of significant numbers of microorganisms anywhere within the urinary tract.

The prevalence of UTI in childhood is second only to infections of the respiratory tract and is a significant cause of hospitalization and morbidity in children. The peak incidence of UTI not caused by structural anomalies occurs between 2 and 6 years of age and, except for the neonatal period, females have a 10 to 30 times greater risk for developing UTI than males. An increased incidence of UTI is observed in adolescents, especially those with evidence of sexual activity (Weir and Lampe, 1984).

Classification

Infection of the urinary tract may be present with or without clinical symptoms. As a result, the site of infection is often difficult to pinpoint with any degree of accuracy. Various terms used to describe urinary tract disorders include the following:

bacteriuria Growth of bacteria in uncontaminated urine (greater than 100,000 colonies/ml)
asymptomatic bacteriuria Significant bacteriuria with no clinical evidence of active infection
symptomatic bacteriuria Significant bacteriuria accompanied by physical symptoms
recurrent UTI Repeated symptomatic episodes, usually caused by entry of new organisms from the perineal-fecal flora (sometimes termed *reinfection*)
relapse of UTI Relapse is persistence of the same organism despite appropriate antibiotic therapy
urethritis Inflammation of the urethra
cystitis Inflammation of the bladder
ureteritis Inflammation of the ureters
pyelonephritis Inflammation of the kidney and upper tract (may be acute or chronic)

Etiology

A variety of organisms can be responsible for UTI. *Escherichia coli* and other gram-negative enteric organisms are most frequently implicated; all are common to the anal, perineal, and perianal region. Other organisms associated with UTI include *Proteus, Pseudomonas, Klebsiella, Staphylococcus aureus, Haemophilus,* and coagulase-negative *Staphylococcus*.

Several factors contribute to the development of UTI in childhood. These include anatomic, physical, and chemical conditions or properties of the host urinary tract.

Anatomic and physical factors. The structure of the lower urinary tract is believed to account for the increased incidence of bacteriuria in females. The short urethra, which measures about 2 cm (3/4 inch) in young females and 4 cm (1½ inches) in mature women, provides a ready pathway for invasion of organisms. In addition, the closure of the urethra at the end of micturition may return contaminated bacteria to the bladder. The longer male urethra (as long as 20 cm [8 inches] in an adult) and the antibacterial properties of prostatic secretions inhibit the entry and growth of pathogens.

The single most important host factor influencing the occurrence of UTI is urinary stasis. Ordinarily urine is sterile, but at 37° C (98.6° F) it provides an excellent culture medium. Under normal conditions the act of completely and repeatedly emptying the bladder flushes away any organisms before they have an opportunity to multiply and invade surrounding tissue. However, urine that remains in the bladder allows bacteria from the urethra to rapidly become established in the rich medium. Incomplete bladder emptying (stasis) may result from reflux (see p. 863 for a discussion of reflux), anatomic abnormalities (especially those involving the ureters), dysfunction of the voiding mechanism, or extrinsic ureteral or bladder compression.

Altered urine and bladder chemistry. Several chemical characteristics of the urine and bladder mucosa help maintain urinary sterility. An increased fluid intake promotes flushing of the normal bladder and lowers the concentration of organisms in the infected bladder. Water diuresis also seems to enhance the antibacterial properties of the renal medulla.

Most pathogens favor an alkaline medium. Normally urine is slightly acidic, but it can be made more acidic by diet (apple juice, large amounts of ascorbic acid, animal protein) or acid-forming drugs. A urine pH of about 5 hampers bacterial multiplication, although the acidification rarely eliminates the bacteriuria. However, it may enhance the therapeutic effectiveness of drugs and of the natural defense mechanisms, as well as help relieve some of the symptoms.

Diagnostic Evaluation

The clinical manifestations of UTIs depend on the age of the child (see box). Presumptive UTI diagnosis can be made by the presence of organisms in the urine. Several factors can alter a urine specimen, and contamination from a specimen by organisms from sources other than the urine is the most frequent cause of false-positive results, such as perineal and perianal flora in bag specimens. More accurate estimates are obtained from clean-catch midstream specimens. Unless the specimen is a first morning sample, a recent high fluid intake may indicate a falsely low organism count. Therefore children should not be encouraged to drink large volumes of water in an attempt to obtain a specimen quickly.

Catheterized specimens are usually excellent as long

Clinical Manifestations of Urinary Tract Infection

Newborns May Have
Fever or hypothermia
Sepsis

Children Less Than 2 Years of Age
Failure to thrive
Feeding problems
Vomiting
Diarrhea
Abdominal distention
Jaundice
Frequent or infrequent voiding
Constant squirming
Irritability
Strong-smelling urine
Abnormal stream
Persistent diaper rash

Children Over 2 Years of Age
Enuresis
Daytime incontinence in toilet-trained child
Fever
Strong or foul-smelling urine
Increased frequency of urination
Dysuria
Urinary urgency
Abdominal pain
Costovertebral angle tenderness (flank pain)
Hematuria
Vomiting (preschoolers)

Adolescents
Lower tract infection:
- Frequency
- Painful urination (small amount of turbulent urine)
- Hematuria
- Fever usually absent

Upper tract infection:
- Fever
- Chills
- Flank pain
- Lower tract symptoms

Urine
- Cloudy
- Hazy
- Thick with noticeable strands of mucus and pus
- Unpleasant fishy smell even when fresh

as the first few millileters are excluded from the collection. Suprapubic aspiration is equally reliable and frequently used for collecting specimens in infants. Specimens obtained for culture should be taken to the laboratory immediately.

Recently developed tests to detect bacteriuria are being used with increased frequency in screening for UTI. The plastic dipstick, Chemstrip, and the agar-coated slide tests are quick and inexpensive alternatives to microscopic examination and, in some instances, are replacing routine culture.

Other tests may be needed to localize an infection site, including ureteral catheterization and bladder washout procedures. Other tests, such as ultrasonography, voiding cystourethrogram (VCUG), intravenous pyelogram (IVP), and cystoscopy, are often performed after the infection subsides to identify anatomic abnormalities contributing to the development of infection and existing kidney changes from recurrent infection.

Therapeutic Management

The objectives of treatment of children with UTI are (1) to eliminate the infection, (2) to detect and correct functional or anatomic abnormalities, (3) to prevent recurrences, and (4) to preserve renal function (Krugman and others, 1985). Antibiotic therapy should be initiated based on identification of the pathogen, the child's history of antibiotic use, and the location of the infection. A variety of antimicrobial drugs are available for treating UTI, but all of them can occasionally be ineffective because of resistance of organisms. Antibacterial compounds used in the management of UTI include (1) systemic penicillins and sulfonamides, which are used for a short, intensive course of therapy; and (2) antiseptic preparations, which are often continued over longer periods to maintain urinary sterility, especially in children with long-term susceptibility to infection, such as those with neurogenic bladder.

If anatomic defects such as primary reflux or bladder neck obstruction are present, surgical correction of these abnormalities may be necessary to prevent recurrent infection. Follow-up study is an important component of medical management, since the relapse rate is high and recurrent infection tends to occur 1 to 2 months after termination of treatment. Even with recurrent infections, renal damage is rare if no anatomic abnormalities complicate the condition. The aim of therapy and careful follow-up in such cases is to prevent morbidity rather than reduce the chance of renal failure. However, the hazard of progressive renal injury is greatest when infection occurs in young children (especially under 2 years of age) and is associated with congenital renal malformations and reflux. Therefore early diagnosis of children at risk is particularly important during infancy and toddlerhood.

Vesicoureteral reflux. Vesicoureteral reflux (VUR) is the backward flow of bladder urine into the ureters that occurs when urine is swept into the ureters during voiding. The urine then flows into the bladder after voiding, where it remains as a reservoir for bacterial growth until the next void (Fig. 26-1). Primary reflux results from congenitally abnormal insertion of ureters into the bladder; secondary reflux occurs as a result of infection.

VUR is managed conservatively with antibacterial therapy and frequent urine cultures and requires a motivated, reliable, and cooperative family. Indications for surgical intervention include significant anatomic abnormality at the ureterovesical junction, recurrent UTI, severe forms of VUR, noncompliance with medical therapy, intolerance to antibiotics, and VUR after puberty in females (Hensle and Burbige, 1986).

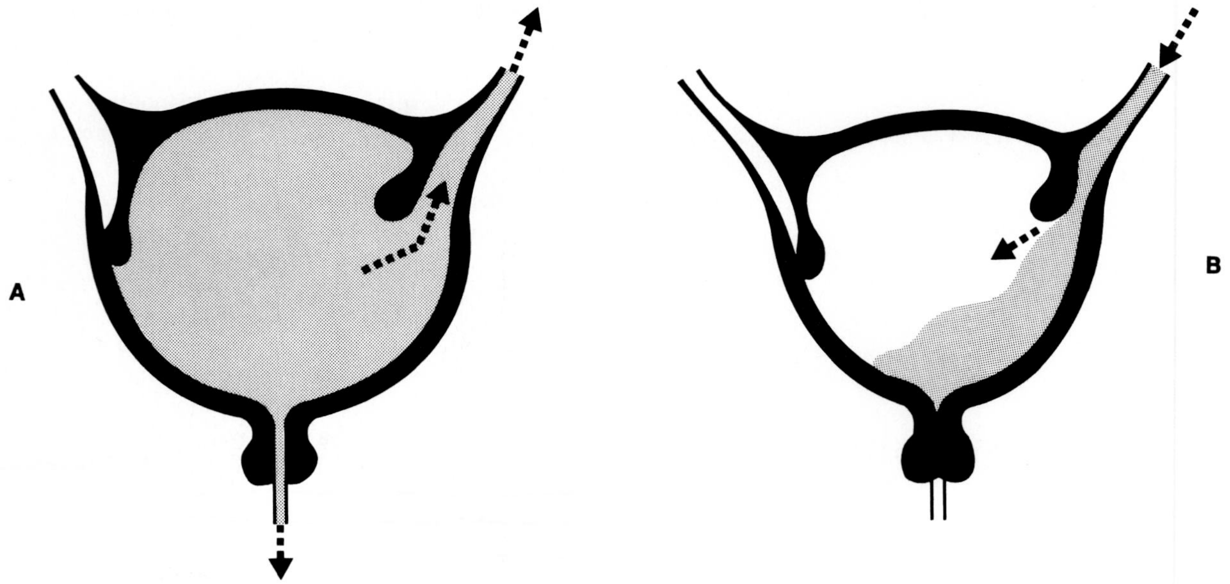

FIG. 26-1 Mechanisms of vesicoureteral reflux. **A,** During voiding, urine refluxes into the ureter. **B,** After voiding, residual urine from the ureter remains in the bladder.

Nursing Considerations

Nurses have an important role in the preventive approaches of UTI, collection of specimens, and teaching families these essential aspects of care.

ASSESSMENT

Since children are not a captive population, mass screening is difficult. However, the annual health examinations should include a routine urinalysis. In addition, nurses should instruct parents to observe regularly for clues suggesting UTI. Unfortunately the signs of UTI are not as evident as those of upper respiratory infection. Therefore many cases go undetected because no one thought to investigate this very common problem.

Since infants and young children are unable to express their feelings and sensations verbally, it is difficult to detect discomfort they may be experiencing from dysuria. A careful history regarding voiding habits and episodes of unexplained irritability may assist in detecting less obvious cases of UTI. Consequently parents should be cautioned to observe for specific clues of UTI in suspected cases, such as checking the diaper every ½ hour, which increases the opportunity for observing the stream for such findings as straining or fretting before voiding begins, signs of discomfort before and during urinating, starting and stopping the stream intermittently, and frequent dripping of small amounts of urine.

When infection is suspected, collecting an appropriate specimen is essential. It is the nurse's responsibility to take every precaution to obtain acceptable clean-voided specimens in order to avoid the use of other collecting procedures except where absolutely indicated.

NURSING DIAGNOSES

Based on a thorough assessment a number of nursing diagnoses become evident. They include but are not limited to those outlined in the accompanying box.

PLANNING

The goals of nursing care for children with UTI are:

1. Prepare children and families for needed tests and procedures
2. Educate parents and children regarding prevention and treatment of infection

IMPLEMENTATION

Frequently additional tests are performed to detect anatomic defects. Children are prepared for these tests as appropriate for their age. Except for intravenous pyelography (IVP), voiding cystography and cystoscopy are usually performed under general anesthesia. However, children who are old enough to understand still need an explanation of the procedure, its purpose, and what they

Nursing Diagnoses: The Child with Urinary Tract Infection

Potential for injury related to possibility of kidney damage from chronic infection
Anxiety related to unfamiliar procedures
Altered family processes related to illness of a child

will experience (see Preparing for procedures, p. 623). Sometimes a simple description of the urinary system is helpful. Especially for preschool children, the nurse must clarify that the urinary tract is separate from any sexual function and that the test is for a problem that they did not cause. It is not uncommon for children to associate blame for perceived wrongdoing (e.g., masturbation) or unacceptable thoughts with the reason for the illness or the tests. For young children under 3 to 4 years of age, the procedure can be explained on a doll. For those who are older, a simple drawing of the bladder, urethra, ureters, and kidneys makes the explanation more understandable.

Children may be treated as outpatients to avoid overnight separation from home for such procedures. In such cases nurses must be careful not to overlook the need for adequate preparation; thus if surgery is subsequently indicated, the child will be able to encounter the impending operation with facts and understanding of the procedures. The preparation will help to decrease his fear and anxiety of more extensive medical-surgical intervention.

Since antibacterial drugs are indicated in UTI, the nurse advises parents of proper dosage and administration. Ampicillin is frequently the drug of choice, but it must be given every 6 hours to maintain high blood levels. This generally requires waking the child during sleep for one dose. Amoxicillin allows for 8-hour intervals, which is more convenient, but the drug is more expensive than ampicillin. When antiseptics such as nitrofurantoin are used for prolonged therapy to maintain urine sterility, parents need an explanation of the drug's continued necessity when no signs of infection are present.* For all children an adequate or increased fluid intake is encouraged.

Prevention. Prevention is the most important goal in both primary and recurrent infection, and most preventive measures are simple to very simple, ordinary hygienic habits that should be a routine part of daily care (see box). For example, parents are taught to cleanse their infant's genital areas from front to back to avoid contaminating the urethral area with fecal organisms. Female children are taught to wipe from front to back after voiding or defecating.

Sexually active adolescent females are advised to urinate as soon as possible after intercourse to flush out bacteria introduced during sexual activity. Children with disabilities involving the bladder are frequently on a prophylactic regimen, such as acidifying agents and prescribed fluid intake. The nurse should reinforce the importance of compliance to parents and responsible children.

Prevention of Urinary Tract Infection

Factors Predisposing to Development	Measures of Prevention
Short female urethra close to vagina and anus	Perineal hygiene—wipe from front to back Avoid tight clothing or diapers; wear cotton panties rather than nylon Check for vaginitis or pinworms, especially if child scratches between legs
Incomplete emptying (reflux) and overdistention of bladder	Avoid "holding" urine; encourage child to void frequently, especially before a long trip or other circumstances where toilet facilities are not available Empty bladder completely with each void Avoid straining at stool
Concentrated and alkaline urine	Encourage generous fluid intake Acidify urine with juices such as apple and a diet high in animal protein

EVALUATION

The effectiveness of nursing interventions is determined by continual reassessment and evaluation of care based on the following observational guidelines and expected outcomes:

1. Question children and families regarding their understanding of the disease and the diagnostic measures required for identifying the presence of infection and/or physical abnormalites
2. Observe and interview family and child regarding preventive practices and observe laboratory reports of urinalyses and cultures for evidence of treatment efficacy

Expected outcomes:

1. The child and family demonstrate an understanding of the illness and diagnostic tests (specify knowledge and means of demonstration)
2. Child and family demonstrate an understanding of preventive practices (specify means of demonstration); child exhibits no evidence of infection

NEPHROTIC SYNDROME

The *nephrotic syndrome* is a clinical state that is defined as massive proteinuria, hypoalbuminemia, hyperlipemia, and edema. The disorder can occur as (1) a primary disease known as *idiopathic nephrosis, childhood nephrosis,* or *minimal change nephrotic syndrome;* (2) a secondary disorder that occurs as a clinical manifestation after or in association with glomerular damage of known or presumed etiology; and (3) a congenital form inherited as an autosomal recessive disorder. The disorder is characterized by increased glomerular permeability to plasma protein, which results in massive urinary protein loss.

*See Home care instructions for giving medications to children. In Wong, D.L., and Whaley, L.F.: Clinical handbook of pediatric nursing, ed 2. St. Louis, 1986, The C.V. Mosby Co.

This discussion is devoted to minimal change nephrotic syndrome (MCNS) because it constitutes 80% of nephrotic syndrome cases.

Pathophysiology

The onset of MCNS can occur at any age but predominantly occurs in children between the ages of 2 and 7 years. It is rare in children younger than 6 months of age, uncommon in infants younger than 1 year of age, and unusual after the age of 8.

The pathogenesis of MCNS is not understood. There may be a metabolic, biochemical, or physiochemical disturbance that causes the basement membrane of the glomeruli to become increasingly permeable to protein, but the cause and mechanisms are only speculative.

The glomerular membrane, normally impermeable to albumin and other proteins, becomes permeable to proteins, especially albumin, which leak through the membrane and are lost in urine (*hyperalbuminuria*). This reduces the serum albumin level (*hypoalbuminemia*), decreasing the colloidal osmotic pressure in the capillaries. As a result, the vascular hydrostatic pressure exceeds the pull of the colloidal osmotic pressure, causing fluid to accumulate in the interstitial spaces (*edema*) and body cavities, particularly in the abdominal cavity (*ascites*). The shift of fluid from the plasma to the interstitial spaces reduces the vascular fluid volume (*hypovolemia*), which in turn stimulates the renin-angiotensin system and the secretion of antidiuretic hormone and aldosterone. Tubular reabsorption of sodium and water is increased in an attempt to increase intravascular volume. The elevation of serum lipids is unexplained. The sequence of events in nephrotic syndrome is diagrammed in Fig. 26-2.

Diagnostic Evaluation

The disease is suspected on the basis of clinical manifestations (see box), especially when weight gain in a previously well child progresses insidiously over a period of days or weeks. The generalized edema develops so slowly that parents may consider it a sign of healthy growth. Although an acute infection may precipitate severe generalized edema (*anasarca*) (Fig. 26-3), the usual course is one of progressive weight gain until either rapid or gradual increase in edema prompts the family to seek medical evaluation. Neurologic examinations are negative, and the sensorium is clear.

Massive proteinuria is reflected in urine excretion of large amounts of protein with high specific gravity proportionate to the concentration of protein. Hyaline casts, fat bodies, and a few red blood cells can be found in the urine of most affected children, although there is seldom gross hematuria. If hypovolemia is not significant and if the child is well hydrated, the glomerular filtration rate is usually normal.

Total serum protein concentrations are lowered, with the albumin fractions significantly reduced and globulins and plasma lipids elevated. Hemoglobin and hematocrit

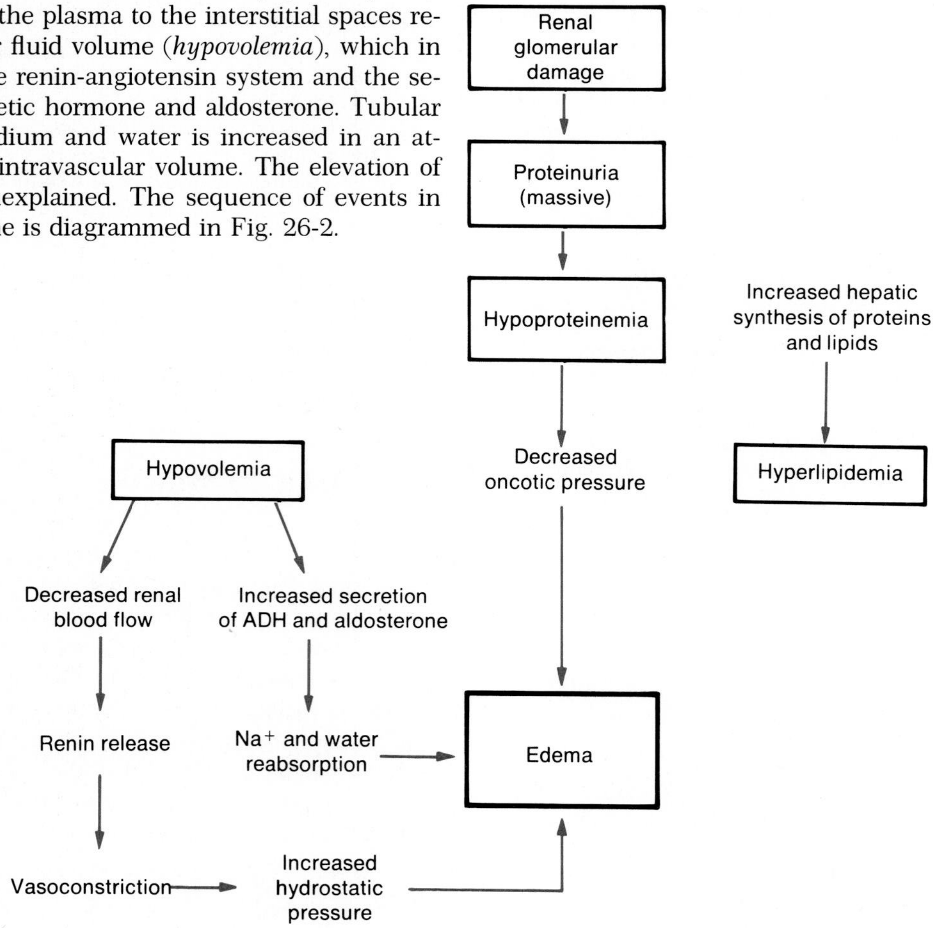

FIG. 26-2 Sequence of events in nephrotic syndrome.

Clinical Manifestations of Nephrotic Syndrome

- Weight gain
- Edema
- Puffiness of face
  - Especially around the eyes
  - Apparent on arising in the morning
  - Subsides during the day
- Abdominal swelling (ascites)
- Respiratory difficulty (pleural effusion)
- Labial or scrotal swelling
- Edema of intestinal mucosal causes:
  - Diarrhea
  - Anorexia
  - Poor intestinal absorption
- Extreme skin pallor (often)
- Irritability
- Easily fatigued
- Lethargic
- Blood pressure normal or slightly decreased
- Susceptibility to infection
- Urine alterations:
  - Decreased volume
  - Darkly opalescent
  - Frothy

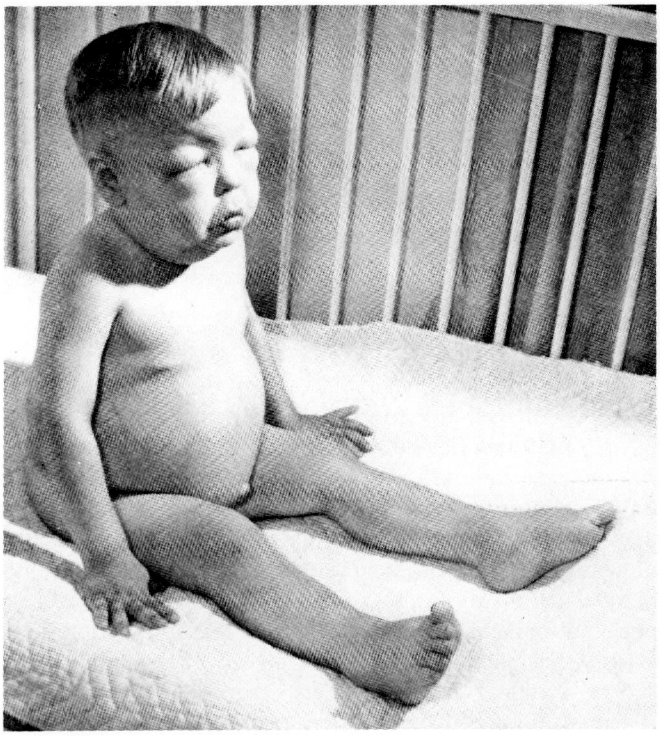

FIG. 26-3 Child with nephrotic syndrome. (From Benz, G.S.: Pediatric nursing, ed. 5, St. Louis, 1964, The C.V. Mosby Co. Courtesy University of Minnesota Photographic Laboratory.)

are usually normal or even elevated as a result of hemoconcentration. Serum sodium concentration is usually low.

Renal biopsy and the appearance of renal tissue under the light and electron microscope provide information regarding the glomerular status and type of nephrotic syndrome, response to drugs, and probable course of the disease. Under the microscope the foot processes of the basement membrane appear fused.

Therapeutic Management

The medical management consists of both general and specific measures. Children with severe symptoms or whose disease is newly recognized are hospitalized for assessment and observation for evidence of infection and response to therapy. During the edema phase the child is often placed on bed rest, but activity is not restricted during remission. Acute and intercurrent infections are treated with appropriate antibiotics, and efforts are made to eliminate possible infection.

The child who is in remission is allowed a regular diet; however, during periods of massive edema, salt is restricted. This is usually tolerated by the child for a time, but it should be adjusted to the child's appetite and must not interfere with nutrient intake. Although edema cannot be removed by a low-sodium diet, its rate of increase may be reduced. Water is seldom restricted (Kim and Grupe, 1986).

Oral corticosteroid (prednisone) therapy is begun as soon as the diagnosis has been established and the course of the disease is fairly predictable. There is little change during the first few days of therapy. In most patients diuresis occurs, urine protein excretion disappears within 7 to 21 days, and other clinical manifestations stabilize or return to normal. In 90% of patients urine returns to normal within 4 weeks; in many patients this occurs as early as 3 or 4 days. After a satisfactory response the dose is tapered gradually, then discontinued.

Most children with nephrotic syndrome have this favorable prognosis. However, children who require frequent courses of steroid therapy are highly susceptible to complications of steroids, such as growth retardation, hypertension, gastrointestinal bleeding, Cushing syndrome, bone demineralization, infections, and diabetes mellitus. Children who do not respond to steroid therapy, children who have frequent relapses, and those in whom the side effects threaten their growth and general health are considered for a course of immunosuppressant drug therapy with an oral alkylating agent, usually cyclophosphamide (Cytoxan), alternating with prednisone. Both drugs are administered for up to 2 months, after which cyclophosphamide is discontinued abruptly and the prednisone is decreased gradually.

One characteristic of the edema of nephrotic syndrome is its usual lack of responsiveness to diuretic agents. Also, the increased susceptibility to infection during the edematous phase of the disease and the lowered resistance associated with corticosteroid therapy are a constant hazard. Therefore a broad-spectrum antimicrobial agent is often administered in an effort to reduce the risk of infection until the initial phase of treatment is completed and the child is receiving reduced dosages of corticosteroids.

Nursing Considerations

Whether nephrotic syndrome occurs as an initial disorder, a recurrent health problem, or a complication of another disorder, the affected child presents a nursing challenge.

ASSESSMENT

Continuous monitoring of fluid retention or excretion is an important nursing function. Strict intake and output records are essential but may be difficult to obtain from very young children. Application of collection bags is highly irritating to sensitive skin that is readily subject to breakdown. Application of diapers or weighing wet pads may be necessary. Other methods of monitoring progress include urine examination for specific gravity and albumin and measurement of daily weight and abdominal girth. Assessment of edema, such as increased or decreased swelling around the eyes and dependent areas, degree of pitting (if noted), and color and texture of skin are part of nursing care. Vital signs are monitored to detect any early signs of complications such as shock or an infective process.

NURSING DIAGNOSES

Constant reassessment and evaluation reveal a number of nursing diagnoses that are relevant to the care of these children and their families (see Nursing Care Plan, pp. 869-870). Others will be apparent in specific situations.

PLANNING

The goals of nursing care of the child with nephrotic syndrome are:

1. Reduce the excretion of urinary protein and maintain a protein-free urine
2. Prevent infection
3. Establish and maintain good nutrition
4. Support and educate child and family

IMPLEMENTATION

Children hospitalized with nephrotic syndrome are placed on bed rest during the edema phase of the disease. They seldom offer resistance since they are usually lethargic and easily fatigued, and their cumbersome edematous bulk is not conducive to movement.

Reducing the excretion of urinary protein primarily involves the administration of corticosteroids. Nurses must be aware of the problems associated with these drugs and be alert to complications from their use.

Infection is a constant source of danger to edematous children and those on corticosteroid therapy. These children are particularly vulnerable to upper respiratory infection; therefore, they must be kept warm and dry, and protected from contact with infected roommates, visitors, and personnel. Vital signs are monitored to detect any early signs of an infective process. Most children are content to lie in the prone position and must be encouraged and helped to turn regularly to prevent tissue breakdown. Areas that are particularly edematous, such as the scrotum, abdomen, and legs, may require support, and skin surfaces should be cleaned and separated with clothing, cotton, or antiseptic powder to prevent intertrigo.

Loss of appetite accompanying active nephrosis creates a perplexing problem for nurses. During this time the combined efforts of nurse, dietitian, parents, and the child are needed to formulate a nutritionally adequate and attractive diet. Salt is usually restricted (but not eliminated) during the edema phase, and fluid restriction (if prescribed) is limited to short-term use during massive edema. A generous protein intake is highly desirable to minimize negative nitrogen balance but is poorly accepted by most children. Every effort should be made to serve attractive meals with preferred foods and a minimum of fuss, but it usually requires a considerable amount of ingenuity and enticement to get the child to eat (see the discussion on Feeding the sick child on p. 640).

As the edema subsides, children are allowed increased activity, which is desirable in order to prevent bone demineralization from immobilization and corticosteroid administration. Although easily fatigued, children usually adjust activities according to their tolerance level. However, they may require guidance in selecting play activities. Suitable recreational and diversional activities are an important part of their care. Once edema fluid has been lost, children are allowed to resume their usual activities with discretion. Irritability and mood swings that accompany the inactivity, disease process, and steroid therapy are not unusual manifestations in these children, and they create an additional challenge to the nurse and the family.

Family support and home care. Continuous support of the child and family is one of the major nursing considerations. Parents are taught to detect signs of relapse and to bring the child for treatment at the earliest indications. Unless the edema and proteinuria are severe or the parents, for some reason, are unable to care for the ill child, home care is preferred. Parents are instructed in testing urine for albumin, administration of medications, diet restrictions (if any), and the common effects of steroid therapy. Parents are also instructed regarding avoiding contact with infected playmates, but the child is permitted to attend school.

The prolonged course of the relapsing form of nephrotic syndrome is taxing to both the child and the family. The up-and-down course of remissions and exacerbations with periodic disruption of family life by hospitalization places a severe strain on the child and the family, both psychologically and financially. Parents and children over 5 or 6 years of age need reassurance regarding this

NURSING CARE PLAN

The Child with Nephrotic Syndrome

Nursing Goals	Nursing Interventions	Expected Patient/Family Outcomes
HP-HMP* **Potential for infection** **Risk factors: lowered body defenses**		
Prevent and control acute infection	Protect child from contact with infected persons Observe medical asepsis Keep child dry and warm Monitor vital signs for early signs of infectious processes Collect specimens, such as urine for culture, blood	Child displays no evidence of infection
N-MP **Potential (intravascular) fluid volume deficit** **Etiology: protein and fluid loss, edema**		
Detect evidence of intravascular fluid loss	Monitor vital signs to detect physical signs Assess pulse quality and rate Take blood pressure Report deviations	Child displays no evidence of hypovolemic shock †Deviations from baseline findings are detected and appropriate interventions are initiated (specify parameters) (see inside front cover for normal variations in vital signs)
N-MP **Fluid volume excess (total body)** **Etiology: impaired renal excretion of water**		
Detect evidence of fluid retention	Assess intake relative to output Measure and record intake and output accurately Weigh daily (or more often if needed) Assess changes in edema Measure abdominal girth at umbilicus Test urine for specific gravity, albumin Collect specimens for laboratory examination	†Child's intake and output are recorded and evaluated Child exhibits no evidence of increased edema (specify parameters)
Prevent fluid retention	Limit fluids as indicated	Child displays no evidence of increased fluid accumulation (specify parameters)
N-MP **Altered nutrition: less than body requirements** **Etiology: loss of appetite**		
Provide good nutrition Stimulate appetite	Offer high-protein, high-carbohydrate diet (restrict sodium during edema) Enlist aid of child, parents, and dietitian in formulation of diet Provide cheerful, clean, relaxed atmosphere during meals Serve small quantities initially to stimulate appetite; encourage seconds Provide special and preferred foods Serve foods in an attractive manner (see p. 640 for Feeding the sick child)	Child consumes an adequate diet (specify amounts)
N-MP **Potential impaired skin integrity** **Risk factors: edema, lowered body defenses**		
Prevent skin breakdown	Provide meticulous skin care Cleanse and powder opposing skin surfaces several times per day Separate opposing skin surfaces with soft cotton Support edematous organs, such as scrotum Cleanse edematous eyelids with warm saline wipes Change position frequently; maintain good body alignment	Skin displays no evidence of redness or irritation

*For an explanation of abbreviations, see p. 20.
†Nursing outcome.

Continued.

NURSING CARE PLAN

The Child with Nephrotic Syndrome—cont'd

Nursing Goals	Nursing Interventions	Expected Patient/Family Outcomes
NDx A-EP Activity intolerance **Etiology: bed rest, fatigue**		
Conserve energy	Maintain bed rest initially Balance rest and activity when ambulatory Plan and provide quiet activities Instruct child to rest when he begins to feel tired	Child engages in activities appropriate to his capabilities
NDx RRP Altered family processes **Etiology: situational crisis (child with a serious illness)**		
Support family	Listen to family Assist family with problem solving Provide education when indicated Provide positive feedback Refer to parent groups See also The child in the hospital, p. 603; Family of the hospitalized child, p. 610	Family members discuss their feelings and anxieties
Prepare family for home care	Instruct family Testing urine for albumin daily Administration of medications Initial signs of relapse Side effects of drugs Prevention of infection Impress on family importance of following prescribed regimen	Family conveys an understanding of the instructions; repeats instructions; demonstrates procedures (specify)
Encourage follow-up care	Maintain contact with family Refer to appropriate persons or agencies for assistance	Family complies with instructions (specify)

Nursing interventions related to medical management

Assist with diagnosis
- Collect specimens as needed
- Assist with diagnostic procedures

Control edema
- Provide salt-restricted diet
- Administer steroids (if prescribed as ordered)
- Administer diuretics if ordered
- Administer salt-poor albumin intravenous infusion if ordered
- Limit intake, if ordered

Ensure adequate nutrition
- Administer supplementary vitamins and iron as ordered

characteristic of the course of the disease, with emphasis on the importance of long-term care to gain their cooperation. A satisfactory response is more likely when relapses are detected and therapy is instituted early, and remissions are prolonged when instructions are carried out faithfully.

EVALUATION

The effectiveness of nursing interventions is determined by continual reassessment and evaluation of care based on the following observational guidelines and expected outcomes:

1. Measure intake and output and examine urine for albumin
2. Monitor vital signs and assess skin for evidence of infection
3. Assess appetite and eating behaviors
4. Observe and interview child and family regarding their understanding of the disease, therapies, and compliance with prescribed regimen

Expected outcomes:
See Nursing Care Plan on pp. 869 to 870.

ACUTE GLOMERULONEPHRITIS

Acute glomerulonephritis (AGN) may be a primary event or a manifestation of a systemic disorder that can range from minimal to severe. Most cases are postinfectious and have been associated with pneumococcal, streptococcal, and viral infections. *Acute poststreptococcal glomerulonephritis (APSGN)* is the most common of the noninfectious renal diseases in childhood and the one for which a cause can be established in the majority of cases. APSGN can occur at any age but affects primarily early school-age children with a peak age of onset of 6 to 7 years. It is uncommon in children younger than 2 years of age, and males outnumber females 2:1 (Jordan and Lemire, 1982).

Etiology

It is now generally accepted that acute glomerulonephritis is caused by a reaction to streptococcal infection with certain strains of the group A β-hemolytic *Streptococcus* with a period of 10 to 14 days between the streptococcal infection and the onset of clinical manifestations. The peak incidence of disease is in the school-age years and corresponds to the incidence of streptococcal infections. Disease secondary to streptococcal pharyngitis is more common in the winter or spring, but, when associated with pyoderma (principally impetigo), it may be more prevalent in later summer or early fall, especially in warmer climates.

Pathophysiology

In the inflammatory process that follows a streptococcal infection, the glomeruli become edematous and infiltrated with polymorphonuclear leukocytes, which occlude the capillary lumen. The resulting decrease in plasma filtration results in an excessive accumulation of water and retention of sodium that expands plasma and interstitial fluid volumes, leading to circulatory congestion and edema. It is unclear whether the decreased glomerular filtration rate, increased capillary permeability, or vascular spasm is responsible for these various manifestations. The cause of the hypertension associated with acute glomerulonephritis is also unexplained.

Diagnostic Evaluation

Typically, affected children are in good health until they experience the streptococcal infection. In some instances there is no history of an infection, or it is only described as a mild cold. The onset of nephritis appears after an average latent period of about 10 days (see box). Since the child appears to be well during this time, the association is not recognized by parents. The edema is relatively moderate and may not be appreciated by someone unfamiliar with the child's normal appearance.

Urinalysis during the acute phase characteristically shows hematuria, proteinuria, and increased specific gravity. The specific gravity is moderately elevated and seldom exceeds 1.02. Proteinuria generally parallels the hematuria, and the content usually shows 3+ or 4+ but is not the massive proteinuria seen in nephrotic syndrome. Gross discoloration of urine reflects its red blood cell and hemoglobin content. Microscopic examination of the sediment shows many red blood cells, leukocytes, epithelial cells, and casts, primarily composed of epithelial and red blood cells. Bacteria are not seen, and urine cultures are negative.

Clinical Manifestations of Acute Poststreptococcal Glomerulonephritis

- Edema
  - Especially periorbital
  - Facial edema more prominent in the morning
  - Spreads during the day to involve extremities and abdomen
- Anorexia
- Urine
  - Cloudy, smoky brown (resembles tea or cola)
  - Severely reduced volume
- Pallor
- Irritability
- Lethargy
- Child appears ill
- Child seldom expresses specific complaints
- Older children may complain
  - Headaches
  - Abdominal discomfort
  - Dysuria
- Vomiting not uncommon
- Mild to moderately elevated blood pressure

Azotemia that results from impaired glomerular filtration is reflected in elevated blood urea nitrogen and creatinine levels in at least 50% of cases. When proteinuria is heavy, there may be changes associated with nephrotic syndrome, that is, transient hypoproteinemia and hyperlipidemia.

Cultures of the pharynx are positive for streptococci in only a few cases, and the numbers are not significantly greater than the normal carrier incidence in many communities. Positive cultures help to establish a diagnosis. Cultures should be obtained from other household members, and persons positive for group A streptococci should receive a course of antistreptococcal therapy.

Some serologic tests may help in the diagnosis of acute glomerulonephritis. The antistreptolysin O (ASO) titer is the most familiar and readily available test for streptococcal infection. It is used to detect the presence of antibodies, which documents a recent infection, especially a rising titer in two samples taken a week apart. Other serologic tests that may aid in diagnosis following streptococcal skin infections are elevated antihyaluronidase (AHase), antideoxyribonuclease B (ADNase-B), and antinicotyladenine dinucleotidase (ANADase) titers.

Since AGN is an immune-complex disease, there is reduced total serum complement activity in the early stages of the disease. Nonspecific acute-phase reactants that reflect acute inflammatory processes, such as the erythrocyte sedimentation rate (ESR), C-reactive protein (CRP), and serum mucoprotein tests, are elevated during the early stages of acute disease and then gradually return to normal as healing takes place. The erythrocyte sedimentation rate is sometimes used as a guide to the progress of the nephritis.

Therapeutic Management

There is no specific treatment for acute glomerulonephritis, and recovery is spontaneous and uneventful in most cases. Bed rest is recommended during the acute phase, but ambulation does not seem to have an adverse effect on the course of the disease once the gross hematuria, edema, hypertension, and azotemia have abated. After diuresis has occurred, ambulation is allowed for those children without hypertension and gross urine abnormalities.

Regular measurement of vital signs, body weight, and intake and output is essential in order to monitor the progress of the disease and to detect complications that may appear at any time during the course of the disease. A record of daily weight is the most useful means to assess fluid balance and is kept for children treated at home as well as for those who are hospitalized. Water restriction is seldom necessary unless the output is significantly reduced.

Dietary restrictions depend on the severity of the edema. A regular diet is permitted in uncomplicated cases, but the intake of sodium is usually limited (no salt is added to foods). Moderate sodium restriction is usually instituted for children with hypertension or edema. Severe sodium restriction is not tolerated well by children and may interfere with caloric intake in these already anorexic youngsters. Foods with substantial amounts of potassium are generally restricted during the period of oliguria. Protein restriction is reserved only for patients with severe azotemia resulting from prolonged oliguria. The anorexia associated with the disease usually limits the protein intake sufficiently.

Antibiotic therapy is indicated only for those children with evidence of persistent streptococcal infections. Significant hypertension is controlled with hydralazine (Apresoline), usually in conjunction with reserpine or furosemide (Lasix). Oral hydrochlorothiazide is used to control mild hypertension, and seizure activity associated with hypertensive encephalopathy requires anticonvulsant therapy.

Nursing Considerations

Nursing care of the child with glomerulonephritis involves careful assessment of the disease status, with regular monitoring of vital signs (including blood pressure), fluid balance, and behavior.

ASSESSMENT

Vital signs provide clues to the severity of the disease and early signs of complications. They are carefully measured, and any deviations are reported and recorded. The volume and character of urine are noted, and the child is weighed daily. Children on restricted fluids, especially those who are not severely edematous or those who have lost weight, are observed for signs of dehydration.

Assessment of the child's appearance for signs of cerebral complications is an important nursing function, since the severity of the acute phase is variable and unpredictable. The child with edema, hypertension, and gross hematuria may be subject to complications, and anticipatory preparations such as seizure precautions and intravenous equipment are included in the nursing care plan.

Nursing Diagnoses: The Child with Acute Glomerulonephritis

Fluid volume excess related to decreased plasma filtration
Activity intolerance related to fatigue
Altered patterns of urinary elimination related to fluid retention and impaired glomerular filtration
Altered family processes related to the child with a renal disorder

NURSING DIAGNOSES

Based on assessment several nursing diagnoses become obvious (see box). Others may be evident in specific situations.

PLANNING

The goals of nursing care for the child with acute glomerulonephritis include the following:

1. Promote rest
2. Provide nutrition and promote appetite
3. Prevent and/observe for complications
4. Support and educate child and family

IMPLEMENTATION

During the acute phase children are generally quite content to lie in bed. Activities should be those that require little expenditure of energy. Since they are generally listless and experience fatigue and malaise, most children voluntarily restrict their activities during the most active phase of the disease. As they begin to feel better and as their symptoms subside, activities are planned to allow for frequent rest periods and avoidance of fatigue.

For most children a regular diet is allowed, but it should contain no added salt. Foods high in sodium and salted treats are eliminated, and parents and friends are advised not to bring items such as potato chips or pretzels. However, the total amount of salt ingested is usually less than prescribed because of the child's poor appetite. Fluid restriction, if included in care, is more difficult, and the amount permitted is evenly divided throughout the waking hours and served in small cups to give the illusion of larger servings. Meal preparation and service require special attention, since the child is indifferent to meals during the acute phase. Again, collaboration with parents and the dietitian and special consideration for food preferences facilitate meal planning.

Children who have mild edema and no hypertension and convalescent children who are being treated at home need follow-up care. Parents are instructed regarding general measures, including activity, diet, and prevention of infection. The children are permitted to be ambulatory but should not attend school or participate in outside games and sports until the risk of complications has passed. Strenuous activity is usually restricted until there is no microscopic evidence of proteinuria or hematuria, which may persist for months.

Health supervision is continued with weekly, followed by monthly, visits for evaluation and urinalysis. Parent education and support in preparation for discharge and home care include education in home management and the need for follow-up care and health supervision.

EVALUATION

The effectiveness of nursing interventions is determined by continual reassessment and evaluation of care based on the following observational guidelines and expected outcomes:

1. Observe child's behavior
2. Monitor dietary and fluid intake; interview family regarding child's diet and appetite
3. Monitor vital signs, intake and output, and observe for signs of complications, such as hypertension, increased intracranial pressure, infection
4. Observe behaviors and interview child and family regarding reaction to the disease and therapies

Expected outcomes:

1. Child plays and rests quietly
2. Child consumes a sufficient amount of appropriate foods
3. Child exhibits no evidence of complications
4. Child and family demonstrate an understanding of the disease and its therapy (specify learnings and methods of demonstration), and they express their feelings and concerns

◆ *Miscellaneous Renal Disorders*

Renal damage occurs as a major or minor complication in many systemic diseases and with varying degrees of severity. In some the renal complications may be the principal cause of death or one of several complications with fatal consequences. In others it may be only a source of discomfort but no direct threat to life.

HEMOLYTIC-UREMIC SYNDROME

Hemolytic-uremic syndrome (HUS) is an uncommon, acute renal disease that occurs primarily in infants and small children between the ages of 6 months and 3 years. It occurs worldwide but is recognized predominantly in white children. Although uncommon, hemolytic-uremic syndrome represents one of the most frequent causes of acute renal failure in children.

In the majority of cases no causative agents have been identified; however, many possible agents or precipitating events have been implicated. These include genetic factors, specific enzyme deficiencies, endotoxins, and reduced platelet aggregation. The appearance of the disease has been associated with rickettsial, viral, pneumococcal, and gastrointestinal disorders. The disease usually follows an acute gastrointestinal or upper respiratory infection and tends to occur in scattered outbreaks in small geographic areas.

Pathophysiology

The primary site of injury appears to be the endothelial lining of the small glomerular arterioles, which become swollen and occluded with deposits of platelets and fibrin clots. Red cells are damaged as they attempt to move through the partially occluded blood vessels. These damaged cells are removed by the spleen, causing acute hemolytic anemia. The platelet aggregation within the damaged blood vessels or the damage and removal of platelets produce the characteristic thrombocytopenia.

Diagnostic Evaluation

The presence of anemia, thrombocytopenia, and renal failure is sufficient for diagnosis (see box). Renal involvement is evidenced by proteinuria, hematuria, and the presence of urinary casts; blood urea nitrogen and serum creatinine levels are elevated. A high reticulocyte count confirms the hemolytic nature of the anemia.

Therapeutic Management

The goals of therapy are early diagnosis and aggressive, supportive care of the acute renal failure and hemolytic

Clinical Manifestations of Hemolytic Uremic Syndrome

Anorexia
Irritability
Lethargy
Marked pallor
Hemorrhagic manifestations:
- Bruising
- Purpura
- Rectal bleeding

Oliguria or anuria (usually)
Central nervous system involvement:
- Convulsions
- Stupor

Signs of acute heart failure (sometimes)

anemia. The most consistently effective treatment of hemolytic-uremic syndrome is peritoneal dialysis, which is instituted in any child who has been anuric for 24 hours or who demonstrates oliguria with hypertension and seizures. Blood transfusions with fresh, washed packed cells are administered for severe anemia but are used with caution to prevent circulatory overload from added volume.

There is no substantial evidence that heparin, corticosteroids, or fibrinolytic agents are beneficial. With prompt treatment the recovery rate is about 95%, but there may be residual renal impairment. Renal impairment or central nervous system injury are the usual causes of death.

Nursing Considerations

Nursing care is the same as that provided in acute renal failure and, for children with continued impairment, includes management of chronic disease.

Clinical Manifestations of Wilms Tumor

Abdominal swelling or mass
- Firm
- Nontender
- Does not extend beyond midline

Hematuria (less than 1/4 of cases)
Anemia secondary to hemorrhage within the tumor
- Pallor
- Anorexia
- Lethargy

Hypertension (occasionally)
Weight loss
Fever
Manifestations resulting from compression of tumor mass
Secondary metabolic alterations from tumor or metastasis
If metastasis, symptoms of lung involvement:
- Dyspnea
- Cough
- Shortness of breath
- Chest pain (sometimes)

WILMS TUMOR

Wilms tumor, or nephroblastoma, is the most frequent intraabdominal tumor of childhood and accounts for almost all renal neoplasms. Its frequency is estimated to be 7.8 per million children less that 15 years of age, and occurs with approximately equal frequency in boys and girls (Leventhal, 1987).

Etiology

Wilms tumor probably arises from a malignant, undifferentiated cluster of primordial cells capable of initiating the regeneration of an abnormal structure. Its occurrence slightly favors the left kidney, which is advantageous because surgically this kidney is easier to manipulate and remove. In about 10% of the cases both kidneys are involved. Although the tumor may become quite large, it remains encapsulated for an extended period of time. There is a hereditary element in some tumors, especially those that are associated with congenital anomalies.

Diagnostic Evaluation

Parents usually first discover the mass while bathing or dressing the child. Abdominal masses vary greatly in size. On palpation of the abdomen, if the tumor is on the right side, it may be difficult to distinguish from the liver, although, unlike that organ, it does not move with respiration (see box for clinical manifestations).

The usual tests include ultrasound (if available) and computed tomography of abdomen and chest. A complete blood count and peripheral smear are done preoperatively to evaluate the degree of anemia, especially in terms of increasing surgical risks. Liver function tests may be performed to assess liver dysfunction from metastasis or any preexisting abnormality that may alter antineoplastic drug metabolism and excretion. Renal function tests determine function of the unaffected kidney.

Therapeutic Management

Excellent survival rates for children with Wilms tumor have been the result of optimum treatment protocols, including surgery, radiation, and chemotherapy. Combined treatment of surgery and chemotherapy with or without radiation is based on the clinical stage and histologic pattern.

Surgery is scheduled as soon as possible after confirmation of a renal mass, usually within 24 to 48 hours after admission. A large transabdominal incision is performed for optimum visualization of the abdominal cavity. The tumor, affected kidney, and adjacent adrenal gland are removed. Great care is taken to keep the encapsulated tumor intact, since rupture can seed cancer cells throughout the abdomen, lymph channel, and bloodstream. The contralateral kidney is carefully inspected for evidence of disease or dysfunction. Regional lymph nodes are inspected and a biopsy is performed when indicated. Any involved structures, such as part of the colon, diaphragm, or vena cava, are removed. Metal clips are placed around the tumor site for exact marking during radiotherapy.

If both kidneys are involved, a partial nephrectomy is performed on the less affected kidney, with a total nephrectomy on the opposite side, and the child is treated with radiotherapy and chemotherapy. When a transplant is feasible, such as from a twin, sibling, or parent, bilateral nephrectomy is considered.

Postoperative radiotherapy is indicated for all children with Wilms tumor except those with stage I disease and favorable histology. Chemotherapy is indicated for all stages. The most effective agents for treating Wilms tumor are actinomycin D, vincristine, and adriamycin. Duration of therapy varies, ranging from 6 to 15 months.

Nursing Considerations

Nursing care of the child with Wilms tumor is similar to that of other cancers treated with surgery, irradiation, and chemotherapy. However, there are some significant differences; these are discussed for each phase of nursing intervention.

Preoperative care. The preoperative period is one of swift diagnosis. Typically surgery is scheduled within 24 to 48 hours of admission. The nurse is faced with the challenge of preparing the child and parents for all laboratory and operative procedures. Because of the little time available, explanations are kept simple and they are repeated often.

There are several special preoperative concerns, the most important of which is that the tumor is not palpated unless absolutely necessary because manipulation of the mass may cause dissemination of cancer cells to adjacent and distant sites. In teaching hospitals in which many medical and nursing students are assigned to one patient, it may be necessary to post a sign on the bed, such as, *Do not palpate abdomen.* This same precaution is extended to parents as soon as Wilms tumor is suspected. Careful bathing and handling are also important in preventing trauma to the tumor site.

Children and parents need preparation for the size of the incision and dressing. An extensive abdominal incision is required to adequately view the internal organs. Postoperatively a large dressing and retention sutures are in place. If the child is unprepared, he may become upset and angry when he sees the surgical area.

In addition to the usual preoperative observations, the nurse carefully monitors blood pressure, since hypertension from excess renin production is a possibility. This is particularly important in young children in whom improperly sized blood pressure cuffs can yield inaccurate readings.

Postoperative care. Despite the extensive surgical intervention necessary in many children with Wilms tumor, the recovery is usually rapid. The major nursing responsibilities are the same as those following any abdominal surgery (see The child undergoing surgery on p. 630). Since these children are at risk for intestinal obstruction from vincristine-induced adynamic ileus, radiation-induced edema, and postsurgical adhesion formation, gastrointestinal activity, such as bowel movements, bowel sounds, distention, vomiting, and pain are carefully monitored.

The nurse also monitors blood pressure for a possible drop after removal of the tumor, urinary output to assess functioning of the remaining kidney, and signs of infection, especially during chemotherapy. Because of the myelosuppression from the drugs, pulmonary hygiene measures are instituted in the immediate postoperative period to prevent lung involvement.

Family support. The postoperative period is frequently difficult for parents. The shock of seeing their child immediately after surgery may be the first realization of the seriousness of the diagnosis. It also marks the confirmation of the stage of the tumor. Again, during this period, the nurse should be with the parents to assure them of the child's recovery after surgery and to assess the parents' understanding of the operative report. They need an opportunity to express their feelings and to realize that they are normal and realistic. The same emotional care discussed in Chapter 18 for families who have a child with a life-threatening disorder is applied to these individuals.

Older children need an opportunity to deal with their feelings concerning the many procedures to which they have been subjected in rapid succession. Play therapy with dolls or puppets or through drawing can be extremely beneficial in helping them adjust to the surgery and hair loss. It is not unusual for children to feel betrayed because they were not adequately prepared for the extent of surgery, the need for additional therapy, or the seriousness of the disorder.

The overall objective in discharge planning is returning the child to his normal preoperative life-style. The nurse emphasizes the usual needs for discipline and moderate protection from infection. Treatment schedules are planned to allow uninterrupted school attendance.

◆ *Renal Failure*

Renal failure is the inability of the kidneys to excrete wastes, concentrate urine, and conserve electrolytes. It can occur suddenly (acute renal failure) in response to inadequate perfusion, kidney disease, or urinary tract obstruction, or it can develop slowly (chronic renal failure) as the result of long-standing kidney disease.

The terms *azotemia* and *uremia* are often used in relation to renal failure. Azotemia is the accumulation of nitrogenous waste within the blood. Uremia is a more advanced condition in which retention of nitrogenous products produces toxic symptoms. Azotemia is not life threatening, whereas uremia is a serious condition that often involves other body systems.

ACUTE RENAL FAILURE

Acute renal failure (ARF) is said to exist when the kidneys suddenly are unable to regulate the volume and composition of urine appropriately in response to food and fluid intake and the needs of the organism. The principal feature of ARF is oliguria* associated with azotemia, acidosis, and diverse electrolyte disturbances. Acute renal failure is not common in childhood, but the outcome depends on the cause, associated findings, and prompt recognition and treatment.

*The definition of oliguria varies extensively in the literature, from 100 to 400 $ml/m^2/24$ hours.

The pathologic conditions that produce acute renal failure caused by glomerulonephritis and hemolytic-uremic syndrome have been discussed in relation to those diseases. Acute renal failure can also develop as a result of a large number of related or unrelated clinical conditions—poor renal perfusion, acute renal injury, or the final expression of chronic, irreversible renal disease. The most common cause in children is transient renal failure resulting from dehydration or other causes of poor perfusion that responds to restoration of fluid volume.

Pathophysiology

ARF is usually reversible, but the deviations of physiologic function can be extreme and mortality in the pediatric age-group is still high. There is severe reduction in the glomerular filtration rate, an elevated blood urea nitrogen level, and a significant reduction in renal blood flow.

The clinical course is variable and depends on the cause. In reversible acute renal failure there is a period of severe oliguria, or a low-output phase, followed by an abrupt onset of diuresis, or a high-output phase, then a gradual return to, or toward, normal urine volumes.

Diagnostic Evaluation

In many instances of acute renal failure the infant or child is already critically ill with the precipitating disorder and the explanation for development of oliguria is readily apparent (see box). When a previously healthy child develops acute renal failure without obvious cause, a careful history is taken to reveal symptoms that may be related to disorders of the urinary tract or regarding exposure to nephrotoxic chemicals, such as ingestion of heavy metals, inhalation of carbon tetrachloride or other organic solvents, or drugs known to be toxic to kidneys. Significant laboratory measurements that are elevated during renal shutdown and that serve as a guide for therapy are blood urea nitrogen and serum creatinine, pH, sodium, potassium, and calcium.

Clinical Manifestations of Acute Renal Failure

Specific:
- Oliguria
- Anuria uncommon (except in obstructive disorders)

Non-specific (may develop):
- Nausea
- Vomiting
- Drowsiness
- Edema
- Hypertension

Manifestations of underlying disorder or pathology

Therapeutic Management

Treatment of acute renal failure is directed toward (1) treatment of the underlying cause, (2) management of the complications of renal failure, and (3) provision of supportive therapy within the constraints imposed by the renal failure.

Treatment of poor perfusion resulting from dehydration consists of volume restoration as described previously in treatment of dehydration. If oliguria persists after restoration of fluid volume or if the renal failure is caused by intrinsic renal damage, the physiologic and biochemical abnormalities that have resulted from kidney dysfunction must be corrected or controlled.

Initially a Foley catheter is inserted to rule out urine retention, to collect available urine for analysis, and to monitor results of mannitol or furosemide administration. The catheter may or may not be removed. Many authorities who believe that it serves little purpose during the oliguric phase and that it predisposes the bladder to infection prefer collection bags for measuring urine output. Others maintain a catheter for hourly urine measurements.

The amount of exogenous water provided should not exceed the amount needed to maintain zero water balance. It is calculated on the basis of estimated endogenous water formation and losses from sensible (primarily gastrointestinal) and insensible sources. No allotment is calculated for urine as long as oliguria persists.

When the output begins to increase, either spontaneously or in response to diuretic therapy, the intake of fluid, potassium, and sodium must be monitored and adequate replacement provided to prevent depletion and its consequences. In some cases enormous amounts of electrolyte-rich urine are passed.

Complications of ARF. The child with acute renal failure has a tendency to develop water intoxication and hyponatremia, which make it difficult to provide calories in sufficient amounts to meet the needs of the child and reduce the tissue catabolism, metabolic acidosis, hyperkalemia, and uremia. If the child is able to tolerate oral foods, concentrated food sources high in carbohydrate and fat but low in protein, potassium, and sodium may be provided. However, many children have functional disturbances of the gastrointestinal tract, such as nausea and vomiting; therefore, the intravenous route is generally preferred and usually consists of highly concentrated carbohydrate solutions in small volumes of water administered by the central venous route.

Control of water balance in these patients requires careful monitoring of feedback information, such as accurate intake and output, body weight, and electrolyte measurements. In general, during the oliguric phase, no sodium, chloride, or potassium is given unless there are other large ongoing losses. Regular measurement of plasma electrolyte, pH, blood urea nitrogen, and creatinine levels is required to assess the adequacy of fluid therapy and to anticipate complications that require specific treatment.

Hyperkalemia is the most immediate threat to the life of the child with acute renal failure. Hyperkalemia can be minimized and sometimes avoided by eliminating potassium from all food and fluid, by reducing tissue catabolism, and by correcting acidosis. Measures employed for the reduction of serum potassium levels are oral or rectal administration of an ion-exchange resin such as sodium polystyrene sulfonate (Kayexalate) and peritoneal dialysis or hemodialysis. The resin produces its effect by exchange of its sodium for the potassium, thus binding potassium for removal from the body. Dialysis removes potassium and other waste products from the serum by diffusion through a semipermeable membrane.

Hypertension is a frequent and serious complication of ARF, and, to detect it early, blood pressure measurements are made every 4 to 6 hours. The most common cause of hypertension in ARF is overexpansion of extracellular fluid and plasma volume together with hypersecretion of renin. Hypertension is controlled with antihypertensive drugs singly or in combination. Other measures that may be used are limiting fluids and salt.

Anemia is frequently associated with acute renal failure, but transfusion is not recommended unless the hemoglobin drops below 6 g/100 ml. Transfusions, if used, consist of fresh, packed red blood cells given slowly to reduce the likelihood of increasing blood volume, hypertension, and hyperkalemia.

Seizures occur rather often when renal failure progresses to uremia and are also related to hypertension, hyponatremia, and hypocalcemia. Treatment is directed to the specific cause, when it is known. More obscure causes are managed with anticonvulsant drugs.

Cardiac failure with pulmonary edema is almost always associated with hypervolemia. Treatment is directed toward reduction of fluid volume, with water and sodium restriction and administration of diuretics.

Outcome. The prognosis of ARF depends largely on the nature and severity of the causative factor or precipitating event and the promptness and competence of management. The outcome is least favorable in children with rapidly progressive nephritis and cortical necrosis. Children in whom ARF is a result of hemolytic-uremic syndrome or acute glomerulitis may recover completely, but residual renal impairment or hypertension is more often the rule. Complete recovery is usually expected in children whose renal failure is a result of dehydration, nephrotoxins, or ischemia.

Nursing Considerations

Nursing care of the infant or child with acute renal failure supports medical care and management. The probability of dialysis must be considered and the necessary equipment made available in anticipation of such an eventuality. Because the child requires intensive observation and, often, specialized equipment, he is usually admitted to an intensive care unit in which needed equipment and trained personnel are available.

Nursing Diagnoses: The Child with Acute Renal Failure

A. Fluid volume excess related to failure of regulatory mechanisms
B. Fluid volume deficit (1) related to active loss
Potential for infection related to diminished body defenses, fluid overload
Altered family processes related to child hospitalized with a serious disorder

ASSESSMENT

Meticulous attention to fluid intake and output is mandatory, including all the physical measurements discussed previously in relation to problems of fluid balance. Monitoring fluid balance and vital signs is a continuous process, and observers are constantly on the alert to recognize signs of complications so that appropriate interventions can be implemented.

NURSING DIAGNOSES

A number of nursing diagnoses are evident following a thorough assessment of the child with ARF (see box). Others will be noted depending on the age of the child, the cause of the renal failure, and any concomitant complications.

PLANNING

The major goals in the care of the child with ARF are to:

1. Monitor fluid and electrolyte status
2. Provide an adequate caloric intake to minimize reduction of protein stores
3. Prevent and/or manage complications
4. Support and educate child and family

IMPLEMENTATION

The major nursing task in the care of the infant or child with ARF is monitoring and assessing fluid and electrolyte balance. Limiting fluid intake requires ingenuity on the part of caregivers to cope with the child who is thirsty. Rationing the daily intake in small amounts of fluid served in containers that give the impression of larger volumes is one strategy. Older children who understand the rationale of fluid limits can help determine how their daily ration should be distributed.

Meeting nutritional needs is sometimes a problem since the child may be nauseated and encouraging concentrated foods without fluids may be difficult. When nourishment is provided by the intravenous route, careful monitoring is essential to prevent fluid overload. In addition, nursing measures, such as maintaining an optimum thermal environment, reducing any elevation of body temperature, and reducing restlessness and anxiety, are employed to decrease the rate of tissue catabolism.

The nurse must be continually alert for changes in behavior that indicate the onset of complications. Infection from reduced resistance, anemia, and general morbidity is a constant threat. Fluid overload and electrolyte disturbances can precipitate cardiovascular complications such as hypertension and cardiac failure. Fluid and electrolyte imbalances, acidosis, and accumulation of nitrogenous waste products can produce neurologic involvement manifest by coma, convulsions, or alterations in sensorium.

Although children with ARF are usually quite ill and voluntarily diminish their activity, infants may become restless and irritable and children are often anxious and frightened. There are frequent, painful, and stress-producing treatments and tests that must be performed. The presence of a supportive, empathetic nurse can provide comfort and stability in a threatening and unnatural environment.

Family support. Providing support and reassurance to parents are among the major nursing responsibilities. The seriousness and emergency nature of acute renal failure are stressful to parents, and most parents feel some degree of guilt regarding the child's condition, especially when the illness is the result of ingestion of a toxic substance, dehydration, or a genetic disease. They need reassurance and a sympathetic listener. They also need to be kept informed of the child's progress and provided explanations regarding the therapeutic regimen. The equipment and the child's behavior are sometimes frightening and anxiety provoking. Nurses can do much to help parents comprehend and deal with the stresses of the situation.

EVALUATION

The effectiveness of nursing interventions is determined by continual reassessment and evaluation of care based on the following observational guidelines and expected outcomes:

1. Carry out frequent assessment of vital signs and behaviors
2. Observe eating behaviors and energy expenditure; monitor intake of protein and calories; carefully monitor intake and output, weigh daily or more often as prescribed
3. Monitor vital signs, sensorium and other neurologic signs; evaluate laboratory results and observe for signs of electrolyte imbalance
4. Observe and interview child and family regarding their understanding of the disease and therapies; encourage child and family to express their feelings and concerns

Expected outcomes:

1. Alterations in vital signs and behavior are detected
2. Child consumes a sufficient amount of appropriate nutrients
3. Evidence of complications is detected early, and appropriate interventions implemented
4. Child and family express their feelings and concerns and demonstrate their understanding of the condition and the therapies (specify knowledge and method of demonstration)

CHRONIC RENAL FAILURE

The kidneys are able to maintain the chemical composition of fluids within normal limits until more than 50% of functional renal capacity is destroyed by disease or injury. Chronic renal insufficiency or failure (CRF) begins when the diseased kidneys can no longer maintain normal chemical structure of body fluids under normal conditions. Progressive deterioration over a period of months or years produces a variety of clinical and biochemical disturbances that eventually culminate in the clinical syndrome known as *uremia*.

A variety of diseases and disorders can result in chronic renal failure. The most frequent causes of CRF are recurrent urinary tract infections, hereditary disorders, chronic pyelonephritis, chronic glomerulonephritis, and glomerulonephropathy associated with systemic diseases such as anaphylactoid purpura and lupus erythematosus. Renal vascular disorders such as hemolytic-uremic syndrome, vascular thrombosis, or cortical necrosis are less frequent causes.

Pathophysiology

Early in the course of progressive nephron destruction the child remains asymptomatic with only minimum biochemical abnormalities. Unless its presence is detected in the process of routine assessment, signs and symptoms that indicate advanced renal damage frequently emerge only late in the course of the disease. Midway in the disease process, as increasing numbers of nephrons are totally destroyed and as most others are damaged in varying degree, the few that remain intact are hypertrophied but functional. These few normal nephrons are able to make sufficient adjustments to maintain reasonable degrees of fluid and electrolyte balance. Definitive biochemical examination at this time will reveal restricted tolerance to excesses or restrictions. As the disease progresses to the terminal stage, because of severe reduction in the number of functioning nephrons, the kidneys are no longer able to maintain fluid and electrolyte balance, and the features of the uremic syndrome appear.

The accumulation of various biochemical substances in the blood, those that result from diminished renal function, produces complications such as:

1. **Retention of waste products,** especially the blood urea nitrogen and creatinine
2. **Water and sodium retention,** which contributes to edema and vascular congestion
3. **Hyperkalemia** of dangerous levels
4. **Metabolic acidosis** of a sustained nature because of continual hydrogen ion retention and bicarbonate loss
5. **Calcium and phosphorus disturbances** resulting in altered bone metabolism, which in turn causes growth ar-

rest or retardation, bone pain, and deformities known as *renal osteodystrophy*

6. **Anemia** caused by hematologic dysfunction including shortened life span of red blood cells, impaired red blood cell production related to decreased production of erythropoietin, prolonged bleeding time, and nutritional anemia
7. **Growth disturbance**, probably caused by such factors as poor nutrition, anorexia, and bone demineralization

Children with chronic renal failure seem to be more susceptible to infection, especially pneumonia, urinary tract infection, and septicemia, although the reason for this is unclear. These children become extraordinarily sensitive to changes in vascular volume that may cause pulmonary overload, cerebral symptoms, hypertension, and cardiac failure.

Diagnostic Evaluation

The diagnosis of CRF is usually suspected on the basis of any number of manifestations, history of prior renal disease, and/or biochemical findings. The onset is usually gradual and the intial signs and symptoms are vague and nonspecific (see box).

Laboratory and other diagnostic tools and tests are of value in assessing the extent of renal damage, biochemical disturbances, and related physical dysfunction (see Table 26-1). Often they can help establish the nature of the underlying disease and differentiate between other disease processes and the pathologic consequences of renal dysfunction.

Therapeutic Management

In irreversible renal failure the goals of medical management are (1) to promote effective renal function, (2) to maintain body fluid and electrolyte balance within acceptable limits, (3) to treat systemic complications, and (4) to promote as active and normal a life as possible for the child for as long as possible. The child is allowed unrestricted activity, and he is allowed to set his own limits regarding rest and extent of exertion. He is encouraged to attend school as long as he is able. When the effort is too great, home tutoring is arranged.

Diet regulation is the most effective means, short of dialysis, for reducing the quantity of materials that require renal excretion. The goal of the diet in renal failure is to provide sufficient calories and protein for growth while limiting the excretory demands made on the kidney, to minimize metabolic bone disease (*osteodystrophy*), and to minimize fluid and electrolyte disturbances. Protein is limited and the proteins allowed should be those high in essential amino acids. Bottle-fed infants are placed on a low-protein, low-electrolyte formula with additional caloric supplements.

Sodium and water are not usually limited, unless there is evidence of edema or hypertension, and potassium is not usually restricted. However, restrictions of any or all three may be imposed in later stages or at any time at which factors cause abnormal serum concentrations.

Dietary phosphorus is controlled to prevent or correct the calcium phosphorus imbalance by the reduction of protein and milk. Phosphorus levels can be further reduced by the oral administration of aluminum hydroxide gel (Amphojel) or tablets that combine with the phosphorus to decrease gastrointestinal absorption and, thus, the serum levels of phosphate. At the same time, serum calcium levels are increased with supplementary calcium preparations, calcium gluconate, calcium carbonate, or calcium lactate.

Metabolic acidosis is alleviated through administration of alkalizing agents such as sodium bicarbonate or a com-

Clinical Manifestations of Chronic Renal Failure

- Early signs:
  - Loss of normal energy
  - Increased fatigue on exertion
  - Pallor, subtle (may not be noticed)
  - Elevated blood pressure (sometimes)
- As the disease progresses:
  - Decreased appetite (especially breakfast)
  - Less interest in normal activities
  - Increased urinary output with compensatory intake of fluid
  - Pallor more evident
  - Sallow, muddy appearance of skin
- Child may complain of:
  - Headache
  - Muscle cramps
  - Nausea
- Other signs and symptoms:
  - Weight loss
  - Facial edema
  - Malaise
  - Bone or joint pain
  - Growth retardation
  - Dryness or itching of the skin
  - Bruised skin
  - Sensory or motor loss (sometimes)
  - Amenorrhea (common in adolescent girls)
- Uremic syndrome (untreated):
  - Gastrointestinal symptoms
    - Anorexia
    - Nausea and vomiting
  - Bleeding tendencies
    - Bruises
    - Bloody diarrheal stools
    - Stomatitis
    - Bleeding from lips and mouth
  - Intractable itching
  - Uremic frost (deposits of urea crystals on skin)
  - Unpleasant "uremic" breath odor
  - Deep respirations
  - Hypertension
  - Congestive heart failure
  - Pulmonary edema
  - Neurologic involvement:
    - Progressive confusion
    - Dulled sensorium
    - Coma (ultimately)
    - Tremors
    - Muscular twitching
    - Seizures

bination of sodium and potassium citrate. Sufficient sources of folic acid and iron should be provided in the diet, and iron losses that may occur should be replaced.

Growth failure is one major consequence of CRF, especially in the preadolescent. These children grow poorly both before and after the initiation of hemodialysis. Some success has been achieved with administration of the anabolic steroid, which has powerful anabolic but weak androgenic properties. *Osseous deformities* that result from renal osteodystrophy, especially those related to ambulation, are troublesome and require correction as soon as feasible. However, until the osteodystrophy is under control, the deformities will recur. *Dental defects* are also common in children with CRF, and the earlier the onset of the disease the more severe are the dental manifestations (including hypoplasia, hypomineralization, alteration in size and shape of teeth, malocclusion, and stomatitis). Therefore, regular dental care is especially important in these children.

Anemia is treated with packed red blood cells, which are given to the child slowly over several hours. Blood transfusions carry the risk of aggravating or precipitating cardiovascular disturbances and also tend to inhibit erythropoiesis.

Hypertension of advanced renal disease may be managed initially by cautious use of a low-sodium diet, fluid restriction, and perhaps diuretics, such as hydrochlorothiazide or furosemide. Severe hypertension requires the use of antihypertensive agents, singly or in combinations.

Intercurrent infections are treated with appropriate antimicrobials at the first sign of infection; however, any drug eliminated through the kidneys is administered with caution. Other complications are treated symptomatically, for example, central acting antiemetics for *nausea*, anticonvulsants for *seizures*, and diphenhydramine (Benadryl) for *pruritus*.

Once symptoms of *uremia* appear in a child, the disease runs its relentless course and results in death in a few weeks, unless waste products and toxins are removed from body fluids by dialysis and/or kidney transplantation. Since these techniques have been adapted for infants and small children, these alternatives are implemented in most cases of renal failure once palliative management is no longer effective.

Dialysis. Dialysis is the process of separating substances in solution by the difference in their rate of diffusion through a semipermeable membrane. Two methods of dialysis are currently available for clinical management of renal failure:

1. **Peritoneal dialysis** wherein the abdominal cavity acts as a semipermeable membrane through which water and solutes of small molecular size move by osmosis and diffusion according to their respective concentrations on either side of the membrane
2. **Hemodialysis** in which blood is circulated outside the body through artificial cellophane membranes that permit a similar passage of water and solutes

As a rule, hemodialysis is reserved for children who have end-stage renal disease (ESRD), since it requires creation of a vascular access and special equipment. Peritoneal dialysis is preferred for children in acute renal failure, because it is usually a temporary therapy, it is generally an emergency procedure, and, therefore, it is more readily available, requires less expertise, and does not require specialized facilities.

Most children show rapid clinical improvement with the implementation of dialysis, although it is directly related to the duration of uremia before dialysis and the extent to which dietary regulations are followed. Growth rate and skeletal maturation usually improve, but recovery of normal growth is infrequent. In many cases sexual development, although delayed, progresses to completion.

Home dialysis. With appropriate implantation or cannulization and proper training and education of both the child and the parents, either peritoneal dialysis or hemodialysis can be performed at home. Time spent in transportation is eliminated, the environment is more pleasant and secure, and the child is able to assume a more active role in the treatment program.

Home dialysis units are available to some children, and the preparation and management for its use are similar to that required for hemodialysis in the hospital. The child is equipped with a dialysis unit that is used with the vascular access established for outpatient dialysis.

The development of satisfactory methods for *continuous ambulatory peritoneal dialysis (CAPD)* and its alternative *continuous cycling peritoneal dialysis (CCPD)* has provided an additional means for managing ESRD at home. It provides more mobility and eliminates the need for intermittent hemodialysis. In both methods commercially available sterile dialysate is instilled into the peritoneal cavity through a surgically implanted indwelling catheter sutured in place. The warmed solution is allowed to enter the peritoneal cavity by gravity and remains a variable length of time according to the procedure used.

In CAPD the dialysate is instilled, the line clamped off, and the empty bag is rolled up and worn attached to the abdomen or thigh or placed in a pocket. The solution is allowed to remain in the peritoneum for 4 to 6 hours. The bag is then unrolled and placed on the floor, the line is unclamped, and the fluid is drained into the bag by gravity. Another heated bag is hung and the process repeated. The process is performed 3 times during the day and once at night.

CCPD is a modification of CAPD and intermittent peritoneal dialysis. The dialysis exchange is performed only at night using an automatic dialysis machine, which controls the timed cycles of inflow and outflow of dialysate. The catheter is opened only at night, although an additional exchange may be prescribed during the day.

Transplantation. Renal transplantation is now an acceptable and effective means of therapy in the pediatric age-group. The criteria for selection are quite liberal, and uniform criteria have not been established among the various centers that specialize in the procedure. Many children with systemic disease and tumors have had successful transplants. On the other hand, there is a high incidence of recurrent disease in the donor kidney in children who receive a transplant for rapidly progressive glomerulonephritis with irreversible renal failure.

In addition transplantation requires the administration of drugs to suppress the immune response and subsequent rejection of the transplant. These drugs are not without hazard. The major problem of immunosuppression is suppression of the body's ability to respond to other antigenic stimuli; thus the child is at risk for overwhelming infection. Corticosteroids carry the disadvantage of producing Cushing syndrome (p. 947), growth retardation, cataracts, fluid and sodium retention, and gastric ulcer. Cyclosporine, a powerful immunosuppressant, causes undesirable hypertension, hirsutism, and nephrotoxicity, a major concern in renal transplants.

Nursing Considerations

The child with chronic renal failure is a prime example of an individual whose life is maintained by drugs and artificial means, and the multiple stresses placed on these children and their families are often overwhelming. The unrelenting course of the disease process is one of progressive deterioration. The affected child progresses from renal insufficiency to uremia and then to hemodialysis and transplantation. As the need for therapy intensifies, the need for supportive nursing care is also intensified. Team effort is more important than ever and involves coordination of personnel from medicine, nursing, social services, dietetics, and psychologic or psychiatric specialties.

ASSESSMENT

Assessment of the child with chronic renal failure is primarily one of observation for signs of complications and evidence of improvement from therapy. Some of the first changes observed are those of physical appearance—fluctuations in weight, pallor, and failure to grow.

NURSING DIAGNOSES

A number of nursing diagnoses become evident upon assessment of the child. The most relevant in the majority of cases are outlined in the Nursing care plan on p. 882. Others will be appropriate to individual children and their families.

PLANNING

The goals of care for the child with CRF, especially one in ESRD, are:

1. Minimize the impact of the disease process
2. Prevent complications
3. Provide support, guidance, and education to the child and family

IMPLEMENTATION

The multiple complications of ESRD are managed according to medical protocols prescribed for the care of those specific problems. However, progressive disease places a number of stresses on the child and his family, including those of a potentially fatal illness (see Chapter 18). There is a continuing need for repeated examinations that often entail painful procedures, side effects, and frequent hospitalizations. Diet therapy becomes progressively more restricted and intense, and the child is required to take a variety of medications. Ever present in all aspects of the treatment regimen is the agonizing realization that without treatment death is the inevitable outcome.

Some specific stresses related to ESRD and its treatment are predictable. When it first becomes apparent that kidney failure is inevitable, both parents and child experience great depression and anxiety. Acceptance is particularly difficult if renal failure progresses rapidly after diagnosis. Denial and disbelief are usually pronounced, especially among the parents. Once the kidney failure is established and once symptoms become progressively more distressing, the initiation of hemodialysis is usually perceived as a positive experience, and, after the initial concerns of implementing the treatment, the child begins to feel better and parental anxiety is relieved for a time.

Initiating a hemodialysis regimen is a traumatic and anxiety-provoking experience for most children, since it involves surgery for implantation of the shunt or fistula. The initial experience with the hemodialysis machine and its implication is frightening to most children. They need reassurance about the nature of the preparations for dialysis and conduct of the treatment.

Adolescents, with their increased need for independence and their urge for rebellion, usually adapt less well. They resent the control and enforced dependence imposed by the rigorous and unrelenting therapy program. They resent being dependent on a machine, their parents, and the professional staff. Depression and/or hostility are common in adolescents undergoing hemodialysis.

The availability of home dialysis has offered a greater degree of freedom for persons undergoing long-term dialysis. The family must learn the technique, and the nurse is responsible for teaching this technique to the family. The family must learn how to take vital signs before and after the dialysis, and they must learn the significance of blood pressure and temperature variations. They need to know how to manage the various aspects of the procedure, how to maintain accurate records, and how to observe for signs of complications that need to be reported to the proper persons.

Body changes related to the disease process, such as skin color, growth retardation, and lack of sexual maturation, are stress provoking. Dietary restrictions are particularly burdensome for both children and parents. Children feel deprived when unable to eat foods previously enjoyed and unrestricted for other family members. Consequently failure to cooperate is not uncommon. Diet restrictions are interpreted as punishment and, since they may not be able to fully understand the purpose of restrictions, some will sneak forbidden food items at every opportunity. Allowing children, especially adolescents,

NURSING CARE PLAN

The Child with Chronic Renal Failure

Nursing Goals	Nursing Interventions	Expected Patient/Family Outcomes
HP-HMP* Potential for infection **Risk factors: diminished body defenses, restricted diet**		
Prevent infection	Avoid contact with infected persons Employ careful medical asepsis	Child exhibits no evidence of infection
N-NP Altered growth and development **Etiology: restricted diet, chronic illness**		
Promote growth	Encourage normal activities for age Engage child in planning diet and schedule of activities	Child attains maximum growth and development potential
N-MP Altered nutrition: less than body requirements **Etiology: restricted diet**		
Prevent dietary deficiencies	Provide foods rich in folic acid and iron Encourage allowable foods that provide basic nutritional needs	Child shows no evidence of deficiencies
Prevent retention of waste products	Provide diet that reduces excretory demands on kidney Limit protein to essential amino acids and no more than required for growth Allow no added salt Discourage foods high in potassium	Child consumes an adequate amount of appropriate foods (specify type and amount)
SP-SCP Body image disturbance **Etiology: chronic illness, impaired growth, perception of being "different"**		
Promote self-care See Nursing Care Plan, The child with chronic illness or disability, p. 531	Teach child about disease and treatment Encourage child to assist in his own care Food selection How he can cooperate during treatment and tests	Child demonstrates an understanding of his disease and complies with therapies
RRP Altered family processes **Etiology: situational crisis (child with a chronic illness)**		
See Nursing Care Plan, The child with chronic illness or disability, p. 531		

Nursing interventions related to medical management

Assess extent of renal dysfunction
- Collect specimens for analysis
  - Urine
  - Blood
- Prepare child for and assist with renal biopsy
- Prepare for and assist with x-ray examinations

Prevent osteodystrophy
- Restrict protein and phosphorus-containing foods in the diet, especially milk and carbonated beverages
- Administer aluminum hydroxide
- Provide supplementary calcium
- Administer alkalizing agents
- Administer supplementary vitamin D

Prevent or treat hypertension
- Monitor fluid intake
- Provide low-sodium diet
- Administer diuretics as prescribed
- Administer antihypertensive agents as ordered

Treat anemia
- Administer supplementary iron
- Administer packed red blood cells periodically as prescribed

Prevent infection
- Administer appropriate antibiotics, as prescribed, at first sign of infection

Remove waste products and toxins from body fluids
- Assist with dialysis procedure

*For an explanation of abbreviations, see p. 20.

maximum participation in and responsibility for their own treatment program is helpful.

After weeks or months of hemodialysis, the parents and child feel anxiety associated with the prognosis and continued pressures of the treatment. The relentless need for treatment interferes with family plans. Transportation to and from the dialysis unit and the time spent on the machine cut into time for outside activities, including school. Shunt and fistula problems are not uncommon and present a common source of aggravation. Eventually most severely affected children face nephrectomy, which predictably causes depression in both the child and family.

The possibility of renal transplantation often comes as a hope for relief from the rigors of hemodialysis and the hated diet restrictions. Except for children with preexisting personality problems or residual physical disabilities, most children and families respond well to kidney transplant and the majority return to normal life within a year after surgery.

The **National Kidney Foundation*** and numerous other agencies provide services and information, including pamphlets, descriptive literature, and easily understandable booklets for children with renal disease, for families of affected children.

EVALUATION

The effectiveness of nursing interventions is determined by continual reassessment and evaluation of care based on the following observational guidelines and expected outcomes:

1. Observe and interview the family regarding their compliance with the medical and dietary regimen
2. Monitor vital signs, growth measurements, laboratory reports, behavior, and appearance
3. Observe and interview child and family regarding their feelings, concerns, and fears; observe reactions to therapies and prognosis

Expected outcomes:

See Nursing Care Plan on p. 882.

◆ *Defects of the Genitourinary Tract*

External defects of the genitourinary tract are usually obvious at birth. Several, such as hypospadias, epispadias, and cryptorchidism, do not necessitate immediate repair but may require one or more staged repairs during early childhood. Others require initial intervention at birth with repeated medical and surgical treatment for several years. The anatomic location of these defects frequently causes more psychologic concern to children and parents than does the actual condition or treatment. Hernias are common in young children and are usually repaired as soon as diagnosis is established.

*2 Park Ave., New York, NY 10016. In Canada the **Kidney Foundation of Canada,** 4060 Ste. Catherine St. W, Suite 555, Montreal, Quebec H3Z 2Z3.

OBSTRUCTIVE UROPATHY

Structural or functional abnormalities of the urinary system that obstruct the normal flow of urine can produce renal disorders. When there is interference with urine flow, the collecting system above the obstruction causes *hydronephrosis* (the collection of urine in the renal pelvis to the point of cyst formation from the distention) with eventual pressure destruction to renal parenchyma, although the dilating ureters form a reservoir that reduces the effect on the kidneys for a long time.

Obstruction may be congenital or acquired, unilateral or bilateral, complete or incomplete, and the manifestations may be acute or chronic. The obstruction can occur at any level of the upper or lower urinary tract (Fig. 26-4). Partial obstruction may not be symptomatic unless there is a water or solute diuresis. Boys are affected more commonly than girls, and malformations should be suspected when patients have some other congenital defects (e.g., prune belly syndrome, chromosome anomalies, hypospadias, anorectal malformations, and aural defects).

Damage to distal nephrons in chronic uropathy alters the ability to concentrate urine, contributing to increased urine flow and metabolic acidosis occurring from de-

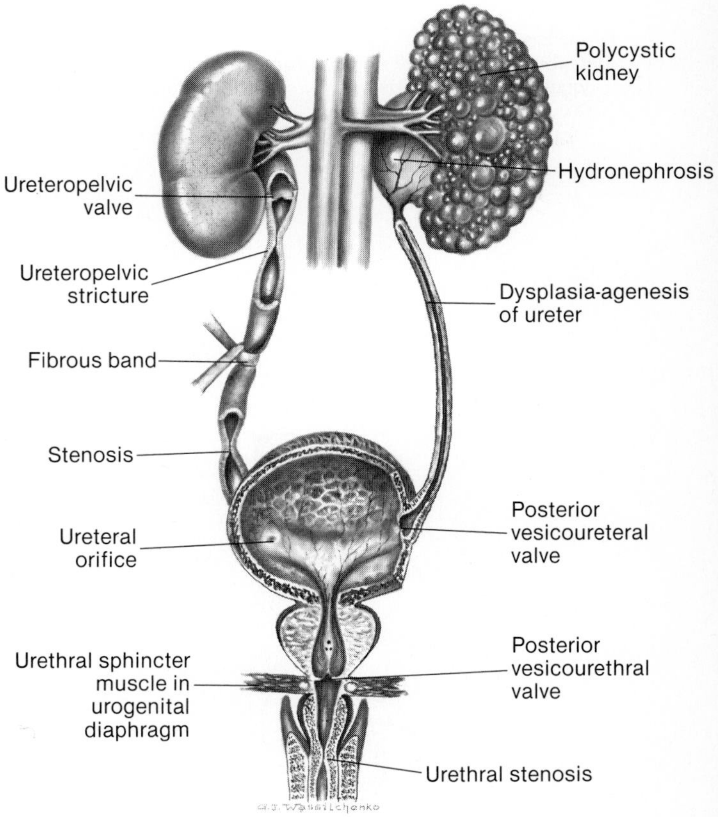

FIG. 26-4 Major sites of urinary tract obstruction.

TABLE 26-2

Defects of the Genitourinary Tract

Defect	Therapeutic Management
Inguinal Hernia Protrusion of abdominal contents through inguinal canal into the scrotum (Fig. 26-5, *B*)	Detected as painless inguinal swelling of variable size Surgical closure of inguinal defect
Hydrocele Fluid in the scrotum (Fig. 26-5, *C*)	Surgical repair indicated if spontaneous resolution not accomplished in 1 year
Phimosis Narrowing or stenosis of the preputial opening of the foreskin	Mild cases: manual retraction of foreskin and proper cleansing of area Severe cases: circumcision or vertical division and transverse suturing of foreskin
Hypospadias Urethral opening located behind the glans penis or anywhere along the ventral surface of the penile shaft (Fig. 26-6)	Objectives of surgical correction: To enable the child to void in the standing position and direct stream voluntarily in usual manner Improve physical appearnace of genitalia Produce a sexually adequate organ
Chordee Ventral curvature of penis, often associated with hypospadias (Fig. 26-7)	Surgical release of fibrous band causing the deformity
Epispadias Meatal opening located on dorsal surface of penis	Surgical correction, usually including penile and urethral lengthening and bladder neck reconstruction (if necessary)
Cryptorchidism Failure of one or both testes to descend normally through the inguinal canal	Detected by inability to palpate testes within the scrotum Medical: administration of human chorionic gonadotropin (older child) Surgical: orchiopexy Objectives of therapy: Prevent damage to undescended testicle Decrease incidence of malignant tumor formation Avoid trauma and torsion Close the inguinal canal Prevent cosmetic and psychologic disability from empty scrotum
Exstrophy of Bladder Eversion of posterior bladder through anterior bladder wall and lower abdominal wall; associated with open pubic arch (Fig. 26-8)	Objectives of surgical correction: Preserve renal function Attain urinary control Adequate reconstructive repair Improve sexual function (esp. in males)
Ambiguous Genitalia Types:	Assignment of gender sex
Masculinized female (female pseudo-hermaphrodite)	Surgical correction if needed; gender assignment—female
Incompletely masculinized male (male pseudo-hermaphrodite)	Gender assignment—female
True hermaphrodite (both ovaries and testes)	Gender assignment depends on predominant characteristics
Mixed gonadal dysgenesis	Gender assignment depends on predominant characteristics

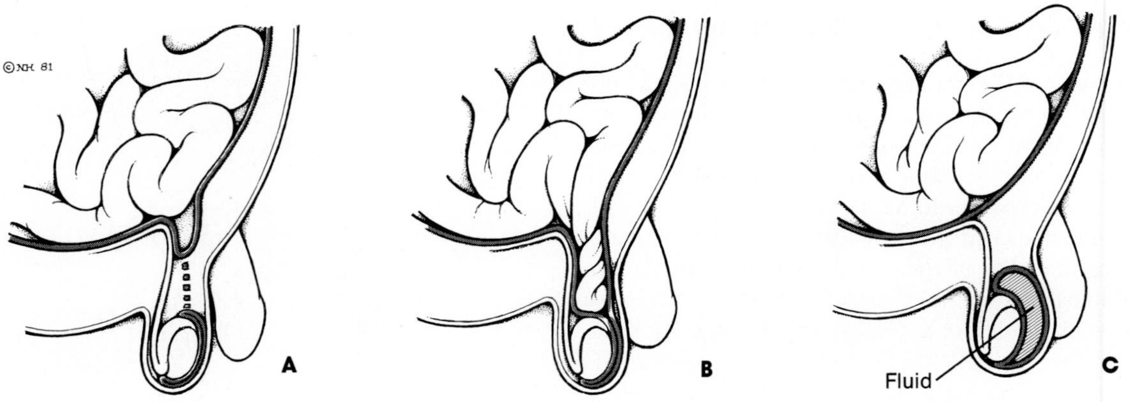

FIG. 26-5 Development of inguinal hernias. **A,** Normal. **B,** Hernia. **C,** Hydrocele.

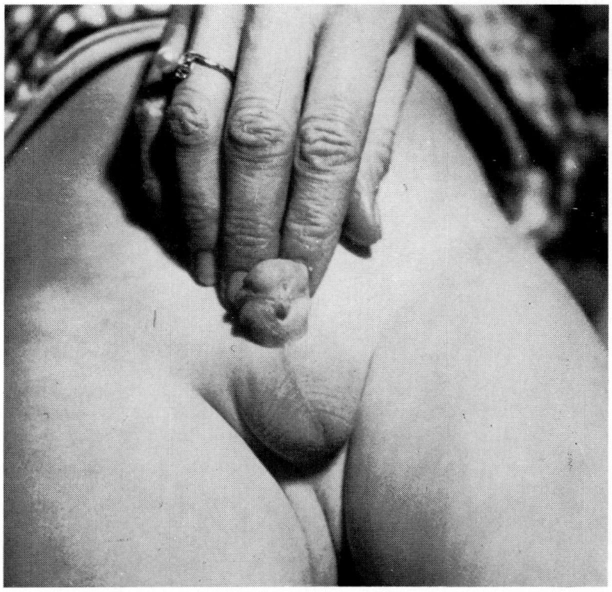

FIG. 26-6 Hypospadias. (Courtesy M.C. Gleason, M.D., San Diego,, CA. From Ingalls, A.J., and Salerno, M.C.: Maternal and child health nursing, ed. 6, St. Louis, 1987, The C.V. Mosby Co.)

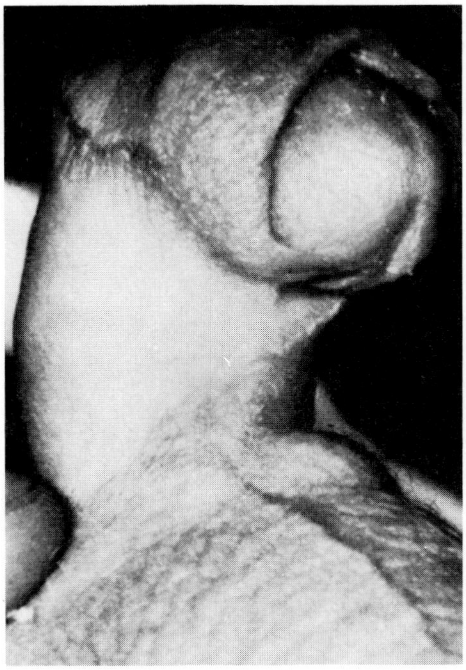

FIG. 26-7 Hypospadias with significant chordee. (From Shirkey, H.C.: Pediatric therapy, ed., 6, St. Louis, 1980, The C.V. Mosby Co.)

creased excretion of acid secondary to impaired ability of the distal nephron to secrete hydrogen ions. Partial obstruction results in progressive loss of renal function as a result of irreversible damage to the nephrons. Pooled urine serves as a medium for bacterial growth; therefore, urinary tract infections further increase the extent of renal damage.

Early diagnosis and surgical correction or bypass procedures, such as ileal conduit or cutaneous ureterostomy that divert the flow of urine, are essential in order to prevent progressive renal damage. Medical complications of acute or chronic renal failure and/or infection are managed as described for those disorders.

Nursing Considerations

Nursing goals in urinary tract obstruction include helping to identify cases, assisting with diagnostic procedures, and caring for children with complications (described elsewhere). Preparing parents and children for procedures is a major nursing responsibility, especially preparation for urinary diversion procedures (see Preparation for procedures, p. 623).

Parents and children need emotional support and counseling during the lengthy management of these disorders. Many children are discharged with ureteral drainage systems in place that must be protected from damage, and the danger of infection is a constant concern. Parents are taught to care for the equipment and recognize the signs of possible obstruction or infection within the system.

Children with external diversional systems will need

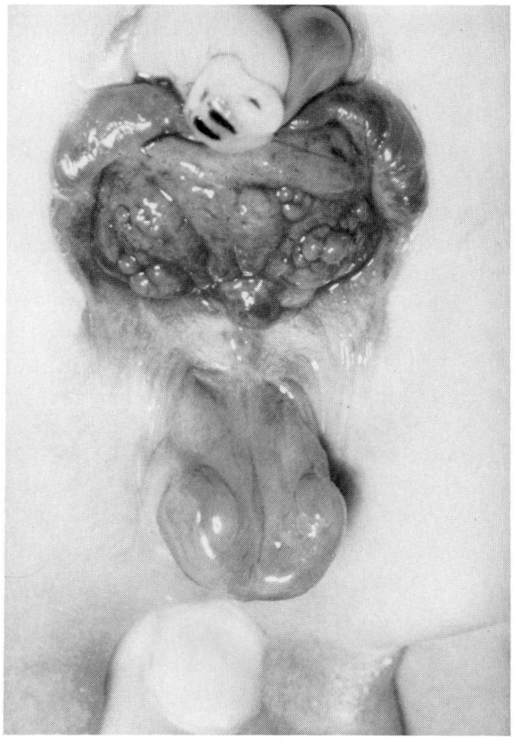

FIG. 26-8 Exstrophy of bladder. (Courtesy E.S. Tank, M.D., Division of Urology, University of Oregon Health Sciences Center, Portland, OR.)

psychologic support and guidance, especially as they reach adolescence and body image concerns assume more prominence. Those with progressive renal deterioration may face the prospect of dialysis and/or transplantation and the emotional aspects that accompany these procedures.

EXTERNAL DEFECTS

Defects of the external genitourinary tract are serious conditions primarily because of the psychologic impact on the child. Satisfactory surgical repair is successful for the more common disorders and is carried out or initiated as early as possible. The major anomalies of the lower genitourinary tract, their description, and their management are outlined in Table 26-2.

Psychologic Problems Related to Genital Surgery

Surgery involving sexual organs can be particularly disruptive to children, especially preschoolers fearing punishment, retaliation, body mutilation, or castration. Some of the problems of hospitalization, separation, and anxiety can be eased by hospital practices that are sensitive to the needs of the child (see Chapter 20).

The body image of a child is largely derived as a result of feedback from the primary caregivers, and parental anxiety regarding an acceptable physical appearance and adequate future sexual competency is readily communicated to an affected child. Therefore children with birth defects are at risk for developing a distorted body image that reflects the caregiver's subtly communicated evaluation of their bodies (Schultz, Klykylo, and Wacksman, 1983). The trend toward repair of visible genital defects is based in large part on these psychologic variables. The earlier a repair can be achieved, the more likely the possibility that the child will develop a normal body image.

During the years from 3 to 6, the phallico-oedipal period, children show a strong interest and concern about the genital area, sex differences, and genital normality or its lack. It is also a time when children are frightened of what they perceive to be threats to their body, especially the sex organs. They also view any untoward happening as a punishment for real or imagined wrongdoing or unacceptable sexual feelings, such as masturbation, sex play, or erotic feelings. Surgical repair is recommended before the development of these fears and anxieties.

Nursing Considerations

Preparing children and their families for diagnostic and surgical procedures (see Preparation for procedures, p. 623) and for home care are major nursing functions. Most postoperative care involves care of the surgical site. Tub baths are discouraged for 1 week following simple surgeries, and the surgical site is kept clean and otherwise protected from infection and inspected for signs of infection. Dressings, if any, are inspected regularly. More complex surgeries require additional care and observation, for example, catheter care for urethral reconstruction and care of urinary diversion stomas and collection devices.

Some older children's activities, such as pushing, lifting, straddle toys, sandboxes, swimming, and rough activities, may be restricted for some types of surgical repairs. Precise restrictions depend on the specific type of surgery. Activities of infants and toddlers are not limited.

In most cases the results of surgery are quite satisfactory. However, in some of the more severe defects, such as exstrophy, and those that require stomas additional emotional interventions may be needed. A major concern of parents and children is related to surgery affecting the genitals directly. Concerns about penile size, ugliness of genitalia, potential ability to procreate, and rejection by peers (especially the opposite sex) are potential fears that require psychologic adjustment, particularly during adolescence.

SUMMARY

Urinary tract infections are a common cause of childhood morbidity. Therefore the single most important aspect in management of urinary tract disorders in children is prevention, including recognizing the presence of anatomic obstruction. Judicious care of streptococcal infections and diseases known to have renal problems as a complication help reduce long-term renal damage and renal failure.

The relentless nature of the progressive renal damage in chronic renal disease can be devastating for children and their families. In addition to the financial and psychologic burden of a chronic illness the children suffer multiple health problems as complications of the disease. Children who are born with a genitourinary anomaly, unless corrected at an early age, also suffer emotional trauma, especially when they reach the developmental stage when the genitals have highly significant psychologic importance.

KEY CONCEPTS

- Common inflammatory disorders of the genitourinary tract include urinary tract infection, nephrotic syndrome, and acute glomerulonephritis.
- Management of UTIs is directed at eliminating infection, detecting and correcting functional or anatomic abnormalities, preventing recurrences, and preserving renal function.
- Vesicoureteral reflux is the retrograde of bladder urine into the ureters.
- Nephrotic syndrome is characterized by increased glomerular permeability to protein with massive urinary loss of protein resulting in hypoproteinemia and edema.
- Management of nephrotic syndrome is aimed at reducing excretion of protein, reducing or preventing fluid retention by tissues, and preventing infection and other complications.
- Common features of acute glomerulonephritis are oliguria, edema, hypertension, circulatory congestion, hematuria, and proteinuria.
- Therapeutic management of acute glomerulonephritis is maintenance of fluid balance, treatment of hypertension, and antibiotic therapy.
- Management of hemolytic-uremic syndrome is aimed at control of complications and hematologic manifestations of renal failure.
- Wilms tumor is the most common nephroblastic tumor of childhood.
- In acute renal failure, management is directed at determining treatment of underlying cause, management of complications of renal failure, and supportive therapy.
- Abnormalities in chronic renal failure are waste product retention, water and sodium retention, hyperkalemia, acidosis, calcium and phosphorus disturbance, anemia, and growth disturbances.
- When the child will need home dialysis, the nurse educates the family on the disease, its implications, the therapeutic plan, possible psychologic effects of the disease, and the treatment and technical aspects of the procedure.
- The major concerns in renal transplantation are tissue matching and prevention of rejection; psychologic concerns involve self-image as related to possible body changes as a result of the effects of corticosteroid therapy.
- Obstructive uropathy is the result of structural or functional abnormalities of the urinary system that obstruct the normal flow of urine.
- The more common defects of the genitourinary tract include phimosis, cryptorchidism, inguinal hernia, hydrocele, and hypospadias.
- Body image concerns and castration anxiety are particularly intense in children with defects in the genital area.

STUDY QUESTIONS AND ACTIVITIES

1 Prepare a plan for teaching prevention of urinary tract infections to (1) a child and (2) a family of a child.
2 Compile a list of laboratory tests used to detect abnormal renal function and the significance of deviations from normal expectations.
3 Describe the physical complications of chronic renal failure.
4 Prepare a teaching plan for a child scheduled for genital surgery.

REFERENCES

Hensle, T.W., and Burbige, K.A.: Vesicoureteral reflux. In Gellis, S.S., and Kagan, B.M., editors: Current pediatric therapy 12, Philadelphia, 1986, W.B. Saunders Co.

Jordan, S.C., and Lemire, J.M.: Acute glomerulonephritis, Pediatr. Clin. North Am. **29:**857-873, 1982.

Kim, M.S., and Grupe, W.E.: The nephrotic syndrome. In Gellis, S.S., and Kagan, B.M.: Current pediatric therapy 12, Philadelphia, 1986, W.B. Saunders Co.

Krugman, S., and others: Infectious diseases of children, ed. 8, St. Louis, 1985, The C.V. Mosby Co.

Leventhal, B.G.: Neoplasms and neoplasm-like structures. In Behrman, R.E., and Vaughan, V.C., III: Nelson textbook of pediatrics, ed. 13, Philadelphia, 1987, W.B. Saunders Co.

Schultz, J.R., KlyKylo, W.M., and Wacksman, J.: Timing of elective hypospadias repair in children, Pediatrics **71:**342-351, 1983.

Weir, M.R., and Lampe, R.M.: Urinary tract infections in children, Am. Fam. Physician **29:**147-153, 1984.

BIBLIOGRAPHY

General

Bielski, M.: Preventing infection in the catheterized patient, Nurs. Clin. North Am. **15:**703-713, 1980.

Chambers, J.K.: Fluid and electrolyte problems in renal and urologic disorders, Nurs. Clin. North Am. **22:**815-826, 1987.

Murphy, L.M., and Cole, M.J.: Renal disease: nutritional implications, Nurs. Clin. North Am. **18:**57-70, 1983.

Nace, G.: Preventing adverse drug reactions in patients with renal failure, J. Nephrol. Nurs. **2:**30-32, 1985.

Orr, M.L.: Drugs and renal disease, Am. J. Nurs. **81:**969-971, 1981.

Pickering, L., and Robbins, D.: Fluid, electrolyte, and acid-base balance in the renal patient, Nurs. Clin. North Am. **15:**577-592, 1980.

Stark, J.L.: BUN/creatinine: your keys to kidney function, Nursing 80 **10**(5):33-38, 1980.

Tichy, A.M.: Renal failure, Crit. Care Update **7**(3):5-18, 1980.

Urinary Tract Infection

Brogna, L., and Lakaszawski, M.L.: The continent urostomy, Am. J. Nurs. **86:**160-163, 1986.

Conti, M.T., and Euthropius, L.: Preventing UTIs: what works? Am. J. Nurs. **87:**307-309, 1987.

Thomas, C.K.: Childhood urinary tract infection, Pediatr. Nurs. **8:**114-119, 1982.

Underwood, M.A.: Urinary tract infections, Crit. Care Q. **3**(3):63-70, 1980.

Renal Diseases

Green, D.M.: The diagnosis and management of Wilms' tumor, Pediatr. Clin. North Am. **32**(3):735-754, 1985.

Renal Failure

Coleman, E.A.: When the kidneys fail, RN **49**(7):28-38, 1986.

Dracopoulos, D.T., and Weatherly, J.B.: Chronic renal failure: the effects on the entire family, Issues Compr. Pediatr. Nurs. **6:**141-146, 1983.

Frauman, A.C., and Lansing, L.: The child with chronic renal failure. I. Change and challenge, Issues Compr. Pediatr. Nurs. **6:**127-133, 1983.

Frauman, A.C., and Lansing, L.: The child with chronic renal failure. II. Developmental habilitation, Issues Compr. Pediatr. Nurs. **6:**135-139, 1983.

Fine, R.N., Salusky, I.B., and Ettenger, R.B.: Therapeutic approach to the infant, child, and adolescent with end-stage renal disease, Pediatr. Clin. North Am. **34:**789-801, 1987.

Korsch, B.: The impact of end-stage renal disease. In Azarnoff, P., and Hardgrove, C., editors: The family in child health care, New York, 1981, John Wiley & Sons.

Lewis, S.M.: Pathophysiology of chronic renal failure, Nurs. Clin. North Am. **16:**501-513, 1981.

Lopes, G.S.: A dietary approach to chronic renal failure, Issues Compr. Pediatr. Nurs. **6:**23-62, 1983.

Rodriguez, D.J., and Hunter, V.M.: Nutritional intervention in the treatment of chronic renal failure, Nurs. Clin. North Am. **16:**573-585, 1981.

Stark, J.L.: How to succeed against acute renal failure, Nursing 82 **12**(12):26-33, 1982.

Stark, J.L., and Hunt, V.: Helping your patient with chronic renal failure, Nursing 83 **13**(9):56-63, 1983.

Tichy, A.M.: Renal failure, Crit. Care Update **9:**7-21, 1982.

Topor, M.: Chronic renal disease in children, Nurs. Clin. North Am. **16:**587-597, 1981.

Tyndall, M.G.: Chronic renal failure: past and future trends, Nurs. Clin. North Am. **16;**489-499, 1981.

Dialysis

Binkley, L.S.: Keeping up with peritoneal dialysis, Am. J. Nurs. **84:**729-733, 1984.

Ceccarelli, C.M.: Hemodialytic therapy for the patient with chronic renal failure, Nurs. Clin. North Am. **16:**531-550, 1981.

Chambers, J.K.: Assessing the dialysis patient at home, Am. J. Nurs. **81:**750-754, 1981.

Chambers, J.K.: Bowel management in dialysis patients, Am. J. Nurs. **83:**1051-1052, 1983.

Davis, V., and Lavandero, R.: Caring for the catheter carefully ... before, during, and after peritoneal dialysis, Nursing 80 **10**(12):67-71, 1980.

Denniston, D.J., and Burns, K.T.: Home peritoneal dialysis, Am. J. Nurs. **80:**2022-2026, 1980.

Duffy, M.M.: Peritoneal dialysis, Crit. Care Update **10**(8):7-22, 1983.

Fear of floating to a renal unit, Nursing 82 **12**(12):42-43, 1982.

Fleming, L.M., and Kane, J.: Step-by-step guide to safe peritoneal dialysis, RN **47**(2):44-47, 1984.

Gross, S.: Teaching young patients—and their families—about home peritoneal dialysis, Nursing 80 **10**(10):72-73, 1980.

How do you manage peritoneal dialysis? Am. J. Nurs. **86:**592-596, 1986.

Kadas, N.: Reducing fluid overload without dialysis, RN **49**(5):27-31, 1986.

Reed, S.B.: Giving more than dialysis, Nursing 82 **12**(4):58-63, 1982.

Sorrels, P.A.J.: Peritoneal dialysis: a rediscovery, Nurs. Clin. North Am. **16:**515-529, 1981.

Williams, J.A.: Hypotension during hemodialysis, Crit. Care Update **10**(6):44-49, 1983.

Transplantation

Cianci, J., Lamb, J., and Ryan, R.K.: Renal transplantation, Am. J. Nurs. **81:**354-355, 1981.

Enthusiastic cyclosporine consensus, Am. J. Nurs. **85:**861-862, 1985.

Golden, D., and others: Understanding the magic of cyclosporine, RN **48**(6):53-54, 1985.

Hazinski, M.F.: Organ donations: what the new "required request" law means to you, Pediatr. Nurs. **6:**415, 1987.

Irwin, B.C.: The renal transplant patient, Crit. Care Update **8**(9):30-41, 1981.

Irwin, B.C.: Renal transplantation, Crit. Care Update **10**(2):28-35, 1983.

McHugh, M.J.: Intensive care aspects of organ transplanation in children, Pediatr. Clin. North Am. **34:**187-201, 1987.

Powers, A.M.: Renal transplantation: the patient's choice, Nurs. Clin. North Am. **16:**551-564, 1981.

Reckling, J.B.: Safeguarding the renal transplant patient, Nursing 82 **12**(2):47-49, 1982.

Rimar, J.M.: Cyclosporine for organ transplantation, MCN **10:**237, 1985.

Structural Defects of Genitourinary Tract

Bernhardt, J.: Percutaneous nephrostomy tubes in the neonate with obstructive uropathy, Neonatal Network **4**(6):51-53, 1986.

DiGrande, A.: The child born with ambiguous genitalia: family assessment and nursing intervention, Issues Compr. Pediatr. Nurs. **7:**307-318, 1984.

Mazur, T.: Ambiguous genitalia: detection and counseling, Pediatr. Nurs. **9:**417-422, 431, 1983.

Pagon, R.A.: Diagnostic approach to the newborn with ambiguous genitalia, Pediatr. Clin. North Am. **34:**1019-1031, 1987.

Stevens, M.S., and Reinitz, M.: Nursing a child through exstrophic bladder reconstruction surgery, MCN **5:**265-270, 1980.

CHAPTER 27

The Child with Cerebral Dysfunction

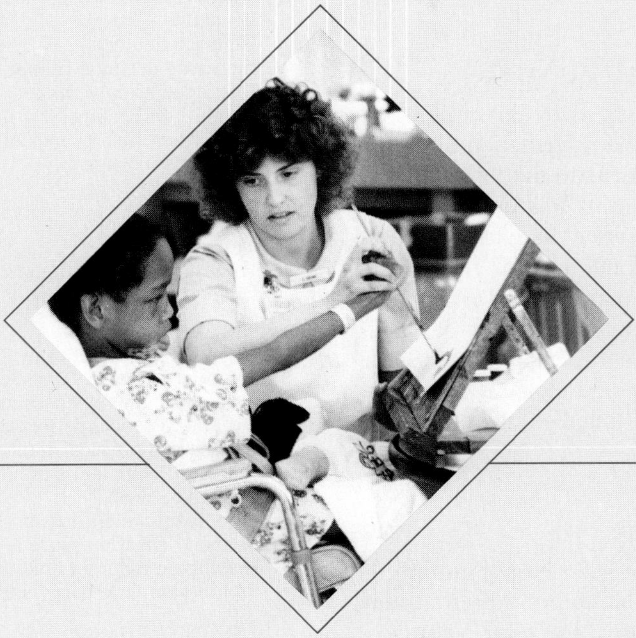

LEARNING OBJECTIVES

On completion of this chapter the reader will be able to:

- Describe the various modalities for assessment of cerebral function
- Differentiate between the stages of consciousness
- Formulate a plan of care for the unconscious child
- Distinguish between the types and serious complications of head injuries
- Describe the nursing care of a child with a tumor of the central nervous system
- Outline a plan of care for the child with bacterial meningitis
- Differentiate between the various types of seizure disorders
- Demonstrate an understanding of the manifestations of a convulsive disorder and the management of a child with such a disorder
- Describe the preoperative and postoperative care of a child with hydrocephalus

The brain is the center for multiple vital body functions. Any disturbance in this regulating, controlling, and communicating mechanism can produce alterations in the way in which the system receives, integrates, and/or responds to stimuli entering the system. These disturbances are reflected in a variety of clinical manifestations, depending on the focus of the disturbance and the integrity of the conducting mechanism. Three major physiologic disturbances create significant cerebral dysfunction: increased intracranial pressure (ICP), hypoxia, and seizure activity. This chapter is concerned with some of the major sources of insult to the brain and the way in which a skilled observer can assess the clinical evidence of neurologic dysfunction and intervene appropriately.

◆ *Cerebral Dysfunction*

Cerebral dysfunction is manifest in a variety of ways and in almost any system in the body and can be the result of a number of etiologies. Therefore accurate observation and assessment are vital to the diagnosis and management. Because it is common to a variety of disorders, alterations in consciousness will be discussed as a concept.

ASSESSMENT OF CEREBRAL FUNCTION

Since the brain is impossible to assess by direct observation and measurement, most of the information about its status is obtained by indirect measurements. Some of these measurements are discussed in relation to numerous aspects of child care; for instance, as part of assessments of health (p. 168), gestational age (p. 185), newborn status (p. 183), mental retardation (p. 543), hypoxic injury (cerebral palsy, p. 1057), and attainment of developmental milestones at each stage of development. Since it has such a prominent place in neurologic dysfunction increased ICP is briefly described followed by assessment techniques and diagnostic tests.

Increased Intracranial Pressure

The brain, tightly enclosed in the solid bony cranium, is well protected but highly vulnerable to pressure that may accumulate within the enclosure. Its total volume—brain, cerebral spinal fluid (CSF), and blood—must remain approximately the same at all times. A change in the proportional volume of one of these components (e.g., increase or decrease in intracranial blood) must be accompanied by a compensatory change in another. In this way the volume and pressure normally remain constant. Examples of compensatory changes are reduction in blood volume, decrease in CSF production, increase in CSF absorption, or shrinking of brain mass by displacement of intracellular and extracellular fluid. Children with open fontanels compensate by skull expansion and widened sutures. However, at any age the capacity for spacial compensation is limited. An increase in ICP may be caused by tumors or other space-occupying lesions, accumulation of fluid within the ventricular system, bleeding, or edema of cerebral tissues. Once compensation is exhausted any further increase in volume will result in a rapid rise in ICP.

Early signs and symptoms of increased ICP are often subtle and assume many patterns (see accompanying box). As pressure increases signs and symptoms become more pronounced and the level of consciousness deteriorates.

Clinical Manifestations of Increased Intracranial Pressure (ICP) in Infants and Children

Infants
Tense, bulging fontanel; lack of normal pulsations
Separated cranial sutures
Macewen (cracked-pot) sign
Irritability
High-pitched cry
Increased occipital-frontal circumference (OFC)
Distended scalp veins
Changes in feeding
Cries when held or rocked
"Setting sun" sign

Children
Headache
Nausea
Vomiting—often without nausea
Diplopia, blurred vision
Seizures

Personality and Behavior Signs
Irritability (toddlers), restlessness
Indifference, drowsiness, or lack of interest
Decline in school performance
Diminished physical activity and motor performance
Increased complaints of fatigue, tiredness; increased time devoted to sleep
Significant weight loss possible from anorexia and vomiting
Memory loss if pressure is markedly increased
Inability to follow simple commands
Progression to lethargy and drowsiness

Late Signs
Lowered level of consciousness
Decreased motor response to command
Decreased sensory response to painful stimuli
Alterations in pupil size and reactivity
Sometimes decerebrate or decorticate posturing
Cheyne-Stokes respirations
Papilledema

Assessment: General Aspects

Children younger than 2 years are difficult to evaluate neurologically. Therefore, most information about infants and small children is gained through observation of their spontaneous and elicited reflex responses, by their development of increasingly complex locomotor and fine motor skills, and by eliciting progressively more sophisticated communicative and adaptive behaviors. Older children are evaluated by the usual methods employed in a neurologic examination, including developmental attainment and abnormalities of gait.

General aspects of assessment that provide clues to the etiology of dysfunction include:

Family history sometimes offers clues regarding possible genetic disorders with neurologic manifestations.

Health history may provide valuable clues regarding the cause of dysfunction, e.g., an injury, short febrile illness, encounter with an animal or insect, ingestion of neurotoxic substances, inhalation of chemicals, a past illness, or known diabetes mellitus.

Physical evaluation of infants includes observation of:
- Size and shape of the head
- Spontaneous activity and postural reflex activity
- Sensory responses
- Attitude—normal flexed posture, extreme extension, opisthotonos, hypotonia

Symmetry in movement of extremities
Excessive tremulousness or frequent twitching movements
Altered expiratory cycle:
  Prolonged apnea
  Ataxic breathing
  Paradoxic chest movement
  Hyperventilation
Skin and hair texture
Distinctive facial features
Presence of a high-pitched, piercing cry
Abnormal eye movements
Inability to suck or swallow
Lip smacking
Asymmetric contraction of facial muscles
Yawning (may indicate cranial nerve involvement)
Muscular activity and coordination

Altered States of Consciousness

Consciousness implies awareness—the ability to respond to sensory stimuli and have subjective experiences. There are two components of consciousness: *alertness,* an arousal-waking state including the ability to respond to stimuli, and *cognitive power,* including the ability to process stimuli and produce verbal and motor responses.

An altered state of consciousness usually refers to varying states of unconsciousness that may be momentary or may extend for hours, days, or indefinitely. *Unconsiousness* is depressed cerebral function—the inability to respond to sensory stimuli and have subjective experiences. *Coma* is defined as a state of unconsiousness from which the patient cannot be aroused even with powerful stimuli (see coma assessment, opposite).

Levels of consciousness. Various terms are used to describe alterations in level of consciousness (LOC) and, since they have not been standardized, are subject to wide range of interpretation. LOC is determined by observations of the patient's responses to his environment. Other diagnostic tests such as motor activity, reflexes, and vital signs are more variable and do not necessarily directly parallel the depth of the comatose state. The most consistently used terms are described as follows:

Sleep (normal unconsciousness)—cyclic (or regularly recurring) physiologic state in which there is absence of alertness, cognition, and voluntary movement that is readily reversible by an auditory, visual, or tactile stimulus.

Confusion—failure to comprehend their surroundings—disorientation relative to time, inability to follow even simple directions, misidentification of persons, short attention span, loss of proper bearings, inability to estimate direction or location, and misinterpretation of events; usually able to give relevant answers to simple questions involving such things as age or location of pain but will give irrelevant and inaccurate answers to more complex questions; may be hyperactive or apathetic and immobile, but alert and arousal responses are intact.

Delirium—a state characterized by confusion, disorientation, fear, irritability, agitation, and hyperactivity; marked by illusions (false interpretation of sensory perceptions), hallucinations (false sensory perceptions), and delusions (false ideas).

Pseudo-wakeful states—demonstrated by wakefulness but inability to follow objects or lights, does not turn eyes toward a noise, and does not speak; in less developed states the patient may follow objects or persons with his eyes, turn slowly toward a sound, and appear about to speak but remain silent.

Comatose states—characterized by diminished alertness that can extend from somnolence or semistupor to deep coma.

Coma assessment. Several scales have been devised in an attempt to standardize the description and interpretation of the degree of depressed consciousness. The most popular of these is the Glasgow Coma Scale (GCS), which consists of a three-part assessment: eye opening, verbal response, and motor response (see box). When assessing level of consciousness in young children it is often useful to have a parent present to help elicit a desired response. An infant or child may not respond in an unfamiliar environment or to unfamiliar voices.

Numerical values are assigned to the levels of response in each category, and the sum of these numeric values provides an objective measure of the patient's LOC. The lower the score, the deeper the coma. A normal person would score the highest, 15; a score of 7 or below is generally accepted as a definition of coma; the lowest score, 3, indicates deep coma.

Neurologic Examination

The purpose of the neurologic examination is to establish an accurate, objective baseline of neurologic information. It is essential that the neurologic examination be documented in a fashion that is able to be reproduced by others. Descriptions of behaviors should be simple, objective, and easily interpreted: "Drowsy but awake and conversationally rational/oriented"; "Sleepy but arousable with vigorous physical stimuli. Pressure to nail base of right hand results in upper extremity flexion/lower extremity extension."

Vital signs. Pulse, respiration, and blood pressure provide information regarding the adequacy of circulation and the possible underlying cause of altered consciousness. Autonomic activity is most intensively disturbed in deep coma and in brain stem lesions.

Body temperature is often elevated, and sometimes the elevation may be extreme. Coma of a toxic origin may produce hypothermia. High temperature is most frequently a sign of an acute infectious process or heat stroke but may be caused by ingestion of some drugs (especially salicylates, alcohol, and barbiturates) or intracranial bleeding. A fever sometimes follows a cerebral seizure.

The *pulse* is variable and may be rapid, slow and bounding, or feeble. *Blood pressure* may be normal, elevated, or at shock levels. The Cushing reflex or pressor response that causes a slowing of the pulse and an increase in blood pressure is uncommon in children; when it occurs, it is a very late sign. Vital signs are also affected by medications. For assessment purposes *changes* in

*Pediatric Coma Scale**

	Score	Over 1 Year	Less Than 1 Year	
Eyes opening	4	Spontaneously	Spontaneously	
	3	To verbal command	To shout	
	2	To pain	To pain	
	1	No response	No response	
		Over 1 Year	**Less Than 1 Year**	
Best motor response	6	Obeys		
	5	Localizes pain	Localizes pain	
	4	Flexion withdrawal	Flexion withdrawal	
	3	Flexion—abnormal (decorticate rigidity)	Flexion—abnormal (decorticate rigidity)	
	2	Extension (decerebrate rigidity)	Extension (decerebrate rigidity)	
	1	No response	No response	
		Over 5 Years	**2-5 Years**	**0-23 Months**
Best verbal	5	Oriented and converses	Appropriate words and phrases	Smiles, coos, cries appropriately
	4	Disoriented and converses	Inappropriate words	Cries
	3	Inappropriate words	Cries and/or screams	Inappropriate crying and/or screaming
	2	Incomprehensible sounds	Grunts	Grunts
	1	No response	No response	No response
Total	3-15			

*Modification of Glasgow Coma Scale.

pulse and blood pressure are more important than the direction.

Respirations are more often slow, deep, and irregular. Slow and deep breathing is often seen in the heavy sleep caused by sedatives, after seizures, or in cerebral infections. Slow, shallow breathing may result from sedatives or narcotics. Hyperventilation (deep and rapid respirations) is usually the result of metabolic acidosis or abnormal stimulation of the respiratory center in the medulla caused by salicylate poisoning, hepatic coma, or Reye syndrome.

Breathing patterns have been described with a number of terms (e.g., apneustic, cluster, ataxic, Cheyne-Stokes). However, it is better to describe what is being observed rather than to place a label on it. The terms are often used and interpreted incorrectly. Periodic and irregular breathing are signs of brain stem (especially medullary) dysfunction. This is an ominous sign that often precedes complete apnea. The *odor* of the breath may provide additional clues; for example, the fruity, acetone odor of ketosis, the foul odor of uremia, the fetid odor of hepatic failure, or the odor of alcohol.

Skin. The skin may offer clues to the cause of unconsciousness. The body surface should be examined for the presence of injury, needle marks, petechiae, bites, and ticks. Evidence of toxic substances may be found on the hands, face, mouth, and clothing—especially in small children.

Eyes. Pupil size and reactivity are assessed (Fig. 27-1). Pinpoint pupils are commonly observed in poisoning, such as opiate or barbiturate poisoning, or in brain stem dysfunction. Widely dilated and reactive pupils are often seen after seizures and may involve only one side. Dilated pupils may also be caused by eye trauma. Widely dilated and fixed pupils suggest paralysis of cranial nerve III secondary to pressure from herniation of the brain through the tentorium. A unilateral fixed pupil usually suggests a lesion on the same side. Bilateral fixed pupils usually imply brain stem damage if present for more than 5 minutes. Dilated and unreactive pupils are also seen in hypothermia, anoxia, ischemia, poisoning with atropine-like substances, or prior instillation of mydriatic drugs.

The description of eye movements should indicate whether one or both eyes are involved and how the reaction was elicited. The sudden appearance of a fixed and dilated pupil is a neurosurgical emergency.

Special tests, usually performed by qualified persons, include the following:

The *doll's head maneuver* is one in which the child's head is rotated quickly to one side and then to the other. Conjugate (paired or working together) movement of the eyes in the direction opposite to the head rotation is normal. Absence of this response suggests dysfunction of the brain stem or oculomotor nerve (cranial nerve III).

The *caloric test,* or oculovestibular response, is elicited by irrigating the external auditory canal with ice water, which normally causes conjugate movement of the eyes toward the side of stimulation. This is lost when the pontine centers are impaired, thus providing important information in assessment of the comatose patient.

Funduscopic examination reveals additional clues. Papilledema, if it develops at all, will not be evident early in the course of unconsciousness because papilledema takes 24

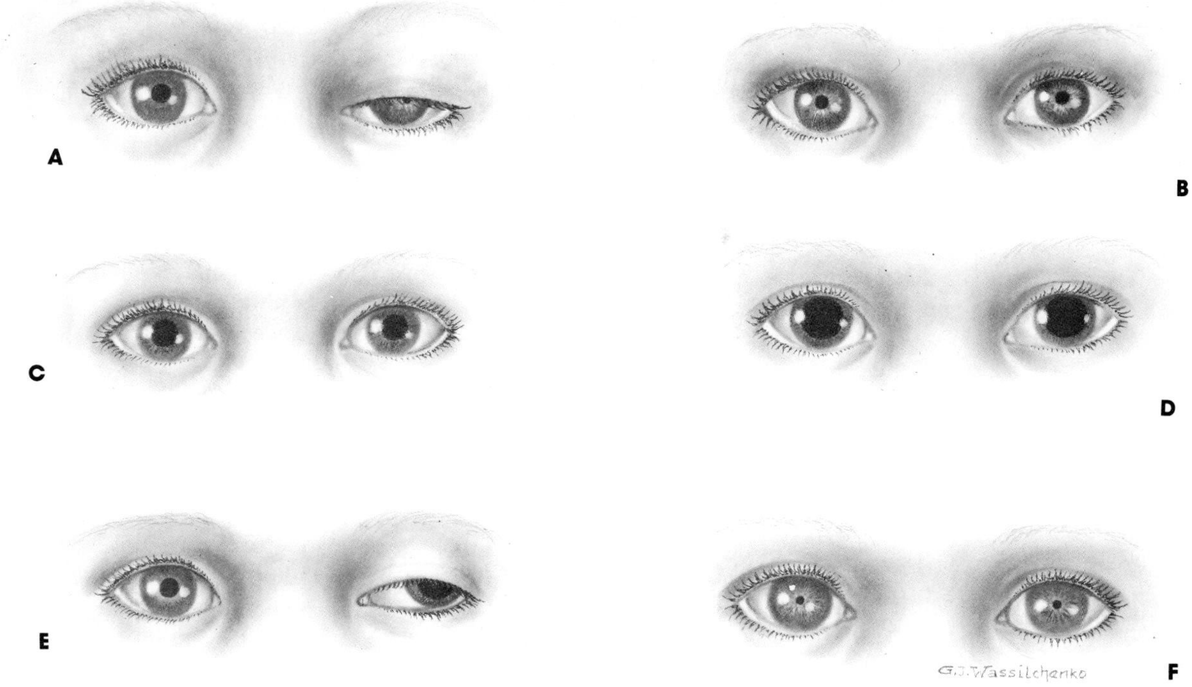

FIG. 27-1 Variations in pupil size with altered states of consciousness. **A,** Ipsilateral pupillary constriction with slight ptosis. **B,** Bilateral small pupils. **C,** Midposition; light fixed to all stimuli. **D,** Bilateral dilated and fixed pupils. **E,** Dilated pupil; left eye abducted with ptosis. **F,** Pinpoint pupils.

to 48 hours to develop. The presence of preretinal (subhyaloid) hemorrhages in children is almost invariably the result of acute trauma with intracranial bleeding, usually subarachnoid or subdural hemorrhage.

Motor function. Observation of spontaneous activity, posture, and response to painful stimuli provides clues to the location and extent of cerebral dysfunction. Even subtle movements (e.g., the outward rotation of a hip) should be noted. Asymmetric movements of the limbs or absence of movement suggests paralysis. In hemiplegia the affected limb lies in external rotation and will fall uncontrollably when lifted and allowed to drop. These observations should be described rather than labeled.

In the deeper comatose states there is little or no spontaneous movement and the musculature tends to be flaccid. There is considerable variability in the motor behavior in lesser degrees of coma. For example, the child may be relatively immobile or restless and hyperkinetic; muscle tone may be increased or decreased. Tremors, twitching, and spasms of muscles are common observations. The patient may display purposeless plucking or tossing movements. Combative or negativistic behavior is not uncommon. Hyperactivity is more common in acute febrile and toxic states than in cases of increased ICP. Convulsions are common in children and may be present in coma from any cause. Any repetitive or convulsive movements should be described.

Posturing. As cortical control over motor function is lost in brain dysfunction, primitive postural reflexes emerge. These are evident in posturing and motor movements directly related to the area of the brain involved. *Decorticate posturing* (Fig. 27-2, *A*) is seen when there is severe dysfunction of the cerebral cortex. Typical decorticate posturing includes adduction of arms at the shoulders, the arms being flexed on the chest with the wrists flexed and the hands fisted, and the lower extrem-

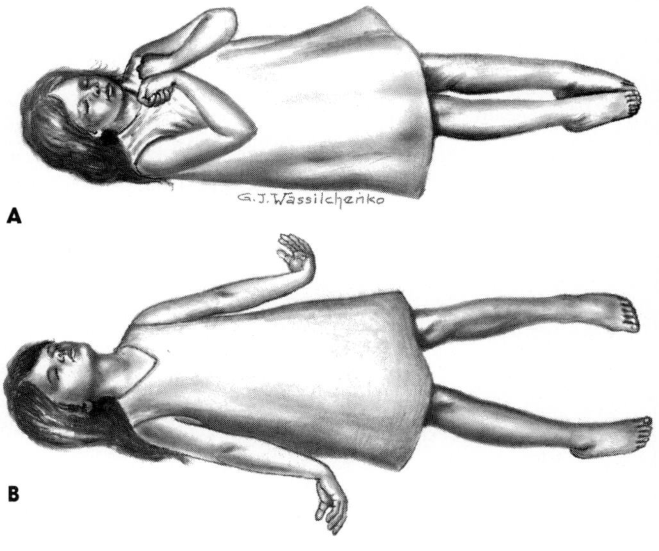

FIG. 27-2 **A,** Decorticate posturing. **B,** Decerebrate posturing.

ities being extended and adducted. *Decerebrate posturing* (Fig. 27-2, *B*), a sign of dysfunction at the level of the midbrain, is characterized by rigid extension and pronation of the arms and legs. The posturing may not be evident when the child is quiet but can usually be elicited by applying painful stimuli, such as a blunt object pressed on the base of the nail.

Reflexes. Testing of some reflexes may be of limited value. In general, the corneal, pupillary, muscle-stretch, superficial, and plantar reflexes tend to be absent in deep coma. The state of reflexes is variable in lighter grades of unconsciousness and depends on the underlying pathologic process and the location of the lesion. Absence of corneal reflexes and presence of a tonic neck reflex are associated with severe brain damage. The Babinski reflex (p. 167) may be of value if it is found to be present consistently in children older than 1 year. A positive Babinski reflex is significant in assessment of pyramidal tract lesions when it is unilateral and associated with other pyramidal signs.

Special Diagnostic Procedures

Numerous diagnostic procedures are used for assessment of cerebral function. Laboratory tests that may help to determine the cause of unconsciousness include blood glucose, urea nitrogen, and electrolyte (pH, sodium, potassium, chloride, calcium, and bicarbonate) tests; clotting studies, hematocrit, and a complete blood count; liver function tests; blood cultures if there is fever; and sometimes studies to detect lead or other toxic substances, such as drugs.

Highly sophisticated tests are carried out with specialized equipment by skilled personnel. Most of these tests are outlined in Table 27-1. Because such tests can be threatening to children, a child will need preparation for, and support and reassurance during, the tests. (See also Preparation for procedures, p. 623).

Children who are old enough to understand require careful explanation of the procedure, why it is being done, what they will experience, and how they can help. School-age children usually appreciate a more detailed description of why contrast material is injected. The importance of lying still for tests, particularly tomography, needs to be stressed. Children unfamiliar with the machines can be shown a picture beforehand.

Tomography requires that the child's head be placed within a special immobilizing device, although for only about 5 to 10 minutes. Chin and cheek pads are sometimes used to prevent the slightest head movement, and

TABLE 27-1

Procedures Used in Cerebral Assessment

Test	Purpose
Lumbar puncture (LP)	Diagnostic—measures spinal fluid pressure, obtains CSF for visualization and laboratory analysis
Subdural tap	Helps rule out subdural effusions
Electroencephalography (EEG)	Measures electric activity of cerebral cortex Detects electric abnormalities—diagnosis of seizures Used to determine brain death
Video EEG	Split-screen simultaneous visualization of whole body, facial, and EEG recording
Computed tomography (CT scan)	Visualized horizontal and vertical cross section of brain at any axis Distinguishes density of various intracranial tissues and structures—congenital abnormalities, hemorrhage, tumors, and demyelinating and inflammatory processes
Nuclear brain scan	Test material accumulates in areas where blood-brain barrier is defective Identifies focal brain lesions (e.g., tumors, abscesses) Positive uptake of material with encephalitis and subdural hematoma Visualizes CSF pathways
Transillumination	Varying degrees of localized glowing may be seen in abnormal fluid accumulation in various areas of head
Echoencephalography	Identifies shifts in midline structures from their normal positions as a result of intracranial lesions May show ventricular dilation
Radiography	Shows fractures, dislocations, spreading suture lines, and craniostenosis Shows degenerative changes, bone erosion, and calcifications
Magnetic resonance imaging (MRI) or nuclear magnetic resonance (NMR)	Permits visualization of morphologic features of target structures Permits tissue discrimination unavailable with many techniques
Positron emission transaxial tomography (PETT)	Detects and measures blood volume and flow in brain, metabolic activity, and biochemical changes within tissues, etc.
Real-time ultrasonography (RTUS)	Allows high-resolution anatomic visualization in variety of imaging planes
Digital subtraction angiography (DSA)	Visualizes vasculature of target tissue Visualizes finite vascular abnormalities

straps are applied to the body to prevent a slight change in body position. The nurse can explain these events to a frightened child by comparing them to an astronaut's preparation for a space flight. It is very important to emphasize to the child that at no time is the procedure painful.

It is helpful for nurses to become acquainted with the equipment and the general environment in which the test will take place so that they can better explain the procedure to the child at his level of understanding. Equipment is often strange and ominous to a child and may be perceived as a frightening monster. It is especially frightening to young children to experience a large mechanical device coming toward them as if to crush or devour them. They need constant reassurance from a trusted companion (Fig. 27-3).

Physical preparation may involve administering a sedative or providing an intravenous access for infusion of contrast material. If so, the child should be helped through the preparation and administration and assured that someone will remain with him (if this is possible). The child will need continual support and reinforcement during the procedures in which he remains conscious. The child's vital signs and physiologic response to the procedure are monitored throughout. Care after the test depends on the nature of the procedure.

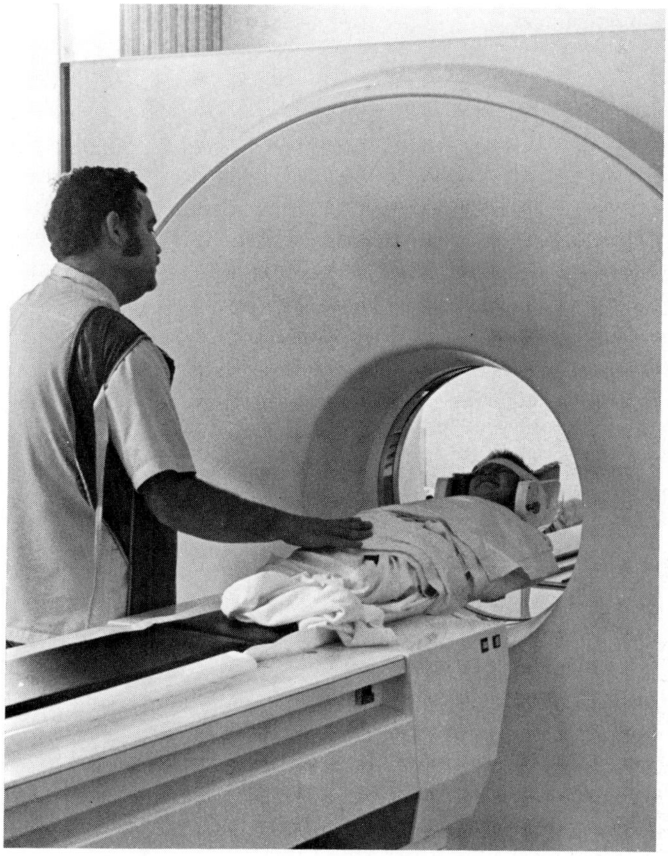

FIG. 27-3 A child reflects stress and a feeling of powerlessness during tomography, even when he is accompanied by a kind and supportive person.

Children who have undergone a procedure with general anesthesia require postanesthesia care, including positioning to prevent aspiration of secretions and frequent assessment of vital signs and LOC. In addition, other neurologic functions, such as pupillary responses, motor strength, and movement, are tested at regular intervals. Any surgical wound resulting from the test is checked for bleeding, cerebrospinal fluid leakage, and other complications. Children who undergo repeated subdural taps should have their hematocrit measured daily to detect any blood loss from the procedure.

The child's emotional reaction to the procedure is also considered. He should be allowed to express his feelings about the experience through verbal expression and the use of therapeutic play.

THE UNCONSCIOUS CHILD

The child who has sustained some manner of cerebral compromise as a result of physical injury, infection, near-drowning, or toxic injury is usually in varying states of consciousness. Regardless of the etiology, the nursing efforts are directed primarily toward detecting possible alterations in condition and preventing further damage to the various systems and tissues. Care of the unconscious child is almost the same no matter what the cause of the condition. The outcome of unconsciousness may be early and complete recovery, death within a few hours or days, persistent and permanent unconsciousness, or recovery with varying degrees of residual mental and/or physical disability.

Therapeutic Management

Emergency measures are directed toward ensuring a patent airway, treating shock, and reducing ICP (if present). Delayed treatment often leads to increased damage. As soon as emergency measures have been implemented—in many cases concurrently—specific therapies for specific causes are initiated, such as antibiotics for infection and glucose for diabetic coma.

Respiratory management. Respiratory effectiveness is the primary concern in care of the unconscious child, and establishment of an adequate airway is *always* the first priority. Carbon dioxide has a potent vasodilating effect and will increase cerebral blood flow and ICP. Cerebral hypoxia that extends longer than 4 minutes almost always causes irreversible brain damage.

Children in lighter stages of coma may be able to cough and swallow, but those in deeper states of coma are unable to handle secretions, which tend to pool in the throat and pharynx. The child is placed in side-lying or partial side-lying position to prevent aspiration of secretions, and the stomach is emptied to reduce the likelihood of vomiting. In infants, blockage of air passages from secretions can happen in seconds. In addition, upper airway obstruction from laryngospasm is a frequent complication in comatose children.

A temporary airway can be used for the child who is suffering a temporary loss of consciousness, such as after a seizure or anesthesia. For children who remain unconscious for a period of time, a nasotracheal or orotracheal tube is inserted to maintain the open airway and facilitate removal of secretions. A tracheostomy is performed in cases in which laryngoscopy for introduction of an endotracheal tube would be difficult or dangerous and when prolonged mechanical ventilation is needed. When the respiratory center is involved, mechanical ventilation is usually indicated.

Blood gas analysis is performed regularly, and oxygen is administered when indicated. Moderately severe hypoxia and respiratory acidosis are often present but not always evident from clinical manifestations. Hyperventilation frequently accompanies unconsciousness and may lead to respiratory alkalosis, or it may represent the body's attempt to compensate for metabolic acidosis. Therefore blood gas and pH determinations are essential guides for electrolyte therapy.

Increased ICP monitoring. Prompt intervention is lifesaving in the comatose patient who has evidence of marked increase in ICP. When increased ICP is the result of accumulation of CSF from obstruction of cerebrospinal fluid flow, a ventricular tap will provide relief quickly and effectively. Evacuation of a hematoma reduces pressure from this source.

ICP monitoring is frequently employed for early detection and observation of progress of ICP. ICP is monitored directly by means of a hollow subarachnoid bolt (Richmond screw) or an intraventricular catheter with fibroscopic sensors that are attached to a monitoring system. In children over 3 years of age this is accomplished through a bur hole. The bolt is stabilized with dressings, but these are not changed or disturbed, even to check the site. The placement of the bolt is not adjusted by anyone except the neurosurgeon who placed the device.

The catheter method involves introduction of a catheter into the lateral ventricle on the nondominant side, if known, or placement in the subdural space. In infants a fontanel transducer can be used to detect impulses from a pressure sensor and convert them to electrical energy (Fig. 27-4). The electrical energy is then converted to visible waves or numerical readings on an oscilloscope. The catheter has the advantage of providing a means of extraventricular (or continuous) drainage to reduce pressure. A drainage bag attached to the system is kept at the level of the ventricles and can be lowered to decrease ICP. Antibiotics are usually instilled into the ventricle once a day, and fluid is obtained for culture.

Nutrition and hydration. Fluids and calories are supplied initially by the intravenous route. An intravenous infusion is started early, and the type of fluid administered is determined by the general condition of the patient. Later, nutrition is provided in a balanced formula given by nasogastric or gastrostomy tube. Hydration is maintained in the same manner. When cerebral edema is a threat, fluids may be restricted to reduce the chance of fluid overload.

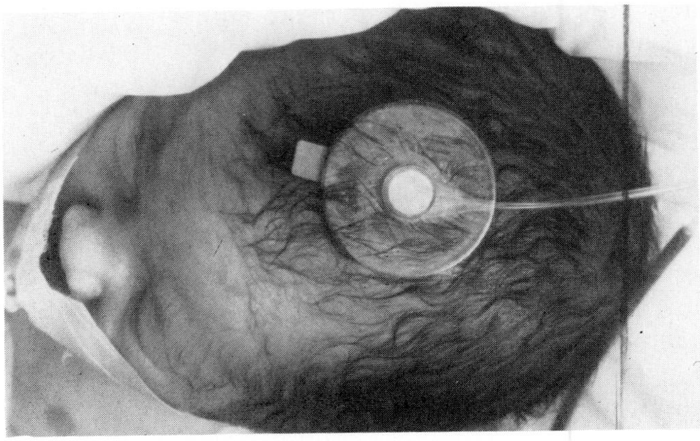

FIG. 27-4 Infant with intracranial pressure monitor.

Medications. The cause of unconsciousness determines specific drug therapies. Children with infectious processes are given antibiotics appropriate to the disease and the infecting organism, and corticosteroids are prescribed for inflammatory conditions and edema. Cerebral edema is an indication for osmotherapy with osmotic diuretics (e.g., mannitol), diuretics (e.g., furosemide), and/or hypertonic glucose solution.

Sedatives are often indicated for extreme restlessness, agitation, and hyperresponsiveness to stimuli. Sedatives or anticonvulsants are prescribed for seizure activity. Deep coma may be induced by administration of barbiturates to diminish activities that might contribute to increased ICP. Paralyzing agents, such as pancuronium (Pavulon), also may be needed to aid in performing diagnostic tests, improving effectiveness of therapy, and reducing risks of secondary complications.

Thermoregulation. Elevated temperature often accompanies cerebral dysfunction, and if fever or hyperthermia is present, measures are implemented to reduce the temperature to prevent brain damage and to reduce metabolic demands generated by the increased body temperature. Antipyretics are the method of choice for fever reduction; cooling devices are used for hyperthermia. Laboratory tests and other methods are used to attempt to determine the cause, if any, of the temperature elevation.

Nursing Considerations

The unconscious child requires continuous nursing attendance with observation, recording, and evaluation of changes in objective signs. These observations provide valuable information regarding the patient's progress. Often they serve as a guide to diagnosis and treatment. Therefore careful and detailed observations are essential for the patient's welfare. In addition, vital functions must be maintained and complications prevented through conscientious and meticulous nursing care.

ASSESSMENT

Continual observation of vital signs, pupillary reaction, and LOC is essential to management of central nervous system disorders. Regular assessment of neurologic signs is a vital part of nursing comatose children. Vital signs are taken and recorded regularly. The frequency depends on the cause of coma and the status and the progression of cerebral involvement. Intervals may be as frequent as every 15 minutes or as long as every 2 hours. Significant alterations are reported immediately. Temperature is taken every 2 to 4 hours, depending on the patient's condition.

The LOC is assessed periodically, including size, equality, and reaction of pupils to light; signs of meningeal irritation, such as nuchal rigidity; and LOC. LOC is assessed by response to vocal commands, spontaneous behavior, resistance to care, and response to painful stimuli; motions of any kind, changes in muscle tone or strength, and body position are noted. Seizure activity is described according to type and length of seizure and body areas involved (see p. 924).

NURSING DIAGNOSES

Nursing diagnoses are determined on the basis of initial and subsequent assessments. Those most often associated with the unconscious child are outlined in the Nursing Care Plan on pp. 900 to 902. Others may be apparent based on specific cases.

PLANNING

The goals of care for the unconscious child include:

1. Maintain respiratory integrity
2. Prevent increasing ICP
3. Provide for basic needs—hygiene, nutrition, hydration, elimination
4. Prevent complications of immobility
5. Support and educate the family

IMPLEMENTATION

Continual neurologic assessment is vital to the management as well as the assessment of the unconscious child. However, many other nursing activities are essential to optimum care.

Respiratory status. Maintaining a patent airway is a primary consideration. Children in lighter stages of coma may be able to cough and swallow, but those in deeper states of coma are unable to handle secretions, which tend to pool in the throat and pharynx. Suctioning is used as often as needed to clear the airway, with care exerted to prevent increasing ICP.

Respiratory status is observed and evaluated regularly. When making an assessment of respirations it is usually best to describe what is observed rather than attempt to place a label to the respirations, because terms are frequently used incorrectly. Signs of respiratory embarrassment may be an indication for ventilatory assistance.

Prevent increasing ICP. Children with elevated ICP are placed on an ICP monitoring device. Nurses caring for patients with intracranial monitoring devices must be acquainted with the system, assist with insertion, interpret the monitor readings, and be able to distinguish between danger signals and mechanical dysfunction. Irrigation and nursing management are the same as for any other line (e.g., arterial or central venous pressure). The neurosurgeon is notified if a satisfactory wave form is not observed.

In cases of high levels of increased ICP, nursing procedures tend to trigger reactive pressure waves in many patients. For example, increased intrathoracic or abdominal pressure will be transmitted to the cranium. Particular care should be taken in positioning these patients to avoid neck vein compression, which may further increase ICP by interfering with venous return. The head of the bed is elevated 15 to 30 degrees (although this is controversial) and the child positioned so that the head is maintained in a midline to facilitate venous drainage and avoid jugular compression. Turning the head from side to side is contraindicated because of the risk of jugular compression. The child can be propped to one side or the other; and the use of an alternating pressure or egg-crate pad reduces the chance of prolonged pressure to vulnerable areas.

Therefore it is important to avoid activities that may increase ICP by causing pain, emotional stress, or crying or those that might trigger a convulsive seizure. Gentle range-of-motion exercises can be carried out but should not be performed vigorously. Nontherapeutic touch can cause an increase in ICP. Any disturbing procedures to be performed should be scheduled to take advantage of therapies that reduce ICP, such as osmotherapy and sedation. Efforts are taken to minimize or eliminate environmental noise. Sudden, loud noises can also contribute to increased ICP.

Nursing Tip: Environmental Noise

Placing earphones over a child's ears has been shown to lower ICP, heart rate, and blood pressure significantly. A greater net decline was achieved when soothing music was played through the earphones (Wincek as reported by Wong, 1988).

Suctioning and percussion are poorly tolerated and are therefore contraindicated unless there are concurrent respiratory problems. Hypoxia and the Valsalva maneuver associated with cough both acutely elevate ICP. Vibration, which does not increase ICP, accomplishes excellent results and should be tried first if treatment is needed. If suctioning is necessary, it should be used judiciously and preceded by hyperventilation with 100% oxygen.

Barbiturate-induced coma requires extensive monitoring, cardiovascular and respiratory support, and ICP monitoring to assess response to therapy. Elevation of ICP and/or heart rate of patients who are being given paralyzing agents or are under sedation may indicate the need for another dose of either or both medications.

An elevated temperature is not uncommon in children with central nervous system dysfunction; therefore, a light covering is sufficient. Vigorous efforts are needed, such as tepid sponge baths or application of a hypothermia blanket, to prevent brain damage from hyperthermia.

Hygienic care. Routine measures for cleansing and maintaining skin integrity are an integral part of nursing care of the unconscious child. Skin folds require special attention to prevent excoriation. Children who are unable to move are prone to develop tissue breakdown and pressure necrosis; therefore, the child is placed on a sheepskin, egg-crate pad, or other resilient surface (alternating pressure mattresses and water-filled mattresses are also used) to prevent pressure on prominent areas of the body. The goal is prevention by regular change of position and inspection of vulnerable areas, such as the ankle, trochanter, and shoulder. Bed linen and any clothing are kept dry and free of wrinkles. Rubbing the back and extremities with lotion or other lubricating preparation stimulates circulation and helps prevent drying of the skin.

Mouth care is performed at least twice daily, since the mouth tends to become dry or coated with mucus. The teeth and mucous surfaces are carefully cleansed and moistened with a soft toothbrush, Toothettes, or gauze saturated with saline. Lips are coated with ointment, petrolatum, or other preparations to protect them from drying, cracking, or blistering.

The deeply comatose child is also prone to eye irritation. The corneal reflexes are absent; therefore, the eyes are easily irritated or damaged by linen, dust, or other substances that may come in contact with them. There is excessive dryness as a result of decreased secretions, especially if the child is undergoing osmotherapy to reduce or prevent brain edema, and incomplete closure of the eyes. The eyes are examined regularly and carefully for early signs of irritation or inflammation. Artificial tears (methylcellulose) are placed in the eyes at frequent intervals. Sometimes eye dressings may be needed to protect the eyes from possible damage.

The hair is combed and styled neatly. Long hair is usually braided and secured with rubber hands. The scalp is kept clean with dry or wet shampoos as needed. The child's head may be shaved for tests or surgical procedures. If so, the hair is saved if possible.

Nutrition and hydration. Initially, unconscious children are fed by intravenous infusion or hyperalimentation. Later, nutrition is provided in a balanced formula given by nasogastric or gastrostomy tube. The nasogastric tube is usually taped in place with care to prevent pressure on the nares. The tube is rinsed carefully after each feeding and is replaced frequently (usually every 24 hours) to prevent bacterial growth and to alternate nostrils to prevent nasal irritation and pressure. Overfeeding is avoided to prevent vomiting, with the danger of aspiration. The stomach contents are aspirated and measured prior to feeding to ascertain the amount remaining in the stomach. If the residual volume is excessive (depending on the size of the child), the dietitian and physician should be consulted regarding alteration of the formula composition to provide the needed calories and nutrients in a smaller volume. The aspirated contents should always be refed to prevent electrolyte loss.

Hydration is maintained in the same manner. When cerebral edema is a threat, the fluids may be restricted to reduce the chance of fluid overload. Skin and mucous membranes are examined for signs of dehydration.

Elimination. A retention catheter is usually inserted in the older child, and a plastic collection bag is placed on the infant or small child. The child who formerly had bowel and bladder control is generally incontinent. The collecting devices help keep the skin clean and provide a means for obtaining an accurate intake and output measurement. If the child remains comatose for a long period of time, the indwelling catheter may be removed and replaced by intermittent catheterization. Stool softeners are usually sufficient to maintain bowel function, but suppositories or enemas may be needed occasionally for adequate elimination.

Positioning and exercise. The unconscious child is positioned to prevent aspiration of saliva, nasogastric secretions, and vomitus and to minimize ICP. The child is positioned as described previously, with a small, firm pillow placed under the head and the uppermost limbs flexed and supported with pillows. The weight of the body should not rest on the dependent arm. In the semiprone position the child lies with the dependent arm at the side behind the body and the opposite side supported on pillows with the uppermost arm and leg flexed and resting on the pillows. This position prevents undue pressure on the dependent extremities. The dependent position of the face encourages drainage of secretions and prevents the flaccid tongue from obstructing the airway.

Normal range-of-motion exercises are carried out to maintain function and prevent contractures of joints. Exercises are performed gently and with full range of motion. A small, rolled pad can be placed in the palms to help maintain proper position of fingers; footboards or boots can be used to help prevent foot-drop, and sometimes splinting may be needed to prevent severe contractures of the wrist, knee, or ankle in decerebrate children.

Medications. Medications are administered as prescribed. Drugs such as antibiotics and corticosteroids may be ordered intravenously during the early days of unconsciousness. When nasogastric or gastrostomy feedings are implemented, most medications are given by this route. It is particularly important to be alert to signs of adverse drug reactions, since many of the side effects or toxic effects of drugs involve observation of changes in behavior or responsiveness, which is rendered invalid by the child's unconscious state.

Stimulation. Sensory stimulation is important in the care of the unconscious child, just as it is in the care of the alert child. For the temporarily unconscious or semiconscious child, sensory stimulation helps to arouse him to the conscious state and orient him in terms of time and place. Unconscious children need sensory stimulation as much as conscious children. Auditory and tactile stimulation are especially valuable. Tactile stimulation is not appropriate for the child in whom it may elicit an undesirable response. However, for other children, tactile contact often has a relaxing and calming effect. When the child's condition permits, holding or rocking the child has a soothing effect on him and provides the body contact needed by young children.

The auditory sense is often present in a state of coma. Hearing is the last sense to be lost and the first sense to be regained; therefore, the child is spoken to as any other child. Conversation around the child should not include thoughtless or derogatory remarks. A radio or record player playing soft music, a music box, or tapes of familiar voices are frequently employed to provide auditory stimulation. Singing the child's favorite songs or reading a favorite story within his hearing is a tactic used to maintain his contact with a familiar world. Above all, it is important to remember that this is a child who has all the needs of any ill child.

Certain behaviors have been observed when children waken from the unconscious state. The stress and anxiety they appear to feel in a strange and unfamiliar environment are consistently expressed in silent and withdrawn behavior. The children respond to basic questioning but do not display their prehospitalization personality and social behavior until they are transferred from the critical care area.

The children awaken disoriented, with no recollection of events that took place during the critical phase of their illness. Strange equipment being introduced while they were unconscious requires explanation. The appearance of other ill children is puzzling and frightening, increasing their anxiety and stress concerning their own situation. They are powerless to control what is happening to them. Nurses can help these children deal with their stress by orienting them to where they are and the circumstances of their being there, describing what is expected of them, and giving them a sense of control whenever possible. Encouraging parents to visit and providing other items associated with home, such as a favorite toy, a photograph, or other item, help them maintain a link with their lives outside the confines of the critical care environment. Understanding and individualized care help children to weather the stresses and tension of this period of crisis (see Chapter 20).

Family support. Dealing with the parents of an unconscious child is especially difficult. They may demonstrate all the guilt, fear, and anxiety of any parent of a seriously ill child. In addition they are faced with the uncertain outcome of the cerebral dysfunction. The fear of death, mental retardation, or other permanent disability is present. Nursing intervention with parents depends on the nature of the pathologic condition, the personality of the parents, and the parent-child relationship prior to injury or illness.

Waking from a coma is a gradual process; however, the child may regain consciousness within a short period of time. If there is little or no residual effect, the child will be dismissed to home care fairly soon. The parents need the most intensive nursing intervention during the period of crisis and uncertainty. During the recovery phase they are given information, information is clarified, and they are encouraged to become involved in the child's care. Often the child's hospitalization is brief; however, some children require extended hospitalization for intensive therapy and rehabilitation

The parents of children who die within hours or days require the support and guidance that the parents of any dying child need to cope with the reality and resolve their grief (see Chapter 18).

Probably the most difficult situations are those that involve children who are unconscious permanently or for an indefinite period. Unlike parents who lose a child through death, the finality is lacking for these parents, often leaving them in a state of suspended grief. The presence of the child renders the parents unable to resolve the loss. Superimposed on the process of grieving for the "lost" child, parents may be faced with difficult decisions. First there is the child whose brain is so severely damaged that his vital functions must be maintained by artificial means. When brain death has been determined according to established criteria, the parents must make the final decision to remove the life-support systems.

Second, there is the child who has survived the illness or injury that produced the brain damage but who is left unconscious permanently. These parents must decide whether to place the child in an extended care facility or make arrangements to care for the child at home. The parents who choose to care for their child at home will need education and support in learning to care for the child, regular follow-up observation and assessment of the home management, and planning for some respite care for the family (see p. 609). Parents need to understand that it is important to plan for periodic relief from the continual care of the child.

EVALUATION

The effectiveness of nursing interventions is determined by continual reassessment and evaluation of care based on the following observational guidelines and expected outcomes:

1. Monitor the child's vital signs, neurologic signs, and behavior

NURSING CARE PLAN

The Unconscious Child

HP-HMP* **Potential for trauma**
Risk factors: physical immobility, depressed sensorium, intracranial pathology

Nursing Goals	Nursing Interventions	Expected Patient/Family Outcomes
Assess neurologic status frequently	Monitor vital signs Check pupillary reaction for size, reaction to light and accommodation, equality of responses Note and describe Voluntary movements of extremities (e.g., purposeful, random) Changes in muscular tone Changes in position of body and/or head Tremor, twitching Seizure activity (e.g., generalized or local) Signs of meningeal irritation (e.g., nuchal rigidity, opisthotonos) Measure OFC of infants Assess status of fontanel—full or sunken, tense or soft	†Signs of neurologic alterations are detected early
Prevent respiratory complications	Position for optimum ventilation Turn frequently—at least every 2 hours Avoid contact with persons with upper respiratory infection Maintain patent airway Remove accumulated secretions promptly Provide good oral hygiene Perform percussion, vibration, and suctioning every 3-4 hours	Child exhibits no evidence of lung dysfunction
Prevent cerebral edema	Elevate head of bed to 15 to 30 degrees Monitor vital signs and neurologic signs to detect early indications of increased intracranial pressure Monitor fluid intake and output Observe for signs of impending overhydration	Child exhibits no signs of increased intracranial pressure
Minimize intracranial pressure	Elevate head of the bed 15 to 30 degrees Avoid positions or activities that increase ICP Pressure on neck veins Flexion or extension of neck Head rotation Valsalva maneuver Painful stimuli Respiratory procedures (especially suctioning) Prevent constipation Provide Quiet, subdued environment Pleasant auditory experiences Therapeutic touch Avoid emotionally stressful conversation (e.g., about pain, condition, prognosis)	†Early signs are detected and appropriate action is initiated Intracranial pressure remains within safe limits Child shows no evidence of increased intracranial pressure
Prevent or control hyperthermia	Assess temperature regularly to detect elevation Remove excess coverings	Body temperature remains within safe limits
Prevent cerebral hypoxia	Position for maximum ventilation Maintain patent airway Position to prevent aspiration: semiprone position; side-lying position Aspirate airway as needed Insert oral airway if indicated Avoid neck hyperextension	Child breathes easily; respirations are within normal limits
Prevent corneal irritation	Patch eyes if indicated Keep lids completely closed Instill "artificial tears"	Corneas remain clear and moist

*For an explanation of abbreviations, see p. 20.
†Nursing outcome.

NURSING CARE PLAN

The Unconscious Child—cont'd

Nursing Goals	Nursing Interventions	Expected Patient/Family Outcomes
Prevent drying and caking of mucous membranes	Provide meticulous mouth care	Mucous membranes remain clean, moist, and free of irritation
Protect from physical injury	Keep side rails up Pad hard surfaces that may injure extremities during spontaneous or involuntary movement	Child remains free of physical injury
Maintain limb flexibility and functions	Perform passive range-of-motion exercises Position to reduce contractures—splint contracting joints if needed	Joints remain flexible and retain full range of motion
N-MP **Potential impaired skin integrity** **Risk factors: immobility, body secretions**		
Maintain skin integrity	Place child on sheepskin, egg-carton pad, or other resilient surface Change position frequently unless contraindicated by increased ICP Protect pressure points (e.g., trochanter, sacrum, ankle, shoulder, occiput) Inspect skin surfaces regularly for signs of irritation, redness, evidence of pressure Cleanse skin regularly, at least once daily Protect skin folds and surfaces that rub together Keep clothing and linen clean and dry Carry out good perineal care under urine collection device Stimulate circulation by gentle rubbing with lotion or other lubricating substance Protect lips with cream or ointment	Skin remains clean and intact
A-EP **Feeding, bathing/hygiene, dressing/grooming, toileting (level 4) self-care deficit** **Etiology: perceptual and cognitive impairment**		
Ensure adequate nutritional intake	Provide nourishment in manner suitable to child's condition	Child obtains sufficient nourishment
Provide hygienic care	Bathe daily or more often, if indicated Dress appropriately Keep hair combed and styled	Child appears clean and as well groomed as possible within limitations of his condition
Provide toileting	Diaper as needed Use collection appliances, if feasible Clean skin well after each elimination	Child's diaper area remains clean and free of irritation
Ensure adequate elimination	Provide sufficient liquid intake, unless contraindicated by cerebral edema or if overhydration is a threat Apply urine collecting device or insert indwelling catheter (if ordered) Provide proper care of catheter	Bowel is evacuated daily
CPP **Sensory/perceptual alterations (visual, auditory, kinesthetic, gustatory, tactile, olfactory)** **Etiology: central nervous system depression, bed rest**		
Assess LOC	Observe and record Change in spontaneous behavior Resistance to care Response to verbal commands Response to noxious stimuli Type of verbalization or crying	Consciousness level is determined
Provide sensory stimulation	Provide tactile stimulation (if it does not evoke undesirable muscle response, e.g., seizures) Provide auditory stimulation by voice, radio, music box, etc. Provide visual stimuli appropriate for age Provide proprioceptive stimulation by rocking, cuddling, etc.	Child receives sensory stimulation appropriate to his age and condition Child appears relaxed and rests quietly

Continued.

NURSING CARE PLAN

The Unconscious Child—cont'd

Nursing Goals	Nursing Interventions	Expected Patient/Family Outcomes
Prevent overstimulation	Avoid stimulation that precipitates undesirable responses Space nursing activities for minimal disturbance	Child exhibits no seizure activity or undue restlessness and agitation
RRP Altered family processes **Etiology: situational crisis (child with a serious illness)**		
Support family	Explain therapies; clarify and reinforce information given to family by physician Interpret child's behaviors and responses Allow expression of feelings and concerns Accept aggressive behavior	Family demonstrates an understanding of child's behaviors, therapies, and probable outcome
Assist in child placement, if indicated	Provide needed information Answer family's questions; encourage expression of feelings Refer to persons or agencies for further information and clarification Support parent's decisions	Family verbalizes feelings and concerns
Arrange for discharge and follow-up care	Teach family techniques and procedures needed in care of child Arrange for follow-up visit by appropriate persons (e.g., public health nurse)	Family demonstrates skills and procedures for child's care

Nursing interventions related to medical management

Maintain patent airway
Administer care of endotracheal tube or tracheostomy if appropriate; have equipment available for emergency insertion if indicated for respiratory distress
Ensure adequate respiration
Assist with insertion of endotracheal tube
Monitor artificial ventilation
Ensure adequate circulation
Assist with establishment of intravenous infusion
Monitor intravenous infusion
Administer intravenous fluids as prescribed
Assist with diagnostic tests
Collect specimens as ordered
Carry out examinations as indicated or ordered, such as urine specific gravity, blood samples
Prepare for and assist with diagnostic procedures, such as lumbar puncture, x-ray examination
Interpret and report results of tests
Provide nutrition and hydration
Monitor intravenous feedings when ordered
Feed prescribed formula by means of nasogastric or gastrostomy tube
Prevent increased ICP
Administer paralyzing agents if prescribed
Prevent cerebral hypoxia
Maintain patent airway
Provide oxygen as indicated by objective signs or as ordered
If on mechanical ventilation:
Monitor for correct settings, proper functioning
Prepare to provide artificial ventilation in case of ventilatory failure; have AmBU bag at hand
Administer medications as ordered to prevent cerebral edema and improve cerebral circulation
Prevent cerebral edema
Monitor intravenous fluids carefully
Administer hyperosmolar fluids as prescribed
Administer corticosteroids as ordered
Weigh daily or as ordered to detect fluid accumulation or reduction
Monitor ICP
Prevent elevated temperature
Administer antipyretics, if prescribed
Apply and monitor hypothermia blanket if indicated or ordered; administer antishivering agents if ordered
Prevent seizures
Administer sedatives or anticonvulsants as prescribed
Ensure adequate elimination
Administer stool softener
Administer suppositories or enema as indicated

2. Observe child's response to nursing activities, therapies, and diagnostic procedures; monitor ICP
3. Observe color, position, and motor activity; measure fluid and nutritional intake and output
4. Monitor status of respiratory, renal, and gastrointestinal systems, skin
5. Observe family behaviors and interview members regarding their understandings and their feelings and concerns

Expected outcomes:
See the Nursing Care Plan on pp. 900 to 902.

HEAD INJURY

Head injury can be defined as any pathologic process involving the scalp, skull, meninges, or brain resulting from mechanical force. Accidental injury is the major single cause of death in the pediatric age-group, and although it cannot be stated with certainty, most of these injuries are probably the result of central nervous system trauma. Rarely does a child attain adulthood without having sustained a significant bump or blow to the head. Most children do not require hospitalization, but a large number are admitted to hospitals for evaluation and treatment.

Etiology

Falls are the leading cause of head injury; motor vehicle–related accidents are the major cause of severe and fatal head injury, especially from improper passenger restraint. Child abuse is a cause of severe head injury in children less than 1 year of age. Vigorous shaking of an infant can cause central nervous system damage, especially a whiplash type of injury and subdural hematoma. Short falls, as from furniture or counters, are also common in this age-group. Lack of a helmet when riding a bicycle and impact injuries in sports are the causes of a significant number of injuries in children over 12 years of age. Adolescents are most often injured in motor vehicle accidents.

The exposed nature of the head renders it particularly vulnerable to external violence, and many of the physical characteristics of children predispose them to craniocerebral trauma. For example, infants are frequently left unattended on beds, in high chairs, and in other places from which they can fall. Because the head of an infant or toddler is proportionately large and heavy in relation to other body parts, it is the most likely to be injured. Incomplete motor development contributes to falls at all ages, and the natural curiosity and exuberance of children frequently place them in situations in which they are likely to incur an injury.

Pathophysiology

The skull forms such an excellent protection for the brain that, although nerve tissue is delicate, a severe blow is usually required to cause significant damage. As a whole, head injuries can be regarded as localized or generalized. In localized injuries the force is spent on a local area of both skull and underlying tissues; in generalized injuries the force is transmitted to the entire skull, causing widespread movement, distortion, and damage. Local injuries frequently cause hemorrhage and infection, but generalized trauma is associated with a higher mortality.

Injury to the brain occurs by way of compression, tearing, or shearing, either singly, in combination, or in succession. When the stationary head receives a blow, the sudden movement causes deformation of the skull and mass movement of the brain. Continued movement of the intracranial contents allows the brain to strike parts of the skull (such as the sharp edges of the sphenoid or the irregular surface of the anterior fossa) or the edges of the tentorium. Although the brain volume remains unchanged, significant distortion takes place as the brain changes shape in response to the force of impact to the skull. This movement can cause bruising at the point of impact *(coup)* and/or at a distance as the brain collides with the unyielding surfaces far removed from the point of impact *(contrecoup)* (Fig. 27-5). Thus a blow to the occipital region can cause severe injury to the frontal and temporal areas of the brain. Sudden deceleration, such as takes place during a fall, causes the greatest cerebral injury at the point of impact.

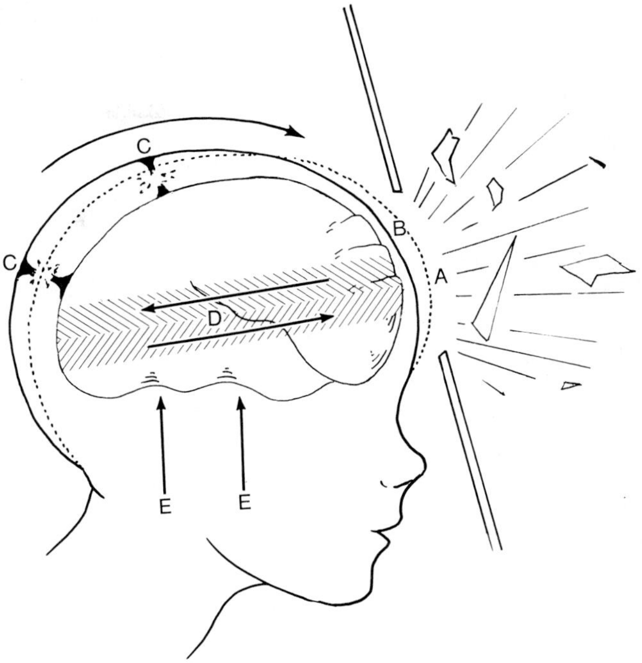

FIG. 27-5 Mechanical distortions of cranium during closed head injury. *A*, Preinjury contour of skull. *B*, Immediate postinjury contour of skull. *C*, Torn subdural vessels. *D*, Shearing forces. *E*, Trauma from contact with floor of cranium. (Redrawn from Grubb, R.L., and Coxe, W.S.: Central nervous system trauma: cranial. In Eliasson, S.G., Prensky, A.L., and Hardin, W.B., Jr., editors: Neurological pathophysiology, New York, 1974, Oxford University Press.)

Another effect of brain movement is shearing stresses, which tear small arteries and cause subdural hemorrhages. Another source of damage occurs when severe compression of the skull causes the brain to be forced through the tentorial opening. This can produce irreparable damage to the brain stem (see Figs. 27-6 and 27-7).

Concussion. The most common head injury is concussion, a transient and reversible neuronal dysfunction, with instantaneous loss of awareness and responsiveness, that results from trauma to the head and that persists for a relatively short time, usually minutes or hours. It is generally followed by amnesia for the moment of the injury and a variable period before the injury.

Contusion and laceration. The terms *contusion* and *laceration* are used to describe visible bruising and tearing of cerebral tissue. Contusions represent petechial hemorrhages along the superficial aspects of the brain at the site of impact (*coup* injury) and/or a lesion remote from the site of direct trauma (*contrecoup* injury). In serious accidents there may be multiple sites of injury. Contusions may cause focal disturbances in strength, sensation, or visual awareness. The degree of brain damage in the contused areas varies according to the extent of vascular injury. Cerebral lacerations are generally associated with penetrating or depressed skull fractures.

Fractures. Compared to that of the adult the immature skull, because of its flexibility, is able to sustain a greater degree of deformation before it incurs a fracture. A great deal of force is required to produce a fracture in the skull of an infant. A fracture may occur with little or no brain damage, or severe and fatal brain injury can take place without fracture. The undersurface of the skull contains grooves in which the meningeal arteries lie. A fracture that runs through one of these grooves may tear the artery and produce severe and damaging hemorrhage.

The types of fractures that occur are:

Linear fractures are those in which the lines of the fracture are predetermined by the site and velocity of the impact as well as the strength of the bone. These are uncommon before 2 to 3 years of age.

Depressed fractures are those in which the bone is locally broken, usually into several irregular fragments that are pushed inward, causing pressure on the brain. The inner portion of the bone is more extensively fragmented than the outer portion, which almost invariably produces tears in the dura. These are uncommon before 2 to 3 years of age. In infants and very young children, the soft, malleable bone may become dented in a peculiar rounded or Ping-Pong ball depression, without laceration of either skin or dura.

Compound fractures consist of laceration of skin that extends to the site of the bony fracture, which can be linear, depressed, or comminuted.

Basilar fractures involve the basilar portion of the frontal, ethmoid, sphenoid, temporal, or occipital bones.

Diastatic fractures are traumatic separations of cranial sutures. These most frequently affect the lambdoid suture and are rarely seen beyond the first 4 years of life. They require no specific treatment.

Complications

The major complications of trauma to the head are hemorrhage, infection, edema, and herniation through the tentorium. Infection is always a hazard in open injuries, and edema is related to tissue trauma. Vascular rupture may occur even in minor head injuries, causing hemorrhage between the skull and cerebral surfaces. Compression of the underlying brain produces effects that can be rapidly fatal or insidiously progressive.

Epidural hemorrhage. The blood accumulates between the dura and the skull to form a hematoma, which, because of the difficulty with which dura is stripped from bone, forces the underlying brain contents downward and inward as the brain expands (Fig. 27-6). Since bleeding is generally arterial, brain compression occurs rapidly. Most often the expanding hematoma is located in the parietotemporal region, forcing the medial portion of the temporal lobe under the edge of the tentorium, where it causes pressure on nerves and blood vessels.

The classic clinical picture of epidural hemorrhage (momentary unconsciousness followed by a normal period, then lethargy or coma) is seldom evident in children (see box on p. 905 for clinical manifestations). The period of impaired consciousness is frequently lacking, and the symptom-free period is atypical because of nonspecific complaints such as irritability, headache, and vomiting. The symptom-free period frequently lasts longer than 48 hours. Clinically significant epidural hematomas are uncommon in children younger than 4 years of age. These differences may be caused by the decreased tendency of the resilient skull to fracture; the ability of blood to escape through widened sutures, an open fontanel, or a fracture; bleeding from smaller vessels with less rapid and massive bleeding; lower systolic blood pressure in children; and possibly the decreased susceptibility of the child's brain to pressure changes.

Subdural hemorrhage. A subdural hemorrhage is bleeding between the dura and the cerebrum, usually as a result of rupture of cortical veins that bridge the subdural space (Fig. 27-7). Unlike epidural hemorrhage, which de-

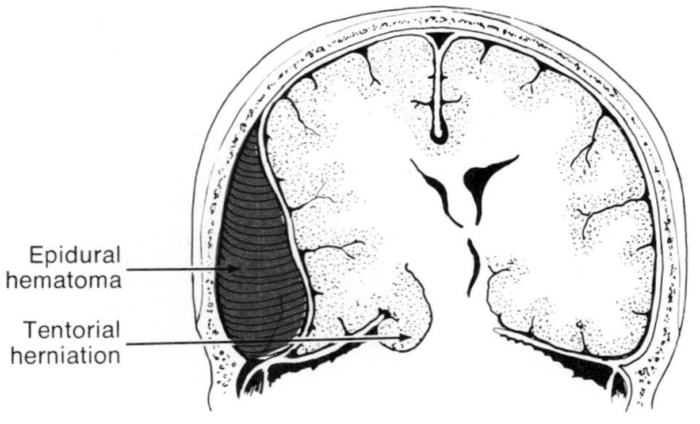

FIG. 27-6 Epidural (extradural) hematoma and compression of portion of temporal lobe through tentorial hiatus.

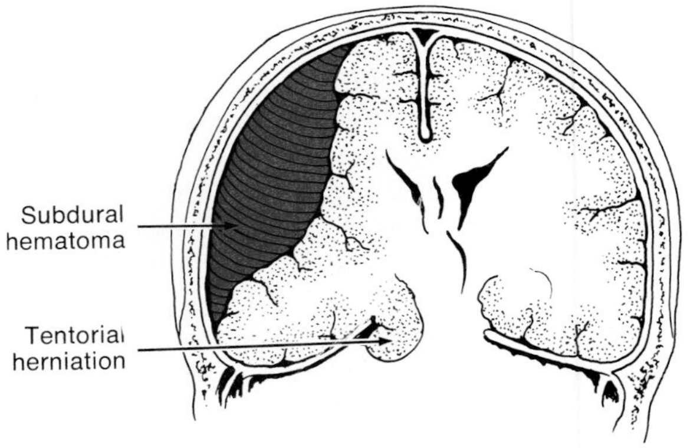

FIG. 27-7 Subdural hematoma.

velops inwardly, subdural hemorrhage tends to develop more slowly and spreads thinly and widely until it is limited by the dural barriers—the falx and tentorium. Subdural hematoma is fairly common in infants, frequently as the result of birth trauma.

Subdural hemorrhage can cause either acute or chronic subdural hematoma. Acute subdural hematoma develops within minutes or hours of injury and is associated with a high mortality and poor prognosis. The clinical course and manifestations of the more common chronic subdural hematoma are variable and depend on the damage sustained by the brain substance and the age of the child. Delayed symptoms are common in children with open fontanels and sutures.

Repeated subdural taps often provide relief in the infant. Surgical evacuation of the hematoma is the treatment of choice in the older child and is frequently required in infants.

Cerebral edema. Some degree of brain edema is expected after craniocerebral trauma. Cerebral edema caused by direct cellular injury or vascular injury induces vascular stasis, anoxia, and further vasodilation. If the progression continues unchecked, ICP exceeds arterial pressure and fatal anoxia ensues and/or the pressure causes herniation of a portion of the brain over the edge of the tentorium, compressing the brain stem and occluding the posterior cerebral arteries.

Clinical Manifestations of Acute Head Injury

Minor Injury
May or may not lose consciousness
Transient period of confusion
Somnolence
Listlessness
Irritability
Pallor
Vomiting (1 or more episodes)

Signs of Progression
Altered mental status (e.g., difficulty rousing child)
Mounting agitation
Development of focal lateral neurologic signs (see p. 891)
Marked changes in vital signs

Severe Injury
Signs of increased ICP (see box on p. 890)
  Increased head size (infant)
  Bulging fontanel (infant)
Retinal hemorrhage
Extraocular palsies (especially cranial nerve VI)
Hemiparesis
Quadriplegia
Elevated temperature (sometimes)
Unsteady gait (older child)
Papilledema (older child)

Associated Signs
Skin injury (to area of head sustaining injury)
Other iinjuries (e.g., to extremities)

Diagnostic Evaluation

A detailed history, both past and present, is essential in evaluating the child with a head injury. It is important to know whether the child suffers from disorders that may produce his symptoms, and events surrounding the injury often supply significant data. It must be determined whether or not the infant or child exhibited alterations in consciousness and any other signs and behaviors exhibited by the child must be noted.

A neurologic examination is performed, including vital signs, ocular signs, motor function, reflexes, and LOC. Less urgent but important additional assessments include examination of the scalp for lacerations and palpation for other abnormalities. Bleeding from the nose or ears (although uncommon in children) needs further evaluation, and a watery discharge from the nose (rhinorrhea) that is positive for glucose (as tested with Dextrostix) suggests leaking of CSF from a skull fracture.

An accurate assessment of clinical signs provides baseline information (see box). Serial evaluations, preferably by a single observer, help to detect changes in the neurologic status. Alterations in mental status, evidenced by increased difficulty in rousing the child, mounting agitation, development of focal lateral neurologic signs, or marked changes in vital signs, usually indicate extension or progression of the basic pathologic process.

Special tests. After a thorough clinical examination, a variety of diagnostic tests are helpful in providing a more definitive diagnosis of the type and extent of the trauma. Where available, computed tomography is especially valuable in diagnosis of neurologic trauma and usually makes other diagnostic procedures unnecessary. It is easily carried out, is noninvasive, and can be repeated serially for reassessment in the patient who remains unconscious or shows progressive neurologic deterioration.

Other tests that might be used include magnetic resonance imaging (where available), skull films, and echoencephalography. Electroencephalography is not particularly helpful for early diagnosis but is useful for defining seizure activity or focal destructive lesions after the acute phase of illness. Lumbar puncture is rarely employed in craniocerebral trauma and is contraindicated in the presence of increased ICP.

In the infant or small child a subdural tap through a fontanel or coronal suture may establish the diagnosis of subdural or epidural hemorrhage. In some centers monitoring intracranial pressure is part of the assessment.

Posttraumatic syndromes. Postconcussion syndrome is a common sequela to brain injury and occurs within minutes to an hour after a minimum head injury (see box). The manifestations vary with the age of the child. The syndrome occurs very frequently in children under 1 year of age. The syndrome in adolescents is similar to that in adults. The duration of manifestations can vary from several days to several months.

Posttraumatic seizures occur in a number of children who survive a head injury. The onset may be in the first 24 hours, usually within the first year, and in most cases

Clinical Manifestations of Posttraumatic Syndrome

Infants
- Pallor
- Sweating
- Irritability
- Sleepiness
- May vomit

Children
- Behavioral disturbances
  - Aggressiveness
  - Disobedience
  - Withdrawal
  - Regression
  - Anxiety
- Sleep disturbances
- Phobias
- Emotional lability
- Irritability
- Altered school performance
- Seizures

Adolescents
- Headache
- Dizziness
- Impaired concentration

Structural Complications
- Hydrocephalus
- Focal deficits
  - Optic atrophy
  - Cranial nerve palsies
  - Motor deficits
  - Diabetes insipidus
  - Aphasia

within 2 years after the injury. Structural complications may occur, and type of residual effect depends on the location and nature of the trauma. True mental retardation occurs only after severe injuries.

Therapeutic Management

The majority of children with mild to moderate concussion who have not lost consciousness can be cared for and observed at home after careful examination reveals no serious intracranial injury. The parents are instructed to check the child every 2 hours to determine any changes in responsiveness. The sleeping child should be wakened to see if he can be roused normally. Parents are advised to maintain contact with the health professional, who usually wishes to examine the child again in 1 or 2 days. The manifestations of epidural hematoma in children do not generally appear until 24 hours or more after injury.

Children with severe injuries, those who have lost consciousness for more than a few minutes, and those with prolonged and continued seizures or other focal or diffuse neurologic signs must be hospitalized until their condition is stable and their neurologic signs have diminished.

The child is maintained on nothing by mouth or restricted to clear liquids, if able to take fluids by mouth, until it is determined that vomiting will not occur. Intravenous fluids are indicated in the child who is comatose or displays dulled sensorium and/or in the child with persistent vomiting. Fluid balance is closely monitored by daily weights, accurate intake and output measurements, and serum osmolality to detect early signs of water retention, excessive dehydration, and states of hypertonicity or hypotonicity.

Restlessness can be satisfactorily managed, if necessary, with mild sedation, and headache is usually controlled with acetaminophen (Tylenol). Anticonvulsants are used for seizure control and frequently in cases of suspected contusion or laceration. Antibiotics are administered if there are lacerations, cerebrospinal fluid leakage, or excessive cerebral tissue damage. Prophylactic tetanus toxoid is given as appropriate (see p. 1072). Cerebral edema is managed as described for the unconscious child. Hyperthermia is controlled with tepid sponges or a hypothermia blanket.

Surgical therapy. Scalp lacerations are sutured after the underlying bone is carefully examined. Depressed fractures require surgical reduction and removal of bone fragments. Torn dura is sutured. "Ping-Pong ball" skull fractures in very young infants ordinarily correct themselves within a few weeks and do not require specific treatment, although they can be reduced by pressure against the bone.

Nursing Considerations

The hospitalized child requires careful neurologic assessment and evaluation (including vital signs) repeated at frequent intervals to provide information needed to establish a correct diagnosis, to reveal signs and symptoms of increased ICP, to determine clinical management, and to prevent many complications.

The child is placed on bed rest, usually with the head of the bed elevated slightly, and appropriate safety measures, such as side rails kept up for older children and seizure precautions for children of all ages, are implemented. The extremely restless child may require that hard surfaces be padded and restraint used to prevent the possibility of further injury. Care is individualized according to the specific needs of the child. The unconscious child is managed as described in the previous section, but most childhood head injuries are those causing momentary stunning or temporary unconsciousness. The child may be restless and irritable, but more often his reaction is to fall asleep when left undisturbed. A quiet environment helps reduce the restlessness and irritability. Bright lights shining directly into the child's face are irritating. This often makes checking the ocular responses more difficult to perform and more aggravating to the child.

Frequent examinations of vital signs, neurologic signs, and LOC are extremely important nursing observations. When possible they should be performed by a single observer in order to better detect subtle changes that may indicate worsening of neurologic status. Pupils are checked for size, equality, reaction to light, and accommodation. After the initial elevations usually seen after injury, the vital signs generally return to normal unless there is brain stem involvement. An axillary measurement of temperature is the safest method, since seizures are not uncommon and vomiting is a frequent response in children, especially when the child is disturbed.

The most important nursing observation is assessment

of the child's LOC. Alterations in consciousness appear earlier in the progression of an injury than alterations of vital signs or focal neurologic signs. Some expected responses may be misinterpreted as deviations from the normal. Frequent examinations of alertness are fatiguing to the child; therefore the child often desires to fall asleep, which may be confused with depressed consciousness. When left alone, the child promptly dozes. It is not uncommon to observe ocular divergence through the partially closed eyelids.

Observations of position and movement provide additional information. Any abnormal posturing is noted as well as whether or not it occurs continuously or intermittently. Are the child's handgrips strong and equal in strength? Are there any signs of decerebrate or decorticate posturing? What is the child's response to stimulation? Is movement purposeful, random, or absent? Are movement and/or sensation equal on both sides or restricted to one side only?

The child may complain of headache or other discomfort. The child who is too young to describe a headache will be fussy and resist being handled. The child who suffers from vertigo will often assume a position and vigorously resist efforts to move him. Forcible movement causes the child to vomit and display spontaneous nystagmus. Seizures, relatively common in children with craniocerebral trauma, may be of any type but are more often generalized regardless of the type of injury. Any seizure activity should be carefully observed and described in detail (see p. 924).

Drainage from any orifice is noted. Bleeding from the ear suggests the possibility of a basal skull fracture. The amount and characteristics of the drainage are observed, and since the auditory canal may be a source of infection, dry, sterile cotton can be placed loosely at the orifice and changed when soiled. Suctioning through the nares is contraindicated, since there is a high risk of secondary infection and the probability of the catheter entering the brain substance through the fracture.

Head trauma is frequently accompanied by other undetected injuries; therefore any bruises, lacerations, or evidence of internal injuries or fractures of the extremities is noted and reported. Associated injuries are evaluated and treated appropriately.

The child with normal LOC is usually allowed clear liquids unless fluid is restricted. If the child has an intravenous infusion, it is maintained as prescribed. The diet is advanced to that appropriate for the child's age as soon as his condition permits. Intake and output are measured and recorded, and any incontinence of bowel or bladder is noted in the child who has been toilet trained.

The child should be observed for any unusual behavior, but behavior should be interpreted in relation to the child's normal behavior. For example, urinary incontinence during sleep would be of no consequence in a child who routinely wets the bed but would be highly significant for one who is always dry. In addition, a child who is subject to nightmares might cry out and demonstrate agitated behavior at night. Parents are valuable resources. Information obtained from parents at or shortly after admission is helpful in evaluating the child's behavior; for example, the ease with which the child is roused normally, his usual sleeping position, how much he sleeps during the day, motor activity of which he is capable (rolling over, sitting up, climbing), hearing and visual acuity, appetite, and manner of eating (spoon, bottle, cup). There would be less concern about a child who falls asleep several times during the day if this particular type of behavior is consistent with his usual behavior.

When the child is discharged, the parents are advised of probable posttraumatic symptoms that may be expected, such as behavioral changes, sleep disturbances, phobias, and seizures. They should understand observations that should be made and how to contact the physician, nurse, or health facility in case the child develops any unusual signs or symptoms. The importance of follow-up evaluation should be emphasized, and it is often advisable to refer the family to a public health agency for home follow-through to be certain that the child receives posthospital evaluation.

The rehabilitation and management of the child with permanent brain injury are beyond the scope of this discussion, but it is an important aspect of care. Rehabilitation of brain-injured children is begun as soon as feasible and usually involves the family and a rehabilitation team. Careful assessment of the child's capabilities, limitations, and probable potential is made as early as possible, and appropriate interventions are implemented to maximize the residual capacities. The **National Head Injury Foundation*** "arose from the mutual frustration and sense of hopelessness experienced by families in their search for appropriate facilities and support to return head-injured loved ones to their maximum functioning potential." It provides information and listings of rehabilitation services and support groups throughout the country.

NEAR-DROWNING

Drowning is not an uncommon accident in childhood. It ranks second as a cause of accidental death in children. About 85% of these children are male and the majority are between ages 10 and 19 years (Spyker, 1985). However, a significant number are children under age 3 years. Most cases are accidental, usually involving children who are helpless in water, such as inadequately attended children in or near swimming pools or infants in bathtubs; small children who fall into ponds, streams, and flooded excavations, usually near home; occupants of pleasure boats who fail to wear life preservers; children who have diving accidents; and children who are able to swim but overestimate their endurance.

*333 Turnpike Rd., Southborough, MA 01772. In Canada, the **Association for the Rehabilitation for the Brain-Injured,** 97 Warwick Dr., S.W., Calgary, Alberta T3C 2R5.

Drowning can take place in any body of water, including such unlikely places as a pail of water. Top-heavy toddlers fall head first into a pail of water, their arms become trapped, and they are unable to free themselves. Hot tubs and whirlpool spas have been implicated in childhood drowning injury. The suction created at the outlet is strong enough to trap even larger children underwater (Monroe, 1982). However, with expeditious treatment many children can be and are being saved. For purposes of this discussion, two terms need clarification:

drowning Death from asphyxia while submerged, regardless of whether fluid has entered the lungs.

near-drowning Survival at least 24 hours after submersion in a fluid medium.

Pathophysiology

The major pulmonary changes that occur in drowning are directly related to the length of submersion (regardless of the type and amount of fluid aspirated), the physiologic response of the victim, and the development and degree of immersion hypothermia. In addition, cerebral recovery depends on the effectiveness of initial resuscitation and subsequent critical care measures to support cerebral salvage.

Physiologic factors that influence the extent of damage from immersion include resistance to asphyxia and anoxia, which shows some individual variation. There is greater resistance with diminishing age; young children can withstand longer periods of submersion. More important is the drowning, or diving, reflex. This neurologic response is triggered by immersion of the face in cold water. Blood is shunted away from the periphery, and the flow is concentrated to the brain and heart predominantly.

The problems created by near-drowning are (1) hypoxia and asphyxiation, (2) aspiration, and (3) hypothermia (except near-drowning in hot tubs). Cardiopulmonary arrest is secondary to asphyxia.

Hypoxia is the primary problem because it results in global cell damage, and different cells tolerate variable lengths of anoxia. Neurons, especially cerebral cells, sustain irreversible damage after 4 to 6 minutes of submersion. The heart and lungs can survive up to 30 minutes. Regardless of the amount of water aspirated, there is arterial hypoxemia (resulting from atelectasis with shunting of blood through the nonventilated alveoli) and a combined respiratory acidosis (resulting from retained carbon dioxide) and metabolic acidosis (caused by buildup of acid metabolites caused by anaerobic metabolism). The pathologic events are directly related to the duration of submersion. The major difficulty is acute ventilatory insufficiency. Approximately 10% of drowning victims die without aspirating fluid but succumb from acute asphyxia as a result of prolonged reflex laryngospasm.

Aspiration of fluid occurs in the majority of drownings. The aspirated fluid results in pulmonary edema, atelectasis, airway spasm, and pneumonitis, which aggravates the hypoxia. It was previously thought that submersion in salt water and fresh water altered the physiologic response to near-drowning. However, there is no clinically significant difference in human survivors and it does not alter the therapy or outcome.

Hypothermia occurs rapidly in infants and children partly because of their large surface area relative to body mass and partly as a result of the cold water itself. Water is an excellent heat conductor and the contact with the skin is increased by struggling. Hypothermia may make resumption or maintenance of cardiac function possible if body temperature is less than 30° C. Profound hypothermia is usually evidence of lengthy submersion.

Therapeutic Management

Resuscitative measures should begin at the scene of a drowning, and the victim should be transported to the hospital with maximum ventilatory and circulatory support. Many victims need care for some time after aspiration of fluid. In the hospital, intensive pulmonary care is implemented and continued according to the needs of the patient.

In general, the management of the near-drowning victim is based on the degree of cerebral insult (see box). The first priority is to restore oxygen delivery to the cells

Clinical Manifestations of Near-Drowning

Directly related to the degree of consciousness following rescue and resuscitation:

Category A: awake (minimum injury)
- Fully conscious
- May have mild hypothermia
- Mild chest radiographic changes
- Mild arterial blood gas abnormalities

Category B: blunted sensorium (moderate injury)
- Obtunded
- Stuporous
- Purposeful response to painful stimuli
- Mild to moderate hypothermia
- Respiratory distress (frequently)
- Chest radiograms abnormal
- Arterial blood gas abnormalities

Category C: comatose (severe anoxia)
- Patient unarousable
- Abnormal response to pain
- Abnormal respiratory pattern
- Seizures
- Shock
- Marked arterial blood gas abnormalities
- Abnormal chest radiograms
- Arrhythmias
- Metabolic acidosis
- Hyperkalemia, hyperglycemia
- Disseminated intravascular coagulation

Also:
- **C1:** decorticate, Cheyne-Stokes respirations
- **C2:** decerebrate, central hyperventilation
- **C3:** flaccid, apneustic or cluster breathing
- **C4:** flaccid, apneic, no detectable circulation

and prevent further hypoxic damage. A spontaneously breathing child will do well in an oxygen-enriched atmosphere; the more severely affected child will require endotracheal intubation and mechanical ventilation. Blood gases and pH are monitored frequently as a guide to oxygen, fluid, and electrolyte therapies.

Category A patients are managed symptomatically with oxygen administration, warming, and symptomatic treatment. Laboratory assessment of electrolytes provides a guide to needed therapy. These children are usually well enough to be discharged in 12 to 24 hours.

Category B patients are admitted to the hospital and treated symptomatically as Category A patients, with regular monitoring of neurologic and respiratory status. The respiratory symptoms predominate and are managed with oxygen therapy, correction of acidosis, and furosemide to stimulate diuresis.

Category C patients require invasive life-support measures. These children do best if they are mechanically ventilated, for at least 12 to 24 hours. Unassisted respiration consumes too much energy, which is best directed to the needs of the brain. More severely affected children are managed as any other unconscious child (see p. 895).

Because of the frequency of complications after near-drowning, any patient should be hospitalized for 12 to 48 hours for observation. If the victim is one of the 10% who do not aspirate water, is rescued and resuscitated before circulatory arrest, and does not suffer damage to the central nervous system, recovery should be complete. The outcome for near-drowning is excellent for most patients in Categories C1 and C2 if they are resuscitated and receive intensive care. The poorest outlook is for children in Category C4, especially when near-drowning is associated with complications.

Aspiration pneumonia is a frequent complication that occurs about 48 to 72 hours after the episode. Bronchospasm, alveolar-capillary membrane damage, atelectasis, abscess formation, and hyaline membrane disease are other complications that occur after aspiration of fluid.

Nursing Considerations

Nursing care depends on whether the child is a near-drowning or a drowning victim. If the child survives, he may need intensive respiratory nursing care with attention to vital signs, mechanical ventilation and/or tracheostomy, blood gas determination, chest therapy, and intravenous infusion. Frequently the child is comatose for an indefinite period and requires the same care as an unconscious child.

Probably the most difficult aspect in the care of the child victim of near-drowning is dealing with the parents, whose guilt reactions are severe. The magnitude of the event is so great that efforts to provide comfort and support are of only limited success. Parents need to hear that everything possible is being done to treat the child, and this message needs to be repeated often.

The parents of the child who is saved from death are also faced with the anxiety of not knowing what the outcome will be, and sometimes they wish for the death of the child. Because their situation generates such intense feelings of loneliness, it is important for families to know that they are not alone. They need to be reminded frequently that there are caring people to assist them both during the crisis and later. Additional sources of support that can be recommended are psychiatric and social work consultants, community services, and religious support. Self-help groups are excellent if these are available in the community.

Nurses often have difficulty relating to the parents if obvious neglect has precipitated the accident and subsequent problems; therefore it is important for those who care for these children and their families to assess their own feelings about the situation as well as the coping abilities and resources of the family. Caring for near-drowning victims and their families requires the nurse to be sensitive to the needs of the child and the family and to recognize his or her own reactions and emotions.

Prevention. Most drownings, particularly of infants or small children, can be prevented with adequate supervision. All children should be taught to handle themselves in the water. Even very young children can learn to do so sufficiently to avoid panic and propel themselves to safety until they can be removed from the water. The American Academy of Pediatrics supports the recommendations of the YMCA regarding guidelines for swimming instruction for children less than 3 years of age. The programs recommended for older infants and toddlers are not those that promise to "waterproof" or "drownproof" the child, which can lead to complacency on the part of parents who believe the child can "swim." Those that offer water enrichment, emphasize water familiarization and water fun, and stress water safety and parent participation are best for very young children. These programs train both parent and child in swimming instruction, safety precautions, and risk awareness.

Water safety and survival training should be required for all school-age children, and nurses can be active advocates in their communities. Nurses are also in a position to emphasize the importance of adequate adult supervision when children are in the water. Young children should never be left unattended when in the water.

◆ *Central Nervous System Tumors*

Two major forms of childhood cancer are derived from neural tissue. Brain tumors are the most common solid tumors that occur in children and are second only to leukemia, the most common cancer in children. Neuroblastomas, tumors that usually arise in the autonomic nervous system or adrenal medulla, are not cerebral tumors but are the most common malignant tumors of infancy and are included here for convenience.

BRAIN TUMORS

The majority of tumors (about 60%) are *infratentorial* (below the tentorium cerebelli), which means that they occur in the posterior third of the brain, primarily in the cerebellum or brain stem. This anatomic distribution accounts for the frequency of symptoms resulting from increased ICP. A smaller number are *supratentorial,* or within the anterior two thirds of the brain, mainly the cerebrum. In adults the majority of tumors are of the latter type.

Neoplasms can arise from any cell within the cranium, and the type of cell in which the tumor has its origin provides a histologic classification for major tumors. The major infratentorial tumors of childhood are *meduloblastoma, cerebellar astrocytoma, brain stem glioma,* and *ependymomas*. Gliomas, arising from glial cells (the supporting structures of the brain), are the most common brain tumors in children.

Clinical Manifestations of Brain Tumors

Headache
Recurrent and progressive
In frontal or occipital areas
Worse on arising, less during day
Intensified by lowering head and straining, such as during bowel movement, coughing, sneezing

Vomiting
With or without nausea or feeding
Progressively more projectile
More severe in morning
Relieved by moving about and changing position

Neuromuscular Changes
Incoordination or clumsiness
Loss of balance (use of wide-based stance, falling, tripping, banging into objects)
Poor fine motor control
Weakness
Hyporeflexia or hyperreflexia
Positive Babinski sign
Spasticity
Paralysis

Behavioral Changes
Irritability
Decreased appetite
Failure to thrive
Fatigue (frequent naps)
Lethargy
Coma

Cranial Nerve Neuropathy
Cranial nerve involvement varies according to tumor location
Most common signs
  Head tilt
  Visual defects (nystagmus, diplopia, strabismus, episodic "greying out" of vision, and visual field defects)

Vital Sign Disturbances
Decreased pulse and respiration
Increased blood pressure
Decreased pulse pressure
Hypothermia or hyperthermia

Other Signs
Seizures
*Cranial enlargement
*Tense, bulging fontanel at rest
Nuchal ridigity
Papilledema (edema of optic nerve)

*Present only in infants and young children.

Diagnostic Evaluation

The signs and symptoms of brain tumors are those of increased ICP and are directly related to their anatomic location and size and to some extent the age of the child. In infants, whose sutures are still open, virtually no early detectable symptoms develop. It is not until spinal fluid obstruction causes markedly increased head size that a lesion may be suspected. Even in older children, clinical manifestations are nonspecific. However, the most common symptoms are headache, especially upon awakening, and vomiting that is not related to feeding and is attributable to increased ICP. The common clinical manifestations of brain tumors are presented in the accompanying box.

Diagnosis of a brain tumor is based subjectively on presenting clinical signs and objectively on neurologic tests. Because the signs and symptoms are vague and easily overlooked, early diagnosis necessitates a high index of suspicion during history taking. A number of tests may be employed in the neurologic evaluation, but the most common diagnostic procedure is computerized tomography, which provides an exact estimation of the location and extent of the tumor. Other tests that may be used include magnetic resonance imaging (where available), angiography, electroencephalography, or lumbar puncture, although the latter is dangerous in the presence of increased ICP.

Therapeutic Management

Treatment may involve the use of surgery, radiotherapy, and chemotherapy. All three may or may not be used, depending on the type of tumor. The treatment of choice is total extirpation of the tumor without residual neurologic damage. Patients with the most complete tumor removal have the greatest chance of survival. Radiotherapy is used to treat most tumors and to shrink the size of the tumor prior to attempting surgical removal. The use of chemotherapy is being employed with increased frequency.

Nursing Considerations

Nursing care of the child with a brain tumor involves the same principles of care regardless of the type of intracranial lesion. Since a brain tumor is a potentially fatal diagnosis, the reader is urged to incorporate the psychologic interventions discussed in Chapter 18 with those included in this section.

ASSESSMENT

A child admitted to the hospital with neurologic dysfunction is often suspected of having a brain tumor, although the actual diagnosis is as yet unconfirmed. Establishing a baseline of data on which to compare preoperative and postoperative changes is an essential step toward planning physical care and preventing complications. It also allows the nurse to assess the degree of physical incapacity and the family's emotional reaction to the diagnosis.

Vital signs, including blood pressure and pulse pressure, are taken routinely and more often when any change is noted. Any sudden variations are reported immediately. It is especially important to note a change in vital signs during or following diagnostic procedures. A routine neurologic assessment is also performed at the same time as vital signs, and head circumference is measured on infants and very young children.

The child is also observed for evidence of headache, vomiting, and any seizure activity. The location, severity, and duration of the headache are noted as well as its relationship to activity and time of day. Behaviors such as lying flat and facing away from light or refusing to engage in play are clues to discomfort in the nonverbal child. The child's gait is observed at least once daily. Head tilt and any other change in posturing are always noted.

NURSING DIAGNOSES

A number of nursing diagnoses will be evident following a thorough assessment of the child and family. Some of these are outlined in the accompanying box. Others may be determined in individual cases.

PLANNING

The goals of nursing care for the child with a brain tumor are:

1. Prepare child and family for diagnostic and/or operative procedures.
2. Prevent postoperative complications.
3. Provide support to child and family.
4. Promote return to normal functioning.

Nursing Diagnoses: The Child with a Brain Tumor

Pain related to increased ICP
Sensory/perceptual alterations (visual, auditory, kinesthetic, gustatory, tactile, olfactory related to altered sensory reception, transmission, and/or integration)
Altered family processes related to situational crisis (child with a serious illness)
Anticipatory grieving related to potential loss of child

IMPLEMENTATION

The suspected diagnosis of a brain tumor is always a crisis event. Despite the fact that some tumors are removed with excellent results, the physician can rarely give definitive answers regarding prognosis until after surgery. Therefore parents and older children require much emotional support to face the diagnostic procedures and a craniotomy.

Prepare child and family for diagnostic/operative procedures. How the child is prepared for the diagnostic tests depends on his age and previous experience. Since most of the tests involve x-ray equipment, the child may be familiar with the procedure. By the time most children are late preschoolers, they know that the head and brain are important parts of their bodies. It may be helpful to have a child draw his concept of the brain in order to clarify misconceptions and base the explanation on his level of understanding.

Although the temptation is to justify the need for surgery by stating that removing the tumor will take away various symptoms, the nurse should refrain from emphasizing this point too strenuously. Postsurgery headaches and cerebellar symptoms, such as ataxia, may be aggravated rather than improved. Surgery may not improve vision. With optic gliomas the child will be blind in one eye. Finally, surgical removal of the mass may be impossible, and after surgery there may be temporary deterioration of functioning. Being honest before surgery most often makes honesty after the operation easier because no false hopes were created.

However, honesty does not negate instilling hope. A truthful explanation regarding the operation is: "The physician will see exactly where the tumor is. If it is small and in one place, it will be removed. If it is large, as much of it as possible will be removed so that some of your symptoms will go away." It is best to deliver information in small amounts to let the child pursue additional answers. For example, some children will ask about what happens when part of the tumor is left in. An honest reply is that, after surgery, the physician will try to shrink the tumor with a special radiation machine and/or drugs. A further explanation of radiation or drug side effects is unwarranted, since the child will be bombarded with information before it is relevant.

Usually the night before surgery the child's head is shaved. This can be traumatic to the child and parents. However, it can be approached in a sensitive, positive way. If the child's hair is long, it should be braided so that the long swatch can be saved. Showing the child how he looks at different stages of the process helps him prepare for the final appearance.

Once the hair is clipped very short or shaved, the child can be given a cap or scarf to wear in order to camouflage the baldness. Every precaution is taken to protect the child from teasing or ridicule by other children before surgery. It is also emphasized that the hair will regrow shortly after the operation. Depending on the child's immediate adjustment to the hair loss, the nurse may introduce the idea of wearing a wig until the hair is grown in, particularly if additional irradiation or chemotherapy is anticipated.

In some hospitals a special technician shaves the scalp to minimize the risk of skin cuts. Sometimes the shaving is done in the operating room with the child under anesthesia. The scalp is shampooed before surgery. During these procedures the child is afforded maximum privacy.

The child is also told about the size of the dressing. Usually the entire scalp is covered to maintain a tight wound closure, even if a small incision is made. Infratentorial head dressings may be attached to the upper back and extend forward on the neck in order to maintain slight extension and alignment as a precaution against wound rupture. Applying a similar dressing or "special hat" to a doll is often a less traumatic way of demonstrating the physical appearance.

The child also needs a brief explanation of how he will feel after surgery and where he will be. Ordinarily he will return to a special intensive care unit, which he may visit beforehand depending on hospital policy. He should be aware that he may be sleepy for some time after surgery and that a headache is likely, although it should last only a few days.

Parents need similar explanations before surgery, especially in terms of special equipment used in the intensive care unit, dressings, and their child's behavior. For example, they should know that it is not unusual for the child to be comatose or lethargic for a few days after surgery. The nurse may wish to encourage less frequent visiting during this period so that parents can rest and be able to support their child when he awakens.

It is also advisable for the nurse to participate in preoperative conferences with the physician and parents. The nurse needs to know what information the parents have been given in order to be able to give further explanations or emotional support when necessary.

Prevent postoperative complications. Usually the surgeon will prescribe specific orders for vital signs, positioning, fluid regulation, and medication. These vary somewhat, depending on the location of the craniotomy. The following are general principles of care for infratentorial or supratentorial surgery. Additional aspects of care that are discussed elsewhere may include care of the child with seizures and care of the unconscious child in terms of neurologic assessment.

Vital signs are taken as frequently as every 15 to 30 minutes until stable. Temperatures taken via rectal or axillary routes are particularly important because of hyperthermia resulting from surgical intervention in the hypothalamus or brain stem and from some types of general anesthesia. To prepare for this reaction, a cooling blanket should be placed on the bed *before* the child returns to the unit so that it is ready for use when needed. The temperature is monitored carefully when any cooling measures are employed, because hypothermia can occur suddenly.

Observations for signs of complications include increased ICP, meningitis, and respiratory tract infection. When temperature is elevated, an infectious process must always be suspected, particularly if the febrile state occurs 1 to 2 days after surgery.

Observations for function are not instituted until the child regains consciousness. However, as soon as possible the nurse should begin testing reflexes, handgrip, and functioning of the cranial nerves. Muscle strength is usually diminished as a result of general weakness after surgery but should improve daily. Ataxia may be significantly worse with cerebellar intervention, but it will slowly improve. Edema near the cranial nerves may depress important functions such as the gag, blink, or swallowing reflex.

The nurse records behavior at regular intervals, noting sleep patterns, response to stimuli, and LOC. Although a child may be comatose for a few days, once he regains consciousness there should be a steady increase in alertness. Regression to a lethargic, irritable state indicates increasing pressure, possibly caused by meningitis.

Dressings are observed for evidence of drainage. If a drain is in place, the physician specifies this, since drainage frequently soaks through the dressing. If soiled, the dressing is reinforced with dry, sterile gauze and the approximate amount of drainage is estimated and recorded. To keep an accurate account of drainage, the soiled area is circled with a pen at regular intervals to recognize continuous bleeding. A colorless drainage, which is most likely CSF, is noted, reported immediately and a culture taken.

Once the child is alert, his arms may need to be restrained to prevent him from removing the dressing. Even a child who has been cooperative before surgery must be closely supervised during the initial stages of regaining consciousness, when disorientation and restlessness are common. Elbow restraints are satisfactory to prevent the hands from reaching the head, although additional restraint may be necessary to preserve an infusion line and maintain a specific position.

Correct positioning after surgery is critical to prevent pressure against the operative site, reduce ICP, and avoid the danger of aspiration. If position is restricted, notice of this is posted above the head of the bed. The child with an infratentorial operation is usually positioned flat and on the side, with pillows placed against his back, not his head, to maintain the desired position. Ordinarily the head and neck are kept in midline with the body and slightly extended.

The head of a child with a supratentorial craniotomy is usually elevated above the heart to facilitate CSF drainage and decrease excessive blood flow to the brain to prevent hemorrhage. Trendelenburg position is contraindicated in both types of surgeries because it increases ICP and the risk of hemorrhage. If shock is impending, the physician is notified immediately, before the head is lowered.

With an infratentorial craniotomy the child is allowed

nothing by mouth for at least 24 hours, or longer if the gag and swallowing reflexes are depressed or he is comatose. With a supratentorial operation, feeding may be resumed soon after the child is alert, sometimes within 24 hours. The child should be fed to conserve energy and minimize movement. If there is any sign of facial paralysis, the child is fed slowly to prevent choking or aspiration. Sometimes gavage feeding is necessary when bodily functions are too depressed to permit safe oral feedings or when the child refuses to eat or drink. Intravenous fluids are continued until fluids are well tolerated. Because of the cerebral edema postoperatively and danger of increased ICP, fluids are carefully monitored.

Although used after most other types of surgery, postoperative analgesics may not be routinely prescribed, because they may mask signs of altered consciousness or body functioning. However, this varies, and if analgesics are ordered, they should be used effectively, preferably on a preventive basis and in sufficient doses.

Headache may be severe and is largely the result of cerebral edema. Measures to relieve some of the discomfort include providing a quiet, dimly lit environment, restricting visitors to a minimum, preventing any sudden jarring movement, such as banging into the bed, and preventing an increase in ICP. The last is most effectively achieved by proper positioning and prevention of straining, such as during coughing, vomiting, or defecating. Bowel movements are monitored to prevent constipation. Stool softeners may be given as soon as liquids are tolerated to facilitate easy passage of stool. Placing an ice bag on the forehead may also provide some headache relief, especially if facial edema is severe.

Support the family. The emotional needs of the family are great when the diagnosis is a brain tumor, and feelings are influenced by the extent of surgery, any neurologic deficits, expected prognosis, and additional therapy. Since few definitive answers can be given before surgery, the surgeon's report is a significant finding that can vary from a completely benign, resected neoplasm to a highly malignant, invasive, and only partially removed tumor. Although parents try to prepare themselves for a potentially fatal diagnosis, it is a shock for them.

Ideally a nurse should be with the family when the physician visits with them to discuss with parents the expected prognosis and plan of therapy. Although parents may hear only a fraction of what they are told, they can begin to put the future into perspective. While some children will be cured, those with residual tumor may die within a relatively short period of time or live for several years. Regardless of the future prospects, the parents' thinking must be directed toward helping the child recover and resume a normal life to his maximum potential.

It is also a time to encourage parents to verbalize their feelings about the diagnosis, the prognosis, and any guilt they may feel regarding not seeking medical help earlier. Often they express tremendous guilt for attributing the insidious onset of symptoms, such as ataxia, visual difficulty, or headache, to minor "complaints" by the child. Any comments that insinuate that the parents should have sought medical advice sooner are avoided, since such remarks only add to the parents' guilt feelings.

During this period the nurse should also discuss with parents what they plan to tell the child. If he was prepared honestly the diagnosis can be expressed in a similar manner, such as, "The physician removed most of the tumor; the rest will be treated with special medicine and x-ray treatments." As the child improves, he will need additional explanation about the treatment (similar to that discussed for leukemia) as well as the reason for any residual neurologic effects, such as ataxia or blindness.

Promote return to optimum functioning. The ultimate goal is a cured child who has maximum functioning. As soon as possible the child should resume his usual activities within his limits, especially returning to school.* Until the skull is completely healed, the child may need to wear a helmet if he engages in any active sport. The school nurse and teacher should confer with the parents to discuss activity restrictions, such as physical education, and the reactions of schoolmates to the child's appearance. Since children often equate brain surgery with "going crazy," it is important to prepare the child for possible remarks to this effect. As one child told a classmate, "It's *your* head they should have fixed, because you're crazy. Can't you see that I'm all better?"

After discharge the family needs continuing medical and emotional support from health personnel. Even with children who are long-term survivors after treatment for a brain tumor, residual disabilities, such as growth retardation, cranial nerve palsies, sensory defects, motor abnormalities, especially ataxia, intellectual deficits, dysphagia, dysgraphia, and behavioral problems, are not uncommon. The high frequency of late effects affirms a decided need for follow-up care despite successful treatment of the tumor.

EVALUATION

The effectiveness of nursing interventions is determined by continual reassessment and evaluation of care based on the following observational guidelines and expected outcomes:

1. Interview the child and family regarding their understanding of scheduled tests and procedures; observe the child's behavior during procedures.
2. Monitor child's vital signs, neurologic signs, and behavior.
3. Interview child and family and observe their behaviors during hospitalization and recovery.
4. Interview child and family regarding activities and interests.

Expected outcomes:

1. The child is able to demonstrate an understanding of the

*Excellent publications, including the pamphlet *When Your Child is Ready to Return to School,* are available from the **Association for Brain Tumor Research**, 2910 West Montrose Ave., Chicago, IL 60618.

tests and procedures and submits to them with a minimum of stress.
2. The child exhibits no evidence of complications.
3. The child and family demonstrate evidence of healthy coping.
4. The family devises and carries out a realistic activity schedule, and the child attends school with reasonable regularity (specify).

NEUROBLASTOMA

Neuroblastoma occurs in about 1 per 10,000 live births, with a slightly higher incidence in males. About half the cases occur in children under 2 years of age, and another fourth occur in children under age 4 years. These tumors originate from embryonic neural crest cells that normally give rise to the adrenal medulla and the sympathetic ganglia. Consequently, the majority of tumors develop in the adrenal gland or the retroperitoneal sympathetic chain. Other sites may be within the head, neck, chest, or pelvis.

Neuroblastoma is a "silent" tumor. In more than 70% of cases, diagnosis is made after metastasis occurs, with the first signs caused by involvement in the nonprimary site, usually the lymph nodes, bone marrow, skeletal system, skin, or liver. Because of the frequency of invasiveness, prognosis for neuroblastoma is poor, and generally the younger the child at diagnosis, the better the survival rates. Also, neuroblastoma is one of the few tumors that demonstrates spontaneous regression, possibly as a result of maturity of the embryonic cell or the development of an active immune system.

Diagnostic Evaluation

The objective of diagnosis is to locate the primary site and areas of metastasis. The signs and symptoms of neuroblastoma depend on the location and stage of the disease. Most presenting signs are caused by compression of adjacent structures (see box). Skull, neck, chest, abdominal, and bone computerized tomographs and a bone marrow test are used to locate a tumor mass and/or metastasis. An intravenous pyelogram may provide evidence of renal involvement.

Urinary excretion of catecholamines is increased in children with adrenal or sympathetic tumors. A 24-hour urine collection analyzed for breakdown products of catecholamine metabolism permits detection of a suspected tumor both before and after therapeutic intervention.

Therapeutic Management

Accurate clinical staging is important for establishing initial treatment. Therefore surgery is employed both to remove as much of the tumor as possible and to obtain biopsies. In early stages, complete surgical removal of the tumor is the treatment of choice. If the tumors are large, partial resection is attempted, with a course of irradiation postoperatively to shrink the tumor in the hope of complete removal at a later date. Chemotherapy, administered in a variety of combinations, is the mainstay of therapy for extensive local or disseminated disease.

Clinical Manifestations of Neuroblastoma

Abdominal Tumors
Firm, nontender, irregular mass
Crosses the midline
Compression of kidney, ureter, or bladder may cause urinary frequency or retention

Distant Metastasis
Ocular:
Supraorbital ecchymosis
Periorbital edema
Proptosis (exophthalmos) from invasion of retrobulbar soft tissue
Lymphadenopathy, especially cervical and supraclavicular
Skeletal: bone pain may or may not be present
Intracranial: neurologic impairment
Thoracic: respiratory obstruction
Spinal cord: varying degrees of paralysis
Adrenal:
Increased catecholamine excretion
Flushing
Hypertension
Tachycardia
Diaphoresis

Widespread Metastasis—Vague Symptoms
Pallor
Weakness
Irritability
Anorexia
Weight loss

Nursing Considerations

Nursing considerations are similar to those discussed for leukemia and brain tumors, including psychologic and physical preparation for diagnostic and operative procedures, prevention of postoperative complications for abdominal, thoracic, or cranial surgery, and explanation of chemotherapy and radiotherapy and their side effects.

Since this tumor carries a poor prognosis for many children, every consideration must be given the family in terms of coping with a life-threatening illness (see Chapter 18). Because of the high degree of metastasis at the time of diagnosis, many parents suffer much guilt for not having recognized signs earlier. Often the guilt is expressed as anger toward professionals for not diagnosing it sooner. Parents need much support in dealing with these feelings and expressing them to the appropriate people.

◆ *Intracranial Infections*

The nervous system and its coverings are subject to infection by the same organisms that affect other organs of the body. However, the nervous system is limited in the ways in which it responds to injury. Infectious processes share virtually the same clinical and pathologic features. They differ primarily in the growth and virulence of the specific organism. It is generally difficult to distinguish between the various etiologic agents by looking at clinical manifestations. Laboratory studies are needed to identify the causative agent. The inflammatory process can affect the meninges *(meningitis)*, the brain *(encephalitis)*, or the spinal cord *(myelitis)*.

The most common infection of the central nervous system is meningitis, which can be caused by a variety of organisms, but the three main types are:

1. **Bacterial,** or pyogenic, caused by pus-forming bacteria, especially the meningococcus, pneumococcus, and influenza bacillus
2. **Tuberculous,** caused by the tubercle bacillus
3. **Viral,** or aseptic, caused by a wide variety of viral agents

Encephalitis is usually caused by a virus, and the discussion is limited to viral encephalitis. Myelitis is not discussed.

BACTERIAL MENINGITIS

Bacterial meningitis is a potentially fatal disease, and although the advent of antimicrobial therapy has had a marked effect on the course and prognosis, it remains a significant cause of illness in the pediatric age-groups. Its importance lies primarily in the frequency with which it occurs in infancy and childhood and the unnecessarily high death rates and residual damage caused by undiagnosed and untreated or inadequately treated cases.

Bacterial meningitis can be caused by any of a variety of bacterial agents. *Haemophilus influenzae* (type B), *Streptococcus pneumoniae,* and *Neisseria meningitidis* (meningococcal) organisms are responsible for bacterial meningitis in 95% of children older than 2 months of age. *H. influenzae* is the predominant organism in children 3 months to 3 years of age but is rare in the infant younger than 3 months of age, who is apparently protected by passively acquired bactericidal substances, and in children older than 5 years of age. The leading causes of neonatal meningitis are the group B streptococci and *Escherichia coli* organisms. *E. coli* infection is seldom seen beyond infancy. Meningococcic (epidemic cerebrospinal) meningitis occurs in epidemic form and is the only form readily transmitted to others. It is transmitted by droplet infection from nasopharyngeal secretions. Although it may develop at any age, the risk of meningococcal infection increases with the number of contacts; therefore, it occurs predominantly in school-age children and adolescents. The highest incidence of meningitis occurs between ages 6 and 12 months.

Pathophysiology

Meningitis appears to occur as an extension of a variety of bacterial infections, probably as a result of the lack of acquired resistance to the various causative organisms. The most common route of infection is by vascular dissemination from a focus of infection elsewhere. Organisms also gain entry by direct implantation after penetrating wounds, skull fractures that provide an opening into the skin or sinuses, lumbar puncture or surgical procedures, and anatomic abnormalities such as spina bifida or foreign bodies such as a ventricular shunt. Once implanted, the organisms spread into the CSF, which serves as a conduit for spread of infection throughout the subarachnoid space.

The infective process is that seen in any bacterial infection—inflammation, exudation, white blood cell accumulation, and varying degrees of tissue damage. The brain becomes hyperemic and edematous, and the entire surface of the brain is covered with a layer of purulent exudate. As infection extends to the ventricles, thick pus, fibrin, or adhesions may occlude the narrow passages, obstructing the flow of CSF.

Diagnostic Evaluation

The clinical manifestations of acute bacterial meningitis depend to a large extent on the age of the child (see box). The picture is also influenced to some degree by the type of organism, the effectiveness of therapy for antecedent illness, and whether it occurs as an isolated entity or as a complication of another illness or injury. Although the onset of symptoms is usually abrupt, it is sometimes slower, frequently preceded by several days of respiratory or gastrointestinal symptoms.

A definitive diagnosis of acute bacterial meningitis is made only by examination of the CSF by means of a lumbar puncture. The fluid pressure is measured and samples are obtained for culture and various immunologic tests. The findings are usually diagnostic. There is generally an elevated white blood cell count, predominantly polymorphonuclear leukocytes, but it may be extremely variable. The glucose level is reduced, generally in proportion to the duration and severity of the infection.

A blood culture is advisable for all children suspected of having meningitis and occasionally proves positive when results of CSF culture are negative. Nose and throat cultures may provide helpful information in some cases.

Therapeutic Management

Acute bacterial meningitis is a medical emergency that requires early recognition and immediate institution of therapy to prevent death and avoid residual disabilities. The initial therapeutic management includes (Committee on Infectious Diseases, 1982):

Isolation
Initiation of antimicrobial therapy
Maintenance of optimum hydration
Maintenance of ventilation
Reduction of increased ICP

Clinical Manifestations of Bacterial Meningitis

Children and Adolescents
Usually abrupt onset
Fever
Chills
Headache
Vomiting
Alterations in sensorium
Seizures (often the initial sign)
Irritability
Agitation
May develop:
- Delirium
- Aggressive or maniacal behavior
- Drowsiness
- Stupor
- Coma

Nuchal rigidity
- May progress to opisthotonos

Positive Kernig and Brudzinski signs
Hyperactive but variable reflex responses
Signs and symptoms peculiar to individual organisms:
- Petechial or purpuric rashes (meningococcal infection), especially when associated with a shocklike state
- Joint involvement (meningococcial and *H. influenzae* infection)
- Chronically draining ear (pneumococcal meningitis)

Infants and Young Children
Classic picture rarely seen in children between 3 months and 2 years of age
Fever
Vomiting
Marked irritability
Frequent seizures (often accompanied by a high-pitched cry)
Bulging fontanel
Nuchal rigidity may or may not be present
Brudzinski and Kernig signs are not helpful in diagnosis
- Difficult to elicit and evaluate in this age-group

Neonatal
Extremely difficult to diagnose
Manifestations vague and nonspecific
Well at birth but within a few days begins to look and behave poorly
Refuses feedings
Poor sucking ability
Vomiting or diarrhea
Poor tone
Lack of movement
Poor cry
Full, tense, and bulging fontanel may appear late in course of illness
Neck usually supple

Nonspecific Signs May Be Present
Hypothermia or fever (depending on the maturity of the infant)
Jaundice
Irritability
Drowsiness
Seizures
Respiratory irregularities or apnea
Cyanosis
Weight loss

Management of bacterial shock
Control of seizures
Control of extremes of temperature
Correction of anemia
Treatment of complications

The child is isolated from other children, usually in an intensive care unit for close observation. An intravenous infusion is started as soon as the lumbar puncture has been completed in order to facilitate the administration of antimicrobial agents, fluids, anticonvulsant drugs, and blood if needed. The child is placed on a cardiac monitor.

Until the causative organism is identified, the choice of antibiotic is based on the known sensitivity of the organism most likely to be the infective agent in any given situation and the probable interactions with the specific patient. Except under special circumstances, the drugs are administered intravenously throughout the course of treatment. The drugs are given in large doses, and the period of therapy is determined by CSF findings (normal glucose level and negative culture) and the child's clinical condition.

Maintaining hydration is a prime concern, and the decision to administer intravenous fluids and the type and amount of fluid are determined by the patient's condition. The optimum hydration involves correction of any fluid deficits followed by maintenance of low levels to prevent cerebral edema. If indicated, measures are employed to reduce ICP as described previously (p. 896).

Complications are treated appropriately, such as aspiration of subdural effusion in infants and heparin therapy for children who develop disseminated intravascular coagulation syndrome. Shock, if it occurs, is managed by restoration of blood volume and maintenance of electrolyte balance. Seizures, which occur in a large number of children, are controlled with anticonvulsants.

Lumbar puncture is carried out as needed to determine the effectiveness of therapy. The patient is evaluated neurologically during the convalescent period and at regular intervals during the succeeding year.

Prognosis is related to a variety of factors: the age of the child, the type of organisms, the severity of the infection, the duration of the illness prior to the onset of therapy, and the sensitivity of the organism to antimicrobial drugs. Sequelae are most commonly seen when the disease occurs in the first 2 months of life and least often in children with meningococcal meningitis.

Prevention. Vaccines are now available for some types of meningococcal infections. Meningococcal vaccine is recommended for household, nursery school, and hospital staff contacts of a primary case caused by type A or type C meningococci. Household contacts may also be treated prophylactically with rifampin. *H. influenzae* type B vaccine is recommended for all children as part of routine immunization (see p. 293).

Nursing Considerations

The first priority of nursing care of a child suspected of having meningitis is to administer the antibiotic as soon as it is ordered. The child is also placed on respiratory isolation for at least 24 hours after antimicrobial therapy is implemented. Nurses should take necessary precautions to protect themselves and others from possible infection. Parents are taught the proper protective procedures and supervised in their application.

The room should be kept as quiet as possible and environmental stimuli kept at a minimum, since most affected children are sensitive to noise, bright lights, and other external stimuli. Most children are more comfortable without a pillow and with the head of the bed slightly elevated. A side-lying position is more often assumed because of nuchal rigidity. The nurse should avoid actions, such as lifting the child's head, that cause pain or increase discomfort. Measures are employed to ensure safety, since the child is often restless and subject to seizures.

The nursing care of the child with meningitis is determined by the child's symptoms and treatment. Observation of vital signs, neurologic signs, LOC, urine output, and other pertinent data is carried out at frequent intervals. The child who is unconscious is managed as described previously (see p. 895), and all children are observed carefully for signs of complications just described, especially signs of increased ICP, shock, or respiratory distress.

Fluids and nourishment are determined by the child's status. The child with dulled sensorium is usually given nothing by mouth. Other children are allowed clear liquids initially and progressed to a diet suitable for their age. Careful monitoring and recording of intake and output are needed to determine deviations that might indicate impending shock or increasing fluid accumulation, such as cerebral edema or subdural effusion.

One of the most difficult problems in nursing care of children with meningitis is maintaining the intravenous infusion for the length of time needed to provide adequate antimicrobial therapy. When possible the heparin-lock device is used to decrease the time the child must spend immobilized for administration of antibiotics. If infants or children require restraining devices to maintain the integrity of the infusion site, these children should be released from the restraints as often as possible to reduce the ill effects of long-term immobilization. The children should be allowed ambulation and other normal activities as soon as their condition allows and as often as feasible. The infusion site is monitored for signs of inflammation as well as for patency. Some medications are highly irritating to veins and may tend to produce phlebitis if the infusion is continued in the same site over a prolonged time. These children are particularly in need of attendance and opportunities for play.

Family support. The sudden nature of the illness makes emotional support of the child and parents extremely important. Parents are very upset and concerned about their child's condition and frequently feel guilty for not having suspected the seriousness of the illness sooner. They need much reassurance that the natural onset of meningitis is sudden and that they acted responsibly in seeking medical assistance when they did. The nurse encourages them to openly discuss their feelings to minimize blame and guilt. They also are kept informed of the child's progress and of all procedures and treatments. In the event that the child's condition worsens, they need the same psychologic care as parents facing the possible death of their child (see Chapter 18).

NONBACTERIAL (ASEPTIC) MENINGITIS

Aseptic meningitis is a benign syndrome caused by a number of agents, principally viruses, and is frequently associated with other diseases, such as measles, mumps, herpes, and leukemia. Enteroviruses and mumps viruses account for a large number of cases.

The onset may be abrupt or gradual. The initial manifestations are headache, fever, malaise, gastrointestinal symptoms, and signs of meningeal irritation that develop a day or two after the onset of illness. Abdominal pain and nausea and vomiting are common; sore throat, chest pain, and generalized muscular aches or pains are found occasionally. There may be a maculopapular rash. These symptoms usually subside spontaneously and rapidly, and the child is well in 3 to 10 days with no residual effects.

Diagnosis is based on clinical features and CSF findings, which include increased lymphocytes, predominantly mononuclear cells. It is important to differentiate this benign disorder from the more serious form of meningitis and to diagnose any disease of which it is a manifestation and treat the patient.

Treatment is primarily symptomatic, such as acetaminophen for headache, moist heat for muscle aches and pains, and positioning for comfort. Antimicrobial agents may be administered and isolation enforced until a definitive diagnosis is made as a precaution against the possibility that the disease might be of bacterial origin.

Nursing care is similar to nursing care of the child with bacterial meningitis.

ENCEPHALITIS

Encephalitis is an inflammatory process of the central nervous system producing altered function of various portions of the brain and spinal cord. Encephalitis can be caused by a variety of organisms, including bacteria, spirochetes, fungi, protozoa, helminths, and viruses. Most infections are associated with viruses, and this discussion will be limited to these etiologic agents.

Etiology

Encephalitis can occur as a result of (1) direct invasion of the central nervous system by a virus or (2) postinfectious involvement of the CNS after a viral disease. Often the specific type of encephalitis in a particular child may not be identified for some time or not at all. The majority of cases of known etiology are associated with the childhood viral diseases. Most other viral infections are those involved with arthropod vectors and those associated with

Clinical Manifestations of Encephalitis

Onset: sudden or gradual	Severe cases:
Malaise	High fever
Fever	Stupor
Headache	Seizures
Dizziness	Disorientation
Apathy	Spasticity
Neck stiffness	Coma (may proceed to death)
Nausea and vomiting	Ocular palsies (may occur)
Ataxia	Paralysis (may occur)
Tremors	
Hyperactivity	
Speech difficulties	

hemorrhagic fevers. The vector reservoir for most agents pathogenic for humans and detected in the United States is the mosquito; therefore most cases of encephalitis appear during the hot summer months.

Diagnostic Evaluation

The clinical features are similar regardless of the agent involved. Manifestations can range from a mild, benign form that resembles aseptic meningitis, lasting a few days and followed by rapid and complete recovery, to a fulminating encephalitis with severe central nervous system involvement (see box).

The diagnosis is made on the basis of clinical findings, circumstances associated with the disease, and (where possible) identification of the specific virus. Some are rarely detected in blood or spinal fluid. Others (such as herpes, mumps, measles, and enteroviruses) may be found in CSF. Serologic diagnosis may be reached by means of a variety of antibody tests, which are performed as soon after onset as possible.

Therapeutic Management

Patients suspected of having encephalitis are hospitalized promptly for skilled nursing care and observation. Treatment is primarily supportive, including conscientious nursing care, control of cerebral manifestations, and adequate nutrition and hydration, with observations and management as for other disorders involving cerebral injury. Follow-up care with periodic reevaluation and rehabilitation are important requisites to survivors with residual effects of the disease.

Nursing Considerations

Nursing care of the child with encephalitis is the same as for any unconscious child and the child with meningitis. Neurologic monitoring, administration of medications, and support to the child and parents are the major aspects of care.

REYE SYNDROME

Reye syndrome (RS) is a disorder defined as toxic encephalopathy associated with other characteristic organ involvement. It is characterized by fever, profoundly impaired consciousness, and disordered hepatic function. The ages of affected children range from 2 months to adolescence, with peak incidences occurring at 6 and 11 years. This syndrome is one of the most common causes of encephalopathy in children.

Etiology

The etiology of the disorder is obscure, but most cases of RS follow a common viral illness, most frequently influenza or varicella. There is evidence to indicate an association between the ingestion of aspirin during the prodromal illness and the occurrence of Reye syndrome. Consequently, the Committee on Infectious Diseases of the American Academy of Pediatrics (1982) recommends that aspirin not be prescribed for children with varicella or those suspected of having influenza.

Pathophysiology

The liver of patients with RS is enlarged, with marked fatty infiltration. There is a reduction in the enzymes that convert ammonia to urea, which is reflected in a hyperammonemia. Brain edema is severe; cerebral dysfunction and death are the result of swollen or damaged cells.

The clinical course of the disease is rapid, and mortality is high (40%), particularly in children younger than 2 years and if convulsions are part of the clinical picture. Fortunately recovery is rapid and complete in those who survive, and residual disability is uncommon.

Diagnostic Evaluation

The onset of the disease is preceded in most cases by prodromal symptoms, including malaise, cough, rhinorrhea, or sore throat. The child appears to be recovering but then develops recurrent, intractable vomiting and central nervous system dysfunction. Various staging criteria have been developed that help to objectively evaluate the patient's progress, to predict a probable outcome, and to evaluate the efficacy of therapies. The clinical manifestations and the staging that is used most frequently are outlined in the accompanying box.

Evidence of liver dysfunction is reflected by elevated serum glutamic-oxaloacetic transaminase (SGOT), serum glutamic-pyruvic transaminase (SGPT), and lactic dehydrogenase (LDH) levels. Liver-dependent clotting factors, such as prothrombin, are diminished. Serum bilirubin and alkaline phosphatase levels are usually unaffected. Elevated ammonia levels establish the diagnosis and tend to correlate with the clinical manifestations and prognosis. In the majority of children blood sugar levels fall to below 50 mg/dl, with reduced insulin levels and dimin-

Staging Criteria for Reye Syndrome

Stage I	Vomiting, lethargy, and drowsiness; liver dysfunction; type I EEG, follows commands, pupillary reaction brisk
Stage II	Disorientation, combativeness, delirium, hyperventilation, hyperactive reflexes, appropriate responses to painful stimuli; evidence of liver dysfunction; type I EEG, pupillary reaction sluggish
Stage III	Obtunded, coma, hyperventilation, decorticate rigidity, preservation of pupillary light reaction and oculovestibular reflexes (although sluggish); type II EEG
Stage IV	Deepening coma, decerebrate rigidity, loss of oculocephalic reflexes, large and fixed pupils, loss of doll's eye reflex, loss of corneal reflexes; minimum liver dysfunction; type III or IV EEG, evidence of brain stem dysfunction
Stage V	Seizures, loss of deep tendon reflexes, respiratory arrest, flaccidity; type IV EEG; usually no evidence of liver dysfunction

ished glucagon response. There is a combined respiratory alkalosis and metabolic acidosis. CSF is normal, if examined. Definitive diagnosis is established by liver biopsy.

Therapeutic Management

The most important aspect of successful management of the child with RS is early diagnosis and aggressive therapy, which is determined by the clinical stage of the disease and the rapidity with which it progresses. For children at stage I, treatment is primarily supportive and directed toward restoring blood sugar levels, controlling cerebral edema, correcting acid-base imbalances, and eliminating factors known to increase ICP. Intravenous administration of hypertonic (10%) glucose solution with added insulin helps to replace glycogen stores, but it is controlled to avoid overhydration. The pH and electrolyte levels are monitored and replaced according to regular assessments. Sometimes corticosteroids are useful. Noninvasive monitoring is adequate to assess status and progress.

Stages II through V require more aggressive measures. The child is admitted to an intensive care unit where invasive support and monitoring are implemented to supplement supportive measures and prevent irreversible brain damage. Since increased ICP kills, the major efforts are directed toward preventing and/or reducing cerebral edema. These include ICP monitoring and administration of intravenous mannitol, urea, or glycol and hypertonic solutions, which cause fluid to move out of edematous tissues. Tracheal intubation, preferably nasotracheal, is performed as soon as possible, and the child is placed on controlled hyperventilation to decrease carbon dioxide levels.

A standard approach is curarization and sedation. Skeletal muscles are paralyzed with administration of *d*-tubocurarine or pancuronium (Pavulon) to prevent any activity, especially coughing, that might increase ICP. Curarization does not affect sensory input including pain sensation; therefore the child's anxiety may be sufficient to cause cerebral hypertension. Exchange transfusions or peritoneal dialysis has been used in some cases to reduce elevated blood ammonia levels.

Nursing Considerations

The child who is acutely ill with RS requires continuous and intensive nursing care. On admission to the hospital numerous procedures and observations must be carried out as quickly as possible. In addition to an appraisal of vital functions and neurologic status, the nurse assists with a lumbar puncture, obtaining blood for laboratory examination, and insertion of various intravenous lines such as peripheral, arterial, and central venous pressure. A retention catheter and a nasogastric tube are inserted, and when respirations are compromised, an endotracheal tube is inserted and attached to a respirator to control respirations. If equipment is available, a pressure monitoring device is inserted for continuous monitoring of intracranial pressure.

Care and observations are implemented as for any child with an altered state of consciousness (p. 897) and increasing ICP. Accurate and frequent monitoring of intake and output is essential for adjusting fluid volumes to prevent both dehydration and cerebral edema. The child paralyzed and in a drug-induced coma is totally dependent on the caregivers, and meticulous vigilance and attention to all biologic needs are mandatory. Since hypovolemic shock is a constant danger in children with controlled fluid intake and osmotic diuresis, vital signs, including central venous pressure and/or cardiac output (balloon-tipped pulmonary artery catheter), are monitored frequently. Arranging for collection of blood gasses and other laboratory data is a nursing responsibility. Because of related liver dysfunction, the nurse must observe for signs of impaired coagulation such as prolonged bleeding and petechiae.

Family support. Parents of children with RS need a great deal of emotional support. They are usually frightened by the child's appearance, the treatment, and the life-threatening severity and suddenness of the illness. Their distress is increased if they believe that their actions may have contributed to a delay in diagnosis. Parents are encouraged to verbalize their guilt feelings and are provided with reassurance that they did not contribute to the child's condition, that the development of the disease cannot be anticipated, and that their care was proper under the circumstances. They need to be kept informed regarding the child's progress, to have diagnostic procedures and therapeutic management explained, and to be given concerned and sympathetic support.

The **National Reye's Syndrome Foundation*** has been established by the parents of a child who died from this disease, in hope of encouraging research on the disease and of educating parents and health professionals.

RABIES

Rabies is an acute infection of the nervous system caused by a virus that is almost invariably fatal. It is transmitted to humans by the saliva of an infected mammal introduced through a bite or skin abrasion. Over 75% of animals reported as rabid have been raccoons. Other animals in order of frequency are skunks, bats, foxes, and groundhogs. The domestic dog, formerly considered a prime source, is relatively well controlled by rabies vaccination programs.

The disease is uncommon in humans, but the highest incidence occurs in children under 15 years of age. The incubation period usually ranges from 1 to 3 months but may be as short as 10 days or as long as 8 months. Only 10% to 15% of persons bitten develop the disease, but once symptoms are present, rabies progresses inexorably to a fatal outcome.

Diagnosis is made on the basis of history and clinical features (see box). Once symptoms appear, treatment is of little avail, but the long incubation period allows time for induction of active as well as passive immunity before the onset of illness. The current therapy for a rabid animal bite consists of thorough cleansing of the wound and inoculation with human rabies immune globulin (RIG) or hyperimmune antirabies serum (ARS) as soon as possible after exposure to provide rapid, short-term passive immunity. Active immunity is conferred by administration of the recently developed human diploid cell rabies vaccine (HDCV). The first dose of the vaccine is given at the same time as the immune globulin and followed by injections at 3, 7, 14, and 21 days. An additional dose in 90 days is recommended by the World Health Organization.

*426 N. Lewis, Bryan, OH 43506. In Canada, **Reye's Syndrome Foundation of Canada,** Children's Hospital of Southwestern Ontario, P.O. Box 5375, London, Ontario N6A 4G5.

Clinical Manifestations of Rabies

Initially:
- General malaise
- Fever
- Sore throat

Excitement phase:
- Hypersensitivity
- Increased reaction to external stimuli
- Convulsions
- Maniacal behavior
- Choking

Severe spasm of respiratory muscles from attempts at swallowing (characteristics from which the term "hydrophobia" was derived):
- Apnea
- Cyanosis
- Anoxia

Nursing Considerations

Parents as well as children are frightened by the urgency and seriousness of the situation. They need anticipatory guidance for the therapy and support and reassurance regarding the efficacy of the preventive measures for this dreaded disease. The vaccine is well tolerated by children, but mass immunization is unnecessary and unlikely to be implemented. Certain circumstances may warrant vaccination, such as when a child is being taken to an area of the world where rabies in stray dogs is still a problem.

◆ *Seizure Disorders*

Convulsive phenomena are among the most frequently observed neurologic dysfunctions in children and can occur with a wide variety of conditions involving the CNS. Generally a *convulsion* is defined as involuntary muscular contractions and relaxation; a *seizure* is a sudden attack. Persons who have a tendency to experience seizures are said to have *epilepsy*. The words are all used synonymously. More specifically, seizure phenomena are characterized by a single attack or recurrent transient attacks of involuntary loss of consciousness, altered motor activity and/or autonomic function, disturbed feelings, or behavior associated with excessive neuronal discharges. These discharges may be focal or diffuse, and the sites of the discharges determine the clinical manifestations observed during the attack.

EPILEPSY

Seizures result from paroxysmal discharges in cortical neurons and are symptoms of abnormal brain function. They are considered to be a symptom of an underlying disease process.

Etiology

Seizure disorders have numerous and varied causes (e.g. tumors, infections, neoplasms). Most are *idiopathic*. Although the cause of idiopathic epilepsy is unknown, genetic factors may in some way alter the seizure threshold to influence neuronal discharge. A seizure disorder also can be *acquired* as a result of brain injury during prenatal, perinatal, or postnatal periods. This injury may be caused by trauma, hypoxia, infections, exogenous or endogenous toxins, and a variety of other factors. Biochemical events (e.g., hypoglycemia, hypocalcemia, and certain nutritional deficiencies) produce seizure activity.

The incidence of causative factors associated with childhood seizures is frequently related to the age of the child. Seizures are more common during the first 2 years of life than during any other period of childhood. In very young infants the most frequent causes are birth injuries, such as intracranial trauma, hemorrhage, or anoxia, and congenital defects of the brain. Acute infections are a frequent cause of seizures in late infancy and early childhood but become an infrequent cause in middle childhood. In children older than 3 years of age the most common factor is idiopathic epilepsy.

Seizure activity is believed to be caused by spontaneous electric discharge initiated by a group of hyperexcitable cells referred to as the *epileptogenic focus*. These cells display increased electric excitability in response to any of a variety of physiologic stimuli, such as cellular dehydration, abnormal blood sugar levels, electrolyte imbalance, fatigue, emotional stress, and endocrine changes. When neuronal excitation from the epileptogenic focus spreads to the brain stem, a generalized seizure develops. Seizures are designated as *focal, focal with rapid generalization,* and *generalized,* on the basis of the characteristic neuronal discharges. In a large proportion of children focal seizures spread to other areas, ultimately becoming generalized with loss of consciousness.

Classification

There are many different types of epileptic seizures and each has unique characteristics. The onset of a seizure is abrupt, paroxysmal, and transitory, and signs are highly variable. The current classification system divides seizures into two major categories: partial seizures and generalized seizures (see box). Some of these are described in the following segment.

Partial seizures. Partial seizures are caused by abnormal electric discharges from epileptogenic foci limited to a more or less circumscribed region of the cerebral cortex. Focal seizures may arise from any area of the cerebral cortex, but the frontal, temporal, and parietal lobes are the ones most often affected. The area of cerebral involvement is reflected by clinical manifestations.

Generalized seizures. Generalized seizures without a focal onset appear to arise in the reticular formation and the clinical observations indicate that the initial involvement is from both hemispheres. Loss of consciousness occurs and is the initial clinical manifestation. Unlike partial seizures that become generalized, there is no aura. Attacks occur at any time, day or night, and the interval between attacks may be minutes, hours, weeks, or even years. Most affected persons first experience seizures in childhood, and children whose seizures begin before age 4 years have mental retardation and behavioral and learning problems more frequently than those whose seizures begin after age 4.

Diagnostic Evaluation

Establishing a diagnosis is critical. The process of diagnosis in a child with a convulsive disorder has two major foci: (1) to ascertain the type of seizure the child has experienced and (2) to attempt to understand the cause of the attacks. The assessment and diagnosis rely heavily on a thorough history, skilled observation, and employment of several diagnostic tests.

During the assessment process it is unusual to observe the child having a seizure; therefore, a complete, accurate, and detailed history should be obtained from a reliable and knowledgeable informant. This history involves prenatal, perinatal, and neonatal periods, including any instances of infection, apnea, colic, or poor feeding, and information regarding any previous accidents or serious illnesses.

History of the seizure(s) should be equally detailed, including the type of seizure or description of the child's behavior during the attack(s), the age at onset, and the time at which the seizure occurs (i.e., early morning, before meals, while awake, or during sleep). Any factors that may have precipitated the seizure are important, including fever, infection, falls that may have caused trauma to the head, anxiety, fatigue, activity (e.g., hyperventilation), and environmental events (exposure to strong stimuli such as bright, flashing lights or loud noises). If the child can describe any sensory phenomena, these are recorded. The duration and progression of the seizure (if any) and the postictal feelings and behavior, such as confusion, inability to speak, amnesia, headache, and sleep, are recorded.

A complete physical and neurologic examination, including developmental assessment of language, learning, behavior, and motor abilities, often provides clues to neurologic disturbances. A family history can offer clues to paroxysmal disorders such as migraine, breath-holding spells, febrile convulsions, or neurologic diseases that may be related to the convulsive disorder.

Laboratory studies that may prove to be of value include a complete blood cell count (for evidence of lead poisoning) and white blood cell count (for signs of infection). Blood and CSF glucose may give evidence of hypoglycemic episodes, and serum electrolytes, blood urea nitrogen, calcium, and other blood studies might indicate metabolic disturbances. Lumbar puncture can confirm a suspected diagnosis of cerebrospinal infection or trauma.

Skull radiograms, computed tomograms, echoencephalograms, brain scans, and other studies help to identify skull abnormalities, separation of sutures, and intracranial calcifications. The electroencephalogram (EEG) is obtained for all children with convulsive manifestations and is the most useful tool for evaluating seizure disorders. The EEG is carried out under varying conditions—with the child asleep, awake, awake with provocative stimulation (flashing lights, noise), and hyperventilating. Stimulation elicits abnormal electrical activity, which is recorded on the EEG.

Variations of the EEG are video recordings and simultaneous polygraphs of the patient during waking and/or sleeping. These techniques can be used concurrently and are especially valuable in differentiating epileptic activity from paroxysmal behavior or nonepileptic motor events.

Classification and Clinical Manifestations of Seizures

I. Partial Seizures

Simple Partial Seizures

Characterized by:
- Localized motor symptoms
- Somatosensory, psychic, autonomic symptoms
- Combination of these
- Abnormal discharges remain unilateral

Manifestations:
- Aversive seizure (most common motor seizure in children)
  - Eye or eyes and head turn away from the side of the focus
  - Awareness of movement or loss of consciousness
- Sylvan seizure
  - Tonic-clonic movements involving the face
  - Salivation
  - Arrested speech
  - Most common during sleep
- Jacksonian march (rare in children)
  - Orderly, sequential progression of clonic movements beginning in a foot, hand, or face and moving or "marching" to adjacent body parts

Special Sensory Seizures

Characterized by various sensations, including:
- Numbness, tingling, prickling, paresthesia, or pain originating in one area (e.g., face or extremities) and spreading to other parts of the body
- Visual sensations or formed images
- Motor phenomena such as posturing or hypertonia
- Uncommon in children under 8 years of age

Complex Partial Seizures (psychomotor seizures)

Observed more often in children from 3 years through adolescence

Characterized by:
- Period of altered behavior
- Amnesia for event (no recollection of behavior)
- Inability to respond to environment
- No loss of consciousness during attack
- Drowsiness or sleep usually follows seizure
- Confusion and amnesia may be prolonged
- Complex sensory phenomena
  - Most frequent sensation—strange feeling in the pit of the stomach that rises toward the throat
  - Often accompanied by:
    - Odd or unpleasant odors or tastes
    - Complex auditory or visual hallucinations
    - Ill-defined feelings of elation or strangeness (e.g., deja vu, a feeling of familiarity in a strange environment)
  - Small children may emit a cry or attempt to run for help
  - May be strong feelings of fear and anxiety, distorted sense of time and self

Patterns of motor behavior:
- Stereotypic
- Similar with each subsequent seizure
- May suddenly cease activity, appear dazed, stare into space, become confused and apathetic, and become limp or stiff or display some form of posturing
- May be confused
- May perform purposeless, complicated activities in a repetitive manner (automatisms), such as walking, running, kicking, laughing, or speaking incoherently, most often followed by postictal confusion or sleep
- May be oropharyngeal activities, such as smacking, chewing, drooling, swallowing, and nausea or abdominal pain followed by stiffness, a fall, and postictal sleep
- Rarely manifests auras such as rage or temper tantrums
- Aggressive acts uncommon during seizure

II. Generalized Seizures

***Tonic-Clonic Seizures* (traditionally known as *grand mal*)**

Most common and most dramatic of all seizure manifestations

Occur without warning

Tonic phase: lasts approximately 10 to 20 seconds

Manifestations:
- Eyes roll upward
- Immediate loss of consciousness
- If standing, falls to floor or ground
- Stiffens in generalized, symmetric tonic contraction of entire body musculature
- Arms usually flexed
- Legs, head, and neck extended
- May utter a peculiar piercing cry
- Apneic, may become cyanotic
- Increased salivation

Clonic phase: lasts about 30 seconds but can vary from only a few seconds to a half hour or longer

Manifestations:
- Violent jerking movements as the trunk and extremities undergo rhythmic contraction and relaxation
- May foam at the mouth
- May be incontinent of urine and feces

As attack ends, movements become less intense, occur at longer intervals, then cease entirely

Therapeutic Management

The objective of treatment of convulsive disorders is to (1) control the seizures or to reduce their frequency, (2) discover and correct the cause when possible, and (3) help the child who has recurrent seizures to live as normal a life as possible. Seizures of a recurrent nature are treated as soon as the diagnosis is established. If the seizure activity is a manifestation of an infectious, traumatic, or metabolic process, the seizure therapy is instituted as a part of the general therapeutic regimen.

It is known that persons predisposed to epilepsy have seizures when their basal level of neuronal excitability exceeds a critical point or threshold; no attack occurs if the excitability is maintained below this threshold. The administration of anticonvulsant drugs serves to raise this threshold and prevent seizures. Consequently the primary therapy for convulsive disorders is the administration of the appropriate anticonvulsant drug or combination of drugs in a dosage that provides the desired effect without causing undesirable side effects or toxic reactions.

Numerous drugs are available for control of seizures. The primary drugs prescribed for partial seizures and/or generalized tonic-clonic seizures are carbamazepine (Tegretol), phenytoin (Dilantin), and mephenytoin. The drug of choice for absences is ethosuximide; next is valproic

Status epilepticus: series of seizures at intervals too brief to allow the child to regain consciousness between the time one attack ends and the next begins
- Requires emergency intervention
- Can lead to exhaustion, respiratory failure, and death

Postictal state:
- Appears to relax
- May remain semiconscious and difficult to rouse
- May awaken in a few minutes
- Remains confused for several hours
- Poor coordination
- Mild impairment of fine motor movements
- May have visual and speech difficulties
- May vomit or complain of severe headache
- When left alone, usually sleeps for several hours
- On awakening is fully conscious
- Usually feels tired and complains of sore muscles and headache
- No recollection of entire event

Absence Seizures **(traditionally called *petit mal* or *lapses*)**

Characterized by:
- Brief loss of consciousness
- Minimal or no alteration in muscle tone
- May go unrecognized because little change in child's behavior
- Abrupt onset; suddenly develops 20 or more attacks daily
- Attack often mistaken for inattentiveness or daydreaming
- Attacks can be precipitated by hyperventilation, hypoglycemia, stresses (emotional and physiologic), fatigue, or sleeplessness

Manifestations:
- Brief loss of consciousness
- Appear without warning or aura
- Usually last about 5 to 10 seconds
- Slight loss of muscle tone may cause child to drop objects
- Able to maintain postural control; seldom falls
- Minor movements such as lip smacking, twitching of eyelids or face, or slight hand movements
- Not accompanied by incontinence
- Amnesia for episode
- May need to reorient self to previous activity

Atonic and Akinetic Seizures **(also known as *drop attacks*)**

Characterized by:
- Onset usually between 2 and 5 years of age
- Sudden, momentary loss of muscle tone and postural control
- Attacks recur frequently during the day, particularly in the morning hours and shortly after awakening

Manifestations:
- Loss of tone causes child to fall to floor violently
  - Unable to break the fall by putting out hand
  - May incur a serious injury to the face, head, or shoulder
- Loss of consciousness only momentary

Myoclonic Seizures

A variety of convulsive episodes
May be isolated as benign essential myoclonus
May occur in association with other seizure forms
Characterized by:
- Sudden, brief contractures of a muscle or group of muscles
- Occur singly or repetitively
- No loss of consciousness or postictal state
- May or may not be symmetric

Infantile Spasms

Also called: infantile myoclonus, massive spasms, hypsarrhythmia, salaam attacks, or infantile myoclonic spasms
Most commonly occur between 3 and 12 months of age
Twice as common in males as in females
Child may have numerous seizures during the day without postictal drowsiness or sleep
Outlook for normal intelligence poor
Manifestations:
- Possible series of sudden, brief, symmetric, muscular contractions
  - Head flexed, arms extended, and legs drawn up
  - Eyes may roll upward or inward
  - May be preceded or followed by a cry or giggling
  - May or may not be loss of consciousness
  - Sometimes flushing, pallor, or cyanosis

Infants who are able to sit but not stand:
- Sudden dropping forward of the head and neck with trunk flexed forward and knees drawn up—the "salaam" or "jackknife" seizure

Less often: alternate clinical forms observed
- Extensor spasms rather than flexion of arms, legs, and trunk and head nodding
- Lightning attacks involving a single, momentary, shocklike contraction of the entire body

acid. The dosage is determined by monitoring serum drug levels. Complete control can be achieved in only 50% to 75% of epileptic children, however, even with careful attention to details of therapy.

Once seizures are controlled, the drug or drugs are continued for a prolonged time. However, periodic reevaluation of the drug is important to assess the continued effectiveness and to alter the dosage if indicated. The dosage will need to be increased as the child grows. When a medication is discontinued, the dosage should be reduced gradually over 1 to 2 weeks. Sudden withdrawal of a drug can cause an increase in the number and severity of seizures, often precipitating status epilepticus. If the time for reducing the medication coincides with puberty or, in younger children, occurs during periods when the child is subject to frequent infections, the drug is continued for a longer period. Repeat EEGs are generally obtained every ½ to 2 years.

When seizure activity is determined to be caused by a hematoma, tumor, or other progressive cerebral lesion, surgical removal is the treatment. Surgery also may be indicated for those who suffer from repetitive, incapacitating seizures that are caused by a focal brain abnormality, if removal of the lesion does not result in significant loss of vital functions, such as speech and movement.

Status epilepticus. Status epilepticus is managed by

Assessment of the Child during a Generalized Convulsive Seizure

OBSERVE SEIZURE

Describe
- Only what is actually observed
- Order of events
- Duration of seizure

Onset
- Significant preseizure events—bright lights, noise, excitement, emotional outbursts
- Behavior
  - Change in facial expression, such as of fear
  - Cry or other sound
  - Stereotyped or automatous movements
  - Random activity
- Position of head, body, extremities
  - Unilateral or bilateral posturing of one or more extremities
  - Body deviation to side
- Time of onset

Movement
- Change of position, if any
- Site of commencement—hand, thumb, mouth, generalized
- Tonic phase, if present—length, parts of body involved
- Clonic phase—twitching or jerking movements, parts of body involved, sequence of parts involved, generalized, change in character of movements
- Lack of movement of any extremity

Face
- Color change—pallor, cyanosis, flushing
- Perspiration
- Mouth—position, deviating to one side, teeth clenched, tongue bitten, frothing at mouth, flecks of blood or bleeding

Eyes
- Position—straight ahead, deviation upward, deviation outward, conjugate or divergent
- Pupils (if able to assess)—change in size, equality, reaction to light and accommodation

Respiratory effort
- Presence and length of apnea
- Presence of stertor

Other
- Involuntary urination
- Involuntary defecation

OBSERVE POSTICTALLY
- Method of termination
- State of consciousness—unresponsiveness, drowsiness, confusion
- Orientation to time, place, persons, and so on
- Sleeping but able to be aroused
- Motor ability
  - Any change in motor power
  - Ability to move all extremities
  - Any paresis or weakness
  - Ability to whistle (if appropriate to age)
- Speech—changes, peculiarities, type and extent of any difficulties
- Sensations
  - Complaint of discomfort or pain
  - Any sensory impairment of hearing, vision
  - Recollection of preseizure sensations, warning of attack
  - Awareness that attack was beginning
- Promote rest
  - Make child comfortable
  - Allow child to rest after seizure
  - Reduce sensory stimuli
  - Record length of postictal sleep
  - Notify physician if seizure is followed by other seizures in rapid succession or if duration of seizure is excessive
- Reduce anxiety
  - Provide calm, relaxed atmosphere

supportive measures, including maintenance of an adequate airway, administration of oxygen, and hydration, and by the intravenous administration of either diazepam or phenobarbital. The child must be closely monitored during administration to detect early alterations in vital signs that may indicate impending cardiac arrest or respiratory depression. Occasionally paraldehyde is administered (intramuscularly or rectally). Patients that do not respond to drug therapy may require the use of intravenous lidocaine, general anesthesia, or a potent skeletal muscle relaxant such as curare.

Nursing Considerations

Nursing care of the child with a convulsive disorder involves assisting with diagnosis, acute care during a seizure, and long-term management, including support of the child and the family and education of the child, family, and community regarding the disorder.

ASSESSMENT

An important nursing function during a convulsion is observing the seizure and describing its pertinent features. Any alterations in behavior and characteristics of the attack such as sensory-hallucinatory phenomena (e.g., an aura), motor effects (e.g., eye movements, muscular contractions, laterality, and complex activities), alterations in consciousness, and postictal state are noted and recorded (see accompanying box and box on pp. 922-923).

Generalized seizures and others with dramatic manifestations are easily detected, but absences may be more difficult to detect. They are easily misinterpreted as inattention. Any unusual behavior, even seemingly inconsequential behavior such as a momentary interruption of activity, staring, or mental blankness, should be described. The more detailed these descriptions, the more

Nursing Diagnoses: The Child with Epilepsy

- Potential for trauma related to sudden and unexpected loss of consciousness
- Body image disturbance related to perception of seizure disorder
- Altered family processes related to chronic disease of a child

valuable they are for assessment. The nurse notes the time that the seizure began and times the length of the seizure. This is especially important if the child becomes cyanotic.

History taking is a vital tool for helping to identify factors that are valuable in establishing a cause of the seizures. Interviewing the child and family helps to elicit problems related to the psychologic impact of the disorder on their lives.

NURSING DIAGNOSES

Several nursing diagnoses that become apparent following an assessment of the child with a convulsive disorder are listed in the accompanying box. Others may be identified in specific cases.

PLANNING

The goals of nursing care for the child with a convulsive disorder are:

1. Protect the child during a seizure
2. Prevent seizures if possible
3. Help the child and family cope with the stigma often associated with the disorder
4. Promote a positive self-image in the child

IMPLEMENTATION

Nurses, when they first witness a child in a generalized cerebral seizure, are often frightened, puzzled, and immobilized. These reactions are normal but can reduce the effectiveness of care for the child and interfere with observations of the event. The child must be protected from injury during the seizure, and nursing observations made during the attack provide valuable information for diagnosis and management of the disorder.

It is impossible to halt a seizure once it has begun, and no attempt should be made to do so. The nurse must remain calm, stay with the child, and prevent him from sustaining any harm during the attack. If possible, the child should be isolated from the view of others by closing a door or pulling screens around him. A seizure can be very upsetting to visitors and to other children and their families. If other persons are present, they should be assured that the affected child is in no danger, and after the attack they can be provided with a simple explanation to meet their needs.

The convulsing child should not be moved or forcefully restrained, and force should not be exerted in an attempt to place a solid object between his teeth. If the child is standing and the nurse is able to reach him in time, or if the child is seated in a chair (including a wheelchair), he should be eased to the floor immediately. After the attack the child should be placed on his side in his bed or a similar place to allow him to sleep until he awakens. If the child is at school or away from his home, the parents should be contacted so that he can be taken home to rest.

EMERGENCY TREATMENT

Seizure

Protect child during seizure:
- Do not attempt to restrain child or use force
- If child is standing or sitting in wheelchair at beginning of attack, ease child down so that he will not fall; when possible, place cushion or blanket under child
- Do not put anything in child's mouth
- Loosen restrictive clothing
- Prevent child from hitting hard or sharp objects that might cause injury during uncontrolled movements
- Remove object(s)
- Pad object(s)
- Move furniture out of way
- Allow seizure to end without interference

When seizure has stopped, check for breathing
If not present, use mouth-to-mouth resuscitation
Check around mouth for evidence of burns or suspicious substances that might indicate poisoning
Remain with child
When child is able to move, seek help

See box for emergency treatment of a child during a generalized seizure.

A child who is known to have convulsive attacks or one who is under observation for seizures will require special precautions. The extent of these measures will depend on the type and frequency of the seizure. The child who is subject to daily seizures should not be permitted to engage in activities in which he might be injured, such as climbing, swimming, or handling sharp implements, and most of these children are advised to wear lightweight protective helmets. Such helmets can be purchased at bicycle shops. These children should have side rails on beds with the hard surfaces padded if there is danger that they could hurt themselves.

A child who has infrequent seizures or who is relatively free of seizures will have few restrictions on his activities. When the child is hospitalized, appropriate precautions should be implemented, such as side rails kept up when the child is sleeping or resting, especially if the seizures are of the grand mal variety, since many of these children are subject to nocturnal attacks. The bed should be protected with a waterproof mattress or sheeting.

Long-term care. Care of the child with a recurrent convulsive disorder involves physical care and instruction regarding the importance of the drug therapy and, probably more significant, the problems related to the emotional aspects of the disorder. There are few diseases that generate as much anxiety among relatives as epilepsy. Fears and misconceptions about the disease and its treatment abound in the lay person's mind. For many it represents the archetype of severe hereditary affliction. Therefore the foci of nursing care are directed toward helping the child and the family to deal with the psychologic and sociologic problems related to the disorder and educating the child, his family, his peers, and the public in general toward a more realistic and liberal view of the disease.

Children subject to seizures are placed on some type of drug therapy. The nurse can help the parents plan the administration of the medication at convenient times in order to disrupt the family routine as little as possible. The most convenient times for administration seem to be with meals or at bedtime. Although the anticonvulsant drugs are available in liquid extracts or emulsions, the tablet form is preferred by neurologists. The unequal distribution of the drug in the solute and the increased likelihood of inaccurate measurements make liquid medication less desirable. For small children the tablet of the proper dosage can be crushed and administered in syrup, jelly, or other palatable substances. Children taking phenobarbital and/or phenytoin should receive adequate vitamin D and folic acid, since deficiencies of both have been associated with these anticonvulsants.

It is important to impress on the family the need to continue the medication regularly without interruption for as long as required. The parents and the child will need to know the common side effects of the drug prescribed and observe for signs that might indicate unfavorable reactions.

The degree to which activities are restricted is individualized for each child and depends on the type, frequency, and severity of the seizures, the child's response to therapy, and the length of time the seizures have been controlled. Normal healthy activities are encouraged for children, and participation in competitive sports is determined on an individual basis. With encouragement most older children can accept the restrictions placed on activities. Contact sports such as football, karate, or wrestling are to be avoided, but basketball, baseball, and tennis are allowed. Climbing trees or an apparatus from which the child might fall and be seriously injured is not usually permitted. The well-controlled epileptic child can ride a bicycle or swim if accompanied by a companion.

Because the child is encouraged to attend school, camp, and other normal activities, the school nurse and the teacher should be made aware of the child's condition and his therapy. They can help to ensure regularity of medication and any special care the child might need. The child's teacher should be instructed regarding care of the child during a seizure so that he or she can act in a calm manner for the welfare of the child and to influence the attitude of the child's classmates.

Family support. Parental attitudes and management of a child with a convulsive disorder are as varied as those of other parents of children with a chronic disorder, and they are subject to the same long-term problems (see Chapter 18). Whether the seizures result from illness, injury, or unknown etiology, the parents may feel guilt, anxiety, and often humiliation. They want to know if it will affect the child's mental capacities. To many persons epilepsy is erroneously associated with mental deficiency. Seizures do frequently accompany other manifestations of severe brain damage from disease or injury, but the majority of children with seizures, like any population of healthy children, display a wide range of intelligence.

Parents also wonder how the illness will affect the child's future and need reassurance that the illness will not shorten the life of the child and that he can attend school, marry, and have children if he chooses. The child will need vocational guidance, and the parents should become familiar with the laws in their state regarding any limitations that might be imposed on the child because of the disorder. They also need reassurance that in this enlightened day and age there is less stigma attached to the disease than there has been in the past.

The child should be reared as any unaffected child with natural concern tempered by the understanding of his need not to be overprotected. Many parents refrain from correcting or punishing the child, especially if they have had the experience of such an emotional stress precipitating an attack. The child must not be made to feel that he is different. Parents should be honest and open about the disorder with the child and with others. Some parents are tempted to try to conceal the nature of the child's illness because of their belief that the disorder is shameful or a disgrace to the family.

Restrictions on the child's activities will be necessary for safety, but this area can be approached in a positive way in terms of what the child *can* do rather than what he cannot do. Sometimes parents curtail the child's activities more than necessary. The child needs to experience the maturing influences of play and work. The **Epilepsy Foundation of America*** is a national organization that works toward and for the welfare of persons with epilepsy and their families, helps with employment and legal problems, and provides education to patients, families, and communities.

The child with epilepsy. The child who is provided the security of a loving family, rewards and punishments no different from those of other children, and support in acquiring self-esteem is more apt to have a positive attitude toward his disease. The child derives his self-concept and self-esteem from his observations of others' reactions to him and his own perception of his capabilities. The suddenness and unpredictability of the attacks and the reactions of others further influence his feelings. When others consider the child to be different, inferior, or an object of ridicule, he comes to view himself as different, inferior, and incapable.

Behavioral problems are common in children with epilepsy and can become more serious than the seizures. Much of the behavior difficulty, especially aggressive or delinquent behaviors, has been attributed to the child's reaction to parental rejection. Feelings of guilt, frustration, depression, and self-negation can contribute to antisocial behaviors.

The child needs to learn about his disease and the role

*4351 Garden City Drive, Landover, MD 20785. In Canada, **Epilepsy Canada,** 2099 Alexandre De Sève, Bureau 27, Montreal, Quebec H2L 4R8.

that the medication plays in contributing to his prolonged well-being. As soon as he is old enough, the child should assume responsibility for taking his own medication and be advised to carry a card or a Medic Alert bracelet with pertinent information about his condition. Planning activities with the child and emphasizing those in which he can engage rather than those in which he cannot participate help the child to succeed and to gain satisfaction in his achievements. The child should be offered opportunities and encouraged to exercise judgment in his daily life.

The adolescent period may prove to be a trying time for the child with epilepsy. Limits imposed on the young person's activities at a time when he desires freedom and independence may bring his disability into sharp focus. For example, some states do not allow persons with epilepsy to obtain a driver's license, even when the disease is controlled; in others there are restrictions on employment and insurance.

Epilepsy should not be a severe impairment to most youngsters, and the nurse, by assuming the role of patient advocate, helping to educate the public regarding the disease, working toward making opportunities available to persons with the disorder, and lobbying for legislation that recognizes the needs of the individual with a seizure disorder, can help to erase the stigma that still remains regarding the disease.

EVALUATION

The effectiveness of nursing interventions is determined by continual reassessment and evaluation of care based on the following observational guidelines and expected outcomes:

1. Observe the child's behavior for evidence of seizure activity and assess the environment for situations that could cause injury to the child in the event of a seizure; interview the family regarding management of the child during a seizure.
2. Interview the child and family regarding compliance with medication.
3. Observe and interview the family regarding their feelings and concerns about and their understanding of the child's disease.
4. Observe the child's interactions with others and interview him about his feelings and concerns about the disease.

Expected outcomes:

1. The child exhibits no evidence of physical injury.
2. The family complies with instructions; the child remains free of seizure activity.
3. The family treats the child as any unaffected child.
4. The child expresses feelings and concerns and demonstrates a healthy view of his disorder and alterations in life-style that it imposes.

FEBRILE SEIZURES

Febrile convulsions are transient disorders of children that occur in association with a fever. They are one of the most common neurologic disorders of childhood, affecting 3% to 5% of children. Most febrile convulsions occur after 6 months of age and usually before age 3 years, with increased frequency in children younger than 18 months. They are unusual after 5 years of age. Boys are affected about twice as often as girls, and there appears to be an increased susceptibility in families, indicating a possible genetic predisposition.

The cause of febrile seizures is still uncertain. In most children the height and rapidity of the temperature elevation seem to be factors. The fever usually exceeds 38.8° C (101.8° F) and occurs during the temperature rise rather than after a prolonged elevation. Sometimes it constitutes the dramatic beginning of an illness. Febrile seizures usually accompany an upper respiratory or gastrointestinal infection, and 25% of children with simple febrile seizures have a recurrence of the seizure with subsequent infections. Since fevers are almost impossible to prevent in children, efforts are directed toward preventing an increase in the temperature.

Treatment consists of controlling the seizure with phenobarbital or diazepam (Valium) in appropriate dosage and reducing the temperature by administration of acetaminophen (Tylenol). Whether or not to implement continuous prophylactic anticonvulsant therapy in children who have experienced their initial febrile convulsion is still controversial. At present, anticonvulsant therapy is recommended for those children with febrile seizures who are at increased risk for developing sequelae.

The chance of developing chronic seizure disorder is increased in children who have a prolonged convulsion, those with focal seizures, those who have a near relative who experiences convulsions, and those with an abnormal EEG. Recurrences are more likely when the first seizure occurs in the first year of life.

◆ *Cerebral Malformations*

Defects of the central nervous system are usually the result of embryologic developmental failures. Some can be attributed to genetic factors; others may be a result of postnatal infections. However, in most cases the etiology is obscure. The defects that will be discussed are abnormalities of neural tube closure and hydrocephalus, characterized by an increase of free fluid in the cranial cavity.

CRANIAL DEFORMITIES

In the normal newborn the cranial sutures are separated by membranous seams several millimeters wide. For the first few hours to 1 to 2 days after birth, the cranial bones are highly mobile, which allows the cranial bones to mold and slide over one another, adjusting the circumference of the head to accommodate to the changing shape and character of the birth canal. The principal sutures in the infant's skull are the sagittal, coronal, and lambdoidal sutures, and the major soft areas at the juncture of these sutures are the anterior and posterior fontanels (see Fig. 8-6).

Following birth, growth of the skull bones occurs in a direction *perpendicular* to the line of the suture and normal closure occurs in a regular and predictable order. Although there are wide variations in the age at which closure takes place in individual children, normally all sutures and fontanels are ossified by the following ages:

8 weeks: posterior fontanel closed
6 months: fibrous union of suture lines and interlocking of serrated edges
18 months: anterior fontanel closed
12 years: sutures unable to be separated by increased ICP

Solid union of all sutures is not completed until very late childhood.

Closure of a suture before the expected time inhibits the perpendicular growth. Since normal increase in brain volume requires expansion, the skull is forced to grow in a direction *parallel* to the fused suture. This alteration in skull growth always produces a distortion of the head shape when the underlying brain growth is normal. The small head with closed and normal shape is the result of deficient brain growth; the suture closure is secondary to this brain growth failure. Failure of brain growth is not secondary to suture closure.

Various types of cranial deformities are encountered in early infancy. These include the enlarged head with frontal protrusion (bossing) characteristic of hydrocephalus, the parietal bossing that is seen in chronic subdural hematoma, the small head, and a variety of skull deformities (see box). Some occur during prenatal development; in others, head circumference is usually within normal limits at birth and the deviation from normal development becomes apparent with advancing age.

Cranial Deformities

Microcephaly: head circumference more than 2 standard deviations below average for age, sex, and gestation; caused by failure of brain development
Management: no treatment available

Craniosynostosis: premature closure of single or multiple sutures of the cranial vault, face, and base of skull
- **Scaphocephaly:** premature closure of sagittal suture causes skull to become elongated in an anteroposterior direction with a high cranial vault and a subnormal transverse diameter
- **Brachycephaly:** premature closure of the coronal sutures causes skull to become shortened in an anteroposterior direction with flattening of occiput and forehead
- **Oxycephaly:** premature closure of both coronal and sagittal sutures causes an excessively high and narrow skull that tapers upward on all sides
- **Plagiocephaly:** unilateral closure of one coronal or lambdoidal suture causes skull to become asymmetric
- **Craniofacial dysostosis** (Crouzon disease): premature closure of any or all cranial sutures, most frequently the coronal, and a typical facial deformity (widely spaced eyes, hypoplastic maxilla, and beaklike nose; tongue appears large and protruding; frequently with exophthalmos)

Management: surgical release of closed sutures; Crouzon disease—surgical correction of major facial deformities

Nursing Considerations

Nursing care of families in which there is a child with a cranial defect involves identifying children with deformities and referring them for evaluation. Since there is no therapy available for children with microcephaly, nursing care is directed toward helping parents adjust to rearing a child with brain damage (see Chapter 19). The care for those who benefit from surgery is the same as for any child who undergoes a surgical procedure. When a child's defect (such as plagiocephaly) can be corrected by the wearing of a helmet to alter the direction of growth, the family must be educated regarding use of the device and general supportive care. Special support is needed for children and families who may find it difficult to adjust to the unfamiliar change in head structure and body image that often accompanies cosmetic surgery for correction of craniofacial abnormalities.

HYDROCEPHALUS

Hydrocephalus is a condition caused by an imbalance in the production and absorption of CSF in the ventricular system. When production is greater than absorption, CSF accumulates within the ventricular system, usually under increased pressure, producing passive dilation of the ventricles.

Pathophysiology

The primary site of CSF formation is believed to be the choroid plexuses of the lateral ventricles, although it is also believed to be produced by the brain parenchyma. CSF circulates throughout the ventricular system, then is absorbed within the subarachnoid spaces by a mechanism that is not entirely clear.

The causes of hydrocephalus are varied, but the result is either (1) impaired absorption of CSF within the subarachnoid space (*communicating hydrocephalus*) or (2) obstruction to the flow of CSF within the ventricles (*noncommunicating hydrocephalus*). A tumor of the choroid plexus rarely causes increased CSF secretion. Any imbalance of secretion and absorption causes an increased accumulation of CSF in the ventricles, which become dilated and compress the brain substance against the surrounding rigid bony cranium. When this occurs before fusion of the cranial sutures, it produces enlargement of the skull as well as dilation of the ventricles (Figs. 27-8 and 27-9).

Most cases of noncommunicating hydrocephalus are a result of developmental malformations. Although the defect usually is apparent in early infancy, it may become evident at any time from the prenatal period to late childhood or early adulthood. Other causes include neoplasms, infections, and trauma. An obstruction to the normal flow can occur at any point in the CSF pathway to produce increased pressure and dilation of the pathways proximal to the site of obstruction.

Developmental defects—for example, Arnold-Chiari

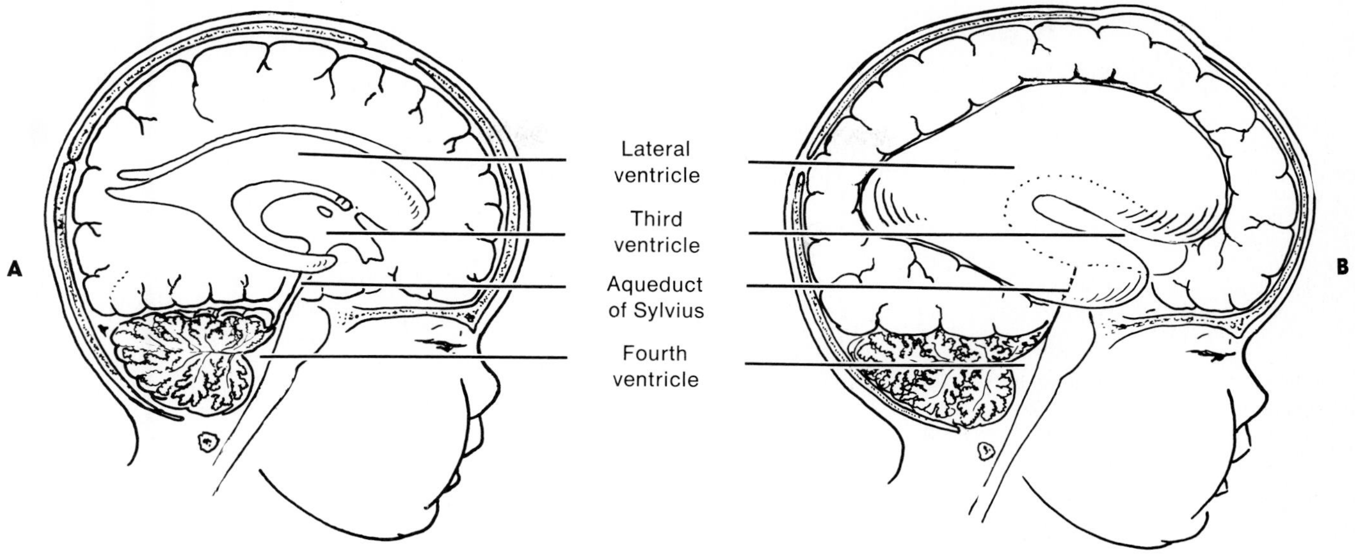

FIG. 27-8 Hydrocephalus: a block in the flow of CSF. **A,** Patent cerebrospinal fluid circulation. **B,** Enlarged lateral and third ventricle caused by obstruction of circulation—stenosis of the aqueduct of Sylvius.

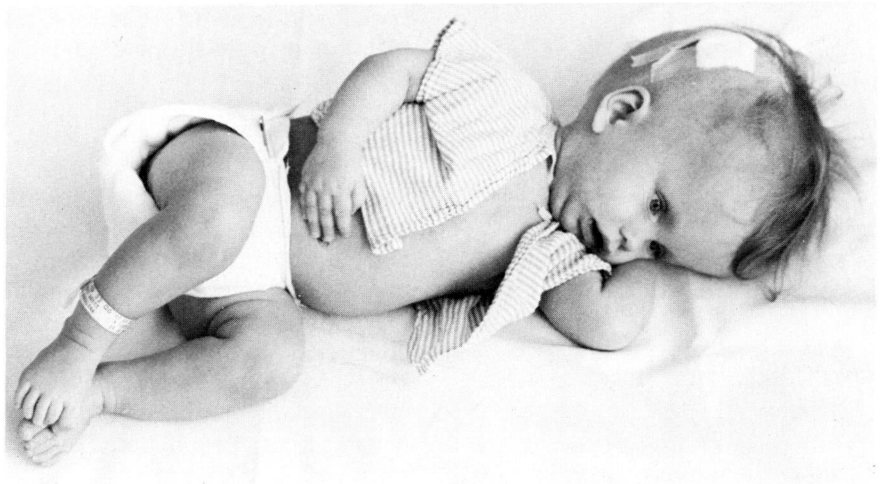

FIG. 27-9 Child with enlarged head caused by hydrocephalus.

malformations, aqueduct stenosis, and aqueduct gliosis—account for most cases of hydrocephalus from birth to 2 years of age. Hydrocephalus is so often associated with myelomeningocele that all such infants should be observed for its development. In the remainder of cases there is a history of intrauterine infection, perinatal hemorrhage, and neonatal meningoencephalitis. In older children hydrocephalus is most often the result of space-occupying lesions, intracranial infections, hemorrhage, or preexisting developmental defects, such as aqueduct stenosis or the *Arnold-Chiari malformation* (a congenital anomaly in which the cerebellum and medulla oblongata extend down through the foramen magnum).

Diagnostic Evaluation

The two factors that influence the clinical picture in hydrocephalus are the time of onset and the presence of preexisting structural lesions. In infancy, before closure of the cranial sutures, head enlargement is the predominant sign, whereas in older infants and children the lesions responsible for hydrocephalus produce other neurologic signs through pressure on adjacent structures before causing CSF obstruction (see box).

In infancy the diagnosis of hydrocephalus is based on head circumference that crosses one or more grid lines on the measurement chart within a period of 2 to 4 weeks and on associated neurologic signs that are present and

Clinical Manifestations of Hydrocephalus

Infancy, early:
- Abnormally rapid head growth
- Bulging fontanels (especially anterior) sometimes without head enlargement:
  - Tense
  - Nonpulsatile
- Dilated scalp veins
- Separated sutures
- Macewen sign ("cracked-pot" sound) on percussion
- Thinning of skull bones

Infancy, later:
- Frontal enlargement or "bossing"
- Depressed eyes
- "Setting sun" sign (sclera visible above the iris)
- Pupils sluggish, with unequal response to light

Infancy, general:
- Irritability
- Lethargy
- Infant cries when picked up or rocked and quiets when allowed to lie still
- Early infantile reflex acts may persist
- Normally expected responses fail to appear
- May display:
  - Change in level of consciousness
  - Opisthotonos (often extreme)
  - Lower extremity spasticity
- Advanced cases:
  - Difficulty in sucking and feeding
  - Shrill, brief, high-pitched cry
  - Cardiopulmonary embarrassment

Childhood:
- Headache on awakening; improvement following emesis or upright posture
- Papilledema
- Strabismus
- Extrapyramidal tract signs (e.g., ataxia)
- Irritability
- Lethargy
- Apathy
- Confusion
- Often incoherence

progressive. However, other diagnostic studies are needed to localize the site of CSF obstruction. Routine daily head circumference measurements are carried out in infants with myelomeningocele and intracranial infections. In evaluation of a premature infant, specially adapted head circumference charts are consulted to distinguish abnormal head growth from rapid head growth that takes place normally.

The signs and symptoms in early to late childhood are caused by increased ICP, and specific manifestations are related to the focal lesion. Most commonly resulting from posterior fossa neoplasms and aqueduct stenosis, the clinical manifestations are primarily those associated with space-occupying lesions.

The primary diagnostic tool for detecting hydrocephalus is computed tomography. Sedation is required since the child must remain absolutely still for an accurate picture to be produced. Diagnostic evaluation of children who have symptoms of hydrocephalus after infancy is

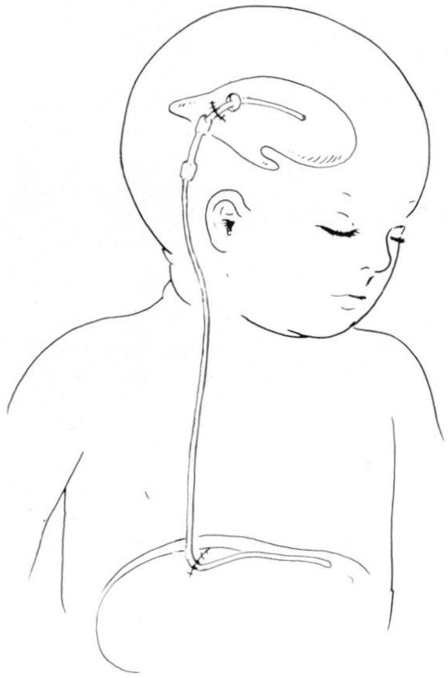

FIG. 27-10 Ventricular peritoneal shunt. Catheter is threaded subcutaneously from small incisions at the sites of ventricular and peritoneal insertions.

similar to that employed in those with suspected intracranial tumor. In the neonate echoencephalography is useful in comparing the ratio of lateral ventricle to cortex.

Therapeutic Management

The treatment of hydrocephalus is directed toward (1) relief of the hydrocephalus, (2) treatment of complications, and (3) management of problems related to the effect of the disorder on psychomotor development. The treatment is, with few exceptions, surgical. This is accomplished by direct removal of an obstruction (such as a tumor) or a shunt procedure that provides primary drainage of the CSF from the ventricles to an extracranial compartment, usually the peritoneum (ventricular peritoneal [VP] shunt) (Fig. 27-10).

Most shunt systems consist of a ventricular catheter, a flush pump, a unidirectional flow valve, and a distal catheter. In all models the valves are designed to open at a predetermined intraventricular pressure and close when the pressure falls below that level, thus preventing backflow of secretions.

The initial shunt is placed at about 3 to 4 months of age and, although there is wide variation, revisions are needed when there are signs of malfunction but are sometimes planned for 18 to 24 months, 4 to 6 years, and when approximately 80% of adult height has been attained (usually 10 to 12 years of age) (Noetzel, 1986). In all mechanisms the initial success rate is relatively high; however, shunts are associated with complications that interfere with continued shunt function or that threaten the life of the child.

The major complications of VP shunts are infection and malfunction. All shunts are subject to mechanical difficulties, such as kinking, plugging, or separation or migration of the tubing. Malfunction is most often caused by mechanical obstruction either within the ventricles from particulate matter (tissue or exudate) or at the distal end from thrombosis or displacement as a result of growth. The child with a shunt obstruction is often first seen in an emergency room with clinical manifestations of increased ICP, frequently accompanied by worsening neurologic status.

The most serious complication, shunt infection, can occur at any time, but the period of greatest risk is 1 to 2 months following placement. A persistent infection requires removal of the shunt until the infection is controlled.

Untreated hydrocephalus or intercurrent illnesses are associated with a 50% to 60% mortality rate. Of the survivors, very few (fewer than 10%) are intellectually normal. Patients with surgically treated hydrocephalus with continued neurosurgical and medical management have a survival rate of about 80%, with the highest incidence of mortality occurring within the first year of treatment. Reports on surviving children vary regarding their intellectual and neurologic status.

Nursing Considerations

Care of the child with hydrocephalus involves both preoperative and postoperative management. It is also important to carefully assess the child with myelomeningocele (p. 1062) for signs of increasing ICP, since hydrocephalus is commonly associated with that anomaly.

ASSESSMENT

Preoperatively the infant with diagnosed or suspected hydrocephalus is observed carefully for signs of increasing ICP. In infants the head is measured daily at the point of largest measurement—the occipitofrontal circumference (OFC) (see p. 134 for technique). To avoid the likelihood of wide discrepancies the point at which the measurements are taken is indicated on the head with a marking pen. Fontanels and suture lines are gently palpated for size, signs of bulging, tenseness, and separation. However, an infant with normal ICP will display bulging under certain circumstances such as straining or crying; therefore such accompanying behavior should be noted. Irritability, lethargy, or seizure activity as well as altered vital signs and feeding behavior may indicate an advancing pathologic condition.

In older children, who are usually admitted to the hospital for elective or emergency shunt revision, the most valuable indicator of increasing ICP is an alteration in the child's LOC and the way in which the child interacts with the environment. Changes are identified by observation and by comparison of present behavior with customary behavior, sleep patterns, developmental capabilities, and habits, all obtained through a detailed history and a baseline assessment. This baseline information serves as a guide for postoperative assessment and evaluation of shunt function.

NURSING DIAGNOSES

Following a thorough assessment nursing diagnoses become apparent. These include, but are not limited to, those listed in the accompanying box.

PLANNING

The goals of nursing care of the child with hydrocephalus include:

1. Prevent complications of hydrocephalus and/or corrective surgery
2. Provide education and emotional support to the family

IMPLEMENTATION

General nursing care of the infant with hydrocephalus may present special problems. Maintaining adequate nutrition often requires flexible feeding schedules to accommodate diagnostic procedures, since feeding before or after handling can precipitate an episode of vomiting. Small feedings at more frequent intervals are often better tolerated than are larger ones spaced farther apart. These infants are often difficult to feed and require extra time and innovation.

The nurse is responsible for preparing the child for diagnostic tests such as tomography and for assisting the physician with procedures such as a ventricular tap, which is often performed to relieve excessive pressure during the preoperative period, and CSF examination. (See Chapter 21 for preparing children for procedures.)

Fortunately, almost all affected children are recognized and treatment is begun early. For those children with significant head enlargement care must be exercised to see that the head is well supported when the infant is fed or moved to prevent extra strain on the infant's neck, and measures must be taken to prevent development of pressure areas. As the hydrocephalus progresses, untreated children become increasingly helpless and prone to the multiple problems of immobility; for example, pressure sores and contracture deformities. Not infrequently infants with irreversible brain damage or with se-

Nursing Diagnoses: The Child with Hydrocephalus

Potential for infection related to presence of mechanical drainage system
Potential impaired skin integrity related to pressure areas, paralysis, relaxed anal sphincter
Altered family processes related to situational crisis (child with a physical defect)

vere developmental defects such as hydranencephaly, in which both cerebral hemispheres fail to develop and are replaced with a membranous sac filled with cerebrospinal fluid, are placed in long-term institutions specially designed for care of these infants.

Postoperative care. Routine postoperative care and observation are instituted. In addition the infant or child is positioned carefully on the unoperated side to prevent pressure on the shunt valve and pressure areas. The child is kept flat to help avert complications resulting from too rapid reduction of intracranial fluid. When the ventricular size is reduced too rapidly, the cerebral cortex may pull away from the dura and tear the small interlacing veins, producing a subdural hematoma. This is not a problem in children with elective shunt revision, since their intraventricular size and pressure have been normal. The surgeon indicates the position to be maintained and the extent of activity allowed. If there is increased ICP, the surgeon will prescribe elevation of the head of the bed and/or that the child be allowed to sit up to enhance gravity flow through the shunt. Sedation is avoided because the LOC is an important observation.

Observation for signs of increased ICP, which indicates obstruction of the shunt, is continued. Neurologic assessment includes evaluation of pupil dilation (pressure causes compression or stretching of the oculomotor nerve, producing dilation on the same side as the pressure) and blood pressure (hypoxia to the brain stem causes variability in these vital signs). Sometimes the valve can be tested for patency and flushed to maintain patency by pumping several times to relieve the pressure. This is done by compressing the reservoir or antechamber of the valve mechanism, thus forcing a bolus of fluid from the reservoir into the distal catheter. Fluid that moves out of the chamber indicates a patent peritoneal catheter; ready refilling of the chamber with CSF is evidence of a patent ventricular catheter. The procedure is repeated when indicated or routinely (a prescribed number of times every hour or two) as ordered. If these measures are unsuccessful, shunt replacement may be required.

Intake and output are carefully monitored. Children are often placed on fluid restriction with nothing by mouth for 24 to 48 hours. The intravenous infusion is closely monitored to prevent fluid overload. Routine feeding is resumed after the prescribed NPO period, but the presence of bowel sounds is determined before feeding children with VP shunts.

Since infection is the greatest hazard of the postoperative period, nurses are continually on the alert for the usual manifestations of CSF infection, which may include elevated vital signs, poor feeding, vomiting, decreased responsiveness, and seizure activity. There may be signs of local inflammation at the operative sites and along the shunt tract. Antibiotics are administered by the intravenous route as ordered, and the nurse may also need to assist the physician with intraventricular instillation. The incision site is inspected for leakage and any suspected drainage is tested for glucose, an indication of cerebrospinal fluid.

Meticulous skin care is continued postoperatively with extra care to prevent tissue damage from pressure. A sheepskin pad underneath the child and a doughnut for the head help prevent pressure on prominent areas. Skin is inspected regularly for any signs of pressure, irritation, or infection.

Family support. Specific needs and concerns of parents during periods of hospitalization are related to the reason for the child's hospitalization (shunt revision, infection, diagnosis) and the diagnostic and/or surgical procedures to which the child must be subjected. Often parents have very little understanding of anatomy; therefore they need further exploration and reinforcement of information that was given to them by the physician and neurosurgeon as well as information about what they can expect. They are especially frightened of any procedure that involves the brain, and the fear of retardation or brain damage is very real and pervasive. Nurses can do much to allay their anxiety by explaining the rationale underlying the various nursing and medical activities such as positioning or testing, and by simply being available and willing to listen to their concerns.

To prepare for the child's discharge and home care, the parents are instructed how to recognize signs that indicate shunt malfunction or infection and how to pump the shunt, if necessary. Active children may have accidents, such as a fall, that can damage the shunt, and the tubing may pull out of the distal insertion site or become disconnected during normal growth.

The management of hydrocephalus in a child is a demanding task for both family and health professionals, and helping a family cope with the child is an important nursing responsibility. It is important to emphasize that hydrocephalus is a lifelong problem and that the child will require evaluation on a regular basis. The overall aim is to establish realistic goals and an appropriate educational program that will assist the child to achieve his optimum potential.

Anticipatory guidance will prepare parents for possible problems and help them to avoid being overprotective of the child. There need be few restrictions placed on the child's activities (mainly contact sports), and the child should be encouraged to live as would any other child of the same age and abilities. Parents need support and encouragement in coping with the child and problems he may encounter in relationships with peers and others. Reactions of other children when the child has a noticeably enlarged head or requires shaving at the times of revision are stress situations for both child and parents. (See Chapter 18 for problems and coping with the child with a disability.)

EVALUATION

The effectiveness of nursing interventions is determined by continual reassessment and evaluation of care based

on the following observational guidelines and expected outcomes:

1. Monitor child's neurologic status (physical signs and behavior), take temperature, examine skin at points of pressure
2. Interview family regarding their feelings and concerns

Expected outcomes:

1. Child remains free from complications of the disorder and surgical correction
2. Famiy discusses their feelings and concerns regarding the child's condition

SUMMARY

Neurologic disorders occur with relative frequency in the pediatric population, and this is an area of nursing practice in which continual nursing assessment is critical. Since the brain cannot be examined directly, information derived from observation of behavior and objective signs provides clues to the location of cerebral lesions. The most serious aspect of brain abnormality is increased ICP regardless of whether the cause is a space-occupying lesion, blood, or accumulation of fluid such as edema or ventricular CSF. Detecting signs of this complication and directing efforts toward reducing the pressure are the primary concerns of nursing care.

KEY CONCEPTS

- LOCs include sleep, confusion, delirium, pseudo-wakeful states, and comatose states.
- Complete neurologic examination takes into account vital signs, posture and movement, eye examination, and reflex testing.
- Nursing care of the unconscious child focuses on respiratory mangement, neurologic assessment, intracranial pressure monitoring, supplying adequate nutrition and hydration, drug therapy, promoting elimination, hygienic care, positioning and exercise, stimulation, and family support.
- Fractures resulting from head injuries may be classified as depressed, compound, basilar, and diastatic.
- Complications of head trauma can include epidural and subdural hemorrhage, cerebral edema, posttraumatic syndromes, and infections.
- Problems resulting from near-drowning include hypoxia and asphyxiation, aspiration, and hypothermia.
- Nursing care of the child with a brain tumor includes observing for signs and symptoms related to the tumor, preparing the child and family for diagnostic tests and operative procedures, preventing postoperative complications, planning for discharge, and promoting a return to optimum health.
- Nursing care of the child with meningitis includes administering antibiotics, preventing spread of infection, reducing environmental stimuli, assessment and physical care, and providing fluid and nutrition.
- Encephalitis may result from direct invasion of the central nervous system by a virus or from involvement of the central nervous system after viral disease.
- There has been a strong association between ingestion of aspirin during prodromal illness and Reye syndrome.
- Seizure disorders may exhibit sensory-hallucinatory phenomena, motor effects, sensorimotor effects, and loss of consciousness.
- Partial seizures are categorized as (1) simple, with unimpaired consciousness, (2) complex, with associated impairment of consciousness, and (3) those with impaired consciousness and that spread to become generalized.
- Generalized seizures are categorized as tonic-clonic, absence, atonic and akinetic, myoclonic, and infantile spasms.
- Long-term care of the child with recurrent convulsive disorders includes physical care and education regarding the importance of drug therapy and problems related to emotional aspects of the disorder.
- Many cranial deformities are amenable to surgical correction.
- Hydrocephalus can be caused by impaired absorption of CSF or obstruction to the flow of cerebrospinal fluid within the ventricles.
- Therapy for hydrocephalus involves relief of the hydrocephalus, prevention and/or treatment of complications, and management of problems related to psychomotor development.

STUDY QUESTIONS AND ACTIVITIES

1 Visit a pediatric intensive care unit and examine the charting record of an unconscious patient.
2 Interview a nurse in the pediatric intensive care unit regarding the ways in which the staff attempt to maintain the unconcious child's orientation and contact with his environment.
3 Investigate the practices that are implemented for the safety of seizure-prone children on the pediatric unit.
4 Consult a textbook on anatomy and outline the flow of cerebrospinal fluid from the area of its formation to its areas of absorption.

REFERENCES

Committee on Infectious Diseases, American Academy of Pediatrics: Aspirin and Reye's syndrome, Pediatrics **69:**810, 1982.
Monroe, B.: Immersion accidents in hot tubs and whirlpool spas, Pediatrics **69:**805-807, 1982.
Noetzel, M.J.: Hydrocephalus. In Gellis, S.S., and Kagan, B.M.: Current pediatric therapy 12, Philadelphia, 1986, W.B. Saunders Co.
Spyker, D.A.: Submersion injury: epidemiology, prevention, and management, Pediatr. Clin. North Am. **32:**113-125, 1985.
Wong, D.: Changing what children hear in the ICU can lower intracranial pressure, Am. J. Nurs. **88:**279-280, 1988.

BIBLIOGRAPHY

General

Benjamin, R., and McKay, R.: Working with a brain-injured child, J. Assoc. Care Child Health **8**(4):99-104, 1980.
Boortz-Marx, R.: Factors affecting intracranial pressure: a descriptive study, J. Neurosurg. Nurs. **17:**89-94, 1985.
Burgess, K.E.: Cerebral depressants: their effects and safe administration, Nursing 85 **15**(8):47-54, 1985.
Burgess, K.E.: Increased I.C.P., Nurs. Life **5**(2):33-48, 1985.
Conway-Rudtkowski, B.L.: Carini and Owens' neurological and neurosurgical nursing, ed. 8, St. Louis, 1982, The C.V. Mosby Co.
Diamond, L.: Triaging pediatric emergencies, Crit. Care Update **7**(2):28-32, 1980.
Gever, L.N.: Mannitol: the osmotic diuretic of choice, Nursing 85 **15**(7):64, 1985.
Hausman, K.A.: Critical care of the child with increased intracranial pressure, Nurs. Clin. North Am. **16:**647-656, 1981.
Hazinski, M.F.: Nursing care of the critically ill child, St. Louis, 1984, The C.V. Mosby Co.
Hinkle, J.L.: Treating traumatic coma, Am. J. Nurs. **86:**551-556, 1986.
Jackson, P.L.: Increased intracranial pressure in infants and young children, Crit. Care Q. **3:**47-59, 1981.
Johnson, L.K.: If your patient has increased intracranial pressure, your goal should be: no surprises, Nursing 83 **13**(6):58-63, 1983.
Mitchell, P.H.: Intracranial hypertension: implications of research for nursing care, J. Neurosurg. Nurs. **12:**145-154, 1980.
Mitchell, P.H., Ozuna, J., and Lipe, H.P.: Moving the patient in bed: effects on intracranial pressure, Nurs. Res. **30:**212-218, 1981.
Oakes, A.R., editor: Critical care nursing of children and adolescents, Philadelphia, 1981, W.B. Saunders Co.
Rimar, J.M.: Pancuronium bromide, MCN **10:**65, 1985.
Robinet, K.: Increased intracranial pressure: management with an intraventricular catheter, J. Neurosurg. Nurs. **17:**95-104, 1985.
Smith, S.L.: Continuous intracranial pressure monitoring: implications and applications for critical care, Crit. Care Nurse **3**(4):42-51, 1983.
Vestal, K.W., editor: Pediatric critical care nursing, New York, 1981, John Wiley & Sons, Inc.

Neurologic Assessment

Engler, M.B., and Engler, M.M.: The hazards of magnetic resonance imaging, Am. J. Nurs. **86:**650, 1986.
Esposito, N., and Westgate, P.: Continuous EEG monitoring in the PICU, J. Pediatr. Nurs. **2:**272-277, 1987.
Ferry, P.C.: Computed cranial tomography in children, J. Pediatr. **96:**961-967, 1980.
Fisher, J.: What you need to know about neurological testing, RN **50**(1):47-53, 1987.
Hellier, A., Ptak, H., and Cerreto, M.: CATS inside my brain: children's understanding of the cerebral computed tomography scan procedure, Child Health Care **14:**211-217, 1986.
Houghey, C.W.: CT scans, Nursing 81 **11**(12):72-77, 1981.
Jackson, P.L.: Assessing increased intracranial pressure in infants and young children, Crit. Care Update **10**(9):8-15, 1983.
Jess, L.W.: Assessing your patient for increased I.C.P., Nursing 87 **17**(6):34-41, 1987.
King, R.C.: Checking the patient's neurological status, RN **45**(12):57-63, 1982.
Kyba, F.N., Ogburn-Russell, L., and Rutledge, J.N.: Magnetic resonance imaging: the latest in diagnostic technology, Nursing 87 **17**(1):45-47, 1987.
Marchette, L., and Holloman, F.: A first-hand report on the new body scanners, RN **48**(11):28-31, 1985.
McManus, J.C., and Hausman, K.A.: Deciphering diagnostic studies: cerebrospinal fluid analysis, Nursing 82 **12**(8):43-47, 1982.
Mills, G.C.: Preparing children and parents for cerebral computed tomography, MCN **5:**403-407, 1980.
Slota, M.C.: Neurological assessment of the infant and toddler, Crit. Care Nurse **3**(5):87-92, 1983.
Slota, M.C.: Pediatric neurological assessment, Crit. Care Nurse **3**(6):106-112, 1983.
Vernberg, K., Jagger, J., and Jane, J.A.: The Glasgow Coma Scale: how do you rate? Nurse Educ. **8**(3):33-37, 1983.
Walleck, C.A.: A neurologic assessment procedure that won't make you nervous, Nursing 82 **12**(12):50-58, 1982.

The Unconscious Child

Mauss-Clum, N.: Bringing the unconscious patient back safely: nursing makes the critical difference, Nursing 82 **12:**34-42, 1982.
Nursing Grand Rounds: Overcoming acute complications in the unconscious patient, Nursing 84 **14**(5):42-45, 1984.
Scherer, P.: Assessment: the logic of coma, Am. J. Nurs. **86:**541-550, 1986.
Stolarik, A.: What the comatose patient can tell you, RN **48**(4):26-33, 1985.
Summers, A.: Billy was totally unresponsive, Am. J. Nurs. **79:**1262-1263, 1979.

Head Injury

Benjamin, R., and McKay, R.: Working with a brain-injured child, J. Assoc. Care Child Hosp. **8**(4):99-104, 1980.
Bowers, S.A., and Marshall, L.F.: Severe head injury: current treatment and research, J. Neurosurg. Nurs. **14:**210-218, 1982.
Derechin, M.E.: Pediatric head injury, Crit. Care. Nurs. Q. **10**(3)12-24, 1987.
Epstein, F.B., and Hamilton, G.C.: Initial approach to the brain-injured patient, Crit. Care Q. **5**(4):12-30, 1983.
Jorden, R.C.: Pathophysiology of brain injury, Crit. Care Q. **5**(4):1-12, 1983.
Kunkel, J.: Nursing management of the head injured patient, Crit. Care Update **8**(3):22-33, 1981.
Lipe, H.P.: Prevention of nervous system trauma from travel in motor vehicles, J. Neurosurg. Nurs. **17:**77-82, 1985.
Meier, E.M.: Evaluating head trauma in infants and children, MCN **8:**54-57, 1983.
Mirr, M.P., Jankowski, K., and Taylon, M.A.: Nursing management for barbiturate therapy in acute head injuries, Heart Lung **12:**52-59, 1983.
Nikas, D.L.: Critical aspects of head trauma, Crit. Care Nurs. Q. **10**(1):19-43, 1987.

Saul, T.G.: Intensive care of the brain-injured patient, Crit. Care Q. **5**(4):82-90, 1983.
Spielman, G.: Metabolic complications associated with severe diffuse brain injury, J. Neurosurg. Nurs. **17:**83-88, 1985.
Stevens, M.: Post-concussion syndrome, J. Neurosurg. Nurs. **14:**239-244, 1982.

Near-Drowning

Blauer, R.E.: Emergency: dealing with drownings . . . you can help keep the near-drowning victim alive, RN **48**(5):41-42, 1985.
Donahue, A.: Beware of the obvious with near-drowning victims, RN **45**(6):41-44, 1982.
Hartsell, M.B.: New technology for safety and research, J. Pediatr. Nurs. **2:**212-213, 1987.
Niggemann, E.H.: Near-drowning, Nursing 83 **13**(7):45, 1983.
Stickler, J.F., and Shawman, T.: A child drowns: a nursing perspective, MCN **6:**324-328, 1981.
Wolf, D.: Near drowning, Crit. Care Update **7**(6):31-35, 1980.

Central Nervous System Tumors

Cleaveland, M.J.: Nursing care in childhood cancer: brain tumor, Am. J. Nurs. **82:**422-425, 1982.
Flaherty, A.M.: Symptom management: nausea and vomiting, Cancer Nurs. **8**(1)[suppl.]:36, 1985.
Hardin, K.: Solid tumors in children, Issues Compr. Pediatr. Nurs.**4**(1):29-47, 1980.
Maul, S.K.: Childhood brain tumors: a special nursing challenge, MCN **9:**123-129, 1984.
Walker, R.W., and Allen, J.C.: Pediatric brain tumors, Pediatr. Ann. **12:**383-391, 1983.
Yasko, J.M.: Holistic management of nausea and vomiting caused by chemotherapy, Topics Clin. Nurs. **7**(1):26-38, 1985.

Intracranial Infections

Dagbjartsson, A., and Ludvigsson, P.: Bacterial meningitis: diagnosis and initial antibiotic therapy, Pediatr. Clin. North Am. **34:**219-230, 1987.
Ferguson, C.K., and Roll, L.J.: Human rabies, Am. J. Nurs. **81:**1175-1179, 1981.
Ferguson, C.K., and Roll, L.J.: Rabies in humans, Crit. Care Nurs. **10**(7):11-16, 1983.
Immunization Practices Advisory Committee: Rabies prevention, MMWR **29:**278, 1980.
Krugman, S., and Katz, S.L.: Infectious diseases of children, ed. 8, St. Louis, 1987, The C.V. Mosby Co.
Nebens, I.A., and Jackson, B.S.: A case of acute fulminating meningococcemia, Am. J. Nurs. **82:**1390-1393, 1982.
Nichols, A.O.: Taking the fear out of rabies treatment, Nursing 83 **13**(6):42-43, 1983.
Rimar, J.M., and Goschke, B.: Fulminant meningococcemia in children, Heart Lung **14:**385-390, 1985.
Spaniolo, A.M., and Antwerp, C.V.: Case study of a child with meningococcemia, J. Pediatr. Nurs. **1:**396-403, 1986.
Wink, D.: Bacterial meningitis in children, Am. J. Nurs. **84:**456-460, 1984.

Reye Syndrome

Belkengren, R.P., and Sapala, S.: Reye syndrome: clinical guidelines for practitioners in ambulatory care, Pediatr. Nurs. **7**(2):26-28, 1981.
Budd, R.A., and Rothwell, R.: Spotting Reye's syndrome while there's still time, RN **46**(12):38-42, 1983.
Dalgas, P.: Reye's syndrome update, MCN **8:**345-349, 1983.
Dunne, R.S., and Perez, R.C.: Reye's syndrome: a challenge not limited to critical care nurses, Issues Compr. Pediatr. Nurs. **5:**253-263, 1981.
Hurwitz, E.S., and others: Public health service study on Reye's syndrome and medications, N. Engl. J. Med. **313:**849-857, 1985.
Jemison-Smith, P., and Hamm, P.: Reye's syndrome, Crit. Care Update **10**(7):54-55, 1983.
Lopez, T., Oleri, L., and Redican, W.: Reye's syndrome; a review of research studies, J. Sch. Health **52:**206-210, 1982.
Martelli, M.E.: Teaching parents about Reye's syndrome, Am. J. Nurs. **82:**260-263, 1982.
Miller, J., and Arsenault, L.: Reye's syndrome, Neurosurg. Nurs. **15:**154-164, 1983.

Seizure Disorders

Austin, J.K., McBride, A.B., and Davis, H.W.: Parental attitude and adjustment to childhood epilepsy, Nurs. Res. **33:**92-96, 1984.
Berkowitz, C.D., and Jones, C.R.: The PNP's role in evaluation and management of febrile seizures, Pediatr. Nurs. **9:**432-434, 1983.
Coughlin, M.K.: Teaching children about their seizures and medications, MCN **4:**161-162, 1979.
Coulter, D.L.: The psychosocial impact of epilepsy in childhood, Child. Health Care **11:**48-53, 1982.
Farley, J.N.: Valproic acid for children with uncontrolled epilepsy, MCN **15:**22, 1982.
Frank, J., and Fischer, R.G.: Drug interactions with carbamazepine, Pediatr. Nurs. **13:**54-55, 1987.
Friedman, D.: Taking the scare out of caring for seizure patients, Nursing 88 **18**(2):52-59, 1988.
Gever, L.N.: Anticonvulsants, Nursing 84 **14:**41, 1984.
McGrath, D.M.: Nursing management of the child in status epilepticus, Issues Compr. Pediatr. Nurs. **5:**2173-2177, 1981.
McGrath, D.M.: Video recording seizure activity in children, MCN **8:**218-220, 1983.
Mills, M.: When a child has surgery for focal epilepsy, MCN **7:**304-308, 1982.
Norman, S.E.: Surgical treatment of epilepsy, Am. J. Nurs. **81:**994-996, 1981.
Norman, S.E., and Browne, T.R.: Seizure disorders, Am. J. Nurs. **81:**985-994, 1981.
Parish, M.A.: A comparison of behavioral side effects related to commonly used anticonvulsants, Pediatr. Nurs. **10:**149-152, 1984.
Santilli, N., and Tonelson, D.: Screening for seizures, Pediatr. Nurs. **7**(2):11-15, 1981.
Sasso, S.S.: Phenytoin for seizure disorders, MCN **9:**279, 1984.
Trekas, J.: Managing epilepsy: don't forget the patient, Nursing 82 **12**(10):63-65, 1982.
Tse, A.M.: Seizures and societal attitudes: a teaching tool for children, siblings, classmates, parents, and classroom teachers, Issues Compr. Pediatr. Nurs. **9:**299-303, 1986.
Tucker, C.A.: Complex partial seizures, Am. J. Nurs. **81:**996-1000, 1981.
Vining, E.P.G., and Freeman, J.H.: Discussion and explanation of seizures to the parents and child, Pediatr. Ann. **14:**737-739, 1985.
Williams, A., Swisher, C., and Bremer, H.L.: Critical care of seizures, Crit. Care Update **8**(7):22-25, 1981.

Cranial Malformations

Arsenault, L.: Delayed onset of symptomatic hydrocephalus related to aqueductal stenosis, J. Neurosurg. Nurs. **15**(5):291-297, 1983.
Bernardo, M.L.: Craniosynostosis: the child's care from detection through correction, MCN **4:**234-237, 1979.
Grant, L.: Hydrocephalus; an overview and update, J. Neurosurg. Nurs. **16**(6):313-318, 1984.
Humphrey, P.A., Britt, P.H., and Peters, C.R.: Craniofacial malformations, Am. J. Nurs. **79:**1230-1234, 1979.
Jackson, P.L.: Ventriculoperitoneal shunts, Am. J. Nurs. **80:**1104-1109, 1980.
Jackson, P.L.: Peritoneal shunting for hydrocephalus, Crit. Care Update **10**(4):33-39, 1983.

CHAPTER 28

The Child with Endocrine Dysfunction

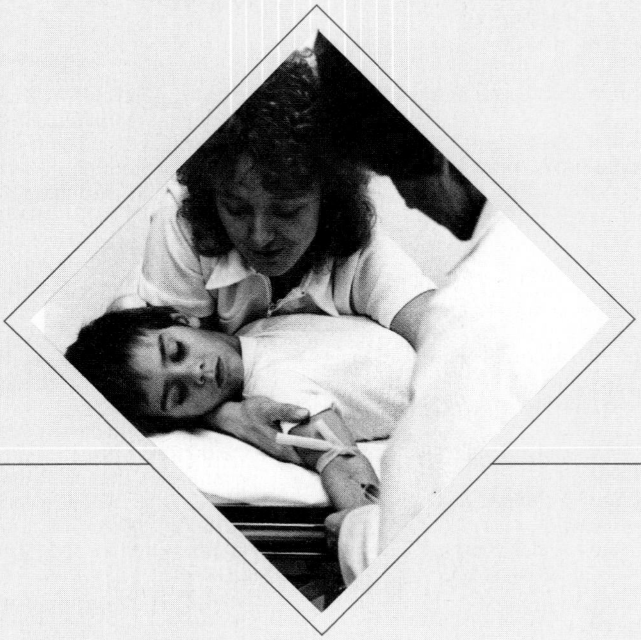

LEARNING OBJECTIVES

On completion of this chapter the reader will be able to:

- Differentiate between the disorders caused by hypopituitary and hyperpituitary dysfunction
- Describe the manifestations of thyroid hypofunction and hyperfunction and the management of children with the disorders
- Distinguish between the manifestations of adrenal hypofunction and hyperfunction
- Differentiate among the various categories of diabetes mellitus
- Discuss the management and nursing care of the child with diabetes mellitus in the acute care setting
- Distinguish between a hypoglycemic and a hyperglycemic reaction
- Design a teaching plan for a child with diabetes mellitus
- Formulate a teaching plan for instructing parents of a child with diabetes mellitus

The major chemical regulators of the body are substances produced and secreted by a diverse group of tissues collectively known as the endocrine system. These substances, the hormones, are synthesized intracellularly and secreted into the circulation, where they are transported to other tissues to stimulate, catalyze, or serve as pacemaker substances for metabolic processes. Together with the closely related but more rapidly reacting nervous system, hormones integrate the various physiologic functions of the body in its adjustment to external and internal environmental demands. Endocrine substances, even in extremely small concentrations, are effective in modifying metabolism, behavior, and development (Table 28-1).

This chapter is primarily concerned with problems stemming from oversecretion or undersecretion of the major hormones or from defective responses in those organs and tissues that are sensitive to these hormones. It is the endocrine system that affects all aspects of body function, including growth, feelings of physical and emotional well-being, and appearance. The endocrine system is largely responsible for the size, shape, texture, and sexual characteristics of the body and, therefore, has a profound influence on body image. Most endocrine disorders are relatively uncommon; however, the most common endocrine disturbance in childhood, diabetes mellitus, is a health problem with lifelong implications, so it will be discussed at length.

◆ *Disorders of Pituitary Function*

The pituitary gland, or hypophysis, is often referred to as the *master gland* because of its role in regulating other endocrine glands. Under the influence of secretions from the hypothalamus, the anterior lobe of the pituitary (adenohypophysis) releases or withholds seven hormones. These hormones control the secretion of hormones from other endocrine glands and influence somatic and sexual development. Because of this relationship a dysfunction observed in target tissues can be the result of malfunction of the hypothalamus, the pituitary gland, or the target gland. If the tropic hormones are involved, the resulting disorder reflects the altered stimulus to the target gland. For example, if thyroid-stimulating hormone is deficient, thyroid hormone is also deficient, and the child displays the manifestations of hypothyroidism. Overproduction of pituitary hormone is thought to be caused by hyperplasia of the pituitary cells or by a primary hypothalamic defect that results in excess production of the hormone's releasing factor.

Deficiencies of the anterior pituitary hormones may be the result of organic defects or of idiopathic etiology and may occur as a single hormonal problem or in combination with other hormonal deficiencies. The clinical manifestations depend on the hormones involved and the age of onset. This discussion is limited to dysfunction related primarily to the secretion of growth hormone.

HYPOPITUITARISM

Hypopituitarism is primarily a disorder associated with deficient secretion of growth hormone (somatotropin). It may be caused by a variety of conditions: developmental defects; destructive lesions such as tumors, trauma, vascular abnormalities, or surgery; a manifestation of certain hereditary disorders; or the result of functional disorders such as anorexia nervosa or psychosocial dwarfism. In more than half of children with hypopituitarism, no lesion is evident and the cause is unknown—*idiopathic hypopituitarism* or idiopathic pituitary growth failure.

Idiopathic hypopituitarism is usually related to growth hormone (GH) deficiency, which inhibits somatic growth in all body cells (Fig. 28-1). The primary site of dysfunction in the syndrome appears to be in the hypothalamus.

TABLE 28-1

Endocrine Glands and Their Function

Gland/Hormone	Primary Effect
Adenohypophysis (anterior pituitary)	
Growth hormone (GH)	Promotes growth of bone and soft tissues
Thyroid-stimulating hormone (TSH)	Stimulates thyroid hormone secretion
Adrenocorticotropic hormone (ACTH)	Stimulates adrenal cortex to secrete glucocorticoids and androgens
Gonadotropins Follicle-stimulating hormone (FSH) Luteinizing hormone (LH)	Stimulate gonads to mature and produce sex hormones and germ cells
Prolactin	Stimulates milk secretion
Melanocyte-stimulating hormone (MSH)	Promotes pigmentation of skin
Neurohypophysis (posterior pituitary)	
Antidiuretic hormone (ADH)	Acts on kidney tubules to reabsorb water
Oxytocin	Stimulates uterine contractions Causes milk-ejection reflex
Thyroid Gland	
Thyroid hormones	Regulate metabolic rate Control rate of body cell growth
Thyrocalcitonin	Influences ossification and development of bone
Parathyroid Glands	
Parathyroid hormone (PTH)	Regulates calcium metabolism
Adrenal Cortex	
Aldosterone	Regulates sodium retention and excretion
Sex hormones	Same as hormones from gonads
Glucocorticoids	Promote metabolism Mobilize body defenses during stress Suppress inflammatory reaction
Adrenal Medulla	
Catecholamines	Produce a sympathetic response
Islands of Langerhans of Pancreas	
Insulin	Promotes utilization of glucose by cells; reduces blood sugar
Glucagon	Increases blood sugar
Somatostatin	Inhibits secretion of insulin and glucagon
Ovaries	
Estrogen	Stimulates ripening of ova Produces female secondary sex characteristics
Progesterone	Prepares uterus for fertilization
Testes	
Testosterone	Stimulates spermatogenesis Produces male secondary sex characteristics

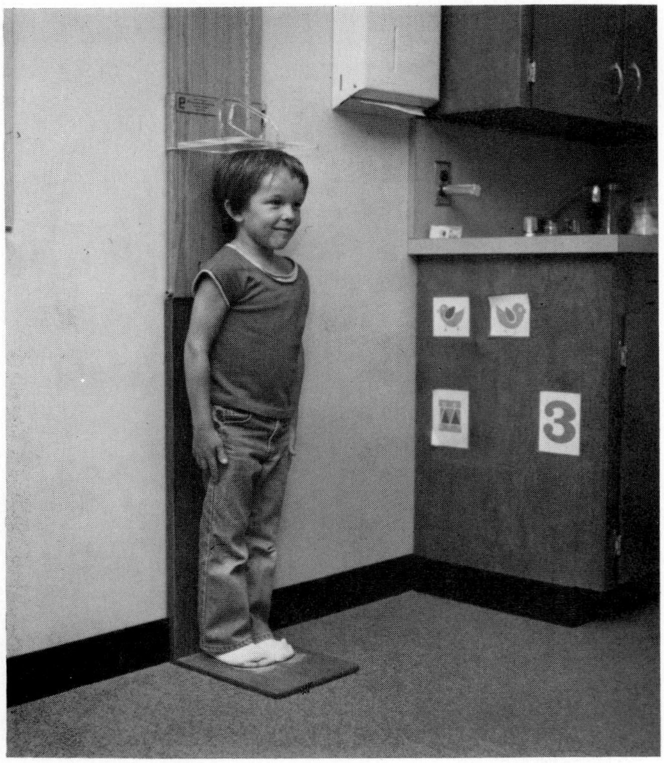

FIG. 28-1 Ten-year-old child with growth hormone deficiency. Height is 42.5 inches.

The extent of idiopathic GH deficiency may be complete or partial, but the cause is unknown. It is frequently associated with other pituitary hormone deficiencies and is seen more frequently in boys than in girls.

Diagnostic Evaluation

Only a small number of children with delayed growth or short stature have hypopituitary dwarfism. In the majority of instances the cause is constitutional delay (see p. 473). Although children with hypopituitarism are normal at birth, they show growth patterns that progressively deviate from the normal growth rate, often beginning in infancy. The chief complaint in most instances is short stature (see box).

A complete diagnostic evaluation should include a family history, a history of the child's growth patterns and previous health status, physical examination, radiographic surveys, and endocrine studies. Definitive diagnosis is based on radioimmunoassay of plasma growth hormone levels. Radiographic examination of the wrist for centers of ossification is an important procedure in evaluating growth. Endocrine studies to detect tropic hormone deficiencies are also performed if there is evidence of hypothyroidism or hypoadrenalism.

Clinical Manifestations of Hypopituitarism

- Presenting complaint—short stature
  - Usually normal growth first year
  - Afterward—slowed growth curve
  - Growth measurements below 5th percentile
- Premature aging common in later life
- Height may be retarded more than weight
- Appear well-nourished
- Skeletal proportions normal
- Tend to be relatively inactive
- Less apt to participate in aggressive, sporting-type activities
- Bone age nearly always retarded but closely related to height age
- Usually primary teeth appear at expected age; eruption of permanent teeth delayed
- Teeth are overcrowded and malpositioned (because of underdeveloped jaw)
- Sexual development usually delayed but normal

Therapeutic Management

Treatment of GH deficiency caused by organic lesions is directed toward correction of the underlying disease process, e.g., surgical removal or irradiation of a tumor. The definitive treatment of GH deficiency is replacement of GH and is successful in 80% of affected children. Children with other hormone deficiencies require replacement therapy to correct the specific disorders. This may involve administration of thyroid extract, cortisone, testosterone, or estrogens and progesterone. The sex hormones are usually begun during adolescence to promote normal sexual maturation.

Nursing Considerations

Nursing care is primarily directed toward assisting in establishing the diagnosis and providing emotional support to the child and family (see also p. 473). Since these children appear younger than their chronologic age, others frequently relate to them in infantile or childish ways. Parents and teachers benefit from guidance directed toward realistic expectations of the child, based on his age and abilities.

Children undergoing hormone replacement require additional support, such as preparation for frequent injections (several times per week). Even when hormone replacement is successful, these children attain their eventual adult height at a slower rate than their peers, so they need assistance in setting realistic expectations regarding improvement. Professionals and families may find education and support from the **Human Growth Foundation.***

PITUITARY HYPERFUNCTION

Excess growth hormone prior to closure of the epiphyseal shafts results in proportional overgrowth of long bones,

*Call 1-800-451-6434.
4720 Montgomery Lane, Bethesda, MD 20814.

until the individual reaches a height of 8 feet or more. Vertical growth is accompanied by rapid and increased development of muscles and viscera. Weight is increased but is usually in proportion to height. Proportional enlargement of head circumference also occurs and may result in delayed closure of the fontanels. Children with a pituitary-secreting tumor may also demonstrate signs of increasing intracranial pressure, especially headache.

If hypersecretion of growth hormone occurs after epiphyseal closure, growth is in the transverse direction, producing a condition known as *acromegaly*. Typical facial features include overgrowth of head, lips, nose, tongue, jaw, and paranasal and mastoid sinuses; separation and malocclusion of the teeth in the enlarged jaw; disproportion of the face to the cerebral division of the skull; increased facial hair; and thickened, deeply creased skin.

Diagnostic Evaluation

Diagnosis is based on a history of excessive growth during childhood and evidence of increased levels of growth hormone. Radiologic studies may reveal a tumor in an enlarged sella turcica, normal bone age, enlargement of bones, such as the paranasal sinuses, and evidence of joint changes. Endocrine studies to confirm excess of other hormones, such as cortisol and sex hormones, are also included in the differential diagnosis.

Therapeutic Management

If a lesion is present, surgical treatment, including cryosurgery or hypophysectomy, may be warranted to remove the tumor whenever feasible. Other therapies that destroy pituitary tissue include external irradiation and radioactive implants. Depending on the extent of surgical extirpation and the degree of pituitary insufficiency, hormone replacement with thyroid extract, cortisone, and sex hormones may be necessary.

Nursing Considerations

The primary nursing consideration is early identification of children with excessive growth rates. Although medical management does not diminish the height already attained, it can retard further growth. The earlier the treatment is begun, the better the chance to attain a normal adult height.

Children with excessive growth rates require as much emotional support as those with short stature. However, girls may suffer from the effects of excessive height much more than boys, who may find the tallness an asset when pursuing sports such as basketball. A compassionate nurse can be very supportive to these children, especially prior to adolescence, when they are larger than their peers. The nurse can emphasize to a tall girl that as boys grow older, they become taller and she will not always be looking down at them. Since early adolescence is a time of idol worship, the nurse can point out marriages of celebrities in which the woman is taller than the man to help the girl gain a perspective that not all heterosexual relationships must follow stereotypic models.

DIABETES INSIPIDUS

The principal disorder of posterior pituitary hypofunction is diabetes insipidus (DI), also known as neurogenic DI. The disease is the result of hyposecretion of antidiuretic hormone (ADH), or vasopressin, which produces a state of uncontrolled diuresis. Primary causes are familial or idiopathic; secondary causes include trauma (accidental or surgical), tumors, granulomatous disease, infections (meningitis or encephalitis), or vascular anomalies (aneurysm). The disorder is not to be confused with *nephrogenic diabetes insipidus,* a rare hereditary disorder caused by unresponsiveness of the renal tubules to the hormone.

Diagnostic Evaluation

The cardinal signs of DI are polyuria and polydipsia. In the older child excessive urination accompanied by a compensatory insatiable thirst may be so intense that the child does little other than go to the toilet and drink fluids. Not infrequently the first sign is enuresis. In the infant the initial symptom is irritability that is relieved with feedings of water but not milk. The infant is also prone to dehydration, electrolyte imbalance, hyperthermia, azotemia, and potential circulatory collapse.

The simplest test used to diagnose this condition is restriction of oral fluids and observation of consequent changes in urine volume and concentration. In diabetes insipidus fluid restriction has little or no effect on urine formation but causes weight loss from dehydration. If this test is positive, the child should be given a test dose of injected aqueous vasopressin (Pitressin), which should alleviate the polyuria and polydipsia. Unresponsiveness to exogenous vasopressin usually indicates nephrogenic diabetes insipidus.

Therapeutic Management

The usual treatment is hormone replacement, either with an intramuscular or subcutaneous injection of vasopressin tannate in peanut oil or via aqueous vasopressin nasal spray. The injectable form has the advantage of lasting for 48 to 72 hours, which affords the child a full night's sleep. However, it has the disadvantages of requiring frequent injections and proper preparation of the drug.

Nursing Considerations

The initial objective of care is identification of the disorder. After confirmation of the diagnosis, parents need a thorough explanation of the condition, with special emphasis on distinguishing the difference between diabetes insipidus and diabetes mellitus. The parents must realize that treatment is lifelong. If the child is to receive the injectable vasopressin (Pitressin), ideally both parents and children over 7 years of age should be taught the correct procedure for preparation and administration of the drug. Once the child is old enough, he should be encouraged to assume full responsibility for his care.

For emergency purposes these children should wear Medic Alert tags. Older children are advised to carry the nasal vasopressin spray with them for temporary relief of symptoms. School personnel should be made aware of the problem in order that the child is granted unrestricted use of the lavatory and drinking water. Failure to permit this may result in embarrassing accidents that often result in the child's unwillingness to attend school.

SYNDROME OF INAPPROPRIATE ANTIDIURETIC HORMONE SECRETION

Hypersecretion of the posterior pituitary antidiuretic hormone (ADH, vasopressin) produces the disorder known as the syndrome of inappropriate ADH secretion (SIADH). SIADH is observed with increased frequency in a variety of conditions, especially those involving infections, tumors, and trauma of the central nervous system.

The manifestations observed are directly related to fluid retention and hypotonicity. Increased secretion of ADH causes the kidneys to reabsorb water, which increases the fluid volume and decreases serum osmolality. When serum sodium levels are diminished to 120 mEq/liter, the child displays anorexia, nausea (and sometimes vomiting), stomach cramps, irritability, and personality changes. With progressive reduction in sodium, other neurologic signs, stupor, and convulsions may be evident. The symptoms disappear when the underlying disorder is corrected. Immediate management consists of restricting fluids.

Nursing Considerations

The first goal of nursing management is recognizing the presence of SIADH from symptoms described in patients at risk. Accurately measuring intake and output, noting daily weight, and observing for signs of fluid overload are primary nursing functions, especially in the child receiving intravenous fluids. Seizure precautions are implemented, and the child and family need education regarding the rationale for fluid restrictions. The rare child with chronic SIADH will be placed on long-term ADH-antagonizing medication and require instructions for its administration.

◆ *Disorders of Thyroid Function*

The thyroid gland secretes two types of hormones: thyroid hormone, which consists of the hormones thyroxine (T_4) and triiodothyronine (T_3), and thyrocalcitonin. The secretion of thyroid hormones is controlled by thyroid-stimulating hormone (TSH) from the anterior pituitary. Consequently hypothyroidism or hyperthyroidism may result from a defect in the target gland or from a disturbance in the secretion of TSH or its releasing factor in the hypothalamus.

Since the functions of T_3 and T_4 are qualitatively the same, the term *thyroid hormone* (TH) will be used throughout the discussion.

The synthesis of thyroid hormones depends on available sources of dietary iodine and tyrosine. The thyroid is the only endocrine gland capable of storing excess amounts of hormones for release as needed. The main physiologic action of thyroid hormone is to regulate the basal metabolic rate and thereby control the processes of growth and tissue differentiation.

Thyrocalcitonin helps maintain blood calcium levels by decreasing the calcium concentration. Its effect is the opposite of parathormone in that it inhibits skeletal demineralization and promotes calcium deposition in the bone.

HYPOTHYROIDISM

Hypothyroidism is one of the most common endocrine problems of childhood. It may be either congenital or acquired and represents a deficiency in secretion of thyroid hormones. Hypothyroidism from dietary insufficiency of iodine is now rare in the United States because the use of iodized salt has permitted a readily available source of the nutrient.

Congenital Hypothyroidism

Screening programs for detecting hypothyroidism in the newborn period have significantly altered the adverse effects of this disorder (see p. 258 for a discussion of congenital hypothyroidism.)

Juvenile Hypothyroidism

Beyond infancy primary hypothyroidism may be caused by a number of defects. For example, a congenital hypoplastic thyroid gland may provide sufficient amounts of TH during the first year or two but be inadequate when rapid body growth increases demands on the gland. Partial or complete thyroidectomy for cancer or thyrotoxicosis can leave insufficient thyroid tissue to furnish hormones for body requirements. Irradiation for Hodgkin disease or other malignancies or infectious processes may be a cause of hypothyroidism. It can also occur when dietary iodine is deficient.

Clinical manifestations depend on the extent of dysfunction and the age of the child at the onset (see box). Since brain growth is nearly complete by 2 to 3 years of age, mental retardation or neurologic sequelae are not associated with juvenile hypothyroidism.

Therapy is thyroid hormone replacement, the same as for hypothyroidism in the infant, although the prompt

Clinical Manifestations of Juvenile Hypothyroidism

Decelerated growth	Constipation
Less when acquired at later age	Sleepiness
Myxedematous skin changes	Mental decline
Dry skin	
Puffiness around eyes	
Sparse hair	

treatment needed in the infant is not required in the child. In children with severe symptoms, the restoration of euthyroidism is achieved more gradually, with administration of increasing amounts of L-thyroxine over 4 to 8 weeks to avoid symptoms of hyperthyroidism that can occur with treatment of chronic hypothyroidism.

Nursing Considerations

The importance of early recognition in the infant has already been discussed in Chapter 9. Cessation or retardation of growth in a child whose growth has previously been normal should alert the observer to the possibility of hypothyroidism. Following diagnosis and implementation of thyroxine therapy, the importance of compliance and periodic monitoring of response to therapy should be stressed to parents. The child should learn to take responsibility for his own health as soon as he is old enough.

GOITER

A goiter is an enlargement or hypertrophy of the thyroid gland. It can be congenital or acquired. Congenital disease usually occurs as a result of antithyroid drugs and/or iodides administered to the mother during pregnancy. The acquired disease can result from increased secretion of pituitary thyrotropic hormone in response to decreased circulating levels of thyroid hormones, neoplastic or inflammatory processes, or dietary iodine deficiency.

Enlargement of the thyroid gland can be mild and noticeable only when there is an increased demand for TH; e.g., during periods of rapid growth. Enlargement of the thyroid at birth can be sufficient to cause severe respiratory distress. Thyroid hormone replacement is necessary to treat the hypothyroidism and reverse the thyroid-stimulating hormone effect on the gland.

Nursing Considerations

Identification of large goiters is facilitated by their obvious appearance. Smaller nodules may be evident only on palpation. Nurses in ambulatory settings need to be aware of the possibility of goiters and report such findings to a physician. If an infant is born with a goiter, immediate precautions are instituted for emergency ventilation, such as supplemental oxygen and a tracheostomy set. Positioning the child with the neck hyperextended often facilitates breathing. Immediate surgery to remove part of the gland may be lifesaving.

When thyroid replacement is necessary, parents have the same needs regarding its administration as discussed for the parents of children who have hypothyroidism (Chapter 9).

LYMPHOCYTIC THYROIDITIS

Lymphocytic thyroiditis (Hashimoto disease, juvenile autoimmune thyroiditis) is the most common cause of thyroid disease in children and adolescents, and it accounts for the largest percentage of juvenile hypothyroidism. It also accounts for many of the enlarged thyroid glands formerly designated as thyroid hyperplasia of adolescence, or "adolescent goiter." The disease is more common in girls than in boys and in white than in black persons. It occurs more frequently after age 6, reaching a peak incidence at adolescence.

Pathophysiology

There is a strong genetic predisposition to the development of autoimmune thyroiditis, although no mode of inheritance has been delineated and the basic stimulus or autoimmune defect is unknown. The disease is characterized by lymphocytic infiltration of the gland, inflammation, and, in many patients, replacement with fibrous tissue. In the early stages there may be only hyperplasia.

Diagnostic Evaluation

The enlarged thyroid gland may be detected by the physician or pediatric nurse practitioner during a routine examination, although it may be noted by parents when the youngster swallows. Most children are euthyroid but some display symptoms of hypothyroidism. Others have signs that suggest hyperthyroidism (see box).

Thyroid function tests are usually normal, although TSH levels may be slightly or moderately elevated. With progressive disease the T_4 decreases, followed by a de-

Clinical Manifestations of Lymphocytic Thyroiditis

Enlarged thyroid gland	May have symptoms of hyperthyroidism
Usually symmetrical	Nervousness
Firm	Irritability
Freely movable	Increased sweating
Nontender	Hyperactivity
Tracheal compression	
Sense of fullness	
Hoarseness	
Dysphagia	

crease in T_3 levels and an increase in TSH. A variety of abnormalities in radioactive iodine uptake may be noted. The majority of children have serum antibody titers to thyroid antigens, but fewer children have a positive red blood cell hemagglutination test. When both tests are used, almost all children with thyroid autoimmunity are detected.

Therapeutic Management

In many cases the goiter is transient and asymptomatic and regresses spontaneously within a year or two. Therapy of nontoxic diffuse goiter is usually simple, uncomplicated, and effective. Oral administration of thyroid hormone depresses thyroid-stimulating hormone, thus decreasing the size of the gland significantly. Surgery is contraindicated in this disorder.

Nursing Considerations

Nursing care consists of identifying the youngster with thyroid enlargement, reassuring the child that the condition is probably only temporary, and reinforcing instructions for thyroid therapy.

HYPERTHYROIDISM

The largest percentage of hyperthyroidism in childhood is caused by *Graves disease.* The peak incidence of the disease occurs between 12 and 14 years of age, but it may be present at birth in children of thyrotoxic mothers. The incidence is five times higher in girls than in boys. The disease is apparently caused by a serum thyroid-stimulating immunoglobulin, but no specific etiology has been identified. There is definitive evidence for familial association; a large number of persons with the disease possess the histocompatibility antigen HLA-B8.

Diagnostic Evaluation

The development of manifestations is highly variable (see box). Manifestations develop gradually with an interval between onset and diagnosis of approximately 6 to 12 months. Diagnosis is established on the basis of increased levels of T_4 and T_3. Thyrotropin (TSH) is suppressed to unmeasurable levels. Other tests are rarely indicated.

Therapeutic Management

Therapy for hyperthyroidism is controversial, but all methods are directed toward retarding the rate of hormone secretion. The three acceptable modes available are (1) the antithyroid drugs, which interfere with the biosynthesis of thyroid hormone, including propylthiouracil (PTU) and methimazole (MTZ, Tapazole); (2) subtotal thyroidectomy; and (3) ablation with radioiodine (^{131}I-iodide).

Thyrotoxicosis. Thyrotoxicosis (thyroid "crisis" or thyroid "storm") may occur from sudden release of the hormone. Although unusual in children, a crisis can be life-threatening. A crisis may be precipitated by acute infection, surgical emergencies, or discontinuation of antithyroid therapy. Treatment in addition to antithyroid drugs is administration of beta-adrenergic blocking agents (propranolol), which provide relief from the disturbing side effects of the reaction.

Clinical Manifestations of Hyperthyroidism (Graves Disease)

Cardinal Signs
- Emotional lability
- Physical restlessness, characteristically at rest
- Decelerated school performance
- Increased appetite, with or without weight loss
- Fatigue

Physical Signs
- Tachycardia
- Increased pulse pressure
- Wide-eyed, staring expression with lid lag
- Tremor
- Goiter (hypertrophy and hyperplasia)
- Warm, moist skin
- Accelerated linear growth
- Heat intolerance (may be severe)
- Hair fine and unable to hold a curl

Thyroid Storm
- Acute onset:
  - Severe irritability and restlessness
  - Vomiting
  - Diarrhea
  - Hyperthermia
  - Hypertension
  - Severe tachycardia
  - Prostration
- May progress rapidly to:
  - Delirium
  - Coma
  - Death

Nursing Considerations

The initial nursing objective is identification of children with hyperthyroidism. Since the clinical manifestations often appear gradually, the goiter and ophthalmic changes may not be noticed and the excessive activity may be attributed to behavioral problems. Nurses in ambulatory settings, particularly those caring for children in school, need to be alert to signs that suggest this disorder, especially weight loss despite an excellent appetite, academic difficulties resulting from short attention span and inability to sit still, unexplained fatigue and sleeplessness, and difficulty with fine motor skills, such as writing.

Much of the child's care during diagnosis and initial medical therapy is related to the physical symptoms. He needs a quiet, unstimulating environment that is conducive to rest, and sometimes hospitalization is necessary during the immediate treatment phase to remove the child from a troubled home. A regular routine is beneficial with frequent rest periods, minimizing the stress of coping with unexpected demands, and meeting the child's needs promptly. Despite the excessive activity of these children, they tire easily, experience muscle weakness, and are unable to relax to recoup their strength.

Emotional lability is often manifest by sudden episodes of crying or elation. Such behavior, together with irritability, disrupts interpersonal relationships, creating difficulties within and outside the home. Heat intolerance may produce considerable family conflict. Since the child prefers a cooler environment than others, he is likely to open windows, complain about the heat, wear minimum clothing, and kick off blankets while sleeping.

Dietary requirements are regulated to meet the child's increased metabolic rate. Although his need for calories is increased, these should be provided in wholesome foods rather than "junk" foods. He may require vitamin supplements to meet his daily requirement. Rather than three large meals, the child's appetite may be better satisfied by five or six moderate meals throughout the day.

Once therapy is instituted, the nurse explains the drug regimen, emphasizing the importance of observing for side effects of antithyroid drugs. Untoward effects of propylthiouracil and related compounds include skin rash, drug fever, enlargement of the salivary and cervical lymph glands, diminished sense of taste, hepatitis, and edema of the lower extremities. Since sore throat and fever accompany the grave complication of leukopenia, these children should be seen by a physician if such symptoms occur. Parents should also be aware of the signs of hypothyroidism, which can occur from overdose of the drugs. The most common indications are lethargy and somnolence.

If surgery is anticipated, iodine is usually administered for a few weeks prior to the procedure. Since oral iodine preparations are unpalatable, they should be mixed with a strong-tasting fruit juice, such as grape or punch flavors, and be given through a straw. Compliance with iodine therapy is essential to avoid the danger of thyroid crisis after sudden discontinuation.

Psychologic preparation of the child for thyroidectomy is similar to that for any other surgical procedure (p. 624). However, of special consideration is the site of the incision. The fear of cutting one's throat is very real and in older children is associated with death. The nurse explains that the throat is not cut, only the skin, to allow for removal of the gland. The child should be prepared for the dressing around the neck and the possibility of an endotracheal or "breathing" tube after surgery.

Postoperative care involves observation for bleeding into the operative site, which can rapidly lead to asphyxiation. The nurse inspects the dressing for bleeding, checks behind the neck for accumulation of draining blood, and reports any signs of hemorrhage or respiratory distress. The child should be positioned with the neck slightly flexed to avoid strain on the sutures and should be taught to support the neck in this position when he sits up.

Another complication is damage to the recurrent laryngeal nerve. If damage is bilateral, airway obstruction will usually occur within a few hours. Although some hoarseness is expected postoperatively, any evidence of increased hoarseness or stridor is reported immediately, and a tracheostomy set is placed at the bedside. Unilateral injury to the nerve causes dysphonia. Although the hoarseness often improves in a few weeks, the child may have a permanent speech defect.

Since hypothyroidism and/or hypoparathyroidism may result, the nurse observes for signs of these conditions. The earliest indication of hypoparathyroidism may be anxiety and mental depression, followed by paresthesia and evidence of heightened neuromuscular excitability, such as the Chvostek sign (spasm of facial muscles elicited by light taps over the area of the facial nerve) and the Trousseau sign (carpal muscle spasm induced by pressure on the principal vessels and nerves of the upper arm) and carpopedal spasm (tetany). The behavioral manifestations, including those of hypothyroidism, must be differentiated from emotional depression as a reaction to the stress of surgery. Each of these conditions may require appropriate chemical replacement, which is discussed with the family prior to discharge.

◆ *Disorders of Parathyroid Function*

The parathyroid glands secrete parathormone (PTH), whose main function, along with vitamin D, is to maintain homeostasis of blood calcium concentration. Parathormone exerts its effect by (1) increasing the release of calcium and phosphate from the bone (bone demineralization), (2) increasing the absorption of calcium and the excretion of phosphate by the kidneys, and (3) promoting calcium absorption in the gastrointestinal tract. The net result of these actions is to increase the plasma calcium concentration while lowering the plasma phosphate concentration.

HYPOPARATHYROIDISM

Two classic forms of hypoparathyroidism are observed during childhood: (1) *idiopathic hypoparathyroidism,* in which there is deficient production of PTH, and (2) *pseudohypoparathyroidism,* in which production of PTH is increased but end-organ responsiveness to the hormone is deficient. The signs or symptoms are similar.

Idiopathic hypoparathyroidism may occur as a component of multi-glandular failure, possibly related to autoimmune phenomena, or from parathyroidectomy (it may follow thyroidectomy). Familial hypoparathyroidism is inherited as an X-linked recessive trait, with early onset in male infants, usually in the first month of life. Pseudohypoparathyroidism is also thought to be inherited as an X-linked dominant trait with variable expressivity. Transient hypoparathyroidism may also be observed in infants born to mothers with the disease or in infants fed a milk formula with high phosphate-to-calcium ratio (see p. 243).

Diagnostic Evaluation

The diagnosis of hypoparathyroidism is made on the basis of clinical manifestations associated with decreased serum calcium and increased serum phosphorus (see box). Levels of plasma PTH are low in idiopathic hypoparathyroidism but high in pseudohypoparathyroidism. End-organ responsiveness is tested by the administration of PTH with measurement of urinary cyclic AMP. Kidney function tests are included in the differential diagnosis to rule out renal insufficiency. Although bone radiographs are usually normal, they may demonstrate increased bone density and suppressed growth.

Therapeutic Management

The objective of treatment is to maintain normal serum calcium and phosphate levels with minimum complications. Acute or severe tetany is corrected immediately by intravenous and oral administration of calcium gluconate and follow-up daily doses to achieve normal levels. When diagnosis is confirmed, vitamin D therapy is begun. Long-term management consists of administration of massive doses of vitamin D; oral calcium supplementation may be useful, although it is not essential.

Clinical Manifestations of Hypoparathyroidism

Pseudohypoparathyroidism
Short stature
Round face
Short, thick neck
Short, stubby fingers and toes
Dimpling of skin over knuckles
Subcutaneous soft tissue calcifications
Mental retardation a prominent feature

Idiopathic Hypoparathyroidism
None of the above physical characteristics observed
Papilledema may be seen
May be mental retardation

Both Types
Dry, scaly, coarse skin with eruptions
Hair often brittle
Nails thin and brittle with characteristic transverse grooves
Dental and enamel hypoplasia
Muscle contractions:
- Tetany
- Carpopedal spasm
- Laryngospasm (laryngeal stridor)
- Muscle cramps and twitching
- Positive Chvostek and/or Trousseau signs

Paresthesias, tingling
Neurologic:
- Headache
- Seizures (generalized, absences, or focal)
- Swings of emotion
- Loss of memory
- Depression
- Confusion can occur

Gastrointestinal:
- Muscle cramps
- Diarrhea
- Vomiting

Retarded skeletal growth

Nursing Considerations

The initial objective is recognition of hypocalcemia. Unexplained convulsions, irritability (especially to external stimuli), gastrointestinal symptoms (e.g., diarrhea, vomiting, abdominal cramps), and positive signs of tetany should lead the nurse to suspect this disorder. Much of the initial nursing care is related to the physical manifestations and includes institution of seizure and safety precautions, reduction of environmental stimuli (e.g., sudden noises or movements, bright lights), and observation for signs of laryngospasm, such as stridor, hoarseness, and a feeling of tightness in the throat. A tracheostomy set and injectable calcium gluconate should be placed near the bedside for emergency use. The administration of calcium gluconate requires precautions against extravasation of the drug.

After initiation of treatment, the nurse discusses with the parents the need for continuous daily administration of calcium salts and vitamin D. Because vitamin D toxicity can be a serious consequence of therapy, parents are advised to watch for signs, which include weakness, fatigue, lassitude, headache, nausea, vomiting, and diarrhea. Early renal impairment is manifest by polyuria, polydipsia, and nocturia.

HYPERPARATHYROIDISM

Hyperparathyroidism is rare in childhood but can be primary or secondary. The most common cause of primary hyperparathyroidism is adenoma of the gland. The most common causes of secondary hyperparathyroidism are chronic renal disease, renal osteodystrophy, and congenital anomalies of the urinary tract. The common factor is hypercalcemia.

Diagnostic Evaluation

Blood studies to confirm the presence of elevated calcium and lowered phosphorus levels are routinely performed. Measurement of PTH, as well as several tests to isolate the cause of the hypercalcemia, such as renal function studies, should be included. Other procedures employed to substantiate the physiologic consequences of the disorder include electrocardiography and radiographic bone surveys (see box for clinical manifestations).

Therapeutic Management

Treatment depends on the cause of hyperparathyroidism. The treatment of primary hyperparathyroidism is surgical

Clinical Manifestations of Hyperparathyroidism

Gastrointestinal
Nausea
Vomiting
Abdominal discomfort
Constipation

Central Nervous System
Delusions
Confusion
Hallucinations
Impaired memory
Lack of interest and initiative
Depression
Varying levels of consciousness

Neuromuscular
Weakness
Easy fatigability
Muscle atrophy (especially proximal muscles of lower limbs)
Tongue twitching
Paresthesias in extremities

Skeletal
Vague bone pain
Subperiosteal resorption of phalanges
Spontaneous fractures
Absence of lamina dura around teeth

Renal
Polyuria
Polydipsia
Renal colic
Hypertension

removal of the tumor or hyperplastic tissue. Treatment of secondary hyperparathyroidism is directed at the underlying contributing cause, thus subsequently restoring the serum calcium balance. However, in some instances the underlying disorder is irreversible, such as in chronic renal failure. In this instance treatment is the same as that for renal osteodystrophy (p. 879).

Nursing Considerations

Since surgical exploration is the major treatment modality, nursing care is similar to that discussed for the child with hyperthyroidism (p. 942).

◆ *Disorders of Adrenal Function*

The adrenal cortex secretes three main groups of hormones collectively called steroids and classified according to their biologic activity: (1) glucocorticoids (cortisol, corticosterone), (2) mineralocorticoids (aldosterone), and (3) sex steroids (androgens, estrogens, and progestins). Alterations in the levels of these hormones produce significant dysfunction in a variety of body tissues and organs. Since the adrenocortical cells are capable of producing any of the steroids, pathologic conditions may result in a deficiency or an excess of more than one type of hormone. However, most are rare in children.

The adrenal medulla secretes the catecholamines epinephrine and norepinephrine. Both hormones have essentially the same effects on various organs as those caused by direct sympathetic stimulation, except that the hormonal effects last several times longer. Catecholamine-secreting tumors are the primary cause of adrenal medullary hyperfunction.

ACUTE ADRENOCORTICAL INSUFFICIENCY

The acute form of adrenocortical insufficiency (adrenal crisis) may result from a number of causes during childhood. Although a rare disorder, some of the more common etiologic factors include hemorrhage into the gland from trauma, fulminating infections, abrupt withdrawal of exogenous sources of cortisone or failure to increase exogenous supplies during stress, or as a result of congenital adrenogenital hyperplasia of the salt-losing type.

Diagnostic Evaluation

There is no rapid, definitive test for confirmation of acute adrenocortical insufficiency. Routine procedures such as measurement of plasma cortisol levels are too time-consuming to be practical. Therefore diagnosis is usually made based on clinical symptoms (see box). Improvement with cortisol therapy confirms the diagnosis.

Therapeutic Management

Treatment involves replacement of cortisol, replacement of body fluids to combat dehydration and hypovolemia, administration of glucose solutions to correct hypoglycemia, and specific antibiotic therapy in the presence of infection. If hemorrhage has been severe, whole blood may be replaced. In the event that these measures do not reverse the circulatory collapse, vasopressors are used for immediate vasoconstriction and elevation of blood pressure. Once the child's condition is stabilized, oral doses of cortisone, fluids, and salt are given, similar to the regimen used for chronic adrenal insufficiency.

Nursing Considerations

Because of the abrupt onset and potentially fatal outcome of this condition, prompt recognition is essential. Vital signs are watched and other observations made to monitor the hyperpyrexia and shocklike state. Seizure precautions are instituted, since convulsions from the elevated temperature are not uncommon. As soon as therapy is instituted, the nurse should monitor the child's response to fluid and cortisol replacement, being alert to too rapid administration of fluids and drugs. Overtreatment with cortisol and sodium chloride can precipitate complications. The nurse should observe for signs of hypokalemia,

Clinical Manifestations of Acute Adrenocortical Insufficiency

- Early symptoms
  - Increased irritability
  - Headache
  - Diffuse abdominal pain
  - Weakness
  - Nausea and vomiting
  - Diarrhea
- Generalized hemorrhagic manifestations (Waterhouse-Friderichsen syndrome)
  - Fever—increases as condition worsens
  - Central nervous system signs
    - Nuchal rigidity
    - Convulsions
    - Stupor
    - Coma
- Shocklike state
  - Weak, rapid pulse
  - Decreased blood pressure
  - Shallow respirations
  - Cold, clammy skin
  - Cyanosis
- Circulatory collapse is the terminal event
- *Newborn*
  - Hyperpyrexia
  - Tachypnea
  - Cyanosis
  - Convulsions
  - Gland may be evident as palpable retroperitoneal mass (hemorrhagic)

Clinical Manifestations of Chronic Adrenocortical Insufficiency

- Muscular weakness
- Mental fatigue
- Pigmentary changes of
  - Previous scars
  - Palmar creases
  - Mucous membranes
  - Hair
- Hyperpigmentation over pressure points (elbows, knees, or waist)
- Less frequently, vitiligo (loss of pigmentation)
- Weight loss
- Hypotension and small heart size
  - Dizziness
  - Syncopal (fainting) attacks
- Irritability, apathy, and negativism
- Signs of hypoglycemia
  - Headache
  - Hunger
  - Weakness
  - Trembling
  - Sweating
- Other signs (seen in some children)
  - Recurrent, unexplained convulsions
  - Intense craving for salt
  - Acute abdominal pain

such as cardiac irregularities and poor muscle control, and should evaluate serum electrolyte levels. Intake and urinary output are measured and recorded.

The sudden, severe nature of this disorder requires considerable emotional support for the child and family. The child may be placed in an intensive care unit, where the surroundings are strange and frightening. Since recovery within 24 hours is often dramatic, the nurse should keep the parents apprised of the child's condition, emphasizing signs of improvement, such as a lowered temperature and elevated blood pressure. If paralysis occurs, the nurse should assure them that this condition is temporary and quickly reversed.

CHRONIC ADRENOCORTICAL INSUFFICIENCY

Chronic adrenocortical insufficiency (Addison disease) is rare in children. When it does occur, it is usually caused by a destructive lesion of the adrenal glands or a neoplasm, or it has an idiopathic cause.

Evidence of this disorder is usually gradual in onset, since 90% of adrenal tissue must be nonfunctional before signs of insufficiency are manifest. However, during periods of stress, when demands for additional cortisol are increased, symptoms of acute insufficiency may appear in a previously well child (see box).

Definitive diagnosis is based on measurements of functional cortisol reserve. The cortisol and urinary 17-hydroxycorticosteroid levels are low and fail to rise, while plasma ACTH levels are elevated with corticotropin (ACTH) stimulation, the definitive test for the disease.

Therapeutic Management

Treatment involves replacement of glucocorticoids (cortisol) and mineralocorticoids (aldosterone). Some children are able to be maintained solely on oral supplements of cortisol (cortisone or hydrocortisone preparations) with a liberal intake of salt. During stressful situations, such as infection, emotional upset, or surgery, the dosage must be tripled to accommodate the body's increased need for glucocorticoids. Failure to meet this requirement will precipitate an acute crisis. Overdosage produces appearance of cushingoid signs.

Nursing Considerations

Once the disorder is diagnosed, parents need guidance concerning drug therapy. They must be aware of the continuous need for cortisol replacement. Sudden termination of the drug because of inadequate supplies or inability to ingest the oral form because of vomiting places the child in danger of an acute adrenal crisis. Ideally the par-

Clinical Manifestations of Cushing Syndrome

Centripetal fat distribution
- Truncal obesity
- Supraclavicular fat pads
- Fat pads on neck and back ("buffalo hump")

Rounded or "moon" face
Muscular wasting
- Thin extremities
- Pendulous abdomen
- Muscle weakness

Thin skin and subcutaneous tissue
Poor wound healing
Increased susceptibility to infection
Decreased inflammatory response
Excessive bruising
Petechial hemorrhages
Facial plethora ("red cheeks")
Reddish purple abdominal striae
Hypertension
Hypokalemia
Alkalosis
Osteoporosis
- Compression fractures of vertebrae
- Kyphosis
- Backache
- Retarded linear growth

Hypercalciuria–renal calculi
Psychoses
- Irritability
- Insomnia
- Euphoria
- Depression
- Frank psychoses

Peptic ulcer
Hyperglycemia
- Glycosuria
- Latent or overt diabetes

Virilization
- Hirsutism
- Acne
- Deepening of voice
- Clitoral enlargement
- Tendency toward male physique in female

Amenorrhea
Impotence

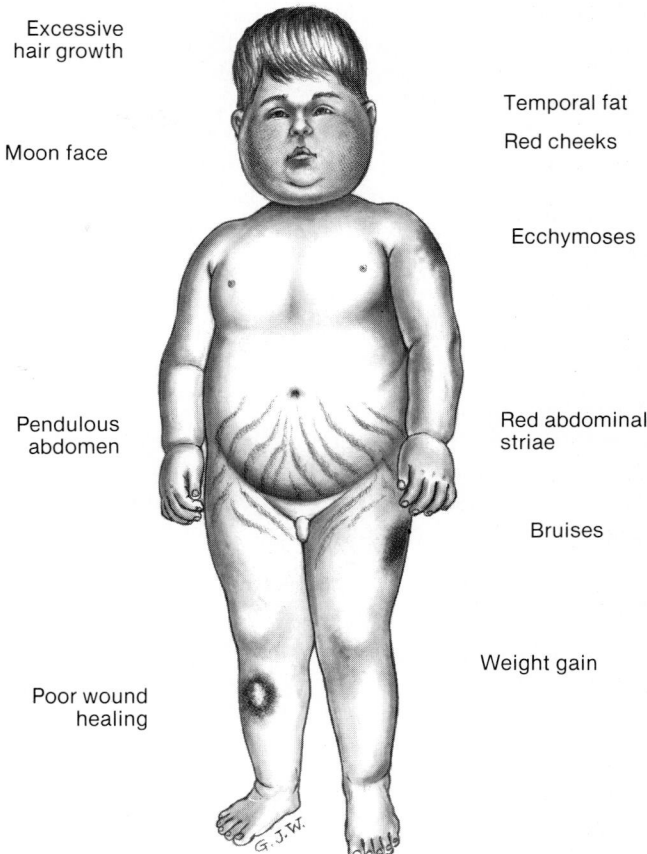

ents should have a prefilled syringe of hydrocortisone in the home, having been instructed in proper technique for intramuscular administration of the drug in case of a crisis. Unnecessary administration of cortisone will not harm the child, but, if needed, may be lifesaving. Any evidence of acute insufficiency should be reported to the physician immediately.

Since the body cannot supply endogenous sources of cortical hormones during times of stress, the home environment should be stable and relatively unstressful. Parents need to be aware that during periods of emotional or physical crisis the child requires additional hormone replacement. The child should wear a Medic Alert tag to permit medical personnel to adjust the requirements during emergency care.

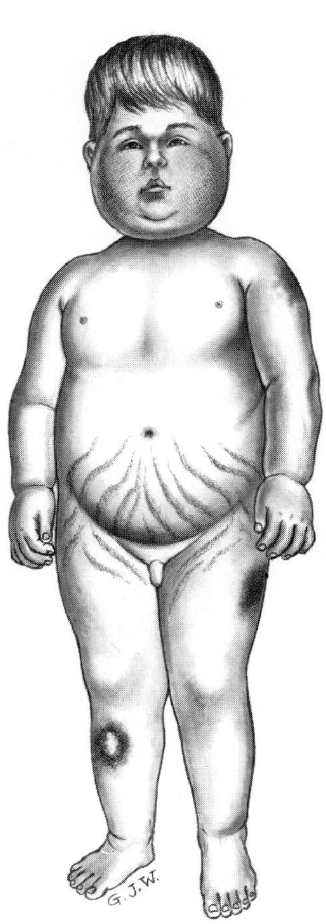

FIG. 28-2 Characteristics of Cushing syndrome.

CUSHING SYNDROME

Cushing syndrome is a characteristic group of manifestations caused by excessive circulating free cortisol. It can result from a variety of etiologies, which generally fall into one of four categories:

1. Pituitary Cushing syndrome with adrenal hyperplasia, usually attributed to an excess of ACTH
2. Adrenal Cushing syndrome with hypersecretion of glucocorticoids, generally the result of adrenocortical neoplasms
3. Ectopic Cushing syndrome with autonomous secretion of ACTH, most often caused by extrapituitary neoplasms
4. Iatrogenic Cushing syndrome, frequently the result of administration of large amounts of exogenous corticosteroids

Cushing syndrome is uncommon in children. When seen it is often caused by excessive or prolonged steroid therapy, which produces a cushingoid appearance (see box and Fig. 28-2).

Diagnostic Evaluation

Several tests are helpful in confirming excess cortisol levels. They include fasting blood glucose levels for hyperglycemia, serum electrolyte levels for hypokalemia and alkalosis, 24-hour urinary levels of elevated 17-hydroxycorticoids and 17-ketosteroids, and radiographic studies of bone for evidence of osteoporosis and of the skull for enlargement of the sella turcica. Administration of an exogenous supply of cortisone normally suppresses adrenocorticotropic hormone production. However, in individuals with Cushing syndrome, cortisol levels remain elevated. This test is helpful in differentiating between children who are obese and those who appear to have cushingoid features.

Therapeutic Management

Treatment depends on the cause. In most cases surgical intervention involves bilateral adrenalectomy and postoperative replacement of the cortical hormones (the therapy for this is the same as that outlined for chronic adrenal insufficiency). If a pituitary tumor is found, surgical extirpation or irradiation may be chosen. In either of these instances, treatment of panhypopituitarism with replacement of growth hormone, thyroid extract, antidiuretic hormone, gonadotropins, and steroids may be necessary for an indefinite period.

Nursing Considerations

Nursing care also depends on the cause. When cushingoid features are caused by steroid therapy, the effects may be lessened with administration of the drug early in the morning and on an alternate-day basis. Giving the drug early in the day maintains the normal diurnal pattern of cortisol secretion. If given during the evening the drug is more likely to produce symptoms because endogenous cortisol levels are already low and the additional supply exerts more pronounced effects. An alternate-day schedule allows the anterior pituitary an opportunity to maintain more normal hypothalamic-pituitary-adrenal control mechanisms.

If an organic cause is found, nursing care is related to the treatment regimen. Although a bilateral adrenalectomy permanently solves one condition, it reciprocally produces another syndrome. Before surgery parents need to be adequately informed of the operative benefits and disadvantages. Postoperative teaching regarding drug replacement is a nursing function.

CONGENITAL ADRENOGENITAL HYPERPLASIA

Disorders caused by excessive secretion of androgens by the adrenal cortex are known variously as *congenital adrenogenital hyperplasia (CAH)*, *adrenocortical hyperplasia (ACH)*, *adrenogenital syndrome (AGS)*, and *congenital adrenocortical hyperplasia (CAH)*. Hyperfunction of the adrenal gland can occur from a number of causes, such as a virilizing adrenal tumor. In children the most common cause is congenital adrenogenital hyperplasia, an inborn deficiency of various enzymes necessary for the biosynthesis of cortisol. CAH is inherited as an autosomal-recessive disorder or may result from a tumor or maternal ingestion of steroids.

Pathophysiology

Interference in the biosynthesis of cortisol during fetal life results in an increased production of adrenocorticotropic hormone, which stimulates hyperplasia of the adrenal gland. Depending on the enzymatic defect, increased quantities of cortisol precursors and androgens are secreted. There are six major types of biochemical defects. In each there is excess production of androgens, which causes ambiguous female genitalia in females and precocious genital development in males. Other forms of CAH do not result in excess production of androgens but cause various degrees of hypoaldosteronism or hyperaldosteronism.

Diagnostic Evaluation

Clinical diagnosis is initially based on congenital abnormalities that lead to difficulty in assigning sex to the newborn (see box) and on signs and symptoms of adrenal insufficiency or hypertension. Definitive diagnosis is confirmed by evidence of increased 17-ketosteroid levels in most types of congenital adrenogenital hyperplasia. Blood electrolytes demonstrate loss of sodium and chloride and elevation of potassium. A karyotype for positive sex determination should always be done in any case of ambiguous genitalia.

Ultrasonography can also be used to visualize the presence of pelvic structures. It is especially useful in CAH to

Clinical Manifestations of Adrenogenital Hyperplasia

Female: masculinization
- Enlarged clitoris (appears as small phallus)
- Fusion of labia (saclike structure resembling a scrotum)
- Vaginal orifice usually closed by fused labia

Male: precocious genital development
- Genital enlargement (macrogenitosomia precox)
- Frequent erections

Untreated: Early sexual maturation
- Enlargement of external sexual organs
- Development of axillary, pubic, and facial hair
- Deepening of voice
- Acne
- Marked increase in musculature (changes toward an adult male physique)
- Accelerated linear growth
- Premature epiphyseal closure (short stature by end of puberty)
- Female:
  - No breast development
  - Females remain amenorrheic and infertile
- Male:
  - Testes remain small

identify the absence or presence of female reproductive organs in a newborn or child with ambiguous genitalia. Because it yields immediate results, it has the advantage of determining the child's gender long before the more complex laboratory results for chromosomal analysis or steroid levels are available.

Therapeutic Management

The initial medical objective is to confirm the diagnosis and assign a sex to the child, usually according to the genotype. In both sexes cortisone is administered to suppress the abnormally high secretions of adrenocorticotropic hormone. If this is begun early enough, it is very effective. Cortisone depresses the secretion of adrenocorticotropic hormone by the adenohypophysis, which in turn inhibits the secretion of adrenocorticosteroids, which stems the progressive virilization. The signs and symptoms of masculinization in the female gradually disappear, and excessive early linear growth is slowed. Puberty occurs normally at the appropriate age.

Since these children are unable to produce cortisol in response to stress, it is necessary to increase the dosage during episodes of infection, fever, or other stresses. Acute emergencies require immediate intravenous or intramuscular administration. Children with the salt-losing type of CAH require aldosterone replacement and supplementary dietary salt.

Depending on the degree of masculinization in the female, reconstructive surgery may be required to reduce the size of the clitoris, separate the labia, and create a vaginal orifice. This should be done after the infant is physically able to withstand the procedure and before she is old enough to be aware of the abnormal genitalia. Plastic surgery is generally done in stages and yields excellent cosmetic results.

Unfortunately, not all children with CAH are diagnosed at birth and raised in accordance with their genetic sex. Particularly in the case of affected females, masculinization of the external genitalia may have led to sex assignment as a male. In males diagnosis is usually delayed until early childhood, when signs of virilism appear. In these situations it is advisable to continue rearing the child as a male in accordance with assigned sex and phenotype. Hormone replacement may be required to permit linear growth and to initiate male pubertal changes. Surgery is usually indicated to remove the female organs and reconstruct the phallus for satisfactory sexual relations. These individuals are not fertile.

Nursing Considerations

The nursing care of the child with CAH and his family is concerned primarily with identifying the child, assigning a correct gender sex, and providing support and assistance.

Of major importance is recognition of ambiguous genitalia in newborns. If there is any question regarding assignment of sex, the parents need to be told immediately to prevent the embarrassing situation of informing family members of the child's sex and then having to change the announcement. As with any congenital defect, the parents require an adequate explanation of the condition and a period of time to grieve for the loss of perfection. Parents need an explanation regarding this disorder that facilitates their explaining it to others. Before confirmation of the diagnosis and sex of the child, the nurse should refer to the infant as "child" or "baby" rather than "he" or "she" and definitely not "it." When referring to the external genitalia, it is preferable to refer to them as sex organs and to emphasize the similarity between the penis/clitoris and scrotum/labia during fetal development. In this way it can be explained that the sex organs were overdeveloped because of too much male hormone secretion. Using a correct vocabulary allows parents to explain the abnormalities to others in a straightforward manner, just as if the defect involved the heart or an extremity.

It is also important to stress that sex assignment and rearing depend on psychosocial influences, not on genetic sex hormonal influences during fetal life. Parents often fear that the infant will retain "male behavioral characteristics" because of prenatal masculinization and will not be able to develop female characteristics. Using the word *hermaphrodite* often confuses parents, because they interpret this term to mean that the child is "half male–half female." Since the prognosis for normal sexual development is excellent after early treatment, the nurse should foster identification with the child as one sex only. It is also beneficial to mention that ambiguous genitalia have no relationship with homosexual or bisexual activity later in life.

As soon as the sex is determined, parents should be informed of the findings and encouraged to choose an appropriate name, and the child should be identified as a male or female, with no reference to ambiguous sex. If the appearance of the enlarged genitalia in a female child concerns the parents, they should be encouraged to discuss their feelings. Suggesting ways to avoid questioning remarks from visitors, such as diapering the child in a separate room, is also helpful. If surgery is anticipated, showing parents before and after photographs of reconstruction helps to reinforce the expected cosmetic benefits.

Nursing considerations regarding cortisol and aldosterone replacement are the same as those that are discussed for chronic adrenocortical insufficiency. A follow-up visit by a public health nurse may be desirable to ensure that parents understand and comply with the treatment regimen. Likewise, nurses in well-child facilities should assume responsibility for guidance and supervision regarding this aspect of care during each visit.

In the unfortunate situation in which sex is erroneously assigned and later diagnosed, parents need a great deal of help in understanding the reason for the incorrect sex identification and the options for sex reassignment and/or medical/surgical intervention. Since children become aware of their sexual identity by 18 months to 2 years of age, it is believed that any reassignment after this period can cause tremendous psychologic conflicts in the child. Therefore sex rearing should be continued as previously established with medical/surgical intervention as required.

A dilemma often arises, however, regarding what the child should know about his condition, especially gender identification. Because the knowledge that one has been reared opposite his genetic gender can initiate profound psychologic problems, it is recommended that the child not be told this fact but rather be given an explanation regarding his physical disabilities, such as infertility, and the need for hormone replacement and plastic surgery. Parents, in turn, must believe that the child has been raised according to his "true sex," which is absolutely honest, since sex is not solely a biologic entity but an expression of multiple environmental influences.

Since the hereditary form of CAH is an autosomal-recessive disorder, parents should be referred for genetic counseling before conceiving another child.

PHEOCHROMOCYTOMA

Pheochromocytoma is an adrenal tumor characterized by secretion of catecholamines. In children this type of tumor is most frequently bilateral or multiple and is generally benign. Often there is a familial transmission of the condition as an autosomal-dominant trait that tends to favor males. The clinical manifestations of pheochromocytoma are caused by an increased production of catecholamines, and they mimic those of other disorders, such as hyperthyroidism, diabetes mellitus, or functional hyperventilation (see box).

Therapeutic Management

Definitive treatment consists of surgical removal of the tumor. In children the tumors may be bilateral, requiring a bilateral adrenalectomy and lifelong glucocorticoid and mineralocorticoid therapy.

Clinical Manifestations of Pheochromocytoma

Hypertension
Tachycardia
Headache
Decreased gastrointestinal activity
  Resultant constipation
Anorexia
Weight loss
Hyperglycemia
Polyuria
Polydipsia
Hyperventilation
Nervousness
Diaphoresis
Signs of congestive heart failure in severe cases

Nursing Considerations

An initial nursing objective is identification of children with this disorder. Preoperative nursing care involves frequent monitoring of vital signs and observing for evidence of hypertensive attacks and congestive heart failure. Urine should be tested at least daily for sugar and acetone. Any signs of hyperglycemia are noted and reported immediately.

The environment should be conducive to rest and free of emotional stress. This requires adequate preparation during hospital admission and before surgery. Parents should be encouraged to room-in with their child and to participate in his care. Play activities need to be tailored to the child's energy level but should not be overly strenuous or challenging, since these can increase metabolic rate and promote frustration and anxiety.

After surgery the child is observed for signs of shock from removal of excess catecholamines. If a bilateral adrenalectomy was performed, the nursing interventions are those discussed for chronic adrenocortical insufficiency.

◆ *Disorders of Pancreatic Hormone Function*

The islands of Langerhans of the pancreas have three major functioning cells:

1. The alpha cells produce glucagon, which increases the blood glucose levels by stimulating the liver and other cells to release stored glucose (glycogenolysis).
2. The beta cells produce insulin, which lowers blood glucose levels by facilitating the entrance of glucose into the cells for metabolism.
3. The delta cells produce somatostatin, which is believed to regulate the release of insulin and glucagon.

The discussion of disorders of pancreatic hormone secretion is limited to diabetes mellitus.

DIABETES MELLITUS

Diabetes mellitus (DM) is a disease of metabolism characterized by a deficiency (relative or absolute) of the hormone insulin, resulting in a metabolic adjustment or physiologic change in almost all areas of the body. It is the most frequent endocrine disorder of childhood, with the peak incidence reached during early adolescence.

Classification

Idiopathic DM can be classified into two major groups and one newly described type:

Insulin-dependent (IDDM), or **type I**—characterized by catabolism and the development of ketosis in the absence of insulin replacement therapy; onset is typically in childhood and adolescence but can be at any age

Non-insulin-dependent (NIDDM), or **type II**—appears to involve resistance to insulin action and defective glucose-mediated insulin secretion; onset is usually after age 40, and there appears to be considerable heterogeneity; affected persons may or may not require daily insulin injections

Maturity-onset diabetes of youth (MODY)—transmitted as an autosomal-dominant disorder in which there is formation of structurally abnormal insulin that has decreased biologic activity

Because DM of childhood is, with few exceptions, the IDDM (or type I) form, the remainder of the discussion will be devoted to this important cause of long-term health problems. However, NIDDM will be included as appropriate for comparison throughout.

Etiology

The clinical syndrome of DM results from a large variety of etiologic and pathogenic mechanisms. IDDM is now believed to be an autoimmune disease that arises when a person with a genetic predisposition is exposed to a precipitating event, such as a viral infection.

Genetic factors. IDDM is not inherited, but heredity is unquestioned as a prominent factor in the etiology. A variety of genetic mechanisms have been proposed, but most authorities favor a multifactorial inheritance or a recessive gene somehow linked to the human lymphocyte antigen (HLA). However, the genetic influence in NIDDM and IDDM appears to differ in several ways. Nearly 100% of offspring of parents who both have NIDDM develop that type of diabetes, but only 45% to 60% of the offspring of both parents who have IDDM will develop the disease. The incidence doubles with every 20% of excess weight, and this figure applies to the young as well as to the older diabetic person.

Autoimmune mechanisms. It is now accepted that an autoimmune process is involved in the great majority of persons who develop IDDM. The current theory is that the presence of the HLA genes causes a defect in the immune system that renders the possessor susceptible to viral infections. In susceptible persons the virus invades the beta cells and initiates an autoimmune process that gradually destroys them. Without beta cells no insulin can be produced. There is also a strong association between IDDM and other autoimmune endocrine disorders, such as thyroiditis and Addison disease.

Viruses. Viruses have been implicated in the etiology of diabetes. Islet cells appear to be particularly susceptible to either direct viral damage or chemical insult. The body reacts to this damaged or changed tissue in an autoimmune phenomenon. Therefore the virus serves as a precipitating factor or "trigger." The Coxsackie group of viruses (especially the Coxsackie B4 virus) has created the most interest, but mumps, cytomegalovirus, Epstein-Barr virus, and infectious hepatitis viruses have all been implicated. However, no specific virus has been clearly documented as the precipitating factor.

Pathophysiology

Insulin is needed to support the metabolism of carbohydrates, fats, and proteins, primarily by facilitating the entry of these substances into the cell, except nerve cells and vascular tissue. With a deficiency of insulin, glucose is unable to enter the cell and its concentration in the bloodstream increases. The increased concentration of glucose *(hyperglycemia)* produces an osmotic gradient that causes the movement of body fluid from the intracellular space to the extracellular space; from there it is then excreted by the kidneys. When the serum glucose exceeds the renal threshold (180 mg/dl), glucose "spills" into the urine, along with an osmotic diversion of water *(polyuria)*, a cardinal sign of diabetes. The urinary fluid losses cause the excessive thirst *(polydipsia)* observed in diabetes. As might be expected, this water washout results in a depletion of other essential chemicals.

Protein is also wasted during insulin deficiency. Since glucose is unable to enter the cells, protein is broken down and converted to glucose by the liver (glucogenesis); this glucose then contributes to the hyperglycemia. Without the use of carbohydrates for energy, fat and protein stores are depleted as the body attempts to meet its energy needs. The hunger mechanism is triggered, but the increased food intake *(polyphagia)* enhances the problem by further elevating the blood glucose.

Ketoacidosis. When insulin is absent, glucose is unavailable for cellular metabolism and the body chooses alternate sources of energy, principally fat. Consequently fats break down into fatty acids, and glycerol in fat cells and liver is converted to ketone bodies (β-hydroxybutyric acid, acetoacetic acid, acetone). The ketone bodies can be used as an alternative source of fuel for glucose, but they are used in the cells at a limited rate. Any excess is eliminated in the urine *(ketonuria)* or the lungs (acetone breath). The ketone bodies are strong acids that lower serum pH, producing *ketoacidosis*.

The respiratory system attempts to eliminate the excess carbon dioxide by increased depth and rate—*Kussmaul respirations*, the hyperventilation characteristic of metabolic acidosis. Excess ketones are excreted by the urine and lungs, producing ketonuria and the characteristic acetone odor to the breath.

Potassium levels are also a problem. With cellular death, potassium is released from the cell into the interstitial spaces, then into the bloodstream and excreted by the kidney, where the loss is accelerated by the osmotic diuresis. The total body potassium is then decreased, even though the serum potassium level may be elevated as a result of the decreased fluid volume in which it circulates. Alteration in serum and tissue potassium can make cardiac arrest a potential problem.

If these conditions are not reversed by insulin therapy in combination with correction of the fluid deficiency and electrolyte imbalance, progressive deterioration occurs, with dehydration, electrolyte imbalance, acidosis, coma, and death. Diabetic ketoacidosis should be diagnosed promptly in a seriously ill patient and therapy instituted.

Long-term complications. Long-term complications of diabetes involve the small as well as larger blood vessels. The principal microvascular complications are nephropathy, retinopathy, and neuropathy. The process appears to be one of *glycosylation*, wherein proteins from the blood become deposited in the walls of small vessels (e.g., glomeruli, retina), where they become trapped by "sticky" glucose compounds (glycosyl radicals). The build-up of these substances over time causes narrowing of the vessels with subsequent interference with microcirculation to the affected areas. With poor control, vascular changes appear as early as 2½ to 3 years after diagnosis; with good control changes have been postponed for 20 or more years.

Mild diabetes. Although most childhood diabetes is recognized during the rapid initial deterioration in carbohydrate metabolism, other cases with more benign disease are being identified with increasing frequency. A few are detected accidentally by urinalysis before overt symptoms are observed. Maturity-onset diabetes of youth (MODY) is sometimes seen in an obese teenager. This type, like NIDDM, can often be controlled with diet restriction. Diabetes is a great imitator; influenza, gastroenteritis, and appendicitis are the conditions most often diagnosed.

Diagnostic Evaluation

Three groups of children who should be considered as possibly diabetic are (1) those who have glycosuria, polyuria, and a history of weight loss or failure to gain despite a voracious appetite; (2) those with transient or persistent glycosuria; and (3) those who display manifestations of metabolic acidosis, with or without stupor or coma. Clinical manifestations of diabetes are outlined in the accompanying box.

Tests used to determine glycosuria are the glucose oxidase tapes (Tes-Tape and Clinistix) or Clinitest tablets. A fasting blood sugar greater than 120 mg/dl is almost certain to be caused by diabetes. Postprandial blood glucose determinations and the traditional oral glucose tolerance tests have yielded low detection rates in children and are not usually necessary for establishing a diagnosis. Serum insulin levels may be normal or moderately elevated at the onset of diabetes; delayed insulin response to glucose indicates the presence of prediabetes.

Ketoacidosis must be differentiated from other causes of acidosis or coma, including hypoglycemia, uremia, gastroenteritis with metabolic acidosis, salicylate intoxication, encephalitis, and other intracranial lesions. Diabetic ketoacidosis is determined by the presence of hyperglycemia (blood glucose measurement equal to or greater than 300 mg/dl), ketonemia (strongly positive), acidosis (pH less than 7.30 and bicarbonate less than 15 mEq/liter), glycosuria, and ketonuria.

Clinical Manifestations of Diabetes Mellitus

- The three polys (cardinal signs of diabetes)
  - Polyphagia
  - Polyuria
  - Polydipsia
- IDDM
  - Weight loss
  - Child may start bed-wetting
  - Irritability and "not himself"
  - Shortened attention span
  - Lowered frustration tolerance
  - Appears overly tired
  - Dry skin
  - Blurred vision
  - Sores that are slow to heal
  - Flushed skin
  - Headache
- NIDDM
  - Overweight
  - Fatigue
  - Frequent infections
- Child will exhibit:
  - Hyperglycemia
    - Elevated blood glucose
    - Glucosuria
  - Diabetic ketosis
    - Ketones as well as glucose in urine
    - No noticeable dehydration
  - Diabetic ketoacidosis
    - Dehydration
    - Electrolyte imbalance
    - Acidosis

Therapeutic Management

The management of the child with IDDM consists of a multidisciplinary approach involving the family, the child (when appropriate), and professionals, including a pediatrician, diabetes nurse educator, and nutritionist. Sometimes psychologic support from a mental health professional is also needed. Communication among the team members is essential and extends to other individuals in the child's life, such as teachers, the school nurse, school guidance counselor, and coach.

The definitive treatment is replacement of insulin that the child is unable to produce. However, insulin needs are affected by emotions, nutritional intake, activity, and other life events, such as illnesses and puberty. Medical and nutritional guidance are primary, but management also includes continuing diabetes education, family guidance, and emotional support.

Insulin therapy. Replacement of insulin is the cornerstone of management of IDDM. Insulin is available in highly purified beef, pork, or beef-pork preparations, and in human insulin manufactured by gene-splicing techniques. It is available in rapid-, intermediate-, and long-acting preparations, and all are packaged in the strength of 100 units/ml. (Other dosages are available for situations where extraordinarily large or small dosages are required.)

The precise dose of insulin needed cannot be predicted. Therefore a regimen of total dosage and the percentage of regular- to intermediate-acting insulin should be determined empirically for each child. The amount of insulin is based on capillary blood sugar levels, which the child or parent tests by means of a drop of blood on a chemically treated test strip (Glucostix, Chemstrip bG) with the aid of a color chart or a glucose monitor (Accu-Chek or Glucometer).

Daily insulin is administered subcutaneously by twice daily injections, by multiple dose injections, or by means of a portable pump. Most children with diabetes can be controlled satisfactorily with a twice daily insulin regimen consisting of a combination of rapid-acting (regular) and intermediate-acting (NPH or Lente) insulin drawn up into the same syringe and injected before breakfast and before the evening meal. The amount of insulin is determined by measurements of the blood glucose after the peak effect of the insulin has occurred. For example, the amount of regular insulin at breakfast is determined by the previous late morning blood glucose measurement. Regular insulin is best given at least 30 minutes before meals to allow sufficient time for absorption. Some children require more frequent administration of insulin. This includes children with difficult-to-control diabetes and during the adolescent growth spurt.

The insulin pump is an electromechanical device designed to deliver fixed amounts of regular insulin continuously, thereby more closely imitating the release of the hormone by the islet cells. The system consists of a syringe to hold the insulin, a plunger, and a mechanism to drive the plunger. The insulin flows from the syringe through a catheter to a needle inserted into subcutaneous tissue (the abdomen or thigh) and the lightweight device is worn on a belt or a shoulder holster. The needle and catheter are changed every 48 hours by the child or parent, using aseptic technique, and taped in place.

Although the pump provides more even insulin release, it has certain disadvantages. It cannot be removed for more than 1 hour, which limits some activities, such as bathing and swimming (it is damaged by water) and like any other mechanical device, it is subject to malfunction. However, the pumps are equipped with alarms that signal problems that may arise, such as run-down batteries, blocked needle or tubing, or a malfunction that allows uncontrollable insulin delivery.

Monitoring. Home blood glucose monitoring (HBGM) has improved diabetes management and is used successfully by children from the onset of their diabetes. By testing their own blood, children are able to change their insulin regimen to maintain their glucose level in the euglycemic range of 80 to 120 mg/dl. Diabetes management depends to a great extent on home glucose monitoring. In general, children tolerate the testing well.

Laboratory measurement of glycosylated hemoglobin (hemoglobin A_{1c}) levels reflects the average blood glucose levels during the previous 2 to 3 months and is of value in assessing glucose control in any person with diabetes. Urine testing, formerly a mainstay of diabetic management, has many limitations; for example, there is poor correlation between simultaneous glycosuria and blood glucose concentrations. However, urine testing can be carried out periodically to detect evidence of ketonuria.

Nutrition. Essentially, the nutritional needs of children with diabetes are no different from those of healthy children, except for deletion of concentrated sugars. Children with diabetes require no special foods or supplements. They need sufficient calories to balance daily expenditure for energy and to satisfy the requirement for growth and development.

In the healthy child, insulin is secreted in response to food intake. Insulin injected subcutaneously, however, has a relatively predictable time of onset, peak effect, duration of action, and absorption rate, depending on the type of insulin used. Consequently the timing of food consumption is regulated to correspond to the time and action of the insulin prescribed. Meals and snacks must be eaten at the same times each day, and the total number of calories and proportions of basic nutrients must be consistent from day to day. The distribution of calories also should be calculated to fit the activity pattern of each child. Alterations in food intake should be made so that food, insulin, and exercise are balanced. Extra food is needed for extra activity.

The food intake is based on a balanced diet that incorporates six basic food groups: milk, meat, vegetables, fat, fruit, and bread. The family may follow the exchange system approved by the American Diabetes Association (ADA) or the point system, based on 75 kcal equaling 1 point. The exchange system indicates the amount (portion size) of each food by volume or weight and is prescribed in terms of the number of exchanges from each food group that constitutes each meal and snack. This ensures day-to-day consistency in total calories, protein, fat, and carbohydrate while allowing a choice from a wide variety of foods.

Concentrated sweets are eliminated. Dietary fiber has become increasingly important in dietary planning because of its influence on digestion, absorption, and metabolism of many nutrients and has been found to diminish the rise in blood sugar after meals.

Exercise. Exercise is encouraged and never restricted unless indicated by other health conditions, because it lowers blood sugar levels. It should be included as part of diabetic management and planned around the child's interests and capabilities. However, in most instances children's activities are unplanned, and the resulting decrease in blood sugar can be compensated for by providing extra snacks before (and, if prolonged, during) the activity. Besides providing a feeling of well-being, regular exercise aids in the body's use of food and often decreases insulin requirements.

Hypoglycemia. Even a well-controlled child may experience mild symptoms of hypoglycemia almost daily, but if the signs and symptoms are recognized early (see Table 28-2) and promptly relieved by appropriate therapy, the child's activity should not be interrupted for more than a few minutes. The most common causes of hypoglycemia are bursts of physical activity without additional food, or delayed, omitted, or incompletely consumed meals.

In the majority of cases, simple concentrated sugar, such as honey, that can be held in the mouth for a short time will elevate the blood glucose level and alleviate the symptoms. The simpler the carbohydrate the more rapidly it will be absorbed. For a mild reaction milk is a good food to use in children. It supplies them with lactose or milk sugar as well as a more prolonged action from the protein and fat (aids in decreased absorption). All children with diabetes should carry with them sugar-containing candy, such as Life Savers or Charms, or some sugar cubes. The rapid-releasing sugar is followed by a complex carbohydrate such as a slice of bread or a cracker.

Glucagon is sometimes prescribed for home treatment of hypoglycemia. It is available as a tablet to be mixed with diluting fluid from its accompanying bottle and is administered intramuscularly or subcutaneously. It functions by releasing stored glycogen from the liver and requires about 15 to 20 minutes to elevate the blood glucose level. Once the child is responsive, the lost glycogen stores are replaced by small amounts of sugar-containing fluid administered frequently until the child feels comfortable about trying solid foods.

The *somogyi effect* should be recognized as a separate response. This phenomenon occurs when the blood glucose level decreases to the point where stress hormones (epinephrine, growth hormone, and corticosteroids) are released, causing an elevation in the blood glucose level. Treatment consists of increasing the amount of food eaten and/or decreasing the insulin.

Illness management. Illness alters diabetes management, and maintaining control is usually related to the seriousness of the illness. As the illness runs its course, the goal of diabetic management is to maintain some glycosuria but keep the urine free of acetone. Because a decreased appetite occurs during illness, a 20% decrease in caloric intake (simpler foods along with fluids and simple sugars) may reduce the need for insulin.

The physiologic and emotional stresses related to surgery require careful adjustment of insulin. Since the child receives intravenous glucose during surgery and the stress of the surgery itself will also raise the blood glucose level, the risk of an insulin reaction (hypoglycemia, hyperinsulinism) is very slight. Regular insulin should be continued until the child is able to tolerate oral feedings and a return to the routine pattern of insulin administration.

Islet cell transplantation. There has been some experimentation with islet cell transplants. Viable insulin-producing cells are injected into the portal vein, where they take root in the liver and eventually produce up to two thirds of the needed insulin. However, because it is an allograft, persons receiving islet cell transplants require immunosuppression, which in itself is a risk factor. The major use of transplants has been in persons who have serious complications, particularly those whose deteriorating kidneys have required renal transplants and who are necessarily on immunosuppression.

Management of ketoacidosis. Diabetic ketoacidosis (DKA), the most complete state of insulin deficiency, is a life-threatening situation. The child should be admitted to an intensive care facility for management, which consists of rapid assessment, adequate insulin to reduce the elevated blood glucose, fluids to overcome dehydration, and electrolyte replacement (especially potassium and bicarbonate).

The preferred method for administering insulin to the child with ketoacidosis is a continuous infusion of low-dose insulin. It has been found that plastic tubing and in-line filters can chemically bind to significant amounts of insulin, thereby reducing the amount of the medication reaching the bloodstream; therefore, an insulin mixture is run through the tubing to saturate the insulin binding sites before beginning the infusion.

Serum potassium levels may be normal on admission, but rapid return of potassium to cells following initiation of fluid and insulin can seriously deplete serum levels, with the attendant risk of cardiac arrhythmias. Vigorous potassium replacement is implemented as soon as the child is voiding sufficiently, and a cardiac monitor is employed as a guide to therapy and to determine changes that might indicate alterations in potassium concentration.

Nursing Considerations

Nurses play a prominent role in diagnosis and management of children with IDDM. Assessing and educating the child and family are almost exclusively a nursing function.

ASSESSMENT

Diabetic management involves a constant state of assessment. Daily monitoring of blood glucose levels, periodic urine analysis for ketones, and observation for signs of hypoglycemia, hyperglycemia, or other complications is part of the daily life of the child with diabetes and his family. Diabetes can be suspected in any child who exhibits the manifestations outlined in the box on p. 952 and the child referred for further assessment and appropriate testing.

The signs and symptoms of hypoglycemia are caused by both increased adrenergic activity and impaired brain function, and it is often difficult to distinguish between hyperglycemia and a hypoglycemic reaction (Table 28-2). Since the symptoms are similar and usually begin with changes in behavior, the simplest way to differentiate between the two is to test the blood glucose level (low in hypoglycemia; elevated in hyperglycemia).

The nurse should also be alert to evidence of complications, although these are usually not manifest until adulthood. Assessment of skin for evidence of breakdown is important, in order that appropriate care can be implemented to facilitate healing and prevent infection. Because illnesses, such as respiratory infections or gastrointestinal upsets, complicate the diabetes management, they should be detected early.

Education is the cornerstone of diabetes management

TABLE 28-2

Comparison of Manifestations of Hypoglycemia and Hyperglycemia

Variable	Hypoglycemia	Hyperglycemia
Onset	Rapid (minutes)	Gradual (days)
Mood	Labile, irritable, nervous, weepy	Lethargic
Mental status	Difficulty concentrating, speaking, focusing, coordinating	Dulled sensorium Confused
Inward feeling	Shaky feeling, hunger Headache Dizziness	Thirst Weakness Nausea/vomiting Abdominal pain
Skin	Pallor Sweating	Flushed Signs of dehydration
Mucous membranes	Normal	Dry, crusty
Respirations	Shallow	Deep, rapid (Kussmaul)
Pulse	Tachycardia	Less rapid, weak
Breath odor	Normal	Fruity, acetone
Neurologic	Tremors Late: hyperflexia, dilated pupils, convulsion	Diminished reflexes Paresthesia
Ominous signs	Shock, coma	Acidosis, coma
Blood:		
Glucose	Low: below 60 mg/dl	High: 250 mg/dl or more
Ketones	Negative	High/large
Osmolarity	Normal	High
pH	Normal	Low (7.25 or less)
Hematocrit	Normal	High
HCO_3	Normal	Less than 20 mEq/L
Urine:		
Output	Normal	Polyuria (early) to oliguria (late)
Sugar	Negative	High
Acetone	Negative	High

and the major responsibility in diabetes nursing care. Whether teaching is conducted on an outpatient basis or in a preparatory, in-depth manner on an inpatient basis, the ability of the individuals involved to learn must be accurately assessed. This includes assessment of the educational background and emotional stability of the individual(s) involved and the use of appropriate measurement tools, such as a pretest or an objective assessment of the learner's educational level.

NURSING DIAGNOSES

A number of nursing diagnoses are prominent in the nursing management of IDDM, and others specific to individual cases become evident. The most common are outlined in the Nursing Care Plan on pp. 960-963.

PLANNING

The goals of nursing care for the child with IDDM are:

1. Educate the child and family about the disease, assessment techniques, and therapy
2. Prevent ill effects from complications of diabetes
3. Promote a positive self-image in the child
4. Provide support to child and family

IMPLEMENTATION

Once the child with diabetes is diagnosed and insulin therapy initiated, the major nursing responsibility is the education of the family and reinforcement of information. One of the first things that should be called to the attention of the parents is the need for the child to wear some means of medical identification, such as the Medic Alert bracelet or necklace.

The parents must supervise and manage the child's therapeutic program, but the child should assume responsibility for self-management as soon as he is capable. Children can learn to collect their own blood for glucose testing at a relatively young age (4 to 5 years), and most should be able to check their blood glucose and administer their own insulin at about 9 years of age. In situations in which the parents are inconsistent and/or unreliable, the child is taught self-care at an earlier age.

A child learns best when sessions are kept short, no more than 15 to 20 minutes. The parents do best in periods of 45 to 60 minutes and, often, longer if they are inquisitive. Education should involve all the senses, and, although visual aids are valuable tools, participation is the most effective method for learning. For example, to teach blood testing, the technique is explained, the procedure is demonstrated, the learner is allowed to perform the procedure, followed by a review of the material by visual aids, and the learning is validated by some testing method that includes a feedback. Varying the presentation with a number of audiovisual materials including motion pictures, slide-tape programs, and books stimulates the senses and helps the individual to learn.

Several organizations are prepared to assist with education and dissemination of knowledge about diabetes. The **American Diabetes Association, Inc.,*** **Canadian Diabetes Association,†** **Juvenile Diabetes Foundation International,‡** and **Juvenile Diabetes Foundation International–Canada§** are valuable resources for a wide variety of educational materials. The **National Diabetes Information Clearinghouse‖** publishes a number of comprehensive annotated bibliogra-

*1660 Duke St., Alexandria, VA 22314.
†78 Bond St., Toronto, Ontario, Canada M5B 258.
‡60 Madison Ave., New York, NY 10010, hotline (800)223-1138.
§4632 Yonge St., Suite 201, Willowdale, Ontario, Canada M2N 5M1.
‖Box NDIC, Bethesda, MD 20205.

phies including "Educational Materials for and about Young People with Diabetes," a compilation of resource materials for children, siblings, parents, teachers, and health professionals, and "Sports and Exercise for People with Diabetes." Highly recommended is a book written for children and parents, *An Instructional Aid on Juvenile Diabetes Mellitus* by L.B. Travis.*

Self-management, the ultimate goal for the child with diabetes, is more likely to occur when the child understands the disease and the care it requires. Properly educated, any family should be able to follow a program of regulated control satisfactorily. The following information will allow the family to manage the daily aspects of care.

Nature of diabetes. The better the parents understand the pathophysiology of diabetes and the function and action of insulin and glucagon in relation to calorie intake and exercise, the better their understanding of the disease and its effect on the child. Parents need answers to a number of questions (voiced or unvoiced), because those answers will provide them with an increased feeling of security in coping with the disease.

Meal planning. Normal nutrition is a major aspect of the family education program. Diet instruction is usually conducted by the nutritionist, with reinforcement and guidance from the nurse (Fig. 28-3). Learning about foods within specific food groups helps in choices. Weights and measures of foods, used as eye-training devices in defining food volumes, should be practiced for about 3 months, with gradual conversion to estimating foods. Members of the family are also guided in reading labels for the nutritional value of foods and food contents.

Lists of popular fast-food items and items served at the major fast-food chains can be obtained from the American Diabetes Association (ADA) to help guide food selections. Children should be advised to use sugar substitutes with moderation in items such as soft drinks. "Sugar-free" chewing gum and candies made with sorbitol are not usually recommended for children with diabetes. Although sorbitol is less cariogenic than other varieties of sugar substitutes, it is an alcohol sugar that is metabolized to fructose and then to glucose. Furthermore, large amounts can cause an osmotic diarrhea. Most dietetic foods contain sorbitol also. They are more expensive than regular foods, and careful reading of labels reveals that the caloric content is the same or even greater.

Insulin. Families need to understand the treatment method and the insulin prescribed, including the effective duration, onset, and peak action. They also need to know the characteristics of the various types of insulins, the proper mixing and dilution of insulins, and how to substitute another type when their usual brand is not available (insulin is a nonprescription drug). Insulin need not be refrigerated but should be maintained at a temperature below 29.4° C (85° F). An extra supply can be kept in the refrigerator.

*Available from the **American Diabetes Association,** P.O. Box 12946, Austin, TX 78711 or a local branch of the association.

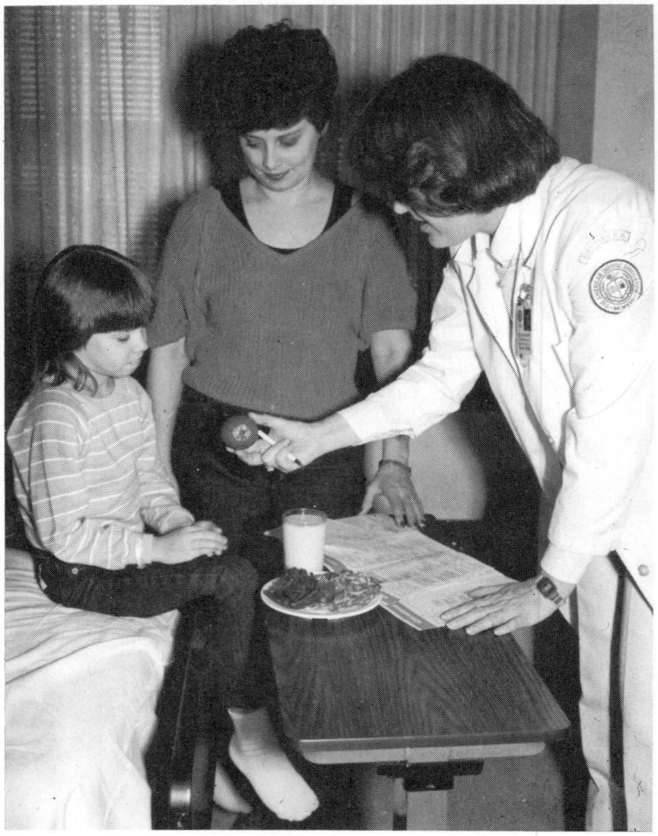

FIG. 28-3 Nutritionist instructs child and family, using food models to explain food exchanges.

Injection procedure. Learning to give the insulin injections is a source of anxiety for the family and the child. It is helpful for the learner to know that this important aspect of care will become as routine as brushing the teeth. First, the basic injection technique is taught, using an orange or similar item for practice. To gain the confidence of the child, the nurse demonstrates the technique by giving a skillful injection to the caregiver, who then returns the demonstration by giving the nurse an injection. With practice family members soon are able to give the insulin injection to the child, and he will trust them. Both parents or other caregivers should participate, and as little time as possible should elapse between instruction and the actual injection, especially with parents and the teenage learner.

Insulin can be injected into any area in which there is skin over muscle with fatty tissue in between (Fig. 28-4). The drug is injected at a 45-degree angle, and the depth of injection is altered according to the thickness of the skin. Usually the smaller the child, the thinner the skin. The pinch technique is the most effective method for obtaining skin tightness to allow easy entrance of the needle into subcutaneous tissues in children. The site selected will sometimes depend on whether the child or parent administers the insulin. The upper arms, thighs, hips, and abdomen are usual injection sites for insulin.

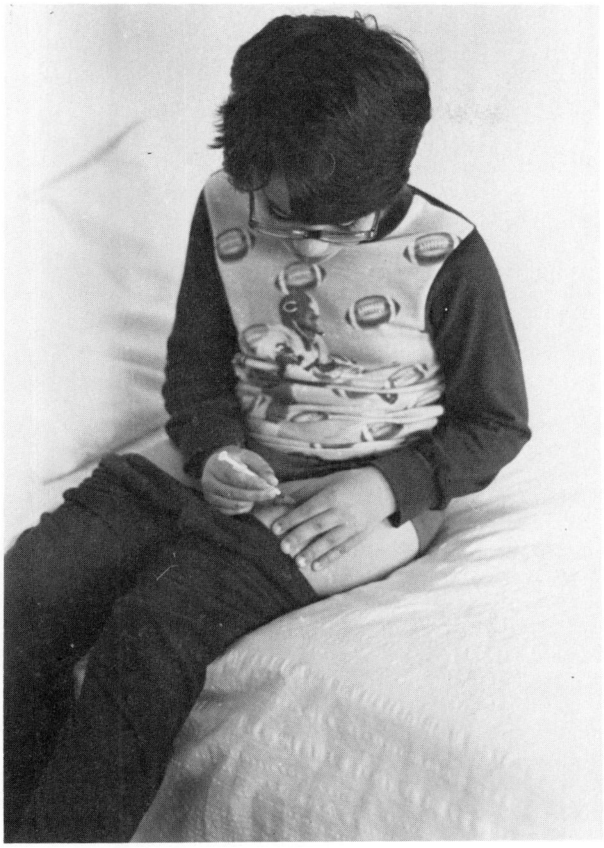

FIG. 28-4 School-age children are able to administer their own insulin.

The child can reach the thighs, abdomen, and part of the hip and arm easily but may require help to inject other sites. For example, a parent can pinch a loose fold of skin on the arm while the child injects the insulin.

Injections are rotated to various areas of the body to enhance absorption, since insulin absorption is slowed by the fat pads that develop in overused areas of injection. The parents and child are helped to work out a rotation pattern, which involves giving about four to six injections in one area (each injection about 1 inch, or the diameter of the insulin vial, from the previous injection) and then moving to another area. In this way injection sites for an entire month can be worked out in advance on a simple chart or illustration, such as an outline of a body or a teddy bear. It is a good idea for the parents each to give one or two shots a week in the areas that are difficult to reach in order to keep in practice.

The teaching includes the proper way to equalize pressure in the bottle by injecting an amount of air equal to the amount of solution withdrawn and removal of air bubbles from the syringe. When insulin dosages are small, an air bubble in the syringe can displace a significant amount of medication. Since the introduction of the low-dose syringe, the risk of incorrect dosage has diminished. Patients who have small doses of mixed insulins are advised and instructed to use these syringes. Insulin syringes should be compared for accuracy, comfort, and strength, and the family and/or child should be able to choose both "their" insulin and "their" syringe from a variety of samples. Use of the same type of syringe (even during hospitalization) is recommended to prevent errors in dosage.

When the child's dosage requires the injection of both short- and intermediate-acting insulin at the same time, most families prefer to mix the two and use a single injection. However, there are some problems associated with this accepted practice, and the family should understand what happens when insulins are mixed. Longer-acting insulins contain ingredients that bind to insulin, allowing for gradual release after injection. Some brands contain extra binding compounds that can bind with regular insulin, converting it to the long-acting type and altering the effect on blood glucose. The degree of alteration depends on the type of longer-acting insulin, the ratio of short- to long-acting insulin, and how long the mixture is allowed to stand before injection.

To obtain the maximum benefit from mixing insulins, the recommended practice is to (1) inject the measured amount of air (equivalent to the dosage) into the longer-acting insulin, (2) inject the measured amount of air into the regular insulin and, without removing the needle, (3) withdraw the regular insulin, and (4) insert the needle (already containing the regular insulin) into the longer-acting insulin and withdraw the desired amount. The mixture should be injected immediately—in less than 5 minutes after mixing (Jenkins and Molitch, 1986).

It has become acceptable practice to reuse disposable needles and syringes up to 7 days. Research has shown that no infection has resulted, and there is a considerable cost saving (Poteet, Reinert, and Ptak, 1987). If this method is approved, it is important to stress the importance of vigorous handwashing before handling any equipment, as well as capping the syringe immediately after use and storing it in the refrigerator to decrease the possibility of infection. The nurse should also teach proper disposal of equipment after use.

Some children are considered candidates for continuous subcutaneous insulin infusion with a portable insulin pump (Fig. 28-5). The child and the parents are taught to operate the device, including the mechanics of the pump, battery changes, and alarm systems. They learn how to load the syringe, insert the catheter, adjust the insulin flow for routine needs and for illnesses, and connect and disconnect the catheter. Nurses who work where the pumps are part of the therapeutic regimen should become familiar with the operation of the specific device being used and the protocol of the regimen.

Glucose monitoring. Nurses should also be prepared to teach and supervise blood glucose monitoring, which is becoming the standard method for assessing glucose levels and an essential component of insulin infusion pump therapy (Fig. 28-6). It provides an accurate assessment of blood glucose levels and can be performed anywhere. It is recommended that every family with a child who has

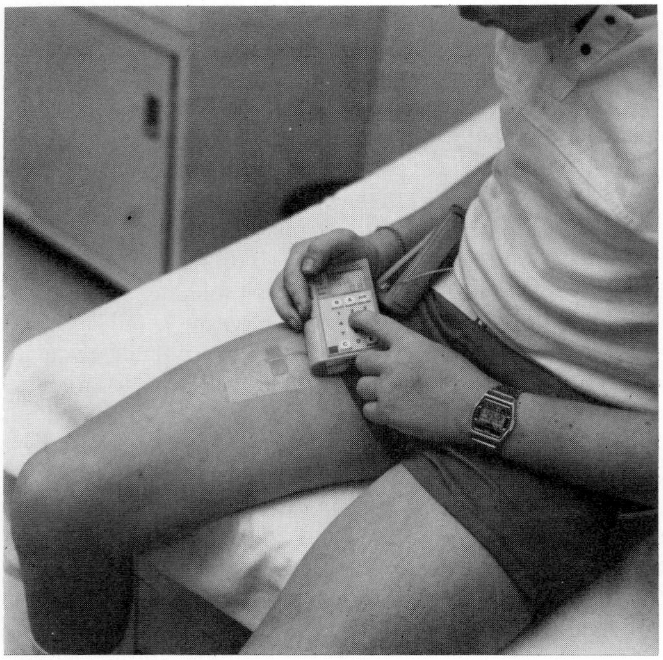

FIG. 28-5 Child programming insulin pump. Note insertion site on anterior thigh and carrying case on belt.

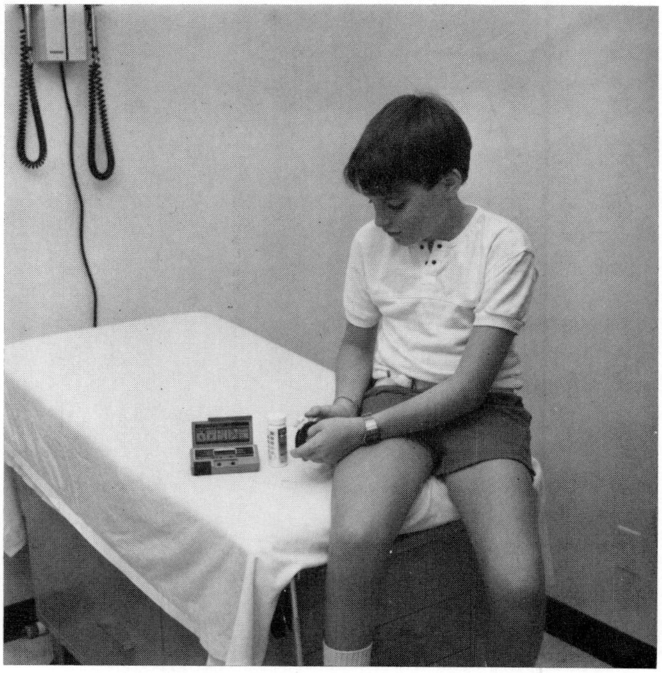

FIG. 28-6 Child using Autolet to obtain blood sample. Gluometer and reagent strips at hand.

type I diabetes have equipment available for home blood glucose monitoring (HBGM). Information on monitoring products can be obtained from the American Diabetes Association or from local representatives of the major suppliers.

Urine testing. Urine testing is easily taught and should include all methods, not just the test to be used for the particular child. Testing for acetone is usually recommended during times of illness or when glucose readings are high. Since moisture will cause changes to take place in both glucose and acetone reagent tablets, families are instructed to discard tablets that are discolored, that have been open for a specified time, or after an expiration date. Also, the potentially toxic tablets should be stored in a safe place away from small children.

Hyperglycemia and hypoglycemia. Severe hyperglycemia is most often caused by illness, growth, or emotional upset. With careful glucose monitoring, any elevation can be managed by adjustment of insulin or food intake. Parents should understand how to adjust food, activity, and insulin at the time of illness or when the child is treated for an illness with a medication known to raise the blood glucose level. The hyperglycemia is managed by increasing insulin soon after the increased glucose is noted.

Hypoglycemia is caused by imbalances of food intake, insulin, and activity. Ideally hypoglycemia should be prevented, and parents need to be prepared to prevent, recognize, and treat the problem. They should be familiar with the signs of hypoglycemia and instructed in treatment, including care of the child with seizures (see p. 924). Hypoglycemia can be managed effectively as outlined in the emergency treatment box.

Hygiene. All aspects of personal hygiene are emphasized for the child with diabetes. The child has not had time to develop the blood vessel disease that causes a decrease in peripheral circulation; therefore, foot care is not as important in the child as it is in the adult with diabetes. However, wearing tennis shoes without socks, wearing sandals, and going barefoot are discouraged. The correct method of nail and extremity care instituted for each particular child (with the guidance of a podiatrist) can begin health practices that last a lifetime. Eyes should be checked once a year, unless the child wears glasses, and then as directed by the ophthalmologist. Regular dental care is emphasized, and cuts and scratches should be treated with plain soap and water unless otherwise indicated.

Exercise. Exercise should be planned (as may be necessary for the sedentary teenager) or observed (as in most active children). If the child is more active at one time of the day than at another, food and/or insulin can be altered to meet the activity pattern of the individual. Food should be increased in the summer, when children tend to be more active. Decreased activity on return to school may require a decrease in food intake. The child who is active in team sports will need additional food intake on the days of activity in the form of a snack about ½ hour before the anticipated activity. Races or other competition may call for a slightly higher food intake than practice times.

Food will usually need to be repeated for prolonged activity periods, often as frequently as every 45 minutes to 1 hour. Families should be informed that if increased food is not tolerated, decreased insulin is the next course of action.

Record keeping. Keeping information about food, insulin, blood glucose measurements, and glucosuria is useful to the physician as well as to the family. Insulin reactions are noted, including the time, severity, treatment, and response to treatment. Dietary variations are noted so that an increased blood glucose or urinary glucose spill can be analyzed in relation to insulin dose, food intake, and activity level.

Self-management. Self-management is the key to close control. Being able to make changes at the time they are needed rather than waiting until the next contact with health professionals is important for self-management and gives the individual and family the feeling that they have control over the disease. As children grow and assume more and more responsibility for self-management, they develop confidence in their ability to manage their disease and in themselves as persons. Self-management techniques to be mastered are the testing of blood and urine and adjustment of insulin and diet with alterations in day-to-day activities and unusual occurrences.

Acute care. Children with diabetes may be admitted to the hospital at the time of their initial diagnosis, during illness or surgery, or during episodes of ketoacidosis—especially the small number who exhibit a degree of metabolic lability, who have repeated episodes of diabetic ketoacidosis. Most children with diabetes are able to keep the disease under control with periodic assessment and adjustment of insulin, diet, and activity as needed under health supervision.

The child with diabetic ketoacidosis requires intensive nursing care. On admission to the hospital an intravenous infusion is started immediately to hydrate the child and to administer insulin, usually as a continuous infusion (see medical management, p. 954). The blood glucose level is monitored at regular intervals, and the insulin administered as ordered.

Sodium, potassium, and bicarbonate levels are monitored and replaced as indicated. Since potassium and sodium reenter the cells rapidly after administration of insulin, depletion of these electrolytes can be a serious consequence. Generally the child is attached to a cardiac monitor for continual assessment of cardiac status, especially when potassium levels are markedly altered.

Careful and accurate records are maintained, including vital signs (pulse, respiration, temperature, and blood pressure), intravenous fluids, electrolytes, insulin, blood glucose level, and intake and output. A urine collection device or retention catheter is used to obtain the urine measurements, which include volume, specific gravity, and glucose and acetone values. The volume relative to the glucose content is important, since 5% glucose in a 300 ml sample is a significantly greater amount than a similar reading from a 75 ml sample. A diabetic flow sheet maintained at the bedside provides an ongoing record of the vital signs, urine and blood tests, amount of insulin given, and intake and output of the patient. The level of consciousness is assessed and recorded at frequent intervals. The comatose child generally regains consciousness fairly soon after initiation of therapy but is managed as any unconscious child during that time.

EMERGENCY TREATMENT

Hypoglycemia

Mild reaction:
Give child food
  Milk, crackers, fruit
Moderate reaction:
Give child simple sugar
  Life Saver, sugar cube
Follow with food

Severe reaction:
Administer glucagon
Follow in 15 to 20 minutes with simple sugar

Family support. In any educational program psychologic needs are just as important as the physical needs of the child. Adjustment to a chronic illness is difficult and follows the grief process (see Chapter 18). A noticeable adjustment cycle occurs during the week-long education course. First, there is interest and perhaps some anger and doubt, followed by denial and accompanied by the overwhelming feeling of "Why me?" There are doubts regarding the ability to absorb so much essential information. Then there are the acceptance and synthesis of material, as the learners realize that they are able to state and demonstrate their understanding of the material.

Children in the years before adolescence probably accept their condition most easily. They are able to understand the basic concepts related to their disease and its treatment. Adolescents appear to have most difficulty in adjusting. Adolescence is a time when there is much stress on being perfect and being like peers, and no matter what others say, having diabetes is being different. If children can accept the difference as a part of life—in other words, that each person has something different about him—then with adequate parental support, they should be able to adjust well.

Camps for children with diabetes and other special groups are very useful. In the special camp these children learn that they are not alone (Fig. 28-7). As a result most children become more independent and resourceful in the nondiabetic camp setting. Most communities have special children's support groups (members of one community group call themselves the "Friskie Frescas"). Useful information about such camps and organizations can be obtained from the ADA. A free list of accredited camps specifically for children and teens with diabetes is also available.*

*Camp Directory, 1660 Duke St., Alexandria, VA 22314.

NURSING CARE PLAN

The Child with Diabetes Mellitus

Nursing Goals	Nursing Interventions	Expected Patient/Family Outcomes
HP-HMP* **Potential for injury** **Risk factors: unconsciousness secondary to cerebral dysfunction, metabolic imbalance**		
Ketoacidosis		
Recognize diabetic ketoacidosis	Be alert to signs of acidosis, especially in children with known diabetes mellitus Observe for evidence of precipitating factors, such as infection, stress, or omission of insulin injections	†Signs of ketoacidosis are detected and appropriate actions initiated
Treat associated problems	Carry out therapeutic regimen as prescribed for infection if present Implement appropriate care for the child who is unconscious (see p. 895)	†Signs of associated problems are detected early and appropriate actions implemented
Detect alterations in status	Maintain meticulous records Assess vital signs frequently Observe for signs of complications, such as cerebral edema, hyperkalemia, or hypokalemia	†Signs of altered status are detected early and appropriate actions initiated
Ensure adequate hydration	Assess state of hydration Monitor fluid intake and output Administer fluids in manner dictated by child's condition	Child exhibits evidence of good hydration
Hypoglycemia		
Recognize signs of hypoglycemia early	Be particularly alert at times when blood glucose levels are lowest Observe for lability of mood, irritability, seizures, and indications of subjective symptoms, such as shaky feeling, headache, hunger, and impaired vision (p. 955) Test for glucose	†Signs of hypoglycemia are recognized
Elevate blood glucose level	Offer readily absorbed carbohydrates, such as orange juice, hard candy, or milk Follow with complex carbohydrate, such as bread or cracker	Child ingests an appropriate carbohydrate Child displays no evidence of hypoglycemia
CPP **Knowledge deficit (diabetic management)** **Etiology: newly diagnosed diabetic**		
Determine the educational needs of child and/or family	Assess the understanding and level of intelligence of the learners Select methods, vocabulary, and content appropriate to the level of the learner	†Appropriate teaching tools are assembled for teaching child and family
Educate child and/or family regarding diabetic management	Allow 3 or 4 days for family and child to begin to adjust to the initial impact of the diagnosis Select an environment conducive to learning Allow ample time for the education process Restrict length of teaching sessions Child—15-20 minutes Parents—45-60 minutes Involve all senses and employ a variety of teaching strategies Provide pamphlets or other supplementary materials	Child and/or family display attitudes conducive to learning

*For an explanation of abbreviations, see p. 20.
†Nursing outcome.

NURSING CARE PLAN

The Child with Diabetes Mellitus—cont'd

Nursing Goals	Nursing Interventions	Expected Patient/Family Outcomes
Teach:		
Nature of the disease	Provide information regarding the pathophysiology of diabetes and the function and actions of insulin and glucagon in relation to caloric intake Answer questions and clarify misconceptions Explain function and expected effects of procedures and tests	Child and/or family demonstrate an understanding of the disease and its therapy (specify indicators)
Meal planning	Enlist the services of a dietitian Emphasize the relationship between normal nutritional needs and the disease Become familiar with the family's food preferences Teach or reinforce the learners' understanding of the basic food groups and the diet plan prescribed (e.g., exchange diet) Help the child and family estimate food weights by volume Suggest low-carbohydrate snack items Guide family in assessing the labels of food products for carbohydrate content Teach or reinforce an understanding of the concept of exchanges Relate carbohydrate equivalents to familiar foods Retain cultural patterns and family preferences as much as possible	Child and/or family demonstrate an understanding of diet planning and food selection (specify indicators)
Insulin	Teach child and family the characteristics of the insulins prescribed for the child Teach the proper mixing of insulins and acceptable substitutions (when the familiar brand is unavailable)	Child and/or family demonstrate an understanding of insulin, its various forms, and action (specify indicators)
Injection procedure	Impress upon the learners that the procedure will be a routine part of the child's life Involve caregivers and the child, if old enough Teach basic techniques using an orange or similar item Use demonstration and return demonstration techniques on another before injecting the child	Child and/or family demonstrate injection technique correctly
	Help family and child work out a set rotational pattern Teach proper care of insulin and equipment	Child and/or family develop a rotation plan
Continuous infusion pump	Teach: Basic pump mechanism Preparing and loading syringe Programming Preparation, injection, and care of injection site	Child and/or family demonstrate correct use of pump and care of injection site
Blood glucose testing	Teach: Blood glucose monitoring and/or use of equipment selected for use Interpretation of results Care and maintenance of equipment	Child and/or family demonstrate the correct use of the glucose monitoring equipment
Urine testing	Teach: All methods of urine testing and interpretation of results Proper care of test materials and equipment	Child and/or family demonstrate urine testing and interpretation
Hygiene	Emphasize the importance of personal hygiene Encourage regular dental care and yearly ophthalmologic examinations Teach proper care of cuts and scratches Teach proper foot care	Family demonstrates an understanding of the importance of proper hygiene
Exercise	Arrange for occupational therapy program that includes physical activity Work with child, family, and others (e.g., coaches) to help plan a home exercise program Reiterate physician's instructions regarding adjustment of food and/or insulin to meet the child's activity pattern; reinforce with examples	Family helps child outline and carry out a regular exercise program

Continued.

NURSING CARE PLAN

The Child with Diabetes Mellitus—cont'd

Nursing Goals	Nursing Interventions	Expected Patient/Family Outcomes
Recognition of hyperglycemia and hypoglycemia	Instruct learners in how to recognize signs of hyperglycemia and hypoglycemia (especially hypoglycemia) Explain the relationship of insulin needs to illness, activity, and intense emotion (either positive or negative) Teach how to adjust food, activity and insulin at times of illness and during other situations that alter blood sugar levels Suggest carrying source of carbohydrate, such as sugar cubes or hard candy, in pocket or handbag Instruct parents and child in how to treat hypoglycemia with food, simple sugars, or glucagon	Family demonstrates an understanding of the signs and management of a hypoglycemic reaction (specify)
Identification	Encourage the acquisition of a means of identification, such as an identification bracelet, that explains the child's condition in case of emergency	Family acquires and child wears identification bracelet
General health status	Avoid exposure to infections	Child exhibits no signs of infection
Record keeping	Help child and family to design a form for keeping records of Insulin administered Blood and urine tests Food intake Marked variation in exercise Illness	Family and child keep an accurate record of insulin administration, glucose testing, etc.
Facilitate: Self-management	Encourage honesty in recording, such as eating a forbidden candy bar Encourage independence in applying the concepts learned in teaching sessions Instruct when to seek assistance from medical personnel	Child takes responsibility for management of his disease commensurate with age and capabilities

NDA SP-SCP Body image disturbance
Etiology: biologic changes (insulin dependency)

Nursing Goals	Nursing Interventions	Expected Patient/Family Outcomes
Promote positive self-esteem	Encourage child to express feelings and concerns Determine assets and strengths Help devise coping strategies for managing areas of concern	Child verbalizes or otherwise expresses his feelings and concerns Child maintains prediagnosis activities and relationships
Promote positive adjustment to the disease	Assist child and family in solving problems associated with each of the child's developmental stages Encourage the child to maintain normal activity pattern Encourage interpersonal relationships with peers Suggest involvement with special groups and facilities for children with diabetes Be alert to signs that may indicate rebellion against the disease, such as nonadherence or other forms of acting-out Be available for consultation when needed	Child interacts with other children according to developmental level Child becomes involved with special group activities

NDA RRP Altered family processes
Etiology: situational crisis (child with a chronic disorder)

See The child with a chronic illness or disability, p. 531

NURSING CARE PLAN

The Child with Diabetes Mellitus—cont'd

Nursing interventions related to medical management

Assist with diagnosis
- Check blood glucose as ordered
- Obtain and check urine specimen for glucose, acetone, and specific gravity as ordered
- Collect 24-hour urine specimen for glucose if ordered
- Order or obtain blood for analysis
- Assist with glucose tolerance test

Replace insulin deficit
- Understand the action of insulin
- Understand the differences in composition, time of onset, and duration of action for the various insulin preparations
- Employ correct techniques when preparing and administering insulin
  - Subcutaneous injection
  - Rotation of sites

Assess status
- General
  - Maintain bedside flow sheet, including vital signs, intake, output, blood glucose, copper reduction test (Clinitest), acetone test (Acetest), and insulin administered (varies according to institution)
- Vital signs
  - Measure vital signs as ordered, usually every 4 hours
- Urine
  - Measure intake and output
  - Test for glucose, acetone, and specific gravity
- Blood glucose
  - Order fasting blood sugar (FBS) daily or as requested
  - Withhold breakfast and insulin until after blood is drawn for test
  - Obtain blood glucose measurements as prescribed

Treat hypoglycemia
- Administer glucagon, if ordered

Ketoacidosis

Replace fluid and electrolyte losses
- Monitor intravenous infusion
- Administer fluids as prescribed

Correct hyperglycemia
- Administer insulin intravenously and subcutaneously as prescribed
- Monitor blood glucose levels every 1-2 hours as ordered
- Monitor urine glucose and acetone every 1-2 hours if ordered

Assess status
- Monitor mental status, level of consciousness
- Monitor serum electrolytes, pH, glucose, and blood gases
- Monitor urine glucose, acetone, specific gravity, and volume frequently
- Attach to cardiac monitor

Parents develop guilt feelings when they have a child with any chronic disease, especially one with a hereditary component. They cope with these feelings in a number of ways. For example, they may be either overprotective or neglectful. Guilt-ridden parents may blame themselves for the disease, consciously or subconsciously. Nevertheless, they must come to realize, through education and counseling, that there was nothing they could have done to prevent the disease and that it was not their fault, since environmental as well as hereditary factors may be involved in the development of the disease.

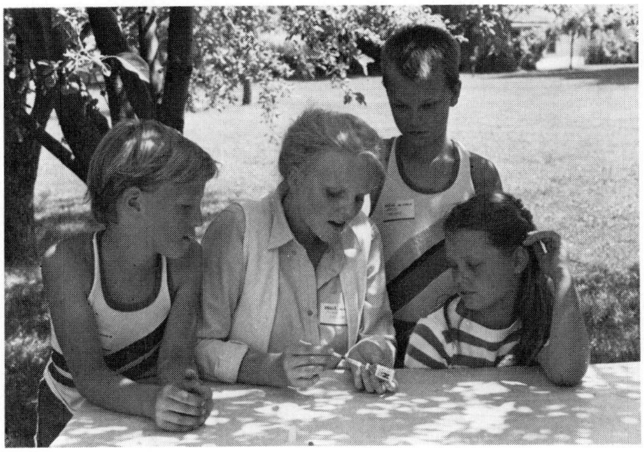

FIG. 28-7 Nurse demonstrates the withdrawal of insulin at a summer camp for children with diabetes.

Problems in the parental response provide a challenge for the nurse to assist through counseling or, if severe enough, to refer the parents to appropriate resources designed to help them alter their behavior. Times should be set aside during the child's health visit or afterward to meet the needs of the parents. Parents should also be included in special sessions to keep them abreast of the child's management, to help them continue to participate in the child's care, and to provide them with an opportunity to express their own feelings concerning their own or their child's adjustment to the disease. The amount of information that they offer at this time can give clues to their level of support of the child and help assist in decisions concerning the therapeutic management of the child. This helps guide the child through the most disruptive time of life—the teenage years.

EVALUATION

The effectiveness of nursing interventions is determined by continual reassessment and evaluation of care based

on the following observational guidelines and expected outcomes:

1. Interview the family to determine their understanding of the disease; have the child and family demonstrate and discuss the needed assessment and therapeutic techniques.
2. Interview the family regarding their understanding of tight control; analyze and evaluate management records.
3. Discuss the child's disease with him.
4. Interview the family and child regarding their feelings and concerns about the disease.

Expected outcomes:
See Nursing Care Plan, pp. 960 to 963.

SUMMARY

Most endocrine disorders are rare in children. Growth hormone deficiency has assumed a prominent place of interest, especially since the introduction of synthetic growth hormone as an available therapy. The most common endocrine disease at all ages is diabetes mellitus, which can occur at any age but is diagnosed with greatest frequency in the preadolescent and early adolescent years. Self-management is the aim of education, and tight control of the disease to prevent complications of the disease is the ultimate goal of care.

KEY CONCEPTS

- The endocrine system has three components: the cell, which sends a chemical message via a hormone; target cells, which receive the message; and the environment through which the chemical is transported from the site of synthesis to the sites of cellular action.
- Generalized tissue alterations can take place as a result of oversecretion or undersecretion of a hormone.
- Disorders that reflect a hormone deficiency can be the result of deficient or absent hormone or end-organ unresponsiveness to the hormone.
- Most hormone-deficiency disorders are managed by replacement of the deficient hormone.
- The pituitary gland stores and releases tropic hormones from the hypothalamus; therefore pituitary dysfunction can be reflected in dysfunction of any of the other endocrine glands.
- Pituitary dysfunction is manifest primarily by growth disturbance.
- The major physiologic action of thyroid hormone is to regulate the basal metabolic rate and control the processes of growth and tissue development.
- Disorders of thyroid hormone include hypothyroidism, autoimmune thyroiditis, goiter, and hyperthyroidism.
- Classic forms of hypoparathyroidism in childhood are caused by deficient parathormone production (idiopathic) or end-organ unresponsiveness (pseudohypoparathyroidism).
- The adrenal cortex secretes three important groups of hormones: glucocorticoids, mineralocorticoids, and sex steroids.
- Disorders of adrenal function include acute or chronic adrenocortical insufficiency, Cushing syndrome, congenital adrenal hyperplasia, and hyperaldosteronism.
- Diminished secretion or absence of the hormone insulin results in diabetes mellitus.
- Diabetes in childhood is classified as insulin-dependent (type I), non-insulin–dependent (type II), and maturity-onset diabetes of youth (MODY).
- Insulin replacement is the basis of diabetes therapy.
- To effectively manage diabetes the child and family need education regarding the nature of the disease, insulin administration, monitoring, hygiene and health practices, and preventing and managing complications.

STUDY QUESTIONS AND ACTIVITIES

1 Using a standard anatomy and physiology textbook, diagram the relationship between pituitary gland secretions and the secretion of thyroid hormones, corticosteroids, mineralocorticoids, and sex hormones, including the pituitary tropic hormones and the feedback mechanisms.
2 How can the nurse help the parents cope with the multiple problems related to the birth of an infant with adrenogenital hyperplasia?
3 Visit the local branch of the American Diabetes Association and determine the services available to families with a child who has diabetes, including information about summer camps, traveling, and consumer products.
4 Outline a plan for teaching the insulin injection procedure to a child and his parents.
5 Contact (through a diabetic clinic or chapter of the diabetes association) the nurse advisor of a local group of teenagers with diabetes and plan to attend a meeting. Observe their discussion of everyday problems and solutions.

REFERENCES

Jenkins, C.A., and Molitch, M.E.: Get the most out of mixing insulin, Diabetes Forecast **39**(1):13-14, 1986.
Poteet, G., Reinert, B., and Ptok, H.: Outcome of multiple usage of disposable syringes in the insulin-requiring diabetic, Nurs. Res. **36:**350-352, 1987.

BIBLIOGRAPHY

General

Hurwitz, L.S.: Nursing implications of selected pediatric endocrine problems, Nurs. Clin. North Am. **15:**525-536, 1980.
Lessick, M.L.: Genetic counseling of families with endocrine disorders, Issues Compr. Pediatr. Nurs. **4**(2):27-40, 1980.
Lippe, B.M.: Short stature in children: evaluation and management, J. Pediatr. Health Care **1:**313-322, 1987.
Wong, D.L.: The significance of dead space in syringes, Am. J. Nurs. **82:**1237, 1982.

Disorders of Pituitary Function

Camuñas, C.: Transsphenoidal hypophysectomy, Am. J. Nurs. **80:**1820-1823, 1980.
Fairchild, R.S.: Diabetes insipidus: a review, Crit. Care Q. **3**(3):111-118, 1980.
McElroy, D.B., and Davis, G.T.: SIADH and the acutely ill child, MCN **11:**193-196, 1986.
Solomon, B.L.: The hypothalamus and the pituitary gland: an overview, Nurs. Clin. North Am. **15:**435-451, 1980.
Stern, M., and Zaiken, H.: Assessing the child with short stature, Pediatr. Nurs. **11:**106-110, 1985.
Stewarts, M.L.K.: When patient has the "other" diabetes, RN **48**(5):54-58, 1985.
Trounson, L.W.: Nursing diagnosis and the syndrome of inappropriate antidiuretic hormone, J. Post Anesth. Nurs. **1:**244-247, 1986.
Zucker, A.R., and Chernow, B.: Diabetes insipidus and the syndrome of inappropriate antidiuretic hormone release, Crit. Care Q. **6**(3):63-74, 1983.

Disorders of Thyroid/Parathyroid Function

Arcangelo, V.P.: Simple goiter, Nursing 83 **13**(3):47, 1983.
Hoffmann, J.T.T, and Newby, T.B.: Hypercalcemia in primary hyperparathyroidism, Nurs. Clin. North Am. **15:**469-480, 1980.
Honigman, R.E.: Thyroid function tests, Nursing 82 **12**(4):68-71, 1982.
Sharkey, P.L., and Meyer, S.A.: Hyperthyroidism, Crit. Care Update **8**(5):12-24, 1981.
Wake, M.M., and Brensigner, J.F., III: The nurse's role in hypothyroidism, Nurs. Clin. North Am. **15:**453-467, 1980.

Disorders of Adrenal Function

Burnett, J.: Congenital adrenocortical hyperplasia: a boy with CAH, Am. J. Nurs. **80:**1304-1305, 1980.
Burnett, J.: Congenital adrenocortical hyperplasia: the syndrome, Am. J. Nurs. **80:**1306-1308, 1980.
Burnett, J.: Congenital adrenocortical hyperplasia: nursing interactions, Am. J. Nurs. **80:**1309-1311, 1980.
Camuñas, C.: Surviving pheochromocytoma, Am. J. Nurs. **83:**887-891, 1983.
Darland, N.W.: Congenital adrenocortical hyperplasia: supportive nursing interventions, J. Pediatr. Nurs. **1**(2):117-123, 1986.
Larson, C.A.: The critical path of adrenocortical insufficiency, Nursing 84 **14**(10):66-69, 1984.
Lee, P.D.K., Winter, R.J., and Green, O.C.: Virilizing adrenocortical tumors in childhood: eight cases and a review of the literature, Pediatrics **76:**437-444, 1985.
New, M.I., and Levine, L.S.: New developments in congenital adrenal hyperplasia, Pediatr. Ann. **10:**346-355, 1981.
Sanford, S.J.: Dysfunction of the adrenal gland: physiologic considerations and nursing problems, Nurs. Clin. North Am. **15:**481-498, 1980.

Diabetes Mellitus

Ahlfield, J.E., Soler, N.G., and Marcus, S.D.: Adolescent diabetes mellitus: parent/child perspectives of the effect of the disease on family and social interactions, Diabetes Care **6:**393-398, 1983.

Alli, C.R., and Crapo, P.A.: Sweetener safety: the bitter debate, Diabetes Forecast **38**(3):34-37, 1985.

Balik, B., Haig, B., and Moynihan, P.M.: Diabetes and the school-aged child, MCN **11:**324-330, 1986.

Banion, C.R., Miles, M.S., and Carter, M.C.: Problems of mothers in management of children with diabetes, Diabetes Care **6:**548-551, 1983.

Bates, S., and Ahern, J.A.: Tight control: what does it mean? Am. J. Nurs. **86:**1256-1258, 1986.

Bobrow, E.S., AvRuskin, T.W., and Siller, J.: Mother-daughter interaction and adherence to diabetes regimens, Diabetes Care **8:**146-151, 1985.

Brown, A.J.: School-age children with diabetes: knowledge and management of the disease, and adequacy of self-concept, Matern. Child Nurs. J. **14**(1):47-61, 1985.

Byrnes, C.A.: What's new in the diabetic diet, Nursing 87 **17**(8):58-59, 1987.

Childs, B.P.: Insulin infusion pumps, Nursing 83 **13**(11):55-57, 1983.

Chrisman, C., and Bennett, J.: Diabetes: new names, new test, new diet, Nursing 87 **17**(1):34-41, 1987.

Christensen, K.S.: Self-management in diabetic children, Diabetes Care **6:**552-555, 1983.

Clarson, C., and others: Self-monitoring of blood glucose: how accurate are children with diabetes at reading Chemstrip bG? Diabetes Care **8:**354-358, 1985.

Connors, M.H.: Blood glucose monitoring in childhood diabetes, Nurse Pract. **9:**30-32, 62, 1984.

Daneman, D., and others: The role of self-monitoring of blood glucose in the routine management of children with insulin-dependent diabetes mellitus, Diabetes Care **8:**1-4, 1985.

DiFlorio, I.A., and Duncan, P.: Design for successful patient teaching, MCN **11:**246-249, 1986.

Dillon, R.: Improved serum insulin profiles in diabetic individuals who massaged their insulin injection sites, Diabetes Care **6:**399-401, 1983.

Donohue-Porter, P.: Insulin-dependent diabetes mellitus, Nurs. Clin. North Am. **20:**191-198, 1985.

Faro, B.: Maintaining good control in children with diabetes, Pediatr. Nurs. **9:**368-373, 1983.

Fendya, D.G., and Flynn, K.: Nursing care for children with hypoglycemia due to hyperinsulinism, MCN **6:**100-105, 1981.

Ferrari, M.: The diabetic child and well sibling: risks to the well child's self-concept, Child. Health Care **15:**141-148, 1987.

Flavin, K., and Haire-Joshu, D.: The pharmacologic repertoire, Am. J. Nurs. **86:**1244-1251, 1986.

Fow, S.M.: Home blood glucose monitoring in children with insulin-dependent diabetes mellitus, Pediatr. Nurs. **9:**439-442, 1983.

Franz, M.J.: Fast food: where's the nutrition? Diabetes Forecast **38**(6):31-34, 1985.

Guthrie, D.W., and Guthrie, R.A.: The disease process of diabetes mellitus, Nurs. Clin. North Am. **18:**617-630, 1983.

Haire-Joshu, D., Flavin, K., and Clutter, W.: Contrasting type I and type II diabetes, Am. J. Nurs. **86:**1240-1243, 1986.

Haire-Joshu, D., Flavin, K., and Santiago, J.V.: Intensive conventional insulin therapy, Am. J. Nurs. **86:**1251-1255, 1987.

Harrigan, J.F., and others: The application of locus of control to diabetes education in school-aged children, J. Pediatr. Nurs. **2:**236-243, 1987.

Heins, J.M., Rosett, J.W., and Davis, S.G.: The new look in diabetic diets, Am. J. Nurs. **87:**196-198, 1987.

Hernandez, C.M.G.: Surgery and diabetes: minimizing the risks, Am. J. Nurs. **87:**788-792, 1987.

Hodges, L.C., and Parker, J.: Concerns of parents with diabetic children, Pediatr. Nurs. **13:**22-24, 68, 1987.

Hoette, S.J.: The adolescent with diabetes mellitus, Nurs. Clin. North Am. **18:**763-776, 1983.

Ingersoll, G.M., and others: Cognitive maturity and self-management among adolescents with insulin-dependent diabetes mellitus, J. Pediatr. **108:**620-623, 1986.

Kiser, D.: The Somogyi effect, Am. J. Nurs. **80:**236-238, 1980.

Krauser, K.L., and Madden, P.B.: The child with diabetes mellitus, Nurs. Clin. North Am. **18:**749-762, 1983.

Lillo, R.: Outpatient management of children with diabetic ketoacidosis, Pediatr. Nurs. **8:**383-385, 1982.

Lipman, T.H.: Assessment of the child with diabetic ketoacidosis, Dimens. Crit. Care Nurs. **6:**82-93, 1987.

Loman, D., and Galgani, C.: Monitoring diabetic children's blood-glucose levels at home, MCN **9:**192-196, 1984.

Miller, B.K., and White, N.E.: An assessment guide for diabetic patients, Crit. Care Update **9**(8):28-34, 1982.

Miller, V.G.: Diabetes: let's stop testing urine, Am. J. Nurs. **86:**54, 1986.

Moorman, N.H.: Acute complications of hyperglycemia and hypoglycemia, Nurs. Clin. North Am. **18:**707-719, 1983.

Moran, M.M.: Diabetes camps: management guidelines, Pediatr. Nurs. **11:**183-186, 1985.

Narins, B.: Products to help with insulin reactions, Diabetes Forecast **39**(5):26, 1986.

Ory, M.G., and Dronenfeld, J.J.: Living with juvenile diabetes mellitus, Pediatr. Nurs. **6**(5):47-50, 1980.

Pond, H.: Parental attitudes toward children with a chronic medical disorder: special reference to diabetes mellitus, Diabetes Care **2:**425-431, 1979.

Robertson, C.: Interpreting blood glucose studies, Nursing 86 **16**(8):64, 1986.

Saucier, C.P.: Self concept and self-care management in school-age children with diabetes, Pediatr. Nurs. **10:**135-138, 1984.

Snyder, A.: The role of school personnel in caring for the child with diabetes, School Nurse **3**(1):8-16, 1987.

Stock, P.L.: Action stat! insulin shock, Nursing 85 **15**(4):53, 1985.

Stock-Barkman, P.: Confusing concepts: is it diabetic shock or diabetic coma? Nursing 83 **13**(6):33-41, 1983.

Tamborlane, W.V.: Teenage trouble with glucose control. It's not all in their heads, Juv. Diabetes Found. Countdown **8**(2):14-17, 1987.

Tauer, K.M.: Physiologic mechanisms in childhood hypoglycemia, Pediatr. Nurs. **9:**341-344, 1983.

Turco, S.J.: Absorption of insulin in infusion containers and tubing, Am. J. Intrav. Ther. Nutr. **9:**44, 1982.

Villeneuve, M.E., Murphy, J., and Mazze, R.S.: Evaluating blood glucose monitors, Am. J. Nurs. **85:**1258-1259, 1985.

White, N.E., and Miller, B.K.: Glycohemoglobin: a new test to help the diabetic stay in control, Nursing 83 **13**(8):55-57, 1983.

Zimmerman, E., and others: Diabetic camping: effect on knowledge, attitude, and self-concept, Issues Compr. Pediatr. Nurs. **10:**99-111, 1987.

CHAPTER 29

The Child with Integumentary Dysfunction

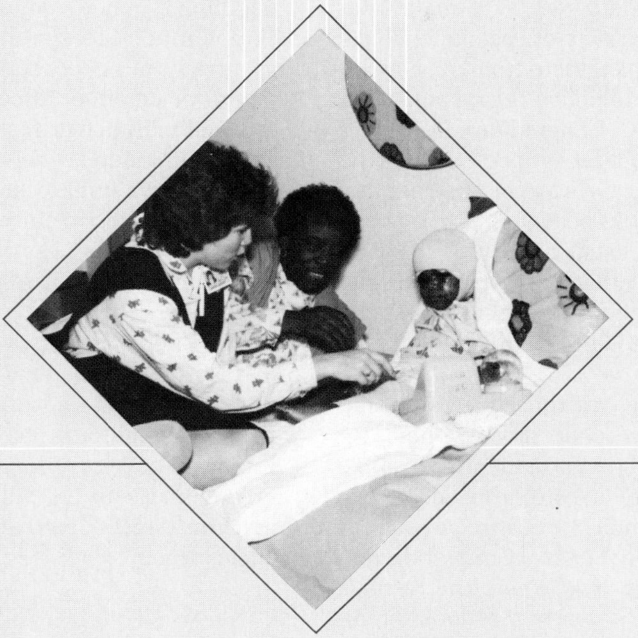

LEARNING OBJECTIVES

On completion of this chapter the reader will be able to:

- Describe the distribution and configuration of the various skin lesions
- Discuss the nursing care related to therapies for skin disorders
- Contrast the manifestations of and therapies for bacterial, viral, and fungal infections of the skin
- Compare the skin manifestations related to age in children
- Outline a plan of care for a child with atopic dermatitis
- Formulate a teaching plan for an adolescent with acne
- Describe the methods for assessing a burn wound
- Discuss the physical and emotional care of a child with a severe burn wound

The skin, the largest organ of the body, is not merely a covering but also a complex structure that serves many functions, the most important of which are to protect the tissues that it encloses and to protect itself. This pliable sheath is a vital shield against the shifting physical and chemical stresses of the environment, and it fulfills that role to the extent that outside changes are not transmitted inward to upset the body's internal equilibrium. The skin is primarily an insulator, not an organ of exchange.

DISORDERS AFFECTING THE SKIN

Diseases of the skin focus sharply on the epidermis, which is the site of many distinctive patterns ranging from the vesiculation of contact dermatitis to common superficial tumors. Clearly visible, these morphologic changes produce the varied patterns on which a dermatologic diagnosis is made.

Lesions of the skin or disorders with skin manifestations can be a result of a wide variety of specific etiologic factors. In general, skin lesions originate from (1) contact with injurious agents, such as infective organisms, toxic chemicals, and physical trauma, (2) hereditary factors, or (3) some external factor that produces a reaction in the skin; for example, allergens. In the case of external factors, the damage is caused by the body's response to the agent rather than by the agent itself. Such responses are highly individualized. An agent that may be harmless to one individual may be damaging to another, and a single agent may produce various types of responses in different individuals.

Among other factors involved in the etiology of skin manifestations is the age of the child. For example, infants are subject to "birthmark" malformations and atopic dermatitis, which appear early in life; the school-age child is susceptible to ringworm of the scalp; and acne is a characteristic skin disorder of puberty. Contact dermatitis, such as poison ivy, is seen only where the noxious agent is a feature of the area. Similarly reactions to animal bites are associated with the animal's life cycle and seasonal activities. Tension and anxiety may produce, modify, or prolong many skin conditions, although this happens less commonly in children.

Pathophysiology

Over half of dermatologic problems are various forms of dermatitis. This implies a sequence of inflammatory changes in the skin that are grossly and microscopically similar but diverse in course and causation. Acute responses produce intercellular and intracellular edema, the formation of intradermal vesicles, and an initial minimum infiltration of inflammatory cells into the epidermis. In the dermis there is edema, vascular dilation, and early perivascular cellular infiltration. The location and manner of these reactions produce the lesions characteristic of each disorder. The changes are reversible, and the skin ordinarily recovers without blemish and completely intact unless complicating factors, such as ulceration from the primary irritant, scratching, and infection, are introduced or underlying vascular disease develops. In chronic conditions permanent effects are seen that vary according to the disorder, the general condition of the affected individual, and available therapy.

Skin of Younger Children

Several characteristics influence skin responses in infants and young children. Their skin is far more susceptible to superficial bacterial infection. They are more likely to have associated systemic symptoms with some infections and are more apt to react to a primary irritant than to a sensitizing allergen. In the infant and small child the epidermis is still loosely bound to the corium. Consequently the layers may easily separate during an inflammatory process to form blisters or during careless handling (such as removal of adhesive tape). The infant's skin is much more prone to developing a toxic erythema as a result of skin eruptions or drug reactions and is subject to maceration, infection, and the sweat retention associated with diaper rash.

The transitional zone between the epidermal layers, which allows fluid to flow from lower layers to outer layers, is less effective in young children than in older children and adults. Consequently the small child's skin chaps more easily. Also, sebaceous glands are very active prenatally, when they produce the protective *vernix caseosa*. The sebaceous activity slowly subsides after birth and continues to decrease throughout infancy. In the newborn period and early infancy, sebaceous secretions may cause minor problems such as "cradle cap" in some infants. The secretion gradually rises in childhood to increase markedly at puberty, when it remains constant and contributes greatly to the disturbing skin problems of adolescence.

Diagnostic Evaluation

One of the more advantageous aspects of skin disorders is that often the diagnosis is readily established after simple, careful inspection. Much can be determined by the distribution, size, morphology, and arrangement of the lesions. Extrinsic causes usually result from physical, chemical, or allergic irritants or from an infectious agent such as bacteria, fungi, viruses, or animal parasites. Skin manifestations can be produced by such intrinsic causes as a specific infection (such as measles or chickenpox), drug sensitization, or other allergic phenomena. Other diagnostic tools are subjective symptoms, history, and medical and laboratory studies.

Lesion. According to the nature of the pathologic process, lesions assume more or less distinct characteristics. Although the names that have been applied to these lesions are of little value in themselves, they are important for descriptive purposes in the processes of record keeping and communication. For example, a reddened area is usually caused by increased amounts of oxygenated blood in the dermal vasculature and is described as *erythema*. Hemorrhages into the skin produce localized discolorations.

Nurses should also become familiar with the more common terms used to describe skin lesions seen in dermatologic conditions:

erythema a reddened area caused by increased amounts of oxygenated blood in the dermal vasculature
ecchymoses (bruises) localized red or purple discolorations

Flat circumscribed area of color changes less than 1 cm in diameter, neither elevated nor depressed and with no alteration in skin texture

Example: Freckle, nevus, measles

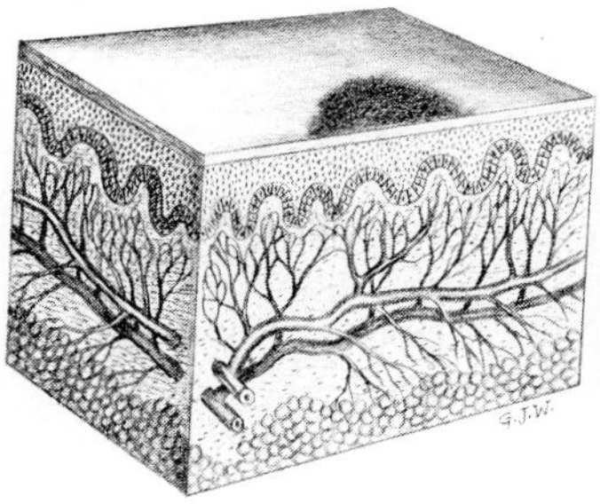

Macule

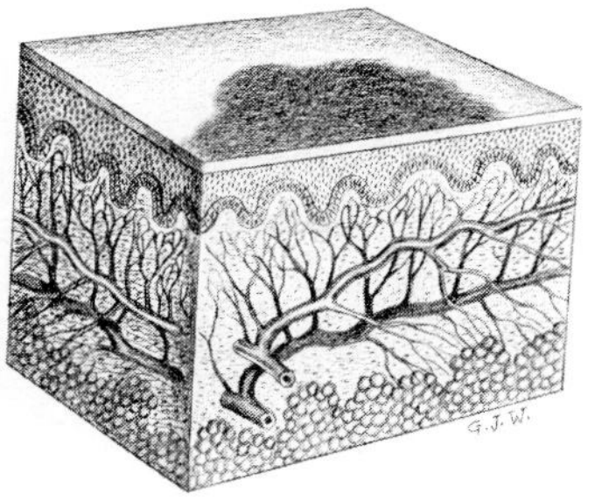

Patch

Flat circumscribed discoloration of skin greater than 1 cm in diameter

Example: Mongolian spot, vitiligo

Small, circumscribed solid elevation of the skin, less than 1 cm in diameter; exists mostly above the plane of the skin surface, and the more superficial it is, the more distinct are the borders

Example: Wart, ringworm

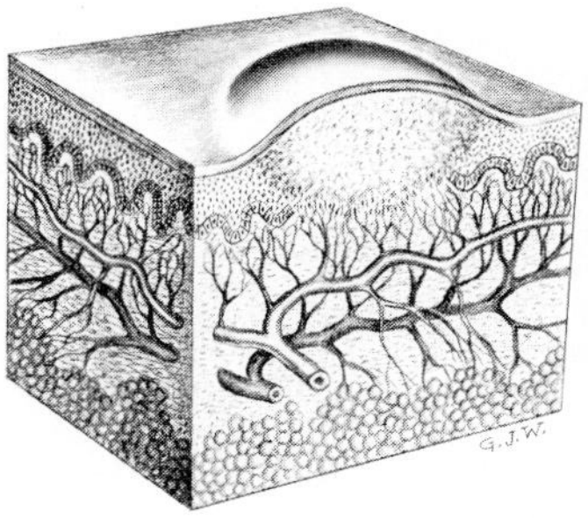

Papule

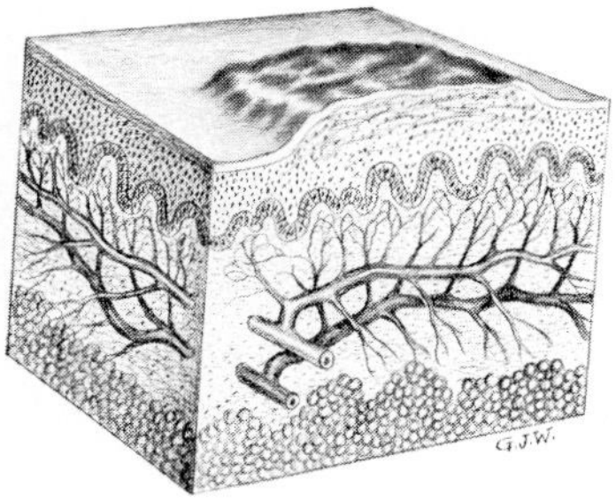

Plaque

Flattened, raised lesion in which the surface area involved is relatively large in relation to its height

Example: Psoriasis

Solid circumscribed elevation, round or ellipsoid, located deep in dermis or subcutaneous tissue

Example: Dermatofibroma

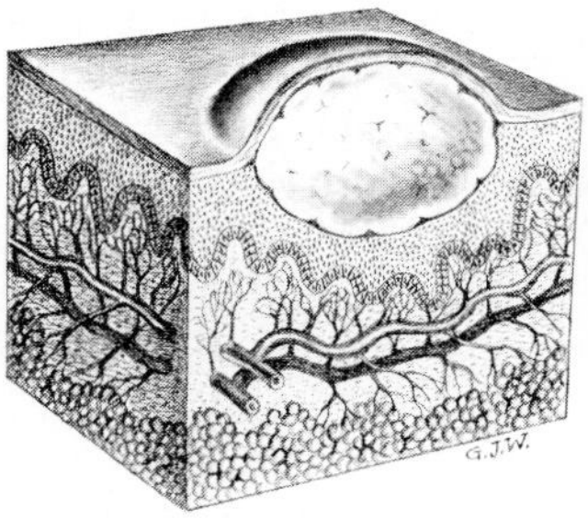

Tumor

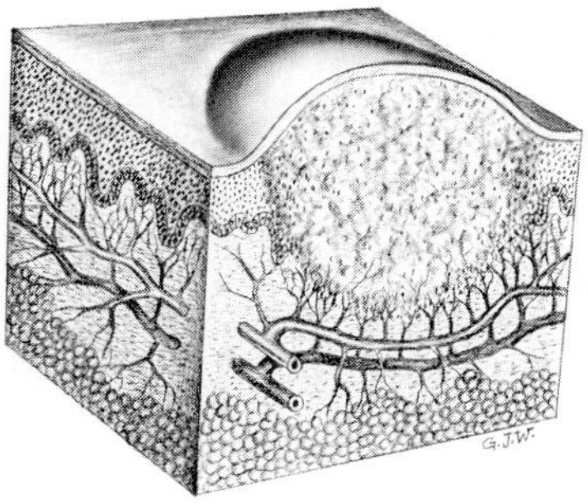

Nodule

Circumscribed infiltration of skin or subcutaneous tissue that is larger (greater than 1 cm in diameter) and deeper than nodule

Example: Cavernous hemangioma

Encapsulated semisolid or fluid-filled mass in dermis or subcutaneous tissue

Example: Epidermoid cyst

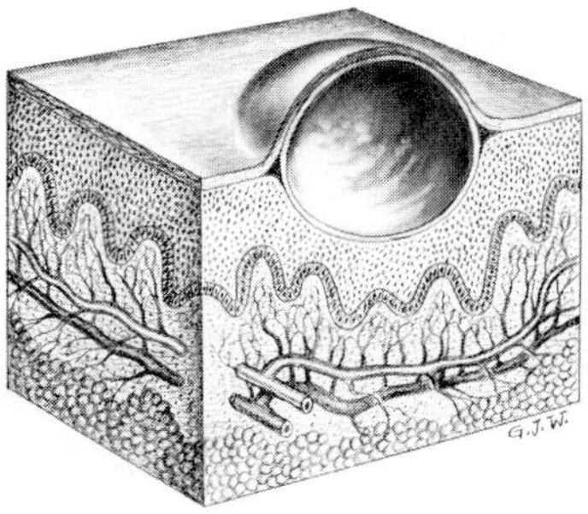

Cyst

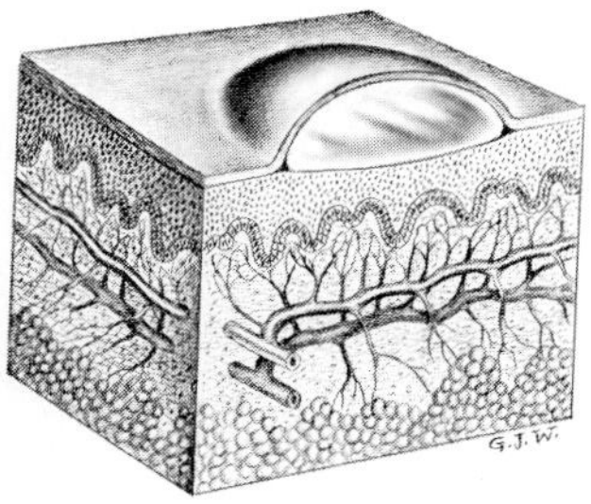

Vesicle

Small (less than 1 cm in diameter), superficial circumscribed elevation of the skin containing serous or blood-tinged fluid

Example: Chickenpox, herpes, poison ivy, dermatitis

FIG. 29-1 Primary skin lesions.

Continued.

Vesicle filled with pus that may or may not be caused by infection

Example: Acne, impetigo, folliculitis

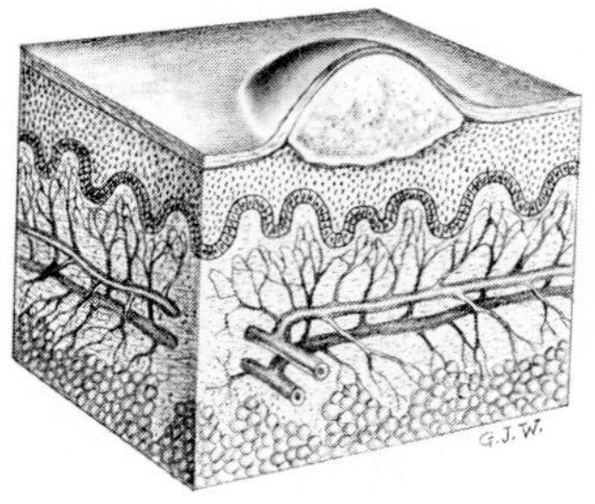

Pustule

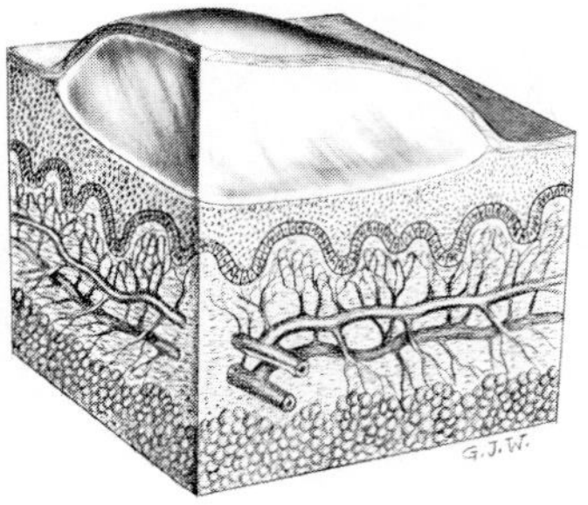

Bulla

Fluid-filled vesicle greater than 1 cm in diameter; a large vesicle; bleb; blister

Example: Second-degree burn

Round or flat-topped and irregularly shaped, evanescent lesions resulting from acute accumulation of edema fluid in upper dermis

Example: Mosquito bites, urticaria

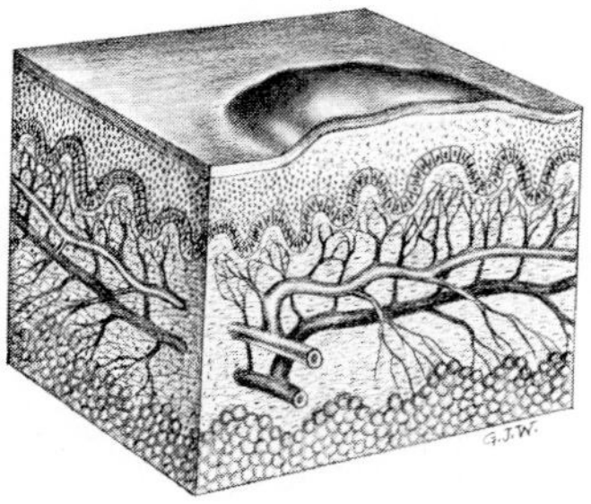

Wheal

FIG. 29-1, cont'd Primary skin lesions.

caused by extravasation of blood into dermis and subcutaneous tissues

petechiae pinpoint, tiny and, sharp circumscribed spots in the superficial layers of the epidermis

primary lesions skin changes produced by some causative factor (Fig. 29-1)

secondary lesions changes that result from alteration in the primary lesions, such as those caused by rubbing, scratching, medication, or involution (Fig. 29-2)

distribution pattern the pattern in which lesions are distributed over the body, whether local or generalized, and specific areas associated with the lesions

configuration and arrangement the size, shape, and arrangement of a lesion or groups of lesions; for example, discrete, clustered, diffuse, or confluent

History and subjective symptoms. Many cutaneous lesions are associated with local symptoms, the most common of which is itching that varies in kind and intensity. Pain or tenderness often accompanies some skin lesions, and other sensations may be described as burning, prickling, stinging, or crawling. Alterations in local feeling or sensation include absence of sensation (anesthesia), excessive sensitiveness (hyperesthesia), or diminished sensation (hypesthesia or hypoesthesia). These symptoms may remain localized or may migrate, may be constant or intermittent, and may be aggravated by a specific activity or circumstance, such as exposure to sunlight.

It is also important to determine whether the child has had an allergic condition such as asthma or hay fever or has had previous skin disease. Atopic dermatitis, often associated with allergies, frequently begins in infancy. It should be determined when the lesion or symptom first became apparent as well as whether it is related to ingestion of a food or other substance, including any medication the child might be taking. It should be kept in mind that the condition may be related to an activity such as contact with plants, insects, or chemicals.

Laboratory studies. When it is suspected that a skin problem might be related to a systemic disease, such as one of the collagen diseases or immune deficiency disease, studies are needed to rule out these possibilities. Microscopic examination of a skin lesion may be essential in many chronic conditions and in pigmented nevi. Cultures in bacterial infections, scrapings for fungal infections, allergic skin testing, and various other laboratory tests (blood count, sedimentation rate) are employed when indicated.

General Therapeutic Management

The major aims of any treatment are to prevent further damage, eliminate the cause, prevent complications, and provide relief from discomfort while tissues undergo healing. Factors that contribute to the dermatitis and may prolong the course of the disease must be eliminated where possible. The most common offenders in pediatrics are environmental factors, such as soaps; bubble baths; shampoos; rough or tight clothing, blankets, or toys; and the natural elements, such as dirt, sand, heat, cold, moisture, and wind. Dermatitis can also be aggravated by home remedies and medications.

Topical therapy. A variety of agents and methods are available for treatment of dermatologic problems. In selecting a therapeutic program the practitioner considers (1) a choice of active ingredient, (2) a proper vehicle or base, (3) the cosmetic effect, (4) the cost, and (5) instruc-

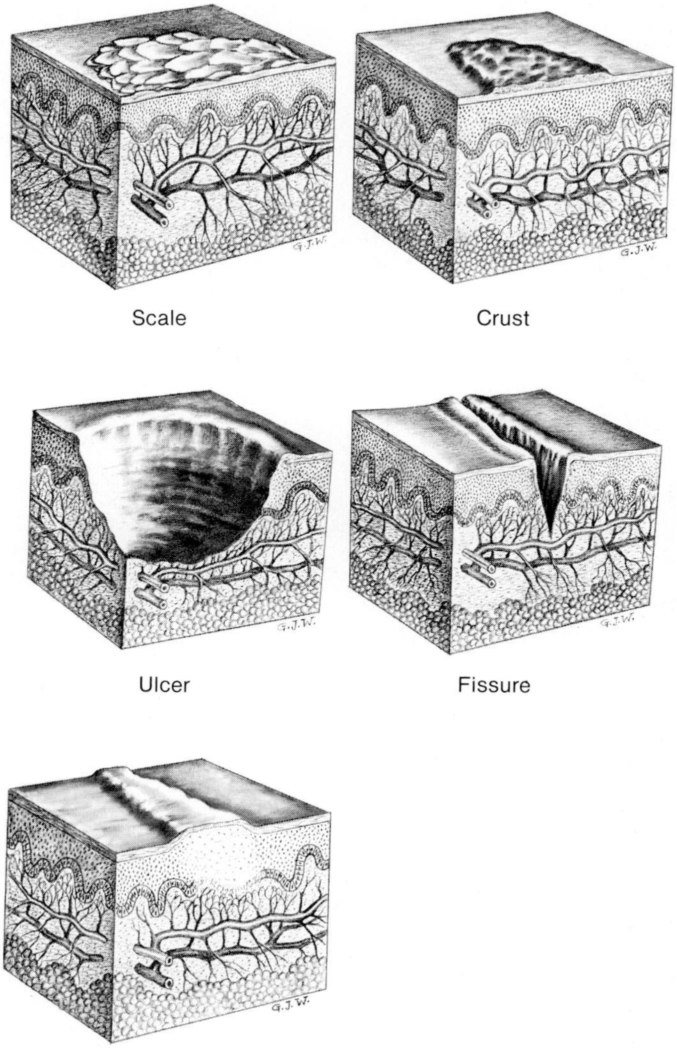

Flakes of dead, cornified tissue being shed from skin
Example: Psoriasis, ringworm
Scale
Crust
Dried masses of serum, pus, dead skin, and debris that can be found surmounting any lesion
Example: Impetigo, other infectious dermatitis
Irregularly shaped, excavation caused by loss of substance with gradual disintegration and necrosis of tissue
Example: Decubiti
Ulcer
Fissure
Deep linear split through epidermis into dermis
Example: Chapping
Permanent dermal changes with production of excess collagen following damage to corium
Example: Vaccination, burns, deep scratches
Scar

FIG. 29-2 Secondary skin lesions.

tions for its use. In addition, several basic concepts are kept in mind. Overtreatment is avoided. For example, when the dermatitis is acute, the applications should be mild and bland to avoid further irritation. Broken or inflamed skin, especially in children, is more absorbent than intact skin, and chemicals that are nonirritating to intact skin may be quite irritating to inflamed skin.

Topical applications may be given to treat the disorder, reduce the itching associated with many diseases, decrease external stimuli, or apply external heat or cold. The emollient action of soaks, baths, and lotions provides a soothing film over the skin surface that reduces external stimuli. Application of heat tends to aggravate most conditions, and its use is usually reserved for reducing specific inflammatory processes, such as folliculitis and cellulitis. Ordinarily applications offer most relief when they are lukewarm, tepid, or cool.

The most frequent means of topical treatment for skin disorders are wet dressings, soaks, lotions and shake solutions, baths, creams and ointments, sprays and aerosols, pastes, powders, occlusive dressings, soaps and shampoos, other topical treatments, and topical glucocorticoid therapy.

Topical corticosteroid therapy. The glucocorticoids exert a local anti-inflammatory effect but are merely palliative, so the medication must be applied until the disease state undergoes a remission or the causative agent is eliminated. Corticosteroids are applied directly to the affected area and can be applied over prolonged periods with continuing effectiveness. As with the use of any steroids, in large amounts they may mask signs of infection and there may be exacerbation of symptoms following termination of the drug.

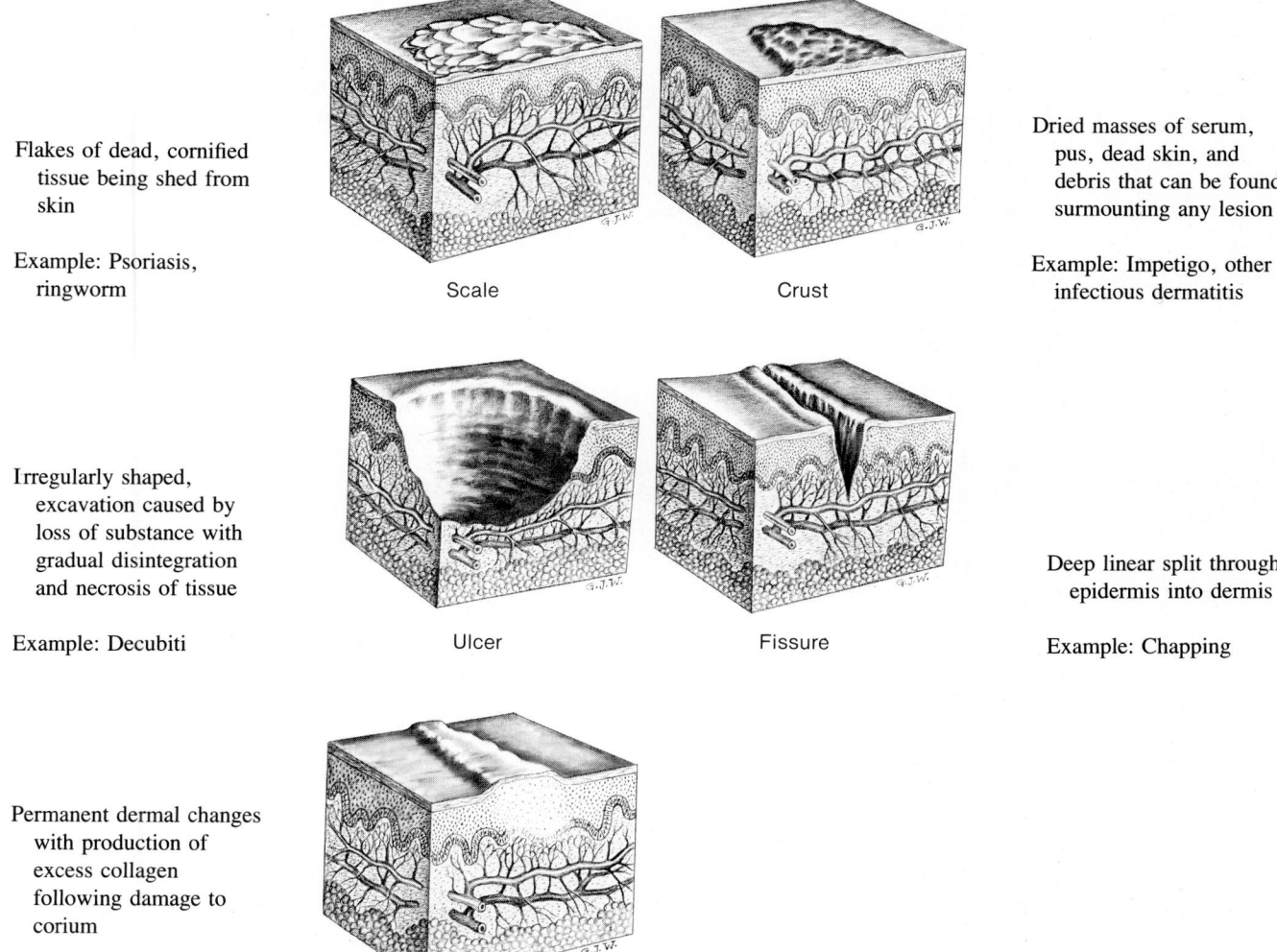

Families should be cautioned that the medication cannot be used for all skin disorders. The concentrations available without prescription are not adequate for some stubborn conditions (e.g., psoriasis) and may cause worsening of inflammation caused by fungus or bacteria. It has also been found that users apply too much topical hydrocortisone; therefore they should be counseled that it is both effective and economical to apply only a thin film and massage it into the skin.

Other topical therapies. Other topical treatments include chemical cautery (especially useful for warts), cryosurgery, electrodesiccation (chiefly used for warts, granulomas, and nevi), ultraviolet therapy (primarily used in psoriasis and acne), and special acne therapies such as dermabrasion and acne "surgery."

Systemic therapy. Therapeutic agents are often used as an adjunct to topical therapy in dermatologic disorders, and those most frequently used therapeutically are the corticosteroids and the antibiotics. Corticosteroid dosage is carefully adjusted and gradually tapered to the minimum that is effective and tolerated. Protracted use may temporarily suppress growth, however.

Antibiotics, which interfere with the growth of microorganisms, are used in severe or widespread skin infections. The danger inherent in the use of antibiotics is their tendency to produce a hypersensitivity in the patient; therefore they are used with caution. Antifungal agents are the only means for treating systemic fungal infections.

Nursing Considerations

Skin disorders present nurses with some of their most challenging problems. In children the identification of skin disorders requires a familiarity with various types of lesions in order to accurately describe them and to advise parents regarding medical consultation. Removal of foreign objects (such as small splinters), mild sunburn, and scratches pose no problem, but lesions, lacerations, and bites need careful evaluation and referral.

ASSESSMENT

To assist in establishing a diagnosis, it is important for nurses to accurately describe any deviation in the character of the skin, using both inspection and palpation. The color, shape, and distribution of the lesions are noted, including absence of pigment (vitiligo). The individual lesions are described according to the accepted terminology and may involve more than one type, such as a maculopapular rash.

To confirm or amplify the findings made by inspection, the skin is gently palpated to detect characteristics such as temperature, moisture, texture, elasticity, and the presence of edema. It should be indicated whether the findings are restricted to the area of the lesion(s) or are generalized.

The child's subjective symptoms provide additional information. Older children are able to describe the condition as painful, itching, or tingling, or they may use other descriptive terms. However, much can be determined by observation of the child's behavior and the parents' account of his reactions. A doubtful diagnosis is frequently confirmed on the basis of history.

The skin is assessed before the treatment or application of medication and reassessed after the treatment is completed. Any observed changes are noted and described. Nursing responsibilities related to specific disorders are discussed in relation to those disorders.

NURSING DIAGNOSES

Nursing diagnoses are identified following an assessment of the child and the skin lesions. The major diagnoses identified for the child with a disorder manifest in the skin are outlined in the Nursing Care Plan, pp. 975 to 976.

PLANNING

The goals of care for the child with a skin condition are:

1. Prevent secondary damage to the lesion(s)
2. Relieve discomfort
3. Educate and support the child and family

IMPLEMENTATION

Since only a few skin diseases are contagious, it is usually not necessary to isolate the affected child unless there is a danger of acquiring a secondary infection. This is usually the child who is receiving large doses of corticosteroids or other immunosuppressant drugs or the child with an immunologic deficiency disorder. If the skin manifestation is caused by a viral exanthem, such as measles or chickenpox, the child should be prevented from exposing other susceptible children to the disease.

Autoinoculation is a constant hazard in some disorders such as impetigo or (to a lesser extent) warts. The cooperation of older children can be obtained, although they may need reminding to stop scratching or rubbing, but smaller and uncooperative children require the use of techniques and devices such as mittens, restraints, or special coverings. These methods, along with general cleanliness and hygiene, also serve to reduce the likelihood of secondary infection of a primary lesion.

Therapeutic programs are usually designed to provide general measures such as rest, protection, and relief of discomfort and specific treatments such as a definitive medication or physical technique. They usually involve some type of topical treatment, and the mode of application depends on the nature and location of the lesion being treated.

Most of the therapeutic regimens are directed toward relief of pruritus, the most common subjective complaint. Cooling applications that reduce external stimuli to the affected part are highly beneficial together with maintenance of cleanliness and good aeration. Clothing and bed linen should be soft and lightweight to decrease the irritation from friction and stimulation. During any type of treatment both affected and unaffected areas of skin are protected from damage and secondary infection.

Nurses and parents are responsible for the application of topical therapeutic agents and the administration of systemic medications. Most topical preparations are ap-

Nursing Tip: Topical Applications

Apply topical applications systematically with the contour of the body surface (not simply up and down).

plied to intact skin with the bare hands. The use of bare hands has the advantage of communicating an attitude of acceptance to the child and the family. It is especially important to wash the hands before and after application of topical therapies. Gloves are worn for applications to nonintact skin.

Wet dressings. Open wet dressings and compresses are probably the mildest form of topical therapy. They cool the skin by evaporation, relieve itching and inflammation, and cleanse the area by loosening and removing crusts and debris. Any of a variety of ingredients, such as the time-honored Burow solution (available without a prescription), can be applied on Kerlix gauze, plain gauze, or (preferably) soft cotton cloths such as freshly laundered handkerchiefs or strips from diaper, sheeting, or pillowcase material.

Dressings immersed in the desired solution are wrung out slightly and applied to the affected area wet but not dripping. They are applied flat and smooth and in such a way that motion is not totally restricted—fingers are wrapped separately and arms and legs are wrapped so that elbows and knees can bend. Dressings are kept in place by Kerlix or other cotton wrap, tubular stockinette, mittens, or socks (two pair—one to hold the dressings in place, the other to take up movement) but are left uncovered. When evaporation begins to dry them, the dressings are removed, rewet in the solution, and reapplied to the area using aseptic technique. The solution is not poured or syringed directly over the dressings. As fluid evaporates, the solution becomes increasingly concentrated, altering the strength of the solution, which may be damaging to sensitive lesions.

Water is the most important ingredient in wet dressings, and evaporation is primarily responsible for the symptomatic relief experienced by the patient. The most common solutions used for wet dressings are aluminum acetate (Burow solution) and normal saline. They are applied to cleanse and disinfect open, oozing, crusting, and/or secondarily infected lesions. Sometimes fresh warm or tepid tap water is used alone or in conjunction with topical steroids.

Fresh solution at room temperature is applied at 2-, 3-, or 4-hour intervals and is allowed to remain on the lesion from 30 minutes to 1½ hours. Wet dressings are seldom continued after about 48 hours. The child must be guarded against chilling during treatment, and no more than one third of the body should be covered at one time. After treatment the skin is dried thoroughly by patting with a towel. Application of lotion or other medication may be ordered at this time.

Occlusive dressings. Used primarily in association with topical steroids, occlusive dressings are usually restricted to treatment of chronic dermatoses. A thin application of ointment or cream is covered with a thin, transparent, pliable plastic film anchored with adhesive. The treatment consists of an 8- to 10-hour period, usually overnight, and covers no more than 10% of the body.

Small children may need some type of restraint, depending on the location of the dressing. Often clothing can be worn that covers the area; for example, leg dressings are covered with pants legs. If the child attempts to remove or disturb the dressings, elbow restraints may be needed. Diversional activities are always a useful nursing tool.

Soaks. When young children are uncooperative in the use of wet dressings, soaks are often employed for removal of crusts and for their mild astringent action, using the same solution employed for wet compresses. Gaining young children's cooperation for hand or foot soaks is difficult unless the procedure is made attractive to them through play (see Nursing tip).

Nursing Tip: Play Activities

Older infants and toddlers delight in playing with brightly colored objects or poker chips scattered over the bottom of the receptacle, and preschoolers can be challenged to hold a floating item beneath the water's surface. These activities require supervision; infants and small children will often place items in their mouths, and children can easily lose control with water play.

Washing dishes, cars, dolls, or doll clothes will occupy many children for quite some time. The older child is able to cooperate but may need something to do during the procedure, such as listening to music or a story or watching television.

Nursing Tip: Soaking an Extremity

Soaking a single extremity (a foot or a hand) can be easily accomplished by placing the solution and the extremity in a plastic sealable bag. The closure is then zipped snugly around the limb. This method for soaking fingers or toes can be highly entertaining to young children (Perelson and Seyler, 1985).

Baths. Baths are especially useful in the treatment of widespread dermatitis, because they evenly distribute the soothing antipruritic and anti-inflammatory effects of the solution, usually oatmeal or mineral oil preparations. The solution is added to a tub of lukewarm water. The temperature of the bath is tepid, and the duration of treatment is usually 15 to 30 minutes. Therapeutic baths are always more interesting when the child is accompanied by toy boats or other items for water play.

Lotions. Lotions are preparations of powder suspended in solution; the container must be well shaken before application. As the liquid evaporates, it cools the skin and provides it with a coating of soothing, lubricating, protective, and drying powder. Lotions are applied evenly over the skin with the hands or gauze. Lotions are frequently applied after wet dressings or soaks but not to oozing surfaces. They are not ordinarily washed off between applications but may be removed by soaking with the solution used for soaks or dressings.

Nursing Tip: Applying Lotion

Children love to be "painted." Therefore lotion applications can be fun when an ordinary paintbrush is used.

Creams and gels. Creams and gels are easily and evenly spread over the skin. Both tend to disappear when rubbed into the skin, and they are less occlusive and esthetically more pleasing than ointments. Creams and gels are nongreasy and readily removed with soap and water. They are applied by placing a teaspoonful of the preparation in the palm of the hand, rubbing it briskly between the hands until the consistency is thin and smooth, and then applying it to the skin area.

Ointments. The major constituent of ointments is oil. The lipid component may consist of animal fats, such as lard or wool fat (lanolin), petrolatum, or vegetable oils. Ointments that contain 20% to 50% water (such as cold cream and Eucerin) vanish on application and are removable with water but leave a greasy sensation to the skin. Absorbent ointments contain no water but will absorb water and are more lubricating than water in oil preparations. They have a greasy sensation and are difficult to remove with soap and water. Water-repellent ointments, such as petrolatum, retain heat for increased absorption of medications but are difficult to remove and can cause maceration when used with an occlusive dressing. If ointment is not absorbed but remains on the skin, too much is being applied. Ointments are not used in hairy, intertriginous, or macerated areas.

Pastes. Pastes are powders mixed with an ointment base. More porous and less occlusive than ointments, they absorb moisture and produce a drying effect. Because they are difficult to apply and must be removed from the skin with mineral oil, pastes are used less frequently than other preparations. They are most easily applied with a tongue depressor and are "buttered" on.

Powders. There is some controversy over the use of powders in pediatrics. They are very effective for soothing, absorbing moisture, and protecting the skin by reducing friction. Since they are chemically inert, their chief use is prophylactic when applied to intertriginous areas. However, powder must be applied in a fine film that does not cake or form lumps when wet, and care must be exerted to prevent the child from inhaling the powder, especially if it contains talc or kaolin. To reduce the risk of inhalation, powder is sprinkled into the palm of the hand and then applied to the skin surface; it is never sprinkled directly onto the patient's skin. The container is placed well out of reach of the child.

Sprays and aerosols. Many active agents are now available suspended in an alcohol-based spray. Such sprays serve as an alternative method of delivering a solution to the skin when direct application is difficult or uncomfortable for the patient. The container must be shaken thoroughly before application and the child's face shielded from the spray to avoid inhalation.

Soaps and shampoos. Germicidal soaps are useful adjunctive therapy for skin infections. Bactericidal agents are found in many of the well-known soaps. Soaps containing hexachlorophene are used with caution to reduce the risk of absorption, especially on broken or denuded areas. When absorbed, large amounts of the drug can cause central nervous system symptoms. Another effective topical microbicide is povidone-iodine (Betadine) skin cleanser, which assists in disinfecting the skin and is effective in eliminating common pathogens, including *Staphylococcus aureus*.

Shampoos that are used in dermatologic skin conditions include tar shampoos for resistant scalp seborrhea and psoriasis and antiparasitic shampoos, such as gamma benzene hexachloride (Kwell) for pediculosis capitis and scabies (see p. 984).

Sunscreening agents. Chemicals that have the capacity to absorb certain wavelengths of light are especially useful in dermatoses when applied to light-exposed areas. They provide skin protection for hours under ordinary circumstances. (For further discussion of sunscreening agents, see Sunburn, p. 1008.)

Home care and family support. Dermatologic conditions always involve the family. Since few situations require hospitalization and children who are hospitalized will complete a therapy program at home, the family must carry out the treatment plan; therefore their cooperation is essential. Regimens that are simple to accomplish in the hospital or office may be frustrating and baffling at home. The family often needs assistance in adapting equipment available in the home to the therapy.

It is important that the child and family be given as detailed explanations as possible about both the expected and unexpected results of treatment, including any ill effects that might occur. If unexplained reactions do develop, the family is directed to discontinue treatment and report the reactions to the appropriate person(s). The use of over-the-counter medicines is discouraged unless this has first been discussed with the attending practitioner and received approval.

Since the skin is the most visible portion of the body, defects in its surface that alter its appearance are sometimes a source of distress to the child and of revulsion and rejection by others. Parents of other children may fear that their children will "catch" the disorder. Occasionally the affected child's own family members will reduce their interaction with him, especially close physical contact, or otherwise demonstrate a distaste for the con-

NURSING CARE PLAN

The Child with a Disorder Affecting the Skin

Nursing Goals	Nursing Interventions	Expected Patient/Family Outcomes
HP-HMP* Potential for infection **Risk factors: infectious agents, damaged skin, mechanical trauma (e.g., scratching)**		
Prevent spread of infection to self and others	Isolate affected child from susceptible individuals if indicated Maintain careful handwashing after caring for child Avoid unnecessary close contact with affected child during infective stage of disease Use correct technique for disposal of dressings, solutions, and other fomites in contact with lesion(s) Teach and reinforce positive habits of hygienic care	Infection remains confined to primary site Child and family comply with preventive measures
Prevent secondary infection	Maintain careful handwashing before handling affected child Wear surgical gloves when handling or dressing affected parts if indicated by nature of lesion Teach child and family hygienic care and medical asepsis Devise methods to prevent secondary infection of lesion in small or uncooperative children	Infection remains confined to primary lesions
Protect healthy skin surface	Teach and impress on child importance of keeping hands away from lesion(s) Help child determine ways of preventing autoinoculation Devise means for keeping small or uncooperative children from spreading infection to other areas Protect healthy skin from maceration by keeping it dry	Skin lesions remain confined to primary sites
Prevent occurrence and/or recurrence	Avoid or reduce contact with agents or circumstances known to precipitate skin reaction Teach child to recognize agents or circumstances that produce reaction	Child avoids precipitating agents
N-MP Impaired skin integrity **Etiology: environmental agents, somatic factors**		
Identify lesion and its cause	Describe skin lesion accurately; use descriptive terminology for type, configuration, and distribution of lesion(s) Describe any associated characteristics such as temperature, moisture, texture, elasticity, and hardness of skin in general or in area of lesion(s) Obtain history of onset, possible precipitating events, and course of development Determine any symptoms associated with disorder such as itching, pain, and fever	†Lesion(s) is accurately described †Associated factors are enumerated
Promote healing	Carry out therapeutic regimens as prescribed or support and assist parents in carrying out treatment plan Prevent secondary infection and autoinoculation Encourage rest Reduce external stimuli that aggravate condition Encourage well-balanced diet	Affected area exhibits signs of healing
CPP Pain **Etiology: skin lesions**		
Relieve discomfort	Assess need for pain medication (see p. 587) Avoid or reduce external stimuli that aggravate discomfort, such as clothing and bed linen Implement other appropriate nonpharmacologic pain reduction techniques (see p. 591)	Child remains calm and exhibits no evidence of discomfort

*For an explanation of abbreviations, see p. 20.
†Nursing outcome.

Continued.

NURSING CARE PLAN

The Child with a Disorder Affecting the Skin—cont'd

Nursing Goals	Nursing Interventions	Expected Patient/Family Outcomes
Promote rest	Plan meals, baths, medications, and treatments around nap or bedtime Make child as comfortable as possible before sleep to enhance restfulness (for example, give sedation and then bathe before bedtime)	Child receives an adequate amount of rest for age
Prevent or minimize scratching	Keep fingernails and toenails short and clean Wrap hands in soft cotton gloves or stockings; pin to shirt cuff Avoid overheating, high humidity, and perspiration Use elbow restraints when absolutely necessary but allow supervised periods of unrestricted movement Encourage exposure to ultraviolet light, but avoid sunburn	Affected areas remain unirritated
ND SP-SCP **Body image disturbance** **Etiology: perception of appearance**		
Promote a positive self-image	Encourage child to express feelings about his appearance and the way he thinks others view him	Child verbalizes feelings and concerns
Provide tactile contact	Hold child Remember that there is no substitute for the stimulation and comfort of human contact Touch and caress unaffected area	Child exhibits signs of comfort Child responds positively to tactile stimulation
Support child	Teach self-care where appropriate Involve child in planning treatment schedules Support and encourage child in efforts to deal with multiple problems that may be associated with disorder, including discomfort, rejection, discouragement, and feelings of self-revulsion Encourage child to maintain usual activities	Child collaborates in determining means for improving appearance Child maintains customary activities and relationships
ND RRP **Altered family processes** **Etiology: situational crisis (child with a skin condition)**		
Support family	Teach family skills needed to carry out therapeutic program Inform family of expected and unexpected results of therapy and a course of action to follow Help devise special techniques to carry out therapy Be aware of overprotectiveness and restrictiveness, which can stifle child's emotional growth Allow and encourage family members, particularly the one who cares for the child most of the time, to express negative feelings, such as anger, frustration, and perhaps guilt Stress that negative feelings are normal, acceptable, and expected but that they must have an outlet in order for family members to remain healthy Encourage family in efforts to carry out plan of care Provide assistance when appropriate Refer to agencies and services that assist with social, financial, and medical problems	Family demonstrates necessary skills (specify) Family demonstrates positive interaction with child Family expresses feelings of frustration and concern Family contacts appropriate agencies (specify)

Nursing interventions related to medical management

Assist with diagnosis
- Participate in special tests, such as collection of specimens for laboratory examination, use of Wood light, or elimination diet

Promote healing
- Carry out therapeutic regimen
  - Topical treatments and applications
- Administer systemic medications as prescribed

Relieve discomfort
- Apply soothing treatments and topical applications as ordered
- Administer medications to relieve discomfort and/or restlessness and irritability

dition, which the child may interpret as rejection. This is seldom a difficulty with dermatitis of short duration, but chronic conditions can create problems in development of a positive self-concept.

EVALUATION

The effectiveness of nursing interventions is determined by continual reassessment and evaluation of care based on the following observational guidelines and expected outcomes:

1. Observe if reasonable care is used in performing nursing activities, and observe lesions and child's reactions to therapies.
2. Employ assessment techniques to identify relief of discomfort as described on p. 587.
3. Reassess skin lesions; observe and interview child and family regarding compliance with therapy.

Expected outcomes:

See Nursing Care Plan for the child with a skin disorder, pp. 975 to 976.

◆ *Infections of the Skin*

Dermatologic infections and other disorders of the skin constitute a significant portion of the complaints that prompt children's visits to offices and clinics. Most such conditions are troublesome ailments and the source of considerable physical and emotional discomfort. For most of the disorders the diagnosis and treatment are relatively simple; for others the management is more complex and puzzling.

BACTERIAL INFECTIONS

Normally the skin harbors a variety of bacterial flora, including the major pathogenic varieties of staphylococci and streptococci. The degree of their pathogenicity depends on the specific organism's invasiveness and toxigenicity, the integrity of the skin, the barrier of the host, and the immune and cellular defenses of the host. Children with immune deficiency states are highly susceptible to bacterial invasion. This includes infants, children with congenital immune deficiency disorders, children in a debilitated condition, those on immunosuppressive therapy, and those with a generalized malignancy such as leukemia or lymphoma.

Because of the characteristic "walling-off" process of the inflammatory reaction (abscess formation), staphylococci are more difficult to attack and the local infected area is associated with an increase in numbers of bacteria all over the skin surface that serve as a source of continuing infection. Staphylococcal infections occur most often in children in the younger age-groups, and the incidence decreases with advancing age. All of these factors emphasize the importance of careful handwashing and cleanliness when caring for infected children and their lesions to prevent spread of the infection and as an essential prophylactic measure when caring for infants and small children. Common bacterial skin disorders are outlined in Table 29-1.

Nursing Considerations

The major nursing functions related to bacterial skin infections are to prevent the spread of infection and to prevent complications. Handwashing is mandatory before and after contact with an affected child. Handwashing is also emphasized to both the child and the family, and the child should be provided with towels separate from other family members. Impetigo contagiosa is easily spread by self-inoculation; therefore the child must be cautioned against touching the involved area. This is difficult to accomplish; distraction or reminders are useful but are not helpful when the child is alone, such as bedtime.

Children and parents are often tempted to squeeze follicular lesions. They must be warned that squeezing will not hasten the resolution of the infection and that there is a risk of making the lesion worse or spreading the infection. No attempt should be made to puncture the surface of the pustule with a needle or sharp instrument.

The child with limited cellulitis of an extremity is usually managed at home on oral antibiotics and warm compresses. The parents are taught the procedures and instructed in administration of the medication. Children with more extensive cellulitis, especially around a joint with lymphadenitis or on the face, are usually admitted to the hospital for parenteral antibiotics. Nurses are responsible for administering the medication, applying compresses, and maintaining the intravenous infusion.

VIRAL INFECTIONS

Viruses are intracellular parasites that produce their effect by using the intracellular substances of the host

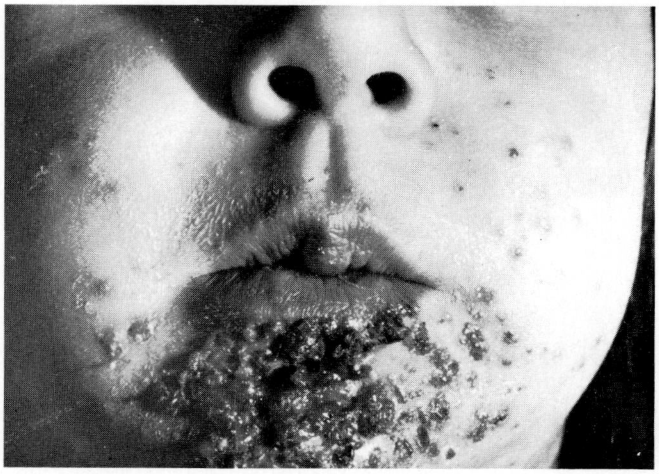

FIG. 29-3 Impetigo contagiosa. (From Stewart, W.D., Danto, J.L., and Maddin, S.: Dermatology: diagnosis and treatment of cutaneous disorders, ed. 4, St. Louis, 1978, The C.V. Mosby Co.)

TABLE 29-1

Bacterial Infections

Disorder/Organism	Manifestations	Treatment	Comments
Impetigo contagiosa (Fig. 29-3)—*Streptococcus, Staphylococcus*	Begins as a reddish macule Becomes vesicular Ruptures easily, leaving superficial, moist erosion Tends to spread peripherally in sharply marginated irregular outlines Exudate dries to form heavy, honey-colored crusts Pruritus common Systemic effects: minimal or asymptomatic	Careful removal of undermined skin, crusts, and debris by softening with 1:20 Burow solution compresses Topical application of bactericidal ointment Systemic administration of oral or parenteral antibiotics (penicillin) in severe or extensive lesions	Tends to heal without scarring unless secondary infection Autoinoculable and contagious Very common in toddler, preschooler
Pyoderma—*Staphylococcus, Streptococcus*	Deeper extension of infection into dermis Tissue reaction more severe Systemic effects: fever, lymphangitis	Soap and water cleansing Wet compresses Bathing with antibacterial soap as prescribed	Autoinoculable and contagious May heal with or without scarring
Folliculitis (pimple), furuncle (boil), carbuncle (multiple boils)—*Staphylococcus aureus*	Folliculitis: infection of hair follicle Furuncle: larger lesion with more redness and swelling at a single follicle Carbuncle: more extensive lesion with widespread inflammation and "pointing" at several follicular orifices Systemic effects: malaise, if severe	Skin cleanliness Local warm moist compresses Topical application of antibiotic agents Systemic antibiotics in severe cases Incision and drainage of severe lesions, followed by wound irrigations with antibiotics or suitable drain implantation	Autoinoculable and contagious Furuncle and carbuncle tend to heal with scar formation A lesion should *never* be squeezed
Cellulitis—*Streptococcus, Haemophilus influenzae*	Inflammation of skin and subcutaneous tissues with intense redness, swelling, and firm infiltration Lymphangitis "streaking" frequently seen Involvement of regional lymph nodes common May progress to abscess formation Systemic effects: fever, malaise	Oral or parenteral penicillin Rest and immobilization of both affected area and child Hot moist compresses to area	Hospitalization may be necessary for child with systemic symptoms

A

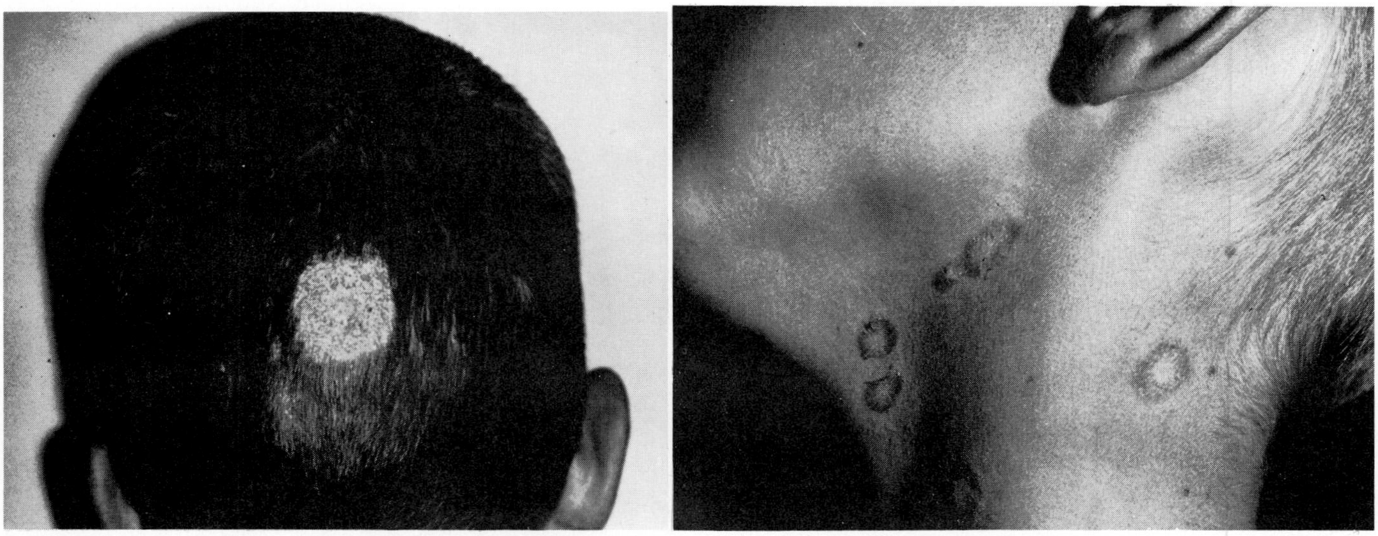

B

FIG. 29-4A, Tinea capitis. **B,** Tinea corporis. Both infections caused by *Microsporum canis*, the "kitten" or "puppy" fungus. (From Stewart, W.D., Danto, J.L., and Maddin, S.: Dermatology: diagnosis and treatment of cutaneous disorders, ed. 4, St. Louis, 1978, The C.V. Mosby Co.)

TABLE 29-2

Viral Infections

Disease	Manifestations	Treatment	Comments
Verruca (warts)	Small, benign tumors Usually well-circumscribed, gray or brown, elevated firm papules with a roughened, finely papillomatous texture Occur anywhere but usually appear on exposed areas such as fingers, hands, face, and soles May be single or multiple Asymptomatic	Not uniformly successful Local destructive therapy, individualized according to location, type, and number—surgical removal, electrocautery, curettage, cryotherapy (liquid nitrogen), caustic solutions (lactic acid and salicylic acid in flexible collodion, retinoic acid, salicylic acid plasters), radiographic treatment Hypnotherapy may be effective	Common in children Tend to disappear spontaneously Course unpredictable Most destructive techniques tend to leave scars Autoinoculable Repeated irritation will cause to enlarge
Verruca plantaris (plantar wart)	Located on plantar surface of feet and, because of pressure, are practically flat; may be surrounded by a collar of hyperkeratosis	Apply caustic solution to wart, wear foam insole with hole cut to relieve pressure on wart; soak 20 min after 2-3 days. Repeat until wart comes out	
Herpes simplex virus type I (cold sore, fever blister)	Grouped, burning, and itching vesicles on inflammatory base, usually on or near mucocutaneous junctions (lips, nose, genitals, buttocks) Vesicles dry, forming a crust, followed by exfoliation and spontaneous healing in 8-10 days May be accompanied by regional lymphadenopathy	Avoidance of secondary infection Burow solution compresses during weeping stages No topical therapy has proved to be effective	Heal without scarring unless secondary infection Aggravated by corticosteroids Positive psychologic effect from treatment
Herpes zoster (shingles)	Caused by same virus that causes varicella (chickenpox) Virus has affinity for posterior root ganglia, posterior horn of spinal cord, and skin; crops of vesicles usually confined to dermatome following along course of affected nerve Usually preceded by neuralgic pain, hyperesthesias, or itching May be accompanied by constitutional symptoms	Symptomatic Salicylates for pain Mild sedation sometimes helpful Local moist compresses Drying lotions may be helpful Ophthalmic variety: systemic corticotropin (ACTH) and/or corticosteroids	Pain in children usually minimal Postherpetic pain does not occur in children Chickenpox may follow exposure; isolate affected child from other children in a hospital May occur in children with depressed immunity; can be fatal
Molluscum contagiosum	Caused by a pox virus Flesh-colored papules with a central caseous plug Usually asymptomatic	Cases in well children resolve spontaneously in about 18 months Treatment reserved for troublesome cases	Common in school-age children Spread by person-to-person contact and by autoinoculation

cells. Composed of only a DNA or RNA core enclosed in an antigenic protein shell, viruses are unable to provide for their own metabolic needs or to reproduce themselves. After a virus penetrates a cell of the host organism, it sheds the outer shell and disappears within the cell, where the nucleic acid core stimulates the host cell to form more virus material from its intracellular substance. In a viral infection the epidermal cells react with inflammation and vesiculation (as in herpes simplex) or by proliferating to form growths (warts).

Most of the communicable diseases of childhood are associated with rashes, and each rash is characteristic. The type of lesion and the configuration of the viral exanthems of rubeola, rubella, and chickenpox are described in Table 14-1. Other common viral disorders of the skin are outlined in Table 29-2.

DERMATOPHYTOSES (FUNGAL INFECTIONS)

The dermatophytoses (ringworm) are infections caused by a group of closely related filamentous fungi that invade primarily the stratum corneum, hair, and nails. These are superficial infections that live on, not in, the skin. They are confined to the dead keratin layers and are unable to survive in the deeper layers. Since the keratin is being desquamated constantly, the fungus must multiply at a rate that equals the rate of keratin production to maintain itself; otherwise the infection would be shed with the discarded skin cells. Common dermatophytoses are outlined in Table 29-3.

Dermatophytoses are designated by the Latin word *tinea,* with further designation related to the area of the body where they are found, for example, tinea capitis (ringworm of the scalp) (Fig. 29-4, *A*). Dermatophyte in-

TABLE 29-3

Dermatophytoses (ringworm)

Disease/Organism	Manifestations	Treatment	Comments
Tinea capitis—*Microsporum audouini, M. canis* (see Fig. 29-4, *A*)	Lesions in scalp but may extend to hairline or neck Characteristic configuration of scaly, circumscribed patches and/or patchy, scaling areas of alopecia Generally asymptomatic, but severe, deep inflammatory reaction may occur that manifests as boggy, encrusted lesions (kerions) Pruritic Diagnosis: fluoresce green under Wood light; check at 2-week intervals Direct examination of scales and culture if doubtful	Oral griseofulvin Oral ketoconazole for difficult cases Selenium sulfide shampoos Topical antifungal agents, e. g., clotrimazole, haloprogin, miconazole; treatment extended for weeks or months—even after subjective symptoms subside	Person-to-person transmission Animal-to-person transmission Rarely, permanent loss of hair *M. audouini* transmitted from one human being to another directly or from personal items; *M. canis* usually contracted from household pets
Tinea corporis—*Trichophyton, Microsporum* (see Fig. 29-4, *B*)	Generally round or oval, erythematous scaling patch that spreads peripherally and clears centrally; may involve nails (tinea unguium) Diagnosis: direct microscopic examination of scales	Oral griseofulvin Local application of antifungal preparation such as tolnaftate, haloprogin, miconazole, clotrimazole	Usually of animal origin from infected pets Majority of infections in children caused by *M. canis* and *M. audouini*
Tinea cruris ("jock itch")—*Epidermophyton floccosum, T. rubrum*	Skin response similar to tinea corporis Localized to medial proximal aspect of thigh and crural fold; may involve scrotum in males Pruritic Diagnosis: same as for tinea corporis	Local application of tolnaftate liquid Wet compresses or sitz baths may be soothing	Rare in preadolescent children Health education regarding personal hygiene
Tinea pedis ("athlete's foot")—*E. floccosum, T. rubrum, T. interdigitale*	On intertriginous areas between toes or on plantar surface of feet Lesions vary: Maceration and fissuring between toes Patches with pinhead-sized vesicles on plantar surface Pruritic Diagnosis: direct microscopic examination of scrapings	Oral griseofulvin Local applications of tolnaftate liquid and antifungal powder containing tolnaftate Acute infections: compresses or soaks followed by application of glucocorticoid cream Elimination of conditions of heat and perspiration by clean, light socks and well-ventilated shoes; avoidance of occlusive shoes	Most frequent in adolescents and adults; rare in children Transmission to other individuals rare despite general opinion to contrary Ointments not successful
Candidiasis (moniliasis)—*Candida albicans*	Grows in chronically moist areas Inflamed area with white exudate, peeling, and easy bleeding Pruritic Diagnosis: characteristic appearance	Amphotericin B or nystatin ointment to affected areas	Common form of diaper dermatitis Oral form common in infants (p. 220)

fections are most often transmitted from one person to another or from infected animals to humans.

Nursing Considerations

When teaching families regarding the care of children with ringworm, it is important to emphasize good health and hygiene. Because of the infectious nature of the disease, several basic hygienic measures are particularly pertinent. Affected children are not to exchange with other children any grooming items, headgear, scarves, or other articles of apparel that have been in proximity to the infected area. Affected children are provided with their own towels and directed to wear protective caps at night to avoid transmitting the fungus to bedding, especially if they sleep with another person. Since the infection can be acquired by animal-to-human transmission, all household pets should be examined for the presence of the disorder. Other sources of infection are seats with headrests, such as theater seats or seats in public transportation.

TABLE 29-4

Systemic Mycoses

Disorder/ Organism	Skin Manifestations	Systemic Manifestations	Treatment	Comments
Actinomycosis—*Actinomyces israelii*	Deep-seated granulomatous nodules and subcutaneous abscesses that drain as chronic fistulas, especially in jaw or neck	General health not affected	Penicillin or other antibiotics Incision and wide debridement of lesions	Acess frequently through a carious tooth or mucous membranes of mouth Uncommon in children Noninfectious
North American blastomycosis—*Blastomyces dermatitidis*	Chronic granulomatous lesions and microabscesses in any part of body Initial lesion is a papule; undergoes ulceration and peripheral spread	Pulmonary symptoms, such as cough, chest pain, weakness, and weight loss May have skeletal involvement, with bone destruction and formation of cutaneous abscesses	Intravenous administration of amphotericin B	Usual portal of entry is lungs Source of infection unknown Noninfectious Pulmonary infections may be mild and self-limiting and require no treatment Progressive disease often fatal
Cryptococcosis—*Cryptococcus neoformans (Torula histolytica)*	Usually on face; acneiform, firm, nodular, painless eruption	Central nervous system (CNS) manifestations; headache, dizziness, stiff neck, and signs of increased intracranial pressure Low-grade fever, mild cough, lung infiltration	Intravenous amphotericin B; may be administered intrathecally for CNS involvement 5-Flurocytosine for meningitis Excision and drainage of local lesions	Acquired by inhalation of dust but may enter through skin Prognosis serious Noninfectious Increased incidence in persons receiving corticosteroids with lymphoreticular malignancies, or type II diabetes
Histoplasmosis—*Histoplasma capsulatum*	Not distinctive or uniform but most appear as punched-out or granulomatous ulcers	General systemic symptoms may include pallor, diarrhea, vomiting, irregular spiking temperature, hepatosplenomegaly, and pulmonary symptoms Any tissue of body may be involved with related symptoms	Intravenous amphotericin B for severe cases Oral ketoconazole	Organism cultured from soil, especially where contaminated with fowl droppings Fungus enters through skin or mucous membranes of mouth and respiratory tract Endemic in Mississippi and Ohio River valleys Disseminated diseases most common in infants and children
Coccidioidomycosis (valley fever)—*Coccidioides immitis*	Erythema nodosum	Primary lung disease usually asymptomatic May be sign of acute febrile illness Disseminated disease is very serious	Intravenous amphotericin B Intravenous miconazole (synthetic imidazole) Intraventricular miconazole plus oral ketoconazole for CNS involvement Surgical resection of persistent pulmonary cavities	Inhalation of aerospores from soil Endemic in southwestern United States Usually resolves spontaneously Increased incidence in dark-skinned races (Filipino, black, Mexican, Asian)

SYSTEMIC MYCOTIC (FUNGAL) INFECTIONS

Mycotic (systemic or deep fungal) infections have the capacity to invade the viscera as well as the skin. The best known of these infections are primarily lung diseases, which are usually acquired by inhalation of fungal spores. These fungi produce a variable spectrum of disease, and some are quite common in certain geographic areas. They are not transmitted from person to person but appear to reside in the soil, from which their spores are airborne. The cutaneous lesions caused by deep fungal infections are granulomatous and appear as ulcers, plaques, nodules, fungating mosses, and abscesses. The course of deep fungal diseases is chronic with slow progression that favors sensitization (Table 29-4).

◆ *Skin Disorders Related to Chemical or Physical Contacts*

Children come in contact with an endless variety of substances and objects in day-to-day activities, including sunshine (see discussion on p. 1008). Some children are troubled very little by these encounters; others are sensitive to many commonplace substances.

CONTACT DERMATITIS

Contact dermatitis is an inflammatory reaction of the skin to chemical substances, natural or synthetic, that evoke a hypersensitivity response or to those agents that cause direct irritation. The initial reaction occurs in an exposed region, most commonly the face and neck, backs of the hands, forearms, male genitalia, and lower legs. Characteristically there is a sharp delineation between inflamed and normal skin early in the reaction that ranges from a faint, transient erythema to massive bullae on an erythematous swollen base. Itching is a constant symptom.

The most frequent offenders are plant and animal irritants, the prototype of which is poison ivy. The common contact dermatitis in infants occurs on the convex surfaces of the diaper area (see discussion on p. 991). Other agents that frequently produce dermatologic responses from contact are animal irritants, such as wool, feathers, and furs; vegetable irritants, such as oleoresins, oils, and turpentine; and chemicals of all kinds, including synthetic fabrics, dyes, metals, cosmetics, perfumes, and soaps.

Several cosmetic products advertised as safe for children include a cream hair relaxer that contains lye and preparations to curl or straighten hair. These products are stronger than those intended for adults because children's hair is more resistant to these attempts. Frequent causes of genital irritation in girls are bubble baths and feminine hygiene products. The list is endless.

The major goal in treatment is to prevent further exposure of the skin to the offending substance. Providing there is no further irritation, the normal recuperative powers of the skin will produce satisfactory results without treatment.

Nursing Considerations

Nurses frequently detect evidence of contact dermatitis during routine physical assessments. Skin manifestations in specific areas suggest limited contact, such as around the eyes (mascara), areas of the body covered by clothing but not protected by undergarments (wool), or areas of the body not covered by clothing (ultraviolet injury). Generalized involvement is more likely to be caused by bubble bath or soap. Often nurses are able to determine the offending agent and counsel families regarding management. However, if the lesions persist, are extensive, or show evidence of infection, medical evaluation is indicated.

POISON IVY, OAK, AND SUMAC

The prototype of plant offenders is poison ivy (also poison oak and sumac) (Fig. 29-5). Contact with the dry or succulent portions of the plant produces localized, streaked or spotty, oozing and painful impetiginous lesions. The offending substance in these plants is an oil, urushiol, that is extremely potent. Sensitivity to urushiol is not inborn but is developed after one or two exposures and may change over a lifetime. All parts of the plants contain the oil, so dried leaves and stems contain the irritant. Even smoke from burning brush piles can produce a reaction.

Animals do not seem to be affected by the oil; however, dogs or other animals that have run or played in the plants may carry the sap on their fur, and animals who eat the plants can transfer the oil in saliva. Shoes, tools, and toys can transfer the oil. Golf balls that have been in the rough also are sources of contact.

The substance begins to take effect as soon as it touches the skin. It penetrates through the epidermis and bonds with the dermal layer, where it initiates an immune response. The full-blown reaction is evident after about 2 days with redness, swelling, and itching at the site of contact. Several days later streaked or spotty blisters oozing serum from damaged cells produce the characteristic impetiginous lesions. The lesions dry and heal spontaneously and itching stops by 10 to 14 days.

Therapeutic Management

Treatment of the lesions includes calamine lotion, soothing Burow solution compresses, and/or Aveeno baths to relieve discomfort. Topical corticosteroid gel is very effective for prevention or relief of inflammation, especially when applied before formation of blisters. Oral corticoste-

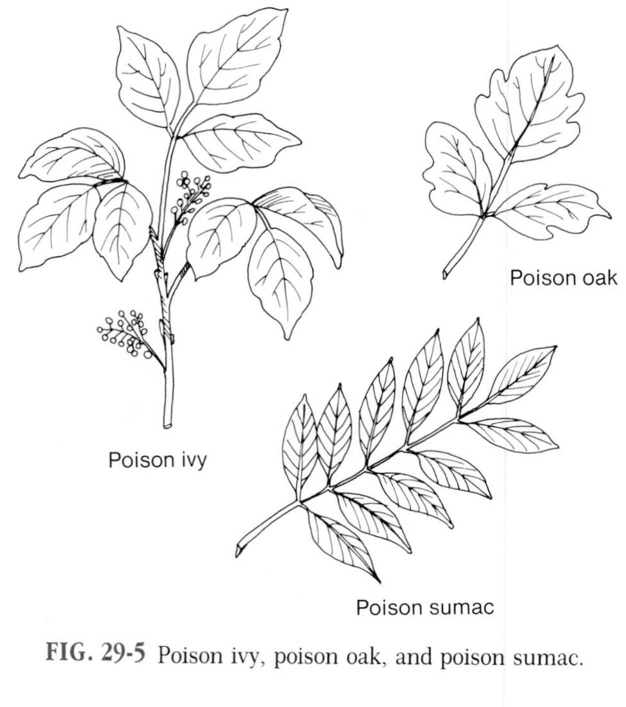

FIG. 29-5 Poison ivy, poison oak, and poison sumac.

roids may be needed for severe reactions, and a sedative such as diphenhydramine (Benadryl) may be ordered.

Nursing Considerations

When it is known that the child has made contact with the plant, the area is immediately flushed (within 15 minutes) with *cold* running water to neutralize the urushiol not yet bonded to the skin. If there is a stream nearby, an effective method is to have the child enter the water (clothes and all) and allow the water to rinse the oil from both skin and clothing. Soap is contraindicated because it removes protective skin oils and dilutes the urushiol, allowing it to spread; also, hard scrubbing irritates the skin. All clothing that has come in contact with the plant is removed with care and thoroughly laundered in hot water and detergent. Every effort should be made to prevent the child from scratching the lesions. Although the lesions do not spread by contact with the blister serum or from scratching, the lesions can become secondarily infected.

Prevention. Prevention is best accomplished by avoidance of contact and removal of the plant from the environment when feasible. All children, especially those known to be sensitive, should be taught to recognize the plant. Information regarding means for destroying plants can be obtained from the U.S. Department of Agriculture or Forestry Service.

Drug Reactions

Adverse reactions to drugs are seen more often in the skin than in any other organ. Cutaneous manifestations can resemble almost any skin disease and can be seen in almost any degree of severity. With few exceptions the distribution of a drug eruption is widespread, since the eruption results from a circulating agent. The onset is sudden and the eruption appears as an inflammatory response with itching. It may be associated with constitutional symptoms, such as fever, malaise, gastrointestinal upsets, anemia, or liver and kidney damage.

Although any drug is capable of producing almost any form of reaction in the susceptible individual, some drugs have a tendency to produce a particular reaction. Individual drug reactions may vary from a single lesion to extensive, generalized epidermal necrosis, such as occurs in Stevens-Johnson syndrome (see box, p. 990). Reactions are also related to the amount of drug administered and the route of administration.

Treatment for cutaneous reactions consists of discontinuation of the drug. In urticarial-type eruptions antihistamines may be ordered, and for widespread and severe lesions corticosteroids are beneficial. Severe anaphylactic reactions are a medical emergency.

TRAUMA AND FOREIGN BODIES

Cuts, scratches, scrapes, and abrasions are all part of growing up. No child escapes them. Small injuries are managed by the parents at home with only a few simple guidelines. Cuts on the face, a gaping cut longer than ¼ inch, or one that bleeds persistently should be evaluated for possible suturing. To prevent possible tattooing, abrasions from which the dirt cannot be removed will require abrading under topical anesthesia (liquid topical anesthetics can be dripped into the wound). Those covering a very large area (over 15% of the body) will need medical attention. There is also a high risk of contamination from a wound sustained in a bicycle injury. Since abrasions are often painful, analgesics such as acetaminophen are advised.

Nursing Considerations

Advice to parents regarding management of small wounds to the skin is often assumed by nurses. Parents are instructed to wash their hands, then wash the wound thoroughly but gently with soap and water for at least 5 minutes, and then rinse the wound well. If possible the wound is left exposed to air, since wounds heal faster without a dressing. However, if the area is one that will probably get dirty, it can be covered with a Band-Aid sterile dressing. Ointments, sprays, alcohol, or Merthiolate is not needed; some sting and can damage normal tissue.

Abrasions are cleaned in the same manner as wounds except that any foreign matter must be removed with clean tweezers and loose skin is cut off with sterile scissors. Small abrasions are left exposed; larger ones are covered with Telfa or other nonstick dressing that is changed in 12 hours and left uncovered after 24 hours. Bruises are managed with ice applications for 20 to 30 minutes.

Puncture wounds that do not require a tetanus booster are soaked in hot water and soap for 15 minutes. Causing the wound to rebleed may be helpful. A Band-Aid can be applied if desired. Puncture wounds of the head, chest, or abdomen or those that could still contain a portion of the puncturing object need to be evaluated.

Parents are cautioned against opening blood blisters or kissing a wound "to make it better." The wound can easily become contaminated from germs in the human mouth. Also, scabs should be allowed to slough off without assistance; picking or early removal may cause scarring. Parents are advised to seek medical help if there is evidence of infection.

Foreign Bodies

Small wooden splinters can be removed by parents with a needle and tweezers that have been sterilized with alcohol or a flame. The area around the sliver is washed with soap and water before attempting the removal. The sliver is exposed with the needle, then grasped firmly by the tweezers and pulled in the same direction in which it entered. Some foreign bodies should have medical evaluation; these include a fishhook, a piece of glass or other

Nursing Tip: Removal of Cactus Spines

Cactus prickles or spines are readily removed by one of several methods:

1. Drop wax from a lighted candle over the affected area (from a sufficient height to avoid burning the skin), then cool by immersion in cold water and lift off to bring the foreign bodies with it.
2. Apply a thin coat of white glue (woodworking or household) to the area, allow to dry about 10 minutes, then apply a second coat. When the second coat becomes dry, peel the layer of glue, along with the cactus spines, from the skin.
3. Apply a thin layer of household glue and cover with gauze. When glue dries, peel off gauze and spines will come with it.
4. Apply a layer of facial gel, allow to dry, then peel off.

Information based on Gelbard, 1984, Putnam and Lawton, 1985, and Martinez and others, 1987.

difficult-to-see object, or a deeply imbedded object, such as a needle in a foot or near a joint.

◆ Skin Disorders Related to Insect and Animal Contacts

Young children are curious by nature and fascinated by the world around them. Schoolchildren's social nature and proximity to other children render them highly susceptible to communicable diseases, including those caused by parasites. Because they spend a great deal of time outdoors and in fields and vacant lots, children often come in contact with insects. Consequently, children are frequently the victims of insects that puncture the skin for the purpose of sucking blood, injecting venom, or laying their eggs. In the process of these activities, substances foreign to the victim may create an allergic sensitivity in that individual to produce pruritus, urticaria, or systemic reactions of greater or lesser degree, depending on the child's sensitivity.

Infestations with insect parasites are relatively common, and those encountered most frequently in childhood are scabies and pediculosis capitis. Body lice infestations are seen less often, and pubic lice (pediculosis pubis, or "crabs") are rare in childhood.

SCABIES

Scabies is an endemic infestation produced by the scabies mite, *Sarcoptes scabiei*. The lesions are created as the impregnated female burrows into the stratum corneum of the epidermis (never into living tissue) to bury her eggs. The inflammatory response and itching occur after the host becomes sensitized to the mite, approximately 30 to 60 days following initial contact. After this time, anywhere the mite has traveled will begin to itch and develop the characteristic eruption (see box). Consequently mites will not necessarily be located at all sites of eruption. The picture is often confusing in infants, who often develop an eczematous eruption; therefore, the observer must look for discrete papules, burrows, or vesicles.

Clinical Manifestations of Scabies

Pruritus
Lesion:
Children—minute grayish brown, threadlike (mite burrows)
Black dot at end of burrow (mite)
Infants—eczematous eruption
Distribution:
Generally in intertriginous areas—interdigital, axillary-cubital, popliteal, inguinal
Children over 2 years of age—primarily hands and wrists
Children less than 2 years—primarily feet and ankles

Nursing Considerations

The treatment of scabies is the application of a scabicide, usually 1% lindane (Kwell) in a vanishing cream base. Nurses instructing families in use of the scabicide should emphasize the importance of following the directions accurately. The lotion is applied to cool, dry skin—not following a hot bath—and left on for the recommended time, usually 4 hours for infants and 6 hours for older children and adults. Since it is a superficial skin disorder, penetration need not be promoted. One liberal application is sufficient, but all persons in the family (including baby-sitters, etc.) should be treated. Parents need to know that, although the mite will be killed, the rash and the itch will not be eliminated until the stratum corneum is replaced, which takes approximately 2 to 3 weeks. Soothing ointments or lotions can be applied for itching.

PEDICULOSIS CAPITIS

Pediculosis capitis (head lice, or "cooties") is an infestation of the scalp by *Pediculus humanus capitis,* a very common parasite, especially in school-age children. The adult louse lives only about 48 hours when away from a human host, and the life span of the average female is only 1 month. The female lays her eggs at night at the junction of a hair shaft and close to the skin, because the eggs need a warm environment. The eggs hatch in approximately 7 to 10 days; the egg is thus about 4 mm from the scalp (but may be farther) at the time of hatching (McLaury, 1983).

Diagnostic Evaluation

Diagnosis is made by observation of the white eggs (nits) firmly attached to the base of the hair shafts (see box). Because of their brief life span and mobility, adult lice are

Clinical Manifestations of Pediculosis

Pruritus (caused by crawling insect and insect saliva on skin)
Nits observable on hair shaft
Distribution:
Occipital area
Behind ears
Nape of neck
Eyebrows and eyelashes (occasionally) (caused by pubic lice)

more difficult to locate. Nits must be differentiated from dandruff, lint, hair spray, and other items of similar size and shape. The nits will fluoresce white under Wood light. Scratch marks and/or inflammatory papules, caused by secondary infection, may also be found on the scalp in the vulnerable areas.

Therapeutic Management

Treatment consists of the application of pediculocidal shampoos and manual removal of nit cases. A number of shampoos are available that are highly effective. A prescription drug, 1% lindane shampoo (gamma benzene hexachloride—Kwell, Scabene), is applied as directed and repeated in 7 to 10 days to kill the hatching nymphs. However, lindane is not effective against nits and, if not used properly, is potentially toxic, especially in infants. Permethrin 1% creme rinse (Nix) kills both lice and nits after one application. Preparations of pyrethrin with piperonyl butoxide (RID or A-200 pyrinate) can be obtained without a prescription and appear to be as effective as lindane.

Nursing Considerations

There are several things that nurses should be aware of in order to successfully manage or assist parents in coping with pediculosis. It should be emphasized that *anyone* can get pediculosis; it has no respect for age, socioeconomic level, or cleanliness. The louse does not jump or fly, but it can be transmitted from one person to another on personal items. Therefore children are cautioned against sharing combs, hats, caps, scarves, coats, and other items used on or near the hair. Children who share lockers are more likely to contract an infestation, and slumber parties place children at risk. Lice are not carried or transmitted by household pets.

Parents should carefully inspect the head of a child who scratches the head more than usual for bite marks, redness, and nits. The hair is systematically spread with two Popsicle sticks or tongue depressors and the scalp observed for any movement that indicates a louse. Lice are visible to the naked eye. The nits, or eggs, appear as tiny whitish oval specks adhering to the hair shaft about ¼ inch from the scalp. The adherent nature of the nits distinguishes them from dandruff, which falls off readily. Empty nit cases, indicating hatched lice, are translucent rather than white and are located more than ¼ inch from the scalp.

If evidence of infestation is found, it is important to perform the treatment according to the directions described on the label of the pediculocide. Parents are advised to read the directions several times in a quiet room before beginning treatment (McLaury, 1983). Instructions on the labels indicate that dead lice and remaining nits are removed with an extra-fine-tooth comb. Most preparations include a comb to dislodge the firmly adhered nits. However, if the comb is ineffective in removing the nit cases, they must be removed with tweezers or between the fingernails.

Nursing Tip: Nit Removal

A dilute vinegar rinse (¼ cup vinegar to 1 quart water) may help to loosen the nits for easier removal.

The child should be made as comfortable as possible during the application process, because the pediculocide must remain on the scalp and hair for several minutes. If eye irritation occurs, the eyes must be flushed well with tepid water.

Nursing Tip: Shampoo

Playing "beauty parlor" during the shampoo is a useful strategy. The child lies supine, with his head over a sink or basin, and covers his eyes with a dry towel or washcloth. This prevents medication, which can cause chemical conjunctivitis, from splashing into the eyes.

Washable items of clothing and bed linen are laundered in hot water and dried in a hot dryer. Combs, brushes, and other items can be soaked in the louse shampoo or lotion for an hour or in very hot water (105° F) for 5 to 10 minutes. All mattresses and upholstered furniture should be vacuumed carefully to remove any living lice or nits that may be attached to fallen hair. Spraying with insecticide is not recommended because of the danger to children and animals. Some advocate placing nonwashable, noncleanable items in a tightly closed plastic bag that remains sealed for 14 days; ova are able to lie dormant for this length of time. Families should also be advised that the pediculocide is relatively costly, especially when several members of the household require treatment.

The psychologic effects of lice infestations can be highly stressful to children. They are influenced by the reactions of others, including their parents, and may be made to feel ashamed or guilty. Parents are strongly cautioned against cutting a child's hair or, worse, shaving a

TABLE 29-5

Skin Lesions Caused by Insect Bites and Stings

Mechanism/Characteristics	Manifestations	Management
Insect Bites—Flies, Gnats, Mosquitoes, Fleas Mechanism: Foreign protein in insects' saliva introduced when skin penetrated for a blood-sucking meal Distribution: Almost everywhere—fleas, mosquitoes, ants Suburbs and rural areas—bees Urban areas—hornets, wasps, yellow jackets	Hypersensitivity reaction Papular urticaria Firm papules; may be capped by vesicles or excoriated Little or no reaction in nonsensitized person	Treatment: Antipruritic agents and baths Antihistamines Prevention of secondary infection Prevention: Avoidance of contact Remove focus, such as treating furniture, mattresses, carpets, and pets, where insects may live Apply insect repellent when exposure is anticipated
Chiggers—Harvest Mite Mechanism: Creeps into skin pores and hair follicles to feed Manifestations: Erythematous papules Intense itching	Same as insect bites May require systemic steroids for extensive bites	Favor warm areas of body, especially intertriginous areas and areas covered with clothing Avoidance of contact, especially in areas of tall grass and underbrush Apply insect repellant when exposure is anticipated
Hymenoptera Stings—Bees, Wasps, Hornets, Yellow Jackets, Fire Ants Mechanism: Injection of venom through stinging apparatus Venom contains histamine, allergenic proteins, and often a spreading factor, hyaluronidase Severe reactions caused by hypersensitivity and/or multiple stings Hypersensitive children should wear identifying tag to indicate allergy and therapy needed; family should keep emergency medication and be taught its administration	Local reaction: small red area, wheal, itching, and heat Systemic reactions: may be mild to severe, including generalized edema, pain, nausea and vomiting, confusion, respiratory embarrassment, and shock	Treatment: Carefully scrape off stinger if present Cleanse with soap and water Apply cool compresses or ice packs Apply common household product, e.g., lemon juice, paste made with aspirin, baking soda, or Adolph's Meat Tenderizer Elevate involved extremity Antihistamines Severe reactions: administer epinephrine, corticosteroids; treat for shock Prevention: Child taught to wear shoes, to avoid wearing bright clothing or perfumed grooming products that might attract the insect, and to avoid places where the insect may be contacted

child's head. Lice infest short hair as readily as long hair, and these actions only compound the child's distress and serve as a continual reminder to peers, who are always ready to taunt another with something out of the ordinary (McLaury, 1983).

Prevention. The increasing incidence of pediculosis in schoolchildren has become a serious concern for school nurses, parents, and community health agencies. School nurses are constantly on the alert for evidence of infestation. The **National Pediculosis Association*** has been organized by a group of parents frustrated by repeated infestations of their children. These parents have developed an approach to the problem that offers hope that vigorous effort on the part of parents and the community will reduce the epidemics in children. Some of their suggestions include encouraging parents to notify others if a child becomes infected and preventing children from reentering school until they are completely free of nits.

*P.O. Box 149, Newton, MA 02161.

INSECT BITES AND STINGS

Bites and stings account for a significant incidence of mild to moderate discomfort, and most are managed by simple symptomatic measures, such as compresses, calamine lotion, and prevention of secondary infection. The major offending creatures, their manifestations, and management are outlined in Tables 29-5 and 29-6.

When an insect stings, its stinger often remains embedded in the skin. For example, bees have barbed stingers that penetrate the skin, and any pressure on the venom sac at the tip of the barb pushes more venom into the skin. Children who have become sensitized to hymenopteran bites may demonstrate a severe systemic response that can be life-threatening. One sting can produce generalized urticaria, respiratory difficulty (from laryngeal edema), hypotension, and death within 1 hour. Intramuscular administration of epinephrine provides immediate relief and must be available for emergency use.

Hypersensitive children need a kit available that contains epinephrine and a hypodermic syringe; they also

TABLE 29-6

Skin Lesions Caused by Arachnids

Mechanism/Characteristics	Manifestations	Management
Black Widow Spider Mechanism: Venom injected through a clawlike appendage; has neurotoxic action Characteristics: Spider is recognized by red or orange hourglass-shaped marking on underside Avoids light and bites in self-defense	Mild sting at time of bite Area becomes swollen, painful, and erythematous Dizziness, weakness, and abdominal pain May produce delirium, paralysis, convulsions, and (if large amount of venom absorbed) death	Treatment: Cleanse wound with antiseptic Apply ice packs Antivenin Muscle relaxant, such as calcium gluconate Analgesics and/or sedatives Prevention: Teach children to avoid places that harbor the spider, e.g., woodpiles
Brown Recluse Spider Mechanism: Venom injected via fangs Venom contains powerful necrotoxin Characteristics: Spider is fawn to dark brown and recognized by fiddle-shaped mark on head Shy; bites only when annoyed or surprised Prefers dark areas where seldom disturbed	Mild sting at time of bite Transient erythema followed by bleb or blister; mild to severe pain in 2-8 hours; purple, star-shaped area in 3-4 days; necrotic ulceration in 7-14 days Systemic reactions may include fever, malaise, restlessness, nausea and vomiting, and joint pain Generalized petechial eruption Wounds heal with scar formation	Treatment: Local application of cool compresses Antibiotics Corticosteroids Relief of pain Wound may require skin graft Some advocate early excision of necrotic area and surrounding tissue Prevention: Teach children to avoid possible nesting sites
Scorpions Mechanism: Sting by means of a hooked caudal stinger that discharges venom Venom of more venomous species contains hemolysins, endotheliolysins, and neurotoxins Characteristics: Usual habitat is southwestern United States	Intense local pain, erythema, numbness, burning, restlessness, vomiting Ascending motor paralysis with convulsions, weakness, rapid pulse, excessive salivation, thirst, dysuria, pulmonary edema, coma, and death Some species produce only local tissue reaction with swelling at puncture site (distinctive) Symptoms subside in a few hours Deaths occur among children under 4 years of age, usually in first 24 hours	Treatment: Delay absorption of venom by application of tourniquets for 10-15 minutes; apply cold with ice packs or submerge in cold water Administration of antivenin Surveillance in PICU Prevention: Teach children to avoid possible nesting sites
Ticks Mechanism: In process of sucking blood, head and mouth parts are buried in skin Characteristics: Feed on blood of mammals Significant in humans because of pathologic organism carried May be vectors of various infectious diseases, such as Rocky Mountain spotted fever, Q fever, tularemia, relapsing fever, Lyme disease, tick paralysis Must attach and feed 1-2 hours to transmit disease Usual habitat is very wooded area	Tick usually attached to skin, head embedded Produce firm, discrete, intensely pruritic nodules at site of attachment May cause urticaria or persistent localized edema	Treatment: Grasp tick with fingers protected by gloves or tissues as close as possible to point of attachment Pull straight up with steady, even pressure Remove any remaining part (e.g., head) with sterile needle Cleanse wounds with soap and disinfectant If bare hands touch tick during removal, wash hands thoroughly with soap and water Prevention: Teach children to avoid areas where prevalent Inspect skin (especially scalp) after being in wooded areas

should wear a Medic Alert bracelet. Families should be reminded to check the expiration date on the kit and to replace an outdated one. Families should determine if a school nurse is available at the school and the school policy regarding administration of drugs. If a school nurse is not present, someone at the school should be designated to inject the epinephrine in case of an emergency.

Most arachnids in the United States are relatively harmless, including tarantulas. Although all spiders produce venom that is injected via fangs, some species are unable to pierce the skin; others produce a venom that is insufficiently toxic to be harmful. Only scorpions and two species of spiders—the brown recluse and the black widow—inject venom deadly enough to require immedi-

TABLE 29-7

Disorders Transmitted by Arthropods

Disorder/Organism/Host	Manifestations	Management	Comments
Rocky Mountain spotted fever—*R. rickettsii* Arthropod: tick Transmission: tick bite Mammal source: wild rodents; dogs	Gradual onset: fever, malaise, anorexia, myalgia Abrupt onset: rapid temperature elevation, chills, vomiting, myalgia, severe headache Maculopapular or petechial rash primarily on extremities (ankles and wrists) but may spread to other areas	Control: protection from tick bite by proper wearing apparel, tick repellent Treatment: Tetracycline or chloramphenicol Vigorous supportive therapy	Usually self-limited in children Onset in children may resemble any infectious disease Severe disease rare in children Children and dogs should be inspected regularly if they play in wooded areas See Table 29-6 for management of ticks
Epidemic typhus—*R. prowazekii* Arthropod: body louse Transmission: infected feces into broken skin Mammal source: humans	Abrupt onset of chills, fever, diffuse myalgia, headache, malaise Maculopapular rash 4 to 7 days later spreading from trunk outward	Control: immediate destruction of vectors Treatment: Tetracycline or chloramphenicol	Patient should be isolated until deloused See discussion on p. 984 for management of pediculosis Excreta from infected lice also in dust—disinfect patient's clothing, bedding, and possessions with DDT and wash in hot water
Endemic typhus—*R. mooseri* Arthropod: rat fleas, or lice Transmission: flea bite; inhaling or ingesting flea excreta Mammal source: rats	Headache, arthralgia, backache followed by fever; may last 9-14 days Maculopapular rash after 1-8 days of fever begins in trunk and spreads to periphery; rarely involves face, palms, soles	Control; eliminate rat reservoir, insect vectors, or both Treatment: Supportive	Fairly common in U.S. Shorter duration than epidemic typhus Mild, seldom fatal illness Difficult to distinguish from epidemic typhus
Rickettsialpox—*R. akari* Arthropod: mouse mite Transmission: mite Mammal source: house mouse	Maculopapular rash following primary lesion at site of bite, fever, chills, headache	Control: eradication of rodent reservoir and mite vector Treatment: Tetracycline or chloramphenicol Supportive	Self-limited nonfatal disease Endemic in New York City Found in many cities in U.S.
Q fever—*Coxiella burnetti* Arthropod: tick Transmission: inhalation of dried, infected material Mammal source: domestic farm animals (cattle, sheep, goats)	Abrupt onset of chills, fever, weakness, and nonspecific symptoms Severe frontal headache often associated with pain upon eye movement After 1 week—cough and chest pains	Control: impossible; exact mode of spread unknown Treatment: Tetracycline or chloramphenicol Supportive	Usually a mild disease Duration 2-3 weeks Endemic in California Milk should be pasteurized Persons who work around farm animals are at risk
Lyme disease—Spirochete *Borrelia burgdorferi* Arthropod: tick Transmission: tick bite Mammal source: rodents, deer	Stage 1: tick bite Stage 2: erythema chronicum migrans, papule at bite site progresses to large circumferential ring with a raised edematous doughnutlike border Stage 3: systemic involvement—cardiac, neurologic, musculoskeletal	Control: protection from tick bite by proper wearing apparel, tick repellent Treatment: Antibiotics Supportive	Regional distribution: Northeast (Massachusetts to Maryland); Midwest (Wisconsin, Minnesota); West (California, Oregon)

ate attention. Children bitten by these arachnids must receive medical attention as soon as possible.

INFECTIONS TRANSMITTED BY ARTHROPODS

The organisms responsible for a number of disorders are transmitted to human beings by way of arthropods—ticks, fleas, and lice (Table 29-7). Rickettsiae are intracellular parasites, similar in size to bacteria, that inhabit the alimentary tract of a wide range of natural hosts. With the exception of Q fever, mammals become infected only through the bites of infected insects (lice and fleas) or arachnids (ticks and mites), both of which serve as both infectors and reservoirs. Rickettsial diseases are more common in temperate and tropical climates and in areas where humans live in association with arthropods. Infection in humans is incidental (except epidemic typhus) and not necessary for the survival of the rickettsial species. However, once the organisms invade a human, they cause a disease that varies in intensity from a benign, self-limiting illness to a fulminating and frequently fatal one.

Lyme disease is a relatively recently recognized disorder caused by a spirochete transmitted by ticks. The disease may first be seen by health professionals in any of three stages: (1) the tick bite at the time of inoculation; (2) development of erythema chronicum migrans (EMC) at the site of the bite; and (3) the most serious stage of the disease, systemic involvement of neurologic, cardiac, and musculoskeletal systems that appears several weeks after the cutaneous phase is completed.

ANIMAL BITES

Contrary to popular conception, children are bitten more often by animals belonging to the family or to neighbors than by strange animals. Boys are bitten more often by dogs; girls are bitten more often by cats. Most dog or cat injuries are to the upper extremities. However, small children are more likely to be bitten or scratched on the head, face, and neck because they tend to put their heads near the animal's head and to flail their arms rather than protecting their heads. The injuries vary from small puncture wounds to complete evulsion of tissue and can be associated with significant crush injury.

Therapeutic Management

General wound care consists of rinsing the wound with copious amounts of water or saline under pressure (syringe) and washing the surrounding skin with mild soap. A clean pressure dressing is applied and the extremity elevated if the wound is bleeding. Medical evaluation is advised since there is danger of tetanus and rabies, although dogs in most urban areas are required to be immunized against rabies. Bites from wild animals, such as squirrels, bats, and raccoons, are potentially dangerous.

Prophylactic antibiotics are indicated for puncture wounds and wounds in areas that may prove to be cosmetically or functionally impaired if infected. Extensive lacerations are sutured. Tetanus toxoid is administered according to standard guidelines (p. 294), and rabies protocol is followed (p. 920). Cat bites become infected more easily than dog bites but no more so than lacerations from other causes. Injuries to poorly vascularized areas such as the hands are more likely to become infected than those in more vascularized areas such as the face; puncture wounds are more apt to become infected than lacerations.

Nursing Considerations

The most important aspect related to animal bites is prevention. Children should be taught the proper behavior around and toward animals, both their own and those of others. Small children should be supervised closely when around animals. Parents who are contemplating a pet, especially a dog, for themselves or their children should receive some advice about the dog that is least likely to be a danger to their children. A categorization of dogs related to their potential interaction with children can be found in the publication *The Right Dog for You.**

HUMAN BITES

Children often acquire lacerations from the teeth of other humans in rough play, during fights, or as victims of child abuse. Many preschool children bite others out of frustration or anger. Because human dental plaque and gingiva harbor pathogenic bacteria, all human bites should receive attention.

If the laceration is less than ¼ inch in length, the wound can be treated at home. The wound is washed thoroughly with soap and water, and a pressure dressing is applied to stop bleeding. Ice applications minimize discomfort and swelling. Increased pain or redness at the wound site is an indication that the child should receive medical attention for antibiotic therapy. Tetanus toxoid is needed if the child is insufficiently immunized. Wounds greater than ¼ inch should receive medical attention.

CAT SCRATCH DISEASE

Cat scratch disease (CSD) is described as a subacute regional adenitis that follows the scratch or bite of an animal, especially a cat (99% of cases). The disease is usually a benign, self-limiting illness that resolves spontaneously in about 2 to 4 months. The diagnosis is made on the basis of three of the following: (1) cat contact (usually a kitten), (2) lymphadenopathy, (3) an inoculation site (a painless, nonpruritic erythematous papule), and (4) a positive CSD skin test (Carithers, 1985). The disease may persist for several months before gradual resolution. In some children the adenitis progresses to suppuration, and a few children may be very ill with various symptoms, including a prolonged high temperature. The treatment is primarily supportive.

◆ *Miscellaneous Skin Disorders*

There are a number of skin lesions caused by extrinsic or intrinsic factors. Some of these are listed in Table 29-8. There are a number of congenital skin disorders, usually inherited as an autosomal-dominant trait. The ichthyoses are a heterogenous group of disorders characterized by scaling that create a challenging problem in treatment. These disorders are not discussed in detail because of their wide variability.

*Tortora, D.F.: The right dog for you, New York, 1980, Simon & Schuster.

TABLE 29-8

Miscellaneous Skin Disorders

Disease/Causative Agent	Local Manifestations	Management	Comments
Urticaria—usually allergic response to drugs or infection	Development of wheals Vary in size and configuration and tend to appear quickly, spread irregularly, and fade within a few hours May be constant or intermittent, sparse or profuse, small or large, discrete or confluent May be acute, chronic, or recurrent in acute attacks	Local soothing and antipruritic applications Antihistamines Epinephrine or ephedrine Cortisone or corticotropin (ACTH) in severe cases Severe upper respiratory involvement may require tracheostomy	Known etiologic agents should be avoided May be accompanied by malaise, fever, lymphadenopathy Severe cases may involve mucous membranes, internal organs, and joints Obstruction to air passages constitutes medical emergency (see p. 733)
Psoriasis—unknown; hereditary predisposition	Round, thick, dry, reddish patches covered with coarse, silvery scales over trunk and extremities; first lesions commonly appear in scalp; facial lesions more common in children than adults Affected cells proliferate at a much more rapid rate than normal cells	Exposure to sunlight, ultraviolet light Topical corticosteroids Tar derivatives Trihydroxyanthracine Keratolytic agents (salicylic acid) Psoralin—ultraviolet A (PUVA)*	Uncommon in children under age 6 yrs Persons are otherwise healthy individuals Coal tar and psoralin act synergistically with ultraviolet light Keratolytic agents enhance absorption of corticosteroids
Intertrigo—mechanical trauma and aggravating factors of excessive heat, moisture, and sweat retention	Red, inflamed, moist, partially denuded, marginated areas, the shape of which is determined by location Appear where opposing skin surfaces rub together, such as intergluteal folds, groin, neck, and axilla Hyperhydrosis and obesity are often factors	Affected areas kept clean and dry Skin folds kept separated with a generous supply of nonmedicated powder Area exposed to air and light Remove excess clothing	A form of diaper irritation Prevent recurrence by keeping susceptible areas clean and dry Frequently associated with overheating from too much clothing
Erythema multiforme (Stevens-Johnson syndrome)—unknown; associated with ingestion of some drugs; often follows upper respiratory infection	Erythematous papular rash Lesions enlarge by peripheral expansion; develop central vesicle Involves most skin surfaces except scalp May extend to mucous membranes, especially oral, ocular, and urethral	Symptomatic and supportive Maintain adequate fluid intake (oral or IV), calorie, and protein Cutaneous hygiene Appropriate treatment of complications Diligent monitoring of urine volume and specific gravity, hemoglobin and hematocrit, serum electrolyte levels, total body weight	Rash often preceded by fever and malaise Complications include renal failure and severe eye disease Respiratory involvement in a number of cases Self-limiting, but recovery may extend for weeks; skin lesions subside without scarring; mucous membrane lesions may persist for months Recurrence rate 20%; mortality as high as 10%
Neurofibromatosis—inherited disorder	Café-au-lait spots, pigmented nevi, axillary freckling Slow-growing cutaneous and subcutaneous neurofibromas	Symptomatic treatment of associated manifestations, e.g., speech defects, seizures, skeletal defects (scoliosis, kyphosis), learning disabilities Surgical removal of troublesome tumors	Autosomal-dominant inheritance pattern High mutation rate

*Use with caution.

◆ Skin Disorders Associated with Specific Age-Groups

Several common and important dermatologic conditions are confined primarily to children in specific age-groups. These conditions include atopic, seborrheic, and diaper dermatitis and the acne of adolescence. The treatment modalities include those previously described. However, there are some special needs and therapies involved with these disorders.

TABLE 29-9

Skin Eruptions in the Diaper Area

Area Involved	Usual Diagnosis/Cause
Convex surfaces involved; folds spared	Contact dermatitis Allergic or irritant dermatitis/ Chemical irritants (urine, feces, detergents, soaps)
Folds involved, sharply demarcated	Intertrigo/Heat, moisture, and sweat retention Seborrheic dermatitis/Inborn trait
Folds involved with satellite lesions	Seborrheic dermatitis with secondary candidiasis/Inborn trait plus *Candida albicans* infection
Perianal	Chemical and mechanical irritation/Chemical irritants (fecal enzymes)
Perianal with satellite lesions	Primary candidiasis/*C. albicans* infection
Band of erythema at diaper margins	"Tide mark" dermatitis/Plastic or rubber border on diaper and sweat retention
Small, sterile vesicopustules	Miliaria "Heat rash," "prickly heat"/Hot, humid climate in diaper area
Vesicles of bullae	Bullous impetigo Herpes (less common)/*Staphylococcus aureus,* herpes simplex

Modified from Jacobs, A.H.: Pediatr. Clin. North Am. **25**(2):209-224, 1978.

DIAPER DERMATITIS

Diaper dermatitis, one of the most common dermatoses in infants, is one of several acute inflammatory skin disorders caused either directly or indirectly by the wearing of diapers. The most common forms are irritant contact dermatitis, intertrigo, miliaria, and candidiasis. The peak age of occurrence is 9 to 12 months of age, and the incidence is higher in bottle-fed than in breast-fed infants.

The eruptions can be observed primarily on convex surfaces, in folds, and at diaper margins, and the lesions can represent a variety of types and configurations (Table 29-9). Diaper dermatitis is caused by prolonged and repetitive contact with an irritant, principally urine, feces, soaps, detergents, ointments, and friction. The increased pH of the urine promotes fecal enzyme activity, and the enzymes also increase the skin permeability to bile salts.

Nursing Considerations

The aims of management of diaper dermatitis are to (1) minimize skin wetness, (2) allow the skin to maintain its normal acidic pH, and (3) minimize the interaction of urine and feces, which greatly increases the activity and irritancy of fecal enzymes.

The most significant factor amenable to therapeutic and preventive intervention is the hot, humid environment created in the diaper area. Changing the diaper as soon as it becomes wet eliminates a large part of the problem, and removing the diaper entirely for extended periods to expose the area to light and air facilitates drying and healing. Occlusive diaper coverings, such as plastic pants, prevent evaporation and should not be used except for brief social occasions. During the nighttime the diaper should be changed at least once, for example, before the parents retire.

After soiling, the perianal area is cleansed. Wiping the area with a wet cloth is usually sufficient to remove urine. However, after stooling, the area (especially skin folds) needs to be thoroughly cleansed, rinsed, and dried. In some instances, especially with diarrheal stools and irritated skin, a sponge bath may be an efficient alternative. Exposing the skin to warm, dry air for a few minutes before putting on the diaper is helpful. Parents should be advised that the use of disposable wet towels can aggravate the problem because the child may be sensitive to one or more agents in the product.

Occasionally an occlusive ointment, such as zinc oxide or petrolatum, applied to *noninflamed* areas will prevent the development of dermatitis, provided good hygiene is also practiced. The ointment is removed during cleansing and reapplied. Because they tend to contribute to sweat retention, ointments are not applied to inflamed areas. The use of talcum powder is of questionable benefit and poses the hazard of accidental aspiration (see p. 300).

The selection and care of diapers are important aspects in preventing inflammation or further irritation. Disposable diapers that contain absorbent gelling material appear to be superior in fluid-handling capabilities to cloth or conventional disposable diapers. The gel binds fluid tightly in the core, and the buffer characteristics of the gel help maintain the normal acidic pH of the skin.

If parents prefer cloth diapers, soft, thoroughly laundered and sterilized diapers are best. Licensed, commercial diaper laundries provide the least irritating diapers. If diapers are laundered at home, they should be soaked in a quaternary ammonium compound (such as Diaparene), washed in hot water with a simple laundry soap (such as Ivory), and run through the rinse cycle twice. Using a dryer enhances diaper softness.

Topical glucocorticoid preparations are sometimes prescribed for stubborn inflammations that do not respond to the simple measures just described. *Candida* infections are treated with nystatin dusting powder, using precautions against the infant's inhaling the powder. Where *Candida* is the causative agent, oral administration of nystatin is advised also since the gastrointestinal tract is usually the source of infection.

ATOPIC DERMATITIS (ECZEMA)

Atopic dermatitis (AD), or eczema, is a common pruritic disease that usually appears in three forms based on the age of the child and the distribution of lesions:

infantile (infantile eczema)—usually begins between 2 and 6 months of age and usually undergoes spontaneous remission by 3 years of age
childhood—may follow the infantile form; it occurs at 2 to 3 years of age
preadolescent and adolescent—begins at about 12 years of age and may continue into the early adult years

The diagnosis of AD is based on a combination of history and morphologic findings (see box). The victims of the disease have a lower threshhold for cutaneous itching, and many authorities believe the dermatologic manifestations appear subsequent to scratching of the intense pruritus. For example, infants will rub their faces against bed linen, and crawling (a form of scratching) results in irritation of knees and elbows. Lesions will disappear if the scratching is stopped.

The majority of children with infantile AD have a family history of atopy (eczema, asthma, or allergic rhinitis), which strongly supports a genetic predisposition. The cause is unknown but appears to be related to abnormal function of the skin, including alterations in sweating, peripheral vascular function, and heat tolerance. The disease is better in humid climates and worse in fall and winter, when homes are heated and environmental humidity is lower. The disorder can be controlled but not cured.

Clinical Manifestations of Atopic Dermatitis

Distribution of lesions:
- Infantile form—generalized, especially cheeks, scalp, trunk, and extensor surfaces of extremities
- Childhood form—flexural areas (antecubital and popliteal fossae, neck), wrists, ankles, and feet
- Preadolescent and adolescent form—face, sides of neck, hands, feet, face, and antecubital and popliteal fossae (to a lesser extent)

Appearance of lesions:
- Infantile form
  - Erythema
  - Vesicles
  - Papules
  - Weeping
  - Oozing
  - Crusting
  - Scaling
  - Often symmetrical
- Childhood form
  - Symmetrical involvement
  - Clusters of small erythematous or flesh-colored papules or minimally scaling patches
  - Dry and may be hyperpigmented
  - Lichenification (thickened skin with accentuation of creases)
  - Keratosis pilaris (follicular hyperkeratosis) common
- Adolescent/adult form
  - Same as childhood manifestations
  - Dry, thick lesions (lichenified plaques) common
  - Confluent papules

Other manifestations
- Intense itching
- Unaffected skin dry and rough
- Black children likely to exhibit more papular and/or follicular lesions than white children
- May exhibit one or more of the following:
  - Lymphadenopathy, especially near affected sites
  - Increased palmar creases (many cases)
  - Atopic pleats (extra line or groove of lower eyelid)
  - Prone to cold hands
  - Pityriasis alba (small, poorly defined areas of hypopigmentation)
  - Facial pallor (especially around nose, mouth, and ears)
  - Bluish discoloration beneath eyes ("allergic shiners")
  - Increased susceptibility to unusual cutaneous infections (especially viral)
- Personality traits often associated with eczema:
  - Active
  - Restless
  - Irritable
  - Aggressive
  - Frequently precocious and bright

Therapeutic Management

The major goals of management are to (1) relieve pruritus, (2) hydrate the skin, (3) reduce inflammation, and (4) prevent or control secondary infection. Most of the general measures for managing AD serve to reduce pruritus as well other aspects of the disease. General management includes avoiding exposure to skin irritants, avoiding overheating, improving skin hydration, and administration of medications such as antihistamines, topical steroids, and (sometimes) mild sedatives as indicated.

Differing philosophies regarding cleansing and hydrating the skin of the child with AD generally embrace two methods—the wet and the dry methods. In the dry method baths are infrequent and skin is cleansed with a nonlipid, hydrophilic agent such as Cetaphil. The wet method consists of frequent baths (up to 4 times per day) followed immediately by the application of a lubricant (while the skin is still damp) to trap moisture in the skin. No soap or a very mild, nonperfumed soap (such as Dove, Lowila, or Neutrogena) is used. Some advocate oil or oilated oatmeal baths with light drying so that a protective, oily film remains on the skin. Showers should be avoided because of their drying effect.

Enhancing skin hydration can be accomplished by application of preparations that occlude the skin to prevent evaporation and retain moisture in the upper skin layers and/or by replacement of natural moisturizing substances in the skin. A variety of emollients containing petrolatum or lanolin have occlusive properties and are prescribed according to the degree of occlusion desired. For the majority of patients lotions applied twice or three times daily maintain satisfactory hydration. The frequency may be increased if greater hydration is required. Creams or ointments provide more occlusion, and those that contain urea or lactic acid improve the binding of water in the skin as well as prevent evaporation of moisture.

Sometimes colloid baths, such as the addition of 2 cups of cornstarch to a tub of warm water, provide temporary relief of itching and may help the child sleep if given before bedtime. Cool wet compresses are soothing to the skin and provide antiseptic protection.

Moderate or severe pruritus is usually relieved by administration of oral antihistamine drugs (hydroxyzine [Atarax] or diphenhydramine [Benadryl]), and the amount is tailored to the individual child. Since pruritus increases at night, a mild sedative may be needed.

Occasional flare-ups require the use of topical steroids to diminish inflammation. Low-, moderate-, or high-potency topical corticosteroids are prescribed, depending on the degree of involvement, the area of the body to be treated, the age of the child, and the type of vehicle to be used (e.g., cream, lotion, ointment). Secondary infection is managed with appropriate antibiotic therapy.

The role of food allergy in the etiology of AD is controversial, and the value of dietary modification is questionable. If there is a clear relationship between ingestion of a certain food and exacerbation of the condition, the offending allergen is eliminated from the diet. A small proportion of children with AD exhibit a sensitivity to eggs, milk, peanuts, soy, wheat, or fish. It is especially important that infants at risk for atopy remain on breast-feedings, with delayed introduction of solid foods for the first 6 months of life.

Nursing Considerations

Long-term treatment of AD is usually established on an outpatient basis. As a result the major burden of responsibility and physical care rests on the parents in the home. A vicious cycle of exacerbations–scratching–infection–irritability–frustration is the usual course unless the initial phase can be altered.

ASSESSMENT

Assessment of the child with AD includes a family history for evidence of atopy, a history of previous involvement, and any environmental or dietary factors associated with the present and previous exacerbations. The skin lesions are examined for type, distribution, and evidence of secondary infection. The parents are interviewed regarding the child's behavior, especially in relation to the child's scratching, irritability, and sleeping patterns. The interview should also include exploration of the family's feelings and methods of coping with the situation.

Nursing Diagnoses: The Child with Atopic Dermatitis

Chronic pain related to intense pruritus
Impaired skin integrity related to eczematous lesions
Potential for infection related to risk of secondary infection of primary lesions
Sleep pattern disturbance related to pruritus
Altered family processes related to child's discomfort and lengthy therapy

NURSING DIAGNOSES

A number of nursing diagnoses identified for the child with AD are outlined in the accompanying box. Others will be apparent in individual cases.

PLANNING

The objectives for nursing care of the child with AD are similar to those for medical management as follows:

1. Relieve pruritus
2. Improve skin hydration
3. Prevent secondary infection
4. Support child and family

IMPLEMENTATION

The child with AD presents a nursing challenge. Controlling the intense pruritus is imperative if the disorder is to be successfully managed, since scratching leads to the formation of new lesions and may cause secondary infection. In addition to the medical regimen other measures can be taken to prevent or minimize the scratching. Fingernails and toenails are cut short, kept clean, and filed frequently to prevent sharp edges. Gloves or cotton stockings may have to be placed over the hands and pinned to shirtsleeves. To prevent any contact with the skin, elbow restraints are sometimes necessary. One-piece outfits with long sleeves and long pants also decrease direct contact with the skin. Whether gloves or restraints are used, the child needs time when he is free from such restrictions. An excellent time to remove any protective devices is during the bath or after receiving sedative or antipruritic medication. Restraints should not be removed during sleep because of the likelihood that the child will scratch while asleep.

Conditions that increase itching should be eliminated when possible. Woolen clothes or blankets, rough fabrics, and furry stuffed animals should be removed. Since heat and humidity cause perspiration, which intensifies the itching, proper dress for climatic conditions is essential. Pruritus is often precipitated by exposure to the irritant effects of certain components of common products such as soaps, detergents, fabric softeners, perfumes, and powders. Most children experience less itching when soft cotton fabrics are worn next to the skin. During cold months, synthetic fabrics (not wool) should be used for overcoats, hats, gloves, and snowsuits.

Clothes and sheets should be laundered in a mild detergent and rinsed thoroughly in clear water (without fabric softeners and antistatic chemicals). Putting the clothes through a second complete wash cycle without using detergent minimizes the amount of residue remaining in the fabric.

Preventing infection is usually secondary to preventing scratching. Personal hygiene is accomplished as described previously. Baths are given as prescribed, the water kept tepid, and soaps (except as indicated) and bubble baths are avoided, as well as the use of oils or powder. Skin folds and diaper areas need frequent cleansing with plain water. If the child is being treated with frequent baths for hydration, it is imperative that the emollient preparation be applied *immediately* following bathing (while the skin is still slightly moist) to prevent drying. A room humidifier or vaporizer may benefit children with extremely dry skin.

Soaks and compresses are applied as directed. Medications for pruritus or infection are administered as directed. The family is given explicit instructions on the preparation and use of soaks, special baths, and topical medications, including the order of application if more than one is prescribed. It is important to emphasize that one thick application of a topical medication is *not* equivalent to several thin applications, and that excessive use of an agent, particularly steroids, can be hazardous. If children have difficulty remaining still for a 10- or 15-minute soak, bath, or dressing application, these can be carried out at naptime or when the child is engrossed in television or a story.

Since adequate rest is also important for these children, who are usually fretful and irritable, planning meals, baths, medications, and treatments during awake periods is paramount. Sleepy, tired children are normally cranky, and such behavior only intensifies the urge to scratch. During periods of irritability, these children tend to be anorectic, which is worsened by restriction of their usual foods.

Diet modification is another source of frustration to parents. When a hypoallergenic diet is prescribed, parents need help in understanding the reason for the diet and guidelines for following it. Since hypoallergenic diets take time before visible effects are apparent, parents need reassurance that this is not an immediate cure.

Family support. Parents can be assured that the lesions will not produce scarring (unless secondarily infected) and that the disease is not contagious. However, the child will be subject to repeated exacerbations and remissions. Spontaneous and permanent remission takes place at approximately 2 to 3 years of age in most children with the infantile disorder.

Perhaps it is because the physical problems seem insurmountable during periods of acute exacerbation that the emotional stress becomes so intense for the family members. They need time to discuss negative feelings and to be reassured that these feelings are expected, normal, acceptable, and healthy, provided there is an emotional outlet to dissipate the invested energy. During acute phases, relieving as much anxiety as possible in both parents and child has a beneficial emotional and physical effect, since stress tends to aggravate the severity of the condition.

EVALUATION

The effectiveness of nursing interventions is determined by continual reassessment and evaluation of care based on the following observational guidelines and expected outcomes:

1. Observe the child's behavior, clothing, and activities
2. Examine the skin surface for evidence of dryness
3. Examine skin lesions for evidence of secondary infection
4. Interview the family and encourage dialog regarding the child and his care

Expected outcomes:

1. The child does not scratch, appears comfortable, and sleeps well
2. The skin appears well hydrated
3. There is no evidence of secondary infection
4. Family members comply with the therapeutic regimen, freely discuss their feelings and concerns, and appear to be coping with the inconveniences imposed by the disorder (specify)

SEBORRHEIC DERMATITIS

Seborrheic dermatitis is a chronic, recurrent, inflammatory reaction of the skin. It occurs most commonly in the scalp (cradle cap) but may involve the eyelids (blepharitis), external ear canal (otitis externa), nasolabial folds, and inguinal region. The cause is unknown, although it is more common in early infancy, when sebum production is increased. The lesions are characteristically thick, adherent, yellowish, scaly, oily patches that may or may not be mildly pruritic. Unlike atopic dermatitis, seborrheic dermatitis is not associated with a positive family history for allergy and is very common in infants shortly after birth. Diagnosis is made primarily on the appearance and location of the crusts.

Nursing Considerations

Cradle cap may be prevented with adequate scalp hygiene. Not infrequently parents omit shampooing the infant's hair for fear of damaging the "soft spots," or fontanels. It is important to discuss how to shampoo the infant's hair and to emphasize that the fontanel is like skin anywhere else on the body—it does not puncture or tear with mild pressure.

When seborrheic lesions are present, parents are taught the appropriate procedure to clean the scalp, which may require a demonstration. Shampooing should be done three to four times a week with a mild soap or commercial shampoo. If an oil is applied, it is massaged into the scalp and allowed to penetrate and soften the crusts and then thoroughly washed out. Using a fine-tooth comb after shampooing helps remove the loosened crusts from the strands of hair. Topical preparations are usually not necessary but if prescribed require the same teaching as discussed for atopic dermatitis.

ACNE

There is one skin disorder that, although not limited to the adolescent age-group, appears predominantly at this time—*acne vulgaris*. Acne is an almost universal occurrence during these years and involves anatomic, physiologic, biochemical, genetic, immunologic, and psychologic factors of significant import.

It is estimated that about 70% of the population will have had acne by the end of the teenage years. Although the disorder can appear before this time, the peak incidence is in late adolescence, at about age 16 to 17 in girls and 17 to 18 years in boys. It is more common in males than in females. The degree to which an individual is affected may range from nothing more than a few isolated comedones to a severe inflammatory reaction. Although the disease is self-limited and not life-threatening, its significance to the adolescent is great, and it is a mistake to underestimate the impact it can have on young persons.

The etiology of acne is still unclear, although a number of factors appear to be related to its development. Its distribution in families and a high degree of concordance in identical twins suggest that hereditary factors predispose to susceptibility to acne. Androgens are implicated, and the disorder seems to be aggravated by emotional stress, winter weather, some stimulant drugs, and the premenstrual period in females. There is no positive evidence that any specific foods are factors, except perhaps in individual youngsters.

Pathophysiology

Acne is a disease that involves the pilosebaceous follicles (the hair follicle and sebaceous gland complex) of the face, neck, shoulders, back, and upper chest—the so-called flush areas of the skin. There are two basic types of lesions seen in acne:

1. **Noninflamed** lesions, called *comedones,* consisting of compact masses of keratin, lipids, fatty acids, and bacteria that dilate the follicular duct, which may be plugged (closed comedones, or whiteheads, with no visible opening) or open (blackheads, with visible dilated openings that are discolored as fatty acids are oxidated by air)
2. **Inflamed** lesions, which result when the follicular wall ruptures to produce papules, pustules, nodules, and cysts (Fig. 29-6). The inflammatory acne is responsible for the destructiveness and propensity for scarring

Secondary invasion by *Staphylococcus albus* can complicate the acne lesion, and adolescents' concern about their appearance tempts them to pick, finger, squeeze, and otherwise manipulate the lesions; this plays an important role in the perpetuation of acne. In addition to the precipitating factors mentioned previously, the application of creams, oils, and some cosmetics that add to the plugging of the follicles may aggravate acne; therefore, only water-based cosmetic agents should be selected to avoid those with greasy or occlusive bases.

Therapeutic Management

There is little evidence that treatment shortens the duration of the entire course of the disease. However, much can be done to control acne, reduce the inflammatory process and scarring, and improve the appearance. No single therapeutic agent is effective in the management of acne except in a few mild cases. It is usually more effective to employ a combination of therapies. The treatment most commonly consists of measures directed toward improving the general health of the youngster, removing comedones, preventing their formation, controlling excessive sebaceous gland activity, controlling infection, and preventing scar formation.

General measures. Improvement of the adolescent's overall health status is part of the general management. Adequate rest, moderate exercise, a well-balanced diet,

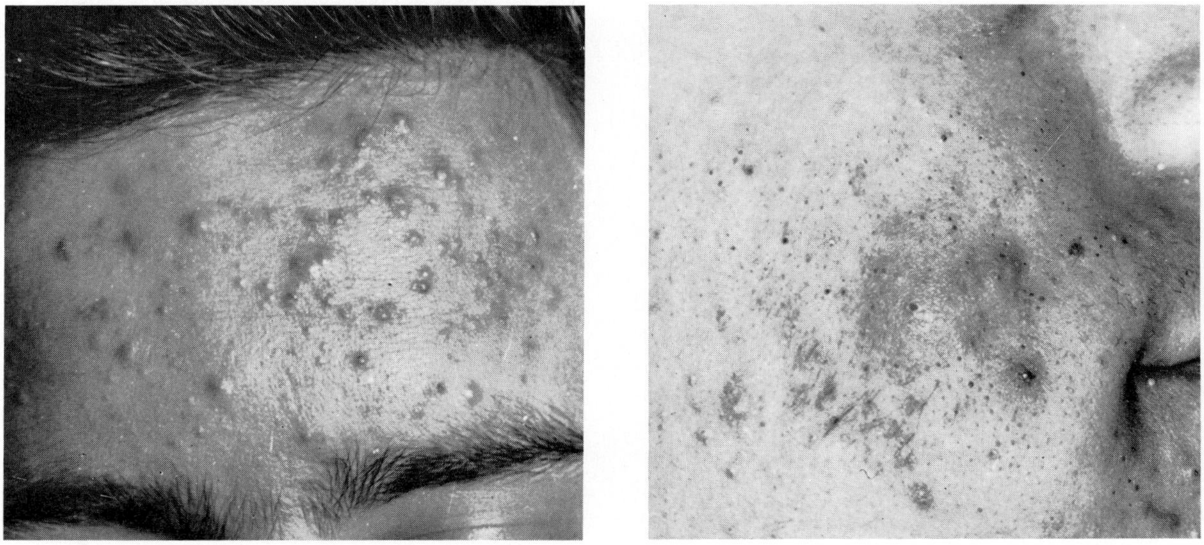

FIG. 29-6 Acne vulgaris. Papular pustules and comedones. (From Stewart, W.D., Danto, J.L., and Maddin, S.: Dermatology: diagnosis and treatment of cutaneous disorders, ed. 4, St. Louis, 1978, The C.V. Mosby Co.)

reduction of emotional stress, elimination of any foci of infection, and correction of constipation (if it exists) are all part of general health promotion. There is no convincing evidence to implicate any single dietary item or combination of foods in the exacerbation of acne, with the possible exception of iodides and bromide in therapeutic amounts. Occasionally a youngster will demonstrate an aggravation of symptoms after each ingestion of a given food. In such instances the food is eliminated for a period of time to assess its influence on the disease.

Medication. There is a wide range of types and combinations of topical agents for the treatment of acne, with selection depending on the type and severity of the lesions. The most effective therapy involves the use of benzoyl peroxide, tretinoin (retinoic acid), or a combination of these. Both agents can cause redness and peeling early in their use; therefore the treatment usually begins with graded increases in concentration and/or frequency of application according to the patient's tolerance. The two drugs should not be applied together, since the benzoyl peroxide may oxidize the retinoic acid and render it impotent.

Since most patients also have some inflammatory lesions accompanying the comedones, a topical antibacterial agent is prescribed. Systemic antibiotic therapy may be needed for some patients who do not respond to topical therapy. Isotretinoin, 13-*cis* retinoic acid (Accutane), a very potent and effective topical agent, is reserved for severe cystic acne because of its side effects. Since the drug has been found to be teratogenic and therefore unsuitable for pregnant women, all sexually active teenagers should be identified before treatment and the drug given only if they use an effective form of contraception during and for 3 to 4 months after completion of treatment (Committee on Drugs, 1983).

Cleansing. Gentle cleansing with a mild cleanser once or twice daily is usually sufficient. Harsh, rough soaps and excessive scrubbing may irritate the skin and cause rupture of the pilosebaceous ducts. For some adolescents hygiene of the hair and scalp appears to be related to the clinical activity of the acne. In these persons acne of the forehead can be improved by brushing the hair away from the forehead and more frequent shampooing.

Nursing Considerations

The adolescent should be encouraged to seek medical treatment for the skin lesions from a sympathetic and understanding dermatologist; however, the extent of physician involvement varies. Self-treatment is extremely common and associated with the many myths related to the cause and treatment of acne. Often it is the nurse who establishes the initial contact with the affected adolescent and is instrumental in the youngster's seeking medical advice and embarking on a course of treatment. It is essential that the youngster with inflammatory lesions obtain medical treatment in order to control the process and reduce the incidence of scarring.

Teenagers need a supportive, caring individual to help them maintain the persistence required to deal with the disorder over such an extended period of time. The adolescent needs education regarding the disease process and instruction in the prescribed therapy. Instruction should be definite and as specific as practical for each individual youngster. A written instruction sheet that describes the etiology and therapeutic regimen is often helpful, and parents should be cautioned against nagging. Adolescents should assume responsibility for following through on the instructions. They need to be cautioned against damaging the skin through too vigorous scrubbing. Several points are emphasized as particularly important: using only those preparations and appliances (such as the ultraviolet light) prescribed for their particular needs; carrying out associated directions, such as hairstyling and shampooing; and, for girls, not leaving cosmetics on the face overnight. Nurses can help girls select proper cosmetic preparations.

Initially the procedures are carried out in the physician's office by the physician or nurse, but a parent or other family member often can be taught to use the extractor. The face is washed with soap and water before and after extraction, and the instrument is cleaned and cared for in the manner directed by the individual physician. This usually means cleaning the extractor with soap and water and then either storing it in alcohol or wiping it with alcohol and storing it in a clean receptacle, such as a dry envelope. The parent is cautioned against using excessive pressure that might bruise the skin. The blackhead that cannot be removed readily should be left until another time. Some dermatologists limit home treatment to removal of blackheads only.

During conversations with teenagers, the nurse can dispel the common myths often associated with acne and allow youngsters to discuss any feelings related to the disorder, such as self-consciousness or anxieties regarding relationships with others. Sometimes, the nurse also can help teenagers explore job or other after-school interests. The acne lesions need not become an excuse to avoid social contacts and activities.

◆ *Thermal Injury*

Thermal injuries are usually attributed to injury from extreme heat sources. Although thermal burns are the most frequent type of burns, harmful effects also occur from exposure to cold or hot environments.

BURNS

Minor burn injuries are experienced by everyone in day-to-day living and are relatively commonplace in nursing practice. Extensive burns, on the other hand, are relatively uncommon; however, they account for some of the most difficult nursing problems encountered in the pediatric age-group. As a cause of accidental death in childhood, burns are outranked only by automobile casualties and drownings. In addition, serious burn injury accounts for a very large number of children who must undergo prolonged, painful, and restrictive hospitalization.

Burns can be caused by thermal, chemical, electric, or radioactive agents. Most burn injuries are caused by thermal agents, principally flame and hot water (including steam), and, to a lesser extent, friction. Chemical burns can be caused by either acids or alkalis, radiation burns by either radiographs or ultraviolet radiation, and electric burns by live wires, transformers, or lightning. The extent of tissue destruction is determined by the intensity of the heat source, the duration of contact or exposure, and the speed with which the heat energy is dissipated by the burned surface. For example, a brief exposure to high-intensity heat, such as a flame, or a longer exposure to a low-intensity heat, such as hot water, can produce similar burn injuries.

Contact burns from heated metal or liquids (such as tar) at extreme temperatures, prolonged immersion in hot water, chemical burns without rinsing with water, and electric burns are all significant in the etiology of severe burn trauma. Chemical agents continue to cauterize the tissues until the injurious agent is chemically united with tissue elements, neutralized, or removed by washing with running water. Electric burns are especially deceptive, since they are characterized by more extensive thrombosis that is not evident until 24 to 36 hours after injury. Their extensive destruction has been described as resembling a crush injury.

Characteristics of Burn Injury

The physiologic responses, therapy, prognosis, and disposition of the injured child are all directly related to the *amount of tissue destroyed;* therefore, the severity of the burn injury is assessed on the basis of the percentage of surface burned and the depth of the burn. Also important in determining the seriousness of the injury are the location of the burn(s), the age of the child, causative agent, the presence or absence of respiratory involvement, the general health of the child, and the presence of any associated injury or condition.

Extent of injury. The extent of a burn is usually expressed as a percentage of total body surface area, which is most accurately estimated by using specially designed age-related charts (Fig. 29-7). Because of the body proportions, especially the head and lower extremities, the standard "rule of nines" charts used for adults are not applicable to small children.

Depth of injury. A thermal injury is a three-dimensional wound and therefore is also assessed in relation to depth of injury. Traditionally the terms *first-*, *second-*, and *third-degree* have been used to describe the depth of tissue injury. However, with the current emphasis on burn healing, these are gradually being replaced by more descriptive terms based on the extent of destruction to the epithelializing elements of the skin (Fig. 29-8).

A

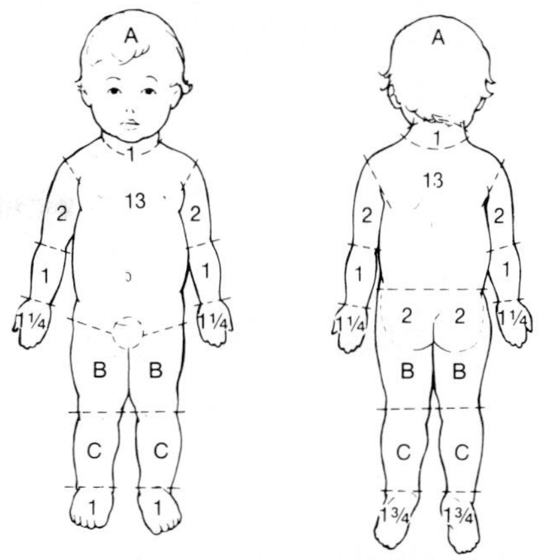

RELATIVE PERCENTAGES OF AREAS AFFECTED BY GROWTH

AREA	BIRTH	AGE 1 YR	AGE 5 YR
A = ½ of head	9½	8½	6½
B = ½ of one thigh	2¾	3¼	4
C = ½ of one leg	2½	2½	2¾

B

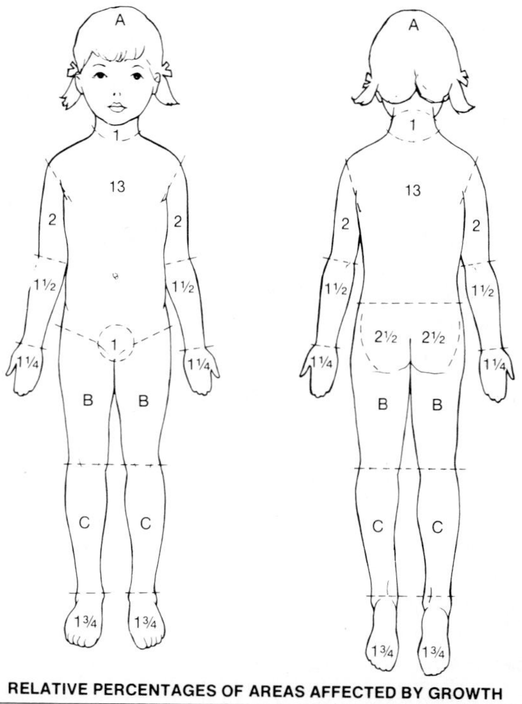

RELATIVE PERCENTAGES OF AREAS AFFECTED BY GROWTH

AREA	AGE 10 YR	AGE 15 YR	ADULT
A = ½ of head	5½	4½	3½
B = ½ of one thigh	4½	4½	4¾
C = ½ of one leg	3	3¼	3½

FIG. 29-7 Estimation of distribution of burns in children. **A,** Children from birth to age 5 years. **B,** Older children.

Superficial (first-degree) burns are usually of minor significance. There is frequently a latent period followed by erythema. Tissue damage is minimal, protective functions remain intact, and systemic effects are rare. Pain is the predominant symptom.

Partial-thickness (second-degree) burns are deeper and involve not only the epithelium but a minimal to sub-

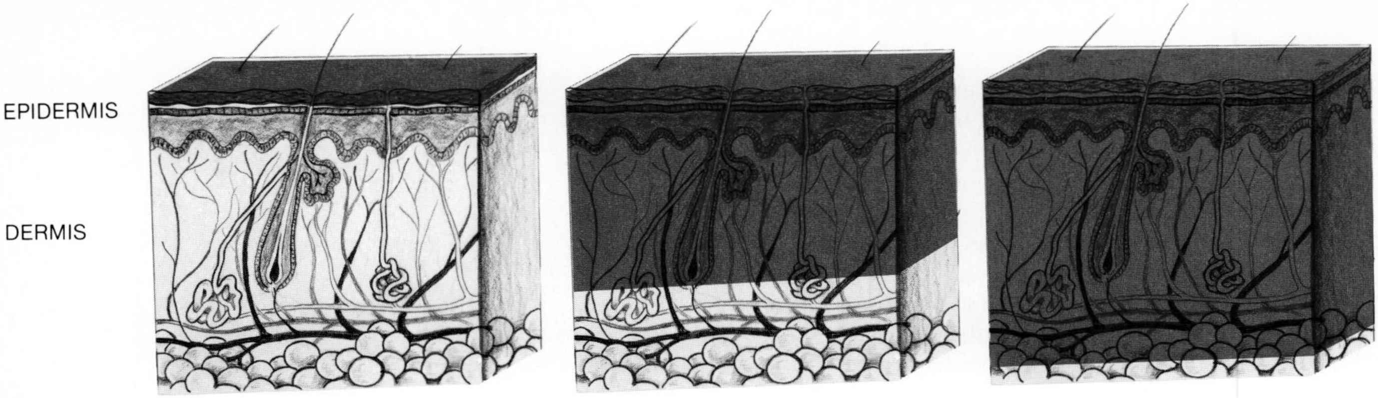

	Superficial (first degree)	Partial-thickness (second degree)	Full-thickness (third degree)
Type of burn	Sunburn; low-intensity flash; brief scald	Scalds; flash flame	Fire; contact with hot objects
Appearance	Dry surface; red; blanches on pressure and refills	Blistered; moist; mottled pink or red, reddened; blanches on pressure and refills	Tough, leathery; brown, tan, black, or red; does not blanch on pressure; dull, dry
Sensation	Painful	Very painful	Little pain

FIG. 29-8 Classification of burn depth.

stantial portion of the corium. The severity of the injury and the rate of healing are directly related to the amount of undamaged corium from which new tissue can regenerate. Superficial partial-thickness burns are often classified with first-degree burns and heal uneventfully. Deep thermal burns, although classified as partial-thickness burns, in many respects resemble full-thickness burns. Whereas superficial burns and superficial partial-thickness burns are painful, deep dermal burns are often anesthetic for the first 1 or 2 days after injury.

Full-thickness (third-degree) burns are serious injuries in which all layers of the skin are destroyed; such burns may involve underlying tissues as well, and they are usually combined with extensive partial-thickness damage. Systemic effects can be life-threatening and involve every organ system in the body. Although a notable characteristic of third-degree burns is lack of sensation at the wound surface, this is misleading. Superficial nerve endings are destroyed in the full-thickness areas, but nerve endings on wound edges are hypersensitive.

Severity of injury. Burns are also assessed on the basis of their severity, which is useful in determining the disposition and management of the patient. Burned patients can usually be distinguished as (1) those with a critical burn, who require the services and equipment of a special burn unit, (2) those with moderate burns, who may be treated in any hospital unit, and (3) those with minor burns, who are able to be treated on an outpatient basis. (See criteria for burn severity in the accompanying box.)

Other factors. Regardless of the amount of tissue destroyed, if inhalation of heated air and/or toxic fumes is suspected, there is risk of airway obstruction developing. Because infants' skin is so thin, it is readily destroyed by thermal agents. Children less than 2 years of age have a significantly higher mortality rate than older children with burns of similar magnitude. Acute or chronic illnesses or superimposed injuries also complicate burn care and response to treatment.

Burn Severity Criteria

Minor Burns

Partial-thickness burns of less than 15% of body surface
Full-thickness burns of less than 2% of body surface

Moderate Burns

Partial-thickness burns of 15% to 25% of body surface
Full-thickness burns of less than 10% of body area, except in small children and when the burns involve critical areas, such as the face, hands, feet, or genitalia

Major or Critical Burns

Burns complicated by respiratory tract injury
Partial-thickness burns of 25% total area or greater
Burns of face, hands, feet, or genitalia, even if they appear to be partial thickness
Full-thickness burns of 10% of body surface or greater
Any child younger than 2 years of age, unless the burn is very small and very superficial
Electric burns that penetrate
Deep chemical burns
Respiratory tract damage
Burns complicated by fractures or soft tissue injury
Burns complicated by concurrent illness, such as obesity, diabetes, epilepsy, and cardiac and renal diseases

Pathophysiology

Thermal injury produces both local and systemic effects that are directly related to the extent of tissue destruction. In superficial burns the tissue damage is minimal. The burning sensation and pain resolve in 48 to 72 hours; the damaged epithelium peels off in small scales or sheets, in 5 to 10 days, leaving no scarring. In partial-thickness burns there is considerable edema and more severe capillary damage. In 3 to 5 days a crust of dried exudate and injured tissue covers the wound to form a protective seal while healing takes place from underneath. With reasonable care, superficial burns heal spontaneously. The crust separates in 10 to 14 days with minimal or no scarring.

Deep-dermal burns heal more slowly. A thin epithelial covering develops in 25 to 35 days, but this type of burn may require several months to heal. Scarring is common, and trauma or infection can easily convert a partial-thickness burn to a full-thickness injury, especially in young children with their normally thinner skin. Fluid loss and metabolic effects may be considerable.

Along with and subsequent to the pathophysiologic response at the site of thermal injury, a number of systemic responses occur. Swelling takes place in and around the wound site as a result of increased capillary permeability and vasodilation. The edema can reach tremendous proportions and, in severe burns, loss of circulating fluid can precipitate shock. Loss of fluid, protein, and electrolytes at the wound surface further complicates the management of these patients.

Other systemic responses to severe burns include anemia, caused by direct heat destruction of red blood cells, hemolysis of heat-damaged red blood cells, and depressed bone marrow; massive protein loss from the burn wound and from gluconeogenesis; and increased metabolism to maintain body heat and provide for the increased energy needs of the body.

Complications. Thermally injured persons are subject to a number of serious complications, both from the wound and from systemic alterations resulting from the wound. The immediate threat to life is asphyxia caused by irritation and edema of the lungs and respiratory passages. In the first 48 to 72 hours the greatest hazard is unremitting shock, followed by possible renal shutdown and potassium excess during the first week. During healing, infection—both local and generalized sepsis—is the primary complication.

Pulmonary problems persist as the major cause of fatality in patients with either thermal burns or an injury to or complications in the respiratory tract. A full range of respiratory insufficiency can occur, including inhalation injury, aspiration in unconscious patients, bacterial pneumonia, pulmonary edema, pulmonary embolus, and post-traumatic pulmonary insufficiency. The most common causative factor in respiratory failure in the pediatric age-group is bacterial pneumonia, which may be secondary to airway injury or contamination from a tracheostomy or acquired through hematogenous spread of bacteria, usually from the burn wound.

EMERGENCY TREATMENT

Burns

Minor Burns

Stop burning process:
- Apply cool water to burn or hold burned area under cool running water

Do not disturb any blisters that form
Do not apply anything to wound
Leave small burns exposed to air
Apply dry, nonstick dressing if risk of damage or contamination
Observe for signs of infection

Major Burns

Stop burning process:
- Flame burns—smother fire
- Place victim in horizontal position
- Roll victim in blanket or similar object—avoid covering head
- Immerse in cool water or any nonflammable liquid

Remove burned clothing
Assess for adequate airway and breathing
- If not breathing, begin mouth-to-mouth resuscitation

Cover wound with clean cloth
Transport to medical aid

Sepsis is the most critical problem in treatment of burns, and it is an ever-present threat after the shock phase. Initially burns are relatively pathogen free, unless the wound is contaminated with potentially infectious material, such as dirt or polluted water. However, dead tissue and exudate provide a fertile field for bacterial growth. Early colonization of the wound surface by a preponderance of gram-positive organisms (primarily staphylococci) changes on about the third postburn day to predominantly gram-negative organisms, particularly *Pseudomonas aeruginosa.* By the fifth postburn day the bacterial invasion is well under way beneath the surface of the wound.

Recurrent or intermittent bleeding resulting from Curling, or stress, ulceration is a major noninfectious complication of burns. Routine antacid administration has reduced the incidence of this complication in recent years, but these superficial, erosive gastric lesions still occur in a number of burn injuries.

Therapeutic Management: Emergency Care

The aims of immediate treatment of thermal injury are to stop the burning process, begin emergency procedures, cover the wound, transport the child to medical aid, and provide reassurance.

In flame burns the chief aim in rescue is to smother the fire, not to fan it. Children tend to panic and run, which only serves to fan the flames and make assistance more difficult. The victim should not run and should not remain standing. The injured child is placed in a horizontal position and rolled in a blanket, rug, or similar article, with care taken not to cover the child's head and face because of the danger of the child's inhaling the toxic fumes. If no covering is available, the child is made to lie down and roll over slowly. If the victim remains in a vertical position, the hair may be ignited or he may inhale flames, heat, or smoke.

Spontaneous cooling of burns by slow immersion in cold water or any nonflammable liquid helps to relieve the pain, inhibit edema formation, and slow the process of heat damage. Ice water or ice packs are contraindicated because the resulting vasoconstriction interferes with capillary perfusion and carries the risk of further damage from cold burn. Unless there is nothing else available, no dirt or sand should be thrown on the burn. In chemical burns it is particularly important to wash the burn with copious amounts of cool running water, except when the chemical irritant is a powder (addition of water causes the caustic agent to spread). Burned clothing is removed to prevent further damage from smoldering fabric or hot beads of melted synthetic material.

As soon as the flames are extinguished, the condition of the victim is assessed. Airway, breathing, and circulation are the priority concerns. The burn wound should be covered with a clean cloth to prevent contamination and to alleviate pain by avoiding air contact. The child with extensive burns is covered to prevent hypothermia. No attempt should be made to treat the burn, including application of topical ointments, oils, or other home remedies.

The child with an extensive burn is not given anything by mouth because of the risk of aspiration and water intoxication. The child is transported to the nearest place where medical aid is available. Providing reassurance and psychologic support to both the parents and the child helps immeasurably during postinjury crisis. Reducing anxiety helps to conserve energy needed to cope with the physiologic and emotional stress of a traumatic injury.

Therapeutic Management: Minor Burns

Treatment of burns classified as minor usually can be managed adequately on an outpatient basis when it is determined that the parents can be relied on to carry out instructions for care and observation. The wound is cleansed and debrided (all foreign material and devitalized tissue removed) with a tepid or cool dilute, nonirritating soap solution and then rinsed with sterile saline solution. Coolness reduces pain and probably reduces edema that can interfere with capillary flow in the area. Because they provide a sterile covering for the wound, intact blisters may or may not be debrided.

Most physicians favor covering the wound with a dry dressing or fine-mesh gauze lightly lubricated with water-soluble antiseptic or antimicrobial cream and then wrapping it with bulky dry gauze dressings. Some physicians prefer that an occlusive dressing be left in place for 7 to 10 days if the dressing remains clean and the child afebrile. The parents are instructed to cleanse the wound with mild soap and tepid water, change the dressings once or twice daily, and return to the office or clinic as directed for wound observation.

If there is a high probability of infection or other complications or if there is doubt about their ability to carry out the directions, the parents may be directed to return daily for dressing change and inspection or a nurse may be assigned to make a home visit for that purpose. Soaking the dressings in tepid water prior to removal will help loosen dressings and debris and reduce the discomfort. Burns about the face are usually treated by exposure, since a protective crust will form in 24 to 36 hours, provided the atmosphere is cool and dry.

A tetanus history is obtained on admission. When there is no history of immunization, human tetanus antitoxin should be administered. Administration of antibiotics for minor burns is controversial. A mild analgesic, such as acetaminophen, is usually sufficient to relieve any discomfort, and the antipyretic effect of the drug helps alleviate the sensation of heat.

Most mild burns heal with little difficulty, but if the wound margin becomes erythematous, gross purulence is noted, or the child develops evidence of systemic reaction, such as fever or tachycardia, hospitalization is indicated.

Therapeutic Management: Major Burns

When a child with serious burns is admitted to the hospital for treatment, a variety of assessments are made and therapies initiated. Of these, the priority concerns are (1) to establish and maintain an adequate airway, (2) to establish a lifeline for fluid resuscitation, and (3) to care for the burn wound. Other needs and therapies, including nutritional support, splinting to prevent contractures, treatment of anemia and hypoproteinemia, and the rehabilitative aspects of burn management, are initiated as appropriate throughout the course of treatment.

Establishment of adequate airway. The first priority of care is airway maintenance. If there is evidence of respiratory involvement, oxygen is administered and blood gases, including carbon monoxide, are quickly determined. If the child exhibits air hunger or otherwise appears in critical condition, an endotracheal tube is inserted to maintain the airway. Since early edema subsides within 24 to 48 hours and many have been managed successfully for longer periods of time without significant damage, nasotracheal intubation is safer and preferred to a tracheostomy.

Frequently, placing the child in a Croupette or under an oxygen hood with a high flow of oxygen and maximum humidity is sufficient to reduce reflex bronchospasm produced by trauma to the bronchial mucosa.

Fluid replacement therapy. The objectives of fluid therapy are to (1) compensate for water and sodium lost to traumatized areas and interstitial spaces, (2) replenish sodium deficits, (3) restore plasma volume, (4) obtain adequate perfusion, (5) correct acidosis, and (6) improve renal function.

Fluid and electrolyte therapy for children in the first 24 hours after a burn injury is still controversial, especially in relation to whether colloid solution should be part of this phase of fluid therapy. Therefore, the composition of the fluid selected varies with the philosophy of the individual physician or the burn unit. Needs are determined by several parameters, such as vital signs, urine volume and character, pulse, adequacy of capillary filling, and state of sensorium.

After diuresis (in 48 to 72 hours) when capillary permeability is restored, colloid solutions such as albumin or plasma are useful in maintaining plasma volume. Oral fluids are usually withheld in the early resuscitative phase but may be administered in 24 to 48 hours. Fluid balance may continue to be a problem throughout the course of treatment, especially during the periods in which there may be considerable evaporative loss from the wound.

Nutrition. The high metabolic requirements and catabolism in severe burns make nutritional needs of paramount importance and often difficult to provide. The diet must provide sufficient protein to avoid protein breakdown, as well as extra calories to help use the proteins, sustain the adaptive hypermetabolism, and spare protein breakdown. Extra calories should be derived from carbohydrates, since fat, although higher in total calories, will not spare protein.

Most burn patients are able to eat, and the child is given oral feedings as soon as possible. Because burned children have poor appetites and the caloric requirements may be as much as two to three times their usual requirements for size and age, the diet is high in calories and protein, supplemented with high doses of vitamins B and C and iron. Nasogastric feedings may be needed to supplement oral intake, and intravenous hyperalimentation has been used to provide a large amount of concentrated glucose and amino acids, especially in infants.

Medication. Controversy also exists regarding the use of antibiotics during the first few days after injury. Some authorities believe that low doses of penicillin should be given prophylactically to all children with serious burns. Others prefer to treat infections only when they become a problem. Elevated temperatures are evaluated and antibiotics administered if no immediate source of the elevation can be identified.

Some form of sedation and analgesia is required in the care of burned children. Morphine sulfate is the drug of choice for severe burn injuries. Morphine has extensive distribution, although it is eliminated rapidly; therefore, more frequent administration is needed for burn management. Acetaminophen with codeine is effective for less severe injury. The use of potent narcotics, such as fentanyl, or short-acting anesthetic agents, such as ketamine, is very effective in eliminating the pain during debridement. See Chapter 20 for a discussion of pain, pain assessment, and pain management.

To facilitate growth and proliferation of epithelial cells, administration of vitamin A is begun early in the postburn period. Zinc sulfate is also administered by some physicians, because zinc stores are depleted during catabolism and it appears to facilitate wound healing and epithelialization.

Care of burn wound. After the initial period of shock and restoration of fluid balance, the primary concern is the burn wound. The objectives of management for epidermal and superficial burns are to prevent infection by providing as aseptic an environment as possible, prevent mechanical trauma, and relieve pain. Occlusive dressings protect the wound from injury and help to reduce pain by minimizing exposure to air. The exposure method allows the wound to dry and is used primarily for mild to moderate face wounds. The objectives for management of full-thickness wounds are prevention of invasive infection, removal of dead tissue, and closure of the wound.

The use of hydrotherapy has reduced the need for surgical debridement under general anesthetic. Debridement is painful and requires some type of analgesia before the procedure (Fig. 29-9). Soaking in the Hubbard tank for 20 to 30 minutes once or twice daily facilitates the loosening and removal of sloughing tissue, eschar, exudate, and topical medications. The mesh gauze serves to entrap exudative slough and is readily removed during the tubbing procedure (Fig. 29-10). Any loose tissue or eschar is carefully trimmed away before redressing.

There are several methods for covering the burn wound, and all meet the objectives of preparation for per-

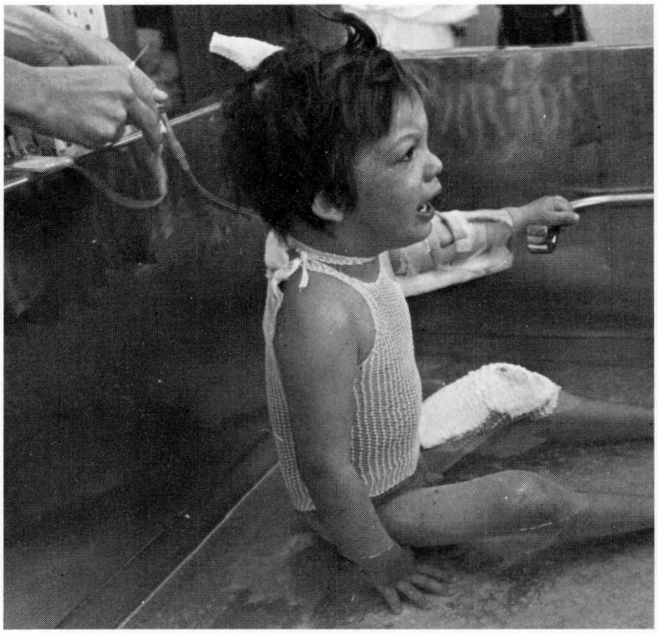

FIG. 29-9 An analgesic is administered prior to removal of dressings and debridement. In this instance the analgesic is injected directly into the intravenous line at the time of tubbing.

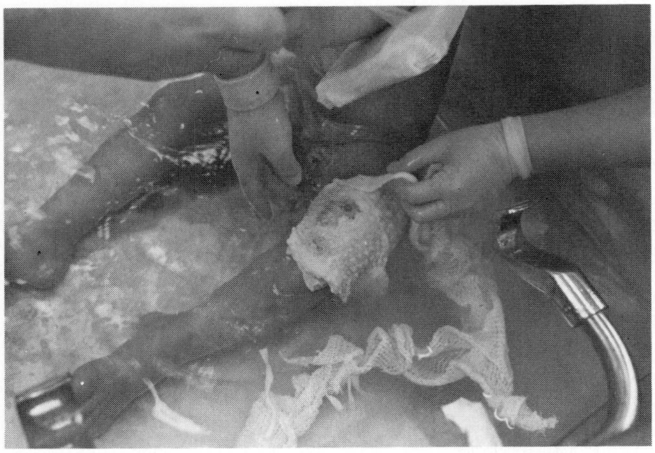

FIG. 29-10 Removal of dressings during tubbing.

manent wound coverage. Four methods are employed in the management of burn wounds:

Exposure—the wounds are left open to the air; crust forms on partial-thickness wounds, eschar forms on full-thickness wounds

Open—a topical antimicrobial ointment is applied directly to the wound surface, but the wound is left uncovered

Modified—ointment is applied directly to wound or impregnated into thin gauze that is applied to the wound; a stretched gauze or net covering secures the area

Occlusive—ointment-impregnated gauze or ointment covered with a gauze layer is placed on the burn wound; multiple layers of bulky gauze are placed over the primary layer and secured with stretched gauze or net

A number of topical agents are employed, but those used most frequently are 0.5% silver nitrate solution, 10% mafenide acetate (Sulfamylon), and 1% silver sulfadiazine (Silvadene). All three are effective bacteriostatic agents, but each has advantages and disadvantages. Less frequently used are 0.1% gentamycin sulfate (Garamycin) and povidone-iodine (Betadine) ointment.

Temporary or permanent coverage of full-thickness wounds is accomplished with grafts. Temporary grafts are those that provide biologic dressings during the acute phase of therapy to protect the wound from bacterial invasion and to minimize fluid loss. Permanent grafting is used to restore cosmetic appearance and to achieve maximum functional capacity. In recent years the early application of temporary biologic dressings to partial-thickness burns, especially in children, has significantly improved burn management and is gaining in popularity.

Grafts are derived from several sources. Permanent grafts, however, are obtained from only two sources and are of two types:

autografts tissues obtained from undamaged areas of the patient's own body

isografts histocompatible tissue obtained from genetically identical individuals, that is, the patient's identical twin

Temporary grafts include:

allografts (homografts) tissues obtained from genetically different members of the same species, living or dead—usually cadavers—that are free from disease

xenografts (heterografts) tissues obtained from members of a different species. At present most xenografts are derived primarily from pigskin, either fresh or frozen

Biologic (pigskin, amnion, cadaver skin), biosynthetic (Biobrane, Biobrin), or synthetic adhesive polyurethane film (Op-Site, Clingfilm, Via-film) dressings are frequently employed as temporary covering until the wound bed has developed sufficient granulation for permanent grafts. Permanent grafting of full-thickness burns is usually accomplished with a split-thickness skin graft. This consists of the epidermis and part of the dermis being removed from an undamaged area by a special instrument, the dermatome, which is designed to excise split-thickness skin. The priority areas for coverage are the face, neck, and areas around joints, especially the hands.

The donor site is dressed with either a xenograft or fine-mesh gauze and left exposed until the graft falls off, in about 10 to 14 days. Dressings are not changed on donor sites to prevent tearing the new, delicate epithelium.

Nursing Considerations

Nursing care is the most important aspect of burn therapy. The care of the severely burned child encompasses a broad range of skills and foci.

ASSESSMENT

Initial assessment of the burned child includes the wound assessments described on p. 997 as well as a comprehensive assessment of his general condition and behaviors. The child with severe and/or extensive burns requires constant observation and assessment, with special attention to signs of complications. Each major phase of care has areas of greatest threat: fluid and electrolyte disturbances (especially shock) in the acute phase, infection in the management phase, and healing and functional disturbances from scar formation in the rehabilitative phases. Respiratory, cardiac, and renal complications may appear early in the postburn period.

NURSING DIAGNOSES

Nursing diagnoses identified for the child with severe or extensive burns are included in the Nursing Care Plan on pp. 1006 to 1008. Additional diagnoses may be ascertained for individual children.

Planning

The aims of nursing care for the burned child are:

1. Relieve pain
2. Facilitate wound healing

THERAPEUTIC DIALOGUE

Burns

A 9-year-old child who has sustained 60% partial- and full-thickness burns from a barbecue fire is talking to the nurse.

CHILD: Why did God punish me like this?
NURSE: What do you mean?
CHILD: Why did God let me get burned when my grandpa was the one who started the grill?
NURSE: Your grandpa wasn't burned?
CHILD: No, only me. And it isn't fair. I was just sitting a little way from the grill.
NURSE: It sounds like you're wondering what you did to deserve this.
CHILD: That's right. God must hate me for letting me get burned.
NURSE: What could you have done to make God hate you?
CHILD: I don't know.
NURSE: Do you think that sometimes things just happen to people, and maybe nobody meant to hurt them?
CHILD: Yes, like in car accidents or plane accidents.
NURSE: So why do you think your accident is any different?
CHILD: I don't know. Do you think it was just bad luck for me but not for my grandpa?
NURSE: Yes, I do. I don't believe anyone is punishing you. These unhappy things just happen, and nobody is to blame.

SUMMARY

This conversation helped the child deal with his guilt and also his resentment toward the grandfather, whom he had refused to see.

3. Provide nutrition
4. Prevent complications
5. Support the child and family

IMPLEMENTATION

The primary emphasis during the initial phases of burn care is on prevention of burn shock. Checking vital signs, monitoring the intravenous infusion, and measuring urinary output are ongoing nursing activities in the hours immediately after injury. The intravenous infusion is started immediately by intracatheter or cutdown and is regulated according to urine output and specific gravity, laboratory data, and objective signs of adequate hydration. Urine volume, measured at least every hour, should be:

20 to 30 ml/hour in a child over 2 years of age
10 to 20 ml/hour in a child less than 2 years of age

The burn wound is treated according to the protocol of the specific burn facility. Extensive wounds may require the use of special beds and other equipment, such as CircOelectric beds, flotation beds, alternating pressure mattresses, and many other devices, depending on the extent and location of the wound.

The course of treatment is often long and emotionally laden for the child, the family, and the nursing staff. The severe pain of the wound and the therapies, the anxiety generated by these experiences, and the conscious and unconscious interpretations of traumatic events contribute to the psychologic reactions frequently observed in burned children. Much of the difficulty encountered in managing burned children is related to these factors. Soon after hospitalization many burned children become irritable, depressed, hostile, and aggressive toward the members of the health team. In his helplessness, the child often resorts to angry outbursts against anything and anybody.

Relieve pain. The burn pain is overwhelming, engulfing, and irrepressible. Consequently, the pain causes anxiety and a feeling of profound helplessness in the child and can produce reactions of confusion, fear, and panic. Compounding the pain is the child's interpretation of it and of the procedures; this is closely related to the developmental level of the child. Many burned children believe their pain is punishment for past misdeeds and therefore deserved. There are often feelings of anger, guilt, and depression, and, as in all illness, regressive behavior. When a child appears to accept his pain and shows little or no aggressive behavior, psychologic consultation is usually in order.

It is always difficult to deal with a child in pain, and to inflict pain on a helpless child is contrary to the empathetic nature of nursing. Adequate management of pain is essential to reduce the discomfort of the burn and the necessary therapeutic procedures. Management of pain consists of (1) choosing the correct analgesic, (2) using sufficient dosage, and (3) observing appropriate timing.

> ### *Nursing Tip: Burn Treatments*
>
> To relieve pain effectively during pain treatments, administer IV narcotics immediately before the procedure but oral nonnarcotics 1 hour before the procedure.

For example, to relieve pain adequately, the *onset* of action of the drug must be considered in order that the peak effect occurs when the treatment is performed (see Nursing tip). An analgesic administered shortly before the procedure will exert its effect *after* the procedure is completed. Management of pain follows the principles described in Chapter 20.

Facilitate wound healing. After the patient's condition is stabilized, the long management phase begins. The nurse has the major responsibility for cleansing, debriding, and applying topical medication and dressings to the burn wound. Because dressing removal is a painful procedure, the child should receive adequate analgesia before the scheduled tubbing. Both nurse and child must recognize it for exactly what it is—a dreadful but absolutely necessary procedure. Because it is painful, the child should know that it is all right to cry when the treatment hurts, but only *when it hurts*. Since it is easy for the child to give way to emotional excesses he cannot control, he needs the firm control of a caring adult. This includes both actual and anticipated hurt. The child needs help to gain and maintain control of his emotions. He benefits from knowing why things are being done to him, how they will help him get better, and how he can contribute. New procedures or changes in routine need to be explained. Children feel comfortable with the known, the routine.

Outer dressings (if any) are removed before the child is placed in the tub, but adherent dressings are more easily removed after soaking in the water. It is helpful to involve the child in the process. Whereas a child will cry and protest vigorously when others remove the dressings, he will remove adherent gauze with a minimum of fuss. In this way he maintains some control of the situation. Loose or easily detached tissue is also removed during hydrotherapy, and the child is encouraged to move about as much as possible to exercise muscles and reduce contracture formation.

Providing something constructive for the child to do during dressing application, such as holding a package of dressings or a roll of Kerlix or simply holding someone's hand, helps him to focus on something other than the procedure. In dressing the wound, it is important that all areas are clean, that medication is amply applied, and that no two burned surfaces touch, such as fingers or toes. Application of the medication can be a painful experience also, especially when mafenide (Sulfamylon) cream is the agent employed. Both nurse and child must understand that there is a painful sensation often described as "burning" that may have special significance for burned children. They must be reassured that the medication is not inflicting further injury and that the sensation is only a transient discomfort.

When occlusive dressings are applied, elastic bandages are worn over dressings to prevent epithelial breakdown, stimulate circulation, and make mobility easier. This is especially important when the child is ambulatory.

Provide nutrition. After the initial phase of care, children are usually allowed oral feedings (unless paralytic ileus persists). Because children frequently lack appetite and their caloric and protein needs are markedly increased, a great deal of encouragement, help, and patience are required on the part of the nursing staff. Consultation with the parents and the dietitian is arranged to determine the best way to provide needed nutrients in foods the child will be more likely to eat. Children who are old enough to participate should be included in the planning.

Nourishing snacks are provided between regularly scheduled mealtimes, and if a child eats better at a time other than a scheduled mealtime, that is the time he should be fed. Most importantly, meals should not be scheduled immediately after a dressing change. Most children are too physically exhausted and too emotionally upset to eat at this time. If they will not eat, tube feeding is necessary, but every effort should be made to encourage oral intake. (See Chapter 21 for suggestions for feeding the sick child.)

Prevent complications. The chief danger in this phase of burn care is infection—wound infection, generalized sepsis, and bacterial pneumonia. All burn patients are treated in a protected environment. Staff and visitors change into "scrub" clothing when entering the burn unit, and those on general units are placed in private rooms. It is important to make accurate ongoing assessments. Wound cultures are obtained at least three times weekly, and a blood culture is indicated in any child with a rectal temperature of 39.5° C (103° F) or higher.

To reduce metabolic expenditure as much as possible, the ambient temperature of the environment is maintained between 28° and 33° C (82.4° to 91.4° F) to avoid both overheating and underheating. An overhead warming unit may be provided to maintain body heat. Heat is often provided by means of a heat cradle over the child, but if employed, the heat source should be situated well away from the child's body. Other methods include using electric heaters, which should be situated 4 to 5 feet away to avoid overheating, and maintaining room temperature sufficiently elevated to reduce evaporative loss.

Antacids are usually administered prophylactically to prevent or minimize the effect of Curling (stress) ulcer, a frequent complication of severe burns, but nurses must be alert for any signs of bleeding.

Because the child is reluctant to move and doing so causes pain or discomfort, stiffness and joint contracture develop easily. In an effort to prevent this complication, the child is encouraged to move whenever feasible and active physiotherapy is included as an essential aspect of burn care. When the child is resting or sleeping, contracture is prevented by proper splinting. The child's natural tendency is to be active, and he will usually move spontaneously unless the pain is severe.

Care for skin graft. Effort in the care of children with skin grafts is directed toward facilitating a "take." Trauma, infection, and bleeding must be avoided for a successful transplantation to occur. When the grafted area is left exposed, the child must be immobilized to prevent the graft from becoming dislodged. Flat surfaces usually pose few problems, but grafts over irregular or mobile areas may require special techniques, such as splints or skeletal traction. Small children may need to be restrained. Sedation might be needed for very restless and/or uncooperative children for the first 2 or 3 days after surgery.

The grafted areas can be left exposed (which allows for easy inspection of the grafts), dressed with occlusive pressure dressings, or secured with sutures attached to normal surrounding skin and tied over the grafted skin to hold it in place. Wet dressings are occasionally applied over lace grafts and kept moist with antimicrobial agents, silver nitrate, or normal saline and then covered with dry absorbent gauze.

Wound contraction and scar tissue formation are normal parts of wound healing. Scar tissue is metabolically active tissue that continually rearranges itself; as a result disabling contractures, deformity, and disfigurement are ever-present possibilities. Physical therapy, splints, and other methods are employed to minimize these long-term effects. Pressure splints and elastic bandages or elasticized (Jobst) garments help reduce scar hypertrophy and are sometimes worn for months after hospitalization (Fig. 29-11). Often, severely burned children must return to the hospital periodically for additional skin grafts and scar revisions, especially to release contractures over joint spaces and for cosmetic considerations. Achievement of optimum results frequently requires years. In the meantime, burn scars are unsightly, and although improvements can be made, hope should not be extended to the parents and child for total cosmetic and functional repair.

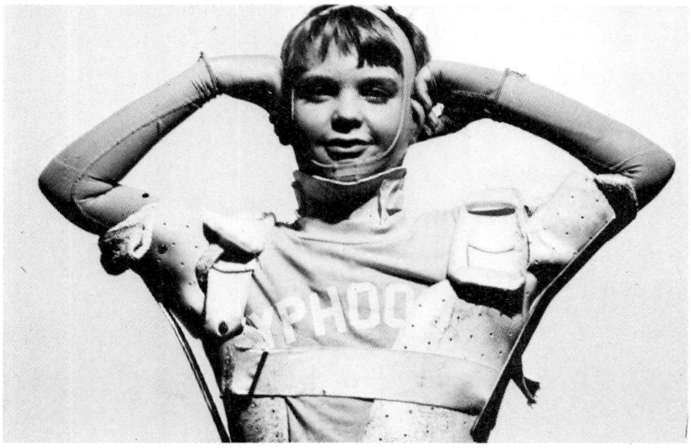

FIG. 29-11 Child in elasticized garment (Jobst) and "airplane" splints.

Support child and family. Throughout the acute phase of care, the child's emotional needs should not be overlooked. The child is frightened, uncomfortable, and often confused. He is isolated from familiar persons and surroundings, and the often overwhelming physical needs at this time are the primary focus of staff and parents. The child needs to be reassured that he is all right and that he will get better.

The child should be encouraged to participate in as many aspects of his care as possible. With illness, children always regress to the developmental level that allows them to deal with the stress. As their condition permits, children can be expected to do things that they were capable of doing for themselves before they were burned, such as oral hygiene, face washing, feeding themselves, and playing. Allowing the child to make choices and to help make decisions about the time of his care and recreational activities makes him feel a part of the team and provides him a measure of control. The child will probably require assistance; however, as the child sees himself contributing to his care, he gains confidence and self-esteem.

The psychologic pain and sequelae of severe burn trauma are as intense as the physical trauma. Each burned child goes through a tremendous amount of pain, often continuous for varying periods, and he also is often separated from his family for extended periods. In addition, there is a continual barrage of painful therapeutic and diagnostic procedures that are inflicted by others. He wonders why this has happened to *him*—what he has done that he should be punished so. Past experiences cannot serve him in this crisis. He does not understand the "ugliness" and disfigurement he sees as his body.

The impact of such severe injury taxes the capabilities of children at all ages, but the young child, who suffers acutely from separation anxiety, and the adolescent, who is developing an identity, are probably most affected psychologically. The toddler cannot begin to comprehend why the parents whom he loves and who have protected him from hurt can leave him in such a dreadful place and allow others to inflict such painful indignities on him.

The adolescent, in the process of achieving independence from his family and seeking to find out who he is in the world, finds himself in a dependent position with a damaged body. Being different from others at a time when conformity and being like his peers are so important is difficult to accept. These children need understanding adults to help them deal with the struggles concerning resentment and other feelings generated by such a catastrophe.

Members of the family, as well as the child, feel the impact of severe burn injury. They are concerned about the child's survival, recovery, and future appearance. Nurses are in the most opportune position to assist parents to cope with the stresses of the child's illness and their feelings of guilt and helplessness. The parents need

NURSING CARE PLAN

The Child with Burns

Management and Rehabilitative Phases of Burn Care

Nursing Goals	Nursing Interventions	Expected Patient/Family Outcomes
NDx HP-HMP* **Potential for infection** **Risk factors: denuded skin, presence of pathogenic organisms**		
Recognize signs of complications	Assess for abdominal discomfort Check for recurrent or intermittent bleeding from GI tract Observe for seizures, alterations in sensorium, behavioral changes Check blood pressure regularly Observe amount, color, specific gravity, and reaction of urine daily or as ordered Record intake and output	†Deviations from baseline findings are detected early and appropriate interventions initiated
Recognize signs of infection	Take vital signs (temperature, pulse, respirations, blood pressure) as ordered Observe for signs of septicemia Observe for signs of pneumonia Carefully cleanse and observe for signs of infection	†Evidence of infection detected early and appropriate interventions implemented
NDx N-MP **Altered nutrition: less than body requirements** **Etiology: increased catabolism, loss of appetite**		
Maintain adequate nutrition and prevent nitrogen loss	Provide high-calorie, high-protein meals and snacks	Child maintains a positive nitrogen balance—no weight loss
Stimulate appetite	Encourage oral feeding Provide foods child likes Allow self-help Provide meals when child is most likely to eat well Provide attractive meals and surroundings Provide companionship at meals Employ "contract" with older children	Child consumes a sufficient amount of nutrients (specify) Child interacts with other children
NDx N-MP **Impaired skin integrity** **Etiology: thermal injury**		
Facilitate wound healing	Keep child from scratching and picking at wound Provide distraction Older child: explain reasons Young child: apply restraining devices as needed Maintain care in handling wound to avoid damaging epithelializing and granulating tissues Offer high-calorie, high-protein meals and snacks Prevent infection	Wound heals without evidence of damage or inflammation
Control bacterial growth on wound	Maintain clean environment Maintain careful handwashing Wear sterile gown, mask, and gloves when handling burn wound Carefully cleanse wound and remove devitalized tissue and eschar Administer good oral hygiene Avoid injury to crusts and eschar Avoid contact with infected persons Assess wound for signs of invasive infection, including redness, purulent drainage, unpleasant odor	Wound displays minimum or no evidence of infection
Protect graft area	Position for minimum disturbance of graft site Restrain if necessary	Skin graft remains intact

*For an explanation of abbreviations, see p. 20.
†Nursing outcome.

NURSING CARE PLAN

The Child with Burns—cont'd

Management and Rehabilitative Phases of Burn Care

Nursing Goals	Nursing Interventions	Expected Patient/Family Outcomes
A-EP Impaired physical mobility (specify level) **Etiology: pain, impaired joint movement**		
Promote optimum functioning (physical)	Carry out range of motion exercises Encourage mobility if child is able to move extremities Ambulate as soon as feasible Splint involved joints at night and rest periods Encourage and promote self-help activities	Joints remain flexible with maximum functional capacity
Minimize scar formation	Position in functional attitude for minimum deformity and optimum function Apply splints as ordered and designed Wrap healing tissue with elastic bandage or dress in elastic garments as ordered Carry out physical therapy	Wound heals with minimum scar formation; joints remain flexible and functional
CPP Pain **Etiology: burn wound, donor graft site**		
Relieve pain	Assess need for pain medication (see p. 587) Implement appropriate nonpharmacologic pain reduction techniques (p. 597)	Child exhibits only minimum evidence of pain
SP-SCP Body image disturbance **Etiology: perception of appearance and mobility**		
Meet emotional needs	Convey positive attitude toward child Encourage parents to visit Encourage as much independence as condition allows Arrange for continued schooling Promote peer contact where possible	Child accepts efforts of family and caregivers Child engages in activities with others according to age and capabilities
Help build self-esteem and a positive self-image	Explore feelings concerning physical appearance Discuss feelings about returning to home and family, school, and friends Provide reinforcement of positive aspects of appearance and capabilities Point out evidence of healing Discuss aids that camouflage disfigurement Wigs Clothing; for example, turtleneck sweaters Makeup Provide recreational and diversional activities Promote constructive thinking in child	Child discusses feelings and concerns regarding appearance and perceived reactions of others Child verbalizes positive suggestions for adjusting to appearance
Promote self-care	Assist with self-care activities as needed Encourage self-care according to capabilities	Child assists with care as able
Prepare child for discharge	Begin early in hospitalization to discuss "going home" Accept regressive behavior where appropriate Help child develop independence and self-help capabilities	Child verbalizes and otherwise demonstrates interest in going home Child engages in self-help activities
RRP Altered processes **Etiology: situational crisis (child with a severe injury)**		
Prepare family for discharge	Teach wound care to caregiver Discuss diet, rest, and activity Explore attitudes toward child's reentry into the family Explore family's concept regarding child's capabilities and the possible restrictions and freedom they will allow	Family demonstrates an understanding of the needs of the child and the impact his condition will have on them
	Help family set realistic goals for themselves, child, and other relatives	Family sets realistic goals for themselves, child, and others

Continued.

NURSING CARE PLAN

The Child with Burns—cont'd

Management and Rehabilitative Phases of Burn Care

Nursing Goals	Nursing Interventions	Expected Patient/Family Outcomes
	Help family acquire needed equipment and supplies	
Participate in follow-up care	Coordinate team management of child and family Arrange for return visits Assess needs of family Arrange for referral to agencies based on need assessment	Family maintains contact with health providers
	Collaborate with school nurse to help with child's reintegration into school and the world of peers Visit school to prepare teacher and peers, if possible See also The hospitalized child, p. 603, and The family of the hospitalized child, p. 610	Child attends school regularly and interacts with age-mates

Nursing interventions related to medical management

Facilitate wound healing
- Administer supplementary vitamins and minerals—vitamins A, B, and C and zinc sulfate
- Apply prescribed topical antimicrobial preparation and dressings (if ordered) to wound
- Obtain wound cultures three times per week to ascertain any increase in wound flora

Relieve pain
- Administer analgesics as needed
- Monitor effectiveness of analgesics using a pain assessment record

Prevent constipation
- Administer stool softeners as needed

Prevent and/or treat complications
- Obtain blood culture of child with temperature of 39.5° C (103° F) or over
- Administer antacids as ordered
- Determine hematocrit
- Send urine specimens for laboratory examination periodically

to be informed of the child's progress and helped in their efforts to cope with their feelings while providing support to the child. The nurse is the person who can help them understand that it is not selfish to look after themselves and their own needs in order that they can better meet the needs of the child. For parents whose response to the illness is too severe or whose response to stress is manifest in destructive behavior, professional help may be needed.

EVALUATION

The effectiveness of nursing interventions is determined by continual reassessment and evaluation of care based on the following observational guidelines and expected outcomes:

1. Observe child's behavior during all aspects of care; listen to verbal cues
2. Observe the burn wound and general condition of the patient
3. Observe child's eating behavior and amount of food consumed; weigh daily or as indicated
4. Inspect the burn wound for signs of infection; take vital signs; observe for evidence of gastric bleeding, respiratory complications, weight loss, hemoglobin level, and neurologic signs
5. Observe the child's and family's behaviors; interview the child and family regarding their feelings and concerns

Expected outcomes:

See Nursing Care Plan, pp. 1006 to 1008.

SUNBURN

Sunburn is a very common skin injury caused by ultraviolet light waves. The sun emits a continuous spectrum of visible and nonvisible light rays that range in length from very short to very long. The shorter, higher-frequency waves are more damaging than longer wavelengths, but much of the light is filtered out as it travels through the atmosphere. Of the light that does filter through, ultraviolet A (UVA) waves are the longest and cause only minimum burning, but they play a significant role in photosensitive and photoallergic reactions. Ultraviolet B (UVB) waves are shorter and responsible for tanning, burning, and most of the harmful effects attributed to sunlight.

Numerous factors influence the amount of UVB exposure. Maximum exposure occurs at midday (11 AM to 3 AM) when the distance from the sun to a given spot on the earth is shortest. There is more exposure at higher altitudes, less when the sky is hazy (although the amount of ultraviolet radiation that does penetrate is easily underestimated); window glass effectively screens out UVB but not UVA rays. Fresh snow and water reflect ultraviolet rays, especially when the sun is directly overhead; some rays are reflected by sand.

Nursing Considerations

Protection from sunburn is the major goal of medical and nursing management, and the harmful effects of the sun on the delicate skin of infants and children is receiving increased attention. The safest time to sunbathe is when the sun is nearest the horizon (before 9 or 10 &Å and after 3 or 4 PM), when rays must travel the greatest distance. When skin is exposed to the sun for more extended periods, a protective covering is advised.

Two types of products are available for sun protection: topical sunscreens, which partially absorb ultraviolet light, and sun blockers, which block out ultraviolet rays by reflecting sunlight. The most frequently recommended sun blockers are zinc oxide and titanium dioxide ointments. Sunscreens are products containing a sun protection factor (SPF) based on evaluation of effectiveness against ultraviolet rays. The SPF is indicated by number, such as 15, which indicates that 15 hours of sun exposure with a sunscreen is equivalent to 1 hour of sun exposure without a sunscreen. The most effective sunscreens are para-aminobenzoic acid (PABA) and para-aminobenzoic acid esters (PABA-esters). PABA is more effective but may stain clothing; PABA-esters are less likely to stain clothing but are less effective than PABA.

Sunscreens are applied evenly to all exposed areas, with special attention to skin folds and areas that might become exposed as clothing shifts. For the best effect, sunscreens are applied about 45 minutes before exposure and should be reapplied in 4 to 6 hours and after swimming or perspiring (this may vary according to the product). Parents are directed to read labels of sunscreen products carefully for the SPF.

Sunburn is usually an epidermal burn, although severe sunburn can be a partial-thickness burn with blister formation. Treatment involves stopping the burning process, decreasing the inflammatory response, and rehydrating the skin. Local application of cool tap water soaks, or immersion in a tepid water bath for 20 minutes or until the skin is cool limits tissue destruction and relieves the discomfort. An oil-in-water moisturizing lotion is then applied. Oil-based products should be avoided, because they can trap irradiant heat in the tissues (Anders and Leach, 1983). Partial-thickness burns are treated the same as those from any heat source (see p. 462 for a discussion of suntanning machines).

COLD INJURY

Cold injuries are most commonly seen in very cold regions. The nature of the heat-regulating mechanisms of the body are such that the inner portion of the body, or core, produces heat, and the periphery, or outer area, conserves or dissipates the heat. When the body attempts to conserve heat, the outer tissues are subjected to low temperatures, and local trauma may result.

Chilblain occurs when extremities, usually the hands, are exposed intermittently to temperatures 30° to 60° F (DeLapp, 1980). The response may vary but is characterized by intense vasodilation that increases the temperature of involved tissues above unaffected tissue and produces edematous, reddish blue patches that itch and burn. As warming takes place, the sensations become more intense, but they ordinarily subside in a few days.

Frostbite results from sufficient exposure to cool the tissues to the point that small ice crystals form in interstitial spaces of superficial and deep structures, resulting in variable degrees of tissue loss and function. The frostbitten part appears white or blanched, feels solid, and is without sensation. Rapid rewarming produces a flush (sometimes deep purple) and a return of sensation, which is extremely painful. In 24 to 48 hours after rewarming, large blisters appear, which begin to reabsorb within 5 to 10 days, followed by formation of a hard black eschar. Superficial injury often heals without incident. Rewarming is accomplished by immersing the part in well-agitated water at 100° to 108° F. Discomfort is managed with analgesics and sedatives. Care of blistered skin is similar to that described for burns. It is seldom possible to estimate the extent of tissue loss until new skin layers are revealed after the eschar layer separates.

SUMMARY

All children at various times suffer some skin disorder. It may be a short-lived, minor inconvenience (such as a viral exanthem, infestation, or minor burn); a temporary but troublesome affliction (such as acne or atopic dermatitis); a lifelong affliction (such as an inherited skin disorder); or a life-threatening condition with permanent disability (such as a major burn). Most of the disorders manifest in the skin can be managed at home or on an outpatient basis. Consequently, an important nursing role is teaching the family how to care for the affected member and helping them to solve problems in areas of frustration and/or concern.

KEY CONCEPTS

- Therapeutic management of skin disorders includes a variety of methods and agents to cool, soothe, and reduce the irritating effects of external stimuli.
- Skin infections can be caused by bacteria, viruses, or fungi.
- Some diseases manifest in the skin are transmitted by arthropod vectors, especially ticks.
- The most common skin infestations of childhood, scabies and pediculosis capitis, can affect children of any age and from any social class.
- Contact dermatitis may involve a primary irritant or a sensitizing agent.
- Adverse reactions to drugs are manifest more often in the skin than in any other body organ.
- The most common skin disorders of infancy are diaper dermatitis, seborrheic dermatitis, and atopic dermatitis.
- Acne, a disorder affecting a large proportion of adolescents, is related to maturation of pilosebaceous follicles and increased androgen secretion.
- Noninflammatory acne is predominantly an obstructive disease characterized by open and closed comedones; lesions of inflammatory acne consist of papules, pustules, nodules, and cysts.
- Burns are caused by thermal, chemical, electric, or radioactive agents.
- Burns are assessed on the extent, depth, and severity of the wound.
- Essentials of emergency care of burn injury include stopping the burning process, covering the burn, transporting the injured child to medical aid, and providing reassurance to child and family.
- Management of minor burns consists of facilitating wound healing, relieving discomfort, and preventing complications.
- Management of major burns consists of facilitating wound healing, relieving discomfort, replacing destroyed skin, preventing and/or treating complications, and providing rehabilitation.
- Sunscreen is recommended for use when the skin is exposed to damaging effects of the sun's rays.
- Thermal injuries to the skin can result from exposure to extreme cold.

STUDY QUESTIONS AND ACTIVITIES

1 Devise a plan for incorporating play into the treatment modalities (e.g., baths, soaks, moist compresses) for a 12-month-old, a 2-year-old, and a 4-year-old child with a dermatologic condition.
2 At a local pharmacy investigate the over-the-counter products available for treating any of the following: acne, skin itching and irritation, superficial fungal infections, and infestations.
3 Design a teaching plan for the prevention and management of pediculosis that would be appropriate for presentation to parents of school-age children.
4 Outline a teaching plan for a teenager with acne.
5 Compute the percentage of body surface area burned for a 2-year-old child with partial-thickness burns to the chest, upper right arm, and face; for a 9-year-old child with burns to the back, back thighs and lower legs, back of arms, and hands.

REFERENCES

Anders, J.E., and Leach, E.E.: Sun versus skin, Am. J. Nurs. **83:**1015-1020, 1983.

Carithers, H.A.: Cat-scratch disease—an overview based on a study of 1,200 patients, Am. J. Dis. Child. **139:**1124-1133, 1985.

Committee on Drugs, American Academy of Pediatrics: New therapy for severe cystic acne, Pediatrics **72:**258-259, 1983.

DeLapp, T.D.: Taking the bite out of frostbite and other cold-weather injuries, Am. J. Nurs. **80:**56-60, 1980.

Gelbard, M.K.: Removal of small cactus spines from the skin, JAMA **252:**3368, 1984.

Martinez, T.T., and others: Removal of cactus spines from the skin: comparative evaluation of several methods, Am. J. Dis. Child. **141:**1291-1292, 1987.

McLaury, P.: Head lice—pediatric social disease, Am. J. Nurs. **83:**1300-1303, 1983.

Perelson, A.M., and Seyler, M.F.: First aid: soaking an injured finger or toe, Emerg. Med. **16:**158, 1985.

Putnam, M.H., and Lawton, M.B.: Resourceful women unmask cactus spine, JAMA **253:**2830, 1985.

BIBLIOGRAPHY

General

Cohen, B.A.: Common dermatoses of childhood, Am. Fam. Physician **32:**186-203, 1985.

Fleming, J.W.: Common dermatologic conditions in children, MCN **6:**346-354, 1981.

Hawkins, K.: Wet dressings, Crit. Care Update **9**(11):24-26, 1982.

Krowchuck, D.P.: Practical aspects of the diagnosis and management of atopic dermatitis, Pediatr. Ann. **16:**57-66, 1987.

Nicol, N.H.: Atopic dermatitis: the (wet) wrap-up, Am. J. Nurs. **87:**1560-1563, 1987.

Rasmussen, J.E.: Recent advances in pediatric dermatology, Child Care Newsletter **5**(2):7-11, 1986.

Rosen, T., Lanning, M.B., and Hill, M.J.: The nurse's atlas of dermatology, Boston, 1983, Little, Brown & Co.

Shalita, A.R.: Principles of infant skin care, Skillman, NJ, 1981, Johnson & Johnson Baby Products Co.

Infections

Caputo, R.V.: Fungal infections in children, Dermatol. Clin. North Am. **4:**137-150, 1986.

Krugman, S., and others: Infectious diseases of children, ed. 8, St. Louis, 1985, The C.V. Mosby Co.

Nortarangelo, P.R., and Dixon, D.M.: Opportunistic systemic mycoses and the critical care patient, Crit. Care Update **10**(5):7-11, 1983.

Rees, P.L., and Dixon, D.M.: Opportunistic mycoses, Am. J. Nurs. **81:**1160-1163, 1981.

Infestations

Clore, E.R.: Lice: ancient pest with new resistance, Pediatr. Nurs. **9:**347-350, 1983.

Clore, E.: Prioderm and permethrin: product update, Progress **1**(2):1, 1985.

Meinking, T.L., and others: Comparative efficacy of treatments for pediculosis capitis infestations, Arch. Dermatol. **122:**267-271, 1986.

Minster, J.: Nursing management of patients with scabies and lice, Nurs. Clin. North Am. **15:**747-756, 1980.

Bites and Stings

Frazier, C.A.: Severe toxic and allergic reactions to insect bites and stings, Crit. Care Update **8**(9):17-24, 1981.

King, R.C., and Giles, J.: Dealing with insect bites, RN **46**(5):53-55, 1984.

Thompson, S.: Summertime and ticks, Am. J. Nurs. **83:**758, 1983.

Wright, J.C.: Severe attacks by dogs: characteristics of the dogs, the victims, and the attack settings, Public Health Rep. **100:**55-61, 1985.

Diaper Dermatitis

Esterly, N.B.: Atopic dermatitis: the challenge of effective management, Child Care Newsletter **1**(2):1-4, 1982.

Gaunder, B.N., and Plummer, E.: Diaper rash: managing and controlling a common problem in infants and toddlers, J. Pediatr. Health Care **1:**26-34, 1987.

Koblenzer, P.J.: Diaper dermatitis: diagnosis and treatment, Child Care Newsletter **1**(3):1-4, 1982.

Acne

Lawlis, G.F., and Achterberg, J.: Acne: the disease and stress, Top. Clin. Nurs. **5**(2):23-31, 1983.

Rasmussen, J.E., and Smith, S.B.: Patient concepts and misconceptions about acne, Arch. Dermatol. **119:**570-573, 1983.

Stone, A.C.: Facing up to acne, Pediatr. Nurs. **8:**229-234, 1983.

Thermal Injury

Acres, C., and Kraft, E.R.: Skin transplantation, Am. J. Nurs. **81:**1466-1467, 1981.

Anders, J.E., and Moeller, P.J.: Topicals: a welter of options calls for refined application techniques, RN **45**(9):33-42, 1982.

Cameron, C.O., Juszczak, L., and Wallace, N.: Using creative arts to help children cope with altered body image, Child Health Care **12:**108-112, 1984.

Conrad, F.L.: Tips for treating corrosive burns, Nursing 83 **13**(2):55-57, 1983.

Dittemore, I.L.: Behavioral responses in the early recovery of a severely burned 4-year-old child, MCN **12:**21-34, 1983.

Fonger, L.: Emergency! First aid for burns, Nursing 82 **12**(9):70-77, 1982.

Gaston, S.F., and Pathak, M.A: Burn wound management, Crit. Care Update **7**(10):5-17, 1980.

Gedrose, J.: When cold can be a killer: prevention and treatment of hypothermia and frostbite, Nursing 80 **10**(2):34-36, 1980.

Hemenway, B.: Major thermal injury: initial assessment and treatment, Emerg. Nurs. **1**(20):1-8, 1981.

Hurt, R.A.: More than skin deep: guidelines on caring for the burn patient, Nursing 85 **15**(6):52-57, 1985.

Kavanagh, C.: Should children participate in burn care? Am. J. Nurs. **84:**601, 1984.

Kenner, C., and Manning, S.: Emergency care of the burn patient, Crit. Care Update **7**(10):24-33, 1980.

Langley, J.: Description and classification of childhood burns, Burns **10:**231, 1984.

LaVoy, K.: Dealing with hypothermia and frostbite, RN **48**(1):53-56, 1985.

Lushbaugh, M.A.: Critical care of the child with burns, Nurs. Clin. North Am. **16:**635-646, 1981.

Luterman, A., Adams, M., and Curreri, P.W.: Nutritional management of the burn patient, Crit. Care Q. **7**(3):34-43, 1984.

Marvin, J.A.: Planning home care for burn patients, Nursing 83 **13**(8):65-67, 1983.

Marvin, J.A., and Einfeldt, L.E.: Infection control for the burn patient, Nurs. Clin. North Am. **15:**833-842, 1980.

McLouglin, E., and others: Project burn prevention: outcome and implications, Am. J. Public Health **72:**241-247, 1982.

Plein, E.M.: Sunscreens, Nurs. Pract. **6:**35, 1981.

Rausch, T.: Minor thermal injury: initial assessment and treatment, Emerg. Nurs. **1**(19):1-8, 1980.

Robertson, K.E., Cross, P.L.J., and Terry, J.C.: Burn care: the crucial first days, Am. J. Nurs. **85:**30-50, 1985.

Robinson, L.A.: Sun exposure and sun protection, Pediatr. Nurs. **8:**272-273, 1982.

Stoddard, F.J.: Coping with pain: a developmental approach to treatment of burned children, Am. J. Psychiatry **139:**736-740, 1982.

Surveyer, J.A., and Clougherty, D.M.: Burn scars: fighting the effects, Am. J. Nurs. **83:**746-751, 1983.

Surveyer, J.A., and Halpern, J.: Age-related burn injuries and their prevention, Pediatr. Nurs. **7**(5):29-34, 1981.

Van Oss, S.: Emergency burn care: those crucial first minutes, RN **44:**45-49, 1982.

Wingate, E.: A nursing perspective on frostbite, Crit. Care Update **10**(1):8-15, 1983.

Wingate, E.: Emergent burn care: a time for life-saving measures, Crit. Care Update **10**(8):49-54, 1983.

Wooldridge, M., and Surveyer, J.A.: Skin grafting for full-thickness burn injury, Am. J. Nurs. **80:**2000-2004, 1980.

UNIT

XIII

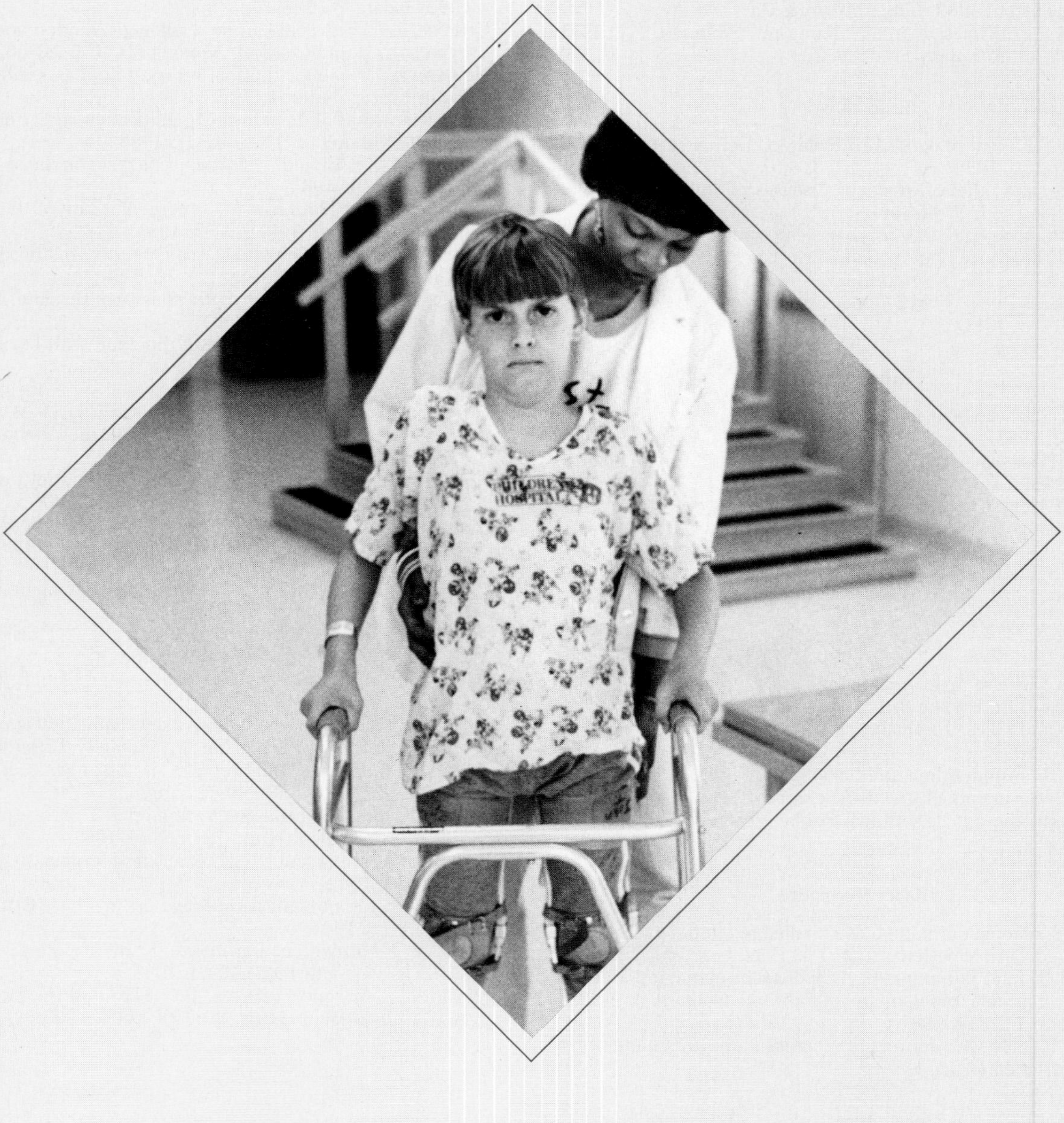

The Child with a Problem That Interferes with Locomotion

Childhood is the time of onset for a variety of physically disabling conditions with hereditary, infectious, or traumatic etiologies. Many disorders that interfere with locomotion are present at birth; others appear later in childhood. Defects in locomotion can be associated with diseases or deficits in the supporting structures (the skeleton), the movement-producing structures (muscles or their innervation), or the articulating structures (joints) of the body. Some of these defects, such as fractures, occur at any age, and others make their appearance at ages characteristic of the specific condition; for example, muscular dystrophy occurs during early childhood and slipped epiphysis at puberty.

Some locomotor disabilities are acquired in an instant (such as amputation or spinal cord injury); others develop over an extended period (such as tuberculosis or progressive muscular atrophy). Some need only short-term therapy (such as fractures); others require long-term therapy and a longer term of adjustment and involve all aspects of daily living (such as spinal cord injuries and cerebral palsy).

The physical limitations may involve only temporary inconvenience, or they may be permanent and require an alternative form of locomotion. Some disabilities are helped by specific treatments; for others therapy is merely supportive. A large number of these disabilities require a health team approach with contributions from a variety of specialists. Concomitant problems associated with permanent disabilities, particularly those acquired in later childhood, are emotional adjustment and alterations in self-image.

Chapter 30, *The Child with Impaired Mobility,* is concerned with disorders that involve the skeleton and articular systems. Also included in this discussion is the collagen disease, systemic lupus erythematosus. Chapter 31, *The Child with Neuromuscular Dysfunction,* deals with disorders that involve muscle dysfunction of either muscular or neurologic origin.

CHAPTER 30

The Child with Impaired Mobility

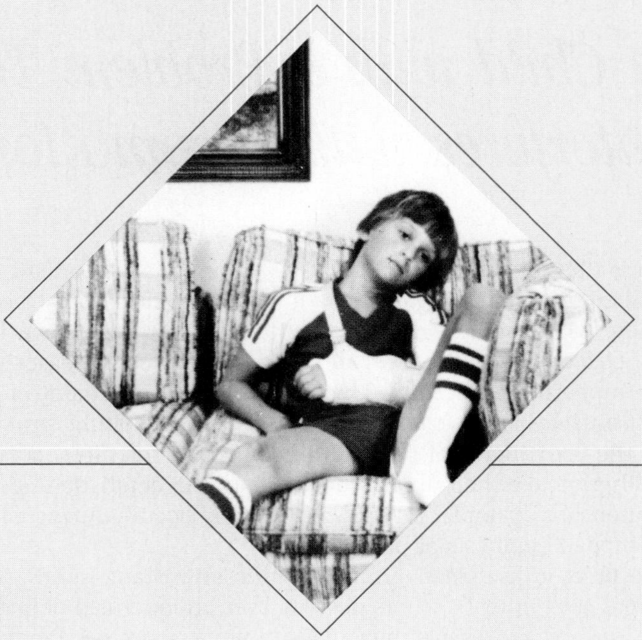

LEARNING OBJECTIVES

On completion of this chapter the reader will be able to:

- Outline a plan for the care of a child immobilized with an injury or a degenerative disease
- Formulate a teaching plan for the parents of a child in a cast
- Explain the functions of the various types of traction
- Devise a nursing care plan for a child in traction
- Differentiate among the various congenital skeletal defects
- Design a teaching plan for the parents of a child with a congenital skeletal deformity
- Describe the therapies and nursing care of a child with scoliosis
- Outline a plan of care for the child with osteomyelitis
- Differentiate between osteosarcoma and Ewing sarcoma
- Describe the nursing care of a child with juvenile rheumatoid arthritis
- Demonstrate an understanding of the management of systemic lupus erythematosus

Disorders that affect the skeletal and associated structures are of congenital, traumatic, infectious, neoplastic, or idiopathic origin. Some disorders, such as fractures, appear at any age, whereas others have a predilection for a particular stage of childhood. For example, there are those disorders detected at birth or shortly thereafter, such as congenital deformities and defects; Legg-Calvé-Perthes disease affects children in middle childhood; and slipped femoral capital epiphysis and scoliosis are characteristic of late childhood and adolescence.

◆ *The Immobilized Child*

Immobilization is a major therapy for injuries to soft tissues, long bones, ligaments, vertebrae, and joints. Restriction of motion for a period of time at the site at which muscle or bone integrity has been disrupted allows tissue and bone to heal. However, prolonged immobilization, whether for therapy or because of disability, can produce severe complications, many of which are preventable. The nurse's awareness and implementation of appropriate actions during this restrictive state can significantly reduce the adverse effects of immobilization. Thus nursing care plans must focus not only on tissue and bone healing but also on regaining functional use of the injured part to the greatest extent possible.

This chapter is concerned with the problem of immobilization as a therapy and some of the more common injuries that require this method of treatment, primarily bone fractures and orthopedic dysfunction.

IMMOBILIZATION

One of the most difficult aspects of illness is the immobility it often imposes on a child. Children's natural tendency to be mobile influences all elements of growth and development—physical, social, psychologic, and emotional. It is also important for expression and for dealing with anxiety and frustration. For these reasons children are immobilized only when necessary and for the shortest time possible.

Physiologic Effects of Immobilization

Functional and metabolic responses to restricted movement can be noted in most of the body systems, all of which have a direct influence on the child's growth and development, because homeostatic mechanisms thrive on normal use and need feedback to maintain dynamic equilibrium. Most of the pathologic changes that take place during immobilization arise from decreased muscle strength and mass, decreased metabolism, and bone demineralization. Some results of immobilization are primary and produce a direct effect; others seem to be more indirect, or secondary. The effects are especially marked in the child who suffers some degree of paralysis.

The major effects of immobilization are outlined briefly in Table 30-1. They are related directly or indirectly to decreased muscle activity, which produces numerous primary changes in both muscular and bone structures with secondary alterations in the cardiovascular, respiratory, metabolic, and renal systems. The major consequences are:

1. Significant loss of muscle strength, endurance, and muscle mass (atrophy)
2. Bone demineralization leading to osteoporosis
3. Loss of joint mobility and contractures

The larger the portion of the body immobilized and the longer the immobilization, the greater the hazards of immobility.

Psychologic Effects of Immobilization

Throughout childhood physical activity is an integral part of daily life and is essential for physical growth and development. It helps children deal with a variety of feelings and impulses and provides a mechanism by which they can exert control over inner tensions. Children respond to anxiety with increased activity. Removal of this power deprives them of necessary input and a natural outlet for their feelings and fantasies.

When a child is immobilized by disease or as part of a treatment regimen, he experiences diminished environmental stimuli with a loss of tactile input and an altered perception of himself and his environment. Sudden or gradual immobilization narrows the amount and variety of environmental stimuli he receives by means of all of his senses: touch, sight, hearing, taste, smell, and proprioception—a feeling of where he is in his environment. This sensory deprivation frequently leads to feelings of isolation and boredom, and of being forgotten, especially by his peers.

Physical interference with the activity of infants and young children gives them a feeling of helplessness. It has also been found that speech and language skills require sensorimotor activity and experience. Children who are restrained by casts, splints, or straps during the first 3 years of life have more difficulty with language than children whose activities are unrestricted.

For the toddler, exploration and imitative behaviors are essential to developing a sense of autonomy; the preschooler's expression of initiative is evidenced by his penchant for vigorous physical activity; the school-age child's development is strongly influenced by physical achievement and competition; and the adolescent relies on mobility to achieve independence. The quest for mastery at every stage of development is related to mobility.

The monotony of immobilization can lead to sluggish intellectual and psychomotor responses, decreased communication skills, increased fantasizing, and even hallucinations and disorientation. The child is likely to become depressed over his loss of ability to function or the marked changes in his body image. He seeks the attention of others by reverting to earlier developmental behaviors, such as wanting to be fed, bed-wetting, and baby talk.

Also, limbs in casts or traction transmit less than normal sensory data. A child who has limited ability to feel others touching him not only experiences less tactile stimuli in a physical sense but is also deprived of warm, loving feelings that arise from being touched. The loss of feeling derived from touch can further add to his sense of being isolated and unwanted.

Children may react to immobility by active protest, an-

TABLE 30-1

*Summary of Physical Effects of Immobilization**

Primary Effects	Secondary Effects
Muscular System	
Decreased muscle strength, tone, and endurance	Decreased venous return and decreased cardiac output Decreased metabolism and need for oxygen Decreased exercise tolerance Bone demineralization
Disuse atrophy and loss of muscle mass	Catabolism Loss of strength
Loss of joint mobility	Contractures, ankylosis of joints
Weak back muscles	Secondary spinal deformities
Weak abdominal muscles	Impaired respiration
Skeletal System	
Bone demineralization—osteoporosis, hypercalcemia	Negative calcium balance Pathologic fractures Calcium deposits Extraosseous bone formation, especially at hip, knee, elbow, and shoulder Renal calculi
Negative calcium balance	Life-threatening electrolyte imbalance
Metabolism	
Decreased metabolic rate	Slowing of all systems Decreased food intake
Negative nitrogen balance	Decline in nutritional state Impaired healing
Hypercalcemia	Electrolyte imbalance
Decreased production of stress hormones	Decreased physical and emotional coping capacity
Cardiovascular System	
Decreased efficiency of orthostatic neurovascular reflexes	Inability to adapt readily to upright position Pooling of blood in extremities in upright posture
Diminished vasopressor mechanism	Orthostatic hypotension with syncope—hypotension, decreased cerebral blood flow, tachycardia
Cardiovascular System—cont'd	
Altered distribution of blood volume	Decreased cardiac workload Decreased exercise tolerance
Venous stasis	Pulmonary emboli and/or thrombi
Dependent edema	Tissue breakdown and susceptibility to infection
Respiratory System	
Decreased need for oxygen	Altered oxygen–carbon dioxide exchange and metabolism
Decreased chest expansion and diminished vital capacity	Diminished oxygen intake Dyspnea and inadequate arterial oxygen saturation; acidosis
Poor abdominal tone and distention	Interference with diaphragmatic excursion
Mechanical or biochemical secretion retention	Hypostatic pneumonia Bacterial and viral pneumonia Atelectasis
Loss of respiratory muscle strength	Poor cough Upper respiratory infection
Gastrointestinal System	
Distention caused by poor abdominal muscle tone	Interference with respiratory movements
No specific primary effect	Difficulty in feeding in prone position; gravitation effect on feces through ascending colon or weakened smooth muscle tone may cause constipation Anorexia
Urinary System	
Alteration of gravitational force	Difficulty in voiding in prone position
Impaired ureteral peristalsis	Urinary retention in calyces and bladder Infection Renal calculi
Integumentary System	
No specific primary effect	Decreased circulation and pressure leading to tissue injury Difficulty with personal hygiene

*Not all problems will be applicable in every situation.

ger, and aggressive behavior, or they may become quiet, passive, and submissive. Often children believe that the immobilization is a justified punishment for misbehavior. Children should be allowed to discharge their anger, but it should be within the limits of safety to their self-esteem and not damaging to the integrity of others. For example, providing an object to attack rather than a person or a valued possession is safe and therapeutic. When a child is unable to express his anger, his aggression is often displayed inappropriately through regressive behavior and outbursts of crying or temper tantrums over insignificant irritations, such as warm milk, a wrinkled collar, or a delay in routine.

Nursing Considerations

The effects of immobilization can be minimized and in many instances prevented by conscientious nursing care. The major goals in care of the immobilized child are to prevent the pathophysiologies associated with immobility and to use measures for regaining function and remobilization within the limitations of the therapeutic regimen or the physical disabilities of the child.

ASSESSMENT

Assessment of the child who is immobilized as a result of an injury or a degenerative disease not only includes the injured part (as a fracture or damaged joint), but also the functioning of other systems that may be affected secondarily—the circulatory, renal, respiratory, muscular, and gastrointestinal systems. In long-term immobilization there may also be neurologic impairment and metabolic changes in electrolytes (especially calcium), nitrogen balance, and general metabolic rate.

Nursing assessment includes psychosocial data as well as physical manifestations, since long-term immobilization has a profound effect on the child and family. Nursing approaches are evaluated frequently and continued, discontinued, or modified to meet the changing problems and goals.

NURSING DIAGNOSES

Nursing diagnoses for the immobilized child are outlined in the Nursing Care Plan on pp. 1018 to 1019. Others will be identified in specific cases.

PLANNING

The goals of care for the immobilized child include those that apply to specific conditions that are discussed in the remainder of the chapter. Some general goals include:

1. Prevent physical complications
2. Prevent psychologic complications
3. Provide appropriate diversional activities
4. Support child and family

IMPLEMENTATION

Frequent position changes help to prevent dependent edema and fluid movement and to stimulate circulation, respiratory function, gastrointestinal motility, and neurologic sensations. Metabolism is increased by activity within the limitations of the disability and capabilities of the child. High-protein, high-calorie foods are encouraged for correction of negative nitrogen balance. This may be difficult to correct by diet, especially if there is loss of appetite. Stimulating the appetite with small servings of attractively arranged, preferred foods may be sufficient.

Adequate hydration promotes bowel and kidney function and helps prevent complications in these systems. It is also a primary measure for managing hypercalcemia, in addition to restricting high-calcium foods.

Children should be encouraged to be as active as their condition and restrictive devices allow. This poses few problems for children, whose innate ingenuity and natural inclination toward mobility provide them with the impetus for physical activity. They need the opportunity, the materials or objects to stimulate activity, and the encour-

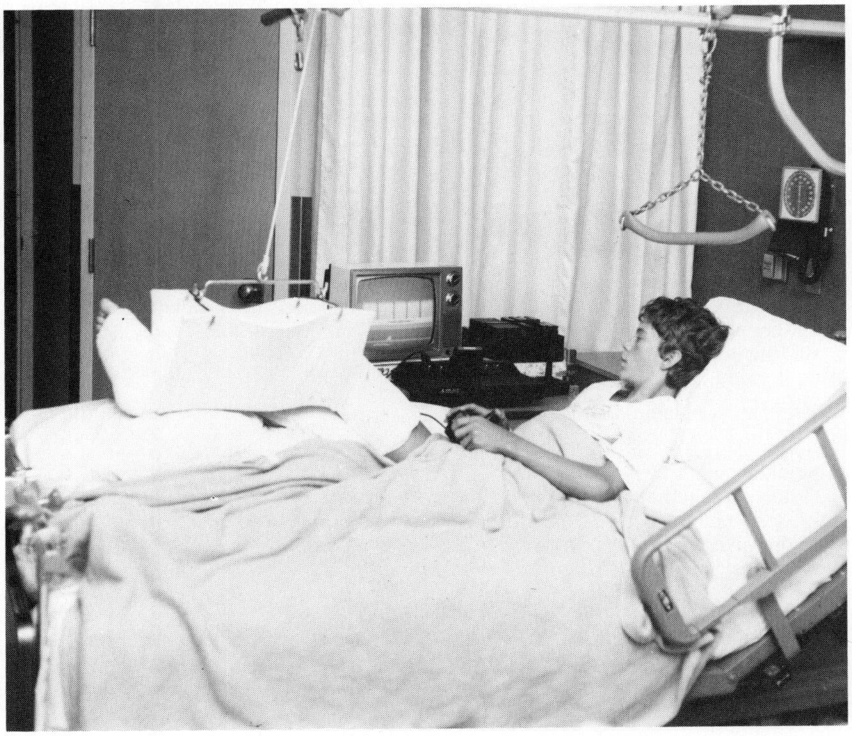

FIG. 30-1 Immobilized child playing a video game.

NURSING CARE PLAN

The Immobilized Child

Nursing Goals	Nursing Interventions	Expected Patient/Family Outcomes
HP-HMP* **Potential for trauma** **Risk factors: immobility, physical disability**		
Prevent falls	Teach correct use of mobilizing devices and/or apparatus Assist with moving and/or ambulating as needed Remove hazards from environment (specify) Modify environment as needed (specify)	Child does not fall
Prevent other injuries (specify)	Implement safety measures appropriate to child's developmental age (specify)	Child exhibits no signs of injury
N-MP **Potential impaired skin integrity** **Risk factors: immobility, therapeutic appliances**		
Maintain skin integrity	Turn and reposition at least every 2 hours Inspect total skin area frequently Eliminate mechanical factors causing pressure, friction, or irritation Keep skin clean and dry	Skin remains clean, intact, and free of irritation
A-EP **Impaired physical mobility (state level)** **Etiology: physical disability, mechanical restrictions**		
Provide mobilization (if appropriate)	Transport child by gurney, stroller, wagon, or other conveyance from confines of room	Child moves from confines of bed
Promote autonomy	Provide mobilizing devices Assist with acquisition of specialized equipment Instruct in use of equipment	Child moves about without assistance
A-EP **Feeding, bathing/hygiene, dressing/grooming, or toileting (specify level) self-care deficit** **Etiology: immobility, physical disability, presence of therapeutic appliance**		
Promote self-help	Allow child to help plan his daily routine and choose from alternatives when appropriate Encourage participation in self-care activities according to developmental level and capabilities Provide devices, equipment, and methods to assist the child in self-care	Child engages in self-help activities to maximum capabilities
Facilitate elimination	Sit in upright position when possible Employ special devices where appropriate (e.g., fracture pan, commode, elevated toilet seat) Carry out bowel training program with hydration, stool softeners, and mild laxatives if needed Provide privacy	Child has daily bowel movement
Stimulate voiding and prevent urinary tract infection	Position as upright as possible to void Hydrate to adequate urinary output for age Stimulate bladder emptying with warm water, running water, striking suprapubic area Catheterize as indicated	No urinary retention noted Child consumes an adequate amount of fluid Child exhibits no evidence of urinary tract infection
Empty bladder	Teach self-catheterization to appropriate children (paraplegia)	Child demonstrates self-catheterization
Promote self-feeding	Serve easy-to-handle foods Make meals as interesting and attractive as possible Offer small bites, semisolid foods, and fluids through a straw for children lying in prone position Include child in food selection and sequence of eating foods served Modify utensils to facilitate self-help	Child assists with meal selection Child assists with feeding as much as possible within limitations

*For an explanation of abbreviations, see p. 20.

NURSING CARE PLAN

The Immobilized Child—cont'd

Nursing Goals	Nursing Interventions	Expected Patient/Family Outcomes
NDX A-EP Diversional activity deficit **Etiology: immobility**		
Provide environmental stimulation	Provide for play activities and diversions Change position of bed in room periodically Promote ambulation (if appropriate) Modify equipment to facilitate use	Child engages in activities suited to age and interest (specify)
Promote social contacts	Encourage interaction with others Encourage visits from family and friends	Child associates with other children and family
NDX SP-SCP Body image disturbance **Etiology: perception of disability, nonintegration of change in body limitations**		
Support child	Allow the child to express feelings regarding immobilization Direct acting-out behavior in constructive directions Employ therapeutic play techniques for teaching and expressing feelings Explain purpose and function of restraining device if used Set realistic limits on behavior Answer questions regarding child's conditions, therapies, and schedules Promote and reinforce his support systems Encourage activities and relationships that foster self-esteem Emphasize good grooming	Child verbalizes feelings and concerns Behavior is within acceptable parameters Child demonstrates an understanding of therapies and expected outcomes Child helps plan activities and schedules
NDX RRP Altered family processes **Etiology: situational crisis (serious injury to child)**		
Support family	Answer questions, explain, and clarify information about the child, his condition, therapy, and behavior Allow for expression of feelings, especially if the child is immobilized as the result of an accidental injury Refer to appropriate agencies and services See also The child in the hospital, p. 603	Family expresses feelings and concerns Family demonstrates an understanding of the child's condition, therapies, and expected outcomes of therapies

agement and participation of others. Those who are unable to move will need passive exercise and movement.

Whenever possible, transporting the child by gurney, stroller, or wagon outside the confines of his room will increase environmental stimuli and provide social contact with others. While hospitalized, the child will benefit from frequent visitors, clocks and calendars, and a program of diversional therapy, which will help him to function in a more normal way (Fig. 30-1). As soon as possible he should wear "street clothes" and resume school and preinjury hobbies. The use of play (see Chapter 20) and any activity that is tolerated (e.g., turning in bed or changing the position of a bed in the room) help to alter the monotony of immobilization and dissipate tension and frustration.

Using dolls to illustrate and explain the restraining method is a valuable tool for small children. Placing a cast, tubing, or other restraining equipment on the doll offers the child a nonthreatening opportunity to express, through the doll, his feelings concerning the restrictions and the nurse, and it provides a means for anticipatory teaching and explanation of needed restraining devices.

One of the most useful interventions to help children cope with immobility is participation in their own care. Self-care to the maximum extent is usually well received by children. They should be encouraged to help plan their daily routine and do as much for themselves as they are able in order to keep muscles active and their interest alive. If feasible, they should be placed where they can benefit from the company of other children who are immobilized, which assures them that they are not singled out for this treatment.

It is important for the child to understand behavioral limitations or rules, and his questions should be answered. For example, he needs to know the reasons for medical, nursing, occupational, and physical therapy and to know that schedules are necessary. In some areas he has a choice; in others he does not. He may or may not be permitted to sleep late, but he can choose his own clothing. Most of a child's activity of daily living is play; therefore therapies that incorporate this concept are more apt to gain his cooperation. Visits from significant persons, such as family members and friends, offer occasions for emotional support and also provide opportunities for learning how to care for the child.

For a child with greatly restricted movement (for example, the quadriplegic child or the child with a large bilateral hip spica cast), nursing care is a challenge. These situations require long-term care either in the hospital or at home, but wherever the care occurs, consistent planning and coordination of activities with professionals and significant others are vital.

Family support and home care. A severely disabled child's needs can be very complex, and family members require time to assimilate the teachings and demonstrations needed to understand his situation and care. Even the child who is confined on a short-term basis can be a challenge for the family, which is usually unprepared for the problems imposed by the child's special needs. Home modification is usually needed for facilitating care, especially when it involves traction, large casts, or extended confinement. Suitable child care may be needed for times when all family members work.

Just as in hospital care, the child at home is encouraged to be as independent as possible and to follow a schedule that approximates his normal life-style as nearly as possible, such as continuing school lessons, regular bedtime, and suitable recreational activities.

EVALUATION

The effectiveness of nursing interventions is determined by continual reassessment and evaluation of care based on the following observational guidelines and expected outcomes:

1. Observe vital signs, skin inspection, neurologic signs, respiratory, gastrointestinal, and renal functioning, effects of and correct functioning of equipment—restraints, traction, cast, braces
2. Observe child's behavior; engage in dialogue to elicit his feelings, concerns, and interests
3. Observe the child's activities and interests
4. Interview child and family regarding their feelings and concerns; observe the family interaction at home, if possible

Expected outcomes
See Nursing Care Plan, pp. 1018 to 1019.

◆ *Traumatic Injury*

Children, with their natural tendency toward active mobility and their limited gross motor coordination, are highly susceptible to physical injury. Cuts, bruises, and contusions are a part of growing up, and fractures occur frequently in the pediatric age-groups.

FRACTURES

Bones fracture when the resistance of bone against the stress being exerted yields to the stress force. Fractures are a common injury at any age but are more likely to occur in children and elderly persons. Because of the characteristics of the child's skeleton, there are some differences in the pattern of fractures, problems of diagnosis, and methods of treatment.

Etiology

Fracture injuries in children are the result of traumatic incidents at home, at school, in a motor vehicle, or in association with recreational activities. Children's everyday activities include vigorous play that predisposes them to injury—climbing, falling down, running into immovable objects, and receiving blows to any part of their bodies.

Aside from automobile accidents, true injuries that cause fractures rarely occur in infancy; therefore, bone injury in children of that age-group warrants further investigation. In any small child radiographic evidence of fractures at various stages of healing are, with few exceptions, the result of physical abuse. Fractures in school-age children are often the result of bicycle-automobile or skateboard injuries. Adolescents are vulnerable to multiple and severe trauma, because they are mobile on bikes and motorcycles and active in sports. Speed and congested surroundings often intensify the impact. Young children and teenagers usually do not calculate risks as they learn to manipulate their environment and achieve developmental goals. Therefore, injuries are a part of most childhood experience.

The Fracture Wound

A fractured bone consists of fragments—the fragment closer to the midline, or the proximal fragment, and the fragment farther from the midline, or the distal fragment. When fracture fragments are separated, the fracture is *complete;* when fragments remain attached the fracture is *incomplete*. The fracture line can be:

transverse crosswise, at right angles to the long axis of the bone
oblique slanting but straight, between a horizontal and a perpendicular direction
spiral slanting and circular, twisting around the bone shaft

The twisting of an extremity while the bone is breaking results in a spiral break. If the fracture does not produce a break in the skin, it is a *simple,* or *closed,* fracture. *Open,* or *compound,* fractures are those with an open wound through which the bone is or has protruded. If the bone fragments cause damage to other organs or tissues (such as the lung or bladder), the injury is said to be *complicated*. When small fragments of bone are broken

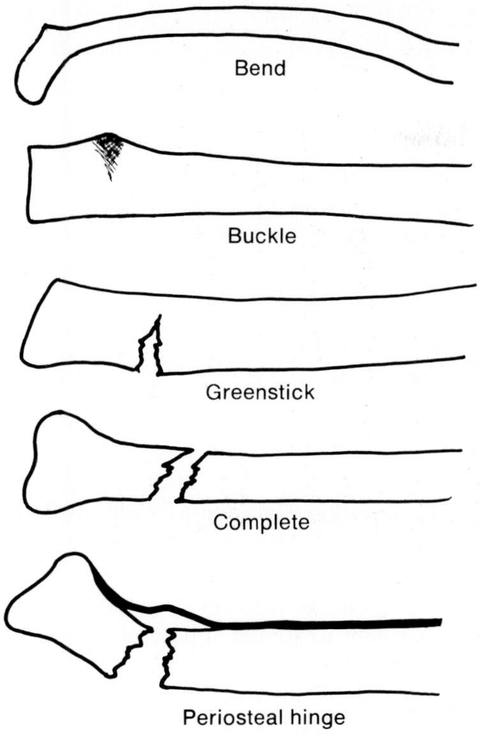

FIG. 30-2 Types of fractures in children.

from the fractured shaft and lie in the surrounding tissue, the fracture is called *comminuted*. This type of fracture is rare in children. The types of fractures seen most often in children are (Fig. 30-2):

bends a child's flexible bone can be bent 45 degrees or more before breaking. However, if bent, the bone will straighten slowly, but not completely, to produce some deformity but without the angulation seen when the bone breaks. Bends occur more commonly in the ulna and fibula, often associated with fractures of the radius and tibia.

buckle fracture compression of the porous bone produces a *buckle,* or *torus,* fracture. This appears as a raised or bulging projection at the fracture site. Torus fractures occur in the most porous portion of the bone near the metaphysis (the portion of the bone shaft adjacent to the epiphysis) and are more common in young children.

green-stick fracture a green-stick fracture occurs when a bone is angulated beyond the limits of bending. The compressed side bends and the tension side fails, causing an incomplete fracture similar to the break observed when a green stick is broken.

complete fracture complete fractures are those that divide the bone fragments. They often remain attached by a periosteal hinge, which can aid or hinder reduction.

Immediately after a fracture occurs, the muscles contract and physiologically splint the injured area. This phenomenon accounts for the muscle tightness observed over a fracture site and the deformity that is produced as the muscles pull the bone ends out of alignment. This muscle response must be overcome by traction or complete muscle relaxation (that is, anesthesia) in order to realign the distal bone fragment to the proximal bone fragment.

EMERGENCY TREATMENT

Fracture

1. Assess extent of injury—5 "Ps"
   - Pain and point of tenderness
   - Pulse—distal to the fracture site
   - Pallor
   - Paresthesia—sensation distal to the fracture site
   - Paralysis—movement distal to the fracture site
2. Determine the mechanism of injury
3. Move injured part as little as possible
   - Cover open wounds with sterile or clean dressing
4. Immobilize the limb, including joints above and below fracture site; do not attempt to reduce fracture or push protruding bone under the skin
   - Soft splint (pillow or folded towel)
   - Rigid splint (rolled newspaper or magazine)
   - Uninjured leg can serve as splint for leg fracture if no splint available
5. Reassess neurovascular status
6. Apply traction if circulatory compromise is present
7. Elevate the injured limb if possible
8. Apply cold to the injured area
9. Call Emergency Transport Team (Service) or transport to medical facility

EMERGENCY TREATMENT

Bone healing and remodeling. Bone healing is characteristically rapid in children because of the thickened periosteum and generous blood supply. When there is a break in the continuity of bone, the osteoblasts are in some way stimulated to maximum activity. New bone cells are formed in immense numbers almost immediately after the injury and, in time, are evidenced by a bulging growth of new bone tissue between the fractured bone fragments. This is followed by deposition of calcium salts to form a *callus*.

Fractures heal in less time in children than in adults. The approximate healing times for a femoral shaft are:

Neonatal period—2 to 3 weeks
Early childhood—4 weeks
Later childhood—6 weeks
Adolescence—8 to 10 weeks

Diagnostic Evaluation

A history is often lacking in childhood injuries. Infants are unable to communicate, and older children are unreliable informants and seldom volunteer information (even under direct questioning) when the injury occurred during forbidden activities. Unless they are witnesses to the injury, parents may misinterpret what the child is trying to say. In cases of child abuse, parents may give false information deliberately in order to protect themselves.

The child exhibits the same manifestations seen in adults (see box). However, often a fracture is remarkably stable because of intact periosteum. The child may even be able to use an affected arm or walk on a fractured leg. However, a fracture should be strongly suspected in a small child who refuses to walk.

Clinical Manifestations of a Fracture

Signs of injury
- Generalized swelling
- Pain or tenderness
- Diminished functional use of affected part

May be
- Bruising
- Severe muscular rigidity
- Crepitus (grating sensation at fracture site)

Radiographic examination is the most useful diagnostic tool for assessing skeletal trauma. The calcium deposits in bone make the entire structure radiopaque. Radiographic films are taken after fracture reduction and, in some cases, may be taken during the healing process to determine satisfactory progress.

Therapeutic Management

The majority of children's fractures heal well, and nonunion is rare. Most fractures are readily reduced by simple traction and immobilization until healing takes place. However, the position of the bone fragments in relation to one another influences the rapidity of healing and the residual deformity. Healing is prompt and complete with end-to-end apposition, but a gap between fragments delays (or prevents) healing. The goals of fracture management are:

1. To regain alignment and length of the bony fragments (reduction)
2. To retain alignment and length (immobilization)
3. To restore function to the injured parts

In children the bone fragments are usually realigned and immobilized by traction or by closed manipulation and casting until adequate callus is formed. Weight bearing on lower extremity fractures and active movement for the purpose of regaining function can begin after the fracture site is stable. The child's natural tendency to be active is usually sufficient to restore normal mobility, and physical therapy is rarely needed. In most cases children's fractures can be managed by closed reduction and plaster immobilization, which is most often provided on an outpatient basis with reevaluation in 7 to 10 days.

Children are most frequently hospitalized for fractures of the femur and the supracondylar area of the distal humerus. If simple reductions cannot be achieved or if a neurovascular problem is detected after injury, observation in a hospital is indicated. Severe contusions with profound swelling cannot be treated with a cast, which would act as a tourniquet on the extremity. A badly maligned fracture requires traction for a period of time before a cast is applied.

The major methods for immobilizing a fracture, casting and traction, are described in the following section in relation to the nursing care involved.

Nursing Considerations

Nurses are frequently the persons who make the initial assessment of a child with a suspected fracture (see Emergency treatment box). The child and his parents are frightened and upset, the child is in pain, and since most fractures are obvious, the parents and (frequently) the child are already convinced of the diagnosis. Therefore, if the child is alert and if there is no evidence of hemorrhage, the initial nursing interventions are directed toward calming and reassuring the child and his parents so that a more extensive assessment can be more easily accomplished.

While maintaining a calm manner and speaking in a quiet voice, the nurse can ask the parents to describe what happened and how they feel about it. Since the child usually arrives with the limb supported in some manner, this time does not delay or endanger the treatment. Initially it is best not to touch the child but to ask him to point to the painful area and to wiggle his fingers or toes. By this time he usually feels relatively safe and will allow someone to gently touch him just enough to feel the pulse and test for sensation. A child's anxiety is greatly influenced by previous experiences with injury and health personnel. However, the child needs to be told what will happen and what he can do to help. The affected limb need not be palpated, and it should not be moved unless properly splinted. If the child is at home or if the physician is not present to examine the child, some type of splint is applied carefully for transport to the hospital and to the radiology department and cast room.

THE CHILD IN A CAST

The completeness of the fracture, the type of bone involved, and the amount of weight bearing influence how much of the extremity must be included in the cast to immobilize the fracture site completely. In most cases the joints above and below the fracture are immobilized to eliminate the possibility of movement that might cause displacement at the fracture site. Four major categories of casts are used for fractures: *upper extremity* to immobilize wrist and/or elbow, *lower extremity* to immobilize ankle and/or knee, *spinal* and *cervical* for immobilization of the spine, and *spica casts* to immobilize the hip and knee.

When a cast is to be applied, it is often the nurse's role to set up the cast materials and to hold the extremity in alignment. In most instances only the cast material is required; however, special cast tables that hold the child's body are used for applying large hip spica casts. If possible the small child should be allowed to play with a doll that has a cast so that he understands what will be done.

For plaster casts a tube of stockinette is first stretched over the area to be casted, and bony prominences are padded with soft cotton sheeting. Dry rolls of gauze impregnated with plaster of Paris are immersed in a pail of tepid water with the open end of the roll downward to allow soaking of the bandage. The wet plaster rolls are put on in a bandage fashion and molded to the extremity. A heat-producing chemical reaction occurs between the plaster and water as the plaster becomes a crystalline gypsum. During application of the cast, the underlying stockinette is pulled over the raw edges of the cast and secured with a layer of wet plaster ½ to 1 inch below the rim to form a smooth, padded edge to protect the skin.

Fiberglass (some available in fashion colors), plastic, and resin materials are also used as casting materials. They are lightweight, dry quickly, can tolerate more contact with water, and can be lightly sponged when they become soiled. Preparation and application of these materials are similar to the application of plaster casts. The temperature of the water varies with the type of material, however.

Nursing Considerations

The complete evaporation of the water from a hip spica cast can take 24 to 48 hours when older types of plaster materials are used. Drying occurs within minutes with new quick-drying substances. The cast must remain uncovered to allow it to dry from the inside out. Turning the child in a plaster cast at least every 2 hours will help to dry a body cast evenly as well as prevent complications related to immobility. A regular fan to circulate air may be helpful during high-humidity weather. Heated fans or dryers should not be used, since they cause the cast to dry on the outside and remain wet beneath or cause burns from heat conduction by way of the cast to the underlying tissue.

A wet cast should be supported by a pillow that is covered with plastic and handled by the palms of the hands to prevent indenting the cast, which can create pressure areas. A dry plaster of Paris cast produces a hollow sound when it is tapped with the finger. If "hot spots" are felt on the cast surface (usually indicating infection beneath the area), this should be reported so a window can be made in the cast to observe the site.

During the first few hours after a cast is applied, the chief concern is that the extremity may continue to swell to the extent that the cast becomes a tourniquet, shutting off circulation and producing neurovascular complications. A measure for reducing the likelihood of this potential problem is to elevate the body part, thereby increasing venous return. If edema is excessive, casts are bivalved, that is, cut to make an anterior and a posterior half that are held together with an elastic bandage. The cast and the involved extremity are observed frequently for neurovascular integrity, and any signs of compromise, such as pain, swelling, discoloration (pallor or cyanosis) of the exposed portions, lack of pulsation and warmth, or the inability to move the exposed part(s), are reported immediately.

If the physician does not form a protective edge with stockinette, the raw edges of the cast can be protected by a "petaled" edge. Small pieces approximately 2 to 3 inches long are cut from 1- or 1½-inch wide adhesive tape. The edges are rounded with scissors, and each of these "petals" is placed over the edge of the cast, each petal slightly overlapping the previous petal to form a smooth, neat edge. It is easier to apply the petal to the underside of the cast first and then bring the unadhered edge to the front, pressing firmly so that the edges remain securely attached. Band-Aids can be used instead of the tape petals for quicker preparation and a slightly padded cast edge.

When casting an extremity that has sustained an open fracture, a window is often left over the wound area to allow for observation and for dressing of the wound. A surgical reduction is usually casted as for a closed fracture. For the first few hours after surgery, there may be substantial bleeding that will soak through the cast. Periodically the circumscribed blood-stained area should be outlined with a ball-point pen or pencil and the time indicated to provide a guide for assessing the amount of bleeding.

Cutting the cast to remove it or to relieve tightness is frequently a frightening experience for a child. He fears the sound of the cast cutter and is terrified that his flesh as well as the cast will be cut. Since it works by vibration, a cast cutter cuts only the hard surface of the cast. This

Guidelines for Cast Care

Keep the casted extremity elevated on pillows or similar support for the first day, or as directed by the physician.
Avoid indenting the cast until it is thoroughly dry.
Observe the extremities (fingers or toes) for any evidence of swelling; discoloration (darker or lighter than a comparable extremity), or foul odor and contact the health professional if noted.
Check movement of the visible extremities frequently.
Follow physician's orders regarding any restriction of activities.
Restrict strenuous activities for the first few days.
- Engage in quiet activities but encourage use of muscles.
- Move the joints above and below the cast on the affected extremity.

Encourage frequent rest for a few days keeping the injured extremity elevated while resting.
Avoid allowing the affected limb to hang down for any length of time.
- Keep an injured upper extremity elevated (e.g., in a sling) while upright.
- Elevate a lower limb when sitting and avoid standing for too long.

Do not allow the child to put anything inside the cast.
- Keep small items that might be placed inside the cast away from small children.

Keep a clear path for ambulation.
- Remove toys, hazardous floor rugs, pets, or other items over which the child might stumble.

Use crutches appropriately if lower limb fracture.
- The crutches should fit properly, have a soft rubber tip to prevent slipping, and be well padded at the axilla.

Alleviate itching underneath cast by using alcohol swabs; cool air blown from a large syringe, fan, or hairdryer (on low or cool setting); or by scratching or rubbing the unaffected extremity.

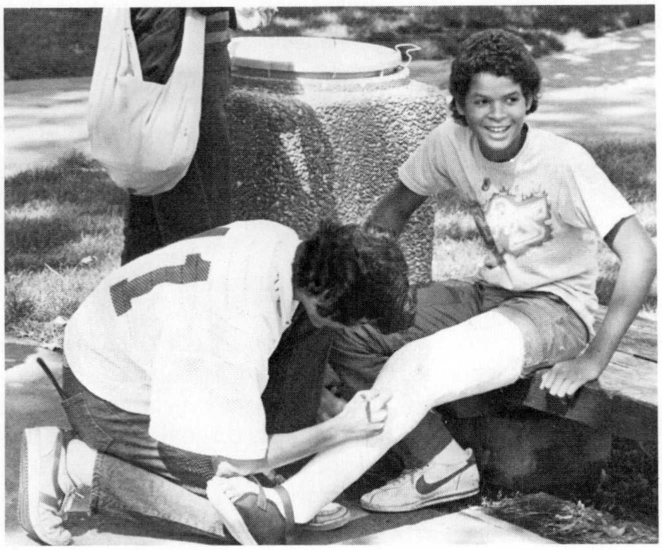

FIG. 30-3A cast serves as an excellent medium for collecting autographs and assorted graffiti.

can be demonstrated on the nurse or person removing the cast. However, the vibration generates heat that may be felt by the child, and this should be explained. Preparation for the procedure will help reduce his anxiety, especially if a trusting relationship has been established between the child and the nurse. Many young children come to regard the cast as part of themselves, which intensifies their fear of removal. Using the analogy of having fingernails or hair cut sometimes helps reduce their anxiety. Children need continual reassurance that all is going well and that their behavior is accepted.

Frequently the child will be discharged to home care after a cast is applied in the emergency room or clinic. Parents need instructions on drying and caring for the cast and on checking for signs and symptoms that indicate that the cast is too tight (see box). They should also be told to take the child to the health professional for attention if the cast becomes too loose, since a loose cast no longer serves its purpose. A cast is a badge of honor for the child and serves as visible evidence of an otherwise invisible injury (Fig. 30-3).

After the cast is removed, the skin surface will be caked with desquamated skin and sebaceous secretions. Simple soaking in a bathtub is usually sufficient for its removal, but it may require a period of several days to eliminate the accumulation completely. Application of olive oil or lotion may provide comfort. Parents and child should be instructed not to pull or forcibly remove this material with vigorous scrubbing, because it may cause excoriation and bleeding.

THE CHILD IN TRACTION

Bone fragments that cannot be aligned initially by simple traction and stabilization with a cast require the extended

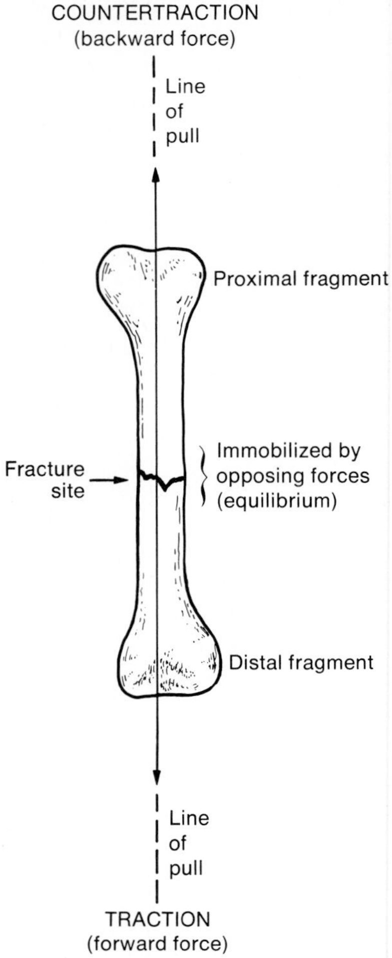

FIG. 30-4Application of traction for maintaining equilibrium.

pulling force offered by continuous traction. Traction may be used for other purposes also:

- To provide rest for an extremity
- To help prevent or improve contracture deformity
- To correct a deformity
- To treat a dislocation
- To allow preoperative or postoperative positioning and alignment
- To provide immobilization of specific areas of of the body
- To reduce muscle spasms (rare in children)

In most of these cases the traction is often applied at night and intermittently during the day. Muscle relaxants may be administered for muscle spasms.

Purposes of Traction

The three essential components of traction management are traction, countertraction, and friction (Fig. 30-4). To reduce or realign a fracture site, *traction* (forward force) is produced by attaching weight to the distal bone fragment; body weight provides *countertraction* (backward force); and the patient's contact with the bed constitutes the *frictional* force. The physician uses these forces to align the distal and proximal bone fragments by adjusting the line of pull upward or downward and adducting or abducting the extremity.

To attain equilibrium, the amount of forward force is adjusted by adding weight to or subtracting weight from the traction, and/or countertraction can be increased by elevating the foot of the bed to create a greater gravitational pull to the backward force. A bed board placed under the mattress of heavy children prevents sagging, which might otherwise change the direction of the forces applied to the fracture.

The three primary purposes of traction for reduction of fractures are:

1. To fatigue the involved muscle and reduce muscle spasm so that bones can be realigned
2. To position the distal and proximal bone ends in desired realignment to promote satisfactory bone healing
3. To immobilize the fracture site until realignment has been achieved and sufficient healing has taken place to permit casting or splinting

The all-or-none law, characteristic of muscle contractibility, influences the complete relaxation. When muscle is stretched, muscle spasm ceases and permits the realignment of the bone ends. The continuous maintenance of traction is important during this phase because releasing the traction allows the muscle's normal contracting ability to again cause a malpositioning of the bone ends.

The realignment of the fragments is a gradual process that is achieved more rapidly in infants, who have limited muscle tone, than in muscular teenagers. The desired line of pull and callus formation are checked periodically by radiographic examination. The traction pull to some degree immobilizes the fracture site; however, adjunctive immobilizing devices such as splints or casts are sometimes used with skeletal traction. In injuries in which there is severe soft tissue swelling or vascular and nerve damage, it is customary to use traction until these complications have been resolved and it is safe to apply a cast. Immobilization with traction will be maintained until the bone ends are in satisfactory realignment, after which a less-confining type of immobilization, usually a cast, will be applied.

Types of Traction (General)

The pull needed for traction can be applied to the distal bone fragment in several ways:

manual traction Traction applied to the body part by the hand placed distally to the fracture site. Nurses frequently provide manual traction during cast application.

skin traction Pull applied directly to the skin surface and indirectly to the skeletal structures. The pulling mechanism is attached to the skin with adhesive material or an elastic bandage. Both types are applied over soft, foam-backed traction straps to distribute the traction pull.

skeletal traction Pull applied directly to the skeletal structure by a pin, wire, or tongs inserted into or through the diameter of the bone distal to the fracture.

Manual traction is used by the physician in uncomplicated arm or leg fractures in which there is little overriding of the bones and minimum muscle pull to overcome. Manual traction is used to realign bone fragments for immediate cast application. Skin traction is applied when there is minimum displacement and little muscle spasticity, but it is contraindicated when there is associated skin damage. Skin traction has specific limits of weight that it can pull without causing tissue breakdown. Skeletal traction is used when significant traction pull must be applied in order to achieve realignment and immobilization. By inserting a pin or wire into the bone, the stress is placed on the bone and not on the surrounding tissue.

The type of traction applied is determined primarily by the age of the child, the condition of the soft tissues, and the type and degree of displacement of the fracture. Fractures most commonly treated by application of traction are those involving the humerus, femur, and vertebrae. The major types of traction for specific fractures are discussed in the following sections.

Upper Extremity Traction

Treatment of fractures of the humerus by traction is accomplished by (1) overhead suspension, in which the arm, bent at the elbow, is suspended vertically by skin or skeletal attachment and traction is applied to the distal end of the humerus, or (2) Dunlop traction.

Dunlop traction. With Dunlop traction (Fig. 30-5), the arm is suspended horizontally, using either skin or skeletal attachment. When skin traction is used, straps are placed on the lower and upper arm with the arm flexed to accomplish pull in two directions: one along the longitudinal direction of the upper arm and one to maintain vertical alignment of the lower arm.

Fractures of the humerus, which usually result from a fall with the arm in extension, frequently involve the supracondylar portion. These fractures are especially at risk for nerve damage and angulation deformities; therefore, they must be reduced carefully, sometimes under anesthesia, and, because of the danger of complications, children with closed reduction of supracondylar fractures are often hospitalized for observation. In severely malaligned fractures, closed reduction under anesthesia is followed by application of skeletal traction for 2 to 3 weeks, after which a long arm cast is applied for an additional 2 to 3 weeks.

Lower Extremity Traction

The severity of the fracturing force and the ability of the muscles to hold the fracture out of alignment will determine the degree of bone fragment displacement. A fracture in the middle third of the shaft results in significant overriding but minimum displacement. In a fracture in the lower one third of the shaft, the pull of the gastrocnemius muscle causes the distal fragment to become downwardly displaced.

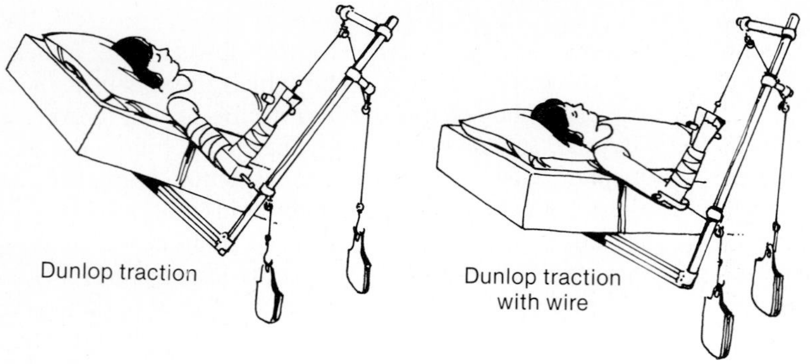

FIG. 30-5 Dunlop traction.

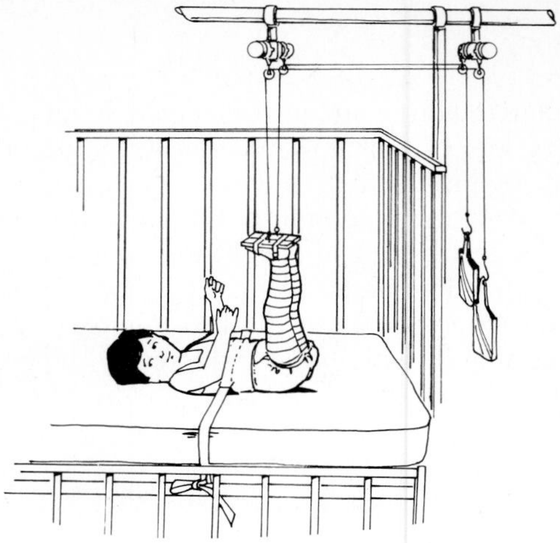

FIG. 30-6 Bryant traction.

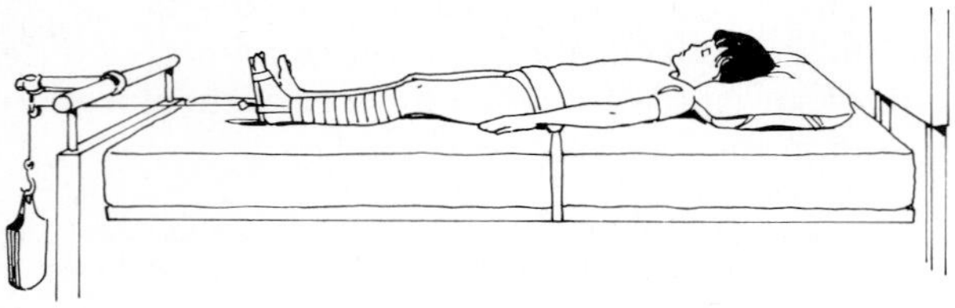

FIG. 30-7 Buck extension traction.

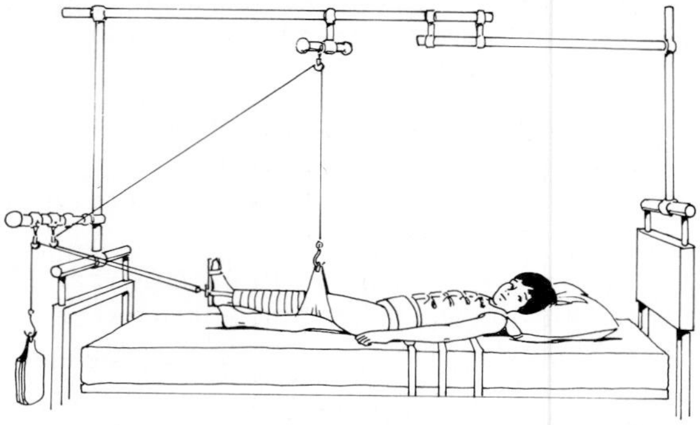

FIG. 30-8 Russell traction.

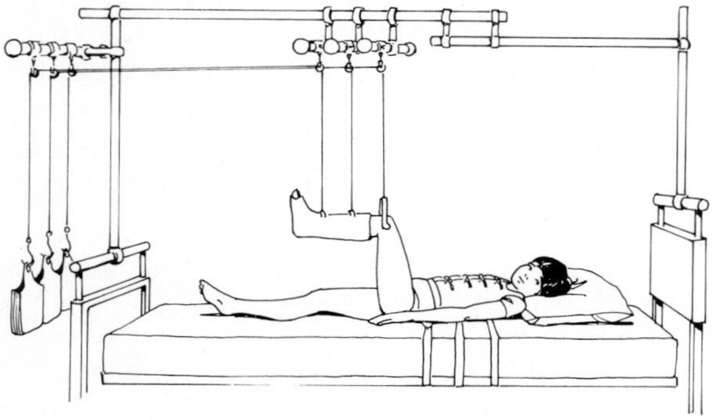

FIG. 30-9 Ninety-degree–ninety-degree traction.

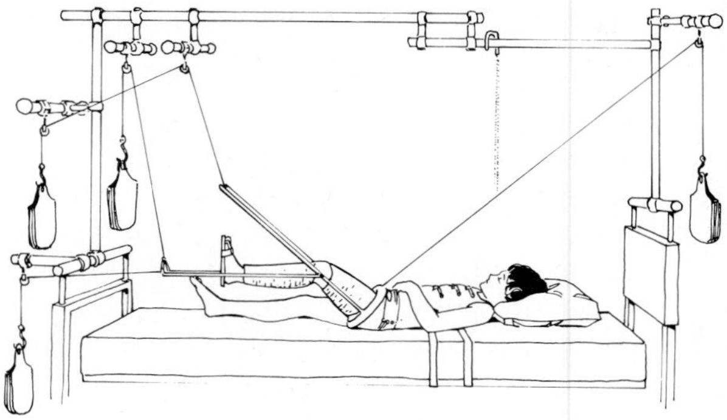

FIG. 30-10 Balance suspension with Thomas ring splint and Pearson attachment.

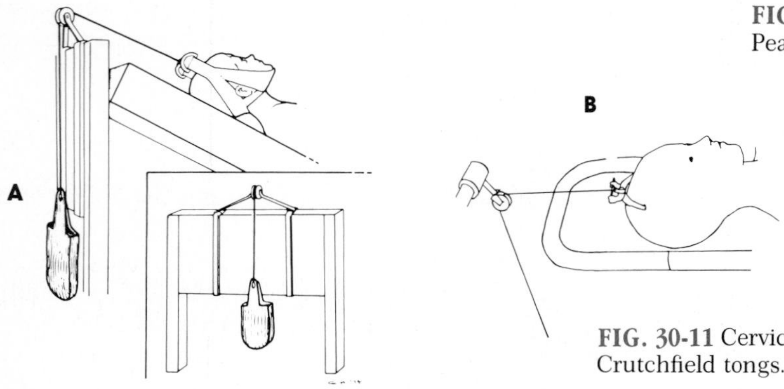

FIG. 30-11 Cervical traction. **A,** With chin strap. **B,** With Crutchfield tongs.

FIGS. 30-5 to 30-11 (Redrawn from Hilt, N.E., and Schitt, E.W.: Pediatric orthopedic nursing, St. Louis, 1975, The C.V. Mosby Co.)

Fractures of the femur can often be reduced with immediate application of a hip spica cast in young children. When traction is required, several types may be used, based on the initial assessment.

Bryant traction. When a traction pulls only in one direction, it is called *running traction*. Bryant traction is this type of traction (Fig. 30-6). Adhesive traction strips are applied to the child's legs and secured with elastic bandages wrapped from the foot to the groin. Both of the child's hips are flexed at a 90-degree angle with the knees in extension and the legs suspended by pulleys and weights. The child's weight supplies the countertraction; therefore the buttocks are slightly elevated off the bed. By applying the same amount of traction to both legs and restraining the torso, the pelvis and hips are prevented from rotating and equal stress is placed on the growing extremities. The ankle bones are protected with stockinette or cotton wadding.

This type of traction is used for children younger than 2 years of age whose weight is not sufficient to provide adequate countertraction without the additional gravitational force. Both legs are suspended, even though only one may be involved. Bryant traction is unsuitable for older children and is usually limited to children who weigh less than 12 to 14 kg (26 to 30 pounds), because of the risk of postural hypertension, and to children without spasticity or contractures of the hamstring muscles.

The youngster is permitted sufficient room between his foot and the traction foot plate to move his foot and prevent ankle problems. The legs must be maintained perpendicular to the trunk, and the buttocks should not be allowed to rest on the mattress. Sometimes the child, especially a very active child, is placed in a jacket restraint to prevent turning and twisting out of alignment.

The child's position needs to be monitored, and the alignment of the fracture is checked by periodic radiographic films with needed traction adjustments made by the physician. Remodeling and callus formation occur rapidly, within 2 to 3 weeks, after which the child is placed in a hip spica cast for an additional 3 to 9 weeks.

A specific complication of overhead traction is impairment of circulation. This is especially a problem in Bryant traction because of the gravitational vascular draining of the elevated extremities, the possible tourniquet effect of the bandages, and the effect of the traction, which can trigger vasospasms.

Buck extension. Buck extension (Fig. 30-7) is a type of skin traction with the legs in an extended position, but it differs from Bryant traction in that the hips are not flexed. The postural hypertension that could develop as a result of Bryant traction is avoided, and this traction allows for greater mobility. Turning from side to side is permitted with care to maintain the involved leg in alignment. Buck extension is used primarily for short-term immobilization or frequently for correcting contracture or bone deformities such as Legg-Calvé-Perthes disease.

Russell traction. Russell traction (Fig. 30-8) uses skin traction on the lower leg and a padded sling under the knee. Two lines of pull, one along the longitudinal line of the lower leg and one perpendicular to the leg, are produced. This combination of pulls allows realignment of the lower extremity and immobilizes the hip and knee in a flexed position. The hip flexion must be kept at the prescribed angle to prevent fracture malalignment, since there is no direct support under the fracture and the skin traction may slip. Special nursing measures include carefully checking the position of the traction so that the amount of desired hip flexion is maintained and damage to the common peroneal nerve under the knee does not produce footdrop.

Ninety-degree–ninety-degree traction. The most common skeletal traction is 90-degree–90-degree traction (Fig. 30-9) in which the lower leg is put in a boot cast and a skeletal Steinmann pin or Kirschner wire is placed in the distal fragment of the femur. From a nursing standpoint, this traction easily facilitates position changes, toileting, and prevention of traction complications.

Balance suspension traction. Balance suspension traction (Fig. 30-10) may be used with or without skin or skeletal traction. Unless used with another traction, the balanced suspension merely suspends the leg in a desired flexed position to relax the hip and hamstring muscles and does not exert any traction directly on a body part. A Thomas splint extends from the groin to midair above the foot, and a Pearson attachment supports the lower leg. Towels or pieces of felt covered with stockinette are clipped or pinned to the splints for leg support. When the child is lifted off the bed, the traction lifts with him without loss of alignment. This traction requires very careful checking of splints and ropes to make certain that no slippage or fraying has occurred. The traction is of great value in an older and heavier child when it is essential to lift the patient for care.

Cervical Traction

The cervical area is a vulnerable site for flexion or extension injuries to muscle, vertebrae, and/or the spinal cord. Cervical muscle trauma without other complications is treated with a cervical soft or hard collar to relieve the weight of the head from the fracture site. Intermittent cervical skin traction might be used with a child halter and weight to decrease muscle spasms (Fig. 30-11).

Cervical traction is usually accomplished by the insertion of Crutchfield or Barton tongs through burr holes in the skull and weights attached to the hyperextended head. As the neck muscles fatigue with constant traction pull, the vertebral bodies gradually separate so that the cord is no longer pinched between the vertebrae. Immobilization until fracture healing can occur is an essential goal of cervical traction. If the injury has been limited to a vertebral fracture without neurologic deficit, a halo cast can be applied to permit earlier ambulation.

Nursing Considerations

Generally the child in traction is hospitalized under the direct care of nurses who develop individualized nursing care plans based on an understanding of correct traction management. Evaluating the therapeutic effects and possible negative consequences is essential to good patient care. Many of the nursing problems associated with a child in traction are related to immobility. However, it is important that nurses understand the basic principles of traction and their role in its maintenance.

Skeletal traction is never released by the nurse, except under certain circumstances, such as the child with Legg-Calvé-Perthes disease or scoliosis. The nurse may remove nonadhesive skin traction. In these cases intermittent traction is periodically released and reapplied as ordered. When skin traction must be constantly maintained, such as in fractures, nurses may occasionally remove and reapply the Ace bandage if this is approved by the attending physician, provided that *someone manually maintains the traction during the rewrapping process*. It is not uncommon for a child to have several types of traction at one time, and each traction must be assessed separately to avoid problems.

When the child is first placed in traction, he may have an increase in discomfort as a result of the traction pull fatiguing the muscle. It has been determined that orthopedic conditions are associated with a higher-than-average number of painful events and a higher percentage of bodily symptoms than other common conditions (Wong and Baker, 1988). Analgesics and muscle relaxants will help during this phase of care and should be administered liberally.

Helping the child cope with the confinement and new experience requires more than medications. An explanation should be given at the child's level of understanding about what is happening and why he must remain in the

Guidelines for Traction Care

Understand Therapy

Understand purpose of traction
Understand function of traction in each specific situation

Maintain Traction

Check desired line of pull and relationship of distal fragment to proximal fragment
- Check whether fragment is being directed upward, adducted, or abducted

Check function of each component
- Position of bandages, frames, splints
- Ropes: in center tract of pulley, taut, no fraying, knots tied securely
- Pulleys
  - In original position on attachment bar; have not slid from original site
  - Wheels freely movable
- Weights
  - Correct amount of weight
  - Hanging freely
  - In safe location

Check bed position—head or foot elevated as directed for desired amount of pull and countertraction
Do not remove skeletal traction or adhesive traction straps on skin traction

Maintain Alignment

Observe for correct body alignment with emphasis on alignment of shoulder, hip, and leg
Check after child has moved
Apply restraints when indicated
Maintain correct angles at joints

Skin Traction

Replace nonadhesive straps and/or Ace bandage on skin traction *when permitted* and/or absolutely necessary, but make certain that traction on limb is maintained by someone during procedure
Assess bandages to ascertain if they are correctly applied (diagonal or spiral), not too loose or too tight, which could cause slippage and malalignment of traction

Skeletal Traction

Check pin sites frequently for signs of bleeding, inflammation, or infection
Cleanse and dress pin sites as ordered
Apply topical antiseptic or antibiotic daily as ordered
Cover ends of pins with protective cord or padding to prevent child's being scratched by pin
Note pull of traction on pin; pull should be even
Check pin screws to be certain that screws are tight in metal clamp that attaches traction apparatus to pin

Prevent Skin Breakdown

Provide sheepskin, egg crate, or alternating pressure mattress underneath hips and back
Make total body skin checks for redness or breakdown, especially over areas that receive greatest pressure (see Nursing tip)
Wash and dry skin at least daily
Stimulate circulation with gentle massage over pressure areas
Change position at least every 2 hours to relieve pressure

Prevent Complications

Assess circular dressings for excessive tightness
Assess restraining devices
- Make certain that they are not too loose or too tight
- Remove periodically and check for pressure areas

Encourage deep breathing frequently with maximum inspiratory chest expansion
Note any neurovascular changes, such as
- Color in skin and nail beds
- Alterations in sensation
- Alterations in motor ability

Take immediate action to correct problem or report to physician if neurovascular changes are found
Record findings of neurovascular changes
Carry out passive, active, or active-with-resistance exercises of uninvolved joints
Note if any tightness, weakness, or contractures are developing in uninvolved joints and muscles
Take measures to correct or prevent further development of weakness, such as applying foot plate to prevent footdrop

> *Nursing Tip: Inaccessible Areas*
>
> A small hand mirror facilitates visualization of inaccessible skin areas.

device, and he should be reassured of the presence of someone who will aid him in adjusting to the traction and coping with the problems of immobilization.

The specific nursing responsibilities for the patient in traction are outlined in the accompanying box.

AMPUTATION

A child may be born with the congenital absence of a body part, have a traumatic loss of an extremity, or need a surgical amputation for a pathologic condition, such as osteogenic sarcoma. With today's surgical technology and the quick thinking of bystanders who save a traumatically amputated body part, some children have had fingers and arms sewn back on with variable degrees of functional use regained. A severed part should be wrapped in a clean cloth or placed in saline if possible and taken to the hospital with the victim.

Surgical amputation or the surgical repair of a permanently severed limb focuses on constructing an adequately nourished stump. A smooth, healthy, padded stump, free of nerve endings, is important in prosthesis fitting and subsequent ambulation. In some situations in which there is no vascular or neurologic deficit, a cast is applied to the stump immediately after the operation and a pylon, metal extension, and artificial foot are attached so that the patient can walk on the temporary prosthesis within a few hours.

Nursing Considerations

Stump shaping is done postoperatively with special elastic bandaging using a figure-8 bandage, which applies pressure in a cone-shaped fashion. This technique decreases stump edema, controls hemorrhage, and aids in developing desired contours so that the child will bear weight on the posterior aspect of the skin flap rather than on the end of the stump. Stump elevation may be used during the first 24 hours, but after this time the extremity should not be left in this position because contractures in the proximal joint will develop and seriously hamper ambulation. Monitoring proper body alignment will further decrease the risk of flexion contractures.

For older children and adolescents, arm exercises and bed pushups, as well as parallel bars, which are used in prosthesis-training programs, help to build up the arm muscles necessary for walking with crutches. Full range of motion exercises of joints above the amputation must be performed several times daily, using active and isotonic exercises. Young children are spontaneously active and require little encouragement.

Depending on the child's age, he or his parents will need to learn stump hygiene, with careful soap and water washing every day and checking for skin irritation, breakdown, or infection. A tube of stockinette or talcum powder is used to slide the prosthesis on more easily. A careful skin check must be done every time the prosthesis is removed, and prosthesis tolerance time must be adjusted to prevent skin breakdown.

For the child who has had an amputation, phantom limb sensation is an expected experience because the nerve-brain connections are still present. Gradually these sensations fade. Preoperative discussion of this phenomenon will aid the child in understanding his "unusual feelings" and in not hiding his experiences from others. Limb pain, especially pain that increases with ambulation, should be evaluated for the possibility of a neuroma at the free nerve endings in the stump. Psychogenic phantom limb pain is a complex problem that involves the child's response to the altered body image and the coping mechanisms he uses to handle the new experience. The problems of amputation, particularly the psychologic aspects, are discussed on p. 1047.

SPINAL CORD INJURIES

Spinal cord injuries with major neurologic involvement are not a common cause of physical disability in childhood. However, there are a sufficient number of children with these injuries who are admitted to major medical centers and, because of the increased survival rate as the result of improved management, nurses are more likely to become involved with such children.

Mechanisms of Injury

In automobile accidents, most spinal cord injuries in children are the result of indirect trauma caused by sudden hyperflexion or hyperextension of the neck, often combined with a rotational force. Trauma to the spinal cord without evidence of vertebral fracture or dislocation is particularly likely to occur in a motor vehicle accident when proper restraints are not used. An unrestrained child becomes a projectile during sudden deceleration and is subject to injury from contact with a variety of objects inside and outside the vehicle.

Falling from heights takes place less often in children than in adults, but vertebral compression from blows to the head or buttocks can occur in water sports (diving and surfing), falls from horses, or other athletic activities. Birth injuries may occur in breech deliveries from traction force on the spinal cord during delivery of the head and shoulders. A number of teenagers receive spinal cord injuries when they are accidentally shot or stabbed in the back. Individuals who use only a lap seat belt restraint are at greater risk of spinal cord injury than those who use a combination lap and shoulder restraint.

The injury sustained can affect any of the spinal nerves, and the higher the injury, the more extensive the damage. The child can be left with complete or partial paralysis of the lower extremities (paraplegia) or sustain damage at a higher level, which leaves him without functional use of all four extremities (quadriplegia). A high cervical cord injury that affects the phrenic nerve paralyzes the diaphragm and leaves the child dependent on a respirator.

Therapeutic Management

In any situation in which spinal cord injury is suspected or a possibility, the child is calmed, reassured, and advised not to move, and no person should be allowed to move him unless able to do so carefully. The child must be lifted gently and without undue haste (preferably by a coordinated team) to avoid twisting or bending the spine. If the child is conscious, he is placed supine on a rigid surface to prevent sagging. Because of the complexity and relative infrequency of these injuries, it is usually recommended that the injured person be transferred to a spinal injury center for care by a team of specially trained professionals.

Nursing Considerations

The nursing care of the paraplegic or quadriplegic child is complex and challenging. As a member of the acute care and rehabilitation teams, the nurse is involved in all aspects of care. Ideally, initial care takes place in a special intensive care unit with personnel trained to handle spinal cord injuries. Nursing management is concerned primarily with prevention of complications and maintenance of function.

Once the acute period is over, the lesion is usually static and nonprogressive, regardless of whether the paralysis is secondary to trauma, congenital defects, infection, treated tumor, or surgery. In the treatment of children with spinal cord injuries, nurses are members of a team that consists of specialists, including physicians from a number of specialty areas, physical and occupational therapists, psychologists, social workers, teachers, and vocational counselors. Each member has a unique contribution to make, and mutual agreement for specific areas of responsibility is determined during regularly scheduled team conferences.

The complexity of the care and the extensive knowledge required are beyond the scope of this volume. The reader who is interested in the multiple problems of spinal cord rehabilitation is directed to the more extensive coverage in Whaley and Wong (1987) or to books that deal exclusively with the problem.

◆ *Congenital Defects*

There are numerous skeletal defects that can be diagnosed at or shortly after birth. The alert nurse is frequently the person who detects the defect and refers the family for correction of the condition. The deviation is often difficult to detect without careful inspection. Therefore, it is imperative that nurses become acquainted with signs of these defects and understand the principles of therapy in order to direct others in the care and management of these children.

CONGENITAL HIP DYSPLASIA

The broad term *congenital hip dysplasia* describes imperfect development of the hip that can affect the femoral head, the acetabulum, or both. More commonly known as *congenital hip dislocation (CHD)* or *congenital dislocated hip (CDH)*, the disorder is apparent at birth and displays various degrees of deformity. The cause of the disorder is unknown, but it is one of the most common congenital defects, with an incidence of about 1:500 to 1:1000 births.

The disorder occurs more frequently in females than in males (7:1) and occurs 25 to 30 times more often in first-degree relatives than in the general population. The concordance in monozygotic twins is 40% but only 3% in dizygotic twins, which suggests that genetic factors play a role in the causation. One fourth of all cases involve

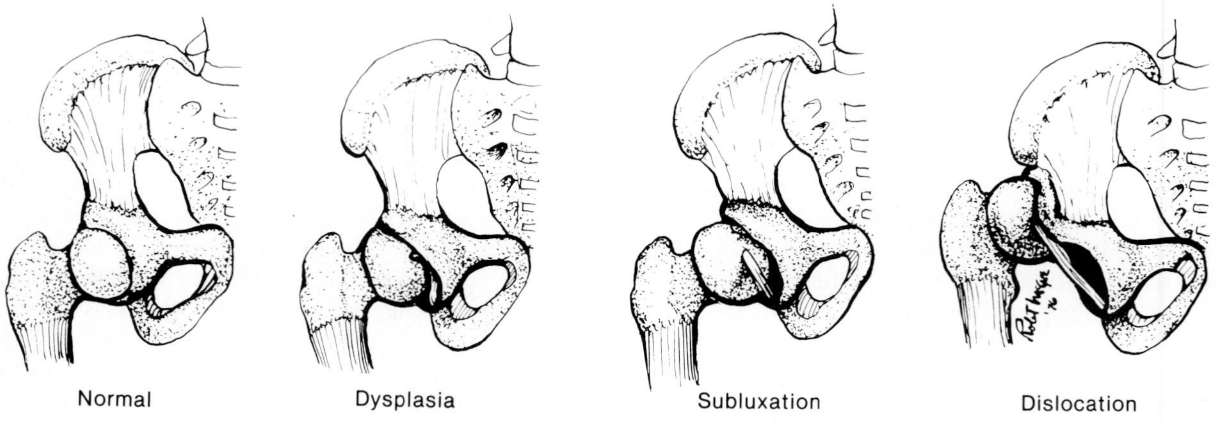

FIG. 30-12 Configuration and relationship of structures in congenital hip deformities.

both hips, and when only one hip is involved, the left hip is affected three times more often than the right. Congenital hip dysplasia is frequently associated with other conditions, such as spina bifida.

Pathophysiology

Three degrees of congenital hip dysplasia can be identified (Fig. 30-12):

acetabular dysplasia (or preluxation) the mildest form, in which there is neither subluxation nor dislocation. The dysplasia reflects an apparent delay in acetabular development evidenced by osseous hypoplasia of the acetabular roof that is oblique and shallow, although the cartilaginous roof is comparatively intact. The femoral head remains in the acetabulum.

subluxation accounts for the largest percentage of congenital hip dysplasias. Subluxation implies incomplete dislocation or dislocatable hip and is sometimes regarded as an intermediate state in the development from primary dysplasia to complete dislocation. The femoral head remains in contact with the acetabulum, but a stretched capsule and ligamentum teres cause the head of the femur to be partially displaced. Pressure on the cartilaginous roof inhibits ossification and produces a flattening of the socket.

dislocation in which the femoral head loses contact with the acetabulum and is displaced posteriorly and superiorly over the fibrocartilaginous rim. The ligamentum teres is elongated and taut.

There appear to be intrauterine, racial, and cultural factors associated with CHD. There is a striking relationship between the development of the dislocation and methods of handling infants. Among the cultures with the highest incidence of dislocation, newly born infants are tightly wrapped in blankets or other swaddling material or are strapped to cradle boards. In cultures such as the Far East, where mothers traditionally carry infants on their backs or hips in the widely abducted straddle position, the disorder is virtually unknown.

Prenatal factors that are considered to influence development of hip abnormalities are maternal hormone secretion and mechanical factors of intrauterine posture. The maternal hormone secretion that produces laxity of the maternal pelvis toward the end of gestation affects the fetal joints as well. There is also reliable evidence to indicate an association between a higher incidence of congenital hip deformities and breech presentations and cesarean section (often necessitated by abnormal intrauterine position). Legs in frank breech position, that is, with the hips acutely flexed and knees extended, is an important factor. Other prenatal factors that contribute to hip dysplasia include twinning and large infant size.

Diagnostic Evaluation

The diagnosis of congenital hip dysplasia should be made in the newborn period if possible since treatment initiated before 2 months of age achieves the highest rate of success (see box). In the newborn period dysplasia usually appears as hip joint laxity rather than as outright dislocation (Fig. 30-13). Subluxation and the tendency to dislocate can be demonstrated by the Ortolani manipulation or the Barlow modification of the maneuver performed by persons skilled in the techniques (Fig. 30-13, *B*, *C*, and *D*). There are cases in which dislocation is not diagnosed by these standard tests, and the disorder may not be apparent at birth. Therefore it is recommended that hip examination be included as part of the well-baby visits until the child begins to walk and the gait is obviously normal.

In older infants and children radiographic examination is useful in confirming the diagnosis. An upward slope in the roof of the acetabulum (the acetabular angle) greater than 40 degrees with upward and outward displacement of the femoral head is a frequent finding in older children. Radiographic examination in early infancy is not reliable because the bones are largely cartilaginous and difficult to visualize. However, sonographic images show the unossified head of the femur and its relationship to the acetabulum; therefore, this test is being used with increased frequency.

Clinical Manifestations of Congenital Hip Dysplasia

Infant:
- Shortening of limb on affected side (Galleazzi sign, Allis sign)
- Restricted abduction of hip on affected side
- Unequal gluteal folds (infant prone)
- Positive Ortolani test
- Positive Barlow test

Older infant and child:
- Affected leg shorter than the other
- Telescoping or piston mobility of joint
  - The head of the femur can be felt to move up and down in buttock when the extended thigh is pushed first toward the child's head and then pulled distally
- Trendelenburg sign
  - When the child stands first on one foot and then on the other (holding onto a chair, rail, or someone's hands) bearing weight on the affected hip, the pelvis tilts downward on the normal side instead of upward as it would with normal stability
- Prominent greater trochanter
- Greater trochanter prominent and appears above a line from the anterior superior iliac spine to the tuberosity of the ischium
- Marked lordosis (bilateral dislocations)
- Waddling gait (bilateral dislocations)

Therapeutic Management

Treatment is begun as soon as the condition is recognized, since early intervention is more favorable to the restoration of normal bony architecture and function. The longer treatment is delayed, the more severe the deformity, the more difficult the treatment, and the less favorable the prognosis. The treatment varies with the age of the child and the extent of the dysplasia.

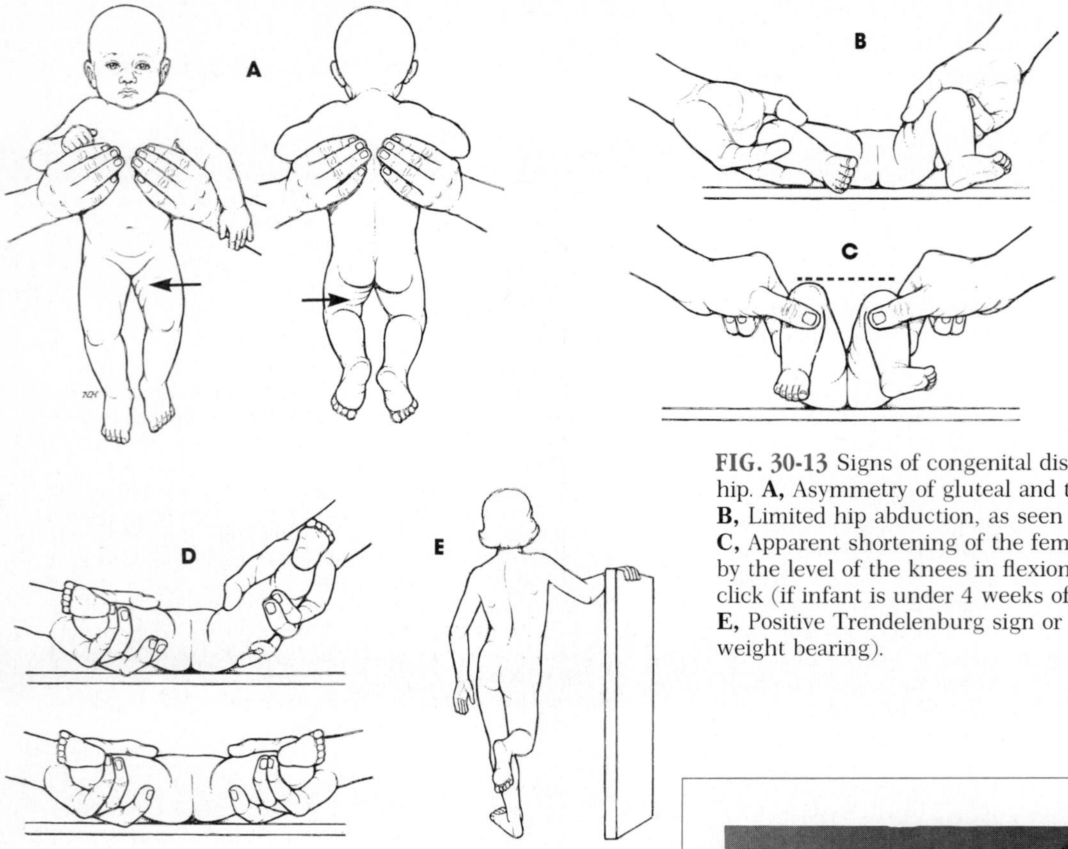

FIG. 30-13 Signs of congenital dislocation of the hip. **A,** Asymmetry of gluteal and thigh folds. **B,** Limited hip abduction, as seen in flexion. **C,** Apparent shortening of the femur, as indicated by the level of the knees in flexion. **D,** Ortolani click (if infant is under 4 weeks of age). **E,** Positive Trendelenburg sign or gait (if child is weight bearing).

Newborn to six months. The hip joint is maintained by splinting with the proximal femur centered in the acetabulum in an attitude of flexion. Of the numerous devices available, the Pavlik harness is the most widely used, and with time, motion, and gravity the hip works into a more abducted, reduced position (Fig. 30-14). The harness is worn full time until the hip is clinically and radiographically stable, usually about 3 to 6 months.

When adduction contracture is present, the hips are slowly and gently stretched to abduction and maintained with a device until stability is attained. When there is difficulty in maintaining stable reduction, a plaster hip spica cast is applied and changed periodically to accommodate the child's growth. After 3 to 6 months, sufficient stability is acquired to allow transfer to a removable protective abduction brace. The duration of treatment depends on development of the acetabulum but is usually accomplished within the first year.

Six to eighteen months. In this age-group the dislocation is not recognized until the child begins to stand and walk, when attendant shortening of the limb and contractures of hip adductor and flexor muscles become apparent. Gradual reduction by traction is followed by plaster cast immobilization, which is maintained until radiographic examination confirms a stable joint. Often soft

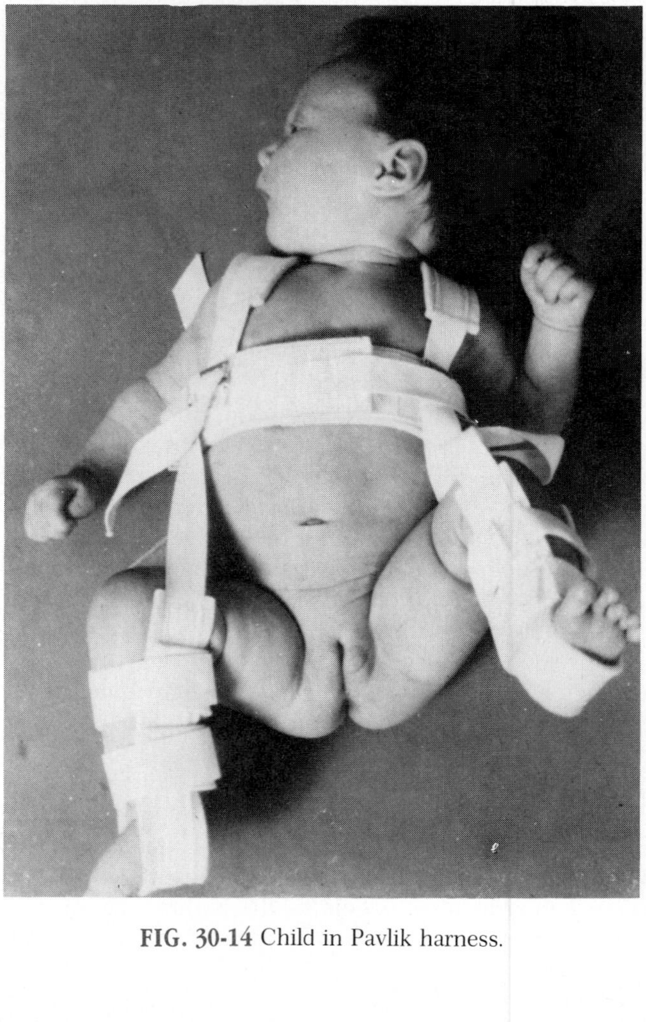

FIG. 30-14 Child in Pavlik harness.

tissue may obstruct and complicate reduction and subsequent joint development. In this case open reduction is performed to remove the obstruction followed by postoperative spica cast immobilization and, after 4 to 6 months, replacement with an abduction splint.

Older child. Correction of the hip deformity in the older child is inherently more difficult than in the preceding age-groups, since secondary adaptive changes complicate the condition. Operative reduction, which may involve preoperative traction, tenotomy of contracted muscles, and any one of several innominate osteotomy procedures designed to construct an acetabular roof, is usually required. After cast removal and before weight bearing is permitted, range of motion exercises help restore movement. Next, rehabilitative measures are instituted. Successful reduction and reconstruction become increasingly difficult after the age of 4 years and are usually impossible or inadvisable over 6 years of age because of severe shortening and contracture of muscles and deformity of the femoral and acetabular structures.

Nursing Considerations

Numerous congenital defects can be identified in the newborn period, and the earlier they are detected the more likely is the therapy to be effective. Nurses always need to be alert to the possibility of a defect in the infants in their care.

ASSESSMENT

Nurses are in a unique position to detect congenital dislocation of the hip in the newborn. During the infant assessment process and routine nurturing activities, the hips and extremities are inspected for any deviations from the normal. Usually only nurses specially trained in the technique are permitted to perform Ortolani and Barlow tests, but any nurse can be alert to other signs, such as leg shortening, gluteal folds, and limited abduction. Diapering, for example, provides an excellent opportunity to observe for limited movement and a wide perineum. These observations are reported to the attending physician, and the ambulatory child who displays a limp or an unusual gait should be referred for evaluation. This may indicate an orthopedic or neurologic problem.

> *Nursing Diagnoses: The Child with Congenital Hip Dysplasia*
>
> Impaired physical mobility related to correction device
> Potential impaired skin integrity related to presence of correction device
> Altered family processes related to care of a child in a corrective device

NURSING DIAGNOSES

Nursing diagnoses identified for the child with congenital hip dysplasia are listed in the accompanying box. Other diagnoses will be apparent in specific situations.

PLANNING

The goals of nursing care for the child in a mechanical device for correction of a congenital hip dysplasia are:

1. Maintain correct position of hip in acetabulum
2. Prevent complications related to wearing corrective device
3. Assist family in adapting routine nurturing activities to accommodate corrective device

IMPLEMENTATION

The major nursing problems in the care of an infant or child in a cast or other device are related to maintenance of the device and adapting nurturing activities to meet the needs of the infant or child. Generally, treatment and follow-up care of these children are carried out in a clinic, physician's office, or outpatient unit. Hospitalization may be necessary for cast application or brace fitting but seldom exceeds 24 to 48 hours. Longer hospitalization is required for open reduction procedures or if the child is hospitalized for a concurrent illness.

The major nursing function is teaching parents to apply and maintain the reduction device. The Pavlik harness allows for easy handling of the infant and usually produces less apprehension in the parent than heavy braces and casts. It is important that parents understand the correct use of the appliance, which may or may not allow for its removal during bathing. When the infant has a harness that is not removed, a sponge bath is recommended and the skin beneath the harness is assessed daily for irritation. Powders and lotions are not used, because they tend to cake or "ball" underneath straps or clothing.

The parents are permitted to pad shoulder straps at pressure points if desired, but unbuckling or removal is determined individually, based on the family's level of understanding and the degree of deformity in the hip. If allowed, the family needs to know how to replace the harness or adjust the buckles if straps become loose. The physician may wish to see the child before any adjustment is attempted.

Casts and braces offer more challenging nursing problems, since they cannot be removed for routine care, although sometimes a brace may be removed for bathing. Care of an infant or small child with a cast requires nursing innovation to reduce irritation and to maintain cleanliness of both the child and the cast, particularly in the diaper area. (See p. 1023 for care of the child in a cast.)

Parents are taught the proper care of the cast (or brace) and are helped to devise means for maintaining cleanliness. A disposable diaper (newborn size) is tucked beneath the entire perineal opening of the cast. A larger (toddler size) diaper can be applied and fastened over the small diaper and cast (Holland, 1983).

Nursing Tip: Reducing Wetness

For heavy wetters or for night use, a sanitary napkin can be placed inside the small diaper for added absorbency. Both diapers are changed at each wetting. Another alternative is the newer diapers with absorbent gel material that holds moisture.

For tightly fitting casts, Op-Site sheeting can be cut into strips as for petalling (p. 1023) and one edge applied to the cast edge and the other directly to the perineum; this forms a continuous, waterproof bridge between the perineum and the cast to prevent leakage. An additional advantage to the use of this transparent dressing material is that it keeps both the skin and cast dry while allowing for observation of skin beneath the dressing.

Older infants and small children may stuff bits of food, small toys, or other items under the cast; parents should be alerted to this possibility so that suitable preventive measures can be instigated.

Feeding the infant in a hip spica cast or brace offers problems of positioning. Very young infants can be fed in the supine position with head elevated, and, with the infant's hips and legs supported on a pillow at the side, the parent can cuddle the infant in his or her arms during feeding. A somewhat similar position can be used for breast-feeding; that is, with the infant supported on pillows or held in a "football" hold facing the mother with the legs behind her. An alternate position is to hold the infant upright on the mother's lap with the legs of the infant astride the mother's leg.

Infants who are able to sit up can be fed in a feeding table or modified high chair. Parents may be able to fashion a tilt board with padded seat or an adjustable chair. The table or chair provides an excellent place for the child to play in an upright position. The child's car seat is also a vital consideration. Modifications can be made on several standard, government-approved car seats (Shesser, 1985), and instructions can be obtained for modification of one model, which has been tested (Feller and others, 1986).* A specially designed car restraint is also available commercially (Fig. 30-15).†

It is important for nurses, parents, and other caregivers to understand that children in corrective devices need to be involved in all the activities of any child in the same age-group. Toys are chosen that can be used in a prone position on the floor or in the seats devised for feeding and other activities. Confinement in a cast or appliance should not exclude children from family (or unit) activities. They can be held astride the lap for comfort and transported to areas of activity. The child may be allowed to walk in a cast or brace.

*Automobile Safety for Children Program, James Whitcomb Riley Hospital for Children, Indiana School of Medicine, 702 Barnhill Drive, P-121, Indianapolis, IN 46223.

†Available from Jerome Koziatek and Associates, Inc., 190 W. Boston Rd., Hinkley, OH 44233-9631.

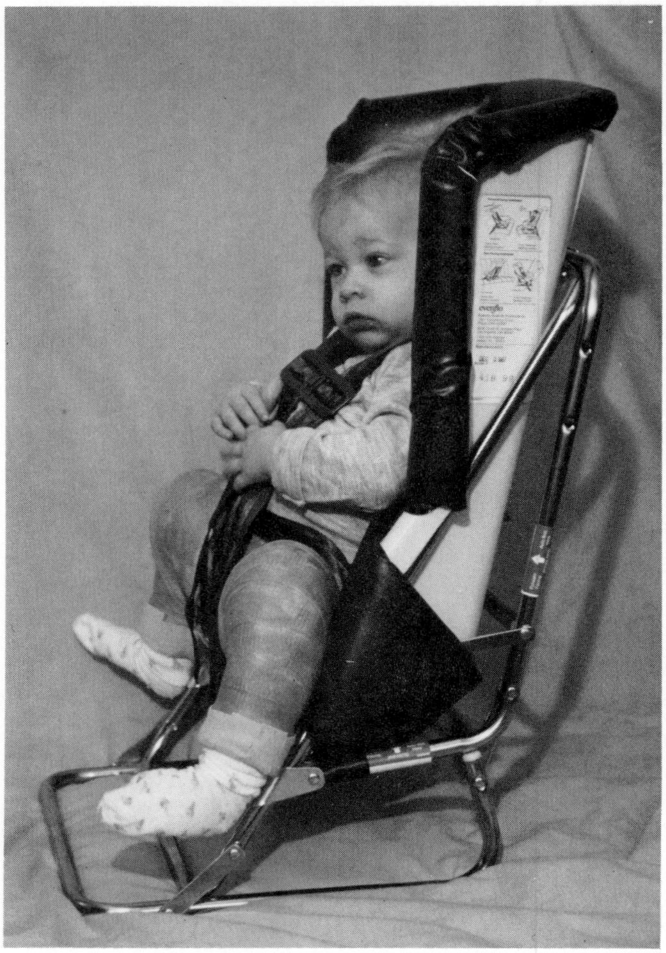

FIG. 30-15 Child in specially designed car restraint (Spelcast®).

EVALUATION

The effectiveness of nursing interventions is determined by continual reassessment and evaluation of care based on the following observational guidelines and expected outcomes:

1. Inspect corrective device regularly
2. Inspect child's skin and circulation regularly
3. Observe family's behavior with child and interview them regarding identified problems and solutions

Expected outcomes:

1. Hip remains in desired position; corrective device is positioned properly
2. Skin remains free of irritation; circulation is unimpaired
3. Family adjusts nurturing activities to accommodate corrective device

CONGENITAL CLUBFOOT

Clubfoot is a general term used to describe a common deformity in which the foot is twisted out of its normal shape or position. Any foot deformity involving the ankle is called *talipes,* derived from *talus,* meaning ankle, and *pes,* meaning foot. Deformities of foot and ankle are con-

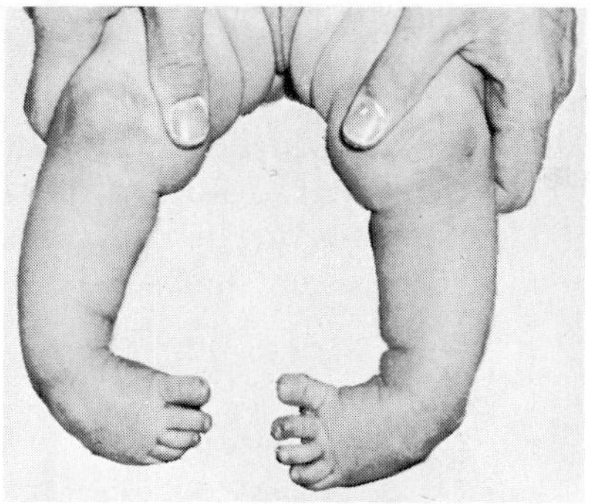

FIG. 30-16 Bilateral congenital talipes equinovarus (congenital clubfoot) in 2-month-old infant. (From Brashear, H.R., Jr., and Raney, R.B.: Shands' handbook of orthopaedic surgery, ed. 9, St. Louis, 1978, The C.V. Mosby Co.)

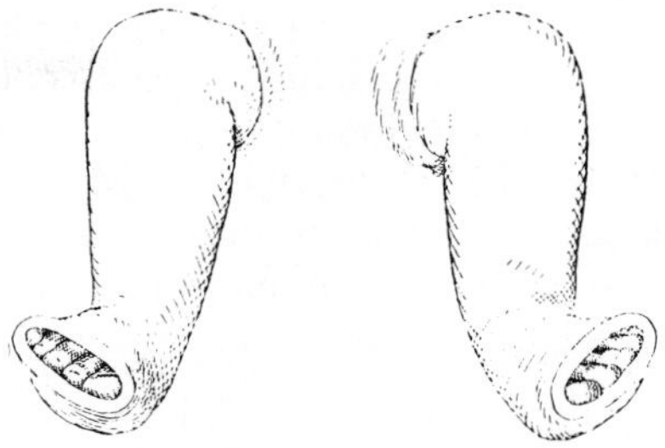

FIG. 30-17 Feet casted for correction of bilateral congenital talipes equinovarus. (From Brashear, H.R., Jr., and Raney, R.B.: Shands' handbook of orthopaedic surgery, ed. 9, St. Louis, 1978, The C.V. Mosby Co.)

veniently described according to the position of the ankle and foot. The more common positions involve the following variations:

talipes varus An inversion or a bending inward
talipes valgus An eversion or bending outward
talipes equinus Plantar flexion in which the toes are lower than the heel
talipes calcaneus Dorsiflexion, in which the toes are higher than the heel

Most clubfeet are a combination of these positions, and the most frequently occurring type of clubfoot (approximately 95%) is the composite deformity *talipes equinovarus,* in which the foot is pointed downward and inward in varying degrees of severity (Fig. 30-16). Unilateral clubfoot is somewhat more common than bilateral clubfoot and may occur as an isolated defect or in association with other disorders or syndromes, such as chromosomal aberrations, arthrogryposis (a generalized immobility of the joints), cerebral palsy, or spina bifida.

The frequency of clubfoot in the general population is 1:700 to 1:1000 live births, with boys affected twice as often as girls. There is a 35% concordance in monozygotic twins, as opposed to a 3% concordance in dizygotic twins, which indicates a hereditary component.

Pathophysiology

The precise cause of clubfoot is unknown. Some authorities attribute the defect to abnormal positioning and restricted movement in utero, although the evidence is not conclusive. Other experts implicate arrested or abnormal embryonic development. Arrested development during this early stage tends to result in a rigid deformity, whereas mechanical pressures from intrauterine position are likely causes of more flexible deformities.

Diagnostic Evaluation

The deformity is readily apparent and easily detected at birth. However, it must be differentiated from some positional deformities that can be passively corrected or overcorrected. The true clubfoot is fixed. Paralytic changes in the lower extremity of children with neuromuscular involvement often produce equinovarus deformity.

Therapeutic Management

Treatment is begun as soon as the deformity is recognized and involves three stages: (1) correction of the deformity, (2) maintenance of the correction until normal muscle balance is regained, and (3) follow-up observation to avert possible recurrence of the deformity. Some feet respond to treatment readily, some respond only to prolonged, vigorous, and sustained efforts, and the improvement in others remains disappointing even with maximum effort on the part of all concerned.

Correction of talipes equinovarus is most reliably accomplished by manipulation and the application of a series of casts begun immediately or shortly after birth and continued until marked overcorrection is reached (Fig. 30-17). Successive casts allow for gradual stretching of tight structures on the medial side and gradual contraction of lax structures on the lateral side of the foot. Manipulation and casting are repeated frequently (every few days for 1 to 2 weeks, then at 1- to 2-week intervals) in order to accommodate the rapid growth of early infancy. The extremity or extremities are casted until the desired result is achieved.

Nursing Considerations

Nursing care of the child with nonsurgical correction of clubfoot is the same as it is for any child who has a cast (p. 1023). The child will spend a considerable time in a corrective device; therefore, nursing care plans include both long-term and short-term goals. Conscientious observation of skin and circulation is particularly important in young infants because of their normally rapid growth rate. Since treatment and follow-up care are handled in the orthopedist's office, clinic, or outpatient department, parent education and support are important in nursing care of these children.

Parents need to understand the overall treatment program, the importance of regular cast changes, and the role they play in the long-term effectiveness of the therapy. Reinforcing and clarifying the orthopedist's explanations and instructions, teaching parents about care of the cast or appliance, including vigilant observation for potential problems, and encouraging parents to facilitate normal development within the limitations imposed by the deformity or therapy are all part of nursing responsibilities.

METATARSUS ADDUCTUS (VARUS)

Metatarsus adductus, or metatarsus varus, is probably the most common congenital foot deformity. In most instances it is the result of abnormal intrauterine positioning and is usually detected at birth. The deformity is characterized by medial adduction of the toes and forefoot, frequently associated with inversion, and convexity of the lateral border of the foot. Unlike talipes equinovarus, with which it is often confused, the angulation occurs at the tarsometatarsal joint, while the heel and ankle remain in a neutral position. This deformity often causes a pigeon-toed gait in the child.

Management depends on the rigidity of the deformity. Correction can usually be accomplished by gentle manipulation and passive stretching of the foot, which the parent is taught to perform. Repeated and consistent stretching is continued for the first 6 weeks, after which the treatment is based on the flexibility of the foot. Those feet that do not respond to the manipulation require orthopedic therapy. If the child is able to actively overcorrect the deformity voluntarily on stimulation, continued stretching is generally sufficient. If the foot cannot be actively or passively overcorrected, the feet are stretched and manipulated and held with casts.

Nursing Considerations

The nursing role primarily involves identifying the defect, so that early therapy and instruction of the parents can be instigated. The nurse teaches the parents how to hold the heel firmly and to stretch only the forefoot; otherwise, undue force on the heel may produce a valgus deformity. If casting is needed, the nurse instructs the parents in cast care and observation (see p. 1023).

SKELETAL LIMB DEFICIENCY

Congenital limb deficiencies, or reduction malformations, are manifest by a variety of degrees of loss of functional capacity. They are characterized by underdevelopment of skeletal elements of the extremities. The range of malformation can extend from minor defects of the digits to serious abnormalities, such as *amelia,* absence of an entire extremity, or *meromelia,* partial absence of an extremity, which includes *phocomelia* (seal limbs), an intercalary deficiency of long bones with relatively good development of hands and feet attached at or near the shoulder or the hips.

In rare instances prenatal destruction of limbs has been reported, but most reduction deformities are primary defects of development (agenesis, aplasia). Therefore, congenital amputations, in the literal sense, are not amputations, since nonexistent limbs cannot be amputated.

Pathophysiology

Limb deficiencies can be attributed to both heredity and environment and can originate at any stage of limb development. Formation of limbs may be suppressed at the time of limb bud formation, or there may be interference in later stages of differentiation and growth. Heredity appears to play a prominent role, and prenatal environmental insults have been implicated in a number of cases, such as the well-publicized thalidomide tragedy of the 1950s, which demonstrated a clear relationship between the time of exposure to the drug and the presence and type of limb deformity.

Therapeutic Management

It is generally agreed that children with congenital limb deficiencies should be fitted with prosthetic devices whenever possible and that such a functional replacement should be applied at the earliest possible stage of development in an attempt to match the motor readiness of the infant. This favors natural progression of prosthetic use. For example, an infant with an upper extremity deficiency is fitted with a simple passive device, such as a mitten prosthesis, between 3 and 6 months of age, when limb exploration is active, sitting is beginning, with the extremities needed for support, and bilateral hand activities are to be encouraged.

Lower limb prostheses are applied when the infant is ready to pull to a standing position. In preparation for prosthetic devices, surgical modification is often necessary to ensure the most favorable use of the device, since severe deformity can interfere with its effective use. Phocomelic digits are preserved for controlling switches of externally powered appliances in upper extremities. Digits (in both upper and lower extremities) provide the child with surfaces for tactile exploration and stimulation. Prostheses are replaced to accommodate growth and increasing capabilities of the child.

Nursing Considerations

Prosthetic application training and habilitation are most successfully carried out in a center that specializes in meeting the special needs of these children, especially the very young children and those with multiple amputations. It involves a team of health professionals and the parents, who must encourage the child in making age-commensurate adjustments to the environment. Although these children need assistance, excessive overprotection may produce overdependency, with later maladjustment to school and other situations.

OSTEOGENESIS IMPERFECTA

Osteogenesis imperfecta (OI) is a group of heterogenous inherited disorders of connective tissue characterized by connective tissue and bone defects. The inheritance pattern is autosomal-dominant in the majority of cases, although the most severe form demonstrates autosomal-recessive inheritance (see Appendix B).

Persons with OI appear to have abnormal precollagen that prevents the formation of collagen, the major component of connective tissue. At present OI is believed to consist of four different variations (see box). Type II, the most severe form of OI, is characterized by multiple intrauterine or perinatal fractures and severe deformity and, often, early death. The brittle nature of the bones renders them easily fractured by the slightest trauma.

The diseases of later onset run a milder course. The tendency to fracture appears later (at variable ages) and disappears after puberty. During childhood the shafts of long bones are slender, with reduced cortical thickness resulting from defective periosteal bone formation. In addition to the features already described, the child with OI has thin skin, hyperextensibility of ligaments, a tendency to recurrent epistaxis, excess diaphoresis, tendency to bruise easily, and mild hyperpyrexia. The disease shows variable expressivity, that is, the number and extent of pathologic features appear in any individual range, from severe to minimal involvement. The incidence of fractures decreases at puberty, when the body's production of hormones helps strengthen bones.

Classification of Osteogenesis Imperfecta (OI)

Type		Characteristics
I*	A	Mild bone fragility; blue sclerae; normal teeth; presenile deafness (age 20-30 years); autosomal-dominant inheritance
	B	Same as A except dentinogenesis imperfecta instead of normal teeth
	C	Same as B; no bone fragility
II		Lethal; stillborn or die in early infancy; severe bone fragility, multiple fractures at birth; 10% of OI cases; autosomal-recessive inheritance
III		Severe bone fragility leads to severe progressive deformities; normal sclerae; marked growth failure; most autosomal-recessive; few autosomal-dominant
IV	A	Mild to moderate bone fragility; normal sclerae; short stature; variable deformity; autosomal-dominant
	B	Same as A except dentinogenesis imperfecta instead of normal teeth; approximately 6% of OI cases

*Two thirds of cases are type I.

Therapeutic Management

The treatment is primarily supportive. Several drugs have been tried but appear to be of limited benefit. Lightweight braces and splints help support limbs, prevent fractures, and aid in ambulation. Physical therapy helps prevent disuse osteoporosis and strengthens muscles, which in turn improves bone density. Exercises are usually simple ones against light resistance or water exercises with swimming. Patients with milder disease are encouraged to participate in appropriate sports. Exercise also gives the child a sense of well-being and confidence in his body (Root, 1984).

Surgery is sometimes used to help treat the manifestations of the disease. Surgical techniques are used to correct deformities that interfere with bracing, standing, or walking. For the child with recurrent fractures, inserting an intermedullary rod provides stability to bones. Unfortunately the rods must be replaced as the child grows, otherwise fractures may occur through the unprotected portion of the bone.

Nursing Considerations

Infants and children with this disorder require careful handling to prevent fractures. They must be supported when they are being turned, positioned, moved, and fondled. Even changing a diaper may cause a fracture in severely affected infants. These children should never be held by the ankles when being diapered but should be gently lifted by the buttocks.

Both parents and the affected child need education regarding the child's limitations and guidelines in planning suitable activities that promote optimum development as well as protect him from harm. Realistic occupational planning and genetic counseling are part of the long-term goals of care. Educational materials and information can be obtained from the **Osteogenesis Imperfecta Foundation, Inc.*** and from the **American Brittle Bone Society.†** These organizations also have a network that can put a family in contact with other families with a similar problem.

◆ *Acquired Defects*

There are a number of skeletal defects that are acquired during the childhood years. Most of these defects are age-related. Nurses caring for children in an ambulatory set-

*P.O. Box 14807, Clearwater, FL 34629-4807.

†Cherry Hill Plaza, 1415 E. Marlton Place, Suite LL-3, Cherry Hill, NJ 08034.

In Canada, the **Canadian Osteogenesis Imperfecta Society,** P.O. Box 607, Stn. V, Toronto, Ontario M8Z 5Y9.

ting should be aware of the possibility of these correctable conditions and be alert to signs that indicate their presence so that corrective therapy can be implemented early.

COXA PLANA (LEGG-CALVÉ-PERTHES DISEASE)

Coxa plana or *osteochondritis deformans juvenilis*, more commonly known as Legg-Perthes or Legg-Calvé-Perthes disease, is a self-limited disorder in which aseptic necrosis of the femoral head produces hip deformation and dysfunction of varying degrees. The disease affects children 3 to 12 years of age, and most cases occur in males between 4 and 8 years of age as an isolated event. In approximately 10% to 15% of all cases the involvement is bilateral, and most of the affected children have a skeletal age significantly below their chronologic age. The male to female ratio is 4:1 or 5:1, and white children are affected 10 times more frequently than black children.

Clinical Manifestations of Coxa Plana

Insidious onset
Intermittent appearance of limp on affected side
Pain:
- Soreness or aching
- In hip, along entire length of thigh, or in vicinity of knee
- Most evident on rising or at end of a long day
- Usually accompanied by joint dysfunction and limited range of motion

Stiffness
Point tenderness over hip capsule
External hip rotation (late sign)

Pathophysiology

The cause of the disease is unknown, but there is a disturbance of circulation to the femoral capital epiphysis that produces an ischemic aseptic necrosis of the femoral head. During middle childhood, circulation to the femoral epiphysis is more tenuous than at other ages and can become obstructed by trauma, inflammation, coagulation defects, and a variety of other causes (Staheli, 1986). The pathologic events seem to take place in four stages:

Stage I: Septic necrosis or infarction of the femoral capital epiphysis with degenerative changes producing flattening of the upper surface of the femoral head—the *avascular stage*.

Stage II: Capital bone absorption and revascularization with fragmentation (vascular resorption of the epiphysis) that gives a mottled appearance on radiographs—the *fragmentation*, or *revascularization, stage*.

Stage III: New bone formation, which is represented on radiographs as calcification and ossification or increased density in the areas of radiolucency; this filling-in process appears to take place from the periphery of the head centrally—the *reparative stage*.

Stage IV: Gradual reformation of the head of the femur without radiolucency and, it is hoped, to a spherical form—the *regenerative stage*.

The entire process may encompass as little as 18 months or continue for several years. The reformed femoral head may be severely altered or appear entirely normal.

Diagnostic Evaluation

The diagnosis of coxa plana is suspected from clinical manifestations (see box) and established by radiographic examination.

Therapeutic Management

Since deformity occurs early in the disease process, the aim of treatment is to keep the head of the femur "contained" in the acetabulum, which serves as a mold to preserve the spherical shape of the head and to maintain a full range of motion. The initial therapy is rest, which helps reduce inflammation and restore motion. Active motion is encouraged. In some cases traction is applied to stretch tight adductor muscles.

Containment can be accomplished by non–weight-bearing devices, such as an abduction brace, leg casts, or a leather harness sling that prevents weight bearing on the affected limb; by various weight-bearing appliances, such as abduction-ambulation braces or casts, after a period of bed rest and traction; and by surgical reconstructive and containment procedures. Conservative therapy must be continued for 2 to 4 years, although braces constructed from lightweight materials allow the child to maintain a nearly normal activity level. Surgical correction, although a relatively recent advance and subject to additional risks (such as anesthesia, infection, and blood transfusion), returns the child to normal activities in 3 to 4 months.

The disease is self-limited, but the ultimate outcome of therapy depends on early and efficient treatment and the age of onset of the disorder. Younger children, whose epiphyses are more cartilaginous, have the brightest prognosis for complete recovery. The later the diagnosis is made, the more damage has occurred before treatment is implemented. In most cases, with good patient compliance, the prognosis is excellent.

Nursing Considerations

Nurses are often the first health professionals to identify affected children and to refer them for medical evaluation. They are also persons on whom the child and his family can rely to help them understand and adjust to the therapeutic measures. Since most care of the child is conducted on an outpatient basis, the major emphasis of nursing care is teaching the family the care and management of the corrective appliance selected for therapy. The family needs to learn the purpose, function, application, and care of the corrective device and the importance of compliance in order to achieve the desired outcome.

One of the most difficult aspects associated with the disorder is coping with a normally active child who feels well but must remain relatively inactive. Suitable activities must be devised to meet the needs of the child in the process of developing a sense of initiative or industry. Activities that meet the creative urges are well received. This is also an opportune time to encourage the child to begin a hobby, such as collections, model building, or crafts.

SLIPPED FEMORAL CAPITAL EPIPHYSIS

Slipped femoral capital epiphysis (SFCE), or coxa vara, refers to the spontaneous displacement of the proximal femoral epiphysis in a posterior and inferior direction. It develops most frequently shortly before or during accelerated growth and the onset of puberty (children between the ages of 10 and 16 years—median age, 13 for boys, 11 for girls) and is most frequently observed in obese children. Bilateral involvement has been reported variously as 16% to 40%.

Pathophysiology

The cause of SFCE is unknown, but it occurs most often in "overlarge" youngsters or very tall, thin, rapidly growing children. There has been some evidence to implicate hormonal factors, such as decreased growth hormone, increased sex hormone, or hypothyroidism. It has also been associated with endocrine abnormalities, renal osteodystrophy, and growth hormone therapy.

The following different varieties of clinical behavior have been observed: (1) an episode of trauma in which the epiphysis is acutely displaced in a previously functional joint; (2) gradual displacement without definite injury, with progressively increased hip disability; (3) intermittent bouts of displacement alternating with periods of well-being with gradual appearance of symptoms associated with ambulation (such as external rotation); and (4) a combined gradual and traumatic displacement, in which there is gradual slippage with further displacement caused by injury.

Diagnostic Evaluation

The disorder is suspected when an adolescent or preadolescent youngster displays clinical signs or complains of pain (see box). The diagnosis is confirmed by radiographic examination.

Therapeutic Management

The treatment varies with the degree of displacement but involves surgical stabilization and correction of deformity. In mild cases simple pin fixation is sufficient. More extensive displacement requires skeletal traction followed by pin fixation or osteotomy. The prognosis depends on the degree of deformity and the occurrence of complications, such as avascular necrosis and cartilaginous necrosis. As in other disorders, early diagnosis and implementation of therapy increase the likelihood of a satisfactory cure.

Clinical Manifestations of Slipped Femoral Capital Epiphysis

- Obese or tall, lanky youngster
- Limp on affected side
- Pain in hip
  - Continuous or intermittent
  - Frequently referred to the groin, anteromedial aspect of thigh, or knee
- Restriced internal rotation on adduction with external rotation deformity
- Loss of abduction and internal rotation as severity increases

Nursing Considerations

Nursing care is the same as that for a child in a cast or a child in traction.

KYPHOSIS AND LORDOSIS

The spine, consisting of numerous segments, can acquire deformation curves of three types: kyphosis, lordosis, and scoliosis (Fig. 30-18).

Kyphosis

Kyphosis is an abnormally increased convex angulation in the curvature of the thoracic spine (Fig. 30-18, *B*). It can occur secondary to disease processes such as tuberculosis, chronic arthritis, osteodystrophy, or compression fractures of the thoracic spine. The most common form of kyphosis is "postural." Children, especially during the time when skeletal growth outpaces growth of muscle, are prone to exaggeration of a tendency toward kyphosis. They assume bizarre sitting and standing positions. This is particularly common in self-conscious adolescent girls who assume a round-shouldered slouching posture in the attempt to hide their developing breasts.

Postural kyphosis is almost always accompanied by a compensatory postural lordosis, an abnormally exaggerated concave lumbar curvature. Treatment consists of postural exercises to strengthen shoulder and abdominal muscles and bracing for more marked deformity. Unfortunately treatment is difficult because of the nature of the adolescent personality. The normal rebellious tendencies of the adolescent, together with continual parental nagging to "stand up straight," often interfere with compliance to a therapeutic regimen. The best approach is to emphasize the cosmetic value of corrective therapy and to place the responsibility on the adolescent for carrying out an exercise program at home with regular visits to

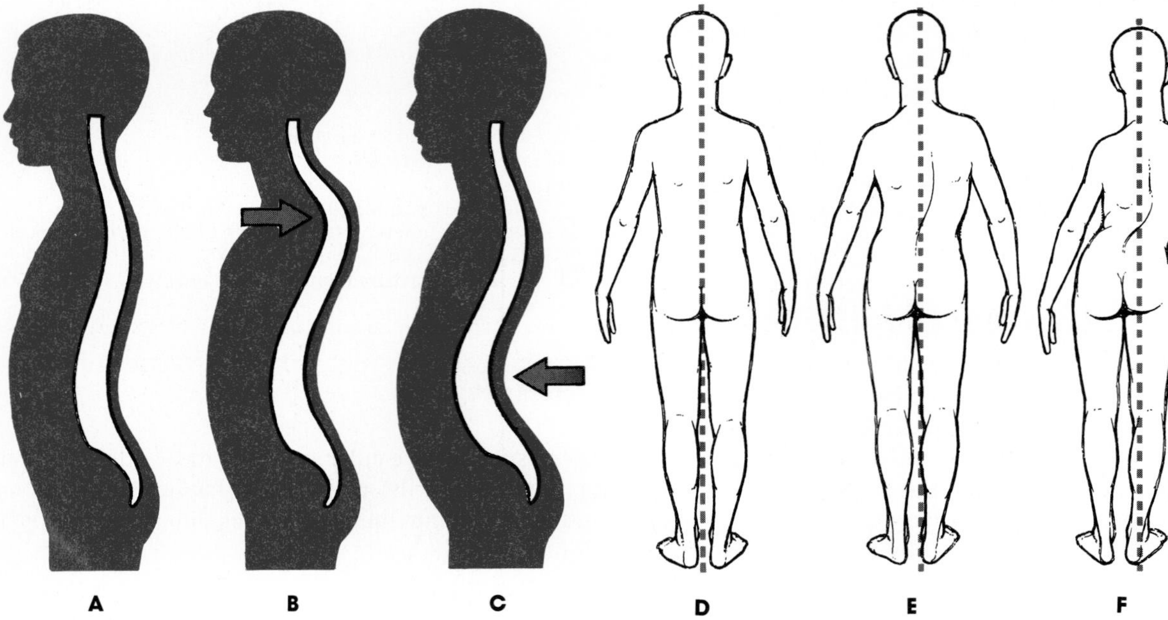

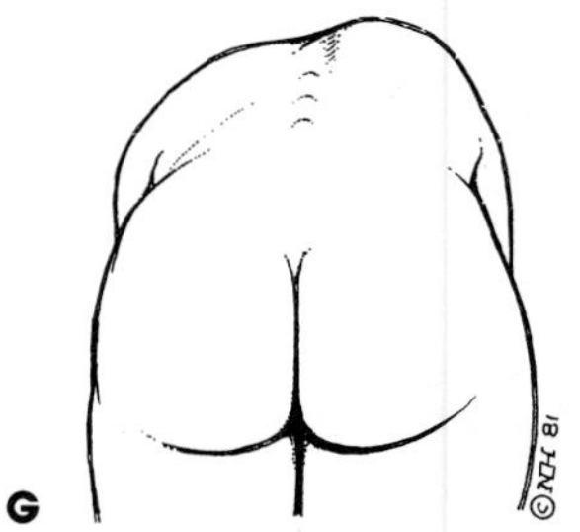

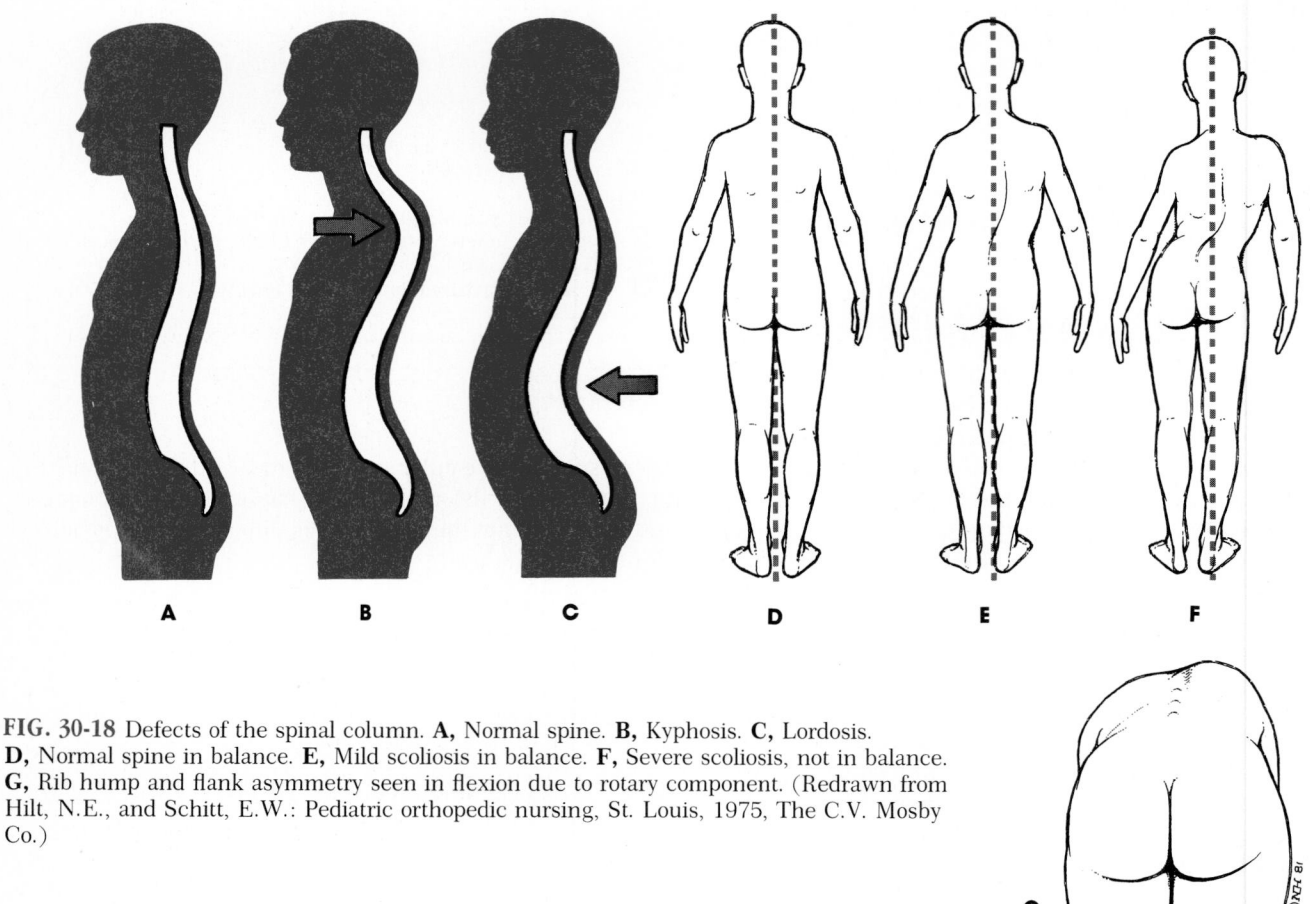

FIG. 30-18 Defects of the spinal column. **A,** Normal spine. **B,** Kyphosis. **C,** Lordosis. **D,** Normal spine in balance. **E,** Mild scoliosis in balance. **F,** Severe scoliosis, not in balance. **G,** Rib hump and flank asymmetry seen in flexion due to rotary component. (Redrawn from Hilt, N.E., and Schitt, E.W.: Pediatric orthopedic nursing, St. Louis, 1975, The C.V. Mosby Co.)

and assessments by a therapist. Most adolescents respond well to selected sports as a supplement to regular exercise. Boys prefer weight lifting (preferably performed from a prone or supine position on a bench) and track sports. Girls respond well to dancing classes (ballet or modern dancing). Swimming is excellent and has the added advantages of exercising all muscles, eliminating gravity, and teaching breath control.

Lordosis

Lordosis is an accentuation of the cervical or lumbar curvature beyond physiologic limits (Fig. 30-18, *C*). It may be a secondary complication of a disease process, the result of trauma, or idiopathic. It is often seen in association with flexion contractures of the hip, obesity, congenital dislocated hip, and slipped femoral capital epiphysis. During the pubertal growth spurt lordosis of varying degrees is observed in teenagers, especially girls. In obese children the weight of the abdominal fat alters the center of gravity, causing a compensatory lordosis. Unlike kyphosis, severe lordosis is usually accompanied by pain.

Treatment involves management of the predisposing cause when possible, such as weight loss and correction of deformities. Postural exercises and/or support garments are helpful in relieving symptoms in some cases; however, these do not usually effect a permanent cure.

SCOLIOSIS

Scoliosis, the most common spinal deformity, is a lateral curvature of the spine usually associated with a rotary deformity that eventually causes cosmetic and physiologic alterations in the spine, chest, and pelvis. It can appear at any age but is most frequent in adolescent girls.

Etiology

Scoliosis can be caused by a number of etiologic agents and may occur spontaneously or in association with other diseases or deformities. Scoliosis can be *structural* or *functional*. Functional, postural, or nonstructural scoliosis is caused by some other deformity, such as unequal leg length, and can be corrected by treating the underlying problem.

Structural scoliosis is characterized by changes in the spine and its supporting structures which cause loss of flexibility and noncorrectable deformity. Structural scoliosis may be congenital or a secondary defect associated with other disorders, especially neuromuscular disease or paralysis. In 70% of cases it is "idiopathic" without apparent cause; however, evidence indicates that it is probably genetic and transmitted as an autosomal-dominant trait with incomplete penetrance or is multifactorial.

Diagnostic Evaluation

Diagnosis is made by observation and radiographic examination. Discomfort is rarely present and there are few outward signs until the deformity is well established. Early detection and treatment are essential to successful management (see also p. 166). The undressed child viewed from the posterior side will often reveal primary curvature and a compensatory curvature that places the head in alignment with the gluteal fold (Fig. 30-18, *E*). In uncompensated scoliosis the head and hips are not in alignment (Fig. 30-18, *F*). In advanced cases with rotary deformity, rib hump and flank asymmetry are observed when the child bends from the waist unsupported by the arms (Fig. 30-18, *G*). Radiographs taken in the standing position establish the degree of deformity.

Therapeutic Management

A thorough examination, history, and assessment of the child are carried out in order to evaluate the status of the deformity, factors contributing to the defect, and factors that may influence the outcome of therapy. Treatment is best undertaken in a center in which a team is available that specializes in management of scoliosis. Current management involves straightening and realignment of the vertebrae by either external (bracing) or internal (surgical) fixation techniques. Bracing is not curative but may slow the progression of the deformity until the spine has reached the more adult size.

Bracing and exercise. Exercises can often help postural scoliosis but are rarely of value with structural defects. Nonoperative treatment by application of a properly constructed and well-fitted external bracing device and close supervision are successful in halting the progression of most curvatures. There are basically two types of braces in use: (1) the Milwaukee brace, an individually adapted steel and leather brace that extends from a chin cup and neck pads to the pelvis, where lumbar pads rest on the hips (Fig. 30-19), and (2) an underarm brace, of which there are numerous varieties, used primarily for lumbar curvatures. The brace is used for minimum curvatures and is worn 23 hours a day but offers little interference with normal activity.

Supplemental exercises are used daily both in and out of the brace to prevent atrophy of spinal and abdominal muscles. The brace is adjusted at regular trimonthly intervals and, when radiographic examinations reveal bone maturity, the child is gradually weaned from the brace over a 1- to 2-year period. The brace is then worn only at night until the spine is absolutely mature.

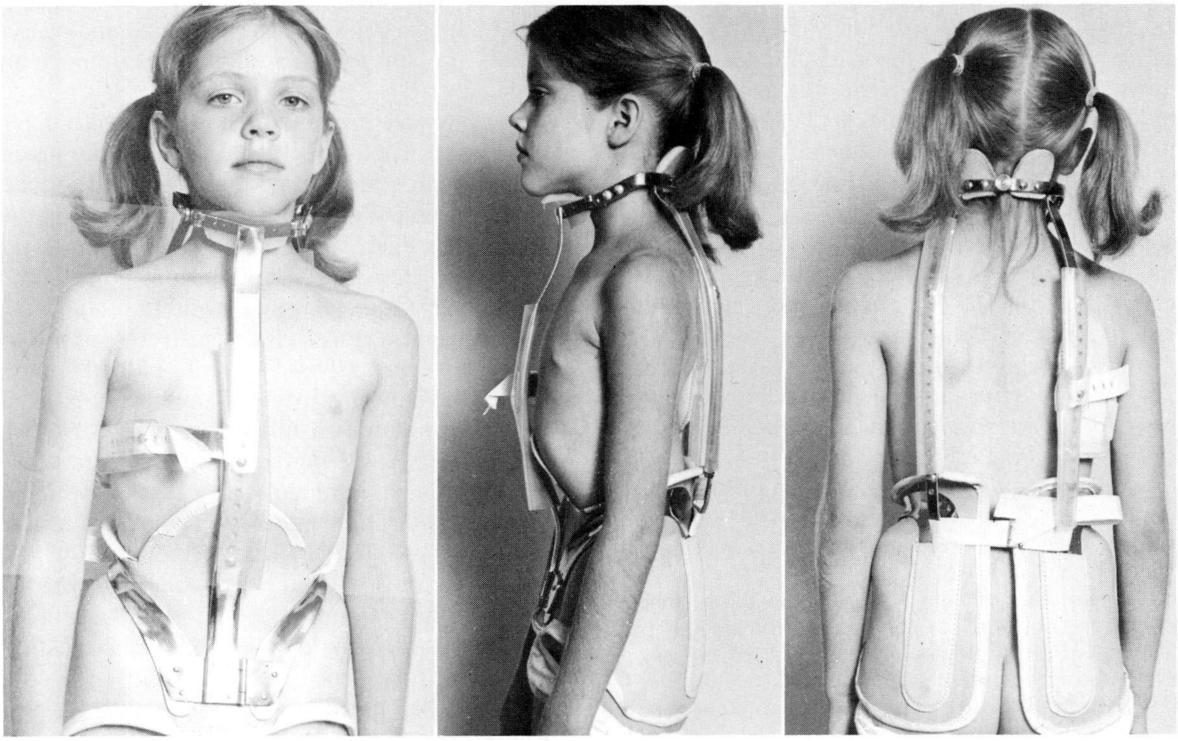

A B C

FIG. 30-19 Milwaukee brace. **A,** Front view. **B,** Side view. **C,** Rear view. (From the clinical material of Dr. Walter P. Blount, Milwaukee, Wis.)

Electrical stimulation. Many young patients with mild to moderate curvatures have an alternative to bracing—electrical stimulation. An electrical stimulator generates an electrical pulse that is transmitted to muscles on the convex side of the curvature. This causes the muscles to contract at regular and frequent intervals, straightening the spine. The devices are worn at night, allowing unrestricted activity during the waking hours. The cost of stimulators taped to the skin compares favorably with the cost of bracing; the cost of surgically implanted stimulators is considerably higher and involves hospitalization for the implant procedure. Not all authorities accept this therapy.

Surgical correction. Surgical intervention may be required for correction. With few exceptions the techniques consist of spinal realignment and straightening by way of external or internal fixation and instrumentation combined with bony fusion (arthrodesis) of the realigned spine. The age of the child and location of the curvature influence the decision for surgery, and any curve that does not respond to more conservative measures requires surgical correction.

For the most severe scoliotic curvatures, traction is often needed for a time before spinal fusion to provide partial correction and more flexibility. Methods incorporating either continuous or intermittent traction are used. One type consists of a leather head halter and pelvic girdle attached to a system of ropes and pulleys that can be manipulated by the patient. More rigid deformities are best managed by skeletal traction techniques.

Skeletal traction is applied to the spine by way of a metal ring, or halo, attached to the skull and pins inserted into either the distal femur or the iliac wings of the pelvis. With halo-femoral traction the child is placed on a special Stryker frame, and progressive traction is applied by weight in twice-daily increments. Halo-pelvic traction is applied by means of turnbuckles, and the child can remain ambulatory. Another alternative is halo-wheelchair traction, applied by means of a pulley system and weights suspended from behind the chair, using the weight of the child's upright body for countertraction.

When surgical intervention is elected, spinal fusion techniques followed by casting for a period of 6 months to a year produce satisfactory results. The surgical techniques for internal vertebral fixation are:

Harrington instrumentation implantation of metal rods by way of clips to hold the vertebrae and bone fragments for permanent fusion; child immobilized on a Stryker frame following surgery

Luque segmental instrumentation a flexible L-shaped metal rod fixed by wires to the bases of the spinous processes; patient can walk within a few days and no postoperative immobilization necessary

Dwyer instrumentation a titanium cable through cannulated screws transfixed to each vertebra; child cared for in bed following surgery

Zielke procedure combination of Harrington and Dwyer procedures

Cotrel-Dubousset procedure a form of bilateral segmental fixation that uses two knurled rods and multiple hooks

Nursing Considerations

Treatment for scoliosis extends over a significant portion of the affected child's period of growth. In adolescents this period is the one in which their identity, physical and psychologic, is formed. For some youngsters much of this time is spent in the hospital setting, immobilized in complex, unattractive appliances. For those treated on an outpatient basis, it means a modified life-style and being "different" from their peers, even though they are usually able to engage in many activities enjoyed by other youngsters.

When a child first faces the prospect of a prolonged period in a brace, cast, or other device, the therapy program and the nature of the device must be explained thoroughly to him and to his parents so that they will have an understanding of the anticipated results, how the appliance corrects the defect, the freedoms and constraints imposed by the device, and what they can do to help achieve the desired goal. The management involves the skills and services of a team of specialists, including the orthopedist, physical therapist, orthotist (a specialist in fitting orthopedic braces), nurse, social worker, and sometimes a pulmonary specialist.

It is difficult for a child to be restricted at any phase of development, but the teenager needs continual positive reinforcement, encouragement, and as much independence as can be safely assumed during this time. Guidance and assistance regarding anticipated problems, such as selection of clothing and participation in social activities, are appreciated by adolescent youngsters. Socialization with peers should be encouraged and every effort expended to help the adolescent feel attractive and worthwhile.

Preoperative care. The child hospitalized for surgical management requires preparation for the procedures involved, which are puzzling and often frightening to the very young patient. The child needs to know what is going to happen and deserves a full explanation of why the procedure is necessary and the potential outcome of the surgery. See care of the child in traction p. 1028.

Postoperative care. Postoperatively patients are monitored in an intensive care unit. They are placed on an egg-crate mattress to prevent pressure areas. The child with Harrington instrumentation will be placed on a Stryker frame, which facilitates care and lessens the possibility of damage to the fusion; it also prevents indwelling instruments from twisting the spine and reduces the possibility of "popping out" the rods. Nurses who work with these appliances should become familiar with their mechanism before assuming responsibility for patient care. The child who is not on a Stryker frame must be carefully logrolled when turned.

In addition to the usual postoperative assessments—of wound, circulation, and vital signs—the neurologic status of the patient's extremities requires special attention. There is usually some degree of paralytic ileus following the procedure; therefore nursing includes care of the nasogastric intubation and assessment for returning bowel function. Urinary retention is common and often requires insertion of an indwelling catheter. Because of the extensive blood loss during the surgical procedure and renal hypoperfusion, observation of urinary output is especially important.

The child usually has considerable pain for the first few days following surgery and requires frequent administration of pain medication, preferably on a regular schedule, as opposed to "as needed." For older children patient-controlled analgesia is a recommended alternative (see p. 597).

All patients are started on physiotherapy as soon as they are able, beginning with range of motion exercises and many of the activities of daily living. Self-care, such as washing and eating, is always encouraged. Some simple physical therapy may be begun during this acute stage. Throughout the hospitalization diversionary activities and contact with family and friends are important parts of nursing care and planning.

The family is encouraged to become involved with the patient's care to facilitate the transition from hospital to home management. Family members learn to apply and care for the brace or learn cast care. Organizations that provide education and services to both families and professionals are the **National Scoliosis Foundation, Inc.*** and the **Scoliosis Association.**† The **Scoliosis Research Society,**‡ an organization of physicians and scientists, has published an excellent book, *Scoliosis: A Handbook for Patients.*

◆ *Infections of Bones and Joints*

Infections of bones and joints are not uncommon and, because of their inaccessibility, are often difficult to treat. Because bones and joints are rigid structures, the inflammatory process is extremely painful. Early detection and therapy significantly shorten the term of treatment and reduce the degree of deformity and disability that often results from infections of these tissues.

OSTEOMYELITIS

Osteomyelitis is an infectious process of bone that can occur at any age but that occurs most frequently between 5 and 14 years of age. It is twice as common in boys as in girls.

Pathophysiology

Osteomyelitis can be acquired from *exogenous* or *hematogenous* sources. Exogenous osteomyelitis is acquired by direct invasion of the bone by direct extension from the outside as a result of a penetrating wound, open fracture, contamination during surgery, or secondary extension from an overlying abscess or burn. Hematogenous spread of organisms from a preexisting focus is the most common source of infection. Frequent infectious foci include furuncles, skin abrasions, impetigo, upper respiratory tract infections, acute otitis media, tonsillitis, abscessed teeth, pyelonephritis, or infected burns.

Any organism can cause osteomyelitis, and there is some relationship between the age of the child and the type of organism responsible. In older children staphylococci are the most common organisms, approximately 80% of which are *Staphylococcus aureus;* in younger children other organisms predominate, especially *Haemophilus influenzae*. In children with sickle cell anemia, *Salmonella* organisms are frequently the responsible agents. Other factors that predispose to development of osteomyelitis are poor physical condition, inadequate nutrition, and surroundings that are not hygienic.

Infective emboli from the focus of infection travel to the small end arteries in the bone metaphysis, where they set up an infectious process that leads to local bone destruction and abscess formation.

Diagnostic Evaluation

The signs and symptoms of *acute* hematogenous osteomyelitis begin abruptly and build up to a maximum intensity during the first few days of the disease, usually less than 1 week (see box). Symptoms often resemble those observed in other disorders involving bones (e.g., leukemia, arthritis). There is marked leukocytosis and an elevated erythrocyte sedimentation rate. Blood culture is usually positive during the early stage, and radiographic findings are often negative or show only soft tissue swelling for 10 to 14 days. After this time the radiographic findings reveal new bone formation. Tomography may reveal bone changes at an early stage.

Most cases involve the femur or tibia and to a lesser extent the humerus and hip. In infants the diagnosis is more difficult because of lack of systemic symptoms, and

Clinical Manifestations of Acute Osteomyelitis

General:
- History of trauma to affected bone (frequent)
- Child appears very ill
- Irritability
- Restlessness
- Elevated temperature
- Rapid pulse
- Dehydration

Local:
- Tenderness
- Increased warmth
- Diffuse swelling over involved bone
- Involved extremity painful, especially on movement
- Involved extremity held in semiflexion
- Surrounding muscles tense and resist passive movement

*P.O. Box 547, Belmont, MA 02178.

†1 Penn Plaza, New York, NY 10019.

‡222 S. Prospect, Suite 127, Park Ridge, IL 60068. The book can be purchased by sending $1.00 to the organization.

it may involve multiple bones or joints because of the difficulty in confining an infectious process in children in this age-group.

In *subacute* hematogenous osteomyelitis, symptoms have been present for a longer period of time, and the child sometimes has been treated with antibiotics, often for another infection, which modifies the clinical symptoms. In some instances the infection may produce a walled-off abscess rather than a spreading infection.

Therapeutic Management

As soon as blood cultures have been drawn, prompt and vigorous intravenous antibiotic therapy is initiated. The choice of antibiotic is influenced by age, and the dosage determined is sufficient to ensure high blood and tissue levels. Since most cases of osteomyelitis in the pediatric age-group are caused by staphylococci, large doses of penicillin G are administered and supplemented by other antibiotics. In children younger than 3 years of age, the infectious agents are more likely to be penicillin-resistant staphylococci or gram-negative organisms; therefore, the agents of choice are usually methicillin, nafcillin, or clindamycin in conjunction with ampicillin. Neonates in whom coliform organisms are likely to be involved are given kanamycin or gentamicin, either intramuscularly or *slowly* by the intravenous route in addition to intravenously administered ampicillin.

Antibiotic therapy is accompanied by local treatment. The child is placed on complete bed rest. Immobilization of the affected extremity, which may require a splint or bivalved cast, is continued throughout therapy to limit the spread of infection and, when it is a complication of a fracture, to maintain alignment of bone fragments.

Opinions differ regarding surgical intervention, but many advocate sequestrectomy (removal of dead bone) and surgical drainage to prevent abscess formation. When surgical drainage is carried out, polyethylene tubes are placed in the wound—one tube instills an antibiotic solution directly into the infected area by gravity, and the other, connected to a suction apparatus, provides drainage.

Nursing Considerations

During the acute phase of illness any movement of the affected limb will cause discomfort to the child; therefore, he should be positioned comfortably with the affected limb supported. Moving and turning are carried out carefully and gently to minimize discomfort. The child may require pain medication or sedation. Vital signs are taken and recorded frequently, and measures are implemented to reduce a significant temperature elevation.

Antibiotic therapy requires careful observation and monitoring of the intravenous equipment and site. Since more than one antibiotic is usually administered, the compatibility of the drugs is determined and care is taken to avoid mixing noncompatible drugs. A double, or piggyback, setup is safest, because there is less opportunity for the two drugs to come in contact with each other. The stability of the drugs, especially ampicillin, is also considered when determining the rate of administration. For long-term antibiotic therapy, the heparin lock is the preferred method of intravenous administration.

The child with an open wound may be placed on complete or wound isolation precautions, depending on the policies of the institution. The wound is managed as prescribed. Antibiotic solution administered directly into the wound is most efficiently accomplished with a regular intravenous infusion setup that is prepared and regulated as any other. The drainage tubes are connected to low Gomco or wall suction for continuous removal. Intake and output are measured and recorded, and the character of the wound drainage is noted. The amount and character of drainage on the wound dressing are also noted.

Casts are sometimes employed for immobilization, and, if so, routine cast care is carried out. The extremity is examined for sensation, circulation, and pain, and the area over the inflammation is usually left open for observation. The affected area, casted or uncasted, is assessed for color, swelling, heat, and tenderness.

The child usually has a poor appetite at first, and he may be subject to vomiting. Nourishment in the form of high-calorie liquids, such as fruit juices, gelatin, and juice bars, should be encouraged until the child begins to feel better. The appetite returns as the acute symptoms subside. During convalescence adequate nutrition must be maintained to aid healing and reconstitution of new bone.

As the child begins to feel better, he becomes interested in his surroundings and relationships. He wishes to move about in bed and is allowed to do so. However, weight bearing on the affected limb is not permitted until healing is well under way in order to avoid pathologic fractures. Diversional and constructive activities become important nursing interventions. The child is usually confined to bed for some time after the acute phase but may be allowed about the unit on a gurney or in a wheelchair when isolation and bed rest are no longer necessary.

As the infection subsides, physical therapy is instituted to ensure restoration of optimum function. The child is usually discharged with oral antibiotics, and his progress is followed closely for some time.

SEPTIC (SUPPURATIVE, PYOGENIC, PURULENT) ARTHRITIS

Infection of the joints, like infection of bone, usually develops through hematogenous dissemination from another focus; occasionally it results from direct extension of a soft tissue infection. Joint infections occur predominantly in males, especially in the adolescent age-group. In infancy, however, the incidence in boys and girls is more nearly equal. Any joint may be involved, but the hip, knee, shoulder, and other large joints are more commonly affected. Usually only one joint is involved.

Clinical Manifestations of Septic Arthritis

History of a traumatic injury to the affected joint (often)
Fever
Involved joint is
- Warm and tender
- Erythematous
- Swollen
- Painful on even gentle pressure
- Superficial joints exquisitely painful
- Deep-seated joints show little superficial evidence

Diagnostic Evaluation

The signs and symptoms of suppurative arthritis, unlike those of osteomyelitis, are usually characteristic (see box). Leukocytosis and an increased erythrocyte sedimentation rate are present but may not be demonstrated in affected infants. The most common pathogens are *Staphylococcus aureus*, group A streptococci, and *Haemophilus influenzae*. Diagnosis is made from blood culture, joint fluid aspirate, and radiographs.

Therapeutic Management

Treatment consists of open surgical drainage of hip and shoulder joint disease and repeated needle aspirations of the joint space in other joints. The goals are (1) to clean the joint to avoid destruction of articular cartilage, (2) to decompress the joint to avoid interference with the blood supply to the epiphysis, (3) to eradicate the infection with adequate antibiotic therapy, and (4) to prevent secondary bone infection and hematogenous spread. Therapy is similar to that for osteomyelitis: intravenous antibiotic therapy, relief of pain, immobilization of the joint, and prohibition of weight bearing until healing is complete.

Nursing Considerations

Nursing care is the same as that for osteomyelitis.

TUBERCULOSIS

Tubercular infection of the bones is acquired by hematogenous dissemination from a primary tubercular focus. The most common sites in infants and small children are the carpals and phalanges and the corresponding bones of the feet. A single bone or several bones may be involved, with spindle-shaped swelling and tenderness as soft tissues are affected. The process, relatively painless, persists with intermittent symptoms for several months and may leave a permanent deformity. The affected areas are immobilized with a splint or cast.

Tuberculosis of Spine (Tuberculous Spondylitis)

In older children the infection attacks the body of one or more vertebrae, destroying the bone, and spreads to all the articular tissues, producing a kyphotic deformity. The lower thoracic spine is most frequently affected (see box for manifestations).

Treatment consists of immobilization until there is no evidence of active infection, followed by spinal fusion. Antimicrobial therapy and drainage of tubercular abscess are standard therapies. The reparative process is slow, but in most instances recovery takes place with little or no deformity.

Clinical Manifestations of Tuberculosis of the Bone

Spinal:
- Insidious onset
- Irritability
- Child complains of persistent or intermittent pain over areas innervated by spinal nerves that arise adjacent to affected vertebrae
- Muscle splinting and pain when there is increased pressure applied to head
- Child assumes position that best eases weight on diseased vertebrae, such as avoiding bending, walking stiffly and carefully on the toes, and resting on the abdomen or across a chair or a lap

Hip:
- Limp that occurs intermittently
- Limp occurs most often on arising in the morning or after exercise
- Pain
- Thigh gradually becomes fixed and adducted with internal rotation
- May be swelling around hip

Tuberculosis of Hip

The hip is the most common joint affected by tuberculosis, but the process usually begins in the epiphysis of the femoral head and then erupts into the joint capsule. There is progressive destruction of the femoral head with accompanying symptoms (see box). There may be abscess formation.

Treatment involves bed rest, traction to reduce muscle spasm, and appropriate drug therapy. Hip fusion may be necessary in severe cases.

◆*Bone Tumors*

Malignant bone tumors represent less than 1% of all malignant neoplasms but are more common in children than adults. The peak ages during childhood are 15 to 19 years. The sexes are affected equally until puberty, at which time the ratio approaches 2:1 in favor of males. This propensity for males, with a peak incidence during adolescence, is thought to be related to the accelerated growth rate of osseous tissue.

GENERAL CONCEPTS

Neoplastic disease can arise from any tissues involved in bone growth. In children the two types that account for 85% of all primary malignant bone tumors are osteogenic sarcoma (osteosarcoma) and Ewing sarcoma. They have several characteristics in common, which are discussed, and then specific information about each tumor is detailed.

Diagnostic Evaluation

A primary objective in diagnosis of bone neoplasm is to rule out causes such as trauma or infection. A history and careful questioning regarding pain help determine the duration and rate of tumor growth (see box). Physical assessment focuses on functional status of the affected area, signs of inflammation, size of the mass, involvement of regional lymph nodes, and any systemic indication of generalized malignancy.

Definitive diagnosis is based on radiologic studies (particularly computerized tomography), radioisotope bone scans, and/or surgical bone biopsy. Radiologic findings are characteristic for each type of tumor: a "sunburst" appearance produced by needlelike bone projections in osteogenic sarcoma; an "onionskin" appearance caused by layers of new bone in Ewing sarcoma. In both types of bone tumors, soft tissue infiltration may be apparent.

At present there is no reliable biochemical test for bone cancers, although elevated alkaline phosphatase levels may occur in osteoid tumors. Several tests may be performed to rule out metastatic disease from other neoplasms; lung tomography is especially important, since pulmonary metastasis is the most common complication of primary bone tumors. Bone marrow aspiration is helpful in diagnosing Ewing sarcoma.

Prognosis

With surgery for osteosarcoma or intensive radiotherapy for Ewing sarcoma combined with chemotherapy, survival statistics are improving for both types of bone cancer. Survival rates depend on the treatment and are influenced by other factors, such as the site of the primary tumor and the presence or absence of metastatic disease at diagnosis. However, approximately 50% of children with either type of bone cancer can expect long-term survival, and various cancer centers are reporting higher percentages (Ettinger, 1983).

Clinical Manifestations of Bone Tumors

- Pain localized at affected site
  - May be severe or dull
  - Often relieved by position of flexion
  - Frequently brought to attention when child
    - Limps
    - Curtails own physical activity
    - Is unable to hold heavy objects

OSTEOGENIC SARCOMA

Osteogenic sarcoma is the most frequently encountered malignant bone cancer in children, with a peak incidence between 10 and 25 years of age. Most primary tumor sites are in the metaphysis of long bones, especially in the lower extremities. More than half occur in the femur, particularly the distal portion, with the rest involving the humerus, tibia, pelvis, jaw, and phalanges.

Therapeutic Management

Optimum treatment of osteosarcoma is controversial. The traditional approach has consisted of radical surgical resection or amputation of the affected area, followed by intensive chemotherapy. Depending on the tumor site, surgery consists of amputation of the affected extremity at least 7.5 cm (3 inches) above the proximal tumor margin or above the joint proximal to the involved bone. With tumors of the distal femur, preservation of the hip joint may be possible. Other procedures include an above-the-knee amputation for tumors of the tibia or fibula, a hemipelvectomy for tumors of the innominate (hip) bone, and a forequarter amputation (removal of arm, scapula, and portion of the clavicle on the affected side) for tumors of the upper humerus. For selected patients, limb salvage procedures are performed; this involves primary tumor resection with prosthetic replacement of the involved bone.

Antineoplastic drugs are often administered singly or in combination and may be employed both before and after surgery. These combined-modality approaches have significantly improved the prognosis in osteosarcoma.

Nursing Considerations

Nursing care depends on the type of surgical approach, and in either instance, preparation of the child and family is critical. Obviously, the family may have more difficulty adjusting to an amputation than a limb salvage procedure. Straightforward honesty is essential to gain the cooperation and trust of the child. The diagnosis of cancer should not be disguised with falsehoods such as "infection." For the child to gradually accept the need for radical surgery, he must be aware of the lack of alternatives for treatment. While the task of informing the child is the responsibility of the physician, the nurse should be present for the discussion or be aware of exactly what is said to the child. The child should be told a few days before surgery, to allow him time to think about the diagnosis and consequent treatment and to ask questions.

Sometimes children have many questions about the prosthesis, limitations on physical ability, and prognosis in terms of cure. At other times they react with silence or with a calm manner that belies their concern and fear.

THERAPEUTIC DIALOGUE

Amputation

Nurse returns to the room of a 17-year-old adolescent with osteogenic sarcoma who has earlier learned that his leg will be amputated tomorrow.

NURSE: I thought that we might talk a bit about the doctor's visit earlier today and your surgery tomorrow.

ADOLESCENT (with anger in his voice): What is there to talk about? I am going to have my leg cut off and be a cripple.

NURSE: You feel angry because your leg will be amputated (nurse uses facilitative responding, see p. 110)

ADOLESCENT: Yes. How would you feel if you knew your leg had to come off?

NURSE: Probably angry, sad, and confused.

ADOLESCENT: Right.

NURSE: That's why I am here. Sometimes talking helps.

SUMMARY

At this time the adolescent was not ready to talk, but after the surgery he asked the nurse several questions about wearing a prosthesis.

Either response is part of the grieving process that accompanies a loss and must be accepted. Children should not be overwhelmed with information. A sound approach is to answer their questions without offering additional information and to show a willingness to talk, with such expressions as, "Anytime you would like to talk or ask questions about the surgery, tell me." The nurse should not push the topic unless the child initiates the discussion. Silence does not always mean nonacceptance. (See Therapeutic dialogue, above).

The child is also informed of the need for chemotherapy. Although it is best to introduce this subject before surgery, since treatment begins as soon as possible postoperatively, caution must be exercised in offering too much information at one time. It is wise to discuss hair loss with emphasis on positive aspects, such as wearing a wig. Since bone tumors affect adolescents and young adults, it is not unusual for them to become angry over all the radical body alterations.

If an amputation is performed, the child is usually fitted with a temporary prosthesis immediately after surgery, which permits early functioning and fosters psychologic adjustment. If this is not done, the child requires stump care, which is the same as for any amputee. A permanent prosthesis is usually fitted within 6 to 8 weeks. During hospitalization the child begins physical therapy to become proficient in the use and care of the device.

Discharge planning must begin early during the postoperative period. Every effort is made to promote normality and gradual resumption of realistic preamputation activities.* Role playing in anticipation of such experiences is very beneficial in preparing the child for the inevitable confrontation by others. Environmental barriers, such as stairs, are assessed in terms of the accessibility of the school and/or home, especially since the child may need to use crutches or a wheelchair before complete healing and prosthetic competency are achieved.

The family and child need a great deal of support in adjusting not only to a life-threatening diagnosis but also to alteration in body form and function. Since loss of a limb requires a grieving process, those caring for the child need to recognize that anger and depression are normal, necessary reactions. Often parents view the anger as a direct affront to them for allowing the amputation, or they view the depression as rejection. These are not personal attacks but the child's attempts to cope with his loss.

EWING SARCOMA

Ewing sarcoma arises in the marrow spaces of the bone rather than from osseous tissue. The principal sites of origin are shafts of long bones (femur, tibia, fibula, humerus, ulna), trunk bones (vertebra, scapula, ribs, pelvis), and skull. The disease occurs almost exclusively in individuals under age 30, with the majority between 4 and 25 years of age.

*Information about special programs for children with amputations such as "Sunshine Skiers," is available from the **Candlelighters Childhood Cancer Foundation**, 1901 Pennsylvania Ave. N.W., Suite 1001, Washington, DC 20006; information about prostheses can be obtained from **National Amputation Foundation, Inc.**, 12-45 150th St., Whitestone, NY 11357; especially recommended is "Sports and Recreation for those with Lower Limb Amputation or Impairment," a copy of which can be obtained free by writing to Dorothy Lester, Publications Dept., Office of Technology Transfer, 5th Floor, Room 20, 103 S. Gay St., Baltimore, MD 21202.

In Canada, **Canadian Amputee Sports Association,** 333 River Road, Vanier, Ontario K1L 8H9; the **Canadian Amputees Foundation,** 2827 Riverside Drive, Ottawa, Ontario K1V 0C4.

Therapeutic Management

Surgical amputation is not routinely recommended but may be considered when the results of radiotherapy render the extremity useless or deformed (such as from retarded growth in young children) or the tumor appears resectable. The treatment of choice is intensive irradiation of the involved bone combined with chemotherapy. A widely used drug regimen includes a group often referred to as VACA: vincristine, actinomycin D, cyclophosphamide, and adriamycin.

Nursing Considerations

The psychologic adjustment to Ewing sarcoma is typically less traumatic than to osteogenic sarcoma because of the preservation of the affected limb. Many families accept the diagnosis with a sense of relief in knowing that this type of bone cancer does not necessitate amputation, and initially they may not be aware of the deleterious effects on the irradiated site. Consequently, they need preparation for the various diagnostic tests, including bone marrow aspiration and surgical biopsy, and adequate explanation of the treatment regimen.

High-dose radiotherapy often causes a skin reaction of dry or moist desquamation followed by hyperpigmentation. The nurse advises the child to wear loose-fitting clothes over the irradiated area to minimize additional skin irritation. Because of increased sensitivity, the area is protected from sunlight and sudden changes in temperature, such as from heating pads or ice packs. The child is encouraged to use the extremity as tolerated. Occasionally an active exercise program may be planned by the physical therapist to preserve maximum function.

The child needs the same considerations as any other patient with cancer in adjusting to the effects of chemotherapy, such as hair loss, severe nausea and vomiting, peripheral neuropathy, and possibly cardiotoxicity. Every effort should be made to outline a treatment plan that allows the child maximum resumption of a normal lifestyle and activities.

◆ *Disorders of Joints*

Many disorders involving the joints have been discussed in relation to other problems of locomotion, such as sprains, dislocations, congenital hip dysplasia, and septic arthritis. This segment is primarily concerned with the inflammatory joint disease, juvenile rheumatoid arthritis, and one of the diseases with joint pain as a manifestation, lupus erythematosus.

JUVENILE RHEUMATOID ARTHRITIS

Clinically and pathologically, juvenile arthritis (JA), or juvenile rheumatoid arthritis (JRA), is an inflammatory disease with an unknown inciting agent. There are two peak ages of onset: between 2 and 5 years of age and between 9 and 12 years of age. Females are affected somewhat more frequently than males. In many instances the disease remains undiagnosed for years.

> *Clinical Manifestations of Juvenile Arthritis*
>
> **Involved joints:**
> - Stiffness
> - Swelling
> - Tenderness
> - Painful to touch or relatively painless
> - Warm to touch (seldom red)
> - Loss of motion
> - Characteristic morning stiffness or "gelling" on arising in the morning or after inactivity

Pathophysiology

The rheumatic process is characterized by a chronic inflammation of the synovium with joint effusion and eventual erosion, destruction, and fibrosis of the articular cartilage. Adhesions between joint surfaces and ankylosis of joints occur if the process persists long enough.

Whether a single joint or multiple joints are involved, the general manifestations (see box) result from edema, joint effusion, and synovial thickening. The limited motion, early in the disease, is the result of muscle spasm and joint inflammation; later it is caused by ankylosis or soft tissue contracture. Infections, injuries, or operations often precipitate a flare-up of the arthritis; therefore prompt recognition and treatment of infections are necessary.

Growth may be retarded during periods of active disease, usually with growth spurts during remissions. In severe long-standing cases growth is significantly retarded. Corticosteroid therapy can be a contributing factor.

JA is a variable disease and is now recognized to pursue three major disease courses: *systemic onset*, *monoarticular* or *pauciarticular* (involving few joints, usually less than five), and *polyarticular* (simultaneous involvement of four or more joints). These groups, including subgroups, and the manifestations associated with each are outlined in Table 30-2.

Diagnostic Evaluation

There are no specific diagnostic tests for JA. The erythrocyte sedimentation rate may or may not be elevated, depending on the degree of inflammation present. Leukocytosis is generally present in the early stages of classic systemic disease. The latex fixation test, the most common test used to detect the presence of rheumatoid factor in adults, is negative in 90% of juvenile cases. Rheumatoid factors are found in some children, usually those with disease of later onset. Antinuclear antibodies are

TABLE 30-2

Characteristics of Juvenile Arthritis Related to Mode of Onset

	Systemic Onset	Pauciarticular	Polyarticular
Percentage of patients	30%	45%	25%
Age at onset	Bimodal distribution 1-3 years of age 8-10 years of age	Type I: less than 10 years Type II: over 10 years	Throughout childhood and adolescence
Sex ratio (F:M)	1.5:1	Type I: almost all F Type II: 1:9	Mostly female
Joints involved	Any Only 20% have joint involvement at time of diagnosis	Usually confined to lower extremities—knee, ankle, and eventually sacroiliac; sometimes elbow	Any joints: usually symmetric involvement of small joints Hip involvement in 50% Spine involved in 50%
Extraarticular manifestations	Fever, malaise, myalgia, rash, pleuritis or pericarditis, adenomegaly, splenomegaly, hepatomegaly	Type I: chronic iridocyclitis; mucocutaneous lesions Type II: acute iridocyclitis; sacroiliitis common; eventual ankylosing spondylitis in many Type III: arthritis only	Systemic signs minimal Possible low-grade fever, malaise, weight loss, rheumatoid nodules, and/or vasculitis

found in three fourths of rheumatoid factor–positive and one fourth of rheumatoid factor–negative children and in pauciarticular type I diseases, but not in children with systemic onset or pauciarticular type II disease.

Radiographic findings are variable, but the earliest manifestations are widening joint spaces followed by gradual evidence of fusion and articular destruction.

Therapeutic Management

There is no specific cure for juvenile rheumatoid arthritis. The major goals of therapy are to preserve joint function, prevent physical deformities, and relieve symptoms without therapeutic harm. Whenever possible the child is treated at home under the supervision of the health team, and intermittent treatment by qualified professionals is administered. Hospitalization may be needed during severe exacerbations or when intercurrent illness warrants. Iridocyclitis, a common complication of JA, requires the attention of an ophthalmologist.

Drugs. Several drugs, given alone or in combination, are effective in suppressing the inflammatory process and relieving pain:

Nonsteroidal antiinflammatory drugs(NSAIDS)—(e.g., aspirin, tolmetin sodium, ibuprofen, and naproxen) daily dose usually divided into four doses

Slower-acting antirheumatic drugs(SAARDS)—(gold, D-penicillamine, and hydroxychloroquine) may be added to the regimen when one or two NSAIDs have been ineffective

Cytotoxic drugs—(e.g., cyclophosphamide, azathioprine, chlorambucil, and methotrexate) reserved for patients with severe debilitating disease and those who have responded poorly to NSAIDs and SAARDs

Corticosteroids—the most potent antiinflammatory agents available; used for life-threatening disease, incapacitating systemic disease (unresponsive to other antiinflammatory therapy), and iridocyclitis; administered in the lowest effective dose, on alternate days (rather than daily), and for the shortest period possible; undesirable chronic side effects

Physical management. Programs of physical management are individualized for each child and designed to reach the ultimate goal—preserving function and/or preventing deformity. Physical therapy is directed toward specific joints, focusing on strengthening muscles, mobilizing restricted joint motion, and preventing or correcting deformities. Occupational therapy assumes responsibility for generalized mobility and performance of activities of daily living.

General treatment or maintenance programs varies; physiotherapists may be involved several times weekly to monthly in management of a home program, or their visits may be limited to infrequent review of the home program for compliance, effectiveness, and need. Normal activities of daily living and the child's natural tendency to be active are usually sufficient to maintain muscle strength and joint mobility.

Exercising in a pool is excellent therapy, since it allows freedom of movement with support and minimum gravitational pull. When joints are inflamed, heavy resistance aggravates the pain; at such times simple isometric or tensing exercises that do not involve joint movement are generally tolerated and should be encouraged. Range of motion exercises are an important aspect of therapy and are continued after evidence of disease has disappeared in order to detect any signs of recurrence.

Most physicians recommend splinting and positioning during rest to help minimize pain and prevent or reduce flexion deformity. Joints most frequently splinted are the knees, wrists, and hands. Positioning during rest is also important. The child rests on a firm mattress with no pillow or a very low one and has no support under the knee.

Nursing Diagnoses: The Child with Juvenile Arthritis

Chronic pain related to joint inflammation
Impaired physical mobility related to joint discomfort and stiffness
Bathing/hygiene, dressing/grooming, feeding, or toileting self-care deficit related to impaired joint mobility
Altered family processes related to a situational crisis (child with a chronic illness)

Loss of extension in the knee, hip, and wrist causes special problems and requires vigilance to detect the earliest signs of involvement and vigorous attention to prevent deformity with specialized passive stretching, positioning, and resting splints.

Nursing Considerations

The child with JA presents a challenge to himself, his family, and the professionals who help them both cope with this prototype of chronic illness.

ASSESSMENT

Nursing the child with JRA involves assessment of the child's general health, the status of involved joints, and the child's emotional response to all ramifications of the disease—discomfort, physical restrictions, therapies, and self-concept.

NURSING DIAGNOSES

Nursing diagnoses and management identified for the child with JA are outlined in the accompanying box. Others will be apparent in individual cases.

PLANNING

The goals of nursing care for the child with JA and his family are:

1. Promote general health
2. Relieve discomfort
3. Prevent physical deformity and preserve joint function
4. Promote self-care
5. Support child and family

IMPLEMENTATION

The effects of this chronic illness are felt in every aspect of the child's life—in physical activities, social experiences, and personality development. Much of the child's adjustment to the stresses and demands of the disease and the level of functioning he achieves are directly related to the reaction and support he receives from his family and the health professionals concerned with his care and management.

The general health of the child must be considered, and it is frequently overlooked as parents and health personnel concentrate on the disease. A well-balanced diet and assessment of nutritional status are integral parts of health supervision. Excessive fatigue and overexertion should be avoided with regular periods of rest, especially during acute flare-ups of arthritis. The child is susceptible to frequent upper respiratory infection, which should receive prompt treatment.

Heat has proved beneficial to children with arthritis. Moist heat is best for relieving pain and stiffness, and the most efficient and practical method for accomplishing this is to place the child in the bathtub. A daily whirlpool bath, paraffin bath, or hot packs may be used as needed for temporary relief of acute swelling and pain. Painful hands or feet can be immersed in a pan of water for 10 minutes two or three times daily in addition to tub baths.

Pool therapy is the easiest method for exercising a large number of joints. Swimming activities strengthen muscles and maintain mobility in larger joints. Most children have access to a therapy pool, although transportation may be a problem for some families. Very small children who are frightened of the water can carry out their exercises in the bathtub.

Posture and body mechanics are important for the child with JA, both when he is at rest and when he is active. He must have a firm mattress to maintain good alignment of spine, hips, and knees and no pillow or a very thin one. The child who is confined to bed either at home or in the hospital may require sandbags, splints, or other types of support to maintain positioning. Lying in the prone position is encouraged to straighten hips and knees; the child can do this, for example, during rest periods or while watching television.

Activities of daily living provide satisfactory exercise for older children to maintain maximum mobility with minimum pain. These children should be encouraged in their efforts and patiently allowed to dress and groom themselves, to assume daily tasks, and to care for their belongings. It is often difficult for stiff fingers to manipulate buttons, comb or brush hair, and turn faucets, but parents and other caregivers should not offer assistance. Also, the child should learn and understand why others do not help him. Many helpful devices, such as Velcro fasteners, tongs for manipulating difficult items, and grab bars installed in bathrooms for safety, can be used to facilitate tasks. A raised toilet seat often makes the difference between dependent and independent toileting, since weak quadriceps muscles and sore knees inhibit the ability to raise the body from a low sitting position.

The child's natural affinity for play offers many opportunities for incorporating therapeutic exercises. Throwing or kicking a ball, hanging from monkey bars, and riding a tricycle (with the seat raised to achieve maximum leg extension) are excellent moving and stretching exercises for preschool children. These are especially important for the very young child whose activities of daily living are physically limited. Parents are instructed in exercises that are designed to fit the needs of the individual child.

The parents are instructed regarding the purpose and correct use of any splints or appliances and the administration of medications, including the value of a regular schedule of administration to maintain a satisfactory drug level in the body. They need to know that aspirin should not be given on an empty stomach, and they must be alert for signs of aspirin toxicity, which include hyperventilation as a sign of acidosis, bleeding from decreased clotting capacity, tinnitus (ringing in the ears) as a sign of cranial nerve VIII involvement, and undue drowsiness that may indicate central nervous system depression.

The **Arthritis Foundation*** and the **Juvenile Arthritis Foundation*** provide services for both parents and professionals, and nurses should refer families to these agencies as an added resource.

Child and family support. Rheumatoid arthritis affects every aspect of the child's daily life. The physical pain and limitations interfere with performance of normal tasks and provision of self-care. There may be school difficulties related to transportation to and from school, stairs, and loss of time as a result of exacerbations and hospitalization. However, school-age children are allowed to attend school, even on days when there may be some pain or discomfort. The aid of the school nurse is enlisted to provide a means for taking prescribed medication and to arrange for rest during the day.

Physical limitations interfere with participation in many activities, both curricular and extracurricular, which limits peer contacts and interaction and increases social isolation. Changes in personality usually accompany juvenile rheumatoid arthritis, as they do in any child with a chronic illness. They may be temporary, such as demanding, irritable behavior, or they may be manifest in more permanent ways, such as passive hostility, uncommunicativeness, and manipulativeness. Efforts should be made to break through the child's defenses and to identify his anxieties, concerns, and conflicts in order to intervene early to prevent the development of permanent personality problems.

Most of the reactions, problems, and concerns of families of a child with JA are those of any family of a chronically ill and/or disabled child. The problems and needs of these families are discussed in Chapter 18, and the reader is directed to this chapter for guidance in planning care.

EVALUATION

The effectiveness of nursing interventions is determined by continual reassessment and evaluation of care based on the following observational guidelines and expected outcomes:

1. Conduct routine assessment of child's general health.
2. Observe child's behavior and employ pain assessment techniques.
3. Observe the child during planned and unplanned activities, assess mobility of joints, and observe the use of prescribed appliances.
4. Observe child's ability to perform activities of daily living.
5. Observe and interview child and family regarding feelings and concerns.

Expected outcomes:

1. Child attains and maintains optimum health status (specify).
2. Child is able to move with minimum or no discomfort.
3. Child engages in activities suitable to his interests, capabilities, and developmental level; joints are mobile, flexible, and free of deformity.
4. Child is involved in self-care activities to his maximum capabilities.
5. Child and family demonstrate an understanding of the child's disease and therapies; they verbalize their feelings and concerns.

*1314 Spring Street, N.W. Atlanta, GA 30309.
In Canada, the **Arthritis Society,** 250 Bloor St. East, Suite 401, Toronto, Ontario M4W 2P2.

SYSTEMIC LUPUS ERYTHEMATOSUS

Systemic lupus erythematosus (SLE), or lupus erythematosus (LE), is a chronic inflammatory disease of the collagen or supporting tissues of the body. It characteristically follows an unpredictable course of remissions and exacerbations. Because connective tissue is found practically everywhere, almost any organ or structure can be affected.

SLE in childhood consists of two basic types: a transient neonatal disease apparently related to maternal pathology and a group of chronic diseases usually having their onset after infancy that correspond to the diseases seen in adults. The major portion of the discussion will be limited to SLE in childhood.

The cause of SLE is not known, although it is believed

Criteria for Diagnosis of Systemic Lupus Erythematosus

1. Butterfly rash
2. Discoid rash
3. Photosensitivity
4. Oral ulcers
5. Arthritis
6. Serositis
7. Renal disorder
8. Neurologic disorder(s) (psychosis, coma, seizures, paresis)
9. Hematologic disorder(s) (anemia, thrombocytopenia, leukopenia)
10. Immunologic disorder(s) (anti-DNA, LE prep, anti-SM, STS)
11. Antinuclear antibody

that some inciting event, such as stress, infection, extreme fatigue, or exposure to various chemicals, drugs, or excessive sunburn triggers a reaction that alters the body's immune response to its own tissues. The disease shows a tendency to occur within families.

Diagnostic Evaluation

Because SLE can affect almost any tissue, the clinical manifestations are variable and the diagnosis is established by the demonstration of any four of 11 diagnostic criteria (see box). However, rapid involvement of vital organs, primarily the kidneys, can herald an accelerated course with minimum or absent involvement of other sites.

Therapeutic Management

The objectives of medical treatment are (1) to reverse the autoimmune and inflammatory processes and (2) to prevent exacerbations and complications. Therapy involves the use of specific and supportive medications and regulation of activity and diet. The principal drugs used to control inflammation are the corticosteroids administered in doses sufficient to suppress symptoms, then tapered to the lowest suppressive dose. Other drugs include the immunosuppressive agent azathioprine (Imuran); antimalarial preparations, which are useful against dermatologic, arthritic, and renal symptoms of the disease; and nonsteroidal antiinflammatory agents which relieve muscle and joint pains and reduce tissue inflammation. Drugs used to control various complications include anticonvulsants, antihypertensives, and antibiotics.

The goal of restricted activity is to prevent a recurrence of the disease. An effective schedule must provide for gradual resumption of pre–lupus erythematosus activity and maximum rest periods, usually 8 to 10 hours of sleep a night and one or two rest times during the day. The most frequently prescribed diet modification, if needed, is moderate or low salt. Low-protein diets may be necessary to prevent elevated nitrogen levels. Weight reduction, if indicated, may help preserve maximum joint function and conserve energy.

Nursing Considerations

The principal nursing goal is to help the child and family adjust to the limitations and treatments of the disease and to prevent exacerbations and complications. Since older female adolescents are the most likely group to be affected, the nurse must be aware of their special needs, such as body image changes, present and future vocational activities, and social relationships. See the principles of adjusting to a chronic illness in Chapter 18.

Family members need an understanding of the disease process to gain an appreciation of the need for regular, uninterrupted drug administration, moderate activity, and any diet modifications that may be imposed. Usually diagnostic tests are performed during hospitalization, which allows the nurse an opportunity to help the child and parents learn about the disease. Several organizations have been formed to help children and families learn about and adjust to the disease. The groups include the **National Lupus Erythematosus Foundation,*** the **Lupus Foundation of America,†** and **Leanon (Lupus Erythematosus Anonymous).‡**

In teaching the child with SLE and his family, the nurse stresses the importance of adequate rest and the need to adhere to the medication schedule. Individuals who are sensitive to the sun must avoid exposure. It is important to emphasize that sun filtered through clouds or reflected from snow, water, or white surfaces (such as cement) can cause a severe reaction. Although clothes can protect most areas of the body, special sunscreening agents are needed on exposed areas such as the face (see p. 1009). A large-brimmed hat helps in partially shading the face.

Affected persons are advised to maintain regular medical supervision and to seek additional attention during periods of stress, illness, or prior to elective surgical procedures, such as dental extraction, because the body may require larger amounts of a drug. People with SLE should carry an identification card or Medic Alert tag emphasizing their dependence on steroids.

SUMMARY

Disorders involving bones and joints profoundly interfere with the natural mobility of children. Consequently, the bulk of nursing problems associated with these disorders is related to the enforced immobility necessitated by therapy. Not only does the therapy involve limited mobility, the length of recovery extends beyond the convalescent period required of most acute disorders. The child's propensity for movement can assist in prevention of some ill effects of immobilization, but it also can complicate some types of therapy. Fortunately a child's infinite optimism, creative capacity, and need for play are the nurses' allies in planning care for children with these challenging nursing problems.

*5430 Van Nuys Ave., Van Nuys, CA 91401.
†11673 Holly Springs Dr., St. Louis, MO 63141.
‡P.O. Box 10243, Corpus Christi, TX 78410.
In Canada, **Lupus Canada,** Box 3302, Station B, Calgary, Alberta T2M 4L8.

KEY CONCEPTS

- Immobility has a profound effect on all aspects of growth and development.
- The major physical consequences of immobilization are loss of muscle strength, endurance, and muscle mass; bone demineralization; loss of joint mobility; and contractures.
- Features of children's fractures not observed in the adult include presence of growth plate, thicker and stronger periosteum, bone porosity, more rapid healing, and less joint stiffness.
- The goals of fracture management are to regain alignment and length of bony fragments, retain alignment and length, and restore function to injured parts.
- The method of fracture reduction is determined by the age of the child, degree of displacement, amount of overriding, amount of edema, condition of skin and soft tissues, sensation, and circulation distal to fracture.
- The primary purposes of traction are to fatigue involved muscles and reduce muscle spasm, position bone ends in desired realignment, and immobilize fracture site until realignment has been achieved to permit casting or splinting.
- Therapeutic management of spinal cord injury is directed toward preventing further neuronal damage, avoiding complications, and maintaining vital functions.
- The development of congenital hip dysplasia appears to be related to intrauterine, genetic, and cultural factors.
- Treatment of clubfoot consists of manipulation and casting to correct the deformity, maintaining the correction, and preventing possible recurrence of the deformity.
- Acquired hip deformities are managed with non–weight-bearing devices (coxa plana) or surgical stabilization (coxa vara).
- Observation for scoliosis is an important part of a routine physical assessment.
- Scoliosis is managed by bracing and exercise, electric stimulation, or surgical correction.
- Bone infections are managed with vigorous antibiotic therapy, immobilization of the affected part, and (sometimes) surgical drainage.
- Osteosarcoma is a neoplasm of bone-forming tissues; Ewing sarcoma is a neoplasm that arises from bone marrow spaces.
- Nursing care of the child with juvenile arthritis consists of promoting general health, relieving discomfort, preventing deformity, and preserving function.
- Lupus erythematosus is a chronic autoimmune disorder that affects the collagen tissues of the body.

STUDY QUESTIONS AND ACTIVITIES

1 Visit a facility where immobilization is a part of therapy. Observe the activities in which children are engaged. Interview one or two children regarding their activities and their attitude toward their immobilization.
2 Visit a "cast room" where casts are applied to broken bones. Investigate the various types of casting materials. Observe and, if possible, arrange to assist with the application of a cast.
3 Visit an orthopedic clinic in which infants with lower extremity or body casts are being treated. Interview a parent or several parents regarding modifications they have implemented to meet the challenge of a child in a cast—for example, hygienic measures, diapering, feeding, or transporting the child.
4 Visit a scoliosis screening clinic and observe the assessment tools and techniques used.
5 Interview a child being treated for scoliosis regarding the therapy and how it has affected his or her day-to-day activities.
6 Devise a schedule of activities for a school-age child with juvenile arthritis.

REFERENCES

Ettinger, L.J.: Osteosarcoma, Pediatr. Ann. **12:**374-382, 1983.

Feller, N., and others: A multidisciplinary approach to developing safe transportation for children with special needs, Orthop. Nurs. **5**(5):25-27, 1986.

Holland, S.H.: Up-to-date home care of a baby in a hip spica cast, Pediatr. Nurs. **9:**114-115, 1983.

Root, L.: The treatment of osteogenesis imperfecta, Orthop. Clin. North Am. **15:**775-790, 1984.

Shesser, L.K.: Car seat modification for children under treatment for congenital dislocated hip, Orthop. Nurs. **4**(6):11-13, 1985.

Staheli, L.T.: The hip. In Gellis, S.S., and Kagan, B.M.: Current pediatric therapy 12, Philadelphia, 1986, W.B. Saunders Co.

Whaley, L.F., and Wong, D.L.: Nursing care of infants and children, ed. 3, St. Louis, 1987, The C.V. Mosby Co.

Wong, D., and Baker, C.: Pain in children: comparison of assessment scales, Pediatr. Nurs. **14**(1):9-17, 1988.

BIBLIOGRAPHY

General

Asher, R.A.J.: The dangers of going to bed, Crit. Care Update **6**(9):4-49, 1983.

Baird, S.E.: Development of a nursing assessment tool to diagnose altered body image in immobilized patients, Orthop. Nurs. **4**(1):47-54, 1985.

Campbell, P.M.: Transportation of the critically ill and injured child, Crit. Care Q. **8**(1):1-12, 1985.

Diamond, L.: Triaging pediatric emergencies, Crit. Care Update **7**(2):28-32, 1980.

Karn, M.A., and Ragiel, C.A.: The psychologic effects of immobilization on the pediatric orthopaedic patient, Orthop. Nurs. **5**(6):12-16, 1987.

Kilcoyne, R.F., and Plumly, T.F.: Infections of bones and joints, Nurse Pract. **8**(3):12, 63, 66, 1983.

Lentz, M.: Selected aspects of deconditioning secondary to immobilization, Nurs. Clin. North Am. **16:**729-737, 1981.

Lyon, S.H.: Critical care of the child with multi-trauma, Nurs. Clin. North Am. **16:**657-670, 1981.

Miller, R.A., and Evans, W.E.: Immediate postop prosthesis, Am. J. Nurs. **87:**310-311, 1987.

Pashley, J., and Wahlstrom, M.L.: Polytrauma: the patient, the family, the nurse, and the health team, Nurs. Clin. North Am. **16:**721-727, 1981.

Ragiel, C.A.: The impact of critical injury on patient, family, and clinical systems, Crit. Care Q. **7**(3):73-78, 1984.

Sigmon, H.D.: Helping your long-term trauma patient travel the road to recovery, Nursing 84 **14**(1):58-63, 1984.

Thomas, D.O.: The ABCs of pediatric emergencies, RN **47**(3):34-41, 1984.

Fractures

Bailey, M.: Emergency! First aid for fractures, Nursing 82 **12**(11):72-79, 1982.

Benz, J.: The adolescent in a spica cast, Orthop. Nurs. **5**(3):22-23, 1986.

Cassels, C.J.: Fundamentals of long bone traction. Part I, Crit. Care Update **10**(3):36-39, 1983.

Cassels, C.J.: Fundamentals of long bone traction. Part II, Crit. Care Update **10**(4):26-31, 1983.

Cassels, C.J.: Fundamentals of long bone traction. Part III, Crit. Care Update **10**(5):38-39, 1983.

Cochran, S.: Action stat! Open fracture, Nursing 87 **17**(5):33, 1987.

Cuddy, C.M.: Caring for the child in a spica cast: a parent's perspective, Orthop. Nurs. **5**(3):17-21, 1986.

Evers, J.A., and Werpachowski, D.: Dealing with fractures, RN **47**(11):53-57, 1984.

Howard, M., and Corbo-Pelaia, S.A.: Psychological aftereffects of halo traction . . . a review of acute care, Am. J. Nurs. **82:**1839-1843, 1982.

Ibrahim, K.: An overview of childhood fractures, Pediatr. Nurs. **10:**57-65, 1984.

Kryschyshen, P.L., and Fischer, D.A.: External fixation for complicated fractures, Am. J. Nurs. **80:**156-159, 1980.

Lane, P.L, and Lee, M.M.: New synthetic casts: what nurses need to know, Orthop. Nurs. **1**(6):13-20, 1982.

Lane, P.L., and Lee, M.M.: Special care for special casts, Nursing 83 **13**(7):50, 1983.

Lane, P.L., and Lee, M.M.: Synthetic materials have changed casts and cast care, Nursing 83 **13**(7):50-51, 1983.

Mather, M.L.S.: The secret to life in a cast, Am. J. Nurs. **87:**56-58, 1987.

Richards, H.: A child with a fractured femur, Nurs. Time **78:**59-62, 1982.

Robinson, J.E., and Marx, L.O.: A nail-safe method, Am. J. Nurs. **85:**158-161, 1985.

Stout, J.A., and Gibbs, K.R.: The child undergoing a leg-lengthening procedure, Am. J. Nurs. **81:**1152-1155, 1981.

Swanson, V.M.: The school-age traction patient: toward better behavior patterns, J. Assoc. Care Child. Hosp. **9**(1):12-14, 1980.

Wassel, A.: Nursing assessment of injuries to the lower extremity, Nurs. Clin. North Am. **16:**739-748, 1981.

Wise, L.B.: A comparison of orthopedic casts: breaking the mold, MCN **11:**174-176, 1986.

Spinal Cord Injuries

Agee, B.L., and Herman, C.: Cervical logrolling on a standard hospital bed, Am. J. Nurs. **84:**314-318, 1984.
Buchanan, L.E.: Emergency! First aid for spinal cord injury, Nursing 82 **12**(8):68-75, 1982.
D'Agnostino, J.: Nursing rehabilitation of the quadriplegic adolescent, J. Assoc. Care Child. Health **9**(3):87-91, 1981.
McConnaughey, L.J.: Spinal cord injury in children, Point View **21**(3):6-7, 1984.
Nurses' hotline helps the spinal cord-injured, Am. J. Nurs. **87:**720-721, 1987.

Congenital Defects

Coleman, S.S.: When a child is born with foot problems, Patient Care **17**(14):68-98, 1983.
Guerrein, A.T.: Osteogenesis imperfecta: a disorder that breaks more than our hearts, MCN **7:**315-318, 1982.
Linley, J.F.: Screening children for common orthopaedic problems, Am. J. Nurs. **87:**1312-1316, 1987.
McLaughlin, S.: Brittle bones or osteogenesis imperfecta, Can. Nurse **78**(2):23, 1983.
Shesser, L., and Kling, T.F.: Practical considerations in caring for a child in a hip spica cast: an evaluation using parental input, Orthop. Nurs. **5**(3):11-15, 1986.
Swagman, A.: Caring for limb-deficient children and their families, MCN **11:**46-52, 1986.
Varni, M.A., and Jaffe, M.: Osteogenesis imperfecta: the basics, Pediatr. Nurs. **10:**29-33, 1984.

Scoliosis

Allard, J.L., and Dibble, S.L.: Scoliosis surgery: a look at Luque rods, Am. J. Nurs. **84:**609-611, 1984.
Anderson, B.: The patient with scoliosis: Carole, a girl treated with bracing, Am. J. Nurs. **79:**1592-1597, 1979.
Brier, L., and Seligson, D.: Care of the patient in the halo, Crit. Care Update **9**(8):38-41, 1982.
Davis, S.E., and Lewis, S.A.: Managing scoliosis: fashions for the body and mind, MCN **9:**186-187, 1984.
Francis, E.E.: Lateral electrical surface stimulation treatment for scoliosis, Pediatr. Nurs. **13:**157-160, 1987.
Gratz, R.R., and Papalia-Finlay, D.: Psychosocial adaptation to wearing the Milwaukee brace for scoliosis; a pilot study of adolescent females and their mothers, J. Adolesc. Health Care **5:**237-242, 1984.
Jacobs-Zacney, J.M., and Horn, M.J.: Nursing care of adolescents having posterior spinal fusion with Cotrel-Dubousset instrumentation, Orthop. Nurs. **7**(1):17-21, 1988.
Morais, T., and others: Age- and sex-specific prevalence of scoliosis and the value of school screening programs, Am. J. Public Health **75:**1377-1380, 1985.
Rutechi, B., and Seligson, D.: Caring for the patient in a halo apparatus, Nursing 80 **10**(10):73-77, 1980.
Thomassen, P.F.: Helping your scoliosis patient walk tall, RN **47**(2):34-37, 1984.
Viviani, G.R., and others: Assessment of accuracy of the scoliosis school screening examination, Am. J. Public Health **74:**497-498, 1984.
Voznak, L.: My life with scoliosis, Orthop. Nurs. **7**(1):22-26, 1988.

Miscellaneous Skeletal Disorders

Benchot, R.J.: The adolescent with slipped capital femoral epiphysis, Point View **19:**6-9, 1982.
Hussey, C.G.: Surviving a handicap in everyday life: how to help, MCN **4:**46-50, 1979.
Malkiewicz,J.: A pragmatic approach to musculoskeletal assessment, RN **45**(11):57-62, 1982.

Bone Tumors

Boren, H.A., and Meell, H.: Adolescent amputee ski rehabilitation program, J. Assoc. Pediatr. Oncol. Nurses **2**(1):16-23, 1985.
Bourne, B.A., and Kutcher, J.L.: Amputation: helping a patient face loss of a limb, RN **48**(2):38-45, 1985.
Gandy, E.D., and Veigh, G.: Help the amputee stand on his own again, Nursing 84 **14**(7):46-49, 1984.
Jaffe, N., and others: Control of primary osteosarcoma with chemotherapy, Cancer **56**(3):461-466, 1985.
Kutcher, J., and Bourne, B.: Postop needs of the amputee, RN **48**(2):46-47, 1985.
Ritchie, J.A.: Nursing the child undergoing limb amputation, MCN **5:**114-120, 1980.
Walters, J.: Coping with a leg amputation, Am. J. Nurs. **81**(7):1349-1352, 1981.

Juvenile Rheumatoid Arthritis

Dickinson, G.B.: A home care program for patients with rheumatoid arthritis, Nurs. Clin. North Am. **15:**403-418, 1980.
Gorman, T.K., and Marsh, M.E.: Arthritis at an early age, Am. J. Nurs. **84:**1472-1477, 1984.
Hangen, M.S., and Lynch, P.A.: Diagnostic tests in pediatric rheumatology: application for nurses, Pediatr. Nurs. **13:**389-393, 1987.
Ignatavicius, D.D.: Meeting the psychosocial needs of patients with rheumatoid arthritis, Orthop. Nurs. **6**(3):16-20, 1987.
Rennebohm, R., and Correll, J.K.: Comprehensive management of juvenile rheumatoid arthritis, Nurs. Clin. North Am. **19:**647-662, 1984.

Systemic Lupus Erythematosus

Ascheim, J.H.: The adolescent and systemic lupus erythematosus: a developmental and educational approach, Issues Compr. Pediatr. Nurs. **5:**293-307, 1981.
Nass, T.: Helping the patient who has lupus, RN **50**(10):69-74, 1987.
White, J.F., and Ziegler, G.L.: Patient management of systemic lupus erythematosus, Crit. Care Update **7**(8):5-15, 1980.

CHAPTER 31

The Child with Neuromuscular Dysfunction

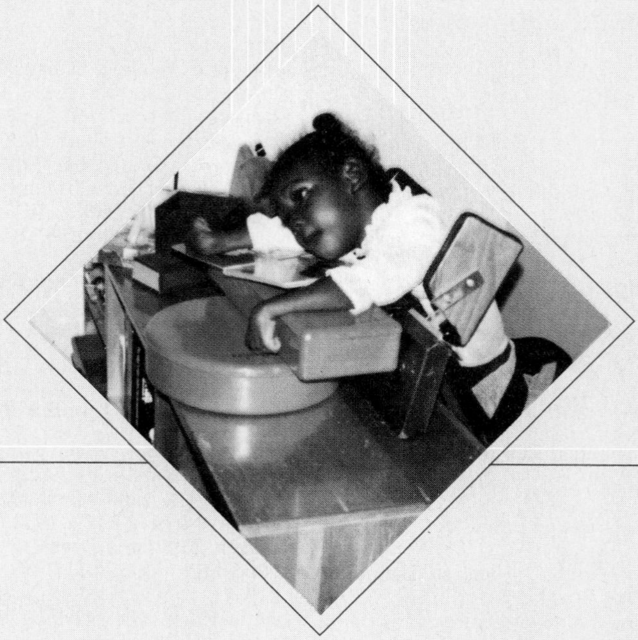

LEARNING OBJECTIVES

On completion of this chapter the reader will be able to:

- Discuss the nursing role in assisting the parents to cope with a child with cerebral palsy
- Formulate a nursing care plan for the preoperative and postoperative care of a child with myelomeningocele
- Discuss the prevention and treatment of tetanus
- Differentiate among the various types of muscular dystrophy
- Outline a plan of care for the child with Guillain-Barré syndrome

Weakness or abnormal muscle performance may result from (1) defects within the muscle itself, (2) defective transmission of nerve impulses to muscles, (3) dysfunction of peripheral motor or sensory nerves, or (4) damage to the central nervous system. Therefore, the identification of the source of muscle dysfunction includes not only the testing of muscle function but also the systematic elimination of possible disorders of neural structures on which muscle function depends for its stimulus. Neuromuscular disorders can be present at birth or acquired from exposure to toxins or infectious organisms.

◆ *Congenital Neuromuscular Disorders*

A number of conditions are observed at birth or during the early years of life. Such conditions include those that are the result of damage to the cerebral cortex (cerebral palsy) and diseases of the anterior horn cells (juvenile spinal muscular atrophy) or muscles (the muscular dystrophies).

CEREBRAL PALSY

Cerebral palsy (CP) is a nonspecific term that is applied to impaired neuromuscular control that results from a nonprogressive abnormality in the pyramidal motor system (motor cortex, basal ganglia, and cerebellum). The etiology, clinical features, and course are variable, and abnormal muscle tone and coordination are the primary disturbances. It is the most frequently occurring permanent physical disability of childhood, and, although the incidence is not known studies suggest that it varies from 1.5 to 5 per 1000 live births.

Various prenatal, perinatal, and postnatal factors contribute to the etiology of CP singly or in combination; these factors include developmental anomalies, infections, cerebral trauma, hypoxia, metabolic disturbances, and toxicoses. Cerebral anoxia, which has long been associated with cerebral damage, is an important cause during the prenatal and perinatal periods.

Pathophysiology

It is difficult to establish a precise location of neurologic lesions based on etiology or clinical signs because there is no characteristic pathologic picture. In some cases there are gross malformations of the brain; in others there may be evidence of vascular occlusion, atrophy, loss of neurons, and degeneration. Anoxia plays the most significant role in the pathology of brain damage, although trauma, neonatal diseases (such as hypoglycemia and kernicterus), trauma, cerebrovascular accident, and prematurity are important factors.

Cerebral palsy has been classified in several ways. The most useful classification is based on the nature and distribution of neuromuscular dysfunction (see box).

Diagnostic Evaluation

The neurologic examination and history are the primary modalities for diagnosis. A thorough knowledge of normal variations of motor development is required for detecting

Clinical Classification of Cerebral Palsy

- Spastic—may involve one side, both sides
  - Hypertonicity with poor control of posture, balance, and coordinated motion
  - Impairment of fine and gross motor skills
  - Active attempts at motion increase abnormal postures and overflow of movement to other parts of the body
- Dyskinetic—abnormal involuntary movement
  - Athetosis—characterized by slow, wormlike, writhing movements that usually involve all extremities, the trunk, neck, facial muscles, and tongue
  - Involvement of the pharyngeal, laryngeal, and oral muscles causes drooling and dysarthria (imperfect speech articulation)
  - Involuntary movements may take on choreoid (involuntary, irregular, jerking movements) and dystonic (disordered muscle tone) manifestations that increase in intensity under emotional stress and around adolescence
- Ataxic
  - Wide-based gait
  - Rapid repetitive movements performed poorly
  - Disintegration of movements of the upper extremities when the child reaches for objects
- Mixed-type—combination of spasticity and athetosis
- Rigid, tremor, and atonic—uncommon types
  - Deformities
  - Lack of active movement

Clinical Manifestations of Cerebral Palsy

- Delayed gross motor development
  - A universal manifestation
  - Delay in all motor accomplishments
  - Increases as growth advances
- Abnormal motor performance
  - Very early preferential unilateral hand use
  - Abnormal and asymmetric crawl
  - Standing or walking on toes
  - Uncoordinated or involuntary movements
  - Poor sucking
  - Feeding difficulties
  - Persistent tongue thrust
- Alterations of muscle tone
  - Increased or decreased resistance to passive movements
  - Opisthotonic postures (exaggerated arching of back)
  - Feels stiff on handling or dressing
  - Difficulty in diapering
  - Rigid and unbending at the hip and knee joints when pulled to sitting position (an early sign)
- Abnormal postures
  - Maintains hips higher than trunk in prone position with legs and arms flexed or drawn under the body
  - Scissoring and extension of legs and with the plantar flexed in supine position
  - Persistent infantile resting and sleeping posture
    - Arms abducted at shoulders
    - Elbows flexed
    - Hands fisted
- Reflex abnormalities
  - Persistence of primitive infantile reflexes
    - Obligatory tonic neck reflex at any age
    - Nonpersistence beyond 6 months of age
  - Persistence or hyperactivity of the Moro, plantar, and palmar grasp reflexes
  - Hyperreflexia, ankle clonus, and stretch reflexes elicited on many muscle groups on fast passive movements
- Associated disabilities (may or may not be present)
  - Subnormal learning and reasoning (mental retardation)
  - Seizures
  - Impaired behavioral and interpersonal relationships
  - Sensory impairment (vision, hearing)

abnormal progress, and a careful history is elicited to detect possible etiologic factors. The alert observer may be suspicious when a child demonstrates some of the manifestations outlined in the accompanying box. The child's spontaneous movements and behavior are observed, including posture, attitude, and muscle size, function, and tone. Persistence of primitive reflexes may be of value, and two offer assistance in diagnoses: the asymmetric tonic neck reflex and the crossed extensor reflex.

Supplemental diagnostic tests may be employed, such as electroencephalography, tomography, screening for metabolic defects, and serum electrolyte values. The possibility that the manifestations are those of slowly progressive degenerative disease or early onset, slowly growing brain tumors must be ruled out.

Therapeutic Management

The goals of therapy for children with cerebral palsy are early recognition and promotion of an optimum developmental course in order that the child may realize his potential within the limits of his brain dysfunction. The disorder is permanent, and therapy is chiefly directed toward treating symptoms and preventing complications.

The broad aims of therapy are (1) to establish locomotion, communication, and self-help; (2) to gain optimum appearance and integration of motor functions; (3) to correct associated defects as effectively as possible; and (4) to provide educational opportunities adapted to the individual child's needs and capabilities. Each child is evaluated and managed on an individual basis. The plan of therapy may involve a variety of settings, facilities, and specially trained persons, including the parents.

Braces are often used to help prevent or reduce deformity, increase the energy efficiency of gait, and control alignment. Other mobilizing devices include wheeled scooter boards that allow the child to propel himself while on his abdomen, wheeled go-carts that provide good sitting balance and serve as early "wheelchair" experience for young children (Fig. 31-1), and special devices that leave the upper extremities free (Fig. 31-2).

Orthopedic surgery may be required to decrease or abolish spastic muscle imbalance. Surgical intervention is usually reserved for the child who does not respond to the more conservative measures, but it is also indicated for the child whose spasticity causes progressive deformities. Surgery is primarily used to improve function and is followed by physical therapy. Surgery is not performed for cosmetic purposes.

Drugs that decrease spasticity have little usefulness in improving function in CP. Antianxiety agents have been used to some extent to relieve excessive motion and tension, particularly in the athetoid child. Skeletal muscle relaxants, such as dantrolene (Dantrium), baclofen, methocarbamol (Robaxin), and diazepam (Valium) may be used on a short-term basis for older children and adolescents. Local nerve block to motor points of a muscle with a neurolytic agent such as phenol solution reduces spasticity temporarily.

Anticonvulsant medications (especially phenobarbital and phenytoin) are prescribed routinely for children who

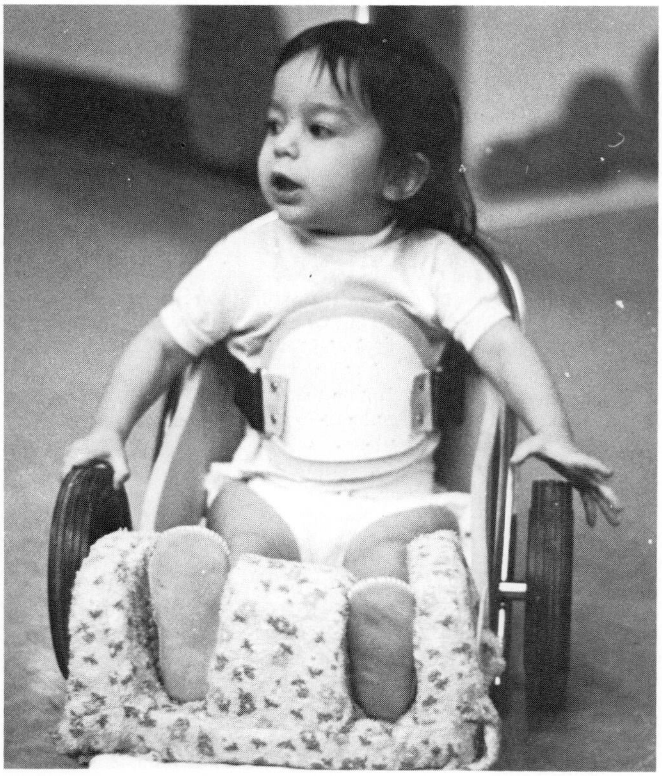

FIG. 31-1 Mobilizing device for a toddler.

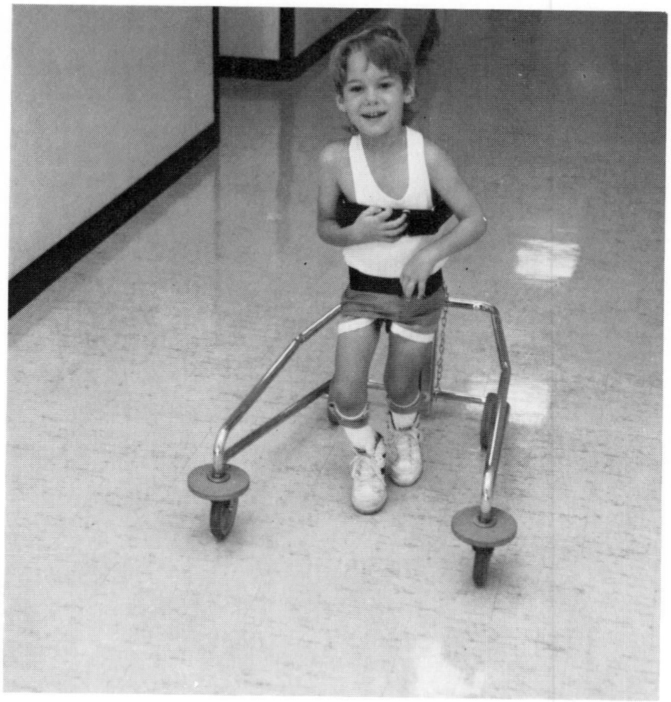

FIG. 31-2 Child in ambulation device that allows arm freedom.

have seizures, and hyperactive, dyskinetic children perform better when given dextroamphetamine or other drugs used for the child with attention deficit disorder. Care of visual and auditory deficits requires the attention of appropriate specialists, and speech therapy involves the services of a speech therapist. Dental care is especially important. Regular visits to the dentist and prophylaxis, including brushing, fluoride, and flossing, should be instituted as soon as the teeth erupt.

A wide variety of technical aids are available to improve the functioning of children with CP. These include electromechanical toys that are manipulated by correct movement of head and trunk, microcomputers combined with voice synthesizers to aid speech, and devices activated and deactivated by a head-stick, tongue, or other voluntary muscle movement over which the child has control (see Fig. 19-4).

Physical therapy is one of the most frequently used conservative treatment modalities. It requires the specialized skills of a qualified therapist with an extensive repertoire of exercise methods who can design a program to stimulate each child to achieve his functional goals.

Nursing Considerations

Nurses in a community setting, especially those in public health, in physicians' offices and clinics, and in schools, are more likely to become involved with a family that has a child with CP. Both the child and the family need the help, support, and encouragement that nurses are prepared to offer, and nurses can be involved in all aspects of the child's management.

ASSESSMENT

The beneficial influences of a habilitation program on both child and family are based on recognition of the disability as early as possible and implementation of treatment. Detection begins at birth, and the nurse should be especially observant for signs of CP in an infant who has a history that includes any of the prenatal and perinatal conditions that predispose to brain damage. An infant in the nursery who displays any sign that may indicate that all is not well—for example, poor feeding, rigidity, tenseness, or hypotonia—merits closer scrutiny and evaluation.

Delayed attainment of developmental milestones is one of the most valuable clues to recognizing cerebral palsy; therefore, slow development in a child is cause for concern. Nurses working with children need to be well acquainted with normal child growth and development and with the tools of assessment. The earlier any deviation from the normal is detected, the better the outlook for therapeutic intervention.

NURSING DIAGNOSES

Nursing diagnoses identified for the child with CP are primarily related to self-help and to facilitating mobility (see Nursing Care Plan, pp. 1061 to 1062). Other diagnoses will be evident in specific cases.

PLANNING

The goals of nursing care for the child with CP and his family are:

1. Establish locomotion and communication
2. Encourage self-help
3. Facilitate acquisition of educational opportunities adapted to the needs and capabilities of the child
4. Promote a positive self-image in the child
5. Support the family in its efforts to meet the needs of the child
6. Care for the child during hospitalization

IMPLEMENTATION

Since children are being treated at an earlier age, parents are participating earlier in treatment programs for their disabled child. They are taught the proper handling and home care of young children with CP and need carefully programmed steps so that their change of role from parent to therapist can be melded into the already established relationship. Nurses reinforce the therapeutic plan and assist the family in devising and modifying equipment and activities to continue the therapy program in the home.

Therapeutic interventions are those that are most appropriate for the specific problem and that best suit the need of the individual child at any given time. Passive range of motion exercises, stretching, and elongation exercises are valuable at any age, even at early ages when the child is unable to cooperate. They are of particular value for postural abnormalities around various joints.

Training in manual skills and activities of daily living proceeds along developmental lines and according to the child's functional level. Sitting, balance, crawling, and walking are encouraged at appropriate ages, accompanied by stimulation of protective extension and equilibrium reactions. Hand activities are begun early to improve motor function and provide the child with sensory experiences and information about his environment. As the child progresses from simple feeding and self-care activities, training is extended to include other tasks, such as cooking or typing, that are within his developmental and functional capabilities. It should be remembered that a child should not be expected to learn a task until he is at the developmental stage at which it would normally be accomplished.

Incorporating play into the therapeutic program often requires a great deal of ingenuity and inventiveness on the part of those involved in the child's care. Objects and toys are chosen to provide needed sensory input, using a variety of shapes, forms, and textures. Nurses can help parents integrate therapy into play activities in natural ways.

Speech training under the supervision of a speech therapist is begun early, before the child learns poor habits of communication. Parents and others can help by following the directions of the speech therapist and by talking to the child slowly and using pictures or handling objects about which the adult is speaking.

As in all aspects of care, educational requirements are determined by the child's needs and potential. Children with mild physical disability, normal intelligence, and no associated learning disability should attend regular school, if possible. Special classes or school facilities designed to meet the special needs of children with disabilities are available in most larger communities. For those who are unable to benefit from formal education, a training program may be appropriate. At any phase or in any setting, education is geared toward the child's assets.

Recreational outlets and after-school activities should be considered for the child who is unable to participate in the regular athletic programs and other peer activities. Some children with CP can compete in athletic and artistic endeavors, and there are many games and pastimes that are suited to their capabilities. Competitive sports are also becoming increasingly available to children with disabilities and offer an added dimension to physical activities.

Recreational activities serve to stimulate children's interest and curiosity, help them adjust to their disability, improve their functional abilities, and build self-esteem. Any accomplishment that helps the child approach a "normal" way of life enhances his self-concept.

Family support. Probably the nursing interventions most valuable to the family are support and help in coping with the emotional aspects of the disorder, many of which are discussed in relation to the child with a disability (Chapter 18). Initially the parents need supportive counseling directed toward understanding the implications of the diagnosis and all the feelings that it engenders. Later they need clarification regarding what they can expect from the child and from health professionals. Having a child with CP implies numerous problems of daily management and changes in family life.

Suggestions are offered at a pace that can be absorbed by the parents to avoid making them feel inadequate in their parenting abilities. The parents are encouraged to define their concerns and these concerns are acknowledged as genuine. The parents are given positive feedback for their observations of the infant, the progress *they* note, and how *they* differentiate the child's needs.

Parents can also find help and solace from parent groups with whom they can share problems and concerns and from whom they can derive comfort and practical information. The national organization, **United Cerebral Palsy Association, Inc.,*** has branches in most communities. The address of the nearest branch can be obtained from a local telephone directory, agency directory, or health department or by writing to the national headquarters. The association provides a variety of services for children and families.

The hospitalized child. CP is not a disorder that requires hospitalization; therefore, when children with cerebral palsy are hospitalized, they are usually admitted for another reason or for corrective surgery. Consequently many nurses are not accustomed to handling these children. Nurses who have never been associated with a child with CP may react in a variety of ways, including fear, revulsion, or overwhelming pity. The basic concept to keep in mind when caring for these children is that they are, first of all, children, who happen to be afflicted with a disorder that limits their capacities in performing some activities of daily living and, for some, in communicating with others.

They should be approached and treated the same as any child in the hospital. The nurse's actions should convey acceptance, affection, and friendliness and promote a feeling of trust and dependability in the child. This is especially true with older children who have normal intelligence but who may have communication problems. Speech impairment is common in children with CP. All too frequently nurses tend to "talk down" to these children and do things for them that they are perfectly capable of doing for themselves, although not as adeptly. This is especially humiliating to a teenager who values his independence and self-esteem.

To facilitate the care and management of the child, the therapy program should be continued, insofar as his condition allows, during the time he is hospitalized. This should be incorporated into his nursing care plan and every effort expended to make certain that the ground that has been so laboriously gained is not lost. Encouraging the parent to room-in and actively participate in the child's care facilitates a continuation of the home therapy program and helps the child adjust to an unfamiliar environment.

EVALUATION

The effectiveness of nursing interventions is determined by continual reassessment and evaluation of care based on the following observational guidelines and expected outcomes:

1. Observe the child's movements and speech
2. Observe the child's activities, especially those related to self-care
3. Interview the family regarding the child's activities and school attendance
4. Observe the child's interactions with others and his choice of activities; interview the child regarding his feelings and concerns
5. Interview the family regarding their feelings and concerns and observe the members' interaction with the child
6. Observe the child's behavior and responses during hospitalization

Expected outcomes:

See Nursing Care Plan, pp. 1061 to 1062.

*66 East 34th St., New York, NY 10016.

In Canada, the **Canadian Cerebral Palsy Association,** 55 Bloor St. East, Suite 301, Toronto, Ontario M4W 1A9.

NURSING CARE PLAN

The Child with Cerebral Palsy

Nursing Goals	Nursing Interventions	Expected Patient/Family Outcomes
NDx HP-HMP* **Potential for trauma** **Risk factors: physiologic disability, neuromuscular impairment**		
Recognize disorder early	Be alert for evidence of motor dysfunction in infant Be alert for associated disabilities Presence of seizures Sensory impairment such as hearing loss, strabismus Hyperactive behavior, marked distractibility, etc.	†Affected infants are detected early
Prevent deformity	Apply and correctly use braces Carry out and teach family to perform stretching exercises Employ appropriate range of motion exercises Perform preoperative and postoperative care for child who requires corrective surgery	Child benefits from appropriate preventive measures (specify measures and child's expected response)
Prevent physical injury	Provide safe physical environment Padded furniture Side rails on bed Sturdy furniture that does not slip Avoid scatter rugs and polished floors Select toys appropriate to age and physical limitations Encourage sufficient rest Use restraints when child is in chair or vehicle Provide child who is prone to falls with protective helmet and enforce its use Institute seizure precautions for susceptible child	Family provides a safe environment for the child (specify)
NDx A-EP **Impaired physical mobility** **Etiology: neuromuscular impairment**		
Establish locomotion	Encourage sitting, crawling, and walking at appropriate ages Carry out therapies that strengthen and improve control Assist child in using reciprocal leg motion when learning to walk Provide incentives to locomotion Ensure adequate rest before attempting locomotion activities Incorporate play that encourages desired behavior Employ aids that facilitate locomotion such as parallel bars, crutches, etc. Prepare child and family for surgical procedures if indicated	Child acquires locomotion within his capabilities (specify)
Promote relaxation	Maintain a well-regulated schedule that allows for adequate rest and sleep periods Be alert for evidence of fatigue, which tends to aggravate symptoms	Child is sufficiently rested
Promote general health	Ensure regular routine health maintenance Physical assessment Dental care Immunizations	Child receives regular health assessments (specify schedule) Child receives appropriate immunizations (specify) and dental care (specify)
Ensure balanced diet	Provide extra calories to meet extra energy demands of increased muscle activity Monitor weight gain Provide vitamin, mineral, and/or protein supplements if eating habits are poor	Child eats a balanced diet Weight remains within acceptable limits (specify)

*For an explanation of abbreviations, see p. 20.
†Nursing outcome.

Continued.

NURSING CARE PLAN

The Child with Cerebral Palsy—cont'd

Nursing Goals	Nursing Interventions	Expected Patient/Family Outcomes
A-EP Feeding, bathing/hygiene, dressing/grooming, or toileting (specify level) self-care deficit **Etiology: neuromuscular impairment**		
Promote self-help	Encourage child to assist in his care as age and capabilities permit Select toys and activities that allow maximum participation by child and that improve motor function and sensory input Avoid undue persistence to accomplish a goal Encourage activities that require both unimanual and bimanual efforts Adapt utensils, foods, and clothing to facilitate self-help, e.g., large-bowled spoon with padded handle, finger foods and foods that adhere to, rather than slip from, utensil, and clothing that opens from front with Velcro closings rather than buttons Assist parents in toilet training the child	Child engages in self-help activities commensurate with his capabilities
RRP Impaired verbal communication **Etiology: neuromuscular impairment**		
Facilitate communication	Enlist services of a speech therapist early Talk to child slowly Use articles and pictures to reinforce speech Use feeding techniques that help facilitate speech, such as using lips, teeth, and various tongue movements Teach and use nonverbal communication methods to dysarthritic child who would benefit, e.g., Blissymbols	Child is able to communicate his needs to caregivers (specify desired communication and means of accomplishment)
SP-SCP Body image or self-esteem disturbance **Etiology: physical disability, appearance**		
Promote a positive self-image	See The Child with Chronic Illness or Disability, p. 531	
Prepare for tests and procedures	Prepare child and family for needed surgical procedures Arrange for hearing and visual tests; assist parents in acquiring corrective devices	Child with correctable defects receives appropriate therapy (specify)
RRP Altered family processes **Etiology: birth of a child with a disability**		
See The Child with Chronic Illness or Disability, p. 531		
Nursing intervention related to medical management		
Prevent convulsions in seizure-prone child Administer anticonvulsant drugs		

SPINA BIFIDA

Spina bifida is the term most often used to describe the more common congenital defects of neural tube closure. Normally the spinal cord and cauda equina are encased in a protective sheath of bone and meninges (Fig. 31-3, *A*). Failure of neural tube closure produces defects that may involve the entire length of the neural tube or may be restricted to a small area. Terms applied to these abnormalities are:

myelodysplasia All-inclusive term that refers to defective development of any part of the spinal cord; usually used to describe abnormalities without gross superficial defects

spinal dysraphia or **spina bifida** Defect in closure of the vertebral column with varying degrees of tissue protrusion through the bony cleft

spina bifida occulta Fusion failure of posterior vertebral arches without accompanying herniation of spinal cord or meninges; usually not visible externally (Fig. 31-3, *B*)

spina bifida cystica Defect in closure with external saccular protrusion through the bony spine with varying degrees of nerve involvement

meningocele Form of spina bifida cystica; consists of a saclike cyst of meninges filled with spinal fluid (Fig. 31-3, *C*, Fig. 31-4, *A*)

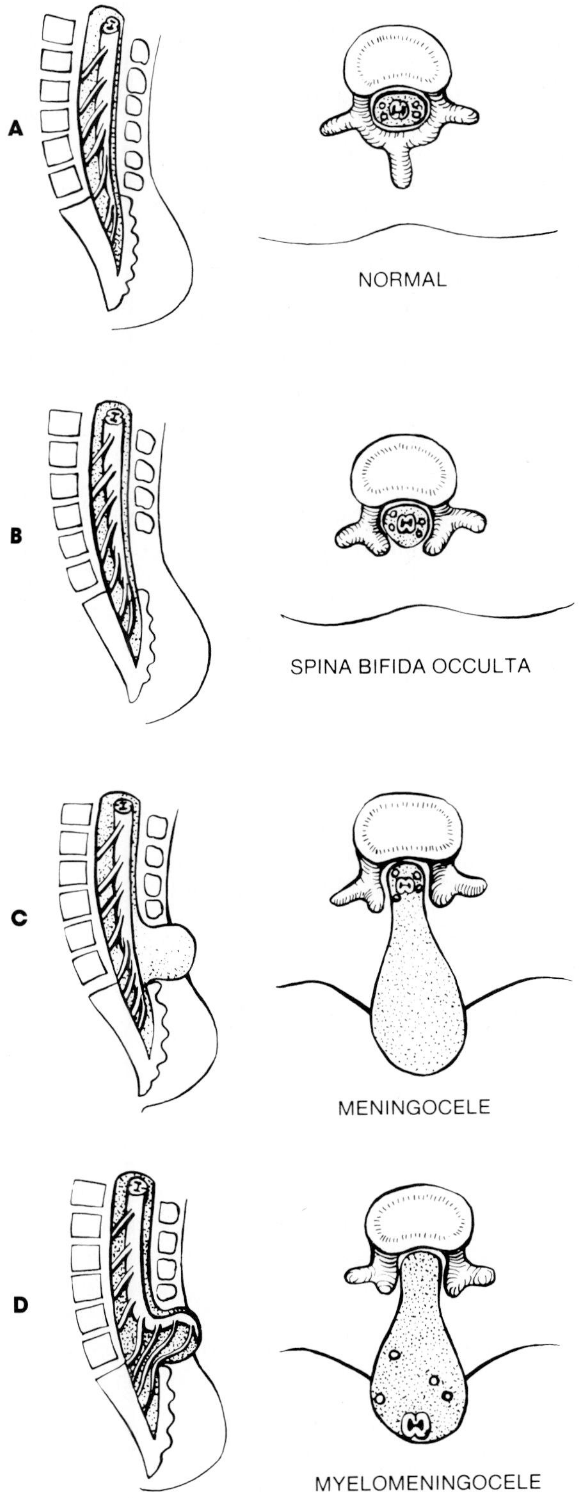

FIG. 31-3 Midline defects of the osseous spine with varying degrees of neural herniations.

myelomeningocele (meningomyelocele) Form of spina bifida cystica; consists of hernial protrusion of a saclike cyst containing meninges, spinal fluid, and a portion of the spinal cord with its nerves (Fig. 31-3, *D*)

More severe neural tube defects are *rachischisis,* a fissure in the spinal column that leaves the meninges and spinal cord exposed, *encephalocele,* herniation of brain and meninges through a defect in the skull that produces a fluid-filled sac in the occipital region, and *anencephaly* (absence of the brain), which consists of only an exposed vascular mass and no bony covering.

The cause of neural tube malformations is unknown, although the increased incidence in families lends support to a genetic influence. There is some speculation regarding a viral cause of spina bifida, since there appears to be an increased incidence of the defect in infants conceived during the early winter months. Radiation and other environmental influences have also been implicated, based on animal experiments. The cystic defect affects 0.2 to 4.2 per 1000 live births.

Pathophysiology

The primary defect in neural tube malformations is believed by most authorities to be a failure of neural tube closure during early development of the embryo. However, there is evidence to indicate that the defects are a result of splitting of the already closed neural tube as a result of an abnormal increase in cerebrospinal fluid pressure during the first trimester of pregnancy. The degree of neurologic dysfunction is directly related to the anatomic level of the defect and thus the nerves involved. Most myelomeningoceles involve the lumbar or lumbosacral area, and hydrocephalus is a frequently associated anomaly.

Diagnostic Evaluation

The diagnosis is made on the basis of clinical manifestations (see box) and examination of the meningeal sac. If the mass can be transilluminated (that is, becomes translucent when a light is held behind it), the defect is probably a meningocele. In these cases neurologic function is rarely disturbed even though the nerve roots are somewhat displaced. If the mass does not transilluminate, it is more likely a myelomeningocele. Supplementary diagnostic measures include plain radiography to disclose the precise bony defect in the symptomatic lesion and to establish the diagnosis in the suspected, nonsymptomatic occult variety. Other spinal tomograms and myelography are used to differentiate between spina bifida occulta and other spinal disorders. Skull tomography helps to establish the presence or absence of hydrocephalus.

Prenatal detection. It is possible to determine the presence of some major open neural tube defects prenatally. Ultrasonic scanning of the uterus and elevated concentrations of alpha-fetoprotein (AFP), a fetal-specific gamma-1 globulin, in amniotic fluid can indicate the

Clinical Manifestations of Spina Bifida

Spina Bifida Cystica
Sensory disturbances usually parallel motor dysfunction
- Below second lumbar vertebra
  - Flaccid, areflexic partial paralysis of lower extremities
  - Varying degrees of sensory deficit
  - Overflow incontinence with constant dribbling of urine
  - Lack of bowel control
  - Rectal prolapse (sometimes)
- Below third sacral vertebra
  - No motor impairment
  - May be saddle anesthesia with bladder and anal sphincter paralysis

Joint deformities (sometimes produced in utero)
- Talipes valgus or varus contractures
- Kyphosis
- Lumbosacral scoliosis
- Hip dislocations

Spina Bifida Occulta
Frequently no observable manifestations
May be associated with one or more cutaneous manifestations
- Skin depression or dimple
- Port-wine angiomatous nevi
- Dark tufts of hair
- Soft, subcutaneous lipomas

May be neuromuscular disturbances
- Progressive disturbance of gait with foot weakness
- Bowel and bladder sphincter disturbances

presence of anencephaly or myelomeningocele. The optimum time for performing these diagnostic tests is between the fourteenth and sixteenth weeks of gestation, before AFP concentrations normally diminish and in sufficient time to permit an elective abortion if chosen.

Therapeutic Management

Management of the child who has a myelomeningocele requires a multidisciplinary approach involving the specialties of neurology, neurosurgery, pediatrics, urology, orthopedics, rehabilitation, and physical therapy, as well as intensive nursing care in a variety of specialty areas. The collaborative efforts of these specialists are focused on (1) the myelomeningocele and the problems associated with the defect—hydrocephalus, paralysis, orthopedic deformities, and genitourinary abnormalities, (2) possible acquired problems that may or may not be associated, such as meningitis, hypoxia, and hemorrhage, and (3) other abnormalities, such as cardiac or gastrointestinal malformations.

Infancy. Initial care involves prevention of infection, neurologic assessment, including observation for associated anomalies, and dealing with the impact of the anomaly on the parents. Although meningoceles are repaired early, especially if there is danger of rupture of the sac, the philosophy regarding skin closure of myelomeningocele varies radically. Most authorities believe that early closure, within the first 24 to 48 hours, offers the most favorable outcome. It not only prevents local infection and trauma to the exposed tissues but avoids stretching of other nerve roots, thus preventing further motor impairment (Reigel, 1982).

Other experts contend that surgical repair is best delayed until after further assessment of neurologic function, intellectual potential, and extent of complications (Charney and others, 1985). This delay increases the ability of the infant to tolerate the surgical procedure, allows for better epithelialization of the sac (thus reducing the risk of infection), and permits easier mobilization of skin for closure.

A variety of plastic surgical procedures can be used for skin closure without disturbing the neural elements or removing any portion of the sac (for example, Fig. 31-4, *B*). The objective is satisfactory skin coverage of the lesion and meticulous closure. Wide excision of the large membranous covering may damage functioning neural tissue. Where the skin over the defect is intact, as often occurs with meningocele, surgical intervention may be performed for cosmetic reasons.

Associated problems are assessed and managed by appropriate surgical and supportive measures. Shunt procedures provide relief from imminent or progressive hydrocephalus (see p. 930). Meningitis, urinary tract infection, and pneumonia are treated with vigorous antibiotic therapy and supportive measures.

Orthopedic considerations. According to most orthopedists, musculoskeletal problems that will affect later locomotion should be evaluated early, and treatment, where indicated, should be instituted without delay. The appropriate members of the health team work together to evaluate the child in regard to the true level of neurologic functioning, and corrective measures are carried out in coordination with the activities of the neurosurgeon. Casting, bracing, traction, and surgical techniques for correction of hip, knee, and foot deformities are employed when they may aid later ambulation.

A variety of devices are available to provide mobility to children with spinal cord lesions, including lightweight braces, special "walking" devices, and custom-built wheelchairs. Corrective procedures, when indicated, are best initiated at an early age so that the child will not lag significantly behind age-mates in developmental progress.

Management of excretory function. Myelomeningocele is one of the most common causes of neurogenic bladder dysfunction in childhood. Ongoing assessment and monitoring of urologic status are lifelong problems in management of the child with or without surgical repair of the spinal defect. Since the majority of these children suffer from incontinence and are subject to recurrent or persistent pyuria, prevention and treatment of renal complications are constant goals.

Treatment of renal problems includes (1) regular urologic care with prompt and vigorous treatment of infections; (2) some type of regular emptying of the bladder, such as intermittent clean catheterization (ICC) taught to and performed by parents, and self-catheterization taught

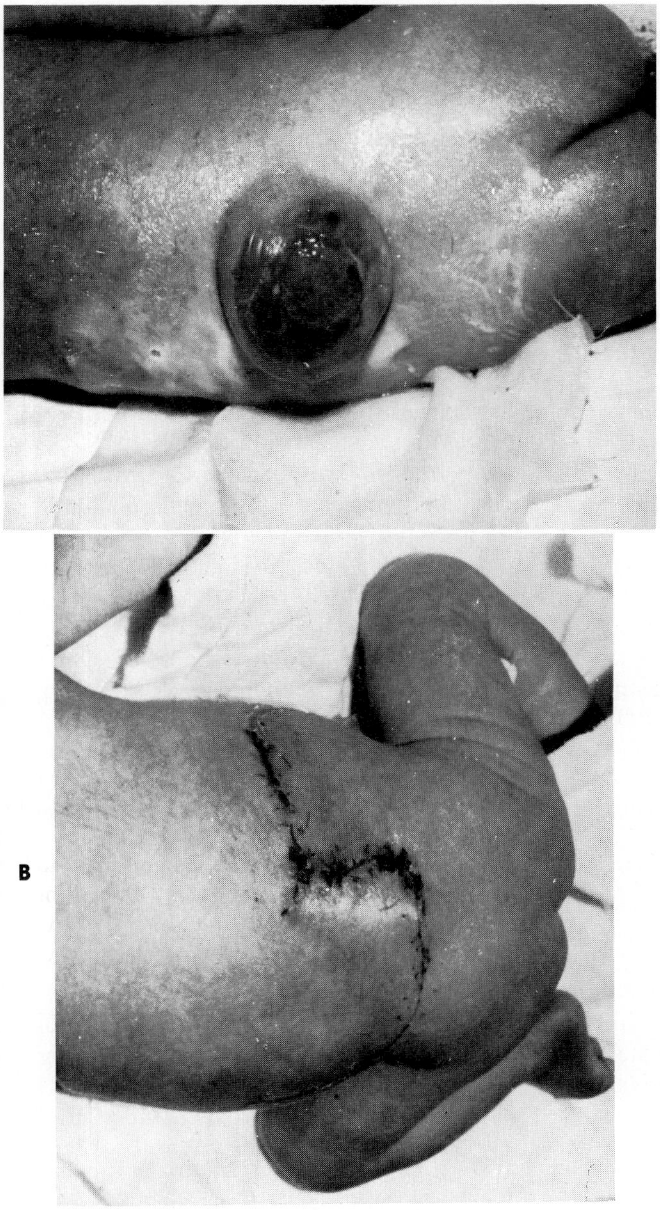

A

B

FIG. 31-4 **A,** Myelomeningocele before surgery. **B,** Same patient after surgery. (Courtesy M.C. Gleason, M.D., San Diego, Calif. From Ingalls, A.J., and Salerno, M.C.: Maternal and child health nursing, ed. 5, 1983, The C.V. Mosby Co.)

to children; (3) medications to improve bladder storage and continence, such as bethanechol (Urecholine), propantheline (Pro-Banthine), phenoxybenzamine (Dibenzyline), and ephedrine; and (4) in many institutions, the surgically implanted artificial urinary sphincter and bladder pacemaker. In cases of intractable severe hydronephrosis or incontinence, urinary diversion, such as a ureteroileostomy, ureterostomy, or cystostomy, may be necessary.

Some degree of fecal continence can usually be achieved in most children with myelomeningocele with diet modification, regular toilet habits, and prevention of constipation and impaction. It is frequently a lengthy process, but biofeedback training is proving to be effective in helping some children to gain control more quickly (Whitehead, Parker, and Masek, 1981).

Nursing Considerations

Care of the infant and child with myelomeningocele requires both immediate and long-term nursing and medical supervision. In the newborn period nursing responsibilities are directed toward preventing infection of and trauma to the fragile cyst, observing for complications, and providing support for and education of parents. Long-term management involves an interdisciplinary team effort to help the child and family with the multitude of problems associated with this disability. This discussion is limited to care of the infant primarily.

ASSESSMENT

At the time of delivery, an examination is performed to assess the intactness of the membranous cyst. Subsequent assessments are directed toward detecting the extent of neurologic deficit and observing for signs of complications. Movement of the extremities or skin response, especially an anal reflex, that might provide clues to the degree of motor or sensory impairment is noted. The head circumference is measured daily (see p. 134), and the fontanels are examined for signs of tension or bulging. The nurse is also alert to early signs of infection, such as elevated temperature (axillary), irritability, lethargy, and nuchal rigidity, and to signs of increased intracranial pressure.

NURSING DIAGNOSES

Nursing diagnoses identified for the infant with spina bifida are listed in the accompanying box. Others will be evident in specific cases and with the child's advancing years.

PLANNING

The goals of nursing care for the infant with myelomeningocele are:

1. Prevent damage to the myelomeningocele sac

Nursing Diagnoses: The Infant with Myelomeningocele

Potential for infection related to presence of infective organisms and nonepithelialized meningeal sac
Potential for trauma related to delicate spinal lesion
Potential impaired skin integrity related to paralysis, unprotected meningeal sac
Altered family processes related to birth of a child with a physical defect

---

2. Prevent complications
3. Support and educate family

IMPLEMENTATION

As the child matures, the problems increase and involve all aspects of daily living. Therefore care is directly related to the child's habilitation at each stage of development.

Prevent damage to the myelomeningocele sac. Before surgical closure the myelomeningocele is prevented from drying by the application of a sterile, moist, nonadherent dressing over the defect. The moistening solution is usually sterile normal saline, although soaks with antibacterial drugs such as silver nitrate or bacitracin are also advocated. Moist dressings are changed frequently (every 2 to 4 hours), and the sac is closely inspected for leaks, abrasions, irritation, or any signs of infection. When an overhead warmer is used, the dressings over the defect require more frequent moistening because of the dehydrating effect of the dry heat.

The sac must be cleansed carefully if it becomes soiled or contaminated. Any opening in the sac greatly increases the risk of infection to the central nervous system. If surgical closure is to be delayed, measures are directed toward facilitating the drying, granulation, and eventual epithelialization of the sac. In this instance the sac is usually left exposed to the air or covered with a dry gauze or nonadherent dressing.

Special measures to toughen the skin or membrane, such as application of a skin sealant, may be indicated, but care must be taken to prevent a dressing from adhering to and damaging the sac. Prolonged use of ointments or moist dressings is usually contraindicated to avoid maceration and breakdown of the tissues. A large doughnut-shaped piece of foam rubber or other spongy material can be fashioned to provide a protective shield for the sac. The edges should be left sufficiently wide to allow for adequate anchoring with strips of bandage or paper tape. A sterile drape, gauze, or other protective cover can form a roof over the opening but should not come in contact with the sac.

One of the most difficult, important, and challenging aspects in the early care of the infant with myelomeningocele is positioning. Before surgery the infant is kept in the prone position to minimize tension on the sac and the risk of trauma. The prone position allows for optimum positioning of legs, especially in cases of associated hip dysplasia. The infant is placed flat with the hips only slightly flexed to reduce tension on the defect. The legs are maintained in abduction with a pad between the knees to counteract hip subluxation, and a small roll is placed under the ankles to maintain a neutral foot position. A variety of aids, including diaper rolls, pads, small sandbags, or specially designed frames and appliances, can be used to maintain the desired position.

Prevent complications. The prone position affects other aspects of the infant's care. For example, in this position the infant is more difficult to keep clean, pressure areas are a constant threat, and feeding becomes a problem. The infant's head is turned to one side for feeding. Fortunately most defects are repaired early, and the infant can be held for feeding as soon as the surgical site is sufficiently healed to permit handling.

Diapering the infant is contraindicated until the defect has been repaired and healing is well advanced or epithelialization has taken place. The padding beneath the diaper area is changed as needed to keep the skin dry and free of irritation. Since the bowel sphincter is frequently affected, there is continual passage of stool, often misinterpreted as diarrhea, which is a constant irritant to the skin and a source of infection to the spinal lesion. This provides another rationale for closure before the infant's first feeding while the meconium is still free of organisms.

Areas of sensory and motor impairment are subject to skin breakdown and therefore require meticulous care. Placing the infant on a soft foam or fleece pad reduces pressure on the knees and ankles. Periodic cleansing, application of lotion, and gentle massage aid circulation. Changing linen is best accomplished by two persons—one changes the linen while the other holds the infant, assuring that the spine is maintained in good alignment without tension in the area of the defect.

Gentle range of motion exercises are sometimes carried out to prevent contractures, and stretching of contractures is performed when indicated. However, these exercises may be restricted to the foot, ankle, and knee joint. Where the hip joints are unstable, stretching against tight hip flexors or adductor muscles, which act much like bowstrings, may aggravate a tendency toward subluxation. In addition, the bones of these infants tend to be fragile and subject to fractures.

Since infants with unrepaired myelomeningocele are unable to be held in the arms and cuddled as unaffected infants are, their need for tactile stimulation is met by fondling, stroking, and other comfort measures. Bright mobiles or other objects can be placed within the infant's view, and other stimulating activities usually provided for infants are appropriate. All infants respond to pleasant sounds (see box on p. 229).

Postoperative care. Postoperative care of the infant with myelomeningocele involves the same basic care as that of any postsurgical infant—monitoring vital signs, monitoring intake and output, nourishment, and observation for signs of infection. Wound management is carried out according to the directions of the surgeon, including close observation for signs of leakage of cerebrospinal fluid. General care is continued as preoperatively.

The prone position is maintained after operative closure, although many neurosurgeons allow a side-lying or partial side-lying position unless it aggravates a coexisting hip dysplasia or permits undesirable hip flexion. This offers an opportunity for position changes, which reduces the risk of pressure sores and facilitates feeding. If permitted by the physician, the infant can be held upright against the body, with care to avoid pressure on the operative site.

Family support and home care. As soon as the parents are able to cope with the infant's condition, they are encouraged to become involved in care. They need to learn how to continue at home the care that has been initiated in the hospital—positioning, feeding, skin care, and range of motion exercises when appropriate. Parents are taught clean catheterization technique when prescribed.* The family needs to know the signs of complications and how to reach assistance when needed. In cases in which the defect has not been repaired, they are taught to care for the lesion.

The long-range planning with and support of parents and child begin in the hospital and extend throughout childhood and even beyond. Long-term care of these children is of uncertain length. Nurses assume an important role as a central member of the health team. As a coordinator the nurse reviews information with the family, takes responsibility for family teaching, and acts as liaison between inpatient and outpatient services. The child will need numerous hospitalizations over the years, and each one will be a source of stress, to which the younger child is especially vulnerable. See Chapter 18 for discussion of the multiple aspects in care of the child with a disability.

Habilitation involves not only solving problems of self-help and locomotion but also the most distressing problem of incontinence, which threatens the child's social acceptability. Assistance with preparing the child and the school regarding the special needs of the child helps provide a better initial adjustment to this broader social experience. The **Spina Bifida Association of America†** is organized to provide services and support for families of children with spinal lesions.

EVALUATION

The effectiveness of nursing interventions is determined by continual reassessment and evaluation of care based on the following observational guidelines and expected outcomes:

1. Inspect the spinal lesion, take appropriate measurements (weight, vital signs, head circumference), observe the child's general health status, and check completed care with preoperative checklist
2. Take vital signs, inspect operative site (or preoperative lesion), inspect skin (especially dependent areas), measure head circumference, and assess range of motion of lower extremities
3. Observe parent-infant interactions, behavior of family members, and interview family members regarding their feelings and concerns

Expected outcomes:

1. The child is physically prepared for surgical repair of the defect
2. The child exhibits no evidence of infection (skin, meningeal, or renal), deformities of extremities, or pressure necrosis; signs of complications (e.g., hydrocephalus, dislocated hip) are detected early and appropriate interventions initiated
3. Family members discuss their feelings and concerns and participate in the infant's care; family makes contact with appropriate community agencies and facilities

PROGRESSIVE INFANTILE SPINAL MUSCULAR ATROPHY (WERDNIG-HOFFMANN DISEASE)

Progressive infantile spinal muscular atrophy (Werdnig-Hoffmann disease) is a disorder characterized by progressive weakness and wasting of skeletal muscles caused by

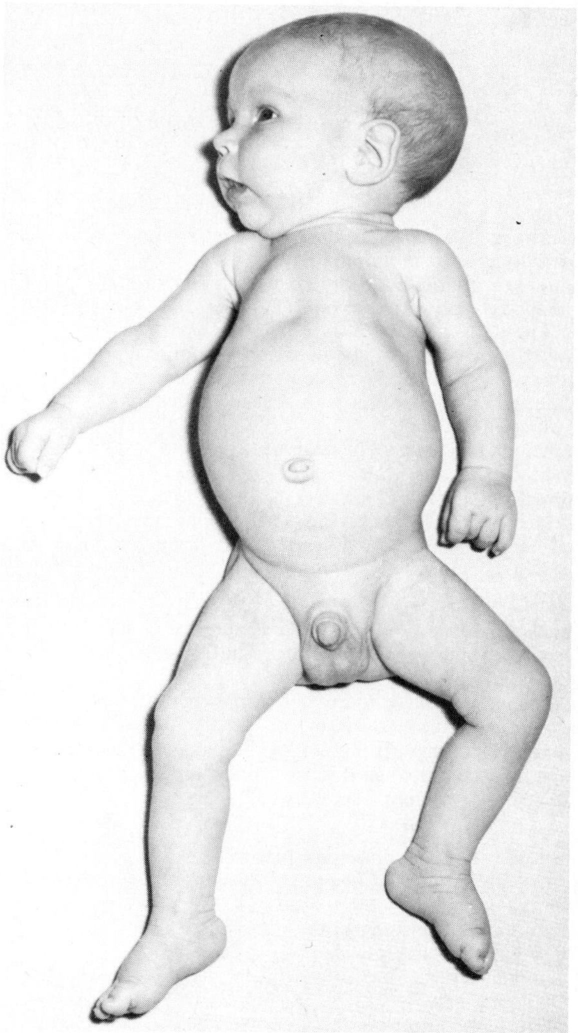

FIG. 31-5 Patient with Werdnig-Hoffman disease lying in typical posture. (From Swaiman, K.F., and Wright, F.S.: The practice of pediatric neurology, ed. 2, St. Louis, 1982, The C.V. Mosby Co.)

*See Wong, D.L., and Whaley, L.F.: Clinical handbook of pediatric nursing, St. Louis, 1986, The C.V. Mosby Co.

†343 S. Dearborn #317, Chicago, IL 60604.

In Canada, the **Spina Bifida and Hydrocephalus Association of Canada,** 633 Wellington Crescent, Winnepeg, Manitoba R3M 0A8.

degeneration of anterior horn cells. It is inherited as an autosomal-recessive trait and is the most common paralytic form of the "floppy infant syndrome" (see p. 221). The site of the pathologic condition is the anterior horn cells of the spinal cord and the motor nuclei of the brain stem, but the primary effect is atrophy of skeletal muscles (Fig. 31-5).

Therapeutic Management

The diagnosis is suspected on the basis of clinical manifestations (see box). It is established from electromyography demonstrating a denervation pattern and is confirmed by muscle biopsy. Treatment is symptomatic and preventive, primarily preventing infection and treating orthopedic problems, the most serious of which is scoliosis. Many children benefit from powered chairs, lifts, special mattresses, and accessible environmental controls. Vigorous antibiotic therapy and pulmonary physical therapy are implemented during upper respiratory infections.

Clinical Manifestations of Werdnig-Hoffmann Disease

Group 1
Disease acquired in utero or during first 2 months of life
Inactivity is most prominent feature
Infant lies in the frog position with legs externally rotated, abducted, and flexed at hips (Fig. 31-5)
Weakness
Limited movements of shoulder and arm muscles
Active movement is usually limited to fingers and toes
Diaphragmatic breathing with sternal retractions
Weak cry and cough
Secretions tend to pool in pharynx
Alert facies
Normal sensation and intellect
Affected infants do not progress to sit alone, roll over, or walk
Early death (usually by 3 years of age) from respiratory failure or infection

Group 2
Disease manifest between 2 and 12 months of age
Early—weakness confined to arms and legs
Later—becomes generalized
Legs usually involved to greater extent than arms
Prominent pectus excavatum
Movements absent during complete relaxation or sleep
Some infants able to sit if placed in position
Life span varies from 7 months to 7 years

Group 3
Onset of symptoms in second year of life
Normal head control and can sit unassisted by 6 to 8 months of age
Thigh and hip muscles weak
Those who manage to walk
- Lumbar lordosis
- Waddling gait
- Genu recurvatum
- Protuberant abdomen
- Ambulation becomes increasingly difficult
- Confined to a wheelchair by second decade

Deep tendon reflexes may be present early but disappear

Nursing Considerations

The infant or small child with extensive paralysis requires frequent change of position to prevent physical injury and complications, especially pneumonia. The pharynx requires frequent suctioning to remove secretions, and feeding must be carried out slowly and carefully to prevent aspiration. These children are intellectually normal, so verbal, tactile, and auditory stimulation are important aspects of care. Supporting them so that they can see the activities around them and transporting them in a buggy for a change of environment provide stimulation and a broader scope of contacts.

Children who are able to sit require proper support and attention to alignment to prevent deformities and other complications. The child with group 3 disease will need attention to education needs and opportunities for social interaction with other children. Parents of a chronically ill or potentially fatally ill child require a great deal of support and encouragement (see Chapter 18). The parents of a child with a genetically transmitted disorder also need to be encouraged to seek genetic counseling.

JUVENILE SPINAL MUSCULAR ATROPHY (KUGELBERG-WELANDER DISEASE)

Juvenile spinal muscular atrophy (Kugelberg-Welander disease, juvenile proximal hereditary muscular atrophy) is also the result of anterior horn cell and motor nerve degeneration. The disease is characterized by a pattern of muscular weakness similar to that of infantile spinal muscular atrophy. Several modes of inheritance have been reported for the disease—autosomal-recessive, autosomal-dominant, and X-linked recessive.

The onset occurs between 2 and 17 years of age with symptoms resembling group 3 infantile spinal muscular atrophy, although proximal muscle weakness (especially of the pelvic girdle) appears later, in early childhood or adolescence, and the progression is slower. Muscles of the lower arms and legs are involved relatively late, and muscles of the trunk and those supplied by the cranial nerves are usually unaffected. The disease runs a slowly progressive course. Some children lose the ability to walk 8 to 9 years after onset of symptoms, but many can still walk after 20 years or more. Many affected persons have a normal life expectancy.

MUSCULAR DYSTROPHIES

The muscular dystrophies (MDs) constitute the largest and most important single group of muscle diseases of childhood. They all have a genetic origin in which there is gradual degeneration of muscle fibers, and they are characterized by progressive weakness and wasting of symmetric groups of skeletal muscles, with increasing disability and deformity. In all forms of MD there is insidious loss of strength, but each type differs in regard to muscle groups affected (Fig. 31-6), age of onset, rate of progression, and inheritance patterns. The most common

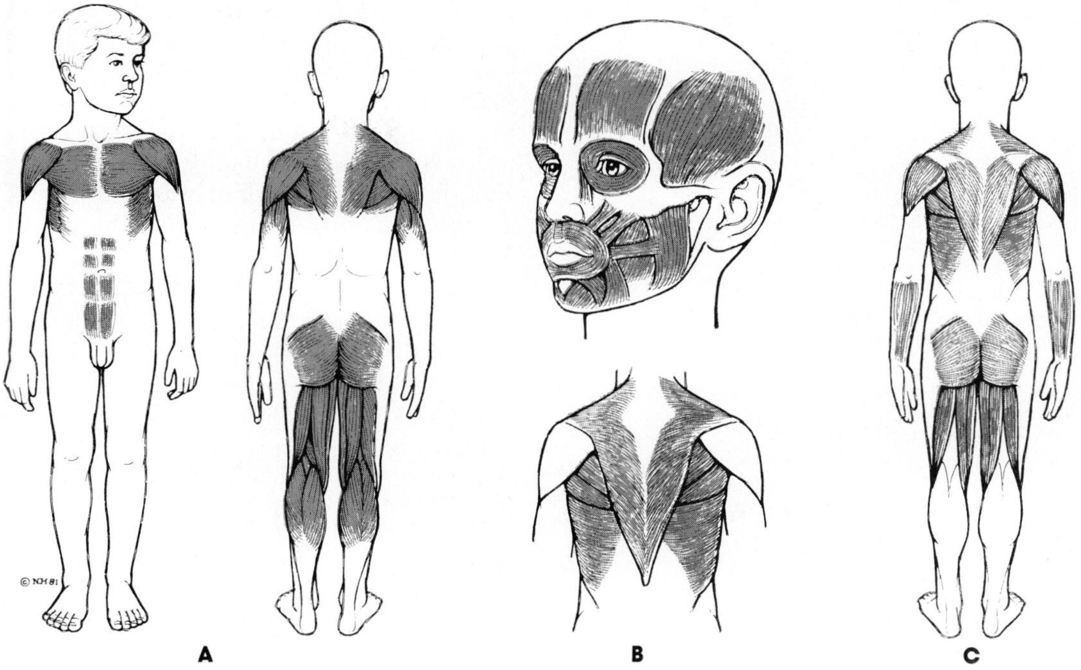

FIG. 31-6 Initial muscle groups involved in the muscular dystrophies. **A,** Pseudohypertrophic. **B,** Facioscapulohumeral. **C,** Limb-girdle.

form, *Duchenne muscular dystrophy,* is considered separately in the next section.

Facioscapulohumeral (Landouzy-Déjérine) muscular dystrophy is inherited as an autosomal-dominant disorder with onset in early adolescence. It is characterized by difficulty raising the arms over the head, lack of facial mobility, and a forward slope of the shoulders. The progression is slow.

Limb-girdle muscular dystrophy is an autosomal-recessive disease of later childhood or adolescence with variable but usually slow progression; it is characterized by weakness of proximal muscles of both pelvic and shoulder girdles.

Treatment of the MDs consists mainly of supportive measures. This includes physical therapy to improve mobility, orthopedic procedures to minimize deformity, and assistance for the affected child in meeting the demands of daily living.

PSEUDOHYPERTROPHIC (DUCHENNE) MUSCULAR DYSTROPHY

The most severe and most common MD seen in childhood is pseudohypertrophic MD. The incidence is approximately 1:3000 to 1:5000 male children (Cohen, 1984), and an X-linked inheritance pattern is identified in 50% of cases (see Appendix B); the remainder appear as sporadic cases and probably represent fresh mutations. As in all X-linked disorders, males are affected almost exclusively. The basic defect in MD is unknown.

Evidence of muscle weakness usually appears during the third year, although there may have been a history of delay in motor development, particularly walking. Difficulty in running, riding a bicycle, and climbing stairs are usually the first symptoms noted. Later, abnormal gait on a level surface becomes apparent. In the early years rapid developmental gains may mask the progression of the disease. Questioning of the parents may reveal that the child has difficulty in rising from a sitting or supine position.

The name *pseudohypertrophy* is derived from muscular enlargement caused by fatty infiltration. Profound muscular atrophy occurs in later stages, and as the disease progresses, contractures and deformities involving large and small joints are common complications. Ambulation usually becomes impossible by 12 years of age. Facial, oropharyngeal, and respiratory muscles are spared until the terminal stages of the disease. Ultimately the disease process involves the diaphragm and auxiliary muscles of respiration, and cardiomegaly is common. The cause of death is usually respiratory tract infection or cardiac failure.

Diagnostic Evaluation

The disease is suspected on the basis of clinical manifestations (see box) and confirmed by serum enzyme measurement, muscle biopsy, and electromyography. The serum creatine phosphokinase, aldolase, and serum glutamic-oxaloacetic transaminase levels are extremely high in the first 2 years of life before onset of clinical weakness. They diminish with muscle deterioration but do not reach normal levels until severe muscle wasting and in-

Clinical Manifestations of Duchenne Muscular Dystrophy

Waddling gait
Lordosis
Frequent falls
Gower sign (child turns onto side or abdomen, flexes knees to assume a kneeling position, then with knees extended gradually pushes torso to an upright position by "walking" the hands up the legs)
Enlarged muscles (especially thighs and upper arms)
 Feel unusually firm or woody on palpation
Later stages
 Profound muscular atrophy
Mental deficiency (common)
 Mild (about 20 IQ points below normal)
 Frank mental deficit present in 25% of cases
Complications
 Contracture deformities of hips, knees, and ankles
 Disuse atrophy
 Obesity

capacitation have occurred. Muscle biopsy reveals degeneration of muscle fibers, with fibrosis and fatty tissue replacement. Electromyography shows decrease in amplitude and duration of motor unit potentials. Ultrasound imaging is assuming a more prominent place in the diagnosis of muscle disease.

Therapeutic Management

There is no effective treatment for childhood muscular dystrophy. Maintaining function in unaffected muscles for as long as possible is the primary goal. It has been found that children who remain as active as possible are able to avoid wheelchair confinement for a longer period of time. Early recourse to a wheelchair accelerates deconditioning and promotes the development of lower extremity contractures. Maintenance of function often includes range of motion exercises, surgery to release contracture deformities, bracing, and performance of activities of daily living (ADL). Genetic counseling is recommended for parents, female siblings, and maternal aunts and their female offspring.

Nursing Considerations

The major emphasis of nursing care is to assist the child and his family to cope with the progressive, incapacitating, and fatal nature of the disease, to help design a program that will afford a greater degree of independence and reduce the predictable and preventable disabilities associated with the disorder, and to help the child and family deal constructively with the limitations the disease imposes on their daily lives.

Working closely with other team members, nurses help the family in developing the child's self-help skills to give the child the satisfaction of being as independent as possible for as long as possible. This requires continual evaluation of the child's capabilities, which are often difficult to assess. It is not always possible to know when the child seeks parental assistance because he wants a little extra attention or because his muscles are overtired. Fortunately most children with muscular dystrophy instinctively recognize this need to become as independent as possible and strive to do so.

Practical difficulties faced by families are physical limitations of housing and mobility. Parents also need help in buying and modifying clothing for their disabled child. It is difficult to find clothing and footwear to wear comfortably in a wheelchair, to fit over contracted limbs, and to fit the obese child. The parent's social activities are also restricted, and the family's activities must be continually modified to the needs of the affected child.

The concentrated efforts and full-time commitment needed to care for these children in the later stages of the disease are frequently reasons why some children are placed in a skilled nursing facility. Helping the parents with this decision and supporting them through their guilt and distress are important nursing functions.

No matter how successful the program or how well the family adapts to the disorder, superimposed on the physical and emotional problems associated with a child with a long-term disability is the constant presence of the ultimate outcome of the disease. All of the manifestations seen in the child with a fatal illness are encountered in these families (see Chapter 18). The guilt feelings of the mother may be particularly pronounced in this disorder because of the mother-to-son transmission of the defective gene.

Nurses can be alert to problems and needs of the families and make necessary referrals when supplementary services are indicated. The **Muscular Dystrophy Association of America, Inc.*** has branches in most communities to provide assistance to families that have a child with muscular dystrophy.

◆*Acquired Neuromuscular Disorders*

Neuromuscular disorders can be acquired. In such cases, the disorder usually is caused by either trauma or infectious agents. Two infectious causes, botulism and tetanus, are discussed later in this chapter. Rhabdomyosarcoma, a tumor derived primarily from muscle tissue, is also considered here, although it is not acquired in the same sense as an infection or an injury.

*810 Seventh Ave., New York, NY 10019.
In Canada the **Muscular Dystrophy Association of Canada,** 150 Eglinton Ave. East, Suite 400, Toronto, Ontario M4P 1E8.

INFECTIOUS POLYNEURITIS (GUILLAIN-BARRÉ SYNDROME)

Infectious polyneuritis, also known as infectious neuronitis or Guillain-Barré syndrome, is probably the most common form of polyneuritis, and it may occur at any age. Although children are less often affected than adults, the incidence in the pediatric age-group appears to be increasing, with higher susceptibility in children between ages 4 and 10 years. Both sexes are affected with equal frequency.

Pathophysiology

The precise etiologic agent is unknown. Since the disease has been associated with a number of viral infections or the administration of vaccines, it has been suggested that it may be a toxic sequela of an original infection, an activated latent virus, or a manifestation of an acute infection. It is an acute polyneuropathy in which motor dysfunction predominates over sensory disturbance and in which there is bilateral facial paresis or paralysis and occasionally weakness of the bulbar and respiratory musculature. Some believe that it may represent a cell-mediated immunologic response directed at the peripheral nerves. Pathologic changes show inflammation and segmented demyelination of peripheral nerves. Nerve conduction is impaired, producing ascending partial or complete paralysis of muscles innervated by the involved nerves.

Diagnostic Evaluation

The paralytic manifestations (see box) are usually preceded by a mild influenza-like illness or sore throat. In 3 to 12 days neurologic symptoms appear. Cerebrospinal fluid analysis reveals an increased protein concentration, but other laboratory studies are noncontributory. The symmetric nature of the paralysis helps differentiate this disorder from spinal paralytic poliomyelitis, which usually affects sporadic muscles.

Clinical Manifestations of Guillain-Barré Syndrome

- Initially:
  - Muscle tenderness
  - Paresthesia and cramps (sometimes)
  - Symmetric muscle weakness
- Paralysis:
  - Begins in periphery
  - Ascends rapidly from lower extremities
  - Frequently involves muscles of trunk, upper extremities, and those supplied by cranial nerves (especially facial)
  - Flaccid paralysis with loss of reflexes
  - May involve facial, extraocular, labial, lingual, pharyngeal, and laryngeal muscles
  - Intercostal and phrenic nerve
    - Breathlessness in vocalizations
    - Shallow, irregular respirations
- Tendon reflexes depressed or absent
- Variable degrees of sensory impairment
- Muscle tenderness or sensitivity to slight pressure
- Urinary incontinence or retention and constipation (frequently)

Therapeutic Management

Treatment of Guillain-Barré syndrome is symptomatic. Corticosteroid therapy has been of benefit in the early stages. Respiratory and pharyngeal involvement require assisted ventilation, frequently with tracheostomy.

Course. The general health of the child and the extent of paralysis influence the outcome of the illness. Almost all deaths are caused by respiratory failure; therefore, early diagnosis and access to respiratory support are especially important. Muscle function begins to return 2 days to 2 weeks after the onset of symptoms, and recovery is complete in most cases. The rate of recovery is usually related to the degree of involvement, which may extend from a few weeks to months. The greater the degree of paralysis, the longer the recovery phase.

Nursing Considerations

Nursing care is essentially supportive and is the same as that required for quadriplegia from any cause. The emphasis of care is on close observation to assess the extent of paralysis and on prevention of complications.

During the acute phase of the disease the child's condition should be carefully observed for possible difficulty in swallowing and respiratory involvement. A respirator with a cardiac monitor attached is kept on standby, and suction apparatus, tracheostomy tray, and vasoconstrictor drugs are kept available at the bedside. Vital signs and level of consciousness are monitored frequently. The child who develops respiratory dysfunction requires the same care as any child who requires mechanical ventilation and who suffers paralysis.

Throughout the recovery phase special emphasis is placed on prevention of complications, including good postural alignment, frequent change of position, and passive range of motion exercises. Children with oral and pharyngeal involvement are usually fed via a nasogastric tube to ensure adequate feeding. Bowel and bladder care is needed to avoid constipation and urine retention. Sensory impairment makes the child susceptible to burns and trophic ulcers.

Physical therapy is limited to passive range of motion exercises during the evolving phase of the disease. Later, as the disease stabilizes and recovery begins, an active physical therapy program is implemented to prevent contracture deformities and facilitate muscle recovery. This may include active exercise, gait training, and bracing.

Throughout the course of the illness, support of the child and parents is paramount. The usual rapidity of the paralysis and the long period of recovery tax the emotional reserves of all family members greatly. The parents and child benefit from repeated reassurance that recovery is occurring and from realistic information regarding the possibility of permanent disability. In the event of a residual disability, the family needs assistance in accepting and adjusting to the loss of function (see Chapter 18).

TETANUS

Tetanus, or lockjaw, is an acute, preventable, and often fatal disease caused by an exotoxin produced by the anaerobic spore-forming, gram-positive bacillus *Clostridium tetani*. The disorder is characterized by painful muscular rigidity primarily involving the masseter and neck muscles. There are four requirements for the development of tetanus: (1) presence of tetanus spores or vegetative forms of the bacillus, (2) injury to the tissues, (3) wound conditions that encourage multiplication of the organism, and (4) a susceptible host.

Tetanus spores are found in soil, dust, and the intestinal tracts of humans and animals, especially herbivorous animals. The organisms are more prevalent in rural areas but are readily carried to urban areas by the wind. The organisms are not invasive but enter the body by way of wounds, particularly a puncture wound, burn, or crushed area. They may enter through a very minor, unnoticed break in the skin, such as a thorn or needle prick, bee sting, or scratch. In the newborn, infection may occur through the umbilical cord, usually in situations in which infants are delivered in contaminated surroundings. The disease has the greatest incidence in months when persons are more involved in outdoor activities. Drug addicts are especially susceptible from poor injection technique and the use of street heroin, which is often mixed with quinine, a protoplasmic poison that favors the growth of the organism.

Pathophysiology

When conditions are favorable, the organisms proliferate and elaborate a potent exotoxin that affects the central nervous system to produce the clinical manifestations of the disease. The ideal conditions for growth of the organisms are devitalized tissues without access to air, such as wounds that have not been washed or kept clean and those that have crusted over, trapping pus beneath.

There are several forms of the disease, but the generalized form is the most common and dangerous. The incubation period for tetanus varies from 1 to 54 days but is generally less than 14 days. The more extensive the injury, the shorter the incubation period and the more severe the symptoms.

The manner of onset varies, but the initial symptoms are usually a progressive stiffness and tenderness of the muscles in the neck and jaw. Eventually all voluntary muscles are affected (see box). As the child recovers from the disease, the paroxysms become less frequent and gradually subside. Survival beyond 4 days usually indicates recovery, but complete recovery may require weeks.

The mortality rate is about 30%, but the disease is almost invariably fatal in the newborn. The incubation period is short with the appearance of symptoms 3 to 10 days following exposure. The first symptom is difficulty sucking, which progresses to total inability to suck, excessive crying, irritability, and nuchal rigidity.

Clinical Manifestations of Tetanus

- Initial symptoms
  - Progressive stiffness and tenderness of muscles in neck and jaw
  - Characteristic difficulty in opening the mouth (trismus)
  - Facial muscle spasm causes risus sardonicus (sardonic smile)
- Progressive involvement
  - Opisthotonos
  - Boardlike rigidity of abdominal and limb muscles
  - Difficulty swallowing
  - High sensitivity to external stimuli (slight noise, gentle touch, or bright light)
    - Trigger paroxysmal muscular contractions that last seconds to minutes
    - Recur with increased frequency until almost continuous
  - Laryngospasm and tetany of respiratory muscles
    - Accumulated secretions
    - Respiratory arrest
    - Atelectasis
    - Pneumonia
- Mentation unaffected
  - Patient alert
- Pain and distress are reflected in
  - Rapid pulse
  - Sweating
  - Anxious expression
- Fever usually absent or only mild

Therapeutic Management: Prevention

Preventive measures are based on the immune status of the affected child and the nature of the injury. Specific prophylactic therapy after trauma is administration of either tetanus toxoid or tetanus antitoxin. Children who have completed the immunization series (see p. 294) are given a tetanus toxoid booster prophylactically if none has been given in the prior 10 years for a clean minor wound or, if there is a heavily contaminated wound, if none has been given in the previous 5 years. Protective levels of antibody are maintained for at least 10 years; therefore passive immunity with antitoxin or tetanus immune globulin is not indicated for the fully immunized child.

The unprotected or inadequately immunized child who sustains a "tetanus-prone" wound (for example, contaminated soil, crush injury, burn, compound fracture, retained foreign body, or a wound unattended for 24 hours) should receive human tetanus immune globulin (TIG). Human tetanus immune globulin is preferred to tetanus antitoxin (TAT) because of its absence of sensitivity reactions and longer half-life. Once the toxin has bound to central nervous system tissue, antitoxin has no effect, but if the binding has taken place only peripherally, administration of human tetanus immune globulin or bovine or horse tetanus antitoxin will prevent binding in the central areas. Concurrent administration of both human tetanus immune globulin and toxoid at separate sites is recommended both to provide protection and to initiate the active immune process. Completion of active immunization is carried out according to the usual pattern.

Therapeutic Management: Treatment

The affected child is best treated in an intensive care facility where close and constant observation and equipment for monitoring and respiratory support are readily available. A quiet environment is preferred to reduce external stimuli. Neonates are placed in an open unit or Isolette to maintain a constant environmental temperature and oxygen supply.

General supportive care, including maintenance of adequate fluid and electrolyte balance and caloric intake, is indicated. Indwelling oral or nasogastric feedings are used whenever possible, but severe laryngospasm may necessitate intravenous alimentation or gastrostomy feeding. Recurrent laryngospasm or excessive accumulation of secretions may require endotracheal intubation.

Antitoxin therapy to neutralize toxins not yet bound to nervous tissue is the most specific therapy for tetanus. Human tetanus immune globulin is preferred, but, if unavailable, tetanus antitoxin is given. Antibiotics are administered to control the proliferation of the vegetative forms of the organism at the site of infection. When the child recovers, active immunization should take place, since the disease does not confer a permanent immunity.

Local care of the wound by surgical débridement and cleansing helps reduce the numbers of proliferating organisms at the site of injury. An antibacterial agent such as pHisoHex or povidone-iodine (Betadine) has proved effective. The cleansing should be repeated several times during the first 48 hours, and deep infected lacerations are usually exposed and débrided.

Sedatives or muscle relaxants are administered to help reduce muscle spasm and prevent convulsions. The most widely used is diazepam (Valium), but phenobarbital, chloral hydrate, the phenothiazines, and paraldehyde may be employed. Patients with severe tetanus and those who do not respond to other sedatives may require the administration of a neuromuscular blocking agent, usually pancuronium bromide (Pavulon) or δ-tubocurarine. Because of their paralytic effect on respiratory muscles, use of these drugs requires mechanical ventilation and constant attendance by trained personnel until muscle spasms are controlled.

Tracheostomy is often indicated and should be performed before severe respiratory distress develops. Administration of corticosteroids has met with success in some instances.

Nursing Considerations

In caring for the child with tetanus, every effort should be made to control or eliminate stimulation from sound, light, and touch. Although a darkened room is ideal, sufficient light is essential in order that the child can be carefully observed; light appears to be less irritating than vibratory or auditory stimuli. The infant or child is handled as little as possible, and extra effort is expended to avoid any sudden and/or loud noise.

Medications are administered as prescribed, and vital signs are observed and recorded at frequent intervals. The location and extent of muscle spasms and assessment of their severity are important nursing observations. Respiratory status is carefully evaluated for any signs of embarrassment, and appropriate emergency equipment is kept available at all times. Muscle relaxants and sedatives that may be prescribed can also cause respiratory depression; therefore the child must be assessed for excessive central nervous system depression. Blood gases are obtained frequently to evaluate the respiratory status. Attention to hydration and nutrition may involve monitoring an intravenous infusion, monitoring nasogastric or gastrostomy feedings, and suctioning oropharyngeal secretions when indicated.

If a potent muscle relaxant such as Pavulon is used, the total paralysis makes oral communication impossible. Therefore all the child's needs must be anticipated and procedures carefully explained beforehand. As the dose of medication is decreased, the child regains movement of the eyelids and facial muscles, which gives him some opportunity to express emotions and indicate choices through a signal system.

Nursing Tip: Communicating during Paralysis

Instructing the child to blink the lids to indicate "yes" or "no" offers a means of communication.

Although most affected children are neonates and receive the nursing care and assessment of any high-risk infant (see Chapter 9), the older child may acquire a tetanus infection. Since the child's mental status is clear, he is aware of what is happening to him and is often in a state of terror. He should not be left alone, and all efforts should be made to reduce his anxiety, which can contribute to muscular spasms. A calm and reassuring manner and sympathetic understanding can help immeasurably in getting the child through this crisis situation.

BOTULISM

Botulism is a serious food poisoning that results from ingestion of the preformed toxin produced by the anaerobic bacillus *Clostridium botulinum*. The most common source of the toxin is improperly sterilized home-canned foods. Nervous system symptoms appear abruptly about

Clinical Manifestations of Botulism

Weakness
Dizziness
Headache
Difficulty talking and speaking
Diplopia
Vomiting
Progressive, life-threatening respiratory paralysis

Infant Botulism

Constipation (a common symptom)
Generalized weakness
Decrease in spontaneous movements
Diminished or absent deep tendon reflexes
Loss of head control
Difficulty feeding
Weak cry
Reduced gag reflex
Progressive respiratory paralysis

12 to 36 hours after ingestion of contaminated food and may or may not have been preceded by acute digestive disturbance (see box).

Treatment consists of intravenous administration of botulism antitoxin and general supportive measures. Toxins vary in protein-binding capacity. Some have a relatively short half-life and do not bind to tissues firmly; therefore therapy is continued until paralysis abates. Other toxins appear to bind irreversibly to nerve endings and are therefore not amenable to neutralization. Respiratory support is often needed and should be available at the bedside, ready for use if indicated.

Infant Botulism

Infant botulism, unlike the disease in older persons, is caused by ingestion of spores or vegetative cells of *C. botulinum* and the subsequent release of the toxin from organisms colonizing the gastrointestinal tract. There appears to be no common food or drug source of the organisms; however, the *C. botulinum* organisms have been found in honey fed to affected infants.

There is wide variation in the severity of the disease, from mild constipation to progressive sequential loss of neurologic function and respiratory failure (see box). The affected infant is usually well before the onset of symptoms, and the most frequently recognized form of the disease is consistent with the "floppy infant syndrome." Botulism toxin exerts its effect by inhibiting the release of acetylcholine at the myoneural junction, thereby impairing motor activity of muscles innervated by affected nerves.

Diagnosis is made on the basis of history, physical examination, and laboratory detection of fecal toxin. Treatment consists of supportive measures, primarily respiratory and nutritional. Botulism antitoxin, used in adults and older children, is not administered to infants. Evidence indicates that the infants recover without it and its therapeutic efficacy is lacking. Furthermore, since the antitoxin is made from horse serum, it may cause serum sickness or anaphylaxis and may induce a lifelong hypersensitivity (Arnon, 1986).

Nursing Considerations

Nursing responsibilities include observing for and reporting signs of muscle impairment and providing intensive nursing care when the infant is hospitalized (see Chapter 9, Nursing care of the high-risk infant). Parental support and reassurance are important. Most infants recover when the disorder is recognized and therapy implemented. Parents should be aware that during recovery patients fatigue easily when muscular action is sustained. This has important implications for timing the resumption of feedings because of the risk of aspiration. Parents should also be advised that normal bowel action may not return for several weeks; therefore a stool softener can be beneficial. Cathartics and enemas are not advised.

Home supervision of the outpatient and education of the parents regarding possible modes of infection (such as use of honey as formula sweetener) are nursing responsibilities. An infant who is recovering from botulism must avoid contact with other infants for about 3 months or until excretion of organisms has ceased.

RHABDOMYOSARCOMA

Soft tissue sarcomas are malignant neoplasms that originate from undifferentiated mesenchymal cells in muscles, tendons, bursae, and fascia or from such cells in fibrous, connective, lymphatic, or vascular tissue. These disorders derive their name from the specific tissue(s) of origin, such as myosarcoma (*myo*—muscle). Rhabdomyosarcoma (*rhabdo*—striated) is the most common soft tissue sarcoma in children. Because striated (skeletal) muscle is found almost anywhere in the body, these tumors occur in many sites, the most common of which are the head and neck, especially the orbit.

The disease occurs in children in all age-groups but most commonly in children younger than 5 years of age. The incidence is approximately 4.4 per million for white children under age 15, but only 1.3 per million for black children in this age-group.

With current treatment protocols survival rates for children with tumors detected at all clinical stages have increased considerably. Data suggest that children who remain disease free for 2 years are probably cured; however, if relapse occurs, the prognosis for long-term survival is extremely poor (Miser and Pizzo, 1985).

Diagnostic Evaluation

The initial signs and symptoms are related to the site of the tumor and compression of adjacent organs (see box). Some tumor locations, particularly the orbit, produce symptoms early in the course of the illness and contribute

Clinical Manifestations of Rhabdomyosarcoma According to Tumor Site

Orbit
Rapidly developing unilateral proptosis
Ecchymosis of conjunctiva
Loss of extraocular movements (strabismus)

Nasopharynx
Stuffy nose (earliest sign)
Nasal obstruction—dysphagia, nasal voice (obstruction of posterior nasal conchae), serous otitis media (obstruction of eustachian tube)
Pain (sore throat and ear)
Epistaxis
Palpable neck nodes
Visible mass in oropharynx (late sign)

Paranasal Sinuses
Nasal obstruction
Local pain
Discharge
Sinusitis
Swelling

Middle Ear
Signs of chronic serous otitis media
Pain
Sanguinopurulent drainage
Facial nerve palsy

Retroperitoneal Area (usually a "silent" tumor)
Abdominal mass
Pain
Signs of intestinal or genitourinary obstruction

Perineum
Visible superficial mass
Bowel or bladder dysfunction (from tumor compression)

to rapid diagnosis and improved prognosis. Other tumors, such as those of the retroperitoneal area, produce no symptoms until they are large, invasive, and widely metastasized. Unfortunately, many of the signs and symptoms attributable to rhabdomyosarcoma are vague and frequently suggest a common childhood illness, such as "earache" or "runny nose." In some instances a primary tumor site is never identified.

Diagnosis begins with a careful examination of the head and neck area, particularly palpation of a nontender, firm, hard mass. The nasopharynx and oropharynx are inspected for any evidence of a visible mass. Radiographic studies are performed to isolate a tumor site, accompanied by chest radiographic examinations, lung tomograms, bone surveys, and bone marrow aspiration to rule out metastasis. A lumbar puncture is indicated for head and neck tumors. An excisional biopsy is performed to confirm histologic type.

Therapeutic Management

Since this tumor is highly malignant, with metastasis frequently occurring at time of diagnosis, aggressive multimodal therapy is recommended. Complete removal of the primary tumor is advocated whenever possible. However, biopsy is required only in certain tumor locations, such as those of the orbit when followed by radiation and chemotherapy. This is a fortunate change, because it avoids the devastating effects of enucleation, amputation, or pelvic exenteration.

High-dose irradiation to the primary tumor is recommended for most tumors, and chemotherapy plays a major role in treatment of all tumors. Drugs that are cytotoxic for rhabdomyosarcoma are vincristine, actinomycin D, and cyclophosphamide (collectively known as VAC), with or without adriamycin.

Nursing Considerations

The nursing responsibilities are similar to those for other types of cancer, especially the solid tumors when surgery is used. Specific objectives include (1) careful assessment for signs of the tumor, especially during well-child examinations; (2) preparation of the child and family for the multiple diagnostic tests; and (3) supportive care during each stage of multimodal therapy. The reader is urged to review Nursing considerations for leukemia in Chapter 25 for physical care of the child, and Chapter 18 for emotional support of the family in the event of a poor prognosis.

SUMMARY

Neuromuscular disease affects muscular strength or coordination, can be congenital or acquired, and may result from dysfunction or damage to the brain (e.g., cerebral palsy), spinal cord cells (e.g., Werdnig-Hoffmann disease), peripheral or cranial nerves (e.g., Guillain-Barré syndrome), myoneural junction (tetanus), or muscles (muscular dystrophy). Any of these interfere with self-care and ambulation permanently or temporarily.

The major aims of care during temporary dysfunction are preventing or coping with life-threatening complications and promoting return to normal functioning. For lifelong disability, either progressive or nonprogressive, the primary goals of care are facilitating optimum functioning within the child's limitations and promoting the best possible way of life for the child and his family.

KEY CONCEPTS

- Clinical manifestations of cerebral palsy include delayed gross motor development, abnormal motor performance, alterations of muscle tone, abnormal postures, and reflex abnormalities.
- Therapy for cerebral palsy takes into consideration the nature of the physical disability, defects associated with the disorder, and interpersonal and social influences encountered by the affected child.
- Care of the infant and child with myelomeningocele is directed toward protecting the meningeal sac, preventing infection and skin breakdown, and observing for signs of complications.
- Werdnig-Hoffmann disease is characterized by progressive weakness and wasting of skeletal muscles caused by degeneration of anterior horn cells of the spinal cord.
- Muscular dystrophies are the largest and most important cause of muscular dysfunction of childhood.
- Major complications of Duchenne muscular dystrophy include joint contractures, disuse atrophy, infections, obesity, and cardiopulmonary problems.
- Nursing care of the child with Guillain-Barré syndrome is directed toward monitoring vital signs, ensuring alignment and positioning, physical therapy, and support of child and family.
- Tetanus occurs when tetanus spores or vegetative bacilli enter a wound and multiply.
- Infant botulism results from the release of toxins from *C. botulinum* colonizing the gastrointestinal tract.
- Rhabdomyosarcoma may occur almost anywhere in the body, but the most common sites are the head and neck.

STUDY QUESTIONS AND ACTIVITIES

1. Visit a school (or class) for children with physical disabilities. Observe the methods and strategies employed to promote ambulation and self-care.
2. Contact the local branches of national organizations providing services to children with physical disabilities (e.g., the United Cerebral Palsy Association and/or the Muscular Dystrophy Association) to determine what services are available to children and their families.
3. Interview a child (or adult) with spina bifida or a family member of a person with the disorder regarding the major difficulties they have encountered or are now encountering because of their disability.
4. Interview a nurse in an intensive care unit regarding the care of children with a disorder that produces temporary respiratory paralysis (e.g., tetanus, botulism, Guillain-Barré syndrome). What kinds of support does the nurse provide for the children and their families?

REFERENCES

Arnon, S.S.: Infant botulism. In Gellis, S.S., and Kagan, B.M.: Current pediatric therapy 12, Philadelphia, 1986, W.B. Saunders Co.

Charney, E.B., and others: Management of the newborn with myelomeningocele: time for a decision-making process, Pediatrics **75:**58-64, 1985.

Cohen, F.L.: Clinical genetics in nursing practice, Philadelphia, 1984, J.B. Lippincott Co.

Miser, J., and Pizza, P.: Soft tissue sarcomas in childhood, Pediatr. Clin. North Am. **32:**779-800, 1985.

Reigel, D.H.: Spina bifida. In McLauren, R.L.: Pediatric psychology, New York, 1982, Grune & Stratton, Inc.

Whitehead, W.E., Parker, L.H., and Masek, B.J.: Biofeedback treatment of fecal incontinence in patients with myelomeningocele, Dev. Med. Child. Neurol. **23:**313-322, 1981.

BIBLIOGRAPHY

General

Bernard, B., and others: Exercise for children with physical disabilities, Issues Compr. Pediatr. Nurs. **5:**99-107, 1981.

Conway-Rutkowski, B.L.: Carini and Owens' neurological and neurosurgical nursing, ed. 8, St. Louis, 1982, The C.V. Mosby Co.

Downey, J.A., and Low, N.L., editors: The child with a disabling illness, ed. 2, Philadelphia, 1984, W.B. Saunders Co.

Hilt, N.E., and Cogburn, S.B.: Manual of orthopedics, St. Louis, 1980, The C.V. Mosby Co.

Hobdell, E.: Hypotonia in infants and children, J. Neurosurg. Nurs. **14**(8):170-172, 1982.

Lenox, A.C.: When motor nerves die, Am. J. Nurs. **83:**540-546, 1983.

Schade, J., and Passo, S.: Needs assessment of parents in pediatric ambulatory care, J. Ambulatory Care Manage. **4:**23-32, 1981.

Scheiner, A.P., and Abroms, I.F.: The practical management of the developmentally disabled child, St. Louis, 1980, The C.V. Mosby Co.

Cerebral Palsy

Barabas, G., and Taft, L.T.: The early signs and differential diagnosis of cerebral palsy, Pediatr. Ann. **15:**203-214, 1986.

Brown, M.S.: How to tell if a baby has cerebral palsy—and what to tell his parents when he does, Nursing 79 **9**(5):88-91, 1979.

Coffman, S.P.: Parents' perceptions of needs for themselves and their children in a cerebral palsy clinic, Issues Compr. Pediatr. Nurs. **6:**67-77, 1983.

Johnson, S.H.: Timmy: a victim of his parents' loving care . . . cerebral palsy, RN **45**(6):60-63, 1982.

Magill, J., and others: The self-esteem of adolescents with cerebral palsy, Am. J. Occup. Ther. **40:**402-407, 1986.

Pilon, B.H., and Smith, K.A.: A parent group for the Hispanic parents of children with severe cerebral palsy, Child. Health Care **14:**96-102, 1985.

Steele, S.: Young children with cerebral palsy: practical guidelines for care, Pediatr. Nurs. **11:**259-267, 1985.

Wolraich, M.L.: Counseling families of children with cerebral palsy, Pediatr. Ann. **15:**239-244, 1986.

Spina Bifida

Birdsall, C.: How do you teach female self-catheterization? Am. J. Nurs. **85:**1226-1227, 1985.

Clark, L.W.: The importance of touch with an anencephalic baby, MCN **7:**336-337, 1982.

Coffman, S.: Description of nursing diagnosis: alteration in bowel elimination related to neurogenic bowel in children with myelomeningocele, Issues Compr. Pediatr. Nurs. **9:**179-191, 1986.

Cohen, F.L.: Neural tube defects: epidemiology, detection, and prevention, JOGNN **16**:105-115, 1987.

Colgan, M.T.: The child with spina bifida, Am. J. Dis. Child. **135:**854-858, 1981.

Crooks, K.K., and Enrile, B.G.: Comparison of the ileal conduit and clean intermittent catheterization for myelomeningocele, Pediatrics **72:**203-206, 1983.

Jeffries, J.S., Killam, P.E., and Varni, J.W.: Behavioral management of fecal incontinence in a child with myelomeningocele, Pediatr. Nurs. **8:**267-270, 1982.

Killam, P.E., and others: Behavioral pediatric weight rehabilitation for children with myelomeningocele, MCN **8:**280-286, 1983.

Macbriar, B.R.: Self-concept of preadolescent and adolescent children with a meningomyelocele, Issues Compr. Pediatr. Nurs. **6:**1-11, 1983.

Macedo, A., and Posel, L.F.: Nursing the family after the birth of a child with spina bifida, Issues Compr. Pediatr. Nurs. **10:**55-65, 1987.

Pinyerd, B.J.: Siblings of children with myelomeningocele: examining their perceptions, MCN **12**(1):61-70, 1983.

Pressman, S.D.: Myelomeningocele: a multidisciplinary problem, J. Neurosurg. Nurs. **13:**333-336, 1981.

Richardson, K., and others: Biofeedback therapy for managing bowel incontinence caused by meningomyelocele, MCN **10:**388-392, 1985.

Sullivan-Bolyai, S., Swanson, M., and Shurtleff, D.B.: Toilet training the child with neurogenic impairment of bowel and bladder function, Issues Compr. Pediatr. Nurs. **7:**33-43, 1984.

Vigliaroto, D.: Managing bowel incontinence in children with meningomyelocele, Am. J. Nurs. **80:**105-107, 1980.

Muscular Dystrophies

Brady, M.H.: Lifelong care of the child with Duchenne muscular dystrophy, MCN **4:**227-230, 1979.

Flynn, I., Schwetz, K., and Williams, D.: Muscular dystrophy: comprehensive nursing care, Nurs. Clin. North Am. **14:**123-132, 1979.

Nursing Grand Rounds: Muscular dystrophy: a nursing point of view, Nursing 80 **10**(1):45-49, 1980.

Guillain-Barré Syndrome

Asmonds, R.J.: Guillain-Barré syndrome: helping the patient in the acute stage, Nursing 80 **10**(8):35-41, 1980.

Jemison-Smith, P., and Hubbell, H.: Guillain-Barré syndrome, Crit. Care Update **10**(6):12-16, 1983.

McBride, M., and Sack, W.: Emotional management of children with respiratory failure in the intensive care unit: a case study, Heart Lung **9:**98-100, 1980.

Mills, N., and Plasterer, H.H.: Guillain-Barré syndrome: a framework for nursing care, Nurs. Clin. North Am. **15:**257-264, 1980.

Samonds, R.J.: Guillain-Barré syndrome: helping the patient in the acute stage, Nursing 80 **10**(8):35-41, 1980.

Samonds, R.J.: Guillain-Barraé syndrome: the acute stage, Crit. Care Update **8**(11):38-44, 1981.

Smith, D.: From student nurse to paralyzed patient, Imprint **26:**40-42, 1979.

Tetanus and Botulism

Miller, D.K.: The challenge of infant botulism, MCN **7:**180-183, 1982.

Research review: Tetanus: controlled, but still hazardous, Immunol. Update **2**(1):2-4, 1980.

Roderick, M.A.: Botulism, Nursing 82 **12**(6):59, 1982.

Roderick, M.A.: Tetanus, Nursing 82 **12**(7):63, 1982.

Sebilia, A.J.: "When was your last tetanus shot?" RN **47**(8):18-24, 1985.

Appendixes

Family Assessment

Family APGAR Questionnaire

PART I

The following questions have been designed to help us better understand you and your family.* You should feel free to ask questions about any item in the questionnaire.

The space for comments should be used when you wish to give additional information or if you wish to discuss the way the question is applied to your family. Please try to answer all questions.

Family is defined as the individual(s) with whom you usually live. If you live alone, your "family" consists of persons with whom you now have the strongest emotional ties.

For each question, check only one box

	ALMOST ALWAYS	SOME OF THE TIME	HARDLY EVER
I am satisfied that I can turn to my family for help when something is troubling me.	☐	☐	☐
I am satisfied with the way my family talks over things with me and shares problems with me.	☐	☐	☐
I am satisfied that my family accepts and supports my wishes to take on new activities or directions.	☐	☐	☐
I am satisfied with the way my family expresses affection and responds to my emotions, such as anger, sorrow, and love.	☐	☐	☐
I am satisfied with the way my family and I share time together.	☐	☐	☐

Comments: ______________________________ (after each question)

A

Scoring: The patient checks one of three choices which are scored as follows: "Almost always" (2 points), "Some of the time" (1) point, or "Hardly ever" (0). The scores for each of the five questions are then totaled. A score of 7 to 10 suggests a highly functional family. A score of 4 to 6 suggests a moderately dysfunctional family. A score of 0 to 3 suggests a severely dysfunctional family.

*According to which member of the family is being interviewed the nurse may substitute for the word "family" either spouse, significant other, parents, or children.

FIG. A-1 Family APGAR questionnaire. **A,** Part I. (Adapted from Smilkstein, G.: The Family APGAR: a proposal for a family function test and its use by physicians, J. Fam. Pract. **6**(6):1231-1239, 1978.)

Family APGAR Questionnaire

PART II

Who lives in your home?* List the persons according to their relationship to you (for example, spouse, significant other,† child, or friend).

RELATIONSHIP	AGE	SEX

Check the column that best describes how you now get along with each member of the family listed.

WELL	FAIRLY	POORLY

If you don't live with your own family, list the persons to whom you turn for help most frequently. List according to relationship (for example, family member, friend, associate at work, or neighbor).

RELATIONSHIP	AGE	SEX

Check the column that best describes how you now get along with each person listed.

WELL	FAIRLY	POORLY

*If you have established your own family, consider your "home" as the place where you live with your spouse, children, or "significant other" (see next footnote for definition): otherwise, consider home as your place of origin, for example, the place where your parents or those who raised you live.

†Significant other is the partner you live with in a physically and emotionally nurturing relationship but to whom you are not married.

B

FIG. A-1, cont'd B, Part II.

APPENDIX B

Patterns of Inheritance

Glossary

congenital The condition is present at birth. The disorder may be brought about by genetic causes, nongenetic causes, or a combination of these.

familial A disorder that "runs in families" or is present in more members of a family than would be expected by chance.

genetic The disorder is caused by a single harmful gene, by several genes, or by a deviation in chromosome number or structure. It may or may not be apparent at birth.

genotype The genetic constitution that determines the physical and chemical characteristics of an individual.

heterozygous Having dissimilar genes at a given position (locus) on a pair of chromosomes.

homozygous Having the same genes at a given position (locus) on a pair of chromosomes.

inherited (heritable, hereditary) Synonymous with genetic, although in the past often used to describe a disorder that appeared in parent and offspring over several generations.

mutation Structural or chemical alteration in genetic material which, when changed, remains unchanged and is transmitted to future generations. Mutations usually occur naturally (*spontaneous*), or can be *induced* by a variety of external agents, or *mutagens,* including temperature, certain chemicals, and radiation.

phenotype The physical or chemical characteristics of an individual, produced by the interaction of the environment on the genotype.

Modifications of Basic Inheritance Patterns

penetrance The regularity with which an inherited trait is manifest in the person who carries the gene. When a gene produces its effect on the phenotype each time it is present in the genotype, it is said to be *fully penetrant* or to exhibit *complete penetrance.* For example, achondroplasia (a form of dwarfism) is always evident whenever the gene is present. If a trait is not recognized in a person who carries the responsible gene, it is said to be *nonpenetrant* in that individual. This phenomenon accounts for what appears to be skipped generations.

variable expressivity The degree of severity of, or the variability in, the manifestations seen in persons of a particular genotype. For instance, polydactyly can be expressed as any number of extra digits, or the extra digits may be fingers in one generation and toes in another. The severity of a disorder may be so mild as to be almost undetected or so severe that the affected individual is totally incapacitated.

pleiotropy The multiple, different, and seemingly unrelated effects associated with a particular disorder; the varied clinical features that constitute a syndrome. For example, Marfan syndrome, a disorder of the elastic fibers of connective tissue, may be manifest in an individual by any or all of the symptoms associated with it—aortic aneurysm, dislocation of the optic lens, or any of a number of skeletal deformities.

linkage Some genes are located too closely together on a chromosome, so that they segregate and migrate together during cell division, and therefore, the characteristics they produce always appear together in the phenotype.

heterogeneity The same or similar manifestations that result from (1) different mutant genes at the same location on a chromosome or (2) mutant genes at different locations on a chromosome (such as the hemophilias that produce defects in coagulation and the muscular dystrophies that produce muscular weakness but which exhibit different inheritance patterns).

		Affected parent	
	Gametes	A	a
Normal parent	a	A a Affected	a a Normal
	a	A a Affected	a a Normal

FIG. B-1 Possible offspring of mating between normal parent, aa, and parent with an autosomal-dominant trait, Aa.

Autosomal dominant inheritance. Characteristics of a condition caused by a dominant gene on an autosome include the following (Fig. B-1):

1. Males and females are affected with equal frequency.
2. Affected individuals will have an affected parent (unless the condition is caused by a fresh mutation).
3. Half the children of a heterozygous affected parent will possess the defective gene, although it may be nonpenetrant.
4. Unaffected children of affected parents will have unaffected children (unless the gene is nonpenetrant).

Autosomal recessive inheritance. Characteristics of a condition caused by a recessive gene on an autosome include the following (Fig. B-2):

1. Males and females are affected with equal frequency.
2. Affected individuals will have unaffected parents who are heterozygous for the trait.
3. There is a one in four chance that any child of two unaffected heterozygous parents will be affected.
4. Two affected parents will have affected children exclusively.
5. Affected individuals married to unaffected individuals will have normal children, all of whom will be carriers.
6. There is usually no evidence of the trait in previous generations—a negative family history.

		Heterozygous parent A/a	
	Gametes	A	a
Heterozygous parent A/a	A	AA Normal	Aa Carrier
	a	Aa Carrier	aa Affected

FIG. B-2 Possible offspring of mating between two parents with a recessive gene, a, on an autosome.

X-linked dominant inheritance. Characteristics of a condition caused by a dominant gene on an X chromosome include the following (Fig. B-3):

1. Affected individuals will have an affected parent.
2. All the daughters but none of the sons of an affected male will be affected.
3. Half the sons and half the daughters of an affected female will be affected.
4. Normal children of an affected parent will have normal offspring.
5. There are no carriers.
6. The inheritance pattern shows a positive family history.

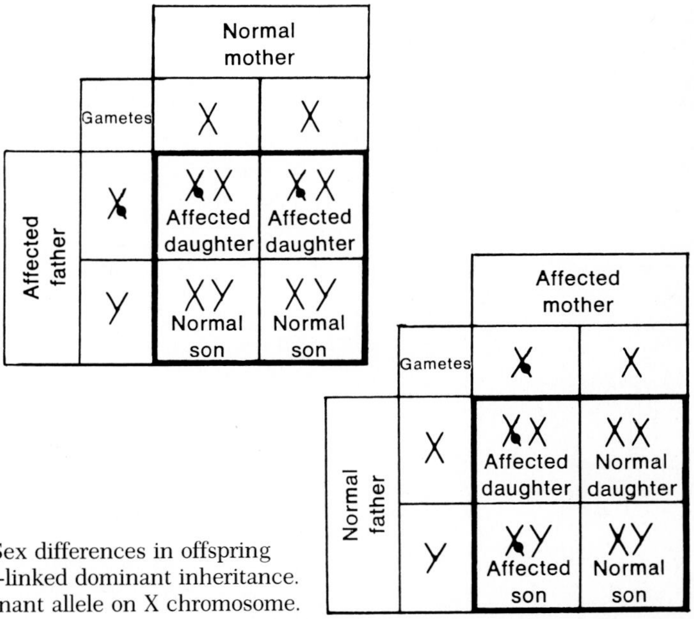

FIG. B-3 Sex differences in offspring ratios in X-linked dominant inheritance. ● = Dominant allele on X chromosome.

X-linked recessive inheritance. Characteristics of a disorder caused by a recessive gene on the X chromosome include the following (Fig. B-4):

1. Affected individuals are principally males.
2. Affected individuals will have unaffected parents (except in the rare possibility that the father is affected and the mother is a carrier).
3. Half of the female siblings of an affected male will be carriers of the trait.
4. Unaffected male siblings of an affected male cannot transmit the disorder.
5. Sons of an affected male are unaffected.
6. Daughters of an affected male are carriers.
7. The unaffected male children of a carrier female do not transmit the disorder.

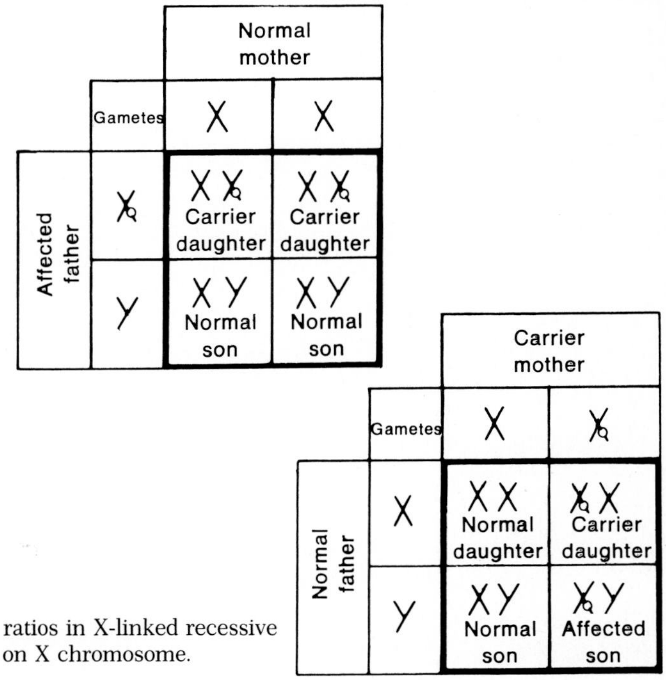

FIG. B-4 Differences in offspring ratios in X-linked recessive inheritance. ○ = Recessive allele on X chromosome.

APPENDIX C

Developmental Assessment

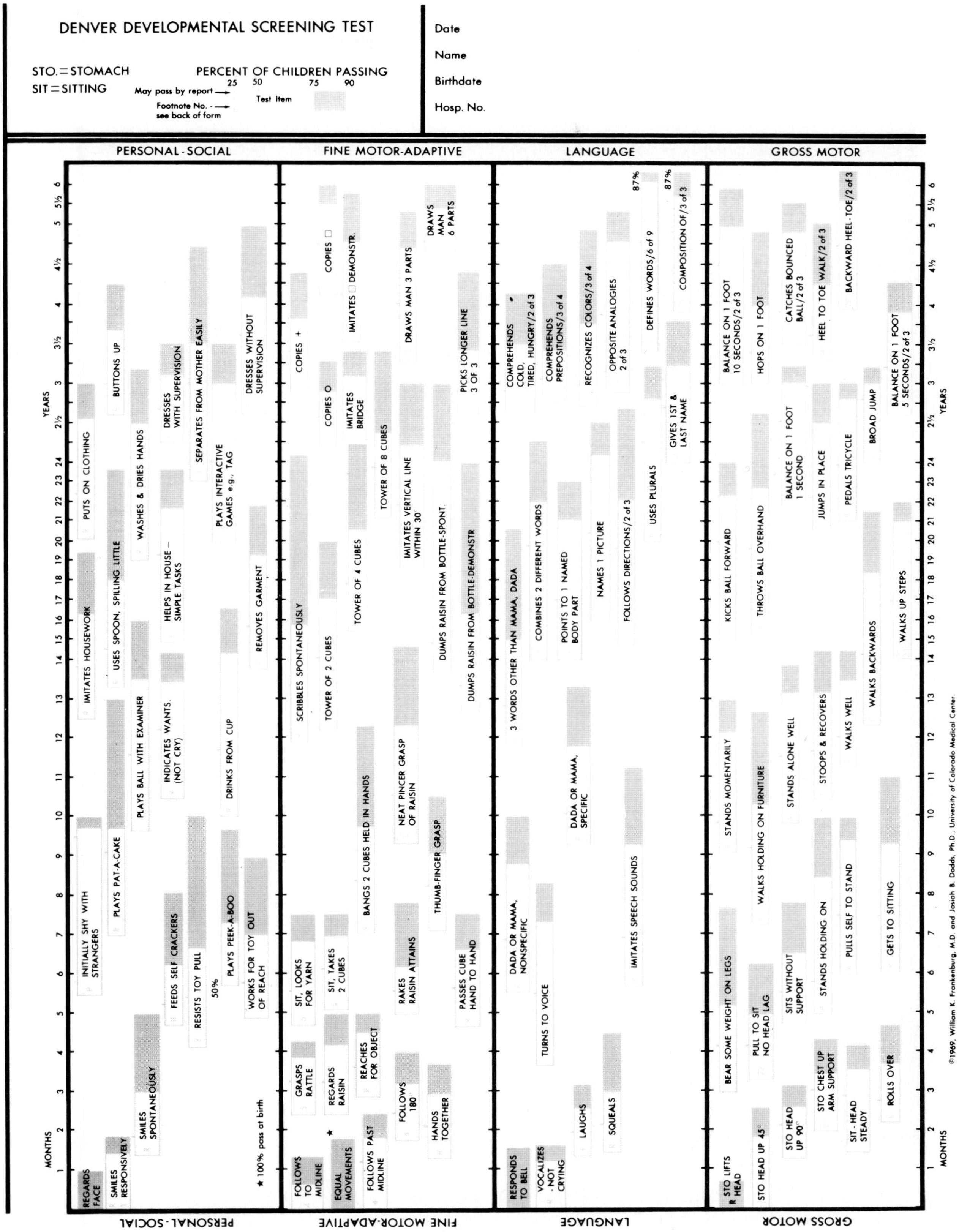

FIG. C-1 A, Denver Developmental Screening Test. (From W.K. Frankenburg and J.B. Dodds, University of Colorado Medical Center, 1969.)

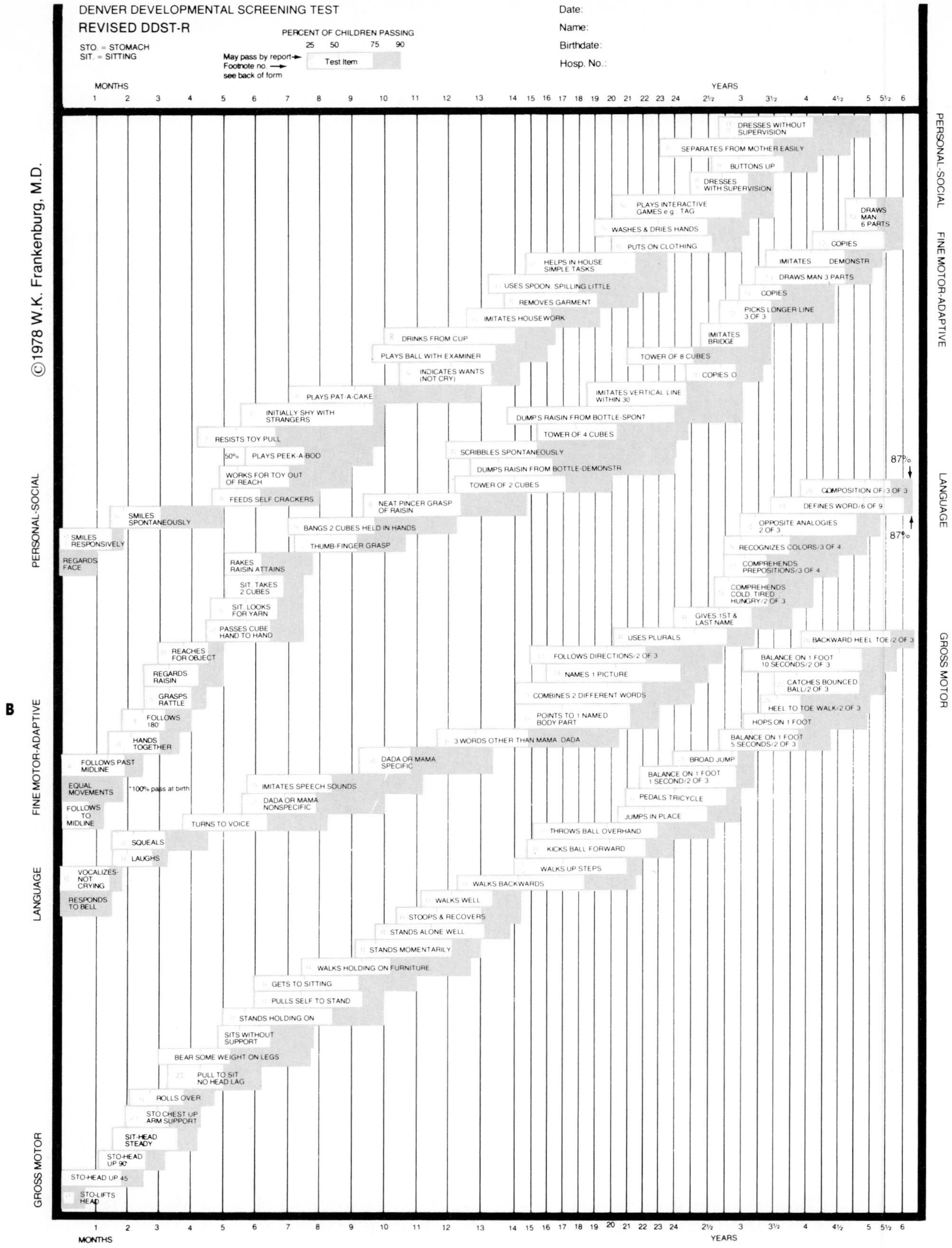

FIG. C-1, cont'd B, DDST revised (DDST-R). Resembling a growth curve, this form places items at lowest age level starting at bottom left and progresses upward to right with increasing age. (**B** from Frankenburg, W.K., Sciarillo, W., and Burgess, D.: The newly abbreviated and revised Denver Developmental Screening Test, J. Pediatr. **99**[6]:995-999, 1981.)

DATE:
NAME:
DIRECTIONS BIRTHDATE:
HOSP. NO.:

1. Try to get child to smile by smiling, talking or waving to him. Do not touch him.
2. When child is playing with toy, pull it away from him. Pass if he resists.
3. Child does not have to be able to tie shoes or button in the back.
4. Move yarn slowly in an arc from one side to the other, about 6" above child's face. Pass if eyes follow 90° to midline. (Past midline; 180°)
5. Pass if child grasps rattle when it is touched to the backs or tips of fingers.
6. Pass if child continues to look where yarn disappeared or tries to see where it went. Yarn should be dropped quickly from sight from tester's hand without arm movement.
7. Pass if child picks up raisin with any part of thumb and a finger.
8. Pass if child picks up raisin with the ends of thumb and index finger using an over hand approach.

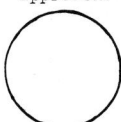

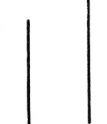

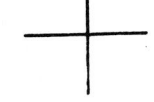

9. Pass any enclosed form. Fail continuous round motions.
10. Which line is longer? (Not bigger.) Turn paper upside down and repeat. (3/3 or 5/6)
11. Pass any crossing lines.
12. Have child copy first. If failed, demonstrate

When giving items 9, 11 and 12, do not name the forms. Do not demonstrate 9 and 11.

13. When scoring, each pair (2 arms, 2 legs, etc.) counts as one part.
14. Point to picture and have child name it. (No credit is given for sounds only.)

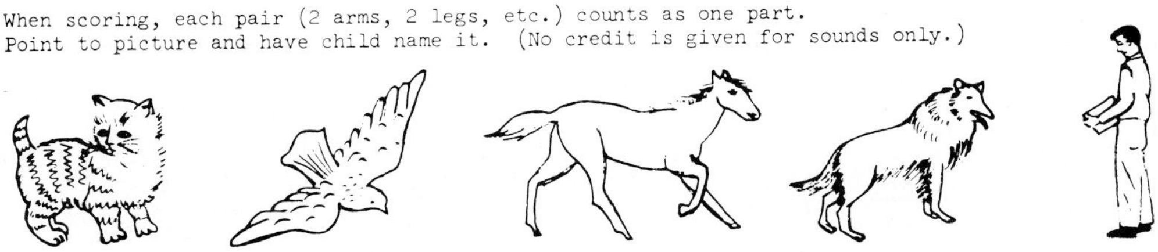

C

15. Tell child to: Give block to Mommie; put block on table; put block on floor. Pass 2 of 3. (Do not help child by pointing, moving head or eyes.)
16. Ask child: What do you do when you are cold? ..hungry? ..tired? Pass 2 of 3.
17. Tell child to: Put block <u>on</u> table; <u>under</u> table; <u>in front</u> of chair, <u>behind</u> chair. Pass 3 of 4. (Do not help child by pointing, moving head or eyes.)
18. Ask child: If fire is hot, ice is ?; Mother is a woman, Dad is a ?; a horse is big, a mouse is ?. Pass 2 of 3.
19. Ask child: What is a ball? ..lake? ..desk? ..house? ..banana? ..curtain? ..ceiling? ..hedge? ..pavement? Pass if defined in terms of use, shape, what it is made of or general category (such as banana is fruit, not just yellow). Pass 6 of 9.
20. Ask child: What is a spoon made of? ..a shoe made of? ..a door made of? (No other objects may be substituted.) Pass 3 of 3.
21. When placed on stomach, child lifts chest off table with support of forearms and/or hands.
22. When child is on back, grasp his hands and pull him to sitting. Pass if head does not hang back.
23. Child may use wall or rail only, not person. May not crawl.
24. Child must throw ball overhand 3 feet to within arm's reach of tester.
25. Child must perform standing broad jump over width of test sheet. (8-1/2 inches)
26. Tell child to walk forward, → heel within 1 inch of toe. Tester may demonstrate. Child must walk 4 consecutive steps, 2 out of 3 trials.
27. Bounce ball to child who should stand 3 feet away from tester. Child must catch ball with hands, not arms, 2 out of 3 trials.
28. Tell child to walk backward, ← toe within 1 inch of heel. Tester may demonstrate. Child must walk 4 consecutive steps, 2 out of 3 trials.

<u>DATE AND BEHAVIORAL OBSERVATIONS</u> (how child feels at time of test, relation to tester, attention span, verbal behavior, self-confidence, etc,):

FIG. C-1, cont'd C, Directions for numbered items of testing form. (From W.K. Frankenburg and J.B. Dodds, University of Colorado Medical Center, 1969.)

A

DENVER ARTICULATION SCREENING EXAM
for children 2 1/2 to 6 years of age

Instructions: Have child repeat each word after you. Circle the underlined sounds that he pronounces correctly. Total correct sounds is the Raw Score. Use charts on reverse side to score results.

NAME

HOSP. NO.

ADDRESS ______________________

Date: __________ Child's Age:________ Examiner: ____________________ Raw Score:_________
Percentile:________ Intelligibility:______________ Result:______________________

1. table	6. zipper	11. sock	16. wagon	21. leaf
2. shirt	7. grapes	12. vacuum	17. gum	22. carrot
3. door	8. flag	13. yarn	18. house	
4. trunk	9. thumb	14. mother	19. pencil	
5. jumping	10. toothbrush	15. twinkle	20. fish	

Intelligibility: (circle one) 1. Easy to understand 3. Not understandable
2. Understandable 1/2 the time. 4. Can't evaluate

Comments:

Date: __________ Child's Age:___________ Examiner:____________________ Raw Score ________
Percentile:__________Intelligibility:______________ Result:______________________

1. table	6. zipper	11. sock	16. wagon	21. leaf
2. shirt	7. grapes	12. vacuum	17. gum	22. carrot
3. door	8. flag	13. yarn	18. house	
4. trunk	9. thumb	14. mother	19. pencil	
5. jumping	10. toothbrush	15. twinkle	20. fish	

Intelligibility: (circle one) 1. Easy to understand 3. Not understandable
2. Understandable 1/2 the time. 4. Can't evaluate

Comments:

Date: ___________ Child's Age: ________ Examiner:__________________ Raw Score__________
Percentile: ___________ Intelligibility:_____________ Result:______________________

1. table	6. zipper	11. sock	16. wagon	21. leaf
2. shirt	7. grapes	12. vacuum	17. gum	22. carrot
3. door	8. flag	13. yarn	18. house	
4. trunk	9. thumb	14. mother	19. pencil	
5. jumping	10. toothbrush	15. twinkle	20. fish	

Intelligibility: (circle one) 1. Easy to understand 3. Not understandable
2. Understandable 1/2 the time. 4. Can't evaluate

FIG. C-2 A, Denver Articulation Screening Examination for children 2½ to 6 years of age. (From A.F. Drumwright, University of Colorado Medical Center, 1971.)

To score DASE words: Note Raw Score for child's performance. Match raw score line (extreme left of chart) with column representing child's age (to the closest previous age group). Where raw score line and age column meet number in that square denotes percentile rank of child's performance when compared to other children that age. Percentiles above heavy line are ABNORMAL percentiles, below heavy line are NORMAL.

PERCENTILE RANK

Raw Score	2.5 yr.	3.0	3.5	4.0	4.5	5.0	5.5	6 years
2	1							
3	2							
4	5							
5	9							
6	16							
7	23							
8	31	2						
9	37	4	1					
10	42	6	2					
11	48	7	4					
12	54	9	6	1	1			
13	58	12	9	2	3	1	1	
14	62	17	11	5	4	2	2	
15	68	23	15	9	5	3	2	
16	75	31	19	12	5	4	3	
17	79	38	25	15	6	6	4	
18	83	46	31	19	8	7	4	
19	86	51	38	24	10	9	5	1
20	89	58	45	30	12	11	7	3
21	92	65	52	36	15	15	9	4
22	94	72	58	43	18	19	12	5
23	96	77	63	50	22	24	15	7
24	97	82	70	58	29	29	20	15
25	99	87	78	66	36	34	26	17
26	99	91	84	75	46	43	34	24
27		94	89	82	57	54	44	34
28		96	94	88	70	68	59	47
29		98	98	94	84	84	77	68
30		100	100	100	100	100	100	100

To Score intelligibility:

	NORMAL	ABNORMAL
2 1/2 years	Understandable 1/2 the time, or, "easy"	Not Understandable
3 years and older	Easy to understand	Understandable 1/2 time Not understandable

Test Result: 1. NORMAL on Dase and Intelligibility = NORMAL

2. ABNORMAL on Dase and/or Intelligibility = ABNORMAL

* If abnormal on initial screening rescreen within 2 weeks. If abnormal again child should be referred for complete speech evaluation.

B

FIG. C-2 cont'd B, Percentile rank. (From A.F. Drumwright, University of Colorado Medical Center, 1971.)

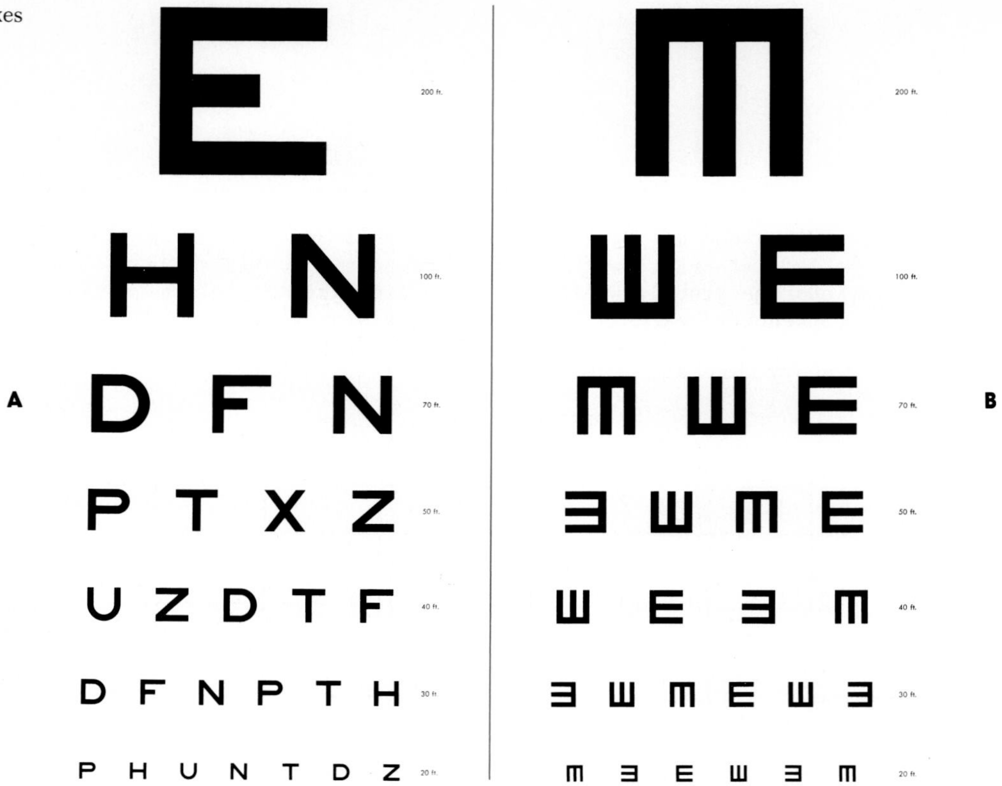

FIG. C-3 Snellen Chart. **A,** Letter (alphabet) chart. **B,** Symbol E chart. (From National Society to Prevent Blindness, Inc., New York.)

DIRECTIONS FOR SNELLEN SCREENING*

Preparation

1. Hang the Snellen chart on a light-colored wall so that the 20- to 30-foot lines are at eye level when children 6 to 12 years old are tested in the standing position.
2. Secure the chart to the wall with double-stick tape on the back side at all four corners. If the chart must be reversed for use of the letter or E chart, secure it at the top and bottom with tacks. Make sure that the chart does not swing when in place.
3. The illumination intensity on the chart should be 10 to 30 footcandles, without any glare from windows or light fixtures. The illumination should be checked with a light meter.
4. Mark an exact 20-foot distance from the chart. Mark the floor with a piece of tape or "footprints" positioned so that the heels touch the 20-foot line.

Procedure

1. Place the child at the 20-foot mark, with the heel edging the line if the child is standing or with the back of the chair placed at the marker if the child is seated.
2. If the E chart is used, accustom the child to identifying which direction the "legs of the E" are pointing. Use a demonstration E card for this purpose.
3. Teach the child to use the occluder to cover one eye. Instruct him to keep both eyes open during the test. Provide a clean cover care for each child and then discard after use.
4. If the child wears glasses, test only with glasses on.
5. Test both eyes together, then right eye, then left eye.
6. Begin with the 40- or 30-foot line and proceed with test to include the 20-foot line.
7. With the child suspected of low vision, begin with the 200-foot line and proceed until the child can no longer correctly read three out of four or four out of six symbols on a line.
8. Use covers on the Snellen chart to expose only one symbol or one line at a time. When screening kindergarten or older children, expose one line but use a pointer to point to one symbol at a time.

*Modified from recommendations in National Society to Prevent Blindness: Children's eye health guide, 1982, New York, The Society.

Recording and Referral

1. Record the last line the child read correctly (three out of four or four out of six symbols).
2. Record visual acuity as a fraction. The numerator represents the distance from the chart, and the denominator represents the last line read correctly. For example, 20/30 means that the child read the 30-foot line at a 20-foot distance.
3. Observe the child's eyes during the testing and record any evidence of squinting, head tilting, thrusting the head forward, excessive blinking, tearing, or redness.
4. Only make referrals after a second screening has been made on children who are potential candidates for referral.
5. Children should be referred for a complete eye examination according to the instructions on p. 146.

Lit. 217

DENVER EYE SCREENING TEST

Name:
Hospital No.:
Ward:
Address:

Vision Tests	1ST SCREENING: DATE: Right Eye Normal	Right Eye Abnormal	Right Eye Untestable	Left Eye Normal	Left Eye Abnormal	Left Eye Untestable	RESCREENING: DATE: Right Eye Normal	Right Eye Abnormal	Right Eye Untestable	Left Eye Normal	Left Eye Abnormal	Left Eye Untestable
1. "E" (3 years and above—3 to 5 trials)	3P	3F	U	3P	3F	U	3P	3F	U	3P	3F	U
2. Picture card (2 1/2 - 2 11/12 yrs.—3 to 5 trials)	3P	3F	U	3P	3F	U	3P	3F	U	3P	3F	U
3. Fixation (6 months - 2 5/12 years)	P	F	U	P	F	U	P	F	U	P	F	U
4. Squinting		yes			yes			yes			yes	

Tests for Non-Straight Eyes	1st Screening: Normal	Abnormal	Untestable	Rescreening: Normal	Abnormal	Untestable
1. Do your child's eyes turn in or out, or are they ever not straight?	NO	YES	U	NO	YES	U
2. Cover Test	P	F	U	P	F	U
3. Pupillary Light Reflex	P	F	U	P	F	U

Total Test Rating (Both Eyes)	1st Screening	Rescreening
Normal (passed vision test plus no squint, plus passed 2/3 tests for non-straight eyes)	Normal	Normal
Abnormal (abnormal on any vision test, squinting or 2 of 3 procedures for non-straight eyes)	Abnormal	Abnormal
Untestable (untestable on any vision test or untestable on 2/3 tests for non-straight eyes)	Untestable	Untestable
Future Rescreening Appointment for Total Test Rating (Abnormal or Untestable)	Date:	Date:

FIG. C-4 Denver Eye Screening Test. (From W.K. Frankenburg and J.B. Dobbs, University of Colorado Medical Center, 1969.)

APPENDIX D

Growth Measurements

Height and Weight Measurements for Boys

	Height by Percentiles						Weight by Percentiles					
	5		50		95		5		50		95	
Age*	cm	Inches	cm	Inches	cm	Inches	kg	lb	kg	lb	kg	lb
Birth	46.4	18¼	50.5	20	54.4	21½	2.54	5½	3.27	7¼	4.15	9¼
3 months	56.7	22¼	61.1	24	65.4	25¾	4.43	9¾	5.98	13¼	7.37	16¼
6 months	63.4	25	67.8	26¾	72.3	28½	6.20	13¾	7.85	17¼	9.46	20¾
9 months	68.0	26¾	72.3	28½	77.1	30¼	7.52	16½	9.18	20¼	10.93	24
1	71.7	28¼	76.1	30	81.2	32	8.43	18½	10.15	22½	11.99	26½
1½	77.5	30½	82.4	32½	88.1	34¾	9.59	21¼	11.47	25¼	13.44	29½
2†	82.5	32½	86.8	34¼	94.4	37¼	10.49	23¼	12.34	27¼	15.50	34¼
2½†	85.4	33½	90.4	35½	97.8	38½	11.27	24¾	13.52	29¾	16.61	36½
3	89.0	35	94.9	37¼	102.0	40¼	12.05	26½	14.62	32¼	17.77	39¼
3½	92.5	36½	99.1	39	106.1	41¾	12.84	28¼	15.68	34½	18.98	41¾
4	95.8	37¾	102.9	40½	109.9	43¼	13.64	30	16.69	36¾	20.27	44¾
4½	98.9	39	106.6	42	113.5	44¾	14.45	31¾	17.69	39	21.63	47¾
5	102.0	40¼	109.9	43¼	117.0	46	15.27	33¾	18.67	41¼	23.09	51
6	107.7	42½	116.1	45¾	123.5	48½	16.93	37¼	20.69	45½	26.34	58
7	113.0	44½	121.7	48	129.7	51	18.64	41	22.85	50¼	30.12	66½
8	118.1	46½	127.0	50	135.7	53½	20.40	45	25.30	55¾	34.51	76
9	122.9	48½	132.2	52	141.8	55¾	22.25	49	28.13	62	39.58	87¼
10	127.7	50¼	137.5	54¼	148.1	58¼	24.33	53¾	31.44	69¼	45.27	99¾
11	132.6	52¼	143.3	56½	154.9	61	26.80	59	35.30	77¾	51.47	113½
12	137.6	54¼	149.7	59	162.3	64	29.85	65¾	39.78	87¾	58.09	128
13	142.9	56¼	156.5	61½	169.8	66¾	33.64	74¼	44.95	99	65.02	143¼
14	148.8	58½	163.1	64¼	176.7	69½	38.22	84¼	50.77	112	72.13	159
15	155.2	61	169.0	66½	181.9	71½	43.11	95	56.71	125	79.12	174½
16	161.1	63½	173.5	68¼	185.4	73	47.74	105¼	62.10	137	85.62	188¾
17	164.9	65	176.2	69¼	187.3	73¾	51.50	113½	66.31	146¼	91.31	201¼
18	165.7	65¼	176.8	69½	187.6	73¾	53.97	119	68.88	151¾	95.76	211

Modified from National Center for Health Statistics (NCHS), Health Resources Administration, Department of Health, Education and Welfare, Hyattsville, MD. Conversion of metric data to approximate inches and pounds by Ross Laborartories.

*Years unless otherwise indicated

†Height data include some recumbent length measurements, which make values slightly higher than if all measurements had been of stature (standing height).

Height and Weight Measurements for Girls

	Height by Percentiles						Weight by Percentiles					
	5		50		95		5		50		95	
Age*	cm	Inches	cm	Inches	cm	Inches	kg	lb	kg	lb	kg	lb
Birth	45.4	17¾	49.9	19¾	52.9	20¾	2.36	5¼	3.23	7	3.81	8½
3 months	55.4	21¾	59.5	23½	63.4	25	4.18	9¼	5.4	12	6.74	14¾
6 months	61.8	24¼	65.9	26	70.2	27¾	5.79	12¾	7.21	16	8.73	19¼
9 months	66.1	26	70.4	27¾	75.0	29½	7.0	15½	8.56	18¾	10.17	22½
1	69.8	27½	74.3	29¼	79.1	31¼	7.84	17¼	9.53	21	11.24	24¾
1½	76.0	30	80.9	31¾	86.1	34	8.92	19¾	10.82	23¾	12.76	28¼
2†	81.6	32¼	86.8	34¼	93.6	36¾	9.95	22	11.8	26	14.15	31¼
2½†	84.6	33¼	90.0	35½	96.6	38	10.8	23¾	13.03	28¾	15.76	34¾
3	88.3	34¾	94.1	37	100.6	39½	11.61	25½	14.1	31	17.22	38
3½	91.7	36	97.9	38½	104.5	41¼	12.37	27¼	15.07	33¼	18.59	41
4	95.0	37½	101.6	40	108.3	42¾	13.11	29	15.96	35¼	19.91	44
4½	98.1	38½	105.0	41¼	112.0	44	13.83	30½	16.81	37	21.24	46¾
5	101.1	39¾	108.4	42¾	115.6	45½	14.55	32	17.66	39	22.62	49¾
6	106.6	42	114.6	45	122.7	48¼	16.05	35½	19.52	43	25.75	56¾
7	111.8	44	120.6	47½	129.5	51	17.71	39	21.84	48¼	29.68	65½
8	116.9	46	126.4	49¾	136.2	53½	19.62	43¼	24.84	54¾	34.71	76½
9	122.1	48	132.2	52	142.9	56¼	21.82	48	28.46	62¾	40.64	89½
10	127.5	50¼	138.3	54½	149.5	58¾	24.36	53¾	32.55	71¾	47.17	104
11	133.5	52½	144.8	57	156.2	61½	27.24	60	36.95	81½	54.0	119
12	139.8	55	151.5	59¾	162.7	64	30.52	67¼	41.53	91½	60.81	134
13	145.2	57¼	157.1	61¾	168.1	66¼	34.14	75¼	46.1	101¾	67.3	148¼
14	148.7	58½	160.4	63¼	171.3	67½	37.76	83¼	50.28	110¾	73.08	161
15	150.5	59¼	161.8	63¾	172.8	68	40.99	90¼	53.68	118¼	77.78	171½
16	151.6	59¾	162.4	64	173.3	68¼	43.41	95¾	55.89	123¼	80.99	178½
17	152.7	60	163.1	64¼	173.5	68¼	44.74	98¾	56.69	125	82.46	181¾
18	153.6	60½	163.7	64½	173.6	68¼	45.26	99¾	56.62	124¾	82.47	181¾

Modified from National Center for Health Statistics, Health Resources Administration, Department of Health, Education and Welfare, Hyattsville, MD. Conversion of metric data to approximate inches and pounds by Ross Laboratories.

*Years unless otherwise indicated.

†Height data include some recumbent length measurements, which make values slightly higher than if all measurements had been of stature.

Growth Standards of Healthy Chinese Children and Adolescents (Urban)*

	Boys				Girls			
Age (months or years)	Weight (kg)	Height (cm)	Head Circumference (cm)	Chest Circumference (cm)	Weight (kg)	Height (cm)	Head Circumference (cm)	Chest Circumference (cm)
Birth	3.27	50.6	34.3	32.8	3.17	50.0	33.7	32.6
1 mo	4.97	56.5	38.1	37.9	4.64	55.5	37.3	36.9
2 mo	5.95	59.6	39.7	40.0	5.49	58.4	38.7	38.9
3 mo	6.73	62.3	41.0	41.3	6.23	60.9	40.0	40.3
4 mo	7.32	64.4	42.0	42.3	6.69	62.9	41.0	41.1
5 mo	7.70	65.9	42.9	42.9	7.19	64.5	41.9	41.9
6 mo	8.22	68.1	43.9	43.8	7.62	66.7	42.8	42.7
8 mo	8.71	70.6	44.9	44.7	8.14	69.0	43.7	43.4
10 mo	9.14	72.9	45.7	45.4	8.57	71.4	44.5	44.2
12 mo	9.66	75.6	46.3	46.1	9.04	74.1	45.2	45.0
15 mo	10.15	78.3	46.8	46.8	9.54	76.9	45.6	45.8
18 mo	10.67	80.7	47.3	47.6	10.08	79.4	46.2	46.6
21 mo	11.18	83.0	47.8	48.3	10.56	81.7	46.7	47.3
24 mo	11.95	86.5	48.2	49.2	11.37	85.3	47.1	48.2
2½ yr	12.84	90.4	48.8	50.2	12.28	89.3	47.7	49.0
3 yr	13.63	93.8	49.1	50.8	13.1	92.8	48.1	49.8
3½ yr	14.45	97.2	49.4	51.5	14.0	96.3	48.5	50.5
4 yr	15.26	100.8	49.7	52.2	14.89	100.1	48.9	51.2
4½ yr	16.07	103.9	50.0	53.0	15.63	103.1	49.1	51.8
5 yr	16.88	107.2	50.2	53.6	16.46	106.5	49.4	52.5
5½ yr	17.65	110.1	50.5	54.4	17.18	109.2	49.6	53.0
6 yr	19.25	114.7	50.8	55.6	18.67	113.9	50.0	54.2
7 yr	21.01	120.6	51.1	57.1	20.35	119.3	50.2	55.5
8 yr	23.08	125.3	51.4	58.8	22.43	124.6	50.6	57.1
9 yr	25.33	130.6	51.7	60.8	24.57	129.5	50.9	58.6
10 yr	27.15	134.4	51.9	62.0	27.05	134.8	51.3	60.7
11 yr	30.13	139.2	52.3	64.3	30.51	140.6	51.7	63.5
12 yr	33.05	144.2	52.7	66.5	34.82	146.6	52.3	67.2
13 yr	36.90	149.3	53.0	68.9	38.52	150.7	52.8	70.3
14 yr	42.03	156.5	53.5	72.4	42.26	153.7	53.1	73.3
15 yr	46.91	162.0	54.3	76.0	45.37	155.5	53.4	75.6
16 yr	50.90	165.6	54.9	78.8	47.43	156.8	53.8	76.6
17 yr	53.11	167.7	55.2	80.8	48.57	157.4	53.9	77.9

Modified from Practical Pediatrics; edited by Peking Children's Hospital, 1979.

*Measurements of rural Chinese children are slightly lower.

NOTE: A comparison of the average growth of American and Chinese children demonstrates than on the standard NCHS growth charts the mean height and weight for Chinese children fall in the 10th percentile, as compared to the mean growth measurements for American children, which comprise the 50th percentile.

Head Circumference Charts

A

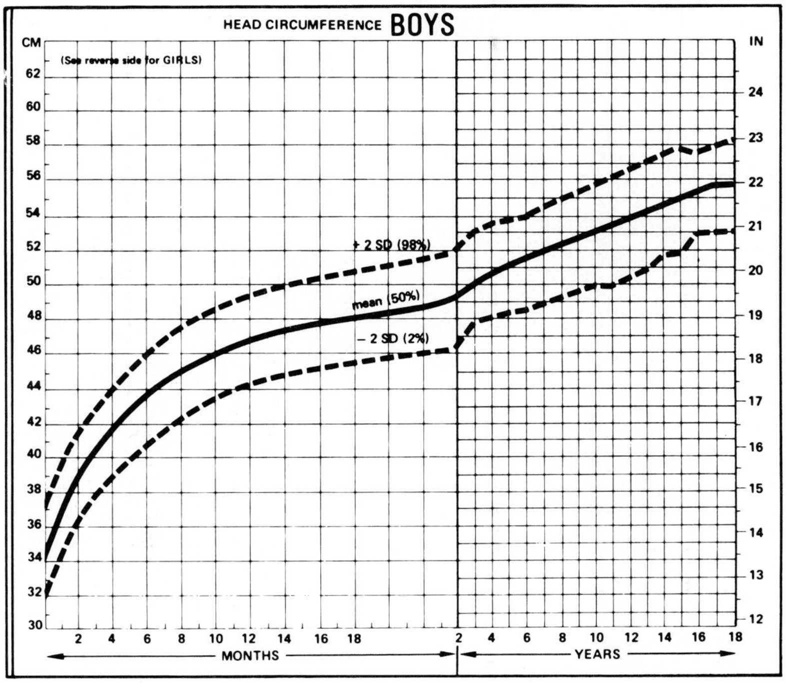

B

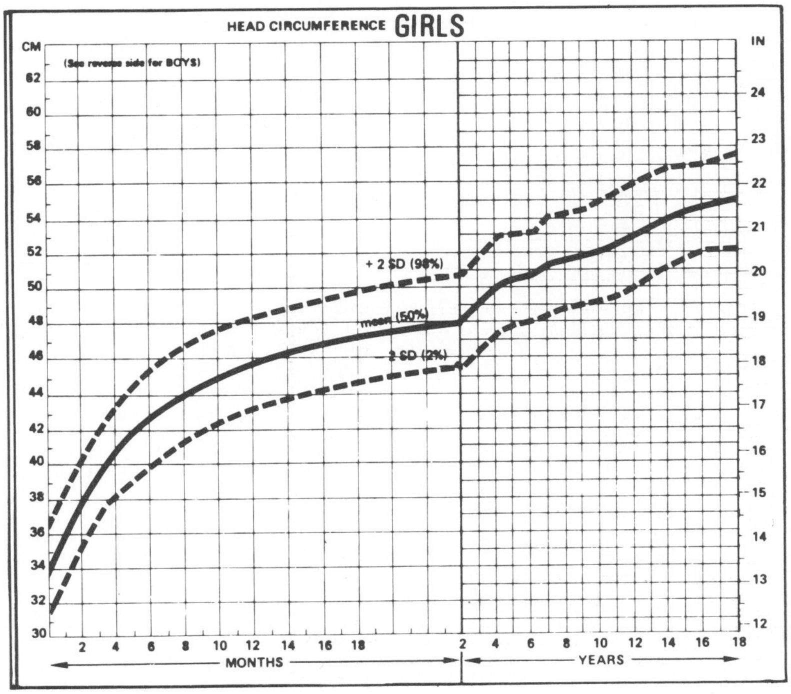

FIG. D-1 Head circumference charts. **A,** Boys; **B,** girls. (From Nelhaus, G.: Composite international and interracial graphs, Pediatrics **41:**106, 1968. Reprinted by permission. Copyright American Academy of Pediatrics, 1968.)

Percentiles for Triceps Skinfold

Age Group (years)	Triceps Skinfold Percentiles (mm) Males 5	25	50	75	95	Females 5	25	50	75	95
1-1.9	6	8	10	12	16	6	8	10	12	16
2-2.9	6	8	10	12	15	6	9	10	12	16
3-3.9	6	8	10	11	15	7	9	11	12	15
4-4.9	6	8	9	11	14	7	8	10	12	16
5-5.9	6	8	9	11	15	6	8	10	12	18
6-6.9	5	7	8	10	16	6	8	10	12	16
7-7.9	5	7	9	12	17	6	9	11	13	18
8-8.9	5	7	8	10	16	6	9	12	15	24
9-9.9	6	7	10	13	18	8	10	13	16	22
10-10.9	6	8	10	14	21	7	10	12	17	27
11-11.9	6	8	11	16	24	7	10	13	18	28
12-12.9	6	8	11	14	28	8	11	14	18	27
13-13.9	5	7	10	14	26	8	12	15	21	30
14-14.9	4	7	9	14	24	9	13	16	21	28
15-15.9	4	6	8	11	24	8	12	17	21	32
16-16.9	4	6	8	12	22	10	15	18	22	31
17-17.9	5	6	8	12	19	10	13	19	24	37
18-18.9	4	6	9	13	24	10	15	18	22	30
19-24.9	4	7	10	15	22	10	14	18	24	34

From Frisancho, A.: New norms of upper limb fat and muscle areas for assessment of nutritional status, Am. J. Clin. Nutr. **34:**2540-2545, 1981.

Percentiles of Upper Arm Circumference

Age Group (years)	Arm Circumference Percentiles (mm) Males 5	25	50	75	95	Females 5	25	50	75	95
1-1.9	142	150	159	170	183	138	148	156	164	177
2-2.9	141	153	162	170	185	142	152	160	167	184
3-3.9	150	160	167	175	190	143	158	167	175	189
4-4.9	149	162	171	180	192	149	160	169	177	191
5-5.9	153	167	175	185	204	153	165	175	185	211
6-6.9	155	167	179	188	228	156	170	176	187	211
7-7.9	162	177	187	201	230	164	174	183	199	231
8-8.9	162	177	190	202	245	168	183	195	214	261
9-9.9	175	187	200	217	257	178	194	211	224	260
10-10.9	181	196	210	231	274	174	193	210	228	265
11-11.9	186	202	223	244	280	185	208	224	248	303
12-12.9	193	214	232	254	303	194	216	237	256	294
13-13.9	194	228	247	263	301	202	223	243	271	338
14-14.9	220	237	253	283	322	214	237	252	272	322
15-15.9	222	244	264	284	320	208	239	254	279	322
16-16.9	244	262	278	303	343	218	241	258	283	334
17-17.9	246	267	285	308	347	220	241	264	295	350
18-18.9	245	276	297	321	379	222	241	258	281	325
19-24.9	262	288	308	331	372	221	247	265	290	345

From Frisancho, A.: New norms of upper limb fat and muscle areas for assessment of nutritional status, Am. J. Clin. Nutr. **34:**2540-2545, 1981.

Table of Normal Laboratory Values

TEST	SPECIMEN	AGE/SEX	NORMAL VALUE	
Ammonia nitrogen	Plasma or serum	Newborn	90-150 µg/dL	
		0-2 weeks	79-129 µg/dL	
		>1 month	29-70 µg/dL	
		Thereafter	15-45 µ/dL	
	Urine, 24 hr		500-1200 mg/d	
Amylase	Serum	Newborn	5-65 U/L	
Beckman; BMD	Urine, timed specimen	>1 yr	25-125 U/L	
			1-17 U/hr	
Antistreptolysin O titer (ASO)	Serum		<166 Todd units	
		School-age children	170-330 Todd units	
Base excess	Whole blood	Newborn	(−10)-(−2) mmol/L	
		Infant	(−7)-(−1) mmol/L	
		Child	(−4)-(+2) mmol/L	
		Thereafter	(−3)-(+3) mmol/L	
Bicarbonate (HCO_3)	Serum	Arterial	21-28 mmol/L	
		Venous	22-29 mmol/L	
			Premature (mg/dL)	**Full-term (mg/dL)**
Bilirubin, total	Serum	Cord	<2.0	<2.0
		0-1 day	<8.0	<6.0
		1-2 days	<12.0	<8.0
		2-5 days	<16.0	<12.0
		Thereafter	<2.0	0.2-1.0
Bilirubin, direct (conjugated)	Serum		0.0-0.2 mg/dL	
Bleeding time	Blood from skin puncture			
Ivy		Normal:	2-7 min	
		Borderline:	7-11 min	
Simplate (G-D)			2.75-8 min	
Blood volume	Whole blood	Male	52-83 mL/kg	
		Female	50-75 mL/kg	
C-reactive protein (CRP)	Serum	Cord	10-350 ng/mL	
		Adult	68-8200 ng/mL	
Calcium, ionized	Serum, plasma, or whole blood	Cord	5.0-6.0 mg/dL	
		Newborn	4.3-5.1 mg/dL	
		24-48 hr	4.0-4.7 mg/dL	
		Thereafter	4.48-4.92 mg/dL or 2.24-2.46 mEq/L	
Calcium, total	Serum	Cord	9.0-11.5 mg/dL	
		Newborn, 3-24 hr	9.0-10.6 mg/dL	
		24-48 hr	7.0-12.0 mg/dL	
		4-7 d	9.0-10.9 mg/dL	
		Child	8.8-10.8 mg/dL	
		Thereafter	8.4-10.2 mg/dL	
	Urine (24 hr)	Ca free diet:	5-40 mg/d	
		Low to average Ca in diet:	50-150 mg/d	
		Average Ca in diet:	100-300 mg/d	
	CSF		4.2-5.4 mg/dL or 2.1-2.7 mEq/L	
	Feces	Average:	0.64 g/d	

Modified from Behrman, R.E., and Vaughan, V.C., III: Nelson textbook of pediatrics, ed. 3, Philadelphia, 1987, W.B. Saunders Co.

Normal Laboratory Values—cont'd

TEST	SPECIMEN	AGE/SEX	NORMAL VALUE
Carbon dioxide, partial pressure (Pco_2)	Whole blood, arterial	Newborn	27-40 mm Hg
		Infant	27-41 mm Hg
		Thereafter: Male	35-48 mm Hg
		Female	32-45 mm Hg
Carbon dioxide, total (tCO_2)	Serum or plasma	Cord	14-22 mmol/L
		Premature (1 week)	14-27 mmol/L
		Newborn	13-22 mmol/L
		Infant	20-28 mmol/L
		Child	20-28 mmol/L
		Thereafter	23-30 mmol/L
Cerebrospinal fluid pressure	CSF		70-180 mm water
Cerebrospinal fluid volume	CSF	Child	60-100 mL
		Adult	100-160 mL
Chloride	Serum or plasma	Cord	96-104 mmol/L
		Newborn	97-110 mmol/L
		Thereafter	98-106 mmol/L
	CSF		118-132 mmol/L
	Urine, 24 hr	Infant	2-10 mmol/d (diet-dependent)
		Child	15-40 mmol/d
		Thereafter	110-250 mmol/d (varies with CL intake)
	Sweat	Normal (homozygote)	0-35 mmol/L
		Marginal (e.g., asthma, Addison disease, malnutrition)	30-60 mmol/L
		Cystic fibrosis	60-200 mmol/L
Cholesterol, total	Serum or plasma	Cord	45-100 mg/dL
		Newborn	53-135 mg/dL
		Infant	70-175 mg/dL
		Child	120-200 mg/dL
		Adolescent	120-210 md/dL
Clotting time (Lee-White)	Whole blood		5-8 minutes (glass tubes) 5-15 minutes (room temp) 30 minutes (silicone tube)
Copper	Serum	Birth-6 mo	20-70 μg/dL
		6 yr	90-190 μg/dL
		12 yr	80-160 μg/dL
		Adult: Male	70-140 μg/dL
		Female	80-155 μg/dL
Creatine kinase (CK, CPK)	Serum	Newborn	68-580 U/L
		Adult: Male	12-70 U/L
		Female	10-55 U/L
		Ambulatory: Male	25-90 U/L
		Female	10-70 U/L
			Higher after exercise
Creatinine	Serum	Cord	0.6-1.2 mg/dL
		Newborn	0.3-1.0 mg/dL
		Infant	0.2-0.4 mg/dL
		Child	0.3-0.7 mg/dL
		Adolescent	0.5-1.0 mg/dL
		Adult: Male	0.6-1.2 mg/dL
		Female	0.5-1.1 mg/dL
	Urine, 24 hr	Infant	8-20 mg/kg/d
		Child	8-22 mg/kg/d
		Adolescent	8-30 mg/kg/d
		Adult	14-26 mg/kg/d
Creatinine clearance (endogenous)	Serum or plasma and urine	Newborn	40-65 ml/min/1.73 m^2
		<40 yr: Male	97-137 ml/min/1.73 m^2
		Female	88-128 ml/min/1.73 m^2

TEST	SPECIMEN	AGE/SEX	NORMAL VALUE	
Eosinophil count	Whole blood, capillary blood		50-350 cell/mm^3 (μL)	
Erythrocyte (RBC) count	Whole blood	cord	3.9-5.5 million/mm^3	
		1-3 d	4.0-6.6 million/mm^3	
		1 wk	3.9-6.3 million/mm^3	
		2 wk	3.6-6.2 million/mm^3	
		1 mo	3.0-5.4 million/mm^3	
		2 mo	2.7-4.9 million/mm^3	
		3-6 mo	3.1-4.5 million/mm^3	
		0.5-2 yr	3.7-5.3 million/mm^3	
		2-6 yr	3.9-5.3 million/mm^3	
		6-12 yr	4.0-5.2 million/mm^3	
		12-18 yr: Male	4.5-5.3 million/mm^3	
		Female	4.1-5.1 million/mm^3	
Erythrocyte sedimentation rate (ESR)	Whole blood			
Westergren (modified)		Child	0-10 mm/hr	
		<50 yr: Male	0-15 mm/hr	
		Female	0.20 mm/hr	
Wintrobe		Child	0-13 mm/hr	
		Adult: Male	0-9 mm/hr	
		Female	0-20 mm/hr	
ZETA			41-54%	
Fat, fecal	Feces (72 hr)	Infant, breast-fed	<1 g/d	
		0-6 yr	<2 g/d	
		Adult	<7 g/d	
Fatty acids, free	Serum or plasma	Adults	8-25 mg/dL	
		Children and obese adults	<31 mg/dL	
Fibrinogen	Plasma	Newborn	125-300 mg/dL	
		Thereafter	200-400 mg/dL	
Galactose	Serum	Newborn	0-20 mg/dL	
		Thereafter	<5 mg/dL	
	Urine	Newborn	≤60 mg/dL	
		Thereafter	<14 mg/dL	
Glucose	Serum	Cord	45-96 mg/dL	
		Premature	20-60 mg/dL	
		Neonate	30-60 mg/dL	
		Newborn, 1 d	40-60 mg/dL	
		Newborn, > 1 d	50-90 mg/dL	
		Child	60-100 mg/dL	
		Thereafter	70-105 mg/dL	
	Whole blood	Adult	65-95 mg/dL	
	CSF	Adult	40-70 mg/dL	
	Urine (quantitative)		<0.5 g/d	
	(Qualitative)		negative	
Glucose tolerance test (GTT), oral	Serum			
Dosages		**Time**	**Normal**	**Diabetic**
Adult: 75 g		Fasting	70-105	>115
Child: 1.75 g/kg of ideal weight up to maximum of 75 g		60 min	120-170	≥200
		90 min	100-140	≥200
		120 min	70-120	≥140
Growth hormone (hGH, Somatotropin)	Plasma Fasting, at rest	Cord	10-50 ng/mL	
		Newborn	10-40 ng/mL	
		Child	<5 ng/mL	
		Adult: Male	<5 ng/mL	
		Female	<8 ng/mL	
Hematocrit (HCT, Hct)	Whole blood	1 d (cap)	48-69%	
		2 d	48-75%	
		3 d	44-72%	
		2 mo	28-42%	
		6-12 yr	35-45%	

Normal Laboratory Values—cont'd

TEST	SPECIMEN	AGE/SEX	NORMAL VALUE
Hematocrit (HCT, Hct)—cont'd		12-18 yr: Male	37-49%
		Female	36-46%
Hemoglobin (Hb)	Whole blood	1-3 d (cap)	14.5-22.5 g/dL
		2 mo	9.0-14.0 g/dL
		6-12 yr	11.5-15.5 g/dL
		12-18 yr: Male	13.0-16.0 g/dL
		Female	12.0-16.0 g/dL
Hemoglobin A	Whole blood		>95% of total
Hemoglobin F	Whole blood	1 d	63-92% HbF
		5 d	65-88% HbF
		3 wk	55-85% HbF
		6-9 wk	31-75% HbF
		3-4 mo	<2-59% HbF
		6 mo	<2-9% HbF
		Adult	<2.0% HbF
Immunoglobulin A(IgA)	Serum	Cord	0-5 mg/dL
		Newborn	0-2.2 mg/dL
		½-6 mo	3-82 mg/dL
		½-6 mo	14-108 mg/dL
		2-6 yr	23-190 mg/dL
		6-12 yr	29-270 mg/dL
		12-16 yr	81-232 mg/dL
		Thereafter	60-380 mg/dL
Immunoglobulin D(IgD)	Serum	Newborn	None detected
		Thereafter	0-8 mg/dL
Immunoglobulin E(IgE)	Serum	Male	0-230 IU/mL
		Female	0-170 IU/mL
Immunoglobulin G(IgG)	Serum	Cord	760-1700 mg/dL
		Newborn	700-1480 mg/dL
		½-6 mo	300-1000 mg/dL
		6 mo-2 yr	500-1200 mg/dL
		2-6 yr	500-1300 mg/dL
		6-12 yr	700-1650 mg/dL
		12-16 yr	700-1550 mg/dL
		Adults	600-1600 mg/dL (higher in blacks)
Immunoglobulin M(IgM)	Serum	Cord	4-24 mg/dL
		Newborn	5-30 mg/dL
		½-6 mo	15-109 mg/dL
		6 mo-2 yr	43-239 mg/dL
		2-6 yr	50-199 mg/dL
		6-12 yr	50-260 mg/dL
		12-16 yr	45-240 mg/dL
		Thereafter	40-345 mg/dL
Iron	Serum	Newborn	100-250 μg/dL
		Infant	40-100 μg/dL
		Child	50-120 μg/dL
		Thereafter, Male	50-160 μg/dL
		Female	40-150 μg/dL
		Intoxicated child	280-2550 μg/dL
		Fatally poisoned child	>1800 μg/dL
Iron-binding capacity, total (TIBC)	Serum	Infant	100-400 μg/dL
		Thereafter	250-400 μg/dL
Lead	Whole blood	Child	<25 μg/dL
		Adult	<40 μg/dL
		Acceptable for industrial exposure	<60
		Toxic	≥100
	Urine, 24 hr		<80 μg/L

TEST	SPECIMEN	AGE/SEX	NORMAL VALUE
Leukocyte count (WBC count)	Whole blood		**× 1000 cells/mm^3 (μL)**
		Birth	9.0-30.0
		24 h	9.4-34.0
		1 mo	5.0-19.5
		1-3 yr	6.0-17.5
		4-7 yr	5.5-15.5
		8-13 yr	4.5-13.5
		Adult	4.5-11.0
	CSF		**× 1000 cells/mm^3** (μL)
		Premature	0-25 mononuclear
			0-100 polymorphonuclear
			0-1000 RBC
		Newborn	0-20 mononuclear
			0-70 polymorphonuclear
			0-800 RBC
		Neonate	0-5 mononuclear
			0-25 polymorphonuclear
			0-50 RBC
		Thereafter	0-5 mononuclear
Leukocyte differential count	Whole blood	Myelocytes	0% 0 Cells/mm^3 (μL)
		Neutrohils—"bands"	3-5% 150-400 Cells/mm^3 (μL)
		Neutrophils—"segs"	54-62% 3000-5800 Cells/mm^3 (μL)
		Lymphocytes	25-33% 1500-3000 Cells/mm^3 (μL)
		Monocytes	3-7% 285-500 Cells/mm^3 (μL)
		Eosinophils	1-3% 50-250 Cells/mm^3 (μL)
		Basophils	0.075% 15-50 Cells/mm^3 (μL)
Mean corpuscular hemoglobin (MCH)	Whole blood	Birth	31-37 pg/cell
		1-3 d (cap)	31-37 pg/cell
		1 wk-1 mo	28-40 pg/cell
		2 mo	26-34 pg/cell
		3-6 mo	25-35 pg/cell
		0.5-2 yr	23-31 pg/cell
		2-6 yr	24-30 pg/cell
		6-12 yr	25-33 pg/cell
		12-18 yr	25-35 pg/cell
		18-49 yr	26-34 pg/cell
Mean corpuscular hemoglobin concentration (MCHC)	Whole blood	Birth	30-36% Hb/cell or g Hb/dL RBC
		1-3 d (cap)	29-37% Hb/cell or g Hb/dL RBC
		1-2 wk	28-38% Hb/cell or g Hb/dL RBC
		1-2 mo	29-37% Hb/cell or g Hb/dL RBC
		3 mo-2 yr	30-36% Hb/cell or g Hb/dL RBC
		2-18 yr	31-37% Hb/cell or g Hb/dL RBC
		>18 yr	31-37% Hb/cell or g Hb/dL RBC
Mean corpuscular volume (MCV)	Whole blood	1-3 d (cap)	95-121 μm^3
		0.5-2 yr	70-86 μm^3
		6-12 yr	77-95 μm^3
		12-18 yr: Male	78-98 μm^3
		Female	78-102 μm^3
Osmolality	Serum	Child, adult:	275-295 mOsmol/kg H_2O
	Urine, random		50-1400 mOsmol/kg H_2O, depending on fluid intake. After 12 hr fluid restriction: >850 mOsmol/kg H_2O
	Urine, 24 hr		≈300-900 mOsmol/kg H_2O
Oxygen, partial pressure (pO_2)	Whole blood, arterial	Birth	8-24 mm Hg
		5-10 min	33-75 mm Hg
		30 min	31-85 mm Hg
		>1 hr	55-80 mm Hg
		1 d	54-95 mm Hg
		Thereafter	83-108 mm Hg
		(Decreased with age)	

Normal Laboratory Values—cont'd

TEST	SPECIMEN	AGE/SEX	NORMAL VALUE
Oxygen saturation	Whole blood, arterial	Newborn	40-90%
		Thereafter	95-99%
Partial thromboplastin time (PTT)	Whole blood (Na citrate)		
Nonactivated			60-85 s (Platelin)
Activated			25-35 s (differs with method)
pH	Whole blood, arterial	Premature (48 hr)	7.35-7.50
		Birth, full term	7.11-7.36
		5-10 min	7.09-7.30
		30 min	7.21-7.38
		>1 hr	7.26-7.49
		1 d	7.29-7.45
		Thereafter	7.35-7.45
		Must be corrected for body temperature	
	Urine, random	Newborn/neonate	5-7
		Thereafter (average ≈6)	4.5-8
	Stool		7.0-7.5
Phenylalanine	Serum	Premature	2.0-7.5 mg/dL
		Newborn	1.2-3.4 mg/dL
		Thereafter	0.8-1.8 mg/dL
	Urine, 24 hr	10 d-2 wk	1-2 mg/d
		3-12 yr	4-18 mg/d
		Thereafter	trace-17 mg/d
Plasma volume	Plasma	Male	25-43 mL/kg
		Female	28-45 mL/kg
Platelet count (thrombocyte count)	Whole blood (EDTA)	Newborn	84-478 × $10^3/mm^3$ (μL)
		(After 1 wk, same as adult)	
		Adult	150-400 × $10^3/mm^3$ (μL)
Potassium	Serum	Newborn	3.9-5.9 mmol/L
		Infant	4.1-5.3 mmol/L
		Child	3.4-4.7 mmol/L
		Thereafter	3.5-5.1 mmol/L
	Plasma (heparin)		3.5-4.5 mmol/L
	Urine, 24 hr		2.5-125 mmol/d varies with diet
Protein			
Total	Serum	Premature	4.3-7.6 g/dL
		Newborn	4.6-7.4 g/dL
		Child	6.2-8.0 g/dL
Electrophoresis			

	g/dL Albumin	α_1-Globulin	α_2-Globulin	β-Globulin	γ-Globulin
Premature	3.0-4.2	0.1-0.5	0.3-0.7	0.3-1.2	0.3-1.4
Newborn	3.6-5.4	0.1-0.3	0.3-0.5	0.2-0.6	0.2-1.0
Infant	4.0-5.0	0.2-0.4	0.5-0.8	0.5-0.8	0.3-1.2
Thereafter	3.5-5.0	0.2-0.3	0.4-1.0	0.5-1.1	0.7-1.2
					Higher in blacks

TEST	SPECIMEN	AGE/SEX	NORMAL VALUE
Total	Urine, 24 hr		1-14 mg/dL
			50-80 mg/d (at rest)
			<250 mg/d after intense exercise
Total	CSF		Lumbar: 8-32 mg/dL
Prothrombin time (PT)			
One-stage (Quick)	Whole blood (Na citrate)	In general	11-15 s (varies with type of thromboplastin)
		Newborn	Prolonged by 2-3 sec
Two-stage modified (Ware and Seegers)	Whole blood (Na citrate)		18-22 sec
RBC count, see erythrocyte count			
Red cell volume	Whole blood	Male	20-36 mL/kg
		Female	19-31 mL/kg

TEST	SPECIMEN	AGE/SEX	NORMAL VALUE
Reticulocyte count	Whole blood	Adults	0.5-1.5% of erythrocytes or 25,000-75,000/mm^3 (μL)
	Capillary	1 d	0.4-6.0%
		7 d	<0.1-1.3%
		1-4 wk	<0.1-1.2%
		5-6 wk	<0.1-2.5%
		7-8 wk	0.1-2.9%
		9-10 wk	<0.1-2.6%
		11-12 wk	0.1-1.3%
Salicylates	Serum, plasma		Therap. conc.: 15-30 mg/dL Toxic conc.: >30
Sedimentation rate, see erythrocyte sedimentation rate			
Sodium	Serum or plasma	Newborn	136-146 mmol/L
		Infant	139-146 mmol/L
		Child	138-145 mmol/L
		Thereafter	136-146 mmol/L
	Urine, 24 hr		40-220 mmol/L (diet dependent)
	Sweat		10-40 mmol/L
		Cystic fibrosis	>70
Specific gravity	Urine, random	Adult	1.002-1.030
		After 12 hr fluid restriction	>1.025
	Urine, 24 h		1.015-1.025
Theophylline	Serum, plasma	Therap. conc.	
		Bronchodilator	8-20 μg/mL
		Prem. apnea	6-13 μg/mL
		Toxic conc.	>20
Thrombin time	Whole blood (Na citrate)		Control time ± 2 sec when control is 9-13 sec
Thyroxine, total (T_4)	Serum	Cord	8-13 μg/dL
		Newborn	11.5-24 (lower in low birth weight infants)
		Neonate	9-18 μg/dL
		Infant	7-15 μg/dL
		1-5 yr	7.3-15 μg/dL
		5-10 yr	6.4-13.3 μg/dL
		Thereafter	5-12 μg/dL
		Newborn screen (filter paper)	6.2-22 μg/dL
Tourniquet test (capillary fragility)			<5-10 petechiae in 2.5 cm circle on forearm (halfway between systolic and diastolic pressure for 5 min); 0-8 petechiae in 6 cm circle (50 torr for 15 min); 10-20 petechiae in 5 cm circle (80 mm Hg)

TEST	SPECIMEN	AGE/SEX	mg/dL M	mg/dL F
Triglycerides (TG)	Serum, after ≥ 12 hr fast			
		Cord blood	10-98	10-98
		0-5 yr	30-86	32-99
		6-11 yr	31-108	35-114
		12-15 yr	36-138	41-138
		16-19 yr	40-163	40-128

TEST	SPECIMEN	AGE/SEX	NORMAL VALUE
Triiodothyronine, free	Serum	Cord	20-240 pg/dL
		1-3 d	200-610 pg/dL
		6 wk	240-560 pg/dL
		Adults (20-50 yr)	230-660 pg/dL

Normal Laboratory Values—cont'd

TEST	SPECIMEN	AGE/SEX	NORMAL VALUE
Triiodothyronine, total (T_3-RIA)	Serum	Cord	30-70 ng/dL
		Newborn	72-260 ng/dL
		1-5 yr	100-260 ng/dL
		5-10 yr	90-240 ng/dL
		10-15 yr	80-210 ng/dL
		Thereafer	115-190 ng/dL
Urea nitrogen	Serum or plasma	Cord	21-40 mg/dL
		Premature (1 wk)	3-25 mg/dL
		Newborn	3-12 mg/dL
		Infant/Child	5-18 mg/dL
		Thereafter	7-18 mg/dL
Uric acid	Serum		
Phosphotungstate		Newborn	2.0-6.2 mg/dL
		Adult: Male	4.5-8.2 mg/dL
		Female	3.0-6.5 mg/dL
Uricase		Child	2.0-5.5 mg/dL
		Adult: Male	3.5-7.2 mg/dL
		Female	2.6-6.0 mg/dL
Urine volume	Urine, 24 hr	Newborn	50-300 mL/d
		Infant	350-550 mL/d
		Child	500-1000 mL/d
		Adolescent	700-1400 mL/d
		Thereafter: Male	800-1800 mL/d
		Female	600-1600 mL/d (varies with intake and other factors)
WBC, see Leukocyte			

APPENDIX F

Recommended Daily Dietary Allowances

Recommended Daily Dietary Allowances (designed for the maintenance of good nutrition of practically all

	Age (years)	Weight kg	Weight lb	Height cm	Height in	Protein (g)	Fat-Soluble Vitamins: Vitamin A (μg RE)[a]	Vitamin D (μg)[b]	Vitamin E (mg α TE)[c]
Infants	0.0-0.5	6	13	60	24	kg × 2.2	420	10	3
	0.5-1.0	9	20	71	28	kg × 2.0	400	10	4
Children	1-3	13	29	90	35	23	400	10	5
	4-6	20	44	112	44	30	500	10	6
	7-10	28	62	132	52	34	700	10	7
Males	11-14	45	99	157	62	45	1000	10	8
	15-18	66	145	176	69	56	1000	10	10
	19-22	70	154	177	70	56	1000	7.5	10
	23-50	70	154	178	70	56	1000	5	10
	51+	70	154	178	70	56	1000	5	10
Females	11-14	46	101	157	62	46	800	10	8
	15-18	55	120	163	64	46	800	10	8
	19-22	55	120	163	64	44	800	7.5	8
	23-50	55	120	163	64	44	800	5	8
	51+	55	120	163	64	44	800	5	8
Pregnant						+30	+200	+5	+2
Lactating						+20	+400	+5	+3

From Food and Nutrition Board, National Academy of Sciences—National Research Council, Washington, D.C., 1980.

*The allowances are intended to provide for individual variations among most normal persons as they live in the United States under usual environment stresses. Diets should be based on a variety of common foods in order to provide other nutrients for which human requirements have been less well defined.

[a]Retinol equivalents. 1 Retinol equivalent = 1 μg retinol or 6 μg β carotene.

[b]As cholecalciferol. 10 μg cholecalciferol = 400 IU vitamin D.

[c]α tocopherol equivalents. 1 mg d-α-tocopherol = 1 α TE.

[d]1 NE (niacin equivalent) is equal to 1 mg of niacin or 60 mg of dietary tryptophan.

[e]The folacin allowances refer to dietary sources as determined by *Lactobacillus casei* assay after treatment with enzymes ("conjugates") to make polyglutamyl forms of the vitamin available for the test organism.

[f]The RDA for vitamin B_{12} in infants based on average concentration of the vitamin in human milk. The allowances after weaning are based on energy intake (as recommended by the American Academy of Pediatrics) and consideration of other factors such as intestinal absorption.

[g]The increased requirement during pregnancy cannot be met by the iron content of habitual American diets nor by the existing iron stores of many women; therefore the use of 30-60 mg of supplemental iron is recommended. Iron needs during lactation are not substantially different from those of nonpregnant women, but continued supplementation of the mother for 2 to 3 months after parturition is advisable in order to replenish stores depleted by pregnancy.

*Estimated Safe and Adequate Daily Dietary Intakes of Additional Selected Vitamins and Minerals**

	Age (years)	Vitamins: Vitamin K (μg)	Biotin (μg)	Pantothenic Acid (mg)	Minerals: Copper (mg)	Manganese (mg)
Infants	0.0-0.5	12	35	2	0.5-0.7	0.5-0.7
	0.5-1.0	10-20	50	3	0.7-1.0	0.7-1.0
Children	1-3	15-30	65	3	1.0-1.5	1.0-1.5
	4-6	20-40	85	3-4	1.5-2.0	1.5-2.0
	7-10	30-60	120	4-5	2.0-2.5	2.0-3.0
Adolescents	11+	50-100	100-200	4-7	2.0-3.0	2.5-5.0
Adults		70-140	100-200	4-7	2.0-3.0	2.5-5.0

From Recommended dietary allowances, Food and Nutrition Board, National Academy of Sciences—National Research Council, Washinton, D.C., 1980.

*Because there is less information on which to base allowances, these figures are not given in the main tables of the RDA and are provided here in the form of ranges of recommended intakes.

†Since the toxic levels for many trace elements may be only several times usual intakes, the upper levels for the trace elements given in this table should not be habitually exceeded.

*healthy people in the United States)**

Water-Soluble Vitamins							Minerals					
Vitamin C (mg)	Thiamin (mg)	Riboflavin (mg)	Niacin (mg NE)[d]	Vitamin B_6 (mg)	Folacin[e] (μg)	Vitamin B_{12} (μg)	Calcium (mg)	Phosphorus (mg)	Magnesium (mg)	Iron (mg)	Zinc (mg)	Iodine (μg)
35	0.3	0.4	6	0.3	30	0.5[f]	360	240	50	10	3	40
35	0.5	0.6	8	0.6	45	1.5	540	360	70	15	5	50
45	0.7	0.8	9	0.9	100	2.0	800	800	150	15	10	70
45	0.9	1.0	11	1.3	200	2.5	800	800	200	10	10	90
45	1.2	1.4	16	1.6	300	3.0	800	800	250	10	10	120
50	1.4	1.6	18	1.8	400	3.0	1200	1200	350	18	15	150
60	1.4	1.7	18	2.0	400	3.0	1200	1200	400	18	15	150
60	1.5	1.7	19	2.2	400	3.0	800	800	350	10	15	150
60	1.4	1.6	18	2.2	400	3.0	800	800	350	10	15	150
60	1.2	1.4	16	2.2	400	3.0	800	800	350	10	15	150
50	1.1	1.3	15	1.8	400	3.0	1200	1200	300	18	15	150
60	1.1	1.3	14	2.0	400	3.0	1200	1200	300	18	15	150
60	1.1	1.3	14	2.0	400	3.0	800	800	300	18	15	150
60	1.0	1.2	13	2.0	400	3.0	800	800	300	18	15	150
60	1.0	1.2	13	2.0	400	3.0	800	800	300	10	15	150
+20	+0.4	+0.3	+2	+0.6	+400	+1.0	+400	+400	+150	[g]	+5	+25
+40	+0.5	+0.5	+5	+0.5	+100	+1.0	+400	+400	+150	[g]	+10	+50

Trace Elements†				Electrolytes		
Fluoride (mg)	Chromium (mg)	Selenium (mg)	Molybdenum (mg)	Sodium (mg)	Potassium (mg)	Chloride (mg)
0.1-0.5	0.01-0.04	0.01-0.04	0.03-0.06	115-350	350-925	295-700
0.2-1.0	0.02-0.06	0.02-0.06	0.04-0.08	250-750	425-1275	400-1200
0.5-1.5	0.02-0.08	0.02-0.08	0.05-0.1	325-975	550-1650	500-1500
1.0-2.5	0.03-0.12	0.03-0.12	0.06-0.15	450-1350	775-2325	700-2100
1.5-2.5	0.05-0.92	0.05-0.2	0.1-0.3	600-1800	1000-3000	925-2775
1.5-2.5	0.05-0.2	0.05-0.2	0.15-0.5	900-2700	1525-4575	1400-4200
1.5-4.0	0.05-0.2	0.05-0.2	0.15-0.5	1100-3300	1875-5625	1700-5100

Index

B

E

G

I

N

Q

R

T

CONVERSION OF POUNDS TO KILOGRAMS FOR PEDIATRIC WEIGHTS

Pounds→ ↓	0	1	2	3	4	5	6	7	8	9
0	0.00	0.45	0.90	1.36	1.81	2.26	2.72	3.17	3.62	4.08
10	4.53	4.98	5.44	5.89	6.35	6.80	7.35	7.71	8.16	8.61
20	9.07	9.52	9.97	10.43	10.88	11.34	11.79	12.24	12.70	13.15
30	13.60	14.06	14.51	14.96	15.42	15.87	16.32	16.78	17.23	17.69
40	18.14	18.59	19.05	19.50	19.95	20.41	20.86	21.31	21.77	22.22
50	22.68	23.13	23.58	24.04	24.49	24.94	25.40	25.85	26.30	26.76
60	27.21	27.66	28.22	28.57	29.03	29.48	29.93	30.39	30.84	31.29
70	31.75	32.20	32.65	33.11	33.56	34.02	34.47	34.92	35.38	35.83
80	36.28	36.74	37.19	37.64	38.10	38.55	39.00	39.46	39.93	40.37
90	40.82	41.27	41.73	42.18	42.63	43.09	43.54	43.99	44.45	44.90
100	45.36	45.81	46.26	46.72	47.17	47.62	48.08	48.53	48.98	49.44
110	49.89	50.34	50.80	51.25	51.71	52.16	52.61	53.07	53.52	53.97
120	54.43	54.88	55.33	55.79	56.24	56.70	57.15	57.60	58.06	58.51
130	58.96	59.42	59.87	60.32	60.78	61.23	61.68	62.14	62.59	63.05
140	63.50	63.95	64.41	64.86	65.31	65.77	66.22	66.67	67.13	67.58
150	68.04	68.49	68.94	69.40	69.85	70.30	70.76	71.21	71.66	72.12
160	72.57	73.02	73.48	73.93	74.39	74.84	75.29	75.75	76.20	76.65
170	77.11	77.56	78.01	78.47	78.92	79.38	79.83	80.28	80.74	81.19
180	81.64	82.10	82.55	83.00	83.46	83.91	84.36	84.82	85.27	85.73
190	86.18	86.68	87.09	87.54	87.99	88.45	88.90	89.35	89.81	90.26
200	90.72	91.17	91.62	92.08	92.53	92.98	93.44	93.89	94.34	94.80

CONVERSION OF POUNDS AND OUNCES TO KILOGRAMS FOR PEDIATRIC WEIGHTS

Pounds	Kilograms	Pounds	Kilograms	Ounces	Kilograms	Ounces	Kilograms
1	0.454	9	4.082	1	0.028	9	0.255
2	0.907	10	4.536	2	0.057	10	0.283
3	1.361	11	4.990	3	0.085	11	0.312
4	1.814	12	5.443	4	0.113	12	0.340
5	2.268	13	5.897	5	0.142	13	0.369
6	2.722			6	0.170	14	0.397
7	3.175			7	0.198	15	0.425
8	3.629			8	0.227		

CONVERSION FACTORS FOR TEMPERATURE*

Celsius	Fahrenheit	Celsius	Fahrenheit	Celsius	Fahrenheit	Celsius	Fahrenheit
34.0	93.2	36.4	97.5	38.6	101.5	41.0	105.9
34.2	93.6	36.6	97.9	38.8	101.8	41.2	106.1
34.4	93.9	36.8	98.2	39.0	102.2	41.4	106.5
34.6	94.3	37.0	98.6	39.2	102.6	41.6	106.8
34.8	94.6	37.2	99.0	39.4	102.9	41.8	107.2
35.0	95.0	37.4	99.3	39.6	103.3	42.0	107.6
35.2	95.4	37.6	99.7	39.8	103.6	42.2	108.0
35.4	95.7	37.8	100.0	40.0	104.0	42.4	108.3
35.6	96.1	38.0	100.4	40.2	104.4	42.6	108.7
35.8	96.4	38.2	100.8	40.4	104.7	42.8	109.0
36.0	96.8	38.4	101.1	40.6	105.2	43.0	109.4
36.2	97.2			40.8	105.4		

*(°C) × (9/5) + 32 = °F
(°F − 32) × (5/9) = °C

°C = temperature in Celsius (centigrade) degrees
°F = temperature in Fahrenheit degrees

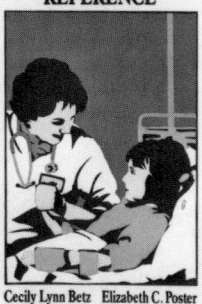

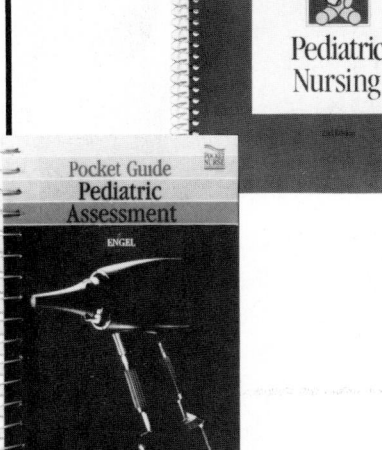

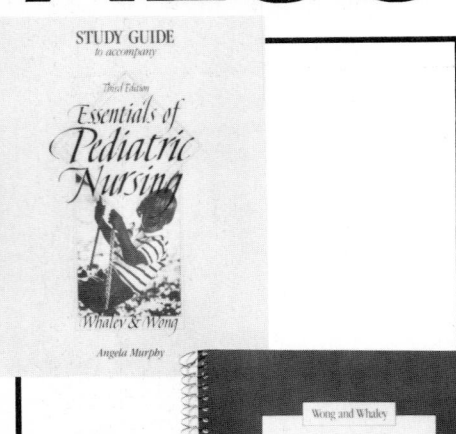